HASCHEK AND ROUSSEAUX'S HANDBOOK OF TOXICOLOGIC PATHOLOGY

FOURTH EDITION

Volume I: Principles and Practice of Toxicologic Pathology

Editors
WANDA M. HASCHEK

COLIN G. ROUSSEAUX

MATTHEW A. WALLIG

BRAD BOLON

Associate Editors
STACEY L. FOSSEY

JOHN H. VAHLE

Illustrations Editor
BETH W. MAHLER

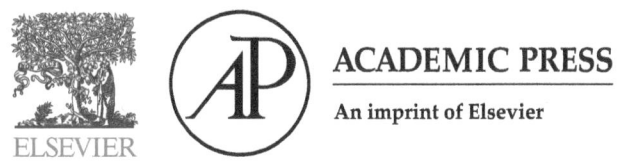

ELSEVIER

ACADEMIC PRESS
An imprint of Elsevier

Academic Press is an imprint of Elsevier
125 London Wall, London EC2Y 5AS, United Kingdom
525 B Street, Suite 1650, San Diego, CA 92101, United States
50 Hampshire Street, 5th Floor, Cambridge, MA 02139, United States
The Boulevard, Langford Lane, Kidlington, Oxford OX5 1GB, United Kingdom

Notices
Knowledge and best practice in this field are constantly changing. As new research and experience broaden our understanding, changes in research methods, professional practices, or medical treatment may become necessary.

Practitioners and researchers must always rely on their own experience and knowledge in evaluating and using any information, methods, compounds, or experiments described herein. In using such information or methods they should be mindful of their own safety and the safety of others, including parties for whom they have a professional responsibility.

To the fullest extent of the law, neither the Publisher nor the authors, contributors, or editors, assume any liability for any injury and/or damage to persons or property as a matter of products liability, negligence or otherwise, or from any use or operation of any methods, products, instructions, or ideas contained in the material herein.

Library of Congress Cataloging-in-Publication Data
A catalog record for this book is available from the Library of Congress

British Library Cataloguing-in-Publication Data
A catalogue record for this book is available from the British Library

ISBN: 978-0-12-821044-4

For information on all Academic Press publications visit our website at
https://www.elsevier.com/books-and-journals

Publisher: Andre Gerhard Wolff
Acquisitions Editor: Kattie Washington
Editorial Project Manager: Billie Jean Fernandez
Production Project Manager: Sreejith Viswanathan
Cover Designer: Matthew Limbert

Typeset by TNQ Technologies

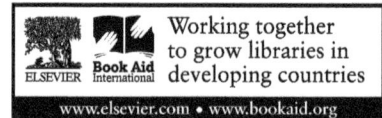

Dedication

To teach is to learn…
(Japanese proverb)

To our families, teachers, colleagues, and friends who have supported us in our journeys through life,
encouraged us when needed, mentored us in our learning, challenged us in our teaching,
joined us in our passion, followed us in our trailblazing,
and inspired us in our scholarly pursuits….

We are grateful for the opportunities we have enjoyed to advance pathology and toxicology as
distinct and blended disciplines, both for our own betterment and in
service to our local and global communities.

Contents

Contributors   xxi
About the Editors   xxiii
Preface to the 4th Edition   xxv

1. Toxicologic Pathology: An Introduction
WANDA M. HASCHEK, COLIN G. ROUSSEAUX,
MATTHEW A. WALLIG AND BRAD BOLON

1. An Overview of Toxicologic Pathology   1
2. What Is Toxicologic Pathology?   3
3. The Basis of Toxicologic Pathology   3
4. Challenges in Toxicologic Pathology   4
   4.1. Core Challenges   4
   4.2. Additional Challenges   6
5. Training and Certification in Toxicologic
   Pathology   8
6. The "Practitioner" of Toxicologic
   Pathology   9
   6.1. Industrial Toxicologic Pathology   9
   6.2. Toxicologic Pathology Related to the
        Environment and Food Safety   10
   6.3. Diagnostic Toxicologic Pathology   10
   6.4. Research in Toxicologic Pathology   11
   6.5. Management Roles in Toxicologic
        Pathology   11
7. Summary   11
References   12

PART 1
Principles of Toxicologic Pathology

2. Biochemical and Molecular Basis of Toxicity
LOIS D. LEHMAN-MCKEEMAN AND
LAURA E. ARMSTRONG

1. Introduction   15
2. General Principles of Xenobiotic
   Disposition   16
   2.1. General Properties of
        Absorption   16
   2.2. Routes of Absorption   19
   2.3. General Principles of
        Distribution   21

2.4. Metabolism: Activation and
     Detoxification   24
2.5. Elimination of Toxicants   30
2.6. Effects of the Microbiome on Absorption,
     Distribution, Biotransformation and
     Elimination   34
3. Interactions of Toxicants with Cellular and
   Molecular Targets   35
   3.1. Covalent Modification
        Chapters 3 and 8   35
   3.2. Stress Responses in Toxicity   36
   3.3. Altered Gene Expression   38
   3.4. Mechanisms of Cell Death   40
4. Idiosyncratic Mechanisms of Toxicity   42
5. Protective Mechanisms, Repair Mechanisms, and
   Adaptation or Failure   42
   5.1. Stress Response Constituents and
        Pathways   42
   5.2. Cell Repair and Adaptation   44
   5.3. Failure to Repair After Toxic Insult   46
6. Summary and Conclusions   47
References   47

3. ADME Principles in Small Molecule Drug Discovery and Development: An Industrial Perspective
ELLEN CANNADY, KISHORE KATYAYAN AND NITA PATEL

1. Introduction   51
2. General ADME Principles   52
3. Discovery Overview   54
4. Absorption, Bioavailability, and PK/TK
   Studies   55
5. Distribution   59
   5.1. Volume of Distribution   59
   5.2. Protein Binding   59
   5.3. Transporter Interactions   59
6. Metabolism   61
   6.1. Overview of Phase I and Phase II
        Metabolism   61
   6.2. Overview of Reactive Metabolites   61
   6.3. Discovery Metabolism   64
7. Excretion   65
8. Physiologically Based PK Modeling   67
9. Development   67
10. Mass Balance Studies   68

11. Tissue Distribution Studies   69
12. Drug Metabolism Studies in
    Development   71
13. Excretion Studies   71
14. Specialized Excretion Studies   73
15. General Timing of Development ADME
    Studies   73
16. Conclusions   74
Acknowledgments   74
References   74

4. Biotherapeutics ADME and PK/PD Principles

DANIELA BUMBACA YADAV, KAPIL GADKAR AND
ISABEL FIGUEROA

1. Introduction   77
   1.1. Monoclonal Antibodies   78
   1.2. Antibody-Based Therapeutics   80
   1.3. Beyond Antibody-Based
        Therapeutics   81
2. Pharmacokinetics of Biotherapeutics   83
   2.1. Monoclonal Antibody PK   84
   2.2. PK of Antibody-Based Therapeutics   90
   2.3. PK of Other Biotherapeutic
        Modalities   92
3. Pharmacodynamics of Biotherapeutics   92
4. PK–PD Modeling and Interspecies
   Scaling   95
5. Summary   96
References   96

5. Principles of Pharmacodynamics and Toxicodynamics

JIN WANG AND DAVID M. STRESSER

1. Introduction: Definition of Pharmacodynamics
   and Toxicodynamics   101
2. Mechanism of Drug Action and Adverse Drug
   Reaction   102
   2.1. Physiochemical Property Based   102
   2.2. Biochemical Based   102
3. Types of Adverse Drug Reaction: Intrinsic (Type
   A) Versus Idiosyncratic (Type B)   104
4. Types of Xenobiotic–Target
   Interaction   106
   4.1. Reversible, Irreversible, Noncompetitive, and
        Allosteric Interaction   106
   4.2. Agonist, Partial Agonist, Antagonist, and
        Inverse Agonist   106
5. Exposure-Dependent Response   107
   5.1. Receptor Occupancy Relationship   107
   5.2. Turnover Model   108
   5.3. Quantal Dose–Effect Model   109
   5.4. Nonmonotonic Dose–Effect   109
6. Response Following Chronic Dosing   110
   6.1. Receptor Downregulation   111
   6.2. Exhaustion of Mediators   111
   6.3. Physiological Adaptation   111
   6.4. Desensitization   111
7. Quantitative Modeling for Pharmacokinetic/
   Pharmacodynamic and Toxicodynamic Data
   Analysis   111
References   112

6. Morphologic Manifestations of Toxic Cell Injury

MATTHEW A. WALLIG AND EVAN B. JANOVITZ

1. Introduction   113
   1.1. Importance of Morphologic Assessment in
        Toxicologic Pathology   113
   1.2. Cell Injury in Context—Structural and
        Functional Components of Cell
        Injury   114
   1.3. Host Reaction to Cell Injury   116
2. Adaptation   116
   2.1. Atrophy   116
   2.2. Hypertrophy   120
3. Irreversible versus Reversible Cell
   Injury   122
   3.1. Cellular Swelling   124
   3.2. Fatty Change—Lipidosis   126
4. Irreversible Cell Injury   127
   4.1. Accidental Cell Death—Necrosis   127
   4.2. Programmed Cell Death   133
   4.3. Consequences of Irreversible Cell
        Injury   139
5. Conclusion   146
References   146

7. The Role of Pathology in Evaluation of Reproductive, Developmental, and Juvenile Toxicity

CHRISTOPHER J. BOWMAN AND WENDY G. HALPERN

1. Introduction   149
2. Reproductive Toxicity Assessment   150
   2.1. Male Reproductive Toxicity
        Assessment   152
   2.2. Female Reproductive Toxicity
        Assessment   159
   2.3. Guidelines   167
3. Pregnancy and Developmental Toxicity   167
   3.1. Embryo–Fetal Development
        Studies   168
   3.2. Pre- and Postnatal Development
        Studies   172

3.3. Enhanced Pre- and Postnatal Development Study in the NHP 174
3.4. Guidelines 176
4. Juvenile Toxicity Assessment 177
4.1. Context for Challenges in Assessing the Neonatal Period 179
4.2. Context for Support of Children: Weaning through Puberty 179
4.3. Postnatal Development of Specific Organ Systems 180
4.4. Models of Disease 188
4.5. Practical Species-Specific Considerations 188
4.6. Guidelines and Regional Legislation 190
5. Conclusions 192
Abbreviations 192
References 193

8. Carcinogenesis: Mechanisms and Evaluation
MARK J. HOENERHOFF, MOLLY BOYLE, SHEROY MINOCHERHOMJI AND ARUN R. PANDIRI

1. Introduction 206
1.1. Prominent Theories of Carcinogenesis 207
1.2. General Features of Carcinogenesis 208
1.3. Cell Growth and Proliferation 210
1.4. Oncogenes and Tumor Suppressor Genes 213
1.5. Apoptosis and DNA Damage Repair 217
1.6. Angiogenesis, Invasion, and Metastasis 218
2. Mechanisms of Chemically Induced Carcinogenesis 219
2.1. Genotoxic Carcinogens 220
2.2. Direct Acting Carcinogens 220
2.3. Indirect Acting Carcinogens 220
2.4. Mechanisms of High-fidelity/Nonmutagenic or Low-fidelity/Mutagenic DNA Repair 222
2.5. DNA Replication and Repair Mechanisms 222
2.6. Consequences of Genotoxicity 224
2.7. Nongenotoxic Carcinogens 224
3. Identification of Carcinogens—Testing Programs and Guidelines 231
3.1. In Vitro Mutagenicity Assays 231
3.2. Chromosomal Aberration Assay 232
3.3. Micronucleus Test 232
3.4. Other DNA Based Assays 232
3.5. Testing Programs and Guidelines 233

3.6. Two-Year National Toxicology Program Rodent Carcinogenicity Bioassay 233
3.7. Carcinogenicity Testing 234
3.8. Current and Future Considerations for Carcinogenicity Testing in Rodents 235
3.9. Conventional Rat Strains for Carcinogenicity Testing 237
3.10. Mouse Models of Carcinogenesis 238
3.11. Transgenic Models for Mutagenicity Testing 240
3.12. The Tg.rasH2 Mouse Model 240
3.13. The $Tp53^{+/-}$ Mouse Model 240
3.14. Hamsters 240
3.15. Zebrafish 241
3.16. Organoids 242
3.17. Clinical Pathology 242
3.18. Histopathology 242
3.19. Carcinogenicity Study Data Interpretation 242
4. Evolving and New Technologies 244
4.1. Gene Expression Analysis 244
4.2. Next Generation Sequencing to Assess Mutagenicity and Genome Instability 244
5. Conclusions 245
Acknowledgments 246
References 247

PART 2
Methods in Toxicologic Pathology

9. Basic Approaches in Anatomic Toxicologic Pathology
TORRIE A. CRABBS AND KEITH NELSON

1. Introduction 257
2. General Considerations in Study Protocol Development 258
3. In-Life Evaluations 265
4. Necropsy 268
5. Fixation and Histologic Procedures 272
6. Specialized Histologic Techniques 275
7. Histopathologic Evaluation 277
7.1. Cause of Death 278
7.2. Nomenclature 279
7.3. Severity Grading 281
8. Artifacts versus Lesions 282
9. Diagnostic Challenges in Anatomic Toxicologic Pathology 284
10. Conclusions 289
References 290

10. Clinical Pathology in Nonclinical Toxicity Testing

A. ERIC SCHULTZE, DANIELA ENNULAT AND
ADAM D. AULBACH

1. Introduction   295
    1.1. Value of Clinical Pathology
         Testing   295
    1.2. The Role of a High-Quality Clinical
         Pathology Laboratory in Toxicity
         Testing   296
    1.3. Samples Submitted to the Clinical Pathology
         Laboratory   302
    1.4. Recommended Test Parameters   303
    1.5. Kinetics   304
    1.6. Controls   305
2. Clinical Pathology Parameters Commonly
   Included in Protocols for General Toxicity
   Studies   305
    2.1. Hematology   305
    2.2. Hemostasis   307
    2.3. Clinical Chemistry   310
    2.4. Urinalysis   315
    2.5. Bone Marrow Evaluation   317
    2.6. Flow Cytometry   318
3. Nonstandard Biomarkers   318
    3.1. Introduction   318
    3.2. Biomarker Assay Kits   318
    3.3. Fit-for-Purpose (Analytical)
         Validation   319
    3.4. Biologic Validation   319
    3.5. Biomarker Application in Nonclinical
         Studies   319
    3.6. Hormones   319
    3.7. Acute Phase Proteins   321
    3.8. Novel Renal Biomarkers   321
    3.9. New Liver Biomarkers   325
    3.10. Heart Biomarkers   327
    3.11. Drug-induced Vascular Injury
          Biomarkers   329
4. Conclusions   330
References   330

11. Special Techniques in Toxicologic Pathology

SHARI A. PRICE, KEVIN MCDORMAN, CURTIS CHAN,
JENNIFER ROJKO, JAMES T. RAYMOND, DANIELLE BROWN, NA LI,
CHRISTINA SATTERWHITE, TRACEY PAPENFUSS AND
JAMES MORRISON

1. Introduction   336
2. Immunohistochemistry   337
    2.1. Introduction   337
    2.2. Applications of Immunohistochemistry in
         Toxicologic Pathology   338

    2.3. Technical Considerations for
         Immunohistochemistry   352
    2.4. Conclusion   356
3. Enzyme Histochemistry   356
    3.1. Introduction   356
    3.2. Applications of Enzyme Histochemistry in
         Toxicologic Pathology   357
    3.3. Technical Considerations for Enzyme
         Histochemistry   357
    3.4. Conclusions   358
4. In Situ Hybridization   358
    4.1. Introduction   358
    4.2. Applications of In Situ Hybridization in
         Toxicologic Pathology   358
    4.3. Technical Considerations for In Situ
         Hybridization   361
    4.4. Conclusions   364
5. Flow Cytometry   365
    5.1. Introduction   365
    5.2. Applications of Flow Cytometry in
         Toxicologic Pathology   369
    5.3. Advantages and Limitations of Flow
         Cytometry   373
    5.4. Conclusions   374
6. Laser Capture Microdissection   374
    6.1. Introduction   374
    6.2. Applications of Laser Capture
         Microdissection in Toxicologic
         Pathology   375
    6.3. Technical Considerations for Laser Capture
         Microdissection   375
    6.4. Limitations   377
    6.5. Conclusions   377
7. Confocal Microscopy   377
    7.1. Introduction   377
    7.2. Applications of Confocal Microscopy in
         Toxicologic Pathology   377
    7.3. Technical Considerations for Confocal
         Microscopy   378
    7.4. Limitations   380
    7.5. Conclusions   380
8. Electron Microscopy   380
    8.1. Introduction   380
    8.2. Applications of Electron Microscopy in
         Toxicologic Pathology   380
    8.3. Technical Considerations for Electron
         Microscopy   381
    8.4. Limitations   382
    8.5. Conclusions   382
9. Stereology   382
10. Digital Pathology   384
11. Conclusions   384
Glossary   384
References   385

12. Digital Pathology and Tissue Image Analysis

FAMKE AEFFNER, THOMAS FOREST, VANESSA SCHUMACHER, MARK ZARELLA AND ALYS BRADLEY

1. Introduction 395
2. Whole-Slide Imaging 396
   2.1. Scanning Modalities 396
   2.2. Scanning in Focus 397
   2.3. Scanning Capacity and Time 398
   2.4. Scanning Magnification 398
   2.5. Scanning Resolution 399
   2.6. Color Preservation 399
   2.7. Image Compression 400
   2.8. Pyramid Representation 401
   2.9. Digital Workflow 401
3. Tissue Image Analysis 406
   3.1. Visual and Cognitive Biases of Manual Slide Review 407
   3.2. Application Areas 407
   3.3. Impact of Preanalytical Variables on Image Analysis 409
   3.4. Manual versus Automated Image Annotations 409
   3.5. The Basics of Quantitative Image Analysis 410
   3.6. Nonquantitative Image Analysis 412
   3.7. Available Tools 412
   3.8. The Pathologist's Role in the Image Analysis Workflow 413
   3.9. Computational Pathology 414
   3.10. Introduction to Artificial Intelligence and Machine Learning in Tissue Image Analysis 414
4. Regulatory Considerations for Digital Pathology Evaluation 416
5. Related Topics 418
   5.1. Stereology 418
   5.2. 3D Reconstruction 419
   5.3. Other Imaging Modalities 419
6. Conclusion 419
References 420

13. In Vivo Small Animal Imaging: A Comparison to Gross and Histopathologic Observations in Animal Models

KATHLEEN GABRIELSON, POLINA SYSA-SHAH, CLAIRE LYONS, DMITRI ARTEMOV, CATHERINE A. FOSS, CHRISTOPHER T. WINKELMANN AND SÉBASTIEN MONETTE

1. Introduction 424
2. Magnetic Resonance Imaging and Magnetic Resonance Microscopy 426

   2.1. Basic Principles of MRI/MRM 426
   2.2. Advantages 428
   2.3. Disadvantages 428
   2.4. Correlation of MRI or MRM to Gross or Histopathological Lesions 429
3. Computed Tomography 430
   3.1. Basic Principles of CT 430
   3.2. Image Information 432
   3.3. Experimental Procedures 432
   3.4. Advantages 433
   3.5. Disadvantages 433
   3.6. CT Imaging in Preclinical Toxicology 434
4. Radionuclide-based Imaging: PET and SPECT 434
   4.1. Basic Physics of PET 434
   4.2. Basic Physics of SPECT 437
   4.3. Comparative Utility of PET and SPECT 437
   4.4. Advantages 437
   4.5. Disadvantages 438
   4.6. Radionuclide-Based Imaging in Preclinical Toxicity Studies 439
5. Optical Imaging 442
   5.1. Basic Principles of Bioluminescence Imaging 442
   5.2. Basic Principles of Fluorescence Imaging 442
   5.3. Advantages 443
   5.4. Disadvantages 444
   5.5. Optical Imaging in Preclinical Toxicity Studies 447
6. Ultrasound 448
   6.1. Basic Physics 448
   6.2. Advantages 451
   6.3. Disadvantages 452
   6.4. Ultrasound Imaging in Preclinical Efficacy Studies 452
7. Translational Application, Safety Assessment, and Drug Screening with In Vivo or Ex Vivo Imaging 453
Abbreviations for Imaging Modalities 453
Acknowledgments 453
References 453

14. Biomarkers: Discovery, Qualification, and Application

MYRTLE A. DAVIS, SANDY ELDRIDGE AND CALVERT LOUDEN

1. Introduction 459
   1.1. Biomarker versus Surrogate 460
   1.2. Qualification versus Validation 460

2. Categories of Biomarkers   460
   2.1. Biomarkers of Tissue Injury/
       Damage   460
   2.2. Biomarkers of Altered Organ
       Function   468
   2.3. Mechanistic Biomarkers   469
   2.4. Biomarkers of Environmental
       Exposure   472
   2.5. Drug Response or Pharmacodynamic
       Biomarkers (See "Principles of
       Pharmacodynamics and Toxicodynamics,
       Vol 1, Chap 5)   473
   2.6. Predictive Biomarkers   474
   2.7. Patient/Clinical Trial Subject
       Selection   475
   2.8. Surrogate Endpoint   476
   2.9. Pharmacogenomic Biomarkers   478
   2.10. Prognostic Biomarkers   478
3. Strategies for Discovery of Biomarkers   481
   3.1. Discovery and Application of Panels of
       Biomarkers   483
4. Methods for Biomarker Measurement and
   Quantitation   483
   4.1. Genomics   485
   4.2. Proteomics   485
   4.3. Metabolomics   485
   4.4. Histocytomics   486
   4.5. Antibody-Based Detection
       Systems   486
   4.6. Multiplexed Assays   486
   4.7. Morphology-Based Methods   486
5. Qualification of Biomarkers: Major
   Considerations   488
References   489

15. Toxicogenomics: A Primer for Toxicologic Pathologists

ARUN R. PANDIRI, PIERRE R. BUSHEL AND
ERIC A. BLOMME

1. Introduction   491
2. Basics of Toxicogenomics   492
3. Overview of Toxicogenomic
   Technologies   493
   3.1. Nucleic Acid-Based -Omics
       Platforms   493
   3.2. Microarray Technologies   495
   3.3. Next-Generation Sequencing
       Technologies   496
   3.4. Protein- and Metabolome-Based -Omics
       Platforms   497
   3.5. Proteomics Technologies   497
   3.6. Metabolomics Technologies   500

4. Key Considerations for Conducting
   Toxicogenomic Studies   500
5. Goals and Applications of Toxicogenomic
   Studies   501
6. Sample Considerations   502
   6.1. Study Planning for -Omics
       Endpoints   502
   6.2. Collection and Processing of the -Omics
       Samples   503
   6.3. Extraction of Biomolecules   504
   6.4. Controls for -Omics Assays   505
   6.5. Study Designs and Statistical
       Considerations   507
   6.6. Software Tools and Databases   509
   6.7. Data Analysis and Interpretation   509
7. Applications of Toxicogenomics   519
   7.1. Predictive Toxicology   519
   7.2. Mechanistic Toxicology   527
   7.3. Carcinogenicity Assessment   529
8. Regulatory Considerations   534
9. Conclusions   536
Glossary   537
Acknowledgments   538
References   538

16. Experimental Design and Statistical Analysis for Toxicologic Pathologists

COLIN G. ROUSSEAUX, KEITH R. SHOCKLEY AND
SHAYNE C. GAD

1. Introduction   546
   1.1. Observations and Measurements   547
   1.2. Data Type and Statistical
       Methods   548
   1.3. Understanding Biological
       Variation   549
   1.4. Biological and Statistical
       Significance   550
2. Considerations Made Before Designing the
   Experiment   553
   2.1. Differing Group Variability   553
   2.2. Involuntary Censoring   553
   2.3. Metaanalysis   553
   2.4. Unbalanced Designs   554
   2.5. Undesirable Variables   554
   2.6. Experimental Unit   554
3. Experimental Design   555
   3.1. Basic Principles of Experimental
       Design   555
   3.2. Detecting Treatment Effects   556
   3.3. Censoring   561
   3.4. Impacts of Sample Size   562

4. Designs Commonly Used in Toxicologic
   Pathology   562
   4.1. Completely Randomized Design   563
   4.2. Completely Randomized Block
        Design   563
   4.3. Matched Pairs Design   563
   4.4. Latin Square Design   564
   4.5. Factorial Design   564
   4.6. Nested Design   564
5. Functions of Statistical Analyses   565
   5.1. Hypothesis Testing and Probability (P)
        Values   566
   5.2. Modeling   566
   5.3. Dimension Reduction   567
6. Prerequisites to Statistical Analysis   568
   6.1. Describing the Data   568
   6.2. Statistical Graphics   570
   6.3. Evaluating Distributional
        Assumptions   576
   6.4. Data Processing   578
7. Statistical Methods   582
   7.1. Statistical Analysis: General
        Considerations   582
   7.2. Hypothesis Testing of Categorical
        Data   588
   7.3. Hypothesis Testing in Single Factor
        Experiments   590
   7.4. Hypothesis Testing in Multifactor
        Experiments   596
   7.5. Analysis of Covariance   597
   7.6. Modeling Trends   599
   7.7. Correlation and Agreement   608
   7.8. Nonparametric Hypothesis
        Testing   610
   7.9. Quantifying Uncertainty   619
   7.10. Methods for the Reduction of
         Dimensionality   620
   7.11. Metaanalysis   624
   7.12. Bayesian Inference   626
8. Interpretation of Results   629
   8.1. Causality versus Association   629
   8.2. Possible Sources of Bias   631
   8.3. Use of Historical Control Data   631
   8.4. Using Scientific Judgment   632
9. Data Analysis Applications in Toxicologic
   Pathology   632
   9.1. Body and Organ Weights   632
   9.2. Clinical Chemistry   634
   9.3. Hematology   634
   9.4. Incidence of Histopathological
        Findings   635
   9.5. Carcinogenesis   636
10. Assumptions of Statistical Tests   638
11. Summary and Conclusions   638
Glossary   645
References   648

PART 3
Animal and Alternative Models in Toxicologic Research

17. Animal Models in Toxicologic Research:
Rodents

PETER J.M. CLEMENTS, BRAD BOLON, ELIZABETH MCINNES,
SYDNEY MUKARATIRWA AND CHERYL SCUDAMORE

1. Introduction   653
2. Rodent Model Selection   655
   2.1. Overview of Species Selection for Toxicity
        Studies   655
   2.2. Rodent Species Used for Special
        Studies   659
   2.3. Rodent Models of Disease and Genetically
        Modified Animals   660
3. Issues in Extrapolation of Rodent Data for Human
   Risk Assessment   661
   3.1. Pharmacologic Translational Relevance and
        Interspecies Pathophysiologic
        Concordance   662
   3.2. Biological and Cell Therapies   665
   3.3. Controlling Variability and Impact of the
        Microbiome in Rodent Studies   665
4. Basic Biological Characteristics of Common Rodent Stocks and Strains   667
   4.1. Outbred Stocks and Inbred Strains of Mice
        and Rats   667
   4.2. Anatomy and Physiology of Rodents Used in
        Toxicologic Research   670
5. Common Pathologic Findings in
   Rodents   675
   5.1. Background Findings in Common
        Species—Mice and Rats   675
   5.2. Background Findings in Uncommon Rodent
        Species   680
   5.3. Considerations in Evaluating Incidental
        Background Findings   682
6. Conclusion   688
Acknowledgments   689
References   689

18. Animal Models in Toxicologic Research:
Rabbit

LYN MILLER WANCKET, ALYS BRADLEY AND
LAUREN E. HIMMEL

1. Introduction   695
2. Model Selection   696
   2.1. Overview of Toxicology Model Species
        Selection   696
   2.2. Issues in Data Extrapolation to
        Human   696
3. Basic Biological Characteristics and Common
   Breeds   696

3.1. Ethics and Animal Welfare
    Considerations   699
4. Regulatory Aspects and Examples of Use of Rabbits in Biomedical Research   699
5. Pharmacokinetic and Toxicity Studies   701
    5.1. Developmental and Reproductive Toxicity
        Studies   701
    5.2. Dermal Irritation/Toxicity Studies   701
    5.3. Intracutaneous and Implantation Safety
        Studies   701
    5.4. Cardiac Safety Studies   702
    5.5. Mucosal Irritation Studies   703
    5.6. Ocular Studies   703
    5.7. Safety Studies Supporting Vaccine
        Development   705
6. Major Disease and Functional Models
    (Other than Safety)   705
    6.1. Antibody Production/Immunological
        Research   705
    6.2. Oncology Disease Models   706
    6.3. Novel Surgical Models   706
    6.4. Medical Device and Regenerative
        Medicine—Functional Studies   706
    6.5. Watanabe Rabbit Model of
        Hypercholesterolemia   707
7. Spontaneous Findings in the Experimental NZW
    Rabbit   709
    7.1. Normal Structures Unique to the
        Rabbit   709
    7.2. Spontaneous Pathology Findings   712
References   715

19. Animal Models in Toxicologic Research: Dog

JOHN R. FOSTER, VASANTHI MOWAT, BHANU P. SINGH,
JENNIFER L. INGRAM–ROSS AND DINO BRADLEY

1. Introduction   722
2. History and Derivation of Beagles   722
    2.1. Genetics of Canines and Background
        for Their Use in Toxicity Testing   722
    2.2. The Evolution of the Laboratory
        Beagle   723
    2.3. Basic Biological Characteristics   723
    2.4. Housing and Care of the Beagle
        Dog   726
3. Use of Dogs in Biomedical Research   727
    3.1. Drug Metabolism, Disposition, and
        Excretion of Drugs/Chemicals in the
        Dog—Comparison with Other
        Species   727
    3.2. Genetic Variability within Beagles and
        Impact on Testing   727
    3.3. Use of the Dog in Drug Discovery and
        Development   728
    3.4. Duration of Studies/Age at Start of Studies
        in Dogs   728
    3.5. Use of the Dog for Assessing Clinical
        Pathology and Pharmacokinetic
        Changes   729
    3.6. Safety Pharmacology Studies in
        Dogs   730
    3.7. Use of Dogs in Developmental Toxicity
        Studies   731
4. Predictivity of Dog Toxicity Data to
    Humans   731
5. Comparative Toxicology of the Dog   732
    5.1. Toxic Responses of the Dog Compared to
        Other Species   732
    5.2. Small-Molecule Kinase
        Inhibitors   733
    5.3. Caffeine   733
    5.4. Theobromine   734
    5.5. Acetaminophen (Paracetamol)   734
    5.6. Aspirin and Ibuprofen   735
    5.7. Vasoactive Drugs   735
6. Spontaneous Background Pathology in the Beagle
    (Refer to Woicke et al., 2021)   735
    6.1. Spontaneous Nonneoplastic Diseases in
        Laboratory Beagles   735
    6.2. Spontaneous Neoplastic Diseases in
        Laboratory Beagles   737
7. Use of the Dog as a Model of Human
    Diseases   737
    7.1. The Dog as an Animal Model of Human
        Cardiovascular Disease   737
    7.2. The Dog as an Animal Model of Human
        Cancer   737
    7.3. The Dog as an Animal Model of Human
        Neurological Diseases   739
8. Regulatory Considerations for Toxicity
    Studies   742
    8.1. Pesticide and Drug Development—Need for
        One-Year Dog Study?   742
9. Ethics of Use of the Dog as a Laboratory
    Animal Species   743
10. Summary   744
References   744

20. Animal Models in Toxicologic Research: Pig

KRISTI HELKE, KEITH NELSON AND AARON SARGEANT

1. Introduction   751
2. Genetics of Pigs and Background for Their Use in
    Research   752

2.1. Breeds   752
2.2. Basic Biological Characteristics   753
2.3. Husbandry Considerations   753
3. Use of Pigs in Toxicological Studies   755
  3.1. Study Design Considerations   755
  3.2. Oral Toxicity Studies   756
  3.3. Intravenous Toxicity Studies   756
  3.4. Subcutaneous Dosing Toxicity
       Studies   757
  3.5. Dermal Toxicity Studies   757
  3.6. Other Routes of Dose
       Administration   759
  3.7. Embryo—Fetal Toxicity Studies   759
  3.8. Juvenile Toxicity Studies   760
4. Pigs as Organ Source for
   Xenotransplantation   761
5. Spontaneous Background Pathology in
   Swine   761
  5.1. Macroscopic Observations   762
  5.2. Microscopic Findings   764
  5.3. Neoplasia in Research Swine   769
6. Use of the Pig as a Model System for Medical
   Devices and of Human Diseases   770
  6.1. Cardiovascular   770
  6.2. Skin   770
  6.3. Renal   771
  6.4. Metabolic Syndrome/Diabetes   771
  6.5. Eye   771
  6.6. Brain   771
  6.7. Immune System   772
  6.8. Cancer   772
  6.9. Genetically Modified Pigs   772
7. Regulatory Aspects   772
8. Ethics and Animal Welfare   773
9. Summary   773
References   774

2.6. The Tamarins (*Saguinus* sp.)   781
2.7. The Vervet and Green Monkeys
     (*Chlorocebus aethiops* ssp. *sabaeus* and
     pygerythrus)   781
2.8. The Capuchin Monkey (*Cebus* sp.)   781
3. Selection of Nonhuman Primates for
   Toxicologic Research and Study Design
   Considerations   782
  3.1. Ethics and Welfare Considerations   782
  3.2. Regulatory Considerations   783
  3.3. Source, Origin, and Genetic
       Variation   784
  3.4. Relevance and Feasibility for Use in Drug
       Development   785
  3.5. Study Design   786
4. Predictivity of Nonhuman Primate Toxicity Data
   to Humans   787
5. Nonhuman Primate Models in Biomedical
   Research (see also (Abee, Mansfield, Tardif, &
   Morris, 2012)   787
  5.1. Nonhuman Primate Models of Human
       Disease   788
  5.2. Models in Pharmacology and Toxicology
       Research   790
6. Background Findings in Nonhuman Primates and
   Use of Historical Control Data   796
  6.1. Incidental Findings in Nonhuman
       Primates   796
  6.2. Environmental, Endemic, and Contagious
       Pathogens   797
  6.3. Findings due to Antidrug
       Antibodies   798
  6.4. Historical Control Data   800
7. Conclusion   801
References   801

21. Animal Models in Toxicologic Research: Nonhuman Primate

JENNIFER A. CHILTON, STEVEN T. LAING AND
ALYS BRADLEY

1. Introduction   777
2. History and Biological Characteristics of
   Nonhuman Primates   778
  2.1. The Cynomolgus Macaque
       (*Macaca fascicularis*)   778
  2.2. The Rhesus Macaque
       (*Macaca mulatta*)   778
  2.3. The Common Marmoset
       (*Callithrix jacchus*)   780
  2.4. The Baboon (*Papio* sp.)   780
  2.5. The Squirrel Monkey (*Saimiri* sp.)   781

22. Animal Models in Toxicologic Research: Nonmammalian

DEBRA A. TOKARZ AND JEFFREY C. WOLF

1. Introduction   811
2. Nonmammalian Animal Taxa   815
  2.1. Invertebrates   815
  2.2. Fish   818
  2.3. Amphibians   825
  2.4. Birds   828
  2.5. Reptiles   830
3. Utilization of Nonmammalian Animals   831
  3.1. Animal Models of Human
       Diseases   831
  3.2. Drug Discovery and Toxicity
       Screening   834
  3.3. Target Animal Safety Studies   837

3.4. Ecotoxicological Testing and Environmental Monitoring 838
4. Study Design Considerations 841
  4.1. Study Design and Implementation 841
  4.2. Subclinical Disease 844
5. Data Extrapolation 847
  5.1. Results Extrapolation and Risk Assessment 847
  5.2. Interspecies Variability 848
  5.3. Knowledge Gap 850
  5.4. Reliability of Published Histopathology Data 851
6. Conclusions 851
Acknowledgments 852
References 853

23. Genetically Engineered Animal Models in Toxicologic Research

LAUREN E. HIMMEL, KRISTIN LEWIS WILSON, SARA F. SANTAGOSTINO AND BRAD BOLON

1. Fundamentals of Genetically Engineered Animal Models 859
  1.1. Methods for Genetic Modification 860
  1.2. Nomenclature Conventions 878
  1.3. Model Selection 879
2. Analysis of Genetically Engineered Animal Models 881
  2.1. Genotyping 881
  2.2. Phenotyping 883
  2.3. Large-Scale Phenotyping 883
  2.4. Directed Phenotypic Characterization for Product Discovery and Development 885
  2.5. Phenotypic Interpretation of Genetically Engineered Animal Models 886
3. Genetically Modified Models for Hazard Identification and Safety Assessment 888
  3.1. Basic Concepts for Using Engineered Animals in Hazard Identification and Safety Assessment 888
  3.2. Absorption, Distribution, Metabolism, and Excretion 889
  3.3. Genotoxicity Testing 892
  3.4. Carcinogenicity Assessment 895
  3.5. Engineered Immunodeficient Models 898
  3.6. Humanized Animal Models 904
4. Limitations in Using Genetically Modified Animals for Hazard Identification and Safety Assessment 913
5. Special Considerations in Safety Assessment of Products Derived from Genetically Engineered Animals 913

  5.1. Biopharming and Xenotransplantation 913
  5.2. Food Products 916
6. Summary 917
Glossary 917
Acknowledgments 918
References 918

24. Alternative Models in Biomedical Research: In Silico, In Vitro, Ex Vivo, and Nontraditional In Vivo Approaches

JINPING GAN, BRAD BOLON, TERRY VAN VLEET AND CHARLES WOOD

1. Introduction 925
2. Nontraditional Models in Toxicity Research 926
  2.1. Overview of In Vitro and Ex Vivo Models 926
  2.2. Overview of In Vivo Models in Alternative Mammalian and Nonmammalian Species 927
  2.3. Overview of In Silico Modeling 928
3. In Vitro and Ex Vivo Models 928
  3.1. Cell Cultures 928
  3.2. Tissue Slices 930
  3.3. Bioprinted Microtissues 934
  3.4. Miniorgans 935
  3.5. Microphysiological Systems ("Organs On Chips") 941
  3.6. Stem Cells and Genetically Modified Cells 943
  3.7. Whole Embryo Culture 945
4. In Silico Models and Data Analytics 946
  4.1. In Silico Predictive Structure–Activity Models 946
  4.2. Pathway-Based Models of Toxicity 947
  4.3. Big Data Analytics in Toxicology Pathology 948
5. In Vivo Models Using Alternative Mammalian and Nonmammalian Species 951
  5.1. Genetically Engineered Animal Models 951
  5.2. Non-mammalian Animal Models 952
6. Regulatory Perspective on Alternative Models 955
7. Conclusions and Perspectives 955
  7.1. Integration of Pathology and Alternative Data Streams 955
  7.2. Context of Use and Qualification Requirements 957
  7.3. Future Directions 958
References 958

PART 4
Practice of Toxicologic Pathology

25. Nomenclature and Diagnostic Resources in Anatomic Toxicologic Pathology

CYNTHIA J. WILLSON, CHARLOTTE M. KEENAN, MARK F. CESTA AND DEEPA B. RAO

1. Introduction 969
2. The Need for Standardized Nomenclature 970
3. Components in Nomenclature 971
   3.1. Terminology for Nonneoplastic Lesions 971
   3.2. Terminology for Neoplastic Lesions 972
4. Challenges in Standardizing Nomenclature 973
   4.1. Training 973
   4.2. Thresholds 974
   4.3. Diagnostic Drift 975
   4.4. Severity Grading 975
   4.5. Lesion Complexity 976
   4.6. Multiple Pathologists 976
5. Recommended Practices 977
   5.1. Training 977
   5.2. Thresholds 977
   5.3. Diagnostic Drift 978
   5.4. Severity Grading 978
   5.5. Lesion Complexity 978
   5.6. Multiple Pathologists 979
   5.7. The Pathology Narrative 979
6. Harmonization of Nomenclature 980
   6.1. International Harmonization of Nomenclature and Diagnostic Criteria 980
   6.2. Standard for Exchange of Nonclinical Data 982
   6.3. National Toxicology Program Nonneoplastic Lesion Atlas 983
   6.4. Other Nomenclature Resources 983
7. Conclusions 983
Acknowledgments 984
References 984

26. Pathology Peer Review

FRANK J. GEOLY, BINDU M. BENNET, JAMES D. FIKES AND JERRY F. HARDISTY

1. Introduction 987
2. Peer Review Timing and Pathology Raw Data 988
   2.1. Pathology Raw Data and Peer Review 989

3. Peer Review Process 990
   3.1. Consultation 990
   3.2. Peer Review: Contemporaneous Peer Review 990
   3.3. Resolution of Disagreements during Contemporaneous Peer Review 997
   3.4. Documentation of Contemporaneous Peer Review 1000
   3.5. Peer Review: Retrospective Peer Review 1001
4. National Toxicology Program Review Process 1003
5. Regulatory Aspects of Pathology Peer Review 1004
   5.1. Regulations for Contemporaneous Pathology Peer Review in China and Japan 1006
6. Use of Digital/Whole-Slide Images in Pathology Peer Review 1006
   6.1. Use of Whole-Slide Images for National Toxicology Program Pathology Working Groups 1007
7. Conclusion 1007
References 1008

27. Pathology and GLPs, Quality Control, and Quality Assurance

KATHLEEN MARIE HEINZ-TAHENY

1. Introduction 1009
2. Overview of Good Laboratory Practice Standards 1010
   2.1. History and Evolution of GLP Standards 1010
   2.2. Objective and Scope 1015
   2.3. FDA GLP General Content 1016
   2.4. Organization of 21 CFR 58 Good Laboratory Practice for Nonclinical Laboratory Studies 1016
3. GLP and Pathology Data 1021
   3.1. Study Pathologist Requirements 1021
   3.2. Histopathology in the GLP Environment 1021
4. Clinical Pathology Assessment in the GLP Environment 1024
5. Ultrastructural Assessment in the GLP Environment 1024
6. Noninvasive Imaging Applications in the GLP Environment 1024
7. In the Spirit of GLP 1025
8. GLP Criticism 1025
   8.1. Academic Research 1025
   8.2. Perspectives on GLP Limitations 1026
9. Conclusions 1026
References 1026

28. Practices to Optimize Generation, Interpretation, and Reporting of Pathology Data from Toxicity Studies

ARMANDO R. IRIZARRY ROVIRA, DAVID GARCIA-TAPIA AND DANIEL J. PATRICK

1. Introduction   1030
2. Practices that Prevent or Mitigate the Introduction of Pathology-Related Issues During Study Design and Protocol Preparation   1031
   2.1. Ensure a Deep Understanding of Regulatory Guidance and Best Practices   1032
   2.2. Clearly Define Realistic Study Goals, Design the Study to Accomplish Those Goals, and Minimize Study Complexity   1035
   2.3. Choose the Appropriate Animal Species, Genetic Background, and/or Disease Model for Toxicity Testing   1037
   2.4. Use Optimal Communication Practices   1039
   2.5. Estimate and Communicate the Number of Potential Target Tissues   1040
   2.6. Develop and Practice Novel or Nonstandard Pathology Procedures and Other Methods Prior to the Start of the Study and Use Accepted Practices for Incorporation of Nonstandard Endpoints   1040
   2.7. Ensure that Study Procedures Are Adequately Described in the Study Protocol or Standard Operating Procedures   1042
   2.8. Plan for Pathology Peer Review   1043
   2.9. Do Not Blind the Study Pathologist   1043
   2.10. Facilitate the Study and Peer Review Pathologists' Workflows   1044
3. Practices that Prevent or Mitigate the Introduction of Pathology-Related Issues Arising During the In-Life Phase   1044
   3.1. Ensure the Proper Training of Personnel, Use of Appropriate Assays, Maintenance of Required Instrumentation, and Use of Quality Assurance Programs   1045
   3.2. Ensure Awareness of Emerging Data from In-Life Time Points and Unscheduled Terminations   1046
   3.3. Mitigate the Impact of Unexpected or Significant Toxicity   1047
   3.4. Scrutinize Impromptu Requests for Samples from Ongoing Studies for Assays that Are Not Critical to the Purpose of the Study   1049
   3.5. Understand When Not to Generate Pathology Data   1049
4. Practices that Prevent or Mitigate Issues Arising from Pathology Assessment and Reporting   1050
   4.1. Ensure Proper Training, Supervision, Procedures, and Protocol Familiarity in the Necropsy, Histology, and Clinical Pathology Laboratories   1050
   4.2. Schedule Adequate Time for Processing and Evaluation   1054
   4.3. Establish Strong Lines of Communication and Freely Share Scientific and Program Information with the Study Pathologist   1057
   4.4. Recommended Practices for Histopathologic Assessment   1060
   4.5. Facilitate Finalization of a Well-Constructed, High-Quality, On-Time Pathology Report   1069
5. Conclusions   1072
Glossary   1072
References   1072

29. Issues in Laboratory Animal Science That Impact Toxicologic Pathology

JEFFREY EVERITT, ANGELA KING-HERBERT, PETER J.M. CLEMENTS AND RICK ADLER

1. Introduction   1078
2. Trends in Global Research Animal Care and Use   1078
3. Regulatory Issues   1081
   3.1. Overview of Rules and Regulations   1081
   3.2. Institutional Animal Care and Use Committee   1083
4. Euthanasia of Research Animals   1083
5. Selection of Animal Models   1084
   5.1. Overview   1084
   5.2. Issues of Translation in Animal Model Selection   1084
   5.3. Genetic Considerations   1086
   5.4. Issues to Consider When Sourcing Animals   1087
   5.5. Use of Specialized Animal Models in Toxicology Research   1088
6. Animal Health Considerations   1089
   6.1. Adventitious Agents   1089
   6.2. Sentinel Monitoring Programs   1090
   6.3. Microbial Effects on Toxicity   1090
7. Microbiome and Microbial Effects on Patho-physiology and Study Outcomes   1091
   7.1. Introduction to the Microbiome   1091
   7.2. Definitions, Natural History, and Characterization   1092

7.3. Association With Development, Immune Status, and Disease Phenotype—Cause or Effect?   1092

7.4. Impact on Efficacy, Biotransformation, and Toxicology   1094

7.5. Impact of Microbiome on Safety Translatability   1095

7.6. Minimizing Experimental Variability and Monitoring Microbiome Status   1095

8. Housing and Husbandry Issues   1096

8.1. Role of Environment in Lesion Production   1096

8.2. Study Design Considerations   1097

9. The Role of Diet in Toxicity Studies   1099

9.1. Introduction   1099

9.2. Types of Diets   1100

9.3. Contaminant Issues   1101

9.4. Dietary Optimization   1101

10. 3R's and In-Life Study Conduct for the Toxicologic Pathologist   1102

11. Description of Animal Studies in Scientific Publications   1103

12. Conclusion   1103

References   1103

Index   1107

Contributors

Rick Adler GlaxoSmithKline, Collegeville, PA, United States

Famke Aeffner Amgen Inc., Amgen Research, Translational Safety and Bioanalytical Sciences, South San Francisco, CA, United States

Laura E. Armstrong Bristol-Myers Squibb Co., Princeton, NJ, United States

Dmitri Artemov Department of Radiology and Radiological Sciences, School of Medicine, Johns Hopkins University, Baltimore, MD, United States

Adam D. Aulbach Inotiv, Maryland Heights, MO, United States

Bindu M. Bennet Nonclinical Safety, Relay Therapeutics, Cambridge, Massachusetts, United States

Eric A. Blomme AbbVie, Chicago, IL, United States

Brad Bolon GEMpath, Inc., Longmont, CO, United States

Christopher J. Bowman Drug Safety Research & Development, Worldwide Research, Development, & Medical Pfizer, Inc., Groton, CT, United States

Molly Boyle Covance Somerset, Somerset, NJ, United States

Alys Bradley Charles River Laboratories Edinburgh Ltd., Tranent, Scotland, United Kingdom

Dino Bradley Janssen Research & Development, McKean Road, Spring House, PA, United States

Danielle Brown Charles River Laboratories, Preclinical Services, Durham, NC, United States

Pierre R. Bushel Biostatistics & Computational Biology Branch, National Institute of Environmental Health Sciences, Durham, NC, United States

Ellen Cannady Eli Lilly and Company, Indianapolis, IN, United States

Mark F. Cesta U.S. National Institute of Environmental Health Sciences, Research Triangle Park, NC, United States

Curtis Chan Charles River Laboratories, Preclinical Services, Reno, NV, United States

Jennifer A. Chilton Charles River Safety Assessment, Reno, NV, United States

Peter J.M. Clements GlaxoSmithKline Research and Development, Ware, Hertfordshire, United Kingdom

Torrie A. Crabbs Experimental Pathology Laboratories, Inc., Research Triangle Park, NC, United States

Myrtle A. Davis Discovery Toxicology, Pharmaceutical Candidate Optimization, Bristol Myers Squib, Princeton, NJ, United States

Sandy Eldridge Toxicology and Pharmacology Branch, Division of Cancer Treatment and Diagnosis, National Cancer Institute, NIH, Bethesda, MD, United States

Daniela Ennulat GlaxoSmithKline, Collegeville, PA, United States

Jeffrey Everitt Duke University School of Medicine, Durham, NC, United States

Isabel Figueroa Preclinical Pharmacokinetics and Drug Metabolism Amgen, South San Francisco, CA, United States

James D. Fikes Biogen, Cambridge, Massachusetts, United States

Thomas Forest Merck & Co, Inc., West Point, PA, United States

Catherine A. Foss Department of Radiology and Radiological Sciences, School of Medicine, Johns Hopkins University, Baltimore, MD, United States

John R. Foster ToxPath Sciences Ltd, Congleton, Cheshire, United Kingdom

Kathleen Gabrielson Departments of Molecular and Comparative Pathobiology and Environmental Health and Engineering, School of Medicine and Bloomberg School of Public Health, Johns Hopkins University, Baltimore, MD, United States

Shayne C. Gad Gad Consulting Services, Raleigh, NC, United States

Kapil Gadkar Denali Therapeutics, South San Francisco, CA, United States

Jinping Gan Bristol-Myers Squibb, Princeton, NJ, United States; HiFiBiO Therapeutics, Cambridge, MA, United States

David Garcia-Tapia Eli Lilly & Company, Indianapolis, IN, United States

Frank J. Geoly Pfizer Worldwide Research, Development, and Medical, Groton, Connecticut, United States

Wendy G. Halpern Safety Assessment Pathology, Genentech, South San Francisco, CA, United States

Jerry F. Hardisty Experimental Pathology Laboratories, Inc., Research Triangle Park, North Carolina, United States

Wanda M. Haschek University of Illinois at Urbana Champaign, Urbana, IL, United States

Kathleen Marie Heinz-Taheny Lilly Research Laboratories — Toxicology, Drug Disposition, and PKPD, Eli Lilly and Company, Indianapolis, IN, United States

Kristi Helke Medical University of South Carolina, Charleston, SC, United States

Lauren E. Himmel AbbVie Inc., Preclinical Safety, North Chicago, IL, United States

Mark J. Hoenerhoff In Vivo Animal Core, Unit for Laboratory Animal Medicine, University of Michigan Medical School, Ann Arbor, MI, United States

Jennifer L. Ingram–Ross Janssen Research & Development, McKean Road, Spring House, PA, United States

Armando R. Irizarry Rovira Eli Lilly & Company, Indianapolis, IN, United States

Evan B. Janovitz Bristol Meyer Squibb Co, Princeton, NJ, United States

Kishore Katyayan Eli Lilly and Company, Indianapolis, IN, United States

Charlotte M. Keenan C.M. Keenan ToxPath Consulting, Doylestown, PA, United States

Angela King-Herbert DNTP Comparative Medicine Group, National Institutes of Environmental Health Sciences, Research Triangle Park, NC, United States

Steven T. Laing Genentech Safety Assessment, South San Francisco, CA, United States

Lois D. Lehman-McKeeman Bristol-Myers Squibb Co., Princeton, NJ, United States

Na Li Charles River Laboratories, Preclinical Services, Morrisville, NC, United States

Calvert Louden Tox-Path-LAM, Janssen Pharmaceuticals R&D, Raritan, NJ, United States

Claire Lyons Department of Molecular and Comparative Pathobiology, School of Medicine, Johns Hopkins University, Baltimore, MD, United States

Kevin McDorman Charles River Laboratories, Preclinical Services, Frederick, MD, United States

Elizabeth McInnes Syngenta, Bracknell, United Kingdom

Lyn Miller Wancket Charles River, Durham, NC, United States

Sheroy Minocherhomji Amgen Inc., Translational Safety & Bioanalytical Sciences, Thousand Oaks, CA, United States

Sébastien Monette Laboratory of Comparative Pathology, Memorial Sloan Kettering Cancer Center, The Rockefeller University, Weill Cornell Medicine, New York, NY, United States

James Morrison Charles River Laboratories, Preclinical Services, Shrewsbury, MA, United States

Vasanthi Mowat Labcorp Clinical & Preclinical Services Ltd, Huntingdon, United Kingdom

Sydney Mukaratirwa Boehringer Ingelheim Pharma GmbH, Biberach, Germany

Keith Nelson Charles River Laboratories, Mattawan, MI, United States

Arun R. Pandiri Molecular Pathology Group, Comparative and Molecular Pathogenesis Branch, Division of the National Toxicology Program, National Institute of Environmental Health Sciences, Durham, NC, United States

Tracey Papenfuss Charles River Laboratories, Preclinical Services, Ashland, OH, United States

Nita Patel Eli Lilly and Company, Indianapolis, IN, United States

Daniel J. Patrick Charles River Laboratories, Mattawan, MI, United States

Shari A. Price Charles River Laboratories, Preclinical Services, Frederick, MD, United States

Deepa B. Rao StageBio, Frederick, MD, United States

James T. Raymond Charles River Laboratories, Preclinical Services, Frederick, MD, United States

Jennifer Rojko Charles River Laboratories, Preclinical Services, Frederick, MD, United States

Colin G. Rousseaux Department of Pathology and Laboratory Medicine, Faculty of Medicine, University of Ottawa, Ottawa, ON, Canada

Sara F. Santagostino Genentech, Inc., South San Francisco, CA, United States

Aaron Sargeant Charles River Laboratories, Spencerville, OH, United States

Christina Satterwhite Charles River Laboratories, Preclinical Services, Reno, NV, United States

A. Eric Schultze Eli Lilly and Company, Indianapolis, IN, United States

Vanessa Schumacher Roche Pharma Research and Early Development, Roche Innovation Center Basel, F. Hoffmann-La Roche Ltd., Basel, Switzerland

Cheryl Scudamore ExePathology, Exmouth, United Kingdom

Keith R. Shockley Biostatistics and Computational Biology Branch, U.S. National Institute of Environmental Health Sciences, Research Triangle Park, NC, United States

Bhanu P. Singh Gilead Sciences, Foster City, CA, United States

David M. Stresser AbbVie Inc., Drug Metabolism and Pharmacokinetics, North Chicago, IL, United States

Polina Sysa-Shah Department of Urology, School of Medicine, Johns Hopkins University, Baltimore, MD, United States

Debra A. Tokarz Experimental Pathology Laboratories, Inc., Durham, NC, United States

Terry Van Vleet AbbVie, North Chicago, IL, United States

Matthew A. Wallig University of Illinois at Urbana Champaign, Urbana, IL, United States

Jin Wang AbbVie Inc., Drug Metabolism and Pharmacokinetics, North Chicago, IL, United States

Cynthia J. Willson Integrated Laboratory Systems, LLC, Cary, Morrisville, NC, United States

Kristin Lewis Wilson Amgen, Inc., South San Francisco, CA, United States

Christopher T. Winkelmann Takeda Pharmaceutical Company Ltd., Cambridge, MA, United States

Jeffrey C. Wolf Experimental Pathology Laboratories, Inc., Sterling, VA, United States

Charles Wood Boehringer Ingelheim, Ridgefield, CT, United States

Daniela Bumbaca Yadav Department of Pharmacokinetics, Pharmacodynamics, and Drug Metabolism Merck & Co., Inc., South San Francisco, CA, United States

Mark Zarella Johns Hopkins University, Department of Pathology, Baltimore, MD, United States

About the Editors

EDITORS

Wanda M. Haschek-Hock, BVSc, PhD, is a Diplomate of the American College of Veterinary Pathologists (DACVP), past Diplomate of the American Board of Toxicology (DABT), Fellow of the International Academy of Toxicologic Pathology (FIATP), and Honorary Member of the Latin American Society of Toxicologic Pathology. She is a Professor Emerita at the University of Illinois College of Veterinary Medicine, Department of Pathobiology. Wanda has over 40 years of experience in comparative, respiratory, and toxicologic pathology with a research focus on natural toxins and food safety. She is a former president of the Society of Toxicologic Pathology (STP) and of the Society of Toxicology's (SOT) Comparative and Veterinary Specialty Section, and has served as an Associate Editor for the journals *Toxicological Sciences* and *Toxicologic Pathology*, as Councilor of the American College of Veterinary Pathologists (ACVP), and as a member of the Board of the American Board of Toxicology (ABT). She served as an Editor for the three editions of the *Fundamentals of Toxicologic Pathology* and *Haschek and Rousseaux's Handbook of Toxicologic Pathology*. She is a recipient of the STP's Lifetime Achievement Award, the SOT Midwest Regional Chapter's Kenneth DuBois Award, and the University of Sydney Faculty of Veterinary Science Alumni Award for International Achievement.

Colin G. Rousseaux, BVSc, PhD, DABT, FIATP, is also a Fellow of the Royal College of Pathology (FRCPath) and Fellow of the Academy of Toxicological Sciences (FATS). He is a Professor (Adjunct) in the Department of Pathology and Laboratory Medicine, Faculty of Medicine, University of Ottawa, Canada. He has 40 years of experience in comparative and toxicologic pathology with a research focus on fetal development and teratology, herbal remedies, and environmental pollutants. He has described, investigated, and evaluated numerous toxicologic pathology issues associated with pharmaceuticals, pesticides, and agrochemicals. He has served on the Editorial Board of *Toxicologic Pathology* and is a former president of the STP. Colin served as an Editor for the three editions of the *Fundamentals of Toxicologic Pathology* and *Haschek and Rousseaux's Handbook of Toxicologic Pathology*.

Matthew A. Wallig, DVM, PhD, DACVP, is a Professor Emeritus in the Department of Pathobiology, College of Veterinary Medicine, the Department of Food Science and Human Nutrition, as well as the Division of Nutritional Sciences at the University of Illinois. His research has focused on the chemoprotective properties and mechanisms of phytochemicals in the diet, in particular those in cruciferous vegetables, soy, and tomatoes. His current interests have expanded to include defining morphologic parameters for diagnostic quantitative ultrasound in pancreatitis, pancreatic and hepatic neoplasia, metastatic disease, and chronic hepatic diseases such as nonalcoholic fatty liver disease (NAFLD) and nonalcoholic steatohepatitis (NASH). Matt has served as an Editor for the last two editions of the *Fundamentals of Toxicologic Pathology* and *Haschek and Rousseaux's Handbook of Toxicologic Pathology*.

Brad Bolon, DVM, MS, PhD, DAVCP, DABT, FIATP, FRCPath, FATS, has worked [sic] as an experimental and toxicologic pathologist in several settings: academia, a contract research organization, pharmaceutical companies (in both biomolecule and traditional small molecule settings), and private consulting. His main professional interests are the pathology of genetically engineered mice (especially embryos, fetuses, and placentas) and toxicologic neuropathology to assess the efficacy and safety of many therapeutic entities (biomolecules, cell and gene therapies, medical devices, and small molecules). He is a former president of the STP and a member of the American College of Toxicology (ACT), British Society of Toxicological Pathology (BSTP), and European Society of Toxicologic Pathology (ESTP). Brad served as an Editor for the 3rd edition of the *Fundamentals of Toxicologic Pathology* and as an Associate Editor for the 3rd edition of *Haschek and Rousseaux's Handbook of Toxicologic Pathology*.

ASSOCIATE EDITORS

Stacey L. Fossey, DVM, PhD, DACVP, DABT, FIATP, is currently a Senior Principal Pathologist at AbbVie, Inc. She has 10 years of experience as a pathologist and toxicologist in pharmaceutical discovery and development across therapeutic modalities and has expertise in skeletal toxicologic pathology. She is currently a Councilor for the STP and has served as an Associate Editor for the journal *Toxicologic Pathology* and as Chair or CoChair for various STP committees.

John L. Vahle, DVM, PhD, DACVP, currently serves as a Senior Research Fellow at Lilly Research Laboratories. He has 25 years of experience as a pathologist and toxicologist supporting pharmaceutical and biotherapeutic safety assessment. John's research interests include carcinogenicity assessments, bone and endocrine toxicology and pathology, and the impact of immunogenicity and immune complex disease on safety assessment of biotherapeutics. He is a former councilor of the STP, past chair of BioSafe, and serves on the International Council for Harmonisation (ICH) Expert Working Group on carcinogenicity testing of pharmaceuticals.

ILLUSTRATIONS EDITOR

Beth W. Mahler is employed by Experimental Pathology Laboratories, Inc., located in Research Triangle Park, NC, and works as a contractor at the U.S. National Institute of Environmental Health Sciences (NIEHS) in the Cellular and Molecular Pathology Branch under the Division of the National Toxicology Program (NTP). She has over 40 years of experience as a certified histologist (HT) in the areas of histology, animal necropsy, embryo collection and sectioning, and digital photomicroscopy. Since 2006, she has served as the Illustrations Editor for the journal *Toxicologic Pathology*. Past illustrative editorship roles include Associate Editor of *Pathology of the Mouse*, edited by Dr Robert R. Maronpot, and Illustrations Editor for the third edition of the *Fundamentals of Toxicologic Pathology* and *Haschek and Rousseaux's Handbook of Toxicologic Pathology*.

Preface to the 4th Edition

Since its inception 3 decades ago, *Haschek and Rousseaux's Handbook of Toxicologic Pathology* has been a comprehensive resource covering fundamental knowledge and skills as well as key technical procedures essential for the proficient practice of toxicologic pathology. The reference has found a home in the libraries of numerous academic, government, and industrial institutions engaged in basic and applied biomedical research around the globe, and in doing so has become an indispensable reference for many toxicologic pathologists, toxicologists, regulators, physicians, biomedical researchers, and students. Indeed, the *Handbook* has been recognized by many as the most authoritative single source of information in the field due to the breadth and depth of coverage.

Prior to publication of the inaugural *Handbook* edition in 1991, information regarding toxicologic pathology had to be gleaned in a piecemeal manner by reading articles in various toxicology and the few toxicologic pathology journals. The success of the one-volume 1st edition and the expanded roles of toxicologic pathologists over time led in due course to the release of updated *Handbook* versions in subsequent years: a two-volume 2nd edition in 2002 and a three-volume 3rd edition in 2013. The many scientific advances, ongoing and extensive collaboration among global societies of toxicologic pathology, and new regulatory guidance that have occurred since release of the 3rd edition indicate that another rendition is necessary to maintain, and indeed enhance, the value of this resource to practitioners of the toxicologic pathology craft. For this reason, the Editors and Associate Editors are pleased to offer this new and expanded *Handbook* to aid your explorations of the toxicologic pathology field.

The 4th edition of *Haschek and Rousseaux's Handbook of Toxicologic Pathology* has been extensively updated to continue its comprehensive coverage. The unrelenting explosion of information in this field has necessitated that this new edition be rendered as a four-volume set.

- Volume 1 covers *"Principles and Practice of Toxicologic Pathology,"* including such key topics as basic concepts in biology, pathology, pharmacology, and toxicology as they intersect in the field of toxicologic pathology (Chapters 2–8); primary methods of investigation in toxicologic pathology (Chapters 9–16); overviews of major models employed in toxicologic research (Chapters 17–24); and essential practices in generating and interpreting toxicologic pathology data (Chapters 25–29). New chapters address absorption, distribution, metabolism, and excretion (ADME) principles for biomolecules; toxicologic pathology considerations in developmental and reproductive toxicity (DART) testing; digital pathology; and various animal models, including rodents, rabbits, dogs, nonhuman primates, and alternative models (e.g., *in silico, ex vivo*).
- Volume 2 encompasses *"Toxicologic Pathology in Safety Assessment"* and *"Environmental Toxicologic Pathology."* These two areas cover the application of toxicologic pathology in developing specific product classes (Chapters 1–12), principles of data interpretation for safety assessment (Chapters 13–17), and the major considerations and agents in environmental toxicologic pathology (Chapters 18–31). New chapters discuss novel therapeutic classes (nucleic acids, cell and gene therapies [including gene editing], and vaccines); agricultural and bulk chemicals; differentiation of adverse from nonadverse effects; and the toxicologic pathology of herbal remedies and animal- and bacterial-derived toxins.
- Volumes 3 and 4 provide deep and broad treatment of *"Target Organ Toxicity"* for major

systems, emphasizing the comparative and correlative aspects of normal biology and toxicant-induced dysfunction, principal methods for toxicologic pathology evaluation, and major mechanisms of toxicity. New chapters (in Volume 3) will cover adipose tissue, non-cardiac muscle and tendon, as well as oral cavity and teeth.

The expanded coverage of nonclinical testing principles and practices, the new material on various models of toxicity, and the toxicologic pathology of novel toxicant classes (especially new therapeutic modalities) will be a particular strength of this new *Handbook* edition and should and will continue to justify its long-standing reputation for excellence. The Editors do accept that information relevant to toxicity research, hazard identification, and risk assessment and management is evergrowing, and they acknowledge that readers may benefit by extending their search for up-to-the-minute information in this area to include other textbooks and journals of toxicology and toxicologic pathology.

We would like to thank the dedicated efforts of the Associate Editors—Stacey Fossey and John Vahle (Volume 1), Katie Heinz-Taheny and Dan Rudmann (Volume 2), Molly Boyle and Mark Hoenerhoff (Volume 3), and Famke Aeffner, Jeff Everitt and Karen Regan (Volume 4); our incomparable Illustrations Editor, Beth Mahler; and the many authors for their outstanding contributions in bringing this book to fruition. In addition, we wish to specifically acknowledge the significant involvement of many leading toxicologic pathologists as essential contributors to this and previous editions; many are now retired and some are deceased including Charles C. Capen, Victor J. Ferrans, Adalbert Koestner, Robert W. Leader, Daniel Morton, John F. Van Vleet, Hanspeter R. Witschi.

Wanda M. Haschek
Colin G. Rousseaux
Matthew A. Wallig
Brad Bolon

Toxicologic Pathology: An Introduction

Wanda M. Haschek[1], Colin G. Rousseaux[2], Matthew A. Wallig[1], Brad Bolon[3]

[1]University of Illinois at Urbana Champaign, Urbana, IL, United States, [2]Department of Pathology and Laboratory Medicine, Faculty of Medicine, University of Ottawa, Ottawa, ON, Canada, [3]GEMpath, Inc., Longmont, CO, United States

OUTLINE

1. An Overview of Toxicologic Pathology	1	6. The "Practitioner" of Toxicologic Pathology	9
2. What Is Toxicologic Pathology?	3	6.1. Industrial Toxicologic Pathology	9
3. The Basis of Toxicologic Pathology	3	6.2. Toxicologic Pathology Related to the Environment and Food Safety	10
4. Challenges in Toxicologic Pathology	4	6.3. Diagnostic Toxicologic Pathology	10
4.1. Core Challenges	4	6.4. Research in Toxicologic Pathology	11
4.2. Additional Challenges	6	6.5. Management Roles in Toxicologic Pathology	11
5. Training and Certification in Toxicologic Pathology	8	7. Summary	11
		References	12

1. AN OVERVIEW OF TOXICOLOGIC PATHOLOGY

Citizens of industrialized societies generally have enjoyed a rising standard of living since the dawn of the Industrial Age in Great Britain during the mid-18th century and in other countries thereafter. This time of widespread economic and social improvements greatly enhanced both individual and communal health, longevity, and productivity. Substantial declines in life-threatening infections and malnutrition reflect not only better hygienic practices and increased food supplies but also the advent of more medical therapies, including drugs with reliable and reproducible efficacy. Concurrent progress in bulk synthetic chemistry led to

fabrication of many new, energy- and time-saving products including fertilizers, pesticides, petrochemical fuels, rubber, and more recently clothing and plastics. The adoption of various chemicals, metals, and mixtures during this period emphasized their utility (efficacy) rather than their potential harmful effects (toxicity).

The large-scale production of chemicals, fuels, and metals in industrializing countries was (and is) accompanied by exposure of people, animals, and the environment to toxic materials in the diet, environment, home, and workplace. Such agents may be introduced purposefully (e.g., chlorine and fluorine added to water), encountered accidentally (e.g., pesticide and solvent residues in soil and water), experienced unavoidably (e.g., automotive and industrial

Haschek and Rousseaux's Handbook of Toxicologic Pathology, Fourth Edition.
https://doi.org/10.1016/B978-0-12-821044-4.00023-6

exhaust particles in air), or consumed deliberately (e.g., alcohol, tobacco smoke). Each individual will be exposed throughout life, often beginning in utero, to a complex and unique "exposome"—a personalized menu of chemicals and metals (Bolon and Haschek, 2020; Krewski et al., 2020)—that collectively has the capacity to alter normal biological activities as well as initiate and sustain unexpected physiological effects. Contaminant exposures in industrialized societies have been linked to such "modern" diseases as cancer (e.g., asbestos in ship workers, soot in chimney sweeps) and hexacarbon neuropathy (in people manufacturing solvents or sniffing glues).

Focus groups and the general public in many industrialized countries soon developed concern over environmental and occupational pollution and the demonstrated potential for a decreased quality of life, eventually leading to legislation to address such issues as the effects of chemical dispersal on people and the environment and the safety of products for consumption (*The Role of Pathology in Product Discovery and Safety Assessment*, Vol 2, Chap 2). Such considerations led to the organized pursuit of toxicology—the study of toxic agents, their harmful effects, and their mechanisms—as a vital means for protecting human, animal, and environmental health (Harrison, Kivuti-Bitok, & Macmillan, 2019; Snyder, Mann, & Bolon, 2010). In industrialized countries, this led to a society-wide enterprise to test new products for toxicity using many endpoints: in-life observations, in vitro screening, and especially evaluation of tissue and fluid samples. The need for a methodical and expert examination of tissues and fluids was the impetus that launched the toxicologic pathology profession as a recognized biomedical specialty.

Toxicologic pathology was practiced nonsystematically to a variable degree in industrialized societies during the 19th and early 20th centuries. More systematic and widespread practice of toxicologic pathology began in the 1970s in many countries in response to the society-wide concerns described above. In the United States, three major factors were responsible for this acceleration. The first was President Richard Nixon's declared "War on Cancer." The second was organization of the U.S. National Toxicology Program to screen environmental chemicals for potential toxicity and carcinogenicity. The third was the increasing demand placed on industrial firms to show that their products were "safe" for humans (or sometimes animals) that might be exposed. This concern was raised by contemporary cases demonstrating that flawed safety testing has a significant economic and social impact, which was shown most clearly by the thousands of infants with limb malformations born in the 1960s to European women who took the antinausea drug thalidomide during early pregnancy. Concern regarding the safety assessment apparatus was amplified by the discovery of fraud in some chemical testing laboratories during the mid-1970s, which resulted in the late 1970s in the release of "Good Laboratory Practice for Nonclinical Laboratory Studies" (GLP) guidance (21 CFR Part 58) by the U.S. Food and Drug Administration (FDA) (*Pathology and GLPs, Quality Control and Quality Assurance in a Global Environment*, Vol 1, Chap 27) to provide more rigor and reproducibility in toxicity study data sets. These FDA GLP guidelines, as well as similar GLP guidance given by other organizations (e.g., the U.S. Environmental Protection Agency, found under 40 CFR 160), provide general direction for optimizing the conduct of many aspects of animal toxicity testing, including toxicologic pathology practices.

Toxicologic pathologists are critical to public health efforts in modern societies, for several reasons. First, toxicologic pathologists typically are experts in integrative ("whole organism") biology, largely due to the veterinary medicine (or medicine) and pathology backgrounds of most practitioners. As such, they can assemble a composite picture incorporating both functional and morphological data to determine a subject's individual health or a treatment group's collective vulnerability following exposure to a novel entity (variously called a "test article" or "test item" or "test substance"). Second, toxicologic pathologists are well versed in comparative biology principles that encompass a range of laboratory animal species as well as humans. This training makes them adept at translating animal data to identify hazards, assess safety, and manage potential risks. Third, toxicologic pathologists work well in a team setting with scientists who are expert in other bioscience disciplines. This ability stems from the broad educational curriculum required to enter the toxicologic pathology field as well as the typical formative experiences encountered by pathologists in training and working at institutions that perform toxicology research (i.e.,

3. THE BASIS OF TOXICOLOGIC PATHOLOGY

multidisciplinary projects requiring an integrated approach followed by regular presentations and reports to multiple audiences with variable levels of expertise in pathology and toxicology). This collaborative ability is essential for an organization's efficient and effective product development program as well as for the individual's own career.

2. WHAT IS TOXICOLOGIC PATHOLOGY?

Toxicologic pathology integrates the disciplines of medicine, pathology, and toxicology. Medical and veterinary medical practitioners study the dynamic basis of health and disease, and are well versed in the normal and abnormal structure (at the cell, tissue, organ, and system levels) and function (in terms of activity and biochemistry) of all elements within the body. Pathologists are biomedical practitioners with extra training and experience in investigating the nature of disease (pathophysiology). As such, pathologists evaluate changes produced in cells, tissues, organs, or body fluids in response to a "challenge," whether that challenge arises internally (e.g., immune mediated, metabolic, or neoplastic cause) or externally (e.g., infectious, physical, or toxic agent). As with other etiologies, most toxic diseases leave significant "signatures" in cells, fluids, and tissues. On the other hand, toxicologists focus on the biochemical basis and metabolism of products with known or unknown toxic potential. While grounded in medicine, pathology, and toxicology, toxicologic pathology also requires familiarity with other related disciplines, such as molecular biology, experimental design, and statistics.

Pathologists are well versed in evaluating manifestations of diseases, whether they affect humans (medical pathologists) or animals (veterinary pathologists). The toxicologic pathologist must master both experimental and comparative pathology in the context of data interpretation and extrapolation from observations in animals to predicting possible responses in target human populations. This perspective differs from those of other pathologists (whether medical or veterinary medical). For example, a diagnostic pathologist examines changes in tissues and body fluids from an individual or small group to define the cause of disease or death in the affected individual or a wider population. Similarly, a forensic pathologist investigates death or disease that is unnatural or "suspicious" in nature. In contrast, the main role of a toxicologic pathologist is to determine the biological significance of changes in form, function, or both as manifested by altered structure of cells and tissues (typically termed "changes" or "findings" or—if judged to be adverse—"lesions") and/or composition of body fluids ("biomarkers") by a test article. Toxicologic pathology is an essential element of hazard identification, dose–response data generation, and risk characterization, which are essential for risk analysis and assessment as well as risk management of human and animal chemical exposure.

Since these activities are largely confined to the industrial setting, toxicologic pathology is sometimes referred to as "industrial" pathology. Indeed, most toxicologic pathologists are employed by industry, be it biopharmaceutical (or other biomedical product), agrochemical, chemical, or contract research organizations (CROs). However, toxicologic pathologists also may work at academic institutions, private research foundations, and regulatory agencies. Finally, many toxicologic pathologists function as independent consultants, typically after completing a stint or an entire career at one of the settings listed above. Thus, toxicologic pathology is a vibrant and far-reaching discipline offering numerous and varied opportunities for scientific engagement and societal service.

3. THE BASIS OF TOXICOLOGIC PATHOLOGY

Toxicologic pathology is founded in the art and science of observation. Detailed descriptions of altered morphology still represent a vital component for understanding tissue changes induced by toxic agents. The quest to understand the causes of disease resulted in efforts to associate lesions with their cause(s). As the discipline of toxicologic pathology has grown, associations have been made between structural lesions, hematologic and serum chemistry findings, and potential etiologic agents or classes.

Observations of altered morphology initially were gained by examining macroscopic changes seen during an autopsy or necropsy (i.e., animal autopsy). With the development of the light microscope and later the electron microscope, morphologic observations could be extended to include changes at the cellular and subcellular levels (*Morphological Manifestations of Toxic Cell Injury*, Vol 1, Chap 6). More recently, special techniques have been developed to quantify subtle structural changes as well as to correlate structural changes in tissues and cells with key functional and molecular changes associated with them (*Special Techniques in Toxicologic Pathology*, Vol 1, Chap 11; *In Vivo Small Animal Imaging: A Comparison to Gross and Histopathologic Observations in Animal Models*, Vol 1, Chap 13). Importantly, enhanced techniques for examination of altered components in blood and other body fluids from living animals have led to the development of biomarkers that can be used to predict the presence and severity of toxic injury (*Biomarkers: Discovery, Qualification, and Application*, Vol 1, Chap 14).

Proficiency in toxicologic pathology now requires a working knowledge of many elements that are more closely related to toxicology than pathology. The most important aspects address what the body does to a chemical (*Biochemical and Molecular Basis of Toxicity*, Vol 1, Chap 2; *ADME Principles in Small Molecule Discovery and Development - An Industrial Perspective*, Vol 1, Chap 3; and *Biotherapeutics ADME and PK/PD Principles*, Vol 1, Chap 4) and what the chemical can do to the body (*Principles of Pharmacodynamics and Toxicodynamics*, Vol 1, Chap 5). From both perspectives, many factors impact those interactions. Examples include the composition or chemical form of the test article, the dose, and the route of exposure; these parameters are different for traditional small molecule chemicals, large biomolecules or macromolecular vectors, cells, implanted materials, and vaccines (see chapters for these specific biomedical product categories in Vol 2). The study design is dictated in part by these factors but also is influenced by biological attributes of various model species (Vol 1: *Animal Models in Toxicologic Research: Rodents*, Chap 17; *Animal Models in Toxicologic Research: Rabbits*, Chap 18; Animal Models in Toxicologic Research: *Dogs*, Chap 19; *Animal Models in Toxicologic Research: Pigs*, Chap 20; *Animal Models in Toxicologic Research*, Chap 21; and *Animal Models in Toxicologic Research*, Chap 22) including race (or breed/strain); individual variations in absorption,

distribution, metabolism, and excretion (ADME); the intended uses of the product; and often the environment in which exposure will occur. Toxicologic pathologists need to be conversant in such disciplines in order to maximize their ability to integrate and interpret data compiled during toxicity studies.

4. CHALLENGES IN TOXICOLOGIC PATHOLOGY

Toxicologic pathology is tasked with gathering data to identify and characterize hazards, evaluate safety, and assess risk associated with toxicant or toxin exposure. When contemplating the implications of these objectives, one is reminded of Albert Einstein's remark, "No amount of experimentation could ever prove me right; a single experiment can prove me wrong." This comment epitomizes the fundamental dilemma of toxicologic pathology data: results may show that a test article has toxic and/or carcinogenic properties, but can never say with certainty that a material is safe (*Experimental Design and Statistical Analysis for Toxicologic Pathologists*, Vol 1, Chap 16).

Toxicologic pathologists regularly encounter a series of challenges during the course of their daily practice. Some of them are related to the unique tasks that comprise the raison d'être for toxicologic pathology as a distinct scientific discipline. Other challenges are related to ancillary knowledge and roles that must be considered by toxicologic pathologists to maximize the value of their work to the entire research endeavor. With experience, proficient practitioners learn to recognize the opportunities for excellence hidden within these challenges.

4.1. Core Challenges

Essential duties of toxicologic pathologists are to evaluate changes in the composition and structure of tissues and fluids of individuals that have been exposed to a potential toxicant. Key duties typically are split between two main subdisciplines: anatomic pathology, which evaluates macroscopic ("gross") and microscopic findings in whole organs and tissues sections as well as organ weights and organ weight ratios (*Basic Approaches in Anatomic Toxicologic Pathology*,

Vol 1, Chap 9), and clinical pathology, which characterizes changes in fluids (e.g., blood, serum, and urine) and isolated cells (blood cells, bone marrow, and tissue squash or touch preparations) (*Clinical Pathology in Nonclinical Toxicity Testing*, Vol 1, Chap 10). Both subdisciplines may be augmented by using molecular pathology procedures to link structural changes with their underlying molecular mechanisms (*Special Techniques in Toxicologic Pathology*, Vol 1, Chap 11; *Toxicogenomics: A Primer for Toxicologic Pathologists*, Vol 1, Chap 15); pathologists, with their expertise in pattern recognition, are well positioned to interpret many forms of omics data. This section considers some of the major challenges inherent in the practice of toxicologic pathology.

Rodent bioassays for determining the potential carcinogenicity of test articles are central to the day-to-day work of many toxicologic pathologists. Historically, such bioassays have relied on 2-year studies in wild-type rats or mice (*Carcinogenesis: Mechanisms and Evaluation*, Vol 1, Chap 8). The general approach involves treating male and female rats and mice at several dose levels over the entire lifetime, followed by pathology evaluation to detect tumor formation. Unfortunately, the results often are equivocal or difficult to interpret due to high numbers of spontaneous neoplasms in the control group or premature removal of ill animals due to background diseases (including obesity due to chronic ad libitum feeding; *Nutrition and Toxicologic Pathology*, Vol 2, Chap 20). Given the high cost and questions regarding the relevance of the rodent cancer bioassay, a search for alternatives continues. Several genetically modified mouse models with genetic mutations predisposing them to chemically induced tumor development may be used in 6-month bioassays (*Genetically Engineered Animal Models in Toxicologic Research*, Vol 1, Chap 23), which can significantly reduce the time and cost required to conduct a carcinogenicity study. For both the 2-year and 6-month systems, toxicologic pathologists are essential researchers in acquiring, interpreting, and communicating the final data.

Anatomic pathology, as applied to generation of macroscopic and microscopic diagnoses, is an interpretive science that provides semiquantitative scores rather than rigorously quantifiable measurements. Accordingly, use of consistent diagnostic terminology (*Nomenclature and Diagnostic Resources in Anatomic Toxicologic Pathology*, Vol 1, Chap 25; International Harmonization of Nomenclature and Diagnostic Criteria for Lesions [INHAND—https://www.toxpath.org/inhand.asp#pubg]) (Mann et al., 2012) and, where warranted, communication of specific criteria for assigning severity scores are of paramount importance in recording observations and formulating interpretations. When the toxicity study is complete, the toxicologic pathologist must be able to synthetize the data into a comprehensive study report or visual representations of key data (Troth et al., 2018) that communicate not only the findings but also the pathologist's interpretation as part of risk assessment. Both anatomic pathology and clinical pathology findings of toxicity studies must be communicated succinctly and accurately (*Preparation of the Pathology Report for a Toxicology Study*, Vol 2, Chap 13; *Interpretation of Clinical Pathology Results in Nonclinical Toxicology Testing*, Vol 2, Chap 14). The pathology report may be part of a product registration package submitted to regulatory or research funding agencies, or may be adapted and submitted for publication in a scientific journal or presentation at a scientific meeting. Accordingly, the language used in the report needs to reflect the audience at which it is aimed. Will it need to be understood by other scientists who are not trained in pathology? Will it need to be understood by nonscientists? Excellent communication skills, both oral and written, are key to the success of toxicologic pathologists.

A particular challenge for toxicologic pathologists is to become proficient in discriminating adverse from both nonadverse test article–related findings and incidental background changes. Adverse findings indicate "harm" to the affected individual, while nonadverse changes are not harmful. Importantly, toxicologic pathologists should communicate that the relevance of their interpretations are confined to the conditions of the study and the choice of test species (Kerlin et al., 2016). In other words, findings in animals cannot automatically be assumed to indicate a similar risk (in terms of lesion kind and severity) to humans but rather represent only a portion of the weight of evidence—along with information on the kinetics, metabolism, lesion progression and reversibility, toxic mechanisms, and variations in species sensitivity for the test article and related substances—needed to define the degree of risk.

The validity of toxicity data is only as good as the quality of that data. Some components of the clinical pathology data set—hematology, serum chemistry, and urinalysis—are quantifiable using automated, calibrated instrumentation, and can be tested in duplicate when necessary to ensure that the final value is accurate. In contrast, anatomic pathology is an interpretive discipline, and histopathologic diagnoses of tissue sections (as well as cytologic diagnoses for isolated cells) depend on practitioners who both share a common biomedical training (i.e., partially objective) and possess individual experience (i.e., partially subjective). Modest differences in diagnostic nomenclature and severity scoring, which occur even between well-trained individuals, are now refined as standard practice by using pathology peer review and/or pathology working groups (*Peer Review*, Vol 1, Chap 26). Pathologists who have viewed the same tissue sections discuss their independent diagnoses to reach a common final diagnosis and interpretation. This approach is one commonly employed means to verify the quality of a toxicologic pathology data set. Judicious use of "blinded" histopathologic evaluation of tissue sections may add clarity to the interpretation. In general, however, a "blinded" assessment should be performed only after scoring criteria have been well defined during an initial open ("nonblinded") examination (Bolon, Caverly Rae, & Colman, 2020; Crissman et al., 2004; Dodd, 1988; Zbinden, 1976).

4.2. Additional Challenges

Proficient practice as a toxicologic pathologist requires a large knowledge base beyond that needed to perform the unique tasks inherent in this discipline. The two principal elements of ancillary information include familiarity with fundamental principles of toxicology proper and a basic appreciation for laboratory animal science as it relates to toxicity testing. A third challenge is to become conversant in nontraditional models to which toxicologic pathology methods might be applied (*Alternative Models in Biomedical Research: In Silico, In Vitro, Ex Vivo, and Non-Traditional In Vivo Approaches.* Vol 1, Chap 24). Finally, toxicologic pathologists need

to be aware of changing scientific and societal perspectives on common toxicity and toxicologic pathology activities, so that they may adjust to any new challenges to the profession that might be forthcoming in the future.

A basic foundation in toxicology is intimately related to toxicologic pathology. Development of toxicant-induced lesions is influenced by many genetic, epigenetic, microbial, environmental, and experimental factors. The toxicologic pathologist needs to understand how factors associated with the test species, animal care and use program, research facility environment, and study conditions and procedures contribute to findings enabling proper evaluation of the results. Species-specific differences in the uptake, metabolism, and excretion of test articles as well as demographic factors such as sex- and aging-related physiological factors make data extrapolation from rodents to humans at best difficult and at worst highly questionable. In many cases, the toxic response observed in a rat to a test article administered at a high dose poorly predicts the action of the same substance in humans following exposure to a low dose. Thus, toxicity studies at best present a worst-case outcome for test article exposure in humans, although toxicity data frequently are not an accurate representation of real-world exposure scenarios. Nonetheless, given the current state of our collective scientific knowledge, the growing number and complexity of test articles, and persistent economic constraints, toxicity testing in animals with a heavy emphasis on toxicologic pathology endpoints is the best tool we have on which to base critical social, political, legislative, and financial decisions affecting humans, animals, and the planetary ecology as a whole.

Familiarity with fundamental concepts in laboratory animal science also is needed to properly perform toxicologic pathology tasks. For example, ongoing efforts to implement the 3Rs ("replacement, reduction, and refinement") to minimize the animal numbers used in toxicity research and testing as well as changes in animal husbandry and environmental enrichment to promote improved animal welfare (*Issues in Laboratory Animal Science that Impact Toxicologic Pathology*, Vol 1, Chap 29) have led to altered study designs. In particular, decreased use of nonrodent species—especially dogs and nonhuman primates—in non-GLP–compliant toxicity studies may yield groups sizes of 1 or 2 animals, which may impact the ability to reach conclusions and perform meaningful statistical analyses (Experimental Design and Statistical Analysis for Toxicologic Pathologists, Vol 1, Chap 16). In contrast, rodent use is increasing due to more frequent utilization of genetically modified mouse and rat models in basic research (Genetically Engineered Animal Models in Toxicologic Research, Vol 1, Chap 23). In many cases, the increasing sophistication of approaches such as remote monitoring systems (e.g., telemetry to assess multiple physiological parameters) and noninvasive imaging methods permits the acquisition of extensive in-life data sets that permit each animal to serve as its own control (by comparing baseline values to those measured following test article exposure). This innovation provides a wealth of ancillary data that the toxicologic pathologist may use to provide a more meaningful integration of functional and structural endpoints and a more useful interpretation of the pathology data set.

A growing emphasis on developing high-throughput screening assays such as in silico calculation and in vitro (cell- and tissue based) methods represents an extension of the 3Rs initiative (Alternative Models in Biomedical Research: In Silico, In Vitro, Ex Vivo, and Non-Traditional In Vivo Approaches, Vol 1, Chap 24) (Bucher, 2013). Importantly, such animal-free platforms represent a key step toward the ultimate stated goal of some regulatory agencies to eliminate animal testing when making product registration decisions (Wheeler, 2019). Toxicity tests with in vitro systems commonly emphasize biochemical evaluations. Conventional anatomic pathology evaluation is feasible for use with in vitro cell culture and tissue mass/slice test systems, and commonly is employed for publication (Bolon et al., 1993) but can be used as an endpoint in product registration (Purcell et al., 2018). The rapidly expanding fields of molecular biology, genomics, and bioinformatics pose a significant challenge to the toxicologic pathologist who must integrate this information into the already complex field of safety evaluation and risk assessment. However, it is this new knowledge that will result in the transformation of generalized to personalized medicine.

Two questions have been raised in recent years regarding the validity of certain toxicity study designs. Major issues include the relevance of the rodent 2-year carcinogenicity bioassay (Carcinogenicity Assessment, Vol 2, Chap 5) and the validity of linear extrapolation using data obtained from inbred animal strains exposed to high chemical doses to predict the impact of low-level human exposure. Comorbidity—the presence of one or more underlying diseases upon which any toxicant-induced lesion(s) are superimposed—may complicate the interpretation of pathology data sets, especially as animals age. These challenges are beginning to be addressed with the advent of mechanistic studies utilizing special molecular pathology techniques (immunohistochemistry [IHC] and in situ hybridization [ISH]), innovative test systems (in vitro models, genetically engineered animals), and new technological approaches (biomarkers, digital image analysis). Such innovations will fundamentally change the manner in which animal-derived data are extrapolated for human risk assessment and risk management in the future.

Finally, economic globalization poses a challenge for toxicologic pathology. The present corporate model is to build organizations in which corporate activities are spread across multiple sites, often in several regions of one country or in different countries of one or several continents. In recent years, companies seeking to discover and develop new products often have outsourced complex testing functions like GLP-compliant safety assessment to CROs that maintain more uniform training standards, diagnostic nomenclature conventions, and operating procedures that are designed to simultaneously address regulatory guidance from many portions of the world. This global synchronicity has been made easier by multinational initiatives seeking to synchronize regulatory testing requirements from multiple regulatory settings (Risk Assessment Vol 2, Chap 16). Successful examples of global cooperation include the International Conference on Harmonisation of Technical Requirements for Registration of Pharmaceuticals for Human Use (ICH) to ensure the quality, efficacy, and safety of new drugs; the INHAND initiative to standardize toxicologic pathology terminology; and the Organisation for Economic

Co-operation and Development (OECD) to standardize testing policies for member nations. A unified standard for training of toxicologic pathologists has been accepted by multiple societies of toxicologic pathology (Bolon et al., 2010), although no formal organization has been incorporated to guarantee that the recommendations are followed. Globalization also creates a need for real-time communication across sites, including advanced capabilities for sharing of large data sets, high-resolution images, and the actual perspective of a tissue section as viewed through a microscope objective (*Digital Pathology and Tissue Image Analysis*, Vol 1, Chap 12). A growing number of hardware and software solutions have been developed that permit such sharing.

5. TRAINING AND CERTIFICATION IN TOXICOLOGIC PATHOLOGY

A toxicologic pathologist typically is a biomedical scientist with extensive training in clinical medicine or veterinary medicine, specialized training in comparative pathology of animals and/or humans, and subspecialization in toxicologic pathology. Most toxicologic pathologists around the world are veterinarians with a veterinary medical degree (DVM or equivalent) and formal pathology training gained through a residency program that generally culminates with board certification in pathology (e.g., Diplomate status in the American or European College of Veterinary Pathologists [ACVP or ECVP, respectively]). In the United States, pathology training focuses on either anatomic pathology or clinical pathology, although some overlap exists both in training and in the ACVP board examinations for these two subspecialties. Very few training institutions provide formal training in toxicologic pathology, per se, although trainees may be exposed to some toxicology courses or undertake short internships in institutions with large toxicity testing programs. Medically trained pathologists (MD or equivalent) are also involved in toxicologic pathology, especially in countries such as China and Japan.

Research training may be obtained through PhD or other postdoctoral programs. Scientists with a doctoral degree (PhD or equivalent) in experimental pathology but no formal medical or veterinary medical training make up a very small group of currently practicing toxicologic pathologists. Global societies of toxicologic pathology have agreed on the training requirements and practical experience considered to be essential for proficient practice as a toxicologic pathologist (Bolon et al., 2010). Many global societies of toxicologic pathology have made basic and advanced education in this discipline a focal point of their outreach activities to members, allied scientists (e.g., toxicologists and regulators), and when warranted the general public (Maronpot and Dagli, 2020).

In many countries, toxicologic pathologists are a subset of individuals with certification as a pathologist. Anatomic pathologists are utilized in toxicologic pathology throughout the world, while clinical pathologists are used as toxicologic pathologists only in some regions (Europe and North America). Toxicologic pathology proficiency typically is achieved by "on-the-job" mentored training (essentially an informal apprenticeship). Formal certification in toxicologic pathology is available in India, Japan, and some European countries (Bolon et al., 2010). This certification may consist of credential review or formal examination. In the absence of a formal toxicologic pathology credential, many toxicologic pathologists demonstrate their familiarity with relevant toxicology principles by obtaining formal certification in toxicology (e.g., Diplomate status through the American Board of Toxicology [ABT] or recognition as a European Registered Toxicologist [ERT]). Individuals who have spent many years practicing toxicologic pathology may be recognized by credential review as a Fellow of the International Academy of Toxicologic Pathology (FIATP) as a means for showcasing their expertise.

The resources needed to meet the challenges faced by toxicologic pathologists are hosted by various professional societies and regulatory agencies around the world. For example, the Society of Toxicologic Pathology (STP, based in North America) regularly defines "best practice" recommendations for essential toxicologic pathology tasks. Such lists are compiled initially by committees of STP members (mainly toxicologic pathologists and toxicologists) with subject matter expertise, are revised using input from multiple STP members as well as members of other global societies of toxicologic pathology and regulatory scientists, and ultimately are published in peer-reviewed journals and also publicly available on the organization's website (https://www.toxpath.org/best-practices.asp). The STP website also hosts many other useful documents including InHAND diagnostic terminology for multiple organ systems and species (https://www.toxpath.org/inhand.asp#pubg) and links to various lesion atlases and sites explaining appropriate measures for tissue collection (https://www.toxpath.org/index.asp, under the "Publications" pull-down menu). The STP, along with the British Society of Toxicological Pathology and European Society of Toxicologic Pathology, sustains the journal *Toxicologic Pathology*, while the Japanese Society of Toxicologic Pathology maintains the *Journal of Toxicologic Pathology*. These two discipline-specific journals as well as several toxicology-oriented journals (e.g., *International Journal of Toxicology*, *Toxicological Sciences*) are valuable sources of current information on toxicologic pathology research topics and current opinion relevant to the discipline. Well-established principles in toxicologic pathology (Greaves, 2012; Sahota et al., 2019; Wallig et al., 2018) and toxicology (Hayes and Kruger, 2014; Klaassen, 2019) may be found in standard reference texts.

6. THE "PRACTITIONER" OF TOXICOLOGIC PATHOLOGY

Toxicologic pathologists serve many roles in protecting human, animal, and environmental health. Many practitioners are involved in hazard identification and characterization for chemicals (*Agro*/Bulk *Chemicals*, Vol 2, Chap 12) or safety assessment of various biomedical products (*Pathology in Nonclinical Safety*, Vol 2, Chap 4). Some toxicologic pathologists are devoted to drug discovery (*Discovery Toxicology and Pathology*, Vol 2, Chap 3), including identification of therapeutic targets and phenotypic analysis of transgenic animals and validation of alternative animal models, or evaluation of drug efficacy (*Overview of Drug Development*, Vol 2, Chap 1). Other scientists in the field are investigating mechanisms of toxicity or dealing with laboratory animal disease surveillance to ensure that animals for toxicity testing are healthy. A "practitioner" of toxicologic pathology utilizes the techniques of this discipline on a daily basis

regardless of the employment sector. The most common practice settings for toxicologic pathologists are discussed below.

6.1. Industrial Toxicologic Pathology

As noted above, the majority of toxicologic pathologists are employed by industry or as consultants to industry. Most toxicologic pathologists in industry participate in regulatory-type (GLP-like or fully GLP-compliant) animal toxicity studies performed in an experimental setting (applied research) to support development of biomedical products (bio/pharmaceuticals, cell and gene therapies, and medical devices) and, to a lesser extent, agricultural and other chemicals. At present, most firms seeking to create and market new products tend to perform key discovery and initial proof-of-concept studies (e.g., molecular discovery, target validation, lead candidate identification, initial efficacy testing in animal disease models, and other studies as appropriate) internally. These discoveries and early development studies often are GLPlike rather than GLP-compliant. Once the best product candidates are identified, firms typically outsource their GLP-compliant, late-stage development studies to CROs with broad experience in performing the full range of animal toxicity studies—general toxicity studies, carcinogenicity studies, and specialized toxicity studies (e.g., developmental and reproductive toxicity [*The Role of Pathology in Evaluation of Reproductive, Developmental, and Juvenile Toxicity*, Vol 1, Chap 7], dedicated neurotoxicity, in vivo mutagenicity).

In biomedical product development, toxicologic pathologists also participate in other aspects of the endeavor, particularly target validation, drug discovery, and investigational toxicology. Experienced practitioners may transition to management, often of a pathology and/or toxicology group but sometimes in more senior executive roles, or to leave corporate organizations to supply their expertise to multiple clients via service as an independent consultant. In developed countries, the optimal qualifications for entry-level industrial toxicologic pathologists include a veterinary medical or medical degree, board certification in veterinary pathology, and a graduate degree (usually a PhD or equivalent) demonstrating research training. This broad background provides the maximum flexibility in moving among different industrial roles.

Industrial toxicologic pathologists play a vital role in risk assessment. Traditionally, toxicologic pathologists have provided diagnoses and interpretations as well as determined a dose–response using observations of whole organs, organ weights, hematoxylin and eosin–stained tissue sections, and standard clinical pathology parameters. The validation and implementation of sophisticated new methods for visualizing altered molecular patterns in relation to tissue lesions as well as new indicators of injury will require toxicologic pathologists to participate more widely in the risk assessment endeavor. In some organizations, toxicologic pathologists often assume an even larger role in product development, serving as Study Director or Program Lead for new compounds or compound classes. In such positions, the impact of their observations, interpretations, and comments will become even greater. Therefore, toxicologic pathologists will need to be ever more knowledgeable regarding proper study design (Practices to Optimize Generation, Interpretation, And Reporting of Pathology Data from Toxicity Studies Vol 1, Chap 29), suitability of statistical analysis, data integration to permit meaningful assessments of health risks (*Risk Assessment*, Vol 2, Chap 16), as well as risk communication and management (*Risk Communication and Management: Building Trust and Credibility with the Public*, Vol 2, Chap 17).

6.2. Toxicologic Pathology Related to the Environment and Food Safety

Pathologists involved in environmental pathology and food safety generally are employed by government agencies, such as bodies regulating agricultural, drug, environmental, food, and other products. However, some pathologists filling these roles work in academia. Increasingly, toxicologic pathology is recognized as a valuable contribution in diagnosing environmental problems, defining background disease prevalence, investigating mechanisms of ecological and food-borne toxicity, and developing alternate (often in vitro or nonvertebrate, or at least non-mammalian, animal) models for evaluating toxicity (*Environmental Toxicologic Pathology,*

Vol 2, Chap 18) (Dagli, Pandiri, & Wolf, 2019). The adverse effects of nutritional constituents and contaminants in food products are also important areas to which the toxicologic pathologist can add value (*Food and Toxicologic Pathology*, Vol 2, Chap 19). Toxicologic pathology also plays an important role in investigating atmospheric, food, and water contaminants such as biological (phycotoxins, mycotoxins, and poisonous plants) and industrial (agrochemicals, air pollutants, and endocrine disruptors) substances, heavy metals, nanoparticulates, and radiation so that the safety of the environment and food supply can be maintained (see chapters for these specific product classes in Vol 2).

6.3. Diagnostic Toxicologic Pathology

Diagnostic pathology identifies the cause of diseases based on morphologic and/or clinical pathology findings as well as an individual's (or group's) history, clinical signs, and ancillary test results. A diagnostic pathology mindset is important in all areas of pathology, both in spontaneous and in experimentally induced disease, and it is no less essential in toxicologic pathology. In experimental studies, it is important to separate out the effects of spontaneous disease and those induced by the experimental agent/test article. Diagnostic pathology skills are necessary to investigate unexpected disease or death in laboratory animal colonies or prior to the termination of a toxicity study, and often are a key asset in differentiating a toxicant-related effect from those associated with a confounding incidental background condition.

In medical and veterinary diagnostic laboratories, toxicologic pathology will continue to be central to diagnosis and prevention of spontaneous, chemically induced diseases. The utility of naturally occurring chemically induced diseases as models for identifying cellular lesions and their molecular pathogeneses should not be underestimated as it is often toxicant-induced cases that add crucial information to understanding mechanisms of toxicity relevant to similar classes of chemicals (sometimes including endogenous metabolic byproducts). One example of this principle was the identification of melamine and cyanuric acid in pet food as the causative agents of acute nephrotoxicity in dogs and cats. Importantly, the extent of melamine metabolism and nephro-toxicity can be modulated by altering the spectrum of microflora in the digestive tract (Zheng et al., 2013), which is consistent with the known ability of the "microbiome" to impact chemical metabolism, efficacy, and toxicity (Koontz et al., 2019; Wilson and Nicholson, 2017).

6.4. Research in Toxicologic Pathology

Toxicologic pathologists participate in research in many settings, including industry (van Tongeren et al., 2011), academia (Turner et al., 2015), and government (Sills et al., 2017). Their unique skills in comparative, descriptive, and experimental pathology permit them to define and tackle problems from many angles, which cannot fail to bring an added dimension to many research areas (Hoenerhoff et al, 2021). Toxicologic pathologists participate in both basic research to understand normal physiological pathways and mechanisms of toxic injury and also applied research to develop new products and fill data gaps that impede risk assessment for new materials.

Research in toxicologic pathology encompasses many different questions and approaches. Associative projects include retrospective studies using archived tissues, prospective cross-sectional surveys, and longitudinal evaluations of disease progression and remission to assess the impact of toxicant-induced changes in initiating and sustaining various diseases. Experiments ranging from simple to complex are designed to test one or more formal hypotheses, ranging from the ability of an agent to produce a toxic disease or recapitulate a known toxic syndrome to an investigation of the mechanisms responsible for any cellular or molecular lesions. New analytical methods (digital image analysis, noninvasive imaging, and stereology); molecular techniques (IHC, ISH, and toxicogenomics); and innovative test systems (in vitro assays and genetically engineered animals) are applicable to addressing many toxicologic pathology questions.

6.5. Management Roles in Toxicologic Pathology

Many scientists involved in product research and development find themselves moving over time toward more managerial roles, where they make decisions on compound development that necessitate the incorporation of techniques for risk management. In fact, they may fill positions in upper management themselves. The toxicologic pathologist is well poised to fill such positions as the management of scientific issues concerning product development is often best served by individuals who are well versed in whole-animal biology and integration of data sets drawn from many disciplines. However, a manager requires more than just a solid toxicologic pathology background to succeed in such a role. Toxicologic pathologists in managerial positions also require strong oral and written communication skills to deal effectively with upper-level managers, regulators, lawyers, and external stakeholders, including prospective investors and the general public. For this reason, polished interactions to accurately and clearly convey benefits and risks as well as mitigate potential stakeholder concerns are an essential prerequisite for success in a managerial role, particularly when it comes to risk management.

7. SUMMARY

Toxicologic pathologists are well suited to play many pivotal roles in discovering and developing new products to promote health, prevent disease, and improve the quality of individual and communal life. Their broad and thorough understanding of anatomic and physiological factors under normal conditions (i.e., the dynamic equilibrium known as "health"), their perspective of biology as an integrative rather than reductive discipline, their ability to reliably convert morphologic observations of whole organs and tissue sections into data suitable for decision-making, and their familiarity with the numerous limitations on the biological significance of such data make the toxicologic pathologist a critical member of the product development process. Practitioners of this unique discipline also are ideally placed to mold or make decisions within the risk assessment–management framework. In conclusion, toxicologic pathologists are key players in protecting human, animal, and environmental health today and will remain so for the foreseeable future (Ettlin, 2013; Maronpot, 2012).

REFERENCES

Bolon B, Barale-Thomas E, Bradley A, et al.: International recommendations for training future toxicologic pathologists participating in regulatory-type, nonclinical toxicity studies, *Toxicol Pathol* 38:984–992, 2010.

Bolon B, Caverly Rae JM, Colman K, et al.: Toxicologic Pathology Forum opinion piece: current use of non-blinded vs. blinded histopathologic evaluation in animal toxicity studies, *Toxicol Pathol* 48, 2020.

Bolon B, Dorman DC, Bonnefoi MS, et al.: Histopathologic approaches to chemical toxicity using primary cultures of dissociated neural cells grown in chamber slides, *Toxicol Pathol* 21:465–479, 1993.

Bolon B, Haschek WM: The exposome in Toxicologic Pathology, *Toxicol Pathol.* 48(6):718–720, 2020, https://doi.org/10.1177/0192623320912403. Epub 2020 Mar 19. PMID: 32191165.

Bucher JR: Regulatory Forum opinion piece: Tox21 and toxicologic pathology, *Toxicol Pathol* 41:125–127, 2013.

Crissman JW, Goodman DG, Hildebrandt PK, et al.: Best practices guideline: toxicologic histopathology, *Toxicol Pathol* 32:126–131, 2004.

Dagli MLZ, Pandiri A, Wolf J, et al.: Global perspective on careers in environmental toxicologic pathology: the 2019 Society of Toxicologic Pathology annual symposium lunchtime career development session, *Toxicol Pathol* 47:1088–1095, 2019.

Dodd DC: Blind slide reading or the uninformed versus the informed pathologist. In Leader RW, Wagner BM, editors: *Comments on toxicology*, London, 1988, Gordon and Breach Science Publishers S.A., pp 81–91.

Ettlin RA: Toxicologic pathology in the 21st century, *Toxicol Pathol* 41:689–708, 2013.

Greaves P: *Histopathology of preclinical toxicity studies: interpretation and relevance in drug safety evaluation*, ed 4, New York, 2012, Academic Press (Elsevier).

Harrison S, Kivuti-Bitok L, Macmillan A, et al.: EcoHealth and One Health: a theory-focused review in response to calls for convergence, *Environ Int* 132:105058, 2019.

Hayes AW, Kruger CL: *Hayes' principles and methods of toxicology*, ed 6, Boca Raton, FL, 2014, CRC Press (Taylor & Francis.

Hoenerhoff MJ, Meyerholz DK, Brayton C, Beck AP: Challenges and opportunities for the Veterinary Pathologist in Biomedical Research, *Vet. Pathol.* 58(2):258–265, 2021, https://doi.org/10.1177/0300985820974005. Epub 2020 Dec 17. PMID: 33327888.

Kerlin R, Bolon B, Burkhardt J, et al.: Scientific and Regulatory Policy Committee: recommended ("best") practices for determining, communicating, and using adverse effect data from nonclinical studies, *Toxicol Pathol* 44:147–162, 2016.

Klaassen CD: *Casarett & Doull's toxicology: the basic science of poisons*, ed 9, New York, 2019, McGraw-Hill Education.

Koontz JM, Dancy BCR, Horton CL, et al.: The role of the human microbiome in chemical toxicity, *Int J Toxicol* 38:251–264, 2019.

Krewski D, Andersen ME, Tyshenko MG, et al.: Toxicity testing in the 21st century: progress in the past decade and future perspectives, *Arch Toxicol* 94:1–58, 2020.

Mann PC, Vahle J, Keenan CM, et al.: International harmonization of toxicologic pathology nomenclature: an overview and review of basic principles, *Toxicol Pathol* 40:7S–13S, 2012.

Maronpot RR: Regulatory Forum opinion piece: the role of the toxicologic pathologist in the postgenomic era: challenges and opportunities, *Toxicol Pathol* 40:1082–1086, 2012.

Maronpot RR, Dagli MLZ: Contemporary activities of toxicologic pathology societies, *Toxicol Pathol* 48:295–301, 2020.

Purcell R, Lynch G, Gall C, et al.: Brain vacuolation resulting from administration of the type II ampakine CX717 is an artifact related to molecular structure and chemical reaction with tissue fixative agents, *Toxicol Sci* 162:383–395, 2018.

Sahota PS, Popp JA, Bouchard PR, et al.: *Toxicologic pathology: nonclinical safety assessment*, ed 2, Boca Raton, FL, 2019, CRC Press (Taylor & Francis.

Sills R, Brix A, Cesta M, et al.: NTP/NIEHS global contributions to toxicologic pathology, *Toxicol Pathol* 45:1035–1038, 2017.

Troth SP, Everds NE, Siska W, et al.: Scientific and Regulatory Policy Committee points to consider: data visualization for clinical and anatomic pathologists, *Toxicol Pathol* 46:476–487, 2018.

Turner PV, Haschek WM, Bolon B, et al.: Commentary: the role of the toxicologic pathologist in academia, *Vet Pathol* 52:7–17, 2015.

Snyder PW, Mann P, Bolon B, et al.: The Society of Toxicologic Pathology and the "One Health" initiative, *Toxicol Pathol* 38:521, 2010.

van Tongeren S, Fagerland JA, Conner MW, et al.: The role of the toxicologic pathologist in the biopharmaceutical industry, *Int J Toxicol* 30:568–582, 2011.

Wallig MA, Haschek WM, Rousseaux CG, et al., editors: *Fundamentals of toxicologic pathology*, ed 3, San Diego, 2018, Academic Press.

Wheeler A: *Directive to prioritize efforts to reduce animal testing [at EPA]*, 2019. https://www.epa.gov/sites/production/files/2019-09/documents/image2019-09-09-231249.pdf. (Accessed 5 March 2020).

Wilson ID, Nicholson JK: Gut microbiome interactions with drug metabolism, efficacy, and toxicity, *Transl Res* 179:204–222, 2017.

Zbinden G:T: The role of pathology in toxicity testing. In *Progress in toxicology*, Berlin, 1976, Springer-Verlag, pp 8–18.

Zheng X, Zhao A, Xie G, et al.: Melamine-induced renal toxicity is mediated by the gut microbiota, *Sci Transl Med* 5:172ra122, 2013 (Erratum: Sci Transl Med 5, 179er3, 2013).

PRINCIPLES OF TOXICOLOGIC PATHOLOGY

Biochemical and Molecular Basis of Toxicity

Lois D. Lehman-McKeeman, Laura E. Armstrong

Bristol-Myers Squibb Co., Princeton, NJ, United States

OUTLINE

1. Introduction	15
2. General Principles of Xenobiotic Disposition	16
2.1. General Properties of Absorption	16
2.2. Routes of Absorption	19
2.3. General Principles of Distribution	21
2.4. Metabolism: Activation and Detoxification	24
2.5. Elimination of Toxicants	30
2.6. Effects of the Microbiome on Absorption, Distribution, Biotransformation and Elimination	34
3. Interactions of Toxicants with Cellular and Molecular Targets	35
3.1. Covalent Modification	35
3.2. Stress Responses in Toxicity	36
3.3. Altered Gene Expression	38
3.4. Mechanisms of Cell Death	40
4. Idiosyncratic Mechanisms of Toxicity	42
5. Protective Mechanisms, Repair Mechanisms, and Adaptation or Failure	42
5.1. Stress Response Constituents and Pathways	42
5.2. Cell Repair and Adaptation	44
5.3. Failure to Repair After Toxic Insult	46
6. Summary and Conclusions	47
References	47

1. INTRODUCTION

This chapter provides an overview of the fundamental principles of toxic mechanisms of injury. It is focused on biochemical, cellular, and molecular mechanisms that contribute to toxicity. Additionally, xenobiotic disposition, representing the integrated action of absorption, distribution, biotransformation, and elimination, plays a central role in the development of toxicity and is often a major determinant of the dose–response relationship for toxicity and the potential for species-specific responses (see *ADME Principles in Small Molecule Drug Discovery and Development—An Industrial Perspective*, Vol 1, Chap 3 and *Biotherapeutic ADME and PK/PD Principles*, Vol 1, Chap 4).

In light of the breadth and variety of target cells, organs, and molecular pathways underlying toxic mechanisms, it is nearly impossible to adequately address the multitude of mechanisms by which toxicants elicit adverse effects. Additionally, many of the chapters that follow will address specific toxicities and pathologies relevant to a particular organ system, as well as methods and approaches for assessing the cellular, biochemical, and molecular pathways that are involved in toxic responses (see *Morphologic Manifestations of Toxic Cell Injury*, Vol 1, Chap 6, *Basic Approaches to Anatomic Toxicologic Pathology*, Vol 1, Chap 9, *Clinical Pathology in Nonclinical Toxicity Testing*, Vol 1, Chap 10, and *Toxicogenomics: A Primer for Toxicologic Pathologists*, Vol 1, Chap 15). Consequently,

MAJOR DETERMINANTS OF TOXIC OUTCOMES

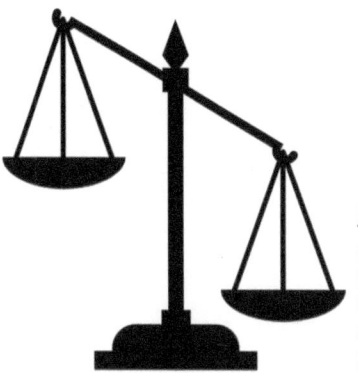

Mechanisms Limiting Toxicity

Protein binding (plasma or tissues)
Elimination: detoxification, excretion
Cellular adaption and repair
Effective response to stress or damage
Exposure allows protection or repair

Mechanisms Increasing Toxicity

Protein interactions including covalent modification
Bioactivation and reactive metabolites
Limited adaptation or repair
Cellular stress and dysfunction
Exposure overwhelms protection or repair

FIGURE 2.1   Schematic representation of the major determinants of toxic outcomes that either limit toxicity or increase toxicity.

this chapter focuses on the fundamental principles that contribute broadly to toxic or pathologic effects. These include the following: (1) characteristics that determine how a toxicant is delivered to its target; (2) the major factors that determine toxic outcome; (3) factors governing whether repair and/or regeneration occur after toxic insult; and (4) the pathological states that manifest when repair mechanisms fail. Examples are provided to illustrate factors that influence the balance between the ability of an organ or cell to adapt to or repair potential toxicity.

The qualitative and quantitative features of the cellular or molecular basis of toxicity are paramount to determining the relative hazard for any toxicant. The dose–response relationship for toxicity also provides a quantitative snapshot of the continuum of effects that contribute to toxicity. Fig. 2.1 provides a general overview of the most critical determinants of toxic mechanisms and serves as the foundation for the content of this chapter.

2. GENERAL PRINCIPLES OF XENOBIOTIC DISPOSITION

The disposition of a xenobiotic is defined as the integrated action of its absorption, distribution, biotransformation, and elimination. The quantitative determination of these properties comprises the field of pharmacokinetics (or toxicokinetics) which is discussed in detail in *ADME Principles in Small Molecule Drug Discovery and Development—An Industrial Perspective*, Vol 1, Chap 3, *Biotherapeutic ADME and PK/PD Principles*, Vol 1, Chap 4, and *Principles of Pharmacodynamics and Toxicodynamics*, Vol 1, Chap 5). Collectively, the disposition and kinetics of a chemical ultimately determine its concentration at a target site for toxicity and contribute to whether adverse effects will occur.

2.1. General Properties of Absorption

A comprehensive overview of basic dispositional parameters and attributes (absorption, distribution, and excretion) is not provided here. Additional relevant information covering absorption, distribution, and excretion can be found in the literature (Klaassen, 2019, (Chapter 5).

Biological Membranes

Cell membranes are comprised of a phospholipid bilayer wherein the polar head groups of the lipids are oriented toward the outer and inner surfaces of the membrane and the lipid tails are oriented inward forming a hydrophobic inner space. Cell membranes are typically 7–9 nm thick, and phosphatidylcholine and phosphatidylethanolamine are the primary phospholipids in the outer and inner leaflets, respectively. They also contain a variety of transmembrane proteins that function as receptors for many endogenous ligands, form pores or ion channels or function in the transport of endogenous and exogenous compounds into and out of cells (discussed below). The processes involved in the passage of compounds across membranes include those that require no energy (e.g., direct passage through pores, filtration, or simple diffusion). Additionally, there are numerous active transport processes, defined as those which require energy utilization to move solutes across membranes and against a concentration gradient.

Simple Diffusion

Diffusion occurs down a concentration gradient, with molecules moving from regions of higher concentration to lower concentration (Fick's law). Large hydrophobic molecules diffuse across the lipid domain of membranes. In contrast, smaller water-soluble molecules can pass through aqueous pores in a process referred to as paracellular diffusion. This is the case for ethanol, and this attribute enables absorption readily across the gastrointestinal (GI) tract and distribution rapidly throughout the body.

Two principal factors that govern the rate of transport across membranes for large organic molecules are lipid solubility and the degree to which a compound is in its nonionized form at physiological pH. Lipid solubility is frequently expressed as the octanol–water partition coefficient (or log P), where a very lipid-soluble molecule has a positive log P. For example, the highly lipophilic compound, 2,3,7,8-tetrachlorodibenzodioxin (TCDD) has a log P of 7.05, whereas the metal salt, lead acetate, has negative log P (-0.63). Ionization is determined by the Henderson–Hasselbalch equation which defines the relationship between the pH and the pK (i.e., the pH at which a weak organic acid or base is 50% ionized). Only the nonionized form of a compound is available for diffusion across membranes. In this manner, a weak base, such as aniline (pK = 5), is 50% ionized at pH 5, but is essentially in its nonionized form at pH 7. Thus, physiological pH favors the absorbance of weak bases more so than weak acids.

Filtration

Filtration is the bulk movement of water across a porous membrane, and any solute that is small enough to pass through membrane pores will flow with it. Overall, filtration is governed by hydrostatic and osmotic pressures along with the pores that allow small molecules to pass through them. Pore sizes are typically 2–7 Å,

and as pressure rises on one side of the membrane, small molecules are forced through the pores. The renal glomerulus is a major site of filtration, and its pores are typically in range of 70–80 Å, allowing numerous solutes and some low molecular weight proteins to be filtered. In some endothelial beds, there are larger pores that form interendothelial gaps to allow larger molecules to move from the plasma to extracellular space. In contrast, such pores are absent in the brain where the blood–brain barrier (BBB) is formed by tight junctions between cells.

Specialized Transport: Active Transport and Facilitated Diffusion (Klaassen and Aleksunes, 2010)

The sequencing of the human genome revealed that there are at least 500 genes likely to function in membrane transport. These systems regulate uptake and efflux of compounds and contribute to the homeostasis of endogenous compounds and xenobiotics, including drug responses and the potential for adverse effects. There are active transporters that utilize energy (typically ATP) to move chemicals against a concentration gradient. They demonstrate some substrate selectivity, with saturation at high concentrations and inhibition by compounds that compete for transport. There is growing evidence that genetic polymorphisms and species differences in transporter function and regulation contribute to interindividual and interspecies differences in toxicity, respectively. Furthermore, transporter activity can influence toxic responses because of saturation or competition for transport which is often the case in drug–drug interactions.

The first ATP-dependent transporter identified to play a role in xenobiotic disposition was a phosphoglycoprotein identified in tumor cells that developed resistance to chemotherapy. The protein was called P-glycoprotein (P-gp) or multidrug resistance protein (MDR1), and subsequently, two forms (Mdr1a and Mdr1b) have been identified in rodents. There are now several transporter families identified that contribute to the disposition of xenobiotics and influence toxicant exposure and outcome. In addition to the MDR family, these include the following: multidrug resistance proteins (MRPs), breast cancer resistance protein (BCRP), bile salt export pump (BSEP), multidrug and toxin extrusion transporters (MATEs), organic anion transporting polypeptides (OATPs), organic anion transporters (OATs), organic cation transporters (OCTs), and peptide transporters (PEPTs). A summary of these gene families is provided in Table 2.1. Additionally, although not summarized here, there is increased interest in these transporters in veterinary practice, with an accumulating body of information on the expression and function of many transport proteins in livestock and animals of veterinary interest (Virkel et al., 2019). A full review of the function of xenobiotic transporters is beyond the scope of this chapter, but examples of how these proteins influence exposure to toxicants or contribute to mechanisms of toxicity will be discussed throughout.

TABLE 2.1   Summary of Major Transporters That Contribute to Xenobiotic Disposition[a,b]

Name	Gene family	Function	Common name	Tissue expression
Multidrug resistance protein; P-glycoprotein	Abcb1	Efflux pump	Mdr1a, 1b	Liver, kidney, brain, small intestine, and skin
Bile salt export pump	Abcb11	Efflux pump for bile salts	Bsep	Liver
Multidrug resistance protein (MRP)	Abcc	Efflux pumps; apical and/or basolateral	Mrp1	Choroid plexus and skin
			Mrp2	Liver, kidney, brain, and small intestine
			Mrp3	Liver, small intestine, and skin
			Mrp4	Liver, kidney, brain, choroid plexus, and skin
			Mrp5	Brain and skin
			Mrp6	Liver
Breast cancer resistance protein (BCRP)	Abcg2	Efflux pump on bile canaliculus	Bcrp	Liver, kidney, brain, and placenta
Organic anion transporting polypeptide (OATP)	Slco	Influx pump; organic anions substrates	Oatp1a1	Liver, kidney, and choroid plexus
			Oatp1a4	Liver, kidney choroid plexus, and brain
			Oatp1b2	Liver
			Oatp 2a1	Kidney
Organic anion transporter (OAT)	Slc22	Uptake of organic anions	Oat1	Kidney
			Oat2	Liver and kidney
			Oat 3	Kidney and brain

(Continued)

TABLE 2.1 Summary of Major Transporters That Contribute to Xenobiotic Disposition[a,b]—cont'd

Name	Gene family	Function	Common name	Tissue expression
Organic cation transporter (OCT)	Slc22	Uptake of organic cations	Oct1	Liver, kidney jejunum, testis, and skin
			Oct2	Kidney, lung, and choroid plexus
			Oct 3	Testis and skin
Organic cation/carnitine transporter	Slc22	Carnitine transport	Octn1	Kidney and skin
		Carnitine transport	Octn2	Kidney, small intestine, and skin
Multidrug and toxin extrusion transporter (MATE)	Slc47	Efflux pump for cations	Mate1	Kidney and liver
		H^+/cation antiporter	MATE2K	Human kidney

[a] Genes listed represent major transporters in rats involved in xenobiotic disposition (except where noted for MATE2K). Several transporter families including those that contribute to nucleoside or peptide transport are not included but are discussed in the text.

[b] Reference: Klaassen CD, Aleksunes LM: Xenobiotic, bile acid, and cholesterol transporters: function and regulation, Pharmacol Rev 62, 1–96, 2010.

The process of facilitated diffusion is also a carrier-mediated process, but it does not require ATP consumption. In facilitated diffusion, a substrate moves with a concentration gradient, and carrier proteins, typically integral membrane proteins, are responsible for the passage of molecules or ions across the membrane. Classically, the transport of glucose occurs by facilitated diffusion. Additionally, the OCT family, which is highly abundant in liver and kidney, moves cations by a facilitated process.

In addition to transporters that contribute to the disposition of xenobiotics, numerous other families are specifically involved in the distribution of important endogenous compounds. These include the glucose transporters described above (gene family SLC5A), nucleoside transporters (gene family SLC29A), and other transporter families involved predominantly in uptake of basic or neutral amino acids, including neurotransmitters, and transporters involved in the distribution of essential elements such as calcium, iron, and copper. The energy requirements of these transporters vary across families, as some, but not all, require ATP.

More importantly, although such transporters are associated with key endogenous nutrients, they can influence exposure to toxicants. For example, lead is a substrate for the facilitated transporters involved in calcium and iron uptake. Furthermore, 1-methyl-4-phenylpyridi-nium selectively targets dopaminergic neurons and leads to Parkinson-like neurotoxicity because its uptake is regulated by the dopamine transporter (SLCA3).

2.2. Routes of Absorption

Absorption from the Gastrointestinal Tract

Absorption can occur all along the GI tract, but as noted earlier, the nonionized fraction is most readily absorbed. Due to the change in pH throughout the GI tract, some weak acids may be absorbed in the acidic pH of the stomach, whereas most weak bases are not absorbed until reaching the more neutral environment of the small intestine. The mammalian GI tract has numerous specialized transport systems for the absorption of nutrients and electrolytes. For example, the absorption of iron depends on the levels of the nutrient in the body and takes place in two steps: Iron first enters the mucosal cells and then moves into the blood. Uptake is relatively rapid, whereas entry into the circulation is slower, leading to accumulation within the mucosal cells as a protein–iron complex (ferritin). When the concentration of iron in blood decreases, it can be liberated from the mucosal stores of ferritin and transported into the blood. Cobalt and manganese (Mn) also utilize and compete with the iron in this transport system, therefore exogenous exposures to the heavy metals can result in changes in iron metabolism and toxicity.

Numerous xenobiotic transporters are expressed in the GI tract, where they function to increase or decrease absorption of these compounds. Influx transporters are predominantly localized on the apical brush border membranes of enterocytes and increase uptake from the lumen into the cells. These include the OATPs, OCTs, and peptide transporters (Pept1). The primary active efflux transporters such as P-gp, Mrp2, and BCRP are also expressed on enterocyte brush border membranes, where they function to excrete their substrates into the lumen. Substrates for efflux transporters show reduced absorption, an action that may limit toxicity. However, these transporters can also limit the oral absorption of drugs. For example, the immunosuppressive drug cyclosporine and chemotherapeutics such as paclitaxel and vincristine are poorly absorbed after oral administration because they are good substrates for P-gp.

The expression patterns of these transporters throughout the duodenum, jejunum, ileum, and colon are not equivalent. P-gp (MDR1) expression in the intestine increases from the duodenum to colon, whereas Mrp2 expression is highest in the duodenum and decreases to undetectable levels in the terminal ileum and colon. BCRP is distributed uniformly throughout the small intestine and colon.

Particles can also be absorbed by the GI epithelium. Particle size is the primary determinant of absorption, and smaller particles are more likely to be absorbed. Absorption of nanoparticles in rats is as high as 30% for particles that are 50 nm in diameter, and nonionized particles are better absorbed than ionized ones.

Absorption into gut-associated lymphoid tissue (e.g., Peyer's patches) and the mesenteric lymph supply is key to systemic absorption. The amount of a chemical that enters the systemic circulation after oral administration depends on the amount absorbed into the cells of the GI tract, the action of transporters on uptake or efflux from the cells, and the potential for biotransformation. An important concept in this regard is presystemic elimination, referred to as a first-pass effect, which is the potential for removal of chemicals before entrance into the systemic circulation. Chemicals that have a high first-pass effect will appear to have lower absorption because they are eliminated as quickly as they are absorbed. Metabolizing enzymes or efflux transporters in the GI tract also contribute to the first-pass effect by limiting the absorption of the chemical to the liver or systemic circulation. A classic example is grapefruit juice that contains a naturally occurring flavonoid, naringin, which directly inhibits P-gp (and cytochrome P450 (CYP) 3A activity, discussed below) (Johnson et al., 2018). As such, drinking grapefruit juice will increase absorption of some xenobiotics because it inhibits their intestinal efflux and metabolism.

Absorption from the Respiratory Tract

Agents that are absorbed by the lungs include gases, vapors of volatile liquids, aerosols, and particulates. The absorption of inhaled gases takes place mainly in the lungs, but they first must pass through the nose where some molecules are retained if they react with cell surface components. Although such actions may reduce systemic exposure or protect the lungs from damage, they also increase the potential for the nose to be adversely affected. Such is the case with formaldehyde and vinyl acetate which cause tumors of the nasal turbinates in rats (Jeffrey et al., 2006). However, with formaldehyde species, differences in respiratory function, including the ability to inhale through both the nose and mouth, contribute to species differences in carcinogenic outcome. Absorption of gases in the lungs is determined primarily by the respiration rate. It differs from GI absorption because most ionized molecules have low volatility and do not achieve significant concentrations in ambient air. Overall, any chemical absorbed by the lungs is removed rapidly by the blood, which moves very quickly through the extensive capillary network.

Absorption of aerosols and particles is determined by the size and water solubility of any chemical in the aerosol. In general, the smaller the particle, the further into the respiratory tree the particle will deposit, resulting in efficient absorption. Particles $\geq 5\,\mu m$ usually are deposited in the nasopharyngeal region, whereas those with diameters of approximately $2.5\,\mu m$ are deposited mainly in the tracheobronchiolar regions, from which they may be cleared by retrograde movement of the mucus layer in the ciliated portions of the respiratory tract (mucociliary escalator). Particles $1\,\mu m$ and smaller travel to the alveolar sacs where they can be readily absorbed in alveoli. Nanoparticles (less than $0.1\,\mu m$ in diameter) are most likely to deposit in the alveolar region where they may be absorbed into the blood or cleared through lymphatics after being scavenged by alveolar macrophages (Medina et al., 2007; Osman et al., 2020). For more information, see *Nanoparticulates*, Vol 2, Chap 31.

Following exposure and deposition, the removal of some particles from the alveoli is relatively inefficient, and the particles may remain indefinitely (e.g., coal dust, asbestos fibers, and carbon nanotubes). The deposition of these types of particles can reduce mucociliary clearance and/or they may be engulfed by alveolar macrophages where they can be retained for years. The long-term sequelae of such deposition is associated with a variety of chronic lung diseases.

Absorption Through the Skin

As the largest organ in the body, skin comes into contact with many chemicals, but exposure is usually limited by its relatively impermeable nature. The stratum corneum is the single most important barrier to preventing fluid loss from the body while also serving to prevent the absorption of xenobiotics. Chemicals move across the stratum corneum by passive diffusion, and in general, diffusion is proportional to their level of lipid solubility and inversely related to molecular weight. Once absorbed across the stratum corneum, the vascular network within the dermis allows these absorbed compounds to enter the body. The skin, particularly keratinocytes, expresses numerous drug metabolizing enzymes and xenobiotic transporters (e.g., Mrp 1, 3, 4, 5, and 6) that can aid or protect against xenobiotic absorption.

Dermal absorption varies widely across species. In general, rodent skin allows greater uptake than human skin, whereas the cutaneous permeability characteristics of guinea pigs, pigs, and monkeys are similar to those in humans. Species differences in dermal absorption of xenobiotics result from several anatomic, physiologic, and biochemical factors. Importantly, the stratum corneum is much thicker in humans than in most laboratory animals. However, the thinner stratum corneum in animals is often compensated for by a relatively thick hair cover, diminishing direct contact of the skin with a xenobiotic. In addition, expression of drug metabolizing enzymes and xenobiotic transporters may contribute to differences in dermal absorption of toxicants across species (Chandra et al., 2015).

2.3. General Principles of Distribution

Once absorbed, a toxicant distributes throughout the body, and this process usually occurs rapidly. The rate of distribution to tissues is determined primarily by blood flow and the rate of diffusion out of capillary beds into a particular organ. The liver is often a major organ for initial distribution given the relatively high blood flow (Table 2.2) and its role in metabolism (discussed below). The final distribution depends on the affinity of a xenobiotic for various tissues, and this factor often determines the target organs of toxicity.

Volume of Distribution

The volume of distribution (Vd) is used to quantify the distribution of a xenobiotic throughout the body. It is defined as the volume (L) in which the amount of compound would need to be uniformly dissolved in order to produce the observed blood concentration. If a chemical is only in the plasma compartment and not distributed into tissues, it would have a higher plasma concentration and a low Vd. In contrast, if a compound distributes throughout the body, it exhibits much lower concentrations in the blood and a high Vd. Some toxicants selectively accumulate in certain parts of the

TABLE 2.2   Estimates of Blood Flow in Liver and Kidney
Across Species

Species	Estimated blood flow (mL/min/kg)		
	Hepatic	Renal	Total
Mouse	90	14	400
Rat	70	5	300
Dog	40	6	120
Monkey[a]	44	2	220
Human	20	1.8	80

[a] *Monkey denotes cynomolgus monkey; all results are estimates (numerous literature sources) for comparative purposes.*
Reference: Lipscomb JC, Poet TS.: In vitro measurements of metabolism for application in pharmacokinetic modeling, Pharmacol. Ther 118, 82–103, 2008.

body as a result of protein binding, active transport, or high solubility in fat.

Storage of Toxicants in Tissues

The most important storage sites for toxicants are plasma, due to protein binding, and tissue depots. The site of disposition and the target organ of a chemical or toxicant can be the same, but toxicants can also accumulate in organs that differ from the site of toxicity. The lung toxicant paraquat or renal toxicants such as adefovir or cis-platinum show selective accumulation in the target organ of toxicity. However, lead is stored in bone but demonstrates toxicity in soft tissues.

Serum albumin, the concentration of which is about 500–600 μM in all species, is a major binding site for compounds in plasma. A second relevant serum protein is α_1-acid glycoprotein that is present in all species but at a much lower concentration than albumin. The degree of binding of chemicals to plasma proteins can determine toxicity because only the unbound fraction can enter tissues. Therefore, a compound that is highly bound to plasma protein may not show toxicity when compared to one that is less extensively bound to plasma proteins. Ironically, a high degree of protein binding can increase the risk of adverse effects resulting from interactions with other highly bound compounds. In particular, severe reactions can occur if a toxicant with a high degree of protein binding is displaced from plasma proteins by another agent, increasing the free fraction of

the compound in plasma. For example, if a strongly bound sulfonamide is given concurrently with an antidiabetic drug, the sulfonamide may displace the antidiabetic drug and induce a hypoglycemic coma. Similarly, interactions resulting from displacement of warfarin can lead to inappropriate blood clotting and deleterious effects. Xenobiotics can also compete with and displace endogenous compounds that are bound to plasma proteins.

The liver and kidney have a high capacity for binding many chemicals. These two organs probably concentrate more toxicants than all the other organs combined, and in most cases, active transport or binding to tissue components is likely to be involved. The heavy metal binding protein metallothionein (MT) sequesters both essential and toxic metals, including zinc (Zn) and cadmium (Cd), with high affinities in the kidney and liver. In liver, Cd is sequestered and bound to MT, preventing its toxicity despite high hepatic levels. In contrast, glomerular filtration of the Cd–MT complex can result in renal toxicity due to proximal tubule damage. For more information, see *Heavy Metals*, Vol 2, Chap 27].

Another protein that sequesters toxicants in the kidney is α2u-globulin. This protein, which is synthesized in large quantities only in male rats, binds to a diverse array of xenobiotics, including metabolites of D-limonene (a major constituent of orange juice) and 2,4,4-trimethylpentane (found in unleaded gasoline). The chemical–α2u-globulin complex is taken up by the kidney, where it accumulates within the lysosomal compartment and damages the proximal tubule epithelial cells. Ultimately, the accumulation of this complex in the kidney, termed α2u-globulin or hyaline droplet nephropathy, is responsible for male rat-specific nephrotoxicity and carcinogenicity.

Adipose tissue is a storage site for chemicals that have a high lipid/water partition coefficient. This is an issue for environmental bioaccumulation and can contribute to low-grade chronic exposure to persistent chemicals. Adipose storage is a critical factor in the toxicity of lipophilic pesticides such as chlordane and dichloro-diphenyl-trichloroethane (DDT), along with the large class of polychlorinated and polybrominated biphenyls, dioxins, and furans (see *Agro/Bulk Chemicals*, Vol **2,** Chap 12] and

Environmental Toxicologic Pathology, Vol 2, Chap 18]). The potential for these compounds to produce toxicity, including carcinogenic, developmental, and endocrine effects, is related to their accumulation and storage in adipose tissue. Although storage in adipose tissue may reduce the amount that reaches target organs, there is a risk that mobilization of lipids from storage sites will increase the concentration of a chemical in blood and the target organ(s) of toxicity (La Merrill et al., 2013).

Bone is an important depot for compounds such as fluoride, lead, and strontium, all of which may be incorporated and stored in the bone matrix. For example, 90% of lead in the body is eventually found in the skeleton, although it is not toxic to bone itself. In contrast, deposition in bone is an important determinant of the toxicity of fluoride and radioactive strontium (see *Bone and Joints*, Vol 3, Chap 4).

Barriers Affecting Distribution

BLOOD–BRAIN BARRIER

Several organs, most notably the brain, have barriers that restrict entry to toxicants. The BBB is formed primarily by endothelial cells with tight junctions between adjacent cells that prevent diffusion of polar compounds through paracellular pathways. Four ATP-dependent transporters also function as part of the BBB including P-gp, Mrp2, Mrp4, and BCRP. These efflux transporters are located on the luminal plasma membrane and prevent distribution to the brain by pumping xenobiotics absorbed into the capillary endothelial cells back out into the blood [see *Nervous System*, Vol 3, Chap 9]).

Genetically modified mice illustrate the importance of transport processes to the maintenance of the BBB and restriction of compounds from the brain. For example, compounds that are substrates for P-gp achieve much higher brain levels in P-gp null (Mdr1a$^{-/-}$/Mdr1b$^{-/-}$) mice relative to wild-type mice. Seminal studies demonstrated that compounds like ivermectin and vinblastine accumulated in the brains of P-gp null mice leading to marked neurotoxicity and increased lethality (Brinkmann and Eichelbaum, 2001; Schinkel et al., 1994).

GUT BARRIER

The gut is a composite of both physical and functional barriers that protect organisms from pathogens while remaining selectively permeable for the absorption of nutrients, electrolytes, and water. The barrier is composed of gut microbiota, mucus, epithelial cells, and gut-associated lymphoid tissue or gut-associated immune cells. Intestinal permeability is described as two major pathways, namely transepithelial/transcellular and paracellular. As discussed previously, major transporters expressed in enterocytes throughout the GI tract, such as P-gp and Mrp2, can alter bioavailability of xenobiotics. A widely used cellular system to assess intestinal permeability of xenobiotics is the Caco-2 cell line, an immortalized line of human colorectal adenocarcinoma cells (Kumar et al., 2010; Wilson et al., 1990). This intestinal system mimics the epithelial barrier by creating an apical brush boarder, tight junctions, and expressing enzymes and transporters within the epithelial monolayer. As in the BBB, passage of molecules through the space between intestinal epithelial cells is controlled by tight junction proteins that are highly regulated, traverse the intestines, and disruption can contribute to disease.

Intestinal barrier dysfunction is often secondary to immune-mediated mechanisms wherein cytokines, released locally as a result of conditions such as inflammatory bowel disease, food allergies, celiac disease, and diabetes, increase permeability and alter absorption of nutrients and drugs. Ethanol metabolism from chronic alcohol consumption has been associated with increased intestinal permeability and endotoxin translocation due to high levels of the metabolite acetaldehyde in the intestine. Both cytokine (e.g., interferon gamma or tissue necrosis factor alpha (TNF-α)) and acetaldehyde treatment disrupt the integrity of tight junctions increasing permeability of the Caco-2 monolayer in vitro. Lastly, xenobiotics such as nonsteroidal antiinflammatory drugs or immunotherapy checkpoint inhibitors demonstrate a multistage process in GI toxicity that alters the integrity of the gut barrier (Tugendreich et al., 2006). For example, adverse intestinal side effects have been observed with grapiprant treatment in dogs and anticytotoxic T-lymphocyte–associated protein-4 (CTLA-4) therapy in humans (Abdel-Rahman et al., 2015; Kirkby Shaw et al., 2016).

PLACENTAL BARRIER

The placenta is a specialized structure that serves to nourish and protect the developing fetus. Although its organization differs markedly across species, the major cellular elements are the syncytiotrophoblast and cytotrophoblast layers (see *Embryo, fetus and placenta,* Vol 4, Chap 11). Xenobiotic transporters are differentially expressed in various cells of the placental unit and contribute to the barrier function that restricts distribution of toxicants to the fetus. Importantly, in most species, BCRP expression is highest in the placenta relative to any other tissue, where it plays a pivotal role in protecting the fetus from exposure to toxicants. Other transporters, namely P-gp and Mrp2, are expressed along with BCRP on the apical border of the syncytiotrophoblast, whereas Mrp1 is localized to the basolateral membranes of these cells and the fetal capillary endothelial cells (Young et al., 2003).

Despite the presence of biotransformation systems and xenobiotic transporters designed to nourish and protect the fetus, the transfer of xenobiotics across the placenta can still occur. One important consequence of placental transfer is that of transplacental carcinogenesis. In this case exposing the mother during gestation increases the likelihood of tumor development in the offspring later in life (see *Carcinogenesis: Mechanisms and Evaluation,* Vol 1, Chap 8). The most well-known transplacental carcinogen in humans is diethylstilbestrol, but other compounds such as the antiviral drug zidovudine and inorganic arsenic induce tumors in mice when exposed to these chemicals only during gestation (Olivero, 2008; Waalkes et al., 2007; Waalkes et al., 2006).

2.4. Metabolism: Activation and Detoxification

Although some xenobiotics are directly toxic (e.g., caustic strong acids or bases, heavy metals, and hydrogen cyanide), many require metabolism to the penultimate toxic moiety. In this regard, the metabolic fate of a xenobiotic can be a critical component of toxic mechanisms, and it contributes to organ and species-specific differences in toxicity. The full range of metabolic reactions and pathways is beyond the scope of this chapter. Additional relevant information covering biotransformation reactions that contribute to toxicity or protect from toxicity can be found in the literature (Klaassen, 2019).

As a general rule, biotransformation (or metabolism) serves to increase the water solubility of a compound and thereby enhance its excretion and limit its toxicity. However, in some cases, biotransformation leads to the formation of a variety of reactive intermediates that can be directly cytotoxic or mutagenic. Examples of such reactive intermediates include electrophiles, free radicals, and redox-reactive intermediates.

Electrophiles are molecules that contain an electron-deficient atom with a partial or full positive charge that can react by sharing electron pairs with an electron-rich atom. Electrophiles include reactive epoxides, arene oxides, aldehydes, quinones, and acyl halides. Examples of compounds that can be activated in this way include acetaminophen (APAP) (to a reactive quinoneimine), aflatoxin (to a reactive epoxide intermediate), ethanol (to acetaldehyde), and chloroform (to a reactive acyl halide, phosgene).

Free radicals are molecules that contain unpaired electrons in their outer orbit. They are reactive because they can accept electrons, transfer that electron to molecular oxygen, and ultimately form the superoxide anion radical ($O_2^{\bullet}$). The hydroxyl radical ($HO^{\bullet}$) is an important toxicological moiety that can be generated from hydrogen peroxide as illustrated in Fig. 2.2. Importantly, this reactive intermediate can be formed by numerous toxic agents that are free radicals or by endogenous sources including NADPH oxidase which is highly abundant in activated macrophages and other cells during toxic or inflammatory reactions. Fig. 2.2 also illustrates the Fenton reaction, a process that generates the hydroxyl free radical. This is an important process catalyzed by transition metals including iron (as illustrated) or by other metals such as copper, chromium, nickel, or Mn (Koppenol and Hider, 2019).

Biotransformation has been described in phases, with Phase I including oxidative, reductive, and hydrolytic reactions. In general, these reactions introduce small changes in the water solubility of the compound. In contrast, Phase II reactions are typically a conjugation reaction wherein a large change in water solubility is introduced through the addition of different types of hydrophilic moieties such as UDP-glucuronic acid (UDPGA) (glucuronidation),

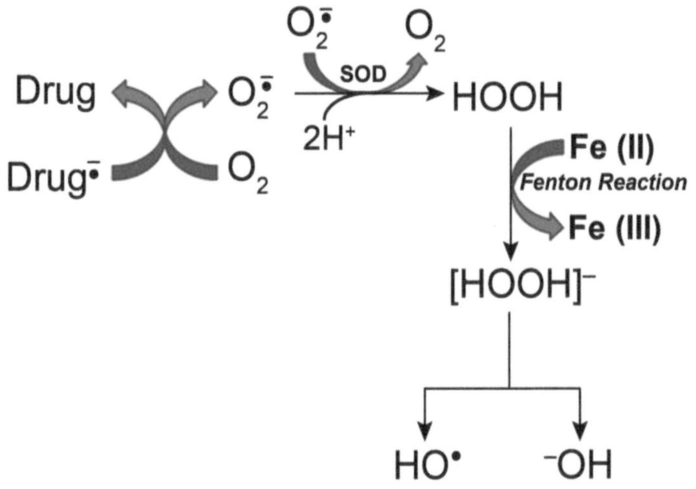

FIGURE 2.2   Formation of the hydroxy radical (HO•) occurs through a reaction involving hydrogen peroxide (HOOH). The generation of free radicals can be a significant contributor to toxicity.

sulfate (sulfation), or the tripeptide glutathione (GSH). The export of conjugated (or other) compounds from cells defines Phase III metabolism, the process by which transporter-mediated efflux contributes to excretion or further metabolism of a xenobiotic. Collectively, the action of these three phases of metabolism typically (but not always) works in concert to prevent toxicity.

Phase I Metabolism

The most important enzymes involved in the Phase I biotransformation of xenobiotics are the CYP450s, a family of more than 50 heme-containing enzymes. Binding of ligands such as oxygen or carbon monoxide (CO) occurs when the iron in the heme moiety is in the reduced ferrous form (Fe^{2+}), and the name CYP 450 was derived from the observation that the CO-saturated protein absorbs light maximally at 450 nm. The basic reaction catalyzed by CYPs is monooxygenation and is summarized by the following equation:

$$Substrate(RH) + O_2 + NADPH + H^+$$
$$\rightarrow Product(ROH) + H_2O + NADP^+$$

Overall, the reactions that are catalyzed by CYPs include the following: (1) hydroxylation of an aliphatic or aromatic carbon; (2) epoxidation across a double bond; (3) oxidation of a heteroatom such as S or N or N-hydroxylation; (4) dealkylation of a heteroatom such as O-, S-, or N-; (5) oxidative group transfer; (6) cleavage of esters; and (7) dehydrogenation.

Given its major role in biotransformation, the liver expresses high levels of a variety of CYPs, and the enzymes involved in xenobiotic metabolism are localized to the endoplasmic reticulum (ER, microsomal fraction). In all species, these enzymes are more highly expressed in the hepatic centrilobular zones (more so than the midzonal or periportal regions), and for this reason, many xenobiotics that are metabolized to reactive intermediates in the liver show toxicity in the centrilobular regions. Additionally, CYPs are localized intracellularly to the smooth ER such that enzyme activity is often studied from the microsomal fraction obtained by differential centrifugation of tissue homogenates.

Of the many CYP families and subfamilies, the CYP3A enzymes are typically the most constitutively abundant in all species. Other enzyme families are more highly expressed in extrahepatic tissues. For example, CYP2F enzymes are more abundant in the lung than liver, particularly in the metabolically competent club cells (nonciliated bronchiolar epithelial cells; formerly called Clara cells). In this manner, toxicants that are metabolically activated in the lung, such as naphthalene or ipomeanol, show marked toxicity in these cells. The major families of CYP enzymes involved in xenobiotic metabolism are summarized in Table 2.3. It should be noted that a variety of CYPs are also critical to or rate limiting in the metabolism of endogenous compounds such as cholesterol, steroid, vitamin D, bile acids, and fatty acids.

Species and sex differences in CYP-mediated metabolism contribute significantly to toxicity. Across species, there are differences in expression of some enzymes and in substrate specificity (Nelson et al., 2004). For example, in rats there are sex-dependent differences in expression of CYP2c enzymes, wherein males express CYP2c11 and females express CYP2c12. Additionally, the CYP2A enzymes differ markedly in substrate specificity, as the human CYP2A6 readily catalyzes 7-hydroxylation of

TABLE 2.3   Cytochrome P450 Enzymes Families and General Function

CYP family	Substrate examples	Tissue distribution (major organs)[a]
CYP1A	Aromatic hydrocarbons	Liver, kidney, lung, and intestine
CYP1A2	Xanthines (caffeine, theophylline), phenacetin, and APAP	Liver, kidney, lung, intestine
CYP1B	Estradiol	Adrenal gland, ovary, testis, and skin
CYP2A	Testosterone (rat), coumarin, and nitrosamines	Liver, testis, skin, and nasal mucosa
CYP2B	Bupropion, 7-benzyloxyresorufin	Liver, kidney, lung, and intestine
CYP2C	Warfarin, diclofenac	Liver, kidney, lung, and intestine
CYP2D	Debrisoquine, codeine, imipramine	Liver, lung, and intestine
CYP2E	Chlorzoxazone, APAP, ethanol,	Liver, lung, kidney, and intestine
CYP2F	Naphthalene, styrene, 3-methylindole	Lung, nasal and mucosa
CYP2J	Arachidonic acid metabolites	Liver, nasal mucosa, lung, kidney, and intestine
CYP3A	APAP, aflatoxin, erythromycin, lovastatin	Liver, lung, and intestine
CYP4A	Fatty acids (omega hydroxylation)	Liver, kidney, and lung
CYP4B	Fatty acids (omega hydroxylation), valproic acid, aromatic amines	Lung, kidney, and liver
CYP7A	Bile acid metabolism	Liver
CYP11A	Cholesterol side-chain cleavage	Adrenal cortex, ovary, testis, and placenta
CYP11B	Steroid 11β-hydroxylation	Adrenal cortex
CYP17	Androgen synthesis	Testis, ovary, and kidney
CYP21	Glucocorticoid synthesis	Adrenal cortex
CYP24	Vitamin D metabolism	Kidney
CYP26	Vitamin A metabolism	Liver and brain

[a] Tissue distribution summarizes the major organs of constitutive expression of CYPs in rats. In most cases, these enzymes are highly abundant in liver, and for those families, the liver is listed first. When the liver is noted, but preceded by other tissues, it is present, but not highly abundant. Some organs that are not listed may also express low levels of CYPs but are not included here (e.g., heart, spleen, and pancreas).

coumarin, and this substrate is used widely to determine CYP2A activity in tissues. In contrast, the rat CYP2a family (e.g., CYP2a1,2, and 3) has only a very low affinity for coumarin, with preference for 7α-hydroxylation of testosterone as a substrate. Moreover, coumarin is hepatotoxic in rats because of the lower capacity to form 7-hydroxycoumarin, a nontoxic metabolite, and greater formation of a toxic epoxide.

Another family of Phase I biotransformation enzymes is the flavin monooxygenases (FMOs). These enzymes, which are also located in the microsomal fraction, catalyze the oxidation of nitrogen, sulfur, or phosphorous in a variety of xenobiotics and are distinguished from CYPs in that they are heat labile (inactivated by heating to 50°C for 1 min) and detergent resistant, whereas as CYPs are inactivated by nonionic detergents. FMOs catalyze the formation of N-oxides from tertiary amines or hydroxylamines from primary or secondary amines, as well as the formation of S-oxides or P-oxides from sulfur- and phosphorous-containing compounds. They play an important role in the metabolism of drugs such as cimetidine as well as endogenous substrates such as trimethylamine.

Other Phase I reactions include hydrolysis, which is important in the biotransformation of esters. A major hydrolytic reaction is that involved in the fate of epoxide intermediates. A wide range of alkene or aromatic compounds can be oxidized by CYPs to epoxides, many of which are potentially reactive. Epoxide hydrolases are enzymes that catalyze the *trans*-addition of water to an epoxide, forming a dihydrodiol metabolite that is generally less reactive than its epoxide precursor. These enzymes are primarily found in the microsomal fraction of virtually all tissues, although a second form is known to exist in the cytosolic fraction. In most cases, formation of the dihydrodiol product represents a detoxification reaction. However, epoxide hydrolases work in concert with CYPs to form bay region diol-epoxides from polyaromatic hydrocarbons, such as

benzo[a]pyrene, the penultimate toxicant for this class of compounds.

Alcohol and aldehyde dehydrogenases are a large family of enzymes that catalyze the oxidation of alcohols to aldehydes and aldehydes to carboxylic acids, respectively (Teschke, 2019). These reactions are classically illustrated by the metabolism of ethanol wherein alcohol dehydrogenase converts ethanol to acetaldehyde which is subsequently oxidized to acetic acid by aldehyde dehydrogenase as follows:

$$CH_3CH_2OH \rightarrow CH_3CHO \rightarrow CH_3COOH$$

A number of metals (such as pentavalent arsenic) or xenobiotics containing aldehyde, ketone, nitro or azo groups are often reduced in vivo. Some enzymes such as alcohol dehydrogenase, aldehyde oxidase, and under reductive conditions (low oxygen tension) CYPs can catalyze reductive reactions. However, it is often difficult to determine whether reduction has occurred enzymatically or by direct interaction with a reducing agent. Furthermore, the reduction of nitro- and azo-containing compounds is generally catalyzed by intestinal microflora particularly in the anaerobic environment of the lower GI tract. This is the case for compounds such as 2,6-nitrotoluene, in which reduction by intestinal bacterial produces mutagenic amine metabolites (discussed below).

There are numerous other enzymes that catalyze the reduction of xenobiotics, many of which are involved in the detoxification of electrophiles. By far, the most important pathway in this regard is GSH conjugation (see below), but an important Phase I enzyme in this class is NAD(P)H oxidoreductase 1 (NQO1). NQO1 catalyzes the reduction of quinones, quinoneimines, nitroaromatics, and azo dyes, and in doing so, diverts these electrophiles away from GSH conjugation so as to protect cells from sulfhydryl depletion while affording detoxification of the reduced metabolites by other Phase II conjugation reactions (glucuronidation and sulfation). This enzyme also functions as an important antioxidant, cytoprotective enzyme, and is highly inducible and regulated by the Keap1/Nrf2 pathway (discussed in more detail below).

Phase II Metabolism

Phase II metabolic reactions are primarily conjugation reactions, generally occurring in the cytosol, with glucuronidation, sulfation, and GSH conjugation being the most important in xenobiotic toxicity. Other conjugation pathways include methylation, acetylation, and amino acid conjugation (e.g., taurine, glycine, or glutamic acid). These pathways are discussed briefly at the end of this section.

Glucuronidation and sulfation require cofactors, namely UDPGA and 3'-phosphoadenosine-5'-phosphosulfate (PAPS), respectively. UDPGA is synthesized from glucose 1-phosphate with concentrations of at least 200 µM detected in the liver. In contrast, the major source of sulfate in PAPS appears to be cysteine, and since free cysteine concentrations are limited, PAPS levels are considerably lower than UDPGA. The availability of the cofactors determines the capacity of the conjugation pathways, in that glucuronidation has a high capacity, whereas sulfation is a low-capacity conjugation pathway. This distinction specifies that sulfation reactions are more likely to become saturated than glucuronidation reactions, most likely from depletion of PAPS.

Glucuronidation and sulfation reactions are catalyzed by UDP-glucuronosyltransferases (UGTs) and sulfotransferases (SULTs), respectively. SULTs, along with most other enzymes catalyzing conjugation reactions, are localized in the cytosol, whereas UGTs are localized to the microsomal fraction. In rats, there are two major families of UGTs (UGT1 and 2) and three predominant families of SULTs (SULT1, 2, and 4). Substrates for both conjugation reactions typically contain functional groups such as alcohols (aliphatic and aromatic), carboxylic acids, and amines although phenolic and aliphatic alcohols are the major substrates for SULTs. Glucuronide and sulfate conjugates markedly increase the water solubility of compounds and facilitate excretion. Although urinary excretion

is favored, glucuronide conjugates are also excreted to a large extent in bile, particularly in rodents. Biliary excretion of glucuronide conjugates is mediated by xenobiotic transporters, particularly Mrp2 and BCRP, and as noted earlier, represent Phase III xenobiotic metabolism.

In most cases, conjugation reactions detoxify xenobiotics and facilitate excretion. However, there are notable cases of increased toxicity or adverse reactions resulting from Phase II metabolism. For example, bilirubin is glucuronidated by reactions catalyzed primarily by UGT1A1. Compounds that compete with bilirubin for conjugation by this enzyme can cause hyperbilirubinemia as a direct consequence of competitive inhibition. Glucuronidation or sulfation of aromatic amines (or the hydroxylamine metabolites of aromatic amines) can increase the potential cellular reactivity and ultimately tumorigenic hazard of these compounds. Additionally, some acyl glucuronides are reactive intermediates that increase the likelihood of toxicity (Bradshaw et al., 2020; Regan et al., 2010). This is the case for a variety of nonsteroidal antiinflammatory drugs.

Finally, there are significant species differences in glucuronidation and sulfation reactions. Most notably, glucuronidation is the major Phase II metabolic pathway in all mammalian species except for cats, and in the cat family, with SULT activity in felines being quite high, a biochemical difference that likely serves to offset their low capacity to form glucuronide conjugates. In rodents, the Gunn rat is a genetic mutant (Wistar strain) that presents with glucuronidation defects resulting from a mutation that renders all enzymes in the UGT1 family functionally inactive.

GSH conjugation is a major pathway involved in the detoxification of electrophilic compounds, thereby reducing damage from these potentially reactive species. GSH is a tripeptide composed of glycine, cysteine, and glutamic acid, with glutamic acid linked to cysteine via a γ-carboxyl group (γ-glutamine–cysteinylglycine). It is a major nonprotein sulfhydryl moiety in most tissues, and in liver, its concentration is extremely high ($\approx$5–10 mM). In light of its high concentration, some compounds can be directly conjugated with GSH, representing a nonenzymatic addition, whereas most reactions are catalyzed by glutathione transferases (GSTs).

GSH conjugates that are formed in liver are often excreted into bile, as they are good substrates for Mrp2. Similarly, GSH conjugates are transported into the blood by Mrp3 and Mrp4. In the kidney, GSH conjugates are often converted to mercapturic acids, a process that involves sequential cleavage of glutamic acid and glycine followed by N-acetylation of the remaining cysteine conjugate (also considered part of Phase III metabolism by some). Accordingly, biliary excretion of GSH-containing metabolites and urinary levels of mercapturates reflect the total conjugation of a compound with GSH.

There is a large family of GSTs classified as alpha, mu, pi, sigma, theta, zeta, and omega forms. The functional enzyme is a dimer, typically comprised of identical subunits, although some forms are heterodimers. The functional activity of GSTs is a major determinant of certain species differences in toxicity, the most notable example of which is the fungal toxicant, aflatoxin B1 (AFB1). Specifically, very low doses of AFB1 are hepatotoxic and tumorigenic in rats but not in mice, even though both species metabolize this fungal contaminant to a highly reactive epoxide (AFB1 8,9-epoxide) at similar rates. The difference in toxic outcome across species is determined by the fact that mice conjugate the 8,9-epoxide with GSH up to 50 times faster than rats. Chemicals that induce GSTs, such as oltipraz or ethoxyquin, increase GSH conjugation and reduce the toxic effects of compounds like AFB1 (Eaton and Gallagher, 1994).

Other conjugation pathways that contribute to xenobiotic fate include methylation, acetylation, and amino acid conjugation reactions. Methylation is generally a minor pathway that differs from most other Phase II reactions in that metabolites formed are typically less water soluble than the parent compound. Methylation requires S-adenosylmethionine as a cofactor, with a variety of methyltransferases responsible for catalyzing the reaction. Although conjugation reactions are typically associated with the fate of organic compounds, methylation is an important pathway for inorganic toxicants such as arsenic. In this case, methylation of arsenic, particularly

the trivalent form (arsenite), results in the formation of methylarsonic acid and dimethylarsinic acid, both of which are more cytotoxic and more genotoxic than arsenite. Species differences in methylation can contribute to arsenic toxicity, as is the case for some primates, as marmosets and chimpanzees do not appear to methylate inorganic arsenic at all.

Acetylation is particularly important for compounds such as aromatic amines and is catalyzed by N-acetyltransferases with acetyl coenzyme A as the required cofactor. These cytosolic enzymes are found in most mammals with the notable exception of dogs (and foxes), which are unable to acetylate xenobiotics. This enzyme family is also characterized by the prevalence of genetic polymorphisms, as "fast" and "slow" acetylators have been described in humans, hamsters, rabbits, and mice (Upton et al., 2001; Walker et al., 2009). Compounds such as p-aminobenzene, isoniazid, and sulfamethazine are recognized substrates for acetylation.

Amino acid conjugation is classically illustrated by the glycine conjugation of benzoic acid to form hippuric acid (hippurate). This reaction, which requires activation of the substrate by conjugation with acetyl CoA, typically occurs in the mitochondria, where numerous acyl-CoA synthetases are present. Bile acids are endogenous substrates for conjugation with glycine or taurine, but this reaction is catalyzed by a family of bile acid–CoA:amino acid N-acetyltransferases that are localized to the microsomal fraction. Marked species differences in the conjugation of bile acids are recognized, as rabbits and pigs form predominantly glycine-conjugated metabolites, whereas rats form predominantly taurine conjugates and humans and primates form both types of conjugates in variable proportions (Thakare et al., 2018a, b).

Phase III Metabolism

Phase III metabolism enables the efflux of hydrophilic conjugates and their excretion in urine, bile, or feces, most of which is accomplished by efflux transporters. These transporters, specifically the ABC-type transporters, are regulated transcriptionally by nuclear receptors (NRs) which include pregnane X receptor (PXR), constitutive androstane receptor (CAR), and FXR (NRs are discussed in the next section). Metabolites, including sulfates, glucuronides, and GSH conjugates, are predominantly excreted by Mrp2 and Mrp1. Competitive inhibition of these efflux transporters can result in toxicity. Many drug–drug interactions resulting in adverse events are due to competitive inhibition and thus are preventable and should not automatically be assumed to be changes in drug metabolizing enzymes. Additionally, genetic deficiencies in transporters can also impact Phase III metabolism of both xenobiotics and endogenous ligands. For example, bilirubin is excreted into bile mainly as glucuronide conjugates, and these conjugates are substrates for MRP2. Dubin–Johnson syndrome is a rare inherited disorder caused by a mutation in the *ABCC2* gene (Mrp2) which manifests as jaundice and hyperbilirubinemia due to an accumulation of bilirubin, as the bilirubin glucuronides are excreted into the bile by Mrp2 (Memon et al., 2016).

The metabolic fate of the widely used analgesic, APAP, prototypically encompasses Phase I and II biotransformation and Phase III metabolism, illustrated in Fig. 2.3. The biotransformation of this compound provides a general summary of biotransformation, conjugation reactions, and the sulfate, glucuronide, and GSH conjugates are substrates for Mrp2

(canalicular) and Mrp3 and Mrp4 (basolateral; see below), with subsequent efflux into bile or plasma, respectively. This figure also illustrates how the biotransformation pathways change with increasing dose of APAP and how metabolic fate limits or ultimately results in toxicity.

2.5. Elimination of Toxicants

The major routes of elimination for xenobiotics are urinary and fecal excretion, with biliary elimination contributing to the net excretion in feces. These routes of excretion are highly dependent on Phase III metabolism (Klaassen and Aleksunes, 2010). Exhalation is another route of excretion, primarily for gases. Compounds are also excreted in body secretions such as sweat, saliva, tears, and breast milk.

Urinary Excretion (Shen et al., 2019)

The kidneys comprise about 4% of total body weight but receive nearly 25% of the cardiac output. The net result is that urinary excretion is a major route of elimination for a diverse group of compounds and electrolytes. Filtration at the glomerulus is driven by pressure differences between the afferent and efferent arteriole, the presence of large pores in the glomerular

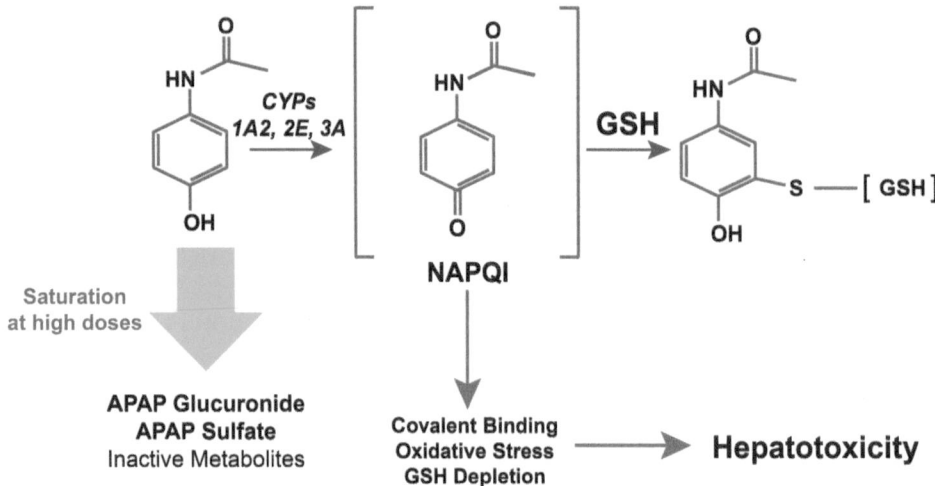

FIGURE 2.3   Outline of the contribution of Phase I and Phase II biotransformation reactions in contributing to the metabolic activation and detoxification of acetaminophen. The major pathway for detoxification is glucuronide and sulfate formation, denoted by the green arrow. A minor detoxification pathway and alternate pathway when saturation occurs at high doses is CYP metabolism to generate the intermediate N-acetyl-p-benzoquinone imine (NAPQI), which is ultimately detoxified by glutathione (GSH) conjugation (*blue arrows*). If high levels of NAPQI are generated via metabolism or GSH is depleted, a build-up of the toxic intermediate leads to hepatotoxicity (*red arrows*).

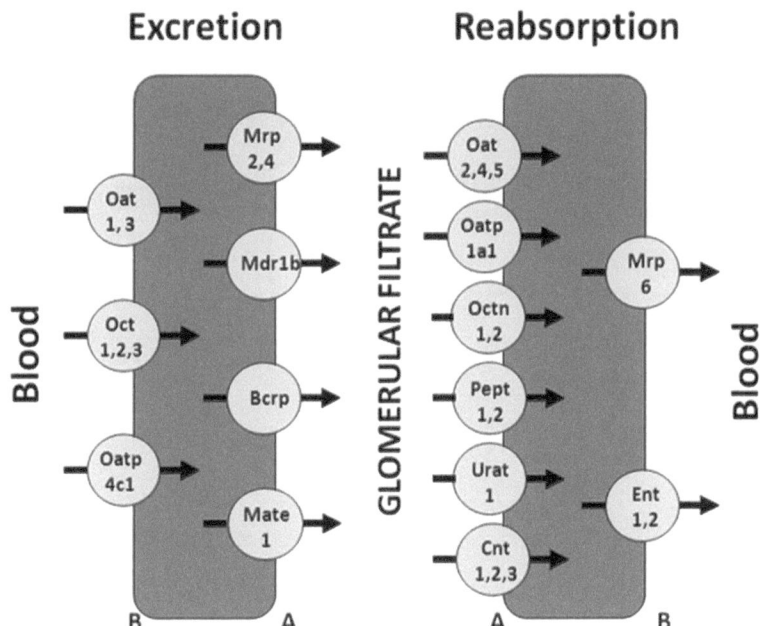

Excretion **Reabsorption**

FIGURE 2.4 Expression and membrane localization of xenobiotic transporters in the rat kidney. Abbreviations: Multidrug resistance protein, P-glycoprotein (MDR), Multidrug resistance protein (MRP), Organic anion transporter (OAT), Organic cation transporter (OCT), Breast cancer resistance protein (BCRP), Organic anion transporting polypeptide (OATP), Multidrug and toxin extrusion transporter (MATE), Organic cation transporters novel (OCTN), Peptide transporter (PEPT), Urate transporter (URAT), Concentrative nucleoside transporters (CNTs), and Equilibrative nucleoside transporter (ENT). (A) apical; (B) basolateral.

capillaries, and the degree of plasma protein binding. The molecular weight limit for filtration is approximately 60 kDa but varies across species. Glomerular filtration rates are determined by the relative number of nephrons (normalized to body weight) and range from a high of approximately 10 mL/min/kg in mice to about 1.8 mL/min/kg in humans (Table 2.2).

Once filtered, a compound may remain in the tubular lumen and be excreted with urine or may be reabsorbed back into the bloodstream. Reabsorption of toxicants occurs primarily in the proximal tubules and is governed by the principles described earlier for passive diffusion (e.g., lipid solubility and ionization). Thus, toxicants with a high log P are reabsorbed more efficiently than polar compounds and ions. The pH of urine is normally slightly acidic (approximately 6–6.5), such that excretion of organic bases is favored, whereas organic acids may be reabsorbed.

Xenobiotics can also be excreted into urine by active secretion, a process that involves uptake across the basolateral cell membrane (from blood) into the epithelial cells of the renal proximal tubule and subsequent efflux from the luminal cell membrane into the tubular fluid. Xenobiotic transporters play an important role in the net secretion, reabsorption, and ultimately

urinary excretion of xenobiotics. Transporters are expressed on the luminal side of the cell, where they contribute to tubular secretion and reabsorption, or are localized to the basolateral membranes, serving to transport xenobiotics to and from the circulation and the renal tubular cells. The expression of major renal transporters involved in xenobiotic disposition is illustrated in Fig. 2.4.

Transporters expressed on the basolateral side of the renal tubular epithelial cells include OATs, OCTs, and selected members of the OATPs (Hagenbuch, 2010). The OAT family mediates the renal uptake of organic acids such as polycyclic aromatic hydrocarbons and is important in the renal exchange of dicarboxylates. In rodents, Oat1 and 3 are localized to the basolateral membranes. Although the OATs play an important role in the physiological exchange of metabolites in the kidney, they can also contribute to the development of renal toxicity. Antiviral drugs cidofovir and adefovir are nephrotoxic, and the target organ for toxicity in these cases is determined by the accumulation of these drugs in the proximal tubule by Oat1. Similarly, Oat5 is reported to transport ochratoxin A, and may play a role in the nephrotoxicity associated with exposure to this mycotoxin.

The OCT family is responsible for the renal uptake of some cations. Substrates for OCTs

FIGURE 2.5 Expression and membrane localization of xenobiotic transporters in rat liver. Abbreviations: Multidrug resistance protein, P-glycoprotein (MDR), Multidrug resistance protein (MRP), Breast cancer resistance protein (BCRP), Bile salt export pump (BSEP), Multidrug and toxin extrusion transporter (MATE), Organic anion transporting polypeptide (OATP), Organic anion transporter (OAT), Organic cation transporter (OCT), Na + −taurocholate cotransporting polypeptide (NTCP). (A) apical; (B) basolateral.

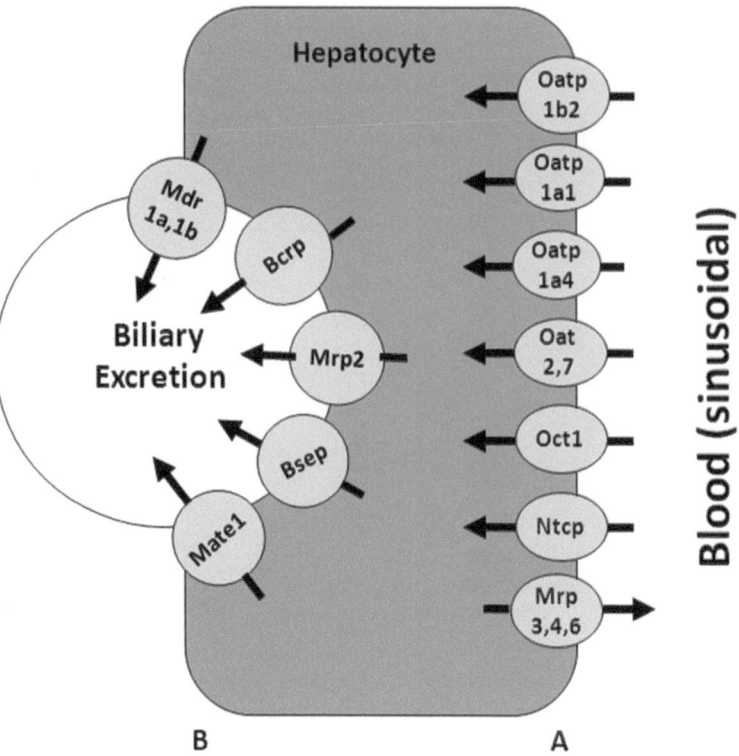

include endogenous compounds such as choline, tetraethylammonium, and cationic drugs including cimetidine and acyclovir. Oct1 and 2 are expressed on the basolateral membranes of the rodent kidney. A second cation transporter is OCTN, and two isoforms, OCTN1 and 2 are localized to the brush border membranes in human and rodent kidney. OCTN2 is particularly important in the renal reabsorption of carnitine.

Peptide transporters, localized to brush border membranes, are important for the reuptake of di- and tripeptides. Pept1 and have been identified in the human and rodent kidney, with Pept1 localized in the upper region of the proximal tubule (pars convoluta) and Pept2 expressed in the lower region (pars recta) of the convoluted tubule.

P-gp, Mrp2, and Mrp4 are also found on the luminal brush border of the proximal tubule, where they contribute to the efflux of xenobiotics into the tubular fluid. BCRP is expressed at high levels in the rat and mouse kidney, where it is localized to the apical brush border of the proximal tubule epithelium. This transporter appears to play an important role in the efflux of certain sulfate conjugates. In contrast, BCRP is not detected in the human kidney, a difference that may contribute to species differences in the urinary excretion of a variety of compounds. Finally, Mate1 is specifically involved in the urinary excretion of cationic compounds.

Fecal Excretion (Jetter and Kullak-Ublick, 2020)

Fecal excretion occurs directly from lack of absorption in the GI tract after oral exposure and by biliary elimination into the GI tract. The factors determining whether a chemical is excreted into bile are not fully understood. A general rule is that low-molecular weight compounds (<325 Da) are poorly excreted into bile, whereas compounds with molecular weights exceeding about 325 Da can be excreted in appreciable quantities. GSH and glucuronide conjugates have a high predilection for excretion into bile. Additionally, rats and mice tend to excrete compounds in bile to a greater degree than other species.

Xenobiotic transporters play a critical role in biliary excretion (Fig. 2.5). The major transporters expressed on the canalicular membrane include P-gp, Mrp2, BCRP, and BSEP and Mate1. P-gp, Mrp2, and BCRP are important in the biliary excretion of a wide range of xenobiotics, whereas BSEP is critical for the secretion of bile and the regulation of bile flow. Mate1 transports cationic compounds.

Mrp2 is extremely important in biliary excretion because it is largely responsible for the transport of organic anions including the glucuronide and GSH conjugates of many xenobiotics. Its role in biliary excretion of toxicants was established in part by the characterization of two naturally occurring mutant strains of rat, the Groningen/Yellow transport deficient (TR⁻) and the Eisai hyperbilirubinemic rat (EHBR), both of which lack functional Mrp2 protein. These rats are phenotypically similar to humans suffering with Dubin–Johnson syndrome (described above). The mutant rats also present with conjugated hyperbilirubinemia, reduced biliary excretion of GSH, and defects in biliary excretion of glucuronide and GSH conjugates of many xenobiotics.

The biliary excretion of xenobiotics mediated by Mrp2, BCRP, and P-gp usually results in increased excretion of toxicants out of hepatocytes and into bile. In doing so, these transporters can reduce the likelihood of toxicity in the liver. However, adverse reactions can occur if the function of these transporters is inhibited. For example, compounds that inhibit the transport function of BSEP cause a net decrease in the biliary excretion of bile acids leading to cholestasis and liver injury. This is the case for troglitazone and to a much greater extent, troglitazone sulfate. A similar mechanism contributes to the cholestasis observed with steroids such as estradiol (Jetter and Kullak-Ublick, 2020; Yang et al., 2013).

Xenobiotic transporters localized to the sinusoidal membranes are also important in determining hepatic concentrations of toxicants and thereby contribute to disposition and biliary elimination. Transporters present on rat sinusoidal membranes include the ABC transport family members, Mrp3, Mrp4, and Mrp6, along with OATPs, OATs, and OCT. The Na^+/taurocholate cotransporting polypeptide is also found on the sinusoidal membrane where it functions in the uptake of bile acids into the liver (Fig. 2.5).

Mrp3 transports many of the same organic anions that are substrates for Mrp2 from the liver into blood. It is also upregulated during cholestasis and in TR⁻ and EHBR rats. The increase in Mrp3 is recognized as a compensatory response that helps to protect hepatocytes from toxic chemicals for cells deficient in Mrp2. Mrp4 is specifically involved in the cellular efflux of purine analogs, nucleoside antiviral drugs, and cyclic nucleotides, including cAMP and cGMP. It has also been shown to be a carrier for some xenobiotics, including conjugated and unconjugated compounds.

Several influx transporters are located on the basolateral membrane of hepatocytes where they contribute to the hepatic uptake of many organic anions. Numerous OATPs are expressed in liver and contribute to the uptake of organic anions including conjugated metabolites. Oatp1b2 is highly expressed in liver and is directly involved in the uptake of the mushroom toxin, phalloidin, and the blue-green algal toxin, microcystin. $Oatp1b2^{-/-}$, mice are resistant to phalloidin and microcystin-induced toxicity as a direct result of reduced hepatic uptake (Choudhuri and Klaassen, 2020). Oat2 is also expressed in liver and transports small organic anions, and Oct1 contributes to the uptake of organic cations. Cations such as metformin are substrates for Oct1. Treatment with metformin can lead to lactic acidosis through alterations in mitochondrial function, and $Oct1^{-/-}$ mice are generally resistant compared to wild-type mice suggesting an important role for this transporter in the elimination and toxic liability of this compound.

An important concept relating to biliary excretion and hepatic disposition is the phenomenon of enterohepatic circulation. This is a cycle in which a compound excreted into bile reenters the intestine to be reabsorbed again and returned to liver. Many compounds excreted into bile are conjugated with UDPGA, sulfate, or GSH, and enzymes found in the intestinal microflora hydrolyze the glucuronide and sulfate conjugates, to facilitate reabsorption from the gut (see *Digestive Tract*, Vol 3, Chap 1]). Reabsorption and uptake into the liver completes a cycle where it can again be metabolized and excreted back into bile. Enterohepatic recycling results in prolongation of the half-life of xenobiotics. Therefore, it is desirable to interrupt this cycle to hasten the elimination of a toxicant from the body.

The toxicity of some compounds can also be directly related to their biliary excretion. The classical example is irinotecan, an anticancer drug that induces severe diarrhea across species. The mechanism for the effect of this drug involves metabolism to an active metabolite that is a good substrate for Mrp2. The excretion into bile mediated by Mrp2 results in high concentrations of the toxic metabolite in the intestinal lumen (de Jong et al., 2007). Modulation of irinotecan is described in more detail in the section discussing the microbiome (see below).

Exhalation

Substances that exist predominantly as a gas at body temperature are eliminated mainly by the lungs. Because volatile liquids are in equilibrium with their gas phase in the alveoli, they may also be excreted via the lungs. The amount of a liquid eliminated via the lungs is proportional to its vapor pressure. A practical application of this principle is seen in the breath analyzer test for determining the amount of ethanol in the body. Highly volatile liquids such as diethyl ether and certain volatile anesthetics (e.g., nitrous oxide) are excreted almost exclusively by the lungs.

No specialized transport systems have been described for the excretion of toxic substances by the lungs. Some xenobiotic transporters, including Mrp1 and P-gp, have been identified in the lung, but overall compounds excreted via exhalation in the lung are most likely to be eliminated by simple diffusion. Therefore, gases with low solubility in blood, such as ethylene, are rapidly excreted whereas chloroform, which has a much higher solubility in blood, is eliminated very slowly by the lungs. Trace concentrations of highly lipid-soluble anesthetic gases such as halothane and methoxyflurane may be present in expired air for as long as 2–3 weeks after a few hours of anesthesia. Undoubtedly, this prolonged retention is due to deposition in and slow mobilization from adipose tissue of these very lipid-soluble agents.

Other Routes of Elimination

Although the urinary system and GI tract are the major routes of excretion for most xenobiotics, some elimination can occur through sweat, saliva, breast milk, and cerebrospinal fluid. Of these minor routes, secretion of toxic compounds into milk is notable because it allows for the materials to be passed from the mother to her nursing offspring or for compounds to be passed from cows to people via dairy products. Many compounds that can accumulate in fat such as aldrin, chlordane, DDT, polychlorinated and polybrominated biphenyls, dibenzo-p-dioxins, and furans are found in milk (Massart et al., 2005).

2.6. Effects of the Microbiome on Absorption, Distribution, Biotransformation and Elimination

An emerging field for understanding mechanisms of toxicity is the gut microbiome (Koontz et al., 2019). Bacteria in the gut can influence or mediate mechanisms of toxicity directly (e.g., action of the bacteria) or indirectly (e.g., influence on host organ function or gene expression), and toxicants can elicit unexpected effects by direct alteration of the composition of the gut flora. In general, the microbiome is composed of obligate anaerobes (e.g., *Bacteroides*, *Clostridium*, *Lactobacillus*, *Escherichia*, and *Bifidobacteria*), and it is estimated that the total microbiome in an average human (70 kg) comprises about 0.2 kg of mass (Sender et al., 2016).

Although there are numerous metabolic reactions carried out by intestinal flora, reductive metabolism is a predominant pathway. For example, nitroreductases specific to the microbiome catalyze the reduction of these compounds to a variety of mutagenic aromatic amines (described above). The role of the intestinal flora is highlighted by the fact that the amine metabolites are not formed in germ-free or antibiotic-treated animals (Claus et al., 2016; Rooks and Garrett, 2016).

Irinotecan, a widely used drug for treating colon cancer, causes significant diarrhea that is directly linked to hydrolysis of a glucuronide conjugate (SN-38), by bacterial β-glucuronidase. Whereas the glucuronide conjugate is nontoxic, formation of the aglycone by the bacterial enzyme is directly associated with dose-limiting diarrhea (Ma and McLeod, 2003). Administration of antibiotics to reduce the gut flora reduces this effect, and ultimately, inhibitors of bacterial β-glucuronidase activity have been developed to modify the gut flora-mediated effect (Bhatt et al., 2020).

Another significant example of microbiome-mediated effects on toxicity was realized when rats received from two different holding rooms at a veterinary supply house showed marked differences in the response to galactosamine. Although the precise mechanism for the differences were not fully explained, profiles of urinary metabolites these rats revealed differences in endogenous metabolites associated with bacterial-mediated reactions (hippuric and chlorogenic acids), and the marked differences in toxicity were eliminated by cohousing the animals to create a more uniform microbiome (Robosky et al., 2005).

Although microbiome-mediated metabolism is a critical determinant of toxicity, gut flora also contributes to the efficacy of some drugs. A most striking example is with antibodies directed against CTLA-4, a widely used immuno-oncology therapy. In germ-free or antibiotic-treated mice, anti-CTLA-4 therapy failed to stop the progression of sarcomas in a mouse tumor model, whereas this therapy was fully effective in conventional mice. It is now recognized that *Bacteroides* species are required for effective anti-CTLA-4 therapy (Vétizou et al., 2015).

From an indirect mechanistic perspective, the microbiome can influence metabolism within the GI tract. Disease states, such as nonalcoholic steatohepatitis, alter expression of genes involved in Phase I, II, and III metabolism. Additionally, in germ-free mice, expression of numerous CYPs was downregulated, whereas expression of phase II conjugation enzymes were decreased, and transporter expression was generally increased (Selwyn et al., 2015). Finally, research in Oatp$^{-/-}$ mice revealed that the predominant phenotypic alteration associated with loss of function of this major hepatic uptake transporter was a change in the intestinal microbiome (Zhang et al., 2012). Overall, the Oatp null mice had nearly 10-times more bacteria in the small intestine when compared to wild-type mice, and bacterial composition was characterized by a marked increase in *Bacteroides* species and a decrease in *Firmicutes*. These changes were associated with altered urinary metabolite profiles and changes in intestinal altered bile acid composition.

Overall, the contribution of the microbiome to effects on xenobiotics is a burgeoning field, and there is much to learn about the contribution of the intestinal flora to species differences in both intended and toxic outcomes. There is no doubt that the microbiome contributes to interspecies differences in toxicity or therapeutic outcome given differences in the composition of gut flora. Finally, the microbiome is likely to contribute to variability in response to xenobiotics as it is influenced by intestinal physiology along with considerable variability driven by diet, overall health status, and the use of antibiotics or probiotics.

3. INTERACTIONS OF TOXICANTS WITH CELLULAR AND MOLECULAR TARGETS

3.1. Covalent Modification (Klaassen, 2019) Chapters 3 and 8

Once delivered to the ultimate target site, toxic compounds and metabolites can elicit numerous adverse effects, and a major example is covalent modification of cellular macromolecules. Covalent adducts are typically formed with cellular nucleophiles including proteins, DNA, RNA, and phospholipids. Covalent modifications impair protein function by altering conformation or structure and ultimately disrupt cellular energy homeostasis and/or signal transduction mechanisms. These effects may activate cell death pathways (discussed below), or in some cases, evoke an immune response. Such adverse effects are exemplified by APAP (Fig. 2.3) wherein metabolic activation leads to reactive intermediates that covalently bind to numerous macromolecules leading to marked hepatocellular necrosis. In most cases, the precise identity of intracellular targets of covalent binding has not been fully characterized. Moreover, although analytical methods have been developed to assess covalent binding and to detect specific modifications in individual peptides or proteins, establishing a causal link between covalent modification and toxic response is far more difficult. In the case of APAP, covalent modification of mitochondrial proteins appears to be an initiating event in the cascade that will lead to cell death.

Covalent binding of xenobiotics to endogenous proteins has also been implicated as a key event in the development of skin sensitization and allergic contact dermatitis. Specifically, the formation of an adducted protein may be recognized as a hapten to ultimately invoke an allergic response. In this regard, in vitro systems using peptide targets that are typically cysteine- or lysine rich have been developed to predict sensitization potential.

Reactive toxicants can also damage DNA. Covalent modification causes nucleotide mispairing during replication, a promutagenic event resulting from incorrect codon formation that alters amino acid sequence and protein function. For example, covalent binding of aflatoxin 8,9-oxide to N-7 of guanine causes it to pair with adenine rather than cytosine forming an incorrect codon and consequently, an incorrect amino acid in the protein. When such genotoxic events induce mutations in critical proto-oncogenes or tumor suppressor genes, cancer risk is increased, and in the case of aflatoxin 8,9-oxide, mutations of the *Ras* proto-oncogene and *p53* tumor suppressor gene are causally related to liver tumor development (discussed below). Some agents also intercalate DNA to cause frame shifts that terminate normal DNA synthesis.

A fundamental principle of covalent binding mechanisms of toxicity is that such adverse effects are often highly dose dependent, and this is readily demonstrated with APAP (Fig. 2.3). Basically, oxidative metabolites will be conjugated with UDPGA or PAPS until these essential cofactors are depleted. As the dose increases and Phase I and II pathways are saturated, GSH conjugation serves as a secondary defense mechanism to bind up reactive metabolites. However, at very high doses, even GSH can be depleted (and transferases saturated) so that cellular macromolecules are now vulnerable to covalent modification and toxicity ensues. Understanding of this mechanistic underpinning can be applied in two important ways. First, trapping reactive metabolites as GSH conjugates is widely used to determine the extent to which a compound is metabolized to potentially toxic intermediates. Additionally, the treatment for APAP overdose in any species is N-acetyl cysteine, a sulfhydryl source that increases hepatic levels of cysteine and replenishes intracellular GSH (Mullins et al., 2020).

Free radicals (described earlier) initiate lipid peroxidation that ultimately alters lipid structure and disrupts membrane integrity. End products include malondialdehyde (MDA) and 4-hydroxynonenal (HNE), and both can contribute to additional toxicity. For illustration, HNE modifies proteins by addition to histidine, cysteine, or lysine residues forming protein adducts or cross-linking proteins (Fig. 2.6). HNE and MDA also react with DNA to generate mutagenic adducts (not illustrated), many of which are detected constitutively. Such adducts can also form with DNA causing DNA damage (e.g., strand breaks) to initiate genotoxic events.

3.2. Stress Responses in Toxicity

There are many different types of stress responses to toxicity, with outcomes that can be fully protective or ultimately overcome with frank toxicity. Additional relevant information covering biotransformation reactions that contribute to toxicity or protect from toxicity can be found in the literature (Jacobs and Marnett, 2010; Klaassen, 2019; Simmons et al., 2009).

A major pathway involved in toxicity is oxidative stress, defined as a disturbance in the redox state of the cell resulting from an imbalance between the production of reactive oxygen species and the cell's ability to detoxify these intermediates or to repair the damage that may result. Examples of oxidative stress include covalent binding to cellular macromolecules, free radical generation, and lipid peroxidation already described. There is increasing evidence that oxidative stress is involved in many conditions, including neurodegenerative diseases, atherosclerosis, and the general process of aging. Additionally, oxidative stress is recognized to contribute to metabolic diseases such as diabetes and nonalcoholic fatty liver disease, and some biomarkers of oxidative stress are applied to evaluating disease severity and progression (Dewidar et al., 2020). Oxidative stress is often detected by measuring cellular levels of MDA (a general marker) or 8-hydroxydeoxyguanosine, a known marker of oxidative DNA damage. Additionally, there are redox-sensitive transcription factors that are activated by oxidative stress and drive expression of cytoprotective genes (Table 2.4 and discussed below).

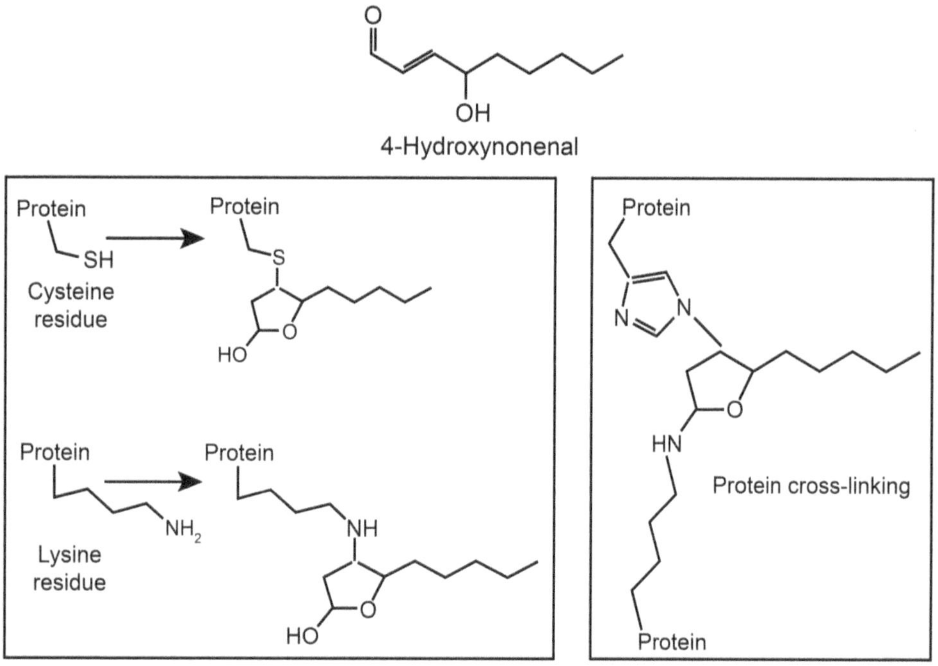

FIGURE 2.6 Illustration of the types of protein adducts that can be formed from 4-hydroxynonenal (HNE), an end product of lipid peroxidation. HNE can adduct proteins or form protein cross-links leading to cellular damage. HNE can also adduct DNA to generate mutagenic adducts (not illustrated).

TABLE 2.4 Common Cellular Stress Response Pathways

Cellular stress mechanism	Transcription factor(s) regulating response	Induced response genes
Oxidative stress	Nrf2	*Heme oxygenase, Quinone Oxidoreductase*
DNA damage	p53	*Growth arrest and DNA damage (GADD)45, mdm2, p21*
Hypoxia	HIF-1	*Vascular endothelial growth factors, erythropoietin*
Heat shock	HSF-1	*Heat shock proteins*
Endoplasmic reticulum stress	XBP-1, ATF4, 6	*Heat shock proteins 90B1, A5, DNAJb9*
Metal stress	MTF-1	*Metallothioneins*
Osmotic stress	NFAT5 (TonEBP)	*Betaine/GABA transporter (SLC6A12) Na-myoinositol transporter (SLC5A3)*
Inflammation	NF-κB	*Interleukin-1, TNF-α*

Abbreviations: Nuclear factor (erthryoid-derived 2)-like (Nrf2); Hypoxia-inducible factor 1 (HIF1); Heat shock transcription factor (HSF-1); X-box binding protein 1 (XBP1); Activating Transcription Factor (ATF); Metal transcription factor 1 (MTF-1); Nuclear Factor of Activated T-cells (NFATF; also known as tonicity enhancer binding protein; TonEBP); Tumor necrosis factor (TNF).

Oxidative stress is also a critical pathway underlying mitochondrial dysfunction and mechanisms of cell death. Importantly, the steady state concentration of superoxide radicals in the mitochondria is at least 5-times higher than cytoplasmic or nuclear levels, and enables the generation of significant levels of the highly toxic $HO^\bullet$ (Fig. 2.2) that can alter mitochondrial function.

There are other important cellular stress responses involved in toxicity, and such mechanisms are associated with histological changes that are secondary to alterations in gene expression or signal transduction pathways (discussed below). These other stress responses are outlined in Table 2.4 and are induced or causal to a variety of mechanisms of toxicities that are outlined here.

(1) DNA damage is associated with chemicals that directly affect DNA sequence or alter the fidelity of DNA replication.

(2) Hypoxia can be caused by any adverse effect that lowers oxygen tension or affects the cellular utilization of oxygen.

(3) Heat shock is a generalized stress response observed with many insults including heavy metals and temperature alterations.

(4) ER stress is elicited by agents that perturb ER function to disrupt essential lipid and protein biosynthesis and normal protein folding.

(5) Metal stress is a specific response elicited by heavy metals secondary to alterations in the homeostasis of essential metals such as Zn and copper.

(6) Osmotic stress is particularly important in the kidney and is evoked by compounds that alter cellular environments by disrupting cellular water or osmolyte movement.

(7) Inflammatory stress or inflammation is a physiologically important pathway that can also exert adverse effects on cells.

3.3. Altered Gene Expression

Toxicants alter gene expression by increasing or decreasing transcriptional activity of numerous targets or by modifying the activity of cellular proteins by posttranscriptional events including changes in phosphorylation state. A major group of ligand-activated transcription factors is the family of NRs that regulate gene expression in response to endogenous hormones and vitamins such as the androgen, estrogen, and glucocorticoid receptors. In general, these receptors remain outside the nucleus when not engaged by ligands but are translocated to the nucleus following ligand interaction where they bind to the consensus sequences in gene promoters and initiate transcriptional activity. Chemicals that interact with these receptors can cause adverse effects by mimicking the action of their endogenous ligands. For example, compounds that can bind to the estrogen receptor can mimic the effects of estrogen, including abnormal developmental programming, inappropriate feminization of male sex organs, or altered mammary proliferation that increases the likelihood of breast cancer. It is speculated that the adverse effects of a variety of environmental compounds, described as endocrine disruptors (e.g., DDT or bisphenol-A; see *Endocrine Disruptors*, Vol 2, Chap 29), are manifested through their ability to engage the estrogen receptor (Baker and Lathe, 2018).

Several NRs, including the Ah receptor (AhR), CAR, PXR, and the peroxisome proliferator–activated receptor α (PPAR α), are widely recognized to control expression of various CYP450 enzymes, UDPGTs, and transporters. Ligands that activate these receptors induce the expression of many genes involved in xenobiotic metabolism and can markedly alter disposition. Examples of compounds that engage these receptors as a primary mechanism of their toxic effects include the following: TCDD and other polyaromatic hydrocarbons that bind to AhR, phenobarbital, and 1,4-bis[2-(3,5-dichloropyridyloxy)] benzene that are ligands for CAR, pregnenolone 16α-carbonitrile, and rifampicin that bind to PXR and phthalate esters that bind to PPARα.

Although the mechanism of transcriptional activation of an NR is generally conserved across species, the downstream effects of this activity often differ significantly among species. For example, in rodents, activation of CAR and PPARα is associated with activation of cell cycle genes leading to marked hepatocellular proliferation and liver tumor development, whereas in humans, no similar liability is observed (Yamada et al., 2020). Gene expression studies in wild-type and humanized mice have shown dramatic variation in both phenotypic changes and AhR-mediated transcriptional activity

(Moriguchi et al., 2003). With over 1000 transcripts upregulated in both models, less than 300 were in common, revealing marked differences in the mechanism by which AhR modulates gene expression across species.

Other important mechanisms underlying altered gene expression patterns are DNA methylation, histone acetylation, and microRNA function (miRNA, discussed below). Briefly, DNA is frequently methylated over time at cytosine residues, and the pattern of this modification, particularly in regulatory regions (e.g., promoters or enhancers), alters gene expression, usually dampening or even silencing it. Methylation patterns in coding sequences and the extent of DNA methylation is inversely correlated to the level of gene expression although this is not an absolute relationship. Such changes are described as epigenetic alterations and represent nongenetic events that alter cellular phenotype. Importantly, epigenetic changes are associated mechanistically with adverse outcomes not only in the developing fetus, but with changes that persist through adulthood. Compounds that exert epigenetic changes via altering constitutive levels of S-adenosylmethionine (major methyl donor) and thus changing the methylation status of DNA include ethanol (a contributing factor to cirrhosis and hepatocellular carcinoma) and inorganic arsenic.

It is suggested that changes in DNA methylation may serve as a long-term "memory" of adverse effects such that toxic changes may be manifested long after the insult occurred. This is the case for chemicals like methoxychlor, a pesticide with estrogenic activity. Male rats exposed in utero to methoxychlor show changes in sperm counts and infertility in adulthood, and these effects were transferrable across three generations of offspring. Such an effect poses a substantial challenge to defining toxicity but represents an area of focused research that will continue to influence our understanding of fundamental mechanisms of toxicity.

Another mechanism of epigenetic regulation is histone acetylation, a process regulated by a critical balance between histone acetyltransferase (HAT) and histone deacetylase (HDAC). These two enzymes contribute to the relaxation and condensation of chromatin structure, respectively, with relaxation associated with greater gene transcription and condensation limiting gene transcription. The antiepileptic drug, valproic acid, is an HDAC inhibitor with adverse developmental effects observed in rodents when pups are exposed during embryonic development (Göttlicher et al., 2001; Wlodarczyk et al., 2012). The inhibition of histone deacetylation impairs neurogenesis and affects brain development leading to learning and memory defects. Histone acetylation can also contribute to disease pathophysiology, as it is well demonstrated that corticosteroids are known to suppress inflammatory genes associated with asthma via inhibition of elevated HAT activity and recruitment of HDACs to the respiratory tree (Barnes et al., 2005).

MiRNAs are small noncoding RNA sequences (21–23 nucleotides) that bind to complementary regions of target messenger RNAs (mRNAs) and repress translation of the mRNA. miRNAs interfere with complementary nucleotide sequences to repress protein synthesis, and over 2500 discovered miRNAs regulate about one third of genes in the human genome (Ha and Kim, 2014). Additional relevant information on the biogenesis of miRNAs and their role in health and disease can be found in the literature (Santulli, 2015).

A major miRNA in liver is miR-122, which comprises about 50% and 70% of the miRNAs in adult mouse and human liver, respectively. miR-122 represses numerous genes involved in lipid biosynthesis and loss of its function may have a role in the development of fatty liver. Similarly, miR-122 is decreased in a carbon tetrachloride (CCl$_4$)–induced model of liver fibrosis in mice. Although the target genes regulated by miR-122 are not fully identified, inflammatory genes such as *Ccl2* (chemokine C–C motif ligand 2; also called macrophage chemoattractant protein 1; MCP1) and the profibrotic Kruppel-like factor 6 are regulated by miR-122 (Murakami and Kawada, 2017).

Renal miR-21 has been shown to be upregulated in models of both acute and chronic injury. It is one of the most highly expressed miRNAs in healthy kidneys, where it is detected in the renal cortex. Kidney injury (e.g., fibrosis) or toxicity is associated with marked increase in miR-21 expression and it is overexpressed in idiopathic pulmonary fibrosis.

miRNAs also contribute to the regulation of drug metabolizing enzymes. For example,

CYP3A4 and CYP2E1 are repressed by miR-27b and miR-378, respectively. Liver-specific miR-122 null mice have higher constitutive concentrations of CYP2E1 and CYP1A2, both of which catalyze the formation of reactive metabolite N-acetyl-p-benzoquinone imine (NAPQI, Fig. 2.3), which renders these mice highly susceptible to APAP-induced toxicity. There is growing interest in clarifying the role of miRNAs in mechanisms of toxicity, as therapeutic modulation of miRNAs is currently not feasible due to the broad array of genes that are regulated by single type of miRNA; thus, off-target effects arise. Therefore, miRNAs are predominantly being assessed for their potential sensitivity and utility as biomarkers of toxicity and diagnostic/prognostic biomarkers of disease (Yokoi and Nakajima, 2013).

3.4. Mechanisms of Cell Death

The major metabolic events associated with toxic cell death pathways include cellular energy status, calcium homeostasis, and mitochondrial changes. A comprehensive review of cell death and its mechanisms is described elsewhere (Orrenius, 2019). The energy state of the cell is regulated by ATP which is essential for the overall maintenance of normal cell morphology and activity. Toxicants disrupt mitochondrial ATP synthesis by affecting numerous steps involved in oxidative phosphorylation or damaging mitochondrial DNA to alter expression of mitochondrial-specific genes.

It is also well established that intracellular calcium levels or alterations in Ca^{2+} compartmentalization are involved in cell death. There is about a 10,000-fold difference between extracellular and cytoplasmic Ca^{2+} levels, and toxicants that increase cytosolic Ca^{2+} levels by stimulating influx or preventing efflux can cause cell death by stimulating a variety of cytotoxic mechanisms resulting in apoptosis by altering expression of ligands or direct toxic effects on the ER and mitochondria. Intracellular Ca^{2+} levels are affected by chemicals that disrupt cell membranes (e.g., detergents, inducers of lipid peroxidation), interfere with Ca^{2+} sequestration in the ER (e.g., lindane), or impair mitochondrial ATP synthesis.

Disruption of mitochondrial function, and particularly mitochondrial permeability transition (MPT), is a critical event in cell death. Biochemical changes that increase MPT include increased Ca^{2+} uptake, low transmembrane potential, generation of reactive oxygen species, and ATP depletion. These events trigger the opening of a permeability transition pore, a large protein complex that traverses both the outer and inner mitochondrial membranes, which ultimately leads to massive swelling of the inner mitochondrial compartment and eventual rupture.

Although necrotic cell death was long considered the ultimate consequence of toxicity, it is now clear that chemical toxicity is associated with multiple modes of cell death. For some toxicants, the mode of cell death is dose dependent, progressing from autophagy at low, toxic doses to apoptosis, and necrosis with increasing dose and severity. It is also clear that these distinct pathways may coexist in a damaged organ. Cell death pathways elicit unique morphological features that are described in more detail in *Morphologic Manifestations of Toxic Cell Injury* Vol 1, Chap 6. The morphologic features are highlighted here with reference to understanding mechanisms of toxicity.

Autophagy

Autophagy is a lysosomal process in which intracellular substrates are degraded within the lysosomal compartment. It is unique among cell death mechanisms in that there is no evidence of chromatin condensation but is characterized by the presence of cytoplasmic vacuoles resulting from engulfment of cellular components. Autophagy is a constitutive and rapid process, and most autophagosomes are very short lived with a half-life of no more than 10 min. It is also distinct from apoptosis and necrosis in that the clearance of "debris" is an intracellular process, and there is no involvement of other phagocytic cells. Autophagy occurs by the engulfment of cellular constituents (i.e., macroautophagy), membrane uptake of smaller amounts of cytoplasm and organelles (i.e., microautophagy), or by chaperone-mediated events that enable specific protein substrates to be taken into the lysosome for degradation. When cells are nutrient deprived (such as during fasting), autophagy is an important mechanism for survival. With respect to toxicity, autophagy is an important mechanism for removing misfolded proteins from cells as occurs through oxidative stress or ER stress as outlined above. ER stress typically results from the accumulation of unfolded proteins in the ER lumen because of oxidative stress or other stressors such as glucose deprivation. The adaptive response is designed to trigger transcriptional activation of a genetic program that will enhance autophagy and the capacity for normal protein folding in the ER. However, if this is excessive or prolonged, ER stress ultimately triggers cell death typically in the form of apoptosis. Compounds such as ethanol suppress autophagy, a deleterious effect that can elicit toxicity by preventing normal intracellular protein trafficking.

Apoptosis

Apoptosis is characterized by homogeneous condensation of chromatin, cytoplasmic shrinkage, nuclear fragmentation, and blebbing of cell membranes. Apoptotic cells ultimately disperse as membrane-enclosed fragments called apoptotic bodies. There are two major pathways that lead to apoptosis in mammalian cells and are referred to as the extrinsic and intrinsic pathways. The extrinsic pathway is a receptor-mediated pathway in which activation of caspases, particularly procaspases 8 or 9, occurs following ligation of membrane receptors (e.g., apoptosis antigen 1 (CD95/Fas), tumor necrosis factor receptor 1). Procaspase 8 is activated directly from receptor ligation through formation of the death-inducible signaling complex. Caspase 8 activates caspase 3, which cleaves target proteins that initiate the morphologic changes of apoptosis. Procaspase 9 is also activated in the extrinsic pathway, after procaspase 8 activation and mitochondrial membrane changes, leading again to activation of caspase 3. In the intrinsic pathway, signals for cell death act directly on mitochondria to stimulate the release of proapoptotic proteins including cytochrome c and APAF-1 (apoptosis activating factor 1), a protein that shuttles CYP c through mitochondrial pores. These together bind procaspase 9 to activate it and form the "apoptosome" that in turn activates caspase 3. This pathway is controlled by B-cell lymphoma 2 (BCL-2) proteins, which regulates the release of CYP c, along with several other intracellular apoptotic regulatory proteins.

Necrosis

Necrotic cell death is comprised of a continuum of effects, culminating in nuclear shrinkage (pyknosis), fragmentation (karyorrhexis), or dissolution (karyolysis). Numerous toxicants have been shown to cause both apoptosis and necrosis, with necrosis occurring at higher doses with more severe toxicity. Furthermore, caspase activation is more likely to be observed in apoptosis usually not in necrosis, and caspase inactivation during apoptosis may redirect the cell to necrosis.

Changes in mitochondria, specifically events causing MPT, are critical in the process of necrosis. MPT occurs when PT pores in the mitochondrial inner membrane are opened to span both inner and outer mitochondrial membranes, leading to leakage of CYP c, depolarization, uncoupling of electron transport from ATP synthesis, and organelle swelling. When the PT pores are opened in all mitochondria, ATP is further depleted, and swelling followed by necrosis results from the lack of energy to maintain ion gradients. MPT is caused by many mechanisms including oxidative stress, and xenobiotics such as salicylic acid increase PT pore opening by a calcium-dependent mechanism.

Necroptosis

Unlike necrosis, necroptosis is a regulated cell death pathway mediated by death receptors, but ultimately results in an inflammatory response, mimicking both apoptosis and necrosis. Classical and nonclassical necrosome complex formation has been recently described in literature (Dhuriya and Sharma, 2018). TNF-α–induced necroptosis results from binding to the TNF receptor and inhibition of caspase 8 results in the formation of a heterodimer between receptor-interacting protein kinase 1 and 3 (RIPK1 and RIPK3), which is considered the necrosome. This necrosome can also directly be formed from interferon signaling through its receptor. The necrosome phosphorylates the mixed lineage kinase domain-like protein (MLKL), and the oligomeric form creates a pore that allows for the chemokine, cytokine, and danger-associated molecular patterns secretion or recruitment of ion channels to the plasma membrane. RIPK3 overexpression promotes the phosphorylation of MLKL and necroptosis. Therefore, these events represent a regulated process that results in unregulated necrotic death. Necroptosis has been demonstrated in models of cisplatin-induced kidney injury (Xu et al., 2015) and APAP-induced hepatotoxicity (Jaeschke et al., 2019). In both cases, a role for necroptosis is supported by the attenuation of tissue injury with the RIPK1 inhibitor, necrostatin-1.

The programs resulting in cell death are evolutionarily conserved and generally consistent across species. The predominance of one type of cell death over another is dictated by factors such as energy requirements, antioxidant status, oxidative stress, calcium homeostasis, ATP concentration, signaling pathways, severity of insult, and tissue-specific factors that govern how specific cell types die.

4. IDIOSYNCRATIC MECHANISMS OF TOXICITY

An idiosyncratic mechanism of toxicity is one that is characterized by its low, frequently rare, incidence and its poor predictability. Idiosyncratic toxicity is most frequently associated with adverse reactions to drugs, and the liver and skin tend to be the most frequently affected organs. Idiosyncratic reactions are distinguished from other adverse reactions because they do not show typical dose–response relationships and concentration dependence. By their very nature, idiosyncratic mechanisms of toxicity exhibit marked species differences, with limited ability to predict human outcome from studies in rodent or nonrodent models. Examples of drugs known to cause idiosyncratic toxicity include isoniazid, ximelagatran, azithromycin, and carbamazepine (Mosedale and Watkins, 2020).

Although idiosyncratic events are poorly understood, there is emerging evidence that nongenetic and genetic factors contribute to toxicity. Genetic factors, such as polymorphisms in drug metabolizing enzymes and drug transporters, and enzymes that reduce oxidative stress have been implicated. Additionally, nongenetic factors such as concurrent infection, inflammation, and pregnancy may play a role. Currently, the most widely supported contributors to idiosyncratic toxicity are immune-mediated effects, particularly those involving the adaptive immune system. For example, the idiosyncratic effects of carbamazepine are strongly correlated to specific human leukocyte antigen allele polymorphisms (Kaniwa and Saito, 2013).

5. PROTECTIVE MECHANISMS, REPAIR MECHANISMS, AND ADAPTATION OR FAILURE

5.1. Stress Response Constituents and Pathways

Table 2.4 summarizes the types of pathways that are activated in response to cellular stress and toxicity. In all cases, activation of transcription factors drives gene expression changes that are designed to protect cells from further damage. There are two major pathways for protection against oxidative stress or DNA damage that are described here.

Keap1–Nrf2 Regulatory Pathway

The transcription factor Nrf2 (NF–E2-related factor 2) plays a central role in the induction of cytoprotective genes in response to oxidative stress and is shown schematically in Fig. 2.7. Additional relevant information on this important path is found in Taguchi and Kensler (Taguchi and Kensler, 2020). Under normal conditions, Nrf2 is bound to Keap1 (Kelch-like ECH-associated protein 1) in the cytoplasm and binding to Keap1 targets Nrf2 for proteosomal degradation in order to maintain low intracellular levels. In the presence of electrophiles or oxidative stress, Keap1 is inactivated by direct modification of reactive cysteine residues, causing the release of active, stabilized Nrf2 that translocates to the nucleus to activate transcription of a variety of antioxidant and detoxification genes. The important characteristic of this pathway is that it is a derepression response. That is, Nrf2 activity is normally repressed by Keap1, and it accumulates in response to cell stress because the constitutive repression of

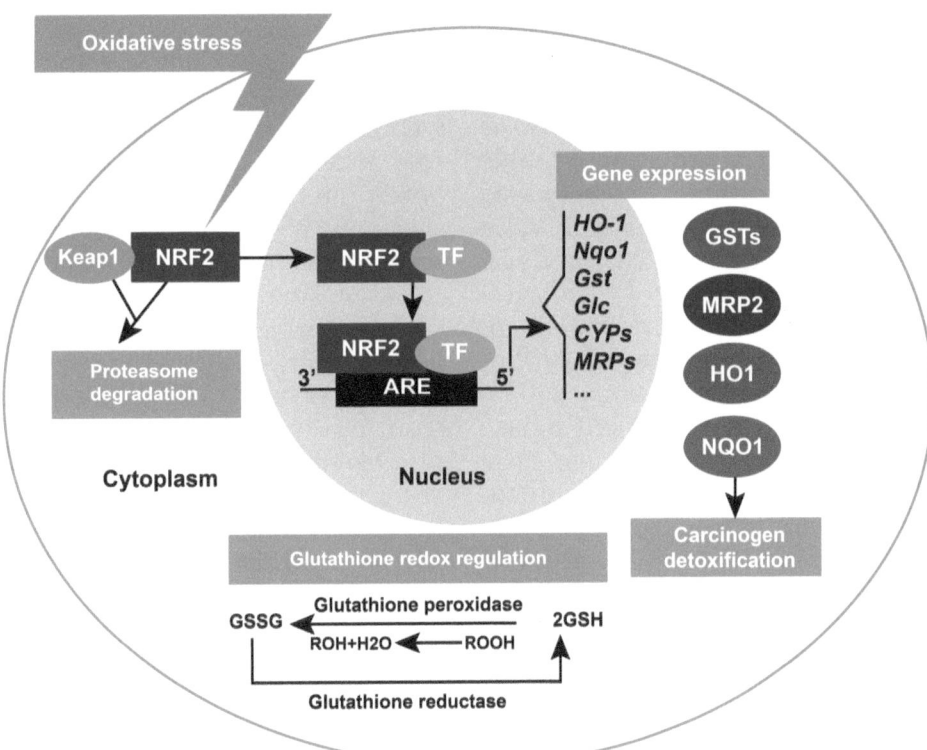

FIGURE 2.7   Nrf2–Keap1 pathway activity in response to oxidative stress. Under normal conditions, Keap1 acts as an adapter between Nrf2 and the ubiquitin ligase Cullin-3 and promotes the proteasomal degradation of Nrf2. Oxidative stress leads to the modification of specific thiols, resulting in dissociation of Nrf2 from Keap1 and translocation of Nrf2 into the nucleus, where Nrf2 binding to the antioxidant response element (ARE) in the regulatory region of a wide array of genes involved in antioxidative responses and xenobiotic disposition leads their transcriptional activation. *Source: Lehman-McKemman LD, Ruepp SU: Biochemical and molecular basis of toxicity In:* Fundamentals of toxicologic pathology, *3 ed, 2018, Elsevier.*

Keap1 is removed. Genes that are activated via the Nrf2 pathway include those involved in xenobiotic disposition (e.g., *GSTs*, *MRPs*, and quinone reductases), protection from electrophiles (e.g., GSH synthesis and superoxide dismutase), and general stress response (e.g., heme oxygenase and thioredoxin).

Some xenobiotics can induce Nrf2, most notably the sulforaphane metabolites derived from broccoli sprouts, along with synthetic compounds oltipraz and butylated hydroxytoluene. Induction of Nrf2 has been shown to protect against the risk of liver cancer associated with exposure to aflatoxin-contaminated food sources. Additionally, Nrf2 induction is protective against lung tumors associated with vinyl carbamate exposure and adverse pulmonary and cardiac effects caused by cigarette smoking. In contrast, some cancer cells activate the Nrf2 pathway as a protective mechanism to enhance cell proliferation and survival (Xue et al., 2020).

The role of GSH as a major cellular nucleophile that protects against a wide array of reactive metabolites has previously been described in detail. GSH is constitutively abundant in essentially all cells, with the highest concentrations in the liver. N-acetylcysteine can be used to increase GSH to help protect against toxicity. In the same manner, some chemicals, including N-ethylmaleamide and buthionine sulfoximine, can be used to intentionally deplete GSH, an action that increases the likelihood of toxicity. Nrf2 also regulates the expression of the enzyme GSH synthetase.

p53 Pathway

The major mechanism involved in protecting against DNA damage is the p53 pathway. Under normal conditions, p53 is bound by Mdm2 (mouse double minute 2), a ubiquitin ligase that targets p53 for proteosomal degradation and prevents its intracellular accumulation. In the presence of DNA damage, p53 is phosphorylated and its binding to Mdm2 is disrupted. Cellular levels of p53 increase dramatically with DNA damage, and with movement to the nucleus, a generalized cellular program to enable DNA repair is transcriptionally activated (Table 2.4). This response includes cell cycle arrest (i.e., G1) to afford more time for DNA repair, along with induction of enzymes enabling this process and increased levels of ribonucleotide reductase to provide deoxyribonucleotides for DNA synthesis. A major p53-dependent gene is the cyclin-dependent kinase inhibitor, *p21*, which plays a critical in cell cycle arrest. Importantly, p53 activation induces Mdm2, serving to terminate p53-dependent programming when DNA repair is complete. Additional information on the regulation, signaling, and transcriptional activity associated with the p53 pathway is found in the literature (Harris and Levine, 2005).

Regulation of p53 is accomplished via a complex and complicated network. In addition to directing cell cycle arrest in response to DNA damage, p53 also contributes to cell senescence and apoptosis, both of which can result from DNA damage or genome instability. The tumor suppressor activities of p53 include activation of apoptosis-promoting genes such as BCL-2–associated protein X and BCL-2 antagonist/killer. The type of response manifested in response to p53 activation also varies in a cell-specific manner. For example, thymocytes typically undergo apoptosis in response to DNA damage, whereas fibroblasts are more likely to undergo senescence. Additionally, apoptosis may be triggered when there is prolonged cell cycle arrest during DNA repair.

Metal Stress Response

MT, a small cytosolic protein that contains 20 cysteine residues (one third of its amino acids) and that has high affinity for essential and toxic metals (Zn, Cu, and Cd), is a major protein involved in cell protection, particularly against heavy metal–induced toxicity. It was originally isolated and identified from the horse kidney to understand what factors contributed to a high burden of Cd in that particular tissue. MT is also a highly inducible protein, and exposure to toxic metals increases transcriptional activity through metal-responsive transcription factor-1

(Table 2.4). Each mole of MT binds up to 7 mol of metal so that with induction, the capacity to bind a toxic metal is increased. Induction of MT is causally related to the development of tolerance to heavy metal toxicity. For example, when an experimental animal is pretreated with Zn, a dose of Cd that would be toxic to an untreated animal shows reduced or no toxicity. This is because increased tissue levels of MT provide a sink to bind the toxic metal and protect cellular organelles. Although MT is most frequently associated with protection from heavy metal toxicity, as a cytosolic source of cysteine residues and sulfhydryl binding sites, it can it also afford protection from other types of cellular stress (Andrews, 2000).

Although the stress response pathways have been described independently, it is clear that toxicity and any form of cell stress can affect multiple pathways concurrently. Thus, transcriptional activation of *Nrf2* may be seen along with MT induction in response to exposure to heavy metals. Furthermore, it is now established that there is some interaction between the p53 and Nrf2 pathways. Specifically, although p21 is a critical component in the p53-dependent pathway, the protective effects of p21 are also dependent on Nrf2. Likewise, induction of the Nrf2-dependent battery of genes is potentiated in the presence of p21, probably through facilitated stabilization of Nrf2.

5.2. Cell Repair and Adaptation

Cell Proliferation

An almost immediate response to tissue injury is that undamaged cells enter the cell cycle to begin the process of tissue repair. It is likely that this process is initiated by mediators released from damaged cells, including a variety of cytokines and growth factors involved in cell replication. In the classical model of liver regeneration following partial hepatectomy, the early regeneration phase is regulated primarily by TNF-α and IL-6. These factors are likely produced from the resident macrophages (i.e., Kupffer cells) rather than from hepatocytes. A variety of other growth factors (e.g., hepatocyte growth factor, transforming growth factor [TGF]-α) increase and drive the cells to proliferate. Additionally, increased expression of genes that function in growth arrest (e.g., *p21*, *GADD45*) is also observed. These genes contribute to terminating the cell cycle, suggesting that there is a tight regulation of the regenerative process.

Tissue-specific stem cells are the primary source of early replication in response to various types of injury and these cells can further differentiate into the mature cell type. This is the case for highly proliferative target organs such as bone marrow and the intestinal mucosa. Hepatic oval cells localized within the portal triad appear to be the source for tissue renewal and repair in the liver. Similarly, Type II pneumocytes and club cells in the lung function to replace the differentiated Type I pneumocyte and bronchiolar epithelium, respectively.

One early feature of repair is that the regenerating tissue is often refractory to additional damage. This phenomenon of tolerance has been illustrated in many tissues. For example, a number of xenobiotics are toxic to the bronchiolar club cells, usually as a result of localized reactive metabolite formation. Chemicals such as naphthalene, coumarin, ipomeanol, and 3-methylindole are activated by CYPs (most frequently Cyp2F enzymes) that are highly expressed in the mouse lung and lead to marked club cell toxicity with accompanying cell proliferation and repair. However, there are two important characteristics of this injury and repair response. The first is that after repeated dosing (i.e., 1–2 weeks), there is no histological evidence of club cell toxicity, compared to marked cell necrosis observed after a single dose. The mechanism(s) underlying this phenomenon are not well understood but are thought to reflect changes in detoxification pathways or altered differentiation of the cells that renders them resistant to toxicity. These events are also typically observed in species that have high levels of pulmonary P450s and abundant club cells (e.g., mouse and rabbit) more so than other species, such as rats and humans (Born et al., 1999; Kültz et al., 2015). Additionally, this example highlights how the time course of histopathological presentation is important to understanding mechanisms of toxicity as the characteristics can change with duration of dosing, and illustrates that if one only evaluates the lung after repeated dosing, there would be little evidence of toxicity.

A variety of xenobiotics, particularly those that activate CAR and PPARα, can also stimulate cell proliferation without evidence of cytotoxicity or cell death (Yamada et al., 2020). In these examples, the effect is primarily observed in liver and is associated with induction of CYPs and peroxisome proliferation, respectively. The stimulus for induction of cell proliferation is not fully understood, but in both cases, $CAR^{-/-}$ and $PPAR\alpha^{-/-}$ mice are refractory to both enzyme induction and increased cell proliferation. As noted earlier, these same effects are not conserved across species, reflecting the complexity of biochemical changes associated with NR activation.

Extracellular Matrix and Fibroblasts

The extracellular matrix (ECM) is composed of collagens, elastin, proteoglycans, and noncollagenous glycoproteins that serve as a major component of the cellular microenvironment with a dynamic structure that contributes to cell–cell and cell–matrix interactions. The regulation of the ECM network exists in an organ-specific manner and is essential during development and maintenance in adults through its roles in cell survival, proliferation, polarity, differentiation, adhesion, and migration. Collagen is the most abundant fibrous protein and is the main structural element of the ECM that provides essential architecture and signaling within tissues via cell adhesion receptors. Integrins are major receptors that facilitate cell adhesion to the ECM and are targeted pharmacologically in the treatment of diseases (e.g., abciximab for acute coronary syndrome, efalizumab for psoriasis, and natalizumab for multiple sclerosis and Crohn's disease). The ECM contributes to the remodeling and repair responses to injury, and is highly influenced by the migration and proliferation of fibroblasts during wound healing (Wynn, 2008). Fibroblasts are cells responsible for the synthesis and secretion of collagenous ECM. They are a major component of the response to injury in both the initiation and resolution (repair mechanisms) phases and have an active role in the inflammatory response. Fibroblasts contribute to cytokine synthesis and secretion, but also respond to them in processes such as wound healing. The cross-talk between fibroblasts and immune cells maintains homeostasis, such that persistent activation of the immune system can also lead to changes in fibroblast function and disorders. This relationship underscores how toxicant-induced injury and human chronic inflammatory disease are major drivers of fibrotic changes. In the lung, accumulated macrophages serve as a key source of profibrotic factors in animals and humans and are known to be in close proximity to fibroblasts during wound healing associated with exposure to different toxicants in animals. Following tissue injury, fibroblasts are stimulated by TGF-β eliciting a profibrotic response via increased synthesis and deposition of collagens I and III, and increased expression of profibrotic genes (e.g., α-smooth muscle actin). Fibroblasts also contribute to the remodeling of the ECM via secretion of matrix metalloproteinases and tissue inhibitor of metalloproteinases. These enzymes play a pivotal role in reepithelialization via matrix degradation and deposition, respectively (Batlle and Massagué, 2019). Another profibrotic factor, connective tissue growth factor (CTGF), is associated with fibrotic pathology and cooperates with TGF-β signaling. Mechanistically, overexpression of CTGF promotes fibrosis in multiple tissues including the kidney, lung, skin, and vasculature. Toxicants known to contribute to fibrosis alter the activation and proliferation of fibroblasts and their secretion of ECM by changing the balance of profibrotic and antifibrotic factors released by the immune cells. Examples of toxicants known to elicit tissue injury, immune response, and subsequent or direct effects on fibroblast signaling include CCl$_4$ which results in hepatic fibrosis, bleomycin-induced pulmonary fibrosis, and aristolochic acid, which induces renal tubulointerstitial fibrosis (Luciano and Perazella, 2015).

5.3. Failure to Repair After Toxic Insult

Repair mechanisms are diverse, cell and organ dependent, and exhibit both time- and exposure-dependent mechanisms. Additional relevant information is presented in more detail in other literature (Klaassen, 2019).

Necrosis

Tissue necrosis is a pathological response that results in loss of organ function due to cell death. Cell death can be caused by external factors such as toxicants and is recognized microscopically by changes in the nucleus as stated previously, including pyknosis, karyorrhexis, and karyolysis (see *Morphologic Manifestations of Toxic Cell Injury* Vol 1, Chap 6). Apoptosis and cell proliferation can interrupt the progression to tissue necrosis. Low-dose exposures to toxicants have been demonstrated to induce apoptosis or early mitotic responses, compared to high-dose exposure where these responses do not occur and therefore necrotic cell death is favored. Some hepatotoxicants such as CCl$_4$ and thioacetamide induce necrosis at high doses, and failure to repair correctly results in eventual development of cirrhosis (Lamas-Paz et al., 2018). Other insults that cause tissue necrosis include interruption of blood supply leading to hypoxia and infections that often induce significant inflammatory responses.

Carcinogenesis

The mechanisms of carcinogenesis are diverse, but most often associated with DNA damage and altered expression of proteins responsible for regulation of cell division or apoptosis. Such changes occur by direct DNA mutation, lack of or reduced ability to repair DNA damage, or transcriptional changes to protooncogenes and/or tumor suppressors by genotoxic and nongenotoxic mechanisms. Genotoxic mechanisms of carcinogenesis require a form of DNA damage that can be achieved by covalent modifications between direct toxicants or metabolic products and DNA, as previously described. Nongenotoxic carcinogens do not cause direct damage to DNA but stimulate sustained cell proliferation via mitogenic growth factors, altered DNA methylation, and miRNA expression. Further information on carcinogenesis is provided elsewhere (see *Carcinogenesis: Mechanisms and Evaluation*, Vol 1, Chap 8), but foundational examples include genotoxic activating mutations of *BRAF* (Miller and Mihm, 2006), that are highly prevalent in human tumors, wherein the mutation promotes neoplastic transformation via sustained activation of the MAP kinase pathway. The key protein in the stress response pathway to DNA damage, p53, can promote carcinogenesis via suppressed DNA repair mechanisms and cell cycle arrest, allowing for DNA amplification via genotoxic and nongenotoxic mechanisms (Harris and Levine, 2005). Diethylstilbestrol, a human and rodent carcinogen, is capable of covalently modifying DNA effecting rapidly dividing cell populations, and it downregulates miRNA-9, which is frequently downregulated in human breast cancer, demonstrating both a genotoxic and nongenotoxic mechanism contributing to carcinogenesis (Hsu et al., 2009; Reed and Fenton, 2013). A classical nongenotoxic chemical is phenobarbital, a known mitogenic compound that increases cell proliferation and alters cell cycle control via multiple mechanisms including the inhibition of p53 signaling (Nelson et al., 2006; Yamada et al., 2020).

Fibrosis

Fibrosis is a reparative process involved in wound healing, but can become chronic and result in excessive ECM, scar formation, and remodeling or destruction of normal tissue architecture. The presence and extent of organ fibrosis due to chronic tissue injury determines progression of diseases, such as chronic kidney disease, nonalcoholic fatty liver disease, and pulmonary fibrosis. Progressive fibrosis phenotypes change mechanical properties of an organ and can lead to loss of function and organ failure (Wynn, 2008). Glomerulosclerosis impairs filtration in the kidney, liver cirrhosis, and portal hypertension that are end-stage features of chronic fibrotic liver diseases, and the vital capacity of the lung is decreased with pulmonary fibrosis. Fibrosis across tissues shares the common features of parenchymal cell injury, persistent macrophage and lymphocyte infiltration, accumulation of the ECM (specifically type-I collagens), accumulation of fibroblasts, and microvascular rarefication. Collagen can be assessed histologically via Masson's trichrome stain or Sirius Red (Direct Red 80) staining.

6. SUMMARY AND CONCLUSIONS

Toxicologic pathologists play a critical role in determining toxic mechanisms of injury using gross and microscopic examination. Additionally, the dose response of a xenobiotic is important as it illustrates the continuum of changes that are observed across a range of dosage levels as it relates to exposure of the compound. Unraveling complex mechanisms of toxicity requires an understanding of the basic principles that govern whether and how a chemical reaches its target

site along with information on how the target organ or target cell responds to the toxicant. Altered gene expression, resulting from direct transcriptional effects, induction of stress response pathways, and epigenetic and miRNA regulation also help to define mechanisms of action. Finally, the biochemical pathways that can help reduce toxicity and facilitate repair when cells are damaged help to determine mechanisms of toxicity. In the end, the understanding of the cellular and molecular changes that lead to toxicity is relevant for addressing species differences, characterizing the potential risk for toxicity to humans resulting from chemical exposure and developing approaches to prevent or treat adverse effects.

REFERENCES

Abdel-Rahman O, ElHalawani H, Fouad M: Risk of gastrointestinal complications in cancer patients treated with immune checkpoint inhibitors: a meta-analysis, *Immunotherapy* 7:1213–1227, 2015.

Andrews GK: Regulation of metallothionein gene expression by oxidative stress and metal ions, *Biochem Pharmacol* 59:95–104, 2000.

Baker ME, Lathe R: The promiscuous estrogen receptor: evolution of physiological estrogens and response to phytochemicals and endocrine disruptors, *J Steroid Biochem Mol Biol* 184:29–37, 2018.

Barnes PJ, Adcock IM, Ito K: Histone acetylation and deacetylation: importance in inflammatory lung diseases, *Eur Respir J* 25:552–563, 2005.

Batlle E, Massagué J: Transforming growth factor-β signaling in immunity and cancer, *Immunity* 50:924–940, 2019.

Bhatt AP, Pellock SJ, Biernat KA, et al.: Targeted inhibition of gut bacterial β-glucuronidase activity enhances anticancer drug efficacy, *Proc Natl Acad Sci U S A* 117:7374–7381, 2020.

Born SL, Fix AS, Caudill D, et al.: Development of tolerance to Clara cell necrosis with repeat administration of coumarin, *Toxicol Sci* 51:300–309, 1999.

Bradshaw PR, Athersuch TJ, Stachulski AV, et al.: Acyl glucuronide reactivity in perspective, *Drug Discov Today* 25(9):1639–1650, 2020.

Brinkmann U, Eichelbaum M: Polymorphisms in the ABC drug transporter gene MDR1, *Pharmacogenomics J* 1:59–64, 2001.

Chandra SA, Stokes AH, Hailey R, et al.: Dermal toxicity studies: factors impacting study interpretation and outcome, *Toxicol Pathol* 43:474–481, 2015.

Choudhuri S, Klaassen CD: Elucidation of OATP1B1 and 1B3 transporter function using transgenic rodent models and commonly known single nucleotide polymorphisms, *Toxicol Appl Pharmacol* 399:115039, 2020.

Claus SP, Guillou H, Ellero-Simatos S: The gut microbiota: a major player in the toxicity of environmental pollutants? *NPJ Biofilms Microbiomes* 2:16003, 2016.

de Jong FA, Scott-Horton TJ, Kroetz DL, et al.: Irinotecan-induced diarrhea: functional significance of the polymorphic ABCC2 transporter protein, *Clin Pharmacol Ther* 81:42–49, 2007.

Dewidar B, Kahl S, Pafili K, et al.: Metabolic liver disease in diabetes - from mechanisms to clinical trials, *Metabolism*, 2020:154299, 2020.

Dhuriya YK, Sharma D: Necroptosis: a regulated inflammatory mode of cell death, *J Neuroinflammation* 15:199, 2018.

Eaton DL, Gallagher EP: Mechanisms of aflatoxin carcinogenesis, *Annu Rev Pharmacol Toxicol* 34:135–172, 1994.

Göttlicher M, Minucci S, Zhu P, et al.: Valproic acid defines a novel class of HDAC inhibitors inducing differentiation of transformed cells, *EMBO J* 20:6969–6978, 2001.

Ha M, Kim VN: Regulation of microRNA biogenesis, *Nat Rev Mol Cell Biol* 15:509–524, 2014.

Hagenbuch B: Drug uptake systems in liver and kidney: a historic perspective, *Clin Pharmacol Ther* 87:39–47, 2010.

Harris SL, Levine AJ: The p53 pathway: positive and negative feedback loops, *Oncogene* 24:2899–2908, 2005.

Hsu PY, Deatherage DE, Rodriguez BA, et al.: Xenoestrogen-induced epigenetic repression of microRNA-9-3 in breast epithelial cells, *Cancer Res* 69:5936–5945, 2009.

Jacobs AT, Marnett LJ: Systems analysis of protein modification and cellular responses induced by electrophile stress, *Acc Chem Res* 43:673–683, 2010.

Jaeschke H, Ramachandran A, Chao X, et al.: Emerging and established modes of cell death during acetaminophen-induced liver injury, *Arch Toxicol* 93:3491–3502, 2019.

Jeffrey AM, Iatropoulos MJ, Williams GM: Nasal cytotoxic and carcinogenic activities of systemically distributed organic chemicals, *Toxicol Pathol* 34:827–852, 2006.

Jetter A, Kullak-Ublick GA: Drugs and hepatic transporters: a review, *Pharmacol Res* 154:104234, 2020.

Johnson EJ, González-Peréz V, Tian DD, et al.: Selection of priority natural products for evaluation as potential precipitants of natural product-drug interactions: a NaPDI center recommended approach, *Drug Metab Dispos* 46:1046–1052, 2018.

Kaniwa N, Saito Y: Pharmacogenomics of severe cutaneous adverse reactions and drug-induced liver injury, *J Hum Genet* 58:317–326, 2013.

Kirkby Shaw K, Rausch-Derra LC, Rhodes L: Grapiprant: an EP4 prostaglandin receptor antagonist and novel therapy for pain and inflammation, *Vet Med Sci* 2:3–9, 2016.

Klaassen CD. *Casarett and Doull's Toxicology: The Basic Science of Poisons, Chapter 5*, ed 9, New York, 2019, McGraw-Hill Education.

Klaassen CD, Aleksunes LM: Xenobiotic, bile acid, and cholesterol transporters: function and regulation, *Pharmacol Rev* 62:1–96, 2010.

Koontz JM, Dancy BCR, Horton CL, et al.: The role of the human microbiome in chemical toxicity, *Int J Toxicol* 38:251–264, 2019.

Koppenol WH, Hider RH: Iron and redox cycling. Do's and don'ts, *Free Radic Biol Med* 133:3–10, 2019.

Kültz D, Li J, Sacchi R, et al.: Alterations in the proteome of the respiratory tract in response to single and multiple exposures to naphthalene, *Proteomics* 15:2655–2668, 2015.

Kumar KK, Karnati S, Reddy MB, et al.: Caco-2 cell lines in drug discovery- an updated perspective, *J Basic Clin Pharm* 1:63–69, 2010.

La Merrill M, Emond C, Kim MJ, et al.: Toxicological function of adipose tissue: focus on persistent organic pollutants, *Environ Health Perspect* 121:162–169, 2013.

Lamas-Paz A, Hao F, Nelson LJ, et al.: Alcoholic liver disease: utility of animal models, *World J Gastroenterol* 24:5063–5075, 2018.

Luciano RL, Perazella MA: Aristolochic acid nephropathy: epidemiology, clinical presentation, and treatment, *Drug Saf* 38:55–64, 2015.

Ma MK, McLeod HL: Lessons learned from the irinotecan metabolic pathway, *Curr Med Chem* 10:41–49, 2003.

Massart F, Harrell JC, Federico G, et al.: Human breast milk and xenoestrogen exposure: a possible impact on human health, *J Perinatol* 25:282–288, 2005.

Medina C, Santos-Martinez MJ, Radomski A, et al.: Nanoparticles: pharmacological and toxicological significance, *Br J Pharmacol* 150:552–558, 2007.

Memon N, Weinberger BI, Hegyi T, et al.: Inherited disorders of bilirubin clearance, *Pediatr Res* 79:378–386, 2016.

Miller AJ, Mihm Jr MC: Melanoma, *N Engl J Med* 355:51–65, 2006.

Moriguchi T, Motohashi H, Hosoya T, et al.: Distinct response to dioxin in an arylhydrocarbon receptor (AHR)-humanized mouse, *Proc Natl Acad Sci U S A* 100:5652–5657, 2003.

Mosedale M, Watkins PB: Understanding idiosyncratic toxicity: lessons learned from drug-induced liver injury, *J Med Chem* 63:6436–6461, 2020.

Mullins ME, Yeager LH, Freeman WE: Metabolic and mitochondrial treatments for severe paracetamol poisoning: a systematic review, *Clin Toxicol*, 2020:1–13, 2020.

Murakami Y, Kawada N: MicroRNAs in hepatic pathophysiology, *Hepatol Res* 47:60–69, 2017.

Nelson DM, Bhaskaran V, Foster WR, et al.: p53-independent induction of rat hepatic Mdm2 following administration of phenobarbital and pregnenolone 16alpha-carbonitrile, *Toxicol Sci* 94:272–280, 2006.

Nelson DR, Zeldin DC, Hoffman SM, et al.: Comparison of cytochrome P450 (CYP) genes from the mouse and human genomes, including nomenclature recommendations for genes, pseudogenes and alternative-splice variants, *Pharmacogenetics* 14:1–18, 2004.

Olivero OA: Relevance of experimental models for investigation of genotoxicity induced by antiretroviral therapy during human pregnancy, *Mutat Res* 658:184–190, 2008.

Orrenius S: Role of cell death in toxicology: does it matter how cells die? *Annu Rev Pharmacol Toxicol* 59:1–14, 2019.

Osman NM, Sexton DW, Saleem IY: Toxicological assessment of nanoparticle interactions with the pulmonary system, *Nanotoxicology* 14:21–58, 2020.

Reed CE, Fenton SE: Exposure to diethylstilbestrol during sensitive life stages: a legacy of heritable health effects, *Birth Defects Res C Embryo Today* 99:134–146, 2013.

Regan SL, Maggs JL, Hammond TG, et al.: Acyl glucuronides: the good, the bad and the ugly, *Biopharm Drug Dispos* 31:367–395, 2010.

Robosky LC, Wells DF, Egnash LA, et al.: Metabonomic identification of two distinct phenotypes in Sprague-Dawley (Crl:CD(SD)) rats, *Toxicol Sci* 87:277–284, 2005.

Rooks MG, Garrett WS: Gut microbiota, metabolites and host immunity, *Nat Rev Immunol* 16:341–352, 2016.

Santulli G: *microRNA: basic science. From molecular biology to clinical practice cham*, Switzerland, 2015, Springer International Publishing.

Schinkel AH, Smit JJ, van Tellingen O, et al.: Disruption of the mouse mdr1a P-glycoprotein gene leads to a deficiency in the blood-brain barrier and to increased sensitivity to drugs, *Cell* 77:491–502, 1994.

Selwyn FP, Cheng SL, Bammler TK, et al.: Developmental regulation of drug-processing genes in livers of germ-free mice, *Toxicol Sci* 147:84–103, 2015.

Sender R, Fuchs S, Milo R: Revised estimates for the number of human and bacteria cells in the body, *PloS Biol* 14:e1002533, 2016.

Shen H, Scialis RJ, Lehman-McKeeman L: Xenobiotic transporters in the kidney: function and role in toxicity, *Semin Nephrol* 39:159–175, 2019.

Simmons SO, Fan CY, Ramabhadran R: Cellular stress response pathway system as a sentinel ensemble in toxicological screening, *Toxicol Sci* 111:202–225, 2009.

Taguchi K, Kensler TW: Nrf2 in liver toxicology, *Arch Pharm Res* 43:337–349, 2020.

Teschke R: Microsomal ethanol-oxidizing system: success over 50 years and an encouraging future, *Alcohol Clin Exp Res* 43:386–400, 2019.

Thakare R, Alamoudi JA, Gautam N, et al.: Species differences in bile acids I. Plasma and urine bile acid composition, *J Appl Toxicol* 38:1323–1335, 2018a.

Thakare R, Alamoudi JA, Gautam N, et al.: Species differences in bile acids II. Bile acid metabolism, *J Appl Toxicol* 38:1336–1352, 2018b.

Tugendreich S, Pearson CI, Sagartz J, et al.: NSAID-induced acute phase response is due to increased intestinal permeability and characterized by early and consistent alterations in hepatic gene expression, *Toxicol Pathol* 34:168–179, 2006.

Upton A, Johnson N, Sandy J, et al.: Arylamine N-acetyltransferases - of mice, men and microorganisms, *Trends Pharmacol Sci* 22:140–146, 2001.

Vétizou M, Pitt JM, Daillère R, et al.: Anticancer immunotherapy by CTLA-4 blockade relies on the gut microbiota, *Science* 350:1079–1084, 2015.

Virkel G, Ballent M, Lanusse C, et al.: Role of ABC transporters in veterinary medicine: pharmaco- toxicological implications, *Curr Med Chem* 26:1251–1269, 2019.

Waalkes MP, Liu J, Diwan BA: Transplacental arsenic carcinogenesis in mice, *Toxicol Appl Pharmacol* 222:271–280, 2007.

Waalkes MP, Liu J, Ward JM, et al.: Enhanced urinary bladder and liver carcinogenesis in male CD1 mice exposed to transplacental inorganic arsenic and postnatal diethylstilbestrol or tamoxifen, *Toxicol Appl Pharmacol* 215:295–305, 2006.

Walker K, Ginsberg G, Hattis D, et al.: Genetic polymorphism in N-acetyltransferase (NAT): population distribution of NAT1 and NAT2 activity, *J Toxicol Environ Health B Crit Rev* 12:440–472, 2009.

Wilson G, Hassan IF, Dix CJ, et al.: Transport and permeability properties of human Caco-2 cells: an in vitro model of the intestinal epithelial cell barrier, *J Contr Release* 11:25–40, 1990.

Wlodarczyk BJ, Palacios AM, George TM, et al.: Antiepileptic drugs and pregnancy outcomes, *Am J Med Genet A* 158a:2071–2090, 2012.

Wynn TA: Cellular and molecular mechanisms of fibrosis, *J Pathol* 214:199–210, 2008.

Xu Y, Ma H, Shao J, et al.: A role for tubular necroptosis in cisplatin-induced AKI, *J Am Soc Nephrol* 26:2647–2658, 2015.

Xue D, Zhou X, Qiu J: Emerging role of NRF2 in ROS-mediated tumor chemoresistance, *Biomed Pharmacother* 131:110676, 2020.

Yamada T, Ohara A, Ozawa N, et al.: Comparison of the hepatic effects of phenobarbital in chimeric mice containing either rat or human hepatocytes with humanized constitutive androstane receptor (CAR) and pregnane X receptor (PXR) mice (hCAR/hPXR mice), *Toxicol Sci* 177(2):362–376, 2020.

Yang K, Köck K, Sedykh A, et al.: An updated review on drug-induced cholestasis: mechanisms and investigation of physicochemical properties and pharmacokinetic parameters, *J Pharmaceut Sci* 102:3037–3057, 2013.

Yokoi T, Nakajima M: microRNAs as mediators of drug toxicity, *Annu Rev Pharmacol Toxicol* 53:377–400, 2013.

Young AM, Allen CE, Audus KL: Efflux transporters of the human placenta, *Adv Drug Deliv Rev* 55:125–132, 2003.

Zhang Y, Limaye PB, Lehman-McKeeman LD, et al.: Dysfunction of organic anion transporting polypeptide 1a1 alters intestinal bacteria and bile acid metabolism in mice, *PloS One* 7:e34522, 2012.

CHAPTER

3

ADME Principles in Small Molecule Drug Discovery and Development: An Industrial Perspective

Ellen Cannady, Kishore Katyayan, Nita Patel

Eli Lilly and Company, Indianapolis, IN, United States

OUTLINE

1. Introduction	51
2. General ADME Principles	52
3. Discovery Overview	54
4. Absorption, Bioavailability, and PK/TK Studies	55
5. Distribution	59
5.1. Volume of Distribution	59
5.2. Protein Binding	59
5.3. Transporter Interactions	59
6. Metabolism	61
6.1. Overview of Phase I and Phase II Metabolism	61
6.2. Overview of Reactive Metabolites	61
6.3. Discovery Metabolism	64
7. Excretion	65

8. Physiologically Based PK modeling	67
9. Development	67
10. Mass Balance Studies	68
11. Tissue Distribution Studies	69
12. Drug Metabolism Studies in Development	71
13. Excretion Studies	71
14. Specialized Excretion Studies	73
15. General Timing of Development ADME Studies	73
16. Conclusions	74
References	74

1. INTRODUCTION

As new medicines are being developed to treat patients, it is important to fully characterize the properties of the new molecular entity (NME) to ensure adequate safety and efficacy. As part of the drug development process, much information is gained about the molecule itself including how the drug is absorbed, distributed, metabolized, and excreted. These "ADME" parameters are evaluated both in vitro and in vivo and are studied in both animal models and humans.

In this chapter, important ADME concepts will be discussed in the context of small molecule drug development, further divided into the discovery phase (defined as the time prior to the

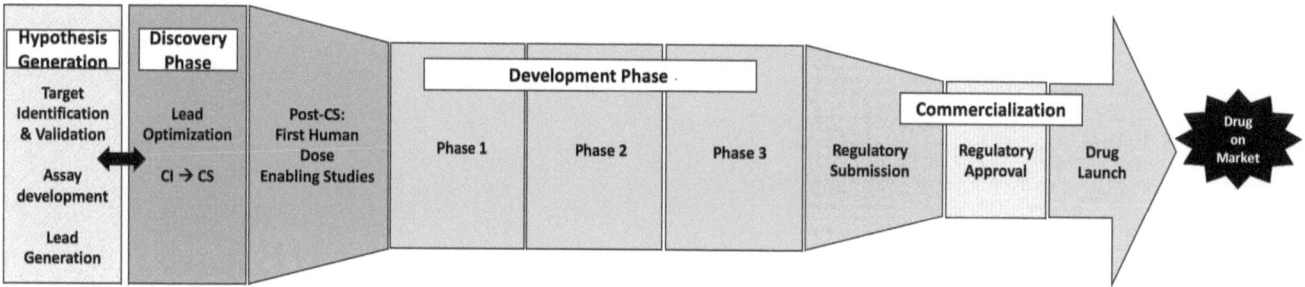

FIGURE 3.1   Drug development paradigm.

conduct of human clinical trials) and the development phase (defined as the time during clinical development, prior to submission and approval of new molecular entities). Prior to these phases, during the early discovery period, much work is done to generate hypotheses, identify, and validate targets, as well as develop a myriad of characterization assays to interrogate compound potency, selectivity, and drug properties in the lead optimization phase. However, this early phase is out of scope for this discussion. The general phases of drug development are depicted in Figure 3.1.

From an ADME-centric view, the goal of the discovery phase is to optimize the structure–activity relationship (SAR) in terms of the balance of pharmacological and toxicological activities. Physical–chemical properties are optimized to support pharmacokinetics (PK)/exposure and metabolism, the presence of reactive intermediate alerts is evaluated, the overall clearance (Cl) pathways are determined at a high level to help predict Cl pathways in humans, and compounds are screened for drug–drug interaction (DDI) risks. At the end of the discovery phase, a single NME is chosen to advance to clinical evaluation in humans. In the development phase, the NME is more fully characterized to support clinical development and ultimately support registration and approval of the new drug by global regulatory agencies. In this chapter, general ADME principles will be reviewed. Additionally, the general types of ADME studies conducted in each of these phases, along with the phase-specific goals of these studies, will also be discussed.

2. GENERAL ADME PRINCIPLES

As previously described, the role of ADME in drug discovery and development is to study the absorption, distribution, metabolism, and excretion of drugs. Both in vitro and in vivo studies are conducted to help guide the early selection of compounds, the appropriate nonclinical toxicology species, and form the basis for clinical studies through dose projections. ADME studies also provide a mechanistic understanding of the link between drug disposition and its effect on pharmacological activity and toxicity.

PK of a molecule describes its plasma concentration versus time profile and can provide a general understanding of its in vivo ADME properties. Two common approaches to understanding the PK of a drug are compartmental analysis and noncompartmental analysis (NCA). Compartmental analysis methods rely on assumptions about interconnected, kinetically homogenous body compartments such as blood and other tissues/organs. This is in comparison to NCA methods, which are less complex, model-independent, and rely almost exclusively on algebraic equations to estimate PK parameters, making this approach an attractive option and the most commonly used approach to determine the exposure of a drug in nonclinical studies. The following list represents some of the most common PK parameters derived from NCA profiles: area under the curve (AUC), maximum plasma concentration (C_{max}), the time at which the maximum plasma concentration occurs (T_{max}), elimination rate constant (k), elimination half-life ($t_{1/2}$), volume of distribution (Vd), Cl, and oral bioavailability (%F). Furthermore, these PK parameters can be affected by various factors. For example, age, gender, pregnancy status, genetics, and nutritional state (e.g., fed vs. fasted) are physiological factors that alter the PK of a drug. Different disease states may also affect the PK of a drug, such as hepatic disease, renal impairment, or diseases that cause inflammation to name a few (Koup, 1989; Morgan, 2009).

PK studies are the most useful when the pharmacological/toxicological response is closely related to the drug concentration in the central compartment. As the plasma drug concentration increases, drug levels will correlate with a subtherapeutic range, the optimal range where the benefits of the drug outweigh the risks/side effects, and eventually reach the toxic range where drug concentrations result in toxicity. Ideally, a drug should have a wide efficacious range in which there is large separation between plasma concentrations that are subtherapeutic and those that cause toxicity. Drugs that exhibit a small degree of separation between subtherapeutic and toxic plasma concentrations have a narrow therapeutic range. These concepts are depicted in Figure 3.2.

From a relatively simple nonclinical in vivo study, discussed in more detail in the sections below, a substantial amount of PK information can be determined for a single molecule. Following a single oral (PO) and intravenous (IV) dose, in which blood samples are typically taken over the course of 24 h after dosing (postdose), a semilog plot of drug concentration versus time can be generated. Multiple PK parameters are derived from this curve including the AUC, C_{max} (for PO administration), and the concentration at time zero (for IV administration). The elimination rate, k, can be calculated from the slope of the log plot, which in turn can be used to calculate the $t_{1/2}$ (= 0.693/k). The $t_{1/2}$ is the amount of time it takes

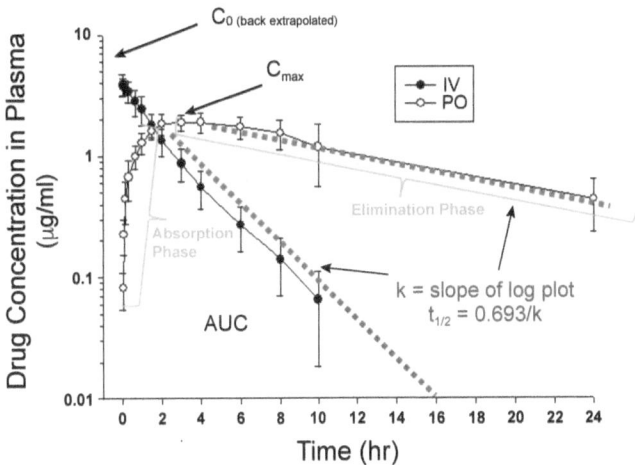

FIGURE 3.3 Derivation of PK parameters from concentration–time profiles after oral or IV dose administration.

for one half of the drug amount to be cleared from the blood or plasma. In general, the assumption is made that it takes five half-lives for compound concentration to either achieve steady state or to be largely eliminated (e.g., 96.875% of the dose) from the body. In Figure 3.3, from a simple in vivo study design where a single PO dose and a single IV dose were administered, followed by extensive postdose blood sampling in which drug concentrations were determined, a lot of insight about the PK properties of a molecule can be gained.

Bioavailability and first-pass metabolism are also important concepts. First-pass metabolism is defined as the loss of drug between the site of administration and systemic circulation on passing through tissues where elimination occurs. Thus, for PO administration, after the drug is absorbed through the intestinal lumen, a portion of the drug can be lost to metabolism by enzymes in the gut wall and the liver, before the remainder of the drug is ultimately delivered to the systemic circulation. The overall PO bioavailability is the percent of drug that successfully enters the systemic circulation and is compared to the IV exposure, since drug is administered directly into the systemic circulation. The overall bioavailability reflects the fraction of drug absorbed through the intestinal lumen, the fraction of drug that is delivered to the portal system, and the fraction of drug that successfully passes through the liver. This process is represented in Figure 3.4.

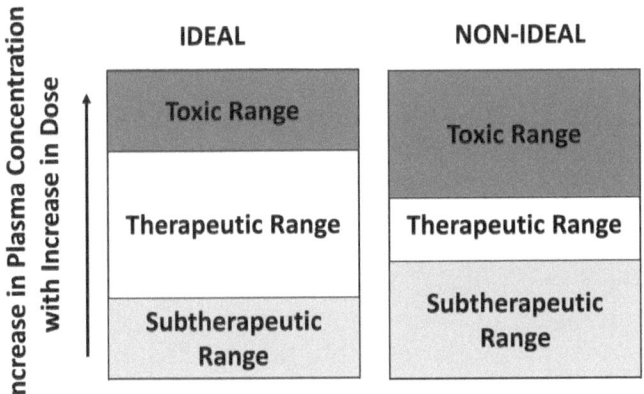

FIGURE 3.2 Comparison of wide versus narrow therapeutic range.

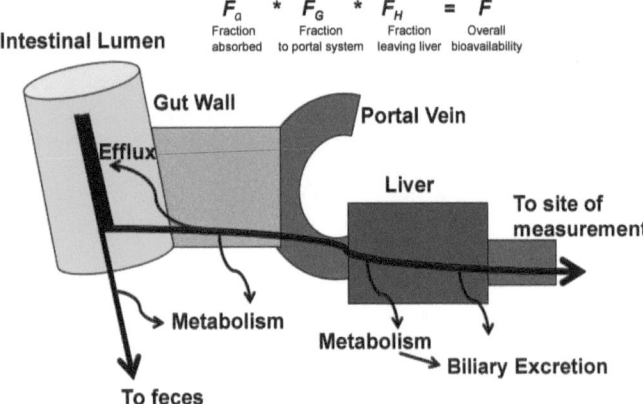

FIGURE 3.4 Drug disposition after oral administration.

These concepts will be discussed in more detail throughout this chapter. Relevant study designs for several types of ADME studies will also be discussed.

3. DISCOVERY OVERVIEW

The goal of the discovery phase of drug development is to identify a series of compounds with pharmacological activity for a given target, characterize these molecules in a myriad of studies across multiple disciplines, and to ultimately decide on the single, best compound to advance into human clinical trials with the most optimal benefit:risk profile based on available data at a particular instance in time. As this can be a daunting task, narrowing the selection from different scaffolds of potentially 1000s of compounds to the ultimate candidate molecule, pharmaceutical companies have created benchmarks using in silico, in vitro, and in vivo databases for decision-making. While the nomenclature may differ across the industry, the general principles are the same. For the sake of discussion within, Candidate Identification (CI) is referred to as the identification of a compound possessing pharmacological activity with optimal drug-like properties to advance to pilot toxicological evaluations and Candidate Selection (CS) is referred to as the ultimate compound chosen to advance to human clinical trials, having demonstrated an acceptable toxicology profile in animals.

ADME properties are thoroughly characterized in compounds that are targeted toward CI or CS using both in vitro and in vivo study data. One of the end goals is to use the available data to translate and predict how the compound is likely to behave in humans while optimizing compounds for demonstration of pharmacology or evaluating toxicology with adequate exposures. Early in discovery, compounds may not advance toward CS due to multiple reasons, including but not limited to the following: lack of potency or lack of selectivity to a given target, inadequate exposure, cardiac toxicity or general toxicity associated with the target itself or with binding to other sites within the body, liabilities such as potential DDI risks by which more than one drug are competing for the same metabolizing enzymes and transporters involved in its clearance, high variability in the ADME parameters and plasma/tissue concentrations, lack of dose response, or an inability to reach target tissues (e.g., brain). Therefore, it is not surprising that there is high and rapid attrition of compounds during this early phase of development. For these reasons, early PK studies in rodents, in conjunction with physicochemical properties, in silico predictions, and in vitro data may be designed to provide a quick answer regarding performance. Multiple CIs may be declared as development teams are unsure of the toxicological outcomes in large animal species or in longer duration rodent toxicology studies, particularly with novel scaffolds that have previously not been studied. After CI, ADME data are collected to more fully characterize the drug to determine whether it is ready for human testing and set the stage for development planning. Thorough in vitro evaluations and PK studies with adequate number of animals, full time course of sampling, and cross-over study designs for such compounds are needed to evaluate clinical candidates.

In recent years, emphasis has also been placed on mechanistic and quantitative understanding of disposition and Cl pathways as they relate to excretion and metabolism/transporter involvement to inform human PK predictions. The data used to understand human ADME properties importantly feed into human PK predictions with uncertainties based on mechanistic understanding of clearance, volume, and absorption properties to inform clinical development. Preclinical evaluations use a combination of physicochemical properties, in vitro, and in vivo metabolism data, as well as PK and excretion data collected in various animal species. Often, scaling methods for metabolic Cl and Vd that are based on in vitro to in vivo extrapolations (IVIVEs) in animals are evaluated to provide confidence for human predicted parameters. In addition, in vivo performance in animals is used as a predictor of that in human to predict extent of renal and biliary excretion. Depending on the properties and performance of the CI molecule, definitive studies to characterize the PK properties of a molecule may include, but are not limited to, bioavailability with the final salt/formulation, dose linearity, and excretion studies in intact and/or bile cannulated animals. Considerations for various in vivo studies include routes of administration: bolus versus infusions, length of infusions to reduce distress to animals, sampling techniques such as dried blood spot (DBS) versus plasma, excreta collection and biomarkers, and tissue distribution into organs of interest (Diehl et al., 2001).

4. ABSORPTION, BIOAVAILABILITY, AND PK/TK STUDIES

Early studies in rodents and nonrodents are utilized to understand the PO versus IV exposures (bioavailability), as well as to derive the previously described PK parameters in order to characterize the overall PK profile of the NME. The rate of absorption and bioavailability is compared across multiple species. The profiles are studied at both lower dose levels in the pharmacological range, as well as at higher dose levels to support the toxicology studies, which are generally designed to maximize compound exposure. Study design considerations are discussed below.

When designing nonclinical PK studies, doses should be low to avoid saturation of Cl pathways if possible, but high enough for drug concentrations to be detected in bioanalytical assays with typical sensitivity. It is good practice to ensure similar conditions for the PO and IV dose to ensure similar conditions for the ADME processes driving exposure in each case. For

example, if the bioavailability is expected to be approximately 30%, the PO dose should be about threefold higher than the IV dose. If the bioavailability is expected to be close to 100%, then the same PO and IV dose should be used. Typical doses for bioavailability studies are 1 mg/kg IV infusion (administered via tail vein in rodents and femoral vein in larger nonclinical species) and 3 mg/kg, PO (administered via oral gavage). Plasma or blood samples are serially collected for long enough to recover most of the area under the concentration–time curve. To facilitate accurate determination of $t_{1/2}$, and hence most other PK parameters, a trough concentration should be targeted that represents approximately two–three half-lives. Additionally, the use of at least four animals in each "arm" of the study allows for evaluation of outliers and characterization of interanimal variability. Cross-over studies with serial blood collections after PO and IV dosing are typically used, and where blood volumes are prohibitive in mice, microbleeding techniques coupled with DBS bioanalysis have been successfully developed and applied (Patel et al., 2016; Wickremsinhe et al., 2016). These methods have also been successfully employed in toxicology studies with no substantial impact on animal health. In fact, microbleeding techniques are sometimes preferred because the toxicokinetic (TK) analysis can be done in the same animals as those on study and are not in a separate "satellite" group of animals. Therefore, the relationship between exposure and effect can be assessed in an individual animal.

IV administration via infusion, rather than a bolus injection, tends to give better estimates of Vd and Cl particularly when the initial distribution phase is very fast and/or when the $t_{1/2}$ is short. Infusions can be short (e.g., few minutes) and do not need to reach steady state. Each has advantages and disadvantages, and several issues need to be considered as described in Table 3.1.

IV dosing can be performed in fed or fasted states, unless the compound has a high extraction ratio in the liver, defined as the proportion of drug "extracted" from the blood or plasma via hepatic clearance as it passes through the liver. In this case, the increase in liver blood flow in the fed state can cause an increase in the extraction ratio. Using formulations that cause irritation or pain should be avoided. The IV

TABLE 3.1   Advantages and Disadvantages of Intravenous Bolus Versus Infusion Administration

Route	Advantages	Disadvantages
Bolus	• Can be done without cannulation/ catheterization, therefore practical for smaller animal models (mice) • Does not require special equipment	• May not capture rapidly falling plasma concentrations • Dosing errors more likely to occur, such as with tail vein administration in small animal models • Can lead to toxicity due to high initial concentrations
Infusion	• Useful particularly for compounds with rapid distribution in which plasma concentrations decline quickly after a bolus and/ or have a short $t_{1/2}$ • Avoids very high initial plasma concentrations	• Concerns about catheter misplacement and potential dosing errors • Requires special equipment, such as infusion lines and pumps • Not practical for smaller animal models such as mice

formulation is preferably delivered as a solution and should have the correct isotonicity and -pH. If high nonspecific binding is expected, one should test if the compound will bind to the tubing or the syringe and consider dose formulation bioanalysis to correct for the actual dose administered. For important CI/CS studies, it is highly recommended that dose formulation bioanalysis is utilized for the IV solutions in order to assure accurate calculations of PK parameters.

PO doses can be administered as solutions or suspensions while avoiding formulations that cause irritation or pain. Solutions are homogenous mixtures in which the particle size is adequately small such that the substance is completely dissolved in the matrix. This makes solutions ideal for dosing. While the particle size in suspensions is larger than those found in solutions and will thus eventually settle, the substance can still be evenly distributed by mechanical means such as mixing, also making suspensions amenable to PO dosing. Parenteral (nonoral) routes of administration tend to be more restrictive as a good understanding of compatibility with site of administration (e.g., subcutaneous) or solubility considerations with IV administration can restrict dose volumes. General dose volume recommendations for exposure studies as well as generally accepted and maximum volumes that can be utilized for each species with various routes of administration in exposure studies are listed in Table 3.2 (Hull, 1995). These guidelines may differ depending on the specific laboratory conducting the study. It is recommended that these volumes should be modified based on limitations of the final formulation chosen (Smith, 1999). For example, while PO dose volumes listed in the table below are considered relevant for aqueous formulations, the drug amount may be limited when using solid dispersions or lipid-based formulations. With such approaches, it is important to consider the compatibility of the formulation, the load of excipients that fit into capsules, and the number of capsules that is practical for species selected.

PK studies using subcutaneous, topical, or inhalation routes are perhaps less frequently conducted as these intended routes of administration are less common than PO routes of administration, particularly for small molecule drug development. Nevertheless, study design considerations are worthy of discussion. For example, for topical/dermal administration, consideration of skin physiology in animals relative to humans is important for translation of PK to human; minipigs may be the best model for skin absorption (Bode et al., 2010). The rate of absorption from subcutaneous administration may be slower than with other parenteral routes. Subcutaneous infusions can be administered with the use of an oily depot or osmotic mini pumps. Topically applying dosing material to skin that is unbroken and free of hair and avoiding application to sites that animals can reach during grooming is recommended. Transdermal dosing is typically accomplished by application of a patch impregnated with the drug of interest. The patch is applied in such a way as to avoid inadvertent ingestion or removal by the animal.

TABLE 3.2   General Dose Volume (mL/kg) Recommendations for Exposure Studies

Species	Recommended oral capsule number (Capsule volume)	Best practice (Maximum possible for repeat dosing)[a] PO Dose volume	Best practice (Maximum possible for repeat dosing)[a] SC Dose volume	Best practice IV Dose volume
Mouse	NA	10 (20)	10 (40)	5
Rat	NA	10 (20)	5 (10)	5
Rabbit	NA	10 (10)	1 (2)	2
Dog	≤3 (10 mL)[c]	5 (10[d])	1 (2)	2.5
Minipig	NA	5 (10)	1 (2)	2.5
Monkey[b]	1 (0.37 mL)	5 (10)	2 (5)	2

[a] *Must pay particular attention to the characteristics of the substance administered if large dose volumes are used.*
[b] *Gavage dosing in monkeys is typically performed via the nasogastric route of administration. Capsule dosing in monkey is possible using a #2 capsule (0.37 mL), which is inserted into the end of an oral gavage tube. The inserted tube is flushed with water to expel the capsule. Experience with repeat dosing in monkeys using a capsule as well as dosing multiple capsules is limited.*
[c] *Gavage is preferred primarily due to the fact that it is much easier for dosing compared to making capsules. Size 11 capsules are used on a case-by-case basis based on scientific rationale (e.g., solid dispersion or an acidic vehicle intended to minimize esophageal exposure to the formulation). Typically use 1–2 capsules and utilize large dogs for studies requiring three capsules.*
[d] *Dose volume of 5 mL/kg is preferred as anecdotally it may decrease emesis, although if the test article is the cause (due to local effects), with the higher concentration it may actually make it worse. A dose volume of 10 mL/kg is acceptable for a dog and this dose volume may be used based on scientific rationale (e.g., need additional volume to make the formulation amenable for dosing).*
NA = not applicable.
From Diehl K-H, Hull R, Morton D, et al: A good practice guide to the administration of substances and removal of blood, including routes and volumes, J Applied Toxicol 21:15–23, 2001; Hull RM: Guideline limit volumes for dosing animals in the preclinical stage of safety evaluation, Human Exp Toxicol 14:305–307, 1995; Smith D: Dosing limit volumes: a European view, Humane Society of the United States Refinement Workshop, New Orleans, 1999.

As compounds advance toward CI, toxicology assessment at high doses necessitates an understanding of dose–exposure relationships. These are in turn used to inform the design of future rodent and nonrodent toxicology studies. Ideally, exposure (AUC and/or C_{max}) should increase in a linear manner with an increase in dose. However, limitations in absorption and potential saturation of Cl may result in lack of dose proportionality in exposure. Examples of dose-proportional, dose-limited, and superproportional increases in exposure are depicted in Figure 3.5.

In addition to dose response, evaluation of the TK allows further understanding of species and sex differences in exposure, as well as the effect of repeated and multiple dosing. Comparing exposures following single and multiple doses gives insight into the extent of accumulation, as well as possible enzyme autoinduction. Autoinduction, where the drug itself increases the

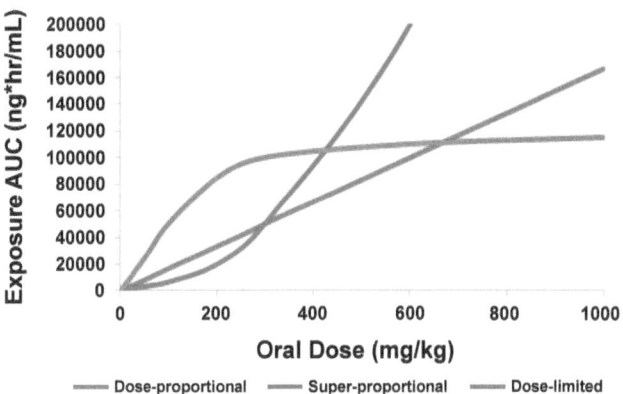

FIGURE 3.5   Illustration of dose-proportional, super-proportional, and dose-limited exposure relationships in toxicology studies.

abundance or activity of the enzymes/metabolic pathways necessary for its own clearance, can have significant impact on multiple dose exposures and jeopardize the evaluation of the

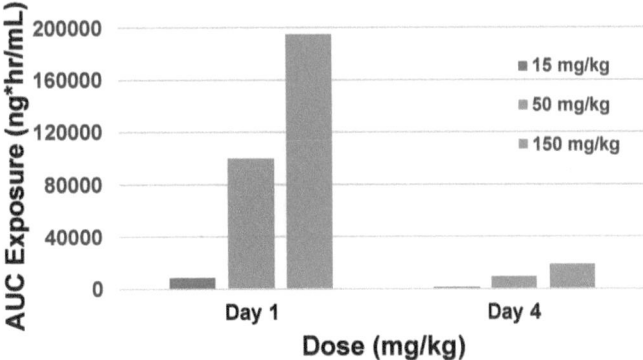

FIGURE 3.6 Reduction in exposure due to auto-induction of unknown metabolic pathways in rats following 4 days of repeat, daily dosing of an NME.

toxicity profile of a compound. In the example depicted in Figure 3.6, following a single dose of 15, 50, or 150 mg/kg in rats, the AUC exposures increase with an increase in dose, as expected. However, after only 4 days of daily dosing, the exposures at each dose level are substantially reduced such that it is impossible to achieve exposures high enough to adequately assess the toxicity profile of the NME. Since autoinduction can be profound, understanding the effects as early as possible in drug discovery is beneficial and may result in the need for a different NME devoid of this liability to be evaluated. Ultimately, the exposure data obtained from the toxicology studies are utilized to determine the margin of safety, which compares the animal exposure data with predicted or observed human exposure data.

Occasionally, the delivery of compound to the systemic circulation for toxicology studies is challenging, due to considerable dose exposure subproportionality in the absence of target organ toxicity. If the limitation in absorption is due to poor permeability, options for enhancing exposures are limited. However, if dissolution rate limited absorption is driving the poor exposure, strategies for overcoming dose-limited absorption such as twice-daily dosing or investigation of methods for enhancing exposures through salt selection or formulation optimization are considered. The dose formulation, as well as the active pharmaceutical ingredient, is often not optimized and fully characterized in early discovery PK studies. Consequently, free bases and carboxylic acids are often administered in

their native state, as an *in situ* salt or as a simple salt form. Prior to CI, salt screening is performed to identify form(s) with optimized solubility that meet criteria for GLP toxicology studies, as well as first-in-man studies, as the NME advances through development. It is not uncommon for the dose form of an NME to evolve from free base to an in situ salt to a salt that is close to the form of the drug that will ultimately be commercially available. In this case, bridging studies to assess the impact of formulation and any formulation changes will be conducted to evaluate their effect on drug exposure. For example, PK studies with salt forms of a drug are necessary to understand the impact of salt form on exposure. In early discovery, formulations used for PO dosing are often standard suspensions. The selection of alternative formulations may be informed by the physicochemical properties of the NME and routine PK studies with standard vehicles. As optimization of both the dose form and formulation occurs to ultimately support the more stringent and regulatory acceptable "good laboratory practice" toxicology studies in development, it may be necessary to conduct bridging studies to compare the PK/TK using prior formulations. The bridging study is conducted in the appropriate species at a dose level relevant to the subsequent study between "arms" that include the prior and subsequent salt form/formulation. The bridging study may be conducted in a parallel or cross-over design with due consideration to adequate washout between study arms. If multiple formulations need to be assessed, a Latin square study design can be utilized to control the variation from different formulations and different experimental runs. If three formulations are tested, with adequate washout periods between runs, each animal receives a different formulation in run one and then rotates to a different formulation in run two, and another rotation in run three.

Finally, in the lead up to CS, PK/TK studies and in silico simulations using commercial software such as Simcyp or GastroPlus can be used to optimize preclinical dose formulations and to model preclinical to clinical translation of absorption. While not the focus of this chapter, these can be powerful tools for predicting the absorption behavior of NMEs in humans.

5. DISTRIBUTION

5.1. Volume of Distribution

The distribution of a compound once introduced in the plasma compartment is important to understand as it contributes to the PK profile and movement of the drug entity across cell membranes and into various tissues and ultimately to the target of interest. The distribution of free drug into tissues depends on membrane permeability by passive diffusion and active transport via membrane transporters present at blood–organ or organ–excretion interfaces. Drug properties such as its lipophilicity (determined by LogP and ionization pKa) that drive cell membrane permeability, along with binding to plasma proteins, dictate how the entity moves from the plasma compartment into various tissues.

The volume of distribution, Vd, is a hypothetical volume that describes the extent of distribution in the body. The Vd seldom represents the true volume of a body compartment. One exception is for drugs that do not widely distribute into tissues (e.g., drugs that are very highly protein bound or hydrophilic). These drugs may exhibit a Vd that is roughly equivalent to the plasma volume. If the Vd is high, the drug can be assumed to be distributed extensively to either a single or multiple tissues.

Physicochemical parameters such as LogP and pKa influence passive permeability across membranes. The higher the lipophilicity (LogP), the greater the partitioning across cell membranes. In addition, for weak acids and bases, the ionization of the compound can influence its ability to partition across the membrane. For example, if the pKa of a weak acid is higher than the pH of the environment, it will predominate as a neutral species and will readily partition across cell membranes. Similarly, if the pKa of a weak base is lower than the pH of its environment, it will predominate as a readily permeable neutral species.

5.2. Protein Binding

The free drug hypothesis states that the free drug concentration at the site of action is the basis of biological activity, such as in vivo efficacy and toxicity. It is also the free drug that moves across membranes and is cleared from the body. Therefore, understanding the protein binding of NMEs is important. Protein binding is usually determined using either ultrafiltration or equilibrium dialysis methods at single concentrations that are incubated with plasma from preclinical species (e.g., mouse, rat, dog, and monkey) and human. The fraction unbound (fu) is determined using sensitive bioanalytical methods such as liquid chromatography–mass spectrometry (LC/MS) in the plasma free compartment. In addition to overall plasma protein binding, it can also be useful to understand the extent of binding to alpha acid glycoprotein (AAG) and human serum albumin, and any concentration dependence of this binding. These are the main plasma binding proteins and they can be saturated, particularly AAG, and may be altered in disease states (e.g., cancer and autoimmune diseases). Different populations such as the very young or pregnant women may also have different concentrations of these proteins and, therefore, may exhibit different binding and PK characteristics for drugs bound to these proteins.

The extent of protein binding across species is used in the translation of animal PK to humans. For instance, some methods for scaling PK parameters such as Vd (Oie and Tozer, 1979) and Cl (Tang and Mayersohn, 2005) from animal to human require consideration of interspecies differences in unbound fraction. The fu is also taken into consideration for projecting the dose that might be efficacious in human based on preclinical data, as well as to assess DDI risks in humans. However, margin of safety calculations typically do not take the fu into account, although whether or not it is appropriate to do so for certain circumstances is often the topic of debate.

5.3. Transporter Interactions

Transporters are proteins that are present in cell membranes and translocate substances across the membrane, in one or both directions. Transporters can play important roles in drug disposition. Not only may they be drug targets themselves, but they may help deliver drugs to a certain site of action. Transporters also have important roles in the absorption, distribution, and clearance of drugs, which can sometimes result in important DDI. Therefore, it is necessary to understand the interaction of an NME with various well-characterized transporters in order to estimate the likely amount of free drug at the site of action and to evaluate the mechanisms involved in Cl and excretion of drug entities. The brain and liver are often target organs of interest for neurological disorders or metabolic diseases, respectively, and the gut, liver, and kidneys are typically involved in the excretion of free drug from the system. These organs are known to express transport proteins such as P-glycoprotein (P-gp), Organic Anion Transporting Polypeptide (OATP), Organic Cation Transporters (OCTs), Multidrug Resistance-associated Protein (MRP), and others that are involved in uptake or efflux of free drug in these tissues (Figure 3.7).

In early discovery, both in vitro and in vivo evaluations are used to determine the role of transporters. In in vitro studies, cell lines (e.g., MDCK, HEPG, or hepatocytes) expressing the transport proteins of interest are incubated with compound to determine flux in the presence and absence of known inhibitors (e.g., digoxin for P-gp), and compound concentrations are measured across two compartments separated by a monolayer of the relevant cells. An in vitro mechanistic MDCK/P-gp study could also be performed to characterize membrane permeability, cell partitioning (% in cell), and potential efflux by P-gp. In vivo assessments are generally conducted to understand the impact of the in vitro results. Organ partitioning or transporter knock-out (KO) and knock-in (KI) studies in rodents are typically conducted in early to mid-stage discovery for structure–activity relationship with organ partitioning. To assess organ partitioning in vivo, mice could be administered an IV bolus dose of compound, with terminal collection of brain and plasma samples used to calculate brain partitioning values (also referred to as Kp,uu values) by dividing unbound brain concentration by unbound plasma concentration. Additional tissues such as heart, fat, brain, lung, kidney, liver, muscle, pancreas, spleen, and whole blood can also be collected to assess Kp,uu depending on the target organ of interest. Spleen or pancreas collection is often used as a control tissue since these organs are well perfused and have relatively low expression levels of known drug transporters; for these tissues, Kp,uu values are usually close to 1. The dose and collection time point(s) of the study should be diligently chosen in order to support the assumption of equilibrium between tissue and plasma while maintaining bioanalytical robustness. Additional insights on the role of transporters in determining the PK of drugs can be obtained by using sophisticated

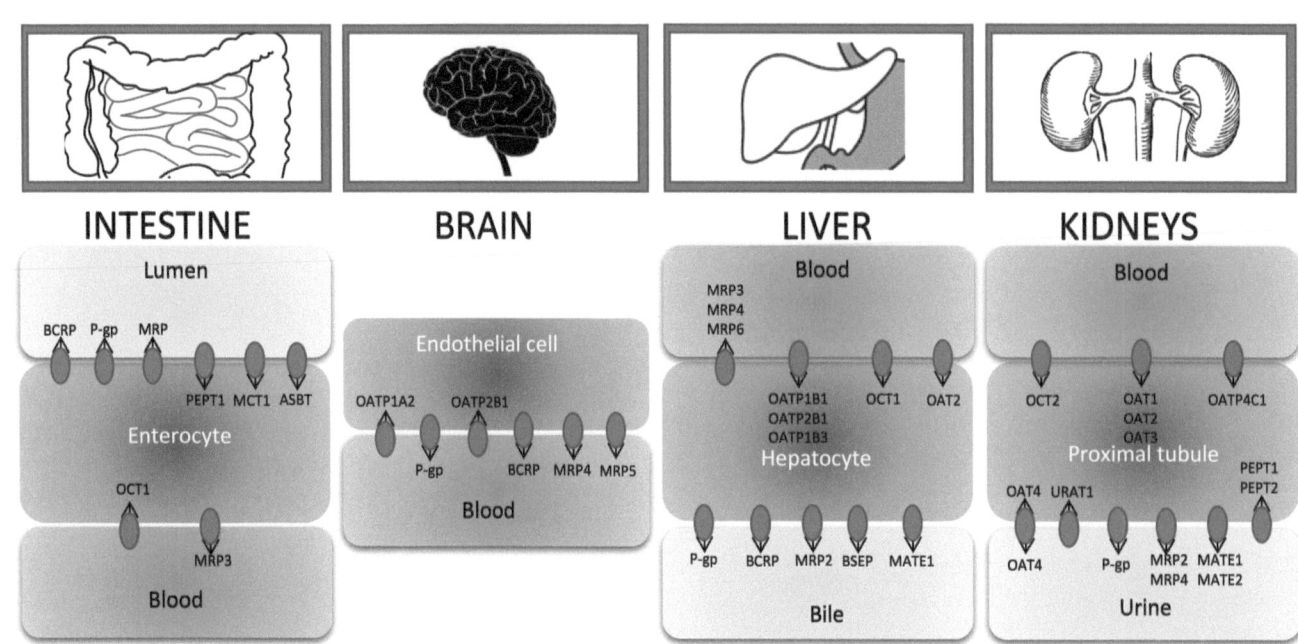

FIGURE 3.7　Representative transporters involved in uptake or efflux of free drug in organs of interest.

transporter KO and KI models. Validated models are commercially available for the following transporters: Mdr1a(/1b) KO rat, Bcrp KO rat, MRP2 KO rat, OATP1a/1b KO mouse, OATP1B1 and OATP1B3 KI mouse, OCT1/2 KO mouse, Mdr1a KO mouse, Mdr1a/1b KO mouse, Bcrp KO mouse, TKO (Mdr1a/1b/Bcrp) KO mouse, Mdr1a/Bcrp KO rat, OCT1 KO rat, OCT2 KO rat, Oat1 KO rat, and Oat3 KO rat. These models can be used for qualitative assessment of the role of transporters in a compound's disposition, along with in vitro transporter data. Work is ongoing to use such assays in a more quantitative sense for translation of transporter effects to human (Morse et al., 2020).

6. METABOLISM

It is important to understand the key metabolic pathways in the Cl of an NME, as well as the enzymes responsible for its metabolism. Modification of these pathways via inhibition or induction (referred to as drug–drug interactions, DDI), or even genetic or environmental factors, can lead to significant differences in drug clearance (Gonzalez et al., 2018). Evaluation of DDIs is focused on understanding human DDI liability, and animal studies are rarely employed. Therefore, this topic is out of scope for this discussion. Nonetheless, understanding the proper context of metabolism in nonclinical species is important in the pharmaceutical setting. Metabolites identified, both qualitatively and quantitatively depending on the stage of development, give insight to the formation of potential human metabolites. Additionally, any metabolic liabilities, such as clues in the molecular structure that could result in potential toxicity, can be identified. A high-level overview of drug metabolism, as well as special considerations for reactive metabolites, will be discussed.

6.1. Overview of Phase I and Phase II Metabolism

Since key goals of small molecule drug development are directed toward good oral absorption and distribution to the site of action through high membrane permeability, most

drugs tend to be lipophilic. Lipophilicity also hinders elimination from the body via biliary and renal pathways. Therefore, most drugs are metabolized to more hydrophilic, or water soluble, entities before elimination from the body occurs. In general, drug metabolizing reactions are divided into two groups: "Phase I" and "Phase II" reactions. Phase I metabolism usually involves oxidation, reduction, and hydrolytic reactions that introduce a polar chemical moiety either by inserting new polar functional groups or unmasking existing functional groups (-OH, -NH2, -SH, COOH). This type of metabolism increases hydrophilicity. Phase II metabolism includes glucuronidation, sulfation, acetylation, glutathione (GSH) conjugation, and conjugation with amino acids. This type of metabolism usually significantly increases hydrophilicity. Phase I reactions are mediated by enzymes such as the cytochrome P450 enzymes (CYPs), flavin monooxygenases, aldehyde oxidases, esterases, and amidases. In humans, the CYP enzymes are the most important enzymes responsible for the metabolism of drugs. The contribution of various Phase I and Phase II reactions responsible in human drug metabolism is depicted in Figure 3.8 (Evans and Relling, 1999).

6.2. Overview of Reactive Metabolites

One of the major concerns of drug safety involves formation of reactive metabolites via metabolism. Idiosyncratic adverse drug reactions (IADRs), including drug-induced liver injury, are a prominent reason for cessation of drug testing in clinical trials, restrictions on use, and the withdrawal of approved drugs (Park et al., 2011; Stepan et al., 2011). One of the many theories for the cause of IADR is the reactive metabolite hypothesis, which proposes that chemically reactive metabolites of drugs can mediate the formation of protein adducts or DNA mutations leading to organ toxicity and/or carcinogenesis. Drug bioactivation is proposed to be the critical step in the process which leads to a reactive metabolite (electrophile) that can bind to cellular macromolecules and potentially lead to IADR. Currently, only circumstantial evidence links reactive metabolites to IADR, and studies in

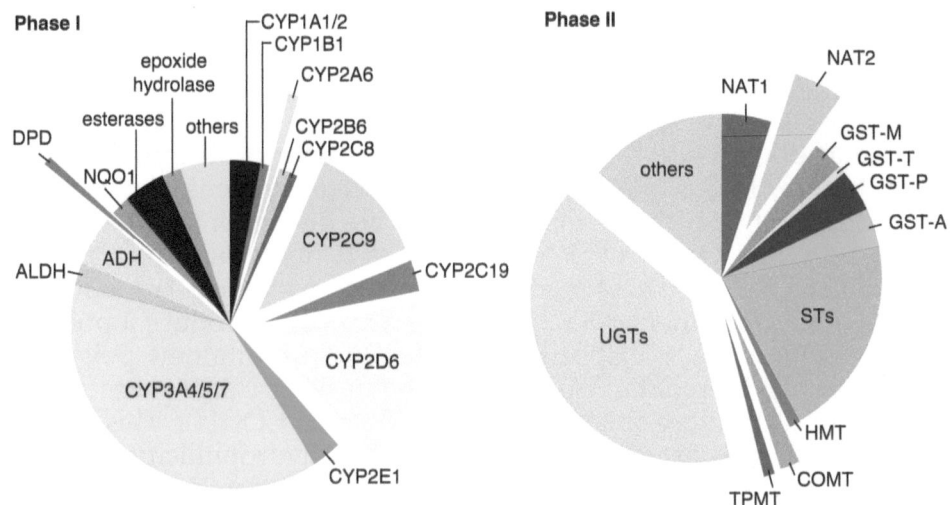

FIGURE 3.8   Phase I and Phase II enzymes involved in drug metabolism. Size of pie piece indicates contribution of enzymes responsible for drug metabolism. Pie piece separated from chart indicates polymorphic enzymes. *Figure 2 from Evans WE, Relling MV: Pharmacogenomics: translating functional genomics into rational therapeutics,* Science *286(5439):487–491, 1999.*

the literature are mostly retrospective and anecdotal (Boelsterli, 2003; LiverTox, 2020; Madyastha and Moorthy, 1989). Regardless, IADR remains a significant safety concern since they often occur at low rates and may be undetectable in early-phase clinical trials, only coming to light once a drug has progressed far into the development process or after the drug is approved and is on the market. Furthermore, they are frequently not foreseen through traditional in vitro or animal safety testing paradigms. Since a priori prediction of IADR is not currently achievable, using a strategy of hazard identification with avoidance of drug candidate molecules that form reactive metabolites or minimization of exposure to a reactive metabolite is recommended (Kalgutkar, 2011).

Reactive metabolites are often short lived and, thus, are not usually detectable in circulating blood/plasma. In vitro approaches are generally employed to examine the bioactivation potential of drug candidates, which may provide some indirect but valuable information for the prediction of potential toxicity. A variety of techniques are available to assess reactive metabolite formation: (1) trapping and characterizing reactive metabolites, (2) evaluation of covalent binding to proteins, and (3) time- and cofactor-dependent CYP450 inhibition. Among these, chemical trapping with GSH is the most widely used in the characterization of reactive

metabolites that form stable adducts. GSH contains a free sulfhydryl group, a soft nucleophile capable of reacting with a broad range of reactive electrophiles, including Michael acceptors, epoxides, arene oxides, nitrenium ions, and alkyl halides. GSH is present virtually in all mammalian tissues and, therefore, serves as a natural scavenger for chemically reactive metabolites. There are several other trapping agents that are used for trapping hard nucleophiles such as cyanide anion for iminium species (Argoti et al., 2005), semicarbazide and methoxylamine for aldehydes (Chauret et al., 1995; Zhang et al., 1996), and dimedone for sulfenic acid intermediates (Dansette et al., 2009). GSH trapping is often conducted in liver microsomes in the presence of NADPH and GSH. The formed GSH adducts are then characterized by LC with tandem MS and/or nuclear magnetic resonance (NMR) spectroscopy (Evans et al., 2004). Observation of a GSH adduct in vitro (in the trapping assay and/or hepatocytes) or in vivo (in preclinical studies) can be interpreted as the potential of a compound to form a reactive metabolite. However, one limitation to the in vitro trapping assay is that it is typically conducted in liver microsomes, and competing non-CYP metabolic or Cl pathways are absent. Therefore, it is important to investigate the metabolism of the compound in a more complete hepatic system (e.g., hepatocytes), as well as to evaluate the metabolism in vivo, in order to put the results of the trapping experiment into perspective. As an example, paroxetine forms GSH adducts and covalently binds to liver microsomes; however, in vivo the quinone metabolites are detoxified via glucuronidation and O-methylation (Haddock et al., 1989).

A number of drugs containing a carboxylic acid moiety have been associated with liver injuries or other related adverse effects and have been either withdrawn from the market or have so-called "black box warnings" on their Food and Drug Administration labels. The toxicity of these drugs, many of which are nonsteroidal antiinflammatory drugs, has been associated with their formation of an acyl glucuronide from the "parent" drug molecule. Glucuronidation is one of the most important pathways of conjugation reactions and is generally considered a detoxification process. In contrast to this traditional view, acyl glucuronide conjugates, formed by esterification of a carboxylic acid moiety on a drug or metabolite with glucuronic acid, have now been recognized as reactive electrophiles (Bailey and Dickinson, 2003; Spahn-Langguth and Benet, 1992). The covalent binding of acyl glucuronides to proteins may occur via two different mechanisms (Figure 3.9). The first is a transacylation mechanism, where a nucleophilic group (–NH2, –OH, or –SH) on a protein attacks the carbonyl group of the acyl glucuronide ester bond, leading to the formation of an acylated protein. The second mechanism of covalent binding to proteins is through glycation. This involves an initial acyl migration followed by a transitional ring opening to form an aldehyde, which can then form a Schiff base with the amino group of a protein. The Schiff base formed from 3- and 4-isomers may further undergo Amadori rearrangement to a more stable 1-amino-2-keto product. Both mechanisms, depicted in Figure 3.9, have been observed and both appear to be important in terms of toxicological consequences arising from acyl glucuronides (Castillo et al., 1995; Ruelius et al., 1986; Sallustio et al., 2000; Shipkova et al., 2003). It has been demonstrated that a correlation exists between the degradation rate of acyl glucuronides and their extent of covalent binding to human albumin in vitro and in vivo (Benet et al., 1993). Furthermore, Sawamura et al. (2010) showed that stability of an acyl glucuronide in phosphate buffer can be used for categorizing drugs as similar or dissimilar to withdraw carboxylic acid drugs. Therefore, stability of an acyl glucuronide in phosphate

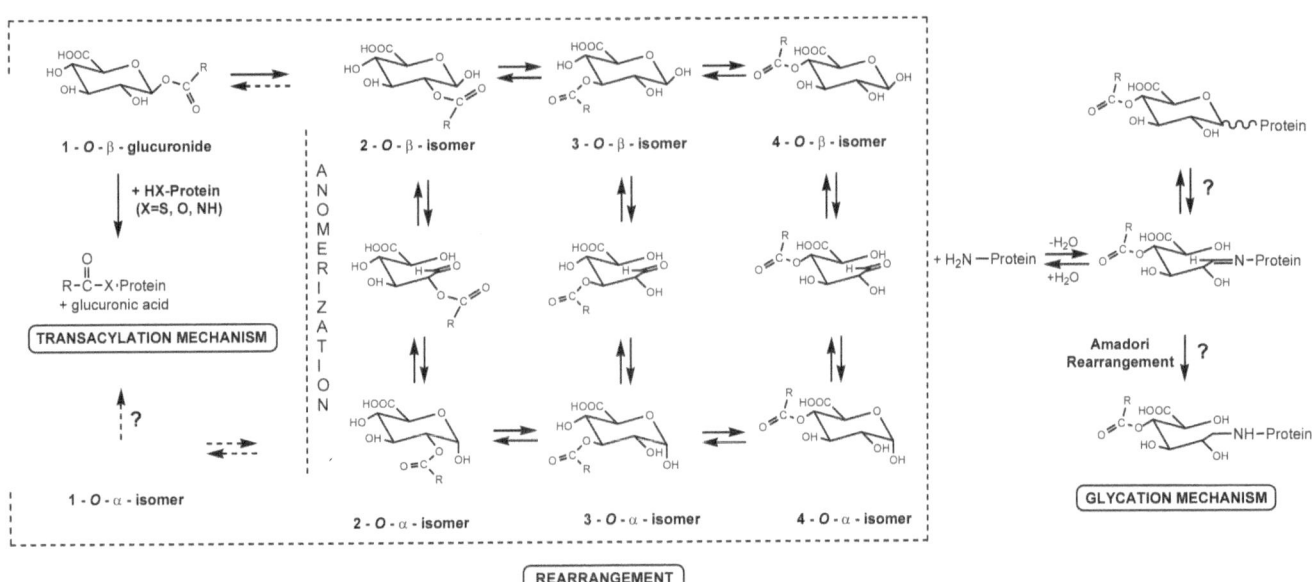

FIGURE 3.9 Mechanisms of covalent binding of acyl glucuronides to proteins. *From Elsevier published journal; Chemico-Biological Interactions; Bailey MJ, Dickinson RG: Acyl glucuronide reactivity in perspective: biological consequences, Chem Biol Interact 145:117–137, 2003. Figure 1 in publication.*

buffer has been now routinely used to evaluate its ability to form reactive metabolites and bind covalently to proteins.

In summary, the presence of chemical substructures that may form reactive metabolites cannot in and of itself predict the type, severity, or incidence of IADR that may occur. Many drugs contain substructures that form reactive metabolites that may cause toxicity, yet they are widely used because of an acceptable benefit: risk ratio and/or exhibit a low body burden of the reactive metabolite (e.g., low dose less than 10 mg or low fraction metabolized via reactive intermediate).

6.3. Discovery Metabolism

During early discovery, one primary focus is to prosecute large numbers of compounds to evaluate metabolic liabilities which lead to high metabolic clearance. The hepatic metabolic Cl of compounds is evaluated in vitro in liver microsomes or hepatocytes by evaluating the rate of disappearance of compound over time. Since liver microsomes are a subfraction of a hepatocyte, data from such preparations can be "scaled up" to the expected intrinsic Cl in a whole liver. Furthermore, using additional parameters such as the fu, liver blood flow, and body weight, a scaled intrinsic Cl can be determined for a preclinical species and then compared to the observed Cl in that same species or a "bottom-up" approach can be used to predict human Cl from in vitro data. Additionally, if Cl of the NME is particularly high, or bioavailability particularly low, this may suggest that impractically high doses would be needed in either animal or human to elicit efficacy or some sort of response; in such cases, additional optimization whereby alternative molecules are selected from a chemical platform or SAR for more "druggable" properties would be warranted. Another focus of metabolism in early discovery is understanding the sites of metabolism or "hot-spots" and whether there are any structural alerts of concern that could result in toxicities and even potentially IADR. Carefully assessing the data from these in vitro studies conducted in liver microsomes and/or hepatocytes allows medicinal chemists to design and synthesize molecules that are less labile and

devoid of metabolic risks that could hinder further drug development. Unfortunately, metabolic liabilities are sometimes not realized for many years into the development process or once the drug is on the market.

During the later stages of discovery, one focus is to characterize the metabolism of the NME of interest across various nonclinical species and to predict human metabolism. In vitro metabolic profiling studies in liver microsomes/hepatocytes of various animals, such as mouse, rat, dog, and monkey, as well as human, give an idea of which metabolites are formed and any species differences in metabolites formed. Hepatocyte coculture where primary cryopreserved hepatocytes are incubated with nonparenchymal, stromal cells may also be an advantageous approach to utilize for compounds that are slowly metabolized or have low Cl (Bonn et al., 2016; Burton et al., 2018). The metabolic profiles in the nonclinical species are ultimately compared to that observed in human liver microsomes/hepatocytes. This information is paramount in determining which nonclinical species, both rodent and nonrodent, should be used in the toxicology studies as the metabolites formed by human should be adequately assessed for safety in the nonclinical toxicology studies. An example of the in vitro metabolic profiles observed across species is represented in Figure 3.10. In this example, peak 6 is the parent drug. The primary metabolite of interest in human is metabolite 4. Of the rodent species, only mouse forms metabolite 4 and thus is the appropriate small animal species to evaluate in toxicology studies. While both large animal species form metabolite 4, monkeys also formed additional metabolites 1, 3, and 5, which are not observed in human hepatocytes and could complicate the interpretation of the toxicology study results. Therefore, dog is the appropriate large animal species to use in toxicology studies.

In addition to the in vitro evaluation of drug metabolism, it is important to understand how the in vitro data translate to the in vivo scenario. The observed in vivo metabolite profiles in animals can confirm formation of metabolites observed in vitro, as well as uncover the involvement of any other metabolism/Cl pathways, such as those pathways that occur extrahepatically at other locations throughout the body that could

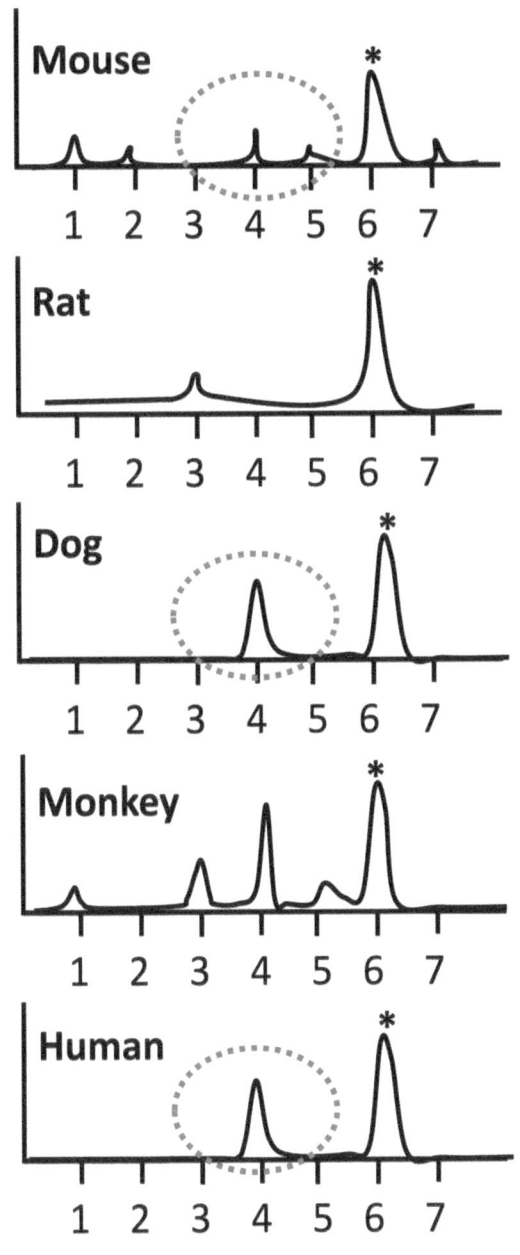

Metabolite Peak Number

FIGURE 3.10 Comparative metabolite profiles of NME incubated in mouse, rat, dog, monkey, and human hepatocytes.

have been missed with in vitro systems. Furthermore, identification of any major circulating metabolites in plasma of animals may raise awareness to potentially major circulating metabolites in humans that could require further characterization during drug development, as well as assessing metabolite coverage for metabolite safety evaluation (FDA, 2020). Ultimately, one

of the major goals is to try to assess translatability to the human, before human ^{14}C data are available (discussed in more detail in "Development" section). In vivo formation of metabolites may be evaluated in multiple types of discovery studies such as bioavailability/PK studies, bile duct cannulated (BDC) studies, pharmacology studies, and toxicology/TK studies. One potential advantage to evaluating in vivo metabolite profiles in plasma samples obtained from the toxicology studies is that since higher dose levels of the NME are investigated, there is a higher likelihood of bioanalytical detection of metabolites. Using plasma samples from animals in repeat-dose toxicology studies also gives additional insight into whether there is any accumulation of the NME and/or its associated metabolites with repeat dosing or if there is potential induction/inhibition of any metabolic pathways. Finally, understanding the potential risks associated with the identification of pharmacologically active metabolites and/or potentially reactive metabolites, such as GSH conjugates or acyl glucuronides, during the discovery phase will help drug development teams make important decisions about advancing molecules to the clinic as they gain a better understanding of the overall benefit:risk profile of the NME.

A list summarizing the typical types of studies performed, including technology applied, and drug metabolism information obtained during the discovery phase are included in Table 3.3.

7. EXCRETION

The final step in evaluating the ADME characteristics of a molecule is to understand how the molecule is ultimately eliminated from the body. Drugs can be excreted into urine, feces, saliva, and breast milk, as well as be exhaled from the lungs. However, excretion into urine and feces via the bile are the most common routes of excretion and are the most amenable to studying in discovery ADME studies. Compounds and their metabolites can easily be analyzed in excreta samples, thus allowing a greater understanding of the fate of a molecule from absorption, through systemic distribution, to metabolism, and finally elimination of the compound.

TABLE 3.3   Types of Metabolism Studies Conducted During Discovery

Study	Animal versus Human	Technology	Information obtained
In vitro Liver microsomes, hepatocytes, Hepatocyte coculture	Mouse, Rat, Dog, Monkey, Human	Nonradioactive/LC/MS	• Qualitative metabolite profiles across species • Preliminary structural information of metabolites (ID) • Not exhaustive
In vivo Exploratory metabolite profiling	Rodents Nonrodents	Nonradioactive/LC/MS	• Quantitation of unchanged drug in urine and bile • Qualitative metabolite profiles in excreta • Qualitative profiles of circulating metabolites • Preliminary structural information of metabolites (ID) • Not exhaustive

During in vivo animal studies, the use of special "metabolism cages" allows for the easy and noninvasive collection of urine and feces. The type of animals used, as well as the number of animals, sex, and species, in addition to dose and dose frequency, route of administration, blood sampling time points, and duration of collections, as well as general urinary markers and animal health parameters, are all aspects for careful consideration in excretion studies. Excretion studies are typically conducted in small animals such as rats or large animals such as dogs or monkeys. In order to avoid confounding data from the PO absorption of the compound, IV administration is usually employed for excretion evaluations. Following IV administration, typically via a short infusion, both blood and urine samples are collected for an extended duration for analysis of drug concentrations. Urine samples are pooled over specific time intervals for evaluation, such as 0–6 h, 6–12 h, 12–24 h, 24–48 h, and 48–72 h. Time intervals are dictated by the known concentration–time profile of the compound, but longer collection periods are recommended for compounds with a particularly long $t_{1/2}$. It is good practice to include determinations of creatinine clearance, as well as urine flow, to understand if any animal is renally compromised or if incomplete sampling has occurred; creatinine Cl can be evaluated as a percent of the glomerular filtration rate (GFR) and should be close to the expected value to be confident in the study output. Renal Cl studies for clinical candidate compounds can inform whether active processes are involved in the excretion of the molecule by comparing the renal Cl to the unbound GFR (plasma fu * GFR). If a drug is renally cleared via passive filtration only, then the renal Cl should not be greater than the GFR, taking into account protein binding, and therefore the proportion of compound that is available in the plasma to be filtered by the kidney. Alternatively, if renal Cl is greater than unbound GFR, then it cannot be accounted for by passive filtration alone and active secretion is inferred. In that case, the involvement of transporters can be assumed. In order to evaluate the contribution of biliary/fecal clearance, specialized studies can be conducted in BDC animals compared to bile duct "intact" animals. As with other excreta matrices, drug concentrations can be determined in the bile and fecal samples, which are typically pooled over defined collection intervals.

Ultimately, the excretion data are utilized for understanding contributions of renal, biliary/

fecal Cl versus hepatic metabolism, and can inform human predictions with the use of appropriate scaling factors (see section on physiologically based PK modeling).

8. PHYSIOLOGICALLY BASED PK MODELING

Prior to the first-in-man study in Phase 1 clinical development, TK data that are derived from early preclinical testing are evaluated relative to predicted human exposures in order to provide an early assessment of exposure multiples that are used to guide first-in-man dosing strategies. Hence, considerable efforts are dedicated to understanding and predicting likely human exposures. Many different tools are available for such predictions but generally may include various scaling techniques and physiologically based pharmacokinetic (PBPK) modeling combined with an in-depth understanding of PK behavior in preclinical species. These approaches rely on a mechanistic understanding of the processes underlying clearance, volume, and absorption properties in vivo.

To generate a human PBPK model, the physicochemical properties of a molecule (permeability, LogP, pKa, molecular weight, etc.) can help guide the approaches used to understand Cl mechanisms such as metabolic, renal, or biliary clearance. A body of evidence approach that combines in vitro data using preclinical and human matrices (e.g., liver microsomes, hepatocytes) along with in vivo PK and excretion data is used to predict human PK. For example, the IVIVE approach is central to Cl predictions and involves the scaling of in vitro intrinsic Cl (determined with microsomal or hepatocyte incubations) to a value for a whole liver or a mean individual, taking into account the microsomal protein or number of hepatocytes per liver, liver weight and body weight, blood flow to the liver, protein binding in plasma and microsomes, and blood to plasma partitioning. Allometric predictions, though empirical, may also be used where animal data are scaled based on body weight and corrected for species differences in protein binding (Tang and Mayersohn, 2005). Vd can be predicted from animal data correcting for plasma protein binding (Oie and Tozer, 1979),

while absorption parameters such as Fa, Fg, and ka are predicted using solubility, permeability, and intestinal metabolism data. The combination of these parameters can then be utilized to predict human PK profiles using simulation software programs (e.g., SimCYP© or Gastro-Plus©) which integrate physiological parameters that are then combined with the physicochemical properties and in vitro evaluations of the drug entity (Davies et al., 2020). These preliminary mechanistic PBPK models are continually refined as new data are available and are useful for designing future studies in the context of safety margins in early and late development. For example, simulations can be performed by modifying physiological parameters to represent specific populations such as pediatric, geriatric, hepatic or renal impairment, and various other diseases. Such analyses in the context of expected exposure multiples in special populations can be useful for risk assessment in these patients.

9. DEVELOPMENT

The goal of ADME studies in the development phase is to more definitively characterize the ADME properties of the NME. As the optimal molecule to be tested in humans has been decided out of potentially thousands of molecules, it is now time to gain a deep understanding of the molecule itself. The data generated in the discovery phase may be confirmed with the use of more robust study designs enabling more definitive characterization of the ADME properties, or new data may emerge resulting in new questions that need to be addressed. Regardless, the ADME package of studies are designed to support global regulatory submissions.

It is necessary to characterize the overall disposition of the NME in both nonclinical and human studies, from absorption through excretion. Although the human study is out of scope for this chapter and will not be discussed, animal ^{14}C studies, or mass balance studies, are the hallmark studies conducted during the development phase to evaluate absorption, PK, distribution, metabolism, and excretion. Being able to quantify and definitively identify metabolites, as well as gain an understanding of the comparative excretion pathways, further enables understanding of potential toxicities and safety implications of the NME. Additionally, depending on the intended patient population for which the drug is being developed, it may be important to conduct specialized distribution studies to determine whether or not a drug crosses the placenta or is excreted into breast milk. Many of these questions can be answered with the help of radiolabel studies.

10. MASS BALANCE STUDIES

The use of radiolabeled material in ADME mass balance studies facilitates quantitation of the PK, metabolic pathways (including metabolite quantification and identification), and routes of excretion of the drug. Therefore, the total fate of the drug-related material is obtained. These studies are typically conducted in the same rodent and nonrodent species as the toxicology studies. The most commonly used isotope is ^{14}C; however, ^{3}H (tritium) may also be used to support these studies (Nijenhuis et al., 2016). Additionally, the advancement of high-field magnets and cryoprobes has enabled the assessment of mass balance and metabolism of some fluorine-containing molecules using ^{19}F-NMR methodologies in both preclinical and clinical studies (Hu et al., 2017; James et al., 2017; Mutlib et al., 2012).

The typical mass balance study design utilizes a single dose of ^{14}C-labeled drug which is administered both orally and intravenously, so that the %F can be calculated. Blood and plasma, as well as urine and feces, are typically collected. In addition, animal studies comparing an intact bile duct versus a cannulated bile duct may be used to understand the role of biliary excretion. Animals are housed in special excretion cages to keep urine and feces separated. As these are not toxicology studies, the administered dose is usually in the pharmacological/efficacious range. However, the radioactivity should have sufficient specific activity, usually in the range of 100–200 µCi. Following dosing, extensive blood sampling allows full characterization of the concentration–time profile. The duration of sample collection should be guided by the known concentration–time profile in the given species as determined in discovery studies.

However, additional, longer duration sample collection should be employed to ensure the concentration–time profile of any metabolites that may have a longer $t_{1/2}$ compared to the parent drug is captured. Generally, samples are collected for several days after the initial dose. Efforts are made to recover as close to 100% of the administered radioactivity as possible. In order to achieve this, the cage is rinsed and washed typically every 24 h. Blood, plasma, urine, bile, and feces, as well as cage wash samples, are then analyzed for total radioactivity by liquid scintillation counting (LSC) methods. The summation of total radioactivity in these tissues and collections should, in theory, be 100%; in practice, some amount of radioactivity is usually lost leading to incomplete recovery. However, a retrospective review by Roffey et al. (2007) showed that overall recovery of radiolabel would often be greater than 90%, 85%, and 80% in rats, dogs, and humans, respectively. These studies still answered the pertinent questions of major Cl and excretion pathways, circulating metabolites, and whether or not any safety issues were identified requiring further risk assessment. If recovery of radioactivity is determined to be too low, residual radioactivity may also be analyzed in the carcass.

Plasma concentrations of the known NME are determined using validated LC/MS/MS methods. The difference in profile between total radioactivity and measured concentrations of the NME will help elucidate the comparative amount of parent drug versus the metabolites. Samples are also profiled for metabolite identification and quantification, discussed in more detail below. Following the analysis of samples, various PK parameters can be calculated. These parameters may include, but are not limited to, AUC, C_{max}, T_{max}, and $t_{1/2}$. When an IV arm is administered, systemic Cl and Vd may also be determined, as well as the %F of the NME. Comparing concentrations in blood versus plasma facilitates an understanding of the association of radioactivity with red blood cells.

The example in Figure 3.11 depicts the concentration versus time curve following a single PO dose administration of ^{14}C-NME. Samples were collected through 120 h postdose. Radioactivity is not preferentially associated with red blood cells, as the curves are similar between radioactivity in blood versus plasma. Additionally,

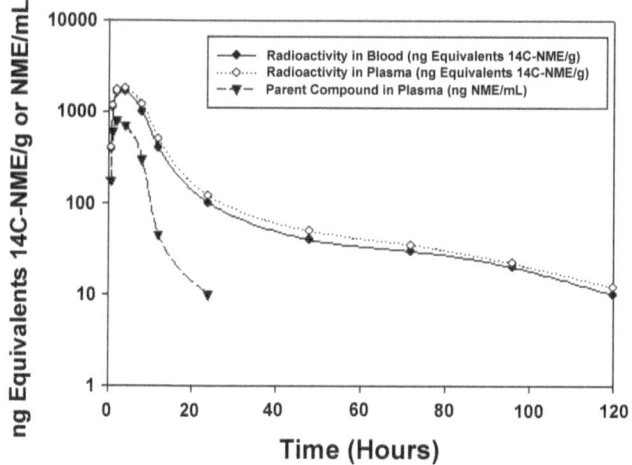

FIGURE 3.11 Concentration–time curve of radioactivity or parent compound NME in blood or plasma following a single, oral dose of ^{14}C-NME.

metabolites in the systemic circulation appear to have a longer $t_{1/2}$ compared to the parent compound, which was not detected after 24 h postdose.

11. TISSUE DISTRIBUTION STUDIES

The general purpose of tissue distribution studies is to assess the overall extent of distribution of the NME and its radiolabeled metabolites within the body. The standard method to generating this information is with the use of quantitative whole-body autoradiography (QWBA; Solon and Kraus, 2002). Using this approach, rats are administered a single PO dose of radiolabeled compound. At designated time points following dosing, blood samples are taken for PK analysis. In addition, animals are euthanized at these same points (typically n = 2/time point) so that the entire body can be evaluated for tissue distribution. The carcass is prepared and embedded into a carboxymethylcellulose block, frozen, and then sagittal whole-body sections are prepared, approximately 20–40 μm thick. The whole-body tissue slices should contain multiple tissues. The amount of radioactivity is then quantitated in the tissue/carcass using autoradiographic techniques. Briefly, mounted whole-body sections are tightly wrapped with Mylar film and exposed on phosphor imaging screens, along with standards to aid in the

calibration, for approximately 4 days. Specified tissues, organs, and fluids are then analyzed, and tissue concentrations are interpolated from each standard curve. PK parameters are then calculated for various tissues. The tissues evaluated are extensive. A list of commonly evaluated tissues is included in Table 3.4.

In general, data from these studies facilitate an understanding of the overall extent of distribution of drug into the tissues. QWBA data allows the investigator to determine if the NME is widely distributed to most or all the tissues or if it is confined to the blood or distributes preferentially to specific tissues. The organs with the most radioactivity can be identified. PK parameters can also be determined for individual organs. For instance, peak concentrations can be determined by evaluating tissues throughout a time course. Additionally, the $t_{1/2}$ of the radiolabel can be determined in specific tissues. It is also important to understand whether the radioactivity penetrates the central nervous system, distributes to reproductive organs, or binds to melanin-containing tissues such as skin or the eyes. Example phosphor images from a QWBA study are shown in Figure 3.12.

When a drug is being developed for women of child-bearing potential, it is also prudent to know if the NME crosses the placenta in these animal studies. An understanding of the placental transfer as well as the lacteal excretion (discussed separately) of radiolabeled NME can be explored in nonclinical species, typically in rats. In these studies, a single dose of ^{14}C-NME is administered to timed-pregnant female rats on day 18 of gestation. Following dosing, blood/plasma is collected for PK analyses and one animal/time point is sacrificed to examine placental transfer and tissue distribution of radioactivity in maternal and fetal tissues by QWBA, as discussed above, although the time course is often shorter in these studies compared to the traditional QWBA study. The presence/absence of radioactivity in fetal tissues will confirm or refute placental transfer of the drug and/or metabolites. Peak radioactivity concentrations can also be determined in fetal tissues, as well as determining how long radioactivity is detectable in these tissues.

TABLE 3.4   Representative List of Standard Tissues Evaluated in the Tissue Distribution Study

Adrenal gland (cortex and medulla)	Eye (lens)	Ovary	Small intestine content
Blood	Harderian gland	Pancreas	Spinal cord
Bone	Kidney (cortex and medulla)	Plasma	Spleen
Bone marrow	Large intestine contents/wall	Pituitary gland	Stomach contents/wall
Brain (cerebrum, cerebellum, medulla)	Liver	Preputial gland	Testes
Brown fat	Lung	Prostate gland	Thymus
Cecum contents/wall	Lymph nodes	Salivary gland	Thyroid gland
Cerebrospinal fluid (within brain ventricles)	Muscle	Seminal vesicles	Urine/urinary bladder
Epididymis	Myocardium	Skin	White fat (renal area)

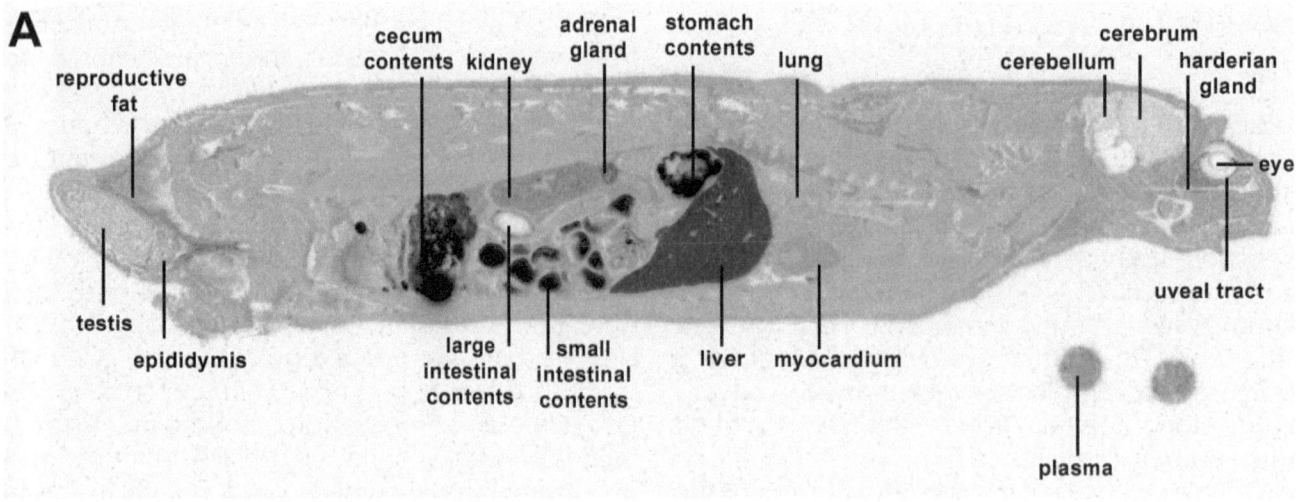

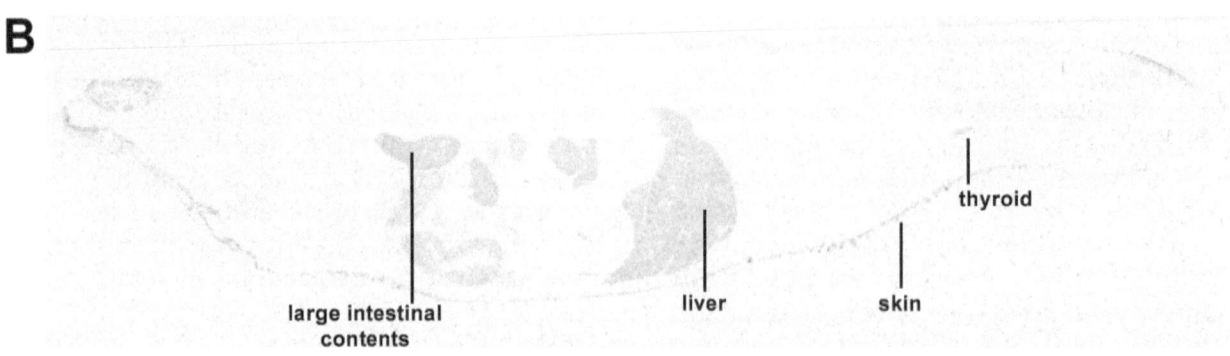

FIGURE 3.12   Quantitative whole-body autoradiography results in a male Long–Evans rat. (A) A phosphor image of a whole-body section 2 h after receiving an oral 125 mg/kg dose of ^{14}C-NME. (B) A phosphor image of a whole-body section 48 h after receiving an oral 125 mg/kg dose of ^{14}C-NME. Retention of drug-related material in target organs of toxicity provide greater insights into understanding of toxic responses. The darker the tissue, the greater the concentration of drug-related material.

12. DRUG METABOLISM STUDIES IN DEVELOPMENT

As part of the mass balance study, the metabolism of an NME is fully characterized in the development phase, both in nonclinical species and in humans. Plasma, urine, feces, and/or bile samples are collected and observed metabolites are characterized using radio-profiling techniques, as well as LC/MS/MS and/or NMR to quantify metabolites and elucidate their structures. More recently, increased use of accelerator mass spectrometry (AMS), an extremely sensitive method for detection of the isotopic ratio, has been noted in certain scenarios (Garner, 2010; Lappin and Stevens, 2008). For instance, the technique is especially useful in cases where only very low doses of radioactivity, or microdoses, can be administered for safety reasons. For compounds where Cl of radioactivity from tissues and/or plasma is very low or there is slow excretion of radioactivity into the excreta, AMS techniques also require extensive sample preparation and can be expensive, factors which may be taken into consideration when applying this technology (Nijenhuis et al., 2016).

While the focus of this chapter is on nonclinical species, understanding whether or not the observed human metabolites above a prespecified threshold are also present in the nonclinical toxicology species is paramount to determine if the safety of these metabolites has been adequately assessed. According to regulatory guidance (FDA, 2020), any human metabolite that exceeds 10% of the total drug-related material in the circulation/plasma at steady state is considered "major" and requires further evaluation to ensure its presence in the nonclinical toxicology species. This is commonly referred to as "metabolite coverage." Metabolite coverage across different species has implications for the interpretation of toxicology data packages. For instance, metabolic coverage and safety assessment in nonrodent species may be adequate for general toxicological studies, but may not provide adequate coverage for reproductive toxicity, genotoxicity, or carcinogenicity studies that are usually evaluated in rodent species. If a human metabolite is considered "unique," such that it is only observed in humans and is not formed by nonclinical species, or is considered "disproportionate," such that the human metabolite is more prevalent in humans compared to nonclinical toxicology species, additional studies may be required to assess the safety of these metabolites. Stand-alone toxicology studies in which the human metabolite of interest is directly administered in nonclinical toxicology studies may be warranted. As these studies can be complicated in terms of determination of appropriate dose to achieve equivalent exposures, and potentially different metabolism pathways may be involved when the parent drug versus metabolite is administered, it is prudent to take advantage of early communication with various global regulatory authorities to garner advice regarding design of such studies.

Finally, it may be necessary to synthesize authentic standards of "major" human metabolites. These metabolites may then be used to develop bioanalytical assays to quantitate the metabolite and to characterize the PK characteristics of the metabolite in other clinical and nonclinical in vivo studies. In vitro, these metabolites may also be tested for pharmacological activity, as well as the potential to be involved in inhibition/induction of drug metabolizing enzymes and transporters.

13. EXCRETION STUDIES

In addition to understanding the PK and metabolism of the NME, the mass balance studies also provide a quantitative analysis of the excretion pathways of the drug. After quantifying the amount of radioactivity in excreta, investigators have a clearer idea of whether the drug and its metabolites are primarily excreted in the urine or the feces and whether biliary excretion is involved in the Cl of the NME. In Figure 3.13A, the cumulative percent of a radioactive dose in urine and feces following a single PO administration of ^{14}C material in bile duct intact rats is depicted. In this example, virtually all of the radioactivity was recovered, and all of the radioactivity was essentially excreted in the feces. Following PO administration of ^{14}C-NME to bile duct intact rats, the mean feces

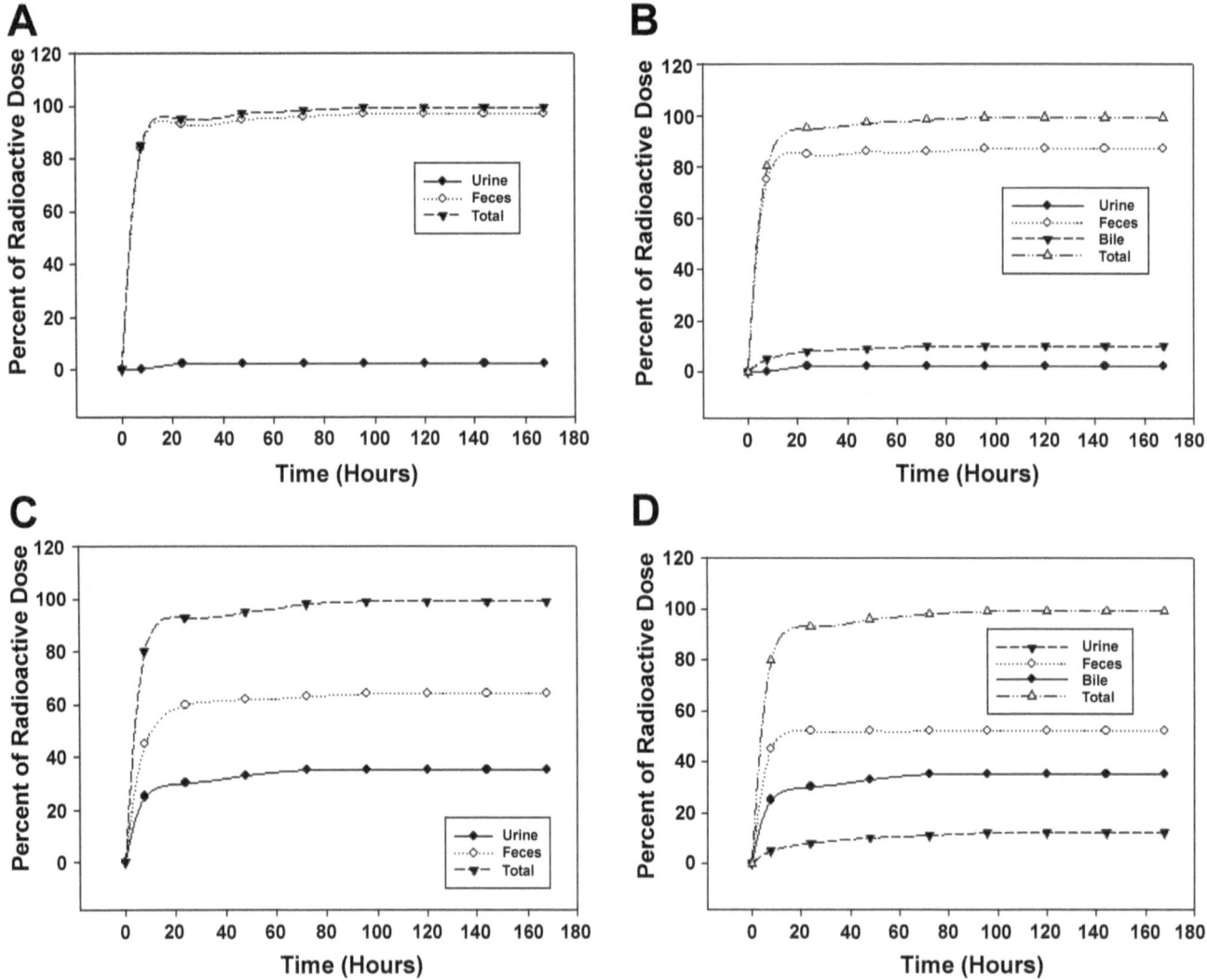

FIGURE 3.13   Mean cumulative percent of radioactive dose in urine, feces, and bile after oral administration of
[14]C-NME to bile duct intact or bile duct cannulated rats.

and urine recoveries represented approximately 97% and 2% of the administered dose, respectively. In this instance, it may be difficult to determine whether the NME was absorbed. That is, did parent drug in feces represent drug that was never absorbed from the gastrointestinal (GI) tract, or was this drug absorbed and then excreted back to the GI tract via biliary Cl or another pathway, such as intestinal secretion. Biliary data are useful to help differentiate between these two possibilities. In Figure 3.13B, in BDC rats, the mean feces, bile, and urine recoveries represented approximately 87%, 10%,

and 2%, respectively. The total radioactivity eliminated in bile and urine following a PO dose indicates that at least 12% of the dose was absorbed, whereas it is likely that the majority of the dose was unabsorbed. In Figure 3.13C, virtually all of the radioactivity was recovered, but the ^{14}C-NME excretion profile is more balanced between feces (approximately 64%) and urine (approximately 35%) in bile duct intact rats compared to the previous examples. In Figure 3.13D, in BDC rats, the mean feces, bile, and urine recoveries represented approximately 52%, 12%, and 35%, respectively. The total radioactivity eliminated in bile and urine following a PO dose indicates that at least 47% of the dose was absorbed.

Furthermore, it is important to understand how excretion and metabolism data are coupled. Whether it is primarily parent drug that is eliminated or metabolite(s), or a mixture of both. Understanding the interplay of these processes provides insight into the overall disposition of the drug. This information may also lead to the conduct of additional in vitro mechanistic studies, as several drug transporters can be involved in both urinary and biliary excretion processes. Drugs that are substrates of these transporters may require further investigation from the perspective of potential DDIs.

14. SPECIALIZED EXCRETION STUDIES

If the NME is being developed for women of child-bearing potential, lacteal excretion of the drug into breast milk is important to understand. Typically evaluated as part of the rat placental transfer study, a single ^{14}C-NME dose is administered to lactating dams who are approximately 12 days postpartum. In addition to blood and plasma, milk samples (n = 3/time point) are collected at various time points, typically out to 24 h postdose. On the day of collection, rats are administered oxytocin to stimulate lactation. Animals are then anesthetized immediately before the start of the milk collection, and milk is collected using a specially constructed milking machine device. Concentrations of radioactivity are then determined in the samples via radioanalysis, such that PK parameters can be calculated. Albeit in rats, and not humans, these studies enable an understanding of whether or not a drug passes into the breast milk and how long it takes for the drug to be cleared from the breast milk. This important information is typically included in drug labels and may help physicians and other health care professionals guide lactating women to determine if it is safe or not to continue breast feeding while taking a particular drug as part of their pharmacotherapy.

15. GENERAL TIMING OF DEVELOPMENT ADME STUDIES

The timing of when to conduct development ADME studies should be tailored to a particular molecule. Thus, it is not a one-size-fits-all approach. However, in general, nonclinical radiolabel mass balance studies are typically conducted during Phase 1 clinical development. As described throughout this chapter, an understanding of the PK characteristics, metabolism, and excretion profiles of a drug in nonclinical species aides in thinking through potential toxicities. The metabolism data are also used to ensure adequate coverage and safety testing of metabolites in the toxicology studies, once the human metabolism data are confirmed in the human ^{14}C study. In addition to tissue distribution data, the QWBA study allows for dosimetry calculations and acceptable limits of radioactivity by humans. Therefore, this study is a prerequisite to the human ^{14}C study. These studies should be done at a time appropriate for the molecule that is under development. Studies may be done sooner or later, depending on what is known about the molecule itself and if any of these studies would help discharge any potential development risks or aid in decision-making. The indication being studied may also dictate when these studies are conducted. Take, for instance, an indication for Alzheimer's disease or certain types of cancer, for which the Phase 2 development may be particularly long, allowing sufficient time to run these studies in parallel with Phase 2. However, for an indication such as pain, an acute infection, or high blood pressure, Phase 2 clinical development may be rather short. In this instance, it may make more sense to conduct these studies sooner in development. In any case, the information should be available by the end of Phase 2 for inclusion in regulatory documents at these milestone discussions.

More specialized studies such as placental transfer and milk excretion are typically conducted in parallel with Phase 3 registration trials. While these studies are conducted in rats, with perhaps uncertain translation to pregnant and lactating human women, the results are nevertheless included in drug labels and used to inform prescribing practice worldwide.

16. CONCLUSIONS

Understanding the ADME principles of small molecule NMEs throughout drug development is important. The ADME discipline is uniquely placed, such that the science can influence studies across the entire development paradigm from early discovery throughout development, including postmarketing commitments.

In early discovery, ADME studies contribute to an understanding of the nonclinical PK and TK characteristics of the NME. The qualitative metabolic profiles generated may also uncover potential metabolic liabilities. Ultimately, the knowledge gained in the discovery phase will aide in the selection of the appropriate rodent and nonrodent species to be used in the toxicology studies to help establish relationships between dose, exposure, and toxicity. Utilizing a myriad of in silico, in vitro, and in vivo approaches aides in the understanding of species differences in PK, TK, metabolism, and excretion. The data generated will ultimately help make predictions about the human ADME properties of the NME to assist in clinical study design.

Throughout the development phase, results from ADME studies may confirm previous findings or may generate new data that lead to additional questions and investigations. In general, the data obtained are more quantitative in nature, such as that generated from radiolabel mass balance studies. TK support continues to be important in chronic dosing studies, reproductive toxicology studies, and carcinogenicity assessments. As development progresses, the margin of safety calculations are refined when longer duration animal exposures and human exposure data in relevant patient populations become available, ensuring adequate patient safety and adverse event monitoring in the clinic. Specialized distribution studies are conducted to gain an in-depth understanding of the NME. As adverse events may arise in both nonclinical and clinical evaluations, addressing the mechanisms underlying such events may rely on a solid characterization of ADME characteristics. Ultimately, the data generated in the development phase are used to support global registration packages as well as label language to safeguard that patients get "the right dose of the right drug at the right time."

Acknowledgments

The following individuals have provided valuable insights to this book chapter: Trent Abraham, Kenneth Cassidy, Gemma Dickinson, Timothy Jones, Bridget Morse, Everett Perkins, Maria Posada, John Vahle, and Lian Zhou.

REFERENCES

Argoti D, Liang L, Conteh A, et al.: Cyanide trapping of iminium reactive intermediates followed by detection and structure identification using liquid chromatography-tandem mass spectrometry (LC-MS/MS), Chem Res Toxicol 18:1537–1544, 2005.

Bailey MJ, Dickinson RG: Acyl glucuronide reactivity in perspective: biological consequences, Chem Biol Interact 145:117–137, 2003.

Benet LZ, Spahn-Langguth H, Iwakawa S, et al.: Predictability of the covalent binding of acidic drugs in man, Life Sci 53(8):141–146, 1993.

Bode G, Clausing P, Gervais F, et al.: The utility of the minipig as an animal model in regulatory toxicology, J Pharmacol Toxicol Methods 62:196–220, 2010.

Boelsterli UA: Diclofenac-induced liver injury: a paradigm of idiosyncratic drug toxicity, Toxicol Appl Pharmacol 192:307–322, 2003.

Bonn B, Svanberg P, Janefeldt A, et al.: Determination of human hepatocyte intrinsic clearance for slowly metabolized compounds: comparison of a primary hepatocyte/stromal cell co-culture with plated primary hepatocytes and HepaRG, Drug Metab Dispos 44:527–533, 2016.

Burton RD, Hieronymus T, Chamem T, et al.: Assessment of the biotransformation of low-turnover drugs in the HμREL human hepatocyte coculture model, Drug Metab Dispos 46:1617–1625, 2018.

Castillo M, Lam YW, Dooley MA, et al.: Disposition and covalent binding of ibuprofen and its acyl glucuronide in the elderly, Clin Pharmacol Ther 57:636–644, 1995.

Chauret N, Nicoll-Griffith D, Friesen R, et al.: Microsomal metabolism of the 5-lipoxygenase inhibitors L-746,530 and L-739,010 to reactive intermediates that covalently bind to protein: the role of the 6,8-dioxabicyclo[3.2.1]octanyl moiety, Drug Metab Dispos 23:1325–1334, 1995.

Dansette PM, Libraire J, Bertho GS, et al.: Metabolic oxidative cleavage of thioesters: evidence for the formation of sulfenic acid intermediates in the bioactivation of the antithrombotic prodrugs ticlopidine and clopidogrel, Chem Res Toxicol 22:369–373, 2009.

Davies M, Jones RDO, Grime K, et al.: Improving the accuracy of predicted human pharmacokinetics: lessons learned from the AstraZeneca drug pipeline over two decades, Trends Pharmacol Sci 41(6):390–408, 2020.

Diehl K-H, Hull R, Morton D, et al.: A good practice guide to the administration of substances and removal of blood, including routes and volumes, J Appl Toxicol 21:15–23, 2001.

Evans DC, Watt AP, Nicoll-Griffith DA, et al.: Drug protein adducts: an industry perspective on minimizing the potential for drug bioactivation in drug discovery and development, *Chem Res Toxicol* 17:3–16, 2004.

Evans WE, Relling MV: Pharmacogenomics: translating functional genomics into rational therapeutics, *Science* 286(5439):487–491, 1999.

Garner RC: Accelerator mass spectrometry in pharmaceutical research and development - a new ultrasensitive analytical method for isotope measurement, *Curr Drug Metabol* 1:205–213, 2000.

Gonzalez FJ, Coughtrie M, Tukey RH: Drug metabolism. In Brunton LL, Hilal-Dandan R, Knollmann BC, editors: *Goodman and Gilman's the pharmaceutical basis of therapeutics*, ed 13, New York, 2018, McGraw Hill. http://access medicine.mhmedical.com.ez1614.infotrieve.com/content.aspx?bookid=2189&sectionid=167889421. (Accessed 1 May 2020).

Haddock RE, Johnson AM, Langley PF, et al.: Metabolic pathways of paroxetine in animals and man and the comparative pharmacological properties of the metabolites, *Acta Psychiatr Scand Suppl* 350:24–26, 1989.

Hull RM: Guideline limit volumes for dosing animals in the preclinical stage of safety evaluation, *Hum Exp Toxicol* 14:305–307, 1995.

Hu H, Katyayan KK, Czeskis BA, et al.: Comparison between radioanalysis and ^{19}F nuclear magnetic resonance spectroscopy in the determination of mass balance, metabolism, and distribution of pefloxacin, *Drug Metab Dispos* 45:399–408, 2017.

James AD, Marvalin C, Luneau A, et al.: Comparison of ^{19}FNMR and ^{14}C measurements for the assessment of ADME of BYL719 (alpelisib) in humans, *Drug Metab Dispos* 45(8):900–907, 2017.

Kalgutkar AS: Handling reactive metabolite positives in drug discovery: what has retrospective structure-toxicity analyses taught us? *Chem Biol Interact* 192:46–55, 2011.

Koup JR: Disease states and pharmacokinetics, *J Clin Pharmacol* 29(8):674–679, 1989.

Lappin G, Stevens L: Biomedical accelerator mass spectrometry: recent applications in metabolism and pharmacokinetics, *Expet Opin Drug Metabol Toxicol* 4:1021–1033, 2008.

LiverTox (website), 2020. https://livertox.nih.gov/aboutus.html. (Accessed 14 April 2020).

Madyastha KM, Moorthy B: Pulegone mediated hepatotoxicity: evidence for covalent binding of R(+)-[14C]pulegone to microsomal proteins in vitro, *Chem Biol Interact* 72:325–333, 1989.

Morgan ET: Impact of infection and inflammatory disease on cytochrome P450-mediated drug metabolism and pharmacokinetics, *Clin Pharmacol Ther* 85(4):434–438, 2009.

Morse BL, Kolur A, Hudson LR, et al.: Pharmacokinetics of organic cation transporter 1 (OCT1) substrates in Oct1/2 knockout mice and species difference in hepatic OCT1-mediated uptake, *Drug Metab Dispos* 48(2):93–105, 2020.

Mutlib A, Espina R, Atherton J, et al.: Alternate strategies to obtain mass balance without the use of radiolabeled compounds: application of quantitative fluorine (^{19}F) nuclear magnetic resonance (NMR) spectroscopy in metabolism studies, *Chem Res Toxicol* 25:572–583, 2012.

Nijenhuis CM, Schellens JHM, Beijnen JH: Regulatory aspects of human radiolabeled mass balance studies in oncology: concise review, *Drug Metab Rev* 48(2):266–280, 2016.

Oie S, Tozer TN: Effect of altered plasma protein binding on apparent volume of distribution, *J Pharmacol Sci* 68:1203–1205, 1979.

Park BK, Boobis A, Clarke S, et al.: Managing the challenge of chemically reactive metabolites in drug development, *Nat Rev Drug Discov* 10:292–306, 2011.

Patel N, Wickremsinhe E, Hui Y, et al.: Evaluation and optimization of micro-sampling methods: serial sampling in a cross-over design from an individual mouse, *J Pharm Pharmaceut Sci* 19(4):496–510, 2016.

Roffey SJ, Obach RS, Gedge JI, et al.: What is the objective of the mass balance study? A retrospective analysis of data in animal and human excretion studies employing radiolabeled drugs, *Drug Metab Rev* 39:17–43, 2007.

Ruelius HW, Kirkman SK, Young EM, et al.: Reactions of oxaprozin-1-O-acyl glucuronide in solutions of human plasma and albumin, *Adv Exp Med Biol* 197:431–441, 1986.

Sallustio BC, Sabordo L, Evans AM, et al.: Hepatic disposition of electrophilic acyl glucuronide conjugates, *Curr Drug Metabol* 1:163–180, 2000.

Sawamura R, Okudaira N, Watanabe K, et al.: Predictability of idiosyncratic drug toxicity risk for carboxylic acid-containing drugs based on the chemical stability of acyl glucuronide, *Drug Metab Dispos* 38:1857–1864, 2010.

Shipkova M, Armstrong VW, Oellerich M, et al.: Acyl glucuronide drug metabolites: toxicological and analytical implications, *Ther Drug Monit* 25:1–16, 2003.

Smith D: *Dosing limit volumes: a European view*, New Orleans, 1999, Humane Society of the United States Refinement Workshop.

Solon EG, Kraus L: Quantitative-whole body autoradiography in the pharmaceutical industry: survey results on study design, methods, and regulatory compliance, *J Pharmacol Toxicol Methods* 46:73–81, 2002.

Spahn-Langguth H, Benet LZ: Acyl glucuronides revisited: is the glucuronidation process a toxification as well as a detoxification mechanism? *Drug Metab Rev* 24:5–47, 1992.

Stepan AF, Walker DP, Bauman J, et al.: Structural alert/reactive metabolite concept as applied in medicinal chemistry to mitigate the risk of idiosyncratic drug toxicity: a perspective based on the critical examination of trends in the top 200 drugs marketed in the United States, *Chem Res Toxicol* 24:1345–1410, 2011.

Tang H, Mayersohn M: A novel model for prediction of human drug clearance by allometric scaling, *Drug Metab Dispos* 33(9):1297–1303, 2005.

US Food and Drug Administration (FDA): *Guidance for industry: safety testing of drug metabolites*, 2020, US Department of Health and Human Services, Food and Drug Administration, Center for Drug Evaluation and Research.

Wickremsinhe ER, Renninger M, Paulman A, et al.: Impact of repeated tail-clip and saphenous vein phlebotomy on rats used in toxicology studies, *Toxicol Pathol* 44(7):1013–1020, 2016.

Zhang KE, Naue JA, Arison B, et al.: Microsomal metabolism of the 5-lipoxygenase inhibitor L-739,010: evidence for furan bioactivation, *Chem Res Toxicol* 9:547–954, 1996.

CHAPTER

4

Biotherapeutics ADME and PK/PD Principles

Daniela Bumbaca Yadav[1], Kapil Gadkar[2], Isabel Figueroa[3]

[1]Department of Pharmacokinetics, Pharmacodynamics, and Drug Metabolism Merck & Co., Inc., South San Francisco, CA, United States, [2]Denali Therapeutics, South San Francisco, CA, United States, [3]Preclinical Pharmacokinetics and Drug Metabolism Amgen, South San Francisco, CA, United States

O U T L I N E

1. Introduction	77		2.3. PK of Other Biotherapeutic Modalities	92
1.1. Monoclonal Antibodies	78		3. Pharmacodynamics of Biotherapeutics	92
1.2. Antibody-Based Therapeutics	80			
1.3. Beyond Antibody-Based Therapeutics	81		4. PK–PD Modeling and Interspecies Scaling	95
2. Pharmacokinetics of Biotherapeutics	83		5. Summary	96
2.1. Monoclonal Antibody PK	84		References	96
2.2. PK of Antibody-Based Therapeutics	90			

1. INTRODUCTION

Large molecules therapeutics, also referred to as biologics or biotherapeutics, are proteins designed to modulate their target(s) pharmacology to achieve therapeutic effect. The key advantage that biotherapeutics offer is their high target specificity, which makes them ideal modalities for targeted therapy. In contrast to small molecules, large molecule therapeutics cannot penetrate cell membranes and therefore must exert their intended effect through extracellular binding in the case of soluble antigens or binding potentially followed by internalization of membrane bound targets. Due to high target specificity, off-target toxicity is rare following the administration of large molecule therapeutics (unlike their small molecule counterparts), and observed toxic events are more frequently associated with exaggerated pharmacology. This specificity stems from a complex structure that usually consists of long sequences of amino acids and molecular weights in the order of several kilodaltons or higher. Because of this complexity, large molecule therapeutics cannot be chemically synthesized and are typically produced by mammalian cells that can perform the posttranslational modifications necessary for correct protein folding, stability, multimer formation, and secretion. As of today, most large molecule therapeutics are antibodies or antibody-based therapeutics; however, other biotherapeutic products, including vaccines, gene and cell therapy, tissue, and other proteins, are emerging as therapeutic alternatives in indications of high unmet needs. For a discussion of ADME and pharmacokinetics/pharmacodynamics (PK/PD) principles of small molecules refer to Chap 3 ADME Principles in Small Molecule Drug Discovery and Development Vol 1, Chap 3, and for a further description of basic principles of Pharmacodynamics and Toxicodynamics refer to Principles of Pharmacodynamics and Toxicodynamics, Vol 1, Chap 5, Principles of Pharmacodynamics and Toxicodynamics. Small peptides (short protein chains of 50 amino acids or less) share some of the properties of large molecules, but their specific pharmacokinetic (PK) and pharmacodynamics (PD) properties are not described here.

1.1. Monoclonal Antibodies

An antibody, also known as an immunoglobulin (Ig), is a large protein produced by the host's immune system in response to a specific antigen. Antibodies are generated to recognize biological substances that are foreign to the host body, such as viruses or bacteria, and can be instrumental to the neutralization and elimination of such substances. The molecular structure of an antibody resembles a distorted Y-shape with two arms conjoined by one region known as the fragment crystallizable (Fc) portion of the antibody. The end of each of these two arms (also referred to as the N-terminus of the antibody) contains the antigen-specific binding sites (Fabs), with two identical sites per antibody molecule. Both arms are joined by a flexible hinge region that enables bivalent binding of the antibody with antigen sites at a range of distances.

Five different antibody classes or isotypes IgA, IgD, IgE, IgG, and IgM can be found in mammals. Ig classes differ in their sequence, number of constant domains, hinge structure, and valency, with the vast majority (70%–85%) of the total antibody pool consisting of the IgG class. IgG antibodies are mostly found in monomeric form and have a molecular weight of approximately 150 kDa. IgGs consist of two identical heavy chains with two identical light chains as shown in Figure 4.1A. The light chain has two domains VL and CL (one variable and one constant among antibodies respectively), both within the Fab region of the antibody. The heavy chain comprises one variable and three constant domains (VH, CH1, CH2, and CH3, respectively), with the first two being in the Fab region and the last two forming the Fc portion of the antibody. There are four IgG subclasses (IgG1, IgG2,

IgG3, and IgG4) each comprising a different heavy chain that imparts different functionalities and capabilities to activate the immune system via effector functions.

One of the key roles of antibodies in the immune system is to trigger immune responses by binding via the Fc domain to specific molecules that could drive chemical cytotoxic responses—such as elements in the complement pathway that result in complement-dependent cytotoxicity (CDC)—or receptors in specialized cells that result in cell killing or cell phagocytosis—as in the case of the antibody-dependent cellular cytotoxicity (ADCC) or antibody-dependent cellular phagocytosis (ADCP) (Figure 4.1B). Mainly, IgG1 and IgG3 can trigger potent effector responses, while the IgG2 and IgG4 subtypes drive weaker effects. Differences in the observed Ig functionality can be explained by the differences in binding affinity to elements of the complement pathway as well as binding affinity to Fc gamma receptors expressed on immune cells that drive the ADCC/ADCP responses. IgGs owe their unusually long half-life to their ability to bind the neonatal Fc receptor, also known as FcRn, in a pH-dependent manner (Figure 4.1C). Serum proteins are continuously taken up by endothelial cells via pinocytosis into the endosome and incorporated into the lysosome for degradation following the fusion of the endosome and lysosome. Binding to FcRn in the slightly acidified environment (pH < 7.0) within the endosome rescues serum IgGs from lysosomal degradation and recycles them back to circulation where they are released at physiological pH (pH > 7.0).

The IgG has been the large molecule format most heavily used in the design and development of therapeutic antibodies because of its extended half-life, ability to modulate the immune system, and relative abundance compared to other Igs. The first generation of therapeutic antibodies were of murine origin. These provided limited therapeutic benefit because the patients' immune systems would recognize these as foreign and generate a human antimouse antibody response that would clear these therapeutics. To overcome this, the following generation of antibody-based therapeutics have focused on making these large molecule therapeutics more "human like." These efforts resulted in chimeric antibodies (structural chimeras made by fusing variable regions from one species like a mouse

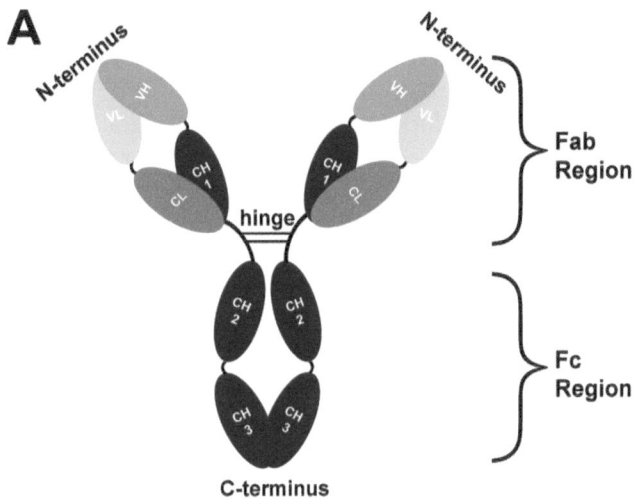

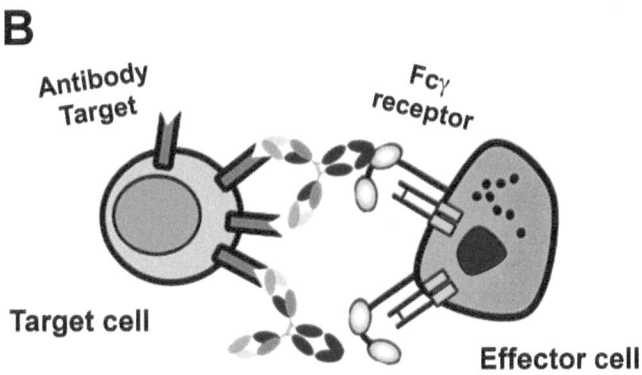

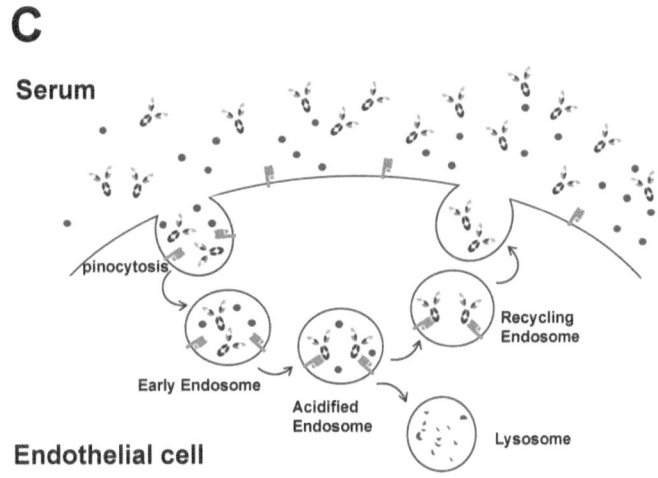

FIGURE 4.1 **Structure and functions of an immunoglobulin molecule.** (A) The structures of the human IgGs resemble a distorted "Y" shape with two identical antigen binding regions and one constant region. The overall antibody structure consists of two identical heavy and light chains with domains (VH, CH1, CH2, CH3, VL, and CL, respectively; heavy chain domains are shown in light and dark shades of blue while light chain domains are shown in light and dark shades of green). (B) The constant region of the antibody can bind to Fc gamma receptors and interact with the immune system to trigger effector functions such as antibody-dependent cell cytotoxicity (ADCC) (represented in this cartoon), antibody dependent cell phagocytosis (ADCP) or complement dependent cell cytotoxicity (CDC). (C) The constant region of the antibody can bind to the FcRn receptor that acts as a salvage mechanism to prevent lysosomal degradation of the circulating IgG resulting in the characteristic long half-life observed for antibodies.

with the constant regions from another species such as a human being) as well as humanized antibodies (where the nonhuman portions of the antibody have been modified to increase similarity of antibody molecules endogenously produced by humans). Further developments in antibody production technology have enabled the generation of fully human antibodies either by using display technologies (e.g., phage, ribosomes, or yeast that display human antibody variable regions) or by using transgenic mice (that is, mice that have been engineered to produce fully human antibodies as part of their normal immune response to foreign agents).

One of the key features that distinguishes antibody-based therapeutics is their high specificity for their intended therapeutic target. Antibodies interact with their intended targets via the complementarity-determining regions located within variable region, area also known as the paratope of the antibody. On the targeted antigen, the specific region that binds to the antibody is known as the target epitope. This interaction can be characterized by the rate of antibody–antigen association (referred to as k_{on}), rate of dissociation (referred as k_{off}), and the ratio between these two (i.e., k_{off}/k_{on}), known as the equilibrium constant or affinity (typically referred as K_D) of the antibody–antigen interactions. Affinity is a critical property in the design of antibodies because it quantitates the strength of the antibody–antigen interaction and can be tuned to optimize the therapeutic performance of the antibody. The affinity value of an antibody has units of concentrations

and the lower the value of K_D, the stronger the antibody–antigen interaction.

Quantitative PK and PD modeling can leverage our knowledge of relevant target properties, such as turnover rate, antigen concentrations under physiological and pathological conditions, and biodistribution, together with the PK and biodistribution properties of the antibody to optimize affinity design goals for antibody-based therapeutics. Figure 4.2 shows an example of an application of a PK/PD model for optimal affinity determination (Bhatt et al., 2018). Here, it is shown that increases in affinity can result in lower clinical doses because of improved antibody potency. However, beyond a certain point, further improvements in the affinity do not produce significant improvements in potency and clinical dose reductions due to limitations in stoichiometry of the antigen. Where this ceiling value in dose lies depends on the properties of the system, such as antigen concentration, turn over, etc., and it is a critical consideration during the design and selection of antibody candidates.

1.2. Antibody-Based Therapeutics

The antibody structure confers multiple advantages to therapeutic molecules, and not surprisingly, the structure of the antibody has been leveraged to test various therapeutic approaches beyond monoclonal antibodies. For example, antibody drug conjugates (ADCs) are a class of antibody-based therapeutics that combines the

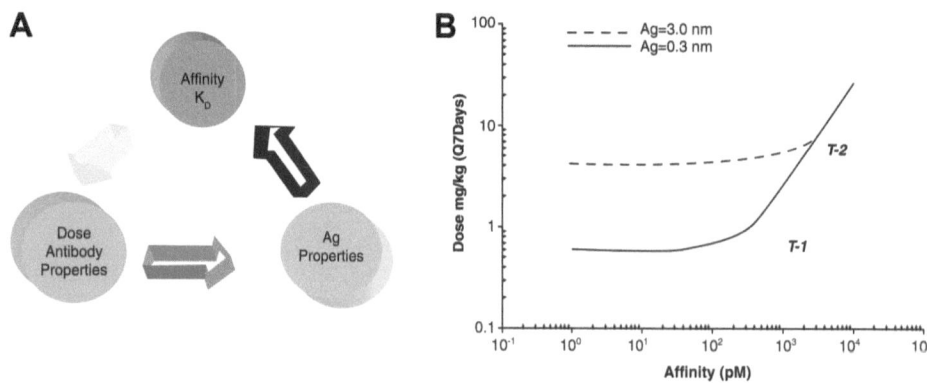

FIGURE 4.2 **Relationship among antibody dose, affinity, and target properties.** (A) Interdependency of antibody and antigen properties and construct affinity. (B) Theoretical relationship between the antibody affinity and dose at different antigen concentrations (the antigen concentrations used were 0.3 nM and 3.0 nM for T-1 and T-2, respectively). *Reprinted from Tabrizi, Mohammad A, Bornstein, Gadi G, Klakamp, Scott L, editors:* Development of antibody-based therapeutics; translational considerations. *Chap 6.*

specificity and prolonged exposure of antibodies with the potent pharmacological activity of small molecules. Most of the existing ADCs being explored in the clinic or approved for clinical use consist of a cytotoxic payload (the small molecule) conjugated to a full-size antibody for the treatment of solid or hematological malignancies (Khongorzul et al., 2020). The antibody acts as a carrier that releases its small molecule cargo selectively upon binding to (and most frequently internalization and catabolism by) target positive cells. Current efforts are extending this concept to other payloads beyond cytotoxic, including antibiotic payload to treat infectious disease (Lehar et al., 2015; Mariathasan and Tan, 2017) and steroid payloads in the immunology field (Brandish et al., 2018; ClinicalTrials.gov, 2019), cardiovascular diseases (Lim et al., 2015), and other disease states (Liu et al., 2016).

Another well-established antibody-based modality is bispecific antibodies, which are a special class of antibodies designed to target two different antigens (one with each of the antibody arms) (Labrijn et al., 2019). These have been most used to tackle mechanistically the disease biology where the combination of the pharmacological activity on different antigens would result in additive or synergistic activity of the constructs in comparison to the monospecific antibody alternative. Moreover, a number of therapeutics in this class have been designed in such a way as to harness the immune system by binding with one arm targeting a cancer cell surface antigen and another arm targeting T-cell receptors to engage the patient's immune system, most commonly through CD3. These bispecific molecules can bridge T-cells to tumor cells through an artificial immunologic synapse, resulting in selective killing of target-expressing tumor cells which, in the case of CD3, occurs independently of the presence of MHC-I or costimulatory molecules. The approach was pioneered by the BiTE molecules (Wolf and Baeuerle, 2002) but has expanded into a plethora of formats during the last few decades (Labrijn et al., 2019).

Fc fusion proteins are another class of antibody-based therapeutic and consist of the Ig Fc fragment domain directly fused to a peptide or protein intended to drive a pharmacological effect. In most existing clinical applications, this approach has been used to replace or enhance the pharmacological action of an endogenous molecule and, many times, this has been achieved leveraging the structure (or a modification thereof) of the endogenous molecule itself (Jafari et al., 2017). Attachment to an Fc domain grants the therapeutic protein many of the advantages of the monoclonal antibody, including improved exposure due to interaction with FcRn. However, the overall resulting PK and biodistribution of Fc-containing constructs varies from molecule to molecule and depends on many factors such as local and global electrostatics charges, hydrophobicity, glycosylation patterns, target-mediated and nonspecific mechanisms, etc.

As mentioned earlier in this chapter, the variable region of antibodies possesses unique properties of high affinity, specificity, and selectivity. The variable region has been explored as a therapeutic alternative where the properties of the Fc backbone are not critical or not desired. The antigen binding fragment (or Fab) is a therapeutic modality comprising only one constant and one variable domain of each light and heavy chain. Due to their smaller size, Fabs are believed to result in better tissue penetration than full-length antibodies. Single-chain variable fragments (commonly referred as scFvs) are even smaller proteins with a peptide linker that connects the variable domain of the heavy and light chain. These smaller proteins can be used as stand-alone therapeutics or as imaging agents; but also their small size has made them amenable to be used as building blocks for multitarget therapy (Bemani et al., 2018).

1.3. Beyond Antibody-Based Therapeutics

Despite the fact that the large majority of large molecule therapeutics consist of monoclonal antibody or antibody-based therapeutics, other protein modalities are also being pursued. Here, we describe some of the most frequent types and formats of biotherapeutics that could be encountered in clinical applications; however, advances in protein engineering have unlocked countless possibilities in terms of how biotherapeutic molecules can be constructed. An exhaustive review of this topic is beyond the scope of this chapter.

Albumin binding therapeutics. The role of FcRn in antibody PK has been described. Similar to IgG, albumin is also rescued from lysosomal degradation by FcRn, giving albumin an extended half-life compared to like proteins in vivo. Protein therapies have taken advantage of this mechanism by generating molecules that can noncovalently bind to endogenous albumin and have potential to exhibit the prolonged half-life while still maintaining the advantages of small proteins in terms of tissue distribution and penetration. Alternatively, another therapeutic strategy involves leveraging the favorable half-life properties of albumin by generating drug with covalent bonds to albumin molecules (via chemical conjugation or genetic fusion). Either of these approaches has demonstrated to be capable of altering the serum half-life (Sleep, 2015; Sleep et al., 2013) as well as the tissue distribution (Baggio et al., 2008; Seijsing et al., 2018; Yao et al., 2004; Yazaki et al., 2008) of the pharmacological agent.

Pegylated proteins. Pegylation refers to the conjugation of drugs to polyethylene glycol molecules as a strategy to modify their PK properties. Mainly, pegylation reduces the renal clearance of the conjugated molecules, resulting in more sustained and constant circulating concentrations which may lead to improved therapeutic effects. Because pegylation can substantially change the physical and chemical properties of the drug, pegylated drugs can exhibit tissue distribution patterns that are dramatically different from that of the parent drug. Moreover, differences in the steric environment around the drug's active site can impact its ability to interact with its intended target, limit the drug's susceptibility to be a substrate for various enzymes, or even change the drug's immunogenic potential (Fishburn, 2008; Hamidi et al., 2006; Harris et al., 2001).

Multimers and other large proteins. Nonantibody–based multimeric structures have also been explored. These structures are most likely sought when the Fc fragment structure would not confer critical advantages and/or when the multimeric structure is believed to be critical for the therapeutic mechanism of action (such as in the case of agonists where the multimeric binding results in superagonistic activity). For local administration, elimination mechanisms in tissue may differ from those after systemic administration and the large size may constitute an exposure advantage. Systemically, these molecules clear fast, so they are typically not utilized for pharmacology that requires sustained engagement of the target.

Gene and Cell Therapy. The concept of gene therapy comprises the use of genes to treat disease. The idea is that genetic material will be delivered into the cells in the target tissues and replace genes that are defective or nonfunctional. The therapeutic gene could aim to replace a mutated gene with a healthy copy, inactivate a gene that is not functioning properly, or introduce new genes which are designed to treat the disease. So far, gene therapy has shown promising success in treating genetic disorders, cancers, and some infectious diseases and is currently being tested for a number of diseases with severe unmet needs. One of the key challenges in gene therapy is how to efficiently deliver the genetic material into target cells and tissues. Currently, genes are typically delivered to cells using a plasmid or a virus. Viruses are specialized agents capable of entering cells and inserting their genetic material; however, there are potential concerns about immune responses and genome manipulation.

Cell therapy entails the use of live cells to treat disease. These cells may be obtained directly from the patient via autologous gene therapy or from a donor via allogenic gene therapy. Different kinds of cells can be used, including hematopoietic stem cells (HSCs), skeletal muscle stem cells, mesenchymal stem cells, lymphocytes, dendritic cells, and pancreatic islet cells depending on the application and disease indication. HSC transplantation is the most frequently used cell therapy and is used to treat a variety of blood cancers and hematologic disorders. Sometimes the cells administered as cell therapy may be genetically altered to treat specific diseases. Such is the case of CAR (chimeric antigen receptor)–T-cells, which is a combination of both gene and cell therapy. Here, T-cells are harvested from a patient and are taken into the laboratory to be genetically modified to become specific to an antigen expressed on a tumor that is not expressed on healthy cells. Then, these modified T-cells are infused back into the patient where they become activated upon binding to the specific antigen, proliferate, and become cytotoxic (Braendstrup et al., 2020; Golchin and Farahany, 2019).

2. PHARMACOKINETICS OF BIOTHERAPEUTICS

The typical concentration–time profiles of systemically administered monoclonal antibodies can be described by two phases; a relatively short distribution phase followed by a relatively long elimination phase (Figure 4.3) (Peletier and Gabrielsson, 2012). Monoclonal antibodies have a relatively long systemic half-life due to their interaction with FcRn, slow clearance, and limited tissue distribution (volume of distribution that approximates that of plasma volume). However, there are many factors that can contribute to the clearance of monoclonal antibodies, either through target- or nontarget–mediated mechanisms. The shape of the concentration–time profile can also change depending on the route of administration and the systemic bioavailability following extravascular administration. The type of assay used to detect the monoclonal antibody (e.g., ligand binding assay vs. total IgG assay) could also yield different PK parameter estimates.

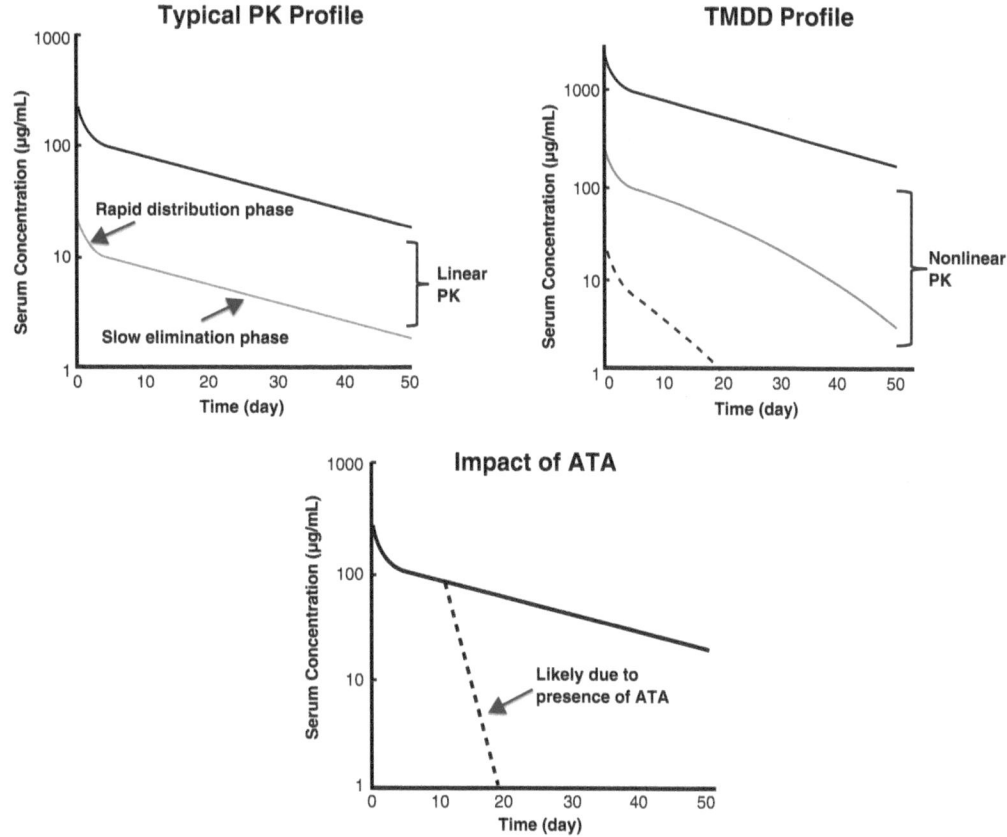

FIGURE 4.3 **Monoclonal antibody concentration–time profile.** Characteristic concentration versus time graphs. The concentration of the antibody is typically presented on a semi-logarithmic scale. A typical concentration–time profile is characterized by a rapid distribution phase and a slow elimination phase. Parallel elimination phases across doses denote linear (dose proportional) PK (top left plot). A TMDD profile is characterized by rapid elimination at lower plasma concentration of antibody that slows as the antibody concentration increases. Nonparallel elimination phases across doses denote nonlinear (dose dependent) PK (top right plot) The presence of antidrug antibodies (ADAs or ATA) causes a rapid drop in plasma concentrations as earlier as 7 days postdose (bottom plot). *Reprinted from Drug discovery today: technologies, Vols 21–22, Kamath A, Translational pharmacokinetics and pharmacodynamics of monoclonalantibodies, pp. 75–83, Copyright (2016), with permission from Elsevier.*

2.1. Monoclonal Antibody PK

Monoclonal Antibody Administration and Absorption

There are numerous routes for antibody administration that are characterized by their own absorption rate and bioavailability. The most common route of administration is intravenous (IV). Absorption refers to the flux of antibody from the administration site into the systemic circulation. When administering antibodies intravenously, the antibody is delivered directly into the systemic circulation, and therefore, there is no absorption phase. As such, the maximum concentration (C_{max}) is always at the earliest sampling time point for IV-administered drugs. Bioavailability is the ratio of the systemic exposure or area under the concentration–time curve (AUC) following extravascular administration to that following IV administration. For IV-administered monoclonal antibodies, the site of administration is the systemic circulation, so this ratio is always 1 and bioavailability is 100%.

Monoclonal antibodies can also be administered extravascularly. The most common extravascular route of administration is subcutaneous (SC). This route of administration is gaining in popularity due to its convenience for patients, and therefore, understanding the factors regulating antibody SC bioavailability is an active area of investigation. There have been several good reviews on this topic (Bittner et al., 2018; Richter et al., 2012; Richter and Jacobsen, 2014; Turner and Balu-Iyer, 2018). Antibodies delivered via SC are deposited in the hypodermis, which is composed primarily of adipose cells with some fibroblast and macrophages (Richter and Jacobsen, 2014). The fibroblasts produce negatively charged extracellular matrix components (ECMs), such as collagen and glycosaminoglycans. Monoclonal antibodies tend to be positively charged under physiological conditions, with isoelectric points (pI) > 8 (Goyon et al., 2017), and can interact with these negatively charged components of the ECM as they move through the interstitial space.

Antibodies primarily move through the interstitial space via convective transport and are largely routed to the lymphatic system for absorption into the systemic circulation. The speed at which monoclonal antibodies do this is dependent upon their physicochemical properties, formulation, and the interstitial environment at the injection site. This process is typically slow, with time to C_{max} typically taking 3–8 days in humans (Richter and Jacobsen, 2014). The bioavailability following SC administration in humans for typical monoclonal antibodies falls within the range of 60%–80% (Richter et al., 2012; Richter and Jacobsen, 2014; Turner and Balu-Iyer, 2018). Recently, in mice, it was shown that hematopoietic cells contribute to IgG catabolism in the SC space and likely play an important role in the <100% bioavailability from this site (Richter et al., 2018). It is challenging to predict the human SC bioavailability from that in preclinical species, and it has been hypothesized that this could be due to species differences in physiology, site of injection, and/or FcRn interactions (McDonald et al., 2010; Richter and Jacobsen, 2014; Turner and Balu-Iyer, 2018; Zheng et al., 2012).

Similar to the SC route of administration, bioavailability from intramuscular (IM) administration is <100% and demonstrates relatively slow absorption into the systemic circulation through the lymphatics (Keizer et al., 2010; Ryman and Meibohm, 2017). Palivizumab is an example of a monoclonal antibody approved for IM administration and it has a T_{max} of ~5 days and a bioavailability of ~70% (Robbie et al., 2013; Zhao et al., 2013). The IM route of administration is far less common in the clinic than IV and SC.

Intravitreal (IVT) administration is primarily used for therapeutics designed for diseases of the eye. Bevacizumab has been administered to humans via this route for the treatment of neovascular age-related macular degeneration and has a T_{max} of ~5 days, with no reported bioavailability (Csaky, 2007). Based on preclinical and clinical data, large protein therapeutics are believed to be cleared primarily from the vitreous through the front of the eye, exiting the aqueous humor via bulk fluid flow through the ciliary body (Missel and Sarangapani, 2019).

Intrathecal (IT) administration is used to treat neurological disorders. Since, the blood–brain barrier limits the amount of antibody that enters the brain parenchyma to ~0.02–0.1% that of the systemic concentration (Banks et al., 2007; Yadav et al., 2017; Yu et al., 2014), IT is an alternative route that may allow for greater exposure in the brain. Administration via IT delivers the antibody into the cerebrospinal fluid (CSF) of patients, and based on the route of CSF flow, the drug can enter the brain parenchyma surrounding the ventricles without having to cross the restrictive blood–brain barrier (Calias et al., 2014; Iliff et al., 2012). Trastuzumab has been successfully delivered to patients with breast cancer brain metastases via the IT route of administration (Colozza et al., 2009). In cynomolgus monkeys, serum concentrations reached C_{max} 24 h following IT administration (Braen et al., 2010), indicating that systemic absorption from this compartment is faster than that from SC, IM, or IVT.

Monoclonal Antibody Distribution

The relatively large size of monoclonal antibodies as well as their physicochemical properties limit the tissue distribution of these proteins, yielding a volume of distribution that approximates plasma volume. As such, in contrast to small molecule therapeutics, the tissue distribution of antibodies is typically not studied in detail. The exit of antibody from the systemic circulation into tissues is primarily driven by convection (Ovacik and Lin, 2018). Once in the tissue interstitial space, the antibody diffuses through the tissue and its movement can be hindered by on-target or off-target interactions. If the antibody target is secreted in the interstitial fluid of the tissue, the antibody can recognize its target and keep flowing through. Conversely, if the target is membrane expressed, the antibody can become associated with the cell or can be internalized following binding. In addition to the target simply being expressed in the tissue potentially causing differences in distribution, the degree of expression, its turnover rate, and the antibody's affinity for the target will also affect distribution (Rudnick et al., 2011). Furthermore, the negatively charged components of the ECM (glycosaminoglycans and proteoglycans) attract the positively charged antibodies and could lead to nonspecific pinocytosis. Convective forces move the antibody through the interstitial space into the lymphatics for reabsorption into the systemic circulation (Ryman and Meibohm, 2017).

The degree of fenestration in the vascular endothelium affects how much antibody can enter a tissue; the more fenestrated or leakier the vasculature, the greater the concentration of antibody in the tissue (Wang et al., 2008). For most tissues, the partitioning of antibodies is 5%–15% that of serum, with the brain and eye being notable exceptions. The brain tends to have a partitioning of 0.02%–0.1%, depending on the species in which it has been assessed (Banks et al., 2007; Yadav et al., 2017; Yu et al., 2014), and the eye tends to be higher with a partitioning closer to 2% (Chirila and Hong, 2016). The exact partitioning of IgGs into specific tissues can be difficult to assess due to varying degrees of blood contamination across the different tissues, although there have been attempts to measure this by various groups utilizing different techniques (Mandikian et al., 2018). The disease state of a given tissue could also change the antibody distribution profile.

Monoclonal Antibody Elimination

Antibodies are cleared by target-mediated mechanisms, nonspecific pinocytosis, specific off-target interactions, and/or antidrug antibodies (ADAs). An antibody that is cleared via target can display nonlinear kinetics. This is evidenced by the nonparallel terminal phases of the concentration–time curves with increasing doses and dose-independent changes in exposure (C_{max} and AUC), as depicted in Figure 4.3. The clearance parameter (CL) also tends to decrease with increasing dose as target becomes saturated and elimination becomes dominated by nonspecific processes. Once target-mediated clearance is saturated, dose-proportional increases in exposure are expected. The degree of target-mediated clearance will depend on the amount of target, its turnover, the affinity of the antibody for the target, and site of expression (soluble vs. membrane bound) (Kamath, 2016). Following binding to the target, some antibody–antigen complexes can be internalized and degraded in the lysosome (Ovacik and Lin, 2018), leading to faster systemic clearance.

Unlike small molecules, bivalent, full-length antibodies are not filtered by the kidney. The main route of nonspecific elimination for monoclonal antibodies is nonspecific pinocytosis and proteolysis by vascular endothelial cells across multiple tissues throughout the body. Nonspecific pinocytosis involves the engulfment of the antibody from the blood vessel lumen or tissue interstitial space by cells (Ryman and Meibohm, 2017). During this process, antibodies can interact with FcRn in a pH-dependent manner, contributing to the relatively long systemic half-life of antibodies (18–25 days in humans) (Ovacik and Lin, 2018; Roopenian and Akilesh, 2007; Ryman and Meibohm, 2017).

Antibodies with little or no target-mediated clearance have linear kinetics characterized by parallel terminal phases of their concentration–time profiles as doses increase, as depicted in Figure 4.3. Antibodies with linear kinetics also have dose-proportional increases in exposure (C_{max} and AUC) and the CL is constant over the dose range. The nonspecific clearance for nonhuman primates and humans is quite predictable with antibodies clearing <8 mL/day/kg in cynomolgus monkeys (Bumbaca Yadav et al., 2015) and <5 mL/day/kg in humans (Deng et al., 2011). Clearance ranges for rodents have not been well defined in the literature.

There are known factors that can alter the nonspecific clearance of antibodies, including charge, hydrophobicity, high mannose (Man) content, FcRn affinity, off-target binding, and immunogenicity (Bumbaca et al., 2012). Typical pI values for antibodies fall in the range of 8–9 (Boswell et al., 2010). More positively charged proteins tend to bind to the negatively charged surfaces of the cells, and therefore, adding positive charge to an antibody by at least one pI unit increases plasma clearance and tissue distribution (Herve et al., 2008; Lee and Pardridge, 2003). On the other hand, reducing the positive charge of antibodies by at least one pI unit can slow its plasma clearance and reduce tissue uptake (Kobayashi et al., 1999). Igawa et al. used site-directed amino acid substitutions to generate antibody variants with a range of pIs in order to more thoroughly investigate the relationship between charge and antibody clearance (Igawa et al., 2010). Specific substitutions were chosen within the surface residues of the heavy chain variable region to modify the pI without affecting the affinity of the antibody. Consistent with earlier reports, variants with lower pI values of 1–2 units had longer half-lives and slower clearance following IV and SC administration into mice and cynomolgus monkeys. Others have changed the framework of the antibody such that a variant having a pI of 8.6

displayed faster clearance in mice than that with a pI of 6.1 (Li et al., 2014). Similar results were obtained when charge modifications were made in the Fv region of two antibodies, trastuzumab and anti-LTa, without altering the pI of either antibody, as seen in Figure 4.4 (Bumbaca Yadav et al., 2015). Sampei et al. also observed this trend in clearance with modifications to Fv charge (Sampei et al., 2013). Taken together, these findings suggest that charge modifications that result in pI changes or that result in charge clustering within specific regions of the antibody can alter the clearance of antibodies.

Monoclonal antibody hydrophobicity is a physical property of the antibody that leads to low affinity for water. One measure of antibody hydrophobicity is its retention time on a hydrophobic interaction chromatography (HIC) column. Lower hydrophobic antibodies elute off the column faster than the higher hydrophobic variants. It has been shown that there is no correlation between HIC retention time and antibody clearance in cynomolgus monkeys (Hotzel et al., 2012). However, there are other literature examples that suggest that antibody hydrophobicity does affect PK.

A study was conducted comparing the PK and tissue distribution of a naked antibody and its ADC counterpart, with the drug conjugated to the antibody increasing the hydrophobicity of the antibody (Boswell et al., 2011). The ADC did indeed have faster systemic clearance and greater liver uptake than the naked antibody in mice. More recently, Dobson et al. showed that an antibody with high hydrophobicity was prone to reversible self-association and had fast systemic clearance in rats and cynomolgus monkeys due to nonspecific interactions with tissues (Dobson et al., 2016). Removing the hydrophobic residues involved in this self-association resulted in an antibody with slower clearance. More data are needed to truly understand the role of hydrophobicity in antibody clearance.

All IgG1 antibodies are N-glycosylated at a conserved site in the CH2 domain of each heavy chain. The majority of the glycans are complex biantennary structures, containing a core oligosaccharide of two N-acetylglucosamine residues (GlcNAc) linked to asparagine 297 via an amide bond and three Man residues. This core structure, depending on the degree of terminal processing, may contain additional terminal sugar residues

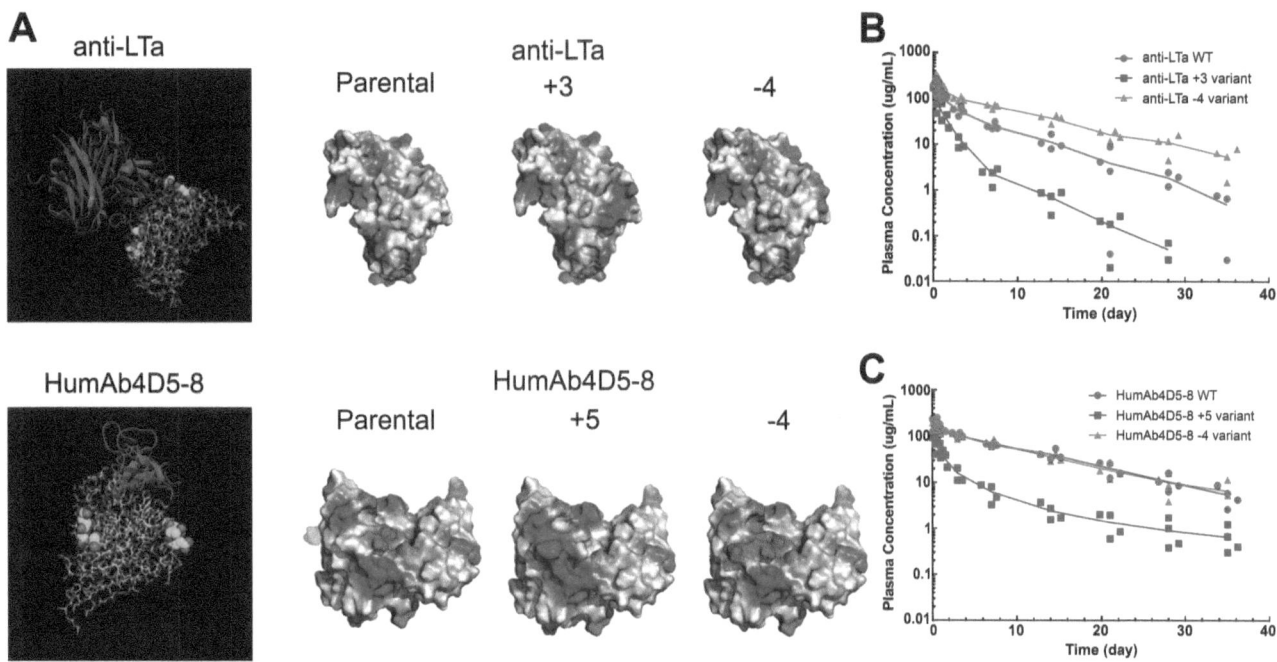

FIGURE 4.4 **Effect of Fv charge on antibody PK.** Modeling of charge variants onto crystal structures determined for complexes of anti-LTα:LTα and humAb4D5-8:HER2. (A) Antibody–antigen structures for anti-LTα (Protein Data Bank code 4MXV) (29) and humAb4D5-8 (Protein Data Bank code 1N8Z) (30) are shown with antigens colored in purple and the antibody Fabs in green. The colored spheres show the location of the amino acids that were mutated to alter Fv charge. (B) Electrostatic surfaces calculated (PyMOL, Shrödinger, Inc.) for Fv portions of modeled charge variants. Positive charge is indicated by blue and negative charge by red. (C) Concentration–time profiles of the parental antibodies and the Fv charge variants following a single IV or SC dose at 10 mg/kg to cynomolgus monkeys. The parental antibodies are depicted in red, and the more positively charge variants are depicted in blue, and the less positively charge variants are depicted in green. Each point represents an individual animal ($n = 4$), and the line represents the average concentration among them. This research was originally published in the Journal of Biological Chemistry. Bumbaca Yadav D, Sharma VK, Boswell CA et al.: Evaluating the Use of Antibody Variable Region (Fv) Charge as a Risk Assessment Tool for Predicting Typical Cynomolgus Monkey Pharmacokinetics. J Biol Chem. 2015; 290: 29732–29741. © Bumbaca Yadav D, Sharma VK, Boswell CA et al.

such as fucose, Man, galactose (Gal), GlcNAc, and N-acetyl neuraminic acid or sialic acid (SA). The oligosaccharides are highly heterogeneous, and recombinant mAbs produced in mammalian cell systems such as the Chinese hamster ovary or mouse myeloma (NS0, SP2/0) typically contain up to 30 or so different types of glycans (Jefferis, 2007). Some therapeutic mAbs may also be glycosylated in the variable domain (Dubois et al., 2008). Antibodies containing 100% Man5 (i.e., high mannose) clear about twofold faster when compared to major glycan forms observed in recombinant antibodies. It has been suggested that the Man5 residues may be accessible to the Man binding protein, asialoglycoproteins, or the Man receptor (Kanda et al., 2006; Wright and Morrison, 1994, 1998; Zhou et al., 2008).

Liver appears to be the major site of catabolism together with skin and muscle for Man5 glycoforms and for mAbs containing terminal Gal (Wright et al., 2000). It has been shown, with an IgG2 antibody, that higher Man forms such as Man7–9 are converted to Man5 by serum mannosidase (Chen et al., 2009). Therapeutic antibodies generally contain low levels of the high-Man glycoforms (~5%). Thus, while a difference in Man5 for therapeutic antibodies may potentially impact their PK in theory, the low Man5 levels are unlikely to produce a meaningful difference in systemic exposure. For example, omalizumab manufacturing lots with varying amounts of Man5 (5%–7%) showed no difference in PK profiles (Harris, 2005).

FcRn is responsible for the relatively long systemic half-life antibodies and there have been many efforts to exploit this interaction for therapeutic benefit. IgG binding to FcRn is pH dependent, with antibodies having high affinity for FcRn at pH 5–6 and low affinity at pH 7 (Roopenian and Akilesh, 2007). If binding affinity for FcRn at pH 6 is increased with little or no increase in affinity at pH 7, then it is possible to reduce systemic clearance and prolong the half-life an antibody, as in Figure 4.5 (Dall'Acqua et al., 2006; Deng et al., 2010; Robbie et al., 2013; Yang et al., 2017; Yeung et al., 2009). If binding affinities at pH 6 and pH 7 are both increased,

then there may not be a detectable change in systemic half-life (Deng et al., 2010; Yeung et al., 2009). If there is a significant increase in binding affinity at pH 7 with little to no increase at pH 6, then the antibody will clear much faster and have a shortened systemic half-life (Igawa et al., 2013; Yang et al., 2017). This last effect has been exploited to generate sweeping antibodies which can lead to the increased clearance of immune complexes (Igawa et al., 2016) Thus, it is important to maintain the balance in affinity at the different pHs in order to ensure the efficient release of antibodies from FcRn.

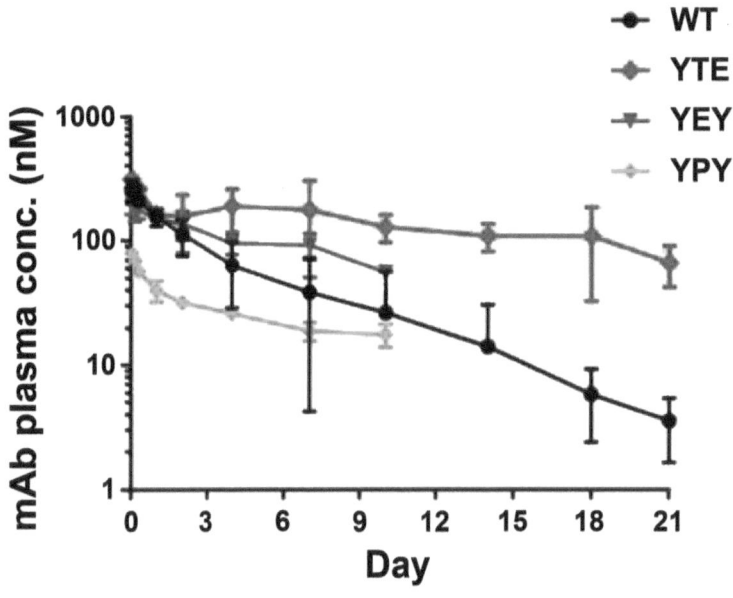

| | | Cyno FcRn | |
Fc variant	Mutations	K_D at pH 7.4 (nM)	K_D at pH 6.0 (nM)
WT	—	>10,000	853 ± 220
YTE	M252Y/S254T/T256E	1110 ± 292	76 ± 23
YEY	M252Y/N286E/N434Y	66 ± 19	4.3 ± 1.6
YPY	M252Y/V308P/N434Y	28 ± 5	2.2 ± 0.9

FIGURE 4.5 **Effect of FcRn affinity modifications on mAb PK.** Plasma concentration–time profiles of pH-dependent antigen binding antibodies in WT, YTE, YEY, and YPY Fc variants in cynomolgus monkeys. The anti-PCSK9 was administered intravenously at single dose of 1.5 mg/kg. Each data point represents the mean ± s.d. (n = 3 each). For the YEY and YPY variants, only data points up to 10 or 14 d are shown due to significant drop in measurable concentrations. The table shows the pH-dependent binding affinities of antibody Fc variants to cyno FcRn. This research was originally published in "Maximizing in vivo target clearance by design of pH-dependent target binding antibodies with altered affinity to FcRn" by Yang TY, Uhlinger DJ, Ayers SA et al. in MAbs in August 2017 by Taylor & Francis Ltd., and is reprinted by permission of the publisher (Taylor & Francis Ltd., http://www.tandfonline.com).

Antibodies can also display specific, off-target binding (to tissue or blood components), which would change their clearance. These antibodies tend to have atypical concentration–time curves that can be monophasic or multiphasic, have more pronounced distribution phases, and/or display nonparallel terminal phases. Further, the antibodies do not always bind the off-target protein in every species; binding is likely dependent upon the species homology of the epitope on the off-target protein and its expression and turnover. Therefore, there can be species differences in PK due to differences in off-target binding. In species in which off-target binding is present, the antibodies tend to clear faster than the species in which there is no off-target binding. Examples of this in the literature include rodent complement 3D binding by a fibroblast growth factor receptor 4–specific antibody (Bumbaca et al., 2011) and fibrinogen binding by an amyloid beta–specific antibody (Vugmeyster et al., 2011).

Immunogenicity, or the development of ADAs, can also contribute to the clearance of monoclonal antibodies (Wang et al., 2008). Most monoclonal antibody therapeutics retain physicochemical properties that are very similar to those of endogenously produced antibodies in order to limit sites that could appear as "foreign" to the immune system; however, even fully human monoclonal antibodies can be immunogenic (Laptos and Omersel, 2018). The type of immune response tends to be polyclonal in nature and affinity can mature over time. ADAs can be neutralizing (inhibiting the activity of the antibody) or nonneutralizing and may have efficacy and/or safety-related ramifications, such as Type IV hypersensitivity (Shankar et al., 2014). Furthermore, ADAs may or may not cause changes in monoclonal antibody exposure (Chirmule et al., 2012). If a change in exposure is observed, it tends to result in a rapid loss in concentration over time and can be observed as early as 7 days postdose (Ovacik and Lin, 2018), as depicted in Figure 4.3. In addition to the physicochemical properties of the antibody, the dose, route of administration, and health of the subject, among other factors, could affect the immunogenic properties of an antibody. Thus, immunogenicity in preclinical species does not usually translate to immunogenicity in patients (Wang et al., 2008). Due to this lack of translatability, there have been many efforts over the years to try to predict clinical immunogenicity risk from in vitro assays, in silico HLA–peptide binding algorithms, and mathematical modeling (Chen et al., 2014a,b; Gokemeijer et al., 2017; Kierzek et al., 2019; Piccoli et al., 2019; Quarmby et al., 2018). The utility of these prediction methods is still to be determined.

Monoclonal Antibody Screening for Acceptable PK Properties

Given the multitude of factors that can negatively affect the exposure of monoclonal antibodies, various assays have been developed to help derisk antibodies early in drug development for PK liabilities. There are assays that have been developed to assess antibodies at high risk for nonspecific binding including the baculovirus assay (Hotzel et al., 2012), FcRn transcytosis assay (Chung et al., 2019; Grevys et al., 2018; Jaramillo et al., 2017), FcRn binding column (Schlothauer et al., 2013), extracellular matrix binding assay (Sampei et al., 2013), and HEK293 cell binding (Datta-Mannan et al., 2015). As charge is a major factor contributing to altered clearance for antibodies, there are also assays designed to assess the risk of electrostatic interactions such as the in silico charge assessment tool (Sharma et al., 2014), heparin binding column (Datta-Mannan et al., 2015; Kraft et al., 2020), 3D homology modeling (Sampei et al., 2013), DNA binding, and insulin binding (Avery et al., 2018). Aggregation propensity can also affect antibody clearance, so there is also an assay that is used to look at the self-association of an antibody called the affinity capture self-interaction nanoparticle spectroscopy assay (Avery et al., 2018). There has also been a link between poor production yields and nonspecific interactions (Wolf Perez et al., 2019). Thus, a combination of nonspecific binding, charge related, and self-association in vitro assays in concert with appropriate in vivo models for assessing PK preclinically has shown to significantly reduce the risk of progressing antibodies with PK liabilities forward into the clinic (Avery et al., 2018; Betts et al., 2018). Historically, antibody PK has translated reasonably well from cynomolgus monkeys to that in humans (Deng et al., 2011; Dong et al., 2011), but there has been some relatively recent work showing the translatability of PK from transgenic mice expressing human FcRn may be even greater (Avery et al., 2016).

Bioanalytical Assays for Assessing Monoclonal Antibody Concentrations

There are several options for detecting monoclonal antibody drug concentration in biological matrices. Understanding what antibody concentration is desired will inform which assay format is the best to select. Figure 4.6 shows the setup for common enzyme-linked immunosorbent assay (ELISA) formats. The free antibody concentration represents the concentration of antibody in the matrix that is not bound to its target or tightly bound to an off-target protein. In order to detect this form of antibody, a bridging assay, antigen capture assay, complementary paired assay, or a competitive assay would suffice. A bridging assay is one in which target or antiidiotypic antibody (anti-Id) is used as the capture and detection reagent. For antigen capture, the target is the capture reagent and anti-Id or antihuman IgG is the detection reagent. In the complementary paired assay, anti-Ids are used for capture and target or antihuman IgG is used for detection. Finally, a competitive assay captures the monoclonal with target or anti-Ids and uses labeled monoclonal for detection (Lee et al., 2011).

The total antibody concentration represents the concentration of antibody in the matrix that is both free and bound to target or another circulating off-target protein. The assay formats that can be used to generate this concentration include a generic bridging assay or a complementary paired assay. The generic bridging assay uses an antihuman IgG for capture and detection. The complementary paired assay uses an anti-CDR antibody for capture and an antihuman IgG for detection. Additionally, the samples can be processed prior to assay analysis in order to aid in the detection of total monoclonal antibody. In one instance, the sample can be preincubated with target. Then that mixture gets added to the capture reagent of antitarget antibody followed by an antihuman IgG or anti-CDR IgG for detection. Alternatively, the sample can be treated with acid to aid in the dissociation of target from the monoclonal, and then the monoclonal can be assayed in any of the assays described for generating the free antibody concentration (Lee et al., 2011).

In addition to selecting which assay format to use to generate the concentration of interest, there is also the option of selecting a platform. Traditionally, antibody drug concentrations are measured using enzyme-linked immunosorbent assays or ELISAs (Ezan et al., 2009; Lee et al., 2011). In an attempt to improve the standard ELISA, a microfluidics platform, The Gyrolab has been developed by Gyros AB (Uppsala, Sweden) and has been gaining popularity due to its small sample requirement and high throughput (Leary et al., 2013; Mora et al., 2010; Yang et al., 2014). The small sample volume required has the added benefit of reducing the number of animals needed for a given study. The sensitivity of this platform seems to be improved over that of traditional ELISAs. Other novel immunoassay platforms with added sensitivity and improved automation that function over the traditional ELISA include Quanterix, Singulex, AlphaLisa, MesoScale Discovery, among others (Comley, 2014).

Besides alternative immunoassay platforms, recently there has been a movement toward using liquid chromatography coupled to mass spectrometry (LC-MS) in order to assess antibody drug concentrations (Faria et al., 2019; Iwamoto and Shimada, 2019; Jenkins et al., 2015). While ELISA requires the intact antibody for detection throughout the assay, LC-MS ultimately digests the monoclonal into peptides and determines its concentration through monitoring the abundance of a specific signal peptide (Ezan et al., 2009). The signal peptide selected determines the specificity and sensitivity of the LC-MS assay; however, in general, sensitivity for biologics in biomatrices is still a challenge that the platform is working to overcome (An et al., 2014).

2.2. PK of Antibody-Based Therapeutics

Other therapeutic modalities have been developed that use variations of the antibody format (see Section 1.2) either through conjugation of cytotoxic drugs (ADCs), the utilization of certain mAb fragments (Fc fusion proteins and scFv), or targeting two antigens, one with each Fab arm (bispecific antibody). The PK of these therapeutics and their similarity to that of antibodies correlates with their size and whether they retain their Fc domain. ADCs, Fc fusion proteins, and bispecific antibodies all contain the Fc domain and, therefore, still retain their ability to bind to FcRn,

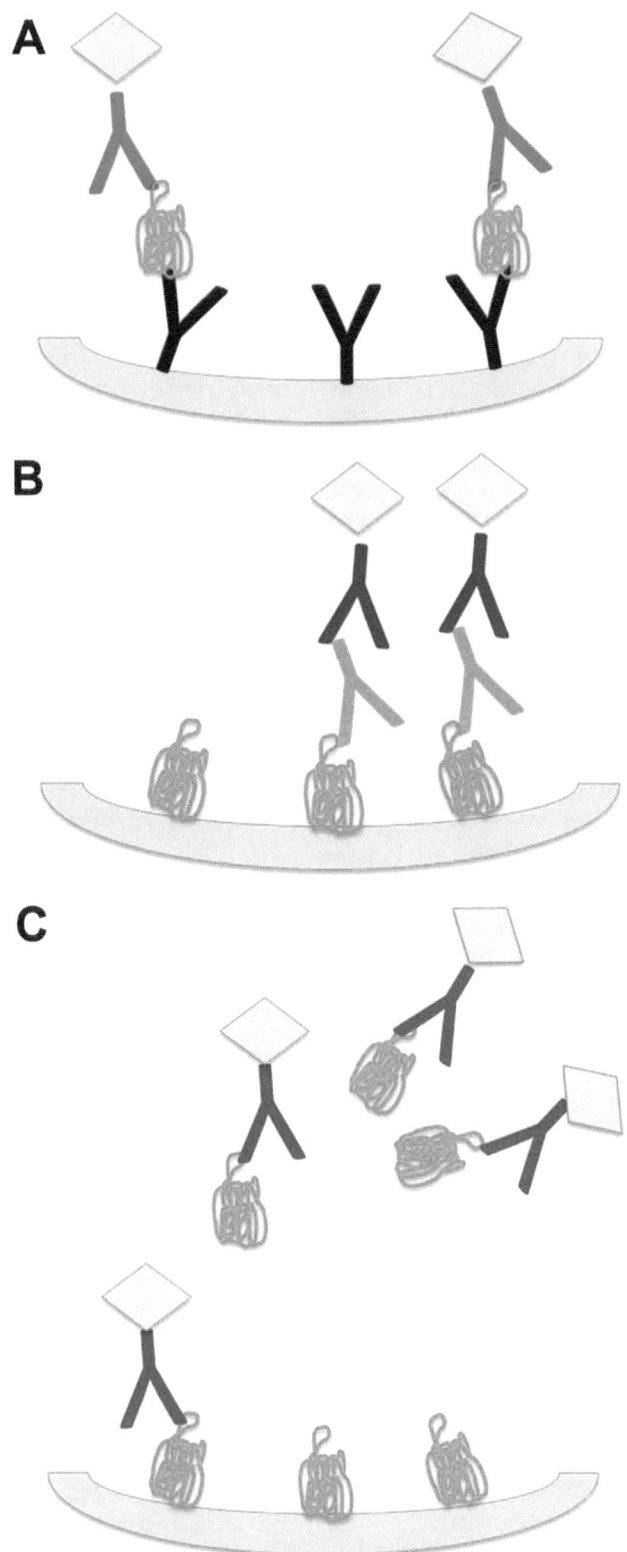

FIGURE 4.6 **Common bioanalytical assay formats.** A complementary paired or sandwich ELISA is depicted in (A). The capture antibody is black, the test material is in blue squiggles, and the labeled detecting antibody is in red. An antigen capture or indirect ELISA is depicted in (B). The target capture is in blue squiggles, the test material is pink, and the labeled detecting antibody is in purple. A competitive ELISA is depicted in (C). The target capture is in blue squiggles and the labeled test material is in blue. *Reprinted from Basic Science Methods for Clinical Reseachers, Drijvers JM, Awan IM, Perugino, CA, Rosenberg IM, Pillai S: Chap 7* - The enzyme-linked immunosorbent assay: the application of elisa in clinical research, *pp. 119–133, Copyright (2017), with permission from Elsevier.*

maintaining relatively long systemic half-lives (Chen and Xu, 2017; Hedrich et al., 2018; Unverdorben et al., 2015). ADCs and bispecific antibodies have PK properties most like that of a traditional monoclonal antibody, including a low volume of distribution (Chen and Xu, 2017; Hedrich et al., 2018). Depending on the degree of hydrophobicity of the cytotoxic drug conjugated to the antibody and how many, an ADC can display faster clearance than its unconjugated antibody counterpart due to enhanced catabolism in the liver (Boswell et al., 2011; Lyon et al., 2015). In a large majority of cases, bispecific antibodies have similar PK as their monospecific antibody counterparts; however, it has been shown that some bispecific antibodies that are larger than monoclonal antibodies can be cleared faster via liver sinusoidal endothelial cells (Datta-Mannan et al., 2016). Fc fusion protein PK is not only driven by the Fc domain but also by the physicochemical properties of the protein to which the Fc is fused in addition to the systemic integrity of the peptide linker itself. These constructs have a relatively long systemic half-life, but not as long as that of a traditional antibody due to lower binding affinity to FcRn. Additionally, for Fc fusion proteins smaller than 150 kDa, they can have greater tissue penetration than mAbs (Li et al., 2016; Liu, 2018). Unlike traditional mAbs, glycosylation greatly impacts the PK of Fc fusion proteins, specifically sialylation. There have been reports showing the correlation of higher SA leading to higher systemic exposure (Liu, 2018). ScFvs, in contrast, are ~30 kDa fragments that do not have Fc domains, and therefore, have relatively short systemic half-lives. Ahamadi-Fesharaki et al. provide a nice review of scFvs currently in Clinical Trials (Ahamadi-Fesharaki et al., 2019). Their small size enables greater tissue distribution than their mAb counterpart and the lack of the Fc provides the added benefit of reducing immunogenicity (Monnier et al., 2013). The structure of the antibody-based therapeutic will influence the selection of the bioanalytical assay format chosen for determining drug concentrations.

2.3. PK of Other Biotherapeutic Modalities

The PK of proteins lacking the FcRn backbone show typically fast clearance with short half-lives unless a half-life extension mechanism has been put in place to improve exposure. In general, small proteins (<60 KDa) are small enough to be excreted by renal filtration (Jia et al., 2009), although the shape and hydrodynamic radius of a drug can also influence renal filtration allowing for larger proteins to pass through (Ruggiero et al., 2010). Beyond that, the catabolism of protein biotherapeutics results in degradation into small peptides and amino acids via target-specific and nontarget–specific mechanisms, with the turnover of nonsalvaged proteins in the order of hours or minutes.

On the other hand, other novel biotherapeutics are often referred as "living drugs" (including, for example, cell and gene therapy) and their exposure is the result of an entire different set of phenomenon including cell population expansion and contractions; and cell persistence (that could be compared to the terminal phase of a typical small or large molecule PK profile) can be as long as months or years in some cases.

3. PHARMACODYNAMICS OF BIOTHERAPEUTICS

The targets for monoclonal antibodies can be plasma soluble proteins or cell surface receptors. The mechanism of action can be broadly classified into the following four categories (as depicted in Figure 4.7) (Lobo et al., 2004; Secher et al., 2018; Wang et al., 2008):

- Antibody binds to soluble protein and prevents binding to their cognate receptors
- Antibody binds to cell surface receptor and blocks binding of endogenous ligand to the receptor
- Agonist activity by antibody binds to cell surface receptor and activating downstream signaling
- Antibody binds to cell surface receptor resulting in cell depletion

Understanding the mechanism of action and the target pharmacology is critical not only in the design of the monoclonal antibody but is also relevant in the preclinical and clinical development for the antibody to achieve the desired therapeutic benefit and minimize safety liabilities. Here we describe these mechanisms with examples for each category.

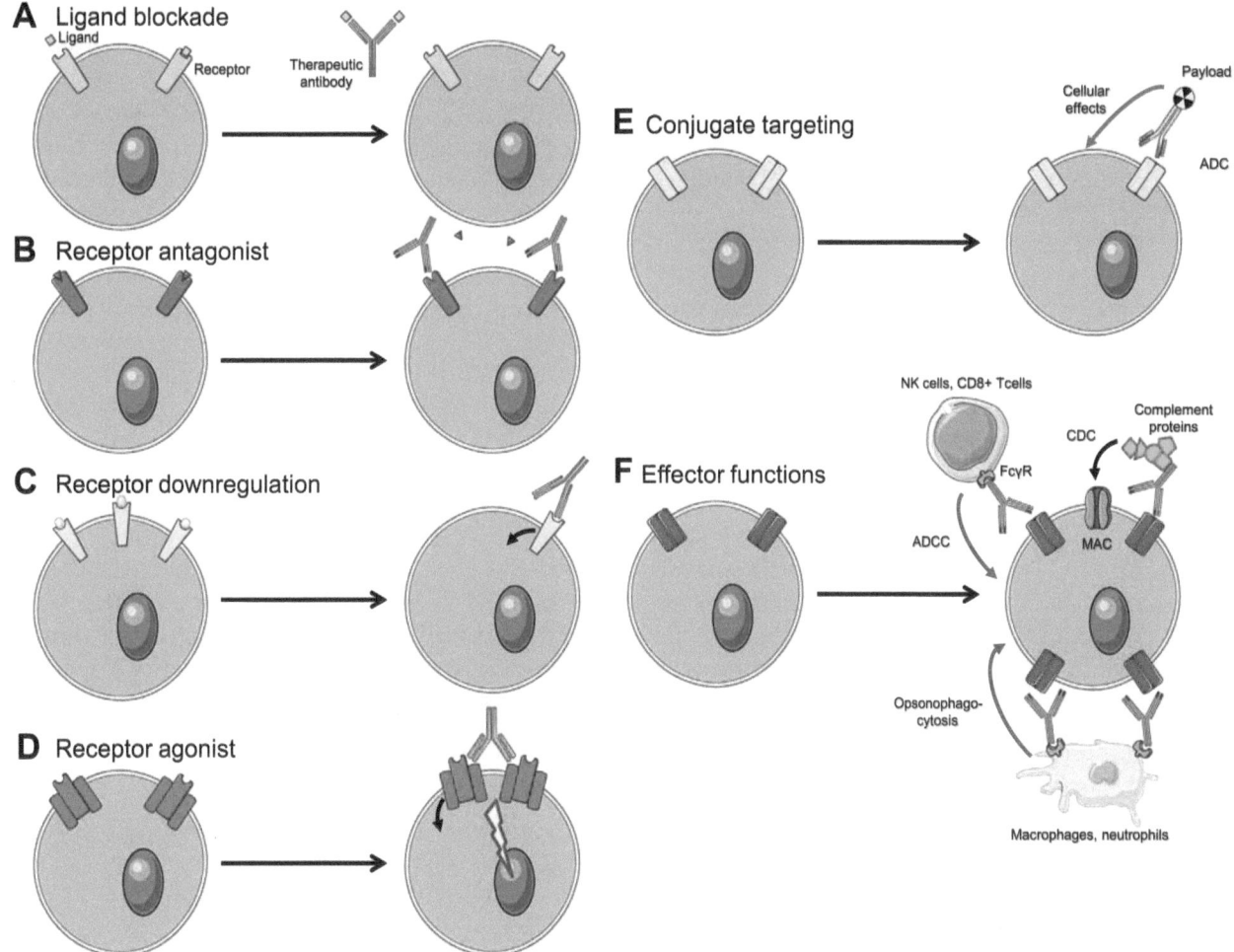

FIGURE 4.7 **Antibody mechanism of action.** (A) Ligand blockade with antibodies will prevent ligands from activating their cognate receptors. (B) Signal transduction by ligands may also be blocked by antibodies that target the cognate receptors and inhibit their activation and function. (C) Ab binding can also result in receptor internalization and downregulation. (D) In contrast, antibodies may act as agonists for specific receptors and induce activation signals. (E) Antibody–drug conjugates (ADCs) use the Ab's specificity to precisely deliver the payload drug (a radio/chemotherapeutic, antibiotic, or cytokine) to the target cell. (F) Binding of antibodies to surface antigens can result in cell depletion via Ab-dependent cell cytotoxicity (ADCC), complement-dependent cytotoxicity (CDC), and opsonophagocytosis. *Reprinted from Pharmacology & Therapeutics, Vol 189, Sécher T, Guilleminault L, Reckamp K, Amanam I, Plantier L, Heuzé-Vourc'h N: Therapeutic antibodies: A new era in the treatment of respiratory diseases?, pp. 149–172, Copyright (2018), with permission from Elsevier.*

Antagonistic antibody against soluble target. In this mechanism of action, the monoclonal antibody binds to a soluble target and prevents it from binding to its cognate receptor. This subsequently prevents receptor activation and downstream signaling. This inhibition leads to the desired therapeutic effect, which is determined by the extent of neutralization of the soluble target and reducing its influence on the underlying pathophysiology.

Typically, soluble targets have fast turnover (in the order of magnitude of minutes to hours) and require close to complete neutralization for therapeutic benefit. As a result of this, the desired binding affinity of the antibody for the target is high (typically $K_d < 100–200pM$). One example of a monoclonal antibody in this category is adalimumab, an approved medication in inflammatory diseases such rheumatoid arthritis, Crohn's disease, ulcerative colitis, and psoriasis and works by neutralizing tumor necrosis factor alpha, a cytokine playing a primary role in the disease inflammation. A second example is ranibizumab that is used for its antiangiogenesis activity in age-related macular degeneration by neutralizing Vascular endothelial growth factor.

Antagonist antibody against cell surface receptor target. This antagonistic mechanism is similar to the previous scenario except that the antibody is designed to bind to a surface receptor instead of the soluble protein. In binding the surface receptor, the antibody blocks the receptor from binding to its natural ligand, preventing activation and downstream signaling. The antibody design should be such that once it binds to the receptor it should be at a site that blocks the natural ligand from binding. Also, the dosing regimen and antibody affinity should be such as to compete with the natural ligand from binding. Moreover, to maximize therapeutic benefit, a high fraction of the receptors is required to be blocked. Thus, for this scenario, both the target receptor dynamics and the dynamics of the receptor's ligand are factors for consideration.

Tocilizumab (anti–IL-6R) is an immunosuppressive drug that is a good example of a monoclonal antibody in this category of mechanism of action. Tocilizumab binds to IL-6R and blocks binding to the natural ligand IL-6 cytokine, which plays an important role in the immune response and is implicated in the pathogenesis of many autoimmune diseases including rheumatoid arthritis. Another example in this category is an immune check point inhibitor anti-PD1 (pembrolizumab and nivolumab). PD1 is a protein on the surface of T-cells that has a role in downregulating the immune system and promoting self-tolerance by suppressing T-cell inflammatory activity to prevent autoimmune diseases. However, this mechanism also prevents the immune system from killing cancer cells. The anti-PD1 antibodies bind the PD1 protein, downregulating its activity and have been approved in several cancer indications.

Agonist antibody against cell surface receptor. In this mechanism of action, the antibody is designed to bind its surface receptor target to lead to activation of downstream signaling. Here, the antibody mimics the role of the physiological ligand of the target receptor. In terms of antibody design and dosing, one important criterion is to keep the activation only on the cells where activity is desired and avoid unregulated increase in activity. Discovery and development of antibodies with agonist mechanisms is challenging, with clinical trials ongoing in oncology indications. A few examples of antibodies in this category include anti-OX40 and anti-GITR.

Antibody binding to surface receptor resulting in cell cytotoxicity. In this scenario, the desired therapeutic effect is depletion of a desired cell. The antibody is designed to bind to a surface receptor target preferentially expressed on the desired cell. Once the antibody binds to the target, the mechanism of killing involves recruitment of complement proteins, phagocytes, or natural killer (NK) cells, which can promote immune-mediated destruction of the cell. Recruitment of immune mediators generally occurs through interactions with the Fc portion of the monoclonal antibody. Fc receptors can modulate the cell killing effects by recruiting effector cells to effect ADCC or ADCP by monocytes, macrophages or NK cells. Fc receptors can also promote cell death via CDC, by activation of the complement cascade after the antibody binds to the target. Some antibodies have features of both ADCC and CDC. Rituximab is a good example in this category. Rituximab is an antibody against cell surface protein CD20, which is expressed primarily on B cells. It is used in the treatment of autoimmune diseases (RA) and lymphoma indications for targeted killing of B cells by both ADCC and CDC mechanisms. In addition to ADCC and CDC activity, rituximab is also shown to induce apoptosis activity by alteration of downstream signaling by the CD20 protein.

In addition to these mechanisms of action, biologics have been designed to explore other mechanisms. ADCs combine monoclonal antibodies specific to surface antigens present on particular tumor cells with highly potent anticancer agents linked via a chemical linker. Another class of biologics is T-cell bispecific antibodies, which are designed to simultaneously bind to T-cells and tumor cell antigens, leading to T-cell activation, proliferation, and tumor cell death. Antibody engineering research continues to modify biologics either to enhance existing mechanisms or to invoke new mechanisms. A detailed overview of these is out of scope for the current section Pharmacokinetic and Pharmacodynamic Modeling and Interspecies translation.

4. PK–PD MODELING AND INTERSPECIES SCALING

The role of PK–PD or PK/PD modeling is to provide quantitative relationships between the exposure of one or more administered drugs (PK) and the anticipated or observed effect or response (PD) in an in vivo system. In the preclinical stages, PK/PD models establish proof of activity of the drug on the desired target. This relationship can be used to understand and quantify the mechanism of action of the drug, and inform lead candidate characterization and selection. In the clinical setting, a key aspect of the PK/PD models is the exploration of the variability in both the PK and PD measurements and more importantly in the relationship between the two. For clinical applications, PK/PD models are primarily used for patient selection and dose optimization for clinical trials.

The simplest forms of PK/PD models include direct (Meibohm and Derendorf, 1997) and indirect response models (Jusko and Ko, 1994) that capture synchronic and delayed effects between PK and PD, respectively. The effect can be agonistic or inhibitory and is represented based on the underlying understanding of the pathways being impacted by the drug. For PD measurements that are the direct target of the drug, target-mediated drug disposition models (Mager and Jusko, 2001) are utilized to represent target engagement by the drug influencing the dynamics of both the drug and the target. There are no limitations in the degree of complexity that is included in PK/PD models. Based on the availability of data and an understanding of the underlying biology that is impacted by the drug, the scope and mathematical implementation of these models are determined to be "fit for purpose" for the desired application. With the increase in complexity, these models may be referred to in the literature as semimechanistic or mechanistic models with an emphasis on capturing the mechanism of action of the drug and its downstream effects in the model. Quantitative systems pharmacology models include the dynamic interactions between drug(s) and a biological system that aims to understand the behavior of the system as a whole, as opposed to the behavior of its individual constituents (Benson and van der Graaf, 2014; Sorger et al., 2011; van Hasselt and van der Graaf, 2015).

One of the most fundamental applications of PK–PD models lies on the interspecies scaling (also referred as interspecies translation) where models built based on one or more preclinical species are "translated" to predict clinical PK–PD relationship. In general, PK and PD of protein therapeutics are translated separately. For PK translation, the two most common approaches used are allometric scaling and the time-invariant methods.

Allometric scaling. The allometric scaling approach to estimate human PK consists of extrapolating PK parameters obtained in preclinical species based on body size and weight. Typical approaches for small molecules use multiple species to make the human predictions. However, for monoclonal antibodies, retrospective analysis has shown that human PK is better predicted based on cynomolgus monkey alone using allometric exponents of 0.85 and 1 for clearance and volume of distribution values, respectively (Deng et al., 2011). Recently, the use of human FcRn expressing mice has shown promise in clinical predictability as well, utilizing allometric exponents of 0.9 and 1 for clearance and volume, respectively (Avery et al., 2016). Prediction for antibody-based therapeutics and other therapeutic proteins many times leverages this same approach; however, less is understood about the validity of this approach for formats beyond monoclonal antibodies.

Species-invariant time method. Another approach that is taken to predict human PK is the species-invariant time method. This methodology provides a prediction of the concentration–time profile in humans based on that of observed in preclinical species and scaling exponents separately chosen based on whether for soluble or for membrane-bound targets. Accordingly, this approach has been successfully used when target-mediated drug disposition is believed to play a role in the overall PK profile; however, this approach must be used with caution since it assumes scalability of target properties (such expression levels, internalization rate, etc.) and antibody properties (such as affinity) across different species (Dedrick, 1973).

Translation of the PD components of PK–PD models must consider different aspects of the biology and pharmacology across species, relevance of preclinical models used to build the PK–PD model and drug candidate properties that can vary from one species to other (Jones and Rowland-Yeo, 2013; Mager and Jusko, 2008; Stroh et al., 2014).

5. SUMMARY

In all, biotherapeutics have unlocked a myriad of therapeutic alternatives for diseases with high unmet needs, enabling pharmacological strategies that would otherwise be not feasible using small molecule approaches. By far, the most utilized format in biologics is the monoclonal antibody or antibody-based therapeutic modality that leverages both the ability of these molecules to interact with the immune system as well as the FcRn-mediated salvage mechanism that results in their characteristic prolonged exposure.

Antibody PK typically can be characterized by a biphasic concentration–time profile with a relatively short distribution phase (that can be explained by their limited tissue distribution into tissues, as illustrated by the volume of distribution approximating that of plasma volume) followed by a relatively long elimination phase (governed by their elimination via nonspecific pinocytosis and proteolysis by the reticuloendothelial system and interactions with FcRn receptor). Many factors that can influence the absorption, distribution, and elimination of monoclonal antibodies include charge, hydrophobicity, Man content, FcRn affinity, target biology, immunogenicity, and subject physiology, among others. Screening assays have been developed in order to help derisk antibodies at risk for poor PK properties early in the drug development process. Beyond antibodies and antibody-based therapeutics, a wide range of therapeutic modalities from small peptides to living cells are being explored with a growing body of preclinical and clinical knowledge being built, as we leverage these therapeutic alternatives. In all, the design and development of these modalities for therapeutic benefit must be driven primarily by the intended mechanism of action. Furthermore, the target pharmacology impacts modality design and development plans. Biotherapeutics continue to be optimized to maximize the therapeutic benefit while maintaining the desired safety profiles. These enhancements could include, but are not limited to, improving target affinity, increasing antibody half-life, and enhancement or elimination of ADCC and CDC activity.

REFERENCES

Ahamadi-Fesharaki R, Fateh A, Vaziri F, et al.: Single-chain variable fragment-based bispecific antibodies: hitting two targets with one sophisticated arrow, *Mol Ther Oncolytics* 14:38–56, 2019.

An B, Zhang M, Qu J: Toward sensitive and accurate analysis of antibody biotherapeutics by liquid chromatography coupled with mass spectrometry, *Drug Metab Dispos* 42: 1858–1866, 2014.

Avery LB, Wade J, Wang M, et al.: Establishing in vitro in vivo correlations to screen monoclonal antibodies for physicochemical properties related to favorable human pharmacokinetics, *mAbs* 10:244–255, 2018.

Avery LB, Wang M, Kavosi MS, et al.: Utility of a human FcRn transgenic mouse model in drug discovery for early assessment and prediction of human pharmacokinetics of monoclonal antibodies, *mAbs* 8:1064–1078, 2016.

Baggio LL, Huang Q, Cao X, et al.: An albumin-exendin-4 conjugate engages central and peripheral circuits regulating murine energy and glucose homeostasis, *Gastroenterology* 134:1137–1147, 2008.

Banks WA, Farr SA, Morley JE, et al.: Anti-amyloid beta protein antibody passage across the blood-brain barrier in the SAMP8 mouse model of Alzheimer's disease: an age-related selective uptake with reversal of learning impairment, *Exp Neurol* 206:248–256, 2007.

Bemani P, Mohammadi M, Hakakian A: ScFv improvement approaches, *Protein Pept Lett* 25:222–229, 2018.

Benson N, van der Graaf PH: The rise of systems pharmacology in drug discovery and development, *Future Med Chem* 6:1731–1734, 2014.

Betts A, Keunecke A, van Steeg TJ, et al.: Linear pharmacokinetic parameters for monoclonal antibodies are similar within a species and across different pharmacological targets: a comparison between human, cynomolgus monkey and hFcRn Tg32 transgenic mouse using a population-modeling approach, *mAbs* 10:751–764, 2018.

Bhatt RR, Haurum JS, Davis CG: Technologies for the generation of human antibodies. In Tabrizi MA, Bornstein GG, Klakamp SL, editors: *Development of antibody-based therapeutics: translational considerations*, New York, NY, 2018, Springer, pp 33–63.

Bittner B, Richter W, Schmidt J: Subcutaneous administration of biotherapeutics: an overview of current challenges and opportunities, *Biodrugs* 32:425–440, 2018.

Boswell CA, Mundo EE, Zhang C, et al.: Impact of drug conjugation on pharmacokinetics and tissue distribution of anti-STEAP1 antibody-drug conjugates in rats, *Bioconjugate Chem* 22:1994–2004, 2011.

Boswell CA, Tesar DB, Mukhyala K, et al.: Effects of charge on antibody tissue distribution and pharmacokinetics, *Bioconjugate Chem* 21:2153–2163, 2010.

Braen AP, Perron J, Tellier P, et al.: A 4-week intrathecal toxicity and pharmacokinetic study with trastuzumab in cynomolgus monkeys, *Int J Toxicol* 29:259–267, 2010.

Braendstrup P, Levine BL, Ruella M: The long road to the first FDA-approved gene therapy: chimeric antigen receptor T cells targeting CD19, *Cytotherapy* 22:57–69, 2020.

Brandish PE, Palmieri A, Antonenko S, et al.: Development of anti-CD74 antibody-drug conjugates to target glucocorticoids to immune cells, *Bioconjugate Chem* 29:2357–2369, 2018.

Bumbaca D, Boswell CA, Fielder PJ, et al.: Physiochemical and biochemical factors influencing the pharmacokinetics of antibody therapeutics, *AAPS J* 14:554–558, 2012.

Bumbaca D, Wong A, Drake E, et al.: Highly specific off-target binding identified and eliminated during the humanization of an antibody against FGF receptor 4, *mAbs* 3:376–386, 2011.

Bumbaca Yadav D, Sharma VK, Boswell CA, et al.: Evaluating the use of antibody variable region (Fv) charge as a risk assessment tool for predicting typical cynomolgus monkey pharmacokinetics, *J Biol Chem* 290:29732–29741, 2015.

Calias P, Banks WA, Begley D, et al.: Intrathecal delivery of protein therapeutics to the brain: a critical reassessment, *Pharmacol Ther* 144:114–122, 2014.

Chen X, Hickling TP, Vicini P: A mechanistic, multiscale mathematical model of immunogenicity for therapeutic proteins: part 1-theoretical model, *CPT Pharmacometrics Syst Pharmacol* 3:e133, 2014a.

Chen X, Hickling TP, Vicini P: A mechanistic, multiscale mathematical model of immunogenicity for therapeutic proteins: part 2-model applications, *CPT Pharmacometrics Syst Pharmacol* 3:e134, 2014b.

Chen X, Liu YD, Flynn GC: The effect of Fc glycan forms on human IgG2 antibody clearance in humans, *Glycobiology* 19:240–249, 2009.

Chen Y, Xu Y: Pharmacokinetics of bispecific antibody, *Curr Pharmacol Rep* 3:126–137, 2017.

Chirila TV, Hong Y: *Handbook of biomaterial properties*, ed 2, 2016, Springer.

Chirmule N, Jawa V, Meibohm B: Immunogenicity to therapeutic proteins: impact on PK/PD and efficacy, *AAPS J* 14: 296–302, 2012.

Chung S, Nguyen V, Lin YL, et al.: An in vitro FcRn- dependent transcytosis assay as a screening tool for predictive assessment of nonspecific clearance of antibody therapeutics in humans, *mAbs* 11:942–955, 2019.

ClinicalTrials.gov: *A study to evaluate the safety, tolerability, pharmacokinetics, and efficacy of ABBV-3373 in participants with moderate to severe rheumatoid arthritis - full text view - ClinicalTrials.gov*, 2019.

Colozza M, Minenza E, Gori S, et al.: Extended survival of a HER-2-positive metastatic breast cancer patient with brain metastases also treated with intrathecal trastuzumab, *Cancer Chemother Pharmacol* 63:1157–1159, 2009.

Comley J: *Immunoassay automation: hands-free platforms set to change the workflow in research labs*, 2014, Drug Discov Workd.

Csaky KG, Gordiyenko N, Rabena MG, Avery RL: Pharmacokinetics of intravitreal bevacizumab in humans, *Investig Ophthalmol Visual Sci* 48:4936, 2007.

Dall'Acqua WF, Kiener PA, Wu H: Properties of human IgG1s engineered for enhanced binding to the neonatal Fc receptor (FcRn), *J Biol Chem* 281:23514–23524, 2006.

Datta-Mannan A, Croy JE, Schirtzinger L, et al.: Aberrant bispecific antibody pharmacokinetics linked to liver sinusoidal endothelium clearance mechanism in cynomolgus monkeys, *mAbs* 8:969–982, 2016.

Datta-Mannan A, Thangaraju A, Leung D, et al.: Balancing charge in the complementarity-determining regions of humanized mAbs without affecting pI reduces non-specific binding and improves the pharmacokinetics, *mAbs* 7:483–493, 2015.

Dedrick RL: Animal scale-up, *J Pharmacokinet Biopharm* 1:435–461, 1973.

Deng R, Iyer S, Theil FP, et al.: Projecting human pharmacokinetics of therapeutic antibodies from nonclinical data: what have we learned? *mAbs* 3:61–66, 2011.

Deng R, Loyet KM, Lien S, et al.: Pharmacokinetics of humanized monoclonal anti-tumor necrosis factor-alpha antibody and its neonatal Fc receptor variants in mice and cynomolgus monkeys, *Drug Metab Dispos* 38:600–605, 2010.

Dobson CL, Devine PW, Phillips JJ, et al.: Engineering the surface properties of a human monoclonal antibody prevents self-association and rapid clearance in vivo, *Sci Rep* 6:38644, 2016.

Dong JQ, Salinger DH, Endres CJ, et al.: Quantitative prediction of human pharmacokinetics for monoclonal antibodies: retrospective analysis of monkey as a single species for first-in-human prediction, *Clin Pharmacokinet* 50:131–142, 2011.

Dubois M, Fenaille F, Clement G, et al.: Immunopurification and mass spectrometric quantification of the active form of a chimeric therapeutic antibody in human serum, *Anal Chem* 80:1737–1745, 2008.

Ezan E, Dubois M, Becher F: Bioanalysis of recombinant proteins and antibodies by mass spectrometry, *Analyst* 134: 825–834, 2009.

Faria M, Peay M, Lam B, et al.: Multiplex LC-MS/MS assays for clinical bioanalysis of MEDI4276, an antibody-drug conjugate of tubulysin analogue attached via cleavable linker to a biparatopic humanized antibody against HER-2, *Antibodies* 8, 2019.

Fishburn CS: The pharmacology of PEGylation: balancing PD with PK to generate novel therapeutics, *J Pharmaceut Sci* 97: 4167–4183, 2008.

Gokemeijer J, Jawa V, Mitra-Kaushik S: How close are we to profiling immunogenicity risk using in silico algorithms and in vitro methods?: an industry perspective, *AAPS J* 19: 1587–1592, 2017.

Golchin A, Farahany TZ: Biological products: cellular therapy and FDA approved products, *Stem Cell Rev Rep* 15:166–175, 2019.

Goyon A, Excoffier M, Janin-Bussat MC, et al.: Determination of isoelectric points and relative charge variants of 23 therapeutic monoclonal antibodies, *J Chromatogr B Analyt Technol Biomed Life Sci* 1065–1066:119–128, 2017.

Grevys A, Nilsen J, Sand KMK, et al.: A human endothelial cell-based recycling assay for screening of FcRn targeted molecules, *Nat Commun* 9:621, 2018.

Hamidi M, Azadi A, Rafiei P: Pharmacokinetic consequences of pegylation, *Drug Deliv* 13:399–409, 2006.

Harris JM, Martin NE, Modi M: Pegylation: a novel process for modifying pharmacokinetics, *Clin Pharmacokinet* 40:539–551, 2001.

Harris RJ: Heterogeneity of recombinant antibodies: linking structure to function, *Dev Biol* 122:117–127, 2005.

Hedrich WD, Fandy TE, Ashour HM, et al.: Antibody-drug conjugates: pharmacokinetic/pharmacodynamic modeling, preclinical characterization, clinical studies, and lessons learned, *Clin Pharmacokinet* 57:687–703, 2018.

Herve F, Ghinea N, Scherrmann JM: CNS delivery via adsorptive transcytosis, *AAPS J* 10:455–472, 2008.

Hotzel I, Theil FP, Bernstein LJ, et al.: A strategy for risk mitigation of antibodies with fast clearance, *mAbs* 4:753–760, 2012.

Igawa T, Haraya K, Hattori K: Sweeping antibody as a novel therapeutic antibody modality capable of eliminating soluble antigens from circulation, *Immunol Rev* 270:132–151, 2016.

Igawa T, Maeda A, Haraya K, et al.: Engineered monoclonal antibody with novel antigen-sweeping activity in vivo, *PloS One* 8:e63236, 2013.

Igawa T, Tsunoda H, Tachibana T, et al.: Reduced elimination of IgG antibodies by engineering the variable region, *Protein Eng Des Sel* 23:385–392, 2010.

Iliff JJ, Wang M, Liao Y, et al.: A paravascular pathway facilitates CSF flow through the brain parenchyma and the clearance of interstitial solutes, including amyloid beta, *Sci Transl Med* 4:147ra111, 2012.

Iwamoto N, Shimada T: Regulated LC-MS/MS bioanalysis technology for therapeutic antibodies and Fc-fusion proteins using structure-indicated approach, *Drug Metabol Pharmacokinet* 34:19–24, 2019.

Jafari R, Zolbanin NM, Rafatpanah H, et al.: Fc-fusion proteins in therapy: an updated view, *Curr Med Chem* 24:1228–1237, 2017.

Jaramillo CAC, Belli S, Cascais AC, et al.: Toward in vitro-to-in vivo translation of monoclonal antibody pharmacokinetics: application of a neonatal Fc receptor-mediated transcytosis assay to understand the interplaying clearance mechanisms, *mAbs* 9:781–791, 2017.

Jefferis R: Antibody therapeutics: isotype and glycoform selection, *Expet Opin Biol Ther* 7:1401–1413, 2007.

Jenkins R, Duggan JX, Aubry AF, et al.: Recommendations for validation of LC-MS/MS bioanalytical methods for protein biotherapeutics, *AAPS J* 17:1–16, 2015.

Jia L, Zhang L, Shao C, et al.: An attempt to understand kidney's protein handling function by comparing plasma and urine proteomes, *PloS One* 4:e5146, 2009.

Jones H, Rowland-Yeo K: Basic concepts in physiologically based pharmacokinetic modeling in drug discovery and development, *CPT Pharmacometrics Syst Pharmacol* 2:e63, 2013.

Jusko WJ, Ko HC: Physiologic indirect response models characterize diverse types of pharmacodynamic effects, *Clin Pharmacol Ther* 56:406–419, 1994.

Kamath AV: Translational pharmacokinetics and pharmacodynamics of monoclonal antibodies, *Drug Discov Today Technol* 21–22:75–83, 2016.

Kanda Y, Yamane-Ohnuki N, Sakai N, et al.: Comparison of cell lines for stable production of fucose-negative antibodies with enhanced ADCC, *Biotechnol Bioeng* 94:680–688, 2006.

Keizer RJ, Huitema AD, Schellens JH, et al.: Clinical pharmacokinetics of therapeutic monoclonal antibodies, *Clin Pharmacokinet* 49:493–507, 2010.

Khongorzul P, Ling CJ, Khan FU, et al.: Antibody-drug conjugates: a comprehensive review, *Mol Cancer Res* 18:3–19, 2020.

Kierzek AM, Hickling TP, Figueroa I, et al.: A quantitative systems pharmacology consortium approach to managing immunogenicity of therapeutic proteins, *CPT Pharmacometrics Syst Pharmacol* 8:773–776, 2019.

Kobayashi H, Le N, Kim IS, et al.: The pharmacokinetic characteristics of glycolated humanized anti-tac fabs are determined by their isoelectric points, *Cancer Res* 59:422–430, 1999.

Kraft TE, Richter WF, Emrich T, et al.: Heparin chromatography as an in vitro predictor for antibody clearance rate through pinocytosis, *mAbs* 12:1683432, 2020.

Labrijn AF, Janmaat ML, Reichert JM, et al.: Bispecific antibodies: a mechanistic review of the pipeline, *Nat Rev Drug Discov* 18:585–608, 2019.

Laptos T, Omersel J: The importance of handling high-value biologicals: physico-chemical instability and immunogenicity of monoclonal antibodies, *Exp Ther Med* 15:3161–3168, 2018.

Leary BA, Lawrence-Henderson R, Mallozzi C, et al.: Bioanalytical platform comparison using a generic human IgG PK assay format, *J Immunol Methods* 397:28–36, 2013.

Lee HJ, Pardridge WM: Monoclonal antibody radiopharmaceuticals: cationization, pegylation, radiometal chelation, pharmacokinetics, and tumor imaging, *Bioconjugate Chem* 14:546–553, 2003.

Lee JW, Kelley M, King LE, et al.: Bioanalytical approaches to quantify "total" and "free" therapeutic antibodies and their targets: technical challenges and PK/PD applications over the course of drug development, *AAPS J* 13:99–110, 2011.

Lehar SM, Pillow T, Xu M, et al.: Novel antibody-antibiotic conjugate eliminates intracellular *S. aureus*, *Nature* 527: 323–328, 2015.

Li B, Tesar D, Boswell CA, et al.: Framework selection can influence pharmacokinetics of a humanized therapeutic antibody through differences in molecule charge, *mAbs* 6: 1255–1264, 2014.

Li Z, Krippendorff BF, Sharma S, et al.: Influence of molecular size on tissue distribution of antibody fragments, *mAbs* 8: 113–119, 2016.

Lim RK, Yu S, Cheng B, et al.: Targeted delivery of LXR agonist using a site-specific antibody-drug conjugate, *Bioconjugate Chem* 26:2216–2222, 2015.

Liu L: Pharmacokinetics of monoclonal antibodies and Fc-fusion proteins, *Protein Cell* 9:15–32, 2018.

Liu R, Wang RE, Wang F: Antibody-drug conjugates for non-oncological indications, *Expet Opin Biol Ther* 16:591–593, 2016.

Lobo ED, Hansen RJ, Balthasar JP: Antibody pharmacokinetics and pharmacodynamics, *J Pharmaceut Sci* 93:2645–2668, 2004.

Lyon RP, Bovee TD, Doronina SO, et al.: Reducing hydrophobicity of homogeneous antibody-drug conjugates improves pharmacokinetics and therapeutic index, *Nat Biotechnol* 33:733–735, 2015.

Mager DE, Jusko WJ: General pharmacokinetic model for drugs exhibiting target-mediated drug disposition, *J Pharmacokinet Pharmacodyn* 28:507–532, 2001.

Mager DE, Jusko WJ: Development of translational pharmacokinetic-pharmacodynamic models, *Clin Pharmacol Ther* 83:909–912, 2008.

Mandikian D, Figueroa I, Oldendorp A, et al.: Tissue physiology of cynomolgus monkeys: cross-species comparison and implications for translational pharmacology, *AAPS J* 20:107, 2018.

Mariathasan S, Tan MW: Antibody-antibiotic conjugates: a novel therapeutic platform against bacterial infections, *Trends Mol Med* 23:135–149, 2017.

McDonald TA, Zepeda ML, Tomlinson MJ, et al.: Subcutaneous administration of biotherapeutics: current experience in animal models, *Curr Opin Mol Therapeut* 12:461–470, 2010.

Meibohm B, Derendorf H: Basic concepts of pharmacokinetic/pharmacodynamic (PK/PD) modelling, *Int J Clin Pharmacol Ther* 35:401–413, 1997.

Missel PJ, Sarangapani R: Physiologically based ocular pharmacokinetic modeling using computational methods, *Drug Discov Today* 24:1551–1563, 2019.

Monnier PP, Vigouroux RJ, Tassew NG: In vivo applications of single chain Fv (variable domain) (scFv) fragments, *Antibodies* 2:193–208, 2013.

Mora JR, Obenauer-Kutner L, Vimal Patel V: Application of the Gyrolab platform to ligand-binding assays: a user's perspective, *Bioanalysis* 2:1711–1715, 2010.

Ovacik M, Lin K: Tutorial on monoclonal antibody pharmacokinetics and its considerations in early development, *Clin Transl Sci* 11:540–552, 2018.

Peletier LA, Gabrielsson J: Dynamics of target-mediated drug disposition: characteristic profiles and parameter identification, *J Pharmacokinet Pharmacodyn* 39:429–451, 2012.

Piccoli S, Mehta D, Vitaliti A, et al.: 2019 White paper on recent issues in bioanalysis: FDA immunogenicity guidance, gene therapy, critical reagents, biomarkers and flow cytometry validation (part 3 - recommendations on 2019 FDA immunogenicity guidance, gene therapy bioanalytical challenges, strategies for critical reagent management, biomarker assay validation, flow cytometry validation & CLSI H62), *Bioanalysis* 11:2207–2244, 2019.

Quarmby V, Phung QT, Lill JR: MAPPs for the identification of immunogenic hotspots of biotherapeutics; an overview of the technology and its application to the biopharmaceutical arena, *Expert Rev Proteomics* 15:733–748, 2018.

Richter WF, Bhansali SG, Morris ME: Mechanistic determinants of biotherapeutics absorption following SC administration, *AAPS J* 14:559–570, 2012.

Richter WF, Christianson GJ, Frances N, et al.: Hematopoietic cells as site of first-pass catabolism after subcutaneous dosing and contributors to systemic clearance of a monoclonal antibody in mice, *mAbs* 10:803–813, 2018.

Richter WF, Jacobsen B: Subcutaneous absorption of biotherapeutics: knowns and unknowns, *Drug Metab Dispos* 42:1881–1889, 2014.

Robbie GJ, Criste R, Dall'acqua WF, et al.: A novel investigational Fc-modified humanized monoclonal antibody, motavizumab-YTE, has an extended half-life in healthy adults, *Antimicrob Agents Chemother* 57:6147–6153, 2013.

Roopenian DC, Akilesh S: FcRn: the neonatal Fc receptor comes of age, *Nat Rev Immunol* 7:715–725, 2007.

Rudnick SI, Lou J, Shaller CC, et al.: Influence of affinity and antigen internalization on the uptake and penetration of Anti-HER2 antibodies in solid tumors, *Cancer Res* 71:2250–2259, 2011.

Ruggiero A, Villa CH, Bander E, et al.: Paradoxical glomerular filtration of carbon nanotubes, *Proc Natl Acad Sci U S A* 107: 12369–12374, 2010.

Ryman JT, Meibohm B: Pharmacokinetics of monoclonal antibodies, *CPT Pharmacometrics Syst Pharmacol* 6:576–588, 2017.

Sampei Z, Igawa T, Soeda T, et al.: Identification and multidimensional optimization of an asymmetric bispecific IgG antibody mimicking the function of factor VIII cofactor activity, *PloS One* 8:e57479, 2013.

Schlothauer T, Rueger P, Stracke JO, et al.: Analytical FcRn affinity chromatography for functional characterization of monoclonal antibodies, *mAbs* 5:576–586, 2013.

Secher T, Guilleminault L, Reckamp K, et al.: Therapeutic antibodies: a new era in the treatment of respiratory diseases? *Pharmacol Ther* 189:149–172, 2018.

Seijsing J, Sobieraj AM, Keller N, et al.: Improved biodistribution and extended serum half-life of a bacteriophage endolysin by albumin binding domain fusion, *Front Microbiol* 9:2927, 2018.

Shankar G, Arkin S, Cocea L, et al.: Assessment and reporting of the clinical immunogenicity of therapeutic proteins and peptides-harmonized terminology and tactical recommendations, *AAPS J* 16:658–673, 2014.

Sharma VK, Patapoff TW, Kabakoff B, et al.: In silico selection of therapeutic antibodies for development: viscosity, clearance, and chemical stability, *Proc Natl Acad Sci U S A* 111:18601–18606, 2014.

Sleep D: Albumin and its application in drug delivery, *Expet Opin Drug Deliv* 12:793–812, 2015.

Sleep D, Cameron J, Evans LR: Albumin as a versatile platform for drug half-life extension, *Biochim Biophys Acta* 1830: 5526–5534, 2013.

Sorger PK, Allerheilligen SRB, Abernethy DR, et al.: *Quantitative and Systems Pharmacology in the Post-genomic Era: New Approaches to Discovering Drugs and Understanding Therapeutic Mechanisms*, NIH White Paper, 2011, pp 1–47.

Stroh M, Duda DG, Takimoto CH, et al.: Translation of anti-cancer efficacy from nonclinical models to the clinic, *CPT Pharmacometrics Syst Pharmacol* 3:e128, 2014.

Turner MR, Balu-Iyer SV: Challenges and opportunities for the subcutaneous delivery of therapeutic proteins, *J Pharmaceut Sci* 107:1247–1260, 2018.

Unverdorben F, Hutt M, Seifert O, et al.: A fab-selective immunoglobulin-binding domain from streptococcal protein G with improved half-life extension properties, *PloS One* 10:e0139838, 2015.

van Hasselt JG, van der Graaf PH: Towards integrative systems pharmacology models in oncology drug development, *Drug Discov Today Technol* 15:1–8, 2015.

Vugmeyster Y, Szklut P, Wensel D, et al.: Complex pharmacokinetics of a humanized antibody against human amyloid beta peptide, anti-abeta Ab2, in nonclinical species, *Pharm Res (N Y)* 28:1696–1706, 2011.

Wang W, Wang EQ, Balthasar JP: Monoclonal antibody pharmacokinetics and pharmacodynamics, *Clin Pharmacol Ther* 84:548–558, 2008.

Wolf E, Baeuerle PA: Micromet: engaging immune cells for life, *Drug Discov Today* 7:S25–S27, 2002.

Wolf Perez AM, Sormanni P, Andersen JS, et al.: In vitro and in silico assessment of the developability of a designed monoclonal antibody library, *mAbs* 11:388–400, 2019.

Wright A, Morrison SL: Effect of altered CH_2-associated carbohydrate structure on the functional properties and in vivo fate of chimeric mouse-human immunoglobulin G1, *J Exp Med* 180:1087–1096, 1994.

Wright A, Morrison SL: Effect of C2-associated carbohydrate structure on Ig effector function: studies with chimeric mouse-human IgG1 antibodies in glycosylation mutants of Chinese hamster ovary cells, *J Immunol* 160:3393–3402, 1998.

Wright A, Sato Y, Okada T, et al.: In vivo trafficking and catabolism of IgG1 antibodies with Fc associated carbohydrates of differing structure, *Glycobiology* 10:1347–1355, 2000.

Yadav DB, Maloney JA, Wildsmith KR, et al.: Widespread brain distribution and activity following i.c.v. infusion of anti-beta-secretase (BACE1) in nonhuman primates, *Br J Pharmacol* 174:4173–4185, 2017.

Yang D, Giragossian C, Castellano S, et al.: Maximizing in vivo target clearance by design of pH-dependent target binding antibodies with altered affinity to FcRn, *mAbs* 9:1105–1117, 2017.

Yang TY, Uhlinger DJ, Ayers SA, et al.: Challenges in selectivity, specificity and quantitation range of ligand-binding assays: case studies using a microfluidics platform, *Bioanalysis* 6:1049–1057, 2014.

Yao Z, Dai W, Perry J, et al.: Effect of albumin fusion on the biodistribution of interleukin-2, *Cancer Immunol Immunother* 53:404–410, 2004.

Yazaki PJ, Kassa T, Cheung CW, et al.: Biodistribution and tumor imaging of an anti-CEA single-chain antibody-albumin fusion protein, *Nucl Med Biol* 35:151–158, 2008.

Yeung YA, Leabman MK, Marvin JS, et al.: Engineering human IgG1 affinity to human neonatal Fc receptor: impact of affinity improvement on pharmacokinetics in primates, *J Immunol* 182:7663–7671, 2009.

Yu YJ, Atwal JK, Zhang Y, et al.: Therapeutic bispecific antibodies cross the blood-brain barrier in nonhuman primates, *Sci Transl Med* 6:261ra154, 2014.

Zhao L, Ji P, Li Z, et al.: The antibody drug absorption following subcutaneous or intramuscular administration and its mathematical description by coupling physiologically based absorption process with the conventional compartment pharmacokinetic model, *J Clin Pharmacol* 53: 314–325, 2013.

Zheng Y, Tesar DB, Benincosa L, et al.: Minipig as a potential translatable model for monoclonal antibody pharmacokinetics after intravenous and subcutaneous administration, *mAbs* 4:243–255, 2012.

Zhou Q, Shankara S, Roy A, et al.: Development of a simple and rapid method for producing non-fucosylated oligomannose containing antibodies with increased effector function, *Biotechnol Bioeng* 99:652–665, 2008.

Principles of Pharmacodynamics and Toxicodynamics

Jin Wang, David M. Stresser

AbbVie Inc., Drug Metabolism and Pharmacokinetics, North Chicago, IL, United States

O U T L I N E

1. Introduction: Definition of Pharmacodynamics and Toxicodynamics   101

2. Mechanism of Drug Action and Adverse Drug Reaction   102
   2.1. Physiochemical Property Based   102
   2.2. Biochemical Based   102

3. Types of Adverse Drug Reaction: Intrinsic (Type A) Versus Idiosyncratic (Type B)   104

4. Types of Xenobiotic–Target Interaction   106
   4.1. Reversible, Irreversible, Noncompetitive, and Allosteric Interaction   106
   4.2. Agonist, Partial Agonist, Antagonist, and Inverse Agonist   106

5. Exposure-Dependent Response   107

5.1. Receptor Occupancy Relationship   107
5.2. Turnover Model   108
5.3. Quantal Dose–Effect Model   109
5.4. Nonmonotonic Dose–Effect   109

6. Response Following Chronic Dosing   110
   6.1. Receptor Downregulation   111
   6.2. Exhaustion of Mediators   111
   6.3. Physiological Adaptation   111
   6.4. Desensitization   111

7. Quantitative Modeling for Pharmacokinetic/ Pharmacodynamic and Toxicodynamic Data Analysis   111

References   112

1. INTRODUCTION: DEFINITION OF PHARMACODYNAMICS AND TOXICODYNAMICS

In simple terms, *pharmacodynamics* (PD) and *toxicodynamics* (TD) describe the relationship between exposure (concentration at the site-of-action) of the drug, toxicant, or toxin (xenobiotic) and the extent of resulting effect on the body over a time course (Toutain, 2009). PD and TD can be evaluated through in vitro, ex vivo, or in vivo studies and endpoints can range from the molecular to the whole organism level.

The adverse effect of a therapeutic drug or toxic agent is determined by its mechanism and duration of action. Together with PK considerations and tissue concentrations, the mechanism of action will determine the tissue sites at which most severe consequences will occur. The combination of either the drug's presence (determined by pharmacokinetic (PK) analyses) and/or its mechanism and duration of action (PD) will determine the nature and degree of altered cellular physiology.

For in vivo studies, PK and PD phases are not always synchronized, such that there may be a delay between the peak of drug concentration (usually measured in plasma) and the observed response. A widely known illustration on this time-dependent PK/PD or TD alteration in vivo is the "hysteresis loop" (Figure 5.1), where the xenobiotic concentration and effect are not in phase. This may be caused by the delay of drug moving from plasma and interstitial fluid to the site-of-action (usually on cell surface or cell interior). Another common mechanism is a delay resulting from the time from target interaction, mRNA synthesis, and finally translation to protein.

2. MECHANISM OF DRUG ACTION AND ADVERSE DRUG REACTION

2.1. Physiochemical Property Based

Examples of drugs that interact through physical or chemical reactions with body fluids or tissues include the osmotic diuretic mannitol and orally administered antacids. Osmotic diuretics, which are not cell permeable, can be filtered into the renal tubules but not reabsorbed. Therefore, they limit the osmosis in the tubular lumen and inhibit the reabsorption of water and electrolytes including sodium and chloride. Antacids like aluminum salts neutralize gastric acid and bind with phosphate in the intestine. These compounds are designed to alter, respectively, *osmolarity* and *pH*, but do not interact directly with cellular processes. Drugs that exert these types of actions are typically older since the mechanism of action of newly discovered drugs is usually based on biochemical reactions, which are discussed at below.

2.2. Biochemical Based

Most xenobiotics cause their effects through biochemical interactions with macromolecules

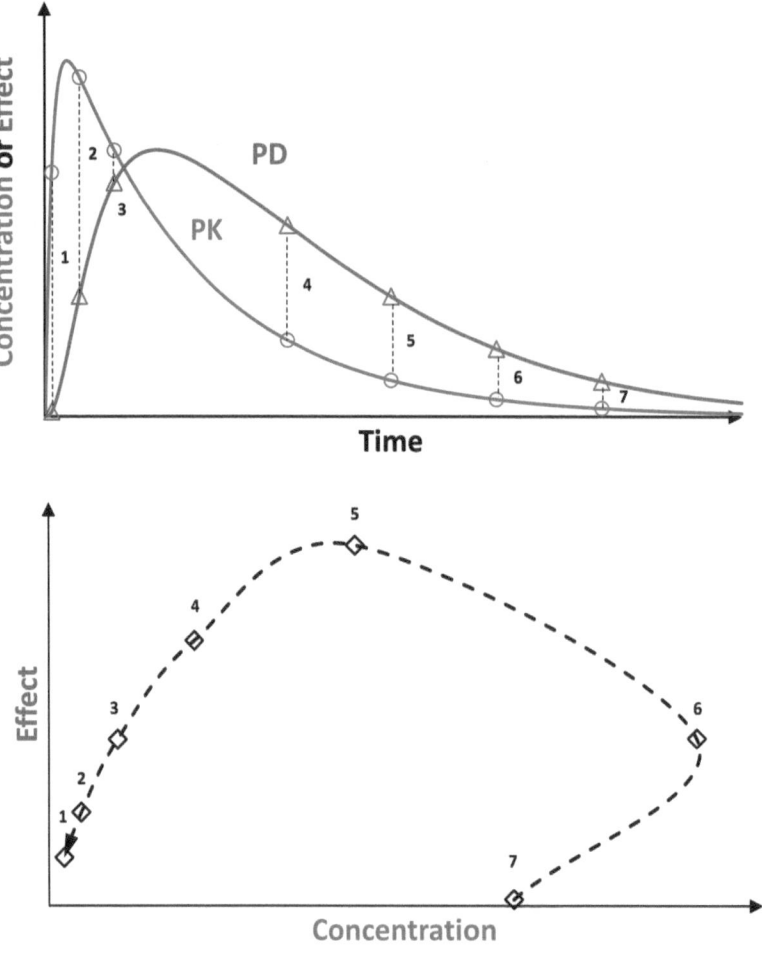

FIGURE 5.1   Plots of concentration (PK) or effect (PD) over the time course (top panel, with selected timepoints 1 through 7). The time delay between the measured concentration and the response onset results in a hysteresis loop in the plot of effect versus concentration, measured at each corresponding timepoint (bottom panel).

that involve normal physiological or pathological process in animals, ectoparasites, or microbial organisms. Those include nonreceptors (e.g., enzymes, ion channel proteins, transporters, nucleic acids, and cell skeleton molecules) and signal transduction receptors.

Action on Nonreceptors

Examples of *enzyme inhibitors* include nonsteroidal antiinflammatory drugs, which inhibit cyclooxygenases during prostanoid synthesis; the anticancer drug methotrexate, which inhibits tetrahydrofolate reductase catalyzing methionine formation; acetylcholinesterase inhibitors like the drug physostigmine or the toxin sarin which prevents the hydrolysis of the neurotransmitter acetylcholine; and digoxin, an inhibitor of sodium (Na^+), potassium (K^+) ATPase in cardiac muscle cells.

Examples of drugs which *interact with DNA* include the anticancer drugs like lomustine (CCNU), which alkylates DNA, and the fluoroquinolones that interact with DNA gyrase resulting in alteration of the three-dimensional structure of DNA leading to reduced bacterial replication and death.

Drugs *interacting with microtubules* include taxanes and vinca alkaloids and anticancer agents that stabilize or destabilize the polymerization of microtubules during cell mitosis. Through this mechanism, the mitotic spindle of the cell is disrupted leading to cell cycle arrest and apoptosis.

Action on Signal Transduction Receptors

Through interaction with a receptor, a drug often alters the receptor protein's three-dimensional structure triggering *signal transduction* processes within the cell resulting in a biological effect (Von Zastrow and Bourne, 2009). Understanding the details of signal transduction leads to understanding of the timeframe and persistence of the biological effect, sometimes long after removal of the agent. Signal transduction mechanisms also underlie the phenomena of the cell's adaptation to *chronic exposure* of the xenobiotic.

Although a complete review of cellular signal transduction is beyond the scope of this chapter, the reader is directed to a web database maintained by the International Union of Basic and Clinical Pharmacology which maintains updated information on signal transduction systems linked with receptors (https://www.guidetopharmacology.org/). This resource is particularly useful because it tracks information about *orphan receptors*, which are receptors proteins identified by genome sequencing and molecular biology with homology to known receptors, but which, to date, have not been unequivocally linked to a known effect.

Signal transduction is usually accomplished with one or more of the following key cellular processes, each of which results in allowing a signal (drug) to move its effect from outside the cell to the intracellular compartment. *Transmembrane receptors* are classified as either *ionotropic* (linked to ion channels) or *metabotropic* (linked to biochemical processes). *Intracellular receptors* include cytosolic and nuclear receptors.

Ionotropic receptors or ligand-gated transmembrane ion channels include γ-aminobutyric acid (GABA) and ionotropic glycine receptors linked to Cl^- channels, nicotinic acetylcholine and glutamate receptors (AMPA [2-amino-3-(5-methyl-3-oxo-1,2- oxazol-4-yl)propanoic acid], kainate, and NMDA [*N*-Methyl-D-aspartate]) linked to Na^+ channels, and serotonin (5HT) 3 receptors are linked to cation currents. There are also subtypes of GABA (GABA$_A$ and GABA$_B$), glutamate, and 5HT receptors that are metabotropic. The human ether-a-go-go related gene codes for a protein subunit, functioning as a voltage-dependent K^+ ion channel that mediates ventricular action potential repolarization. Inhibition of this channel by drugs such as terfenadine and dofetilide may lead to QT prolongation and arrythmias such as torsades de pointes. *Metabotropic receptors* either act directly or indirectly as signal transduction enzymes, or are linked to enzymes that have an extracellular domain recognizing a drug and an intracellular domain that catalyzes a biochemical response. *Transmembrane metabotropic receptors* include the following:

G-COUPLED RECEPTORS

a. **Gs-stimulatory**, e.g., coupled to adenylate cyclase—increases intracellular cyclic AMP resulting in activation of protein kinase A, which phosphorylates proteins associated with cellular action. Examples include glucagon, thyrotropin, adrenocorticotropic hormone, β-adrenergic, and dopamine 1(D_1 and D_5 subtypes).

b. **Gi/o-inhibitory**—inhibits adenylate cyclase or closes Ca^{++} and opens K^+ channels. Examples: α_2-adrenergic, muscarinic acetylcholine (M_2 and M_4 subtypes), dopamine (D_2, D_3 and D_4 subtypes), serotonin ($5HT_1$), and $GABA_B$.

c. **Gq-coupled to phospholipase C-β**—increases formation of inositol triphosphate (IP_3) and diacylglycerol (DAG). IP_3 increases intracellular Ca^{++} and DAG activates protein kinase C that phosphorylates proteins associated with cellular action.

RECEPTORS WITH ASSOCIATED ENZYMATIC ACTIVITY

a. **Plasma membrane kinase–linked receptors:** Enzyme activity is part of the receptor's intracellular domain. *Tyrosine kinase* (TK) or *serine kinases* (SKs) phosphorylate a cellular substrate including other kinases that phosphorylate proteins associated with cellular action often through altered gene transcription. Examples include insulin (via TK), IGF-1 (via TK), TGF-β (via SK), and other growth factors.

b. **Cytosolic kinase–linked receptors:** *Janus kinase* (JAK; a TK) is phosphorylated by the activated plasma membrane receptor. JAK then phosphorylates transcription (STAT) proteins, which form dimers when phosphorylated and move into the nucleus acting as nuclear transcription factors.

c. **Guanylyl cyclase (GC) linked:** Plasma membrane receptors have GC activity and the cyclic GMP formed activates *protein kinase G* that phosphorylates proteins associated with cellular action. *Nitric oxide* (NO) can also directly activate cytosolic GC. Examples include atrial natriuretic factor and NO (including that stimulated by M_3 muscarinic agonists in vascular endothelium).

INTRACELLULAR RECEPTORS (NUCLEAR OR CYTOSOLIC)

Compounds that permeate plasma membranes can bind to cytosolic and/or nuclear receptors, which in turn bind to a *DNA response element*, which then results in inhibition or activation of mRNA and protein transcription. Some hormone receptors act as homodimers (e.g., glucocorticoid receptor) and some as heterodimers (e.g.,

thyroid hormone with retinoic acid receptors) as they interact with the DNA response element. Agents with effects through nuclear receptors generally have a lag time up to several hours associated with new protein synthesis, and their effect can persist for as long as days after removal of the agent because of slow turnover of proteins associated with the effect. Examples include lipid-soluble xenobiotics (e.g., rifampin, polychlorinated biphenyls) or hormones (e.g., thyroid hormone, glucocorticoids, mineralocorticoids, vitamin D, vitamin A) or analogues.

3. TYPES OF ADVERSE DRUG REACTION: INTRINSIC (TYPE A) VERSUS IDIOSYNCRATIC (TYPE B)

There are two types of adverse drug reactions: intrinsic (type A) and idiosyncratic (type B). Type B reactions, which by definition rarely happen, are nondose dependent and cannot be described by a mass–action relationship. The cause of idiosyncratic toxicities is often attributed to immune-mediated mechanisms (Roth and Ganey, 2010). Due to their low incident frequency, idiosyncratic toxicities cannot be properly characterized in preclinical studies or clinical trials and are discovered only after many thousands of patients have taken these medications.

Type A reactions are dose (concentration) dependent and predictable. This type of adverse effect is usually an extension of the therapeutic effect (see Figure 5.2). The rest of this chapter will focus on the type A reactions. In most cases, xenobiotics act on biological macromolecules. For the sake of the following discussion, drug interaction with these macromolecules will be collectively characterized according to *receptor theory* to explain the dose nonlinear interactions leading to xenobiotic exposure response.

The structural specificity of drug–target(s) interaction predicts the clinical selectivity of drug action. More precisely, the ability of receptors to recognize and respond to a given xenobiotic is based upon the three-dimensional structure of the binding pocket. Absolute specificity is uncommon. In fact, for those involved in nonclinical phases of drug development, it is important to screen for binding (*affinity* and

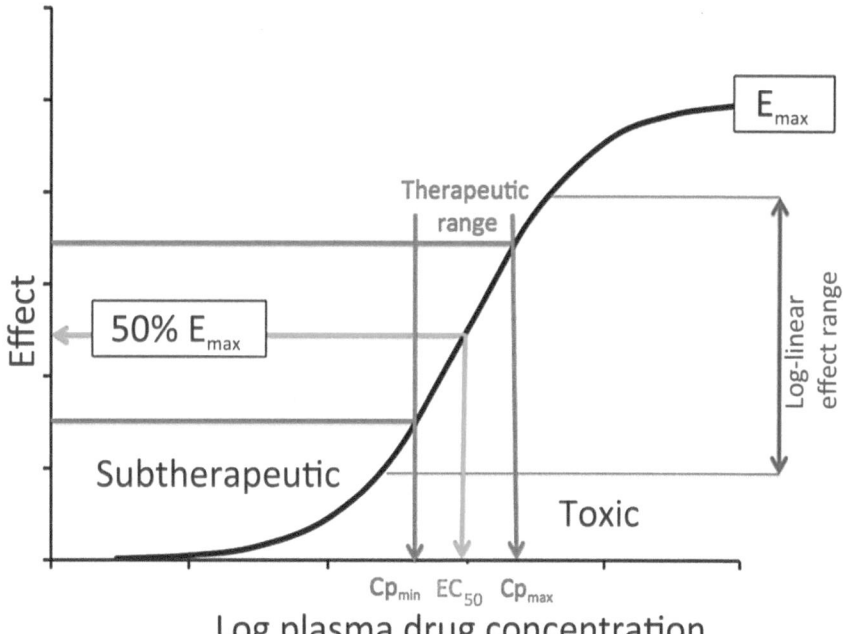

FIGURE 5.2 Classical relationship between dose and concentration determining the efficacy and safety of a therapeutic drug. E_{max}, maximal theoretical effect; EC50, effective concentration producing 50% of E_{max}; Cp_{min}, minimum therapeutic concentration of a drug; Cp_{max}, maximal therapeutic or minimum toxic effect of a drug; log-linear range, approximately linear portion of the log dose–effect curve. *Figure reproduced from Haschek and Rousseaux's: Handbook of toxicologic pathology, ed 3. In Haschek WM, Rousseaux CG, Wallig MA, editors: 2013, Academic Press, p 62. Figure 3.2, with permission.*

capacity, see more detailed discussion in Section 5.1) and activity to a variety of receptor types that may be expressed in a variety of tissues to help predict therapeutic and potentially adverse effects. Drug companies often externalize off-target safety pharmacology profiling screens to commercial suppliers.

Most drugs interact with a variety of receptors with varying affinities. However, eventually, it is important to evaluate the drug's effect in vivo, as relative tissue effects, integrated tissue responses, and counterresponses to a drug are difficult to predict accurately. When a drug's dosage and concentration is increased, *off-target* effects may occur on lower affinity receptors in the same or other tissues and may contribute to adverse effects. For example, when used as a therapeutic, dopamine stimulates renal dopaminergic D_1 receptors to induce renovascular dilation at low dosage infusion rates, then stimulates cardiac β_1-adrenergic receptors at intermediate rates causing tachycardia as a side effect, and at even higher dosage infusion rates stimulates arterial α_1-receptors causing vasoconstriction

and counteracting the renovascular dilatory effect.

By definition, drugs or toxins will generate biological effects when dosed to an organism. Among them, efficacy is defined as a "desired" therapeutic effect, and toxicities are "undesired." For an effect mediated by a single receptor, the log dose–effect relationship parallels that of the log dose receptor binding relationship (Figure 5.2). Efficacy should be distinguished from the term *potency*, a term used to compare the affinity among ligands that bind to the same receptor. The greater the maximal effect (E_{max}) of a drug, determined by the signal transduction systems in a cell per unit receptor occupied, the greater is the efficacy of that drug. The more potent compound has a lower Kd (dissociation constant, a term describing the concentration of free drug when 50% of the total molecules of receptors forms the drug–receptor complex) or lower EC_{50}, defined as the concentration causing 50% of E_{max}. EC_{50} represents the middle of the linear part of the log dose (concentration)–response curve, with the slope steepness representing its sensitivity, often termed n, or the Hill coefficient. More details about the quantitative dose-dependent relationship will be discussed later in this chapter (Section 5).

4. TYPES OF XENOBIOTIC–TARGET INTERACTION

4.1. Reversible, Irreversible, Noncompetitive, and Allosteric Interaction

If the xenobiotic competes with the substrate or endogenous ligand through binding to the active site, it is defined as competitive interaction. These interactions can be reversible or irreversible. Increasing the concentration of substrates will fully reverse the reversible binding of the xenobiotic, but will not reverse irreversible binding, since the latter involves the formation of covalent bonds. With irreversible binding, enzyme function will be restored only after synthesis of new enzyme. Both reversible and irreversible competitive inhibitors increase the Km (Michaelis–Menten constant), but only the irreversible inhibitor decreases the Vmax (maximal catalytic rate) in enzyme kinetic studies.

If the xenobiotic competes with the substrate or endogenous ligand through binding to other site(s) apart from the active site, it is defined as noncompetitive interaction. A noncompetitive ligand and the substrate may both bind to the enzyme at the same time. Allosteric binding is the most common scenario of noncompetitive interaction. It alters the conformation or shape of the active site and subsequently decreases the affinity (km) of substrates or competitive binding ligands and the catalytic capacity (V_{max}) of enzyme.

4.2. Agonist, Partial Agonist, Antagonist, and Inverse Agonist

Agonists

A *full agonist* is a drug that achieves the maximal biological effect at its maximally effective concentration (Negus, 2006). Empirically, this compound has the *highest intrinsic efficacy* possible at the time of its maximal concentration. A *partial agonist* is a drug for which the E_{max}, and therefore the *intrinsic efficacy, is less* than that of a full agonist. It is important to note that a partial agonist may be more potent than a full agonist

with regards to having higher receptor binding affinity, and therefore induce a greater biological effect at a given concentration than a full agonist. A classic example of a partial agonist is buprenorphine, a mu opioid partial agonist whose activity can be compared with morphine, a pure mu agonist. In fact, buprenorphine interacts with the mu opioid receptor with about 30-fold higher affinity but results in lower E_{max} than morphine.

Antagonists

Antagonists are any compounds that act to counteract a specific biological action. However, in terms of receptor interaction, they are defined as compounds that do not cause a biological effect alone and, therefore, have *zero intrinsic efficacy*. For a pure antagonist, its biological effect is only seen in the presence of an agonist. Antagonists are generally divided into those that are *competitive antagonists*; that is, they interact reversibly with the receptor and, in a concentration-dependent and affinity-dependent manner, block the binding of an agonist. Most clinically used antagonists are of a competitive type. In the presence of a competitive antagonist, an increased dosage or concentration of an agonist can completely reverse the effect of the antagonist. The log dose–response curve for the agonist appears only to shift to higher concentrations (See Figure 5.3). An example of a competitive antagonist is atenolol for the β1-adrenergic receptor.

Noncompetitive antagonists are compounds that allosterically or irreversibly bind with a receptor protein to block the effect of an agonist. Increasing the concentration of an agonist does not reverse the effect of a noncompetitive antagonist through mass action principles. Allosteric binding alters the conformation of active site on receptors or enzymes and affects the binding of specific substrates. For irreversible antagonists that might covalently alter a receptor, the effect is indistinguishable from *receptor downregulation*. An example of an irreversible antagonist is phenoxybenzamine which covalently links with the alpha-adrenergic R binding site, and an example of an allosteric inhibitor is the benzodiazepine diazepam which binds noncompetitively to the Cl⁻ channel normally activated by GABA resulting in enhancing the effect of GABA on channel Cl⁻ conductance and, therefore, enhancing membrane hyperpolarization.

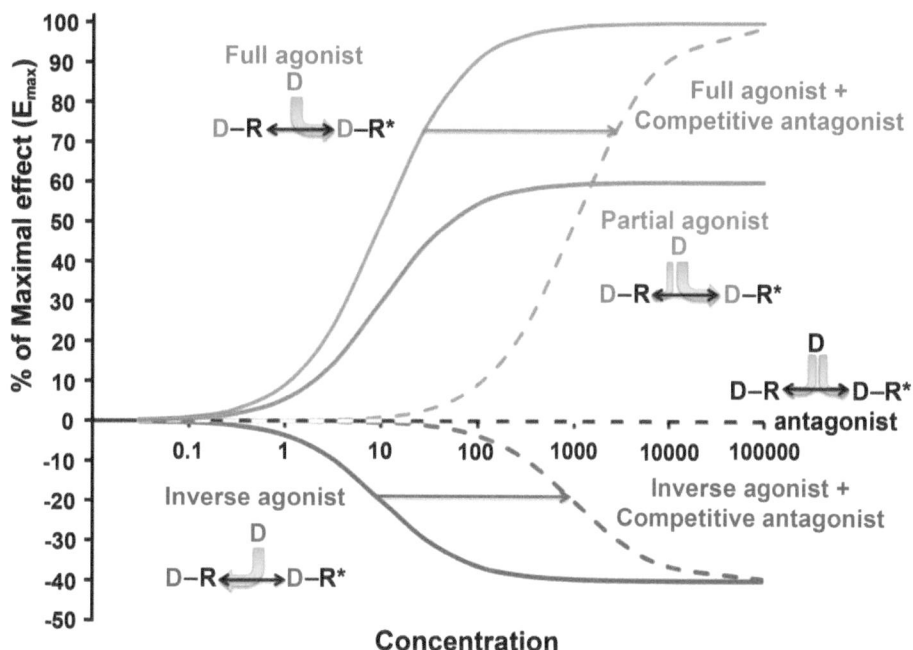

FIGURE 5.3 Summary of Log Dose–Effect Curves for Full Agonist, Antagonist, Partial Agonist, and Inverse Agonists according to Reversible Two-State Receptor Theory. R and R* represent the equilibrium between resting (R) and activated (R*) receptor forms. *Figure reproduced from Haschek and Rousseaux's: Handbook of toxicologic pathology, ed 3. In Haschek WM, Rousseaux CG, Wallig MA, editors: 2013, Academic Press, p 71. Figure 3.10, with permission.*

Inverse agonists are compounds that interact with receptor signal transduction systems that have a constitutive level of activity, and through interaction with the receptor, *reduce the activity in the direction opposite of that of a pure agonist* (de Ligt et al., 2000). Historically, some inverse agonists were previously clinically characterized as pure antagonists. Constitutive activation has been demonstrated for GABA, cannabinoid, histamine, and 5HT receptors.

Some Histamine 1 (H_1) antagonists, such as mepyramine, have been shown to also be inverse agonists, which can downregulate H_1 receptor synthesis (Mizuguchi et al., 2012). As such, compared to the pure or "neutral" H_1 antagonists (e.g., oxatomide), the inverse agonists may have greater clinical potency at alleviating allergic symptomatology.

5. EXPOSURE-DEPENDENT RESPONSE

5.1. Receptor Occupancy Relationship

The vast majority of drugs (D) interact reversibly with their cellular protein targets, hereafter called receptors (R) (Rang, 2006). Drugs combine with their receptors at a rate dependent on the concentration of the drug and receptor, and the resulting drug–receptor complex breaks down at a rate proportional to the number of complexes formed (see Figure 5.4).

The mass action relationship between a drug and a receptor is defined by the strength or affinity of binding. This property can be quantitatively defined by the equilibrium association constant or, more commonly, its inverse, the equilibrium Kd. Kd is used more frequently because of its concentration units, and it describes the midrange of concentrations over which the receptor "operates" in detecting circulating or local concentrations of a physiological signal or xenobiotic.

It is more common to express binding data by starting with the equation for Kd in Figure 5.4 and expressing bound drug ([DR] as a function of free drug ([Dfree]) resulting in the saturation equations shown below. Illustrating the relevance and similarity of drug–receptor binding equations to those describing drug–effect relationships, the homologous equation for the latter is also shown.

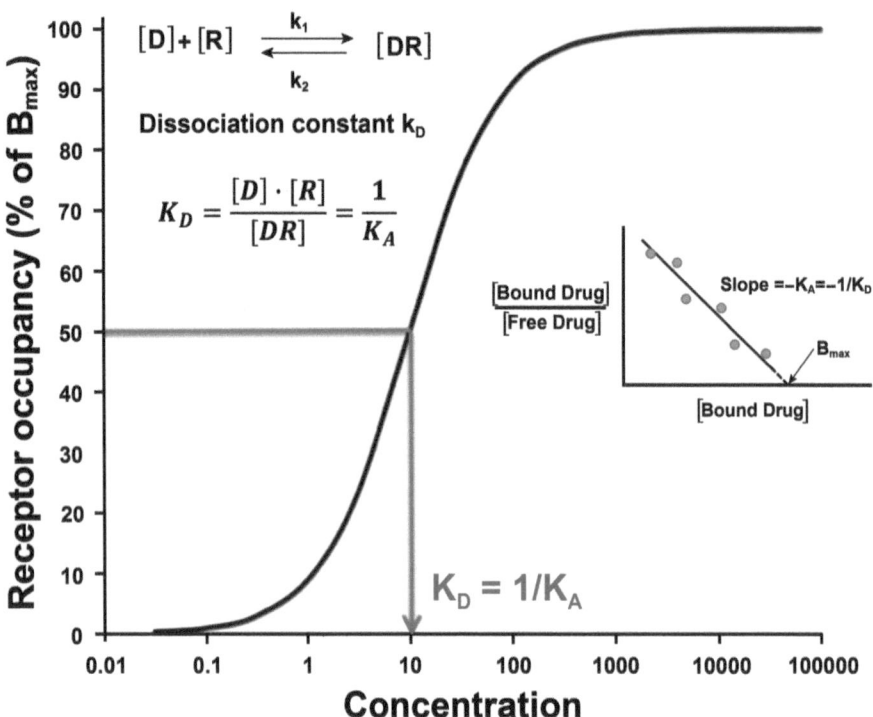

FIGURE 5.4 Sigmoidal log concentration–receptor occupancy curve. In an ideal single-receptor experiment, the receptor occupancy will rise from a threshold to maximum in a concentration range of about 100-fold, and the inflection of the sigmoidal curve is observed at (approximately) the equilibrium dissociation constant (KD) if the experimental conditions are ideal. KD is the inverse of the equilibrium association constant (KA). Inlet: The Scatchard plot of a ligand interacting with a single receptor with a finite binding capacity (B_{max}) and an equilibrium dissociation constant KD is displayed. *Figure (main and inset) reproduced from Haschek and Rousseaux's: Handbook of toxicologic pathology, ed 3. In Haschek WM, Rousseaux CG, Wallig MA, editors: 2013, Academic Press, p 65. Figures 3.6 and 3.8, with permission.*

$$\text{Bound drug } [DR] = \frac{B_{max} \cdot \left[D_{free} \right]}{\left[D_{free} \right] + K_D}$$

$$\text{Effect} = \frac{E_{max} \cdot \left[D_{free} \right]}{\left[D_{free} \right] + EC_{50}}$$

5.2. Turnover Model

In most living organisms, the components of the body are generally maintained at a steady state (homeostasis) through the continuous degradation and regeneration processes. The rate of turnover for any particular component ranges from microseconds (e.g., neurotransmitter) to years (e.g., organ). The simple direct

E_{max} model is sufficient to describe a situation of instant pharmacologic effect (no time delay observed between the exposure and response), where turnover processes are adequately rapid. However, if target turnover is the rate-limiting step or in a range similar to the inhibitor's residence time (the reciprocal of its dissociation rate), the indirect response model (Figure 5.5) becomes useful. In this model, the production (k_{in}) and degradation or loss (k_{out}) processes cooperatively contribute to the observed PD effects. On top of that, a feedback loop can be added to reflect common mechanisms which regulate the production or degradation process based on certain effector components (e.g., hormone levels, white blood cell count) (Jusko, 2013).

For irreversible inhibitors, which deactivate the target enzyme after binding, the target turnover rate plays a key role to determine the extent

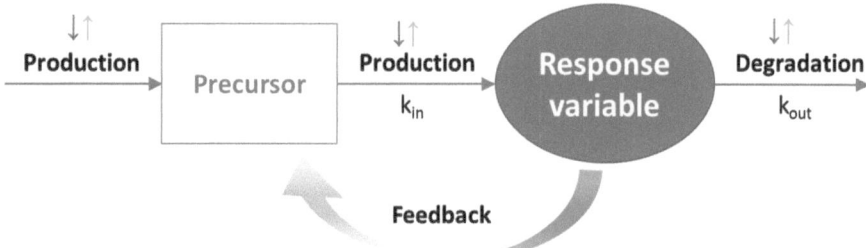

FIGURE 5.5   Indirect response model. The response variable is affected by processes including the formation of precursor, production or degradation of response variable, and feedback loop which regulates other processes. k_{in} and k_{out} are the rate constant for the production and degradation process of response variable, respectively. Drugs or toxins can inhibit or stimulate any of these steps.

and duration of effect after the inhibitor has been eliminated from the system. For example, acalabrutinib (Calquence) is a covalent Bruton's tyrosine kinase (Btk) inhibitor to treat certain B-cell lymphomas. Its PK half-life is less than 2 h, but the Btk occupancy was maintained well above 90% in plasma through 100 mg dosing twice daily due to the relatively slow turnover of this kinase. Notably, for irreversible inhibitors, interindividual variability in target turnover rate can lead to variable response observed in the clinic.

5.3. Quantal Dose–Effect Model

To this point, it has been assumed that dose–effect curves are graded. In some situations, the pharmacological/toxicological effect is an all-or-none (quantal) phenomenon (See *The Use of Statistics in Toxicologic Pathology*, Chap 15). Examples might be when the endpoint is the occurrence of arrhythmias, seizures, or even mortality. In this case, it is more relevant to know the population statistics regarding such a quantal event. For example, the dose might be plotted against the cumulative percent occurrence of the therapeutic effect and a second plot of the dosage against the cumulative incidence of adverse effects. For example, with a β_1-adrenergic receptor agonist, the *quantal therapeutic endpoint* might be achievement of a 20% increase in heart rate, and for the toxic effects, the incidence of premature ventricular contractions. Such a plot is shown in Figure 5.6. In this plot, the *median effective dosage (ED_{50})* is the dosage at which 50% of the subjects have cumulatively demonstrated the therapeutic effect. Likewise, the *median toxic dosage (TD_{50})* is the dosage at

which 50% of the subjects demonstrate the toxic effect. If the toxic effect is death, the median lethal dose is termed LD_{50}. In modern nonclinical safety studies, the LD_{50} is rarely an endpoint because of animal welfare considerations. The ratio of TD_{50}/ED_{50} represents a useful way to characterize the *therapeutic index (TI)* for a therapeutic compound.

5.4. Nonmonotonic Dose–Effect

Standard toxicology testing generally involves the evaluation of relatively high concentrations of a compound to establish a threshold below which no adverse effects are observed. As more low-dose toxicology studies are performed with compounds suspected of disruption of the endocrine or neurotransmitter systems, it has become apparent that not all dose–response curves are characterized by graded responses from low concentrations to toxic at higher concentrations. Instead, the dose–response is best represented as an inverted "U-shaped" curve (Figure 5.7).

For example, at the cellular level, growth of estrogen-dependent human breast cancer cells in culture has been shown to increase their replication rate in response to increasing estradiol concentrations reaching a maximal response with higher concentrations then slowing growth and eventually leading to direct cytotoxicity. The lowest concentration range reflects the physiological response to estrogen and is dependent upon the presence of estrogen receptors. The high-dose effects are not estrogen dependent. Inverted "U-shaped" dose–response curves have also been described in animal and human cognitive functions such as spatial working memory. In fact,

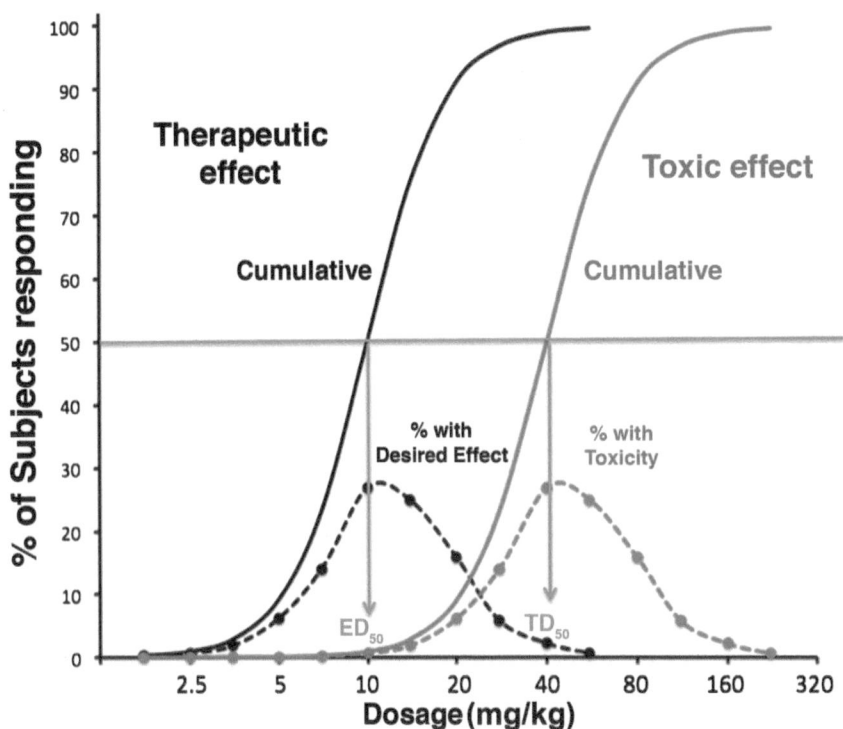

FIGURE 5.6 Classical appearance of dose titration study evaluating the therapeutic index of a drug. The solid lines represent the cumulative percentage of patients showing either the Therapeutic Effect (*black*) or Toxic Effect (*red*). The dotted lines represent the proportion of subjects showing signs at a given dosage. The safety margin may be characterized by the ratio of TD50/ED50. *Figure reproduced from Haschek and Rousseaux's: Handbook of toxicologic pathology, ed 3. In Haschek WM, Rousseaux CG, Wallig MA, editors: 2013, Academic Press, p 72. Figure 3.11, with permission.*

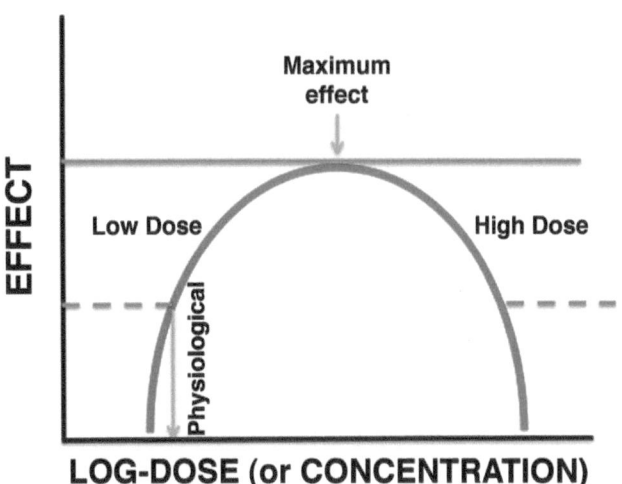

FIGURE 5.7 Classical appearance of an inverted U-shaped dose–response curve: The curve shows no threshold response and shows a maximum beneficial or toxic effect with low concentrations demonstrating an effect or toxicity, which is lost at higher concentrations. This particular example also shows physiological concentrations, which might be achieved under normal physiological conditions (e.g., plasma estradiol or synaptic dopamine concentrations). *Figure reproduced from Haschek and Rousseaux's: Handbook of toxicologic pathology, ed 3. In Haschek WM, Rousseaux CG, Wallig MA, editors: 2013, Academic Press, p 74. Figure 3.12, with permission.*

D_1 receptor agonist stimulation or direct dopaminergic neuron stimulation in the prefrontal cortex has demonstrated that too little or too much D_1 receptor stimulation will impair spatial working memory (Vijayraghavan et al., 2007). As a therapeutic example of the need to achieve optimal drug doses, methylphenidate (Ritalin) is used to treat attention deficit hyperactivity disorder. Methylphenidate is a catecholamine reuptake inhibitor and therefore increases dopamine in dopaminergic synapses in the prefrontal cortex. For each patient, the optimal amount of the drug may vary, but overdoses lead to reduced attention and increased agitation. Of increasing significance for safety assessment, for some toxicities described by an inverted "U-shaped" dose–effect curve, there is no threshold of adverse effect upon which to establish a no adverse effect level of a toxin (Hill et al., 2018).

6. RESPONSE FOLLOWING CHRONIC DOSING

The body has different adaptive mechanisms following the administration of multiple doses of a xenobiotic. Responses observed may be hypo- or hyperactivity. We will focus on the former, which is more common. *Tolerance* is the general term for *response change* after chronic dosing. When it occurs over a relatively short timeframe (hours to days), the term *tachyphylaxis* is used, and usually this is associated with the phenomenon of receptor *desensitization* (see below). However, the mechanism leading to tolerance after chronic dosing may be difficult to distinguish in the individual patient unless a complete dose–response study is performed, which is generally impractical.

6.1. Receptor Downregulation

With some *G-protein–coupled receptors* (GPCRs), including *β-adrenergic receptors* (BARs), more chronic stimulation leads to trafficking of the phosphorylated receptor to lysosomes which *effectively reduces the available number of receptors* (downregulation) available on the plasma membrane and reduces B_{max} and E_{max} in receptor binding and effect studies, respectively.

6.2. Exhaustion of Mediators

The action of a drug given chronically can be reduced by the *exhaustion of mediators* of receptor action. For example, tyramine and amphetamine lead to the release of synaptic catecholamines. Chronic administration may lead to the eventual depletion of catecholamine stores.

6.3. Physiological Adaptation

Several physiological mechanisms unrelated to a specific receptor transduction system may also impact the observed effect in the whole organism. For example, when diuretics are used as antihypertensives, they reduce whole body Na^+ concentrations and blood pressure. In response, the renin–angiotensin–aldosterone system may be activated resulting in increased renal Na^+ retention, angiotensin, and aldosterone, counteracting the beneficial diuretic effect.

6.4. Desensitization

When GPCRs are stimulated, the cellular response may diminish over seconds or minutes, even when the agonist remains present. Exemplified by the BAR, *rapid desensitization* is usually associated with receptor phosphorylation. The alteration of the receptor caused by agonist binding leads the receptor to both activate and be a substrate for G-coupled receptor protein kinases (GRKs). The activated GRK phosphorylates serine residues on the carboxy terminus of the receptor protein.

The presence of phosphoserine residues attracts binding by the protein β-arrestin. Binding by β-arrestin decreases the receptor's affinity for Gs, thereby reducing the response to the receptor agonist and desensitizing the system temporarily. In a desensitized state, the dose–effect curve would be shifted in parallel to higher concentrations (to the right), and the apparent EC_{50} would be higher. When the agonist is removed, cellular phosphatases reverse the effect of GRK. For the BAR, β-arrestin also increases the rate of endocytosis of receptors. The liganded receptor stimulates the formation of clathrin-coated membrane vesicles that invaginate and are moved intracellularly to form the early endosome. Endosomes contain high levels of receptor phosphatases, which then recover normal receptor structure, allowing it to be returned to the plasma membrane, and recovery of sensitivity to short-term agonist stimulation.

Homologous desensitization occurs only when the stimulated receptor is affected and is mediated by receptor-specific kinases. *Heterologous desensitization* may occur when unrelated receptors share a similar signal transduction mechanism, such as adenylate cyclase, and is usually mediated by PKA, which is not receptor specific.

7. QUANTITATIVE MODELING FOR PHARMACOKINETIC/ PHARMACODYNAMIC AND TOXICODYNAMIC DATA ANALYSIS

The importance of PK/PD/TD data analysis in drug development is being increasingly recognized in many aspects from preclinical to late phase clinical trials. With meaningful experimental data, mathematical models can be developed and extrapolated to describe, explain, and predict the xenobiotic exposure and effect behaviors. Applications of such models allow quantification and simulation of drug–system interactions for both therapeutic and toxic responses. In recent years, traditional PK/PD/TD data analysis has been refined with two additional subsets: quantitative system pharmacology (QSP) and pharmacometrics. QSP modeling integrates fundamental knowledge about structural, molecular, and cell biology. It focuses on the interplay among all relevant modules in a biological system relying on known mechanisms ("bottom-up approach"). Pharmacometrics often applies statistics and stochastic simulation through computation programming. It focuses on quantifying the extent of variability and uncertainty around the defined output.

Developing quantitative models involves iterative learning and confirming. Experimental data useful for model development include that which informs on dynamic changes of response at varied dose or concentration levels under multiple conditions (e.g., different target expression levels and disease stages). To establish mathematical model structures, assumptions must be examined thoroughly while integrating the best knowledge about the xenobiotic of interest, key mechanisms, physiology, and disease progression. During this process, any new data or knowledge that may alter the assumptions will necessitate reevaluations of the established quantitative model.

Applications of quantitative PK/PD/TD modeling in drug development include but are not limited to (1) target selection and characterization; (2) preclinical candidate study design optimization; (3) human dose or therapeutic margin projection; (4) prediction of exposure, tissue distribution, and responses in special population (e.g., patients with kidney impairments, pediatrics, and elderly group) that would impact adjustments in dose level/frequency or label recommendations; and (5) guiding risk/benefit evaluation and outcome prediction based on preclinical or early clinical results (Marshall et al., 2019). Among these applications, toxicology and pathology data are essential to inform the risk/benefit-related decision-making with assistance of quantitative modeling. For example, modeling-based approaches have enabled evaluation of QT liability by integrating study results from dog and human, helped to optimize the design of oncology drug combination studies to derisk the occurrence of neutropenia, and permitted assessing the therapeutic window between bleeding (risk) and thrombosis prevention (benefit) of an anticoagulant drug.

REFERENCES

Hill CE, Myers JP, Vandenberg LN: Nonmonotonic dose-response curves occur in dose ranges that are relevant to regulatory decision-making, *Dose Res* 16(3), 2018.
International union of basic and clinical pharmacology (IUPHAR) committee on receptor nomenclature and drug classification website. https://www.guidetopharmacology.org/. (Accessed 27 April 2020).
Jusko WJ: Moving from basic toward systems pharmacodynamic models, *J Pharm Sci* 102(9):2930–2940, 2013.
de Ligt RAF, Kourounakis AP, Ijzerman AP: Inverse agonism at G protein-coupled receptors: (Patho)physiological relevance and implications for drug discovery, *Br J Pharmacol* 130:1–12, 2000.
Marshall S, Madabushi R, Manolis E, Krudys K, Staab A, Dykstra K, Visser SAG: Model-informed drug discovery and development: current industry good practice and regulatory expectations and future perspectives, *CPT Pharmacometrics Syst Pharmacol* 8(2):87–96, 2019.
Mizuguchi H, Shohei S, Hattori M, Fukui H: Inverse agonistic activity of antihistamines and suppression of histamine 1 H1 receptor gene expression, *J Pharmacol Sci* 118:117–121, 2012.
Negus SS: Some implications of receptor theory for in vivo assessment of agonists, antagonists and inverse agonists, *Biochem Pharmacol* 71:1663–1670, 2006.
Rang HP: The receptor concept: pharmacology's big idea, *Br J Pharmacol* 247:S9–S16, 2006.
Roth RA, Ganey PE: Intrinsic versus idiosyncratic drug-induced hepatotoxicity–two villains or one? *J Pharmacol Exp Ther* 332(3):692–697, 2010.
Toutain P-L: Mechanisms of drug action and pharmacokinetics/pharmacodynamics integration in dosage regimen optimization for veterinary medicine. In Riviere JE, Papich MG, editors: *Veterinary pharmacology and therapeutics*, 9th Ed., Ames, IA, 2009, Wiley-Blackwell, pp 75–96.
Vijayraghavan S, Wang M, Birnbaum SG, Williams GV, Arnsten AFT: Inverted-U dopamine D1 receptor actions on prefrontal neurons engaged in working memory, *Nat Neurosci* 10(3):376–384, 2007.
Von Zastrow M, Bourne HR: Drug receptors and pharmacodynamics. In Katzung BG, Masters SB, Trevor AJ, editors: *Basic and clinical pharmacology*, 11th ed., New York, N.Y., 2009, McGraw-Hill, pp 15–35.

Morphologic Manifestations of Toxic Cell Injury

Matthew A. Wallig[1], Evan B. Janovitz[2]

[1]University of Illinois at Urbana Champaign, Urbana, IL, United States, [2]Bristol Meyer Squibb Co, Princeton, NJ, United States

O U T L I N E

1. Introduction   113
   1.1. Importance of Morphologic Assessment in Toxicologic Pathology   113
   1.2. Cell Injury in Context—Structural and Functional Components of Cell Injury   114
   1.3. Host Reaction to Cell Injury   116

2. Adaptation   116
   2.1. Atrophy   116
   2.2. Hypertrophy   120

3. Irreversible versus Reversible Cell Injury   122

   3.1. Cellular Swelling   124
   3.2. Fatty Change—Lipidosis   126

4. Irreversible Cell Injury   127
   4.1. Accidental Cell Death—Necrosis   127
   4.2. Programmed Cell Death   133
   4.3. Consequences of Irreversible Cell Injury   139

5. Conclusion   146

References   146

1. INTRODUCTION

1.1. Importance of Morphologic Assessment in Toxicologic Pathology

Microscopic morphologic assessment is a major component of experimental toxicity studies using laboratory animal models. To realize the full value of these studies, toxicologic pathologists should accurately classify all adverse findings and provide a cogent interpretation including a plausible pathogenesis (see *Nomenclature and Diagnostic Resources in Anatomic Toxicologic Pathology*, Vol 1, Chap 25). Cell injury is a common manifestation of chemically induced toxicity. It can occur as a primary event or as sequelae to a variety of predisposing conditions such as inflammation or ischemia, which are also common manifestations of chemically induced toxicity.

Macroscopic morphological changes are evident when large numbers of cells are injured. Standard light microscopic evaluation of formalin-fixed tissue sections, stained by hematoxylin and eosin (H&E), remains the gold standard for classifying cell injury at the cellular level. In chronic studies, sequelae to cell injury include reactive hyperplasia or tissue atrophy and fibrosis that infer earlier cell injury. Unraveling the pathogenesis of such findings may require meticulous evaluations of tissues and cells in short term in vivo studies, or in vitro cell or tissue models that provide the opportunity to investigate initiating events of cell injury in isolation. Utilizing special techniques such as immunohistochemistry, transmission electron microscopy, or digital image analysis may better define molecular mechanisms, identify target organelles, or quantify the extent of injury by classifying a tissue response to cell injury. Ultimately, articulating the sequence of morphologic changes can generate testable hypotheses that define the mechanism of toxicity and potentially refine risk assessment.

This chapter will serve as an overview of the basic histologic and ultrastructural features that reflect cell injury and cell death as well as the sequelae to such processes. Biochemical and molecular changes that underlie these morphologic alterations are discussed in a previous chapter (See *Biochemical and Molecular Basis of Toxicity*, Vol 1, Chap 2). Injuries that modify the genetic makeup of a cell to produce disturbances in cell cycle and tissue growth are discussed in detail in a succeeding chapter (See *Carcinogenesis: Mechanisms and Evaluation*, Vol 1, Chap 8). More advanced techniques of analysis, whether for determining adaptive responses, cell injury or cell death, will be covered succeeding sections of this volume (see Vol 1, Part 2, *"Methods in Toxicologic Pathology"*).

1.2. Cell Injury in Context—Structural and Functional Components of Cell Injury

Living cells are complex structures comprising an interdependent array of many essential components including organelles, fluids, proteins, electrolytes, signaling molecules, and plasma membrane receptors. Although injury to any one of these components can ultimately result in death of the entire cell, some are particularly critical for cell survival: the plasma membrane is the site of osmotic, electrolyte, and water regulation and receptor–ligand signal transduction; the mitochondrion is the site of aerobic respiration and adenosine triphosphate (ATP) generation; the rough endoplasmic reticulum (rER) is the site of most protein synthesis and calcium storage; and the nucleus, where DNA transcription occurs. The biochemical consequences of damage to these structures have been discussed in a previous chapter (see

Biochemical and Molecular Basis of Toxicity, Vol 1, Chap 2). Other structures, such as lysosomes, peroxisomes, secretory granules, microtubules, microfilaments, and even the extracellular matrix (ECM), may be initially altered in cell injury, depending on the mechanism of action of the injurious agent, but alterations in these structures just as often reflect penultimate secondary changes rather than the proximate cause of cell death.

The onset and progression of cell injury depends on the nature of the noxious insult, including its severity and duration. If injury to the cell is mild and not persistent, recovery is usually rapid and complete; a morphologic manifestation may be absent or imperceptible although a transient functional disruption and/or a brief biochemical alteration may be detectable. For example, transient release of alanine aminotransferase from hepatocytes into plasma after administration of a mild hepatotoxic compound for a short period of time may not correlate to damage microscopically or even ultrastructurally. At the other extreme, a potent hepatotoxic compound may cause such widespread hepatic necrosis after the initial spike in serum levels of the toxicant or toxin. The cause of the massive lysis of hepatocytes cannot be determined as the xenobiotic is no longer detectable in serum due to its relative short half-life at the time of necropsy. However, the lesion is obvious even at the macroscopic level. More information on clinical pathology parameters in toxicity testing can be found in the chapter *Clinical Pathology in Nonclinical Toxicity Testing*, Vol 1, Chap 10.

If cells in a tissue are injured, and the compound suspected of causing the damage is still detectable in blood or tissue, a presumptive etiologic diagnosis is possible. But with chronic tissue injury, such as glomerulosclerosis or retinal atrophy, the etiology may remain undetermined.

Furthermore, cell injury can be manifested exclusively by functional deficits without perceptible morphologic manifestations if the death of the individual cell occurs very rapidly after exposure or insult (e.g., in a matter of minutes). Such injury could even result in death of the animal. The complete disruption of oxidative phosphorylation in acute cyanide toxicity due to inhibition of cytochromes (CYPs) in the mitochondrial respiratory chain is such an example (Miller and Zachary, 2017a, 2017b; ATSDR, 2006).

The metabolic rate of a cell has a significant effect on lesion development. Cells with high metabolic activity are generally more sensitive to noxious injury than cells with low energy needs. For example, neurons are quite sensitive to hypoxia, while fibroblasts are quite resistant. Metabolically active cells absolutely depend on a continuous supply of oxygen (O_2) and functional mitochondria to generate ATP for sustaining cell function. Toxic injuries that break the links between O_2 diffusion from inhaled air across pulmonary alveoli to the O_2-carrying erythrocytes in blood vessels to the interstitium to the cell and finally to mitochondria, where oxidative phosphorylation and ATP generation occur, can subsequently injure cells with high energy needs. Adequate cellular ATP is necessary to maintain normal structure and function of many vital specialized cell populations, such as neurons. These cells require energy to sustain membrane integrity and polarity as well as neurotransmitter production. Similarly, myocardial cells require energy for myofilament contraction/relaxation and Ca^{+2} transport, and renal tubular epithelial cells which require energy for transport of fluids, electrolytes, and metabolites. Even small changes in cellular O_2 tension leading to mildly decreased ATP production can cause serious alterations in essential functions of these cell types, with severe consequences for survival. Shifting to anaerobic glycolysis is inefficient for production of adequate ATP and leads to lactic acidosis. By contrast, cells with low metabolic activity, such as fibroblasts and adipocytes, are resistant to low O_2 supply and can tolerate hypoxic conditions. Hence, these connective tissue elements can play prominent roles in regeneration and scarring after tissue damage.

Highly specialized cells are not only sensitive to hypoxia, they are generally more sensitive to toxic insult than connective tissue cells. The latter, such as fibroblasts, possess greater adaptability to a variety of conditions, assuming an assortment of different roles due to their relatively undifferentiated nature and broad functional capabilities. These cells can tolerate anaerobic conditions and many types of toxic insults. In contrast, highly specialized cells,

such as retinal rods and cones, must expend abundant energy to maintain their membranes in conformations capable of trapping photons; hence, they are exquisitely sensitive to injury.

The specialized functions of a tissue cell may predispose it to a particular type of noxious insult. Specific receptors on a particular cell population may render it susceptible to insults that would not impact neighboring cell types. For instance, cells expressing the Fas receptor (FasR) may undergo apoptosis when Fas ligand binds to it, whereas cells without this receptor will be unaffected. Some cells may accumulate toxins because they have specific transporters that facilitate their uptake. For example, the nephrotoxicity of gentamicin, and similar aminoglycoside antibiotics, depends on the organic cation transport system that leads to accumulation in lysosomes. Lysosomes eventually rupture, triggering changes that lead to cell injury and then cell death (Mingeot-Leclercq and Tulkens, 1999).

Toxicity may be further enhanced if the target cell is incapable of metabolic detoxification or metabolizes the toxin to a more reactive chemical species. Phase I metabolism, especially by certain members of the CYP450 family, is particularly important in bioactivation of xenobiotics to toxic intermediates. For example, the presence in the hepatocyte of CYP 2E1 makes it uniquely susceptible to damage by acetaminophen, which is bioactivated to a highly reactive quinone imine by this CYP isozyme (McGill and Jaeschke, 2013).

The "innate" ability of a cell to counter an injurious stimulus can be critical for resisting a toxic insult. For example, cells with high levels of antioxidants are typically resistant to oxidative injury. The liver, which receives 60% of its blood supply directly from the gastrointestinal tract through the portal vein, can generally tolerate a remarkably high level of potential noxious agents originating from the gut. This tolerability is attributed to high concentrations of antioxidants such as reduced glutathione and the vitamins C and E, and a broad array of phase I and phase II detoxification enzymes within hepatocytes. Of course, metabolizing enzymes are a "double-edged sword" since otherwise innocuous compounds may be metabolized highly bioactive, toxic intermediates which deplete glutathione and then bind to innate proteins or nucleic acids. Cells lacking high concentrations of endogenous antioxidants and/or antioxidant enzymes or missing the appropriate quantities or combinations of phase I and phase II enzymes can be especially prone to toxic injury. This vulnerability is heightened if cells tasked with detoxification, like the hepatocyte or the bronchiolar exocrine (club) cell in the lung, fail to detoxify harmful substances before they reach the general circulation.

1.3. Host Reaction to Cell Injury

Host reaction to injured or dead cells often plays a key role in the morphologic manifestation of toxic cell injury. The inflammatory reaction to injured cells can amplify the original toxic injury to a more substantial lesion or even a life-threatening condition. Thus, what may be a relatively mild and recoverable injury can progress to a severe, nonresolving lesion. For example, acute necrotizing pancreatitis induced by acinar cell toxins is exacerbated by activated neutrophils attracted by released zymogen granules. Neutrophils release a variety of preformed and de novo generated chemicals that indiscriminately destroy even previously unaffected cells in the vicinity of the original injury.

It is important to consider that the inflammatory reaction to "programmed" cell death such as apoptosis or other related forms of death is muted or even absent altogether. With necrosis and other forms of mechanistically related cell death, the inflammatory reaction is provoked by leakage of normally sequestered intracellular contents [e.g., cytochrome c from mitochondria, partially degraded cell components (e.g., cross-linked fragments of damage membranes), cytoplasmic enzymes, and signaling proteins from disintegrating cells]. This process especially attracts neutrophils, the "first responders" of the acute inflammatory response. In contrast, apoptosis and related forms of cell death proceed in an orderly sequence of cell senescence preserves membrane integrity. The sequestration of intracellular materials within the debris ("apoptotic bodies") permits macrophages to scavenge potential proinflammatory products before they can be released.

All the aforementioned factors and more contribute to the varied susceptibility of different cells and tissues to injury. Regardless of the type

of injury or the factors present that mitigate or exacerbate that injury, a given cell population has only a limited number of responses available for survival and repair.

2. ADAPTATION

A cell exists within a narrow range of physiochemical conditions necessary to maintain a viable state. Thus, a cell, even a highly specialized one, dedicates much of its resources toward maintaining this internal environment. Ion gradients, intracellular pH, and cytosolic osmolarity are vigorously controlled by the cell, even at the cost of its own specialized functions. A cell threatened with a loss of these basic conditions will often jettison its specialized structures and cut back on its specialized functions, regardless of whether these functions are critical to the survival or the host at large. Substantial deviations from homeostasis lead to death of the cell. Less substantial deviations may lead to a new, usually reduced, level of function or metabolic activity in an attempt compromise between overall cell survival and specialized cell function. The response of a cell to disrupted homeostasis while maintaining some degree of function and avoiding death is called adaptation.

2.1. Atrophy

Atrophy is an adaptive change characterized as a generally visible reduction in the size (volume) of a cell, tissue, or organ. Cell atrophy can simply result from "lack of use" (i.e., reduced demand for the specialized function or product of the affected cell type), such as occurs in skeletal muscle fibers after denervation or with immobilization. The lack of muscle contraction leads to a reduction in sarcoplasmic contractile proteins which is evident microscopically as a decrease in myofiber diameter (Fig. 6.1).

Atrophy can also result from a lack of hormone stimulation. Deficiencies in pituitary trophic hormones, such as thyroid stimulating hormone (TSH) or adrenocorticotropic hormone, lead to atrophy of thyroid follicular and adrenal cortical epithelial cells, respectively, resulting in atrophy of that portion of each gland where unstimulated cells reside. This type of atrophy, in which cells simply disappear from a tissue, is sometimes

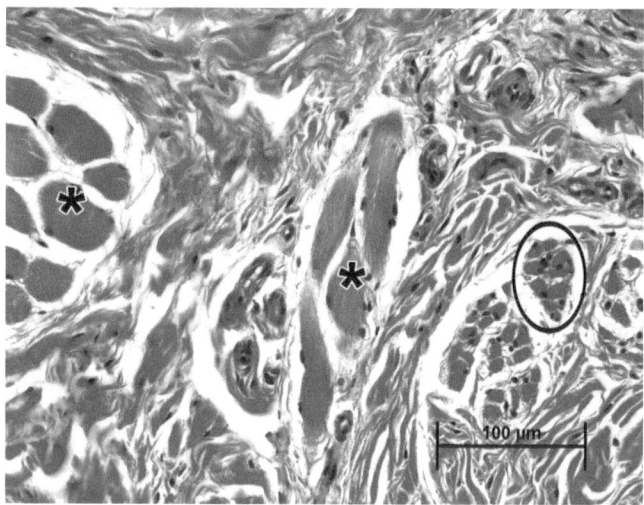

FIGURE 6.1 Atrophy due to loss of cellular mass. Photomicrograph of skeletal muscle from the tongue of a young horse. Portions of the tongue atrophied secondary to impairment of the regional blood supply. Affected muscle bundles (*circled*) are reduced in size, as are individual myofibers. Normal fibers are indicated by an *asterisk*. Hematoxylin and eosin. *Figure reproduced from Haschek WM, Rousseaux CG, Wallig MA, editors:* Handbook of toxicologic pathology, *ed 3, Academic Press, 2013, Figure 4.1, p. 80, with permission.*

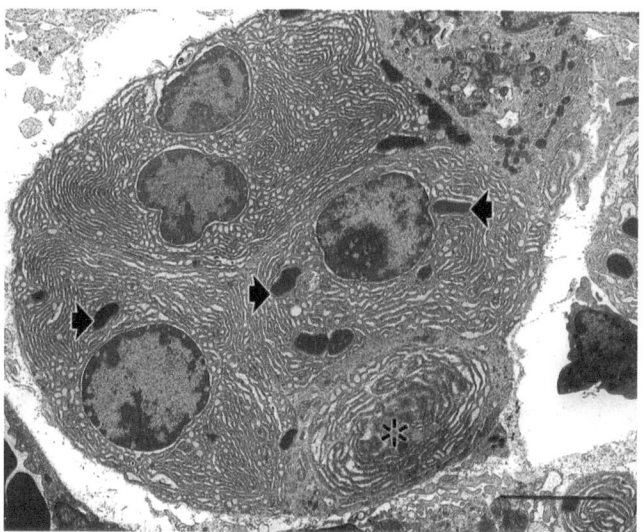

FIGURE 6.2 Atrophy due to loss of cellular mass. Electron photomicrograph of an atrophic pancreatic acinus from a male Fischer 344 (F344) rat after a bout of edematous pancreatitis induced by the phytochemical crambene. Acinar cells are reduced in size, lack polarity, are devoid of granules, and have few mitochondria (*arrows*). An autophagic vacuole containing acinar cell cytoplasm (*asterisk*) is present in one cell. Bar = 10 μm. *Figure reproduced from the Haschek WM, Rousseaux CG, Wallig, editors:* Handbook of toxicologic pathology, *ed 2, Academic Press, 2002, Figure 2, p. 43, with permission.*

termed numerical atrophy. This process occurs by a programmed process of cell death termed apoptosis (see below). The severity of atrophic changes is dependent on both the degree and duration of stimulus withdrawal. Profound or complete loss of stimulation for an extended period of time can lead to large scale autophagy and even cellular senescence.

Cell atrophy can also result from an insufficient supply of energy or substrates required to maintain structure and function even with no change in demand for its products or function. For example, pressure from an adjacent tumor can disrupt normal circulation leading to hypoxia or insufficient delivery of glucose for ATP generation or amino acids to maintain structural proteins. Cells that are capable of surviving in such an adverse environment will generally undergo atrophy. Cells in the immediate vicinity of the tumor may be compressed and distorted by physical displacement.

At the subcellular level, an atrophied cell is not only reduced in size but also may lack organellar features typical for a fully functional cell of that particular phenotype (Fig. 6.2).

Cellular atrophy is typically accomplished by a process termed autophagy. Autophagy has two major forms that can be observed morphologically—microautophagy and macroautophagy (Parzych and Klionsky, 2014; Kumar et al., 2015a). Although these autophagocytic processes may be observable by light microscopy and transmission electron microscopy, the changes observed are dependent upon which adaptive process occurs and at what stage the particular autophagocytic process is in when the cell is assessed morphologically.

Microautophagy

The term "microautophagy" represents a cellular process utilized mainly for getting rid of excess soluble protein product either free within the cytosol, sequestered within ER or within secretory granules (e.g., zymogen in pancreatic acinar cells). The process is apparently mediated by direct uptake by the lysosome of the targeted protein using an endocytosis-like process or by fusion of a protein-laden endosome with the lysosome, leading to activation of lysosomal proteases and degradation of the discharged protein (Setembre et al., 2011). Given the relatively small size of a lysosome, autophagolysosomes may be difficult to visualize histologically, at least in early stages. They have been characterized as being small, indistinct basophilic, sometimes eosinophilic 1–2 micron bodies usually without a well-defined vacuole or halo around them. These bodies may eventually coalesce and condense into dark intensely hyperbasophilic or hypereosinophilic residual bodies (see below).

Macroautophagy

Macroautophagy is a more discernible change associated with the sequestration and degradation of large portions of cytoplasm, including organelles like mitochondria. The process is initiated by the appropriate stress inducer leading to the de novo formation of an induction membrane, derived from ER, that elongates in circular fashion to sequester the targeted cytoplasm within an "autophagosome" (or autophagic vacuole), which then fuses ultimately with lysosomes where the appropriate enzymes are activated for degradation of the sequestered contents (Papadopolus and Meyer, 2017). The autophagosome and autophagolysosome are generally discernible by light microscopy (Fig. 6.3), even in early stages of formation, when newly enveloped organelles may still be largely intact and recognizable within a discrete circular membrane-bound vesicles. As degradation proceeds, organelles lose their distinctive structural features and the content of the vesicles tends to become paler, less discrete, or even disappear over time. Amorphous vesicles containing electron-dense granular material often represent residual bodies, an end stage of the autophagolysosome that contains nondegradable phospholipid and protein–phospholipid end products. The presence of residual bodies not only can reflect an adaptive response to injury or decreased biochemical demand but also can be a reflection of xenobiotic-induced phospholipidosis (see below).

Other Forms of Autophagy

Autophagy can be so severe that the cell undergoes death in a modified form of apoptosis, termed autophagic cell death (Nikoletopoulous et al., 2013). In this case, the ultrastructural and

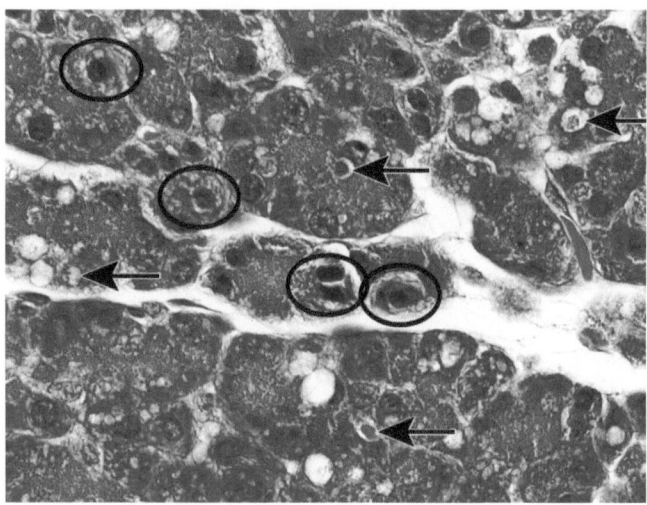

FIGURE 6.3 Macro- and microautophagy in a rat pancreas 4 hours after IV administration of caerulein. Many macroautophagic vacuoles (*arrows*) contain sequestered zymogen granules. Also present are numerous acinar cells in various stages of single-cell necrosis/programmed cell death (*circles*).

histologic morphology of the affected cell has some features of apoptosis, with the added features of numerous autophagic vacuoles but often not the nuclear features of apoptosis (see Table 6.2 below for more description). Cells undergoing autophagic cell death are generally not removed by macrophage ingestion and are filled with autophagic bodies (see below).

The end result of large-scale autophagy of any type, especially secondary to cell injury, may be the formation of residual bodies. These are typically composed of nondegradable complex structural (i.e., membrane associated) lipids and lipoproteins that collectively in the past have been termed lipofuscin or ceroid (wear and tear) pigments (Fig. 6.4). Residual bodies are particularly common in longer lived metabolically active cells that have a high turnover of membrane components, such as striated muscle cells, neurons, and hepatocytes (Yin, 1996).

Atrophic cells often lose some, or all, of their specialized structures such as microvilli, cilia, contractile apparatuses, or secretory granules. In the extreme, an atrophic cell may not be recognizable as a specialized cell at all (Fig. 6.5). As mentioned above, under light microscopy with standard H&E staining an atrophic cell is typically small with a reduced amount of cytoplasm that may contain eosinophilic droplets, reflective of retained autophagosomes,

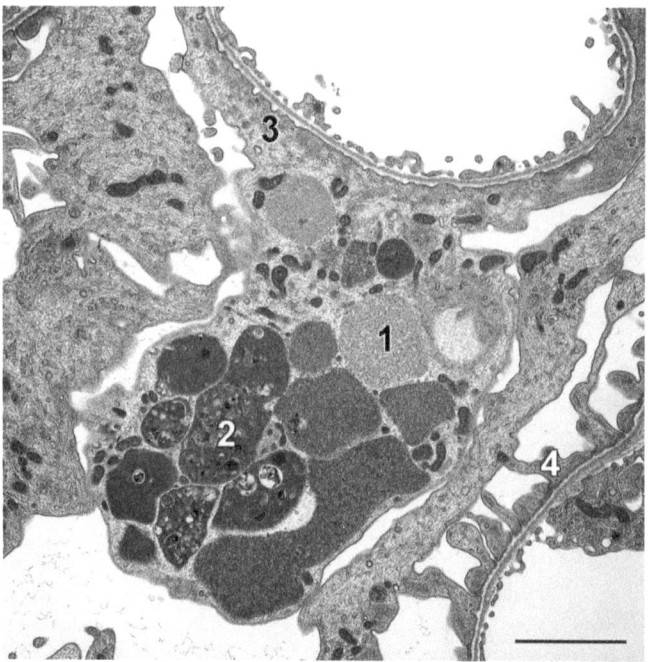

FIGURE 6.4 Residual bodies. Electron photomicrograph of the renal glomerulus from a rat with xenobiotic-induced damage to podocytes. Note the degenerate podocyte with enlarged phagolysosomes (1) and residual bodies (2). Also note diffuse fusion of blunted podocyte foot processes (3), in contrast with the distinct and elongate processes (4) of an adjacent, normal podocyte. Bar = 2 μm. *Figure reproduced from Haschek WM, Rousseaux CG, Wallig MA, editors:* Handbook of toxicologic pathology, *ed 3, Academic Press, 2013, Figure 4.3, p. 81, with permission.*

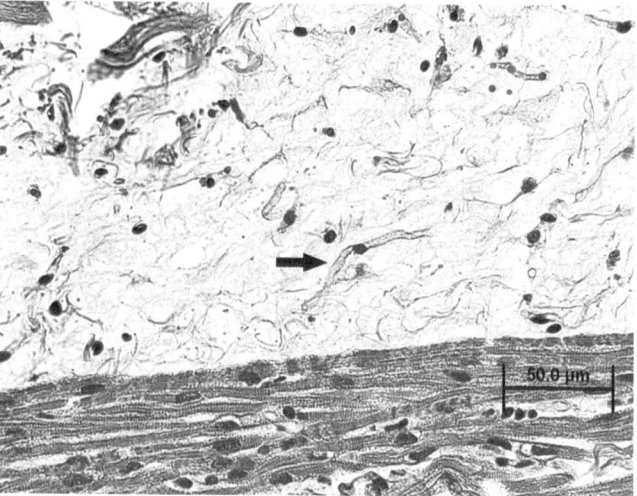

FIGURE 6.5 Atrophy due to loss of cellular mass. Photomicrograph of epicardial adipose tissue from a severely emaciated sheep. The *arrow* points to a severely atrophied adipocyte that no longer retains its normal morphologic features (i.e., round contour with large, central, clear cytoplasmic fat droplet). Note the abundant pale ground substance between the atrophied adipocytes. Hematoxylin and eosin. *Figure reproduced from Haschek WM, Rousseaux CG, Wallig MA, editors:* Handbook of toxicologic pathology, *ed 3, Academic Press, 2013, Figure 4.4, p. 82, with permission.*

autophagolysosomes, or red-brown or golden-brown pigment granules which represent residual bodies filled with lipofuscin and ceroid pigment. Grossly, an atrophic organ may simply appear small and pale, such as thyroid glands as a sequela to prolonged lack of TSH stimulation, or may reflect the underlying etiology such as with shrunken, irregularly contoured, gray, and firm kidneys as a sequela to chronic interstitial inflammation and fibrosis.

Tissue or organ atrophy can also result from a decrease in the overall *number* of cells, subsequent to cell death, e.g., by apoptosis or necrosis or related processes (discussed in more detail below), or insufficient cell replacement after loss of normal cells. The macroscopic and microscopic features of atrophic tissue often reflect the mechanism of cell death. When cell loss has occurred via widespread apoptosis or

related phenomena, tissue macrophages may be prominent within the atrophic tissue (Fig. 6.6). Vacuoles, representing phagolysosomes or residual bodies containing remnants of dead cells in various stages of degradation, may be evident within surviving cells or within nearby tissue macrophages. Apoptotic bodies may be observed (Fig. 6.7), but once apoptosis has waned, residual inflammation, never profound to begin with, is usually absent. Grossly, atrophic organs resulting from loss of cell numbers may be indistinguishable from atrophic tissue resulting from reduction in cell mass but when subtle may only be revealed by reductions in absolute or relative organ weight.

Tissue or organ atrophy resulting from overt cell necrosis is evident with light microscopy by evidence of remaining swollen (injured), dead, or lysed cells, often with obvious damage to interstitium and stroma and residual active vascular inflammatory response (i.e., engorged vessels with rounded endothelium) (Fig. 6.8). Where patent capillary beds do remain, inflammatory cell infiltrate is typical, being

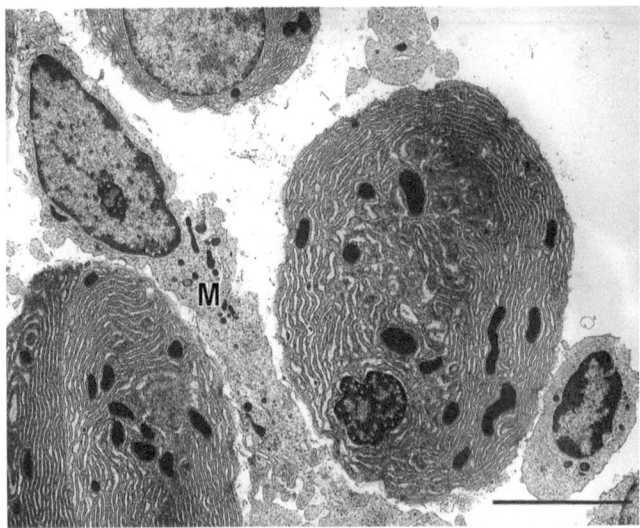

FIGURE 6.6 Atrophy due to loss of cells. Electron photomicrograph of a single remaining atrophied pancreatic acinar cell from a Fischer 344 (F344) rat treated with crambene, resulting in extensive apoptosis of most acinar cells. A tissue macrophage (**M**) is present near the atrophied cell. Bar = 10 μm. *Figure reproduced with permission from the Haschek WM, Rousseaux CG, Wallig MA, editors: Handbook of toxicologic pathology, ed 2, Academic Press, 2002, Figure 3, p. 44, with permission.*

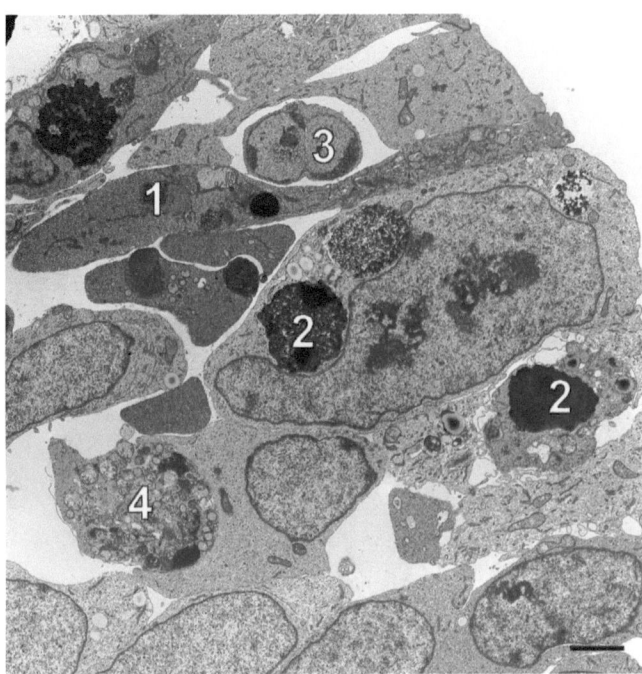

FIGURE 6.7 Atrophy due to loss of cells. Electron photomicrograph of neuroepithelium from the forebrain of a mouse embryo in which xenobiotic-induced organ atrophy has occurred. Note numerous shrunken cells with increased electron density of the cytoplasm, characteristic of apoptosis (1). Note also that many cells contain clumps of condensed chromatin (2). In one cell, peripherally clumped, crescent-shaped chromatin caps a portion of the remaining nucleus (3). An apoptotic cell with degenerate organelles has been phagocytized (4). Bar = 2 μm. *Figure reproduced from Haschek WM, Rousseaux CG, Wallig MA, editors: Handbook of toxicologic pathology, ed 3, Academic Press, 2013, Figure 4.6, p. 83, with permission.*

suppurative in early stages, mixed with neutrophils and macrophages during intermediate stages and predominantly macrophagic in later stages. Chronically, after necrotic cells are removed, fibrosis evident grossly as tissue firmness and pallor will ensue.

2.2. Hypertrophy

Hypertrophy is an adaptive increase in the mass of a cell, tissue, or organ that does not result from cell proliferation, i.e., hyperplasia. The most common example of hypertrophy in toxicologic pathology is xenobiotic induction of hepatocyte metabolizing enzyme systems. The generalized expansion of hepatocyte size may be sufficient to allow leakage of hepatic enzymes to produce elevations in serum transaminases and predispose the hepatocyte to necrosis when rodents such as mice with severely enlarged livers are manipulated for dosing.

Hypertrophy is commonly a metabolic response to increased demand for the specialized function provided by the particular cell population affected. Endocrine cells responsive to trophic hormones often undergo hypertrophy when stimulated by the appropriate hormonal ligand. Hypertrophy of pituitary gonadotrophic adenohypophyseal cells in response to gonadotropin-releasing hormone from the hypothalamus at the onset of puberty is a classic example. By light microscopy, hypertrophy appears as an increase in the volume of cytoplasm which may appear more granular and exhibit cytoplasmic changes in staining intensity (e.g., become paler or darker) if accompanied by organelle hyperplasia. The nuclei of hypertrophied cells are often enlarged, with a prominent nucleolus. By transmission electron microscopy, hypertrophied cells are usually replete with morphologically normal organelles, although

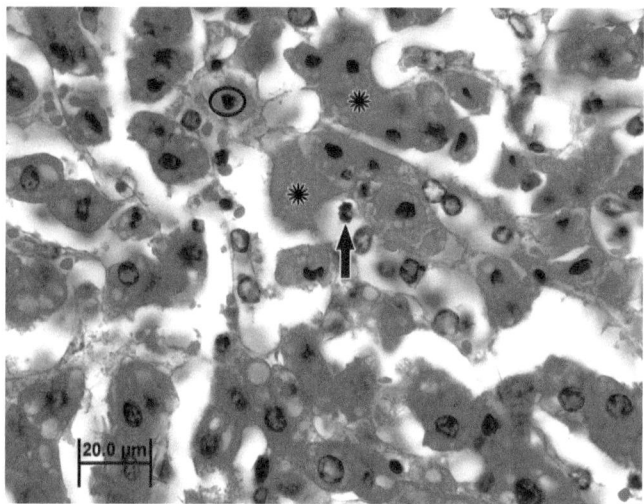

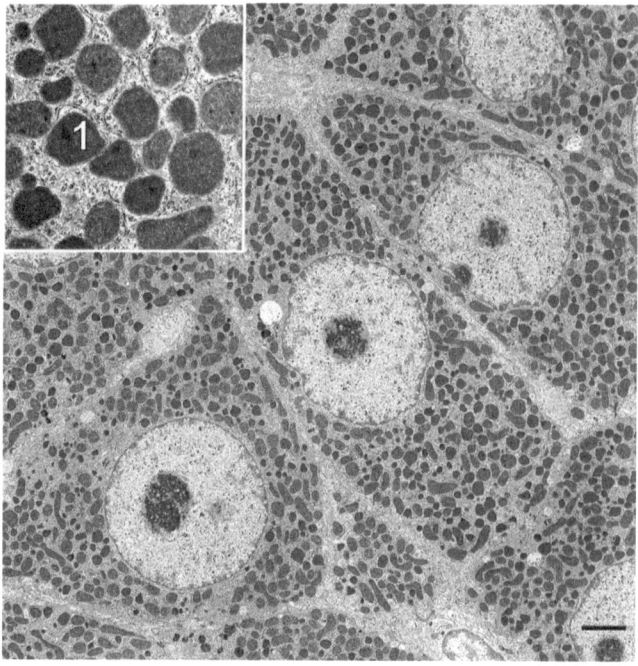

FIGURE 6.8 Necrosis. Photomicrograph of liver from a cow that died of endotoxemia. Foci of necrosis were present throughout the liver. The starburst indicates a hypereosinophilic, swollen hepatocyte with an irregular profile and has most likely ruptured. Encircled is an irregularly shrunken nucleus typical of pyknosis (i.e., nuclear condensation and shrinkage), a change associated with necrosis. The arrow indicates a neutrophil attracted to the partially degraded cellular material released from the dying cell. Less severely affected, viable hepatocytes are present in the lower right hand corner of the image. Hematoxylin and eosin. *Figure reproduced from Haschek WM, Rousseaux CG, Wallig MA, editors:* Handbook of toxicologic pathology, *ed 3, Academic Press, 2013, Figure 4.7, p. 83, with permission.*

FIGURE 6.9 Organellar hypertrophy. Electron photomicrograph of hepatocytes from a rat treated with a peroxisome proliferator–activated receptor (PPAR)-alpha agonist, leading to a dramatic increase in the numbers of electron-dense granules (peroxisomes) in the cytoplasm. Bar = 2 μm. Inset: peroxisomes are identifiable by the presence of a distinctive nucleoid (1). *Figure reproduced from Haschek WM, Rousseaux CG, Wallig MA, editors:* Handbook of toxicologic pathology, *ed 3, Academic Press, 2013, Figure 4.8, p. 84, with permission.*

certain organelles (e.g., peroxisomes, ER, or microfilaments) may be enlarged as well as more numerous (Cheville, part 2, 2009). Diffuse but subtle cellular hypertrophy may be imperceptible by standard light microscopy but can be discerned grossly by organ weight increases or morphometry if necessary.

In toxicologic pathology, hepatocyte peroxisome proliferation is the classic, although now somewhat historical, example of organelle hyperplasia causing cellular and organ hypertrophy. Xenobiotics that agonize peroxisome proliferator–activated receptors (PPARs, especially PPAR-alpha) on the nuclear membrane induce activation of particular transcription factors that subsequently lead to such widespread proliferation of peroxisomes that hepatocytes are noticeably enlarged, with abundant granular eosinophilic cytoplasm (Fig. 6.9).

Although not necessarily considered hypertrophy by every pathologist, phospholipidosis is another common cause of xenobiotic-induced cellular enlargement due to organelle accumulation. Cationic amphiphilic compounds accumulating in lysosomes can alter degradation of phospholipid-rich membranes (Breiden and Sandhoff, 2020). With standard processing for light microscopy, most of the retained lipid-soluble breakdown products dissolve leaving abundant, finely vacuolated, or "moth-eaten" appearing cytoplasm. During processing for transmission electron microscopy, the lipids are retained so "vacuoles" appear as enlarged discrete membrane-bound bodies containing laminated whorls of partially degraded membranes, termed "myelin whorls." (Fig. 6.10) In cases such as this, where there has been microautophagy (see above), the

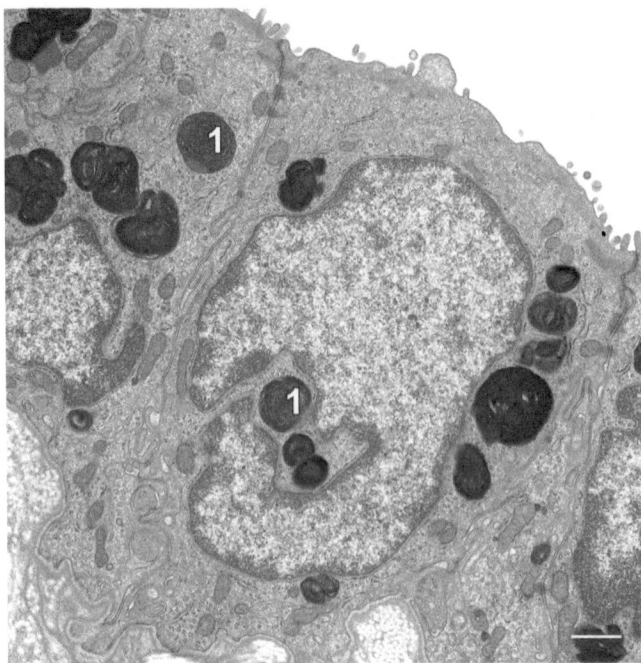

FIGURE 6.10 Phospholipid accumulation. Electron photomicrograph of biliary epithelium from a rat treated with a xenobiotic that induces phospholipidosis. Note the numerous enlarged, electron-dense lysosomes expanded by lamellar or myelinoid bodies (1). These bodies are the ultrastructural hallmark of phospholipidosis. Bar = 1 μm. *Figure reproduced from Haschek WM, Rousseaux CG, Wallig MA, editors:* Handbook of toxicologic pathology, *ed 3, Academic Press, 2013, Figure 4.9, p. 84, with permission.*

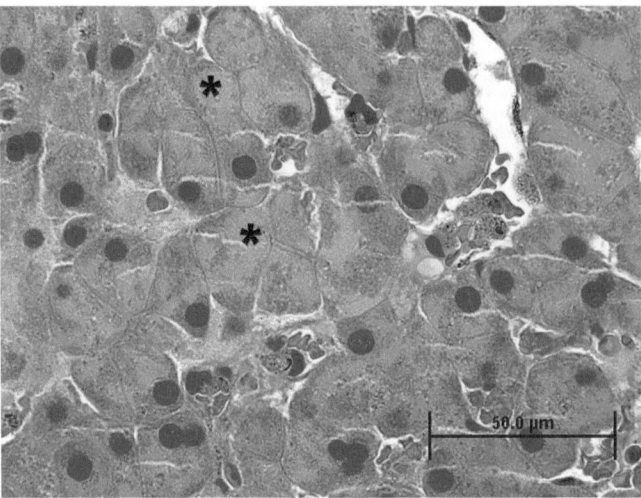

FIGURE 6.11 Pathologic hypertrophy. Photomicrograph of liver from a dog treated for a prolonged period of time with oral phenobarbital to control convulsions. The enlarged hepatocytes contain an increased quantity of pale, hyaline cytoplasm (*asterisks*) due to profound expansion of the smooth endoplasmic reticulum. Hematoxylin and eosin. *Figure reproduced from Haschek WM, Rousseaux CG, Wallig MA, editors:* Fundamentals of toxicologic pathology, *ed 2, Academic Press, 2007, Figure 2.3, p 13, with permission.*

hypertrophy observed microscopically overlaps with the morphologic changes associated with autophagy observed ultrastructurally.

Generally, cellular or even organ hypertrophy is not overtly injurious per se, especially in the short term, and its presence merely reflects a physiologic response to an increased demand on a tissue for its specialized function. However, organelle proliferation can interfere with other cellular functions, leading to so-called pathologic hypertrophy; this is fairly common in toxicologic pathology. For example, hypertrophy of smooth endoplasmic reticulum (sER) of hepatocytes chronically exposed to phenobarbital or other anticonvulsant drugs (Fig. 6.11). Hypertrophy of sER is not necessarily pathologic; however, the sheer volume of sER may crowd out cytosol and other essential organelles that will impair other hepatocyte functions such as urea production or bile excretion leading to liver dysfunction

if hepatocytes are affected globally. In investigative toxicologic pathology, treatment of experimental animals with 1-aminobenzotriazole used to inhibit phase I metabolism (Ortiz de Montellano, 2018) can lead to nonpathologic hypertrophy of affected hepatocytes secondary to mild sER hypertrophy (Fig. 6.12).

3. IRREVERSIBLE VERSUS REVERSIBLE CELL INJURY

Cell injury is any physical or chemical insult that results in the loss of a cell's capacity to maintain homeostasis, in either a normal or adaptive state. In toxicologic pathology, cell injury is often in the context of exposure to a noxious stimulus that prevents the cell from maintaining its physiologic parameters within survivable limits. Defining these limits for an injured cell (i.e., point of no return), at the biochemical level, is a complex undertaking. However, it is clear that alteration of mitochondrial membrane permeability leading to leakage of the electron transport chain enzyme cytochrome c into the

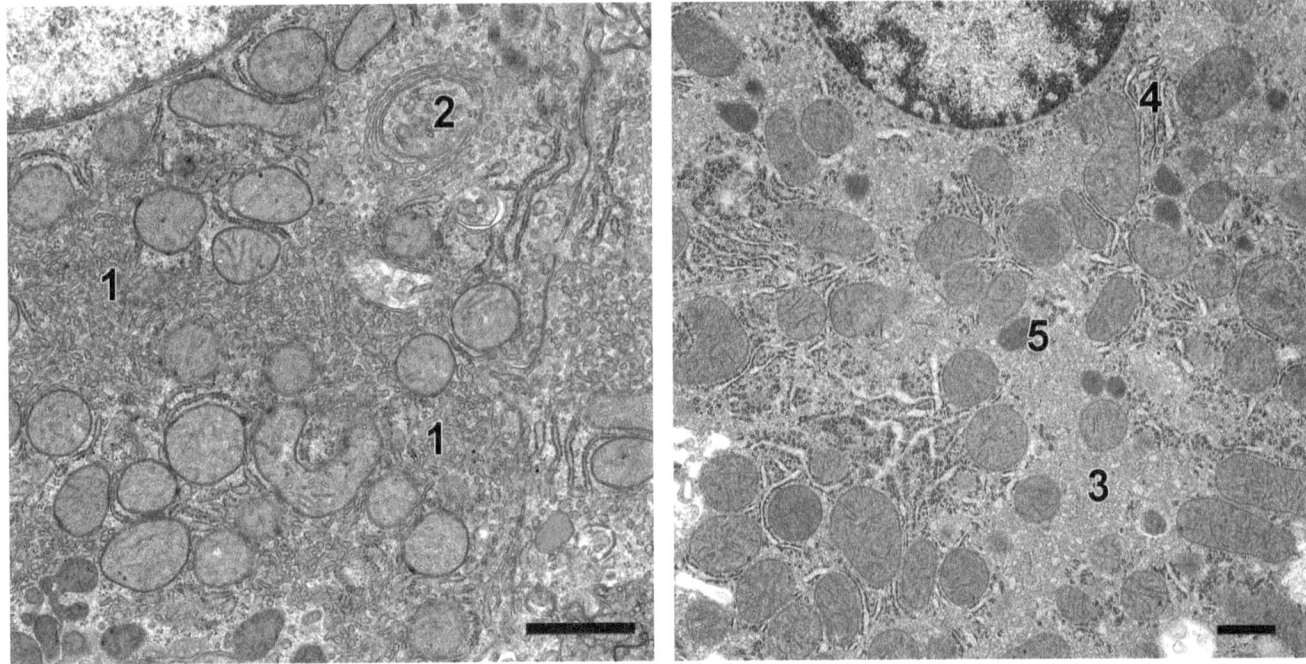

FIGURE 6.12   Adaptive hypertrophy with organellar hyperplasia. Electron photomicrograph of a hypertrophic centrilobular hepatocyte from a rat treated with a xenobiotic (1-aminobenzotriazole) that induces smooth endoplasmic reticulum proliferation (left panel), compared to a normal centrilobular hepatocyte from a control rat (right panel). Note numerous profiles of smooth endoplasmic reticulum (1) and a prominent Golgi complex (2) in the hepatocyte from the treated rat. This contrasts with the normal complement of smooth (3) and rough (4) endoplasmic reticulum, and other organelles such as peroxisomes (5), in the hepatocyte from the control rat. Bar = 1 μm. *Figure reproduced from Haschek WM, Rousseaux CG, Wallig MA, editors:* Handbook of toxicologic pathology, *ed 3, Academic Press, 2013, Figure 4.8, p. 85, with permission.*

cytosol is a critical step for both necrosis (*accidental* cell death) and apoptosis (*programmed* cell death). The escape of cytochrome c from the mitochondrion is a nonrecoverable event.

It should be kept in mind that in many forms of programmed cell death, cell injury per se often is not discernible due to the signal-driven mechanisms by which these processes are initiated. Injury indeed may be present but is generally of a subtle nature and the cell is given the signal to die before the typical cellular changes associated with overt or severe cell injury manifest. Therefore, there may be little "morphologic warning" that the cell is going to die. And so, there is no phase of reversible cell injury that can be identified morphologically prior to death since these processes are rapid, irreversible, and affect cells individually. The following paragraphs therefore will deal with cellular injury associated with direct toxicant-induced injury and recovery therefrom.

Recognizing whether an injured cell is destined to die as compared to one that will survive can be challenging via light microscopy. There is a time lag between those biochemical events that inevitably lead to cell death and the morphological manifestations of necrosis. With transmission electron microscopy, morphologic changes of irreversible cell injury are generally evident somewhat earlier than with light microscopy. Fortunately, it is rarely necessary for a toxicologic pathologist to be concerned with the potential fate of an individual cell because other cells within the affected tissue will typically manifest the morphologic features of irreversible cell injury.

Reversible cell injury simply indicates that the affected cell has the potential to survive following a noxious insult. A reversibly injured cell may be morphologically recognizable by a variety of changes depending on its phenotype. For example, specialized cells may lose their phenotypic structures such as cilia from respiratory epithelium. More generally, reversibly injured cells may exhibit classic morphologic features of cell "degeneration" such as swelling and pallor in the acute phase of injury, lipid accumulation (lipidosis), and autophagy in later phases as recovery becomes manifest (Miller and Zachary, 2017a).

Two classic morphologic features of reversible cell injury are cell swelling and fatty change, but both can progress to cell death.

3.1. Cellular Swelling

Cellular swelling is an early degenerative change that occurs in many types of acute cell injury. It may be a prelude to more drastic changes or may resolve as the cell restores homeostasis and then adapts and repairs the damage.

By standard light microscopy, cell swelling is characterized by expanded, pale cytoplasm; the cell nucleus and/or adjacent cells may be displaced, but most often it remains in its characteristic location within the particular cell. Occasionally, cell swelling associated with reversible cell injury may resemble hypertrophy. While special histochemical stains or electron microscopy may be necessary to distinguish between these processes, microscopic evaluation of the affected tissue overall is usually sufficient to allow for accurate interpretation. By electron microscopy, cell swelling is usually characterized by dilution of cytoplasmic elements and dispersion of organelles; dilated cisternae of both rER and sER may also be evident (Cheville, part 1, 2009). Rarely, extreme organelle hyperplasia/hypertrophy may lead to swelling so that both processes occur simultaneously. As cell swelling progresses, clear spaces or vacuoles may form in the cytoplasm; these usually represent dilated portions of the ER and/or Golgi apparatus. If severe enough, cisternae may rupture and "cytoplasmic lakes" may form. Solubilized or denatured protein that accumulates in these "lakes" is eosinophilic and appears as so-called hyaline droplets. This type of change is termed "vacuolar degeneration" or "vacuolar change." Diffuse cytoplasmic swelling with minimal vacuolation is also termed "ballooning degeneration" or "cloudy swelling" (Fig. 6.13).

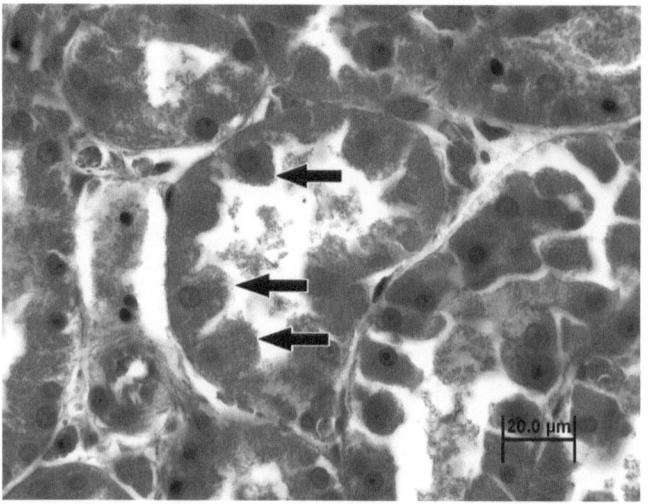

FIGURE 6.13   Cell swelling. Photomicrograph demonstrating swollen renal tubular epithelial cells from a dog in septic shock. Note the bulging of the apical portions of the cells (*arrows*), loss of brush border, and elevation of the nuclei away from their normal basal positions in the affected cells. Hematoxylin and eosin. *Figure reproduced from Haschek WM, Rousseaux CG, Wallig MA, editors:* Fundamentals of toxicologic pathology, *ed 2, Academic Press, 2007, Figure 2.3, p 13, with permission.*

The nucleus of reversibly injured cells is often morphologically normal but may undergo chromatin clumping, rarefaction, and peripheral nucleolar migration as an indication of more severe cell injury. Chromatin clumps as the pH of the cell decreases, postulated to be a protective change, sequestering DNA from potentially degradative enzymes.

Swelling occurs when the cell loses its ability to maintain the balance between cytosolic influx of sodium (Na^+) ions and water and efflux of potassium (K^+) ions. This morphologic change reflects the influx of excessive water as a consequence of ineffective membrane ATPases required to actively exchange Na^+ for K^+. The optimum osmotic gradient is lost, and water follows Na^+ into the cell cytoplasm. Pathophysiologically, cell swelling can result from direct damage to these ATP-dependent "pumps," an inadequate supply of ATP substrate, or due to an overwhelming influx of Na^+ after direct damage to the plasma membrane. Cytoplasmic vacuoles may also form directly from the ER if the Na^+/K^+ ATPases in the ER membrane are sufficiently functional to import excess Na^+

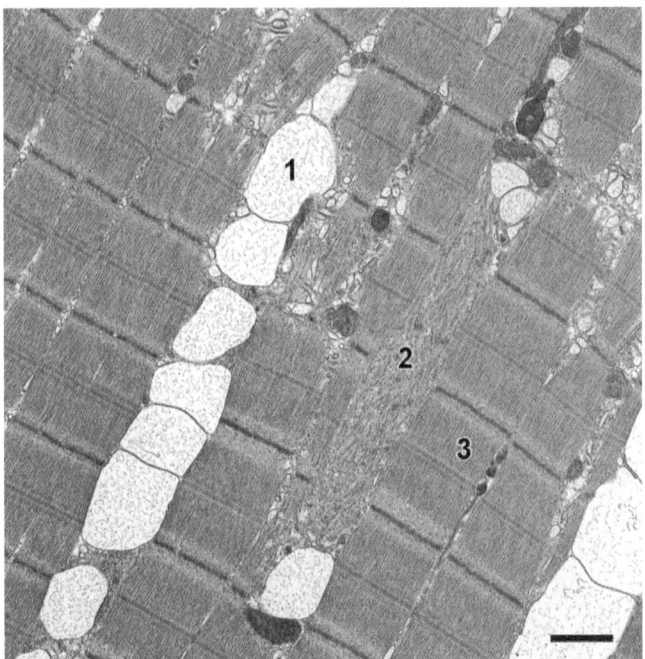

FIGURE 6.14 Vacuolar change. Electron photomicrograph of rat skeletal muscle damaged by a xenobiotic. Note the degenerate myofibers with markedly dilated sarcoplasmic reticulum containing amorphous granular material (1) and disaggregated myofibrils (2). Contrast with normal sarcomeres in adjacent myofibers (3). Bar = 1 μm. *Figure reproduced from Haschek WM, Rousseaux CG, Wallig MA, editors:* Handbook of toxicologic pathology, *ed 3, Academic Press, 2013, Figure 4.13, p. 87, with permission.*

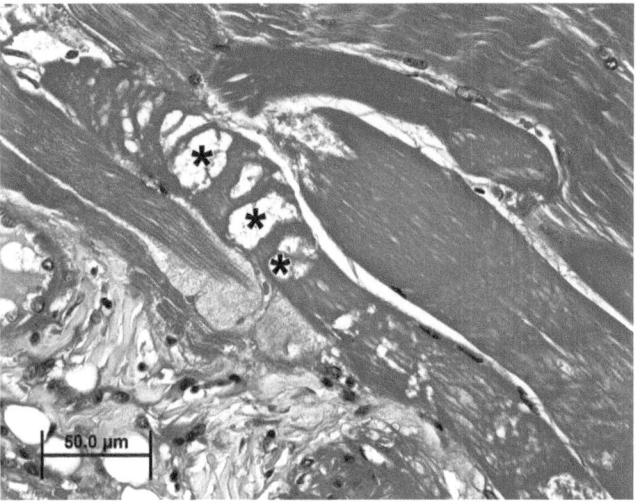

FIGURE 6.15 Vacuolar change. Photomicrograph of injured gluteal muscle of a horse. In addition to swelling, the sarcoplasm of affected myofibers contains clear vacuoles (*asterisks*) as well as separation of myofibrils with loss of striations. Hematoxylin and eosin. *Figure reproduced from Haschek WM, Rousseaux CG, Wallig MA, editors:* Handbook of toxicologic pathology, *ed 3, Academic Press, 2013, Figure 4.8, p. 88, with permission.*

(followed by water) out of the cytoplasm into ER cisternae (Fig. 6.14).

The morphologic changes associated with cell swelling are also due to the influx of calcium (Ca^{++}) via the diminished capacity or function of the ATP-dependent Na^+/Ca^{++} exchange pumps. The dissociation of cytoskeletal elements and the loss of intercellular junctions that result from excessively high cytosolic levels of free Ca^{++} lead to additional loss of normal shape and a tendency for the cell to assume a rounded profile (Fig. 6.15).

Cell swelling is not lethal per se but may indicate an early phase of a lethal process. In other words, a lethally injured cell may have been fixed at the stage of cell swelling before irreversible biochemical and morphological changes manifest. Alternative interpretations for what appears as cell swelling or vacuolar change by light microscopy include hepatocytes with glycogen accumulation, commonly observed when liver samples are obtained from animals in the fed state. Glycogen is typically stored within the hepatocyte cytosol as aggregates recognized by electron microscopy as electron-dense rosettes. A large portion of these rosettes dissolve during processing for light microscopy, leaving behind swollen hepatocytes with clear or feathery cytoplasm that resembles vacuolar change but is not an indication of cell injury. Partially degraded complex carbohydrates that accumulate within neuronal lysosomes with inherited or acquired lysosomal enzyme deficiency such as swainsonine toxicosis (locoism) in sheep can also appear as vacuolar degeneration, with the vacuoles actually being accumulations of partially degraded glycogen or other carbohydrate breakdown products within autophagolysosomes (Li et al., 2012). In principle, such acquired lysosomal storage diseases are reversible following withdrawal of the toxic etiology; however, resolution may be incomplete in highly specialized cells such as neurons.

3.2. Fatty Change—Lipidosis

Fatty change, also termed fatty degeneration, lipidosis, or steatosis, is a second manifestation of reversible cell injury. It occurs in cells that are capable of storing and metabolizing lipids, usually in the form of triglycerides, and is especially common in hepatocytes. However, this change can also affect myocardial cells and renal tubular epithelium. Whether fatty change represents a degenerative (cell injury) or adaptive change (storage) depends on the pathogenesis although severe fatty change can lead to irreversible cell injury regardless of etiology if sufficient displacement of organelles with disruption of function occurs.

Excessive influx or inadequate efflux of triglycerides will lead to accumulation of lipid droplets throughout the cytoplasm. Mitochondrial dysfunction can lead to insufficient β-oxidation of triglycerides and accumulation of triglycerides, typically in the sER adjacent to affected mitochondria. Inadequate protein synthesis secondary to a noxious insult or hypoxia can result in a deficiency of apolipoproteins for lipid transport or oxidative enzymes necessary for β-oxidation of fatty acids; consequently, lipid droplets accumulate initially near mitochondria. Cells with lipidosis can be swollen enough to impinge on the surrounding stroma to the point of occluding vascular supply. Lipid droplets may be so abundant or large that organelles necessary for normal cell function are compromised.

By electron microscopy, fatty change is characterized by accumulation of spherical, often homogenous, cytoplasmic inclusions of varying electron density. These arise from the smooth sER, forming between the inner and outer membrane leaflets. Hence lipid droplets are usually surrounded by a single layer of phospholipids derived from the outer membrane leaflet of the sER (Fig. 6.16). Lipid droplets occur in a wide range of sizes. They can be relatively small and dispersed, so-called "microvesicular" lipidosis, which often occurs in the context of an acute insult (Fig. 6.17). Lipid droplets can also be quite large, so-called "macrovesicular" lipidosis, occupying almost the entire cell and displacing organelles, including the nucleus, peripherally (Fig. 6.18); this type of fatty change typically requires a longer time to develop.

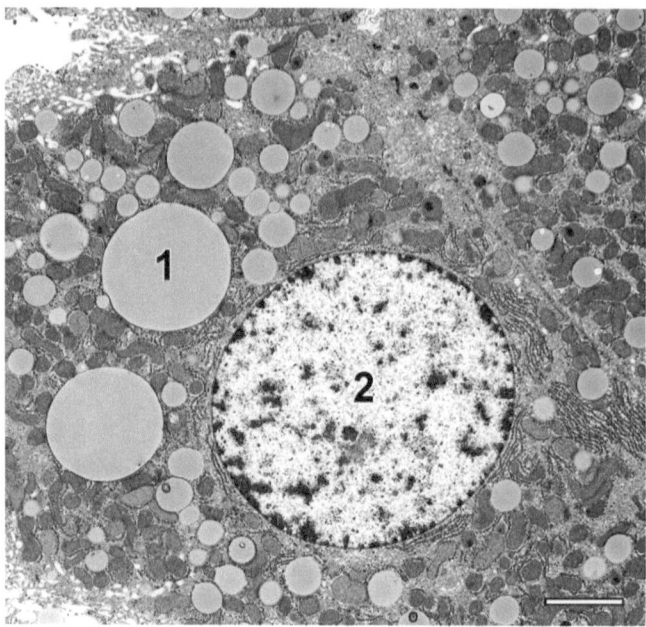

FIGURE 6.16   Lipidosis. Electron photomicrograph of xenobiotic-induced lipidosis in a mouse hepatocyte. Note that numerous, variably sized, membrane-bound lipid droplets (1) are widely dispersed throughout the cytoplasm. Also note that lipid droplets are smaller than the nucleus (2). Bar = 2 μm. *Figure reproduced from Haschek WM, Rousseaux CG, Wallig MA, editors:* Handbook of toxicologic pathology, *ed 3, Academic Press, 2013, Figure 4.15, p. 89, with permission.*

Microscopically, cells that have undergone lipidosis are noticeably swollen, with one large to many numerous, variably sized, perfectly round, clear spaces compressing the residual cytosol and nucleus to the periphery of the cell. Lipid droplets dissolve when tissue is routinely processed for light microscopy but are easily recognized. If confirmation of their lipid component is necessary, frozen sections can be stained with Oil Red O (i.e., with lipid appearing as orange droplets), Sudan black (black droplets), or osmium tetroxide (black droplets).

Macroscopically, an unfixed liver with fatty change is easily recognized as one of the classic lesions in pathology. A fatty liver is orange to yellow, evenly reticulated with a distinct lobular pattern, friable, and greasy. Lipidosis in the heart or kidney appears as pale white to yellow areas. In the heart, lipidosis may occur in the myocardium bordering an infarct where mitochondrial β-oxidation pathways are impaired. In the kidney, triglycerides may accumulate in renal tubular

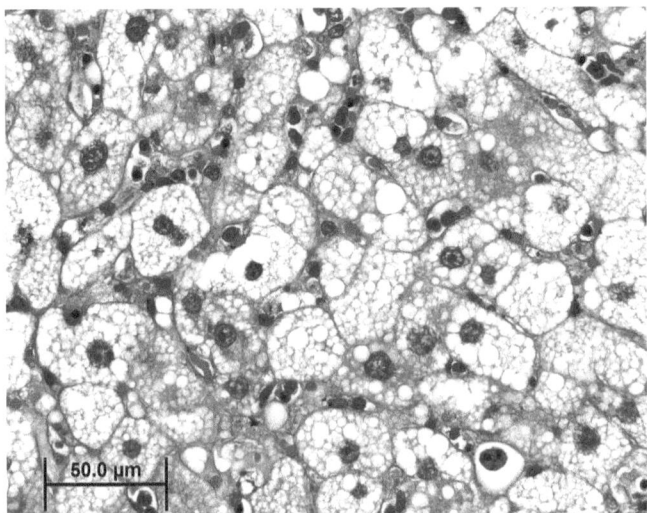

FIGURE 6.17 Microvesicular lipidosis. Photomicrograph of liver from a cat with acute hepatic lipidosis. Most hepatocytes contain many variably sized but usually small vacuoles dispersed throughout the cytoplasm. Hematoxylin and eosin. *Figure reproduced from Haschek WM, Rousseaux CG, Wallig MA, editors:* Handbook of toxicologic pathology, *ed 3, Academic Press, 2013, Figure 4.16, p. 89, with permission.*

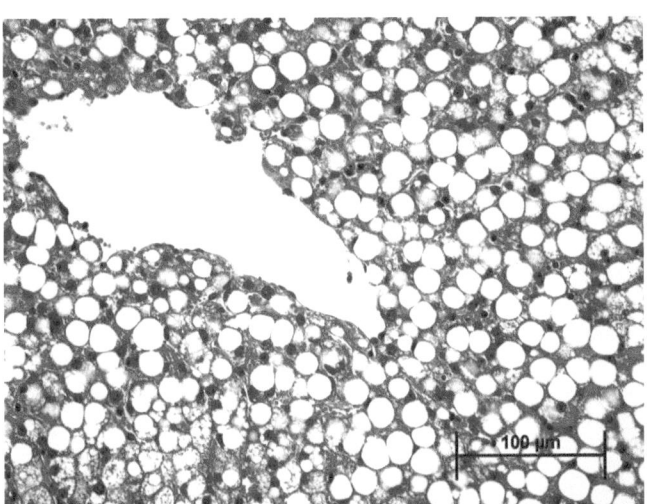

FIGURE 6.18 Macrovesicular lipidosis. Photomicrograph of liver from a goat with chronic hepatic lipidosis as a consequence of pregnancy toxemia. Most hepatocytes contain one large lipid vacuole. Other structures (e.g., nuclei) are displaced to the periphery of the cell, and often indented by the encroaching vacuoles. Hematoxylin and eosin. *Figure reproduced from Haschek WM, Rousseaux CG, Wallig MA, editors:* Fundamentals of toxicologic pathology, *ed 2, Academic Press, 2007, Figure 2.4, p 14, with permission.*

epithelium in the context of hyperlipidemia with diabetes mellitus. In tissue rich in "structural lipids" (e.g., membrane phospholipids, glycolipids, membrane protein–lipid complexes, myelin), scavenger macrophages sequester these relatively indigestible lipids in discrete round phagocytic vacuoles to which lysosomes fuse to empty their proteolytic content. A prototypic instance of this is necrosis of infarcted central nervous system (CNS) tissue, especially white matter, with the recruitment of numerous foamy "gitter cells" to remove the lipid-rich debris (see *Nervous System*, Vol 3, Chap 9). Some structural lipids, in particular damaged ones that have formed as a result of injury and can be relatively indigestible, comprise residual bodies which appear morphologically as darkly pigmented ceroid or lipofuscin and ultrastructurally as electron dense, sometimes whorled membrane-bound structures (see above). On occasion, engorged foamy macrophages may degenerate and elicit phagocytosis by adjacent macrophages; this type of lipid accumulation within macrophages is considered in most cases a normal cell function but reflective of damage to parenchymal tissue cells in the vicinity.

4. IRREVERSIBLE CELL INJURY

4.1. Accidental Cell Death—Necrosis

Irreversible cell injury leading to necrosis denotes the "point of no return" from which a damaged cell is incapable of recovery and is committed to die. Functionally, this occurs when the physiology of an irreversibly injured cell is disrupted enough that homeostasis cannot be maintained. Once a cell has reached this state, cell death whether via a passive process (i.e., necrosis) or an active process (i.e., apoptosis) is inevitable. The dead cell ultimately degrades, ruptures and dissolves, or is phagocytized.

Defining the precise physiologic criteria necessary for a cell to become irreversibly injured is virtually impossible, but cells in this state exhibit morphologic features which can clearly indicate the lethal aspect of the injury. In some instances, such features reveal the pathogenesis or even etiology of the noxious insult and these may provide the only clues to why the cell was in the process of dying (Table 6.1). The morphologic

TABLE 6.1　Necrosis versus Apoptosis

Characteristic	Necrosis	Apoptosis
Gross changes	Grossly evident with disruption of normal tissue structure and detail, scarring if long term	Minimal or atrophy without scarring
Histologic changes	Whole fields of cells affected	Individual cells scattered throughout the affected tissue
	Hypereosinophilia	Hyperbasophilia or hypereosinophilia
	Loss of cell borders with irregular fragmentation	Formation of round bodies, often within a clear halo
	Irregular chromatin clumping, pyknosis, karyorrhexis, and/or karyolysis; rupture of nuclear envelope	Chromatin condensation into caps or crescents, within round nuclear bodies; preservation of nuclear envelope
Ultrastructural changes	Swelling and loss of surface structures with blebbing and loss of apical portions of cytoplasm	Condensation followed by rapid zeiosis (budding)
	Rarefaction of cytoplasm followed by condensation after death	Condensation of cytoplasm followed by rarefaction after ingestion by phagocytes
	Swelling and loss of organellar morphology	Preservation of organellar morphology
	Low-amplitude swelling of mitochondria followed by high-amplitude swelling and rupture	Preservation of mitochondrial ultrastructure
	Rupture and degradation of internal and external membranes with bursting of the cell and leakage of cell contents	Preservation of internal and external membranes with preservation of membrane around apoptotic bodies
	Irregular clumping and degradation of chromatin; disintegration of nuclear envelope	Migration of uniformly degraded chromatin to margins of nuclear envelope; preservation of nuclear envelope
Sequelae	Release of intracellular enzymes into extracellular milieu	Retention of intracellular enzymes within the apoptotic bodies
	Release of proinflammatory cell breakdown products (e.g., DAMPs)	No release of proinflammatory products
	Ingress of neutrophils followed by macrophages	Ingestion by tissue macrophages or adjacent parenchymal cells
	Active inflammation with scarring	Atrophy with stromal collapse but *no* scarring

Table modified from Haschek WM, Rousseaux CG, Wallig MA, editors: Fundamentals of toxicologic pathology, *ed 2, Academic Press, 2007, Table 2.1, p. 16.*

progression of a dead cell's breakdown and removal can be termed generically as "necrosis," regardless of the mechanism of cell death (Elmore et al., 2016).

Generally, the process of postnecrotic cell degradation can be recognized by various gross or light microscopic features after lethal cell injury. Viable tissue surrounding necrotic cells will exhibit a host reaction, such as hemorrhage or inflammation, which allows a pathologist to distinguish antemortem from postmortem cell death. The latter, also termed autolysis, encompasses many of the end-stage physiologic and some of the morphologic manifestations of antemortem cell death. Importantly, autolysis affects large contiguous portions of whole organs, while necrosis typically affects distinct areas. Autolysis proceeds at different rates depending on internal and external factors. For example, autolysis of intestinal mucosa is rapid because bacteria are already present and abdominal viscera retain their warmth after death. In contrast, autolysis of the brain may be quite slow, especially if the ambient temperature is low since heat rapidly dissipates from the skull.

Ultrastructural features of necrosis mimic some of those that characterize reversible cell injury, including cytoplasmic swelling and rarefaction of the cytosol, dilation of the ER or formation of cytoplasmic lakes, loss or deformation of specialized structures such as microvilli, dissociation from adjacent cells, or ECM. Subcellular (ultrastructural) changes of lethal cell injury may be evident hours before they are recognizable histologically (Cheville, part 2, 2009).

Plasma membrane alterations are an early indication of lethal injury. These include loss of microvilli and cilia (Fig. 6.19), disruption of intercellular junctions with separation of gap junctions, degradation of the *maculae densae* and *zonulae adherentes*, and loss of the terminal cytoskeletal web. As the cell swells and the intricate substructure of the plasma membrane is disturbed, cytoplasmic blebs, or outpouchings, may form on the surfaces of lethally injured cells (Fig. 6.20). Such cytoplasmic fragments may detach from the bulging surface of the swollen cell and slough into an adjacent lumen or interstitial space, where they eventually lyse and release their contents which include enzymes and proinflammatory chemicals.

These enzymes and proinflammatory cell products include damage-associated molecular pattern molecules (DAMPs) which trigger inflammatory and immunologic responses; however, these responses are generally mild in comparison to the responses invoked by an infectious agent (discussed below). DAMPs include both proteins and nonprotein substances that

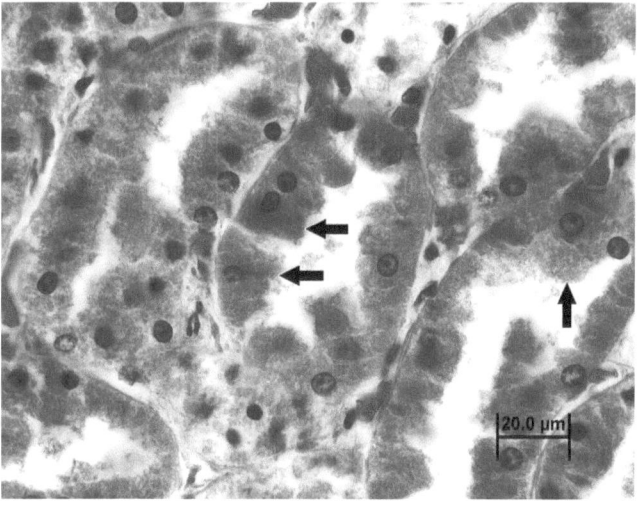

FIGURE 6.19 Loss of specialized structures after injury. Photomicrograph of injured renal tubular epithelial cells in a cat with lily (*Lilium longiflorum*) toxicosis, with loss of microvillous borders (arrows) and swelling of the cytoplasm. Hematoxylin and eosin. *Figure reproduced from Haschek WM, Rousseaux CG, Wallig MA, editors:* Handbook of toxicologic pathology, *ed 3, Academic Press, 2013, Figure 4.18, p. 92, with permission.*

are normally sequestered within a viable cell or are part of the ECM. Intracellular DAMP proteins include heat shock proteins, S-100, and the chromatin-associated protein high mobility group box 1; nonprotein DAMPs include ATP, adenosine, uric acid, and DNA itself. ECM-derived DAMPs include hyaluronan fragments and heparin sulfate.

Lethal cell injury commonly leads to cell swelling with disruption of plasma membrane integrity. Cell swelling often reflects loss of function of energy-dependent, membrane-bound ion exchange proteins, but it also may reflect enzymatic digestion of the plasma membrane by phospholipases activated by uncontrolled Ca^{+2} influx from the extracellular fluids. Other causes of plasma membrane injury include damage by free radicals generated by dysfunctional mitochondria and noxious agents that are directly damaging to plasma membrane phospholipids (Fig. 6.20). By electron microscopy, portions of partially degraded, bilayered plasma membrane, characteristically roll into laminated electron-dense myelin whorls (Fig. 6.10).

Mitochondria exhibit a variety of dramatic morphologic changes during the process of

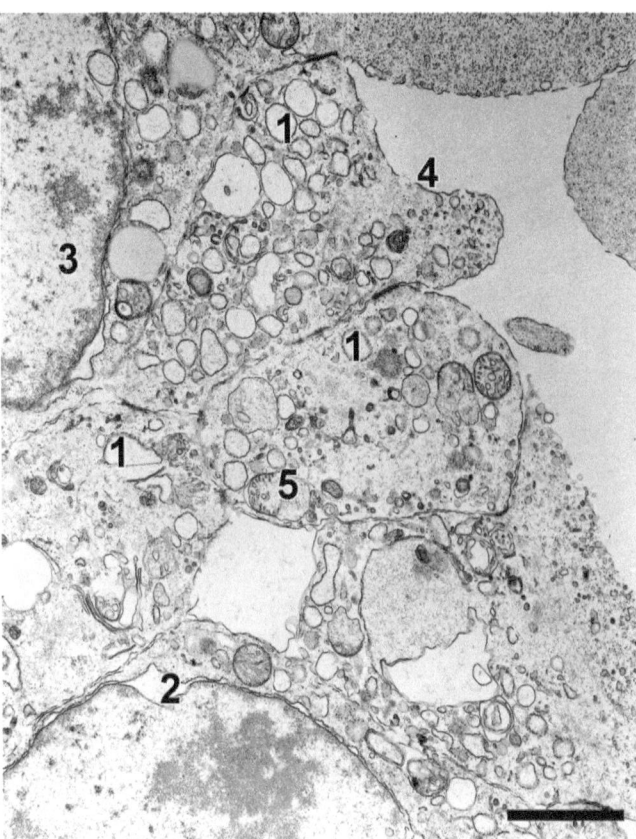

FIGURE 6.20 Necrosis. Electron photomicrograph of a necrotic neuroepithelial cell in a rat embryo with ischemia secondary to xenobiotic-induced toxicity to the dam. Note the widespread dilatation of the cyto-cavity network, including the endoplasmic reticulum (1) and nuclear envelope (2), dissolution of nuclear chromatin (i.e., karyolysis) (3), cytoplasmic bleb formation with loss of plasma membrane integrity (4), and swollen mitochondria with lysis of the cristae (5). These ultrastructural changes of end-stage cell death are not specific as they also occur with postmortem autolysis. Bar = 2 μm. *Figure reproduced from Haschek WM, Rousseaux CG, Wallig MA, editors:* Handbook of toxicologic pathology, *ed 3, Academic Press, 2013, Figure 4.19, p. 92, with permission.*

necrosis. These organelles first undergo a form of distension termed "low-amplitude" swelling, which develops as ATP production diminishes and ATP-dependent ion pumps in the mitochondrial outer membrane become incapable of maintaining water balance. Low-amplitude swelling refers to expansion of the outer mitochondrial compartment as water and electrolytes flow from the inner compartment and

sequester in the intermembranous space. Concurrently, the inner mitochondrial compartment condenses, becoming electron dense when observed ultrastructurally. This state is recoverable if the noxious insult halts.

With persistent and severe injury, electron-dense deposits within mitochondria, termed "flocculent densities" and composed of degraded mitochondrial matrix and membrane proteins (Itkonen and Collan, 1983), become sites for calcium phosphate deposition as Ca^{+2} homeostatic mechanisms fail. Over time, these enlarge (Trump et al., 1984). These mineralized structures are not readily dissolved/degraded and can remain in a recovered mitochondrion as evidence of previous damage.

High-amplitude mitochondrial swelling is an indication of that the necrotic processes have progressed to the point of no return. It is characterized by massive swelling of both inner and outer compartments, loss of cristae (cristolysis), and accumulation of precipitated mineral and protein (Fig. 6.20). As the inner mitochondrial compartment expands to contact the outer compartment, an irreversible state termed mitochondrial permeability transition (MPT) ensues.

Once MPT begins, ATP-generating particles on the inner mitochondrial membrane detach, ATP production ceases, and adenine nucleotide transporter (ANT) is released. ANT binds to the mitochondrial matrix protein cyclophilin D. This complex binds to an outer membrane ion transport protein, the voltage-dependent anion channel forming the MPT pore which allows the passage of small molecules between the mitochondrial matrix and the cytosol.

One of the smallest and earliest proteins to leak out through the MPT pores is the electron transport chain protein, cytochrome c, which is only lightly tethered to the inner mitochondrial membrane. At this stage as well, Ca^{+2} salt precipitates are prominent, especially when vascular perfusion replenishes Ca^{+2} and phosphate into the extracellular interstitial fluid surrounding the injured cells. With MPT pore formation, the mitochondrial outer membrane ruptures, and the mitochondrion is no longer viable. For most cell types, necrosis quickly follows, with complete depletion of energy storage and failure of energy production.

Coincident with the morphologic and functional deterioration of mitochondria that portends imminent necrosis, water continues to accumulate in the cytoplasm, and the cell enlarges by bulging into the lumen (e.g., renal tubular epithelial cell) or becoming spherical. Distension of the rough and smooth ER may reflect a temporary accommodation for the excess fluid; however, ER fragmentation typically ensues as ribosomes detach from the rough ER and adaptive protein synthesis ceases. Recovery is now impossible. Once organelle membranes rupture and release lysosomal enzymes, degradation of cellular components accelerates leaving condensed cellular remnants. The sequence of cell swelling followed by condensation is characteristic of necrosis. In contrast, cell death by apoptosis is characterized initially by condensation followed by fragmentation and ingestion by adjacent cells or macrophages (Table 6.1).

In the nucleus, morphologic changes of irreversible cell injury are manifested mainly by changes in chromatin and the nuclear membrane. Chromatin condenses and forms irregular clumps along the nuclear membrane. This is considered a consequence of decreasing nuclear pH that occurs during the process of necrosis. The nuclear membrane pores break down, severing normal connections between the nucleus and the cytocavitary network (e.g., rER, sER, and Golgi). After the nuclear membrane ruptures, the nucleus typically shrinks and condenses, a morphologic hallmark of necrosis termed pyknosis, while the swollen cytosol and enlarged perinuclear space impinge on the nucleus (Fig. 6.21). Eventually, the nuclear membrane breaks down completely, leading to rarefaction of the remaining nucleoplasm and dispersion of the aggregated bits of degraded chromatin attached to membrane fragments, which characterizes karyorrhexis, another morphologic hallmark of necrosis (Fig. 6.21). Eventually, the entirety of chromatin, nucleoplasm, and nuclear membrane is completely degraded, termed karyolysis (Fig. 6.21).

Once an irreversibly injured cell is no longer physiologically active, lysosomes swell and leak their enzymes into the cytosol, thus triggering autolysis. Because lysosomal enzymes require sequestration to prevent their leakage and activity in a viable cell's cytoplasm, lysosomal

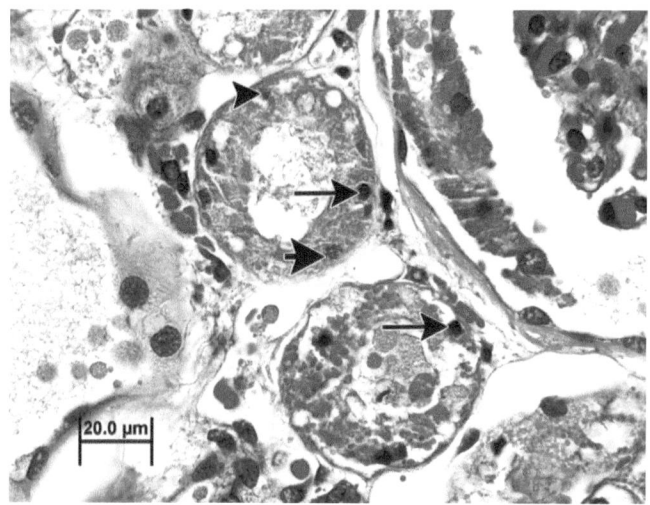

FIGURE 6.21 Nuclear changes associated with necrosis. Photomicrograph of renal tubules from a dog with raisin toxicosis. Pyknosis (nuclear consolidation [*thin arrows*]), karyorrhexis (nuclear fragmentation [*large thick arrow*]), and karyolysis (*arrowhead*) are present in necrotic tubular cells. Hematoxylin and eosin. *Figure reproduced from Haschek WM, Rousseaux CG, Wallig MA, editors:* Handbook of toxicologic pathology, *ed 3, Academic Press, 2013, Figure 4.20, p. 94, with permission.*

membranes are relatively resilient to noxious stimuli. Typically, their constituent enzymes are released into the cytosol quite late in the process of necrosis. However, there are examples of primary lysosomal damage leading to cell injury (e.g., hepatotoxicity occurs when excessive amounts of copper accumulate in hepatocyte lysosomes predisposing to increased lysosomal membrane permeability). Release of enzymes and highly oxidative cupric cations into the cytosol then leads to uncontrolled degradation of cell constituents (Aits and Jäättelä, 2013).

When degradation of cell components by lysosomal enzymes nears completion, the cell is clearly recognizable by light microscopy as necrotic (Table 6.1). The morphology of necrosis is quite stereotypic although it does vary depending on special biochemical, functional, or structural characteristics specific to a particular cell type, tissue, or organ. Most necrotic cells are characterized by the presence of diffusely hypereosinophilic cytoplasm as a consequence of coagulated basic proteins that bind to the acidic eosin stain. The cytoplasm may become "glassy" in appearance, i.e., hyalinized. Eosinophilia is also enhanced by the loss of normally basophilic-staining nucleic acids, such as ribosomal RNA, which bind to the hematoxylin stain and appear basophilic microscopically.

Cytoplasmic granules, representing mitochondria laden with Ca^{+2} precipitates, may also be observed by light microscopy. As the degradation of a necrotic cell progresses, its cytoplasm becomes "moth eaten" and fragmented. In tissues with a large influx of Ca^{+2}, a necrotic cell's cytoplasm may calcify or mineralize, yielding a strongly staining basophilic, stippled, fragmented, or even crystalline appearance (Fig. 6.22). The morphologic progression of necrosis as manifested in the injured cell cytoplasm and nucleus does not necessarily occur in a predictable sequence, so several different permutations are possible. Viable tissue adjacent to necrotic cells typically reacts to the injury with an inflammatory response.

The macroscopic, i.e., gross, characteristics of necrotic tissue are almost as diverse as the number of specialized tissues. The nature of the lethal injury, and the reaction of surrounding viable tissues to the damage, can complicate

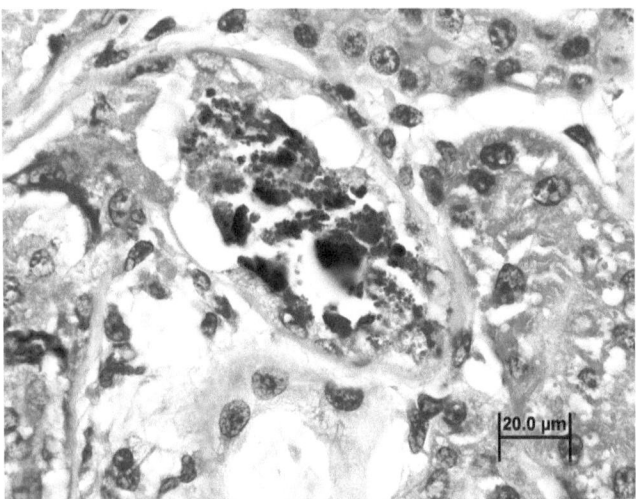

FIGURE 6.22   Postnecrotic mineralization. Photomicrograph of a necrotic renal tubule from a cat with lily (*Lilium longiflorum*) toxicosis. Mineralized necrotic tubular epithelium appears as angular deposits of blue-violet granules (center of the image). Hematoxylin and eosin. *Figure reproduced from Haschek WM, Rousseaux CG, Wallig MA, editors:* Handbook of toxicologic pathology, *ed 3, Academic Press, 2013, Figure 4.21, p. 94, with permission.*

interpretation of the gross pathology further. Necrotic tissue is often pale, friable, and shrunken, especially if its blood supply was lost antemortem. If blood supply was maintained, necrotic tissue may become swollen, soft, and dark as a consequence of dilated vasculature and exuded blood-derived fluid. A clear indication of antemortem necrosis is a discrete area of pallor demarcated by a dark red rim which represents hemorrhage and congestion, often with some degree of inflammation, in response to the necrotic tissue.

Necrotic tissue can be classified based on gross and histologic characteristics. With coagulation or coagulative necrosis, the affected tissue retains its basic structural features so that the necrotic cells remain discernible by light microscopy. Necrotic cells are lightly eosinophilic but lack detail, so they appear ghost- or shadow like. Coagulation necrosis is generally acute and therefore seen with many toxicities. Cells with few lysosomes may be prone to coagulation necrosis because a primary source for enzymes that accelerate the degradative process is less available. The inflammatory response in viable tissue surrounding areas of coagulation necrosis may be somewhat dampened with toxicant-induced injury since DAMPs are required to trigger a substantial inflammatory response. Proinflammatory proteins, such as active complement fragments and antigen–antibody binding, are also typically not a prominent feature of classical toxicant-induced injury. With the development of new protein-based therapeutics, the potential for autoimmune and hypersensitivity reactions is higher, and these reactions, even without direct injury to tissue, may trigger an inappropriate and harmful inflammatory response (see *Protein Pharmaceutical Agents*, Vol 2, Chap 6).

Liquefactive necrosis occurs when neutrophils and activated macrophages infiltrate necrotic tissue, adding their extensive lytic enzyme pools to the process of tissue degradation. This is common with bacterial infections and is related to pathogen-associated molecular patterns (PAMPs), molecular motifs—usually of microbial origin—that activate Toll-like receptors, and other pattern recognition receptors like NOD-1, C-type lectin, scavenger, RNA helicase and complement on neutrophils, macrophages, dendritic cells, and other immune cells (Takeuchi and Akira, 2010). Activated neutrophils characteristically release their lysosomal enzymes into the extracellular milieu, accelerating tissue digestion and producing a lesion that is typically soft and semiliquefied. Some lipid-rich tissues, particularly the CNS, undergo liquefactive necrosis and denatured lipids become greasy or oily.

Caseous necrosis is the term used when necrotic tissue has the consistency of dry cheese and is most common with chronic infections where persistent PAMPs are present. Necrotic tissue is typically pale yellow or light green, sometimes with a white tint, quite soft or pasty, and friable but generally does not spontaneously fall apart.

4.2. Programmed Cell Death

Alternatively, cell death may occur in a "programmed" manner in which cell injury may be very minor or not be present at all. Rather, the binding of a particular ligand to its corresponding receptor on the cell surface may occur, triggering one or more biochemical pathways that induce the cell to die, to "commit suicide" as it were, in a defined sequential manner. Various types of programmed cell death have been identified biochemically although the morphological endpoints are generally subtle and not much different from one another, particularly at the light microscopic level (Table 6.2). In most cases, programmed cell death is a single-cell phenomenon, unlike necrosis, which tends to be locally extensive affecting many cells in a given area. There may or may not be evidence of preexisting injury, especially with apoptosis. Most forms of programmed cell death (e.g., paraptosis, cell death with autophagy) have many characteristics of apoptosis, while others, such as necroptosis and pyroptosis, share similar morphologic changes with necrosis although as an individual cell response (see below).

Apoptosis

Cell death by apoptosis contrasts with cell death by necrosis in a variety of important morphologic manifestations and molecular pathways and is a fairly common response to toxicant-induced injury, especially at low dose levels of toxicity (Elmore, 2007). At a basic morphologic level, apoptosis is characterized by cell condensation and fragmentation with preservation of organellar integrity until very late in the process, while necrosis is characterized by cell swelling and overt deterioration of organellar integrity. Apoptosis is not only morphologically orderly but also tightly regulated biochemically. Even though apoptosis is quite common, it tends to be morphologically less conspicuous than necrosis because it rapidly progresses once triggered and apoptotic cells are quickly ingested by adjacent parenchymal cells or resident tissue macrophages. In addition, apoptosis typically affects only a small fraction of a cell population at any one time. Apoptosis has a variety of causes and triggering mechanisms which progress along generally common biochemical pathways. While generally stereotypic, apoptosis is manifested somewhat uniquely in some specialized cells or tissue.

The ultrastructural morphology of apoptosis is quite distinctive and clearly contrasts with necrosis (Table 6.1). Initially, a cell undergoing apoptosis detaches from adjacent cells or stroma and rapidly condenses into a spherical body losing any specialized surface structures. Secretory cells disgorge their storage granules as they condense. Initial dilation of ER may be observed as sodium ions and water are pumped into ER lumina prior to condensation of the cytoplasm. As the cytosol condenses, organelles are drawn closer together. Portions of the cell pinch off into spherical, membrane-bound fragments or apoptotic bodies, a process termed zeiosis (Fig. 6.23). The integrity of the plasma membrane is generally preserved, even after fragmentation, so organelles such as mitochondria may be visible within detached apoptotic bodies (Fig. 6.23). Ribosomes may even remain attached to the rER.

Nuclear changes during apoptosis occur before, during, or after cytoplasmic changes like zeiosis. While the nuclear envelope is preserved until after the apoptotic cell is ingested and degraded, the nucleolus segregates from the chromatin which uniformly condenses into crescent-shaped or smooth-edged clusters along the nuclear envelope. The nucleus may also undergo zeiosis, forming small, round to oval bodies of densely packed chromatin enveloped by an intact nuclear membrane. After phagocytosis by adjacent cells, apoptotic cells or bodies swell and degrade within phagolysosomes

TABLE 6.2 Cell Death Terminology

Process	Morphologic characteristics	Early events	Cascading events	Late events
Necroptosis Single-cell necrosis	Swelling of cytoplasm and organelles Disruption of plasma membrane integrity Leakage of cell contents Fragmentation of chromatin	Calpain dependent Caspase independent	TNFR RIPk-1 → RIPK-3/ MLKL (necrosome) → PARP-1 and JNK/JNK activation	Release of DAMPs followed by an acute inflammatory response
Apoptosis	Cell shrinkage, fragmentation into membrane-bound bodies, rapid phagocytosis by adjacent cells	BCL-2 dependency BH3 activation	Cytochrome c release	APAF1 Caspase activation
Cell death by autophagy	Massive cytoplasmic vacuolization Numerous membrane-lined vacuoles containing remnants of organelles Cytoplasmic blebs with intact plasma membrane Nuclear structure maintained	Cathepsin dependent Caspase independent Lysosome activation Enhanced autophagy Mitochondrial dysfunction leading to ATP depletion and ion imbalance	Enhanced cell stress responses leading to BECLIN, ULK, and Atg complexes necessary for autophagosome formation	Release of DAMPs followed by an acute inflammatory response
Cell death by lysosome activation	Varies depending on degree of lysosome hyperactivity, can resemble necroptosis, cell death by autophagy, pyroptosis, or apoptosis	Excessive or asynchronous activation of lysosomal proteases including cathepsins	Varies depending on degree of lysosomal hyperactivity	Varies depending on which cell processes predominate
Parthanatos	Nuclear condensation with zeiosis ("blebs") Cell contraction followed by degradation	PARP-1 activation Release of AIF from mitochondria	DNA damage → PARP-1 activation → PAR release AIF release	Release of lipid-derived inflammatory mediators and DAMPs

	Morphological features	Biochemical features	Signaling pathway	Consequences
Pyroptosis	Plasma membrane zeiosis ("blebs") Cytoplasmic vacuolization Cell swelling and rupture Nuclear condensation and fragmentation Described mainly as a macrophage phenomenon	Caspase 1 dependent Caspase 4/5 also involved Inflammasome mediated	DAMP/PAMP binding to PRR → inflammasome formation → caspase 1 activation → gasdermin D plasma membrane pore	Release of proinflammatory mediators including IL-1β, lipid derived, followed by acute inflammation after ingestions of pathogens
Pyronecrosis	Resembles pyroptosis but limited to macrophages Cell lysis	Inflammasome mediated Regulated by NLRP3 Caspase independent	Activation of NRLP 3 by ASC	IL1β release Neutrophil recruitment
Ferroptosis	Shrinkage of cell with intact membrane; shrinkage of mitochondria or loss of individual mitochondria; nuclear morphology intact	Increased cytoplasmic Fe^{+2} → release of ROS Activation of MAPK pathways Depletion of glutathione	Membrane lipid peroxidation	Release of DAMPs with minimal inflammation
NETosis	Neutrophil-derived extracellular traps (NETs) Strands of tangled nuclear material and cytoplasmic granules, including lysosomes	NOX3, ROS, and PKC dependent	Neutrophil activation → respiratory burst → ROS especially H_2O_2 → PKC activation → eventual chromatin unwinding and release	Activation and release of inflammatory mediators

AIF, Apoptosis-inducing factor; *APAF-1*, Apoptotic protease activating factor 1; *ASC*, Apoptosis-associated speck-like protein containing a caspase recruitment domain (also known as PYCARD); *Atg*, Autophagy-related protein; *BCL-2*, B-cell lymphoma 2; *BECLIN*, Coiled-coil moesin-like BCL2-interacting protein; *BH3*, Bcl homology 3 domain; *DAMPs*, Damage-associated molecular pattern molecules; *IL-1β*, Interleukin-1 *beta*; *JNK*, c-Jun N-terminal kinases; *MAPK*, Mitogen-activated protein kinase(s); *MLKL*, Mixed lineage kinase domain-like pseudokinase; *NOX*, NADPH oxidase(s); *NRLP*, NLR family pyrin domain-containing 3; *PAMP*, pathogen-associated-molecular patterns; *PAR*, Poly ADP Ribose; *PARP-1*, Poly (ADP-ribose) polymerase 1; *PKC*, Protein kinase C; *PRR*, Pattern recognition receptor(s); *RIPK-1&3*, Receptor-interacting serine/threonine-protein kinases 1&3; *ROS*, Reactive oxygen species; *TNFR*, Tumor necrosis factor receptor; *ULK*, Unc-51-like autophagy activating kinase.

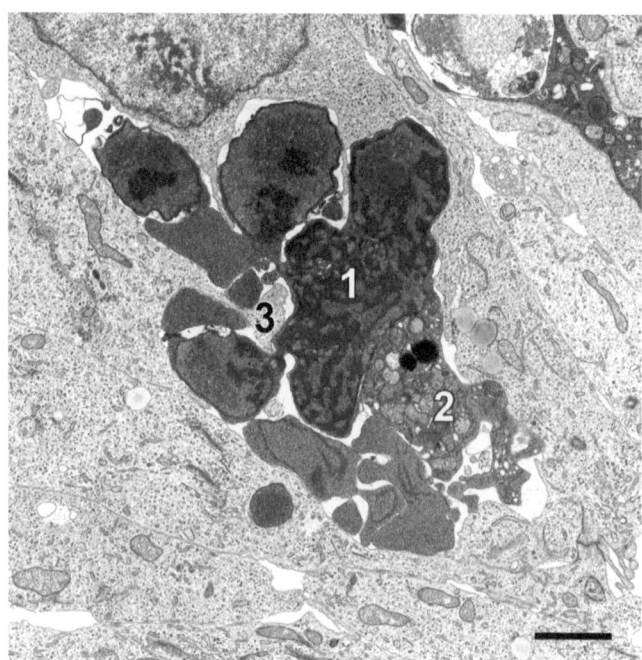

FIGURE 6.23   Apoptosis. Electron photomicrograph of xenobiotic-induced apoptosis in the forebrain of a rat embryo. Note the shrunken and fragmented cell with condensed chromatin (1), and several mitochondria concentrated in the reduced volume of condensed (more electron dense) cytoplasm (2). Note also the partial phagocytosis of this apoptotic cell by cytoplasmic extensions of an adjacent normal cell (3). Bar = 2 μm. *Figure reproduced from Haschek WM, Rousseaux CG, Wallig MA, editors:* Handbook of toxicologic pathology, *ed 3, Academic Press, 2013, Figure 4.22, p. 96, with permission.*

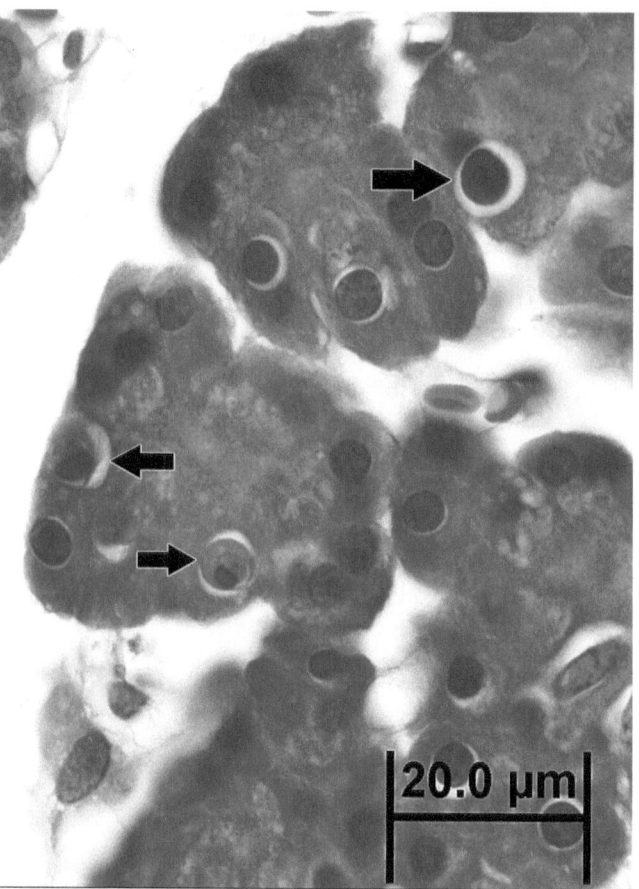

FIGURE 6.24   Apoptosis. Photomicrograph of pancreas from a Fischer 344 (F344) rat 12 h after treatment with the pancreatic toxicant crambene. Arrows point to apoptotic exocrine acinar cells, with their characteristic pericellular halo and round shape (indicative of cell contraction) as well as shrunken, condensed nuclei. Hematoxylin and eosin. *Figure reproduced from Haschek WM, Rousseaux CG, Wallig MA, editors:* Handbook of toxicologic pathology, *ed 3, Academic Press, 2013, Figure 4.23, p. 97, with permission.*

where their remnants are indistinguishable from those of a necrotic cell.

By light microscopy, the morphology of an apoptotic cell is quite distinctive (Table 6.1). A key feature is that an apoptotic cell almost always appears isolated, reduced in size, spherical, and intensely stained. In H&E-stained tissue sections, an apoptotic cell is very often demarcated by a wide clear halo. Its well-defined round nuclear remnants are darkly stained by hematoxylin and its cytoplasm by eosin. Apoptotic bodies have clearly defined cell boundaries, reflective of their intact plasma membranes and the nuclear envelope is generally clearly defined as well. The surrounding halo may actually be a phagocytic vacuole (Fig. 6.24). A particularly characteristic nuclear feature of apoptosis occurs when chromatin condenses as a crescent- or cap-shaped mass along one edge of the nuclear envelope.

Because apoptosis is a rapid process and apoptotic cells are efficiently removed, apoptotic cells are rarely numerous. Even in tissues with toxicologically significant apoptosis, only 1%–2% of the total cell population are recognizable as being apoptotic morphologically, although immunohistochemical and/or imaging modalities may identify many more cells in the preapoptotic phase of the process (see below).

Apoptosis can be triggered by a wide variety of physiologic or toxicologic mechanisms

(Cavalcante et al., 2019). Injured cells with minimal overt morphologic evidence of injury and that still retain enough function to forestall overt necrosis can be simulated to undergo apoptosis. The mechanism underlying this form of apoptosis is caspase 9-mediated, reflecting progressive loss of mitochondrial function and is referred to as an intrinsic pathway of apoptosis. Examples of toxicologic injury leading to this pathway include oxidative stress with decreased sulfide–disulfide ratios (e.g., reduced glutathione/oxidized glutathione balance), disrupted ion gradients, or structural damage to proteins on the inner mitochondrial membrane. Excessive DNA damage that cannot be readily or rapidly repaired in the G1 phase of the cell cycle can also trigger this pathway via p53, which normally inhibits antiapoptotic proteins (e.g., Bcl-xL and Bcl-2). MPT pores, i.e., contact points between inner and outer mitochondrial membranes, are not a prominent feature of mitochondrial-mediated apoptosis but nevertheless are essential for apoptosis to occur. MPT pores form through dimerization and activation of proapoptotic proteins, such as Bax and Bak, from the cytosol and/or outer mitochondrial membrane. As with necrosis, mitochondrial cytochrome c passes through the pores and binds to apoptotic protease activating factor 1 (Apaf-1), a protein that is docked to antiapoptotic proteins such as Bcl-2 (Singh et al., 2019). The Apaf-1/cytochrome c complex forms a hexamer that binds to precaspase 9, also located on the outer mitochondrial membrane, to form the apoptosome leading to activation of caspase 9 via proteolytic cleavage of precaspase 9 already present in the cytosol. This "initiator" caspase in turn activates via proteolytic cleavage cytosolic effector (executioner) caspases (3, 6, and 7) already present in cytosol precaspases. The most important and predominant precaspase in most cell types is caspase 3 (i.e., the master molecule) for induction of most of the structural and morphologic changes associated with classical apoptosis.

Another mechanism of apoptosis is receptor mediated and is triggered when ligands such as Fas or tumor necrosis factor-*alpha* (TNF-α) bind to its corresponding receptor (FasR or TNFR, respectively), a homodimer which trimerizes with FasR to form a "death-inducing signaling complex" (DISC) that spans the cell membrane.

Intracellular attachments to DISC include receptor-specific proteins with death domains (e.g., FADD or TRADD), to which is bound precaspase 8. When activation/assembly of the receptor complex occurs, precaspase 8 is cleaved, and active caspase 8 is released into the cytosol where it activates caspase 3 as well as the proapoptotic protein Bid (to tBid), which then binds to Bcl-2 on the outer mitochondrial membrane causing it to release bound proapoptotic Bax and/or Bak to induce formation of the MPT pores to release cytochrome c and ultimately activate caspase 9. Therefore, although the FasL mechanism of apoptosis is initiated outside mitochondria, they are critical in completing the process. Caspase 10 is another important receptor-linked caspase. This caspase is of greater significance in some mammalian species than caspase 8, in contrast to humans where caspase 8 is of primary importance in signal-induced apoptosis. Caspase 10 interacts in the same way with DISC as does caspase 8 (Shalini et al., 2015).

Although not completely understood, another apoptotic mechanism of toxicologic relevance is initiated by activation of caspase 12 when the severity of ER stress exceeds the injured cell's adaptive capacity to compensate, e.g., through NFκB (Tabas and Ron, 2011). ER stress is manifested by accumulation of misfolded or unfolded proteins within cisternae with subsequent induction of sensor proteins. Then, there is release of Ca^{+2} into the cytosol to activate the enzyme calpain, leading to activation of precaspase 12 on the cytosolic side of the ER. Changes in redox status toward a more oxidized state as well as inadequate ATP are also contributors to ER stress. Caspase 12, once activated and released, attaches to the cytoplasmic side of the endoplasmic reticular membrane. It then activates caspase 3 leading to apoptosis. Also activated are the CCAAT enhancer-binding protein, homologous protein CHOP transcription factor, and the c-Jun N-terminal kinase pathways, commonly referred to as JNK pathways, that inhibit antiapoptotic Bcl-2 and activate proapoptotic Bak and Bax to involve mitochondria and the activation of caspase 9. Caspase 12-mediated apoptosis is morphologically indistinguishable from the classical and receptor-mediated induced apoptosis.

Activated caspase 3 initiates a variety of downstream events that mediate the morphological changes of apoptosis. The substrates that are cleaved by caspase 3 are so vast that it has been difficult to determine which of them are primary to initiating the morphological changes and which are secondary (Porter and Jänicke, 1999). However, substrates considered primary include those that promote degradation of the cytoskeleton, via cleavage of β-catenin, fodrin, actin, lamin, and gel-solin, and the inactivation of several cell cycle pathways such as protein kinase b/Akt. Caspase 3 also activates proapoptotic proteins such as scramblase which promotes eversion of phosphatidyl serine (PS) from the inner plasma membrane leaflet to the outer leaflet. Caspase 3 regulates the fate of the genome during apoptosis via caspase-activated DNAase, an endonuclease that cleaves DNA into 180 base pair units. It also inactivates certain key enzymes involved in DNA repair (e.g., PARP-1, DNA phosphokinase C, and topoisomerases I and II). Indirectly, histones are released from the nucleosome further exposing DNA to degradation. In this way, caspase 3 is also linked to *p53*-initiated apoptosis when toxicant-induced injury to the genome overwhelms DNA repair mechanisms.

It should be noted that caspases require ATP, high levels of cellular glutathione in order to keep the enzymes in correct configuration for activity, and appropriate concentrations of Ca^{2+}. Insufficient concentrations of either glutathione (to maintain appropriate redox status) or ATP or excessively high concentrations of Ca^{2+} will lead to inactivation or nonactivation of caspases, preventing apoptosis and indirectly altering other types of programmed cell death where caspases may be involved initially (see below). Although morphologic criteria for apoptosis are well characterized by light and electron microscopy, ancillary biochemical and imaging analyses (e.g., cytosolic cytochrome c, positive TUNEL immunohistochemistry, or positive immunohistochemistry for cleaved caspase 3) are often preformed to confirm the morphologic diagnosis of apoptosis (See *Special Techniques in Toxicologic Pathology*, Vol 1, Chap 11).

Toxicant-induced injury to a tissue rarely leads exclusively to either apoptosis or necrosis; these two manifestations of cell death often occur simultaneously, and with careful microscopic examination of the lesions, morphologic evidence of both can often be observed. Less severely injured cells, such as those that maintain those functional elements necessary to complete the apoptotic process because they were exposed to a lower dose of the toxicant or are closer to an intact blood supply near the edge of a lesion, tend to undergo apoptosis.

Single-Cell Necrosis and Programmed Cell Death

In some cases, an individual cell may die by a process that morphologically does not resemble apoptosis but instead resembles classic necrosis. This has been described as "single-cell necrosis" and can be seen at lower doses of certain toxicant-induced injury (e.g., acetaminophen), in certain viral diseases (e.g., yellow fever in the liver) and especially in epithelial neoplasms (e.g., liver, prostate, pancreas, mammary). Also, as additional molecular mechanisms involved in cell death are discovered, a large list of various types of cell death, based on biochemical and/or signaling pathways as well as etiologic triggers, have been described and characterized (See *Biochemical and Molecular Basis of Toxicity*, Vol 1, Chap 2). However, the morphologic alterations ("endpoints") that can be observed microscopically are subtle and often not clearly unique, resembling necrosis or apoptosis or some combination of both (see below). Since most of these newly characterized forms of cell death do involve unique but often overlapping signaling pathways, they have been classified as forms of programmed cell death, even though some of these forms (e.g., necroptosis/single-cell necrosis, autophagic cell death) (Fig. 6.3) have some morphologic features more consistent with classic necrosis than apoptosis (Salvesen and Walsh, 2014; Louhimo et al., 2016; Xie et al., 2016; Zhang et al., 2014, 2018), while others resemble a combination of necrosis and apoptosis (e.g., pyroptosis; Fink and Cookson, 2005; Frank and Vince, 2019), while still others (e.g., ferroptosis; Xie et al., 2016) mechanistically and morphologically appear to represent a slower less explosive type of classic necrosis (See Table 6.2 for these and additional types of programmed cell death). Further complicating the issue is that these processes tend to occur on a single-cell basis, at least initially, potentially leading an inexperienced pathologist to mistake an individually dead cell as an example of classic apoptosis. In addition, since individually dead cells are often rapidly ingested and/or degraded by resident tissue macrophages or adjacent parenchymal cells, this degradation may be misinterpreted as the primary process. The International Harmonization of Nomenclature and Diagnostic Criteria Working Group on cell death has recommended using the term "apoptosis/single-cell necrosis" when true single-cell necrosis and apoptosis occur concurrently or when these other types of cell death are suspected to be present as well (Elmore et al., 2016).

Since some of these biochemical pathways of cell death only occur in certain cell types in response to certain etiologies in specific situations (see below), these new classifications have yet to be fully accepted by the community of pathologists, especially since their morphologic endpoints often overlap extensively with classic necrosis and apoptosis. In addition, some forms of cell death are limited to cells of the innate immune system (e.g., pyroptosis, pyronecrosis, and ferroptosis) and inflammatory cells (e.g., NETosis), and as such figure more prominently in infectious diseases (e.g., SARS-coronavirus, Shi et al., 2019) rather than toxicologic insults. Table 6.2 addresses some of the more frequently described examples of programmed cell death, their mechanism of action, and main morphologic features. There are a variety of review articles, some conflicting in certain areas, that describe in depth the various morphological, biochemical, and molecular signaling features of these types of cell death (Kroemer and Levine, 2008; Kroemer et al., 2009; Belizário et al., 2015; Satoh et al., 2013).

4.3. Consequences of Irreversible Cell Injury

Necrosis

In most instances, necrosis elicits an inflammatory response, as do certain forms of programmed cell death (e.g., necroptosis, autophagic cell death), the extent and nature of which depends on a variety of factors, the most obvious being the time elapsed between the initial injury and the actual pathologic evaluation. For example, inflammation will not be observed in

the heart when sudden death results from acute myocardial infarction. Alternatively, when death occurs several days after the infarct was formed, an inflammatory response is often quite remarkable. Another determining factor is the extent of the injury and the number of cells that die, as well as the process by which they die. Because individual cells, rather than whole populations of cells, die in certain forms of programmed cell death, acute inflammation will be more muted than in situations where entire contiguous cell populations are injured and die. Another factor contributing to the intensity of the inflammatory response is whether DAMPs alone or DAMPs and PAMPs are released (see below).

Neutrophils are generally the first inflammatory cell type to infiltrate an area of necrosis. Macrophages, from differentiated blood-derived monocytes and resident precursors, typically predominate within a few days (Fig. 6.25). Neutrophils play a critical role in the progressive morphogenesis of a necrotic lesion since they can (and often do) release enzymes into the ECM during phagocytosis of necrotic cell remnants, often resulting in indiscriminate degradation of stroma and lysis of

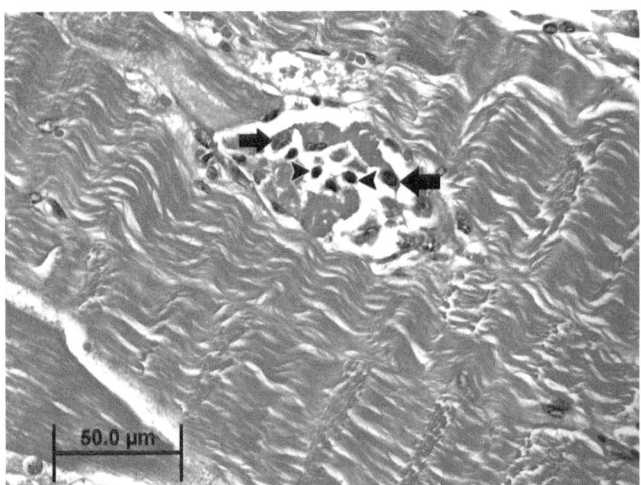

FIGURE 6.25 Postnecrotic inflammation. Photomicrograph of gluteal muscle of a horse with extensive myonecrosis. Neutrophils (*arrowheads*) and macrophages (*large arrows*) are infiltrating and phagocytosing the remnants of a necrotic myocyte. Hematoxylin and eosin. *Figure reproduced from Haschek WM, Rousseaux CG, Wallig MA, editors:* Handbook of toxicologic pathology, *ed 3, Academic Press, 2013, Figure 4.24, p. 99, with permission.*

viable cells, i.e., "innocent bystanders," including adjacent neutrophils themselves. This process has been termed NETosis (Mesa and Gloria Vasquez, 2013) and is triggered by DAMPs, reactive oxygen species, and cytokines such as IL-8. If the neutrophil is sufficiently overstimulated, an internal signal is generated that leads to activation of nuclear DNases degrading its nuclear chromatin, which is then extruded as a fine meshwork. Lysosomal granules are often attached to the meshwork. This "netotic cell death" (Table 6.2) is most profound if PAMPs such as lipopolysaccharide LPS are present. Processes such as netotic cell death can exacerbate the severity of the initial injury. During the process of activation, migration, chemotaxis, and phagocytosis, neutrophils also produce soluble mediators of inflammation (e.g., IL-1 IL-8, TNF-α) that attract more neutrophils, and eventually macrophages, to the site of injury.

In cases of lethal cell injury due to necrosis or related phenomena, when supporting stroma is retained and not substantially damaged following injury, the inflammatory response tends to be muted. For example, inflammation subsequent to gastric erosion is generally less intense than that associated with a gastric ulcer, and the latter is more likely to result in a scar.

Complete structural restoration of injured tissue is predicated on the supporting architectural stroma. For example, following a toxic injury, the basement membrane of an injured epithelial tissue must remain intact or, if damaged, be adequately resynthesized before the epithelium can effectively regenerate. Typically, this type of tissue restoration proceeds from the lateral or deep margins of a resolving necrotic lesion where vascular ingrowth, if needed, initiates. Incomplete tissue restoration, often referred to as repair, may be identified microscopically as fibrosis long after the initial injury, even if overall organ function is maintained.

In most tissues, extensive damage that cannot be resolved by parenchymal regeneration leads to fibrosis (i.e., scar formation), a process characterized by replacement of lost functional parenchymal tissue with nonfunctional stroma. In contrast to normal supporting stroma, which comprises Type IV collagen, elastin, and laminin within an abundant gelatinous glycosaminoglycan

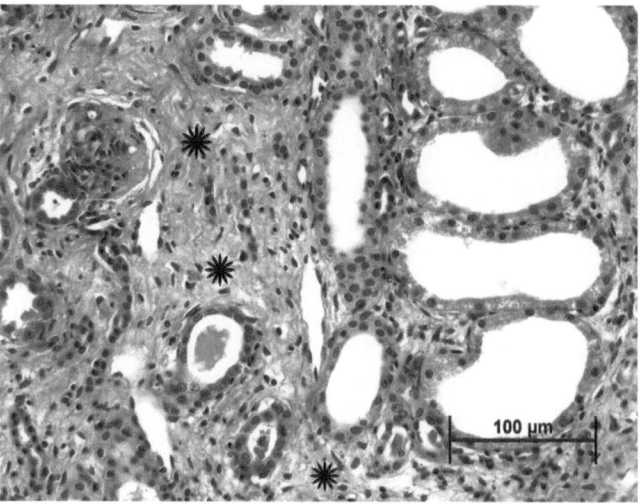

FIGURE 6.26   Postnecrotic fibrosis. Renal cortex from a dog following a bout of severe, widespread renal necrosis due to ethylene glycol intoxication. Tubules lined by flattened, incompletely differentiated epithelium are entrapped within extensive dense collagen matrix (interstitial scar tissue [starbursts]). Hematoxylin and eosin. *Figure reproduced from Haschek WM, Rousseaux CG, Wallig MA, editors:* Handbook of toxicologic pathology, *ed 3, Academic Press, 2013, Figure 4.25, p. 100, with permission.*

ground substance, fibrotic tissue is predominantly composed of Type I collagen which, as it condenses with time, is generally unfavorable to restoration of functional parenchyma (Fig. 6.26). Extensive fibrosis leads to permanent loss of function in the affected tissue. In some organs, such as the liver or kidney, a substantial reserve capacity provides a buffer between multifocal fibrosis and organ failure, but progressive or recurring injury eventually erodes this capacity.

The specialized function and structure of some organs dictates the nature of an inflammatory response to a toxic injury. For example, necrotic pancreatic acinar cells release proteases which further damage already compromised adjacent acinar cells and also stimulate a dramatic influx of neutrophils. A vicious cycle can ensue with neutrophils inciting further acinar cell necrosis so that a localized lesion can rapidly progress to an extensive one. The presence of "interstitial" stromal cells such as stellate cells in liver and pancreas can promote replacement of lost parenchyma by dense collagenous tissue. These cells, presumably of pericyte or myofibroblast origin, can undergo transformation from a storage (e.g., Vitamin A in liver) or a supportive role to an active fibroblastic one.

The intensity of the inflammatory response also depends on the degree of tissue vascularization. Injury to well vascularized tissue, such as the pulmonary parenchyma, often elicits a stronger inflammatory cell infiltrate than it does to a poorly vascularized tissue, such as articular cartilage. However, a better blood supply can also lead to faster and more complete tissue repair.

Secondary or opportunistic infections can complicate the inflammatory response to a toxicant-induced lesion. Bacteria are an additional source of toxins that cause cell injury, inhibit regeneration, and attract more inflammatory cells especially neutrophils. Those tissues with a so-called barrier function, such as the skin and gastrointestinal tract, are at particular risk for opportunistic bacterial infections following a toxic insult. Hematogenous dissemination of bacteria from the damaged intestinal mucosa can lead to secondary hepatitis or even septicemia.

The process leading to repair initially mirrors that of parenchymal regeneration. The initial neutrophil-predominant response is followed by a macrophage-predominant one. Macrophages, derived from circulating monocytes and resident macrophage precursors, first transform into M1 inflammatory macrophages to sustain and maintain the inflammatory response as long as necessary. These macrophages are actively phagocytic, generate hydroxy free radicals and nitric oxide for additional killing if needed, and actively secrete proinflammatory mediators, including IL-1β, IL-6, IL-8 (CXCL8), IL-12, and TNF-α among others.

Resolution begins when macrophages encounter apoptotic neutrophils at the site of injury and inflammation. After ingesting an effete neutrophil, a macrophage will convert into an M2 phenotype. M2 macrophages scavenge cell debris and other effete neutrophils as well as secrete antiinflammatory mediators such as IL-10, which stimulates conversion of other M1 macrophages at the site. Any monocytes entering the tissue from the bloodstream also become M2 in phenotype. Additional mediators released by these M2 scavenger macrophages include Lipoxin A4 and Resolvin E1, which serve to terminate neutrophil activation. Additionally, a variety of cytokines and chemokines are elaborated that drive the repair process. Tissue repair is defective in mice depleted of resident macrophages or lacking certain macrophage functions. Transforming growth factor-beta (TGF-β), also produced by M2 macrophages, is important in signaling to other macrophages in the area as well as new macrophages to transform into or remain in the M2 phenotype and not become activated M1 types.

Besides TGF-β, the numbers of macrophage-derived chemokines are enormous. Of particular importance for repair are platelet-derived growth factor, epithelial growth factor (EGF), and fibroblast growth factors. Epithelial cells, fibroblasts, and endothelial cells are also sources of chemokines. Chemokine-mediated activation of fibroblasts at the site of tissue injury temporally coincides with the influx of macrophages, typically within a few days after the initial injury (Fig. 6.27). These fibroblasts produce a matrix rich in fibronectin, hyaluronan, glycosaminoglycans, and Type III collagen, a matrix that serves as a scaffold for fibroblasts and capillary-forming endothelial cells. The matrix is also well hydrated, and therefore conducive to diffusion of O_2 and amino acids. Many fibroblasts express smooth muscle actin and acquire a contractile function. These myofibroblasts promote contraction of tissue under repair, accelerating lesion resolution but sometimes resulting in tissue distortion.

Vascular endothelial growth factor (VEGF) is another important chemokine. VEGF is secreted by a variety of cell types under hypoxic conditions and stimulates budding of endothelial cells from intact adjacent capillaries into the area of tissue injury. The purpose of this response is obvious—to reestablish the blood supply required for supplying essential nutrients to regenerating parenchymal cells and proliferating fibroblasts. O_2 and a ready supply of amino acids as well as Vitamin C are especially important for collagen synthesis. Provided tissue injury has ceased; endothelial buds form tubular structures that merge with the intact capillary network and interweave with newly deposited collagen fibers. TGF-β also plays an important role in vascularization by promoting the differentiation of pericyte and smooth muscle precursor that follow the endothelial

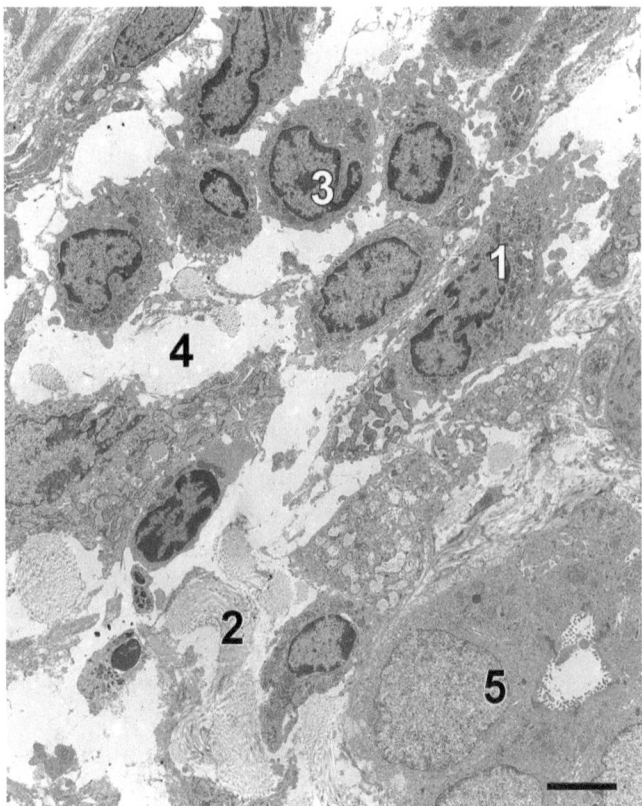

FIGURE 6.27 Postnecrotic fibrosis. Electron photomicrograph of portal triad from a rat with xenobiotic-induced periportal hepatic damage leading to fibrosis. Note the increase in fibroblasts (1), increased deposition of collagen fibers (2), and influx of macrophages (3) within the interstitial space, which is expanded by edema fluid (clear spaces [4]). Epithelial cells lining a bile duct (5) are enlarged, indicating a hypertrophic response due to increased cell mass. Bar = 5 μm. *Figure reproduced from Haschek WM, Rousseaux CG, Wallig MA, editors:* Handbook of toxicologic pathology, *ed 3, Academic Press, 2013, Figure 4.26, p. 101, with permission.*

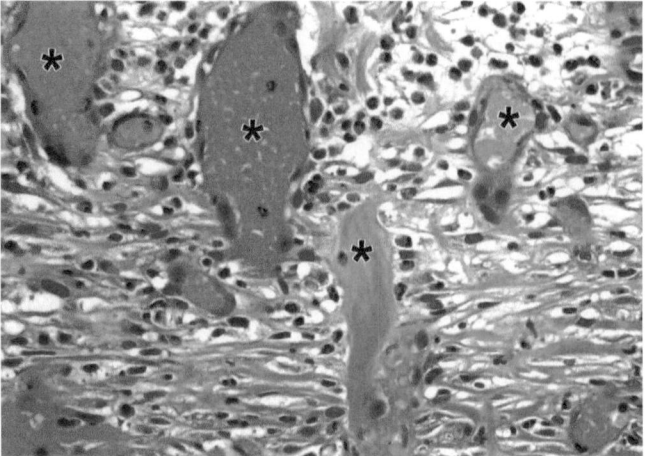

FIGURE 6.28 Classic "gridiron" pattern of granulation tissue from a lip ulcer in a dog. Engorged capillaries (*asterisks*) extend toward the surface of the ulcer within an edematous matrix containing numerous inflammatory cells near the surface (upper portion of image) and fibroblasts and collagen fibers at right angles to capillaries in deeper portions of the tissue toward the bottom. This histomorphologic arrangement translates grossly to the classic glistening, red, cobblestone appearance of granulation tissue.

cells into the newly forming fibrous tissue. By light microscopy, interwoven neocapillaries and immature collagen fibers present a "basket-weave" pattern within a sparsely collagenous pale matrix-rich stroma. This newly formed tissue is often termed granulation tissue because grossly, especially in open cutaneous wounds, it has a rough, "granular" cobblestone appearance on the surface (Ackermann, 2017). Neocapillaries are porous, allowing protein-rich plasma to leak into the well-hydrated ECM; hence, young granulation tissue in particular is typically pink, gelatinous, friable,

and easily induced to bleed (Fig. 6.28). Another characteristic feature of granulation tissue is "contraction," which serves to decrease the surface area/volume of the injury if there is a space-occupying defect. This is mediated by TGF-β released by macrophages in the area of injury. The TGF-β serves to trigger the conversion of fibroblasts to contractile myofibroblasts containing actin and myosin. Myofibroblasts bind to newly deposited collagen fibers and contract, decreasing the surface area which must be filled in with additional ground substance and collagen. The presence of myofibroblasts is very important in wound healing. Contraction, if not too distortional, may aid in parenchymal regeneration since it decreases the area for recovery typically by epithelial cells.

If the parenchymal cell population is capable of regeneration, there is hyperplasia along the viable edges of the injury, due to the release of EGF and other growth factors by macrophages, endothelial cells, and parenchymal cells themselves (Fig. 6.29). TGF-β plays a vital role in signaling to both mesenchymal and epithelial stem cells that are dividing in response to growth factors to stop dividing and differentiate

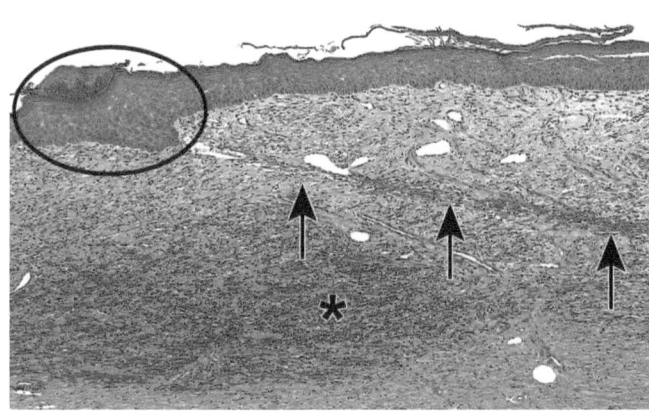

FIGURE 6.29 Healing skin incision from the ear of a dog 10 days after closure. The incision line (*arrows*) has been bridged by newly formed collagen and residual dilated capillaries are present on either side of the incision. The surface of the incision has been reepithelialized and thickened; mildly hyperplasic epidermis (*encircled*) with attached residual dried blood (i.e., a "scab") is present. Residual hemorrhage (*asterisk*) is present peripheral to the incision site.

into their ultimate "adult" phenotype (Weiss et al., 2019). As stated above, however, if there is extensive disruption of the basement membrane, loss of the underlying linker molecules (e.g., laminin and fibronectin) that attach the parenchymal cells to the stroma, and destruction of supportive elastin and collagen III, regeneration may not be complete or an alternative type of parenchymal cell that is more resistant to injury may replace the original cell population. This is known as metaplasia (see below). It must also be noted, as above, that the type of cell injured and lost may have the most profound impact on the type of healing. Some cell populations and complex tissue structures, such as renal glomerular components, myocardium, neurons, retinal rods and cones, and Sertoli cells, are incapable regenerating themselves once injured lethally.

Granulation tissue is more liked to result in scar formation than parenchymal cell regeneration in cases where injury is extensive and/or the preexisting stroma is damaged, but over time and under appropriate conditions, it may be partially remodeled, and partial resolution with some degree of parenchymal regeneration is possible. With Type I collagen "maturation"

(a general term for cross-linking leading to condensation with loss of ground substance, capillaries, and reduced vascularization), tissue contraction proceeds beyond that mediated by myofibroblast function and the lesion can be recognized grossly as a firm, tough, white scar. This scar tissue serves as a near-permanent barrier to regeneration.

The observation that fibrosis is present in a tissue is strong evidence that substantial injury to that tissue has occurred in the past. The histomorphology of the fibrotic tissue as well as its extent can provide a clue as to how far in the past injury may have happened. Loose, richly vascularized collagenous tissue replete with ground substance, capillaries, fibroblasts, and loosely arranged collagen fibers with or without residual macrophages may indicate injury a week to several weeks old; whereas, a densely collagenous, poorly vascularized tissue with few fibrocytes and widespread distortion of the typical tissue architecture indicates an injury many weeks to months (or more) old. A combination of "new" at the core of a lesion and "old" fibrotic tissue along the edges of a lesion can be observed, especially if active inflammation is still present, and usually indicates persistent injury with repeated attempts at repair.

Apoptosis

In contrast to necrosis and related types of programmed cell death, which usually provoke a notable inflammatory response, the tissue response to apoptosis and related forms of programmed cell death (e.g., pyroptosis, parthanatos) is generally quite benign. One explanation for this difference is that apoptotic cells do not release quantities of DAMPs sufficient to attract or activate inflammatory cells, in particular neutrophils and blood-derived monocytes. Instead, the membranes of the apoptotic bodies are targeted for rapid phagocytosis by adjacent parenchymal cells and resident tissue macrophages (Figures 6.30 and 6.31). The molecular basis for this targeting is complex and appears to depend on several factors. PS is normally confined to the inner leaflet of the plasma membrane by a β-catenin bridge to the actin cytoskeleton. During zeiosis, PS everts to the outer leaflet of the plasma membrane. Macrophages loosely bind to externalized PS, along

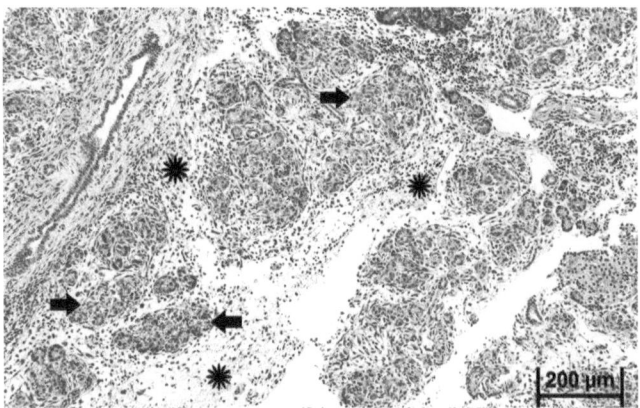

FIGURE 6.30 Postapoptotic atrophy. Photomicrograph of atrophied acinar pancreas in a Fischer 344 (F344) rat 4 days after extensive apoptosis due to administration of the pancreatic toxicant crambene. Small acini (*arrows*) containing shrunken, nonfunctional acinar cells are scattered throughout the section. Numerous histiocytic macrophages (starbursts) occupy the loose preexisting lobular stroma between acini. Hematoxylin and eosin. *Figure reproduced from Haschek WM, Rousseaux CG, Wallig MA, editors:* Handbook of toxicologic pathology, *ed 3, Academic Press, 2013, Figure 4.27, p. 102, with permission.*

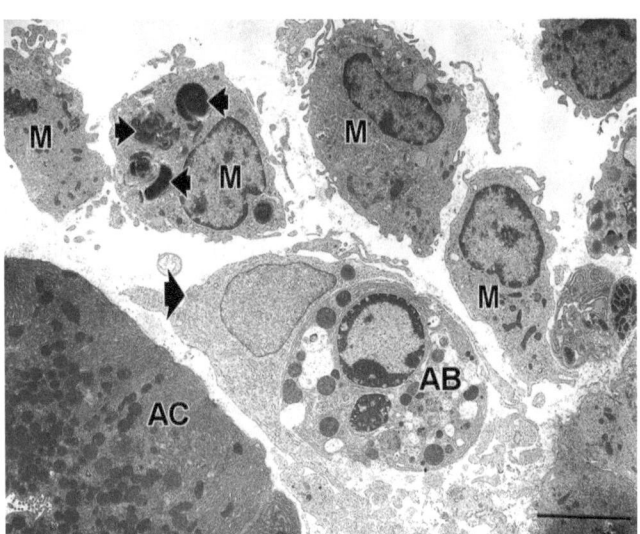

FIGURE 6.31 Sequela to apoptosis. Electron photomicrograph of a macrophage (*large arrow*) ingesting an apoptotic body (AB) within the pancreas of a Fischer 344 (F344) rat in which extensive apoptosis has occurred. Tissue macrophages (M) containing ingested apoptotic bodies (*small arrows*) appearing as inclusions are present as well. Intact pancreatic acinar cells (AC) are also present. Bar = 15 µm. *Figure reproduced with permission from the Haschek WM, Rousseaux CG, Wallig MA, editors:* Fundamentals of toxicologic pathology, *ed 2, Academic Press, 2007, Figure 4.28, p 102.*

with "immature" glycans, facilitating phagocytosis of apoptotic bodies. Other external macromolecules apparently recognized by macrophages include lysophosphatidyl choline, calreticulin, and annexin. Macrophage receptors, such as lectin-type oxidized LDL receptor 1 and platelet glycoproteins IIIa (CD61), appear necessary for binding to apoptotic cells. Phagocytosis of an apoptotic body after engulfment by a macrophage has been described as a "big gulp" to contrast with the "zipper" type of engulfment that typically precedes phagocytosis of bacteria. The latter is characterized by tight binding of the macrophage membrane to specific ligands on the bacterial membrane. The "big gulp" mode of phagocytosis is thought to involve three sequential signaling pathways: Ras-related C3 botulinum toxin substrate 1, Cluster of differentiation 91/Low-density lipoprotein receptor–related protein 1 → Engulfment adaptor PTB domain-containing 1 → ATP-binding cassette transporter A, and Engulfment and Cell Motility.

The precise mechanisms involved in digestion of the apoptotic body are uncertain, but the overall process depends on gradual acidification and protease degradation of the phagosome. IL-10 synthesis and release by macrophages which have engulfed apoptotic bodies partially explains the dampened inflammatory response to apoptosis. IL-10 inhibits synthesis of proinflammatory cytokines such as interferon-gamma, IL-2, IL-3, TNF-α, and granulocyte/macrophage colony stimulating factor. The net effect is blockage of antigen presentation by those macrophages with engulfed apoptotic bodies. Furthermore, while apoptotic bodies remain in their phagosomes, macrophages have markedly reduced phagocytic capability. In total, phagocyte-derived release of intracellular inflammatory chemokines (e.g., those that enhance endothelial permeability and activate or attract neutrophils) is minimal.

It must be noted, however, that in other forms of programmed cell death that result in morphologic changes similar to apoptosis, both caspase dependent (e.g., pyroptosis) and caspase independent (e.g., parthanatos, pyronecrosis), there is release of inflammatory mediators, especially IL-1, on a limited basis presumably to alert the innate immune system in response to injury/infection.

Widespread apoptosis within a tissue eventually leads to atrophy (Fig. 6.26). Once the cause of apoptosis is addressed, e.g., by removing a noxious insult or adding a trophic hormone, full regeneration is usually achievable provided a residual precursor cell population survives. Regeneration potential is particularly high in tissues with constant cell turnover such as lymph nodes, intestinal mucosal epithelium, and liver. However, in those tissues with so-called permanent cell populations, such as the retina, significant apoptosis will result in a permanent lesion (e.g., retinal atrophy) with some loss of function. The presence of an intact stroma, albeit often "collapsed" due to loss of cells that once occupied space within it, is another factor which allows for rapid regeneration and restoration of function once the cause of the apoptosis is removed.

Hyperplasia

As part of the regenerative process subsequent to widespread cell loss, cell proliferation is necessary and often recognizable temporarily as compensatory hyperplasia. However, compensatory hyperplasia can predispose to an ominous molecular event, namely the permanent establishment, i.e., fixation, of genetic mutations which can lead to neoplasia. Hyperplasia in this context is discussed in a later chapter (See *Carcinogenesis: Mechanisms and Evaluation*, Vol 1, Chap 8). Tissues vary widely in their capacity for compensatory hyperplasia. Tissues with labile cell populations which remain mitotically active through the lifetime of the animal and which can rapidly replace any losses include lymph nodes, bone marrow, epidermis, and intestinal crypt epithelium; tissues with stable cell populations, populations which retain the capacity to undergo mitosis but which generally do not remain mitotically active unless stimulated to do so during regeneration, include bronchial/bronchiolar epithelium, Type II pneumocytes, hepatocytes, biliary epithelium, and renal tubular epithelium. Tissues containing labile cells are most likely to undergo extensive hyperplasia under the appropriate stimulus followed by those with stable cell populations retaining precursor cells with the capacity to reenter the active cell cycle. Adequate stromal and vascular support are needed for appropriate regeneration of both. Initiation and maintenance of a hyperplastic response among surviving parenchymal cells is mediated at the molecular level by a myriad of protein and small molecule ligands interacting with an array of receptors and downstream signal transduction pathways (Kumar et al., 2015b).

Some of these proteins and small molecules are tissue specific, such as hepatocyte growth factor, and others are nonselective, such as EGF and TGF-β. Compensatory hyperplasia can result in peculiar lesions such as hyperplastic nodules with cirrhosis or hyperplastic polyps with chronic colitis. While such lesions are benign, they can harbor genetic mutations such as those that may arise from exposure to mutagenic toxins and predispose to carcinomas.

Metaplasia

A less common response to tissue injury than hyperplasia, but quite important from a disease perspective, is metaplasia. Metaplasia is generally defined as the replacement of mature fully specialized cells with mature but less specialized cells. It occurs in certain tissues when conditions for complete regeneration are suboptimal, particularly in the context of persistent but relatively limited injury. Classic examples are squamous metaplasia of bronchial epithelium in response to chronic injury by tobacco smoke and intestinal metaplasia of the esophageal mucosa in response to chronic injury by gastric acid reflux. Acinar to ductal metaplasia is seen with chronic injury and/or inflammation in tissues such as pancreas, mammary gland, and salivary glands. In all of these examples, metaplastic cells are more resistant to the inciting injury than the normal specialized cell population. Metaplastic tissue is a stop-gap measure for regeneration, having less functional efficiency than normal tissue. Metaplastic tissue arises in the context of hyperplasia since the new cell type must arise from a precursor stem cell type and then proliferate. Therefore, metaplastic tissue is also predisposed to neoplastic transformation (Giroux and Rustgi, 2017). In fact, metaplastic tissue is generally more likely to undergo neoplastic transformation than hyperplastic tissue (e.g., pancreatic acinar–ductal metaplasia in mice). This is not surprising since the process of metaplasia requires activation of signaling pathways and genes normally suppressed in the affected cell type and suppression of signaling pathways and genes normally active in the original phenotype. These pathways and new gene products will vary according to the type of metaplasia induced. For example, in acinar–ductal metaplasia in the pancreas, the normal pancreas transcription factor 1A complex, also known as PTF1A, is suppressed, while the Paired Related Homeobox 1 SRY-Box Transcription Factor 1, more commonly referred to as [PRRX]-SOX9, is induced. The Kirsten rat sarcoma and the Mitogen-activated protein kinase–Extracellular Receptor Kinase pathways, commonly referred to as KRAS and MAPK-ERK, respectively, are involved as well. By contrast, the ciliated to squamous epithelium transition in bronchial mucosa after chronic injury due to cigarette smoke involves the signal transducer and activator of transcription 3 among other factors. The signaling pathways and gene induction patterns in metaplasia at this point are complex and not completely understood, but in many cases, activation of proliferation pathways associated with neoplasia is part of the process. Finally, metaplastic cells may metabolize xenobiotics through substantially different enzymatic pathways than normal specialized cells. The nature of such metabolites, for example, whether they form protein or DNA adducts, can impact the eventual pathologic outcome of a metaplastic lesion. Metaplasia is further discussed in the next chapter (See *Carcinogenesis: Mechanisms and Evaluation*, Vol 1, Chap 8).

5. CONCLUSION

The morphologic features of an injured cell are complex but generally stereotypic and often independent of the inciting etiology. Occasionally, they are distinctive enough to provide an indication of the pathogenesis, particularly when the time course of subcellular changes is known. The terminology used to classify, and subclassify, the stages and manifestations of cell injury is in constant flux as modern molecular techniques are used to correlate morphology, including ultrastructural pathology, with biochemical alterations (See *Nomenclature and Diagnostic Resources in Anatomic Toxicologic Pathology*, Vol 1, Chap 25).

This chapter provided a synopsis of concepts in cell injury formulated from observations and experiences communicated since the early 20th century and that are widely accepted by pathologists. No synopsis can be complete because the number of variables, including those that can render injured cells more or less sensitive to noxious stimuli, is impossible to estimate. The succeeding chapters in this book will focus on many of these variables including those that are dependent on the mechanism of toxicity and on the organ system affected.

REFERENCES

Ackermann MR: Wound healing and angiogenesis. In Zachary J, McGrath MD, editors: *Pathologic basis of veterinary disease*, ed 6th, St. Louis, MO, 2017, Elsevier (Mosby), pp 121–132. Section 1, Chapter 3.

Aits S, Jäättelä M: Lysosomal cell death at a glance, *J Cell Sci* 126:1905–1912, 2013.

ATSDR (Agency for Toxic Substances and Disease Registry): *Toxicological profile for cyanide. Centers for disease control*, Atlanta, GA, 2006, U.S. Department of Health and Human Services, Public Health Service, pp 25–129. Section 3: Health Effects, https://www.atsdr.cdc.gov/ToxProfiles/tp.asp?id=72&tid=19.

Belizário J, Vieira-Cordeiro L, Enns S: Necroptotic cell death signaling and execution pathway: lessons from knockout mice, *Mediators Inflamm* 2015:128076, 2015. https://doi.org/10.1155/2015/128076. Epub 2015 Sep 27. PMID: 26491219.

Breiden B, Sandhoff KL: Emerging mechanisms of drug-induced phospholipidois (review), *Biol Chem* 401(1):31–46, 2020.

Cavalcante GC, Schaan AP, Cabral GF, Santana-da-Silva MN, Pinto P, Amanda F, Ribeiro-dos-Santos A: A cell's fate: an overview of the molecular biology and genetics of apoptosis (review), *Int J Mol Sci* 26(3):246–252, 2019.

Cheville NF: Structural basis of cell injury of acute cell injury. In Cheville N, editor: *Ultrastructural pathology: the comparative cellular Basis of disease*, 2nd, Ames, IA, 2009a, Wiley-Blackwell, Part 1, pp 3–73.

Cheville NF: Organellar pathology. In Cheville N, editor: *Consequences of acute cell injury: necrosis, recovery and hypertrophy*, Ames, IA, 2009, Wiley-Blackwell Part 2, pp 75–198. Ultrastructural pathology: the comparative cellular basis of disease. ed 2nd.

Elmore S: Apoptosis: a review of programmed cell death, *Toxicol Pathol* 35(4):495–516, 2007.

Elmore SA, Dixon D, Hailey JR, Harada T, Herbert RA, Maronpot R, Nolte T, Rehg JE, Rittinghausen S, Rosol TJ, Satoh H, Vidal JD, Willard-Mac CL, Creasy DM: Recommendations from the INHAND apoptosis/necrosis working group, *Toxicol Pathol* 44(2):173–188, 2016.

Fink SL, Cookson BT: Apoptosis, pyroptosis, and necrosis: mechanistic description of dead and dying eukaryotic cells, *Infect Immun* 73(4):1907–1916, 2005.

Frank D, Vince JE: Pyroptosis versus necroptosis: similarities, differences, and crosstalk (review article), *Cell Death Differ* 26:99–114, 2019.

Giroux V, Rustgi AK: Metaplasia: tissue injury adaptation and a precursor to the dysplasia-cancer sequence (review), *Nature Rev Cancer* 17:594–604, 2017.

Kroemer G, Levine B: Autophagic cell death: the story of a misnomer, *Nat Rev Mol Cell Biol* 9(12):1004–1010, 2008.

Itkonen P, Collan Y: Mitochondrial flocculent densities in ischemia: Digestion experiments. *Acta Pathol Microbiol Immunol Scand A* 91(6):463–468, 1983. https://doi.org/10.1111/j.1699-0463.1983.tb02779.x.

Kroemer G, Galluzzi L, Vandenabeele P, Abrams J, Alnemri ES, Baehrecke EH, Blagosklonny MV, El-Deiry WS, Golstein P, Green DR, Hengartner M, Knight RA, Kumar S, Lipton SA, Malorni W, Nuñez G, Peter ME, Tschopp J, Yuan J, Piacentini M, Zhivotovsky B, Melino G: Classification of cell death: recommendations of the nomenclature committee on cell death 2009, *Cell Death Differ* 16(1):3–11, 2009.

Kumar V, Abbas A, Aster JC: Autophagy. In Kumar V, Abbas AK, Aster JC, editors: *Robbins and Cotran pathologic bass of disease*, ed. 9th, 2015a, pp 60–61. Philadelphia, PA, Chapter 2.

Kumar V, Abbas AK, Aster JC: Tissue repair. In Kumar V, Abbas AK, Aster JC, editors: *Robbins and Cotran pathologic bass of disease*, ed. 9th, 2015b, pp 100–110. Philadelphia, PA, Chapter 3.

Louhimo JH, Steer ML, Perides G: Necroptosis is an important severity determinant and potential therapeutic target in experimental acute pancreatitis, *Cell Mol Gastroenter Hepatol* 2(4):519–535, 2016.

Li Q, Wang Y, Moldzio R, Lin W, Rausch WD: Swainsonine as a lysosomal toxin affects dopaminergic neurons, *J Neural Transm* 119(12):1483–1490, 2012.

McGill MR, Jaeschke H: Metabolism and disposition of acetaminophen: recent advances in relation to hepatotoxicity and diagnosis, *Pharm Res* 30(9):2174–2187, 2013. https://doi.org/10.1007/s11095-013-1007-6.

Mesa MA, Gloria Vasquez G: NETosis (review article), *Autoimmun Dis* 2013:1–7, 2013. https://doi.org/10.1155/2013/651497. | Article ID 651497.

Miller MA, Zachary JF: Cellular adaptation, injury and death: reversible injury. In Zachary J, McGrath MD, editors: *Pathologic basis of veterinary disease*, ed 6th, St. Louis, MO, 2017a, Elsevier (Mosby), pp 10–12. Section 1, Chapter 1.

Miller MA, Zachary JF: Hematogenous pigments. In Zachary J, McGrath MD, editors: *Pathologic basis of veterinary disease*, ed 6th, St. Louis, MO, 2017b, Elsevier (Mosby), pp 37–38. Section 1, Chapter 1.

Mingeot-Leclercq M-P, Tulkens PM: Aminoglycosides: nephrotoxicity, *Antimicrob Agents Chemother* 43(5):1003–1012, 1999.

Nikoletopoulou V, Makarki M, Polikaras K, Tavanarakis N: Crosstalk between apoptosis, necrosis and autophagy (review), *Biochim Biophys Acta* 1833:3448–3459, 2013.

Ortiz de Montellano PR: 1-Aminobenzotriazole: a mechanism-based cytochrome P450 inhibitor and probe of cytochrome P450 biology, *Med Chem (Los Angeles)* 8(3):038, 2018.

Papadopoulos C, Meyer H: Detection and clearance of damaged lysosomes by the endo-lysosomal damage response and lysophagy, *Curr Biol* 27:R1330–R1341, 2017.

Parzych KR, Klionsky DJ: An overview of autophagy: morphology, mechanism, and regulation, *Antioxid Redox Signal* 20(3):460–473, 2014.

Porter AG, Jänicke RU: Emerging roles of caspase-3 in apoptosis (review), *Cell Death Diff* 6:99104, 1999.

Salvesen G, Walsh CM: Functions of Caspase 8: the identified and the mysterious, *Sem Immunol* 26(3):246–252, 2014.

Satoh T, Kambe N, Matsue H: NLRP3 activation induces ASC-dependent programmed necrotic cell death, which leads to neutrophilic inflammation, *Cell Death Dis* 4:1–10, 2013. https://doi.org/10.1038/cddis.2013.169. e644.

Settembre C, Di Malta C, Assunta Polito V, Garcia Arencibia M, Vetrini F, Erdin S, Uckac Erdin S, Huynh, Medina D, Colella P, Sardiello M, Rubinsztein D, Ballabio A: TFEB links autophagy to lysosomal biogenesis, *Science* 332:1429–1433, 2011.

Shalini S, Dorstyn L, Dawar S, Kumar S: Old, new and emerging functions of caspases, *Cell Death Diff* 22:526–539, 2015.

Shi C-S, Nabar NR, Huang N-N, Kehrl JH: SARS-Coronavirus open reading frame-8b triggers intracellular stress pathways and activates NLRP3 inflammasomes, *Cell Death Discov* 5:101–112, 2019.

Singh R, Letai A, Sarosiek K: Regulation of apoptosis in health and disease: the balancing act of BCL-2 family proteins (review), *Nature Rev – Mol Cell Biol* 20:175–193, 2019.

Tabas I, Ron D: Integrating the mechanisms of apoptosis induced by endoplasmic reticulum stress, *Nat Cell Biol* 13(3):184–190, 2011.

Trump BF, Berezesky IK, Sato T, Laiho KU, Phelps PC, DeClaris N: Cell calcium, cell injury and cell death, *Environ Hlth Perspect* 57:281–287, 1984.

Takeuchi O, Akira S: Pattern recognition receptors and inflammation (leading edge review), *Cell* 140:805–820, 2010.

Weiss DJ, English K, Krasnodembskaya A, Isaza-Correa JM, Hawthorne IJ, Mahon BP: The necrobiology of mesenchymal stromal cells affects therapeutic efficacy, *Front Immunol* 10(1–12):1228, 2019.

Xie Y, Hou W, Song X, Yu Y, Huang J, Sun X, Kang R, Tang D: Ferroptosis: process and function (review), *Cell Death Diff* 23:369–379, 2016.

Yin D: Biochemical basis of lipofuscin, ceroid and age pigment-like fluorophores (review article), *Free Radicals Biol Med* 22(6):871–888, 1996.

Zhang Y, Chen X, Gueydan C, Han J: Plasma membrane changes during programmed cell deaths (review), *Cell Death Diff* 23:369–379, 2018.

Zhang L, Zhang J, Shea K, Lin X, Tobin G, Knapton A, Sharron S, Rouse R: Autophagy in pancreatic acinar cells in caerulein-treated mice: immunolocalization of related proteins and their potential as markers of pancreatitis, *Toxicol Pathol* 42:435–457, 2014.

CHAPTER

7

The Role of Pathology in Evaluation of Reproductive, Developmental, and Juvenile Toxicity

Christopher J. Bowman[1], Wendy G. Halpern[2]

[1]Drug Safety Research & Development, Worldwide Research, Development, & Medical Pfizer, Inc., Groton, CT, United States, [2]Safety Assessment Pathology, Genentech, South San Francisco, CA, United States

OUTLINE

1. Introduction   149

2. Reproductive Toxicity Assessment   150
   2.1. Male Reproductive Toxicity Assessment   152
   2.2. Female Reproductive Toxicity Assessment   159
   2.3. Guidelines   167

3. Pregnancy and Developmental Toxicity   167
   3.1. Embryo–Fetal Development Studies   168
   3.2. Pre- and Postnatal Development Studies   172
   3.3. Enhanced Pre- and Postnatal Development
        Study in the NHP   174
   3.4. Guidelines   176

4. Juvenile Toxicity Assessment   177

4.1. Context for Challenges in Assessing the
     Neonatal Period   179
4.2. Context for Support of Children: Weaning
     through Puberty   179
4.3. Postnatal Development of Specific Organ Systems 180
4.4. Models of Disease   188
4.5. Practical Species-Specific Considerations   188
4.6. Guidelines and Regional Legislation   190

5. Conclusions   192

Abbreviations   192

References   193

1. INTRODUCTION

Developmental and reproductive toxicity (DART) studies represent an important component of the toxicology programs supporting both the development of novel therapeutics and the evaluation of environmental, agricultural, and industrial chemicals. Reproductive toxicity generally refers to adverse effects on fertility and sexual function in adult males and females, while developmental toxicity refers to effects on the viability, structure, growth, or function of a developing embryo, fetus, or offspring (Figure 7.1). For pharmaceuticals, the inclusion of a dedicated juvenile animal study (JAS), while not always warranted, has also become more common with regional legislation in the US and EU mandating exploration of pediatric relevance during drug development.

An understanding of DART is necessary to inform the labeling and use of pharmaceuticals in fertile, pregnant, lactating, and pediatric patients, as well as the regulation and use of

Haschek and Rousseaux's Handbook of Toxicologic Pathology, Fourth Edition.
https://doi.org/10.1016/B978-0-12-821044-4.00031-5

149

environmental chemicals. In addition, in 2020, both the International Council for Harmonisation (ICH) S5(R3) Guideline on Detection of Reproductive and Developmental Toxicity for Human Pharmaceuticals (ICH, 2020a) and the ICH S11 Guideline for Nonclinical Safety Testing in Support of Development of Pediatric Pharmaceuticals (ICH, 2020b) were adopted. These guidelines will influence multiple aspects of DART including the future inclusion and use of pathology endpoints when DART or JAS studies are warranted for development of pharmaceuticals. Existing guidance and experience in other areas such as diagnostic reproductive and developmental pathology, as well as agrochemical and environmental toxicity assessment, also contribute to our overall understanding. A review of relevant guidance documents is provided within each subsection of this chapter and is summarized in Tables 7.1 and 7.5.

We will explore the role of the pathologist in the design, execution, and interpretation of DART and JAS and define some of the issues that distinguish these studies from more standard toxicology testing in this chapter. One important aspect is that pathology endpoints are not uniformly included in DART studies and have historically been variable in juvenile

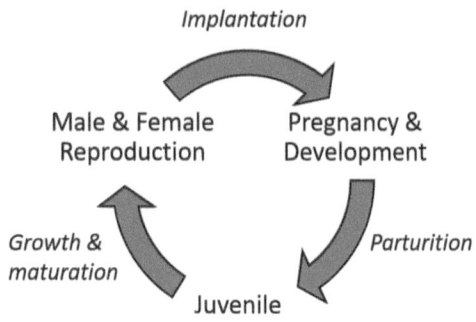

FIGURE 7.1   Stages of reproduction and development. Developmental and reproductive toxicity (DART) studies represent an important component of the toxicology programs supporting both the development of novel therapeutics and the evaluation of environmental, agricultural, and industrial chemicals. Reproductive toxicity generally refers to adverse effects on fertility and sexual function in adult males and females, while developmental toxicity refers to effects on the viability, structure, growth, or function of a developing embryo, fetus, or offspring following maternal exposure. Juvenile toxicity generally refers to effects of direct exposure during postnatal development up to sexual maturity.

toxicity studies as well (Halpern et al., 2016). Therefore, the historical and background pathology data are often sparser for pregnant or young animals, and a working knowledge of reproductive and developmental physiology is a critical aspect of interpretation of pathology endpoints in the setting of DART and JAS.

Important aspects of reproductive and developmental toxicity testing often come relatively late in the overall safety assessment of a bio/pharmaceutical product or environmental chemical. Prior to designing a study, a thorough assessment of available information should be conducted. In addition to available toxicity and toxicokinetic data available for a specific molecule, it is important to review literature on modulation of the target pathway, including with other molecules, as well as potential for off-target effects with the molecule of interest. For chemicals regulated nationally by the United States Environmental Protection Agency (US EPA), and internationally by Organisation for Economic Co-operation and Development (OECD), there is guidance including descriptions of validated study designs, some of which are specifically relevant to reproduction and development (See Table 7.1). Finally, the specific needs or considerations of the target patient population for a bio/pharmaceutical, or the population at risk for an environmental chemical, should be considered. These are important factors in developing a Weight-of-Evidence (WoE) approach for both the need for a study and ultimately the design of such a study, if needed. Pathology endpoints may be prospectively included or added for cause if there are unexpected findings or outcomes on the study. Overall, the pathologist can be a critical contributor to the interpretation and application of these data to human hazard and risk assessment.

2. REPRODUCTIVE TOXICITY ASSESSMENT

The purpose of a reproductive toxicity assessment is to identify the potential of a molecule to impact male and female fertility. This assessment includes consideration of all available information on potential risks based on known effects and/or known physiological targets of the molecule, relevance in the human population, and

TABLE 7.1 Regulatory Guidance for DART Testing

Source[a]	Title	General utility
ICH	• S5(R3): Detection of reproductive and developmental toxicity for human Pharmaceuticals (ICH, 2020a)	• Harmonized nonclinical guidance for developmental and reproductive toxicity (primary resource)
	• S6(R1): Preclinical safety evaluation of biotechnology-derived Pharmaceuticals (ICH, 2011)	• Approach to DART for biopharmaceuticals; description of ePPND
	• M3(R2): Guidance on nonclinical safety studies for the conduct of human clinical trials and marketing authorization for Pharmaceuticals (ICH, 2009a)	• Timing of DART testing
	• S9: Nonclinical evaluation for anticancer Pharmaceuticals (ICH, 2009b)	• Approach to DART testing for oncology
EPA	• OCSPP guideline 890.1500: Pubertal development and thyroid function in the intact Juvenile/Peripubertal male Rats (EPA, 2009a)	• In vivo mammalian tests for chemical endocrine disruption
	• OCSPP guideline 890.1450: Pubertal development and thyroid function in the intact Juvenile/Peripubertal female Rats (EPA, 2009b)	
	• OPPTS guideline 870.3700: Prenatal developmental toxicity Study (EPA, 1998a)	• In vivo mammalian tests for reproductive and developmental toxicity
	• OPPTS guideline 870.3800: Reproduction and fertility Effects (EPA, 1998b)	
	• OPPTS guideline 870.6200: Neurotoxicity screening Battery (EPA, 1998c)	• In vivo mammalian tests for developmental neurotoxicity
	• OPPTS guideline 870.6300: Developmental Neurotoxicity (EPA, 1998d)	
FDA	• Testicular toxicity: Evaluation during drug Development (FDA, 2018)	• Combined guidance for nonclinical and clinical male reproductive safety assessment of drugs
	• Reproductive and developmental toxicities— Integrating study results to assess Concerns (FDA, 2011)	• Guidance on integration of DART data
	• Oncology pharmaceuticals: Reproductive toxicity testing and labeling Recommendations (FDA, 2019)	• Regional recommendations for DART testing in oncology
OECD	• Test no. 414: Prenatal developmental toxicity Study (OECD, 2018a)	• Primary reproductive and toxicity tests for chemicals
	• Test no. 416: Two generation reproduction toxicity Study (OECD, 2001)	
	• Test no. 421: Reproduction/Developmental toxicity Screening (OECD, 2016a)	• Screening reproductive and toxicity tests for chemicals
	• Test no. 422: Combined repeated dose toxicity study with Reproduction/Developmental toxicity Screening (OECD, 2016b)	
	• Test no. 426: Developmental neurotoxicity Study (OECD, 2007)	• Used when there is a concern for developmental neurotoxicity
	• Test no. 443: Extended one generation reproductive toxicity Study (OECD, 2018b)	• Alternative reproductive and toxicity tests for chemicals

[a] All source links current as of November 2020 are provided in the reference list according to the originating institution or organization.

potential for recovery. Typically, most molecules will also be evaluated in repeat-dose toxicity studies in animals that include macroscopic and microscopic examinations of male and female reproductive tissues and potential effects on organ weights. These data from repeat-dose toxicity studies together with background information can provide a WoE assessment for the potential to adversely impact male or female fertility. In most cases, there is also an expectation to experimentally evaluate the potential of a molecule to impact functional aspects of male and female fertility if possible. Figure 7.2 illustrates an example of when these different study types are typically conducted at different stages of drug development, noting that clinical development of therapeutics starts based on repeat-dose toxicity data and functional fertility data are acquired later in development. In all cases, the reproductive toxicity assessment should consider applicable regulatory guidelines, utilize robust scientific approaches to experimental design (See *Experimental Design and Statistical Analysis for Toxicologic Pathologists*, Vol 1, Chap 16) in relevant test systems, and then develop an integrated interpretation of the available information.

2.1. Male Reproductive Toxicity Assessment

Specific experimental considerations for assessing the potential for toxicity to male fertility include the selection of an appropriate animal model, the stage of sexual maturity of the test system, appropriate dose selection to avoid confounding toxicity such as body weight loss, sensitivity of the test system for detection and recovery, and selection of various endpoints of male reproduction. Many of these considerations apply to both general toxicity studies and functional fertility (mating) studies. Many of the endpoints are interrelated; thus, interpretation of the potential for test article–related toxicity to male fertility should consider each endpoint in the context of the other aspects of male reproduction.

General Considerations
SPECIES SELECTION

Although no specific nonclinical species best predicts male infertility, species selection should be justified. Mammalian species should be used and if applicable, should express the pharmacological target; this is especially important if the target is present in the human male reproductive system. Ideally, the same species and strain used in the repeat-dose toxicity studies are utilized for functional fertility studies in order to minimize animal use since pharmacokinetics and metabolism have already been well characterized and can be used for dose setting. See *ADME Principles in Small Molecule Drug Discovery and Development—An Industrial Perspective* Vol 1, Chap 3 and *Biotherapeutic ADME and PK/PD Principles* Vol 1, Chap 4. In addition, use of the same species for repeat-dose toxicity and functional fertility studies allows for better correlation and

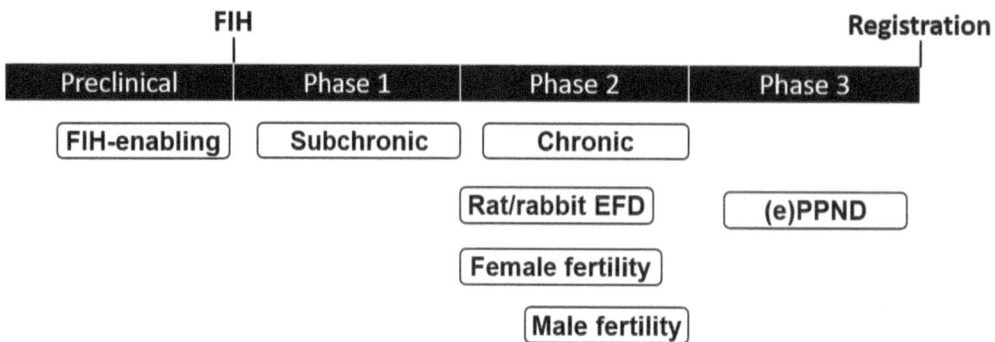

FIGURE 7.2 Representative timing of toxicity studies relevant for DART assessment. First-in-Human (FIH)-enabling study in mature animals supports safety assessment of reproductive tissues in clinical trial subjects. Embryo–fetal development (EFD) and female fertility studies support enrollment of women of child-bearing potential. Male fertility study supports male reproductive safety in Phase 3 population. Enhanced (e) or stand-alone pre- and postnatal development (PPND) study supports registration and labeling.

integration of the overall effects on the male reproductive system. Rodents are the default test system for functional fertility studies with the rat most often used followed by the mouse. Nontraditional species for functional fertility studies include the rabbit, guinea pig, and hamster. Functional fertility studies are not recommended for nonhuman primates (NHPs) or dogs due the practical challenges with low background fertility, limited number of cycles per year (female dog), and relatively long gestation length. Table 7.2 summarizes differences in key male reproductive considerations among standard toxicology species. When there is concern for male reproductive toxicities not specific to the testis, the effects can be better characterized using surrogate fertility endpoints such as sperm assessment and hormones. In addition, sensitivity of specific cell types can be investigated in vitro and support in vivo studies of reproductive toxicology (Chapin et al., 2014; Komeya et al., 2019; Parks Saldutti et al., 2013), specifically the testis and, in the future, potentially more complex models capable of organ-to-organ hormonal signaling during reproduction (Alves-Lopes and Stukenborg, 2018; Baert et al., 2020).

SEXUAL MATURITY

A critical component of experimental test systems to appropriately evaluate potential effects on male fertility is that the test system should be sexually mature. The Society of Toxicologic Pathology (STP) recently endorsed Best Practices for the recording and reporting of sexual maturity status (Vidal et al., 2021). An immature or developing testis can in many ways resemble types of testicular toxicity and at best confound an otherwise adequate assessment of test item–related toxicity (Foley, 2001; Goedken et al., 2008; Lanning et al., 2002). Based on microscopic evaluation of the male reproductive tract including sperm evaluation, the Wistar and Sprague Dawley rat are considered sexually mature by 10 weeks of age (Campion et al., 2013). As such, because male reproductive safety in first-in-human (FIH) studies is typically supported by repeat-dose toxicity studies, it is important to include sexually mature animals in those studies. For functional fertility studies, however, it is common to mate rats between 12 and 24 weeks of age, as that seems to represent peak reproductive capacity in most rat strains. When

younger or older rats are used, there is more variability as animals first mature, and then as they age, their reproductive capacity appears to slowly decline (Auroux et al., 1985; Blazak et al., 1985; Jarak et al., 2018; Saksena et al., 1979; Takakura et al., 2014). Based on microscopy of the testis, it is recommended that mice be older than 7 weeks of age at termination (Lanning et al., 2002).

Sometimes a male reproductive toxicant will not be apparent in a rodent but will present in a nonrodent species, either as part of routine safety evaluation (Losco et al., 2007) or, as is often the case with biologics, the NHP as the only pharmacologically relevant species. Regardless, if the repeat-dose study is the only evaluation of the reproductive tract, it is important that the evaluation of potential effects on male reproduction be done using sexually mature dogs or NHPs. Mature animals are typically used in subchronic or chronic studies and not necessarily FIH studies unless there is a specific cause for concern. It is recommended that dogs be older than 9 months of age at necropsy for an appropriate evaluation of potential testicular toxicity (James and Heywood, 1979; Lanning et al., 2002). Unlike rodents, and to some extent dogs, determination of sexual maturity in male NHPs based on age, body weight, and/or testicular volume is insufficient to predict sexual maturation (defined by testicular histopathology) (Luetjens and Weinbauer, 2012). However, the presence of sperm in a single semen sample unequivocally demonstrates capacity for complete spermatogenesis and is recommended to support selection of male NHPs when the evaluation needs to include an assessment of toxicity to the male reproductive system (Luetjens and Weinbauer, 2012).

CONFOUNDING FACTORS

There are confounding factors that can affect interpretation of potential effects on male reproduction. In addition to the maturity status previously described, nonspecific toxicity such as stress and/or effects resulting in decreased body weight and/or food consumption can complicate otherwise clear signals of male reproductive toxicity. This type of nonspecific stress introduced by feed restriction can result in suppression of the hypothalamic–pituitary–gonad (HPG) axis, gonadotrophin releasing hormone (GnRH), and downstream effects on the male rodent reproductive system such as decreased testosterone, organ

TABLE 7.2   Male Reproductive Milestones Across Species (For Additional Detail, See (Vidal et al., 2021))

Species	Age at preputial separation	Adrenarche	Spermarche	Age at adult reproductive function	Spermatogenic cycle length[a]	Serial semen sampling	Fertility testing (mating study)
Mouse	4–5 weeks	N/A	4–5 weeks	~7 weeks	~9 days	No	Yes
Rat	6–7 weeks	2–3 weeks	~7 weeks	~10 weeks	~13 days	No	Yes
Rabbit	~10 weeks	N/A	14–15 weeks	~4 months	~11 days	Yes	Rare
Beagle dog	N/A	~3 months	~8 months	>9 months	~14 days	Yes	No
Cynomolgus monkey	N/A	3–6 months	2.5–4 years	>4 years	~10 days	Yes	No
Human	N/A	~7 years	10–15 years	>16 years	16 days	Yes	N/A

[a] Completion of spermatogenesis from differentiated type A spermatogonia through spermatozoal release is generally 4–4.5 times the length of the cycle.

weights (decreased seminal vesicles and prostate, but not testis), atrophy of accessory sex organs, and/or testicular degeneration (Chapin and Creasy, 2012; Everds et al., 2013; O'Connor et al., 2000; Rehm et al., 2008).

A specific analysis looking at the value of organ-to-body weight ratio or organ-to-brain weight ratios confirmed that relative testis weights are not useful determinants of toxicity in the rat (Bailey et al., 2004). Interestingly, these effects on the morphology of male reproductive tissues do not seem to negatively impact functional fertility in the rat (Chapin et al., 1993a) and only variably so in the mouse (Chapin et al., 1993b). In general, the reproductive system of dogs and NHPs appears less sensitive to effects of nonspecific stress compared with rodents, although dogs may show atrophy of the prostatic epithelium, and NHPs may have decreased testicular size, weight, and spermatogenesis (Everds et al., 2013; Gondos et al., 1970; Niehoff et al., 2010).

BLOOD–TESTIS BARRIER

A unique aspect of male reproductive physiology is the blood–testis barrier (BTB) and blood–epididymis barrier (BEB). These barriers are an interaction of the structural, physiological, and immunological components (Mital et al., 2011; Mruk and Cheng, 2015) and can be important considerations in test article–related toxicity and potential species-specific sensitivity. Although both barriers are important for sperm maturation, little is known about the BEB (Cyr et al., 2018) compared with the expanding research on the BTB (Setchell, 2008; Su et al., 2011). Specifically, drug biodistribution at the BTB is influenced by transporters such as breast cancer resistance protein on endothelial cells (Qian et al., 2013), transferrin on Sertoli cells (Setchell, 2008), and P-glycoprotein on several different cell types (Setchell, 2008; Su et al., 2011), and these can impact reproductive function (Mruk et al., 2011).

Testing Endpoints

Evaluation of potential effects on male reproduction can include many possible endpoints in standard nonclinical toxicity testing such as organ weights, macroscopic, and microscopic examination of tissues in the male reproductive tract, sperm assessment, systemic biomarkers, and fertility indices. In terms of detecting possible effects, organ weights and histopathology are sufficient to detect effects on sperm production, but mating trials (fertility indices) are optimal for detecting other functional effects unrelated to sperm production such as sperm maturation, behavior, libido, etc (Ulbrich and Palmer, 1995). Addition of other endpoints such as sperm assessment and hormone measurements does not change the ability to detect an effect but certainly can be useful to characterize such an effect once identified, and its potential impact to the human risk assessment (Cappon et al., 2013; Ulbrich and Palmer, 1995).

ORGAN WEIGHTS

There are specific recommendations by the STP for which organ weights should be collected and in which species (Sellers et al., 2007). Specifically, testes should be weighed in all repeat-dose toxicity studies of all species, epididymides and prostate glands should be weighed in all rat studies (and case by case in nonrodent and mouse studies), and thyroid and pituitary gland weights should be collected for all species except mice. As described earlier, organ weights of male reproductive tissues are most appropriate in sexually mature animals. Seminal vesicle (with or without fluid) weights in male rodents provide similar information as prostate weights, but if done consistently or together with the prostate (commonly referred to as the accessory sex organ/glands) can provide a sensitive indication of androgen status (O'Connor et al., 2000). While slight changes in male reproductive organ weights in the absence of other effects may not be the cause for concern (particularly in nonrodent species) (Cappon et al., 2013), specific changes (even unilaterally) can significantly contribute to a better understanding and interpretation of observations in other endpoints including macroscopic and microscopic changes, as well as sperm assessment and fertility indices (Lanning et al., 2002).

MACROSCOPIC AND MICROSCOPIC EVALUATION

In addition to macroscopic examination, there are specific recommendations by the STP as to which tissues should be collected and microscopically evaluated for all repeat-dose toxicity studies (Bregman et al., 2003). These include testes, epididymides, prostate gland, seminal vesicles, and pituitary gland, which serve as a critical part of the evaluation for potential effects on the male reproductive system. A robust microscopic evaluation of the male reproductive tract requires consistent and appropriate trimming and fixation of these tissues, as reviewed by the STP (Creasy, 2003; Lanning et al., 2002; Latendresse et al., 2002). Standardized terminology (See *Nomenclature and Diagnostic Resources in Anatomic Toxicologic Pathology*, Vol 1, Chap 25) and lesion characterization is important and has been published for the female reproductive system with the rat and mouse (Creasy et al., 2012). Just as important as a qualitative, stage-aware, evaluation of spermatogenesis is an integrated assessment of all the reproductive tissues (Creasy, 2001; Vidal and Whitney, 2014) and appropriate recognition of immature tissues (e.g., testis) relative to a potential lesion in nonrodent species such as NHP (Dreef et al., 2007; Halpern et al., 2016).

SPERM ASSESSMENT

Sperm assessment is required for some chemical toxicity testing (e.g., extended one-generation study) but is not routinely required for toxicity screening of pharmaceuticals. Regardless, evaluation for potential effects on sperm counts, motility, and morphology can be triggered to further characterize male reproductive toxicity and is one of the few endpoints that can be evaluated in clinical trials. Figure 7.3 illustrates rat sperm on a slide that is used by computer-assisted sperm analysis to count sperm and calculate percent motility.

Sperm assessment is an important complementary endpoint for male reproductive assessment that falls between effects on male fertility (functional mating) and morphologic changes in male reproductive tissues. In rodents, sperm assessment is usually conducted from testicular tissue and/or cauda epididymis or *vas deferens* collected at necropsy (Campion et al., 2013). Sperm assessment can be a more sensitive measure of effects on spermatogenesis than fertility in rodents because there is a large sperm reserve in these species such that as much as a 90% decrease in sperm count may still result in normal fertility (Blazak et al., 1993; Meistrich, 1982; Takayama et al., 1995). As such, without sperm evaluation, a posttesticular effect on

sperm maturation may be missed in rodents (Marien et al., 2016).

For effects on spermatogenesis in the testis, microscopic evaluation is considered the most sensitive endpoint (Cappon et al., 2013; Creasy, 2001; Vidal and Whitney, 2014). In rabbits, dogs, and NHP, serial semen samples can be collected before, during, and after dose administration in a toxicity study, allowing onset and recovery of effects on sperm to be characterized (Chellman et al., 2009; Clarke et al., 2015; Dostal et al., 2001; Lerman et al., 2009; Takagi et al., 2001; Teo et al., 2004; Williams et al., 1990). In all species, sperm assessment can be conducted in all types of studies as an optional endpoint,

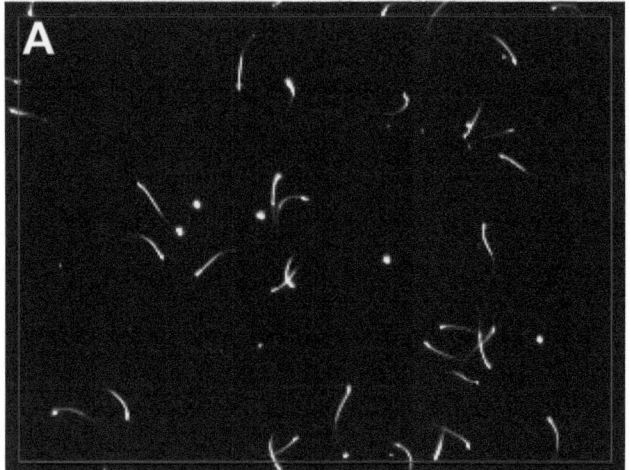

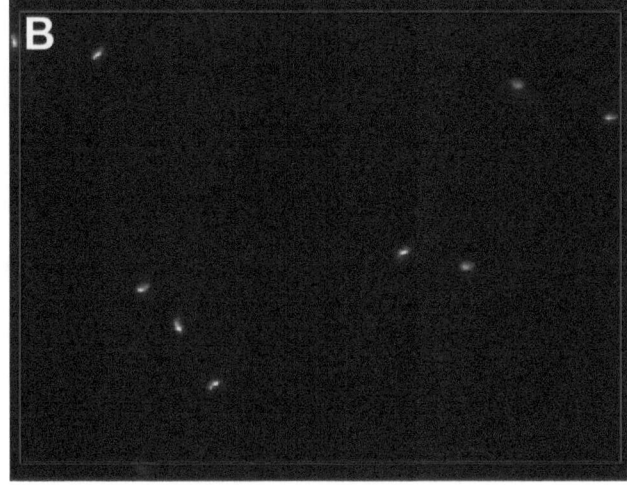

FIGURE 7.3   Rat sperm evaluation using the Hamilton Thorne TOX IVOS sperm analysis system. Blue square is measured field. (A) Viable rat sperm motility (vas deferens). (B) Fixed rat sperm concentration (epididymal), sperm DNA with IDENT stain. *Photo Credit: Charles River Laboratories, Ashland, Ohio, USA.*

including standard repeat-dose toxicity studies and/or fertility studies.

BIOMARKERS

There are few practical biomarkers of male reproductive health that can be measured in blood. These include hormones and more novel markers such as sperm mRNA transcripts as indicators of testicular damage. As a general screen for detecting male reproductive toxicity in nonclinical species, effects on circulating hormones can be difficult to interpret (Chapin and Creasy, 2012). In particular, some hormones are subject to wide variability due to pulsatility of secretion, diurnal rhythms, and stress; as such, it is critical to factor this into the design of any study including these endpoints, as statistical power to detect changes can be limited (Cappon et al., 2013; Chapin and Creasy, 2012). There have been several reviews describing changes in luteinizing hormone (LH), follicle-stimulating hormone (FSH), inhibin, testosterone, or prolactin, as well as how different "fingerprints" correlate to different microscopic changes in the male reproductive tract (Chapin and Creasy, 2012; O'Connor et al., 2002). One commonly observed change in hormones associated with testicular damage is decreased testosterone, which can be secondary to decreased GnRH and/or LH, or through a direct effect on Leydig cell steroidogenesis. This type of effect can occur quickly, as demonstrated in a 7-day study with a neurokinin 1, 2, and 3 receptor antagonist (Enright et al., 2010). After many years of anecdotally using inhibin B as a biomarker of testicular damage, a robust assay was evaluated by many companies and compounds with equivocal results in that approximately half of the exposures demonstrated inhibin B as a lagging biomarker requiring significant testicular damage (Chapin et al., 2013). In an effort to identify additional biomarkers of testicular damage, it was found that sperm mRNA transcripts are sensitive indicators of both Sertoli and germ cell damage, while sperm DNA methylation changes are not (Dere et al., 2016). The lack of a premonitory biomarker of male reproductive toxicity limits clinical management of potential risk and thus large therapeutic margins and/or mechanistic understanding are often needed to assure safety.

MATING TRIALS

As mentioned earlier, the minimum amount of data needed to detect the majority of potential effects on male reproduction using animal models are organ weights and histopathology, but mating trials (fertility indices) are needed to detect other functional effects unrelated to testicular sperm production such as posttesticular sperm maturation, behavior, libido, and fecundity (Ulbrich and Palmer, 1995). It is this latter endpoint of fertility that evaluates the relatively complicated process of gamete maturation and successful delivery via the ejaculate to complete the mating process (copulatory performance) leading to presumptive fertilization of the released oocyte in the female partner, and blastocyte implantation in the uterine wall confirming pregnancy. Mating trials are most often conducted in dedicated fertility studies with treated males and females, or, in the case of male fertility studies, with treated males mated to treatment-naïve females (Barrow, 2009; Lerman et al., 2009). However, it is also possible to do mating trials with treated males on repeat-dose toxicity studies coupled with treatment-naïve females (Mitchard et al., 2012). These options are described later under different study types.

The vast majority of mating trials are conducted in rats, but similar designs can be conducted in mice, rabbits (Breslin et al., 2015), or guinea pigs (Rocca and Wehner, 2009). Mating trials are not practical in dogs or NHPs, so surrogate endpoints of fertility (e.g., sperm assessment) may be used in addition to organ weights and histopathology to fully characterize male reproductive toxicity in those species. In a rodent reproductive toxicity study, functional fertility is evaluated by pairing the treated male with a female for a set period of time, typically 2–3 weeks, until evidence of mating is confirmed by copulatory plug in the vagina or sperm present in a vaginal smear. The animals are unpaired, and the mated female is allowed to progress through gestation. The female is either subject to Cesarean section or allowed to deliver, but the primary fertility endpoint is usually to confirm pregnancy status and then to evaluate the number of viable and nonviable conceptuses or pups relative to the number of implantation sites.

In addition to confirming pregnancy, mating trials can inform the viability of the offspring which can be a sensitive endpoint of male (rodent) reproductive toxicity. The limited apical endpoints calculated in rodent mating trials include time to mating and several different types of reproductive indices such as mating index ([number males with evidence of mating (or females confirmed pregnant)/total number of males used for mating] × 100) and fertility index ([number of males siring a litter/total number of males used for mating] × 100).

As mentioned earlier, evaluation of potential effects on male reproduction ideally consists of data from repeat-dose toxicity studies as well as a functional fertility study that includes a mating trial. It is the integration of all available data across studies and species, accounting for differences in design and species, that should provide a complete evaluation of male reproductive safety of a test item.

Study Types

REPEAT-DOSE TOXICITY STUDIES

Microscopic evaluation of male reproductive tissues is a critical component in all repeat-dose toxicity studies (Creasy, 2001), and specific chapters in this Edition will cover the specific pathologies in these tissues (see *Male Reproductive Tract*, Vol 4, Chap 9). While testicular toxicity can be detected in a short-term study, effects may not fully manifest acutely, or may become more severe with a longer duration of dosing. There are many different targets of toxicity within the testis including interstitial cells (Leydig cells), Sertoli cells, and perhaps most challenging are the spermatogonia, spermatocytes, and spermatids.

The sensitivity to detect the primary cell type affected by a specific toxicant can be challenging; testicular toxicity often simply manifests as seminiferous tubule degeneration and atrophy identified at necropsy and histologically. However, the severity of the damage and cell types impacted can dictate whether the lesion will recover and how long it will take to recover. It is not uncommon in short-term studies for the recovery animals to actually have more severe testicular pathology, as it can take time for affected cell types to manifest as damaged tubules. It is also possible for unilateral testicular toxicity to be secondary to efferent duct toxicity, which can

be useful to identify because it appears to be a rat-specific lesion that is not relevant for humans (La et al., 2012).

It is more difficult to detect male reproductive toxicity other than testicular damage in repeat-dose studies unless other endpoints are included such as sperm assessment and/or in the case of rodents, mating trials (Chapin et al., 1998; Chellman et al., 2009; Clarke et al., 2015; Dostal et al., 2001; Mitchard et al., 2012; Morrissey et al., 1988; Takagi et al., 2001). If the rodent or rabbit are not biologically or pharmacologically relevant and there is a concern for male reproductive toxicity not involving the testis, the addition of sperm assessment can be the most reasonable way to evaluate those potential effects in dogs and NHPs. In fact, ICH S6(R1) describes the scenario for when NHPs are the only pharmacologically relevant species as described earlier (ICH, 2011).

MALE FERTILITY STUDY

Ideally, the evaluation of testicular morphology in repeat-dose toxicity studies is complemented by a study including a mating trial typically conducted in a male fertility study in rodents. The key feature of a male fertility evaluation is a mating trial, but also can include male reproductive organ weights, microscopic evaluation of the male reproductive tract, sperm assessment, or other endpoints, if warranted.

Historically, the male fertility study included dosing for a full 8–10 weeks prior to mating to encompass the full developmental period of spermatogenesis on the impact to mating and fertility. However, current ICH S5(R3) guidance supports a minimum of 2 weeks of dosing prior to mating for detecting potential effects on male mating and fertility, provided no effects on male reproductive organs were observed in previous repeat-dose toxicity studies of at least 2 weeks duration and that testicular microscopic examination was conducted in a "stage-aware" manner (ICH, 2020a; Lanning et al., 2002). The 2-week dosing period prior to mating was justified by a detailed review of known male reproductive toxicants demonstrating that organ weights and microscopic examination detected the majority of male reproductive toxicants (Ulbrich and Palmer, 1995), and by demonstrating that most testicular toxicants could be detected microscopically after only 2–4 weeks of dosing (Sakai et al., 2000; Takayama et al., 1995). Importantly, 2 weeks of dosing prior to mating in a fertility study can detect posttesticular effects on sperm, accessory male organ function, male libido, and male copulatory function. This duration is further supported by the approximate 2-week posttesticular transit time in rats as it is these posttesticular sperm that are ejaculated during the subsequent mating period.

If a functional evaluation of sperm that have been exposed during testicular spermatogenesis is needed (based on findings observed in repeat-dose toxicity studies), then the period of time prior to mating can be extended. Key examples of male reproductive toxicity in the absence of overt effects on testicular weights or histopathology include alpha-chlorohydrin and ornidazole that cause male infertility via effects on sperm maturation (motility and capacitation) in the epididymis (Jones and Cooper, 1999; Takayama et al., 1995).

There are some other examples where lack of testicular toxicity and 2 weeks of dosing prior to mating do not detect male reproductive toxicity in the rat. One example is the dihydrotestosterone inhibitor, finasteride, where no testicular histopathology was observed, and no effect on fertility was observed after 6 or 12 weeks of dosing; effects on male rat fertility were only observed at 24 weeks or longer of dosing (Wise et al., 1991). Another example is a nicotinic acetylcholine receptor agonist that caused profound effects on male fertility after 11 weeks of dosing, but did not cause changes in testicular histopathology, sperm counts, or sperm motility after 6 months of dosing in rats; follow-up investigations revealed that only increased preimplantation loss was observed after 14 days of dosing, with no fertility effect after 5 or 14 days of dosing with the nicotinic acetylcholine receptor agonist (Powles-Glover et al., 2015). The nicotinic acetylcholine receptor agonist example highlights that an extended premating period may have better sensitivity to detect the magnitude of male fertility effects, particularly posttesticular effects, such as those targeting epididymal and ejaculated sperm.

2.2. Female Reproductive Toxicity Assessment

Unlike male reproduction, female reproduction has distinct phases (see *Female Reproductive Tract*, Vol 4, Chap 10). Those phases associated with evaluation of potential effects on infertility will be discussed in this section and generally include reproductive aspects of the nonpregnant female (normal ovulation and cycling) and the events leading up to uterine implantation of the blastocyst (mating, conception, and implantation) (Figure 7.1). Evaluation of potential effects on offspring (developmental toxicity) and on phases of gestation from implantation through delivery and lactation will be discussed later under pregnancy and developmental toxicity.

General Considerations

SPECIES SELECTION

Much like the male, specific experimental considerations for evaluating potential effects on female fertility include selection of an appropriate animal model, the stage of sexual maturity of the test system, controlling for confounding effects, and selection/use of appropriate endpoints associated with female fertility. These considerations apply to in vivo testing, including both general toxicity and functional fertility (mating) studies. Importantly, many of the considerations and endpoints of reproduction are interrelated, and therefore, data interpretation should be done within the context of the other aspects of female reproductive function. Discrete aspects of cell and organ function can also be investigated in vitro and support in vivo studies of reproductive toxicology, specifically the ovary (Stefansdottir et al., 2014; Xu et al., 2020) and, in the future, potentially more complex models capable of organ-to-organ hormonal signaling during reproduction (Xiao et al., 2017).

Many aspects of female reproduction are conserved across species; thus, toxicity to reproductive tissues can be evaluated as part of general toxicity testing. General toxicity testing does not typically include evaluation of reproductive function, and therefore, stand-alone functional fertility studies are used to supplement repeat-dose toxicity testing. Therefore, rodents are the default test system for functional fertility studies with the rat most often used followed by the mouse. Although mating trials in NHP are impractical, the female NHP reproductive cycle (endocrinology and physiology) is very similar to human and has been very useful for understanding effects on female fertility (Gougeon, 1996; Jabbour et al., 2006; Van Esch et al., 2008b). Nontraditional species for functional fertility studies include the rabbit, guinea pig, and hamster. In most species (including NHP), surrogate fertility endpoints such as estrous cycling and hormones can be used to improve evaluation of potential effects on female fertility. Table 7.3 summarizes differences in key female reproductive milestones among standard toxicology species.

SEXUAL MATURITY

Robust evaluation of potential effects on female fertility should be done in female animals of reproductive potential. If the animals are not yet sexually mature (still in puberty) or too old (reproductively senescent), cyclicity and fertility can be inconsistent and is likely to confound interpretation of test item–related effects. As such, documentation of sexual maturity is important (Vidal et al., 2021).

In rats, there is some variability in maturation of estrous cyclicity up to 8 weeks old with morphological maturity by 10 weeks old. However, it is common practice to conduct the mating trial in a functional fertility study using female rats at least 12 weeks of age. Importantly, female rats should cycle normally (4–5 days per cycle) between 3 and 6 months of age. Although abnormal estrous cycles can occur occasionally between 3 and 6 months of age, the number and duration of abnormal cycles start increasing further around 6 months of age, and soon thereafter, fertility indices start decreasing, including embryo loss (Ishii et al., 2012; Mitchard and Klein, 2016). Age-related reproductive senescence in rats usually progresses into a state of persistent diestrus with some percent of rats also going through a protracted estrous stage during the progression to persistent diestrus (LeFevre and McClintock, 1988). Normal reproductive senescence is generally considered a consequence of age-related changes in the HPG axis and exhaustion of oocyte stores in the ovary (Cooper et al., 1986).

In the beagle dog, first estrous occurs between 8 and 14 months old, and they cycle only 1–2 times

per year (Rehm et al., 2007b) making evaluation of any surrogate female fertility endpoints in the dog impractical, although microscopic evaluation of female reproductive organs is appropriate if they are sexually mature.

In the cynomolgus macaque (NHP), most females are sexually mature by 4 years of age and weighing at least 3 kg, but, as with male NHPs, age and body weight are imperfect likely due to biological variability in response to a variety of environmental factors (Mecklenburg et al., 2019). Since female NHPs can cycle normally approximately every 28 days, it is possible to monitor cycling in NHPs in controlled conditions to confirm sexual maturity with high confidence prior to the start of a toxicity study (Mecklenburg et al., 2019). Regardless of the animal model, understanding whether the animals in the experiment are sexually mature is critical to a valid assessment of potential effects on female fertility, whether done as part of a functional fertility study or in a general toxicity study where microscopic evaluation of the reproductive tract is the primary endpoint.

CONFOUNDING FACTORS

In addition to the maturity status of the animal model, there are other potentially confounding factors that can interfere with interpretation of potential effects on female fertility. These other factors include nonspecific toxicity such as stress and/or effects resulting in decreased body weight and/or food consumption, housing conditions, and a combination of these stressors. In the adult female, the most sensitive reproductive endpoint affected by stress is irregular cycling and possibly fewer corpora lutea. With increased stress such as that induced by notable effects on body weight and/or food consumption or in situations where stress has induced hormonal perturbations, several effects including persistent cycling disruption (e.g., diestrus), fewer corpora lutea, and reduced fertility have been observed (Everds et al., 2013; Terry et al., 2005).

Although lower ovarian and uterine organ weights may occur with stress, these can be difficult to distinguish from inherent variability due to stage of the reproductive cycle and sampling of these tissues. Microscopic observations consequent to food restriction in female rodents include decreased or absent corpora lutea, increased follicular atresia in the ovary, and evidence of atrophy

TABLE 7.3 Female Reproductive Milestones Across Species (For Additional Detail, See (Vidal et al., 2021)

Species	Age at vaginal opening	Adrenarche	Age at first estrous cycle or Menarche	Age at adult reproductive function	Length of estrous or menstrual cycle	Gestation length
Mouse	~4 weeks	N/A	~5 weeks	7 weeks	4–5 days	21 days
Rat	~5 weeks	N/A	6–7 weeks	10 weeks	4–5 days	23 days
Rabbit	~4 weeks	N/A	N/A	4–5 months	N/A (induced)	35 days
Beagle dog	~3 weeks	~3 months	8–14 months	>12 months	4–6 months	63 days
Cynomolgus monkey	N/A	3–6 months	3–4 years	>4 years	~4 weeks	~160 days
Human	N/A	~7 years	8–13 years	>14 years	~4 weeks	~39 weeks

in the uterus and vagina (Chapin et al., 1993a; Chapin et al., 1993b). In general, reproductive effects consequent to dietary restriction appear more pronounced in mice than rats. The effects of stress and/or effects resulting in decreased body weight and/or food consumption on reproductive parameters in dogs are not well characterized. This effect is likely due to the common use of immature dogs in general toxicity studies and the protracted duration of the estrous cycle reducing the sensitivity of detecting cycle alterations even for mature dogs (Chandra and Adler, 2008; Everds et al., 2013).

In addition to dietary alterations, in the NHP model, exercise and housing changes can result in changes in female reproductive parameters. Of particular importance to toxicity studies, the social status of female NHPs, such as a change of cage-mates and moving/shipping of animals (Adams et al., 1985; Weinbauer et al., 2008), can alter cycling. An altered social status can be a problem if introduced at the beginning of a toxicity study where measurement of cyclicity is an endpoint (Bussiere et al., 2013). These changes are usually transient and can be controlled by allowing sufficient time to return to normal cycling, which is usually about 3 months (Weinbauer et al., 2008). A larger than expected impact on the female reproductive axis can occur when these minor stressors occur in combination as compared with individual stressors alone (Williams et al., 2007).

Evaluation for potential effects on female fertility includes cyclicity, fertility indices (including implantation), systemic biomarkers, and standard toxicity testing endpoints of organ weights, macroscopic, and microscopic examination of tissues in the female reproductive tract. Most of these endpoints can be evaluated in a general toxicity study using nonpregnant females, but a mating trial with males is needed to detect potential effects on time to mating, tubal transport, implantation, and development of preimplantation stages of embryonic development. As in the male, many reproductive endpoints have biological relationships (Mehta et al., 1986), such that while some endpoints may be redundant, many are complementary and interpretation of potential effects on female fertility should account for those interdependencies in determining the biological importance of any findings.

Testing Endpoints

ORGAN WEIGHTS

Female reproductive organ weights can have marked variability due to normal interanimal reproductive cycling and age, and thus, as recommended by the STP, are not included as tissues for routine weighing in repeat-dose general toxicity studies (Sellers et al., 2007). If ovary weights are collected in rodents, it is recommended that it be done in study of less than 6 months duration due to variability attributed to reproductive senescence. When NHP are the only pharmacologically relevant species, and in the absence of a reproductive cause for concern based on literature, mature female reproductive organ weights and microscopic examination are considered sufficient evaluation for potential effects on female fertility (ICH, 2011).

MACROSCOPIC AND MICROSCOPIC EVALUATION

Macroscopic examination of the female reproductive tract may detect effects but is generally less sensitive than microscopic evaluation. Therefore, due to the limitations of female reproductive organ weights and macroscopic evaluation, the primary evaluation for potential effects on the female reproductive tract in general toxicity studies largely depends upon microscopic evaluation.

The STP-recommended core tissue list for microscopy includes mammary gland, ovary, uterus, and vagina (Bregman et al., 2003). Oviduct and clitoral gland are not included on the list, since toxicities in these tissues would be expected to be accompanied by clinical or macroscopic findings that are not found in humans (clitoral gland), and/or effects are adequately represented by other tissues (oviduct) (Bregman et al., 2003). As mentioned previously, it is critical to account for the stage of sexual maturity in the microscopic evaluation. A recent review provides key physiology and morphologic features for distinguishing and documenting stages of puberty, sexual maturity, and reproductive senescence (Vidal, 2017).

In order to determine toxicity to the female reproductive tract, it is important to understand the stage of the reproductive cycle in each individual animal to understand deviations from normal across those tissues (Li and Davis, 2007; Westwood, 2008). In addition, the STP recommends a two-tier approach to evaluation of the rodent ovary in general or reproductive toxicity testing (Regan et al., 2005). The first-tier evaluation includes all major components of the ovary including follicles, *corpora lutea*, stroma, interstitium, vasculature, and, specifically, a qualitative assessment of primordial and primary follicles together with the entire reproductive tract and all complementary reproductive data, e.g., organ weight, cycling. The second-tier evaluation might include quantitative assessment of small follicles and is triggered on a case-by-case basis depending on the value it brings to the risk assessment. Special stains facilitate follicle counting (Muskhelishvili et al., 2005; Picut et al., 2008), and even an automated method for counting *corpora lutea* (Hu et al., 2020).

Although female cyclicity is protracted in the dog, understanding normal microscopic changes in immature and mature tissues associated with the estrus cycle is mandatory for detecting a treatment-related effect versus normal anatomic variability (Rehm et al., 2007b).

Characterization of microscopic changes in the female NHP is well documented, specifically the ovary (Buse et al., 2008), uterine endometrium (van Esch et al., 2008a), and spontaneous and common lesions (Cline et al., 2008; Cooper and Gabrielson, 2007). Lastly, as with much of pathology, standardized terminology (see *Nomenclature and Diagnostics Resources in Anatomic Toxicologic Pathology*, Vol 1, Chap 25) and lesion characterization is important and has been published for the female reproductive system with the rat and mouse (Dixon et al., 2014).

BIOMARKERS

There are many systemic biomarkers of female reproductive function to consider owing to the hormonal control of cycling and reproduction in most animal models. These include ovarian hormones (progesterone and estrogen), pituitary hormones (LH and FSH) and many others including prolactin, kisspeptin, thyroid hormones, and uterine cytokines (Clarkson et al., 2008; Dittrich et al., 2011). Despite multiple options, these systemic biomarkers should not be used as a general screen for detecting female reproductive toxicity in standard toxicity studies using females without synchronized cycles

(Andersson et al., 2013). Instead, purposefully designed and statistically powered studies are recommended if understanding potential ovarian and pituitary hormone changes are needed for safety assessment (Andersson et al., 2013). In such cases, a solid understanding of the HPG axis is needed to inform appropriate study design (see *Practices to Optimize Generation, Interpretation, and Reporting of Pathology Data from Toxicity Studies*, Vol 1, Chap 28), coordination of hormone sampling with evaluation of cycling patterns, as well as an understanding of species-specific responses associated with various pathologies. Mechanisms of hormone changes can impact synthesis of hormones, regulation of hormone release and storage, hormone transport and clearance, recognition and binding to biological receptors, postreceptor activation, interactions with other endocrine axis, and/or communication with the central nervous system (CNS) (Bretveld et al., 2006).

Systemic biomarkers may not always represent local signaling. One such example is local immune function (including innate and adaptive immunity) in the female reproductive tract regulated by circulating estrogen and progesterone (Wira et al., 2015), as well as the role and balance of cytokines in successful implantation (Paulesu et al., 2010). Prolactin is a hormone with many seemingly disparate actions. For example, hyperprolactinemia has been shown to cause infertility by suppressing LH and GnRH (Grattan and Kokay, 2008). Interestingly, prolactin receptor knock-out mice are infertile with irregular cyclicity which is but one illustration that both hyper- and hypoprolactinema can disrupt reproductive function. Although drugs can induce this state via similar mechanisms in rodents and human, key interspecies difference in prolactin physiology need to be considered when extrapolating effects across species (Hargreaves and Harleman, 2011).

CYCLE EVALUATION

Instead of measuring individual hormones, monitoring estrous or menstrual cycling in animals can provide an integrated assessment of the hypothalamic–pituitary–ovarian reproductive function. Cycling as an endpoint can be added to virtually any rodent toxicity study, but, as mentioned earlier, should be done in sexually mature animals, not during puberty and not as reproductive senescence begins. Evaluation in the mouse or rat is relatively noninvasive as both have short, regular estrous cycles that can easily be monitored by examining cytology from a daily vaginal smear (Goldman et al., 2007; Vidal and Filgo, 2017). Some considerations unique to the mouse are that vaginal smears can be more difficult to obtain, and that the presence of males in adjacent cages can facilitate normal cycling.

Rabbits are induced ovulators so do not cycle spontaneously and are therefore not amenable to assessing cyclicity in standard studies. In the dog first estrus may occur any time between 8 and 14 months old and under controlled conditions will only occur once or twice a year (monoestric), and thus cycling is not a practical endpoint of evaluation in the dog.

In the NHP, cycling as an endpoint depends on the species of monkey. Cynomolgus monkeys are the most commonly used NHP for reproductive assessments as they have regular monthly cycles that can be relatively easily monitored with daily vaginal swabs to detect menses, but they can be susceptible to changes in housing and social groups, so when evaluated as a reproductive endpoint, the study design should allow for 3–6 months baseline normalization (Bussiere et al., 2013; Mecklenburg et al., 2019; Weinbauer et al., 2008). Unfortunately, only about 50% of NHP cycle normally when housed individually, but when group housed can be up to 80% normal cycling (Mecklenburg et al., 2019). Marmosets do not have external signs of cyclicity but can be monitored by regular measurements for progesterone. Rhesus monkeys exhibit seasonal variations in cyclicity, and thus are less commonly used for reproductive assessments.

Unlike microscopic confirmation of estrous stage at a single timepoint, monitoring cycling during a study allows for evaluation of onset, duration, and recovery of toxicity, which can provide important mechanistic insight regarding reproductive biology and toxicity. When assessment of cyclicity is coupled with additional endpoints such as microscopic examination and/or mating, a more complete picture of reproductive function and potential for infertility can be provided.

MATING TRIALS

Additional endpoints for evaluation of potential effects on female fertility are generally associated with functional mating trials, which are in addition to normal cycle progression. These endpoints include ovulation (*corpora lutea* counts), time to mate, calculation of reproductive indices (mating and fertility), and implantation confirming successful development of preimplantation stage of the embryo. Presence and number of viable embryos implanted in the uterus is the expected confirmation of pregnancy and measure of successful fertility. Empty uteri can be stained with ammonium sulfide to detect implantation scars and confirm implantation (Figure 7.4). The vast majority of mating trials are conducted in rats, but similar designs can be conducted in mice, rabbits (Breslin et al., 2015, 2017a), or guinea pigs (Rocca and Wehner, 2009).

A rodent mating trial as part of a female fertility study is typically conducted by pairing the treated female with a male for a set period of time, typically 2–3 weeks, until evidence of mating is confirmed by copulatory plug in the vagina or

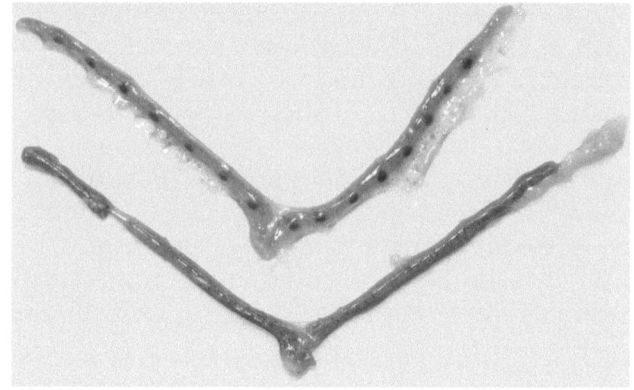

FIGURE 7.4 Ammonium sulfide–stained uterus. Uterine implantation sites with early resorptions, late resorptions, dead or live fetuses or embryos can typically be visualized by the naked eye. However, if an implantation site resorbs very early, it can be hard to detect visually. Therefore, if there are no visual implantation sites, it is possible to more definitively confirm no implantation sites by staining the uterus with 10% ammonium sulfide. This photograph illustrates an empty uterus (top) with implantation sites only visible following staining, as compared to a non pregnant uterus (bottom). *Photo Credit: William Nowland, Pfizer Inc., Groton, CT, USA.*

sperm present in a vaginal smear. The animals are unpaired, and the mated female is allowed to progress through gestation. The female is either subject to Cesarean section or allowed to deliver. The primary fertility endpoint includes pregnancy confirmation, enumeration of *corpora lutea*, implantation sites, and number of viable and nonviable conceptuses or pups relative to the number of implantation sites. In addition to confirming pregnancy, a mating trial can inform the viability of the offspring which can be a sensitive endpoint of female (rodent) reproductive toxicity. The limited apical endpoints calculated in rodent mating trials include time to mating and several different types of reproductive indices such as mating index ([number females with evidence of mating (or females confirmed pregnant)/total number of females used for mating] × 100) and fertility index ([number of pregnant females/total number of females used for mating] × 100). Mating trials are most often conducted in dedicated fertility studies with treated females and males, or, in the case of female fertility studies, where treated females are mated to treatment-naïve males (Barrow, 2009; Lerman et al., 2009). Mating trials are not practical in dogs or NHPs, so microscopic evaluation of the female reproductive tract is the primary evaluation which in the NHP can be supplemented by including cycle monitoring.

Study Types

REPEAT-DOSE TOXICITY STUDIES

Although there is a perception that subtle ovarian toxicity may be hard to detect by histology alone, there are many examples where such toxicity has been observed, and even 2 weeks of dosing in rodents may be sufficient for evaluation ovarian toxicity by careful microscopic evaluation. One exception is cytotoxic compounds such as alkylating agents that may take longer than 2 weeks to manifest ovarian toxicity (Sanbuissho et al., 2009). Specific chapters in this Edition will cover the specific pathologies in female reproductive tissues (see *Female Reproductive Tract*, Vol 4, Chap 10; *and Mammary Gland*, Vol 4, Chap 8).

One example of ovarian toxicity detectable by microscopic examination is tamoxifen, which increased the number of large atretic follicles, increased interstitial cells, and resulted in absence of newly formed *corpora lutea* in both

2- and 4-week rat studies, although findings were detectable at a lower dose in the 4-week study (Tsujioka et al., 2009). Another example is medroxyprogesterone acetate (MPA) that increased large atretic follicles and decreased *corpora lutea* after both 2 and 4 weeks of dosing in rats (Ohtake et al., 2009). These microscopic findings in the repeat-dose rat studies for both tamoxifen and MPA correlated to estrus cycle disruption and decreased pregnancy in fertility studies, supporting that microscopic examination after 2 weeks dosing duration could be sufficient to detect ovarian toxicity due to endocrine disruption (Ohtake et al., 2009; Tsujioka et al., 2009).

Other reviews have offered similar concordance, but with a few exceptions, dependent on the mode of action (Chapin et al., 1998; Dent, 2007). As indicated, microscopic examination can detect morphological effects on the ovarian follicles, but there is evidence that some toxicants may elicit their effects without clear morphologic changes detectable by microscopy; these include altered follicular hormone biosynthesis and somatic cell–germ cell interaction in viable follicles. Such physiological perturbations may impair fertility and have long-range effects on both mother and offspring (Hirshfield, 1997). Although not routinely included in repeat-dose toxicity studies, it could be argued that addition of cycle monitoring in sexually mature rats could increase sensitivity of detection and serve as a useful functional and dynamic measure of potential infertility.

Specific examples of ovarian toxicants in rats and/or mice include 4-vinyl-1-cyclohexene diepoxide (Flaws et al., 1994; Hoyer and Sipes, 2007), polyaromatic hydrocarbons (Mattison et al., 1983), Dimethylbenz[a]anthracene (Sobinoff et al., 2011), and acrylamide (Aldawood et al., 2020). Atrazine is a well-studied example that targets hypothalamic control of pituitary–ovarian function (Cooper et al., 2000) and has served as an example of early reproductive senescence. The gamma-secretase inhibitor, avagacestat, induces ovarian follicular degeneration and atrophy as well as hypertrophy and hyperplasia of granulosa and thecal cells in both rats and dogs (Simutis et al., 2019). An example of a dog study with female reproductive toxicity with microscopic evaluation was with the selective estrogen receptor modulator idoxifene, where estrogenic effects were observed in the ovary, uterus, and vagina, but antiestrogenic effects were seen in the endometrial and mammary glands (Rehm et al., 2007a). Although it is possible to do mating studies with NHPs, it is not considered feasible for evaluation of potential effects on fertility. Therefore, as with dogs, detection of potential female infertility effects in NHPs principally relies on repeat-dose studies using sexually mature animals. As described earlier, body weight and age are not strong indicators of maturity, but appropriate prestudy monitoring of monthly cycles can provide confirmation of maturity and baseline information important for detection of potential effects indicative of reduced fertility. One such example is the reversible effects on cycling and hormones by interferon alpha-2b (Enright et al., 2009). Other examples of repeat-dose toxicity studies in mature NHPs where cycling or reproductive hormones endpoints were incorporated include an anti-IL17A monoclonal antibody (mAb) and an anti-IL12/23p40 mAb (Clarke et al., 2015; Enright et al., 2012a) In these studies, the lack of effects helped to establish a low risk of female reproductive toxicity. Lastly, some conservation of effects is illustrated by danazol, which suppresses LH and FSH in males, but also inhibits normal cycling in both female rats and NHPs (Butterstein et al., 1997).

FEMALE FERTILITY STUDY

While normal folliculogenesis, ovulation, and cycling are important for fertility, other aspects associated with functional fertility leading up to uterine implantation of the blastocyst (mating, conception, and implantation) can also be affected. The current standard approach to evaluation of functional fertility and various study designs for pharmaceuticals are described in ICH S5(R3), and have been reviewed (Lerman et al., 2009).

One example of a study in which findings occurred in the absence of morphologic change is a study where reduction of live litter size in rats occurred; however, there were no ovarian effects detected with microscopic assessment of ovaries after up to 4 weeks of dosing in either rat or monkey (Xie et al., 2018). Another example is a histone deacetylase inhibitor, where there were no effects in female rat reproductive tissues

occurred in 4- and 13-week repeat-dose toxicity studies, but an increase in *corpora lutea* and post-implantation loss was reported in a female rat fertility study, and a decrease in *corpora lutea* in the 26-week rat repeat-dose toxicity study (Wise et al., 2008).

An interesting example regarding time-dependent severity of ovarian toxicity is methoxychlor: with 20 days of dosing in mice, followed by 30 days recovery, there was increased atresia and reduced primordial and total follicle numbers, but without effects on functional fertility; after another 30 days recovery (60 days total), there were no microscopic differences as compared with controls, and no effect on functional fertility, thus indicating full recovery (Tannenbaum and Flaws, 2015).

Octamethylcyclotetrasiloxane is an example where, starting with prolonged estrous, reduced fertility and reduced litter size were seen in a two-generation rat inhalation study (Siddiqui et al., 2007). Additional investigative studies narrowed down the critical exposure window to the time of ovulation and fertilization, due to suppression of the preovulatory LH surge for this specific female infertility effect (Meeks et al., 2007; Quinn et al., 2007).

While effects on female reproduction described in the section above include the reproductive aspects of the nonpregnant female (normal ovulation and cycling) and the events leading up to uterine implantation of the blastocyst (mating, conception, and implantation), the totality of effects on female reproduction also include events during pregnancy from implantation through delivery and lactation in addition to potential effects on offspring (developmental toxicity). These latter events are described below as part of pregnancy and developmental toxicity.

It is important to note that the ultimate manifestation of toxicity on female reproduction is a decrease in the number of normal young born, described as female total reproductive capacity (Bishop et al., 1997). This term has been described for its capacity to detect a range of toxicities to female reproduction including mutagenic and cytotoxic mechanisms, but also other mechanisms of female infertility as described above.

2.3. Guidelines

The regulatory requirements for the evaluation of potential effects on male and female reproduction have evolved over many decades, with different approaches designed to determine reproductive and developmental effects at human relevant exposures. These exposures span chronic environmental exposures of industrial and commercial chemicals to purposeful exposures to potential or marketed therapeutics.

Guidelines evaluating the potential reproductive toxicity of environmental exposures to industrial chemicals and pesticides include exposure throughout the reproductive cycle including different life stages (Table 7.1). Historically, evaluation of reproductive toxicity was done using the multigeneration reproduction study (OECD, 2001), and more recently, the OECD extended one-generation reproduction toxicity study (EOGRT) (OECD, 2018b) and the National Toxicology Program (NTP) modified one-generation reproduction study (Foster, 2014). In addition, potential effects on fertility for pesticides and environmental chemicals have been evaluated in nonmammalian test systems as part of the EPA Series 890 Endocrine Disruptor Screening Program (EDSP). For the EPA and OECD studies listed in Table 7.1, evaluation of male and female fertility is but one aspect of many assessment endpoints that also include developmental toxicity.

For pharmaceuticals, guidelines have evolved over the years (Collins, 2006) to the current state where reproductive toxicity assessment for regulatory purposes is governed by guidelines established by the ICH (Table 7.1). ICH S5(R3) is the primary reference describing regulatory expectations of reproductive toxicity assessment of pharmaceuticals, including study designs to address different life stages (such as gametogenesis, mating, conception, and implantation), different study design options to evaluate functional fertility, relevant study endpoints, and considerations for different modalities and patient populations (ICH, 2020a). ICH M3(R2) describes in general terms the scope and timing of nonclinical safety studies in animals to support clinical trials and marketing authorization including the duration of repeat-dose toxicity studies in two mammalian species (one nonrodent) and the timing of male and female fertility studies relative to clinical trials and marketing (ICH, 2009a). ICH S6(R1) describes specific considerations of biotechnology-derived pharmaceuticals including the importance of evaluation only in pharmacologically relevant species (ICH, 2011). When relevant species are limited to NHPs, a mating study is not warranted as part of the fertility evaluation. In this situation, evaluation of reproductive tissues (organ weight and histopathological examination) should be done in repeat-dose studies of at least 3 months duration using sexually mature animals with additional assessments (e.g., sperm) recommended if there is a specific male reproductive concern. ICH S9 is the nonclinical guideline for anticancer pharmaceuticals and simply states that a fertility and early embryonic development study is not warranted for pharmaceuticals indicated in advanced cancer patients, and that the basis of fertility risk is the evaluation of reproductive tissues in repeat-dose toxicity studies (ICH, 2009b). Overall, these guidelines summarize the timing and types of assessments to be evaluated to inform the human risk assessment for specific patient populations.

3. PREGNANCY AND DEVELOPMENTAL TOXICITY

The purpose of pregnancy and developmental toxicity assessments is to identify the potential of a molecule to impact pregnancy, lactation, and offspring following maternal exposure (Figure 7.1). Key aspects of these assessments include all available information on the pharmacological target during pregnancy and development, risk of off-target toxicity, and context of use (relevance in the human population); if the available WoE evaluation provides the necessary information to communicate human risk, then experimental data may not always be necessary (Bowman and Chapin, 2016; Rocca et al., 2018). If experimental data are needed, these typically include separate embryo–fetal development (EFD) evaluations and/or a pre- and postnatal development (PPND) study. Figure 7.2 illustrates an example of how these different studies inform potential risk of reproductive toxicity over the course of drug development.

The EFD assessment is focused on evaluation of adverse effects on the pregnant female and the development of the embryo and fetus following maternal exposure during the period of major organogenesis (implantation to closure of the hard palate). The PPND study includes evaluation of adverse effects on the pregnant and lactating female and development of the offspring generally following maternal exposure from implantation through weaning. Although the EFD study includes fetal external, visceral, and skeletal morphological evaluation, microscopic examination is not required or routinely included in with EFD or PPND studies but can aid study interpretation when added for cause; for example, microscopic examination of maternal or offspring gross lesions may be warranted (Halpern et al., 2016). When conducted in the NHP for biopharmaceuticals, the risk of teratogenic effects during organogenesis is considered relatively low; therefore, a modified design combining elements of both the EFD and PPND is often used, referred to as the "enhanced design" PPND (ePPND), and microscopic evaluation of the offspring is common. For specific considerations associated with microscopic evaluation of the developing conceptus and the placenta, see *Embryo, Fetus and Placenta*, Vol 4, Chap 11.

3.1. Embryo–Fetal Development Studies

In the absence of a sufficient WoE from the literature to communicate a risk of fetal harm in labeling, the conduct of an EFD study is critical to minimize reoccurrence of a thalidomide-like birth defect tragedy. The EFD study is designed to evaluate the effects on pregnancy and prenatal development following maternal exposure during the period of major organogenesis (generally considered the period between implantation to closure of the hard palate).

The EFD study has also been referred to as a Segment II study, a prenatal developmental toxicity study, and a teratology study. The results of the EFD study inform the fetal risk of human exposure in the first trimester of gestation, a point prior to some women knowing they are pregnant. No single nonclinical species best predicts human risk resulting in the recommended approach of EFD studies in two species, one rodent and one nonrodent. The two-species EFD approach has adequately identified the potential of human developmental toxicity since the thalidomide tragedy (Brown and Fabro, 1983; Schardein et al., 1985). While rat, mouse, and rabbit are the most routine EFD species, nonroutine species include the NHP (Bowman et al., 2010) and minipig (Pique et al., 2018). Rarely used are the hamster, guinea pig (Rocca and Wehner, 2009), and dog (Holson et al., 2015). All species have a low background incidence of rare malformations and variations, so historical control data at the test facility can be a critical component of data interpretation of morphological changes that occur at a low incidence. Use of routine species typically allows for a more accurate differentiation from background findings as they are informed by a more robust historical control database. While the dosing paradigm of targeting exposure between implantation and closure of the hard palate is consistent for EFD studies across species, the specific gestation dosing days are different due to species-specific differences in these developmental milestones (Wise et al., 2009).

There are several types of EFD evaluations for different purposes, but the dosing paradigm is the same. Dose range-finding (DRF) studies in pregnant animals are recommended to establish tolerance in pregnant animals, particularly when there are no previous data with the test item in a species such as rabbit. DRF studies are not standardized and range from simple maternal toxicity studies in five to eight females per group with limited fetal evaluation to dose escalation studies with full fetal evaluation and blood taken to determine systemic exposures.

Following an analysis evaluating the predictivity of DRF studies (Okahashi et al., 2010), ICH M3(R2) introduced the preliminary EFD (pEFD) study to facilitate enrollment of women of child-bearing potential (WOCBP) into clinical trials prior to completion of definitive EFD studies (ICH, 2009a). The pEFD study is basically a DRF study with at least six pregnant animals under Good Laboratory Practices-like conditions with fetal external and visceral morphological examinations and exposure data. The definitive or pivotal EFD study has a minimum of 16 litters per group and includes fetal skeletal examination and maternal exposure data (ICH, 2020a; Wise et al., 2009).

Fetal exposure is not routinely measured for small molecules, but for molecules where fetal exposure cannot reasonably be understood based on available information (e.g., unmodified IgG monoclonal antibodies), it can be helpful to measure fetal exposure if results are unexpected and/or to confirm fetal exposure when no effects are observed. Fetal exposure or placental transfer is dependent on a number of factors including physiochemical properties and binding to a number of biological receptors involved in passage between maternal and fetal circulation. As described in ICH S5(R3), there is also interest that alternative developmental toxicity assays may supplement, defer, and/or replace in vivo EFD studies in certain circumstances (ICH, 2020a), but to date, these assays using stem cells, zebrafish, and rodent embryo culture have not generally been used for regulatory purposes (Clements et al., 2020).

Testing Endpoints

The objective of the definitive EFD study is to assess maternal toxicity and to evaluate potential effects on embryo–fetal lethality, intrauterine growth, and fetal morphological development. Clinical observations, body weight, body weight gain, food consumption, and blood collection for bioanalytical and toxicokinetic analysis are the typical in-life observations. In addition, clinical pathology or other pharmacodynamic markers could be evaluated in maternal or fetal samples for cause, to confirm expected pharmacology, and/or to evaluate potential effects in pregnancy. There are relatively few published examples of clinical pathology or other markers contributing to interpretation of an EFD study (Campion et al., 2015; Katavolos et al., 2018; Wise et al., 1988). It is important to be aware of potential differences in any additional endpoints (e.g., clinical pathology) between early and late gestation and whether pregnant or not (Honda et al., 2008; Liberati et al., 2004; Mizoguchi et al., 2010; Wells et al., 1999); as such control data and/or historical control data can be critical for interpretation of such endpoints.

Required postmortem evaluations include maternal macroscopic evaluation (including placenta and any gross lesions) and Cesarean section with collection of gravid uterine weights, enumeration of *corpora lutea*, implantation sites, and live and dead conceptuses, and early and late resorptions. Body weight, sex, and external, visceral, and skeletal evaluation is completed for all fetuses if possible. Although maternal gross lesions and/or target tissues may be collected and preserved, they are not typically evaluated microscopically unless there is a specific rationale that informs interpretation of the study for risk assessment purposes. When collecting maternal tissues for possible pathologic evaluation, it is important to collect corresponding tissues from control animals.

The most technical aspect of these studies is the fetal evaluations. These fetal evaluations are specialized evaluations that require very specific training and provide a detailed morphological evaluation of all external, visceral, and bone structures. There are several techniques used to examine visceral structures, including fresh (Stuckhardt and Poppe, 1984), frozen (brain) (Astroff et al., 2002), or free-hand sections (Wilson, 1973) gross examinations following fixation. Typically, these fetal evaluations do not include microscopic examination.

A recent comparison between fresh and fixed evaluation of brain and eye illustrated the value of fresh examination (Ziejewski et al., 2015). Evaluations of the skeletal bones are typically performed following an alizarin red staining procedure (Redfern and Wise, 2007). Although not yet accepted as a replacement for alizarin red staining, microCT is being evaluated as an alternative to sometimes tedious bone staining procedures (Solomon et al., 2018; Wise and Winkelmann, 2009a, b). Fetal cartilage can also be evaluated using an alternative staining procedure that includes alcian blue (Redfern et al., 2007), but is not required for evaluation of potential therapeutics although it is done for environmental/industrial chemicals. Terminology used to describe alterations can be variable among laboratories although there are published lexicons based on international scientific discussions (Makris et al., 2009) and future electronic data submissions to FDA will likely standardize fetal terminology.

All laboratories independently classify all fetal anomalies as malformations, variations, and in some cases, additional categories such as incomplete ossification. There is no strict standardization of how specific anomalies are classified as the adversities of many specific malformations and variations are not well understood but have been the subject of scientific debate for many years and continues to this day (Solecki et al., 2013, 2015).

Generally, permanent structural changes likely to adversely affect survival or health are considered malformations and developmental variations are those expected to occur within the normal population under investigation and are unlikely to adversely affect survival or health (including those findings that may be transient). Each endpoint/fetal observation is tabulated and statistically analyzed on a litter basis since fetuses are not directly dosed. Litter-based calculations (e.g., litter percent postimplantation loss, live litter size, fetal percent per litter of specific anomalies) help normalize uneven litter sizes across animals and provide a more appropriate comparison across animals, groups, and studies. Hopefully, apparent by the complicated procedures described above, having EFD studies conducted by personnel and laboratories with years of experience can be critical for appropriate and defined criteria for data collection, and to reduce potential for technical error that could compromise data interpretation.

Data Interpretation

Assuming the fetal evaluations and other aspects of study conduct are of high quality, the next challenging step is appropriate interpretation of EFD study data to ensure the data can be used for human risk assessment as these data are routinely included in product labeling as human data are typically unavailable.

An interpretation of both maternal and embryo–fetal toxicity should be completed and if possible, define the no adverse effect level (NOAEL) for each based on dose and maternal systemic exposure at that dose (Harris and DeSesso, 1994). While dose selection often targets some maternal toxicity at the high dose, the desire is to avoid severe maternal toxicity to minimize potential confounding impact on evaluation of fetal toxicity. Maternal toxicity may include mortality, adverse clinical signs, effects on body weight, and/or food consumption as well as gross observations at necropsy.

While it can be difficult to define maternal toxicity, it can be even more challenging to

understand the impact of maternal toxicity on developmental toxicity. Selective developmental toxicities are those effects in the absence of maternal toxicity. Often developmental effects are observed in the presence of maternal toxicity, but it is difficult to attribute fetal effects to maternal toxicity as it is common to see severe maternal toxicity with no fetal effects as well. Therefore, much effort has been spent over the years to manage fetal risk evaluation in the context of maternal toxicity (Beyer et al., 2011; Chernoff et al., 2008; Schardein, 1987).

Feed restriction studies in pregnant rats and rabbits have been done to understand the potential for developmental effects of reduced maternal food consumption (Nitzsche, 2017). In pregnant rats, reduced food consumption can result in reduced fetal weight and minor changes in skeletal development but not fetal viability or malformations (Fleeman et al., 2005). Feed restriction in pregnant rabbits can result in abortions, reduced fetal weight, and alterations in fetal bone ossification (e.g., unossified sternebra, metatarsals, metacarpals, or caudal vertebrae) but not fetal malformations (Cappon et al., 2005). While these feed restriction studies provide useful context, pharmacologically induced weight loss can differ mechanistically and can present even greater challenges in separating effects of maternal toxicity from specific developmental toxicity.

Abortions in rabbits can be a direct effect on pregnancy maintenance, attributed to nonspecific maternal toxicity (such as reduced food consumption), or they can also be considered secondary to a really small litter size (Adams, 1970). Rabbits are not typically used in the rest of a toxicity testing program, so there is always a possibility of unexpected (maternal) toxicities. One known consideration with rabbits is that a major part of their digestion occurs in the caecum and appears dependent on gram-positive intestinal flora; therefore, antibiotics or other test items that alter the flora can lead to reduced food consumption and subsequently abortions, embryo–fetal lethality (resorptions), and reduced fetal weights (Clark et al., 1986; Frohberg et al., 1979). Because humans normally have a gram-negative intestinal flora, rabbits are not a human-relevant species for oral antibiotics targeting gram-positive flora.

It is well accepted that developmental toxicity is a threshold response, below which there is no developmental toxicity. A NOAEL in an EFD study is unlikely to define that threshold but does provide information under the conditions of the study that the threshold is higher than the NOAEL, but below the Lowest Observed Adverse Effect Level. Identifying a NOAEL for developmental toxicity requires appropriate interpretation of biologically related endpoints and redundant measures/calculations of Cesarean section and fetal examination data to confidently understand which changes are related to test item administration compared to the biological range of normal in the specific test species and strain at that test facility under their procedures (Chahoud and Paumgartten, 2005; Ryan et al., 1991).

In addition to understanding the relationships between effects on specific stages of development (e.g., early resorptions) and measures encompassing all stages of in utero development (e.g., live litter size), it is important to recognize that dose–response relationships exist within and between endpoints and across dose groups. Specifically, as endpoints such as embryo–fetal lethality increase, there may be concomitant decrease incidence of malformations at that dose due to the severity of the malformation. Therefore, higher incidence of malformations at the next lower dose should not be readily dismissed due to lack of higher incidences of malformations at the higher dose. Since there is background incidence of specific fetal anomalies in each species population and due to the rare nature of many of these anomalies, the concurrent control group in an EFD study should ideally be complemented with historical control data in that species and strain at the test facility. Strain-specific historical control data are important as apparent isolated increased incidence of an observation in one strain will not necessarily be test item related in another strain (Noritake et al., 2013; Posobiec et al., 2016).

For interpretation of fetal morphology data and relevance to humans, understanding the biological plausibility and species-specific understanding of specific organ system developmental biology is important (DeSesso, 2017; DeSesso and Scialli, 2018). As mentioned earlier, the biology underpinning the adversity and difference between malformations and developmental variations is not always clear and interpretation has changed over the years as the science of developmental biology has advanced. Specific challenges include the classification and risk assessment of bent long bones and various skeletal anomalies (Carney and Kimmel, 2007; Kimmel et al., 2014; Kimmel and Wilson, 1973).

There are also complicating factors such as litter effect, largely ascribed to the observation that fetuses within a particular litter experience a similar maternal environment as their littermates but different from those in other litters. A litter effect may also reveal confounding results based on maternal or paternal genetics as has been shown with ribs (Green, 1939), omphalocele (Tobin et al., 2019), and hydrocephalus (Bruni et al., 1988). Another complicating factor can be the introduction of fixation artifacts depending on the fixative used in head and eye examinations. It has been shown that the use of Bouin's fluid can introduce folded retinas that can be distinguished from the developmental anomaly of folded retinas but only following magnetic resonance imaging or microscopic examination (French et al., 2008).

One of the unique features of the EFD study design is the developmental window of exposure between implantation of the embryo and closure of the hard palate. There are dynamic changes in pregnancy, the placenta, and the developing embryo/fetus itself during this period of major organogenesis. It is critical to provide exposure throughout implantation of the embryo and closure of the hard palate to adequately meet the objective of the study because the sensitivity to detect effects on each developing organ system depends on exposure during specific periods of time and in short gestation species that sensitive window can be a single dose on a single day. There are several published examples illustrating which dosing days are critical for specific malformations induced by various compounds (Campion et al., 2012a, b; Cappon et al., 2003a, b; White and Clark, 2008). There is also an interesting example regarding critical windows of pregnancy, specifically gestation days 7–9 in the rat when essential histiotrophic nutrition to the embryo is provided via the inverted yolk sac. A case study with a hemoglobin-based oxygen carrier revealed developmental toxicity in the rat due to interference with yolk sac transport capacity and subsequent deficient embryo nutrition during that window (Stump et al., 2015). Because the biology of the inverted yolk sac is not present in dogs or humans, developmental toxicity studies in dogs were conducted to confirm and support that the rat developmental toxicity was not relevant to humans (Holson et al., 2005, 2015).

3.2. Pre- and Postnatal Development Studies

Based on current regulatory guidance, specifically ICH S5(R3) for human pharmaceuticals, the PPND toxicity study is designed to assess maternal toxicity following exposure during gestation, parturition, and lactation as well as impact to the offspring including viability, altered growth and development, and functional deficits such as sexual maturation, reproductive capacity, sensory functions, motor activity, and learning and memory (ICH, 2020a). The study is conducted primarily in rodents, most often the rat although mouse can be a suitable alternative if there are compound-specific factors indicating the rat is not appropriate. There is also some experience in the rabbit if neither rodent model is relevant (Breslin et al., 2017b). A version of the PPND study can be conducted in the NHP and is discussed in more detail in a later section of this chapter.

Testing Endpoints

The PPND study design itself typically includes one control group and three groups of pregnant females administered different dose levels in order to assess the dose responsiveness and allow determination of a NOAEL. Pregnant females are dosed starting at implantation, continuing through pregnancy, parturition, and lactation. The offspring are evaluated preweaning and postweaning until sexual maturity, followed by an evaluation of reproductive capacity (Bailey et al., 2009). The approximate duration of the in-life portion of rodent PPND study is four–five months. While DRF studies can be conducted to minimize uncertainty in early postnatal survival, often the rodent EFD study can serve as sufficient information for dose selection for a PPND study. For the pivotal PPND study, the group size should target at least 16 litters, similar to the EFD study, so often 20 pregnant females/group is used. The endpoints are typically broken into maternal (F0) data, litter data, and offspring (F1) data.

As described in Table 7.4, maternal evaluations include clinical observations, body weight, body weight gain, food consumption, and macroscopic findings at necropsy including number of former implantation scars in the uterus. Litter data include gestation length, evidence of dystocia (parturition difficulties), maternal care of pups, live litter size, pup survival, pup clinical signs including presence of milk bands (evidence of normal nursing), pup body weights and body weight change, and preweaning landmarks of development and reflex ontogeny such as eye opening, pinna unfolding, surface righting, and response to light. Postweaning offspring endpoints evaluated include landmarks of sexual maturation (vaginal opening and preputial separation), functional tests that assess sensory functions, motor activity, and learning and memory, and lastly reproductive performance that includes F1 female cycling data, mating, and fertility indices usually ending with F1 male gross necropsy and female Cesarean section at mid or end of gestation for confirmation of F2 viability.

There is little guidance regarding the specific functional tests that should be conducted; but pragmatically, those tests with some confidence and capability to detect changes (Crofton et al., 2008) and are available at select laboratories with experience and historical control in your test system are preferred. In addition, clinical pathology, toxicokinetic, or pharmacodynamic markers could be evaluated in maternal or pup samples for cause, to confirm expected pharmacology, and/or to evaluate potential effects in pregnancy, lactation, or in offspring. In rodent and rabbit PPND studies, there are typically no scheduled tissue collections in F0 or F1 unless for cause. However, at the gross necropsy for both F0 and F1 animals, routinely any gross lesions will be collected along with corresponding control tissue for possible microscopic examination.

Data Interpretation

The PPND study is a large study with many data points, as such there is a propensity for differences to arise between the control and treated population, whether spurious and/or test item

TABLE 7.4   Minimum (e)PPND Endpoints

		Rat PPND	NHP ePPND
Maternal	Group size	At least 16 litters	14–16 pregnant females
	Administration period	GD 6 to LD 20 (approximately 5 weeks)	GD 20 to parturition (approximately 5.5 months)
	Clinical observations/ mortality	At least once daily	At least once daily
	Body weight	At least 2x weekly	At least 1x weekly
	Food consumption	At least 1x weekly until midlactation	Qualitative optional
	Exposure assessment	Optional	Yes
	Parturition observations	GD 21 until complete	Document day of completion, and preserve placenta if possible
	Necropsy	LD 21, uterine implantation sites, retain any gross findings and corresponding control	Optional
Offspring	Clinical observations/ mortality	Daily from PND 0	Daily from PND 0, including "external morphological evaluation"
	Body weight	At birth, 2x weekly preweaning, 1x weekly postweaning	Weekly
	Preweaning evaluations	Reflex and landmarks (e.g., eye opening, pinna unfolding, surface righting, auditory startle, air righting, and response to light)	Battery of morphological, physical, and neurobehavioral test at appropriate intervals including grip strength, mother–infant interactions, and skeletal evaluation (e.g., X-ray)
	Exposure assessment	Optional	Yes
	Selection of postweaning animals	PND 21, at least 1 male and 1 female per litter	Not applicable
	Sexual maturation	Vaginal opening (females), preputial separation (males)	Not applicable
	Postweaning functional test	Sensory, motor, and learning and memory	Not applicable
	Reproductive performance	At 12 weeks of age, initiate mating trials within same group (1 male:1 female), midgestation Cesarean section	Not applicable
	Necropsy	Female, midgestation Cesarean section following mating (females), male gross necropsy after female evaluation	At minimum 1-month postpartum but often longer depending on aim of any postnatal evaluations, "visceral" evaluation, retain tissues for possible future examination

ePPND, enhanced PPND; *GD*, Gestation Day; *LD*, Lactation Day; *PND*, Postnatal Day; *PPND*, pre- and postnatal developmental.

related. There are many confounding factors to be aware of, many of which have been discussed earlier including the impact of maternal toxicity. For example, in a feed restriction study (gestation day 7 through lactation), F1 body weights were reduced, puberty was delayed, sperm counts were down, and estrous cycle length was increased for those pups maintained on a restricted diet (Carney et al., 2004). All effects observed were reversible but illustrate the sensitivity of some endpoints to general toxicity.

Unfortunately, many of these endpoints (e.g., body weight and developmental landmarks) are crude apical endpoints influenced by any number of factors and it may require additional investigative studies to better understand a potential relationship with the test article to meaningfully inform human risk assessment. As with EFD studies, many of the endpoints in a PPND study are related, especially when additional calculated, rather than measured, endpoints are included. Pup survival indices for different postnatal windows are one example of calculated endpoints that correlate and correspond to other endpoints including live litter size, number of pup deaths, and number of former uterine implantation sites.

Data interpretation of changes or differences attributed to the test article need to consider the full data set of interrelated datapoints together with available historical control data. One of the more complicated set of endpoints and related statistical analyses to interpret is the functional data of sensory, motor, and learning and memory. These data can be highly variable, and the different behavioral paradigms tested can be different among different test facilities. Once again, having an experienced study director and test facility with a long history and validated testing paradigms with positive control studies and historical control data can go a long way to facilitate appropriate interpretation of these data and their potential impact on these safety assessment (Tyl et al., 2008).

For pharmaceuticals, the PPND study is typically conducted just prior to registration and thus the information is not used to support clinical trials but to inform the label about potential long-term risk to offspring if the product is used during pregnancy. It is not often that these studies reveal novel toxicities unrelated to those observed in EFD studies because PPND studies are essentially a lengthy extension of the EFD study in that they both start dosing at implantation with the PPND study continuing dosing through lactation.

One of the primary objectives of both the EFD and PPND studies is evaluation of potential effects on the offspring. A common observation is low fetal weights in an EFD study that translate to low birth weights in offspring at the same dose and either the pups recover or exhibit exacerbated toxicity with continued exposure. An instructive example to be aware of is the developmental toxicity of angiotensin converting enzyme (ACE) inhibitors. Rat EFD studies have generally failed to detect developmental toxicity, but in humans, ACE inhibitors cause fetal hypotension, renal tubular dysplasia, anuria-oligohydramnios, growth retardation, hypocalvaria, and death when used in the second and third trimesters of human pregnancy (Sedman et al., 1995). However, when ACE inhibitors are dosed in late pregnancy and lactation in rats, offspring did demonstrate adverse effects including death during lactation. The lesson is that the critical period of renin synthesis is outside the period of major organogenesis that is studied in a rat EFD study and thus only detectable in the PPND study. This ACE inhibitor example also illustrates the importance of the PPND study in that the rodent and to some extent rabbit gestation is so short relative to human gestation that the offspring are born somewhat premature compared with human. As such, some organ systems that are formed in utero in humans are still developing peripostnatally in rodents, as exemplified by the ACE inhibitor example.

3.3. Enhanced Pre- and Postnatal Development Study in the NHP

In the situation where the test item is a biopharmaceutical and the NHP is the only pharmacologically relevant species, a combined EFD and pre- and postnatal study approach has been adopted and has gained regulatory endorsement as described in the ICH S6(R1) and ICH S5(R3) harmonized guidelines. This "PPND Study, Enhanced Design," or "ePPND" takes advantage of the relatively low incidence of directly teratogenic effects with large molecules, as well as the active transfer of antibodies across the primate placenta in the third trimester. The study design also acknowledges the relatively high rate of fetal/neonatal losses in laboratory macaques, and so is designed to enable meaningful results from a single study to reduce NHP use overall. This ePPND strategy is important given the limited number of breeding macaques available for study and the low fecundity with a single offspring. Specific study design recommendations for the ePPND have been described (Chellman et al., 2009; Jarvis et al., 2010; Weinbauer et al., 2011, 2013), with some recommendations recently revised based on accumulated experience (Grossmann et al., 2020; Luetjens et al., 2020). Table 7.4 provides a list of minimal ePPND endpoints alongside a rodent PPND study.

One topic of continued discussion is that of appropriate group size. The recent ICH S5(R3) suggests a minimum group size of 16 pregnant dams and acknowledges that this remains statistically underpowered for NHPs based on the low fecundity and high fetal and neonatal losses; in contrast, the ICH S6(R1) recommends a design with at least six to eight surviving offspring through the first week postnatal. Additional limitations include the fact that the F1 offspring are not evaluated through sexual maturity or for reproductive function. Finally, the pregnant females are enrolled onto the study, usually over a period of months, and there is variability in gestation length, leading to complex study operations.

Testing Endpoints

In an ePPND study design, the dosing phase is initiated once pregnancy can be confirmed via ultrasound, and dosing continues through natural delivery. In the cynomolgus monkey, pregnancy is usually confirmed at 18–20 days gestation, and the normal gestation is 162 days ±2 weeks. During gestation, pregnancy is periodically monitored via ultrasound for fetal survival, and the study protocol should specify the approach to pathology for fetal death and/ or aborted fetuses. In the event of unscheduled necropsy of fetuses, the gross exam encompasses many features of the external and soft tissue examinations of a typical EFD study. However, fetal losses through death or abortion can occur at any time, and control fetuses are not usually collected in parallel. Therefore, the interpretation of pathology data from these early losses, when they occur, is generally based on pathologist experience. Importantly, there is no routine gross or histologic examination of the placenta in the ePPND study design, as it is often consumed or traumatized postpartum, although the placenta should be evaluated from early Cesarean sections. In cases where a direct placental effect leads to substantial fetal losses, it can be helpful to schedule a subset of remaining pregnancies for Cesarean section to evaluate the close-to-term fetus and placentae from both control and treated groups (Prell et al., 2018).

In the immediate postnatal phase of an ePPND, the developmental assessment of offspring continues with external and physical exam, weekly body weights, and radiography on or after PND 28 to assess skeletal development and identify any skeletal malformations. This early postnatal developmental period also typically includes an assessment of neonatal reflexes and maternal–offspring behavior, as well as survival of offspring. A limited number of paired pharmacokinetic samples from the lactating female and offspring are also often collected beginning on or about day 7 postnatal to assess placental transfer. In general, monoclonal antibodies are effectively transferred, but highly engineered or conjugated antibodies, as well as many other recombinant proteins, do not effectively cross the placenta (Bowman et al., 2013; DeSesso et al., 2012). If needed, an interim report with study results through the first month postnatal can be sufficient to enable appropriate inclusion of WOCBP in clinical trials, similar to an EFD study.

Many of the remaining endpoints in an ePPND study focus on the growth and development of the postnatal offspring. Often, these will be specific to the expected pharmacology and established toxicity profile of the test item. These can include periodic clinical pathology from the pregnant/lactating female and offspring, weekly body weights of offspring to monitor growth, and can include biomarkers of pharmacodynamic effects from the dam and offspring. For immunomodulators, immune function testing on the offspring is often conducted with a T-cell–dependent antigen response (TDAR). The exact timing of the TDAR, and number of antigens tested, will depend on the study design and specific concerns related to the anticipated immunopharmacology. For the pathologist, it is important to consider the expected immunostimulatory consequences of the TDAR when evaluating immune tissues from the offspring.

Learning assessments are typically reserved for a situation where there is a specific mechanistic concern. Common testing approaches include a modified Wisconsin General Testing Apparatus object discrimination test, which includes habituation, learning and reversal phases, or a finger maze, which utilize both training and recall phases (Cappon et al., 2012; Inoue et al., 2014; Makori et al., 2013). For both of these, the initial training or habituation begins at 9 months of age, and therefore requires a postnatal study duration of 12 months. Neither of these assessments is specifically or routinely expected for an ePPND. In general, the duration of postnatal evaluation of offspring is variable for an ePPND and can be as short as 1 month, with most lasting until about 6 months postnatal.

The final stage of the study is the necropsy of the offspring, which allows gross assessment of visceral anomalies and malformations, as well as collection of tissues for potential microscopic evaluation. Due to the rolling enrollment of pregnant dams onto the study and variability in parturition day, scheduled necropsies on, for example, postnatal day 180, might actually be a few animals necropsied per day or every few days over a period of months to meet that schedule.

There is no requirement for histopathology, and it varies by study from none, to target tissues, to a full tissue list comparable to that for general toxicity testing (Halpern et al., 2016). Publications of ePPND studies highlight some of the different ways that these studies can be conducted, including variations on approaches to pathology (Bowman et al., 2015; Boyce et al., 2014; Enright et al., 2012b; Vaidyanathan et al., 2011), and additional perspective can be gleaned from publications of similar studies conducted prior to the establishment of the ePPND study type (Auyeung-Kim et al., 2009; Martin et al., 2007). Also, especially for programs where there is extended exposure and/or pharmacodynamic effects of the test

item, the detailed evaluation of developmental effects on offspring can also be relevant to the support of pediatric patients, potentially precluding the need for a dedicated JAS (Martin and Weinbauer, 2010).

Overall, ePPNDs are designed to meet the needs of individual programs to inform the risk assessment for pregnant women and their fetuses and offspring when NHPs are the only pharmacologically relevant species. Given some of the limitations described above, these studies are most useful in detecting large effects and enabling communication of a potential hazard. Once a mechanistic hazard has been identified, these studies provide limited additional benefit with regard to quantitative risk assessment. For these reasons, a WoE approach has been proposed for developmental toxicity assessment for biopharmaceuticals (Rocca et al., 2018).

3.4. Guidelines

Regulatory requirements for assessment of potential effects on pregnancy and PPND have evolved over many decades, with different approaches and testing designed to assess human relevant exposures. Similar to assessments of reproductive toxicity, these span chronic environmental exposures of industrial and commercial chemicals to purposeful exposures to potential or marketed therapeutics.

Guidelines evaluating the potential developmental toxicity of environmental exposures to industrial chemicals and pesticides include screening studies (OECD, 2016a,b), exposure during pregnancy alone (OECD, 2018a; EPA, 1998a) and throughout the reproductive cycle including different life stages using the multigeneration reproduction study (OECD, 2001; EPA, 1998b) and more recently the extended one-generation study (OECD, 2018b), and the NTP modified one-generation reproduction study (Foster, 2014) (Table 7.1). For these larger reproduction studies, evaluation of developmental toxicity is but one aspect of many assessment endpoints.

For pharmaceuticals, the tragedy of thalidomide-induced birth defects in the late 1950s led the FDA in 1966 to propose Segment I (fertility and general reproduction), Segment II (teratogenicity), and Segment III (perinatal) testing protocols for reproductive toxicity (Kim and Scialli, 2011). Later, these segmented study protocols were harmonized to the current state where reproductive toxicity assessment for regulatory purposes is governed by guidelines established by the ICH (Table 7.1). ICH S5(R3) is latest revision of the primary reference describing regulatory expectations of reproductive toxicity assessment of pharmaceuticals, including study designs to address different life stages such as pregnancy and PPND, and considerations for different modalities and patient populations (ICH, 2020a).

Specifically, these guidelines direct EFD studies in two species (rodent and nonrodent) where possible; however, the most recent version of the guideline provides for alternative approaches for EFD assessment such as single-species EFD if evidence of malformations or embryo lethality is demonstrated (ICH, 2020a). ICH M3(R2) describes the timing of EFD and PPND studies to support clinical trials and marketing in humans including region-specific provisions for pEFD studies in two species to support enrollment of WOCBP in clinical trials (ICH, 2009a). ICH S6(R1) describes specific considerations of biotechnology-derived pharmaceuticals including evaluation only in pharmacologically relevant species and the ePPND study design in NHPs that encompasses endpoints addressed by both EFD and PPND study designs (ICH, 2011). ICH S5(R3) is aligned with ICH S6(R1), including the recommendation that studies in pregnant NHPs should only be conducted when they are the only pharmacologically relevant species. ICH S9 is the nonclinical ICH guideline for anticancer pharmaceuticals where there is no requirement for a PPND study and the EFD assessment can be based on whatever study demonstrates malformations or embryo lethality even if from a DRF study in one species (ICH, 2009b). A more recent FDA guideline describes reproductive toxicity testing and labeling recommendations for oncology pharmaceuticals (FDA, 2019).

Overall, these guidelines summarize the timing and types of pregnancy and developmental toxicity assessments to be evaluated to inform the human risk assessment for specific patient populations (see *Risk Assessment*, Vol 2, Chap 16). Figure 7.2 illustrates representative timings of different study types conducted over the course of drug development to support clinical trials and marketing. Importantly, it is recognized that while the above-described approaches work well to inform human risk, there is interest in evaluating other approaches that use less animals as reflected in the recent revision of ICH S5R3 (ICH, 2020a) and multistakeholder workshops (Brannen et al., 2011; Scialli et al., 2018).

4. JUVENILE TOXICITY ASSESSMENT

One of the primary goals in conducting a JAS is to better understand specific effects on growth and development, including those that might not be evident from general toxicity studies. Effects of potential toxicants on children or juvenile animals may be different from those seen in adult humans or animals. These differences can be generally due to differential drug or chemical exposure when absorption, distribution, metabolism, excretion (ADME) pathways are immature, or to sensitivity of developing target organ systems. In general, the impact and safety of chemicals are evaluated in multigenerational DART studies, and thus the vast majority of dedicated JAS are conducted to support pediatric use of therapeutics.

To some extent, effects can be anticipated based on a combination of known chemical or product attributes and the established toxicity profile, so a careful review of available data is the first step to understanding whether or not a JAS is warranted. In particular, DART studies described earlier in this chapter that include postnatal assessments of the offspring can be highly relevant. For example, specific or unique developmental effects can begin prenatally for drug or chemical compounds that cross the placenta, so gross and microscopic evaluation of offspring from a PPND study can be informative. When the test item is administered to the dam during pregnancy, though, it can be important to evaluate the exposure achieved in the offspring to better understand any findings as they relate to exposure.

In studies designed with direct dosing of juvenile animals, the exposure may change in the early postnatal period as different aspects of ADME pathways mature. For example, exposures after oral administration to the rat can be quite high perinatally, in part, because the neonatal gastrointestinal (GI) tract is open to nonspecific absorption of large and small molecules, while pathways for hepatobiliary metabolism and clearance, as well as renal excretion, are not yet fully developed and functional. Therefore, an assessment of pathology findings must consider the dose and exposure relationships, especially in neonates (De Schaepdrijver et al., 2019).

There can also be effects that are related to target tissue sensitivity rather than exposure differences. For example, any effect on skeletal growth will be magnified during periods of the most rapid bone elongation yet might not be seen in an animal growing more slowly, and would not be detectable in a mature animal with a closed growth plate. Likewise, different aspects of CNS functionality and maturation can extend even into adulthood, although the major developmentally appropriate structural changes of the CNS are mostly complete by weaning, as has been reviewed (Bolon et al., 2006). Finally, cumulative effects related to duration of exposure can also be affected by the concurrent maturation of the animal, and vice versa, necessitating consideration of a number of approaches to study design. References that address study design considerations such as the text *Pediatric Nonclinical Drug Testing* (Hoberman and Lewis, 2012) and published reviews (Cappon et al., 2009; Morford et al., 2011) can provide additional context for different types of drugs that might benefit from a JAS to support pediatric use.

When a JAS is conducted, pathology endpoints are one critical endpoint to assess impact on growth and development. Specific considerations for both scheduled and unscheduled necropsies, as well as clinical pathology and histopathology, are discussed below. Depending on the expected target tissues, as well as gross findings and organ weights, the microscopic pathology can range from a limited assessment of tissues undergoing morphological changes during postnatal development, to a standard comprehensive tissue list, or even an expanded tissue assessment for a specific cause. For the pathologist, it is important to keep in mind that juvenile animals are allocated to the study without extensive prestudy health screening, so there is the potential for greater background congenital findings than are typically seen in general toxicity studies. When animals are dosed in the preweaning period, especially, there is greater potential for background morbidity and mortality than is typically seen in general toxicity studies, and this can be enhanced in test article groups if there is even slight stress or discomfort.

For the pathologist evaluating postnatal development, it can be challenging to understand normal morphology at a given time interval unless it is routinely examined in that species and strain of animal. A few important resources to help recognize developmentally typical histology include textbooks such as the *Atlas of Histology of the Juvenile Rat* (Parker and Picut, 2016) and dedicated chapters in general resources such as *Pathology of the Mouse: A Reference and Atlas* (Maronpot, 1999); *Comparative Anatomy and Histology: A Mouse, Rat and Human Atlas* (Treuting, 2018); *The Minipig in Biomedical Research* (McAnulty et al., 2011); *the Nonhuman Primate in Biomedical Research* (Bluemel et al., 2015); *and Fundamental Neuropathology for Pathologists and Toxicologists* (Bolon and Butt, 2011) as well as reviews such as a recent review of developmental milestones of the C57Bl/6 mouse (Zalewska, 2019).

Importantly, no animal model can completely reflect the developmental differences and sensitivities relevant to children. Of these, toxicologic effects on premature infants and neonates can be especially difficult to model nonclinically. When exposure to a chemical or drug results in different toxicity profile in an immature animal compared to that of a mature animal, species-specific development must be considered before directly extrapolating the findings to human safety assessment. Because of this, the nonclinical support for pediatric medicines begins with a WoE approach, rather than a "check box" study design. There can be a number of potential approaches that will depend on factors such as the known effects of the test compound, as well as the potential pediatric population. In this process, it is helpful for the pathologist to engage early and, as needed, contribute to study design and endpoints. Ultimately, the data from these studies can be a useful tool for appropriate labeling and use of both chemicals and medicines.

4.1. Context for Challenges in Assessing the Neonatal Period

In many ways, the neonate represents both the population of greatest concern, and the most difficult to effectively study and model nonclinically for translational safety assessment. At the time of birth, there are a number of critical transitions that occur: the lungs inflate with air for the first time and initiate oxygen exchange; this is accompanied by changes in circulatory changes initiating the shift away from the fetal shunting with the abrupt elimination of umbilical blood flow; likewise, within the first hours, both the GI system and the renal system must begin the lifelong process of nutrient absorption and waste elimination.

The neonate is dependent on an environment suitable for thermoregulation, maintenance of hydration, and an initial exposure to immunologic and sensorimotor stimuli, as well as functional reflexes that enable respiration, suckling, and elimination. Problems with these functional and acute transitions can be rapidly fatal and cause a medical emergency. Emergency neonatal care is challenging, with a relatively high rate of adverse outcomes and extensive off-label use of medicines as compared to other hospital settings. While it is not possible to draw a causal relationship between the two, there is room for improvement in our nonclinical safety assessment of medicines used in neonates to better optimize dose, schedule, and monitoring.

All of the birth transitions described above are common to mammalian neonates, but specific organ system development is not synchronized across species relative to the birth event. Many species are altricial, with less developed offspring born in a relatively helpless condition, whereas other species are precocial and are more developmentally advanced at the time of birth. The altricial species, such as rats, have had a relatively short gestation and are born as part of a large litter; the energy invested in gestation and maternal care is therefore divided across a number of individual offspring, favoring the strongest to grow quickly and reach their own reproductive potential. In contrast, precocial species have invested more energy in a longer gestation and more focused maternal care on individual offspring.

Different species are advanced or delayed in slightly different ways, depending on needs. For example, ruminants and equids are relatively large and need to be able to stand and even run within hours after birth, piglets must be able to stand and walk within the first few days postnatal, while NHPs must be able to cling to their dam from birth; all of these are born with a more structurally sound musculoskeletal system than humans or altricial species which have limited independent mobility as neonates.

The differences between species have toxicologic relevance both in interpreting toxicity within a species and, for JAS, in the relevant translatability to human development. Humans are not typical of either altricial or precocial species, but rather share features of both: few offspring, long gestation, postnatal reliance on maternal care, and important postnatal development of several organ systems. In assessing the translation and relevance of toxicologic pathology in neonates, it is especially important to consider species-specific differences in postnatal development. The subsequent postnatal organ system development section reviews at a high level some of those differences and provides selected references for additional detail.

4.2. Context for Support of Children: Weaning through Puberty

Nonclinical support for assessing safety for pediatrics during childhood presents a different type of challenge. In the postweaning period, many of the ADME differences are less prominent, and many organ systems are relatively quiescent, or have largely completed structural development. Functional refinement continues especially for the CNS, and the tissues of the immune system reflect both development and experience. However, the variability in achievement of developmental milestones across individuals of many species during this period also attests to the flexibility built into the system, despite the relatively high metabolic activity and sustained growth for most species. Thus, the value and relevance of a JAS for human risk assessment is not as readily linked to specific and monitorable milestones or pathology, and the context of the risk is also important to consider. For example, continuous or intermittent exposures to environmental and agrochemicals can be relevant over a broad age range. In contrast, a pharmaceutical is typically administered at a specific recommended dose to achieve a pharmacologically active exposure. However, a pharmaceutical might be intended to treat medical conditions that affect patients over a narrow or a broad age range, and might be used for a short, intermittent, or chronic treatment duration. For these reasons, where feasible, the treatment period in a JAS often covers the full spectrum of development, starting with the youngest intended patient population.

In addition, for JAS conducted in rodents, as many are, the scheduled necropsy endpoints are typically in young adult animals. Therefore, the morphology of the tissues is essentially the same as that for short-term general toxicity studies. Likewise, the historical control data for young adult animals can be relevant for blood samples collected for clinical pathology at the time of scheduled necropsy, although concurrent controls are the strongest comparator in looking for potential treatment effects. For these studies, the primary value of a JAS would be to address a specific concern, for example, to understand an effect on growth where exposure is expected to be chronic during childhood, or where there is a concern regarding initiation or completion of puberty. Importantly, it is difficult to assess a specific "age range" for comparison for this period. In humans, the period of childhood starts between 2 and 4 years of age and continues through onset of puberty, in most cases, sometime between 9 and 14 years of age. The comparable period in the rat only lasts a few weeks, assuming weaning at 3 weeks of age and initiation of puberty by postnatal day 35 in females and 42 in males, with completion of puberty by 9–10 weeks of age in most strains. In contrast, both dogs and macaques have a protracted period of childhood-like development between weaning and puberty. This period in the dog is generally about 6 months in duration, although full skeletal maturity is not reached until about 18 months of age. In macaques, the period between weaning and maturity can be highly variable, but is generally about 2–3 years, with growth plate closure occurring between 3 and 5 years in females and 5–7 years in males. However, much of the critical structural postnatal development has been

completed by the time of weaning. During the postweaning period, there is both extensive growth as well as refinement of function across organ systems, but most tissues are histologically mature, excepting those of the reproductive tract and skeleton. Functional assessments in this period have focused on assessment of immunologic responsiveness, locomotion, and learning and memory. Many general toxicity studies are conducted with dogs or macaques that have not completed puberty. For this reason, a - dedicated JAS is less commonly needed in these species. Historically, specific requests to better understand developmental neurotoxicity (DNT), developmental immunotoxicity (DIT), and DART have all been drivers toward the conduct of JAS to support risk assessment for children and adolescents. Some additional detail for these is provided in the following section on postnatal organ system development.

4.3. Postnatal Development of Specific Organ Systems

As has been introduced above, postnatal development can differ between species, between different organ systems, and also within organ systems. Figure 7.5 broadly illustrates various paths toward maturation over time in developing animals or humans. These are not a strict and specific guide, but rather a perspective that some postnatal organ system maturation processes will rapidly achieve the structure and function of the mature tissue, whereas others proceed slowly, intermittently, or after a quiescent period. Because of these differences, it is useful to keep in mind some general features of development for each organ system.

Cardiovascular and Pulmonary

The cardiovascular and pulmonary system both undergo immediate postnatal changes at birth in all mammals, as well as important postnatal development in many species (Hew and Keller, 2003; Zoetis and Hurtt, 2003). The first breath of air occurs concomitantly with separation from the maternal unit. The pulmonary vascular pressure changes, as does load on the left and right heart, along with the vasoconstriction of the umbilical vessels—all of which lead to a shift away from fetal shunting. Adequate

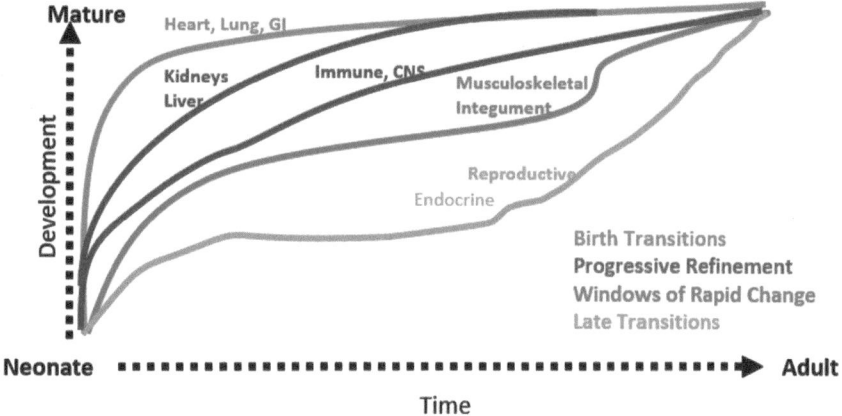

FIGURE 7.5 Postnatal organ system maturation. Different organ systems mature postnatally at different rates, which are not constant between birth and achievement of structural and functional maturity. The neonatal transition curve represents organ systems which must quickly establish function, and tissue morphology in these is often histologically comparable to adults shortly after birth, although the timing may vary between species. In some organ systems such as the CNS, there are substantial structural changes postnatally, as well as a protracted functional refinement extending even beyond sexual maturity. Although inconsistent across species, windows of structural or functional maturation can also occur ("growth spurts"). Finally, the reproductive system components are often in place at or shortly after birth, but in mammals, there are substantial structural and functional changes that occur concomitant with puberty. Overall, care is needed when considering maturation timelines between species, between organ systems, or even within organ systems.

oxygenation within a few minutes after birth is required for survival. For the pathologist, neonatal losses that are not witnessed can be categorized as stillbirth versus early postnatal death based on evidence of lung inflation, or lack thereof. In terms of toxicology, the neonate can be more sensitive to, and potentially with longer term consequences from, cardiac and pulmonary toxicants as compared to older life stages.

The heart goes through a metabolic transition in the neonatal period, which is accompanied by maturation of ion channel conduction and expansion of myocardiocytes (Hausner, Elmore, & Yang, 2019). At this early stage, there is greater potential for arrhythmias, with a relatively high heart rate, despite relatively low cardiac output and systemic blood pressure. Thus, importantly, although there can be increased potential for toxicity from cardioactive drugs during the neonatal and infancy period, there is also a need for them, and therefore some accumulated experience. One example is the effective use of sotalol for pediatric supraventricular tachyarrhythmias, despite an increased risk of QTc prolongation in neonates attributed to the lower density of hERG channels in the neonatal

myocardium (Laer et al., 2005; Mulla, 2010). In humans, the electrocardiogram normalizes by about 5 years of age, but angiogenesis and growth continue into the teenage years. In most nonclinical species, the postnatal cardiovascular development period progresses similarly, achieving adult-like histology by weaning, but with some continued expansion of the sarcoplasm and metabolic capacity through puberty (Hausner, Elmore, & Yang, 2019; Hew and Keller, 2003; Parker and Picut, 2016).

In contrast, the developmental "age" of the lungs at birth is variable across species. Not surprisingly, the lungs of altricial animals like rats and puppies are less fully developed than those of more precocial species like macaques. This reflects the general alignment between lung maturity and mobility of the neonate. Even in species with less developed lungs, alveolarization and lung maturation progresses fairly rapidly. In the rat, alveolarization is complete by weaning, and the lung has an adult histology by PND 28 (Parker and Picut, 2016). In general, the pig and macaque are not considered good models for postnatal developmental toxicity of the respiratory tract because they have close to adult structure and function at birth. Although not routinely used in toxicity testing in general, the neonatal lamb lung physiology is considered relevant in the study of some neonatal diseases such as Respiratory Syncytial Virus infection (Derscheid and Ackermann, 2013). These infectious disease models also highlight the fact that these very young animals can be more likely to develop pneumonia, especially for large animal species. If pulmonary lesions are observed in preweaning animals in a JAS, it is important to distinguish between a direct lung toxicity versus an indirect effect such as an increased incidence or severity of bacterial or viral pneumonia secondary to immunomodulation or general stress.

Gastrointestinal Tract

Like the heart and lungs, the GI tract needs to be functional at birth for the survival of offspring. However, there are also number of critical postnatal development processes that occur, especially in the period between birth and weaning. In JAS, it is important to be cognizant of the species differences in GI development, especially for orally administered compounds. The structural and functional postnatal development of the GI tract across species has been reviewed (Downes, 2018; Neal-Kluever et al., 2019; Walthall et al., 2005), with some emphasis on differences relevant to ADME features (Neal-Kluever et al., 2019). One way to look at the neonatal and postnatal GI tract is that it changes according to the changing needs of the offspring. For example, milk of different species has different relative amounts of proteins, carbohydrates, and fats, and the initial digestive apparatus for each reflects that. Very rapidly growing species like rat pups need to absorb nutrients efficiently; in the first 2 weeks postnatal, there is minimal enzymatic digestion, and also the proximal intestine is highly permeable to large molecules, including protein growth factors and antibodies. Once the pups start exploring other foods, the gastric and pancreatic enzymes follow suit, and by weaning, they are able to continue the rapid growth trajectory. In contrast, the neonatal piglet is much more similar to the human neonate in terms of gastric and digestive function (Downes, 2018), and is often used for studies of human formulas and milk replacers (Guilloteau et al., 2010). Another feature of the neonatal gut is the rapid postnatal

expansion of the microbiome, which will again be species and environment specific. Necrotizing enterocolitis remains an acute and life-threatening neonatal emergency in humans and other large animal species but is uncommon in rodents in a laboratory setting.

Many features of maturation work together to achieve a functional and adaptive GI tract almost immediately following birth. However, the transporters, hepatic type I and II metabolic capacity, and expanded length and surface area of the intestine mature progressively and over a longer period. From a pathology perspective, it is important to keep in mind the potential cumulative impact of chronically reduced nutrient intake or absorption during periods of active growth. More acutely, dysbiosis and naturally occurring infectious diseases may be more prevalent and have greater impact on juvenile animals. Also, juveniles may have an increased, decreased, or similar response to different hepatotoxins, typically linked to a combination of hepatic metabolic capacity and maturation of both biliary/fecal and renal clearance mechanisms (Allegaert and van den Anker, 2019; de Zwart et al., 2008; Zhang et al., 2019; Van Groen et al., 2021).

Renal System

There are critical aspects of both structural and functional postnatal renal system development that can contribute to both acute organ system susceptibility to toxicity and chronic pathological consequences. The postnatal development of the renal system has been recently reviewed, highlighting differences across species as well as relative susceptibilities of the renal system to toxicity during postnatal development (Bueters et al., 2020; Frazier, 2017; Seely, 2017). For example, in the rodent, rabbit and dog, nephrogenesis continues into the postnatal period, while in humans and NHPs it has largely been completed by term birth. However, in all species, there is postnatal elongation of tubules and establishment of concentrating ability. For some species, like rodents, urine concentrating ability precedes development of maximal glomerular filtration rate, while in others, such as humans, both develop concurrently. Because of this, juvenile rodents can be highly susceptible to nephrotoxic injury. This is particularly true during the preweaning period, where pups are growing rapidly and even brief periods of inadequate suckling can result in dehydration, thus further exacerbating renal injury. In young pups, there may be relatively scant overt evidence of renal disease other than poor growth.

At the time of necropsy, it is not unusual to see chronic progressive renal disease in affected animals. This does not always follow a clear dose dependency, as confounders such as pup size at study start, suckling efficiency, and maternal care can contribute, for example, to dehydration. Postnatal development of the renal system also contributes to refinement of blood pressure regulation through the renin–angiotensin system, as well as to erythrocyte production through local production of erythropoietin.

Developmental Neuropathology

In evaluation of developmental toxicity, there has always been interest and focus on the development and refinement of structure and function of the nervous system. In addition, this occurs in most species over a relatively long period and involves many distinct components. Of these, particular attention has been paid to developmental aspects and relevance of postnatal reflexes and acoustic startle, blood–brain barrier (BBB) function, neuronal apoptosis, myelination, establishment of signaling pathways, pain perception and modulation, locomotion, and learning and memory. There are recent publications from both the US FDA (Fisher et al., 2019) and the EMA (van der Laan et al., 2019) that highlight regulatory experience for assessment of neurotoxicity in JAS. Both of these reviews acknowledge the value of neuropathology endpoints from JAS, while also recognizing that neurobehavioral and cognitive effects do not always have a structural correlate. Approaches and challenges for the evaluation of structural and functional neuropathology endpoints across species in JAS have also been reviewed (Bolon et al., 2006; Garman et al., 2016; Li et al., 2017; Sharma et al., 2016; Watson et al., 2006; Wood et al., 2003).

Pathology of the CNS in JAS might reflect (1) findings due to a failure or delay in structural refinement leading to altered morphology, (2) findings due to infectious agents with neuropathologic effects, (3) consequences of maturation of BBB function leading to increased drug or chemical residence time or concentration in the brain. The first of these may reflect a direct or indirect effect. Examples of direct effects could include such as inhibition of apoptosis or delay in myelination. Indirect effects might include neuronal degeneration and necrosis due to hypoglycemia when insulin is studied in nondiabetic animals, or disruption of appropriate hormone support for growth and maturation of signaling pathways, as with learning and memory deficits seen with some inhibitors of thyroid function (Inoue et al., 2014). The latter two are linked to the importance of relating systemic findings on endocrine or immune tissues, some of which can be subtle, to the neuropathology seen.

Assessment of gross and microscopic pathology is an important component of the evaluation of potential DNT, but is not straightforward to apply. For example, a "comprehensive" assessment could require exploration of several windows of exposure during development, and also potentially several windows of evaluation. Using this approach, a single study could potentially include thousands of animals and is not considered an appropriate experimental approach. Rather, there are two general approaches that have been widely applied for chemicals and drugs with particular neurodevelopmental concern: (1) continuous sustained exposure with assessment at the end of the juvenile period to detect any persistent structural or neurobehavioral effects, or (2) acute exposures to support a specific population such as neonates. For the latter, it is likely that at least two assessments could be needed to evaluate both acute structural changes and also persistent or permanent effects on learning and memory.

As an example, a juvenile rodent toxicity study might involve exposures over a period generally reflective of postnatal development, such as PNDs 7–10 through PNDs 63–70, with a series of general in-life assessments (feeding behaviors, mobility, growth, socialization), as well as timed assessments for acoustic startle and sexual maturation. A subset of pups might be necropsied at weaning (~PND 22), another subset at the end of the treatment period, and a third subset after a treatment-free recovery period. For the third subset, and often also the second, a learning and memory assessment is often incorporated into the design. This approach is aligned with the STP best practice recommendations for developmental neuropathology (Bolon et al., 2006), and has been broadly applied to better understand effects of environmental and agrochemicals, especially those with potential for continuous exposure over a lifetime. It is also generally aligned with the recommendations in the ICH S11, although for most medicinal products an early necropsy interval at the time of weaning is not specifically warranted. With accumulated information, the optimized practices continue to evolve, resulting in further resources for the practicing pathologist (Garman et al., 2016; Sharma et al., 2016).

There are also some drug classes, such as anesthetic agents and sedatives, where there is an identified concern for acute effects during the critical period of synaptogenesis and myelination. In particular, increased apoptosis of both neurons and glia, as well as persistently impaired learning and memory performance, has been identified in animal studies. Many of these agents are also highly lipid soluble and can impair active myelination, especially in the early postnatal period. Thus, for these agents, studies of neonatal exposure (PND 6–7) have been conducted with stereotactic evaluation of apoptosis using sections stained immunohistochemically for activated caspase 8, as described for rats given sevoflurane (Zhou et al., 2016), or neonatal macaques given isoflurane for as little as 3 h (Noguchi et al., 2017). Because the stain for activated caspase 8 highlights the full cell body, differential effects on glia and neurons can be discerned in the acute phase.

While many studies with anesthetic agents have been conducted in the rat, results from these studies can be difficult to translate to a risk assessment paradigm for human infants. In part, this reflects potentially different sensitivity to inducers of apoptosis, as well as the more extensive postnatal myelination in the rat. These differences have led to further emphasis on studies in macaques by some investigators, although the data from macaque studies can also be difficult to translate, especially when results are conflicting (Zhou et al., 2015a, b). In sum, a consensus on appropriate study design and interpretation for translatability has not been reached for these agents (Jevtovic-Todorovic et al., 2017).

In humans, most CNS myelination is complete at birth, in contrast to the rat where it is predominantly postnatal. Sections of key anatomic areas

such as the cortex, hippocampus, cerebellum, and pons can be stained with Luxol fast blue and cresyl violet to highlight patterns of myelination. It can also be useful to review the timing and progression of myelination in the rat as has been described in detail (Downes and Mullins, 2014). One example of a dose-dependent effect on myelination, including reversibility in the rat, is that of vigabatrin, a gamma-aminobutyric acid (GABA) analog (Rasmussen et al., 2015). Not surprisingly, pharmaceuticals that are active in the CNS, such as anticonvulsants, anesthetics and sedatives, and those specifically targeting GABA or N-methyl-D-aspartate pathways, have been closely scrutinized for potential developmental effects.

Of all advancements in toxicologic developmental neuropathology, improved understanding of the maturation of the BBB deserves specific mention. The BBB was long regarded as a structural layer of protection that functions to exclude potentially neurotoxic chemicals and drugs, and that "immaturity" resulted in increased permeability and sensitivity to drugs and toxins in neonates. In contrast, it is now recognized that the BBB structure is largely mature even during fetal development, but there are shifts in function related to the demands of the growing brain (Saunders et al., 2018; Schmitt et al., 2017). These depend on age-related blood pressure and cerebral blood flow, which then contribute to CSF production and residence time. Likewise, the BBB is responsible for enabling the supply of necessary nutrients and growth factors to the growing brain, and this is reflected in transporter activities. Thus, brain exposure to a drug or chemical can change markedly during postnatal development, e.g., with initially high concentration and low clearance due to low organic anion transporter activity or longer CSF residence time, but then brain concentrations can drop to near undetectable levels by weaning as the functionality becomes more adult like.

Finally, the development of the eye and maturation of visual acuity should be noted, and has been recently reviewed (Van Cruchten et al., 2017). Importantly, retinal development is largely complete in primates at term birth but continues postnatally in rodents. Also, the neural connections that establish vision require stimulation, which begins in primates and pigs at birth, but is delayed in species born with closed eyes, such as rodents, rabbits, and dogs. In all species, there are postnatal adaptations to refine and advance visual function.

Immune System

Most mammals are born with the structural foundation of a competent immune system, but also a reliance on passive immunity during the initial postnatal period (DeWitt et al., 2012a; Holsapple et al., 2003; Kuper et al., 2016; Parker et al., 2015; Skaggs et al., 2019). In rodents, rabbits, and primates, maternal immunoglobulin is actively transported across the placenta to provide the offspring with some immunity starting at birth, but in dogs, piglets, ruminants, and equids, there is limited or no placental transfer of immunoglobulin, and consumption of immunoglobulin-rich colostrum in the first hours after birth is critical in these species. With failure of passive immunity, the young of these species are at high risk of perinatal infections.

The postnatal development of the immune system has been systematically reviewed across species (Hew and Keller, 2003). In addition, more recent comprehensive reviews of immune system development across species have been conducted with emphasis on translatability to human risk assessment (Kuper et al., 2016; Skaggs et al., 2019). These reviews highlight the fact that the bulk of structural development of the immune system in nonrodents occurs during gestation; however, it is acknowledged that there is postnatal maturation of immunocompetence as well as establishment of immune memory (DeWitt et al., 2012a). The rat immune system lags behind humans and NHPs somewhat, and it is generally recommended that, for example, a TDAR assessment be conducted on or after PND 45 to ensure that the system is capable of responding adequately to evaluate potential treatment effects.

As detailed in other chapters of this book, the assessment of the immune system occurs with varying levels of detail, with some endpoints only added for cause. These might include, for example, cage side observations and physical examination for evidence of active infections, clinical pathology with differential hematology, flow cytometry for specific leukocyte subsets, organ weight for the thymus and spleen, and gross and microscopic assessment of primary and distributed lymphoid tissues. Some studies will also include a functional evaluation of the immune system, with evaluation of a TDAR, effector cell activation with Natural Killer cell and cytotoxic T-lymphocyte assays, and/or assessment of a delayed-type hypersensitivity response, and the pathology assessment can be expanded to include immunohistochemistry for specific leukocyte subsets.

Functional evaluation of the immune system is a standard component of the EOGRTS and DNT assessments for chemicals and pesticides (Burns-Naas et al., 2008; DeWitt et al., 2012b; Weinstock et al., 2010). A TDAR assessment is often included as part of the ePPND study for drugs, with harmonized guidance for immunotoxicity testing for drugs provided in the ICH S8 guidance (Immunotoxicity Studies for Human Pharmaceuticals). For additional detail, recommendations for the conduct of TDAR for drugs and chemicals are also available (Lebrec et al., 2014).

As a side note, the stimulation of the immune system through the conduct of a TDAR will result in substantial expansion of lymphocytes in the spleen and lymph node. For this reason, the pups allocated to the TDAR test endpoint are generally separate from those allocated to pathology endpoints. However, in the situation of a large animal JAS that includes TDAR or other immune function testing, there are not separate cohorts of animals, so it is necessary to evaluate the morphology of immune system tissues in the context of that stimulation.

Pathology findings of the immune system in a JAS most commonly include expansion or depletion of lymphocyte subsets, altered lymphocyte trafficking, and/or increased incidence or severity of naturally occurring infections or neoplasms. In practice, many trafficking and cell subtype population effects both reflect the expected and intended pharmacologic effects and tend to be reversible after a postdose period of adequate duration. Immunologic assessments are often primarily conducted in growing animals, and comparable data from adults are not always available, but comparable results have been reported. One example is that of tofacitinib, a janus kinase inhibitor, which was studied in both juvenile and adult rats and monkeys, with similar reversible findings seen at both age groups, although B-lymphocyte effects were only seen in the rat (Collinge et al., 2018).

As in studies with older animals, the tissues of the immune system in JAS are often affected when the animal is substantially stressed. If an animal declines or dies while on study, the immune tissues can be affected, and tissues from concurrent untreated controls can be helpful to understand the developmentally appropriate morphology (Parker et al., 2015). However, even with controls, in the case of moribundity or mortality, it can sometimes be challenging to distinguish nonspecific stress effects from those of specific immunotoxicity.

Naturally occurring infections in juvenile animals are generally more frequent and more severe than those seen in adult animals in toxicity studies. This reflects the fact that the immune system is seeing these agents for the first time and is also consistent with the frequency of illnesses due to viruses and bacteria in human children. Immunomodulation can affect the outcome of such infections, either by inhibiting or enhancing the inflammatory and immune response. In addition, pathology findings from sporadic infections that occur in individual animals can complicate the interpretation of the study, especially in large animals.

For studies conducted in rodents, colony and study husbandry conditions are relatively well controlled, and many are specific pathogen free. At the other extreme, most macaques used in toxicology studies harbor a number of endemic and persistent viruses, many of which are transmitted, and can result in a transient acute disease phase, during the juvenile period between 6 and 18 months of age. Most of these viruses are highly prevalent in colonies, and older monkeys are largely asymptomatic, so routine serologic screening is limited to viruses of specific concern, such as the pathogenic simian retroviruses. When evaluating findings in a macaque JAS, it is helpful to keep potential infectious agents in mind, and there are a number of helpful reviews on the topic of sporadic infections and diseases of macaques (Mansfield et al., 2014; Sasseville and Mansfield, 2010).

Assessment of Growth

Juvenile animal studies provide the ideal setting to assess potential effects of a compound on growth. Growth itself can reflect both increases in body mass, as well as elongation and maturation of long bones to establish the mature length or height. In a JAS, growth is typically assessed using a combination of measurements, including body weight and long bone length. Body weight is evaluated longitudinally during the study, while measurement of long bone length is typically conducted only at the time of necropsy. For some species such as the pig or dog, additional serial measurements such as withers height can also contribute. In general, if effects on body weight or growth have already been identified in toxicity studies with older animals, it can be assumed that such effects would be more pronounced in younger and more rapidly growing animals.

Importantly, when an effect on growth is identified from these measures, the pathology assessment can help determine whether it reflects a direct effect on the musculoskeletal system, a secondary or indirect effect on other organ systems, or a combination of the two. For example, the endocrine system plays a critical role in bone growth, so endocrine disruptors and thyrotoxicants are likely to have a notable impact. Likewise, overall growth is dependent on effective ingestion and absorption of calories and nutrients via the GI tract. In some cases, pathology of the GI tract can help explain a growth effect, but it is also important to note that effects on appetite or GI motility might not result in overt histopathology. However, gross pathology can identify reduced GI content and/or liquid fecal content, which, when accompanied by decreased food consumption or observation of diarrhea, can aid interpretation. Some effects on bone, such as osteodystrophy, might also reflect a downstream effect of primary renal or parathyroid disease. Finally, when there are direct effects on bone formation and skeletal growth, they should be assessed as reversible, as with a delay in ossification, or irreversible, as with overt dysplasias, or with premature closure of the growth plate. Some aspects of postnatal bone maturation across species have been reviewed (Zoetis et al., 2003).

Reproductive System

Male and female reproductive studies have been described in detail earlier in this chapter, and the assessment of potential effects on structure and function is also relevant to postpubertal adolescents. Thus, if reproductive toxicity has been already identified in general toxicity studies, there is no specific need to replicate those findings in a JAS. Likewise, it is often reasonable to assume that the general toxicity studies are sufficient to support the inclusion of adolescents in clinical trials without a dedicated JAS.

For animals used in toxicity testing, the juvenile period is defined by the completion of puberty; however, puberty is a process, not an event, and there are periods of transition at both onset and completion. In a dedicated JAS, one objective can be to determine whether or not the physiologic events that prepare for and initiate puberty have proceeded as expected. In practice, this is possible in relatively short (2–3 month) studies of rats or mice but requires longer study duration (6–8 months) in minipigs, and up to 12–14 months of age in dogs, to ensure maturation of spermatogenesis in males. Of note, it is not practical to assess puberty in a macaque JAS, as it would require a multiyear study.

The postnatal development of the reproductive system includes several phases, beginning perinatally, and there are detailed reviews of this process across species for both males and females (Beckman and Feuston, 2003; Howroyd et al., 2016; Laffan et al., 2018; Marty et al., 2003; Peter et al., 2016; Picut et al., 2014, 2015a, b), with the greatest level of detail available for rats. The gonads are considered a core tissue for histologic assessment in JAS for both drugs and chemicals, but this assessment must also consider other aspects of development including growth, behavior, and hormones. Of these, hormones are not usually directly measured in a JAS, but patterns of postnatal hormones have been established for some species and can be a useful reference (Bell, 2018). The pharmacologic activity of drugs must also be considered in interpreting study findings. For example, dabrafenib is a BRAF kinase inhibitor used in oncology, and a rat JAS identified premature vaginal opening as one treatment effect. Through a series of investigational studies, it was demonstrated that there was no effect on reproductive maturation, but rather, drug-related hyperkeratosis of the vaginal epithelium resulted in premature vaginal opening (Posobiec et al., 2015).

Differences in maturation processes across species must be considered for appropriate interpretation. For example, both rats and primates undergo a transient "minipuberty" shortly after birth; at this point, the HPG axis is already established, but it takes a quick "test run" for pulsatile hormone secretion, and then takes a break during the "early childhood" phase.

POSTNATAL MATURATION OF TESTES IN MALES

There are important differences between male humans and rats with regard to expansion of spermatogonia and Sertoli cells and also the formation of the BTB. There is an extensive expansion of both spermatogonia and Sertoli cells that occurs prior to the testosterone surge that initiates spermatogenesis and puberty. In the rat, this occurs between postnatal days 5–15, whereas in humans a similar expansion does not occur until late childhood (Picut et al., 2015b). This expansion is then followed by increased testosterone, and formation of the BTB. The function of the BTB includes (1) establishment of physical tight junctions between the Sertoli cells at the level of the leptotene spermatocytes, (2) functional transporters to create an appropriate "spermatogenic bath" of hormones, minerals, and essential nutrients, and (3) exclusion of the immune system as an immune privileged site to prevent autoimmunity (Mital et al., 2011; Mruk and Cheng, 2015). The rat BTB forms between postnatal day 16–18, whereas the primate BTB remains structurally and functionally immature until just before puberty (Marty et al., 2003); thus, the rat may under or overpredict testicular toxicity for some drugs or chemical toxicants (Whitney, 2012). Unlike most large animals, there is no period of reproductive quiescence recognized in rodents; spermatogenesis is initiated in parallel with formation of the BTB, although it takes several weeks to reach spermiation and spermarche.

INITIATION OF PUBERTY AND CYCLING IN FEMALES

In females, the general procession of events begins with hormonal changes of the ovaries, pituitary, and adrenal glands, and re-initiation of pulsatile hormone release, followed by physical phenotypic changes such as vaginal opening and mammary gland development. Initial cycles are irregular and often anovulatory, but eventually progress to regular estrus or menstrual cycling, as has been reviewed (Laffan et al., 2018). One species difference noted between humans and macaques is that of adrenarche, or the expansion of the zona reticularis in the adrenal cortex and with the initiation of sex steroid production. In humans, this occurs in late childhood, prior to the onset of puberty, whereas in macaques, it occurs much earlier in the preweaning period (Conley et al., 2012).

Endocrine Disruptors

The EPA EDSP includes guidance for testing to evaluate potential for endocrine disruption by pesticides and environmental chemicals. With regard to juvenile animal studies, these include in vivo thyroid and pubertal assays in the rat as well as evaluation of amphibian metamorphosis. These studies are conducted in rats exposed to the test compound for a period just after weaning (~PND 22) and through the initiation of puberty (~PND 42 for females and 53 for males). The study design and results from the program to date and a subsequent STP pathology working group were reviewed in 2013, a review of assessment of histopathology endpoints (Keane et al., 2015). The data collected in these studies from all animals include body weights, serum chemistry (including BUN and creatinine), organ weights (adrenal glands, kidneys, liver, pituitary glands, thyroid glands), and hormones (total T4 and serum TSH). In males, additional data include age at preputial separation, testis, epididymis, seminal vesicle and ventral prostate organ weights, and serum testosterone. In females, additional data include age at vaginal opening, age at first estrus, estrous cyclicity, and uterine and ovarian organ weights.

Histopathology includes evaluation, when present, of the thyroid glands, kidneys, uterus, ovaries, testis, and epididymis. In general, the histologic assessment of both ovaries and testis is qualitative, and the terms used should be consistent with those used in other studies (Creasy, 1997; Dixon et al., 2014; Keane et al., 2015). Overall, the data from studies already completed through the EDSP have identified or confirmed a number of key pathways involved in toxicities related to endocrine disruption. However, it is not feasible to test all potential chemicals using in vivo assays. Thus, the path forward also focuses on establishing clear documentation of Adverse Outcome Pathways of known relevance to environmental, animal, and human risk (Browne et al., 2017).

4.4. Models of Disease

Disease models used to understand the pharmacology of therapeutic interventions can also contribute to our understanding of toxicity related to postnatal development. The pathology of the disease model must be well characterized so that both potential benefit and disease-related toxicity can be understood. This paradigm has been most commonly applied in the area of genetic models of genetic diseases, as with spinal muscular atrophy and cystic fibrosis. Another example is that of type 1 diabetes. At present, there are numerous marketed forms of insulin, most of which include guidance for pediatric use in the label. Of course, administration of insulin to a healthy animal at a multiple of the intended clinical dose results in toxicity; in a young animal, the hypoglycemia can result in seizures and death, with concomitant neuronal necrosis. Therefore, there is little value in conducting such a study, and a separate JAS or animal model is rarely needed now for insulin analogs. In this case, the effects of hypoglycemia are well established and important to acknowledge, with the risk assessment for patients derived in part from the safety profile of the earliest insulin analogs studied in models of diabetes. For enzyme replacement therapies used for lysosomal storage diseases, there can be safety concerns regarding immunogenicity against the replacement protein or gene product in the disease model, and there also are concerns regarding toxicity related to the accumulated lysosomal enzyme substrates once the enzymatic activity is restored. Neither of these would be reflected by studies in healthy animals.

4.5. Practical Species-Specific Considerations

Rodents (Rat, Mouse)

The laboratory rat is the most commonly studied species for juvenile animal toxicity testing. The widespread use of the rat provides a deep experience base, and aids the interpretation of findings that may be unique to development, and therefore only seen in a JAS. Although it is recognized that the rat imperfectly models human postnatal development, the developmental processes, with a few exceptions, follow the same general patterns. Although there are some notable maturation differences across species, they are largely understood. The rat and mouse also have the advantage of scale: that is, a relatively large study can be conducted in a relatively small area and over a short period of time while still covering the full juvenile development period. Also, since rats are born relatively premature, early dosing can also be relevant to support safety for premature infants. Finally, if a genetic or disease model is used for a JAS, it will often be in a mouse. Thus, there are increasing JAS conducted with mice, attesting to the value of these models. However, the mouse physiology and pathology are also different from the rat, so species- and strain-relevant literature can aid in appropriate interpretation (Webster et al., 2020; Zalewska, 2019)

Rabbits

As described earlier in this chapter, the rabbit is often included as a second species in EFD studies, and in the specialized areas of ocular and immunotoxicity, but it is rarely used as a nonrodent species for general toxicity testing. For JAS, the rabbit might be considered in special cases based on pharmacologic relevance. Like the dog, rabbit litters are typically not fostered, and interventions usually exclude the neonatal period to avoid maternal rejection or cannibalism by the doe. The kits eyes open at about PND 10, but weaning does not occur until 6–8 weeks of age. Around the time of introduction of solid food through weaning, the kits are also more susceptible to enteritis, which can be fatal. In general, pathology interpretation for JAS in rabbits will rely heavily on concurrent controls, as neither extensive historical control pathology data nor comprehensive reference atlases for postnatal development are available for this species. For this reason, it can be useful to include an untreated sentinel litter to provide an age- and sex-matched tissue control if there is a need for unscheduled necropsy and pathology evaluation of individuals. Finally, the rabbit is not a good species for assessment of postnatal developmental toxicity of the female reproductive tract, as they are induced ovulators, so poorly suited to assessment of progression to functional sexual maturity in the absence of mating.

Swine

Historically, neonatal pigs have been used extensively to evaluate safety of human milk replacers and formulas, and the minipig is gaining popularity as a species for JAS. Both of these uses are in large part due to relevance of the neonatal porcine GI tract to that of neonatal humans (Downes, 2018). Although not routinely used in general toxicity studies, the minipig should be considered, if pharmacologically relevant, in the rare instance that a large animal juvenile toxicity study is warranted. Swine have a predictable gestation length and relatively large litters, which can be fostered to achieve balanced litter size and sex distribution in a JAS. There is no passive transfer of immunoglobulins in utero, so it is important to ensure that the piglets get adequate colostrum prior to allocation to a study. Also, parenteral routes of exposure and frequent blood collections can be somewhat challenging, but overall, they are relatively easy to work with. The pathology of natural diseases in domestic pigs is well described, and there are some resources for minipigs as well (McAnulty et al., 2011). Young pigs are susceptible to a number of bacterial and viral diseases during the period of most active growth. While not a comprehensive list, some of the more commonly seen diseases in pigs include coliform and clostridial enteritides in neonates; rotaviral and coronaviral enteritis and porcine circovirus disease syndrome primarily affecting weanlings; and Staphylococcal exudative dermatitis, swine dysentery due to Brachyspira hyodysenteriae, and "diamond skin disease" due to Erysipelothrix rhusiopathiae, which can affect pigs of all ages, but often with more severe disease in younger pigs. The use of specific pathogen-free breeding colonies and optimized husbandry can minimize, but not fully eliminate, the risk of infectious disease outbreaks. In older piglets, there can be some challenges in predicting the timing of onset of puberty and progression to sexual maturity, which most likely reflecting the importance of environmental cues during maturation. For example, females housed in a single sex environment will maintain anovulatory cycles for a longer period, whereas presence of a mature boar can accelerate this process (Peter et al., 2016).

Dogs

The dog is infrequently used for JAS, and typically chosen to address a pharmacokinetic or metabolism deficiency of the rodent, or when a potential toxicity of developmental concern has been identified in older dogs. The postnatal ontogeny of canine organ systems, as well as the pathology of developing pups, are largely derived from the primary veterinary literature for companion animal care and diagnostic pathology. Specific attention to the neonate and CNS development is critical for successful evaluation (Lavely, 2006; Lawler, 2008). In most studies with dogs, the dosing period is delayed until the second week postnatal to allow the pups to get colostrum and adequately bond with the dam. Litters are not typically fostered, so flexibility regarding sex balance is needed. In all studies with litters, but especially in rabbits and dogs which retain an intact genetic litter, attention and recording of maternal care behavior can also be helpful. Laboratory dogs that come from SPF colonies should have few infectious agents.

Nonhuman Primates

Within the scope of laboratory animal species used for toxicity testing, NHPs represent the phylogenetically closest relative to humans. Of these, the cynomolgus monkey, *Macaca fascicularis*, is one of the most common NHP species studied, but is not routinely appropriate for JAS unless there is a clear need for a study and other species are not relevant or appropriate. In a recent FDA review, NHPs were only requested for JAS with highly specific biopharmaceuticals, and where there was no relevant species alternative. In general, JAS with NHP have included postweaning monkeys of 9–15 months of age (Chellman et al., 2009), or have looked in isolation at the neonatal period to understand drug disposition and toxicity. NHP have also been studied for some pediatric-first indications for diseases that cannot be readily studied clinically in adults. In some cases, a JAS is requested in order to better understand effects on cognition through learning and memory tests (Cappon et al., 2012; Inoue et al., 2014). There are a number of challenges in the use of NHP for JAS, starting with the litter size of 1 for macaques, and the

requirement for maternal care especially over the first 3–6 months postnatal. Marmosets are smaller, and frequently twin, but they require both the dam and sire to care for the infants, so there is a similar ratio of adults to juveniles. Importantly, although the dam is not dosed directly, she remains part of the test system during the preweaning period. As noted earlier in the DIT section, the first 12–18 months postnatal is a period when many young macaques are introduced to endemic viruses such as lymphocryptovirus, rhesus rhadinovirus, cytomegalovirus, and polyomavirus, and they are also susceptible to community spread of bacterial pathogens such as *Shigella flexneri* leading to dysentery, or *Moraxella catarrhalis* leading to epistaxis.

4.6. Guidelines and Regional Legislation

As with DART testing, there are both international and regional guidance documents to clarify current regulatory expectations, and the US and EU also have legislation in support of pediatrics. The guidance typically pertains to pediatric drug development, as with the recently posted Step 4 ICH S11, or to environmental and agrochemical safety assessment relevant to children, as in the OECD and EPA guidelines. A detailed review of existing guidelines is beyond the scope of this chapter, but a few guidelines specifically relevant to the juvenile period of birth through puberty are summarized in Table 7.5 below. Each of the guidelines in the table can be found through the ICH, FDA, EPA, or OECD websites, as listed in the references.

There is a battery of testing guidelines from the EPA and OECD to better understand the safety of pesticides and toxic chemicals, and a subset of these are relevant to developmental or juvenile toxicity testing. However, there are also some differences between similar guidelines (e.g., for assessment of DNT) that prevent full alignment within a single study design. A workshop addressed similarities and differences between the guidelines with the intent to clarify objectives and initiate a path toward better harmonization of DNT (Li et al., 2017). This review includes perspectives from several pathologists with specific expertise in

TABLE 7.5   Regulatory Guidance for Juvenile Animal Testing

Source[a]	Title	General utility
ICH	• S11: Nonclinical safety testing in support of development of Pediatric Pharmaceuticals (ICH, 2020b)	• Harmonized nonclinical guidance for pediatric medicines (primary resource)
FDA	• Nonclinical safety evaluation of pediatric drug Products (FDA, 2006)	• Regional nonclinical guidance for pediatric medicines, USA
EMA	• Need for nonclinical testing in Juvenile animals on human pharmaceuticals for Pediatric Indications (EMA, 2008)	• Regional nonclinical guidance for pediatric medicines, EU
MHLW	• Guideline on the nonclinical safety study in Juvenile animals for Pediatric Drugs (MHLW, 2012)	• Regional nonclinical guidance for pediatric medicines, Japan
EPA	• OPPTS guideline 890.1500: Pubertal development and thyroid function in the intact Juvenile/Peripubertal male Rats (EPA, 2009a) • OPPTS guideline 890.1450: Pubertal development and thyroid function in the intact Juvenile/Peripubertal female Rats (EPA, 2009b) • OPPTS guideline 870.6200: Neurotoxicity screening Battery (EPA, 1998c) • OPPTS guideline 870.6300: Developmental Neurotoxicity (EPA, 1998d)	• Primary in vivo mammalian tests for pesticides and hazardous substances on endocrine disruption • Resources when concern for developmental neurotoxicity (may be incorporated into a reproductive toxicity study)
OECD	• Test no. 416: Two generation reproduction toxicity Study (OECD, 2001) • Test no. 426: Developmental neurotoxicity Study (OECD, 2007) • Test no. 443: Extended one generation reproductive toxicity Study (OECD, 2018b)	• Primary resources for reproductive and developmental toxicity of chemicals • In vivo mammalian tests for pesticides and hazardous substances on developmental neurotoxicity • Alternative reproductive and developmental toxicity test for chemicals

[a] All source links current as of November 2020 are provided in the reference list according to the originating institution or organization.

developmental neuropathology and is an excellent resource for further understanding of the history and scientific objectives of both the OECD and US EPA guidelines. It is a useful companion to the comprehensive recommended best practices endorsed by the STP (Bolon et al., 2006) and subsequent efforts to optimize translational relevance (Sharma et al., 2016).

Importantly, although the studies described in OECD and EPA guidelines are relevant to safety assessment for children, there are only few stand-alone studies, such as those for pubertal development and thyroid function, where exposure is limited to delivery of the test substance to juvenile animals. These are included in the EPA 890 series of studies used to evaluate potential for endocrine disruption. The EOGRTS (OECD, 2018b) has been touted as a replacement for the Two-Generation Reproductive Toxicity Study (OECD, 2001), although the scale and duration of the two are similar when immunotoxicity and/or neurotoxicity endpoints are added. For agrochemicals such as pesticides, the Two-Generation Reproductive Toxicity Study (OECD, 2001) remains fairly standard, with additional attention and concern related to potential thyroid effects in pregnant dams that could have effects on neural development in offspring.

For medicinal products, the recently adopted ICH S11 guidance on Nonclinical safety testing in support of development of pediatric pharmaceuticals has been agreed by ICH member countries and is expected to eventually fully replace regional guidance documents (Table 7.5). Importantly, the ICH S11 guidance clarifies expectations both regarding the WoE approach to determine the need for a study and specific aspects of study design while still retaining flexibility for appropriate program-specific adaptations (ICH, 2020b).

At a high level, many of these guidelines emphasize the value of juvenile toxicity testing to cover the knowledge gap left after considering data from PPND and general toxicity studies or to enable early pediatric use of a medicinal product even before the PPND data are available.

For each of the EPA or OECD guidelines, there are specific recommendations for clinical, gross, and histopathologic assessments, as well as organ weights. For medicinal products, the ICH S11 provides guidance that allows some flexibility in the approach to pathology endpoints in JAS (ICH, 2020b). For animals allocated to pathology endpoints, it is recommended that blood is collected for terminal clinical pathology, and that a complete necropsy is performed, including gross examination, organ weights, and preservation of tissues. For histopathology, there are several major tissues listed as "core": bone/marrow, brain, GI tract, heart, kidney, liver, lung, ovary, and testis. Overall, these are tissues that are expected to be both generally informative and potentially sensitive to developmental effects. In addition, histopathology should include both gross lesions and previously identified target organs. Finally, additional expanded pathology assessments may be warranted depending on the expected or observed pharmacology and toxicity.

5. CONCLUSIONS

DART testing falls under the category of specialized toxicity studies conducted to inform both environmental health regulations and human risk assessment for appropriate support of clinical trials in the case of drugs and labeling for both drugs and chemicals. Likewise, dedicated JAS are generally conducted to support a specific pediatric population. These complex studies often incorporate assessments that are not part of a standard toxicity study. Therefore, when clinical, gross, and histopathology are included, they should be interpreted in the context of the results from those other endpoints. Pathology is often limited to a specific subset of reproductive tissues. In EFD studies, the focus is on morphologic development of the fetus with external, skeletal, and gross soft tissue evaluations, and pathology endpoints would be limited in scope and only conducted for cause. Postnatal development can be assessed from several study types described herein: EOGRT, ePPND, and JAS.

In addition, some chemicals, such as pesticides, are screened for potential endocrine disruption that could impact initiation and progression through puberty. The pathologist must be well informed of typical developmental progression and milestones across organ systems and species. There can also be challenges to pathology interpretation, especially in rapidly growing immature animals, as there can be increased sporadic natural disease and mortality as compared to the prescreened healthy young adult animals used more typically in toxicity studies. In general, a strong partnership between pathologist and reproductive toxicologist is needed in the design, conduct, and interpretation of these important studies.

ABBREVIATIONS

ACE Angiotensin converting enzyme
ADME Absorption, distribution, metabolism, excretion
BCRP Breast cancer resistance protein
BTB Blood–testis barrier
CNS Central nervous system
DART Developmental and reproductive toxicity
DIT Developmental immunotoxicity
DNT Developmental neurotoxicity
DRF Dose range-finding
EDSP Endocrine Disruptor Screening Program
EFD Embryo–fetal development
EOGRTS extended one-generation reproductive toxicity study
ePPND Enhanced pre- and postnatal development
FDA Food and drug administration
FSH Follicle-stimulating hormone
GABA Gamma-aminobutyric acid
GFR Glomerular filtration rate
GI Gastrointestinal
GLP Good laboratory practices
GnRH Gonadotrophin releasing hormone
HPG Hypothalamic–pituitary–gonad

ICH International Council for Harmonisation
JAS Juvenile animal study
LH Luteinizing hormone
LOAEL Lowest observed adverse effect level
mAb monoclonal antibody
NHP Nonhuman primate and cynomolgus monkey
NMDA N-methyl-D-aspartate
NOAEL No observed adverse effect level
OECD Organisation for Economic Co-operation and Development
pEFD Preliminary EFD
PGP P-glycoprotein
PPND Pre- and postnatal development
STP Society of Toxicologic Pathology
TDAR T-cell–dependent antigen response
US EPA United States Environmental Protection Agency
WGTA Wisconsin general testing apparatus
WOCBP Women of child-bearing potential
WoE Weight of evidence

REFERENCES

Adams CE: Maintenance of pregnancy relative to the presence of few embryos in the rabbit, *J Endocrinol* 48:243–249, 1970.

Adams MR, Kaplan JR, Koritnik DR: Psychosocial influences on ovarian endocrine and ovulatory function in *Macaca fascicularis, Physiol Behav* 35:935–940, 1985.

Aldawood N, Alrezaki A, Alanazi S, et al.: Acrylamide impairs ovarian function by promoting apoptosis and affecting reproductive hormone release, steroidogenesis and autophagy-related genes: an in vivo study, *Ecotoxicol Environ Saf* 197:110595, 2020.

Allegaert K, van den Anker J: Ontogeny of phase I metabolism of drugs, *J Clin Pharmacol* 59(Suppl 1):S33–S41, 2019.

Alves-Lopes JP, Stukenborg JB: Testicular organoids: a new model to study the testicular microenvironment in vitro? *Hum Reprod Update* 24:176–191, 2018.

Andersson H, Rehm S, Stanislaus D, et al.: Scientific and regulatory policy committee (SRPC) paper: assessment of circulating hormones in nonclinical toxicity studies III. female reproductive hormones, *Toxicol Pathol* 41:921–934, 2013.

Astroff AB, Ray SE, Rowe LM, et al.: Frozen-sectioning yields similar results as traditional methods for fetal cephalic examination in the rat, *Teratology* 66:77–84, 2002.

Auroux M, Nawar NN, Rizkalla N: Testicular aging: vascularization and gametogenesis modifications in the Wistar rat, *Arch Androl* 14:115–121, 1985.

Auyeung-Kim DJ, Devalaraja MN, Migone TS, et al.: Developmental and peri-postnatal study in cynomolgus monkeys with belimumab, a monoclonal antibody directed against B-lymphocyte stimulator, *Reprod Toxicol* 28:443–455, 2009.

Baert Y, Ruetschle I, Cools W, et al.: A multi-organ-chip co-culture of liver and testis equivalents: a first step toward a systemic male reprotoxicity model, *Hum Reprod* 35:1029–1044, 2020.

Bailey GP, Wise LD, Buschmann J, et al.: Pre- and postnatal developmental toxicity study design for pharmaceuticals, *Birth Defects Res B Dev Reprod Toxicol* 86:437–445, 2009.

Bailey SA, Zidell RH, Perry RW: Relationships between organ weight and body/brain weight in the rat: what is the best analytical endpoint? *Toxicol Pathol* 32:448–466, 2004.

Barrow PC: Reproductive toxicity testing for pharmaceuticals under ICH, *Reprod Toxicol* 28:172–179, 2009.

Beckman DA, Feuston M: Landmarks in the development of the female reproductive system, *Birth Defects Res B Dev Reprod Toxicol* 68:137–143, 2003.

Bell MR: Comparing postnatal development of gonadal hormones and associated social behaviors in rats, mice, and humans, *Endocrinology* 159:2596–2613, 2018.

Beyer BK, Chernoff N, Danielsson BR, et al.: ILSI/HESI maternal toxicity workshop summary: maternal toxicity and its impact on study design and data interpretation, *Birth Defects Res B Dev Reprod Toxicol* 92:36–51, 2011.

Bishop JB, Morris RW, Seely JC, et al.: Alterations in the reproductive patterns of female mice exposed to xenobiotics, *Fundam Appl Toxicol* 40:191–204, 1997.

Blazak WF, Ernst TL, Stewart BE: Potential indicators of reproductive toxicity: testicular sperm production and epididymal sperm number, transit time, and motility in Fischer 344 rats, *Fundam Appl Toxicol* 5:1097–1103, 1985.

Blazak WF, Treinen KA, Juniewicz PE: Application of testicular sperm head counts in the assessment of male reproductive toxicity. In Chapin RE, Heindel JJ, editors: *Methods in toxicology*, San Diego, 1993, Academic Press, Inc., pp 86–94.

Bluemel J, Korte S, Schenck E, et al., editors: *The nonhuman primate in nonclinical drug development and safety assessment*, Boca Raton, FL, 2015, Academic Press.

Bolon B, Butt MT: *Fundamental neuropathology for pathologists and toxicologists*, Hoboken, New Jersey, 2011, John Wiley & Sons, Inc.

Bolon B, Garman R, Jensen K, et al.: A 'best practices' approach to neuropathologic assessment in developmental neurotoxicity testing–for today, *Toxicol Pathol* 34:296–313, 2006.

Bowman CJ, Breslin WJ, Connor AV, et al.: Placental transfer of Fc-containing biopharmaceuticals across species, an industry survey analysis, *Birth Defects Res B Dev Reprod Toxicol* 98:459–485, 2013.

Bowman CJ, Chapin RE: Goldilocks' determination of what new in vivo data are "just right" for different common drug development scenarios, Part 1, *Birth Defects Res B Dev Reprod Toxicol* 107:185–194, 2016.

Bowman CJ, Chmielewski G, Oneda S, et al.: Embryo-fetal developmental toxicity of figitumumab, an anti-insulin-like growth factor-1 receptor (IGF-1R) monoclonal antibody, in cynomolgus monkeys, *Birth Defects Res B Dev Reprod Toxicol* 89:326–338, 2010.

Bowman CJ, Evans M, Cummings T, et al.: Developmental toxicity assessment of tanezumab, an anti-nerve growth factor monoclonal antibody, in cynomolgus monkeys (*Macaca fascicularis*), *Reprod Toxicol* 53:105–118, 2015.

Boyce RW, Varela A, Chouinard L, et al.: Infant cynomolgus monkeys exposed to denosumab in utero exhibit an osteoclast-poor osteopetrotic-like skeletal phenotype at birth and in the early postnatal period, *Bone* 64:314–325, 2014.

Brannen KC, Fenton SE, Hansen DK, et al.: Developmental toxicology: new directions workshop: refining testing strategies and study designs, *Birth Defects Res B Dev Reprod Toxicol* 92:404–412, 2011.

Bregman CL, Adler RR, Morton DG, et al.: Recommended tissue list for histopathologic examination in repeat-dose toxicity and carcinogenicity studies: a proposal of the society of toxicologic pathology (STP), *Toxicol Pathol* 31:252–253, 2003.

Breslin WJ, Hilbish KG, Cannady EA, et al.: Fertility and embryo-fetal development assessment in rats and rabbits with Evacetrapib: a cholesteryl ester transfer protein inhibitor, *Birth Defects Res* 109:513–527, 2017a.

Breslin WJ, Hilbish KG, Cannady EA, et al.: Prenatal and postnatal assessment in rabbits with Evacetrapib: a cholesteryl ester transfer protein inhibitor, *Birth Defects Res* 109:486–496, 2017b.

Breslin WJ, Hilbish KG, Martin JA, et al.: Developmental toxicity and fertility assessment in rabbits with tabalumab: a human IgG4 monoclonal antibody, *Birth Defects Res B Dev Reprod Toxicol* 104:117–128, 2015.

Bretveld RW, Thomas CM, Scheepers PT, et al.: Pesticide exposure: the hormonal function of the female reproductive system disrupted? *Reprod Biol Endocrinol* 4:30, 2006.

Brown NA, Fabro S: The value of animal teratogenicity testing for predicting human risk, *Clin Obstet Gynecol* 26:467–477, 1983.

Browne P, Noyes PD, Casey WM, et al.: Application of adverse outcome pathways to U.S. EPA's endocrine disruptor screening program, *Environ Health Perspect* 125:096001, 2017.

Bruni JE, Del Bigio MR, Cardoso ER, et al.: Hereditary hydrocephalus in laboratory animals and humans, *Exp Pathol* 35:239–246, 1988.

Bueters R, Bael A, Gasthuys E, et al.: Ontogeny and cross-species comparison of pathways involved in drug absorption, distribution, metabolism, and excretion in neonates (review): kidney, *Drug Metab Dispos* 48:353–367, 2020.

Burns-Naas LA, Hastings KL, Ladics GS, et al.: What's so special about the developing immune system? *Int J Toxicol* 27:223–254, 2008.

Buse E, Zöller M, Van Esch E: The macaque ovary, with special reference to the cynomolgus macaque (*Macaca fascicularis*), *Toxicol Pathol* 36:24S–66S, 2008.

Bussiere JL, Moffat G, Zhou L, et al.: Assessment of menstrual cycle length in cynomolgus monkeys as a female fertility endpoint of a biopharmaceutical in a 6 month toxicity study, *Reg Toxicol Pharmacol* 66:269–278, 2013.

Butterstein GM, Mann DR, Gould K, et al.: Prolonged inhibition of normal ovarian cycles in the rat and cynomolgus monkeys following a single s.c. injection of danazol, *Hum Reprod* 12:1409–1415, 1997.

Campion SN, Bowman CJ, Cappon GD, et al.: Developmental toxicity of lersivirine in rabbits when administered throughout organogenesis and when limited to sensitive windows of axial skeletal development, *Birth Defects Res B Dev Reprod Toxicol* 95:250–261, 2012a.

Campion SN, Carvallo FR, Chapin RE, et al.: Comparative assessment of the timing of sexual maturation in male Wistar Han and Sprague-Dawley rats, *Reprod Toxicol* 38:16–24, 2013.

Campion SN, Davenport SJ, Nowland WS, et al.: Sensitive windows of skeletal development in rabbits determined by hydroxyurea exposure at different times throughout gestation, *Birth Defects Res B Dev Reprod Toxicol* 95:238–249, 2012b.

Campion SN, Han B, Cappon GD, et al.: Decreased maternal and fetal cholesterol following maternal bococizumab (anti-PCSK9 monoclonal antibody) administration does not affect rat embryo-fetal development, *Reg Toxicol Pharmacol* 73:562–570, 2015.

Cappon GD, Bailey GP, Buschmann J, et al.: Juvenile animal toxicity study designs to support pediatric drug development, *Birth Defects Res B Dev Reprod Toxicol* 86:463–469, 2009.

Cappon GD, Bowman CJ, Hurtt ME, et al.: Object discrimination reversal as a method to assess cognitive impairment in nonhuman primate enhanced pre- and postnatal developmental (ePPND) studies: statistical power analysis, *Birth Defects Res B Dev Reprod Toxicol* 95:354–362, 2012.

Cappon GD, Cook JC, Hurtt ME: Relationship between cyclooxygenase 1 and 2 selective inhibitors and fetal development when administered to rats and rabbits during the sensitive periods for heart development and midline closure, *Birth Defects Res B Dev Reprod Toxicol* 68:47–56, 2003a.

Cappon GD, Fleeman TL, Chapin RE, et al.: Effects of feed restriction during organogenesis on embryo-fetal development in rabbit, *Birth Defects Res B Dev Reprod Toxicol* 74:424–430, 2005.

Cappon GD, Gupta U, Cook JC, et al.: Comparison of the developmental toxicity of aspirin in rabbits when administered throughout organogenesis or during sensitive windows of development, *Birth Defects Res B Dev Reprod Toxicol* 68:38–46, 2003b.

Cappon GD, Potter D, Hurtt ME, et al.: Sensitivity of male reproductive endpoints in nonhuman primate toxicity studies: a statistical power analysis, *Reprod Toxicol* 41:67–72, 2013.

Carney EW, Kimmel CA: Interpretation of skeletal variations for human risk assessment: delayed ossification and wavy ribs, *Birth Defects Res B Dev Reprod Toxicol* 80:473–496, 2007.

Carney EW, Zablotny CL, Marty MS, et al.: The effects of feed restriction during in utero and postnatal development in rats, *Toxicol Sci* 82:237–249, 2004.

Chahoud I, Paumgartten FJ: Relationships between fetal body weight of Wistar rats at term and the extent of skeletal ossification, *Braz J Med Biol Res* 38:565–575, 2005.

Chandra SA, Adler RR: Frequency of different estrous stages in purpose-bred beagles: a retrospective study, *Toxicol Pathol* 36:944–949, 2008.

Chapin R, Weinbauer G, Thibodeau MS, et al.: Summary of the HESI consortium studies exploring circulating inhibin B as a potential biomarker of testis damage in the rat, *Birth Defects Res B Dev Reprod Toxicol* 98:110–118, 2013.

Chapin RE, Creasy DM: Assessment of circulating hormones in regulatory toxicity studies II. Male reproductive hormones, *Toxicol Pathol* 40:1063–1078, 2012.

Chapin RE, Gulati DK, Barnes LH, et al.: The effects of feed restriction on reproductive function in Sprague-Dawley rats, *Fundam Appl Toxicol* 20:23–29, 1993a.

Chapin RE, Gulati DK, Fail PA, et al.: The effects of feed restriction on reproductive function in Swiss CD-1 mice, *Fundam Appl Toxicol* 20:15–22, 1993b.

Chapin RE, Sloane RA, Haseman JK: Reproductive endpoints in general toxicity studies: are they predictive? *Reprod Toxicol* 12:489–494, 1998.

Chapin RE, Winton TR, Nowland WS, et al.: Primary cell cultures for understanding rat epididymal inflammation, *Birth Defects Res B Dev Reprod Toxicol* 101:325–332, 2014.

Chellman GJ, Bussiere JL, Makori N, et al.: Developmental and reproductive toxicology studies in nonhuman primates, *Birth Defects Res B Dev Reprod Toxicol* 86:446–462, 2009.

Chernoff N, Rogers EH, Gage MI, et al.: The relationship of maternal and fetal toxicity in developmental toxicology bioassays with notes on the biological significance of the "no observed adverse effect level", *Reprod Toxicol* 25:192–202, 2008.

Clark RL, Robertson RT, Peter CP, et al.: Association between adverse maternal and embryo-fetal effects in norfloxacin-treated and food-deprived rabbits, *Fundam Appl Toxicol* 7: 272–286, 1986.

Clarke DO, Hilbish KG, Waters DG, et al.: Assessment of ixekizumab, an interleukin-17A monoclonal antibody, for potential effects on reproduction and development, including immune system function, in cynomolgus monkeys, *Reprod Toxicol* 58:160–173, 2015.

Clarkson J, d'Anglemont de Tassigny X, Moreno AS, et al.: Kisspeptin-GPR54 signaling is essential for preovulatory gonadotropin-releasing hormone neuron activation and the luteinizing hormone surge, *J Neurosci* 28:8691–8697, 2008.

Clements JM, Hawkes RG, Jones D, et al.: Predicting the safety of medicines in pregnancy: a workshop report, *Reprod Toxicol* 93:199–210, 2020.

Cline JM, Wood CE, Vidal JD, et al.: Selected background findings and interpretation of common lesions in the female reproductive system in macaques, *Toxicol Pathol* 36: 142s–163s, 2008.

Collinge M, Ball DJ, Bowman CJ, et al.: Immunologic effects of chronic administration of tofacitinib, a Janus kinase inhibitor, in cynomolgus monkeys and rats - comparison of juvenile and adult responses, *Reg Toxicol Pharmacol* 94:306–322, 2018.

Collins TF: History and evolution of reproductive and developmental toxicology guidelines, *Curr Pharmaceut Des* 12: 1449–1465, 2006.

Conley AJ, Bernstein RM, Nguyen AD: Adrenarche in nonhuman primates: the evidence for it and the need to redefine it, *J Endocrinol* 214:121–131, 2012.

Cooper RL, Goldman JM, Rehnberg GL: Neuroendocrine control of reproductive function in the aging female rodent, *J Am Geriatr Soc* 34:735–751, 1986.

Cooper RL, Stoker TE, Tyrey L, et al.: Atrazine disrupts the hypothalamic control of pituitary-ovarian function, *Toxicol Sci* 53:297–307, 2000.

Cooper TK, Gabrielson KL: Spontaneous lesions in the reproductive tract and mammary gland of female nonhuman primates, *Birth Defects Res B Dev Reprod Toxicol* 80: 149–170, 2007.

Creasy D, Bube A, de Rijk E, et al.: Proliferative and non-proliferative lesions of the rat and mouse male reproductive system, *Toxicol Pathol* 40:40S–121S, 2012.

Creasy DM: Evaluation of testicular toxicity in safety evaluation studies: the appropriate use of spermatogenic staging, *Toxicol Pathol* 25:119–131, 1997.

Creasy DM: Pathogenesis of male reproductive toxicity, *Toxicol Pathol* 29:64–76, 2001.

Creasy DM: Evaluation of testicular toxicology: a synopsis and discussion of the recommendations proposed by the society of toxicologic pathology, *Birth Defects Res B Dev Reprod Toxicol* 68:408–415, 2003.

Crofton KM, Foss JA, Hass U, et al.: Undertaking positive control studies as part of developmental neurotoxicity testing: a report from the ILSI Research Foundation/Risk Science Institute expert working group on neuro-developmental endpoints, *Neurotoxicol Teratol* 30:266–287, 2008.

Cyr DG, Dufresne J, Gregory M: Cellular junctions in the epididymis, a critical parameter for understanding male reproductive toxicology, *Reprod Toxicol* 81:207–219, 2018.

De Schaepdrijver LM, Annaert PPJ, Chen CL: Ontogeny of ADME processes during postnatal development in man and preclinical species: a comprehensive review, *Drug Metab Dispos* 47:295, 2019.

de Zwart L, Scholten M, Monbaliu JG, et al.: The ontogeny of drug metabolizing enzymes and transporters in the rat, *Reprod Toxicol* 26:220–230, 2008.

Dent MP: Strengths and limitations of using repeat-dose toxicity studies to predict effects on fertility, *Regul Toxicol Pharmacol* 48:241–258, 2007.

Dere E, Wilson SK, Anderson LM, et al.: From the cover: sperm molecular biomarkers are sensitive indicators of testicular injury following subchronic model toxicant exposure, *Toxicol Sci* 153:327–340, 2016.

Derscheid RJ, Ackermann MR: The innate immune system of the perinatal lung and responses to respiratory syncytial virus infection, *Vet Pathol* 50:827–841, 2013.

DeSesso JM: Vascular ontogeny within selected thoracoabdominal organs and the limbs, *Reprod Toxicol* 70:3–20, 2017.

DeSesso JM, Scialli AR: Bone development in laboratory mammals used in developmental toxicity studies, *Birth Defects Res* 110:1157–1187, 2018.

DeSesso JM, Williams AL, Ahuja A, et al.: The placenta, transfer of immunoglobulins, and safety assessment of biopharmaceuticals in pregnancy, *Crit Rev Toxicol* 42:185–210, 2012.

DeWitt JC, Peden-Adams MM, Keil DE, et al.: Current status of developmental immunotoxicity: early-life patterns and testing, *Toxicol Pathol* 40:230–236, 2012a.

DeWitt JC, Peden-Adams MM, Keil DE, et al.: Developmental immunotoxicity (DIT): assays for evaluating effects of exogenous agents on development of the immune system, *Curr Protoc Toxicol* 51(1):18.15.1–18.15.14, 2012b.

Dittrich R, Beckmann MW, Oppelt PG, et al.: Thyroid hormone receptors and reproduction, *J Reprod Immunol* 90:58–66, 2011.

Dixon D, Alison R, Bach U, et al.: Nonproliferative and proliferative lesions of the rat and mouse female reproductive system, *J Toxicol Pathol* 27:1S–107S, 2014.

Dostal LA, Juneau P, Rothwell CE: Repeated analysis of semen parameters in beagle dogs during a 2-year study with the HMG-CoA reductase inhibitor, atorvastatin, *Toxicol Sci* 61:128–134, 2001.

Downes N, Mullins P: The development of myelin in the brain of the juvenile rat, *Toxicol Pathol* 42:913–922, 2014.

Downes NJ: Consideration of the development of the gastrointestinal tract in the choice of species for regulatory juvenile studies, *Birth Defects Res* 110:56–62, 2018.

Dreef HC, Van Esch E, De Rijk EP: Spermatogenesis in the cynomolgus monkey (*Macaca fascicularis*): a practical guide for routine morphological staging, *Toxicol Pathol* 35:395–404, 2007.

Enright BP, Compton DR, Collins N, et al.: Comparative effects of interferon alpha-2b and pegylated interferon alpha-2b on menstrual cycles and ovarian hormones in cynomolgus monkeys, *Birth Defects Res B Dev Reprod Toxicol* 86:29–39, 2009.

Enright BP, Leach MW, Pelletier G, et al.: Effects of an antagonist of neurokinin receptors 1, 2 and 3 on reproductive hormones in male beagle dogs, *Birth Defects Res B Dev Reprod Toxicol* 89:517–525, 2010.

Enright BP, Tornesi B, Weinbauer GF, et al.: Male and female fertility assessment in the cynomolgus monkey following administration of ABT-874, a human Anti-IL-12/23p40 monoclonal antibody, *Birth Defects Res B Dev Reprod Toxicol* 95:421–430, 2012a.

Enright BP, Tornesi B, Weinbauer GF, et al.: Pre- and postnatal development in the cynomolgus monkey following administration of ABT-874, a human anti-IL-12/23p40 monoclonal antibody, *Birth Defects Res B Dev Reprod Toxicol* 95:431–443, 2012b.

EMA: *Guideline on the need for non-clinical testing in juvenile animals of pharmaceuticals for paediatric indications (EMEA/ CHMP/SWP/169215/2005)*, 2008. Retrieved from: https:// www.ema.europa.eu/en/documents/scientific-guideline/ guideline-need-non-clinical-testing-juvenile-animals-phar maceuticals-paediatric-indications_en.pdf.

EPA: *OPPTS 870.3700 prenatal developmental toxicity study (EPA-712-C-98-207)*, 1998a. Retrieved from: https://www.regulati ons.gov/document?D=EPA-HQ-OPPT-2009-0156-0017.

EPA: *OPPTS 870.3800 reproduction and fertility effects (EPA-712-C-98-208)*, 1998b. Retrieved from: https://www.regulati ons.gov/document?D=EPA-HQ-OPPT-2009-0156-0018.

EPA: *OPPTS 870.6200 neurotoxicity screening battery (EPA-712-C-98-238)*, 1998c. Retrieved from: https://www.regulati ons.gov/document?D=EPA-HQ-OPPT-2009-0156-0041.

EPA: *OPPTS 870.6300 developmental neurotoxicity (EPA-712-C-98-239)*, 1998d. Retrieved from: https://www.regulations. gov/document?D=EPA-HQ-OPPT-2009-0156-0042.

EPA: *OPPTS 890.1500 pubertal development and thyroid Function in intact juvenile/peripubertal male rats assay (EPA 740-C-09-012)*, 2009a. Retrieved from: https://www.regulations. gov/document?D=EPA-HQ-OPPT-2009-0576-0010.

EPA: *OPPTS 890.1450 pubertal development and thyroid function in intact juvenile/peripubertal female rats assay (EPA 740-C-09-009)*, 2009b. Retrieved from: https://www.regulations. gov/document?D=EPA-HQ-OPPT-2009-0576-0009.

Everds NE, Snyder PW, Bailey KL, et al.: Interpreting stress responses during routine toxicity studies: a review of the biology, impact, and assessment, *Toxicol Pathol* 41:560–614, 2013.

FDA: *Nonclinical safety Evaluation of pediatric drug products (2003D-0001)*, 2006. Retrieved from: https://www.fda. gov/media/119658/download.

FDA: *Reproductive and developmental toxicities-integrating study results to assess concerns (FDA-1999-N-0082)*, 2011. Retrieved from: https://www.fda.gov/media/72231/download.

FDA: *Testicular toxicity: evaluation during drug development (FDA-2015-D-2306)*, 2018. Retrieved from: https://www. fda.gov/media/117948/download.

FDA: *Oncology pharmaceuticals: reproductive toxicity testing and labeling recommendations (FDA-2017-D-2165)*, 2019. Retrieved from: https://www.fda.gov/media/124829/download.

Fisher Jr JE, Ravindran A, Elayan I: CDER experience with juvenile animal studies for CNS drugs, *Int J Toxicol* 38:88–95, 2019.

Flaws JA, Doerr JK, Sipes IG, et al.: Destruction of preantral follicles in adult rats by 4-vinyl-1-cyclohexene diepoxide, *Reprod Toxicol* 8:509–514, 1994.

Fleeman TL, Cappon GD, Chapin RE, et al.: The effects of feed restriction during organogenesis on embryo-fetal development in the rat, *Birth Defects Res B Dev Reprod Toxicol* 74:442–449, 2005.

Foley GL: Overview of male reproductive pathology, *Toxicol Pathol* 29:49–63, 2001.

Foster PM: Regulatory Forum opinion piece: new testing paradigms for reproductive and developmental toxicity–the NTP modified one generation study and OECD 443, *Toxicol Pathol* 42:1165–1167, 2014.

Frazier KS: Species differences in renal development and associated developmental nephrotoxicity, *Birth Defects Res* 109:1243–1256, 2017.

French J, Halliday J, Scott M, et al.: Retinal folding in the term rabbit fetus-developmental abnormality or fixation artifact? *Reprod Toxicol* 26:262–266, 2008.

Frohberg H, Gleich J, Unkelbach HD: Reproduction toxicological studies on cefazedone, *Arzneimittelforschung* 29:419–423, 1979.

Garman RH, Li AA, Kaufmann W, et al.: Recommended methods for brain processing and quantitative analysis in rodent developmental neurotoxicity studies, *Toxicol Pathol* 44:14–42, 2016.

Goedken MJ, Kerlin RL, Morton D: Spontaneous and age-related testicular findings in beagle dogs, *Toxicol Pathol* 36:465–471, 2008.

Goldman JM, Murr AS, Cooper RL: The rodent estrous cycle: characterization of vaginal cytology and its utility in toxicological studies, *Birth Defects Res B Dev Reprod Toxicol* 80:84–97, 2007.

Gondos B, Zemjanis R, Cockett AT: Ultrastructural alterations in the seminiferous epithelium of immobilized monkeys, *Am J Pathol* 61:497–518, 1970.

Gougeon A: Regulation of ovarian follicular development in primates: facts and hypotheses, *Endocr Rev* 17:121–155, 1996.

Grattan DR, Kokay IC: Prolactin: a pleiotropic neuroendocrine hormone, *J Neuroendocrinol* 20:752–763, 2008.

Green EL: The inheritance of a rib variation in the rabbit, *Anat Rec* 74:47–60, 1939.

Grossmann H, Weinbauer GF, Baker A, et al.: Enhanced normograms and pregnancy outcome analysis in nonhuman primate developmental toxicity studies, *Reprod Toxicol* 95:29–36, 2020.

Guilloteau P, Zabielski R, Hammon HM, et al.: Nutritional programming of gastrointestinal tract development. Is the pig a good model for man? *Nutr Res Rev* 23:4–22, 2010.

Halpern WG, Ameri M, Bowman CJ, et al.: Scientific and regulatory policy committee points to consider review: inclusion of reproductive and pathology end points for assessment of reproductive and developmental toxicity in pharmaceutical drug development, *Toxicol Pathol* 44:789–809, 2016.

Hargreaves A, Harleman J: Preclinical risk assessment of drug-induced hypo- and hyperprolactinemia, *J Appl Toxicol* 31:599–607, 2011.

Harris SB, DeSesso JM: Practical guidance for evaluating and interpreting developmental toxicity tests, *J Hazard Mater* 39:245–266, 1994.

Hausner E, Elmore SA, Yang X: Overview of the components of cardiac metabolism, *Drug Metab Dispos* 47(9):673–688, 2019.

Hew KW, Keller KA: Postnatal anatomical and functional development of the heart: a species comparison, *Birth Defects Res B Dev Reprod Toxicol* 68:309–320, 2003.

Hirshfield AN: Overview of ovarian follicular development: considerations for the toxicologist, *Environ Mol Mutagen* 29:10–15, 1997.

Hoberman AM, Lewis EM: *Pediatric non-clinical drug testing; principles, requirements, and practices*, Hoboken, NJ, 2012, John Wiley & Sons, Inc.

Holsapple MP, West LJ, Landreth KS: Species comparison of anatomical and functional immune system development, *Birth Defects Res B Dev Reprod Toxicol* 68:321–334, 2003.

Holson JF, Stump DG, Pearce LB, et al.: Mode of action: yolk sac poisoning and impeded histiotrophic nutrition–HBOC-related congenital malformations, *Crit Rev Toxicol* 35:739–745, 2005.

Holson JF, Stump DG, Pearce LB, et al.: Absence of developmental toxicity in a canine model after infusion of a hemoglobin-based oxygen carrier: implications for risk assessment, *Reprod Toxicol* 52:101–107, 2015.

Honda T, Honda K, Kokubun C, et al.: Time-course changes of hematology and clinical chemistry values in pregnant rats, *J Toxicol Sci* 33:375–380, 2008.

Howroyd PC, Peter B, de Rijk E: Review of sexual maturity in the minipig, *Toxicol Pathol* 44:607–611, 2016.

Hoyer PB, Sipes IG: Development of an animal model for ovotoxicity using 4-vinylcyclohexene: a case study, *Birth Defects Res B Dev Reprod Toxicol* 80:113–125, 2007.

Hu F, Schutt L, Kozlowski C, et al.: Ovarian toxicity assessment in histopathological images using deep learning, *Toxicol Pathol* 48:350–361, 2020.

ICH: *M3(R2): Guidance on nonclinical safety studies for the conduct of human clinical trials and marketing authorization for pharmaceuticals*, 2009a. Retrieved from: https://database.ich.org/sites/default/files/M3_R2__Guideline.pdf.

ICH: *S9: nonclinical evaluation for anticancer pharmaceuticals*, 2009b. Retrieved from: https://database.ich.org/sites/default/files/S9_Guideline.pdf.

ICH: *S6(R1): preclinical safety evaluation of biotechnology-derived pharmaceuticals*, 2011. Retrieved from: https://database.ich.org/sites/default/files/S6_R1_Guideline_0.pdf.

ICH: *S5(R3): detection of reproductive and developmental toxicity for human pharmaceuticals*, 2020a. Retrieved from: https://database.ich.org/sites/default/files/S5-R3_Step4_Guideline_2020_0218_1.pdf.

ICH: *S11: nonclinical safety testing in support of development of paediatric pharmaceuticals*, 2020b. Retrieved from: https://database.ich.org/sites/default/files/S11_Step4_FinalGuideline_2020_0310.pdf.

Inoue A, Arima A, Kato H, et al.: Utility of finger maze test for learning and memory abilities in infants of cynomolgus monkeys exposed to thiamazole, *Congenit Anom (Kyoto)* 54:220–224, 2014.

Ishii M, Yamauchi T, Matsumoto K, et al.: Maternal age and reproductive function in female Sprague-Dawley rats, *J Toxicol Sci* 37:631–638, 2012.

Jabbour HN, Kelly RW, Fraser HM, et al.: Endocrine regulation of menstruation, *Endocr Rev* 27:17–46, 2006.

James RW, Heywood R: Age-related variations in the testes and prostate of beagle dogs, *Toxicology* 12:273–279, 1979.

Jarak I, Almeida S, Carvalho RA, et al.: Senescence and declining reproductive potential: insight into molecular mechanisms through testicular metabolomics, *Biochim Biophys Acta Mol Basis Dis* 1864:3388–3396, 2018.

Jarvis P, Srivastav S, Vogelwedde E, et al.: The cynomolgus monkey as a model for developmental toxicity studies: variability of pregnancy losses, statistical power estimates, and group size considerations, *Birth Defects Res B Dev Reprod Toxicol* 89:175–187, 2010.

Jevtovic-Todorovic V, Bushnell PJ, Paule MG: Introduction to the special issue "Developmental neurotoxicity associated with pediatric general anesthesia: preclinical findings", *Neurotoxicol Teratol* 60(1), 2017.

Jones AR, Cooper TG: A re-appraisal of the post-testicular action and toxicity of chlorinated antifertility compounds, *Int J Androl* 22:130–138, 1999.

Katavolos P, Prell R, Zane D, et al.: Resolution of unexpected pregnancy-related findings in a rat embryofetal development and toxicokinetic study of monoclonal antibodies specific for hCMV, *Birth Defects Res* 110:1347–1357, 2018.

Keane KA, Parker GA, Regan KS, et al.: Scientific and regulatory policy committee (SRPC) points to consider: histopathology evaluation of the pubertal development and thyroid function assay (OPPTS 890.1450, OPPTS 890.1500) in rats to screen for endocrine disruptors, *Toxicol Pathol* 43:1047–1063, 2015.

Kim JH, Scialli AR: Thalidomide: the tragedy of birth defects and the effective treatment of disease, *Toxicol Sci* 122:1–6, 2011.

Kimmel CA, Garry MR, DeSesso JM: Relationship between bent long bones, bent scapulae, and wavy ribs: malformations or variations? *Birth Defects Res B Dev Reprod Toxicol* 101:379–392, 2014.

Kimmel CA, Wilson JG: Skeletal deviations in rats: malformations or variations? *Teratology* 8:309–315, 1973.

Komeya M, Yamanaka H, Sanjo H, et al.: In vitro spermatogenesis in two-dimensionally spread mouse testis tissues, *Reprod Med Biol* 18:362–369, 2019.

Kuper CF, van Bilsen J, Cnossen H, et al.: Development of immune organs and functioning in humans and test animals: implications for immune intervention studies, *Reprod Toxicol* 64:180–190, 2016.

La DK, Creasy DM, Hess RA, et al.: Efferent duct toxicity with secondary testicular changes in rats following administration of a novel leukotriene A(4) hydrolase inhibitor, *Toxicol Pathol* 40:705–714, 2012.

van der Laan JW, van Malderen K, de Jager N, et al.: Evaluation of juvenile animal studies for pediatric CNS-targeted compounds: a regulatory perspective, *Int J Toxicol* 38(6): 456–475, 2019.

Laer S, Elshoff JP, Meibohm B, et al.: Development of a safe and effective pediatric dosing regimen for sotalol based on population pharmacokinetics and pharmacodynamics in children with supraventricular tachycardia, *J Am Coll Cardiol* 46:1322–1330, 2005.

Laffan SB, Posobiec LM, Uhl JE, et al.: Species comparison of postnatal development of the female reproductive system, *Birth Defects Res* 110:163–189, 2018.

Lanning LL, Creasy DM, Chapin RE, et al.: Recommended approaches for the evaluation of testicular and epididymal toxicity, *Toxicol Pathol* 30:507–520, 2002.

Latendresse JR, Warbrittion AR, Jonassen H, et al.: Fixation of testes and eyes using a modified Davidson's fluid: comparison with Bouin's fluid and conventional Davidson's fluid, *Toxicol Pathol* 30:524–533, 2002.

Lavely JA: Pediatric neurology of the dog and cat, *Vet Clin North Am Small Anim Pract* 36:475–501, 2006.

Lawler DF: Neonatal and pediatric care of the puppy and kitten, *Theriogenology* 70:384–392, 2008.

Lebrec H, Molinier B, Boverhof D, et al.: The T-cell-dependent antibody response assay in nonclinical studies of pharmaceuticals and chemicals: study design, data analysis, interpretation, *Reg Toxicol Pharmacol* 69:7–21, 2014.

LeFevre J, McClintock MK: Reproductive senescence in female rats: a longitudinal study of individual differences in estrous cycles and behavior, *Biol Reprod* 38:780–789, 1988.

Lerman SA, Hew KW, Stewart J, et al.: The nonclinical fertility study design for pharmaceuticals, *Birth Defects Res B Dev Reprod Toxicol* 86:429–436, 2009.

Li AA, Sheets LP, Raffaele K, et al.: Recommendations for harmonization of data collection and analysis of developmental neurotoxicity endpoints in regulatory guideline studies: Proceedings of workshops presented at society of toxicology and joint teratology society and neurobehavioral teratology society meetings, *Neurotoxicol Teratol* 63:24–45, 2017.

Li S, Davis B: Evaluating rodent vaginal and uterine histology in toxicity studies, *Birth Defects Res B Dev Reprod Toxicol* 80: 246–252, 2007.

Liberati TA, Sansone SR, Feuston MH: Hematology and clinical chemistry values in pregnant Wistar Hannover rats compared with nonmated controls, *Vet Clin Pathol* 33:68–73, 2004.

Losco PE, Leach MW, Sinha D, et al.: Administration of an antagonist of neurokinin receptors 1, 2, and 3 results in reproductive tract changes in beagle dogs, but not rats, *Toxicol Pathol* 35:310–322, 2007.

Luetjens CM, Fuchs A, Baker A, et al.: Group size experiences with enhanced pre- and postnatal development studies in the long-tailed macaque (*Macaca fascicularis*), *Primate Biol* 7: 1–4, 2020.

Luetjens CM, Weinbauer GF: Functional assessment of sexual maturity in male macaques (*Macaca fascicularis*), *Regul Toxicol Pharmacol* 63:391–400, 2012.

Makori N, Watson RE, Hogrefe CE, et al.: Object discrimination and reversal learning in infant and juvenile non-human primates in a non-clinical laboratory, *J Med Primatol* 42:147–157, 2013.

Makris SL, Solomon HM, Clark R, et al.: Terminology of developmental abnormalities in common laboratory mammals (version 2), *Birth Defects Res B Dev Reprod Toxicol* 86:227–327, 2009.

Mansfield KG, Sasseville VG, Westmoreland SV: Molecular localization techniques in the diagnosis and characterization of nonhuman primate infectious diseases, *Vet Pathol* 51:110–126, 2014.

Marien D, Bailey GP, Eichenbaum G, et al.: Timing is everything for sperm assessment in fertility studies, *Reprod Toxicol* 64:141–150, 2016.

Maronpot RR: *Pathology of the mouse: Atlas and reference*, 1, Vienna IL, 1999, Cache River Press.

Martin PL, Oneda S, Treacy G: Effects of an anti-TNF-alpha monoclonal antibody, administered throughout pregnancy and lactation, on the development of the macaque immune system, *Am J Reprod Immunol* 58:138–149, 2007.

Martin PL, Weinbauer GF: Developmental toxicity testing of biopharmaceuticals in nonhuman primates: previous experience and future directions, *Int J Toxicol* 29:552–568, 2010.

Marty MS, Chapin RE, Parks LG, et al.: Development and maturation of the male reproductive system, *Birth Defects Res B Dev Reprod Toxicol* 68:125–136, 2003.

Mattison DR, Shiromizu K, Nightingale MS: Oocyte destruction by polycyclic aromatic hydrocarbons, *Am J Ind Med* 4: 191–202, 1983.

McAnulty PA, Dayan AD, Ganderup N-C, et al., editors: *The minipig in biomedical research*, 2011, CRC Press, Taylor & Francis Group.

Mecklenburg L, Luetjens CM, Weinbauer GF: Toxicologic pathology forum*: opinion on sexual maturity and fertility assessment in long-tailed macaques (*Macaca fascicularis*) in nonclinical safety studies, *Toxicol Pathol* 47:444–460, 2019.

Meeks RG, Stump DG, Siddiqui WH, et al.: An inhalation reproductive toxicity study of octamethylcyclotetrasiloxane (D4) in female rats using multiple and single day exposure regimens, *Reprod Toxicol* 23:192–201, 2007.

Mehta RR, Jenco JM, Gaynor LV, et al.: Relationships between ovarian morphology, vaginal cytology, serum progesterone, and urinary immunoreactive pregnanediol during the menstrual cycle of the cynomolgus monkey, *Biol Reprod* 35:981–986, 1986.

Meistrich ML: Quantitative correlation between testicular stem cell survival, sperm production, and fertility in the mouse after treatment with different cytotoxic agents, *J Androl* 3:58–68, 1982.

MHLW: *Guideline on the nonclinical safety study in juvenile animals for pediatric drugs (MHLW/PFSB/ELD PFSB/ELD notification 1002 No.5)*, 2012. Retrieved from: https://www.mhlw.go.jp/web/t_doc_keyword?keyword=%E5%B9%BC%E8%8B%A5&dataId=00tb8792&dataType=1&pageNo=1&mode=0.

Mital P, Hinton BT, Dufour JM: The blood-testis and blood-epididymis barriers are more than just their tight junctions, *Biol Reprod* 84:851–858, 2011.

Mitchard T, Jarvis P, Stewart J: Assessment of male rodent fertility in general toxicology 6-month studies, *Birth Defects Res B Dev Reprod Toxicol* 95:410–420, 2012.

Mitchard TL, Klein S: Reproductive senescence, fertility and reproductive tumour profile in ageing female Han Wistar rats, *Exp Toxicol Pathol* 68:143–147, 2016.

Mizoguchi Y, Matsuoka T, Mizuguchi H, et al.: Changes in blood parameters in New Zealand White rabbits during pregnancy, *Lab Anim* 44:33–39, 2010.

Morford LL, Bowman CJ, Blanset DL, et al.: Preclinical safety evaluations supporting pediatric drug development with biopharmaceuticals: strategy, challenges, current practices, *Birth Defects Res B Dev Reprod Toxicol* 92:359–380, 2011.

Morrissey RE, Lamb JC, Schwetz BA, et al.: Association of sperm, vaginal cytology, and reproductive organ weight data with results of continuous breeding reproduction studies in Swiss (CD-1) mice, *Fundam Appl Toxicol* 11:359–371, 1988.

Mruk DD, Cheng CY: The mammalian blood-testis barrier: its biology and regulation, *Endocr Rev* 36:564–591, 2015.

Mruk DD, Su L, Cheng CY: Emerging role for drug transporters at the blood-testis barrier, *Trends Pharmacol Sci* 32: 99–106, 2011.

Mulla H: Understanding developmental pharmacodynamics: importance for drug development and clinical practice, *Paediatr Drugs* 12:223–233, 2010.

Muskhelishvili L, Wingard SK, Latendresse JR: Proliferating cell nuclear antigen–a marker for ovarian follicle counts, *Toxicol Pathol* 33:365–368, 2005.

Neal-Kluever A, Fisher J, Grylack L, et al.: Physiology of the neonatal gastrointestinal system relevant to the disposition of orally administered medications, *Drug Metab Dispos* 47: 296–313, 2019.

Niehoff MO, Bergmann M, Weinbauer GF: Effects of social housing of sexually mature male cynomolgus monkeys during general and reproductive toxicity evaluation, *Reprod Toxicol* 29:57–67, 2010.

Nitzsche D: Effect of maternal feed restriction on prenatal development in rats and rabbits - a review of published data, *Regul Toxicol Pharmacol* 90:95–103, 2017.

Noguchi KK, Johnson SA, Dissen GA, et al.: Isoflurane exposure for three hours triggers apoptotic cell death in neonatal macaque brain, *Br J Anaesth* 119:524–531, 2017.

Noritake K, Ikeda T, Ito K, et al.: Study for collecting background data on Wistar Hannover [Crl:WI(Han)] rats in embryo-fetal development studies–comparative data to Sprague Dawley rats, *J Toxicol Sci* 38:847–854, 2013.

O'Connor JC, Cook JC, Marty MS, et al.: Evaluation of Tier I screening approaches for detecting endocrine-active compounds (EACs), *Crit Rev Toxicol* 32:521–549, 2002.

O'Connor JC, Davis LG, Frame SR, et al.: Evaluation of a Tier I screening battery for detecting endocrine-active compounds (EACs) using the positive controls testosterone, coumestrol, progesterone, and RU486, *Toxicol Sci* 54: 338–354, 2000.

OECD: *Test No. 416: two-generation reproduction toxicity (OECD guidelines for the testing of chemicals, section 4)*, 2001. Retrieved from: https://doi.org/10.1787/9789264070868-en.

OECD: *Test No. 426: developmental neurotoxicity study (OECD guidelines for the testing of chemicals, section 4)*, 2007. Retrieved from: https://doi.org/10.1787/9789264067394-en.

OECD: *Test No. 421: reproduction/developmental toxicity screening test (OECD guidelines for the testing of chemicals, section 4)*, 2016a. Retrieved from: https://doi.org/10.1787/9789264264380-en.

OECD: *Test No. 422: combined repeated dose toxicity study with the reproduction/developmental toxicity screening test (OECD guidelines for the testing of chemicals, section 4)*, 2016b. Retrieved from: https://doi.org/10.1787/9789264264403-en.

OECD: *Test No. 414: prenatal developmental toxicity study (OECD guidelines for the testing of chemicals, section 4)*, 2018a. Retrieved from: https://doi.org/10.1787/9789264070820-en.

OECD: *Test No. 443: extended one-generation reproductive toxicity study (OECD guidelines for the testing of chemicals, section 4)*, 2018b. Retrieved from: https://doi.org/10.1787/97892641 85371-en.

Ohtake S, Fukui M, Hisada S: Collaborative work on evaluation of ovarian toxicity. 1) Effects of 2- or 4-week repeated-dose administration and fertility studies with medroxyprogesterone acetate in female rats, *J Toxicol Sci* 34(Suppl 1):SP23–29, 2009.

Okahashi N, Ikeda T, Kai S, et al.: The predictivity of preliminary embryo-fetal development (EFD) studies: results of a retrospective survey in Japanese pharmaceutical companies, *J Toxicol Sci* 35:21–31, 2010.

Parker G, Picut C, editors: *Atlas of histology of the juvenile rat*, Boston, MA, 2016, Elsevier.

Parker GA, Picut CA, Swanson C, et al.: Histologic features of postnatal development of immune system organs in the Sprague-Dawley rat, *Toxicol Pathol* 43:794–815, 2015.

Parks Saldutti L, Beyer BK, Breslin W, et al.: In vitro testicular toxicity models: opportunities for advancement via biomedical engineering techniques, *ALTEX* 30:353–377, 2013.

Paulesu L, Bhattacharjee J, Bechi N, et al.: Pro-inflammatory cytokines in animal and human gestation, *Curr Pharmaceut Des* 16:3601–3615, 2010.

Peter B, De Rijk EP, Zeltner A, et al.: Sexual maturation in the female Gottingen minipig, *Toxicol Pathol* 44:482–485, 2016.

Picut CA, Dixon D, Simons ML, et al.: Postnatal ovary development in the rat: morphologic study and correlation of morphology to neuroendocrine parameters, *Toxicol Pathol* 43:343–353, 2015a.

Picut CA, Remick AK, Asakawa MG, et al.: Histologic features of prepubertal and pubertal reproductive development in female Sprague-Dawley rats, *Toxicol Pathol* 42:403–413, 2014.

Picut CA, Remick AK, de Rijk EP, et al.: Postnatal development of the testis in the rat: morphologic study and correlation of morphology to neuroendocrine parameters, *Toxicol Pathol* 43:326–342, 2015b.

Picut CA, Swanson CL, Scully KL, et al.: Ovarian follicle counts using proliferating cell nuclear antigen (PCNA) and semi-automated image analysis in rats, *Toxicol Pathol* 36:674–679, 2008.

Pique C, Marsden E, Quesada P, et al.: A shortened study design for embryo-fetal development studies in the minipig, *Reprod Toxicol* 80:35–43, 2018.

Posobiec LM, Cox EM, Solomon HM, et al.: A probability analysis of historical pregnancy and fetal data from Dutch belted and New Zealand white rabbit strains from embryo-fetal development studies, *Birth Defects Res B Dev Reprod Toxicol* 107:76–84, 2016.

Posobiec LM, Vidal JD, Hughes-Earle A, et al.: Early vaginal opening in juvenile female rats given BRAF-inhibitor dabrafenib is not associated with early physiologic sexual maturation, *Birth Defects Res B Dev Reprod Toxicol* 104:244–252, 2015.

Powles-Glover N, Mitchard T, Stewart J: Time course for onset and recovery from effects of a novel male reproductive toxicant: implications for apical preclinical study designs, *Birth Defects Res B Dev Reprod Toxicol* 104:91–99, 2015.

Prell RA, Dybdal N, Arima A, et al.: Placental and fetal effects of Onartuzumab, a Met/HGF signaling antagonist, when administered to pregnant cynomolgus monkeys, *Toxicol Sci* 165:186–197, 2018.

Qian X, Cheng YH, Mruk DD, et al.: Breast cancer resistance protein (Bcrp) and the testis–an unexpected turn of events, *Asian J Androl* 15:455–460, 2013.

Quinn AL, Dalu A, Meeker LS, et al.: Effects of octamethylcyclotetrasiloxane (D4) on the luteinizing hormone (LH) surge and levels of various reproductive hormones in female Sprague-Dawley rats, *Reprod Toxicol* 23:532–540, 2007.

Rasmussen AD, Richmond E, Wegener KM, et al.: Vigabatrin-induced CNS changes in juvenile rats: induction, progression and recovery of myelin-related changes, *Neurotoxicology* 46:137–144, 2015.

Redfern BG, David Wise L, Spence S: An alternative Alcian Blue dye variant for the evaluation of fetal cartilage, *Birth Defects Res B Dev Reprod Toxicol* 80:171–176, 2007.

Redfern BG, Wise LD: High-throughput staining for the evaluation of fetal skeletal development in rats and rabbits, *Birth Defects Res B Dev Reprod Toxicol* 80:177–182, 2007.

Regan KS, Cline JM, Creasy D, et al.: STP position paper: ovarian follicular counting in the assessment of rodent reproductive toxicity, *Toxicol Pathol* 33:409–412, 2005.

Rehm S, Solleveld HA, Portelli ST, et al.: Histologic changes in ovary, uterus, vagina, and mammary gland of mature beagle dogs treated with the SERM idoxifene, *Birth Defects Res B Dev Reprod Toxicol* 80:225–232, 2007a.

Rehm S, Stanislaus DJ, Williams AM: Estrous cycle-dependent histology and review of sex steroid receptor expression in dog reproductive tissues and mammary gland and associated hormone levels, *Birth Defects Res B Dev Reprod Toxicol* 80:233–245, 2007b.

Rehm S, White TE, Zahalka EA, et al.: Effects of food restriction on testis and accessory sex glands in maturing rats, *Toxicol Pathol* 36:687–694, 2008.

Rocca M, Morford LL, Blanset DL, et al.: Applying a weight of evidence approach to the evaluation of developmental toxicity of biopharmaceuticals, *Regul Toxicol Pharmacol* 98:69–79, 2018.

Rocca MS, Wehner NG: The Guinea pig as an animal model for developmental and reproductive toxicology studies, *Birth Defects Res B Dev Reprod Toxicol* 86:92–97, 2009.

Ryan LM, Catalano PJ, Kimmel CA, et al.: Relationship between fetal weight and malformation in developmental toxicity studies, *Teratology* 44:215–223, 1991.

Sakai T, Takahashi M, Mitsumori K, et al.: Collaborative work to evaluate toxicity on male reproductive organs by repeated dose studies in rats–overview of the studies, *J Toxicol Sci* 25(Spec No):1–21, 2000.

Saksena SK, Lau IF, Chang MC: Age dependent changes in the sperm population and fertility in the male rat, *Exp Aging Res* 5:373–381, 1979.

Sanbuissho A, Yoshida M, Hisada S, et al.: Collaborative work on evaluation of ovarian toxicity by repeated-dose and fertility studies in female rats, *J Toxicol Sci* 34(Suppl 1):SP1–22, 2009.

Sasseville VG, Mansfield KG: Overview of known non-human primate pathogens with potential to affect colonies used for toxicity testing, *J Immunotoxicol* 7:79–92, 2010.

Saunders NR, Dziegielewska KM, Mollgard K, et al.: Physiology and molecular biology of barrier mechanisms in the fetal and neonatal brain, *J Physiol* 596(23):5723–5756, 2018.

Schardein JL: Approaches to defining the relationship of maternal and developmental toxicity, *Teratog Carcinog Mutagen* 7:255–271, 1987.

Schardein JL, Schwetz BA, Kenel MF: Species sensitivities and prediction of teratogenic potential, *Environ Health Perspect* 61:55–67, 1985.

Schmitt G, Parrott N, Prinssen E, et al.: The great barrier belief: the blood-brain barrier and considerations for juvenile toxicity studies, *Reprod Toxicol* 72:129–135, 2017.

Scialli AR, Daston G, Chen C, et al.: Rethinking developmental toxicity testing: evolution or revolution? *Birth Defects Res* 110:840–850, 2018.

Sedman AB, Kershaw DB, Bunchman TE: Recognition and management of angiotensin converting enzyme inhibitor fetopathy, *Pediatr Nephrol* 9:382–385, 1995.

Seely JC: A brief review of kidney development, maturation, developmental abnormalities, and drug toxicity: juvenile animal relevancy, *J Toxicol Pathol* 30:125–133, 2017.

Sellers RS, Morton D, Michael B, et al.: Society of Toxicologic Pathology position paper: organ weight recommendations for toxicology studies, *Toxicol Pathol* 35:751–755, 2007.

Setchell BP: Blood-testis barrier, junctional and transport proteins and spermatogenesis, *Adv Exp Med Biol* 636:212–233, 2008.

Sharma AK, Morrison JP, Rao DB, et al.: Toxicologic pathology analysis for translational neuroscience: improving human risk assessment using optimized animal data, *Int J Toxicol* 35:410–419, 2016.

Siddiqui WH, Stump DG, Plotzke KP, et al.: A two-generation reproductive toxicity study of octamethylcyclotetrasiloxane (D4) in rats exposed by whole-body vapor inhalation, *Reprod Toxicol* 23:202–215, 2007.

Simutis FJ, Sanderson TP, Pilcher GD, et al.: Investigations on the relationship between ovarian, endocrine, and renal findings in nonclinical safety studies of the gamma-secretase inhibitor avagacestat, *Toxicol Sci* 171(1):98–116, 2019.

Skaggs H, Chellman GJ, Collinge M, et al.: Comparison of immune system development in nonclinical species and humans: closing information gaps for immunotoxicity testing and human translatability, *Reprod Toxicol* 89:178–188, 2019.

Sobinoff AP, Mahony M, Nixon B, et al.: Understanding the Villain: DMBA-induced preantral ovotoxicity involves selective follicular destruction and primordial follicle activation through PI3K/Akt and mTOR signaling, *Toxicol Sci* 123:563–575, 2011.

Solecki R, Barbellion S, Bergmann B, et al.: Harmonization of description and classification of fetal observations: achievements and problems still unresolved: report of the 7th Workshop on the Terminology in Developmental Toxicology Berlin, 4–6 May 2011, *Reprod Toxicol* 35:48–55, 2013.

Solecki R, Rauch M, Gall A, et al.: Continuing harmonization of terminology and innovations for methodologies in developmental toxicology: report of the 8th Berlin workshop on developmental toxicity, 14–16 May 2014, *Reprod Toxicol* 57:140–146, 2015.

Solomon HM, Murzyn S, Rendemonti J, et al.: The use of micro-CT imaging to examine and illustrate fetal skeletal abnormalities in Dutch Belted rabbits and to prove concordance with Alizarin Red stained skeletal examination, *Birth Defects Res* 110:276–298, 2018.

Stefansdottir A, Fowler PA, Powles-Glover N, et al.: Use of ovary culture techniques in reproductive toxicology, *Reprod Toxicol* 49:117–135, 2014.

Stuckhardt JL, Poppe SM: Fresh visceral examination of rat and rabbit fetuses used in teratogenicity testing, *Teratog Carcinog Mutagen* 4:181–188, 1984.

Stump DG, Holson JF, Harris C, et al.: Developmental toxicity in rats of a hemoglobin-based oxygen carrier results from impeded function of the inverted visceral yolk sac, *Reprod Toxicol* 52:108–117, 2015.

Su L, Mruk DD, Lee WM, et al.: Drug transporters and blood–testis barrier function, *J Endocrinol* 209:337–351, 2011.

Takagi H, Kurihara A, Inoue T, et al.: Investigation of usefulness of sperm analyses in dogs for male fertility study, *J Toxicol Sci* 26:313–321, 2001.

Takakura I, Creasy DM, Yokoi R, et al.: Effects of male sexual maturity of reproductive endpoints relevant to DART studies in Wistar Hannover rats, *J Toxicol Sci* 39:269–279, 2014.

Takayama S, Akaike M, Kawashima K, et al.: Studies on the optimal treatment period and parameters for detection of male fertility disorder in rats–introductory summary, *J Toxicol Sci* 20:173–182, 1995.

Tannenbaum LV, Flaws JA: Exposure duration-dependent ovarian recovery in methoxychlor-treated mice, *Birth Defects Res B Dev Reprod Toxicol* 104:238–243, 2015.

Teo SK, Denny KH, Stirling DI, et al.: Effects of thalidomide on reproductive function and early embryonic development in male and female New Zealand white rabbits, *Birth Defects Res B Dev Reprod Toxicol* 71:1–16, 2004.

Terry KK, Chatman LA, Foley GL, et al.: Effects of feed restriction on fertility in female rats, *Birth Defects Res B Dev Reprod Toxicol* 74:431–441, 2005.

Tobin M, Gunaji R, Walsh JC, et al.: A review of genetic factors underlying craniorachischisis and omphalocele: inspired by a unique trisomy 18 case, *Am J Med Genet* 179:1642–1651, 2019.

Treuting PM: *Comparative anatomy and histology: a mouse, rat and human Atlas.* 2 (vol. 1). 2018, Academic Press, an Elsevier Imprint.

Tsujioka S, Ban Y, Wise LD, et al.: Collaborative work on evaluation of ovarian toxicity. 3) Effects of 2- or 4- week repeated-dose toxicity and fertility studies with tamoxifen in female rats, *J Toxicol Sci* 34(Suppl 1):SP43–51, 2009.

Tyl RW, Crofton K, Moretto A, et al.: Identification and interpretation of developmental neurotoxicity effects: a report from the ILSI Research Foundation/Risk Science Institute expert working group on neurodevelopmental endpoints, *Neurotoxicol Teratol* 30:349–381, 2008.

Ulbrich B, Palmer AK: Detection of effects on male reproduction- A literature survey, *J Am Coll Toxicol* 14:293–327, 1995.

Vaidyanathan A, McKeever K, Anand B, et al.: Developmental immunotoxicology assessment of rituximab in cynomolgus monkeys, *Toxicol Sci* 119:116–125, 2011.

Van Cruchten S, Vrolyk V, Perron Lepage MF, et al.: Pre- and postnatal development of the eye: a species comparison, *Birth Defects Res* 109:1540–1567, 2017.

van Esch E, Cline JM, Buse E, et al.: The macaque endometrium, with special reference to the cynomolgus monkey (*Macaca fascicularis*), *Toxicol Pathol* 36:67S–100S, 2008a.

Van Esch E, Cline JM, Buse E, et al.: Summary comparison of female reproductive system in human and the cynomolgus monkey (*Macaca fascicularis*), *Toxicol Pathol* 36:171S–172S, 2008b.

Van Groen BD, Nicolai J, Van Cruchten S, et al.: Ontogeny of hepatic transporters and drug metabolizing enzymes in humans and in nonclinical species, *Pharmacol Rev* 73:597–678, 2021.

Vidal JD: The impact of age on the female reproductive system, *Toxicol Pathol* 45:206–215, 2017.

Vidal JD, Colman K, Bhaskaran M, et al.: Scientific and regulatory policy committee best practices: socumentation of aexual maturity by microscopic evaluation in nonclinical safety studies, *Toxicol Pathol*, 2021. https://doi.org/10.1177/0192623321990631. In press.

Vidal JD, Filgo AJ: Evaluation of the estrous cycle, reproductive tract, and mammary gland in female mice, *Curr Protoc Mouse Biol* 7:306–325, 2017.

Vidal JD, Whitney KM: Morphologic manifestations of testicular and epididymal toxicity, *Spermatogenesis* 4:e979099, 2014.

Walthall K, Cappon GD, Hurtt ME, et al.: Postnatal development of the gastrointestinal system: a species comparison, *Birth Defects Res B Dev Reprod Toxicol* 74:132–156, 2005.

Watson RE, Desesso JM, Hurtt ME, et al.: Postnatal growth and morphological development of the brain: a species comparison, *Birth Defects Res B Dev Reprod Toxicol* 77:471–484, 2006.

Webster JD, Santagostino SF, Foreman O: Applications and considerations for the use of genetically engineered mouse models in drug development, *Cell Tissue Res* 380:325–340, 2020.

Weinbauer GF, Fuchs A, Niehaus M, et al.: The enhanced pre- and postnatal study for nonhuman primates: update and perspectives, *Birth Defects Res C, Embryo Today Rev* 93:324–333, 2011.

Weinbauer GF, Luft J, Fuchs A: The enhanced pre- and postnatal development study for monoclonal antibodies, *Methods Mol Biol* 947:185–200, 2013.

Weinbauer GF, Niehoff M, Niehaus M, et al.: Physiology and endocrinology of the ovarian cycle in macaques, *Toxicol Pathol* 36:7s–23s, 2008.

Weinstock D, Lewis DB, Parker GA, et al.: Toxicopathology of the developing immune system: investigative and development strategies, *Toxicol Pathol* 38:1111–1117, 2010.

Wells MY, Decobecq CP, Decouvelaere DM, et al.: Changes in clinical pathology parameters during gestation in the New Zealand white rabbit, *Toxicol Pathol* 27:370–379, 1999.

Westwood FR: The female rat reproductive cycle: a practical histological guide to staging, *Toxicol Pathol* 36:375–384, 2008.

White TE, Clark RL: Sensitive periods for developmental toxicity of orally administered artesunate in the rat, *Birth Defects Res B Dev Reprod Toxicol* 83:407–417, 2008.

Whitney KM: Testicular histopathology in juvenile rat studies, *Syst Biol Reprod Med* 58(1):51–56, 2012.

Williams J, Gladen BC, Schrader SM, et al.: Semen analysis and fertility assessment in rabbits: statistical power and design considerations for toxicology studies, *Fundam Appl Toxicol* 15:651–665, 1990.

Williams NI, Berga SL, Cameron JL: Synergism between psychosocial and metabolic stressors: impact on reproductive function in cynomolgus monkeys, *Am J Physiol Endocrinol Metab* 293:E270–E276, 2007.

Wilson JG: *Environment and birth defects* (vol. 3). New York, 1973, Academic Press.

Wira CR, Rodriguez-Garcia M, Patel MV: The role of sex hormones in immune protection of the female reproductive tract, *Nat Rev Immunol* 15:217–230, 2015.

Wise LD, Buschmann J, Feuston MH, et al.: Embryo-fetal developmental toxicity study design for pharmaceuticals, *Birth Defects Res B Dev Reprod Toxicol* 86:418–428, 2009.

Wise LD, Clark RL, Minsker DH, et al.: Use of hematology and serum biochemistry data in developmental toxicity studies, *Teratology* 37:502–503, 1988.

Wise LD, Minsker DH, Cukierski MA, et al.: Reversible decreases of fertility in male Sprague-Dawley rats treated orally with finasteride, a 5 alpha-reductase inhibitor, *Reprod Toxicol* 5:337–346, 1991.

Wise LD, Spence S, Saldutti LP, et al.: Assessment of female and male fertility in Sprague-Dawley rats administered vorinostat, a histone deacetylase inhibitor, *Birth Defects Res B Dev Reprod Toxicol* 83:19–26, 2008.

Wise LD, Winkelmann CT: Evaluation of hydroxyurea-induced fetal skeletal changes in Dutch belted rabbits by micro-computed tomography and alizarin red staining, *Birth Defects Res B Dev Reprod Toxicol* 86:220–226, 2009a.

Wise LD, Winkelmann CT: Micro-computed tomography and alizarin red evaluations of boric acid-induced fetal skeletal changes in Sprague-Dawley rats, *Birth Defects Res B Dev Reprod Toxicol* 86:214–219, 2009b.

Wood SL, Beyer BK, Cappon GD: Species comparison of postnatal CNS development: functional measures, *Birth Defects Res B Dev Reprod Toxicol* 68:391–407, 2003.

Xiao S, Coppeta JR, Rogers HB, et al.: A microfluidic culture model of the human reproductive tract and 28-day menstrual cycle, *Nat Commun* 8:14584, 2017.

Xie J, Funk J, Bopst M, et al.: An innovative investigative approach to characterize the effects observed in a combined fertility study in male and female rats, *Regul Toxicol Pharmacol* 95:339–347, 2018.

Xu J, Wang Y, Kauffman AE, et al.: A tiered female ovarian toxicity screening identifies toxic effects of checkpoint kinase 1 inhibitors on murine growing follicles, *Toxicol Sci* 177:405–419, 2020.

Zalewska A: Developmental milestones in neonatal and juvenile C57Bl/6 mouse - indications for the design of juvenile toxicity studies, *Reprod Toxicol* 88:91–128, 2019.

Zhang Y, Mehta N, Muhari-Stark E, et al.: Pediatric renal ontogeny and applications in drug development, *J Clin Pharmacol* 59(Suppl 1):S9–S20, 2019.

Zhou L, Wang Z, Zhou H, et al.: Neonatal exposure to sevoflurane may not cause learning and memory deficits and behavioral abnormality in the childhood of Cynomolgus monkeys, *Sci Rep* 5:11145, 2015a.

Zhou X, Li W, Chen X, et al.: Dose-dependent effects of sevoflurane exposure during early lifetime on apoptosis in hippocampus and neurocognitive outcomes in Sprague-Dawley rats, *Int J Physiol Pathophysiol Pharmacol* 8:111–119, 2016.

Zhou ZB, Yang XY, Yuan BL, et al.: Sevoflurane-induced down-regulation of hippocampal oxytocin and arginine vasopressin impairs juvenile social behavioral abilities, *J Mol Neurosci* 56:70–77, 2015b.

Ziejewski MK, Solomon HM, Rendemonti J, et al.: Comparison of a modified mid-coronal sectioning technique and Wilson's technique when conducting eye and brain examinations in rabbit teratology studies, *Birth Defects Res B Dev Reprod Toxicol* 104:23–34, 2015.

Zoetis T, Hurtt ME: Species comparison of lung development, *Birth Defects Res B Dev Reprod Toxicol* 68:121–124, 2003.

Zoetis T, Tassinari MS, Bagi C, et al.: Species comparison of postnatal bone growth and development, *Birth Defects Res B Dev Reprod Toxicol* 68:86–110, 2003.

Carcinogenesis: Mechanisms and Evaluation

Mark J. Hoenerhoff[1], Molly Boyle[2], Sheroy Minocherhomji[3], Arun R. Pandiri[4]

[1]In Vivo Animal Core, Unit for Laboratory Animal Medicine, University of Michigan Medical School, Ann Arbor, MI, United States, [2]Covance Somerset, Somerset, NJ, United States, [3]Amgen Inc., Translational Safety & Bioanalytical Sciences, Thousand Oaks, CA, United States, [4]Molecular Pathology Group, Comparative and Molecular Pathogenesis Branch, Division of the National Toxicology Program, National Institute of Environmental Health Sciences, Durham, NC, United States

OUTLINE

1. Introduction — 206
  1.1. Prominent Theories of Carcinogenesis — 207
  1.2. General Features of Carcinogenesis — 208
  1.3. Cell Growth and Proliferation — 210
  1.4. Oncogenes and Tumor Suppressor Genes — 213
  1.5. Apoptosis and DNA Damage Repair — 217
  1.6. Angiogenesis, Invasion, and Metastasis — 218

2. Mechanisms of Chemically Induced Carcinogenesis — 219
  2.1. Genotoxic Carcinogens — 220
  2.2. Direct Acting Carcinogens — 220
  2.3. Indirect Acting Carcinogens — 220
  2.4. Mechanisms of High-fidelity/Nonmutagenic or Low-fidelity/Mutagenic DNA Repair — 222
  2.5. DNA Replication and Repair Mechanisms — 222
  2.6. Consequences of Genotoxicity — 224
  2.7. Nongenotoxic Carcinogens — 224

3. Identification of Carcinogens—Testing Programs and Guidelines — 231
  3.1. In Vitro Mutagenicity Assays — 231
  3.2. Chromosomal Aberration Assay — 232
  3.3. Micronucleus Test — 232
  3.4. Other DNA Based Assays — 232
  3.5. Testing Programs and Guidelines — 233

3.6. Two-Year National Toxicology Program Rodent Carcinogenicity Bioassay — 233
3.7. Carcinogenicity Testing — 234
3.8. Current and Future Considerations for Carcinogenicity Testing in Rodents — 235
3.9. Conventional Rat Strains for Carcinogenicity Testing — 237
3.10. Mouse Models of Carcinogenesis — 238
3.11. Transgenic Models for Mutagenicity Testing — 240
3.12. The Tg.rasH2 Mouse Model — 240
3.13. The Tp53$^{+/-}$ Mouse Model — 240
3.14. Hamsters — 240
3.15. Zebrafish — 241
3.16. Organoids — 242
3.17. Clinical Pathology — 242
3.18. Histopathology — 242
3.19. Carcinogenicity Study Data Interpretation — 242

4. Evolving and New Technologies — 244
  4.1. Gene Expression Analysis — 244
  4.2. Next Generation Sequencing to Assess Mutagenicity and Genome Instability — 244

5. Conclusions — 245

References — 247

Haschek and Rousseaux's Handbook of Toxicologic Pathology, Fourth Edition.
https://doi.org/10.1016/B978-0-12-821044-4.00013-3

We foresee cancer research as an increasingly logical science, in which complexities are manifestations of a small set of underlying organizing principles.Hanahan and Weinberg, 2011

1. INTRODUCTION

Cancer is a major cause of morbidity and mortality throughout the world, caused by the accumulation of genetic and epigenetic alterations in genes regulating cell growth and proliferation, and is influenced by a wide array of extrinsic (e.g., environment, diet, lifestyle factors) and intrinsic (e.g., age, sex, host genetics) factors. As humans reach their sixth decade, they face an exponentially increased risk for developing cancer. Similarly, treatment of preclinical species such as rats with either a single or multiple doses of a carcinogen(s) can increase the susceptibility to chemically induced neoplasms. When adequately tested, compounds that have been shown to be carcinogenic in humans also cause cancer in laboratory animals, and in each instance at the same location in animals and humans (Huff, 1993). Additionally, many chemically induced cancers in animals occur through similar molecular mechanisms as in humans (Hoenerhoff et al., 2009). In fact, approximately 30 compounds first shown to cause cancer in animals were linked to some form of human cancer, including estrogen, formaldehyde, vinyl chloride, radon gas, and asbestos, among others (Kemp, 2015). Therefore, identifying potential human carcinogens in rodent bioassays has been a major focus of the field of toxicologic pathology.

Animal and human cancers are fundamentally similar and frequently share morphological, biological, and molecular features. The first demonstration that a chemical could cause cancer in animals was made in 1918 by two Japanese pathologists, Yamagiwa and Ichikawa, who showed that with chronic exposure of the skin (pinna) to coal tars, rabbits developed squamous cell carcinomas (Yamagiwa & Ichikawa, 1918). These findings not only confirmed Percival Pott's strong epidemiological observations in 1775 of increased rates of cutaneous scrotal cancer in chimney sweeps (Pott & Cancer, 1775) but also demonstrated that chronic exposures were necessary for the induction of some cancers.

Numerous chemicals have been shown to transform cells in vitro and to be carcinogenic in animals. A variety of occupational causes of cancer had been documented, and numerous very potent carcinogens have been identified from chemicals produced by fossil fuels or other industrial compounds. In 1531, Paracelsus described the *"mala metallorum"* among miners for silver and other metals, including uranium, which was later interpreted as radiation-induced lung cancer (Kang et al., 2019). Early reports by Hill in 1761, which called attention to the association of "immoderate use of snuff" and the development of *"polypusses"* (Redmond Jr., 1970), later received experimental confirmation by Roffo in 1931 when he induced skin cancer in rabbits following dermal exposure to tobacco-derived tar (Roffo, 2006). Similarly, in 1775, Pott attributed scrotal skin cancers to prolonged exposure to soot in chimney sweeps (Pott & Cancer, 1775), and on the basis of this observation, the Danish Chimney Sweeps Guild ruled that its members must bathe daily. No public health measure since that time has so successfully controlled a form of cancer.

Cellular pathologists such as Muller and Virchow argued that cancer was related to a form of chronic irritation. This view was supported by experimental studies in mouse skin where wounding seemed to play a tumorigenic role (Balkwill & Mantovani, 2001). Chronic inflammation induced by a number of infectious agents and toxins has been implicated in the development of a number of human and animal cancers. Nobel laureates Drs. Robin Warren and Barry Marshall were credited with determining that infection with *Helicobacter pylori* was a common cause of gastric inflammation and ulcers in man (Marshall, 2008). Some skeptical scientists were not convinced until Dr. Marshall developed gastritis soon after drinking a Petri dish of the bacteria (Marshall et al., 1985). In subsequent years, it was shown that chronic helicobacter gastritis is associated with the development of gastric lymphomas and carcinomas, and thereby, *H. pylori* is listed as a human carcinogen by the International Agency for Research on Cancer (IARC) (International Agency for Research on Cancer I, 1994). Likewise, certain strains of mice (including A/JCr and B6C3F1/N) with chronic *Helicobacter hepaticus* hepatitis develop significantly higher rates of liver cancer compared to uninfected controls (Diwan et al., 1997). Additionally, in conjunction with epidemiologic studies, numerous animal studies have confirmed chronic aflatoxin B1 (AFB1) exposure and infection with hepatitis B or hepatitis C virus as a cause of hepatocellular carcinoma in humans secondary to chronic hepatitis and hepatocellular damage (Loeb & Harris, 2008). Utilizing animal studies, numerous other compounds have shown a link to carcinogenesis through induction of chronic inflammation as an inciting factor.

1.1. Prominent Theories of Carcinogenesis

Our understanding of cancer biology is evolving rapidly. Conceptual views of carcinogenesis are formed by the piece-by-piece discovery of key elements of the complex biological puzzle that this disease entails; however, the search for a comprehensive theory of carcinogenesis has not been forthcoming, and investigation into several theories on the origin and pathogenesis of neoplasia still dominates much of the field of cancer research. Three predominant theories on the origin of carcinogenesis include the Somatic Mutation Theory (SMT), the Cancer Stem Cell (CSC) Theory, and the Tissue Organizational Field Theory (TOFT) (Loeb & Harris, 2008; Loeb, 2016; Venkatesan et al., 2017).

The SMT, which has dominated the last 60 years of cancer research, is based on the premise that cancer originates when a normal somatic cell successively accumulates multiple mutations in genes controlling cell proliferation and the cell cycle (Sonnenschein & Soto, 2008). The transformed cell then passes the mutation to its progeny, generating malignant clones. The longer a population of somatic cells persists, or the higher rate of cell turnover in a given tissue, the higher the likelihood of mutations occurring in that population over time. Then, as the mutated cells proliferate, there is a finite probability that some of them will sustain at least a second mutation. As the process of successive mutation and proliferation continues, cells eventually sustain enough genetic alterations to undergo neoplastic transformation. The accumulation of successive mutations would be expected to increase as a function of age and of the degree of cell proliferation, and finally clones acquire additional mutations until

a subclone arises with the ability to invade and metastasize. The SMT has been refined over the years to include alterations in oncogenes, tumor suppressor genes, DNA repair genes, apoptosis genes, and epigenetic mechanisms, and has been the prevalent means to explain the process of neoplastic transformation and progression (Loeb, 2016).

The CSC hypothesis was first proposed over 150 years ago, which stated that dormant embryonic components exist in adult tissues that may be later induced to become tumorigenic (Reya et al., 2001). According to the CSC theory of carcinogenesis, a distinct subpopulation of cancer stem cells has the capacity to generate a tumor and sustain its growth. Cancer stem cells perpetuate tumorigenesis through the process of self-renewal, in which a stem cell pool maintains its numbers through symmetric and asymmetric division. In symmetric cell division, the progeny is identical to the initial stem cell; in asymmetric division, one of the two progeny is identical to the initial stem cell, whereas the other cell is a committed progenitor cell, which undergoes cellular differentiation. Through the tightly regulated process of self-renewal, normal stem cells are able to function over the lifespan of the host, and thus their longevity and continued mitotic activity make them a significant target and potential reservoir for the accumulation of the numerous genetic mutations needed for transformation. Through the ability to self-renew, a small population of carcinogenic stem cells within a neoplasm has the ability to maintain malignant clones. Finally, two major factors affecting tumor response to therapy and cancer mortality are chemoresistance and metastasis. The CSC hypothesis considers that a tumor is composed largely of transformed but poorly proliferative tumor cells, and that only a small proportion, the highly carcinogenic cancer stem cell subset, is able to form a new tumor or metastasize, or show enhanced chemoresistance.

The TOFT, a relatively new theory on the origin of carcinogenesis, is based on the premise that cancer is a result of tissue organization, and that proliferation is the default state of a host cell (Sonnenschein & Soto, 2008). A tissue-based theory rather than a cellular-based one as is the SMT, the TOFT, proposes that carcinogens cause a disruption in the interactions of cells that maintain normal tissue homeostasis, repair, and tissue organization, and that alteration in the microenvironment relaxes normal forces that maintain tissue order, allowing parenchymal cells to proliferate and migrate. The TOFT states that the normal state of the cell is one of proliferation and migration; that is, the interaction of the physical and biochemical forces of the stromal microenvironment keeps the cell in a resting state, and if this interaction is dysregulated in any way, this leads to release of these forces normally keeping cells in check, and they revert to their natural state of proliferation and migration, thus resulting in uncontrolled growth (tumorigenesis) and migration (metastasis).

These prevailing theories do not necessarily discount one another but may coexist in overlapping space and time. For example, the CSC hypothesis does not discount the SMT, but rather accepts the contribution of genetic instability, mutation, and epigenetic factors that influence the evolution of heterogeneity in a malignancy; however, in this case, the target of the genetic or epigenetic alterations is the stem cell, rather than the somatic cell. In the case of the TOFT, there is increasing support that cancer is also due to abnormalities in the microenvironment as well as tissue organization, in addition to mutations in oncogenes and tumor suppressor genes. Stromal alterations resulting in increased genomic instability and eventual accumulation of genetic mutations in parenchymal cells or overexpression of stromal enzymes such as matrix metalloproteinases inducing reactive oxygen species (ROS) or free radicals inducing DNA damage span the gap between the SMT and the TOFT. In any case, a single path forward to explain the origin of carcinogenesis remains elusive and may likely involve components of multiple predominant theories.

1.2. General Features of Carcinogenesis

Genomic Instability: Initiation, Promotion, and Progression

Cancer develops as the result of the accumulation of numerous mutations over an extended period of time, resulting in progressive genomic instability and increasingly severe genomic alterations (Kumar et al., 2015). For neoplastic transformation of a normal cell to occur, heritable changes involving multiple, independent genes are required. In early studies, it was first observed that a long latent period could elapse from exposure to carcinogens to the development of cancer. In 1941, skin carcinogenesis experiments by Rous and Kidd showed that if dermal exposure to chemical carcinogens was interrupted, induced tumors would regress, only to reappear if the exposure was readministered (Rous & Kidd, 1941). It seemed, therefore, that a reversible process was taking place in those cells that did not attain the complete neoplastic state. These cells had undergone what Rous called "initiation."

During initiation, a normal cell undergoes an irreversible change that becomes fixed in the genome, making this cell more susceptible to transformation (Kumar et al., 2015). This change usually involves mutation of a proto-oncogene, tumor suppressor gene, or genes important for DNA repair. Initiation operationally implies that there is alteration to cellular DNA at one or more sites in the genome, which is converted to a stable biological lesion during DNA replication. Thus, if a round of cell replication occurs before the DNA damage is repaired, the lesion in the DNA is regarded as "fixed." Initiation is additive, and the yield of neoplasms is dose dependent. In other words, increasing the dose of an initiator increases the incidence and multiplicity of neoplasms and shortens the latency to neoplastic transformation. Since initiation requires fixation of a mutation in the genome by a round of cell proliferation, it is also influenced by cell cycle, with more rapidly dividing cells being more susceptible to initiating events. Mutations may either be "driver" mutations, which promote tumorigenesis and contribute to the development of a malignancy when accumulated over time, or "passenger" mutations, which may be numerous, and are generally not essential for transformation, but can still contribute to carcinogenesis through influencing cancer cell fitness, immunologic responses, and altered epigenetic mechanisms (Aparisi et al., 2019; McFarland et al., 2017; Pon & Marra, 2015). As a result of genomic instability and defective DNA repair mechanisms, by the time a cell acquires the number of driver mutations necessary for transformation, it may bear hundreds of acquired mutations which ultimately lead to neoplastic transformation over time. Initiated cells may remain functionally and phenotypically normal for a prolonged time before driven toward full conversion to a malignant neoplasm, often months in animals and years in humans.

Mutational events occur frequently in specific regions or key sequences of DNA that are hypermutagenic, i.e., are prone to mutation. Although mutations in genes occur frequently across the genome, there is a significant variation in somatic mutation rates in certain areas of DNA due to regional differences in DNA mismatch repair (MMR) (Supek & Lehner, 2015). Certain regions of DNA that are more critical for cellular functions have higher rates of and more efficient repair, whereas those regions that encode for housekeeping or noncritical functions have less efficient repair. Mutations in these regions contribute to genomic instability. Conversely, certain classes of genes cluster in regions with high mutation rates, or "hot spots," indicate that the region is prone to mutational events. Genes in "hot spots" tend to encode for dynamic processes such as cell signaling and immune responses, which can evolve in function to adapt to various stimuli (Chuang & Li, 2007). In terms of carcinogen exposure, frequencies of single-nucleotide polymorphisms (SNPs), single- and double-strand breaks (SSBs/DSBs), DNA adduct formation, oxidative damage, and DNA–DNA and DNA–protein cross-linking, chromosomal rearrangements, and changes in gene copy number are associated with exposure to various exogenous mutagens (Barnes et al., 2018; Rogozin et al., 2018). Adduct formation is a classic manifestation of chemical carcinogenesis, as many mutagenic chemicals are metabolized to reactive electrophiles that covalently bind and damage DNA (Barnes et al., 2018). In some cases, patterns of mutation and adduct formation are specific for carcinogen exposure. For example, DNA adducts are observed with various classes of carcinogens including the aromatic amines, polycyclic aromatic hydrocarbons, tobacco-specific nitrosamines, alkylating agents, aldehydes, volatile carcinogens, and oxidative damage (Ma et al., 2019). One example of a carcinogen-specific mutation due to adduct formation is that of AFB1 mycotoxin–induced hepatocellular carcinoma. In aflatoxicosis, the intermediate AFB1-8,9-epoxide reacts with guanine bases in DNA, forming adducts resulting in a specific transversion mutation at codon 249 in exon 7 of *TP53*. Guanine is susceptible to adduct formation because electrophilic carcinogens often target nucleophilic moieties in DNA, including nitrogen and oxygen in guanine (Barnes et al., 2018). Another DNA lesion associated with direct damage from a specific carcinogen is the formation of pyrimidine, or thymine, dimers. This lesion is induced directly by ultraviolet light as well as secondary to oxidative damage, in which pyrimidine dimers form (most often) between two thymine bases, interfering with DNA and RNA polymerases and inhibiting replication of the chromosome (Ikehata & Ono, 2011).

During the process of promotion, certain factors allow initiated cells to clonally expand. Tumor promoters enhance the development of neoplasms from a background of initiated cells by promoting cell growth and proliferation, interfering with normal apoptotic mechanisms, or through inflammatory or stromal mediators within the microenvironment that serve to provide a permissive environment for tumor growth. The temporal sequence of promoter administration is critical to the operational definition of promotion (Figure 8.1). The agent must be administered after initiation and cause enhancement of the neoplastic process to be considered a promoter (Pitot, 2007). In contrast to initiating events, effects of promoters are reversible, and promoters are generally nongenotoxic but influence or alter gene expression through various epigenetic mechanisms (see section below). Some promoters are believed to produce their effect by interaction with receptors in the cell membrane, cytoplasm, or nucleus (e.g., hormones, dioxin, phorbol ester, polychlorinated biphenyls). Alternatively, some hydrophilic and hydrophobic promoting agents exert their effect through their molecular orientation at cellular interfaces. Other promoters are mitogenic, stimulating DNA synthesis and enhanced cell proliferation. This may occur directly or indirectly by targeting cells with a shortened G1 phase, thereby giving them a selective proliferative advantage. Tumor promotion may be modulated by several factors, such as age, sex, diet, and hormone balance. Age- and sex-associated modulations in hormonal levels of estrogens, progesterone (PR), and androgens have been implicated as potential promoters of breast cancer on the basis of epidemiologic studies.

FIGURE 8.1 **Initiation–promotion models in chemical carcinogenesis.** The temporal sequence of administration of initiators and promoters is critical in the progression of neoplastic development. Administration of an initiator with continuous promoter exposure (A) or promoter exposure after initiation delay (B) results in a maximal tumor response, whereas a single administration of initiator without promoter (C), continual promoter administration without initiation (D), exposure to initiator following promoter priming (E), or inconsistent or minimal exposure to promoter following initiation (F) results in a reduced to minimal tumor response. Data demonstrated as a qualitative example of each of the conditions provided. *Modified from Pitot HC: Adventures in hepatocarcinogenesis,* Annu Rev Pathol 2:1–29, 2007.

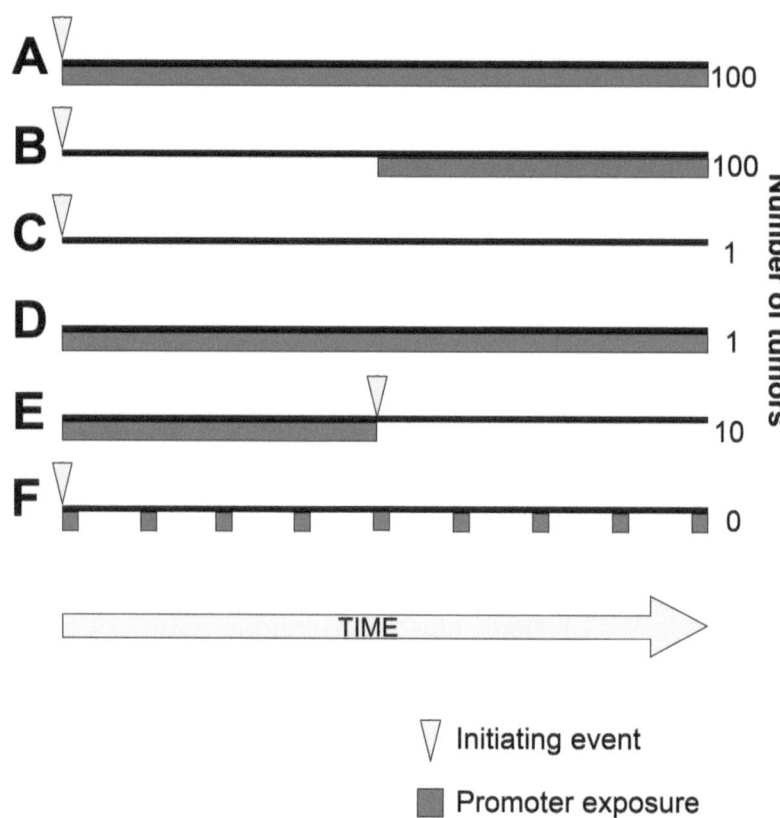

Experimental studies have shown repeatedly that these hormones, in addition to pituitary prolactin, serve to promote mammary tumors in rats initiated with mammary carcinogens.

Progression is that part of the multistep neoplastic process associated with the development of an initiated cell into a biologically malignant cell population. Progression is used frequently to signify the stages whereby a benign proliferation becomes malignant one, or where a neoplasm develops from a low grade to a high grade of malignancy. During progression, neoplasms show progressively increased invasive properties, develop the ability to metastasize, and have alterations in biochemical, metabolic, and morphologic characteristics. Tumor cell heterogeneity is an important characteristic of tumor progression. Expression of this heterogeneity includes antigenic and protein product variants, ability to elaborate angiogenesis factors, emergence of chromosomal variants, development of metastatic capability, altered metabolism, and decreased sensitivity to radiation or chemotherapeutics. The development of tumor heterogeneity may come about as a consequence of additional genomic changes, or as a result of altered epigenetic regulatory mechanisms. More than likely, genetic and epigenetic events subsequent to initiation operate in a nonmutually exclusive manner during progression, possibly in an ordered cascade of latter events superimposed on earlier events.

1.3. Cell Growth and Proliferation

The pivotal role of cell proliferation in all phases (e.g., initiation, promotion, progression) of the multistep process of carcinogenesis is inextricably linked to positive and negative cell cycle control mechanisms as influenced by oncogenes, tumor suppressor genes, growth factors and their cognate receptors, hormones and their receptors, and the action of exogenous agents (e.g., chemicals and viruses) on cell cycle control. Uncontrolled cellular proliferation is a hallmark of neoplasia, and many cancer cells demonstrate genetic alterations that regulate their cell cycles directly.

The prevailing model of the cell cycle is that of a series of transitions at which certain criteria must be met before the cell proceeds to the next phase (Figure 8.2). The cell cycle is composed of an S (DNA synthesis) and an M (mitotic)

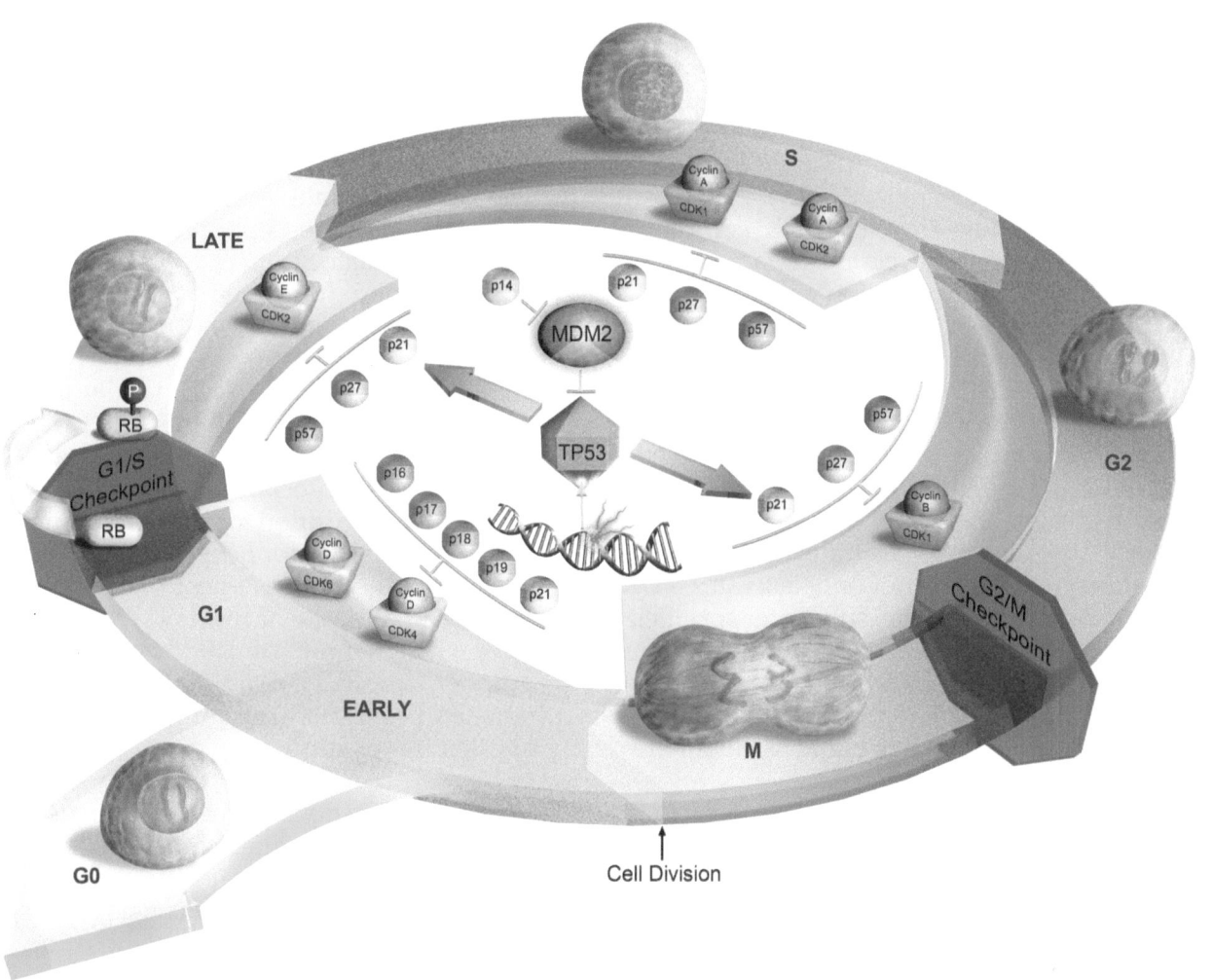

FIGURE 8.2   Cell cycle regulation. The cell cycle is composed of four phases, organized around the synthesis (S) of DNA and mitosis (M), separated by two intermediate gap phases, G1 and G2. During G1, or "growth" phase, the cell increases protein and organelle production in preparation for either differentiation and quiescence (G0), or continuation of cell cycle through the G1/S checkpoint into S phase. The S phase is the phase in which DNA synthesis occurs, ultimately resulting in duplication of the chromosomes. The S phase is followed by the second gap phase, G2, which is a phase of massive protein synthesis and rapid cell growth in preparation for mitosis. Once the cell cycle progresses through the G2/M cell cycle checkpoint, the cell enters mitosis and divides. Cell cycle progression is heavily regulated through the actions of cyclins, cyclin-dependent kinases (CDKs), cyclin-dependent kinase inhibitors (CDKIs) and two critical cell cycle checkpoint regulators, retinoblastoma (RB) and TP53. The association of cyclins with their respective CDKs drives the cell cycle forward, and the actions of CDKIs oppose the progression of the cell cycle by inhibiting binding of cyclins and CDKs. During early G1, a growth factor–dependent phase, association of cyclin D with CDK4/6 drives the cell cycle, while CDKIs p16, p17, p18, and p19 oppose cell cycle progression. In late G1, the cell cycle continues with cyclin E and CDK2 binding, which is opposed by the CKDIs p21, p27, and p57. Following the G1/S checkpoint, the S phase is driven by cyclin A binding with CDK1/2, with inhibition by p21, p27, and p57. Once in G2, the cycle progresses through the actions of cyclin B binding with CDK1, with inhibition by p21, p27, and p57. Once past the G2/M checkpoint, the cell undergoes mitosis. To maintain genomic integrity, the DNA sequence is assessed at the cell cycle checkpoints and the cell cycle halted if DNA errors or damage is detected. At the G1/S checkpoint, inhibition of RB phosphorylation halts the cell cycle before DNA synthesis ensues, preventing DNA damage from becoming fixed in the genome. At the G2/M checkpoint, TP53 induces cell cycle arrest through regulation of the CDKI p21, to prevent errors in the DNA from progressing through mitotic division. TP53 can be activated by numerous factors including DNA damage, cellular stress and injury, or hypoxia, and is inhibited at the protein level by MDM2, which targets it for degradation. The CDKI p14 provides a negative feedback loop inhibiting MDM2 function, to prevent degradation of TP53.

phase, separated by two gap phases (G1 and G2). Progression through the cell cycle is tightly controlled by a group of heterodimeric protein kinases comprising a cyclin as a regulatory element and a catalytic subunit known as a cyclin-dependent kinase (CDK). There are many combinations of cyclin/CDK complexes, and each phase of the cycle is characterized by a specific pattern of expression and activity.

Five major classes of mammalian cyclins (termed A–E) have been described. Cyclins C, D1–3, and E reach their peak of synthesis and activity during the G1 phase and regulate the transition from G1 to S phase. However, cyclins A and Bl–2 achieve their maximal levels later in the cycle, during the S and G2 phases, and are regarded as regulators of the transition to mitosis. Association with cyclins not only activates CDKs but also determines their substrate specificity. Depending on the cyclin partner and therefore the cell cycle stage, different key target molecules are phosphorylated. These events occur in a highly regulated temporal sequence that is maintained through a series of checkpoints.

The importance of DNA damage leading to the DNA damage response (DDR) and consequently cell cycle checkpoint activation is obvious. Replication of a damaged template would certainly result in irreversible chromosomal aberrations and a high mutation rate. Three major checkpoints are thought to be particularly important following DNA damage and have been established at the middle to end of G1 (preceding DNA replication), at G2 (preceding mitosis), and during mitosis (preceding chromosome segregation in anaphase).

Loss of the G1 checkpoint triggers genomic instability at the time of interaction of unrepaired DNA with the DNA replication machinery, leading to deletion-type mutations and aberrant gene amplification. Inactivation of the G1 checkpoint serves as an initiation step that makes the cell susceptible to unregulated growth (initiation), increasing the probability of subsequent genetic alterations and establishing the fully developed neoplastic phenotype. Control at the G1 checkpoint is dependent on cyclin D1 (degraded at the G1/S transition) and cyclin E (degraded in mid-S phase). Overexpression of either cyclin D1 or cyclin E and subsequent activation of the cyclin D1 and cyclin E/CDK complexes result in entry into S phase and decreased G1 time.

Cyclin D1 is overexpressed in many human cancers, including breast and nonsmall cell lung carcinomas, sarcomas, melanomas, B-cell lymphomas, and squamous cell carcinomas of the head and neck. Cyclin D1/CDK4 complexes act to phosphorylate retinoblastoma (RB), the product of the RB susceptibility gene. RB exerts a negative regulatory effect on gene expression through complex formation with DNA-binding proteins, including members of the E2F family. In nondividing or G0 (arrested) cells, hypophosphorylated RB is bound to E2F family members, leading to repression of E2F-mediated transcription. Upon phosphorylation by cyclin/CDK complexes, RB dissociates from E2F proteins, leading to transcription of genes promoting S phase entry. Thus, hypophosphorylated RB maintains cells in G1, whereas phosphorylation inactivates RB and allows exit from G1 (Figure 8.2). In humans, inactivation of RB is observed most commonly in RBs, osteosarcomas, carcinoid tumors, and nonsmall cell lung cancers.

Another tumor suppressor gene, TP53, is necessary for G1 phase arrest after DNA damage (Figure 8.2). Mutations at the TP53 locus are the most frequent genetic alterations associated with cancer in humans. The majority of TP53 mutations involve several highly conserved regions within the DNA-binding core. Loss of TP53 function allows synthesis of damaged DNA and increases the incidence of selected types of mutations. These increased incidences have been shown after a variety of DNA damage insults, such as ionizing radiation (strand breaks), alkylation by methyl-methane sulfonate, ultraviolet irradiation (photodimers), and a variety of environmental carcinogens. Thus, one of the major roles of TP53 is to ensure that, in response to genotoxic damage, cells arrest in G1 and attempt to repair their DNA before it is replicated.

The wild-type TP53 protein is normally kept at very low steady-state cellular levels by its relatively short half-life. However, it is stabilized and accumulates in the nucleus of cells undergoing or following DNA damage, or in cells responding to certain forms of stress. After DNA damage, TP53 binds a consensus-binding site and activates the transcription of several downstream genes, including P21. The P21 gene belongs to a family of negative cell cycle regulators, which function as CDK inhibitory molecules. Genes that encode these proteins are designated cyclin-dependent kinase inhibitor genes. These negative regulators form stable complexes with cyclin/CDK units and inactivate them. *P21* inactivates cyclin E/CDK2, cyclin A/CDK2, and cyclin D/CDK4/6 complexes, thereby inhibiting RB phosphorylation and preventing progression of the cell cycle during the late stages of G1 and beyond (Figure 8.2).

The TP53 protein also activates the proapoptotic *BAX* gene, which is involved in the regulation of apoptosis. Apoptosis is a cell suicide mechanism that leads to programmed cell death in response to DNA damage, preventing replication of cells that have sustained a degree of genetic damage beyond repair (see *Biochemical and Molecular Basis of Toxicity*, Vol 1, Chap 2 and *Morphologic Manifestations of Toxic Cell Injury*, Vol 1, Chap 6). The TP53 protein regulates its own function through the activation of the *MDM2* gene, which acts as a negative regulator, inhibiting wild-type *TP53* transcriptional activity through an autoregulatory feedback loop.

An RB-binding site has also been identified at the carboxy-terminal domain of MDM2 that interacts with RB and restrains its function. Thus, overexpression of *MDM2* inactivates both TP53 and RB, demonstrating a potential link between these genes in cell cycle regulation, apoptosis, and tumor progression. With the loss of both TP53 and RB, E2F activation stimulates unchecked cellular proliferation, leading to the emergence of neoplastic cell growth. The high rate and mutation pattern of *TP53* and *RB* in primary tumors have rendered them prototype tumor suppressor genes. Furthermore, detection of *TP53* and *RB* mutations and altered expression of their encoded products appear to be of clinical prognostic significance when identified in specific cancers. Additional gene products activated in response to DNA damage include transcription factors, growth factors, growth factor receptors, and enzymes and proteins associated with inflammation and tissue injury and repair.

1.4. Oncogenes and Tumor Suppressor Genes

As a result of progressive DNA damage and subsequent mutations, activating alterations in various oncogenes that drive cell proliferation, and inactivation of tumor suppressor genes that suppress proliferation, swing the balance toward increased proliferation, and ultimately to neoplastic transformation and progression (Kumar et al., 2015). Oncogenes are dominant-acting structural genes that encode for protein products capable of transforming the phenotype of a cell. Oncogenes were first identified as part of the genetic makeup of retroviruses, which function to transform virally infected cells and produce neoplasia in the host. It was later learned that transforming oncogenes are normal structural genes captured from eukaryotes previously infected by a retrovirus, rather than intrinsic viral genes. While the viral gene is referred to as a viral oncogene, the homologous gene in the host genome is called a cellular oncogene or a proto-oncogene (Vats & Emami, 1993). As the genomes of various mammalian and submammalian species were examined, it was found that homologues to the retroviral oncogenes were present in species as diverse as yeast, fruit flies, amphibians, birds, and mammals. The high degree of evolutionary conservation of these proto-oncogenes suggested that they served important normal functions in the cell. Proto-oncogenes encode for proteins that are important in cell growth, development, and differentiation. An activated proto-oncogene is referred to as an oncogene and may be altered quantitatively or qualitatively. Quantitative alteration results in overexpression of the normal gene, and qualitative alteration results from an activating mutation, both of which result in either inapporopriate expression or overexpression. Activation can occur in several ways, including through acquisition of point mutations, deletions, or gene fusions within the coding sequence of the proto-oncogene, leading to altered levels or schedule of expression of the normal protein product or in expression of an abnormal protein.

The activation of proto-oncogenes in spontaneous and chemically induced neoplasia has received considerable attention over the years. A variety of activated oncogenes have been documented in rodent neoplasms that play a role in the development of human cancers (Table 8.1). From some experimental studies, it appears that certain types of oncogenes are activated by carcinogen treatment and that this activation is sometimes an early event in tumor induction. Other studies with human and rodent neoplasms suggest that oncogene activation is involved later in the carcinogenic process, specifically

TABLE 8.1　Common Human Oncogenes, Mode of Activation, and Their Associated Tumors

Category	Proto-oncogene	Mode of activation	Associated human tumor
GROWTH FACTORS			
Platelet-derived growth factor-β (PDGF-β) chain	PDGFB	Overexpression	Astrocytoma
Fibroblast growth factors	HST1	Overexpression	Osteosarcoma
	FGF3	Amplification	Gastric, bladder, breast, melanoma
Transforming growth factor-alpha (TGF-a)	TGFA	Overexpression	Astrocytomas
Hepatocyte growth factor (HGF)	HGF	Overexpression	Hepatocellular carcinoma, thyroid cancer
GROWTH FACTOR RECEPTORS			
Epithelial growth factor (EGF) receptor family	ERBB1 (EGFR)	Mutation	Lung adenocarcinoma
	ERBB2 (HER)	Amplification	Breast carcinoma
FMS-like tyrosine kinase 3	FLT3	Point mutation	Leukemia
Receptor for neurotrophic factors	RET	Point mutation	Multiple endocrine neoplasia 2A and B
PDGF receptor	PDGFRB	Overexpression, translocation	Gliomas, leukemias
Receptor for KIT ligand	KIT	Point mutation	GIST, seminomas, leukemias
ALK receptor	ALK	Translocation, fusion gene	Lung adenocarcinoma, lymphomas
		Point mutation	Neuroblastoma
PROTEINS INVOLVED IN SIGNAL TRANSDUCTION			
GTP-binding (G) proteins	KRAS, HRAS, NRAS	Point mutation	Colon, lung, pancreatic, bladder, kidney, melanoma, bone marrow
	GNAQ	Point mutation	Uveal melanoma
	GNAS	Point mutation	Pituitary adenoma, other endocrine tumors

(Continued)

TABLE 8.1 Common Human Oncogenes, Mode of Activation, and Their Associated Tumors—cont'd

Category	Proto-oncogene	Mode of activation	Associated human tumor
Nonreceptor tyrosine kinase	ABL	Translocation, point mutation	Chronic myelogenous, acute lymphoblastic leukemia
RAS signal transduction	BRAF	Point mutation, translocation	Melanomas, leukemias, colon carcinoma, others
Notch signal transduction	NOTCH1	Point mutation, translocation Gene rearrangement	Leukemias, lymphomas, breast carcinoma
JAK/STAT signal transduction	JAK2	Translocation	Myeloproliferative disorders, acute lymphoblastic lymphoma
NUCLEAR REGULATORY PROTEINS			
Transcriptional activators	MYC	Translocation	Burkitt lymphoma
	NMYC	Amplification	Neuroblastoma
CELL CYCLE REGULATORS			
Cyclins	CCND1(Cyclin D1)	Translocation	Mantle cell lymphoma, multiple myeloma
		Amplification	Breast and esophageal cancers
Cyclin-dependent kinase	CDK4	Amplification or point mutation	Glioblastoma, melanoma, sarcoma

Modified from Kumar V., et al.: Robbins and Cotran pathologic basis of disease, Philadelphia, 2015, Elsevier Saunders. Used with permission.

during tumor progression. One important gene frequently mutated in several types of rodent and human cancer is the proto-oncogene *RAS*. The encoded protein for *RAS* is a G-coupled membrane protein and growth regulator that cycles between an inactive GDP-bound and active GTP-bound state. When *RAS* is mutated, hydrolysis of GTP to GDP is blocked, and *RAS* is stuck in a constitutively activated state, leading to activation of downstream cellular growth and proliferation pathways, gene transcription, and promotion of the cell cycle (Kumar et al., 2015). Another proto-oncogene, c-*MYC*, is commonly dysregulated and overexpressed in a variety of human and rodent cancers due to amplification or rearrangement. The *MYC* gene mediates fundamental cellular functions including metabolic processes, regulation of growth and proliferation, cell cycle progression, and regulation of differentiation, apoptosis, and stem cell regulation (Stefan & Bister, 2017). Dysregulation of *MYC* is commonly associated with neoplastic development and progression and is a hallmark of most human cancers.

Tumor suppressor genes also play a critical role in carcinogenesis (Table 8.2). These genes are regulatory genes that normally function to inhibit the activity of structural genes responsible for growth. As such, when intact, they have a function opposite to that of oncogenes and might effectively oppose the action of an oncogene. While proto-oncogenes have to be

TABLE 8.2   Select Human Tumor Suppressor Genes and Their Associated Cancers

Gene	Function	Sporadic cancers
INHIBITORS OF MITOGENIC SIGNALING PATHWAYS		
Adenomatous polyposis coli (APC)	Inhibitor of WNT signaling	Stomach, colon, pancreatic carcinoma, melanoma
Neurofibromin-1 (NF1)	Inhibitor of RAS/MAPK signaling	Neuroblastoma, juvenile myeloid leukemia
Merlin/neurofibromin-2 (NF2)	Cytoskeletal stability, hippo pathway signaling	Schwannoma, meningioma
Patched-1 (PTCH1)	Inhibitor of hedgehog signaling	Basal cell carcinoma, medulloblastoma
Phosphatase and tensin (PTEN)	Inhibitor of PI3K/AKT signaling	Diverse cancers, especially carcinomas and lymphoid
SMAD2, SMAD4	TGFβ signaling pathway, MYC/CDK inhibition	Frequently mutated in colonic and pancreatic carcinoma
INHIBITORS OF CELL CYCLE PROGRESSION		
Retinoblastoma (RB)	Inhibitor of G 1/S transition of cell cycle	Osteosarcoma, breast, colon, lung carcinomas
CDKN2A (p16/INK4a, p14/ARF)	Inhibition of CDKs (p16), activation of p53 (p14)	Pancreatic, breast, and esophageal, melanoma, leukemias
INHIBITORS OF "PROGROWTH" PROGRAMS OF METABOLISM AND ANGIOGENESIS		
von Hippel–Lindau (VHL) protein	Inhibitor of HIF1-α	Renal cell carcinoma
Liver kinase B1 (STK11)	Activator of AMPK kinases; suppresses cell growth	Diverse carcinomas (5%–20% of cases, depending on type)
SDHB, SDHD	TCA cycle, oxidative phosphorylation	Paraganglioma
INHIBITORS OF INVASION AND METASTASIS		
E-cadherin (CDH1)	Cell adhesion, inhibition of cell motility	Gastric carcinoma, lobular breast carcinoma
ENABLERS OF GENOMIC STABILITY		
p53 protein (TP53)	Cell cycle arrest, apoptosis from DNA damage	Most human cancers
DNA REPAIR FACTORS		
Breast cancer-1/2 (BRCA1/2)	Repair of double-stranded breaks in DNA	Rare
MSH2, MLH1, MSH6	DNA mismatch repair	Colonic and endometrial carcinoma

(Continued)

TABLE 8.2   Select Human Tumor Suppressor Genes and Their Associated Cancers—cont'd

Gene	Function	Sporadic cancers
UNKNOWN MECHANISMS		
Wilms tumor-1 (WT1)	Transcription factor	Wilms tumor, certain leukemias
Menin (MEN1)	Transcription factor	Pituitary, parathyroid, and pancreatic endocrine tumors

Modified from Kumar V., et al.: Robbins and Cotran pathologic basis of disease, *Philadelphia, 2015, Elsevier Saunders. Used with permission.*

activated to influence carcinogenesis, inactivation of both alleles of suppressor genes must occur for the transformed phenotype to be expressed. Inactivation can be achieved by chromosome loss, gene deletion, recombination, gene conversion, point mutation, or epigenetic silencing (see below). According to Knudson's two-hit hypothesis, loss of both alleles of a tumor suppressor gene either through direct genomic alterations or through epigenetic silencing is required to develop a cancer phenotype (Kumar et al., 2015). This hypothesis was developed by Alfred Knudson in 1971, through studies of RB in children (Knudson, 1971). These studies resulted in the discovery of tumor suppressor genes and their role in tumorigenesis. Knudson observed that RB was either an inherited or acquired neoplasm that likely developed through two mutational events. In the inherited form, the first "hit" was present already at birth but did not result in disease because the second allele was functional. The second "hit" occurred as an acquired event resulting in loss of heterozygosity (LOH), and subsequently development of RB at an early age. In the acquired form, an individual is born with two normal alleles for the *RB1* gene, and in order for disease to occur, both alleles must be lost, which explained a later onset of disease in these individuals. In addition to RB, mutation of *RB* occurs in most osteosarcomas and small cell lung cancers in humans, and is a component of the INK4A/Cyclin D1/RB/E2F regulatory pathway that is inactivated in most cancers (Dyson, 2016). Exceptions to the two-hit hypothesis for tumor suppressor genes include inactivation of a normal allele by genomic imprinting, an epigenetic process involving histone and DNA methylation which is established, or "imprinted," in the genome and maintained through mitotic division, or by dominant-negative mechanisms as is proposed for the *TP53* tumor suppressor gene, which is the most frequently mutated gene in human cancers (Kastenhuber & Lowe, 2017). The phosphatase and tensin (PTEN) tumor suppressor gene plays a significant role in the control of cell growth, proliferation, and survival. It is the most commonly mutated gene in sporadic human cancer, and loss of function of PTEN is associated with tumorigenesis in rodents as well as humans; several mouse models have been developed to study the pathogenesis of various human tumors mediated by alterations in this tumor suppressor gene (Hollander et al., 2011). Another tumor suppressor gene that has been targeted to model human cancer is the adenomatous polyposis coli (*APC*) gene. Genetically engineered mice (GEM) (ApcMin/+) with loss of one allele of the *APC* gene are commonly used as a model of human colorectal tumorigenesis, often in combination with other mutations in genes associated with intestinal carcinogenesis in humans (Jackstadt & Sansom, 2016).

As such, multiple tumor suppressor genes are often altered during neoplastic progression, in line with the understanding that cancer development involves perturbation of several levels of growth control. Taken together, activation of multiple oncogenes in concert with the loss of function of various tumor suppressor genes through genetic or epigenetic modification, influenced by a variety of endogenous and exogenous stimuli, ultimately culminates in the complex process of neoplastic transformation and progression.

1.5. Apoptosis and DNA Damage Repair

Current data strongly suggest that cell death may be as essential as cell proliferation in carcinogenesis. The ratio between cell birth and counterbalancing cell death determines tumor growth. Two forms of cell death may be seen in cancer development: necrosis and apoptosis. Necrosis typically occurs when a developing cancer outgrows its blood supply. In contrast, apoptosis is an energy-dependent process that involves active gene transcription and translation. In preneoplastic lesions, apoptosis is the predominant form of cell death. Chemicals, nutrient deprivation, certain cytokines, growth factors, and tumor suppressor genes may trigger enhanced apoptosis (Elmore, 2007).

As a result of either endogenous or exogenous DNA damage and genomic instability, a normal cell can either undergo successful DNA repair and return to normal state or if DNA repair is not successful, cells can either undergo apoptosis or survive, resulting in fixed mutations in its DNA structure (Kumar et al., 2015). This leads to functional alterations in oncogenes and tumor suppressor genes, impairment of apoptosis, and ultimately the formation of a malignant tumor. Apoptosis is a protective response to transformation; when DNA damage occurs that cannot be repaired, the affected cells undergo apoptosis to prevent fixation of DNA damage into the genomic sequence. However, in cancer cells that have defective DNA repair mechanisms, DNA damage not corrected becomes fixed in the genome, and this contributes to further genomic instability (Kumar et al., 2015). Thus, apoptosis is a barrier that must be surmounted for cancer to develop and progress, and any abnormalities in the function of genes responsible for normal apoptosis pathway function can predispose to neoplastic transformation.

Apoptosis occurs through two primary mechanisms; the intrinsic and extrinsic apoptosis pathways (Pfeffer & Singh, 2018), *Biochemical and Molecular Basis of Toxicity*, Vol 1, Chap 2 and *Morphologic Manifestations of Toxic Cell Injury*, Vol 1, Chap 6. In the intrinsic (mitochondrial) pathway, cells, which sustain irreparable internal injury due to DNA damage, cellular injury, or stress, undergo apoptosis through release of cytochrome C from the inner mitochondrial membrane in a TP53-dependent fashion, triggering activation of downstream initiator (Caspase 9) and effector (Caspase 3) caspases, leading to the morphologic changes typical of apoptosis. Tumor cells may evade the intrinsic apoptosis pathway and escape cell death through dysfunction of the TP53 pathway or upregulation of prosurvival (*BCL2, BCL-XL*) or inhibition of proapoptosis (*BAX, BAK*) mitochondrial genes (Hata et al., 2015).

In the extrinsic pathway, external signals such as an immune cell response function by activation of death signaling cascades to mediate cell death due to defects in viability. To evade the extrinsic apoptosis pathway, tumor cells may survive through interference with death receptor (e.g., Fas/FasL) function or binding, resulting in defective Caspase 8 function and inactivation of the apoptosis signaling complex. Interference with the intrinsic or extrinsic pathways leads to inhibition of apoptosis and faulty DNA repair, resulting in fixation of additional mutations in the genome over time, and neoplastic transformation and progression (Pfeffer & Singh, 2018).

Tumor cells can also evade apoptosis through inhibition of senescence. Senescence is the process by which cells exit the cell cycle, stop dividing, and become quiescent. Senescence is prevented by the function of telomeres, which are regions of repetitive nucleotide sequences at the ends of each chromosome (Bernal & Tusell, 2018). Each time a cell divides, a small amount of each telomere is lost; as telomeres shorten, the cell ages and eventually stops dividing once the telomeres are completely lost. At this point, the cell enters senescence and may die as a normal part of cellular aging. Telomerase is an enzyme that functions to preserve the telomere, adding nucleotides to the ends of chromosomes to preserve the structural integrity of the telomere. Some cancer cells function to escape senescence through induction of telomerase expression, thereby avoiding cell death through telomere-mediated senescence and apoptosis. Additionally, cancer cells may induce expression of embryonic growth pathways, stem cell genes, and developmental mediators that prevent senescence, allowing them to continue to proliferate (Safa, 2016).

1.6. Angiogenesis, Invasion, and Metastasis

In order for a tumor to survive, it has to be able to grow and proliferate, which requires a sufficient supply of oxygen and nutrients. This requires the acquisition of an independent blood supply. Tumor cells acquire a blood supply through numerous signaling molecules, cytokines, and chemokines, growth factors such as vascular endothelial growth factor, platelet-derived growth factor, and fibroblast growth factor family members, matrix metalloproteinases, integrins and their receptors, and endothelial cells and endothelial progenitor cells, to induce the formation of new blood vessels (Quail & Joyce, 2013), in the form of angiogenesis, neovascularization, or vasculogenic mimicry (Furuya et al., 2005). These processes are driven by tumor cell signaling within the extracellular matrix (ECM) via a number of angiogenic factors. Angiogenesis is defined as the formation of new blood vessels from preexisting vessels, as quiescent endothelial cells become activated when stromal, tumor, and immune cell–derived proangiogenic factors are secreted into the tumor site, leading to proliferation, migration, degradation of the ECM, and tube formation from existing capillaries. Neovascularization is the formation of new blood vessels from bone marrow progenitor cells, with no involvement of preexisting vasculature; bone marrow–derived endothelial precursor cells are recruited to the tumor site and differentiate into endothelial cells, forming de novo capillaries. Finally, vasculogenic mimicry is the formation of channels within tumors by motile tumor cells (rather than endothelial cells) that act as blood channels to feed the tumor. And so, through various mechanisms, tumors can induce their own blood supply through systemic signaling to the bone marrow (neovascularization), or local proangiogenic signaling to promote vascular ingrowth from preexisting vasculature (angiogenesis), or invasive properties of the tumor itself to form vascular channels through vasculogenic mimicry.

In order to develop an invasive and metastatic phenotype, a tumor cell must acquire a number of important features, including epithelial–mesenchymal transition (EMT), ability to escape anoikis (anchorage-dependent apoptosis) and survive in the circulation, and evasion of the immune system. EMT is the process by which an epithelial tumor cell develops a mesenchymal phenotype necessary for migration, especially during local invasion and metastasis. During this process, cells gradually lose expression of epithelial-type proteins (e.g., cytokeratins, E-cadherin, claudins, desmoplakin) that anchor them to the basement membrane and acquire mesenchymal-type proteins (e.g., vimentin, fibronectin, collagen I/III, α-smooth muscle actin) that allow them to reorganize their cytoskeleton, degrade ECM, and migrate through tissue (Angadi et al., 2016). Having obtained an EMT phenotype, tumor cells subsequently need mechanisms to survive outside of the

supporting basement membrane, within the circulation, and at a distant site. Normal epithelial cells that lose integrity of tight junctions or detach from the supporting basement membrane undergo anoikis or anchorage-dependent apoptosis. Obviously, for neoplastic epithelial cells to migrate, this cannot happen. Therefore, tumor cells develop mechanisms to escape anoikis, through increasing genetic instability, intratumoral hypoxia, EMT, and activation of stem cell pathways, in order to survive in the ECM and circulation (Paoli et al., 2013). Finally, to survive migration through the stroma, into and out of the vasculature, within the circulation, and for survival and establishment at the distant site, metastatic tumor cells require the ability to evade the immune system. Evasion of the immune system is accomplished by tumor cells through three primary mechanisms: (1) downregulation or shedding of strong tumor associated antigens that allow the immune system to recognize them, (2) upregulation of antiapoptotic (e.g., *BCL2*) or growth factor (e.g., human epidermal growth factor receptor-2 genes, and (3) induction of an immunosuppressive tumor microenvironment through tumoral expression of antiinflammatory cytokines (e.g., transforming growth factor-beta, interleukin-10) and other molecules that interfere with adaptive immunity. Through these complex and intricate mechanisms, cancer cells are able to survive and migrate in the ECM and systemic circulation, evade host antitumor mechanisms, and undergo growth and proliferation at distant sites to establish metastatic disease.

2. MECHANISMS OF CHEMICALLY INDUCED CARCINOGENESIS

Carcinogenesis is a multistep process and involves the transformation of normal cells into cancer cells triggered by initial events including mutagenesis and genome instability which can promote selective proliferation of the mutated cell leading to neoplasia over time (McGranahan & Swanton, 2017; Tomasetti et al., 2017). Chemicals/xenobiotics that can promote carcinogenic risk have been extensively studied and can be subdivided into two major classes, namely genotoxic carcinogens that can directly interact with the DNA duplex and nongenotoxic carcinogens that indirectly mutate the genome (Table 8.3).

TABLE 8.3   Features of Direct and Indirect Acting
Carcinogens

Feature	Genotoxic (direct) carcinogens	Nongenotoxic (indirect) carcinogens
Mutagenic	X	
DNA reactive	X	
Dose-dependent tumorigenicity	X	X
Nonmutagenic		X
DNA nonreactive		X
Pathway-based mutagenicity		X
Inhibition of DNA repair proteins		X
Oxidative stress		X
Tissue specificity		X
Species specificity		X

2.1. Genotoxic Carcinogens

Genotoxic carcinogens are DNA reactive, leading to damage and ensuing mutation of the genome. Numerous genotoxic carcinogens have been identified with established mechanisms of action including urethane, benzo[a]pyrene (BaP), N-ethyl-N-nitrosourea (ENU), 2-acetylaminofluorene, and diaminobenzamide. Genotoxic carcinogens can mutate the genome either with metabolic activation (i.e., parent compound needing metabolism to engage the DNA duplex) or without this occurring (e.g., compounds that bind the DNA duplex without a need for metabolism).

2.2. Direct Acting Carcinogens

Compounds that do not require metabolic activation to induce mutagenesis associated with cancer risk are known as direct acting carcinogens. Direct acting carcinogens are highly electrophilic and bind DNA with high affinity due to the nature of their chemical structure and composition. Additional factors that promote DNA reactivity of agents include nucleophilicity properties, accessibility of the DNA, and van der

Waals forces that regulate electrostatic interactions between an agent and DNA (Swenson, 1983). These properties render such mutagenic compounds carcinogenic as tumors can potentially form in exposed tissues. The potential of mutagenic compounds to cause cancer depends not only on the replicative capacity of the exposed tissue but also membrane permeability of the exposed cell, the rate of interaction between carcinogen and the DNA duplex, intracellular free radicals triggered by the mutagen, and stability of the chemical itself. Direct acting carcinogens include nanoparticles (Rim et al., 2013; Wan et al., 2017), epoxides (Wade et al., 1979), chemotherapeutics (Benedict et al., 1977; Szikriszt et al., 2016), alkyl halides, and esters (Sobol et al., 2007). The Ames bacterial reverse mutagenicity test (Ames et al., 1973) assesses mutagenesis in the bacterial strains *Salmonella typhimurium* and/or *Escherichia coli* and has been used successfully for decades. It is able to identify the mutagenic capacity of most direct acting electrophilic carcinogens that do not require additional metabolic activation (for example, using S9 fraction of rat liver homogenate) (Zeiger, 2019; Kirkland et al., 2011). Even so, false positives and false negatives are known to have occurred due to the artificially high doses of the chemical and factors involving the mitogenic responses and mutagenicity for a chemical/xenobiotic established using the Ames test and that may not necessarily translate to carcinogenic potential (Walmsley & Billinton, 2011).

2.3. Indirect Acting Carcinogens

Metabolic activation and transformation of a parent compound (procarcinogen) by liver enzymes is a key determinant of the carcinogenic potential of many xenobiotics. Cytosol and microsome fractions (e.g., S9) obtained from rat liver homogenates are most often used together with a compound in the standard in vitro genetic toxicology battery comprising the Ames test (determines whether there has been mutagenicity), micronucleus test (assesses aneugenicity), the COMET assay (detects DNA breakage and damage), or chromosomal aberration (clastogenicity) tests (Table 8.4). Pivotal work done by Miller et al. involving indirect genotoxic nonelectrophilic carcinogens p-Dimethylaminoazobenzene and

TABLE 8.4 OECD Testing Guidelines for Mutagenicity, Clastogenicity, and Aneugenicity Tests

Guideline no.	Description	Assay condition	References
471	Bacterial reverse mutagenicity test		(OECD, 2020)
473	Mammalian chromosomal aberration test	In vitro	(OECD, 2016a)
476	Mammalian cell gene mutation tests using the Hprt and Xprt genes		(OECD, 2016d)
474	Mammalian erythrocyte micronucleus test		(OECD, 2016b)
475	Mammalian bone marrow chromosomal aberration test	In vivo	(OECD, 2016c)
487	Mammalian cell micronucleus test		(OECD, 2016e)

Hprt, hypoxanthine-guanine phosphoribosyltransferase.
Xprt, xanthine phosphoribosyltransferase.

BaP showed a requirement for metabolism of the parent compound associated with its carcinogenic potential (Miller & Miller, 1947, 1981; Miller, 1951). Xenobiotics may also promote mutagenicity and/or cancer risk following persistent signal transduction pathway activation/inhibition, oxidative damage, disequilibrium in ROS within the cell, errors in machinery required for replication/repair of the DNA duplex, or alterations in the mammalian epigenome or chromatin structure/function (Klaunig et al., 2011; Moggs & Terranova, 2018; Macheret & Halazonetis, 2015; Minocherhomji et al., 2015; Kerr et al., 1992). Several signal transduction pathways and those that function via various upstream kinases, including the phosphatidylinositol 3-kinase delta (PI3Kδ), p38 kinases, mitogen-activated protein kinases (MAPK), c-Jun N-terminal kinases, and extracellular signal-regulated kinases, can be influenced by either agonistic or antagonistic effects of xenobiotics (Klaunig et al., 2011; Compagno et al., 2017; Timblin & Bergman, 1997; Klaunig et al., 1998). An imbalance of such pathways can be directly linked with perturbed downstream mechanisms that may promote mutagenicity of the DNA duplex. Recent reports examining the mutagenic capability of PI3Kδ inhibition by xenobiotics and endogenous aldehydes provide direct evidence for xenobiotics traditionally classified as "nonmutagenic" that can promote mutagenesis and increase genome instability by pathway activation in normal mammalian genomes (Compagno et al., 2017; Garaycoechea et al., 2018). Persistent PI3Kδ inhibition results in triggering of the activation-induced deaminase (AID), leading to increased off-target AID-dependent mutagenicity (Compagno et al., 2017). Furthermore, activation or inhibition of signal transduction pathways by an imbalance in ROS can lead to perturbation in expression of genes whose function is required for cellular processes including DNA duplication, mitochondrial function, apoptosis/programmed cell death, or differentiation (Henkler et al., 2010; Lu et al., 2014; Minocherhomji et al., 2012; Shen et al., 2013; Ning et al., 2014).

2.4. Mechanisms of High-fidelity/Nonmutagenic or Low-fidelity/Mutagenic DNA Repair

Direct acting carcinogens are strong electrophiles that can readily bind genomic DNA and form DNA adducts, induce DNA cross-links, or induce other forms of DNA damage including SSBs or DSBs. Cells are proficient in the repair of DNA lesions (Table 8.5); however, the capacity to repair these lesions in an error-free manner can be dependent on the persistence of the damage at the impacted region of the genome or underlining inherent repair capacity impacted by heritable mutations in certain genes (e.g., BRCA1/2) and their involvement in high-fidelity DNA repair mechanisms (Abaji et al., 2005; West, 2003).

High-fidelity DNA repair pathways including error-free homologous recombination (HR) (Jasin & Rothstein, 2013), the Fanconi Anemia (FA) pathway (Nalepa & Clapp, 2018), MMR (Jiricny, 2013), base excision repair (BER) (Krokan & Bjørås, 2013), and classical non-homologous end joining (NHEJ) (Rodgers & McVey, 2016) suppress error-prone mutagenic repair of DNA lesions and promote genomic stability. However, persistence of the lesion(s) as a result of sustained carcinogen exposure can lead to an exhaustive state that activates error-prone DNA repair pathways that serve to promote cell viability albeit at a cost of increased mutagenicity and genomic

instability (Rodgers & McVey, 2016). Similarly, genome editing therapeutics including CRISPR–Cas9 and TALENs can promote off-target mutations or structural changes in the genome following the erroneous repair of induced double-strand break replication intermediates (Rodgers & McVey, 2016; Cox et al., 2015). This balance of DNA repair capacity is further impacted when there is an underlying genetic defect or mutation in genes that function as tumor suppressors (Vineis, 2004). For example, individuals having inherited mutations in the BRCA1 or BRCA2 tumor suppressor genes are at an increased risk of developing breast and/or ovarian cancers (Scully, 2000). Therefore, exposure of individuals having these underlying genetic defects could predispose them further to cancers at a faster rate than their wild-type counterparts following carcinogen-induced DNA damage because of salvage/backup error-prone DNA repair pathway activation. Salvage DNA repair pathways including alternative non-HR (Bennardo et al., 2008; Bothmer et al., 2010), single-strand annealing (Rodgers & McVey, 2016), microhomology-mediated break-induced repair (MMBIR) (Fitzgerald et al., 2017), or mitotic DNA synthesis (MiDAS) (Minocherhomji et al., 2015) are activated under conditions of persistent drug-induced replication stress. The activation of these carcinogen-induced error-prone mechanisms can lead to mutations at tumor suppressor genes and increased fitness of preneoplastic cells to clonally expand and form tumors over time (Venkatesan et al., 2017) as evidenced by the effects of known carcinogens including urethane, ENU, and BaP that are well established to induce tumors (Riley et al., 1994; Hecht et al., 1994; Gurley et al., 2015). Additionally, blocking of PI3Kδ by the small molecule inhibitors idelalisib or duvelisib, compounds that are not directly mutagenic, has recently been shown to increase expression of the AID in mice which leads to increased AID-induced random mutagenesis and ultimately gives rise to plasma cell tumors (Compagno et al., 2017).

TABLE 8.5   DNA Repair Pathways and Fidelity

DNA repair fidelity	DNA repair pathways
High fidelity (error free)	Homologous recombination (HR)
	Fanconi anemia (FA) pathway
	Nucleotide excision repair (NER)
	Base excision repair (BER)
	Mismatch repair (MMR)
Low fidelity (error prone)	Non-homologous end joining (NHEJ)
	Alternative nonhomologous end joining (Alt-NHEJ)
	Break-induced replication (BIR)
	Microhomology-mediated break-induced replication (MMBIR)

2.5. DNA Replication and Repair Mechanisms

Cells are proficient for the repair of DNA damage resulting from exogenous or endogenous stressors. However, persistent DNA damage and stress can inundate the capacity to carry out high-fidelity DNA repair and activate mutagenic DNA repair pathways that serve to maintain cell viability, albeit at a cost of increased genome instability that can give rise to human diseases/disorders including cancers, premature aging, neurological abnormalities, and immunodeficiency syndromes (Iyama & Wilson, 2013; Norbury & Hickson, 2001; Taylor et al., 2019).

Homologous Recombination

HR is an intrinsic essential process that has a critical role in the cell through the replication and repair of the DNA duplex. HR is the predominant pathway used by cells to repair DNA DSBs. Following DNA damage, the DDR ensures high-fidelity DNA repair pathway activation. Following DSB resection, the HR machinery promotes synapse formation that leads to the intertwining of the homologous donor regions (template) and priming/initiation of DNA synthesis (Wright et al., 2018). This process resolves the DSB in an error-free manner and without the formation of mutations.

Non-homologous end Joining

NHEJ involves the joining of two broken ends of chromosomal regions either from the same chromosome or different chromosomes (Lieber, 2010). NHEJ can repair DSBs in an error-free manner only when the broken/blunt-ended DNA ends are ligated without deletions/insertions. NHEJ also has cell essential roles in generating diversity at the T-cell receptor and immunoglobulin [V(D)J recombination and class switch recombination] loci. Individuals that have inactivating mutations in NHEJ proteins are increasingly immunodeficient and can be sensitive to ionizing radiation. Alternative NHEJ is an erroneous backup pathway to canonical NHEJ under conditions of stress or when NHEJ is disabled as a result of mutations in genes that function in NHEJ.

Excision Repair Pathways

Excision repair pathways including base excision repair, nucleotide excision repair and mismatch repair, remove DNA adducts or chemically modified bases that arise within the double stranded DNA duplex as a result of

spontaneous mutations, errors during DNA repair or damage (Krokan & Bjørås, 2013; Lindahl, 1993). Recognition and removal of the damaged base occurs by excision repair machinery through short or long patch repair mechanisms. These excision repair pathways have major protective roles against the development of cancers.

Fanconi Anemia Pathway

The FA pathway is critical in the repair of interstrand cross-links (ICLs) that form within the double-stranded DNA duplex (Ceccaldi et al., 2016). ICLs inhibit the progression of the DNA replication fork during genome duplication or transcription. ICL repair or bypass is critical for cell viability and continued proliferation. Individuals having dysfunctions/mutations in any one gene involved in the FA pathway (e.g., FANCA) have an increased predisposition to cancers. Components of the FA pathway have important roles in cytokinesis, replication fork protection, and DNA repair.

Break-induced Replication

Break-induced replication (BIR) is a highly mutagenic salvage DNA repair process that can lead to complex chromosomal aberrations and genome instability (Rodgers & McVey, 2016; Kramara et al., 2018). Under normal conditions, BIR fails to get activated as error-free pathways are more prevalent. However, following cellular or replicative stress, cells can activate salvage pathways including BIR to maintain viability, albeit at a cost of genome instability. BIR-mediated repair of collapsed replication forks in mammals involves RAD51 and/or RAD52 in a BRCA2-dependent manner. Regions in the genome, including common fragile sites (CFSs) and telomeres that frequently undergo "breakage" under conditions of increased cellular/replication stress and perturbed DNA synthesis, require BIR-like processes for replication/repair. MiDAS, a BIR-like process, is a salvage repair pathway that is activated in early mitosis at CFSs and telomeres to maintain cellular viability and leads to the appearance of chromosome aberrations/breaks (clastogenicity), a phenomenon that is exacerbated in cancer cells (Minocherhomji et al., 2015; Bhowmick et al., 2016; Dilley et al., 2016).

Microhomology-Mediated Break-induced Replication

The MMBIR pathway involves the erroneous replication/repair of regions of the genome that share regions of the genome with short tracks of homology (microhomology). Repetitive regions of the genome that can be repaired based on their microhomology can lead to complex chromosomal rearrangements associated with genome instability. MMBIR is predominantly active when loci need repair in the G1 or G2 phases (nonreplicative phases) of the cell cycle and following persistent endogenous or exogenous stressors, including ROS, radiation, and DNA damaging agents.

2.6. Consequences of Genotoxicity

DNA lesions that are caused by either endogenous mechanisms or via persistent exposure to carcinogens or mutagens can lead to numerous genomic and cellular outcomes if left unrepaired or repaired by erroneous DNA repair pathways. These include mutations, genome instability, micronucleus formation, chromosome aberrations/breaks, and chromosome nondisjunction in mitosis. Avoidance of these results is key in the maintenance of genome stability, cellular viability, and inhibition of carcinogenesis.

2.7. Nongenotoxic Carcinogens

Several chemicals that are negative in traditional genotoxicity assays still cause cancer through nongenotoxic modes of action (MOAs). Even though these chemicals do not directly interact with DNA, they do influence several steps in chemical carcinogenesis such as oxidative damage, indirect DNA damage, cytotoxicity, altered gene expression, transcription factor activation, epigenetic alterations, immune suppression, increased proliferation, and decreased apoptosis. In general, based on the current risk assessment paradigm, nongenotoxic carcinogens have a threshold dose below which there is no potential for carcinogenicity unlike genotoxic carcinogens, where there is no apparent theoretical threshold (linear no-threshold model). Thresholds of toxicological concern are an important consideration in risk assessment since genotoxic chemicals are considered to pose a risk

of cancer over a lifetime exposure of chemicals, even when the doses are extremely low, especially related to food additives. The topic of thresholds for carcinogens is controversial and beyond the scope of this chapter. However, the reader is encouraged to refer to reviews on the topic (Clewell et al., 2019; Kobets & Williams, 2019; Neumann, 2009; Nohmi, 2018). Some of the common modes of nongenotoxic carcinogenesis are related to nuclear receptors, hormones, oxidative damage, cytotoxicity, immune suppression, and epigenetic alterations.

Receptor-Mediated Modes of Action

Nuclear receptors bind to lipophilic endogenous or exogenous ligands to regulate the transcription of several genes involved in cellular homeostasis but are also associated with diseases such as cancer when dysregulated. Nuclear receptors are conserved in animals and are encoded by about 50 functional genes (48 in humans, 47 in rats, and 49 in mice). All nuclear receptors have the same basic structure/function with a variable C-terminal ligand binding domain, conserved N-terminal DNA-binding domain, and various transactivation domains (Evans & Mangelsdorf, 2014).

Aryl Hydrocarbon Receptor

The AhR belongs to basic helix–loop–helix/Per–Ahr nuclear translocator (ARNT)–Sim transcription factor families. In the absence of ligands, the AhR is located in the cytoplasm as part of a protein complex comprising heat shock protein (HSP)90, p23, and AhR-interacting protein. AhR may be activated by numerous endogenous ligands, such as indirubin, kynurenine, equilenin, and arachidonic acid metabolites, or exogenous ligands, such as 2,3,7,8-tetrachlorodibenzo-p-dioxin (TCDD), polycyclic aromatic hydrocarbons, and phytochemicals such as flavonoids and indole-3-carbinol (I3C). Upon ligand activation, the AhR is activated, detaches from the cytoplasmic complex, and translocates to the nucleus. The nuclear AhR complex is a heterodimer containing the AhR and Arnt proteins, and the molecular mechanism of AhR action is associated with binding of the heterodimer to dioxin-responsive elements in regulatory regions of Ah-responsive genes. The classical AhR target genes include cytochrome P450 *(Cyp)1a1, Cyp1a2,* and *Cyp1b1.* Based on the potency of AhR activation, it can result in a carcinogenic response such as by TCDD or an anticarcinogenic response such as by I3C (Safe, 2001). AhR activators that result in tumor formation may function as complete carcinogens or tumor promoters based on their potency of activation. As indicated earlier, TCDD is not genotoxic but its fairly long half-life and ability to bioaccumulate results in sustained activation of the AhR and its downstream targets that in turn cause sustained oxidative stress, and subsequent DNA damage and mutations. In addition, AhR activation leads to induction of CYP1A1 that can metabolize procarcinogens such as BaP to reactive intermediates that can cause DNA and protein adducts resulting in mutagenesis and neoplasia. Hence, TCDD is considered a complete carcinogen where tumors can be initiated and promoted by the similar mechanism (International Agency for Research on Cancer I, 2018).

Several structurally related halogenated aromatic hydrocarbons such as polychlorinated dibenzodioxins and polychlorinated biphenyls are referred to as dioxin-like compounds (DLCs). They activate AhR and cause similar pleotropic responses as TCDD but at varying potencies. Regulatory agencies have developed toxicity equivalence factors (TEFs) for measuring the potency of DLCs, with TCDD as the index chemical. Exposures to mixtures of DLCs are calculated as a simple weighted sum of the individual quantities multiplied by their respective TEFs to yield the equivalent dose in units of TCDD exposure (Van den Berg et al., 2006). This allowed the regulators to assess risk associated with exposures to mixtures that activate AhR. Even though AhR expression is conserved across species, its effects are modulated by various factors including genetic polymorphisms, ligand selectivity and affinity, differences in coactivators, and downstream signaling pathways. In addition, these factors also contribute to interspecies and interindividual variation in responses. The human and mouse AhRs exhibit significant differences in ligand specificity that may differentially (both higher or lower depending on the ligand) influence carcinogenesis, and as a result, the mouse model may overpredict or underpredict human carcinogenesis (Murray et al., 2014).

AhR activators also cross-talk with other nuclear receptors, such as the estrogen receptor (ER), androgen receptor (AR), and retinoic acid receptor-β, and modulate the pathology driven by them. For example, both TCDD and I3C inhibit estrogen-induced breast and endometrial cancer. Several tumors express aberrantly high levels of AhR or its targets such as CYP1B1 and lead to differing prognosis depending on the tumor type. For example, high levels of nuclear AhR lead to poor prognosis in lung squamous cell carcinomas, whereas in breast cancer, it is inversely correlated with the histologic grade. Therefore, modulation of the AhR may be considered as a therapeutic approach in some human cancers (Safe, 2001).

Constitutive Androstane Receptor/Pregnane-X-Receptor

Constitutive androstane receptors/pregnane-X-receptors (CARs/PXRs) are xenobiotic and endobiotic receptors within the nuclear receptor subfamily 1 and belong to the zinc finger class of transcription factors. Both CAR and PXR are low-affinity xenosensors with a variety of functions related to metabolism, transport, and clearance of xenobiotics. CARs/PXRs share several common agonists and most of the drugs or environmental xenobiotics simultaneously activate CAR/PXR. As a result, in the context of chemical carcinogenesis, the biology of CAR/PXR is generally examined in tandem.

CAR, in contrast to other nuclear receptors, is constitutively active in the absence of a ligand and is regulated by both agonists and inverse agonists (binds to the same receptor as an agonist but induces opposite pharmacological effects as an agonist). The inactive phosphorylated CAR located in the cytosol is part of a multiprotein complex that contains HSP90 and the cytoplasmic CAR retention protein. CAR may be activated directly by binding to ligands such as (6-(4-chlorophenyl)imidazo(2,1-b) (1,3)thiazole-5-carbaldehyde O-(3,4-dichlorobenzyl)oxime) (CITCO) for human CAR, 1,4-bis[2-(3,5-dichloropyridyloxy)]benzene (TCPOBOP) for mouse CAR, or indirectly by phenobarbital or phenytoin. Upon TCPOBOP or CITCO binding, CAR is dephosphorylated by protein phosphatase 2 (PP2A). However, the indirect CAR activators competitively bind to EGFR and activate steroid receptor coactivator 1 which dephosphorylates RACK-1 that in turn stimulates PP2A to dephosphorylate CAR. This dephosphorylated CAR is translocated from the cytosol into the nucleus and binds to phenobarbital-responsive enhancer module either as a monomer or together with the retinoid X receptor (RXR) and regulates the downstream targets related to xenobiotic or endobiotic metabolism such as CYP2B, CYP2C, and CYP3A subfamilies, sulfotransferases, and glutathione S-transferases. In humans, PXR is also referred to as steroid and xenobiotic sensing nuclear receptor. Compared to CAR, PXR has a broader substrate specificity due to its flexible ligand-binding pocket and is activated by a range of xenobiotics such as steroids, antibiotics (rifampicin), bile acids, SR12813, paclitaxel, tamoxifen, hyperforin, and a variety of botanicals. Similar to CAR, activated PXR heterodimerizes with RXR and binds to hormone responsive elements on the DNA and regulates the expression of a variety of downstream targets including CYP2B, CYP2C, CYP3A, UGT1A1, glutathione S-transferase, OATP2, MDR1, and 5-AAS.

CAR/PXR activators increase the expression of several xenobiotic responsive genes and are morphologically manifested as centrilobular hepatocellular hypertrophy and hepatomegaly. This is a transient adaptive response to combat the xenobiotic-induced stress. However, prolonged consistent activation of CAR results in oxidative stress causing the progression to hyperplasia and neoplasia. Unlike genotoxic carcinogens, they do not bind to DNA or cause DNA damage but do cause increases in cell proliferation and decreased apoptosis (Huang et al., 2005). CAR/PXR knock-out mouse models have demonstrated unequivocally that consistent activation of these nuclear receptors results in hepatocellular carcinogenesis. However, the translational relevance of CAR-induced hepatocellular tumors in rodents is highly controversial (Elcombe et al., 2014; Felter et al., 2018). Several publications based on humanized CAR/PXR mouse models and chimeric mouse models with humanized livers suggest that CAR activation results in hepatocellular hypertrophy and hepatomegaly but not hyperplasia, implying decreased cancer risk in humans (Ross et al., 2010; Yamada et al., 2014; Haines et al., 2018). Epidemiological data from epileptic patients

receiving phenobarbital over their lifetime did not show clear evidence of increased risk for the development of hepatocellular tumors (La Vecchia & Negri, 2014). However, other lines of experimental data support the translational relevance of CAR-induced hepatocellular carcinogenesis. CAR activation is known to be either a tumor promoter or inhibitor based on the context. In mice, phenobarbital inhibits hepatocellular tumors with constitutively activated MAP kinase signaling (Lee et al., 1998; Moennikes et al., 2000) and promotes development of these tumors with activating β-catenin (*Ctnnb1*) mutations (Aydinlik et al., 2001). It has been shown that human and mouse hepatocellular carcinomas with mutated *Ctnnb1* share several common molecular features. It is possible that the lack of clear evidence of increased hepatocellular tumors in epileptic patients may be due to a combination of tumor promotion and inhibition effects of phenobarbital as observed in rodent models. A recent study demonstrated an unequivocal increase in hepatocellular tumors in epileptic patients treated with phenytoin (Hung et al., 2016), an indirect CAR activator similar to phenobarbital. Thus, hepatocellular tumors due to chronic CAR activation may still be a risk for humans.

Peroxisome Proliferator–Activated Receptors

Peroxisome proliferator–activated receptors (PPARs) are structurally similar type II nuclear receptors that are located in the nucleus. In mammals, there are three distinct PPARs (e.g., PPAR alpha (PPAR-α), PPAR-β, and PPAR-γ) each with distinct functions and different tissue distribution. PPAR-α is expressed in the liver, kidney, heart, macrophages, and adipose tissue and is involved in lipid metabolism, peroxisome proliferation, and hepatocellular carcinogenesis. PPAR-β/δ is located in the brain, adipose, and skin, and increases lipid metabolism. PPAR-γ isoforms are expressed in various tissues including heart, intestine, adipose tissue, kidney, and macrophages and are involved in glucose homeostasis, adipogenesis, and lipid storage. PPARs are located in the nucleus and in the cytosol in association with corepressors such as histone deacetylases, silencing mediator of retinoid and thyroid receptors, and nuclear receptor corepressors. Upon ligand binding, PPARs dissociate from their corepressors and heterodimerize with RXR-a and bind to peroxisome proliferator hormone response elements in DNA and activate a variety of genes that play a role in energy metabolism and cellular development and differentiation. PPARs are molecular targets for a number of endogenous ligands (e.g., free fatty acids, eicosanoids, vitamin B3), marketed drugs (e.g., fibrates, benzbromarone), as well as environmental contaminants such as plasticizers (e.g., phthalates), herbicides (e.g., 2,4-dichlorophenoxyacetic acid), and industrial chemicals (e.g., trichloroethylene, perchloroethylene, perfluoro-n-octanoic acid).

Ligand activation of PPAR-α results in the upregulation of peroxisomal acyl-CoA oxidase and increases H_2O_2 that cause oxidative stress. Excess oxidative stress can lead to DNA damage and subsequent neoplasia. In addition, downstream targets of PPAR-α signaling also promote carcinogenesis by enhancing cell proliferation and inhibiting apoptosis. Several PPAR-α agonists are known to pose a carcinogenic risk in rodents, and similar risks in humans are not unequivocally understood but a majority of the published data suggest the risk of cancer in humans due to PPAR-α agonists may be low (Corton et al., 2018). Species differences in PPAR-α expression may explain some of the differences in tumor incidences since rodents and humans have disparate number of peroxisomes and may have different downstream gene targets. However, risk assessment of environmental exposures to chemicals that activate PPAR-α is not straight forward since several compounds that activate PPAR-α may also activate other nuclear receptors or have other alternate MOAs. For example, di(2-ethylhexyl) phthalate, a PPAR-α agonist in wild-type mice, activates the CAR receptor in PPAR-α null mice and potentially activates PPAR-α–independent pathways causing liver tumors in the PPAR-α null mice (Ito et al., 2007; Ren et al., 2009). Thus, risk assessment based solely on one particular mode of action may be inadequate in protecting human health. PPAR-α agonists cause a tumor triad in rats comprising of hepatocellular tumors, exocrine pancreatic tumors, and Leydig cell tumors. However, the MOAs in inducing tumors in these diverse organs may not be similar and further studies are needed to address this issue.

Hormonal Mechanisms

The nuclear steroid hormone receptor family is comprised of ER α and β, PR, AR, glucocorticoid receptor, and mineralocorticoid receptor. These nuclear receptors belong to a larger family of about 50 nuclear receptors that also include other hormone receptors such as thyroid hormone receptor, and vitamin D3 receptor. All of these receptors function as transcription factors and activate unique downstream targets that play various roles in carcinogenesis. In the following sections, the most common hormonally induced carcinogenic MOAs will be discussed, such as ERs and ARs.

Estrogen Receptor Agonists

ERs exist as ERα and ERβ and differentially respond to estrogen signaling. ERs play distinct roles in maintaining the physiological homeostasis in a variety of tissues such as the female and male reproductive system, central nervous system, cardiovascular system, bone, liver, lung, kidney, and adipose tissue. ERα is uniquely expressed in the liver and hippocampus, whereas ERβ is expressed in prostate, vagina, and cerebellum.

ERα promotes cell proliferation, whereas ERβ opposes ERα and inhibits ERα-driven cell proliferation. In general, ERα and ERβ have similar signal transduction pathways but, depending on the coactivators and corepressors, their functions differ. ERs exist as a single monomer in the cytosol complexed with the heat shock protein complex (HSPC). Ligand binding causes receptor transformation leading to dissociation of ER monomers from the HSPC and leads to formation of ER dimers. The ER dimers translocate into the nucleus and bind to estrogen response element and activate several downstream genes depending on the presence of coactivators/corepressors within specific tissues.

ERs are promiscuous receptors that can interact with a wide range of agonists/antagonists with structures similar to estradiol. Agents that modulate ERs include endogenous ligands (e.g., estrone, estradiol, and estriol), synthetic estrogens (e.g., diethylstilbestrol (DES), ethinylestradiol, tamoxifen, raloxifene), and phytoestrogens (e.g., genistein, daidzein, and miroestrol). In addition, several environmental contaminants such as polychlorinated biphenyls, polycyclic aromatic hydrocarbons, bisphenol A, and organochlorine pesticides can also interact with ERs with varying affinities. Some of the above compounds and their related orthologues are called selective estrogen receptor modulators (SERMs) and exhibit agonist or antagonist activity based on the ERα/ERβ ratio in a specific tissue and tissue- and context-specific recruitment of specific coactivators or corepressors. Due to these factors, tamoxifen is an ER agonist in bone and uterus and an ER antagonist in breast tissue—hence used in adjuvant endocrine therapy for breast cancer. Raloxifene is similar to tamoxifen in its activity profile but exhibits greater activity in bone and less in the uterus, hence used in the prevention of osteoporosis (Deroo & Korach, 2006).

Cumulative exposure to chemicals that can increase or decrease ER activity can cause or modulate neoplasia in organs with ER expression. Chronic exposure to SERMS or nonselective estrogen modulators increases the risk of cancer through multiple, often overlapping, nongenotoxic and genotoxic MOAs (Yue et al., 2005). Activation of ER mediated transcription leads to increased cell proliferation, thereby increasing DNA replication errors and acquisition of unrepaired detrimental mutations that subsequently lead to neoplasia. The other mechanism involves formation of quinolone metabolites of estradiol that are genotoxic and form DNA adducts and result in mutations and neoplasia. As indicated earlier, ER activation may result in increased proliferation or apoptosis depending on the tissue context and the presence of coactivators and corepressors. A significant body of work on DES and other estrogen mimics have demonstrated that ER-driven carcinogenesis may be conserved across species. Some of the DES-induced cancers occur even in the second generation without direct exposure and this is considered due to epigenetic effects (Newbold et al., 2006). The target sites may vary due to species differences in metabolism, coactivators/repressors, and other factors. In general, the target sites of neoplasia due to ER activation as observed in all mammals include mammary tissue, uterus, cervix, vagina, ovary, testes, prostate, and liver.

Androgen Receptor Modulators

AR is a nuclear receptor in the cytosol that is activated by androgenic hormones such as testosterone and dihydrotestosterone or any other structurally similar chemical. Upon ligand binding, AR dissociates from the HSPC, translocates into the nucleus to form dimers, and binds to the androgen response elements in DNA resulting in the transcription of several target genes such as insulin-like growth factor 1 receptor. Similar to ERs, effects of AR activation are regulated by coactivators in a tissue-dependent manner. In addition, ARs can also indirectly influence gene expression by interacting with signal transduction proteins such as MAPKs. AR is abundantly expressed in male and female reproductive organs and to varying extent in liver, kidney, urinary bladder, muscle, skin, and adipose tissue. AR ligands include endogenous agonists such as testosterone, dihydrotestosterone, androstenedione and androstenediol, and synthetic agonists (e.g., nandrolone, stanozolol, and methyltestosterone).

AR signaling plays an important role in modulating tumorigenesis and metastases of several cancers including those of the prostate, urinary bladder, kidney, lung, liver, and breast. Interestingly, AR plays distinct and contrasting roles in each of the above cancers; for example, it promotes tumorigenesis in prostate, kidney, urinary bladder, lung, and liver but suppresses metastases in prostate and liver cancers while promoting this process in lung, urinary bladder, and kidney cancers (Chang et al., 2014).

Cytotoxicity

Low levels of persistent cytotoxicity have been reported to cause tumorigenesis in many chemical carcinogenicity rodent models. Regenerative hyperplasia following cytotoxicity will increase the chance of replication errors, and if left uncorrected, could result in tumor development. Classic examples of chemicals leading to cytotoxicity and subsequent neoplasia include chloroform, carbon tetrachloride, thioacetamide, melamine, saccharin, and ethanol. Some of these cellular injuries are mediated directly by the chemical or its metabolite. For example, chloroform is metabolized to phosgene by CYP2E1 in the liver and phosgene is cytotoxic, ultimately resulting in liver and kidney tumors. Another cell injury mechanism that causes tumors is persistent irritation with repeated tissue injury leading to subsequent neoplasia. This is seen with extremely high doses of saccharin, where amorphous calcium phosphate precipitates in the urinary bladder result in chronic irritation and neoplasia of the urothelium (Cohen et al., 2000). One essential feature of this mode of action is that the cytotoxicity should be persistent, along with evidence of cellular damage. Since cytotoxicity is dose dependent, the resulting carcinogenicity is assumed to have a threshold similar to other nongenotoxic carcinogens. Although cytotoxicity is implicated as a mode of action for carcinogenicity, it is frequently associated with other MOAs such as genotoxicity, inflammation, oxidative stress, nuclear receptor activation, and methylation changes (Hernandez et al., 2009). Therefore, with regards to risk assessment, a threshold-based approach (if the development of tumors is purely due to cytotoxicity) or a default linear low-dose extrapolation may be used based on the supportive data presented.

Immune Suppression

A persistent decrease in the ability of the immune system to effectively respond to foreign antigens related to tumor cells may contribute to neoplasia. Exposure to immunosuppressive chemicals or drugs, ionizing radiation, or exposure to certain pathogens such as human immunodeficiency virus-1 (HIV-1) can indirectly "promote" tumor cell clones induced by previous chemical exposures or increase the risk of cancers in individuals exposed to oncogenic viruses (Chen et al., 2018). Patients that have received tissue or organ transplants and are administered immunosuppressive therapies are more susceptible to cancers due to manifestation of occult or subclinical cancers that were inhibited by the normally functioning immune system. Some immunosuppressive drugs such as cyclophosphamide, chlorambucil, and azathioprine can cause cancer due to their genotoxic metabolites. However, other immunosuppressive agents such as cyclosporine, prednisone, and tacrolimus increase the risk of tumors mainly due to their immunosuppressive effects. Interestingly, people exposed to HIV-1 or immunosuppressive drugs suffer from a similar spectrum of neoplastic conditions such as B-cell non-Hodgkin's lymphoma (secondary to Epstein–Barr infection) and Kaposi sarcoma (Kane, 2019).

While it is known that most immunosuppressive drugs and chemicals are known human carcinogens, they are not known to be unequivocal carcinogens in the routine rodent bioassays unless those chemicals or their metabolites were genotoxic. As a result, purely immunosuppressive drugs such as cyclosporine were negative in a traditional rodent cancer bioassay; however, in a study where the animals were exposed to a genotoxic carcinogen and then exposed to cyclosporine, there were trends of increased incidences of cancer (Johnson et al., 1984). Nontraditional rodent bioassays using $Tp53^{+/-}$ transgenic mice or the AKR mouse strain (which develops lymphomas and leukemia due to the presence of endogenous AK retrovirus) may be useful in testing immunosuppressive agents for carcinogenicity (Alden et al., 2011). In terms of risk assessment of purely immunosuppressive drugs without other concomitant carcinogenic MOAs such as genotoxicity, a threshold is considered (Ryffel, 1992). However, if there is an accompanying genotoxic mode of action, then a linear dose response without a threshold is considered for risk assessment.

Epigenetic Mechanisms

Epigenetic mechanisms do not alter DNA sequence but nevertheless modulate gene expression. Epigenetic alterations may be mediated through changes in chromatin packaging, histone modification, DNA methylation, imprinted genes, and noncoding RNAs (ncRNAs). Chromatin packaging determines the accessibility of transcription factors to DNA for downstream signaling. Chromatin is a tightly coiled nucleoprotein complex comprised of nucleosomes with 147 base pairs (bps) linear DNA wrapped around an octamer of histone proteins containing duplicates of four core histones H2A, H2B, H3, and H4. Chromatin packaging may be further altered by modifications of the histone proteins including acetylation, methylation, ubiquitinylation/sumoylation (addition of small ubiquitin-like modifiers), phosphorylation, and ADP-ribosylation. In general, histone acetylation decreases the affinity of histone proteins for DNA and causes relaxation of the chromatin packaging, leading to increased transcriptional activation. Similarly, other histone modifications can have a myriad of effects either alone or in combination with other proteins in epigenetically influencing gene regulation.

DNA methylation is one of the more commonly studied epigenetic effects in cancer. DNA methyl transferases (DNMTs) transfer a methyl group from S-adenyl methionine onto the C-5 position of cytosine to convert it into 5-methylcytosine. The majority of DNA methylation occurs on cytosines that precede a guanine nucleotide or at CpG (5′-cytosine-phosphate-guanine-3′) sites. DNA methylation is necessary to silence retroviral elements, regulate tissue specific gene expression, genomic imprinting, and X-chromosome inactivation. CpG islands are genomic regions with 300–3000 bp of CpG dinucleotide repeats located near approximately 60% of the promoters in mammalian genes, and differential methylation of the CpG islands or near the islands (shores) regulates gene expression. In transcriptionally inactive states, the promoter regions are hypermethylated leading to repression of gene expression; however, when the promoter regions are hypomethylated, the gene expression is active. In general, global hypomethylation has been linked to increasing malignancy in several cancers, but there are instances where global hypomethylation suppresses certain cancers, including those of the liver and intestine (Yamada et al., 2005). However, when the methylation status of the milieu of genes involved in cancer development is examined closely, tumor suppressor genes may be hypermethylated and oncogenes hypomethylated, causing a respective decrease and increase of corresponding gene expression (Plass & Soloway, 2002). Transcriptional silencing of genes leading to progression of cancer is more commonly influenced by epigenetic effects such as methylation and miRNA-mediated effects than by mutations. In addition, mutations can also affect genes that modify the epigenome, such as mutations in *DNMT1* in colon cancer and *DNMT3A* in hematologic malignancies (Zhang & Xu, 2017).

Genomic imprinting is an epigenetic mechanism involving the expression of only one parental allele, rather than the usual expression of both parental alleles of a gene. A classic example of loss of imprinting occurs in Wilm's tumor, a pediatric embryonic renal tumor, involving the imprinted genes *IGF2/H19* locus on chromosome 11. H19 is an ncRNA that can function like a tumor suppressor gene, whereas insulin growth factor-2 (IGF2) is a growth factor highly expressed in tumor cells. In normal cells, paternal H19 expression is silenced by promoter methylation and maternal H19 is unmethylated, leading to the expression of paternal IGF2 and maternal H19 alleles and maintenance of the IGF2 heterozygosity. However, in cancer cells, maternal H19 is methylated as well, leading to LOH of IGF2 and expression of both parental alleles of IGF2 and increased tumor growth (Steenman et al., 1994). Several other oncogenes and tumor suppressor genes that function through imprinting have been identified and this phenomenon also occurs in other cancers such as hepatoblastoma, gliomas, colorectal cancer, cervical carcinoma, and rhabdomyosarcoma (Joyce & Schofield, 1998).

ncRNAs are functional RNAs that are not translated into proteins but regulate gene expression at the transcriptional and posttranscriptional levels. These ncRNAs include small ncRNAs [(19–31 nucleotides) such as miRNAs (microRNA), piRNAs (PIWI-interacting RNA)], midsize ncRNAs (~20–200 nucleotides) such as SnoRNAs (small nucleolar RNA), and the long noncoding RNA (lncRNA, >200 nucleotides). MiRNAs primarily function as negative regulators of gene expression at the posttranscriptional level. PiRNAs are involved in silencing retrotransposons, transcript degradation and regulating chromatin formation, and other transcriptional and posttranscriptional silencing. SnoRNAs guide chemical modification, posttranscriptional modification, and maturation of other RNAs such as rRNA, tRNA, and snRNA and are involved in methylation and pseudouridylation. lncRNAs have numerous functions and interfere with the transcriptional machinery by acting as molecular scaffolds and modifying chromatic complexes. In contrast to miRNAs, lncRNAs are not conserved between species and their expression is tissue and context specific. Each of these ncRNAs regulates normal physiological homeostasis and also plays a role in diseases such as cancer. Many of the ncRNAs influence carcinogenesis by functioning as either oncogenes or tumor suppressors and can serve as biomarkers. In particular, the role of miRNAs has been extensively evaluated in various cancers and they are used as biomarkers as well as potential therapeutic oncology targets (Hayes et al.,

2014). A discussion on this topic is beyond the scope of this chapter; however, excellent reviews are available on this topic (Lin & Lin, 2017; Slack & Chinnaiyan, 2019).

Pharmaceuticals, dietary components, and environmental exposure to chemicals can result in epigenomic alterations that can influence carcinogenesis. A case study examining the epigenome (i.e., global methylation and histone acetylation) of monozygotic twins has demonstrated that with increasing age the epigenome became different between the twins, suggesting a significant role of the environment and lifestyle factors in shaping the epigenome (Fraga et al., 2005). Some of these exposures can have long-lasting effects on the epigenome including transgenerational effects. A classic example of transgenerational effects on the epigenome was demonstrated with DES-exposed murine dams where increased susceptibility to uterine tumors was passed from the maternal lineage to subsequent generations of male and female descendants (Newbold et al., 2006). DES-related transgenerational epigenetic effects related to infertility, breast cancer, and vaginal epithelial alterations were reported in daughters exposed to DES in utero (Hoover et al., 2011). The Dutch famine birth cohort study also demonstrated transgenerational effects where, not surprisingly, children born during the famine had lower birth weight, but the children of these children born during bountiful times also had lower birth weight and were at higher risk for metabolic diseases (Painter et al., 2008). It has been demonstrated that maternal malnutrition related to methionine, choline, and folate deficiency has contributed to epigenetic alterations in the progeny and their subsequent progeny. These studies support the premise that environmental and lifestyle factors influence the epigenome and may be a contributing etiological factor in increased cancer incidences.

A recent study documented epigenomic alterations (e.g., methylation, histone modification, and ncRNA) in 12/28 IARC group 1 genotoxic chemical carcinogens and these include 1,3-butadiene, 4,4'-methylenebis(2-chlorobenzenamine), 4-aminobiphenyl, aflatoxins, benzene, benzidine, BaP, formaldehyde, sulfur mustard, vinyl chloride, "occupational exposure during coke production," and "occupational exposure as a painter" (Chappell et al., 2016). In addition to the above chemicals, other environmental exposures that alter the epigenome and may potentially contribute to chemical carcinogenesis include metals (e.g., arsenic, cadmium, chromium, nickel, and mercury) and endocrine disrupters (e.g., DES, bisphenol A, and vinclozolin). Chemical carcinogenesis exclusively driven by epigenetic alterations is rare as it is usually a combination of genetic and epigenetic changes that drives the process. In some cases, the epigenetic alteration may be a bystander effect or may be the primary driving event. Despite evidence linking epigenetic alterations with chemical-induced carcinogenesis, epigenetic data do not conclusively link exposure with cancer. In some cases, epigenetic alterations may serve as biomarkers of genotoxic and nongenotoxic carcinogenic MOAs and may support risk assessment especially if these biomarkers are thoroughly validated.

3. IDENTIFICATION OF CARCINOGENS—TESTING PROGRAMS AND GUIDELINES

Several preclinical in vitro and in vivo established model systems have been used to identify the carcinogenic and genotoxic potential of xenobiotics. Collectively, these assays are classified based on their duration and can range from a few days to up to 2 years. Shorter-term mutagenicity assays, including the Ames bacterial reverse mutagenicity assay, chromosomal aberration assay, and the micronucleus test, typically range in duration from a few days to a few weeks. Medium-term assays such as transgenic in vivo mutation assays can last up to a year, and longer term chronic rodent carcinogenicity bioassays can comprise exposure periods of 6–24 months in duration.

3.1. In Vitro Mutagenicity Assays

The Ames test, originally developed by Bruce Ames in the 1970s (Ames et al., 1973, 1975), has been extensively used in both *S. typhimurium* and *E. coli* strains. These strains lack histidine (*hisT*) and the capacity to repair damaged DNA. Exposure of these strains to mutagenic compounds at varying concentrations while grown in media lacking hisT can promote mutagenesis of genes including at the hisT gene which may reverse the dysfunctional gene (and resulting protein product) to a functional state, thereby reestablishing bacterial proliferation. The resulting mutant colonies are termed "revertants" because of their functional *hisT* gene that enables them to synthesize hisT and survive. Both direct and indirect (i.e., chemicals that require metabolic activation) mutagens can be identified using the Ames test. Indirect mutagens are incubated with rat liver homogenate (termed S9) which promotes metabolic activation and conversion of the compound giving rise to the active mutagenic form.

Genetically modified strains of *S. typhimurium* are routinely used in genetic toxicology testing. The TA98, TA1537, and TA1538 strains are used to detect frameshift mutations, whereas the TA100 and TA1535 strains detect SNPs (i.e., point mutations). Exposure of these strains to a range of concentrations of the test compound or positive controls (e.g., sodium azide, 9-Anthracenecarboxylic acid, BaP) with or without the S9 fraction allows detection of dose-dependent mutagenesis.

In vitro mammalian cell assays have also been established and assess mutagenicity in Chinese hamster ovary (CHO) cells or the L5178Y mouse lymphoma cell line. Mutagens are identified in CHO cells following mutation of the hypoxanthine-guanine phosphoribosyltransferase gene (Johnson, 2012). Exposure of the L5178Y mouse cell lines to mutagens can promote resistance to trifluorothymidine. The assay is based on identification of forward mutations in the heterozygous thymidine kinase gene locus (Clive et al., 1983).

3.2. Chromosomal Aberration Assay

Chromosomal aberrations including breaks that appear as 4′,6-diamidino-2-phenylindole (DAPI)-negative breaks during metaphase in mitosis are a common feature of aneuploid cancer cells (Ozery-Flato et al., 2011; Solomon et al., 1991). The mechanism of chromosome breakage has recently been identified. Drug-induced stress promotes late stage replication of vulnerable loci during the cell cycle including CFSs and telomeres which use the error-prone MiDAS pathway to promote viability (Minocherhomji et al., 2015;

Dilley et al., 2016). As a result, MiDAS enhances the appearance of DAPI-negative chromosome breaks in metaphase. Another chromosome aberration is sister chromatid exchanges (SCEs) that detect the interchange between two sister chromatids of a given chromosome or at a homologous locus within a chromosome (Latt et al., 1981). This can be measured using incorporation of bromodeoxyuridine or 5-ethynyl-2′-deoxyuridine to cells in culture together with the xenobiotic being tested (Stults et al., 2014). The Bloom syndrome helicase, together with topoisomerase IIIα, limits the formation of SCEs (Wu & Hickson, 2003), and elevated instances of SCEs are a hallmark of cells obtained from Bloom syndrome patients that are predisposed to all cancers (Chaganti et al., 1974).

3.3. Micronucleus Test

The micronucleus test quantifies the occurrence of extranuclear bodies that form during mitosis, which contain damaged or misaligned whole chromosomes or chromosomal fragments. The micronucleus test is carried out in cells following exposure to a test article or positive control (e.g., mitomycin C, cyclophosphamide) and with or without S9 fraction. The in vitro micronucleus test can be performed either in CHO cells, Epstein–Barr virus–transformed human lymphoblast cell lines, or in human peripheral blood lymphocytes obtained from healthy volunteers (Doherty, 2012). Micronuclei are quantified in binucleated cells either using an imaging-based assay or a flow cytometry assay following a cytokinesis block (e.g., using cytochalasin B) after cells have undergone mitosis. The in vivo micronucleus assay can quantify the occurrence of micronuclei in all dividing cells and is routinely carried out in cells obtained from the bone marrow following repeat doses of test article or a positive control in rats (Hayashi, 2016; Mavournin et al., 1990).

3.4. Other DNA Based Assays

DNA damage can be quantified using the COMET assay that measures the incidence of DNA breaks in affected cells (Vasquez, 2010), either in vitro or in vivo. Additionally, the unscheduled

DNA synthesis assay measures a cell's ability to perform NER (Kelly & Latimer, 2005).

3.5. Testing Programs and Guidelines

Regulatory guidelines for mutagenicity testing have been established by the Organisation for Economic Co-operation and Development (OECD, 2020) as shown in Table 8.4.

3.6. Two-Year National Toxicology Program Rodent Carcinogenicity Bioassay

The United States National Cancer Institute (NCI) formally initiated animal testing programs in the 1970s to identify potential carcinogens and to establish safe levels of exposure. The NCI Carcinogenesis Bioassay Program was succeeded by the National Toxicology Program (NTP), whose mission is to coordinate federal toxicology programs and to refine the toxicity and carcinogenicity tests (Kemp, 2015). Approximately 25% of substances that are causally or strongly associated with human cancer were first identified as carcinogens in animals including estrogen, formaldehyde, DES, DDT, vinyl chloride, 2,3,7,8-TCDD, radon gas, beryllium, asbestos, 4- aminobiphenyl, bis(chloromethyl)ether, and 1,3 butadiene (Huff, 1993; Rall, 2000).

At the NTP, the current strategy for identifying the potential carcinogenicity of chemicals involves systemic exposure of male and female F1 hybrid of inbred mouse strains (B6C3F1/N) and an outbred rat strain to multiple (typically 3) dose levels of chemicals for 2 years to replicate lifetime exposure (Fung et al., 1995; Institute, 1980). The NTP also uses genetically engineered mouse models (GEMMs) in shorter-term hypothesis-driven cancer studies (Pritchard et al., 2003). If an agent is observed to produce characteristics of carcinogenicity (tumor progression, incidences, multiplicity) above background levels in control animals not given the test article, the agent is regarded as a carcinogen in the context of that study. These agents are considered as potential human carcinogens based on the cumulative weight of evidence. Other studies, such as genetic toxicology, chemical disposition and metabolism (toxicokinetics), reproductive toxicity, teratology, behavioral testing, immunotoxicity, and molecular pathology, frequently complement contemporary two-year carcinogenicity studies. As previously discussed, in vitro and in vivo genotoxicity tests are conducted for each chemical (Kemp, 2015) to classify chemical carcinogens into two broad categories, genotoxic and nongenotoxic. The pathology evaluation for both neoplastic and nonneoplastic lesions involves rigorous peer review (Sills et al., 2019; Ward et al., 1995) and any carcinogenic response is categorized according to NTP levels of evidence (Table 8.6). For more information, see *Pathology Peer Review,* Vol 1, Chap 26.

Epidemiologic studies that clearly show a causal association between chemical exposure and an increased risk for the development of cancer provide the strongest evidence for identifying carcinogens (Toporcov & Wunsch Filho, 2018). For most suspected carcinogens, it is often difficult or impossible to quantify the amount and duration of exposure in humans or even to associate the exposure with a disease that may not appear for decades. The animal bioassay identifies agents that are potentially hazardous to human health and must be considered along with as many scientifically based analyses that are known such as the dose response, comparative species metabolism, ability to extrapolate between species, mechanisms of cancer induction, genotoxicity of the agent, amount of agent in the environment, number of people exposed, and strength of the epidemiologic evidence to formulate the strongest weight-of-evidence–based conclusion (see *Practices to Optimize Generation, Interpretation, and Reporting of Pathology Data from Toxicity Studies,* Vol 1, Chap 28).

While chemical carcinogenesis bioassays in animals have long been recognized and accepted as predictors of potential cancer hazards to humans, the bioassay has been subject to critique regarding its limitations (Doe et al., 2019). The predictivity, cost, duration, reproducibility, and resources of the bioassay have been questioned. Furthermore, it has been argued that the carcinogenic potential must be defined by potency and include consideration of the modes/mechanisms of action as determinants of cancer formation and prevention in humans. Additionally, it has been proposed that a range of in vitro and shorter-term in vivo assays can be used to evaluate carcinogenic potential, identify effects which may lead directly or indirectly to DNA damage or increases in cell division, and set

TABLE 8.6 US National Toxicology Program Levels of Evidence (LOE) of Carcinogenic Activity

Clear evidence of carcinogenic activity	Dose-related (i) increased number of malignant neoplasms, (ii) increased number of both malignant and benign neoplasms, or (iii) marked increase in number of benign neoplasms if there is an indication from this or other studies of the ability of such tumors to progress to malignancy
Some evidence of carcinogenic activity	Chemical-related increased incidence of neoplasms in which the strength of the response is less than that required for clear evidence
Equivocal evidence of carcinogenic activity	Marginal increase in number of neoplasms that may be chemically related
No evidence of carcinogenic activity	

US National Toxicologic Program, used with permission.

exposure limit values (Cohen et al., 2019; ICH I.C.o.H, 2012).

3.7. Carcinogenicity Testing

Governmental organizations have traditionally conducted their studies to determine if environmental exposure to a chemical can be harmful under any circumstances, whereas the pharmaceutical industry pilots their tests to determine if a compound is reasonably safe while considering the indication, patient/exposure population, and other compound-specific factors (risk–benefit analysis). For more information, see *Risk Assessment*, Vol 2, Chap 16. For pharmaceuticals, explicit regulatory requirements for carcinogenicity assessments of new chemical entities (NCEs) are described in International Conference on Harmonisation (ICH) guidance documents (ICH Guidelines M3, S1A, S1B, S1C, S2A, S2B and S6) (ICH I.C.o.H, 1996; ICH I.C.o.H, 1997; ICH I.C.o.H, 2008; ICH I.C.o.H, 2010; ICH I.C.o.H, 2012; ICH I.C.o.H., 2012). A two-year rat study and either a two-year mouse or an alternative six-month transgenic mouse carcinogenicity study for small molecule compounds are required for pharmaceuticals that would be dosed in humans for 6 months or longer, or in a frequent and intermittent manner (cumulative lifetime exposure over 6 months) (Sistare et al., 2011).

Archetypal carcinogenicity studies are not traditionally executed for biopharmaceuticals (large molecules) due to use and clinical indication parameters which may render carcinogenicity studies unnecessary, absence of cross-reactivity in rodents, or failure to maintain exposure due to immunogenicity and subsequent rapid clearance; however, exceptions have been reported (Chouinard et al., 2016). Instead, carcinogenicity potential for biopharmaceuticals is commonly estimated using knowledge of target biology, knock-out and/or overexpression information from rodents, and results from general toxicity studies. Immune suppression or mitogenic activity could suggest heightened risk (Vahle et al., 2010), but a case-by-case often hypothesis-driven approach is exercised when assessing the cancer risk of a biopharmaceutical.

The FDA regards chronic feeding studies as the only definitive method for establishing the carcinogenicity of food additives. One factor prompting additional testing for carcinogenicity of food additives includes positive mutagenicity data, but other data may also warrant further study of these compounds (e.g., the intended level of usage is high or when possible carcinogenicity is suspected because of the structure or known biological activity of the additive). Similarly, additives which are used in food packaging and as food processing aids may also undergo carcinogenicity testing (US National Research Council Committee on Diet N. and Cancer, 1983). If carcinogenicity in laboratory animals is established, a chemical is generally regarded as a human carcinogen. Epidemiological studies are not practical because the use of food additives is so extensive that establishment of an unexposed control group would be unattainable. As a result, regulatory agencies limit the presence of known carcinogens in food to the lowest feasible levels, frequently prohibiting any level of an established carcinogenic food additive (FDA U.F.a.D.A., 2002; FDA U.F.a.D.A., 2019).

When assessing possible cancer risk posed by an agrochemical or pesticide, the EPA uses a weight-of-evidence approach and considers factors such as tumor findings in humans and laboratory animals, an agent's chemical and physical properties, its structure–activity relationships as compared with other carcinogenic agents, and studies addressing potential carcinogenic processes and mode(s) of action, either in vivo or in vitro. Data from epidemiologic studies are generally preferred for characterizing human cancer risk (EPA, 2005).

3.8. Current and Future Considerations for Carcinogenicity Testing in Rodents

Current standardized carcinogenicity studies in rodent include at least 50 animals per sex per dose group in three separate treatment groups and in a concurrent control group, usually for 18–24 months depending on the rodent species tested (OECD O.f.E.C.a.D., 1981). The highest dose level in these studies is generally selected to provide the maximum ability to detect treatment-related carcinogenic effects while not compromising the outcome of the study through excessive toxicity or inducing inappropriate toxicokinetics (e.g., overwhelming absorption or detoxification mechanisms). The purpose of including two or more lower dose levels is to provide data to information on dose response. Similar protocols are used by many laboratories worldwide (EPA, 2005). The shortcomings of the rodent bioassay in predicting human cancer risk continue to be debated, mostly due to biological differences between rodents compared to humans and the scarcity of mechanistic data attained from such studies. A two-year rodent carcinogenicity study for an NCE takes about 3 years from start to finish, involves hundreds of animals, and is a massive undertaking in terms of financial resources. Sistare et al. (2011) have proposed that human cancer risk assessment would not be adversely affected by the elimination of rat carcinogenicity studies for novel small pharmaceuticals that (1) lack specific

histopathological risk factors for neoplasia such as hyperplasia, foci of cellular alterations, or chronic inflammation in a 26-week toxicity study in adult rats, (2) lack evidence for genotoxicity, and (3) lack evidence for hormonal perturbation (Sistare et al., 2011). These criteria can predict with 80% accuracy a negative outcome of the two-year rat carcinogenicity study for these compounds. The approach is termed the "Negative for Endocrine, Genotoxicity, and Chronic Study Associated Histopathological Risk factors for Carcinogenicity in the Rat" (NEG CARC Rat) testing paradigm (Figure 8.3). Utilizing this prediction model with new pharmaceuticals could improve drug development timelines by decreasing the number of rat carcinogenicity studies by 40%–50%, and thereby supporting the 3Rs initiative (reduce, refine, reuse). Completion of nonclinical studies could be hypothetically shortened by 2–3 years and registration timelines could be reduced depending on the clinical phases. The estimated total of $3.75M in industry and regulatory resources committed per single rodent carcinogenicity study would be spared (Sistare et al., 2011).

The same dataset used by Sistare et al. (2011) to propose the NEG CARC Rat was complemented with study results from an additional 73 pharmaceuticals (255 compounds in total) and used to analyze the relationship of the carcinogenicity study outcome with pharmacological properties (van der Laan et al., 2016). The authors found that certain drug classes were associated with tumor patterns in specific tissues in rats indicating that pharmacological properties are a determining element for the carcinogenic MOA of many compounds. Therefore, the MOA of a certain pharmaceutical could be used in conjunction with NEG CARC Rat to forecast the positive or negative outcome of a two-year carcinogenicity study, potentially negating the need to perform it (Corvi et al., 2017).

A principal impediment to regulatory adoption of the NEG CARC Rat arises from the definition of the three short-term toxicologic criteria (mentioned above), and how they could be applied, potentially in isolation, to determine the necessity of a two-year rat study. Another concern is the presumption that false-negative carcinogens would not have implications for patient safety. When an unanticipated cancer

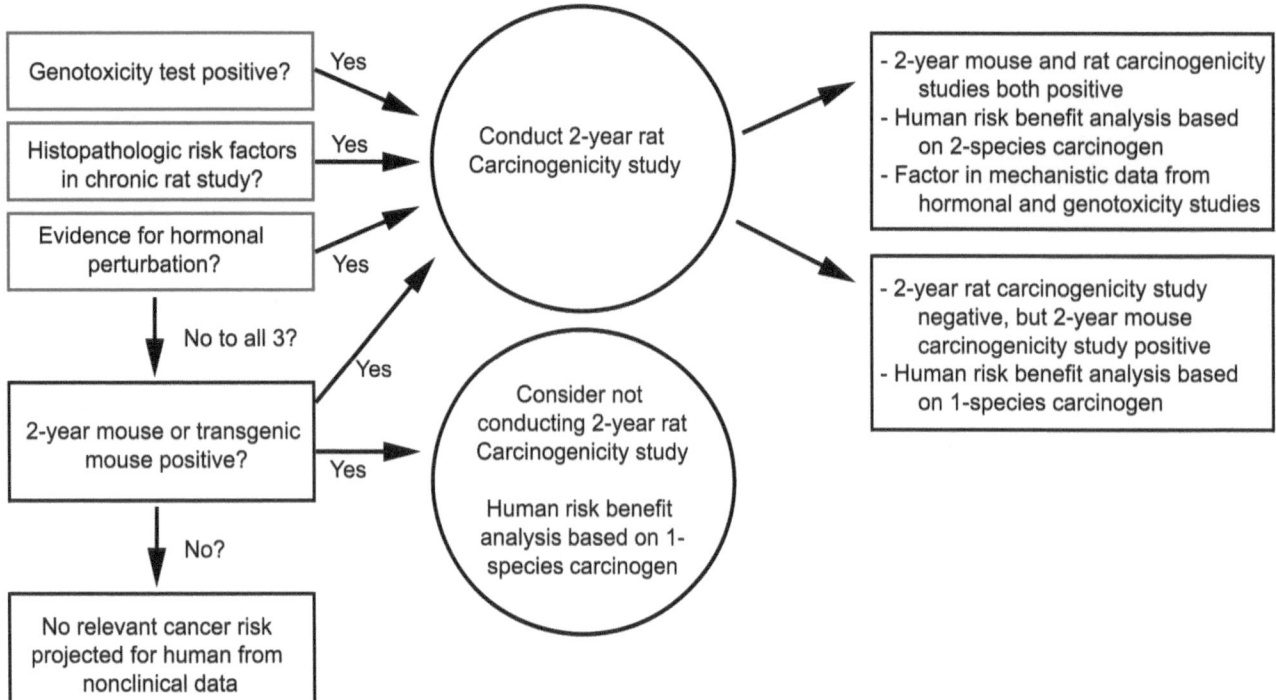

FIGURE 8.3   Negative for endocrine, genotoxicity, and chronic study–associated histopathologic risk factors for carcinogenicity in the rat (NEG CARC Rat) assessment map. If any of the three prediction criteria (*blue boxes*) are positive, a two-year rat carcinogenicity study will be conducted. If all three criteria are negative, the carcinogenicity assessment of the pharmaceutical candidate can be completed with the conduct of a two-year or transgenic mouse carcinogenicity study. If the mouse study is negative, then no relevant cancer risk for humans is anticipated from nonclinical data. If the mouse study is positive when all three criteria for conducting a two-year rat carcinogenicity study are negative, the decision to conduct a two-year rat carcinogenicity study will need to be considered depending on program-specific elements such as magnitude of the neoplastic signal(s) in the mouse study and other factors and/or the exposure margins.

signal has been revealed during phase 3 clinical trials or thereafter, the results of rodent carcinogenicity studies are frequently reexamined to assess the plausibility of the clinical finding and relationship to the test article. Additional discussions are ongoing between regulatory agencies and pharmaceutical associations as part of an expert working group of the ICH. It is thought that more accurate predictions of carcinogenic potential for rodents and potentially for human subjects could be made by considering pharmacologic properties along with the toxicologic endpoints described in NEG CARC Rat. For example, in silico models and short-term toxicologic endpoints would be interpreted in the context of the drug's pharmacology and toxicokinetics in assessing whether a reasonable prediction could be made regarding carcinogenic risk (Bourcier et al., 2015).

The posted ICH RND (ICH I.C.o.H., 2017) proposes that the cancer risk of a new

pharmaceutical can be predicted with sufficient certainty to be classified into one of several categories (Table 8.7). For the prediction categories 1, 3a, and 3b, a request for waiving the two-year rat carcinogenicity study would be justified since the expected study results do not add perceived value to human risk assessment. In order to probe this rationale, industry stakeholders have been urged to present a Carcinogenicity Assessment Document (CAD) to Drug Regulatory Authorities (DRAs) in the ICH regions for all investigational pharmaceuticals with ongoing or planned two-year rat carcinogenicity studies with a weight-of-evidence prediction of the carcinogenic potential (Table 8.8) prior to knowing the outcome of the carcinogenicity testing.

For successful completion of this prospective evaluation, a dataset of at least 20 studies for category 3 (i.e., CAD + study report) should be evaluated. Based on the degree of accuracy of predictions and concurrence between

TABLE 8.7 International Agency for Research on Cancer (IARC) Classification

Category	Description	Request to waive two-year rat study justified?
Category 1	Highly likely to be tumorigenic in humans such that a product would be labeled accordingly and two-year rat, two-year mouse, or transgenic mouse carcinogenicity studies would not add value	Yes
Category 2	The available sets of pharmacologic and toxicologic data indicate that tumorigenic potential for humans is uncertain and rodent carcinogenicity studies are likely to add value to human risk assessment. S1B guidance (ICH S1B, 1997) describes options for rodent carcinogenicity testing	No
Category 3a	Highly likely to be tumorigenic in rats but not in humans through prior established and well-recognized mechanisms known to be irrelevant for human, such that a two-year rat study would not add value	Yes
Category 3b	Highly likely not to be tumorigenic in either rats or humans such that no two-year rat study is needed. A study in a transgenic mouse could prove useful for justifying a category 3 assignment	Yes

biopharmaceutical companies and DRAs, defined weight-of-evidence provisions and ICH guideline modifications may be established to predict human cancer risk as an alternative to two-year rat carcinogenicity studies (Corvi et al., 2017).

3.9. Conventional Rat Strains for Carcinogenicity Testing

Carcinogenicity studies are intended to predict cancer risk and are therefore generally executed to provide near-lifetime exposures up to the maximum tolerated dose that would allow dosing for this period of time. Currently, the main rat strains used for the registration package of a new clinical entity are Sprague Dawley (SD) and Wistar Han rats, with the Fischer 344 rat now used less frequently by many organizations (Weber, 2017). Primary considerations for selecting which outbred strain for a two-year study include longer survival, low background spontaneous tumor rate and organ system predilections, and carcinogenic sensitivity. The known mechanism of carcinogenesis of the test article and how it may affect the particular strain chosen in terms of strain predilection to different MOAs is particularly useful when determining human relevance. Other considerations may

include availability, fecundity, experience with the strain, and similarity to humans (e.g., metabolic pathways, general pathophysiology, and known expression of the target) (King-Herbert & Thayer, 2006).

In general, the incidence of spontaneous tumors in SD rats is higher than in Wistar rats. This is related mainly to the higher incidences of pituitary gland adenomas (in females, up to approximately 70% in SD rats vs. 64% in Wistar rats) and mammary gland neoplasms, especially fibroadenomas (in females, up to approximately 72% in SD rats vs. 22.3% in Wistar rats). Thyroid follicular tumors are recorded at higher mean incidences in Wistar strains (up to approximately 5% in Wistar rats), as are vascular neoplasms in lymph nodes (approximately 9% in Wistar rats) and thymoma (up to 4% in Wistar rats). Malignant lymphomas and renal tumors (especially the amphophilic-vacuolar renal tubule tumor in SD rats and the renal tubular adenoma and nephroblastoma in Wistar rats) are not unusual in younger adult animals (Weber, 2017). Strain-specific historical data for carcinogenicity studies may differ somewhat between pathology laboratories, but is available in many literature reviews (Weber, 2017; Bertrand et al., 2014; Blankenship et al., 2016; Brix et al., 2005; Keenan et al., 2002) (see *Animal Models in Toxicologic Research: Rodents,* Vol 1, Chap 17).

TABLE 8.8   Weight-of-Evidence Factors for Consideration in a Carcinogenicity Assessment Document (ICH, 2016)

1. Knowledge of intended drug target and pathway pharmacology, secondary pharmacology, and drug target distribution in rats and humans

2. Genetic toxicology results

3. Histopathologic evaluation of repeated dose rat toxicology studies, especially chronic studies

4. Exposure margins in chronic rat toxicology studies

5. Metabolic profile

6. Evidence of hormonal perturbation

7. Level of immune suppression

8. Special studies and endpoints

9. Results of nonrodent chronic toxicity study

10. Transgenic mouse carcinogenicity study (not required, but contributory if conducted)

3.10. Mouse Models of Carcinogenesis

Animal models created through genetic engineering, graft transplantation, and viral, chemical, or physical induction have advanced cancer research from the bench to the bedside. These models have become progressively advanced and enabled scientists to study molecular mechanisms of cancer and integrate this knowledge into highly specific and effective treatment modalities (Yee et al., 2015). The murine model has been conventionally used for basic and nonclinical studies of cancer. Syngeneic, GEM, and xenograft mice are explained in Figure 8.4 and in *Genetically Engineered Animal Models in Toxicologic Research*, Vol 1, Chap 23. In syngeneic models, tumors are established in immune-competent mice using cells from the same strain with identical genetic background, so that these isografts (isologous grafts) are not rejected. Because syngeneic mice have intact immune systems, the antitumor immune response can be evaluated and there is a minimal risk for graft rejection. In syngeneic

models, factors such as the tumor microenvironment, epithelial–stromal cell interactions, tumor-secreting factors, immune cell infiltration, and vasculature can be investigated. However, because this model is derived from the animal system, the biology of the tumor may not fully correlate with the corresponding human cancer (House et al., 2014).

GEM are immune-competent mice with defined genetic alterations introduced using RNA interference, inducible gene expression, viruses, or DNA recombination techniques. The GEMMs that result enable exploration into the role of genetic alterations in cancer development by identifying which genes are necessary for progression, regression, and/or resistance to treatment. Gene expression can be controlled and directed, and even limited to the tissue of interest using a tissue-specific promoter to introduce the distinct genetic alteration. Alternatively, gene expression can be engineered to occur throughout the organism using germ-line mutations. Regulation of gene expression in the presence or absence of tetracycline and its receptor allows for inducible gene expression systems, permitting amplification or suppression of a gene of interest. GEMMs are resource intensive but are excellent tools for studying early tumorigenesis and genetic events leading to tumor initiation, maintenance, and relapse and therefore, target validation, treatment response, and chemoprevention (House et al., 2014).

In xenograft rodent models, human tumor cells are transplanted heterotopically under the skin (subcutaneous), into the abdominal cavity (intraperitoneal), into the blood (intravenous), or into the tissue of origin (orthotopic) of an immunocompromised host, typically an athymic nude or severe combined immunodeficiency (SCID) mouse. While intraperitoneal, intravenous, and orthotopic injections can simulate metastasis, subcutaneously injected cells are generally limited to localized tumor formation at the injection site (House et al., 2014). Patient-derived xenograft (PDX) models are created by directly transferring tumor fragments from individual patients via orthotopic or intraperitoneal injection into immune-deficient mice to create "xenopatients" or tumor grafts. Successful engraftment is higher in SCID mice compared to nude mice, likely due to the lack of T- and B-cell responses and subsequent suppression of both cellular and humoral

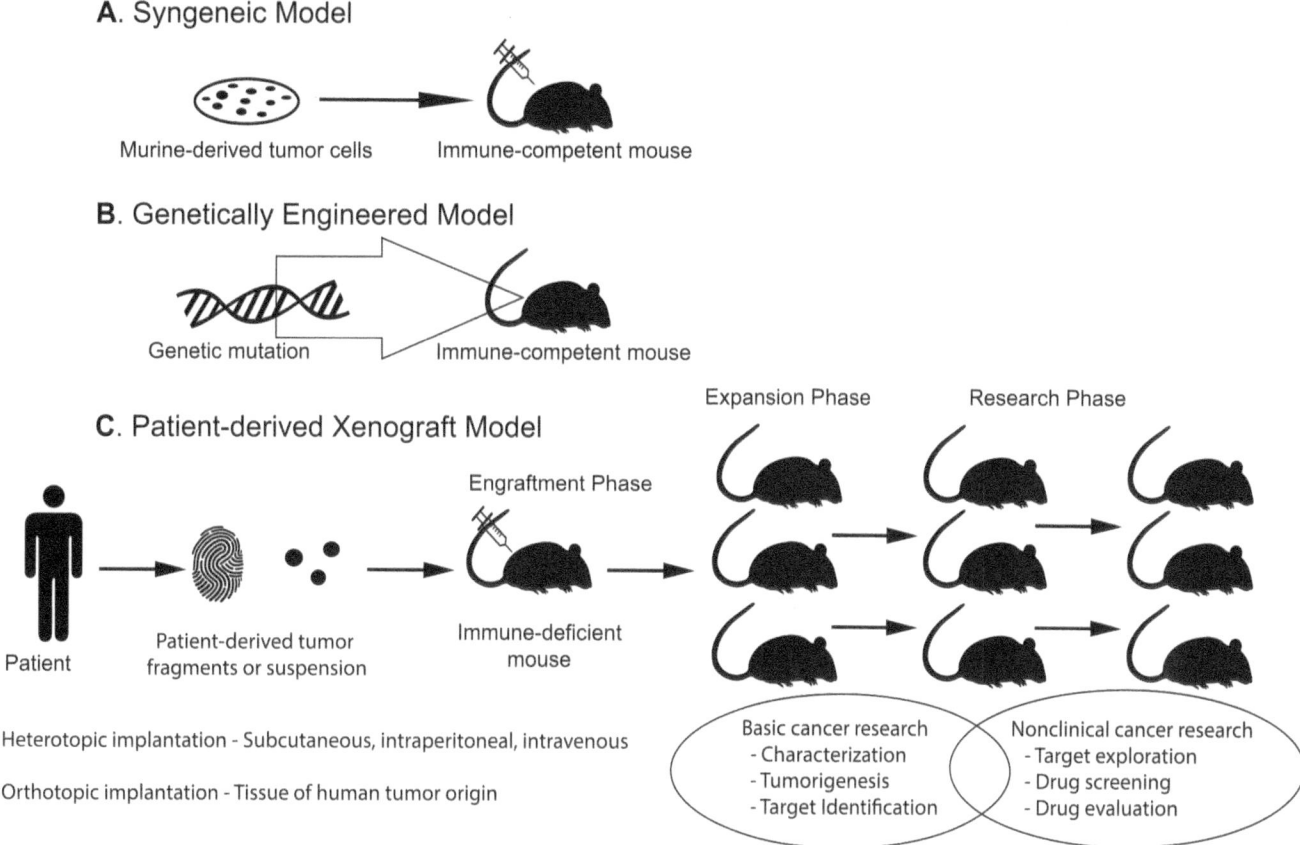

A. Syngeneic Model

Murine-derived tumor cells   Immune-competent mouse

B. Genetically Engineered Model

Genetic mutation   Immune-competent mouse

C. Patient-derived Xenograft Model

Expansion Phase   Research Phase

Engraftment Phase

Patient   Patient-derived tumor fragments or suspension   Immune-deficient mouse

Heterotopic implantation - Subcutaneous, intraperitoneal, intravenous

Orthotopic implantation - Tissue of human tumor origin

Basic cancer research
- Characterization
- Tumorigenesis
- Target Identification

Nonclinical cancer research
- Target exploration
- Drug screening
- Drug evaluation

FIGURE 8.4   Mouse models in cancer research. In the syngeneic model (A), murine-derived tumor cells are implanted into immune-competent mice. In the genetically engineered model (B), a genetic mutation is introduced using various techniques in immune-competent mice. In the patient-derived xenograft (PDX) model (C), tumors from cancer patients are fragmented or digested into a single-cell suspension and then transplanted into immunodeficient mice for engraftment. Once grown, the tumors are transplanted into secondary recipients for tumor expansion. The expanded tumors can then be cryopreserved or transplanted into tertiary recipient mice for cancer research of the type of origin. Specifically, tumors can be transplanted into sites other than those from which the tumors are derived (heterotopic transplantation) or directly into the corresponding tissue type where they originated (orthotopic transplantation). The successfully established PDX models are to be used in basic cancer research and nonclinical studies.

immunity. Tumor grafts preserve the histomorphology, immunophenotype, and clonal heterogeneity of the original tumor. Generating a mouse model using a tumor graft is labor intensive and expensive and mice are immunocompromised, which makes evaluation of the native immune responses challenging. PDX models have enhanced the field of personalized medicine (House et al., 2014; Perez et al., 2016).

The six-month transgenic mouse carcinogenicity study is now frequently used as an alternative to the two-year mouse carcinogenicity bioassay, with the rasH2 model used most often (see *Animal Models in Toxicologic Research: Rodents*, Vol 1, Chap 17 *and Genetically*

Engineered Animal Models in Toxicologic Research, Vol 1, Chap 23). Regulatory agency approval should be attained prior to using a transgenic mouse model as a replacement for a conventional two-year mouse bioassay. Before the carcinogenicity study, a 28-day range-finding study with full tissue histopathology in the same parental strain (e.g., CByB6F1) of the intended transgenic mouse should be completed in wild-type mice, as the presence of transgenes (or inactivated genes) is not expected to influence the subchronic toxicity or pharmacokinetics of a compound (French et al., 2010; Jacobson-Kram et al., 2004; Morton et al., 2002; Storer et al., 2010).

Genetically engineered rodent models are attractive alternatives to conventional rat and mouse strains because of their low incidence of background neoplastic and nonneoplastic lesions, high survival rate, smaller size, shorter study duration, fewer number of animals required per study, and hence lesser quantities of compound required. Conducted according to ICH S1B guidelines (ICH I.C.o.H, 1997), Tg.rasH2 and $p53^{+/-}$ are accepted as primary models for carcinogenicity testing by the Committee for Proprietary Medicinal Products (CPMP), FDA, and the Japanese Ministry of Health, Labour and Welfare. Due to a large number of false-positive outcomes observed in studies submitted for regulatory approval, the Tg.AC model is no longer recommended as an alternative to the two-year bioassay (Storer et al., 2010) (see *Genetically Engineered Animal Models in Toxicologic Research*, Vol 1, Chap 23; and *Carcinogenicity Assessment*, Vol 2, Chap 5).

3.11. Transgenic Models for Mutagenicity Testing

MutaMouse (*lacZ* transgenic mice) and Big Blue (*lacI* transgenic rat or mouse) models have been used for mutagenicity testing of compounds (see *Genetically Engineered Animal Models in Toxicologic Research*, Vol 1, Chap 23). The MutaMouse and Big Blue rodent assays assess mutagenesis indirectly at the *lacZ* or *lacI* transgenes, respectively, that are incorporated into the mouse/rat genome as a surrogate of in vivo mutagenesis following chemical exposure for a given duration of time (Lambert et al., 2005). The *Pig-a* endogenous gene assay has also recently been developed to assess mutagenicity of chemicals following exposure in vivo. The *Pig-a* gene mutation assay is a useful biomarker of in vivo mutagenesis and most commonly performed using cells obtained from rat blood (Olsen et al., 2017).

3.12. The Tg.rasH2 Mouse Model

Tg.rasH2 hemizygous transgenic mice carry multiple copies of the human *c-Ha-ras* gene with their own promoter and enhancer. This model can be used for both genotoxic and nongenotoxic compounds. The percentage of tumor-bearing animals at the end of a six-month study approximates 25% in *Tg.rasH2*, and approximately 70%–80% for two-year mouse studies, respectively (Paranjpe et al., 2013). Nonneoplastic lesions that are commonly observed in the Tg.rasH2 mouse are skeletal muscle myopathy, vascular anomalies, and mesenteric arterial thrombosis (Paranjpe et al., 2013). The vascular anomalies are most commonly noted in the uterus. There may be some association between the vascular anomalies and progression to hemangiosarcomas, the most common spontaneous tumor of the Tg.rasH2 mouse (Paranjpe et al., 2017) (see *Genetically Engineered Animal Models in Toxicologic Research*, Vol 1, Chap 23).

The study design for transgenic mouse carcinogenicity studies generally includes a positive control group dosed with urethane or *N*-methyl-*N*-nitroso-urea to demonstrate the validity of the test system's susceptibility to a carcinogen and to ensure the use of the proper transgenic mouse strain (Shah & He, 2015). Because of its widespread use in the industry, large historical control databases and corresponding publications have been generated (Morton et al., 2002; Paranjpe et al., 2013; Paranjpe et al., 2014).

3.13. The $Tp53^{+/-}$ Mouse Model

The $Tp53^{+/-}$ mouse model has one copy of the wild-type allele and one copy of a null allele. The hemizygous knock-out animals have a very low incidence of spontaneous tumors up to 9 months of age. At approximately 18 months, however, survival is reduced to about 50% due to an increase in the incidence of tumors primarily $CD4^{+}CD8^{+}$ T-cell lymphomas and some sarcomas (Garcia & Attardi, 2014). Use of the $Tp53^{+/-}$ model is usually limited to mutagenic (genotoxic) compounds, as this model is less effective for the identification of nongenotoxic carcinogens and not highly responsive to positive control material such as *p*-cresidine (Storer et al., 2010).

3.14. Hamsters

Hamsters are infrequently selected as the species for carcinogenicity studies (see *Animal Models in Toxicologic Research: Rodents*, Vol 1, Chap 17). The reasons for this include the fact that the hamster lung has proved to be particularly resistant to inhaled materials known to be carcinogenic in the rat (Mohr & Dungworth, 1988). Additionally, the hamster is the preferred rodent species chosen for PPAR-α carcinogenicity studies, as the hamster is less susceptible to enzyme-induced hepatic tumors (Choudhury et al., 2000). The Syrian golden hamster cheek pouch carcinogenesis model was formerly used to study the development of premalignant and malignant human oral cancers, especially squamous cell carcinomas (Gimenez-Conti & Slaga, 1993). However, its recent use has not been reported in the literature.

3.15. Zebrafish

More recently, the *Danio rerio* (zebrafish) has gained traction as an additional cancer model due to its small size, numerous progeny, inexpensive husbandry, and quick maturation. An extensive assay catalog can be executed in the zebrafish from target discovery, target validation, toxicity studies, to the generation of tumors for corresponding in vivo efficacy tests and related areas can be studied using various applications (Table 8.9) (Lee et al., 2005; Letrado et al., 2018) (see *Animal Models in Toxicologic Research: Non-mammalian*, Vol 1, Chap 22). The zebrafish model can be established by carcinogen treatment (generally genotoxic), transgenic regulation, and the transplantation of mammalian tumor cells (Morton et al., 2002). Since zebrafish are poikilotherms, it is not ideal to evaluate some cancer phenotypes in the liver, kidney, and lungs (Howenstein & Sato, 2010) or certain therapies (e.g., immunotherapies) (Repasky et al., 2013) that are at least partially dependent on mammalian homeostatic temperature. Other limitations include some nonconserved organs (including the mammary and prostate glands) and small genome size as compared to humans (White et al., 2013).

With respect to carcinogenicity studies, spontaneous tumors of zebrafish are histologically similar to those of humans and have comparable gene expression profiles. Zebrafish serve as attractive cancer models for several reasons. They are relatively transparent, enabling monitoring of tumor progression, angiogenesis, and metastasis, and depending upon study objectives, different life stages of zebrafish may be leveraged. For

TABLE 8.9 Applications of Zebrafish in Cancer Research

Area of cancer research	Application
Multigenic screening of cancer genes	By injecting plasmids with genes of interest into embryos and monitoring for accelerated tumor onset in adult fish, oncogenic potential of candidate cancer genes can be established
Chemical genetic screening	Using early embryonic phenotypic markers in 96-well plates, chemical libraries can be screened in live zebrafish embryos
Modeling metastatic behavior	Through the injection of GFP-labeled tumor cells in transparent zebrafish, tumor metastasis can be monitored in vivo
Studying epigenetic mechanisms	Investigation of epigenetic mechanisms contributing to cancer phenotypes by using core biochemical techniques (i.e., ChIP-seq, methyl-seq, RNA-seq) along with zebrafish lines and antibodies

ChIP, chromatin immunoprecipitation; *GFP*, green fluorescent protein.

example, in tumor xenograft studies, embryos are sometimes used when a project requires speed, imaging, or high-throughput screening, with tumor formation following implantation of tumor cells possible in as little as 2 days (Letrado et al., 2018; Taylor & Zon, 2009). Furthermore, use of embryos for xenograft studies does not require immune suppression since functional B- and T-lymphocytes do not develop until 3–4 days following fertilization (Taylor & Zon, 2009). Adult zebrafish tend to offer a more realistic in vivo cancer model for the study of mechanisms of tumorigenesis rather than screening, since they are mature and all organs are fully developed. Compared to embryos, xenograft tumor establishment following transplantation in adult zebrafish usually requires approximately 2–4 weeks and necessitates immunosuppression with drugs (dexamethasone) or irradiation (Taylor & Zon, 2009).

3.16. Organoids

The contemporary development of three-dimensional organoid cultures has facilitated long-term propagation of stem cells in an in vitro physiological setting while recapitulating the architecture and distinct functions or genomic alterations of a specific organ or tumor type, respectively. Organoids could serve as an alternative platform for modeling carcinogenesis and also support and improve other applications in cancer research including personalized medicine strategies, regenerative medicine/transplantation therapy, and drug development. Modeling of the immune system has been challenging, but cocultures of organoids and lymphocytes have been developed for potential application in immunotherapy. Several recent publications can be accessed for additional reference (Drost & Clevers, 2018; Kuo & Curtis, 2018; Tuveson & Clevers, 2019; Xu et al., 2018) (see *Carcinogenicity Assessment*, Vol 2, Chap 5).

3.17. Clinical Pathology

While clinical pathology parameters are routinely included in shorter-term repeat-dose toxicity studies, there is no consistent approach to clinical pathology testing in carcinogenicity studies in the guidance from major regulatory organizations. Recommendations for clinical pathology testing in carcinogenicity studies are summarized in Table 8.10. Routine clinical pathology testing in carcinogenicity studies is most suitably used to aid in hematopoietic neoplasia diagnosis and characterization. In general, for two-year rodent carcinogenicity studies, it is recommended that clinical pathology testing be limited to collection of blood smears at scheduled and unscheduled necropsies and examination if histopathologic evaluation deems appropriate (Young et al., 2011).

3.18. Histopathology

The Society of Toxicologic Pathology's recommended tissue list is intended to be an essential compilation (Table 8.11) which can be applied to two-year carcinogenicity studies as well as repeat-dose toxicity studies (Bregman et al., 2003). Route of administration is also important when determining the tissues appropriated for microscopic examination. Several tissues are not universally included depending on the type of study and route of exposure because carcinogenicity rarely occurs in certain tissues, including optic nerve, nasal cavity, diaphragm, and certain salivary glands. However, nasal cavity is routinely examined in inhalation studies and some transgenic carcinogenicity studies. Furthermore, carcinogenicity is often correlated to macroscopic observations. In this regard, microscopic examination would be routinely conducted on gross lesions including masses. The accessory male reproductive organs are adequately represented by prostate and seminal vesicle; therefore, routine examination of the coagulating gland, which is not present in man, would likely be of negligible worth. There are additional tissues found in rodents that do not have human equivalents (e.g., Zymbal's glands, extraorbital lacrimal glands, and clitoral/preputial glands), and carcinogenic responses therein would have uncertain consequence to humans (Bregman et al., 2003).

The recommended tissue list in six-month transgenic mouse carcinogenicity studies is more extensive and includes sternal bone and marrow, rectum, and nasal cavity (Paranjpe et al., 2014). Exudative inflammation of the nasal cavity has been noted in Tg.rasH2 mice administered vehicle and/or test article via oral gavage, particularly when the vehicle and/or test article is an irritant (e.g., in the form of a salt with a low pH and/or a test article with increased viscosity). Additionally, Tg.rasH2 mice are generally much smaller than conventional two-year mice and their small esophageal size may play a role in causing rapid and repeated gastric reflux, resulting in nasal lesions (Paranjpe et al., 2017).

3.19. Carcinogenicity Study Data Interpretation

Several publications provide guidance on interpretation of carcinogenicity study data, including descriptions of statistical methods (Boorman et al., 2003; FDA U.F.a.D.A.C., 2001; Elmore & Peddada, 2009; Morton, 2002; Morton et al., 2002) (see *Experimental Design and Statistical Analysis for Toxicologic Pathologists*, Vol 1, Chap 16 and *Carcinogenicity Assessment*, Vol 2, Chap 5). The multiplicity of statistical tests of

TABLE 8.10 Summary of Major Regulatory Recommendations for Clinical Pathology Testing in Carcinogenicity Studies

Agency	Guideline	Version	Compounds	Sampling month of study	Recommendation
Environmental Protection Agency	OPPTS 870, 4200	8/1998	Agrochemicals	12, 18, scheduled termination	Blood smear[a]
Ministry of Agriculture, Forestry and Fisheries	MAFF no. 12 nousan 8147, chapter 2-1-15	11/2000	Agrochemicals	All terminations	Blood smear[b]
European Economic Community	67/548/EEC, annex V B32	5/1988	Chemicals	12, 18, scheduled termination	Blood smear[c]
Ministry of Economy, Trade and Industry	CSCL, notification form 10	4/2004	Chemicals	Scheduled termination	Blood smear and clinical chemistry, coagulation, and urinalysis as necessary
Organisation for Economic Co-operation and Development	451	9/2009	Chemicals	At discretion of the study director	At discretion of the study director
U.S. Food and Drug Administration	Redbook 2000, Chapter IV.C.6	1/2006	Food additives	0.5, 3, 6, 12, 18, scheduled termination	Complete blood cell count, clinical chemistry, coagulation, and urinalysis[d]
Ministry of Health, Labour and Welfare	Guidelines for toxicity studies of drugs manual	6/1905	Drugs	All terminations	Complete blood cell count[b]
European Medicines Agency	CPMP/SWP/2877/00	7/2002	Drugs	Interim/Scheduled termination	Complete blood cell count, clinical chemistry, coagulation, and urinalysis

[a] Differential leukocyte counts performed for control and high-dose groups at scheduled termination. If changes observed or other data indicate a need, then differential leukocyte counts done for other groups and/or on 12- and 18-month blood smears.
[b] Examine blood smears if a "blood disorder" or hematopoietic tumors suspected.
[c] Differential leukocyte counts performed for control and high-dose groups; if appropriate, differential leukocyte counts performed for other groups.
[d] If changes at 12 or 18 months, then measurements at scheduled termination are conducted.
Adapted from Young JK., et al.: Best practices for clinical pathology testing in carcinogenicity studies. Toxicol Pathol 39(2):429–434, 2011.

significance for both trends and pairwise comparisons needs to be considered when assessing the carcinogenic potential of a test article, and it is essential to make method adjustments for the differences in mortality among treatment groups. There are numerous statistical formulae addressing the multifaceted complexities of a carcinogenicity study. Many methods rely on information regarding tumor lethality (Hoel & Walburg Jr., 1972; Peto et al., 1980; Tarone, 1975), but statistical methods for analyzing tumor incidence rates at multiple terminations (rather than cause of death and tumor lethality) are also available (Ahn & Kodell, 1995; Ahn et al., 2002; Berlin et al., 1979; Dewanji & Kalbfleisch, 1986; Dinse, 1988; Lu & Malani, 1995; Portier & Dinse, 1987; Williams & Portier, 1991). It should be noted that multiple terminations are not common due to expense and study design convolution.

The most apt comparator is always the control group in a given study, but historical control data to classify tumors as rare or common and other information related to biological relevance can also be helpful (*Animal Models in Toxicologic Research: Rodents,* Vol 1, Chap 17). Rare tumors are analyzed with more lenient statistical paradigms (FDA U.F.a.D.A.C., 2001) by means of a higher *P*-value. The pathologist plays a key role in determining how carcinogenicity study data are analyzed using the weight-of-evidence approach. For example, it may be appropriate to combine systemic neoplasms from the same cell type present in various sites throughout the body (e.g., hemangiomas and hemangiosarcomas). Sources for historical control data include the research organization where the study was conducted (data within 5 years), electronic databases (RITA R.o.I.T.A.-d.R, 2019), and peer-reviewed publications. Terminology for nonneoplastic and neoplastic findings should conform to the International Harmonization of Nomenclature and Diagnostic Criteria recommendations (*Nomenclature and Diagnostic Resources in Anatomic Toxicologic Pathology,* Vol 1, Chap 25).

4. EVOLVING AND NEW TECHNOLOGIES

4.1. Gene Expression Analysis

Numerous approaches have been applied recently to assess changes in the global gene expression profiles following administration of xenobiotics in vitro and in vivo. The most frequently used techniques range from low-throughput to high-throughput assays including real-time polymerase chain reaction (RT-PCR microarray analysis) and next generation sequencing (NGS)–based RNA sequencing (RNA-Seq) of total RNA (Alexander-Dann et al., 2018; Bourdon-Lacombe et al., 2015). RT-

PCR assesses locus-specific changes to gene expression using primers that specifically bind to a given region within the genome. Although this assay can be multiplexed with respect to the number of samples analyzed with a given primer pair, it is limited by its throughput and capacity. Microarrays have a more favorable high-throughput capability and can leverage multiple probe sets to assess gene expression. Microarrays have been successfully used to assess gene expression changes following treatment with xenobiotics in both ex vivo and in vitro and in vivo settings (Bourdon-Lacombe et al., 2015). In particular, gene expression changes associated with drug-induced liver injury and mitochondrial dysfunction have been assessed (Bourdon-Lacombe et al., 2015; Jaeschke et al., 2002; Jolly et al., 2004), as well as numerous chemicals and dietary compounds evaluated for chemical carcinogenesis (e.g., aflatoxins, BaP, and cyclophosphamide) (Blackshear et al., 2015; Hayes et al., 2016; Hoenerhoff et al., 2013; International Agency for Research on Cancer I, 2019).

In contrast, approaches that leverage NGS-based platforms including RNA-Seq are able to assess genome-wide changes in gene expression (including messenger RNAs, miRNAs, and ncRNAs) in an unbiased high-throughput and highly sensitive manner (Rao et al., 2018). RNA-Seq is able to provide a richer dataset as compared to microarray profiling and is able to differentiate between expression of protein-coding genes, isoforms, and tissue-specific isoforms and more accurately captures the dynamic range of the quantitative changes in gene expression (Rao et al., 2018).

4.2. Next Generation Sequencing to Assess Mutagenicity and Genome Instability

Mutagenicity testing is a standard step in determining the genotoxic and carcinogenic potential of test compounds as part of the genetic toxicology battery. While assays in the current testing process have been used successfully for decades, they fail in their capability to identify low-frequency mutations and chromosomal rearrangements which represent hallmarks of genome instability. Recent advancements in NGS and the use of paired-end sequencing

TABLE 8.11 Society of Toxicologic Pathology's Recommended Core Tissue List for Two-Year Rodent Carcinogenicity Studies

• Adrenal glands	• Pancreas
• Aorta	• Parathyroid glands
• Bone with marrow (femur including articular cartilage)	• Peripheral nerve
• Brain	• Pituitary gland
• Cecum	• Prostate gland
• Colon	• Salivary gland
• Duodenum	• Seminal vesicle
• Epididymides	• Skeletal muscle
• Esophagus	• Skin
• Eyes	• Spinal cord
• Gallbladder (mouse only)	• Spleen
• Harderian glands	• Stomach
• Heart	• Testes
• Ileum	• Thymus
• Jejunum	• Thyroid glands
• Kidneys	• Trachea
• Liver	• Urinary bladder
• Lung	• Uterus
• Lymph node(s)	• Vagina
• Mammary gland (females only)	• All macroscopic lesions, including masses
• Ovaries	

From Bregman CL., et al.: Recommended tissue list for histopathologic examination in repeat-dose toxicity and carcinogenicity studies: a proposal of the Society of Toxicologic Pathology (STP). Toxicol Pathol 31(2):252–253, 2003.

adapters have allowed for the identification of both low-frequency single nucleotide variants (Hiatt et al., 2013; Kinde et al., 2011; Revollo et al., 2018; Salk et al., 2018; Schmitt et al., 2012) and larger chromosomal rearrangements in mammalian genomes (Compagno et al., 2017; Garaycoechea et al., 2018; Minocherhomji et al., 2020). Duplex sequencing is an error-corrected NGS-based platform that uses ligated barcodes on both strands of the DNA duplex (Salk et al., 2018; Schmitt et al., 2012; Salk & Kennedy, 2020). Genomic DNA is sheared using standard protocols (e.g., sonication) followed by barcode and adapter ligation, sequencing and single and duplex consensus sequence assembly of the two strands to determine whether a mutation is present on either one (false positive) or both strands of the DNA duplex (true positive) (Figure 8.5). This method is able to identify true positive mutations at the locus of interest and the region with genomic DNA that is queried, in addition to identifying mutagen-specific signatures and spectra (for example, $T > A$ or $C > G$).

Other NGS-based methodologies including PCR-free paired-end whole genome sequencing (WGS) are able to identify larger chromosomal rearrangements in the genome (Minocherhomji et al., 2020; Eisfeldt et al., 2019; Suzuki et al., 2014). PCR-free paired-end WGS is becoming a cost-effective way of quantifying genome instability endpoints, including inter- and intra-chromosomal translocations, deletions, amplifications, inversions, and insertions in an unbiased genome-wide manner.

Collectively, error-corrected and paired-end NGS methodologies will be able to identify mutations in any tissue without having a need for transgene reporter assays such as the Muta-Mouse and the Big Blue mouse assays (Morrison & Ashby, 1994). A paradigm shift in the extent to which low-frequency mutations and other features of genomic instability can be identified is underway, and newer error-corrected and paired-end NGS-based methods are being used to address fundamental gaps in the genetic toxicology battery for detection of changes that represent important hallmarks of cancer cells (Hanahan & Weinberg, 2011) and key characteristics of carcinogens (Smith et al., 2016). Further characterization of these mutagenicity assays is needed where genetic toxicity is being evaluated as part of the dataset guiding regulatory decisions (Heflich et al., 2020; White et al., 2020).

5. CONCLUSIONS

Oncogenes and tumor suppressor genes influence a myriad of factors including cell growth and proliferation, apoptosis, DNA damage

FIGURE 8.5 **Experimental work-flow and outline of paired end error-corrected duplex sequencing.** Sheared T-tailed genomic DNA is ligated with adapters (1 and 2) and barcodes (A and B) followed by next generation sequencing and bio-informatic analysis to detect true positive mutations (*blue dot*) present in both the forward and reverse strands. Random differences in single strands (*yellow dot*) and false positive mutations (*red dot*) which are present only in one single strand are disregarded.

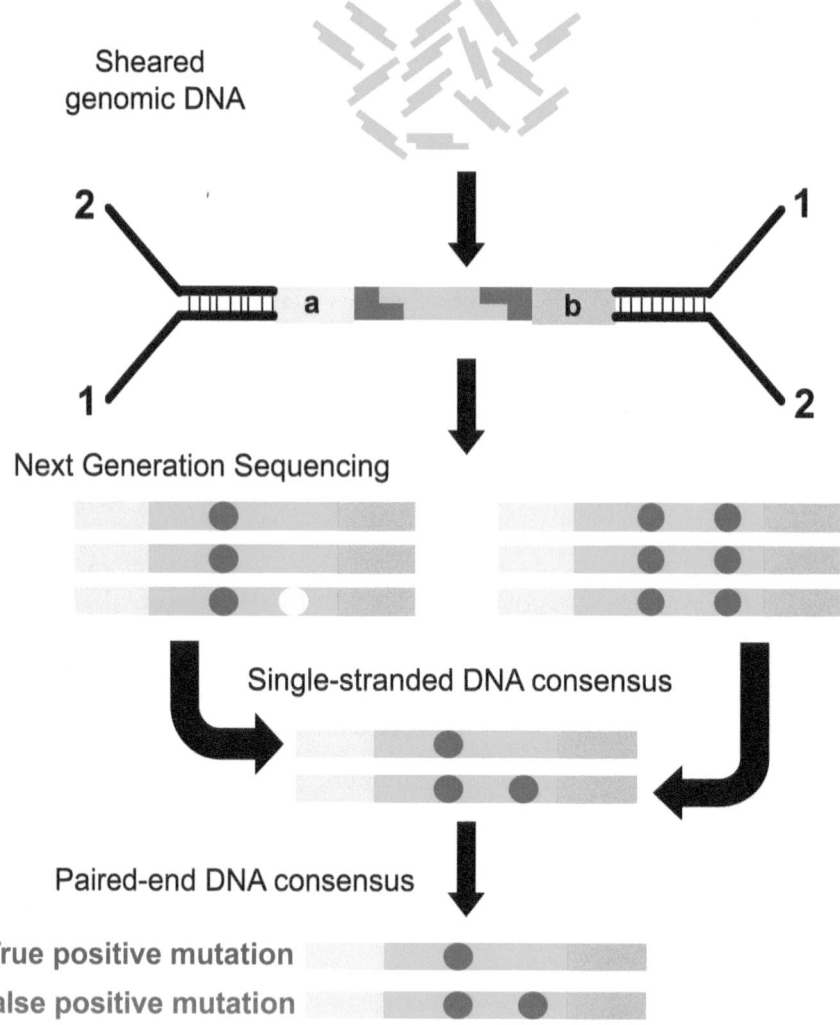

repair, and epigenetic regulation of gene expression and are part of a complex and intertwined balance within the cell. Aberrations of critical genes associated with cellular growth and differentiation determine the propensity of that cell to undergo transformation as a result of DNA damage and mutation. Furthering our understanding of the mechanisms of carcinogenesis and drug development relies on discovery pathology. How those mechanisms are related to cancer development in the face of exposure to potentially carcinogenic compounds is driven by safety assessment pathology and hazard identification. The identification of carcinogens, as well as the evaluation of the efficacy of cancer therapeutics, depends on the combined use of numerous in vitro assays, in vivo animal models, and testing paradigms, combining the expertise of basic scientists, toxicologists, and toxicologic pathologists, among other disciplines. The development and use of new technologies in drug development and cancer assessment will continue to expand our understanding of these diseases, with the ultimate goal of improving human health.

Acknowledgments

The authors would like to thank David Sabio and Experimental Pathology Laboratories for assistance with figure generation.

REFERENCES

Abaji C, Cousineau I, Belmaaza A: BRCA2 regulates homologous recombination in response to DNA damage: implications for genome stability and carcinogenesis, *Canc Res* 65(10):4117–4125, 2005.

Ahn H, Kodell RL: Estimation and testing of turner incidence rates in experiments lacking cause-of-death data, *Biom J* 37(6):745–763, 1995.

Ahn H, Moon CS, Kodell RL: Attribution of tumor lethality and estimation of time to onset of occult tumors in the absence of cause-of-death information, *Appl Stat* 49:157–169, 2002.

Alden CL, et al.: A critical review of the effectiveness of rodent pharmaceutical carcinogenesis testing in predicting for human risk, *Vet Pathol* 48(3):772–784, 2011.

Alexander-Dann B, et al.: Developments in toxicogenomics: understanding and predicting compound-induced toxicity from gene expression data, *Mol Omics* 14(4):218–236, 2018.

Ames BN, et al.: Carcinogens are mutagens: a simple test system combining liver homogenates for activation and bacteria for detection, *Proc Natl Acad Sci U S A* 70(8):2281, 1973.

Ames BN, McCann J, Yamasaki E: Methods for detecting carcinogens and mutagens with the Salmonella/mammalian-microsome mutagenicity test, *Mutat Res* 31(6):347–364, 1975.

Angadi PV, et al.: Immunoexpression of epithelial mesenchymal transition proteins E-cadherin, beta-catenin, and N-cadherin in oral squamous cell carcinoma, *Int J Surg Pathol* 24(8):696–703, 2016.

Aparisi F, et al.: Passenger mutations in cancer evolution, *Cancer Rep Rev* 3:1–8, 2019.

Aydinlik H, et al.: Selective pressure during tumor promotion by phenobarbital leads to clonal outgrowth of beta-catenin-mutated mouse liver tumors, *Oncogene* 20(53):7812–7816, 2001.

Balkwill F, Mantovani A: Inflammation and cancer: back to Virchow? *Lancet* 357(9255):539–545, 2001.

Barnes JL, et al.: Carcinogens and DNA damage, *Biochem Soc Trans* 46(5):1213–1224, 2018.

Benedict WF, et al.: Mutagenicity of cancer chemotherapeutic agents in the Salmonella/microsome test, *Cancer Res* 37(7 Pt 1):2209–2213, 1977.

Bennardo N, et al.: Alternative-NHEJ is a mechanistically distinct pathway of mammalian chromosome break repair, *PLoS Genet* 4(6):e1000110, 2008.

Berlin B, Brodsky J, Clifford P: Testing disease dependence in survival experiments with serial sacrifice, *J Am Stat Assoc* 74(365):5–14, 1979.

Bernal A, Tusell L: Telomeres: implications for cancer development, *Int J Mol Sci* 19(1), 2018.

Bertrand L, Mukaratirwa S, Bradley A: Incidence of spontaneous central nervous system tumors in CD-1 mice and Sprague-Dawley, Han-Wistar, and Wistar rats used in carcinogenicity studies, *Toxicol Pathol* 42(8):1168–1173, 2014.

Bhowmick R, Minocherhomji S, Hickson ID: RAD52 facilitates mitotic DNA synthesis following replication stress, *Mol Cell* 64(6):1117–1126, 2016.

Blackshear PE, et al.: Gene expression of mesothelioma in vinylidene chloride-exposed F344/N rats reveal immune dysfunction, tissue damage, and inflammation pathways, *Toxicol Pathol* 43(2):171–185, 2015.

Blankenship B, et al.: Findings in historical control Harlan RCCHan: WIST rats from 104-week oral gavage studies, *Toxicol Pathol* 44(7):947–961, 2016.

Boorman G, et al.: Assessment of hyperplastic lesions in rodent carcinogenicity studies, *Toxicol Pathol* 31(6):709–710, 2003.

Bothmer A, et al.: 53BP1 regulates DNA resection and the choice between classical and alternative end joining during class switch recombination, *J Exp Med* 207(4):855–865, 2010.

Bourcier T, et al.: Improving prediction of carcinogenicity to reduce, refine, and replace the use of experimental animals, *J Am Assoc Lab Anim Sci* 54(2):163–169, 2015.

Bourdon-Lacombe JA, et al.: Technical guide for applications of gene expression profiling in human health risk assessment of environmental chemicals, *Regul Toxicol Pharmacol* 72(2):292–309, 2015.

Bregman CL, et al.: Recommended tissue list for histopathologic examination in repeat-dose toxicity and carcinogenicity studies: a proposal of the society of toxicologic pathology (STP), *Toxicol Pathol* 31(2):252–253, 2003.

Brix AE, et al.: Incidences of selected lesions in control female Harlan Sprague-Dawley rats from two-year studies performed by the National Toxicology Program, *Toxicol Pathol* 33(4):477–483, 2005.

Ceccaldi R, Sarangi P, D'Andrea AD: The Fanconi anaemia pathway: new players and new functions, *Nat Rev Mol Cell Biol* 17(6):337–349, 2016.

Chaganti RS, Schonberg S, German J: A manyfold increase in sister chromatid exchanges in Bloom's syndrome lymphocytes, *Proc Natl Acad Sci U S A* 71(11):4508–4512, 1974.

Chang C, et al.: Androgen receptor (AR) differential roles in hormone-related tumors including prostate, bladder, kidney, lung, breast and liver, *Oncogene* 33(25):3225–3234, 2014.

Chappell G, et al.: Epigenetic alterations induced by genotoxic occupational and environmental human chemical carcinogens: a systematic literature review, *Mutat Res Rev Mutat Res* 768:27–45, 2016.

Chen L, et al.: Exosomes derived from HIV-1-infected cells promote growth and progression of cancer via HIV TAR RNA, *Nat Commun* 9(1):4585, 2018.

Choudhury AI, et al.: Species differences in peroxisome proliferation; mechanisms and relevance, *Mutat Res* 448(2):201–212, 2000.

Chouinard L, et al.: Carcinogenicity risk assessment of romosozumab: a review of scientific weight-of-evidence and findings in a rat lifetime pharmacology study, *Regul Toxicol Pharmacol* 81:212–222, 2016.

Chuang JH, Li H: Similarity of synonymous substitution rates across mammalian genomes, *J Mol Evol* 65(3):236–248, 2007.

Clewell RA, Thompson CM, Clewell 3rd HJ: Dose-dependence of chemical carcinogenicity: biological mechanisms for thresholds and implications for risk assessment, *Chem Biol Interact* 301:112–127, 2019.

Clive D, et al.: Specific gene mutations in L5178Y cells in culture, *Mutat Res* 115(2):225–251, 1983.

Cohen SM, et al.: Calcium phosphate-containing precipitate and the carcinogenicity of sodium salts in rats, *Carcinogenesis* 21(4):783–792, 2000.

Cohen SM, et al.: Chemical carcinogenicity revisited 3: risk assessment of carcinogenic potential based on the current state of knowledge of carcinogenesis in humans, *Regul Toxicol Pharmacol* 103:100–105, 2019.

Compagno M, et al.: Phosphatidylinositol 3-kinase delta blockade increases genomic instability in B cells, *Nature* 542(7642):489–493, 2017.

Corton JC, Peters JM, Klaunig JE: The PPARalpha-dependent rodent liver tumor response is not relevant to humans: addressing misconceptions, *Arch Toxicol* 92(1):83–119, 2018.

Corvi R, et al.: Moving forward in carcinogenicity assessment: report of an EURL ECVAM/ESTIV workshop, *Toxicol In Vitro* 45(Pt 3):278–286, 2017.

Cox DBT, Platt RJ, Zhang F: Therapeutic genome editing: prospects and challenges, *Nat Med* 21(2):121–131, 2015.

Deroo BJ, Korach KS: Estrogen receptors and human disease, *J Clin Invest* 116(3):561–570, 2006.

Dewanji A, Kalbfleisch JD: Nonparametric methods for survival/sacrifice experiments, *Biometrics* 42(2):325–341, 1986.

Dilley RL, et al.: Break-induced telomere synthesis underlies alternative telomere maintenance, *Nature* 539(7627):54–58, 2016.

Dinse GE: Estimating tumor incidence rates in animal carcinogenicity experiments, *Biometrics* 44(2):405–415, 1988.

Diwan BA, et al.: Promotion by Helicobacter hepaticus-induced hepatitis of hepatic tumors initiated by N-nitrosodimethylamine in male A/JCr mice, *Toxicol Pathol* 25(6):597–605, 1997.

Doe JE, et al.: Chemical carcinogenicity revisited 2: current knowledge of carcinogenesis shows that categorization as a carcinogen or non-carcinogen is not scientifically credible, *Regul Toxicol Pharmacol* 103:124–129, 2019.

Doherty AT: The in vitro micronucleus assay, *Methods Mol Biol* 817:121–141, 2012.

Drost J, Clevers H: Organoids in cancer research, *Nat Rev Cancer* 18(7):407–418, 2018.

Dyson NJ: RB1: a prototype tumor suppressor and an enigma, *Genes Dev* 30(13):1492–1502, 2016.

Eisfeldt J, et al.: Comprehensive structural variation genome map of individuals carrying complex chromosomal rearrangements, *PLoS Genet* 15(2):e1007858, 2019.

Elcombe CR, et al.: Mode of action and human relevance analysis for nuclear receptor-mediated liver toxicity: a case study with phenobarbital as a model constitutive androstane receptor (CAR) activator, *Crit Rev Toxicol* 44(1):64–82, 2014.

Elmore SA, Peddada SD: Points to consider on the statistical analysis of rodent cancer bioassay data when incorporating historical control data, *Toxicol Pathol* 37(5):672–676, 2009.

Elmore S: Apoptosis: a review of programmed cell death, *Toxicol Pathol* 35(4):495–516, 2007.

EPA: *Guidelines for carcinogen risk assessment*, U.E.P.A.E. Risk Assessment Forum.

Evans RM, Mangelsdorf DJ: Nuclear receptors, RXR, and the big bang, *Cell* 157(1):255–266, 2014.

FDA, U.F.a.D.A.: *Guidance for industry: preparation of food contact notifications for food contact substances (toxicology regulations)*, F.a.D.A. US Department of Health and Human Services, Office of Food Additive Safety (OFAS), Center for Food Safety and Applied Nutrition (CFSAN), Editor, 2002.

FDA, U.F.a.D.A.: *CFR - Code of federal regulations Title 21, regulation of carcinogenic compounds used in food-Producing animals*, F.a.D.A. Department of Health and Human Services, Editor, 2019.

FDA, U.F.a.D.A.C.: *Statistical aspects of the design, analysis, and interpretation of chronic rodent carcinogenicity studies of pharmaceuticals*, U.D.o.H.a.H. Services, Editor, Rockville, MD, 2001, Center for Drug Evaluation and Research, pp 1–44.

Felter SP, et al.: Human relevance of rodent liver tumors: key insights from a Toxicology Forum workshop on non-genotoxic modes of action, *Regul Toxicol Pharmacol* 92:1–7, 2018.

Fitzgerald DM, Hastings PJ, Rosenberg SM: Stress-induced mutagenesis: implications in cancer and drug resistance, *Annu Rev Cancer Biol* 1:119–140, 2017.

Fraga MF, et al.: Epigenetic differences arise during the lifetime of monozygotic twins, *Proc Natl Acad Sci U S A* 102(30):10604–10609, 2005.

French JE, et al.: Panel discussion: alternative mouse models for carcinogenicity assessment, *Toxicol Pathol* 38(1):72–75, 2010.

Fung VA, Barrett JC, Huff J: The carcinogenesis bioassay in perspective: application in identifying human cancer hazards, *Environ Health Perspect* 103(7–8):680–683, 1995.

Furuya M, et al.: Pathophysiology of tumor neovascularization, *Vasc Health Risk Manag* 1(4):277–290, 2005.

Garaycoechea JI, et al.: Alcohol and endogenous aldehydes damage chromosomes and mutate stem cells, *Nature* 553(7687):171–177, 2018.

Garcia PB, Attardi LD: Illuminating p53 function in cancer with genetically engineered mouse models, *Semin Cell Dev Biol* 27:74–85, 2014.

Gimenez-Conti IB, Slaga TJ: The hamster cheek pouch carcinogenesis model, *J Cell Biochem Suppl* 17F:83–90, 1993.

Gurley KE, Moser RD, Kemp CJ: Induction of lung tumors in mice with urethane, *Cold Spring Harb Protoc* 2015(9), 2015. pdb.prot077446.

Haines C, et al.: Comparison of the effects of sodium phenobarbital in wild type and humanized constitutive androstane receptor (CAR)/pregnane X receptor (PXR) mice and in cultured mouse, rat and human hepatocytes, *Toxicology* 396–397:23–32, 2018.

Hanahan D, Weinberg RA: Hallmarks of cancer: the next generation, *Cell* 144(5):646–674, 2011.

Hata AN, Engelman JA, Faber AC: The BCL2 family: key mediators of the apoptotic response to targeted anticancer therapeutics, *Cancer Discov* 5(5):475–487, 2015.

Hayashi M: The micronucleus test-most widely used in vivo genotoxicity test, *Genes Environ* 38:18, 2016.

Hayes SA, et al.: Renal cell carcinomas in vinylidene chloride-exposed male B6C3F1 mice are characterized by oxidative stress and TP53 pathway dysregulation, *Toxicol Pathol* 44(1):71–87, 2016.

Hayes J, Peruzzi PP, Lawler S: MicroRNAs in cancer: biomarkers, functions and therapy, *Trends Mol Med* 20(8):460–469, 2014.

Hecht SS, Isaacs S, Trushin N: Lung tumor induction in A/J mice by the tobacco smoke carcinogens 4-(methylnitrosamino)-1-(3-pyridyl)-1-butanone and benzo[a]pyrene: a potentially useful model for evaluation of chemopreventive agents, *Carcinogenesis* 15(12):2721–2725, 1994.

Heflich RH, et al.: Mutation as a toxicological endpoint for regulatory decision-making, *Environ Mol Mutagen* 61(1):34–41, 2020.

Henkler F, Brinkmann J, Luch A: The role of oxidative stress in carcinogenesis induced by metals and xenobiotics, *Cancers* 2(2):376–396, 2010.

Hernandez LG, et al.: Mechanisms of non-genotoxic carcinogens and importance of a weight of evidence approach, *Mutat Res* 682(2–3):94–109, 2009.

Hiatt JB, et al.: Single molecule molecular inversion probes for targeted, high-accuracy detection of low-frequency variation, *Genome Res* 23(5):843–854, 2013.

Hoel DG, Walburg Jr HE: Statistical analysis of survival experiments, *J Natl Cancer Inst* 49(2):361–372, 1972.

Hoenerhoff MJ, et al.: A review of the molecular mechanisms of chemically induced neoplasia in rat and mouse models in National Toxicology Program bioassays and their relevance to human cancer, *Toxicol Pathol* 37(7):835–848, 2009.

Hoenerhoff MJ, et al.: Hepatocellular carcinomas in B6C3F1 mice treated with Ginkgo biloba extract for two years differ from spontaneous liver tumors in cancer gene mutations and genomic pathways, *Toxicol Pathol* 41(6):826–841, 2013.

Hollander MC, Blumenthal GM, Dennis PA: PTEN loss in the continuum of common cancers, rare syndromes and mouse models, *Nat Rev Cancer* 11(4):289–301, 2011.

Hoover RN, et al.: Adverse health outcomes in women exposed in utero to diethylstilbestrol, *N Engl J Med* 365(14):1304–1314, 2011.

House CD, Hernandez L, Annunziata CM: Recent technological advances in using mouse models to study ovarian cancer, *Front Oncol* 4:26, 2014.

Howenstein MJ, Sato KT: Complications of radiofrequency ablation of hepatic, pulmonary, and renal neoplasms, *Semin Intervent Radiol* 27(3):285–295, 2010.

Huang W, et al.: Xenobiotic stress induces hepatomegaly and liver tumors via the nuclear receptor constitutive androstane receptor, *Mol Endocrinol* 19(6):1646–1653, 2005.

Huff J: Chemicals and cancer in humans: first evidence in experimental animals, *Environ Health Perspect* 100:201–210, 1993.

Hung DZ, et al.: Association between antiepileptic drugs and hepatocellular carcinoma in patients with epilepsy: a population-based case-control study, *Brain Behav* 6(11):e00554, 2016.

ICH, I.C.o.H: *S1A the need for long-term rodent carcinogenicity studies of pharmaceuticals*, F.a.D.A. US Department of Health and Human Services, Center for Drug Evaluation and Research (CDER) and Center for Biologics Evaluation and Research (CBER), Editor, 1996.

ICH, I.C.o.H: *S1B testing for carcinogencity of pharmaceuticals*, F.a.D.A. US Department of Health and Human Services, Center for Drug Evaluation and Research (CDER) and Center for Biologics Evaluation and Research (CBER), Editor, 1997, pp 1–7.

ICH, I.C.o.H: *S1C(R2) dose selection for carcinogenicity studies of pharmaceuticals*, F.a.D.A. US Department of Health and Human Services, Center for Drug Evaluation and Research (CDER) and Center for Biologics Evaluation and Research (CBER), Editor, 2008.

ICH, I.C.o.H: *M3(R2) nonclinical safety studies for the conduct of human clinical trials and marketing authorization for pharmaceuticals*, F.a.D.A. US Department of Health and Human Services, Center for Drug Evaluation and Research (CDER) and Center for Biologics Evaluation and Research (CBER), Editor, 2010.

ICH, I.C.o.H: *S1: rodent carcinogenicity studies for human pharmaceuticals*, F.a.D.A. US Department of Health and Human Services, Center for Drug Evaluation and Research (CDER) and Center for Biologics Evaluation and Research (CBER), Editor, 2012.

ICH, I.C.o.H: *S2(R1) genotoxicity testing and data interpretation for pharmaceuticals intended for human use*, F.a.D.A. US Department of Health and Human Services, Center for Drug Evaluation and Research (CDER) and Center for Biologics Evaluation and Research (CBER), Editor, 2012.

ICH, I.C.o.H.: *S6(R1) preclinical safety evaluation of Biotechnology-derived pharmaceuticals*, F.a.D.A. US Department of Health and Human Services, Center for Drug Evaluation and Research (CDER) and Center for Biologics Evaluation and Research (CBER), Editor, 2012.

ICH, I.C.o.H.: *Regulatory testing paradigm of carcinogenicity in rats S1, status report*, 2017, pp 1–5.

Ikehata H, Ono T: The mechanisms of UV mutagenesis, *J Radiat Res* 52(2):115–125, 2011.

Institute NC: *Reports of NCI bioassays of chemical for possible carcinogenicity*, National Cancer Institute Technical Report Series.

International Agency for Research on Cancer, I: Schistosomes, liver flukes and *Helicobacter pylori*. IARC working group on the evaluation of carcinogenic risks to humans. Lyon, 7–14

June 1994, *IARC Monogr Eval Carcinog Risks Hum* 61:1–241, 1994.

International Agency for Research on Cancer, I: *2,3,7,8-tetrachlorodibenzo-para-dioxin, 2,3,4,7,8-pentachlorodibenzofuran, and 3,3',4,4',5-pentachlorobiphenyl*, I. Monographs, Editor, 2018, pp 339–378.

International Agency for Research on Cancer, I: Preamble. In *IARC Monogr eval Carcinog risks Hum*, 2019. Lyons, France.

Ito Y, et al.: Di(2-ethylhexyl)phthalate induces hepatic tumorigenesis through a peroxisome proliferator-activated receptor alpha-independent pathway, *J Occup Health* 49(3):172–182, 2007.

Iyama T, Wilson 3rd DM: DNA repair mechanisms in dividing and non-dividing cells, *DNA Repair* 12(8):620–636, 2013.

Jackstadt R, Sansom OJ: Mouse models of intestinal cancer, *J Pathol* 238(2):141–151, 2016.

Jacobson-Kram D, Sistare FD, Jacobs AC: Use of transgenic mice in carcinogenicity hazard assessment, *Toxicol Pathol* 32(Suppl 1):49–52, 2004.

Jaeschke H, et al.: Mechanisms of hepatotoxicity, *Toxicol Sci* 65(2):166–176, 2002.

Jasin M, Rothstein R: Repair of strand breaks by homologous recombination, *Cold Spring Harb Perspect Biol* 5(11):a012740, 2013.

Jiricny J: Postreplicative mismatch repair, *Cold Spring Harb Perspect Biol* 5(4):a012633, 2013.

Johnson FE, et al.: Effect of cyclosporine on carcinogenesis induced in rats by N-methyl-N'-nitro-N-nitrosoguanidine, *J Surg Res* 37(3):180–188, 1984.

Johnson GE: Mammalian cell HPRT gene mutation assay: test methods, *Methods Mol Biol* 817:55–67, 2012.

Jolly RA, et al.: Microvesicular steatosis induced by a short chain fatty acid: effects on mitochondrial function and correlation with gene expression, *Toxicol Pathol* 32(Suppl 2):19–25, 2004.

Joyce JA, Schofield PN: Genomic imprinting and cancer, *Mol Pathol* 51(4):185–190, 1998.

Kane AB: Inflammation; Part 2. Mechanisms of carcinogenesis. In Baan RA, Stewart BW, Straif K, editors: *IARC scientific publications*, Lyon, France, 2019, IARC, pp 165–174.

Kang JK, Seo S, Jin YW: Health effects of radon exposure, *Yonsei Med J* 60(7):597–603, 2019.

Kastenhuber ER, Lowe SW: Putting p53 in context, *Cell* 170(6):1062–1078, 2017.

Keenan C, et al.: The north american control animal database: a resource based on standardized nomenclature and diagnostic criteria, *Toxicol Pathol* 30(1):75–79, 2002.

Kelly CM, Latimer JJ: Unscheduled DNA synthesis: a functional assay for global genomic nucleotide excision repair, *Methods Mol Biol* 291:303–320, 2005.

Kemp CJ: Animal models of chemical carcinogenesis: driving breakthroughs in cancer research for 100 years, *Cold Spring Harb Protoc* 2015(10):865–874, 2015.

Kerr LD, Inoue J, Verma IM: Signal transduction: the nuclear target, *Curr Opin Cell Biol* 4(3):496–501, 1992.

Kinde I, et al.: Detection and quantification of rare mutations with massively parallel sequencing, *Proc Natl Acad Sci U S A* 108(23):9530–9535, 2011.

King-Herbert A, Thayer K: NTP workshop: animal models for the NTP rodent cancer bioassay: stocks and strains–should we switch? *Toxicol Pathol* 34(6):802–805, 2006.

Kirkland D, et al.: A core in vitro genotoxicity battery comprising the Ames test plus the in vitro micronucleus test is sufficient to detect rodent carcinogens and in vivo genotoxins, *Mutat Res* 721(1):27–73, 2011.

Klaunig JE, et al.: The role of oxidative stress in chemical carcinogenesis, *Environ Health Perspect* 106(Suppl 1):289–295, 1998.

Klaunig JE, et al.: Oxidative stress and oxidative damage in chemical carcinogenesis, *Toxicol Appl Pharmacol* 254(2):86–99, 2011.

Knudson Jr AG: Mutation and cancer: statistical study of retinoblastoma, *Proc Natl Acad Sci U S A* 68(4):820–823, 1971.

Kobets T, Williams GM: Review of the evidence for thresholds for DNA-reactive and epigenetic experimental chemical carcinogens, *Chem Biol Interact* 301:88–111, 2019.

Kramara J, Osia B, Malkova A: Break-induced replication: the where, the why, and the how, *Trends Genet* 34(7):518–531, 2018.

Krokan HE, Bjørås M: Base excision repair, *Cold Spring Harbor Perspect Biol* 5(4):a012583, 2013.

Kumar V, et al.: *Robbins and Cotran pathologic basis of disease*, Philadelphia, 2015, Elsevier Saunders.

Kuo CJ, Curtis C: Organoids reveal cancer dynamics, *Nature* 556(7702):441–442, 2018.

La Vecchia C, Negri E: A review of epidemiological data on epilepsy, phenobarbital, and risk of liver cancer, *Eur J Cancer Prev* 23(1):1–7, 2014.

Lambert IB, et al.: Detailed review of transgenic rodent mutation assays, *Mutat Res* 590(1–3):1–280, 2005.

Latt SA, et al.: Sister-chromatid exchanges: a report of the GENE-TOX program, *Mutat Res* 87(1):17–62, 1981.

Lee LM, et al.: The fate of human malignant melanoma cells transplanted into zebrafish embryos: assessment of migration and cell division in the absence of tumor formation, *Dev Dyn* 233(4):1560–1570, 2005.

Lee GH, Ooasa T, Osanai M: Mechanism of the paradoxical, inhibitory effect of phenobarbital on hepatocarcinogenesis initiated in infant B6C3F1 mice with diethylnitrosamine, *Cancer Res* 58(8):1665–1669, 1998.

Letrado P, et al.: Zebrafish: speeding up the cancer drug discovery process, *Cancer Res* 78(21):6048–6058, 2018.

Lieber MR: The mechanism of double-strand DNA break repair by the nonhomologous DNA end-joining pathway, *Annu Rev Biochem* 79:181–211, 2010.

Lin C-P, Lin H: Noncoding RNAs in cancer development, *Annu Rev Cancer Biol* 1:163–184, 2017.

Lindahl T: Instability and decay of the primary structure of DNA, *Nature* 362(6422):709–715, 1993.

Loeb LA, Harris CC: Advances in chemical carcinogenesis: a historical review and prospective, *Cancer Res* 68(17):6863–6872, 2008.

Loeb LA: Human cancers express a mutator phenotype: hypothesis, origin, and consequences, *Cancer Res* 76(8):2057–2059, 2016.

Lu T-H, et al.: Arsenic induces reactive oxygen species-caused neuronal cell apoptosis through JNK/ERK-mediated mitochondria-dependent and GRP 78/CHOP-regulated pathways, *Toxicol Lett* 224(1):130–140, 2014.

Lu Y, Malani HM: Analysis of animal carcinogenicity experiments with multiple tumor types, *Biometrics* 51(1):73–86, 1995.

Ma B, Stepanov I, Hecht SS: Recent studies on DNA adducts resulting from human exposure to tobacco smoke, *Toxics* 7(1), 2019.

Macheret M, Halazonetis TD: DNA replication stress as a hallmark of cancer, *Annu Rev Pathol* 10:425–448, 2015.

Marshall BJ, et al.: Attempt to fulfil Koch's postulates for pyloric Campylobacter, *Med J Aust* 142(8):436–439, 1985.

Marshall B: *Helicobacter pylori*–a Nobel pursuit? *Can J Gastroenterol* 22(11):895–896, 2008.

Mavournin KH, et al.: The in vivo micronucleus assay in mammalian bone marrow and peripheral blood. A report of the U.S. Environmental Protection Agency Gene-Tox Program, *Mutat Res* 239(1):29–80, 1990.

McFarland CD, et al.: The damaging effect of passenger mutations on cancer progression, *Cancer Res* 77(18):4763–4772, 2017.

McGranahan N, Swanton C: Clonal heterogeneity and tumor evolution: past, present, and the future, *Cell* 168(4):613–628, 2017.

Miller JA, Miller EC: The metabolism and carcinogenicity of p-dimethylaminoazobenzene and related compounds in the rat, *Cancer Res* 7(1):39–41, 1947.

Miller EC, Miller JA: Searches for ultimate chemical carcinogens and their reactions with cellular macromolecules, *Cancer* 47(10):2327–2345, 1981.

Miller EC: Studies on the formation of protein-bound derivatives of 3,4-benzpyrene in the epidermal fraction of mouse skin, *Cancer Res* 11(2):100–108, 1951.

Minocherhomji S, et al.: Replication stress activates DNA repair synthesis in mitosis, *Nature* 528(7581):286–290, 2015.

Minocherhomji S, et al.: Biomarkers of genome instability in normal mammalian genomes following drug-induced replication stress, *Environ Mol Mutagen* 61(8):770–785, 2020.

Minocherhomji S, Tollefsbol TO, Singh KK: Mitochondrial regulation of epigenetics and its role in human diseases, *Epigenetics* 7(4):326–334, 2012.

Moennikes O, et al.: Lack of phenobarbital-mediated promotion of hepatocarcinogenesis in connexin32-null mice, *Cancer Res* 60(18):5087–5091, 2000.

Moggs J, Terranova R: Chromatin dynamics underlying latent responses to xenobiotics, *Toxicol Res* 7(4):606–617, 2018.

Mohr U, Dungworth DL: Relevance to humans of experimentally induced pulmonary tumors in rats and hamsters. In Mohr U, et al., editors: *Inhalation toxicology*, Berlin, 1988, Springer-Verlag, pp 209–232.

Morrison V, Ashby J: A preliminary evaluation of the performance of the Muta Mouse (lacZ) and Big Blue (lacI) transgenic mouse mutation assays, *Mutagenesis* 9(4):367–375, 1994.

Morton D, et al.: The Tg rasH2 mouse in cancer hazard identification, *Toxicol Pathol* 30(1):139–146, 2002.

Morton D, et al.: The Society of Toxicologic Pathology's recommendations on statistical analysis of rodent carcinogenicity studies, *Toxicol Pathol* 30(3):415–418, 2002.

Morton D: Statistical methods for carcinogenicity studies, *Toxicol Pathol* 30(3):403–414, 2002.

Murray IA, Patterson AD, Perdew GH: Aryl hydrocarbon receptor ligands in cancer: friend and foe, *Nat Rev Cancer* 14(12):801–814, 2014.

Nalepa G, Clapp DW: Fanconi anaemia and cancer: an intricate relationship, *Nat Rev Cancer* 18(3):168–185, 2018.

Neumann HG: Risk assessment of chemical carcinogens and thresholds, *Crit Rev Toxicol* 39(6):449–461, 2009.

Newbold RR, Padilla-Banks E, Jefferson WN: Adverse effects of the model environmental estrogen diethylstilbestrol are transmitted to subsequent generations, *Endocrinology* 147(6 Suppl):S11–S17, 2006.

Ning B, et al.: Toxicogenomics and cancer susceptibility: advances with next-generation sequencing, *J Environ Sci Health C Environ Carcinog Ecotoxicol Rev* 32(2):121–158, 2014.

Nohmi T: Thresholds of genotoxic and non-genotoxic carcinogens, *Toxicol Res* 34(4):281–290, 2018.

Norbury CJ, Hickson ID: Cellular responses to DNA damage, *Annu Rev Pharmacol Toxicol* 41:367–401, 2001.

OECD. *Test No. 471: Bacterial Reverse Mutation Test, OECD Guidelines for the Testing of Chemicals, Section 4*, Paris, 2020, OECD Publishing, https://doi.org/10.1787/9789264071247-en (Accessed 19 August 2021).

OECD, O.f.E.C.a.D.: *Guidelines for testing of chemicals*, Paris, France, 1981, Carcinogenicity Studies.

OECD: *Test No. 473: In Vitro Mammalian Chromosomal Aberration Test, OECD Guidelines for the Testing of Chemicals, Section 4*, Paris, 2016a, OECD Publishing, https://doi.org/10.1787/9789264264649-en (Accessed 19 August 2021).

OECD: *Test No. 474: Mammalian Erythrocyte Micronucleus Test, OECD Guidelines for the Testing of Chemicals, Section 4*, Paris, 2016b, OECD Publishing, https://doi.org/10.1787/9789264264762-en.

OECD: *Test No. 475: Mammalian Bone Marrow Chromosomal Aberration Test, OECD Guidelines for the Testing of Chemicals, Section 4*, Paris, 2016c, OECD Publishing, https://doi.org/10.1787/9789264264786-en (Accessed 19 August 2021).

OECD: *Test No. 476: In Vitro Mammalian Cell Gene Mutation Tests using the Hprt and xprt genes, OECD Guidelines for the Testing of Chemicals, Section 4*, Paris, 2016d, OECD Publishing, https://doi.org/10.1787/9789264264809-en (Accessed 19 August 2021).

OECD: *Test No. 487: In Vitro Mammalian Cell Micronucleus Test, OECD Guidelines for the Testing of Chemicals, Section 4*, Paris, 2016e, OECD Publishing, https://doi.org/10.1787/9789264264861-en (Accessed 19 August 2021).

Olsen AK, et al.: The Pig-a gene mutation assay in mice and human cells: a review, *Basic Clin Pharmacol Toxicol* 121(Suppl 3):78–92, 2017.

Ozery-Flato M, et al.: Large-scale analysis of chromosomal aberrations in cancer karyotypes reveals two distinct paths to aneuploidy, *Genome Biol* 12(6):R61, 2011.

Painter RC, et al.: Transgenerational effects of prenatal exposure to the Dutch famine on neonatal adiposity and health in later life, *BJOG* 115(10):1243–1249, 2008.

Paoli P, Giannoni E, Chiarugi P: Anoikis molecular pathways and its role in cancer progression, *Biochim Biophys Acta* 1833(12):3481–3498, 2013.

Paranjpe MG, et al.: Historical control data of spontaneous tumors in transgenic CByB6F1-Tg(HRAS)2Jic (Tg.rasH2) mice, *Int J Toxicol* 32(1):48–57, 2013.

Paranjpe MG, et al.: Incidence of spontaneous non-neoplastic lesions in transgenic CBYB6F1-Tg(HRAS)2Jic mice, *Toxicol Pathol* 41(8):1137–1145, 2013.

Paranjpe MG, et al.: Trend analysis of body weight parameters, mortality, and incidence of spontaneous tumors in Tg.rasH2 mice, *Int J Toxicol* 33(6):475–481, 2014.

Paranjpe MG, et al.: Progression of serosal vascular proliferative lesions to hemangiosarcomas in the uterus of the 26-week Tg.rasH2 mice carcinogenicity studies, *Int J Toxicol* 36(1):29–34, 2017.

Paranjpe MG, et al.: Tg.rasH2 mice and not CByB6F1 mice should Be used for 28-day dose range finding studies prior to 26-week Tg.rasH2 carcinogenicity studies, *Int J Toxicol* 36(4):287–292, 2017.

Paranjpe MG, Denton MD, Elbekai RH: The 26-week Tg.rasH2 mice carcinogenicity studies: microscopic examination of only select tissues in low- and mid-dose groups, *Toxicol Pathol* 42(7):1153–1157, 2014.

Perez M, Navas L, Carnero A: Patient-derived xenografts as models for personalized medicine research in cancer, *Cancer Transl Med* 2(6):197–202, 2016.

Peto R, et al.: Guidelines for simple, sensitive significance tests for carcinogenic effects in long-term animal experiments, *IARC Monogr Eval Carcinog Risk Chem Hum Suppl* (2 Suppl):311–426, 1980.

Pfeffer CM, Singh ATK: Apoptosis: a target for anticancer therapy, *Int J Mol Sci* 19(2), 2018.

Pitot HC: Adventures in hepatocarcinogenesis, *Annu Rev Pathol* 2:1–29, 2007.

Plass C, Soloway PD: DNA methylation, imprinting and cancer, *Eur J Hum Genet* 10(1):6–16, 2002.

Pon JR, Marra MA: Driver and passenger mutations in cancer, *Annu Rev Pathol* 10:25–50, 2015.

Portier CJ, Dinse GE: Semiparametric analysis of tumor incidence rates in survival/sacrifice experiments, *Biometrics* 43(1):107–114, 1987.

Pott P, Cancer S: *Chirurgical observations relative to the cataract, the polypus of the nose, the cancer of the scrotum, the different kinds of ruptures, and the modification of the toes and feet*, 1775, pp 63–68.

Pritchard JB, et al.: The role of transgenic mouse models in carcinogen identification, *Environ Health Perspect* 111(4):444–454, 2003.

Quail DF, Joyce JA: Microenvironmental regulation of tumor progression and metastasis, *Nat Med* 19(11):1423–1437, 2013.

Rall DP: Laboratory animal tests and human cancer, *Drug Metab Rev* 32(2):119–128, 2000.

Rao MS, et al.: Comparison of RNA-seq and microarray gene expression platforms for the toxicogenomic evaluation of liver from short-term rat toxicity studies, *Front Genet* 9:636, 2018.

Redmond Jr DE: Tobacco and cancer: the first clinical report, 1761, *N Engl J Med* 282(1):18–23, 1970.

Ren H, et al.: Evidence for the involvement of xenobiotic-responsive nuclear receptors in transcriptional effects upon perfluoroalkyl acid exposure in diverse species, *Reprod Toxicol* 27(3–4):266–277, 2009.

Repasky EA, Evans SS, Dewhirst MW: Temperature matters! and why it should matter to tumor immunologists, *Cancer Immunol Res* 1(4):210–216, 2013.

Revollo JR, et al.: Genome-wide mutation detection by inter-clonal genetic variation, *Mutat Res Genet Toxicol Environ Mutagen* 829–830:61–69, 2018.

Reya T, et al.: Stem cells, cancer, and cancer stem cells, *Nature* 414(6859):105–111, 2001.

Riley DJ, et al.: Susceptibility to tumors induced in mice by ethylnitrosourea is independent of retinoblastoma gene dosage, *Cancer Res* 54(23):6097–6101, 1994.

Rim KT, Song SW, Kim HY: Oxidative DNA damage from nanoparticle exposure and its application to workers' health: a literature review, *Saf Health Work* 4(4):177–186, 2013.

RITA, R.o.I.T.A.-d.R: *Continuous advancement of rodent tumor data acquisition and interpretation*[cited 2019 November 1]; Available from, https://reni.item.fraunhofer.de/reni/public/rita/.

Rodgers K, McVey M: Error-prone repair of DNA double-strand breaks, *J Cell Physiol* 231(1):15–24, 2016.

Roffo AH: The carcinogenic effects of tobacco. Monatsschrift Fur Krebsbekampfung Vol. 8, Issue 5, 1940, *Bull World Health Organ* 84(6):497–502, 2006.

Rogozin IB, et al.: Mutational signatures and mutable motifs in cancer genomes, *Brief Bioinform* 19(6):1085–1101, 2018.

Ross J, et al.: Human constitutive androstane receptor (CAR) and pregnane X receptor (PXR) support the hypertrophic but not the hyperplastic response to the murine non-genotoxic hepatocarcinogens phenobarbital and chlordane in vivo, *Toxicol Sci* 116(2):452–466, 2010.

Rous P, Kidd JG: Conditional neoplasms and subthreshold neoplastic states : a study of the tar tumors of rabbits, *J Exp Med* 73(3):365–390, 1941.

Ryffel B: The carcinogenicity of ciclosporin, *Toxicology* 73(1):1–22, 1992.

Safa AR: Resistance to cell death and its modulation in cancer stem cells, *Crit Rev Oncog* 21(3–4):203–219, 2016.

Safe S: Molecular biology of the Ah receptor and its role in carcinogenesis, *Toxicol Lett* 120(1–3):1–7, 2001.

Salk JJ, Kennedy SR: Next-generation genotoxicology: using modern sequencing technologies to assess somatic mutagenesis and cancer risk, *Environ Mol Mutagen* 61(1):135–151, 2020.

Salk JJ, Schmitt MW, Loeb LA: Enhancing the accuracy of next-generation sequencing for detecting rare and subclonal mutations, *Nat Rev Genet* 19(5):269–285, 2018.

Schmitt MW, et al.: Detection of ultra-rare mutations by next-generation sequencing, *Proc Natl Acad Sci U S A* 109(36): 14508–14513, 2012.

Scully R: Role of BRCA gene dysfunction in breast and ovarian cancer predisposition, *Breast Cancer Res* 2(5):324–330, 2000.

Shah P, He YY: Molecular regulation of UV-induced DNA repair, *Photochem Photobiol* 91(2):254–264, 2015.

Shen H, et al.: Aflatoxin G1-induced oxidative stress causes DNA damage and triggers apoptosis through MAPK signaling pathway in A549 cells, *Food Chem Toxicol* 62:661–669, 2013.

Sills RC, et al.: National toxicology program position statement on informed ("Nonblinded") analysis in toxicologic pathology evaluation, *Toxicol Pathol* 47(7):887–890, 2019.

Sistare FD, et al.: An analysis of pharmaceutical experience with decades of rat carcinogenicity testing: support for a proposal to modify current regulatory guidelines, *Toxicol Pathol* 39(4):716–744, 2011.

Slack FJ, Chinnaiyan AM: The role of non-coding RNAs in oncology, *Cell* 179(5):1033–1055, 2019.

Smith MT, et al.: Key characteristics of carcinogens as a basis for organizing data on mechanisms of carcinogenesis, *Environ Health Perspect* 124(6):713–721, 2016.

Sobol Z, et al.: Genotoxicity profiles of common alkyl halides and esters with alkylating activity, *Mutat Res* 633(2):80–94, 2007.

Solomon E, Borrow J, Goddard AD: Chromosome aberrations and cancer, *Science* 254(5035):1153–1160, 1991.

Sonnenschein C, Soto AM: Theories of carcinogenesis: an emerging perspective, *Semin Cancer Biol* 18(5):372–377, 2008.

Steenman MJ, et al.: Loss of imprinting of IGF2 is linked to reduced expression and abnormal methylation of H19 in Wilms' tumour, *Nat Genet* 7(3):433–439, 1994.

Stefan E, Bister K: MYC and RAF: key effectors in cellular signaling and major drivers in human cancer, *Curr Top Microbiol Immunol* 407:117–151, 2017.

Storer RD, et al.: An industry perspective on the utility of short-term carcinogenicity testing in transgenic mice in pharmaceutical development, *Toxicol Pathol* 38(1):51–61, 2010.

Stults DM, Killen MW, Pierce AJ: The sister chromatid exchange (SCE) assay, *Methods Mol Biol* 1105:439–455, 2014.

Supek F, Lehner B: Differential DNA mismatch repair underlies mutation rate variation across the human genome, *Nature* 521(7550):81–84, 2015.

Suzuki T, et al.: Precise detection of chromosomal translocation or inversion breakpoints by whole-genome sequencing, *J Hum Genet* 59(12):649–654, 2014.

Swenson DH: Significance of electrophilic reactivity and especially DNA alkylation in carcinogenesis and mutagenesis, *Dev Toxicol Environ Sci* 11:247–254, 1983.

Szikriszt B, et al.: A comprehensive survey of the mutagenic impact of common cancer cytotoxics, *Genome Biol* 17:99, 2016.

Tarone RE: Tests for trend in life table analysis, *Biometrika* 62: 679–682, 1975.

Taylor AMR, et al.: Chromosome instability syndromes, *Nat Rev Dis Primers* 5(1):64, 2019.

Taylor AM, Zon LI: Zebrafish tumor assays: the state of transplantation, *Zebrafish* 6(4):339–346, 2009.

Timblin BK, Bergman LW: Elevated expression of stress response genes resulting from deletion of the PHO85 gene, *Mol Microbiol* 26(5):981–990, 1997.

Tomasetti C, Li L, Vogelstein B: Stem cell divisions, somatic mutations, cancer etiology, and cancer prevention, *Science* 355(6331):1330–1334, 2017.

Toporcov TN, Wunsch Filho V: Epidemiological science and cancer control, *Clinics* 73(Suppl. 1):e627s, 2018.

Tuveson D, Clevers H: Cancer modeling meets human organoid technology, *Science* 364(6444):952–955, 2019.

US National Research Council Committee on Diet, N., and Cancer: Directions for research. In *Diet, nutrition, and cancer: directions for research*, Washington DC, 1983, National Academies Press.

Vahle JL, et al.: Carcinogenicity assessments of biotechnology-derived pharmaceuticals: a review of approved molecules and best practice recommendations, *Toxicol Pathol* 38(4): 522–553, 2010.

Van den Berg M, et al.: The 2005 World Health Organization reevaluation of human and Mammalian toxic equivalency factors for dioxins and dioxin-like compounds, *Toxicol Sci* 93(2):223–241, 2006.

van der Laan JW, et al.: Critical analysis of carcinogenicity study outcomes. Relationship with pharmacological properties, *Crit Rev Toxicol* 46(7):587–614, 2016.

Vasquez MZ: Combining the in vivo comet and micronucleus assays: a practical approach to genotoxicity testing and data interpretation, *Mutagenesis* 25(2):187–199, 2010.

Vats TS, Emami A: Oncogenes: present status, *Indian J Pediatr* 60(2):193–201, 1993.

Venkatesan S, et al.: Treatment-induced mutagenesis and selective pressures sculpt cancer evolution, *Cold Spring Harb Perspect Med* 7(8), 2017.

Venkatesan S, Birkbak NJ, Swanton C: Constraints in cancer evolution, *Biochem Soc Trans* 45(1):1–13, 2017.

Vineis P: Individual susceptibility to carcinogens, *Oncogene* 23(38):6477–6483, 2004.

Wade MJ, Moyer JW, Hine CH: Mutagenic action of a series of epoxides, *Mutat Res* 66(4):367–371, 1979.

Walmsley RM, Billinton N: How accurate is in vitro prediction of carcinogenicity? *Br J Pharmacol* 162(6):1250–1258, 2011.

Wan R, et al.: Cobalt nanoparticles induce lung injury, DNA damage and mutations in mice, *Part Fibre Toxicol* 14(1):38, 2017.

Ward JM, et al.: Peer review in toxicologic pathology, *Toxicol Pathol* 23(2):226–234, 1995.

Weber K: Differences in types and incidence of neoplasms in Wistar han and Sprague-Dawley rats, *Toxicol Pathol* 45(1):64–75, 2017.

West SC: Molecular views of recombination proteins and their control, *Nat Rev Mol Cell Biol* 4(6):435–445, 2003.

White R, Rose K, Zon L: Zebrafish cancer: the state of the art and the path forward, *Nat Rev Cancer* 13(9):624–636, 2013.

White PA, Long AS, Johnson GE: Quantitative interpretation of genetic toxicity dose-response data for risk assessment and regulatory decision-making: current status and emerging priorities, *Environ Mol Mutagen* 61(1):66–83, 2020.

Williams PL, Portier CJ: Analytic expressions for maximum likelihood estimators in a nonparametric model of tumor incidence and death, *Commun Stat Theor Methods* 21(3):711–732, 1991.

Wright WD, Shah SS, Heyer W-D: Homologous recombination and the repair of DNA double-strand breaks, *J Biol Chem* 293(27):10524–10535, 2018.

Wu L, Hickson ID: The Bloom's syndrome helicase suppresses crossing over during homologous recombination, *Nature* 426(6968):870–874, 2003.

Xu H, et al.: Organoid technology and applications in cancer research, *J Hematol Oncol* 11(1):116, 2018.

Yamada Y, et al.: Opposing effects of DNA hypomethylation on intestinal and liver carcinogenesis, *Proc Natl Acad Sci U S A* 102(38):13580–13585, 2005.

Yamada T, et al.: Human hepatocytes support the hypertrophic but not the hyperplastic response to the murine non-genotoxic hepatocarcinogen sodium phenobarbital in an in vivo study using a chimeric mouse with humanized liver, *Toxicol Sci* 142(1):137–157, 2014.

Yamagiwa K, Ichikawa K: Experimental study of the pathogenesis of carcinogens, *J Cancer Res* 3:1–29, 1918.

Yee NS, et al.: Animal models of cancer biology, *Cancer Growth Metastasis* 8(Suppl 1):115–118, 2015.

Young JK, et al.: Best practices for clinical pathology testing in carcinogenicity studies, *Toxicol Pathol* 39(2):429–434, 2011.

Yue W, et al.: Tamoxifen versus aromatase inhibitors for breast cancer prevention, *Clin Cancer Res* 11(2 Pt 2):925s–930s, 2005.

Zeiger E: The test that changed the world: the Ames test and the regulation of chemicals, *Mutat Res* 841:43–48, 2019.

Zhang W, Xu J: DNA methyltransferases and their roles in tumorigenesis, *Biomark Res* 5:1, 2017.

METHODS IN TOXICOLOGIC PATHOLOGY

CHAPTER

9

Basic Approaches in Anatomic Toxicologic Pathology

Torrie A. Crabbs[1], Keith Nelson[2]

[1]Experimental Pathology Laboratories, Inc., Research Triangle Park, NC, United States, [2]Charles River Laboratories, Mattawan, MI, United States

OUTLINE

1. Introduction	257	7.1. Cause of Death	278
2. General Considerations in Study Protocol Development	258	7.2. Nomenclature	279
		7.3. Severity Grading	281
3. In-Life Evaluations	265	8. Artifacts versus Lesions	282
4. Necropsy	268	9. Diagnostic Challenges in Anatomic Toxicologic Pathology	284
5. Fixation and Histologic Procedures	272		
6. Specialized Histologic Techniques	275	10. Conclusions	289
7. Histopathologic Evaluation	277	References	290

1. INTRODUCTION

Traditionally trained veterinary and medical pathologists often encounter unanticipated challenges during their transition from diagnostic pathology to the regulatory-driven environment of toxicologic pathology. During their initial years of training and diagnostic effort, pathologists typically serve both clinical and public health functions. Pathologists in diagnostic, hospital, or private laboratory settings serve the clinical community to support therapeutic approaches and disease prognoses. These laboratories are generally governed by internal work practices and procedures that are based on professionally recognized best practices and for the most part experience a limited degree of governmental oversight and influence on individual anatomic pathologist activities. The specific work practices of veterinary pathologists in these environments are seldom dictated by the extensive regulations that mandate proper management and storage of data, quality assurance review, peer review, animal welfare standards, organizational structure and personnel, and study design that are commonly encountered by toxicologic pathologists in the regulatory environment common to the biomedical and agrochemical industries. In addition, various animal species and different spectra of spontaneous background and induced lesions can be encountered in toxicologic pathology venues

Haschek and Rousseaux's Handbook of Toxicologic Pathology, Fourth Edition.
https://doi.org/10.1016/B978-0-12-821044-4.00019-4

that are not commonly observed in the traditional training or diagnostic setting.

This chapter will provide a basic introduction to the fundamental considerations, practices, and techniques involved in the proficient generation and interpretation of anatomic pathology data from repeat-dose nonclinical or other animal toxicity studies. Basic aspects of protocol development, necropsy, and tissue fixation will be covered as well as the recording of macroscopic (gross) and microscopic (histopathologic) findings and confounding factors (such as sexual dimorphism and artifacts) that can hinder interpretation. Several of these topics will only be mentioned briefly as they are discussed in greater detail in other chapters (see *Nomenclature and Diagnostic Resources in Anatomic Toxicologic Pathology*, Vol 1, Chap 25, *Pathology Peer Review*, Vol 1, Chap 26, and *Practices to Optimize Generation, Interpretation, and Reporting of Pathology Data from Toxicity Studies*, Vol 1, Chap 28).

2. GENERAL CONSIDERATIONS IN STUDY PROTOCOL DEVELOPMENT

Before any toxicity study can get underway, a study protocol must be developed. U.S. Food and Drug Administration (FDA) and U.S. Environmental Protection Agency (EPA) guidance documents state that "each study shall have an approved written protocol that clearly indicates the objectives and all methods for the conduct of the study" (US EPA, 1998a, b; US FDA, 2002). The Organisation for Economic Co-operation and Development (OECD) also recommends that "a written plan should exist prior to the initiation of the study" (OECD Organisation for Economic Co-operation and Development, 2018). Although the guidelines from the three agencies exhibit slight differences in content, all three organizations provide very similar guidance. Briefly, all study protocols should include a descriptive title and statement of the purpose of the study; identification and formulation of the test and control articles (or test items) by name, chemical abstract number, or code number; justification for dose selection; the name of the sponsor and the name and address of the testing facility; and the number, body weight, sex, source, species, strain, substrain, and age of the test animals (see *Pathology and GLPs, Quality Control and Quality Assurance,*

Vol 1, Chap 27). The toxicologic pathologist should be familiar with the protocol requirements of the various regulatory agencies as they will work with study directors, who are typically toxicologists, to support development of the pathology portions of study protocols or study plans.

During the initial stages of developing a study protocol, a number of issues must be addressed so that the ensuing stream of materials and data will meet regulatory requirements, follow established Good Laboratory Practice (GLP) guidelines, and provide reliable data capable of supporting the risk assessment process. These issues include clearly understanding the purpose of a given study; selecting an appropriate test system (i.e., animal species and strain), taking into consideration appropriate animal care and use; incorporating the 3Rs principles (Replacement, Reduction, and Refinement); ensuring appropriate sampling to meet regulatory needs and to satisfy the scientific questions of the study; and addressing key husbandry factors, to name a few. Study protocols should be reviewed by multiple stakeholders and departments involved with the design and conduct of the study to ensure that all parties and separate workgroups have clear direction and that the protocol-directed work is appropriate, necessary, and feasible.

The results of most toxicity studies are included as part of a data package submission to a regulatory agency, such as the U.S. FDA, U.S. EPA, European Medicines Agency, U.K. Medicines and Healthcare Products Regulatory Agency, South Korea's Ministry of Food and Drug Safety, or Japan's Ministry of Health, Labor, and Welfare. These agencies among others are charged with ensuring the safety and efficacy of pharmaceuticals, agrochemicals, medical devices, and food additives as well as numerous other products in their respective host countries. These data packages are part of the review process for these various chemicals and devices.

In the United States, toxicity studies that are included in regulatory submissions must be conducted under the auspices of the GLPs Act of 1975. These practices were adopted by the European Union and Japan as a consequence of the International Council on Harmonisation of Technical Requirements for Pharmaceuticals for Human Use (ICH). GLPs specific to the FDA are detailed in Title 21 CFR (Code of Federal Regulations) Part 58 and are discussed in another chapter of this text, as GLPs are specific to the US EPA Federal Insecticide, Fungicide, and Rodenticide Act (FIFRA, detailed in Title 40 CFR Part 160) and Toxic Substances Control Act (TSCA, detailed in Title 40 CFR Part 792) as well as GLPs specific to the OECD (detailed in OECD Organisation for Economic Co-operation and Development, 1998) (see *Pathology and GLPs, Quality Control and Quality Assurance,* Vol 1, Chap 27). GLP guidelines ensure that a study is conducted in a standardized, documented manner, consistent with global regulatory requirements. These practices result in the conduct of a well-designed and properly performed scientific study, with clearly defined expectations and procedures that will consistently yield high-quality, reproducible, and reliable data sets. However, these guidelines were not designed to dictate the most appropriate type of study for a given test article. Given the breadth of potential test articles, combined with the heightened safety standards of global regulatory agencies, the most appropriate study to characterize the toxicity of a compound must be designed with respect to known target pharmacology and test article–related potential liabilities even though, particularly in the early stages of drug development, the full toxicokinetic and toxicologic profile may not be known. In developing an appropriate toxicity study protocol, the study scientists must always ask "What major question(s) is this particular study expected to answer?" Examples of important questions may include but certainly are not limited to the following: What is the expected clinical dosing route and frequency? Is the compound acutely or chronically toxic according to previous investigations? Is there a dose–response to the toxicities, and do they resolve after dosing cessation? Does the test article induce proliferative changes that might lead to neoplasia? What are the expected effects on an individual at a given age range (e.g., juvenile as compared to skeletally or sexually mature animals)? Is the effect in a laboratory animal species of potential relevance to humans? What are the mechanisms of a particular effect in a single organ or across multiple related tissues?

No single safety study is able to answer all possible questions. Therefore, when developing a study protocol, it is important to focus on specific key questions and consider how the one study will fit into the final regulatory package, given that the package will have been assembled using data from multiple studies that addressed numerous different (though sometimes overlapping) questions. As scientists attempt to gain as much information as possible from a single study in order to reduce animal use and budgets, forethought concerning the information that needs to be conveyed by the final integrated registration package is becoming increasingly important during the design process of individual studies. In addition, GLP studies must comply with the requirements of the regulatory agencies that will evaluate the submission. Depending on the regulatory agency, study requirements may vary according to the species, strain, age, route and frequency of administration, dose range, number of animals per group, study length, and potential need for ancillary data types (e.g., dedicated testing for immunotoxicity, juvenile toxicity, neurotoxicity, or other specialized system-specific endpoints). Thorough knowledge of the requirements of and experience with various regulatory agencies will help preclude costly delays at the time of regulatory package submission, especially in the increasingly frequent desire to seek product registration in multiple parts of the globe.

Husbandry-related factors, such as light exposure (both duration and intensity), temperature, sound, diet, and environmental enrichment, all have the potential of influencing the results of the study or data interpretation, and therefore should be addressed in the study protocol or within facility Standard Operating Procedures (SOPs) or study-specific technical documents in order to assure consistency in experimental manipulations among all study groups (see *Issues in Laboratory Animal Science that Impact Toxicologic Pathology,* Vol 1, Chap 29). These environmental or husbandry-related factors should be recorded, with records available for the pathologist or other contributing scientists to refer to when interpreting findings. For example, extensive retinal degeneration can occur in rats exposed to excessive ambient illumination. Recommended ambient light levels for rodents (20–25 lux for nonpigmented strains and below 60 lux for pigmented strains) are significantly below those recommended for human working conditions (up to 500 lux in laboratory spaces). Therefore, it may be common for rodents to be inadvertently exposed to high light levels in studies with extensive human interaction. Therefore, if only high-dose animals are routinely housed on the upper shelves of cage racks, where light levels are highest, the degree of retinal degeneration could appear to be dose related (De Vera Mudry et al., 2013; Peirsen et al., 2018). Additionally, long photoperiods in rodent rooms can cause atrophy of the ovaries, Harderian glands, and adrenal glands, in addition to anestrus, any of which could erroneously be attributed to a test substance (González, 2018; Hoffman, 1970). Variations in temperature and sound can cause biologically significant changes such as immunosuppression, hormonal changes, alteration in phenotypic manifestation of musculoskeletal development, cardiovascular parameters, and other physiologic stress responses in animals (Castelhano-Carlos and Baumans, 2009; Gamble, 1982; Hankenson et al., 2018; Rubin, 2017).

Another husbandry-related factor that can impact anatomic pathology data is diet. Previous studies have documented a direct correlation between average caloric consumption and the incidence of several commonly recognized spontaneous degenerative diseases in rodents, including such conditions as chronic progressive nephropathy, progressive cardiomyopathy, and pancreatic islet fibrosis, as well as some neoplasms (pituitary and mammary tumors) (Abdo and Kari, 1997; Dillberger, 1994; Keenan et al., 2000; Kemi et al., 2000; Nold, Keenan, Nyska, & Cartwright, 2001; Pellizon and Ricci, 2020; Rao, 2002). Furthermore, caloric consumption is inversely correlated with survival in 2-year rodent carcinogenicity studies (see *Issues in Laboratory Animal Science that Impact Toxicologic Pathology*, Vol 1, Chap 29, *Carcinogenicity Assessment*, Vol 2, Chap 5, and *Nutrition and Toxicologic Pathology*, Vol 2, Chap 20) (Abdo and Kari, 1997). More importantly, feeding diets with different compositions has been demonstrated to alter physiological responses to some test articles. Animals fed a calorie-restricted diet have been shown to be more robust, with demonstrable tolerance to known carcinogens as well as reduced sensitivity to shorter-term toxicity when compared with ad libitum-fed, overweight animals (Hart et al., 1995; Ingram and de Cabo,

2017; Keenan et al., 1996, 1999, 2000; Kemi et al., 2000). Consequently, all toxicity studies of a given test article should be performed using the same diet. Utilizing diets with different compositions or nutrient sources across the spectrum of toxicity studies conducted for the same test article could alter the microbiome, resulting in variability in pathology or toxicokinetic findings. This in turn could lead to conflicting data that could confound data interpretation and potentially lead to repetition of inconclusive studies.

The animal species and strain, as well as the number of animals per sex per dose group, may be determined by customs of the particular laboratory, 3Rs considerations, animal availability (particularly with nonhuman primates [NHPs]), and statistical considerations. Also, the number of treatment groups and the age of the animals should be appropriate to comply with both regulatory and scientific standards. The criteria for selection of an appropriate animal model should weigh a number of factors. It is critical that the animal test system is sensitive to the test article being studied. In this regard, the test animal must exhibit properties relevant to the interaction of the test article (e.g., the target of the test article is expressed in the animal model and the test article is shown to bind to the target, such as in the case of a monoclonal antibody) and the test article must induce a functional pharmacologic response (e.g., as shown by assessment of pharmacodynamic [PD] biomarkers). Species sensitivity may be determined in part by single-dose or short-term repeat-dose exploratory toxicity studies where pharmacokinetic (PK) and PD endpoints are assessed as well as tolerability (ICH S6(R1) Guideline, 2011) (see *Volume 1, Part 1: Principles of Toxicologic Pathology*). Moreover, the PK and metabolic pathways of the test article in the animal model should be well characterized and their comparability to the test article effects in humans should be explored. In addition, the availability of historical control data for parameters measured in animals during the course of a study, such as body weight gain, food consumption, clinical pathology values, and the incidences and severities of background/spontaneous lesions and neoplasia, could be valuable in the recognition of a test article–related effect. Other criteria should include the commercial availability of the animal model, as well as the accessibility of appropriate housing and reagents (e.g., antibodies to quantify protein levels in fluids or detect their localization in tissue sections) that might be needed to probe certain classes of functional and structural effects. Furthermore, investigators should have extensive experience with the husbandry, dosing, and evaluation of the test species.

The number of dose groups should be established during protocol development. Generally, repeat-dose general toxicity studies require a minimum of three test article–treated groups (i.e., low, mid, and high) and at least one control group (usually untreated or vehicle treated), under the same conditions and testing regimen as test article–dosed animals. The lack of control groups, although sometimes advocated by those seeking to reduce the cost of testing and extent of animal use, should be avoided. In the absence of concurrent control animals, data will often be more difficult to interpret, statistical comparisons (for organ weights and clinical chemistry and hematology values) will not be possible, and the study design may not be accepted by regulatory agencies. This is particularly pronounced in nonrodent studies, where individual animal variation (e.g., in genetic background, weight, immune status, responsiveness to compound, social stress–associated changes, etc.) is generally greater than in commonly used rodent stocks and strains. To some degree, this could be ameliorated by including control animals during the in-life phase which could be utilized to obtain clinical pathology values, body weight evaluations, clinical observations, and the like; however, as opposed to euthanizing them for necropsy and histopathology evaluation, they could be recovered and returned to a colony group for use in future studies. This does not provide for concurrent controls in the histopathology or organ weight evaluations of the study, so deliberate consideration should be taken in utilizing this specific approach. The doses for these studies are generally established by prior single-dose or short-term (≤4 weeks) repeat-dose exploratory toxicity studies. Ideally, the high dose should result in evidence of toxicity but not generate more than 10% mortality, with the middose resulting in only slight toxicity and the low dose producing no test article–related effects. This spectrum of dose-dependent effects permits the determination of a No Observed Adverse Effect Level (NOAEL) and/or No Observed Effect Level (NOEL) as measures of the extent to which a test article induces adverse (NOAEL) or any (NOEL) findings in an exposed organism. The meaning and significance of NOAEL and NOEL in risk assessment will be discussed elsewhere in this text (see *Interpreting Adverse Effects*, Vol 2, Chap 15).

The age of the test species used in repeat-dose toxicity studies is fairly standard for routine studies. Unless other factors dictate another time point, exposure in conventional studies is initiated during young adulthood in rodents or during late adolescence in nonrodents. For example, in rodent studies, initiation of test article administration at 6–8 weeks of age will comply with essentially all regulatory guidelines for products destined for administration to adult animals or humans. Exception to this timing in rodents is required for test articles with potential acute reproductive effects (where initial dosing may begin in older animals to ensure full sexual maturity) or where the products are destined for administration to a pediatric or juvenile population (where initial dosing often is initiated prior to weaning) (see *The Role of Pathology in Evaluation of Reproductive, Developmental, and Juvenile Toxicity*, Vol 1, Chap 7) (Picut et al., 2015; Picut and Parker, 2017). Nonrodents have longer lives and mature more slowly than rodents. Accordingly, it is acceptable to regulatory agencies to initiate dosing in studies using dogs or minipigs at approximately 4–6 months of age even though animals at this age are often peripubertal rather than fully mature. In like manner, cynomolgus macaques are generally approximately 2–3 years of age at study initiation; at this age, there are a high number of reproductively immature or peripubertal animals, particularly males. Histologically, male cynomolgus macaques may not be reproductively mature until 4–5 years of age; body weight and testicular weights can be additional indicators of maturity (Halpern et al., 2016; Picut and Remick, 2017). For female macaques, reproductive maturity, with regular ovulatory cycling, may not occur until approximately 4 years of age (Halpern et al., 2016; Vidal, 2017). More mature nonrodent animals may be used for specific study purposes, though such studies are more expensive due to the increased husbandry costs incurred by maintaining animals as they age. For all of the larger animal species, full reproductive maturation in a consistent majority of the population may not be observed at these recommended ages for treatment initiation, so studies reliant on evaluating test article effects in reproductively mature specimens may need to source animals months to years older than these general guidelines, depending on the species (Halpern et al., 2016; Picut and Remick, 2017; Vidal, 2017) (see Table 9.1 and Vol 1, Part 3: *Animal and Alternative Models in Toxicologic Research*).

The proper selection of controls is an important aspect of study design as well. Different study types will require different controls. A standard repeat-dose study in a well-characterized rodent strain will generally require concurrent controls of the same strain, with equal numbers for each sex, all within a 20% body weight range. Animals should be assigned to control and test article–treated groups in a stratified random manner (i.e., ensuring that each treatment group contains a randomized array of animals from separate batches or birthdates or other possible differentiating factors) to minimize bias. For some studies, there may be separate negative control groups for sham-dosed, neutral agent (water or physiologic saline)–dosed, and/or vehicle-dosed groups. In injection studies, an adjuvant-only control group may also be utilized, though this is not required for regulatory purposes if the adjuvant is already well characterized (see *Vaccines*, Vol 2, Chap 9). Additionally, for some studies, such as transgenic mouse carcinogenicity studies, positive control groups (i.e., exposed to a known carcinogenic

agent) may be incorporated to provide internal validation that the model remains responsive (see *Carcinogenicity Assessment*, Vol 2, Chap 5). Finally, juvenile toxicity studies require careful planning for inclusion of control animals that are to be euthanized at planned and unexpected necropsies in order to allow age-matched comparison of evolving histologic features (see *The Role of Pathology in Evaluation of Reproductive, Developmental, and Juvenile Toxicity*, Vol 1, Chap 7). Careful selection of controls can greatly enhance the ability of the pathologist and other scientists to interpret possible test compound–related findings.

The purpose of a given animal study should be taken into account when formulating the study protocol. Studies may be performed to address a range of questions. Therefore, study procedures, sample collections, and all other study parameters need to be aligned with the primary purpose of the study. Some study types, such as dose range-finding studies or lead optimization studies, do not generally require large numbers of animals, extensive sampling, recovery periods, or numerous anatomic pathology or clinical pathology endpoints as they are focused on providing information for supporting future, more comprehensive (i.e., Investigational New Drug-enabling) studies. Such preliminary studies may be designed to include investigative endpoints that will not be incorporated in later GLP-compliant toxicity studies but that are needed for product registration. Subchronic (usually 3–6 months) and chronic (usually 9–18 months) studies should have sufficient numbers of animals across a range

TABLE 9.1　Age of Reproductive Maturation – Nonrodent Species

Species	Male	Female	References
Rabbit	4–6 months	4–6 months	Frame et al. (1994)
Dog (Beagle)	9–10 months	8–10 months	Goedken et al. (2008)
Minipig (Göttingen)	4–5 months	4–7 months	Peter et al., (2016); Howroyd et al. (2016)
Nonhuman primate (cynomolgus macaque)	4–5 years	4 years	Picut and Remick, (2017); Vidal (2017)

of dose levels in order to characterize toxicity even in the face of early attrition due to unscheduled deaths. Generally, in standard GLP-compliant toxicity studies, a minimum of 10 rodents/sex/dose group and 3–4 nonrodents/sex/dose group are enrolled for shorter-term studies (≤6 months); group numbers may be increased by 50% or more for longer studies, especially in rodents. These numbers also may be increased in instances where a subtle or infrequent finding is expected. Recovery intervals may be included in the study (Pandher et al., 2012; Perry et al., 2013; Sewell et al., 2014). Additional animals can be included specifically for serial collection of blood for PK analysis; however, tissues from these animals are typically only examined macroscopically at necropsy and do not undergo histopathologic evaluation. The collective focus of these studies should be evaluation of test article toxicity to facilitate the translatability of these findings to inform human risk. Carcinogenicity studies are conducted in rodents and are meant to determine the potential of a compound under life time exposure to induce neoplastic changes. Numbers of animals for these studies are selected to ensure that there is survival of a sufficient numbers of animals for adequate statistical analysis. Thus, a two-year carcinogenicity study typically is loaded with 60–80 rodents/sex/dose group. For a six-month transgenic mouse carcinogenicity study, where the model has an engineered or spontaneous genetic predisposition to early development of neoplasia, initial animal numbers will be lower (generally 25/sex/group) as age-related mortality should be limited (see *Carcinogenicity Assessment*, Vol 2, Chap 5). It is obvious that a single study plan cannot cover all potential study types, nor can all questions of interest be addressed in a single study.

Another important component of study protocol development is the choice of anatomic pathology endpoints. For instance, the list of essential organs weights to collect and tissues to be saved and processed for histopathologic examination as well as preparation to appropriately preserve samples for other study purposes (e.g., electron microscopy, immunohistochemistry [IHC], etc.) must be compiled in advance of the actual necropsy. Major regulatory agencies and professional organizations have developed guidelines of recommended organ weights,

tissues, and other toxicologic pathology endpoints that should serve as a template for study scientists tasked with designing toxicity studies. For example, after reviewing guidelines from regulatory agencies in the United States, European Union, and Japan, working groups of the Society of Toxicologic Pathology (STP) have formulated "best practice" recommendations for organ weight collection and protocol-specified tissue lists (Bregman et al., 2003; Crissman et al., 2004; Michael et al., 2007; Sellers et al., 2007). In addition to these general recommendations, the standard tissue list in the protocol should be modified to collect tissues appropriate to the design and objective of the study and reflect potential target-related pharmacology. Reasonable examples of study-specific tissue list modification would be addition of the nasal cavity, larynx, and tracheobronchial lymph nodes when evaluating an inhalation study; inclusion of injection/infusion and/or surgical sites as well as draining lymph nodes for parenteral injection, medical device, or surgical intervention studies; or the inclusion of the site(s) of application for a skin paint (dermal toxicity) study. This modification of the tissue list may also extend to increased sampling (sometimes termed "enhanced histopathology" or "expanded histopathology" by regulatory agencies) of organs and tissues to further characterize and assess findings at a specific site of interest; examples include ocular studies where specific areas are targeted for test article delivery or injection studies where the site of injection may be imperfectly visualized on gross examination. The protocol tissue list also should include tissues that are known or suspected targets of the test article, similar agents in the same chemical class, or that act via the same target molecule. Studies with test articles that are expected to alter the immune system should include collection and examination of lymph nodes, spleen, thymus, and related lymphoid tissues. If a test article or class effect is not known in advance, then it typically is reasonable to conduct a complete necropsy and save a - thorough list of tissues even if many of them are archived without histopathological examination. This approach will preclude the loss of valuable data given that the necropsy is a one-time event and that tissues, once discarded, cannot be retrieved. Appropriate collection and preservation of tissues is critical to ensure accurate high-quality sampling and interpretation of the anatomic pathology data set.

Selection of appropriate clinical pathology parameters is another essential step in the development of a study protocol. This choice is particularly critical in shorter studies as hematology, clinical chemistry, and urinalysis results may be sensitive indicators of toxicity (see *Clinical Pathology in Nonclinical Toxicity Testing*, Vol 1, Chap 10). As an example, changes in clinical chemistry values may provide an early indication of hepatic injury (see *Liver and Gallbladder*, Vol 3, Chap 2). The early identification of hepatic injury can be a challenging but decisive event in pharmaceutical compound development. A retrospective study has demonstrated that approximately 10% of marketed human pharmaceuticals that have either been withdrawn or labeled with a "black box" warning over the past several decades have been as a result of hepatic injury reported as a postmarketing adverse event (FDA U.S. Food and Drug Administration, 2009; Lasser et al., 2002). Current recommendations advise measuring the activities of two serum aminotransferase enzymes, alanine aminotransferase (ALT) and aspartate aminotransferase (AST), as the most sensitive and specific indicators of hepatocellular injury in rats, dogs, and NHPs (Boone et al., 2005; FDA U.S. Food and Drug Administration, 2009; Tomlinson et al., 2016). ALT is also considered to be a specific and sensitive test of hepatocellular injury in humans, suggesting that results of nonclinical studies may be predictive of potential hepatic injury in human patients. As with any single parameter, AST values must be used as part of the overall assessment of liver toxicity, including correlation with histopathologic observations in subchronic and chronic toxicity studies. To aid in identifying the clinical pathology parameters that will optimize early recognition of cellular injury, study scientists should be knowledgeable with any potential test article–related toxicities either by perusing data sets from exploratory toxicity studies or by predicting possible effects based on the activities of similar agents in the same class of compounds. Anatomic toxicologic pathologists may analyze, interpret, and communicate routine clinical pathology data from standard toxicity studies or may work

with a board-certified veterinary clinical pathologist to discuss findings from their respective analyses and align on how pathology conclusions are to be communicated to the Study Director. More specialized clinical pathology tests typically are evaluated by a clinical pathologist due to their greater familiarity with unusual assays and artifacts that might result from sampling and/or analytical complications.

Biomarkers also may be of use in demonstrating test article–related effects. Certainly, classical clinical pathology parameters such as hematology, blood chemistry, and urinalysis are the most basic of the biomarkers that are routinely included in the toxicologic pathology portions of study designs. However, additional biomarkers such as gene expression (see *Toxicogenomics: A Primer for Toxicologic Pathologists*, Vol 1, Chap 15) or noninvasive imaging (see *In Vivo Small Animal Imaging: A Comparison to Gross and Histopathologic Observations in Animal Models*, Vol 1, Chap 13) may be incorporated in animal studies to address specific potential findings or to provide more translatable and easily monitored signals for clinical trials. Biomarkers may be used to assess functional responses, direct tissue injury, or to localize toxic insults. Biomarkers are an ever-expanding field of development and may be used to evaluate PD responses, efficacy, or toxicity across a wide range of organ systems, including renal, cardiovascular, musculoskeletal, and nervous systems; hormonal changes; immune function and acute phase reactants; coagulation factors; growth factors; and other metabolic disturbances, to name a few. Biomarker responses vary in timing, as well as among test articles and across species. For example, certain biomarkers of cardiotoxicity may elevate acutely, while others will only elevate over days to weeks, and rodents have different acute phase proteins than humans and other mammals. Some biomarkers may exhibit diurnal variation or fluctuation as a result of feeding or light cycles (Benavides et al., 1998; Matsuzawa 1999; Minematsu et al., 1995). These factors need to be taken into consideration when designing studies utilizing biomarkers or when interpreting biomarker data. Incorporation of biomarkers into the study design should be done in a careful and considered manner, under consultation with a board-certified veterinary clinical pathologist or other subject matter expert to ensure that the correct samples are taken at the optimal time, and the correct panel of biomarkers is used. Avoidance of a random, broad-based ("shotgun") sampling approach is wise as the potential for producing confounding or nonsensical data—often without sufficient context to aid in its interpretation—is present in the absence of a clearly targeted investigation. As with clinical pathology data, biomarker data should be interpreted in consultation with the study anatomic and clinical pathologists in order to understand changes in the context of the whole animal.

Much has been written about animal welfare issues and their potential impact in toxicologic pathology (see *Issues in Laboratory Animal Science that Impact Toxicologic Pathology*, Vol 1, Chap 29). Increased awareness of animal welfare and the regulatory oversight supplied by the U.S. Department of Agriculture (USDA) and equivalent ex-U.S. agencies as well as through organizations such as the American Association for Accreditation of Laboratory Animal Care have generally resulted in improved treatment of laboratory animals. No study can be legally initiated without the prior approval of the detailed study design by an Institutional Animal Care and Use Committee (IACUC). Failure to adhere to animal welfare regulations or lack of appropriate IACUC oversight can result in severe consequences for a research facility and the acceptability of its studies for regulatory submission. In addition, animal welfare concerns have intensified research into ways to utilize fewer animals, such as using transgenic mice in short-term bioassays as well as alternative methods of testing such as in silico (computer based), in vitro (isolated cells or tissue portions), or in vivo testing in nonstandard species (The NICEATM-ICCVAM Five Year Plan, 2008). These advances are expected to lessen our dependence on the use of large numbers of laboratory animals in the future; indeed, the EPA has expressed an ambition to reduce in vivo testing to essentially zero in the next two decades (Wheeler, 2019). Toxicologic pathologists may be involved in the application and interpretation of alternative models of toxicity including cultured cells, microphysiologic systems ("organs on a chip"), organoids, and tissue slices (see *In Silico, In Vitro, Ex Vivo, and Non-Traditional In Vivo Approaches in Toxicologic Research*, Vol 1, Chap 24).

3. IN-LIFE EVALUATIONS

Toxicity studies in laboratory animals may vary from single-dose acute studies to both short- and long-term repeat-dose studies. Results from acute toxicity studies are generally used to estimate doses for short-term repeat-dose studies that may vary from one to 4 weeks in duration. Long-term repeat-dose studies that extend to 3 months are considered to be subchronic, and those that proceed from 6–12 months or more are regarded as chronic studies. Repeat-dose studies of 24-month duration in rodents are considered to inform on carcinogenicity risk as they largely span the lifetime of mice and rats (OECD Organisation for Economic Co-operation and Development, 2014; Committee for Proprietary Medicinal Products CPMP, 1999, Committee for Proprietary Medicinal Products CPMP, 2000; Wilson et al., 2008).

Prior to the initiation of any toxicity study, it is important to assess the health of every animal. Following any quarantine period necessitated by shipment from another facility, all animals should be subjected to a thorough health screening prior to study initiation. This assessment minimally must include a physical examination by trained veterinary staff and baseline total body weight measurement. Ophthalmologic examination, clinical pathology assessment, and pathogen screening are highly recommended. Any animal deemed to be unhealthy should be removed from the study; consequently, it is recommended to acquire at least 10% more animals than will be needed to fill the study groups. In addition, in rodent studies, a sentinel group of 5–10 animals of each sex should be established in the room along with the study animals to monitor for pathogens. Sentinel animal serum antibody titers for species-specific pathogens of concern should be measured at the initiation of the study and at the end of the in-life phase, and sometimes at interim time points for longer-term studies or experiments with immunocompromised animals. In the event of a suspected pathogen, sentinels may be used to measure antibody titers and/or euthanized for gross and histologic examination to assess for evidence of infection without disturbing the animals on study (see *Issues in Laboratory Animal Science that Impact Toxicologic Pathology*, Vol 1, Chap 29).

Upon arrival at a testing facility, each animal should receive a unique individual animal identification number that will be linked to the animal throughout its tenure at that facility. Additional alternate identification numbers may be assigned for use within a specific study, based on group number, sex, or similar parameters, with individual animal study-specific identification numbers assigned after the establishment of groups based on uniform body weight distribution. This unique animal number is used to identify all hematology and clinical chemistry samples, tissues, and all other data (e.g., body weight, organ weights, food consumption, clinical observations, etc.) collected and recorded from the animal during and following the in-life portion of the study. This number is permanently coupled with the animal to preclude misidentification of samples as well as to support the restoration of the study for peer review purposes or in the event of a quality assurance audit. There are a number of methods used to apply these unique animal identification numbers. The most up-to-date method, and one that is becoming virtually ubiquitous in modern laboratory animal facilities, is subcutaneous microchip implantation. This technique facilitates electronic recording of the animal identification numbers into a database for permanent storage, thus minimizing the potential for errors when hand-recording data. This method is well established with few notable side effects. Migration of the transponder microchip within the subcutis has been noted to occur, and there is some evidence to suggest that transponder-associated soft tissue sarcomas can develop in some species (e.g., rats and dogs), potentially complicating carcinogenicity study results unless the potential for this background neoplasm is taken into account during study design (Albrecht, 2010; Elcock et al., 2001; Greaves et al., 2013). Older identification methods used in rodents include toe clipping (a small portion of the toe is removed in a specified coded manner), ear punching (small holes in the ear are punched in a specified coded manner), ear tags, and tattooing (at the base of the tail or digits). Similar methods have been used in larger animals, such as tattooing (of the inner pinnae of the ear or the armpit), ear punching/clipping, or ear tags. These methods are currently much less accepted and may

require IACUC approval prior to implementation.

Following the allocation of unique individual identification numbers, all animals must be randomized into study groups. Proper randomization is essential to minimize bias and improve the recognition of statistical differences between groups in the study. Popular approaches to accomplishing this are through the use of random number tables or generators.

Several parameters are commonly measured and recorded throughout the in-life phase of a study. Each animal should be observed at least twice daily by laboratory animal staff for overt signs of toxicity, moribundity, and mortality. Ideally, observations should be made once in the morning with a subsequent surveillance in the evening. During these inspections, animals should be observed for changes in hair coat, posture, behavior, mobility, and activity. In the event of suspected toxicity, the animal should be removed from the cage for a more detailed physical examination. These examinations should record the date, approximate time, severity, and duration of observed changes in the skin, eyes, mucous membranes, and respiration. Marked changes in motor function, excretory function (e.g., increased or decreased urine output; changes in fecal color, consistency or amount), respiration, and moribundity should prompt an examination by a laboratory animal veterinarian. Severe signs of toxicity, such as profound ataxia, tremors, or seizures; respiratory distress; reduced body temperature; hemorrhage; severe weight loss (>10% compared to controls in 1 week for rodents or dogs or >6% for NHPs) (Chapman et al., 2013); or other signs of ongoing pain or distress, could lead to outcomes such as temporary cessation of treatment (i.e., a dosing holiday), removal of the animal from the study, or humane euthanasia. All clinical signs of toxicity should be uniformly recorded using a glossary of terms that are defined by an approved SOP. The terms should be simple and descriptive, using minimal medical or diagnostic terminology.

The body weight should be measured at least once a week for short-term studies. In chronic studies, body weight is generally measured weekly for the first 13 weeks and then monthly thereafter. A weekly measurement is recommended because rapid body weight loss is one of the most sensitive clinical indicators of a test article effect during the in-life phase of the study. It may reflect declining health and may be prodromal to death. Rapid body weight loss may be due to decreased feed and/or water consumption, disease, dental maladies, or specific toxic effects. Severe, rapid body weight loss can also prompt the removal of an animal from a study. Importantly, changes in body weight not related to test article treatment can impact the interpretation of organ weight data at the conclusion of a study.

Food consumption is another important parameter that should be measured regularly during the in-life phase of a study. In rodents, it is generally measured once per week during the entirety of subchronic studies and the first 3 months of chronic studies; food consumption may be measured less frequently after the first 3 months. The accurate measurement of food consumption is critical for studies in which the test article is administered in the diet given that amount of food consumed and the dietary concentration of the test material are used to calculate the dose of test article consumed by the animals on study. As mentioned above, the amount of food consumed may be an excellent indicator of animal health as reduced levels could indicate a test article effect. Reduced food consumption may also be the consequence of an unpalatable diet (possibly as a result of the addition of the test article) or poor dental health. Food consumption data should be correlated with body and organ weight data during study interpretation.

All animals should receive an ophthalmologic examination prior to study initiation, as well as at the completion of the dosing period (see *Eye*, Vol 3, Chap 10). These examinations should be performed by a trained veterinary ophthalmologist experienced in examination of the test species. Slit lamp examination and the use of an indirect ophthalmoscope are two commonly used methods. Animals are excluded from the study prior to initiation if retinal atrophy; corneal, retinal, or lens dysplasia; or other confounding ophthalmic findings are observed. This avoids possible confusion when having to determine whether ocular findings in the dosing phase are preexisting or potentially test article related in both the ophthalmologic examination and the pathology examination. The outcome of such ophthalmologic assessments typically

should be made available to the anatomic pathologist before eye sections are evaluated.

Hematology, clinical chemistry, and urinalysis are important clinical pathology data sets that inform on the general health of the test animal and are capable markers of test article effect (see *Clinical Pathology in Nonclinical Toxicity Testing*, Vol 1, Chap 10 and *Interpretation and Reporting of Clinical Pathology Results in Nonclinical Toxicity Testing*, Vol 2, Chap 14, for a detailed discussion of clinical pathology endpoints in toxicity testing) (Tomlinson et al., 2013). In addition to the routine clinical pathology endpoints used for safety monitoring, novel biomarkers of organ function and injury may be included (e.g., urinary biomarkers of renal tubular injury) as well as markers of drug PD and efficacy (see *Biomarkers: Discovery, Qualification and Application*, Vol 1, Chap 14). Study scientists should identify the clinical pathology parameters of interest prior to the beginning of the study and select the collection site that will provide the most consistent results, keeping in mind that sampling site selection may (1) affect future ability to evaluate those tissues clinically or microscopically or (2) limit collection of further clinical pathology samples as trauma associated with collection may obscure possible findings (Nemzek et al., 2001). In addition, the effect of serial blood sampling as well as the sample size that can be obtained for a given time interval should be considered. The recommended blood volume for nonterminal blood sampling is 55–70 mL/kg for all species, which limits the sample size for smaller species (Diehl et al., 2001). An important point to consider when planning blood collection (and the choice of plasma or serum) for clinical pathology analysis is that these samples should not be obtained after animals have been dosed in intravenous administration studies, in order to avoid sample dilution; after animals have been handled for behavioral or other physical manipulations that might stress the animals; or after they have been bled for PK measurements, as the prior bleedings will affect both hematology and clinical chemistry parameters. Additionally, collection of clinical pathology samples in animals given dosing holidays (skipped doses), that have had midstudy dose reductions, or that were added to treatment groups during the course of a study will generally limit the ability to interpret clinical pathology data generated from these animals, as it may well result in a lack of clear controls for the affected groups. Certainly, these manipulations are occasionally required to allow assessment of reversibility, toxicity, tolerability, or other parameters, but clinical pathology data assessment may be compromised as a result.

In rodent GLP toxicity studies, clinical pathology assessments are usually performed for 10 animals of each sex per group and should be performed for all animals in nonrodent toxicity studies. Clinical pathology measurements are recommended to be conducted at least once during the course of 2- to 6-week studies for nonrodent species (typically within 7 days of dosing initiation). For rodent and nonrodent subchronic and chronic studies,[1] clinical pathology parameters should be measured at the termination of the dosing phase. These endpoints may also be measured prior to study initiation or at interim stages (typically at 4 weeks in subchronic studies and 13 weeks in chronic studies) to evaluate the progression of test article effects. Clinical pathology measurements may also be conducted during and at the end of the recovery period, if included in the study.

4. NECROPSY

Necropsy is a pivotal process in any toxicity study as it is one of the few events that cannot be repeated, in contrast with blood collection, which can be redone. Tissues and samples that are not collected, are inadvertently damaged as a result of mishandling, or are improperly fixed can result in a permanent loss of data that variably impacts the interpretation of the study. Therefore, careful planning, detailed SOPs, and familiarity with the study protocol (including any amendments) in addition to a coordinated team approach utilizing well-trained necropsy technicians and pathologists are all necessary components for completion of a successful necropsy. While the study protocol takes precedence, institutional SOPs that standardize

practices (e.g., performing euthanasia, collecting and fixing tissues, obtaining organ weights, describing gross lesions, and trimming tissues) are necessary to ensure consistency and to eliminate variables that could subsequently complicate the interpretation of macroscopic observations, organ weight changes, and/or microscopic findings.

Necropsies can be conducted at scheduled intervals (i.e., predetermined interim time points or at the end of the dosing or recovery phases) or at unscheduled time points throughout the course of the study (i.e., when animals are found dead or humanely euthanized due to clinical signs or severe moribundity). Postmortem autolysis, the partial or complete destruction of cells or tissues following death due to self-produced enzymes, can result in a loss of cellular detail, thereby impairing histopathologic examination and interpretation. A study in neonatal Wistar rats determined that delays as short as 30 min can result in histological evidence of autolysis (Scheifele et at., 1987). Therefore, necropsies should be performed as quickly as possible following the death or euthanasia of an animal, preferably beginning within 5 min. Study animals found dead during nonoperational hours should be immediately refrigerated at 4°C (never frozen) until a necropsy can be performed as ice crystals that form during freezing destroy microscopic features of cells and tissues.

The initial steps to a productive necropsy will vary depending on the species, size of the study, and availability of well-trained necropsy technical support. In large studies that require multiple days to complete, the order of necropsy should be randomized among dose groups, as it minimizes the potential for systematic technical errors to mask or exacerbate test article–related effects by distributing procedure-related consequences across the groups (including controls). For example, if animals are euthanized sequentially (i.e., all control males on Day 1 of necropsy, followed by low-, mid-, and high-dose males on subsequent days), a technical error on any single day, such as improper calibration of a balance or misformulation of a fixative, could result in the loss of organ weight data or reduced tissue

---

[1]The authors differentiate *chronic* studies (6–12 months) from *carcinogenicity* studies (generally 24 months). The utility of measuring clinical pathology values at the termination of carcinogenicity studies is debatable and is not recommended as a standard procedure in current best practices (Young et al., 2011).

quality, respectively, for an entire group or inaccurate attribution of a test article effect to a group. In addition, randomization minimizes the effects of fasting on clinical pathology parameters, organ weights, and tissue architecture. For instance, the amount and distribution of hepatocellular glycogen can vary depending upon the length of the fasting, thereby affecting liver weights and histopathologic features of hepatocytes (Chatamra et al., 1984; Li et al., 2003; Rothacker et al., 1988); an artifactual dose–group relationship could result if the animals were not euthanized in random order. Though still preferred, randomization of necropsy order is less crucial in smaller studies as they can be completed in a short period of time.

Careful consideration must be given when deciding upon the appropriate method of euthanasia for a toxicity study. Several acceptable methods are available; however, the preferred method will vary depending upon the capability of the facility, the purpose of the study, and the species and age of the animal used (see *Issues in Laboratory Animal Science that Impact Toxicologic Pathology*, Vol 1, Chap 29). The method of euthanasia should adhere to the guidelines established in the American Veterinary Medical Association Guidelines on Euthanasia (AVMA, 2020) and the *Guide for Care and Use of Laboratory Animals* (National Research Council, 2011), with review and approval of the euthanasia method in the study protocol by the local IACUC. Regardless of the method chosen, it should seek to induce a loss of consciousness and rapid death with little to no pain, distress, or anxiety to the animal; be reliable; be easy to perform consistently with minimal risk of injury and/or emotional distress to the technician; and reduce the production of confounding tissue artifacts. It is essential that personnel are appropriately trained and able to perform the procedure in a professional, compassionate manner.

In general, inhalant (e.g., carbon dioxide) or noninhalant (e.g., sodium pentobarbital) chemicals are preferred to physical methods (e.g., cervical dislocation, decapitation). Carbon dioxide inhalation is the most commonly utilized technique for the euthanasia of small laboratory animals, while the preferred method for dogs, NHPs, and other small nonrodents (e.g., rabbits, Göttingen minipigs) is intravenous injection of a barbituric acid derivative, such as sodium pentobarbital.

Since gross and histopathologic parameters can be altered depending upon the method of euthanasia chosen, the study objectives must be taken into consideration when determining the appropriate method. For example, the use of barbiturates in dogs or Göttingen minipigs can result in variable degrees of splenic congestion which could affect interpretation of gross observations and organ weight data. Therefore, if the spleen is an organ of interest and/or test article–related effects are expected in blood-forming, blood-storing, and/or lymphoid organs, alternative methods of euthanasia may need to be considered during generation of the study protocol. In rodents, focal alveolar hemorrhage can occur in the lungs of animals euthanized via carbon dioxide asphyxiation; such regions need to be differentiated from genuine test article effects.

Following euthanasia, animals are commonly exsanguinated prior to necropsy. This not only serves as a secondary (insurance) method of euthanasia, but improves the microscopic quality of certain tissues, such as the liver and spleen, by removing most of the blood. Failure to exsanguinate can result in increased organ weights compared to historical ranges, while inconsistent exsanguination can result in variability in organ weights among animals, particularly in liver and kidney (Kanerva et al., 1982; Sullivan, 1985).

In order to minimize tissue artifacts associated with postmortem autolysis, dissection should begin within 5 min of euthanasia and ideally be completed within 20 min; larger nonrodent species may require the implementation of technical teams in order to meet this time frame. In addition to autolysis, prolonged postmortem intervals have been associated with increased relative and absolute liver organ weights and hepatocellular centrilobular vacuolization with delays of only 25 min (Li et al., 2003).

The goal of the necropsy is to create a detailed individual animal record that documents all essential findings of the event in a simple, concise, and unambiguous manner. The necropsy record must include the animal's unique individual animal number, time and date of death, method of euthanasia, body weight, organ weight data, macroscopic (gross) tissue findings, a checklist of the saved tissues, and signature lines for all personnel of the prosection team, which generally consists of a prosector, an assistant who weighs tissues, and a supervising pathologist; the "weigher" and pathologist may interact with multiple prosectors serially during a single necropsy session. It is important to thoroughly plan and communicate the duties of each member of the team well before the day of necropsy. Careful planning of the necropsy details can save time (and ultimately cost by eliminating the need to potentially rerun a study) and prevent the aggravation of inadequate supplies, missing specimens, or incorrectly preserved samples. A simple but often overlooked method of facilitating a smooth necropsy is to ensure that each member of the team reads and thoroughly understands the necropsy portion of the study protocol, prior to initiating the necropsy. Some institutions formally document this understanding by requiring delegated personnel to sign statements to this effect.

Each member of the prosection team will have a specific set of assigned duties that should be defined in the study laboratory's SOPs and best practices. A skilled prosector is responsible for the examination, removal, and trimming of the organs identified on the protocol-specified tissue list. In some instances, especially studies that involve larger nonrodent species, one or more "trimmers" may assist the prosector, either by dissecting a subset of tissues or by trimming organs prior to weighing. The "weigher" is responsible for ensuring that the weight of all protocol-specified organs is uniformly measured on a validated scale and in accordance with SOP guidelines; one weigher is often capable of recording organ weights from several prosection teams at the same time. A "recorder" may be required if the necropsy data are manually written. The recorder's task is to document all weights, as well as any other findings, such as macroscopic observations. Depending on the study design and the resources of the study laboratory, this role may be fulfilled by the trimmer or another individual on the necropsy team. While it is not a regulatory requirement that a pathologist be present at the necropsy, one should be available to provide expertise on the identification and nomenclature of gross findings, in addition to assisting with any other important aspects of the necropsy process. Although trained necropsy prosectors are capable of recognizing an abnormal tissue, they

are generally not trained in assessing its significance or selecting the appropriate descriptive terminology for a particular lesion or set of lesions. When there are several teams of prosectors working during a necropsy, it is the pathologist's responsibility to record the macroscopic findings from all animals. Ultimately, the pathologist must sign the necropsy record for each animal and is legally bound to the accuracy of its content.

It is crucial to assure that all protocol-required tissues, in addition to any gross lesions, are collected at necropsy. There are several ways to ensure that this occurs. The necropsy record should contain a list of all of the protocol-specified tissues. These tissues should be harvested in the same order for each animal. The use of a tissue collection template (typically a card with an area marked for all required tissues) under a sheet of plastic, a clear plastic tray with dividers, or an ice cube tray labeled for various tissues is recommended as it helps to ensure that all required tissues are collected from each animal. It is also recommended that two technicians be involved in placement of the tissues into their appropriate fixative. The first technician (a prosector or trimmer) verifies the tissues with the recorder (the second technician) as they are placed in their appropriate fixative one tissue at a time. The recorder subsequently checks off the tissue on the necropsy record as it is being placed in the proper fixative by the first technician. To prevent loss or misidentification during processing for histopathologic examination, small tissues may need to be placed in labeled cassettes. Flaccid organs and tissues, such as open segments of the gastrointestinal tract, skin, skeletal muscle, and nerve, should be placed on a dry piece of stiff white blotter paper or card stock to prevent curling. It is important to remember that collection of protocol-specified tissues typically includes the identification and retrieval of all macroscopic findings irrespective of the location of the finding (Bregman et al., 2003). During the necropsy process, it is crucial that the collected tissues do not dry out prior to their immersion in fixative. Drying can adversely affect the quality of tissue preservation and result in artifacts, such as shrinkage and fractures. To prevent this, tissues can be sprayed with isotonic saline (phosphate buffered or "physiologic" [0.9%

NaCl]) or gently covered with saline-soaked gauze while on the necropsy table or in the collection tray. It is critical that tap water not be used as its hypotonicity can result in the production of tissue artifacts, such as cell swelling (Taqi et al., 2018).

Prosectors must be appropriately trained in and experienced with proper tissue handling techniques to ensure that they understand how to correctly manipulate unfixed tissues during the collection process. Excessive manipulation of tissue, such as increased digital pressure; trauma caused by crushing, puncture, or squeezing of tissues with dissection instruments; or distortion due to pulling or stretching, can create artifacts that confound histopathologic examination. For example, markings caused by forceps can be seen in the liver, lung, and other parenchymatous organs, and nerve fiber deformation can be seen in nervous tissue such as brain, spinal cord, and sciatic nerve that have been aggressively pulled/stretched during removal (McLaurin, 1982).

Necropsy data can either be manually written or electronically recorded. While manual recording of data on a necropsy record is acceptable, it is fraught with potential challenges such as illegible characters, general uncleanliness (due to smudged ink or fixative spots), and an increased risk of missing or misplaced data. It is currently common practice to employ commercially available electronic pathology data management programs such as Provantis (Instem) or Pristima (Xybion). These programs possess specific modules that allow critical information, such as animal identification number, body and organ weights, and gross findings, to be recorded into an online database. When properly validated, these programs have features that help to prevent the loss of data by prompting the user to verify that all listed tissues and organ weights of interest have been recorded prior to proceeding to the necropsy of the next scheduled animal.

Documentation of gross findings is a critical stage in study evaluation. Generally, all gross abnormalities should be recorded. In some cases, normal physiological changes should be documented as well; an example of this is dilatation of the uterine horns in mice and rats during proestrus and estrus. Although this is a normal change, the degree may be affected by

compounds, such as endocrine modulators, and therefore should be recorded in order to determine if there is a test article–related effect. However, the recording of various gross findings is left to the discretion of the laboratory based upon their internal best practices. It is important that gross findings are described rather than merely diagnosed, as an official diagnosis requires microscopic examination. Gross descriptions should include the following: location/distribution, number, shape, size (as maximal or three dimensions), color, consistency, and any additional special features (e.g., presence of a capsule) that characterize the finding. While gross findings can be recorded manually, this may result in variations in descriptive terminology of comparable gross findings. Therefore, the use of commercial pathology data management programs allows for the advanced creation of a consistent and uniform glossary of descriptive terminology. For more information on pathology nomenclature, please consult *Nomenclature and Diagnostic Resources in Anatomic Toxicologic Pathology*, Vol 1, Chap 25).

Total body weight and select organs weights are routinely collected for scheduled necropsies from GLP-compliant toxicity studies, in addition to some other animal studies. Organ weights from found dead or dying (moribund) animals are typically not collected as they are considered of limited value given the absence of matched concurrent control data and differences in nutritional status, exsanguination, and tissue congestion and edema. The STP recommends that the brain, liver, kidneys, heart, adrenal glands, and testes be weighed in all repeat dose GLP toxicity studies of 7 days to 1-year duration; organ weights from acute, single-dose studies are considered of limited value and they are not recommended for carcinogenicity studies, including alternative mouse bioassays (Sellers et al., 2007). Additional organs, such as thyroid/parathyroid glands, ovaries, spleen, uterus, thymus, and lung, also may be included depending on the species, mechanism of action of the test article, and institutional preference. However, it is important to note that interpretation of data derived from these ancillary organs can be complicated due to residual blood (spleen, lung); age-related involution (thymus); hormone-related cyclical changes (ovaries, uterus); and difficult prosection (thyroid/

parathyroid glands in mice). In general, organ weights of reproductive tissues are most valuable in sexually mature animals due to the fact that variability in age, sexual maturity, and cycle stage can complicate or limit interpretation, especially in nonrodent species. While the STP recommends that the testes from all species be weighed in repeat dose general toxicity studies, weights for the epididymides and prostate are only recommended in rat studies; in nonrodent and mouse studies, weights can be considered on a case-by-case basis (Sellers et al., 2007). Organs should be weighed as soon as possible following removal from the test animal but should be trimmed free of fat and connective tissue first. Paired organs are often weighed together. For some organs, such as brain and thyroid/parathyroid glands, there is an advantage to waiting to weigh them until after they have been fixed as this can aid in minimizing the creation of handling artifacts that might confound the histopathologic evaluation. When weighing a given organ, the fixation status of that organ (fresh or fixed) should be consistent for all animals within the study.

Organ weight data must be normalized to facilitate proper interpretation. This is typically done by expressing absolute organ weight relative to either total body weight or brain weight. Normalized ("relative") organ weights eliminate the influence of normal variations in animal growth on organ weight data; however, these relative data have limitations that must be taken into account during analysis and interpretation. For example, body weight loss can impact body-to-organ weight ratios as it can result in an apparent false-positive test article effect on organ weights. Therefore, the body-to-organ weight approach is generally considered less reliable than comparing organ weight data to brain weight; brain weight remains relatively constant in mature, nonsenescent adult animals and is generally not affected by changes in body weight (Bailer et al., 2004). The brain must be collected similarly for all animals when normalizing organ weights to brain weight in rodent studies, by either always including or excluding intact olfactory bulbs, as the paired bulbs account for 6%–7% of the entire brain weight in common stocks and strains of these species (Bolon et al., 2013). When interpreting organ weight data, it is recommended to consider both absolute organ weights and organ weight ratios (organ weight: body weight and/or organ weight: brain weight). Whenever possible, an attempt should be made to correlate organ weight changes with histopathologic findings. However, dramatic changes in organ weight are often necessary before histomorphologic evidence is observed; subtle changes in organ weight are generally not associated with histopathologic changes. For example, in the liver, microscopic evidence of hepatocellular hypertrophy and/or increased liver enzymes often require liver weight increases of up to 20% relative to the controls before it can be appreciated (Amacher et al., 2006). Similarly, dose-related changes in kidney weight commonly occur without histopathological changes.

5. FIXATION AND HISTOLOGIC PROCEDURES

The preparation of tissues for microscopic examination begins the moment tissues are exposed to fixative. The appropriate fixative will depend upon the type of study, the endpoints to be examined, the major organs, and the preferred method of fixation (i.e., immersion, inflation, or perfusion). Proper fixation is perhaps the most critical aspect of ensuring high-quality tissue sections for histopathologic analysis.

Immersion is the most frequent technique used for routine toxicity studies. This method is favored because it is rapid, requires no specialized training, and necessitates minimal to no tissue preparation (e.g., slicing encapsulated solid organs or cracking large bones to expose the marrow cavity). Tissues are simply placed in the fixative solution.

Inflation is the preferred method of fixation for the lungs. It is also often used for hollow organs of rodents, such as the digestive tract and urinary bladder, to ensure that the delicate mucosal linings are fixed quickly. Inflation of these organs results in better fixation and prevents the formation of artifacts, such as atelectasis (collapse of the alveoli) in the lung or thickened epithelium in the empty urinary bladder, both of which could be difficult to differentiate from test article–related histopathologic changes. The ideal method to inflate the lungs is to infuse fixative at 20 mm water pressure and then submerge the trachea and lungs in fixative for 48 h; this procedure is more commonly utilized in larger nonrodent species, such as dogs and NHPs. In rodents and other smaller nonrodent species (e.g., rabbits), the lungs are more commonly inflated by inserting a 14- to 18-gauge blunt needle into the trachea, either with the lungs in situ or following removal of the "pluck" (which consists of the tongue, pharynx, larynx, esophagus, trachea, mainstem bronchi, and lung removed *en bloc*), and then slowly inflating the lungs (without measuring pressure) until their normal inspiratory volume is achieved (as indicated by full expansion of the organ). The amounts of fixative needed for rodents are approximately 1–2 mL for adult mice and 2–4 mL for adult rats. For either method in rodents, some facilities will ligate the trachea (approximately 0.5–1.0 cm cranial to the lung) following inflation to maintain the fixative within the expanded alveolar spaces; however, high-throughput necropsy laboratories may skip this step. The digestive tract typically is inflated by flushing from one cut end, and the urinary bladder is inflated through the urethra.

Perfusion is the preferred method for some special target organ toxicity studies, such as dedicated neurotoxicity studies where the brain and spinal cord are the primary focus of the necropsy. This method typically involves whole body intravascular infusion of fixative by placing a catheter in the left ventricle of the heart; a slit is then made in the right atrium to permit blood drainage (Bolon & Butt, 2014). It is important to note that weights of some organs (especially the spleen) may be affected by this technique. Some facilities limit such organ weight concerns by clamping the aorta just distal to the carotid arteries, thereby performing a head-only perfusion (Musigazi et al., 2018).

Unfortunately, a universal fixative that provides optimum fixation for all tissues and procedures does not exist. For most routine animal studies, aldehyde-based cross-linking fixatives like neutral buffered 10% formalin (NBF) will be the fixative of choice. NBF is widely available, economical, and provides good general fixation for most organs. Exceptions include the eyes and testes, which have a thick outer wall/capsule that requires immersion in a fixative that achieves deeper penetration, such as Davidson's solution, modified Davidson's solution, or Bouin's solution (Latendresse et al., 2002); while Zenker's fixative also provides deeper penetration than NBF, it is infrequently used since it contains toxic components (mercuric chloride and potassium dichromate) that make disposal difficult and expensive. In addition to immersion, NBF is also typically the fixative of choice for inflation of lungs and hollow organs. However, whole body perfusion for evaluation of the central nervous system commonly utilizes methanol-free 4% formaldehyde (often called 4% paraformaldehyde [PFA]) because the methanol included in commercially available NBF formulations as a stabilizing agent can extract lipids from the parenchyma of the brain and spinal cord, inducing artifactual vacuolation in the white matter of these tissues. Mixtures of PFA and glutaraldehyde (e.g., Karnovsky's and Trump's fixatives) are also used for whole body perfusion, especially where tissue collection for electron microscopy is a primary study endpoint, as the PFA provides quick penetration and fixation, while the glutaraldehyde provides better molecular cross-linking and ultrastructural preservation (McDowell and Trump, 1976). Coagulating fixatives (e.g., alcohols, acetone) are seldom used for animal toxicity studies although they may be employed for special purposes, such as preserving tissue without destroying delicate molecules that will be detected by *in situ* molecular pathology procedures (e.g., IHC).

NBF can be purchased premixed or made in the laboratory from concentrated formaldehyde. The latter requires that the correct percentage of formaldehyde and buffers be used in order to ensure proper tissue fixation (Luna, 1992). The relatively low cost, safety, and convenience of premixed NBF makes it preferable for high-throughput necropsy facilities. It is worth noting that a small amount of eosin is added by some laboratories to provide a small amount of color in the solution, thereby ensuring that tissues are not inadvertently placed in water.

To allow for adequate fixation of immersed tissues, tissues need to be trimmed to ≤1/2 cm in thickness and placed in a vessel that contains at least a 10:1 ratio of fixative to tissue. It is good practice to change the NBF after 24–48 h, especially if there is a large amount of tissue or substantial blood release in the container, as this ensures adequate penetration of fixative into the tissue. Tissues that are going to be examined on a transmission electron microscope (TEM) need to be trimmed into small cubes that are no more than $1 \, mm^3$ and then quickly fixed in a solution containing glutaraldehyde (Carson, 1997); in practice, fast fixation is often done by mincing tissues in a few drops of fixative. There are a number of formulations for TEM fixatives, some of which (e.g., Karnovsky's fixative) produce acceptable results for light microscopy as well. With the increasing demand for IHC, the length of time a tissue spends in fixative has become extremely important as prolonged exposure to NBF or other aldehydes results in extensive cross-linking of S-bonds. This cross-linking can result in decreased penetration of the immunoprobes and thus reduced sensitivity of the IHC procedures. For this reason, if IHC is anticipated, it is recommended that tissues be transferred from formalin to 70% ethanol within 48 h of necropsy and/or be trimmed and embedded as quickly as possible following necropsy (Carson, 1997). It is important to note that lipid-rich tissues like brain and spinal cord should not be left for extended periods of time in 70% ethanol since the alcohol can widely produce artifactual vacuoles throughout white matter tracts (Luna, 1992). Therefore, it is important that these tissues not be left in alcohol baths on automated tissue processors over the weekend.

Although NBF is relatively stable and has a long shelf life, certain situations can cause fixative degradation. One such example is freezing. This can occur during the winter months if NBF is shipped in unheated trucks or left for extended periods of time on loading docks. Freezing causes the formaldehyde within the solution to crystallize and precipitate out, resulting in a diluted solution. Subsequent use of the unknowingly diluted solution can result in inadequate fixation. A related problem includes the shipment of fixed tissues in times of weather extremes. Tissues can either end up freezing in the winter or baking in summer. Therefore, prior to shipping irreplaceable specimens to a distant location, one should always consider the upcoming weather and conduct detailed communication and planning between the labs.

Although overnight courier services have improved their shipping options, the unpredictability of nature can occasionally stymie someone's best efforts. With increasing regulations for transporting hazardous materials, it may become more difficult to ship fixed tissues by air. This could result in longer transit times as well as extra paperwork (especially if crossing national borders) and more complex coordination between institutions. Some shippers have also implemented strict regulations with regard to shipments that contain fixatives or fixed tissues. These regulations can include what types of container are acceptable and whether secondary containment (e.g., bagging) and/or spill control measures (e.g., adsorbent padding) are necessary. Therefore, it is critical that the specific requirements of the shipper be met prior to sending samples to a distant laboratory. Some contract laboratories provide a courier service for tissue pickup. This method is beneficial in that it provides control (and documentation) of temperature and time in transit and allows for a strict chain of custody for all materials. It is generally not advisable to ship fixed specimens over the weekend as environmental storage conditions at the shipping and receiving docks may not be suitable and could inadvertently result in the materials being damaged or misplaced.

Fixed tissues must be further processed to permit embedding, a process which is necessary to stabilize cell and tissue structure. This step is typically undertaken using a series of graded alcohols (starting at 50% or 70% and then increasing gradually to 100%) followed by organic solvents (e.g., toluene or xylene) to gradually remove water from the fixed tissue. The sections then are infiltrated with an embedding medium that is miscible with the solvents, most often paraffin wax for general toxicity studies. These steps are generally performed on automated processors in modern histology laboratories. A generic tissue processing scheme can be used for most animal tissues; however, for some tissues (e.g., brain, nerve, and skin), the number and length of the various steps may need to be adjusted to produce better sections (Fortin et al., 2020; Suvarna, Layton, & Bancroft, 2019). Once the infiltrated tissues have been embedded in the appropriate medium, they are mounted on a microtome for sectioning. For general toxicity studies, paraffin-embedded tissues are usually cut at thicknesses ranging from 4 to 8 μm. Use of plastic embedding media (soft [glycol methacrylate] or hard [epoxy resin]) permits acquisition of thinner sections (1–2 μm) but requires special microtomy equipment to cut the harder material.

Once the tissues have reached the histology laboratory for processing, there are several potential areas where problems can arise. Therefore, it is critical that efforts be put into place to minimize the possible introduction of artifactual changes. It should be the primary goal of the laboratory to produce consistent sections from organ to organ, animal to animal, and group to group within a study, and ideally across studies over time. Control of techniques and processes in the histology laboratory are essential to produce tissue sections that are consistent and of high quality. This can be achieved by proper training of the histotechnicians and detailed documentation of the histology laboratory's practices and procedures in the laboratory's SOPs.

It is also critical to have quality control measures in place that verify that all required tissues and gross lesions are present, and that the quality of the tissues and resulting sections are adequate. It is important to attempt to eliminate any introduction of group-based (systematic) bias. Many laboratories process tissues in group order, as this can make documentation easier; however, this approach can create a false treatment-related effect should a processing artifact occur that affects only one group. A solution to this is "counterbalancing," which involves processing the animals in either replicate order (i.e., process one animal from each group before moving to the second animal of any group) or in random order to ensure that each processing run includes one or more animals from each treatment group.

Another potential area where tissues can be improperly prepared for examination is during the embedding process. This step is when tissues are infiltrated with paraffin wax and then placed into blocks of wax to facilitate sectioning. It is important that cassettes contain tissues of similar firmness. Placing bone (firm) and lung (soft) in the same cassette could cause the microtome knife to "hesitate" during sectioning. This would produce force-induced artifacts, such as chatter marks, due to the differences in the tissue composition and density. In addition, cassettes should not be stuffed with tissue since the lids of overfilled cassettes will impress a grid-like pattern of grooves onto the surface of soft organs (e.g., brain, liver, and lung) that distorts structures in the final tissue sections.

Additional problem areas in the histology laboratory can be traced to faulty equipment (e.g., inaccurate temperature or vacuum control) or a lack of training by the operators. For example, if tissue blocks are not properly chilled and rehydrated before they are sectioned, the resulting tissue ribbons can stretch or tear, resulting in artifactual fracturing of the sections. Artifacts (e.g., staining precipitation over sections, use of expired reagents) can also occur during the staining process (Chlipala et al., 2020). A comprehensive consideration of histological processing and procedures is beyond the scope of this book, but further details may be found in other reference texts (Coolidge & Howard, 1979; Suvarna, Layton, & Bancroft, 2019).

6. SPECIALIZED HISTOLOGIC TECHNIQUES

There are several tissues that require specific expertise in processing to ensure that high-quality sections are obtained for microscopic evaluation. Examples of these tissues include bone, brain, eye, lung, larynx, nasal cavity, thyroid, and urinary bladder. (For more information on specialized techniques for tissue collection and preparation, see the organ-specific chapters in Volumes 3 and 4.)

Trimming and embedding methods for the lungs depend not only on the species but also the type of study (e.g., inhalation vs. oral gavage). For rats and mice, the technique for proper trimming and embedding of the lung has been described (Kittle et al., 2004). In general, inhalation studies often demand a more thorough evaluation of the respiratory tract; therefore, it is pertinent that all levels of the tracheobronchial tree (tracheal bifurcation, mainstem bronchi, bronchioles, alveolar ducts, and alveoli), in addition to the interstitial tissue, vasculature, and pleura, be adequately represented in tissue sections. In mice, lung lobes are often submitted *in toto* in one cassette, whereas in rats, the right and left lung lobes are separated at the level of the tracheal bifurcation and placed whole into two separate cassettes. Alternatively, horizontal sections may be taken through each of the five rat lung lobes (one left, four right) and embedded separately. In larger animals in which the lung lobes are too large to submit whole, representative samples of specific lung lobes, as clearly defined in the study protocol or facility SOPs, are embedded and trimmed.

Although the larynx and nasal cavity are not routinely included as protocol-required tissues for most studies, they are often included in inhalation studies. Since certain regions of the larynx, such as the ventral diverticulum (pouch), the epithelium overlying the ventral submucosal glands at the base of the epiglottis, and the tip of the arytenoid cartilages, are the most sensitive to inhaled toxicants, it is critical that the larynx be embedded in such a manner to allow for consistent histologic examination of these particular areas. The technique for proper trimming and embedding of the larynx has been described (Lewis, 1992; Renne et al., 1992; Sargartz et al., 1992). Similarly, the tissues of the nasal cavity require special trimming and embedding in order to produce consistent sections. The nasal cavity is a complex tissue with multiple anatomic regions of interest, lined by four different types of epithelium: squamous, respiratory, transitional, and olfactory. Each epithelial type has a specific species-dependent distribution and differential susceptibility to various classes of toxicants. Therefore, sections must be consistently trimmed and embedded, to accurately assess common changes, such as epithelial metaplasia. Multiple schemes for trimming nasal sections of rodents have been described (Mery et al., 1994; Uriah and Maronpot, 1990; Young, 1981).

The orientation of some tissues, such as the thyroid glands in rodents and the urinary bladder in mice, can affect histologic interpretation. The thyroid glands can be embedded either longitudinally or in cross-section. Longitudinal sections are typically taken when the glands are separated from adjacent tissues for weighing, whereas cross-sections are taken *in situ* to simultaneously include cross-sections of the esophagus and trachea. Since C-cells exhibit a greater prominence near the center of the thyroid gland, the incidence of proliferative changes involving C-cells in a longitudinal section could appear to be greater than would be appreciated in a cross-section that was taken off the midline. This tissue-specific variation in cell distribution can affect study results, especially if different embedding orientations are used for different phases in the study (i.e., interim and terminal necropsies). In mice, the orientation of the urinary bladder can also have an effect on histopathologic interpretation. For many years, the routine section of urinary bladder was a cross-section, taken through the middle portion of the bladder. A unique lesion, submucosal mesenchymal proliferation of the urinary bladder of aging mice, has been described in several strains (Halliwell, 1998). Since this lesion invariably occurs in the trigone region of the bladder, smaller lesions that are not easily observed grossly may be missed if a midorgan cross-section is taken. For this reason, many laboratories have modified their SOPs so that a longitudinal section of mouse urinary bladder, to include the area of the trigone, is collected.

Specialized knowledge is also required during trimming and embedding of nervous tissue, especially the brain due to its considerable anatomic variation in three dimensions over short distances. In general, coronal (i.e., transverse) brain sections (in rodents) or hemisections (in larger animals) are preferred, for two main reasons. In rodents, complete coronal sections allow for assessment of whether findings are unilateral or bilateral, symmetrical or asymmetrical. More importantly, for all species, the various neuroanatomic atlases used by pathologists to identify distinct brain domains predominantly show images in the coronal orientation (for representative examples, refer to following atlases for the rat, dog, and NHP, respectively: Paxinos & Watson, 2007; Palazzi, 2011; Paxinos, Petrides, Huang, & Toga, 2008). At a minimum, three sections of the rodent brain are typically evaluated for routine studies: one at the level of the optic chiasm; one at the level of the hippocampus; and one at the level of the cerebellum and brain stem (medulla oblongata). However, current National Toxicology Program (NTP) and STP recommendations suggest evaluating six to seven coronal sections (Rao, Little, Malarkey, Herbert, & Sills, 2011, Rao, Little, & Sills, 2014; Bolon, Garman, Jensen, Krinke, & Stuart,

2006, 2013), and this strategy is now a common request to sponsors from regulatory agencies. In addition, dedicated neurotoxicity studies are best conducted with additional sections depending upon the compound, expected site(s) of toxicity, and/or observations of clinical signs or behavioral changes. Several such expanded trimming and embedding schemes have been described (Garman, 2003; Pardo et at., 2012; Bolon, 2018). Paraffin embedding is typically sufficient for the central nervous system (Bolon et al., 2013), but some regulatory agencies require hard plastic (resin) embedding for at least one nerve cross-section (reviewed in Bolon et al., 2018).

In many instances, especially during sectioning of the larynx, nasal cavity, and brain, the ability of tissue trimmers and histotechnicians to identify defined external and internal anatomic landmarks is crucial to obtaining equivalent sections among animals in all groups. Therefore, training programs must be in place to ensure that histotechnicians are proficient at identifying these established landmarks.

Bone and teeth typically require decalcification (the process of removing calcium salts) prior to sectioning. Rib or sternum is recommended for nonrodents, while distal femur (with an articulating surface) and sternum are recommended for rodents (Bregman et al., 2003). It should be noted that undecalcified specimens can be sectioned, but special equipment, procedures, and embedding media (e.g., plastic) are needed. Numerous decalcifying methods and commercially available solutions (e.g., Formical, Decal, or Immunocal) are available (Fossey et al., 2016). Selection of a decalcifying solution is predominantly influenced by balancing the desired speed of processing with the need for preservation of antigenic epitopes. Solutions with chelating agents (e.g., EDTA [ethylenediaminetetraacetic acid]) decalcify at a slower speed but elicit less disruption of delicate antigens compared to acid solutions; combinations of acids and chelators (e.g., Formical) represent a reasonable compromise between increased processing speed and molecular preservation. It is important to note that poor hematoxylin and eosin (H&E) staining quality is not related to the speed of decalcification but rather to the length of time the tissue remains in decalcifying solution following complete decalcification. For example, overexposure of specimens to an acid decalcifying solution results in reduced staining quality by 10% for every 2 additional hours the tissue remains in the solution (Luna, 1992).

Prior to decalcification, specimens are collected at necropsy, trimmed free of attached soft tissues (e.g., skeletal muscle, tendons, ligaments, skin), and initially fixed in NBF for one to several days, depending upon the species and specimen collected. After immersion in the decalcification solution, the specimens should be transferred to fresh demineralizing solution every 24–48 h until the completely decalcified bone can be easily cut with a sharp blade; failure to completely decalcify a specimen can result in torn, incomplete sections and damage to the microtome blade. Once the tissues are decalcified, they are rinsed in running water, embedded in paraffin, sectioned at 4–8 µm, and stained. For most routine toxicity studies, H&E is generally used as the main or only stain for bone. However, some specialized investigations may require special stains (e.g., von Kossa or Goldner's trichrome when alterations of bone mineralization are suspected, *in vivo* fluorochrome labeling for histomorphometric assessment of bone formation rates, toluidine blue or safranin O/fast green to assess matrix integrity of articular cartilage) or IHC (e.g., anti-cathepsin K or anti-von Willebrand factor) (Fossey et al., 2016).

7. HISTOPATHOLOGIC EVALUATION

Once the tissues have been processed and sections have been prepared and stained, the next phase is microscopic examination and subsequent interpretation of the results. Evaluation and interpretation are both critically important steps in the safety assessment of a test article and, thus, should be performed by a well-trained, experienced pathologist who is knowledgeable with respect to the test species. There are several facets of microscopic analysis that influence the success of this phase. In order to identify and define the fundamental elements of the histopathologic examination and the appropriate techniques needed to minimize observational bias, best practice recommendations for toxicologic histopathology have been published by the STP (Crissman et al., 2004; Schafer et al., 2018).

Prior to microscopic review, the study pathologist should review the protocol in addition to all relevant data derived from the in-life phase of the study. Clinical observations, gross findings, clinical chemistry, hematology, and urinalysis as well as body and organ weight data should be carefully examined for the presence of any potential test article–related effects. Review of these data will provide insight to the pathologist with respect to potential target organs and aid in the identification of test article–related lesions during the microscopic evaluation.

The study protocol includes a list of the tissues that are to be reviewed by standard bright-field microscopy. Additional lists may be included if other modalities (e.g., IHC, TEM) are to be employed. Regardless of species, all protocol-required tissues, including macroscopic observations, are typically reviewed with standard bright-field microscopy from all animals that were found dead or were euthanized in moribund condition during the course of the study. Studies involving dogs and NHPs typically include examination of all protocol-required tissues from all animals in all dose groups. In contrast, rodent studies typically only require an initial review of high-dose and control group animals, with only select organs (e.g., target organs identified in the high-dose animals and macroscopic observations) being reviewed in the lower-dose animals. Since target organs are typically not identified until completion of the initial review, it is highly recommended that all tissues from all dose groups be processed to paraffin blocks at the same time as the control and high-dose groups as this expedites subsequent sectioning and staining of tissues identified as target organs in the lower-dose groups. Some institutions process all tissues from animals in all groups to slides to further speed any later need to assess sections from lower-dose groups and also as a means of avoiding tinctorial shifts in staining intensity that could preclude a coded ("blinded") evaluation of target tissues. The objectives for reviewing the target organs in the lower-dose groups are to confirm whether or not subtle changes are actually related to test article exposure and to identify the NOAEL and/or NOEL.

The order in which slides and/or dose groups are examined is a matter of preference for the individual study pathologist. The approach may be guided by study design (i.e., are there multiple control or high dose groups); previous knowledge of the test article (e.g., mechanism of action or results from previous studies that involved the same test article or compounds with a similar mechanism of action); or results from the current study (e.g., clinical observations, early deaths, or changes in organ weight, body weight, or clinical pathology parameters).

Pathologists often evaluate slides from the control groups first, as this allows the pathologist to determine the range and extent of background changes. Some pathologists will examine all animals in the control group before moving to the high-dose group, whereas others may opt to review only a portion of the control animals followed by several (but not all) of the high-dose animals. With the latter approach, the pathologist typically moves back and forth between the control and high-dose animals until all required tissues from the cohorts have been examined. This approach not only allows the study pathologist to maintain the boundaries of "normal" throughout the microscopic examination, thus enhancing the likelihood of detecting subtle test article effects, but also aids in minimizing "diagnostic drift" (i.e., shifts in diagnostic terminology that can occur over time, especially during longer studies).

The pathologist may opt to review all tissues from an animal before moving on to the next animal as it enables him/her to obtain an encompassing overview of the animal's health and appreciate any pathologic processes that may be affecting multiple organ systems. This method is particularly useful in long-term (i.e., carcinogenicity) studies where comorbidities are common. Conversely, if test article effect(s) and/or target organ(s) are known prior to reviewing the slides, the study pathologist may find it beneficial to initially examine the affected target organ(s) from control and treated animals separately from the remaining tissues, which can be reviewed following the initial investigation of the affected tissues. This approach aids in consistent application of severity grading schemes across dose groups and detection of subtle test article–related effects. The study pathologist should be responsible for choosing the slide evaluation strategy that best suits the circumstances.

7.1. Cause of Death

Identifying the cause of death (COD) for individual animals that are found dead and/or euthanized in moribund condition during the course of a toxicity or carcinogenicity study is necessary to comprehensively interpret results from the study. However, there is significant controversy among toxicologic pathologists as to whether the COD in such studies can accurately be determined. The STP addressed this concern by stating the following: "Identification of the cause of death in individual animals (not to be confused with classification of neoplasms as Fatal or Incidental) adds significant value to the interpretation of carcinogenicity studies. Causes of death may include neoplasm, cardiomyopathy, chronic renal disease, trauma, and infectious conditions. Whenever possible, pathologists should identify cause of death for animals dying or euthanized before scheduled necropsy as a means to interpret causes of differential mortality and comorbidities among groups" (Long, 2004).

Furthermore, the STP has formulated recommendations to guide the determination of COD in toxicity and carcinogenicity studies. In summary, these recommendations include the following:

(1) The pathologist is responsible for identifying the COD and/or morbidity in animals that die or are euthanized prior to scheduled necropsy in toxicology studies, including carcinogenicity studies. The assignment of COD is an interpretive diagnosis.

(2) The pathologist should have and use all available information (e.g., hematology, clinical chemistry, body weight, clinical observations, and gross and microscopic findings) for each animal to determine the COD.

(3) The COD should be identified for individual animals based on the primary (most severe) disease process leading to morbidity or mortality in that animal. The definition of COD used by the World Health Organization in its guidelines for mortality and morbidity coding (WHO, 1993) is applicable: "the disease or injury which initiated the train of morbid events leading directly to death, or the circumstances of accident or violence which produced the fatal injury." The COD may not be the proximate (final) event leading to death but should be the overall process that leads to the proximate cause. If

there are multiple potential CODs, the pathologist should decide which process(es) most likely led to mortality. More than one COD may be designated if the pathologist feels that each cause contributed significantly to morbidity or mortality.

(4) The pathologist should determine whether overall mortality, and any differences in mortality among groups, is the result of test article administration. The pathology interpretation should include a clear statement regarding whether mortality in the test animals was related to test article exposure.

(5) If the COD cannot be determined, this should be stated as "COD undetermined" or "COD not determined from the available information."

(6) A high incidence of deaths with undetermined cause during a toxicity study should prompt an early critical review of the data to discriminate potential test article effects from other possible contributing factors (e.g., husbandry or technical errors).

7.2. Nomenclature

Many of the practices involved in the proper microscopic evaluation of a regulatory toxicity study vary from the typical anatomic pathologist's initial diagnostic training and experiences (Bolon et al., 2010; American College of Veterinary Pathologists ACVP, 2020) Typically, a diagnostic pathologist is mandated to describe and diagnose lesions as individual findings (regardless of the primary pathologic process) and has the liberty to use a broad range of morphologic terms to describe a lesion or disease process. However, given that histopathologic data from toxicity studies are typically reviewed by regulatory scientists who are not trained in pathology, it is considered best practice to use consistent diagnostic terms that are generally accepted. Global initiatives such as the INHAND (International Harmonization of Nomenclature and Diagnostic Criteria) project undertaken by the global toxicologic pathology community have helped to standardize diagnostic nomenclature and criteria for laboratory animals (see *Nomenclature and Diagnostic Resources in Anatomic Toxicologic Pathology*, Vol 1, Chap 25). The goal of the

INHAND project is to produce publications for each organ system that provide a uniform descriptive nomenclature for classifying microscopic lesions observed in laboratory animals of multiple species during nonclinical studies. These INHAND terms now form the foundation for the approved set of diagnostic descriptors required by some regulatory agencies (e.g., the SEND [Standard for Exchange of Nonclinical Data] initiative of the FDA).

It is important for the pathologist to use consistent diagnostic terminology and severity grades across all animals in a group, all groups in a phase, and all phases within a study (Schafer et al., 2018). Variation in the application of diagnostic terminology and/or criteria over time is referred to as "diagnostic drift." Such drift is a major problem for toxicologic pathologists, and it can negatively impact the interpretation of study data, especially in chronic toxicity and carcinogenicity studies that can involve large numbers of animals ($\geq$400) and take several months (~6) to evaluate. One approach to minimizing diagnostic drift is to establish a "diagnostic dictionary" that lists common terms and morphologic criteria established by the pathologist during the early phases of histopathologic evaluation of a study; many institutions have had their pathologist team generate a common dictionary for use in all toxicity studies. At the end of a study, this dictionary can then be reviewed to identify any duplications, inappropriate terminology, and/or terminology that is inconsistent with previous studies with the same/similar test articles(s); key terms may be extracted from the dictionary and added to the pathology report as a glossary to provide additional clarity for regulatory reviewers. In addition, the pathologist should review the important target organs/histologic findings from any early death animals as these animals could have been reviewed quite some time ago. Having a peer review conducted on the study is an additional approach to reduce diagnostic drift; this is just one of many beneficial reasons to consider peer reviews of toxicity and carcinogenicity studies (see *Pathology Peer Review*, Vol 1, Chap 26 and *Practices to Optimize Generation, Interpretation, and Reporting of Pathology Data from Toxicity Studies*, Vol 1, Chap 28).

Unlike diagnostic pathology (which typically uses interpretive diagnoses), toxicologic pathologists are encouraged to use descriptive diagnostic terms. Such descriptive terms enable microscopic findings to be recorded in a consistent, objective manner that can be easily tabulated and allows for comparison between dose groups. The use of interpretive diagnoses could falsely lead to implication of a particular pathogenesis or impact on the function of an organ based on what is known about the spontaneous disease (Mann et al., 2012). As a consequence, toxicologic pathology diagnoses typically identify the organ first (e.g., liver, skin), followed by the subsite, if applicable, and then the major pathologic process (e.g., hypertrophy, necrosis, inflammation). Additional qualifiers that specify distribution (e.g., focal, multifocal, diffuse); duration (e.g., acute, subchronic, chronic); and/or character (e.g., hemorrhagic, granulomatous) of the histopathologic finding can be added as necessary to provide clarity. As an example, chronic inflammation of the liver would be recorded as "liver – inflammation, chronic" in toxicologic pathology data sets as opposed to "chronic hepatitis," which is typically used in the diagnostic pathology setting. When appropriate, similar histomorphologic changes or multiple changes that represent components of a single pathologic process should be combined under one diagnostic term that captures the primary pathologic process. This approach yields more consistent data that are amenable to statistical analysis and, therefore, provides clarity for study interpretation. For example, multiple lesions recorded separately as "liver – inflammation, chronic"; "liver – inflammation, chronic active"; and liver – inflammation, suppurative" may be part of an inflammatory continuum that would be best captured under a single diagnosis of "liver – inflammation." Recording these lesions separately dilutes the incidence of an overarching inflammatory process, which could mask a possible test article effect.

Since diagnostic qualifiers can add accuracy and deeper identification of a specific site/subsite within an organ, in some instances, they warrant inclusion in the morphologic diagnosis. An excellent example of this is hepatocellular hypertrophy. If the hypertrophy is the result of suspected or confirmed induction of cytochrome P450 enzymes following exposure to a test article, the finding should be recorded as "liver, centrilobular – hypertrophy," as opposed to "liver – hypertrophy." The reason for the more specific localization is that it more accurately describes the observed histopathologic change and also provides mechanistic insight regarding the primary pathologic process. While other qualifiers are sometimes necessary, they should only be used by the study pathologist if it is absolutely necessary to distinguish distinctly separate processes or pathologic events. For example, the separate diagnoses of "liver – necrosis, coagulative" and "liver – necrosis, suppurative" may be acceptable as it is apparent that they are manifestations of two distinct processes. However, the separate categorization of "liver – necrosis, coagulative, focal" and "liver – necrosis, coagulative, multifocal" is unwarranted because the separate diagnoses for the variable lesion distribution dilute the incidence of the primary process of coagulative necrosis.

The pathologist is often required to determine the value of diagnosing secondary lesions. For example, focal compression of the brain is a common secondary manifestation of large pituitary adenomas in rats. This expected tissue displacement generally does not necessitate an additional diagnosis. However, mineralization secondary to severe nephropathy may justifiably add value to the study's data and deserves a distinct diagnosis since it may indicate either primary or secondary parathyroid involvement.

Furthermore, the duration and intent of the study will impact the toxicologic pathologist's diagnostic strategy. The objectives of short-term studies are to identify possible toxic test article effects at elevated dose or exposure levels and determine the appropriate dose or exposure levels for the succeeding longer-term studies. Therefore, in short-term studies ($\leq$3 months), it is essential to document and quantify discrete histomorphologic changes regardless of the underlying pathologic process. This is dissimilar to the diagnostic approach usually employed for chronic studies ($\geq$6 months), which usually require the combination of component histomorphologic changes within the diagnosis of the primary pathologic process. For instance, the pathologist evaluating sections of the kidney from a 3-month rat study may reasonably diagnose "kidney – infiltrate, mononuclear cell";

"kidney – basophilia, tubule"; and "kidney – casts, hyaline" as separate entities. However, in a chronic study, it is preferred to aggregate these linked components within the composite diagnosis of "kidney – nephropathy, chronic progressive" as the primary lesion. Given the large number of animals and tissues reviewed in a chronic study, it would be inefficient and confusing (especially in the data tables) to separately categorize these components.

7.3. Severity Grading

In order to convert histopathologic findings from nominal data ("Is a change present or not?") into ordinal data that can be statistically analyzed, a severity grade must be assigned. Severity grades are measures that take into account a combination of the extent (prevalence of subordinate components), distribution (e.g., focal, multifocal, diffuse), and actual degree (severity) of the process. A five-level scale ("normal" plus four levels of lesion severity) is generally acceptable for regulatory toxicity studies; however, some pathologists and organizations prefer the use of a six-level scale ("normal" plus five levels of lesion severity). The five-level scale assigns lesion severity designations of minimal, mild, moderate, and marked with the numerical correlates of +1, +2, +3, and +4, respectively. With the six-level scale, "severe" is added as an additional severity grade and is assigned a numerical correlate of +5. Regardless, the chosen scale should be clearly documented in the study protocol and pathology report. While severity grades are assigned to many histopathologic findings, severity grading is inappropriate for some common findings, such as liver foci, fractures, foreign bodies, developmental malformations, parasites, cysts, and neoplasms. These types of findings are generally not graded and instead simply recorded as "Present."

In some instances, it is appropriate to document the specific criteria used when grading a particular lesion. An excellent illustration of this would be skin paint studies which often require that the study pathologist outline their standards for grading such changes as hyperkeratosis, epidermal hyperplasia (acanthosis), and melanocyte hyperplasia. An example of a scale for grading the severity of epidermal hyperplasia (acanthosis) might be the following:

Normal – epidermis ranges from one to two cell layers thick.

Minimal – epidermis ranges from three to four cell layers thick.

Mild – epidermis ranges from five to six cell layers thick.

Moderate – epidermis is greater than six cell layers thick but lacks rete peg formation.

Marked – epidermis is greater than six cell layers thick with the presence of rete peg formation.

8. ARTIFACTS VERSUS LESIONS

There are a number of changes or findings that can occur during tissue collection/processing that may initially appear to be treatment-related histopathologic changes but are actually tissue artifacts. Familiarity with these changes can help the pathologist separate genuine effects from artifact. These artifacts typically fall into one of three major classes: fixation or handling artifacts, processing artifacts, and sectioning artifacts. Several examples were mentioned previously; additional examples are discussed below.

Although it is well known that animal tissues should only be refrigerated prior to necropsy and fixation, occasionally tissues are frozen. This occurs either due to a procedural error or due to unacceptable/unexpected environmental conditions during shipping. Since animal tissues are largely water, ice crystals form when the tissues are frozen. These crystals cause major disruption to the cells and tissues that will appear microscopically as large empty spaces where the ice crystals once resided. Similarly, if the fixative used to preserve the tissue was either chilled or frozen, evidence of fixative crystals may appear in the resultant slides (Fig. 9.1).

Centrilobular hepatocellular vacuolation can occur following a prolonged interval between euthanasia/death and prosection. This is an artifact that is believed to be associated with the leakage of serum from the central vein into the adjacent hepatocytes (Li et al., 2003). This change is microscopically similar to that of true centrilobular vacuolation, a histopathologic change

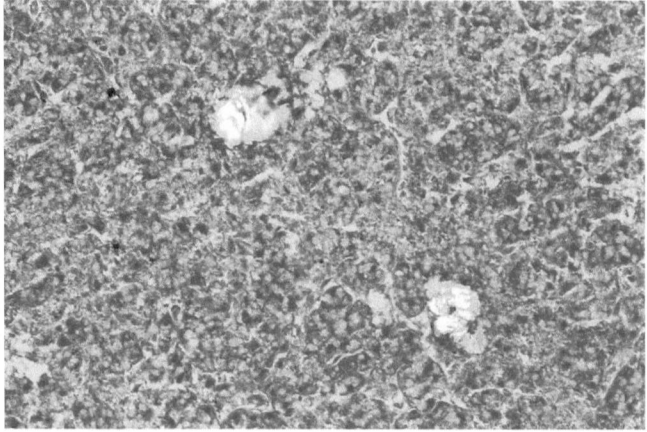

FIGURE 9.1   Liver – Formalin crystals. Crystals form due to the use of chilled or frozen formalin. *Figure reproduced from Haschek WM, Rousseaux CG, Wallig MA, editors:* Handbook of toxicologic pathology, *ed 2, 2002, Academic Press, Figure 1, p 193, with permission.*

that results from lipid accumulation in the hepatocytes following exposure to numerous test articles. In both instances, liver weights may be increased.

There are several potential artifacts that can occur in the lungs if they are improperly handled during necropsy. For example, when the lungs are manually infused with fixative using a syringe inserted in the trachea, excessive force can result in a widening of the space around the vessels in the pulmonary parenchyma. This change mimics the appearance of perivascular edema. However, true edema generally has some amount of eosinophilic proteinaceous fluid surrounding the vessels (Figures 9.2 and 9.3). On the other hand, poorly infused lungs have an atelectatic appearance that microscopically resembles interstitial pneumonia. In addition, interpretation of any true alveolar changes is drastically hindered by the collapse (Fig. 9.4).

Carelessness during necropsy can also result in the formation of artifacts. For example, the misuse of forceps during necropsy can result in "pinch" (or "crush") artifacts. This trauma does not resolve during processing. Additionally, aggressive removal of the brain can result in the insertion of bone from the calvarium into the brain tissue. These bone fragments not only nick the edge of the microtome knife but can result in distortion of the neural tissue if the microtome moves the fragments around during cutting. Another common histological

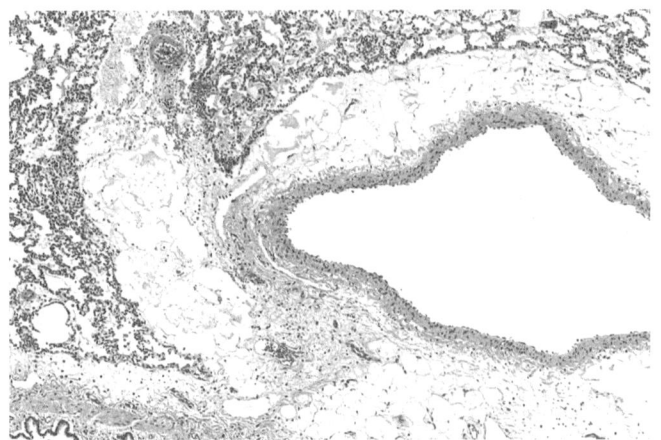

FIGURE 9.2 Lung – Pulmonary edema. Note the presence of eosinophilic proteinaceous fluid in the perivascular space. *Figure reproduced from Haschek WM, Rousseaux CG, Wallig MA, editors:* Handbook of toxicologic pathology, *ed 2, 2002, Academic Press, Fig. 2, p 194, with permission.*

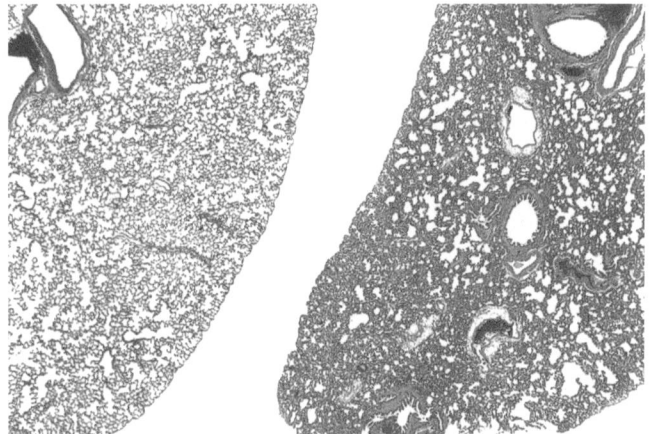

FIGURE 9.4 Lung. The lobe on the left was correctly infused. The lobe on the right was not infused. Note the atelectatic (collapsed) appearance of the alveoli in the right lung lobe. *Figure reproduced from Haschek WM, Rousseaux CG, Wallig MA, editors:* Handbook of toxicologic pathology, *ed 2, 2002, Academic Press, Fig. 4, p 195, with permission.*

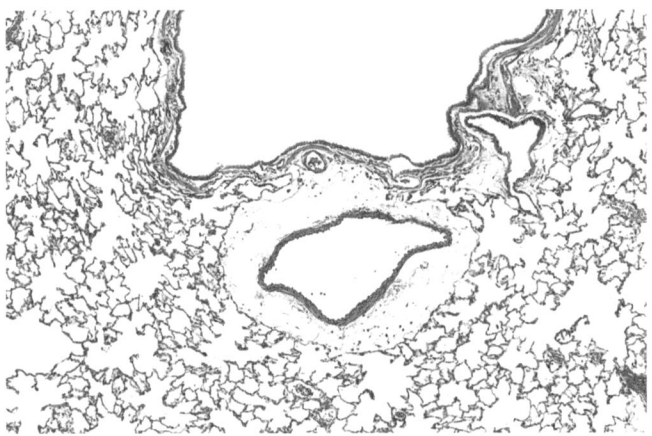

FIGURE 9.3 Lung – "Artifactual" edema. Note the lack of proteinaceous fluid. The widening of the perivascular space is artifactually induced due to excessive pressure during infusion. *Figure reproduced from Haschek WM, Rousseaux CG, Wallig MA, editors:* Handbook of toxicologic pathology, *ed 2, 2002, Academic Press, Fig. 3, p 194, with permission.*

artifact of the brain associated with handling is that of the presence of contracted, intensely stained neurons, which are referred to as "dark neurons." This finding can easily be misinterpreted as dying or degenerating neurons, while in actuality they are a result of postmortem manipulation or trauma to unfixed, ischemic brain tissue (Jortner, 2006).

An additional handling artifact that has been observed in the brain is that of a vacuolated

appearance to the trigeminal nerve tracts. This change results if the trigeminal nerve tracts are stretched during removal of the brain from the skull (Fig. 9.5). Similar artifacts can occur in the spinal cord. Stretching of the myelinated spinal nerve roots during removal from the vertebral column can result in the appearance of swollen axons (McLaurin, 1982). Processing artifacts (vacuoles in white matter tracts) have been reported in the brain and spinal cord when tissues are left in alcohol for prolonged periods of time. For example, if the brain and spinal cord are placed on the tissue processor on a Friday afternoon, the actual processing does not generally begin until Sunday. This results in the tissues sitting in alcohol (the first stage on the processor) for the entire weekend. The prolonged exposure to alcohol results in the appearance of vacuoles in the white matter tracts of the brain and spinal cord (Fig. 9.6) which must be distinguished from a true neurotoxic effect. Since artifactual vacuoles do not occur if the tissues are only left in alcohol overnight, this artifact can be eliminated if tissues are only processed on weekdays (i.e., Monday–Thursday). An alternative solution is the addition of an extra step at the beginning of the processing protocol in which the sections sit in NBF, as opposed to alcohol, until the dehydration process starts (Bolon et al., 2013).

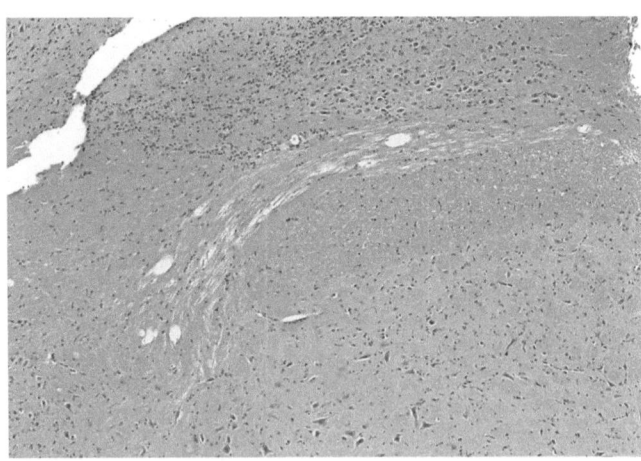

FIGURE 9.5 Brain – Artifactual vacuolization of the trigeminal nerve tracts. This artifact is the result of stretching of the nerve roots during removal of the brain from the skull. *Figure reproduced from Haschek WM, Rousseaux CG, Wallig MA, editors: Handbook of toxicologic pathology, ed 2, 2002, Academic Press, Fig. 5, p 195, with permission.*

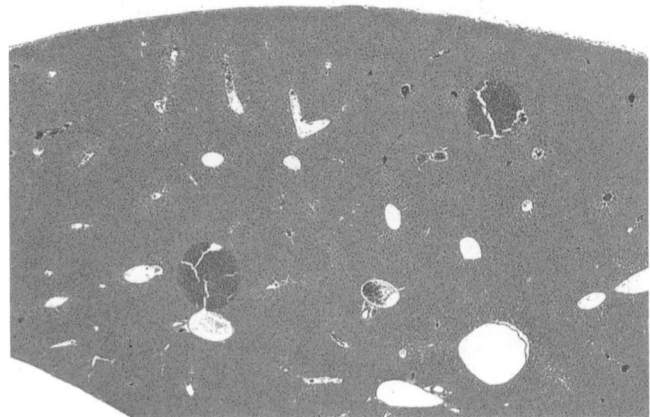

FIGURE 9.7 Liver. Air trapped during sectioning results in the formation of round basophilic circles. These areas can easily be confused with basophilic foci. *Figure reproduced from Haschek WM, Rousseaux CG, Wallig MA, editors:* Handbook of toxicologic pathology, *ed 2, 2002, Academic Press, Fig. 7, p 197, with permission.*

application of coverslips, slides also can become contaminated with spores, pollen, dust, dirt, and cotton fibers that become entrapped under the coverslip. In addition, the mounting media used to attach the coverslips can become contaminated. Furthermore, the over or under use of mounting media can produce artifacts. Artifacts and variability in staining are factors that must be considered when conducting analysis of digital images generated from scanned tissue sections (see *Digital Pathology and Tissue Image Analysis*, Vol 1, Chap 12).

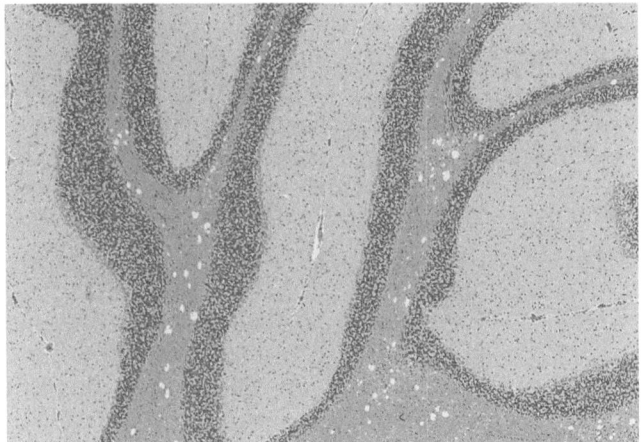

FIGURE 9.6 Brain – Artifactual vacuolization of the white matter. This artifact is the result of prolonged immersion in alcohol. *Figure reproduced from Haschek WM, Rousseaux CG, Wallig MA, editors:* Handbook of toxicologic pathology, *ed 2, 2002, Academic Press, Fig. 6, p 196, with permission.*

Artifacts can also be introduced during sectioning and cover slipping. If air becomes trapped between the tissue and surface of the slide, the tinctorial quality of the tissue will be affected, resulting in the appearance of basophilic circles. Although these circles are quite regular in shape, they must be differentiated from basophilic foci in the liver of rats or mice (Fig. 9.7). During

9. DIAGNOSTIC CHALLENGES IN ANATOMIC TOXICOLOGIC PATHOLOGY

In addition to tissue artifacts that can accidentally be interpreted as lesions by the unwary pathologist, there are a number of true changes that require previous experience in order to properly interpret them during the course of a study evaluation. This section will introduce several examples of diagnostic challenges that can be encountered during the course of study evaluation. Examples will include lesions in animals undergoing unscheduled mortality, rare or poorly understood lesions, differentiation between hyperplasia and neoplasia, sexual dimorphism, and changing terminology for necrosis. The peer review process (Morton et al., 2010) and use of toxicologic pathology literature and diagnostic resources (such as lexicons of harmonized diagnostic nomenclature [e.g., https://www.goreni.org/] and atlases demonstrating normal features and common lesions [e.g., https://ntp.niehs.nih.gov/nnl/]) can support successful identification and interpretation of these lesions.

Animals with unscheduled mortality include any animal that is found dead or is euthanized in moribund condition during the course of a study rather than at a scheduled necropsy time. These deaths could be due to direct toxicity, a procedural error, old age, neoplasia, trauma, or infectious diseases. Unfortunately, in many instances, the COD is not able to be determined following review of available data. Diagnostic challenges are often due to (1) autolysis, (2) the lack of age-matched controls, and (3) the possibility for diagnostic drift during evaluation. Autolysis begins immediately after death. It is a common finding in animals that are found dead or when there was a delay between euthanasia/death and necropsy. Pathologists are relatively comfortable recognizing this change and differentiating it from a test article effect. While autolysis can greatly hinder the ability to histologically evaluate many tissues, attempts should still be made to extract as much information as possible.

With the increased popularity of reproductive and juvenile toxicity studies, the lack of age-matched controls for animals with early mortality can create a diagnostic challenge. In some cases, these animals are extremely young. While most pathologists are comfortable with the histologic features of organs from young adult and aged laboratory animals, there is less familiarity with the evolving anatomic structures of younger animals. Many organs histologically continue to mature postnatally; therefore, one must be able to differentiate immature but normal histologic features from true chemical- or drug-related effects. The testes are an example of this principle. Multinucleated giant cells are common in the normal testes of immature animals; however, increased numbers can indicate Sertoli cell injury (Picut et al., 2015). Similarly, hypospermatogenic tubules are common in young dogs which must be distinguished from degeneration/atrophy associated with toxicity (Picut and Remick, 2017). Fortunately,

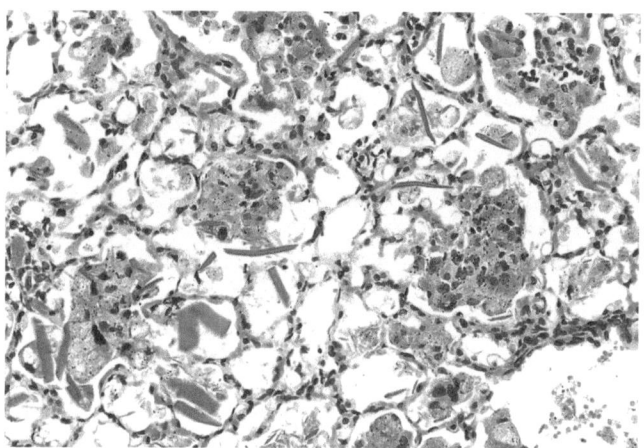

FIGURE 9.8 Lung – Eosinophilic crystals. Crystals are present both within macrophages and the alveolar spaces and have been shown to be composed of Ym1 protein. *Figure reproduced from Haschek WM, Rousseaux CG, Wallig MA, editors:* Handbook of toxicologic pathology, *ed 2, 2002, Academic Press, Fig. 8, p 197, with permission.*

numerous atlases and publications have been published over the past few years that describe postnatal and juvenile histology (Parker and Picut, 2016; Picut & Remick, 2019).

An example of a poorly understood lesion is that of the presence of angular eosinophilic crystals in the lungs of mice (Fig. 9.8). These have previously been recorded as eosinophilic macrophage pneumonia or eosinophilic crystalline pneumonia. These crystals are present both within macrophages and free in the alveolar spaces. While they were originally reported in "moth-eaten mice" (i.e., mice that were heterozygous for the moth-eaten gene [me/me]) (Ward, 1978), they are commonly noted in the respiratory tract of numerous mouse strains (Guo et al., 2000). Recent work by Hoenerhoff et al. (2006) determined that the crystals were composed of YM-1 or T-lymphocyte–derived eosinophil chemotactic factor. The significance of these crystals and their relationship to treatment remains unclear.

Another example of a poorly understood lesion involves the perisinusoidal stellate cells (Ito cells) in the liver. The function of these cells is unclear but is likely associated with vitamin A storage. When there is significant deposition of lipid in the liver, the morphologic appearance of these cells often becomes clouded (i.e., the cytoplasm assumes a hazy pale appearance).

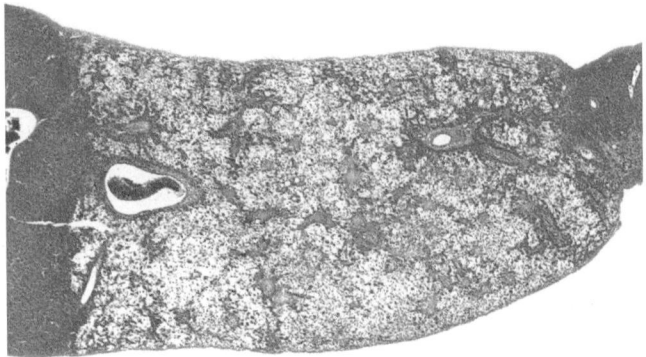

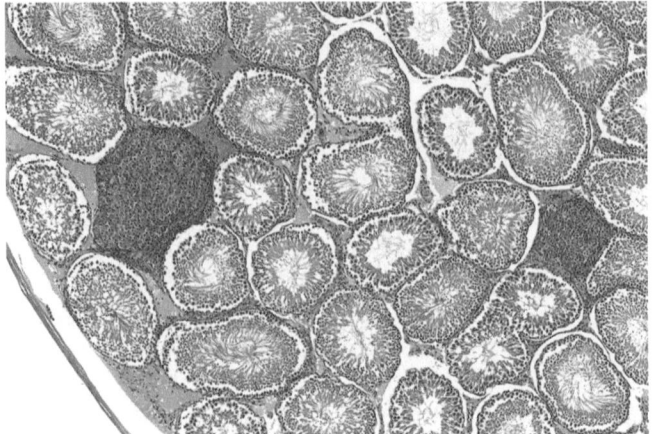

FIGURE 9.9   Liver – Ito cell tumor. This tumor arises from stellate (perisinusoidal) cells and has currently only been reported in mice. *Figure reproduced from Haschek WM, Rousseaux CG, Wallig MA, editors: Handbook of toxicologic pathology, ed 2, 2002, Academic Press, Fig. 9, p 198, with permission.*

FIGURE 9.10   Testes – Proliferation of interstitial (Leydig) cells. Lesions could be diagnosed either as adenomas (U.S. National Toxicology Program [NTP] criteria) or hyperplasia (Society of Toxicologic Pathology [STP] criteria). *Figure reproduced from Haschek WM, Rousseaux CG, Wallig MA, editors: Handbook of toxicologic pathology, ed 2, 2002, Academic Press, Fig. 10, p 199, with permission.*

On rare occasions, these cells can become neoplastic (Dixon et al., 1994). Ito cell tumors have only been reported in mice (Fig. 9.9).

For some lesions, the lines between hyperplasia, atypical hyperplasia, benign neoplasia, and malignancy are blurred. In other instances, the criteria initially used to diagnose a particular lesion may have changed as more was learned about its biological behavior. It is important to remember that histopathologic evaluation represents a single point in time of a lesion that may actually be just a component of a continuous spectrum. Therefore, terminology may sometimes be considered ambiguous by an outside observer, especially one without formal training and experience in pathology. Examples of each of these instances are discussed below. The process of proliferation often represents a continuum in which there is no distinct morphologic change that clearly delineates a difference between hyperplasia and neoplasia. For these types of lesions, diagnostic criteria to distinguish between the not-quite-neoplastic and neoplastic lesions are sometimes somewhat arbitrary. For example, interstitial cell proliferation in the testes distinguishes between hyperplasia and neoplasia differently depending on which recommended nomenclature and diagnostic criteria are followed (Fig. 9.10). In the United States, the NTP has determined that any interstitial cell proliferation greater than one seminiferous tubule in diameter constitutes a benign neoplasm (adenoma), whereas several European authorities as well as the STP recommend that interstitial cell proliferation must be at least three seminiferous

tubules in diameter before it should be called an adenoma (Creasy et al., 2012). Adding to the confusion is the fact that a cross-section of a proliferative lesion may not be through the greatest diameter of the focus. Therefore, the lesion may appear smaller than it actually is and thus would be incorrectly diagnosed. Given these varying diagnostic criteria, problems can arise if interstitial cell proliferative lesions were originally diagnosed using one set of criteria, but peer reviewed using a different set of criteria. This difference in criteria could result in a change regarding the interpretation of a lesion's significance. In the lung, the distinction between type II epithelial hyperplasia and an alveolar/bronchiolar adenoma can be difficult because the hyperplastic cells that line the alveolar septae in more severe cases of hyperplasia can form clusters resembling small adenomas. One suggested criterion is that if more than three contiguous alveoli are filled with proliferating cells, it should be diagnosed as an adenoma. Others will diagnose an adenoma when there is no perceptible interconnecting alveolar wall architecture within the mass of proliferating epithelial cells. On the other end of the spectrum, some pathologists are only comfortable diagnosing an alveolar/bronchiolar carcinoma when the mass shows evidence of local invasion by penetrating through the pleura; however, most pathologists would not require that much

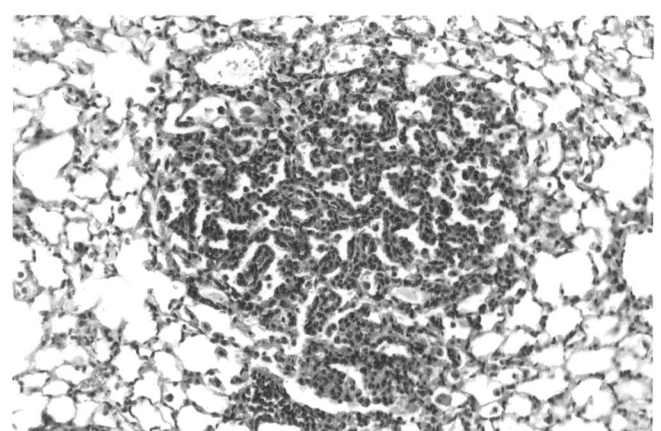

FIGURE 9.11 Lung – Bronchioloalveolar hyperplasia. While this lesion is quite large, alveolar architecture is maintained and the lining cells form a single layer (rather than the multilayered appearance characteristic of neoplasms). *Figure reproduced from Haschek WM, Rousseaux CG, Wallig MA, editors:* Handbook of toxicologic pathology, *ed 2, 2002, Academic Press, Fig. 11, p 199, with permission.*

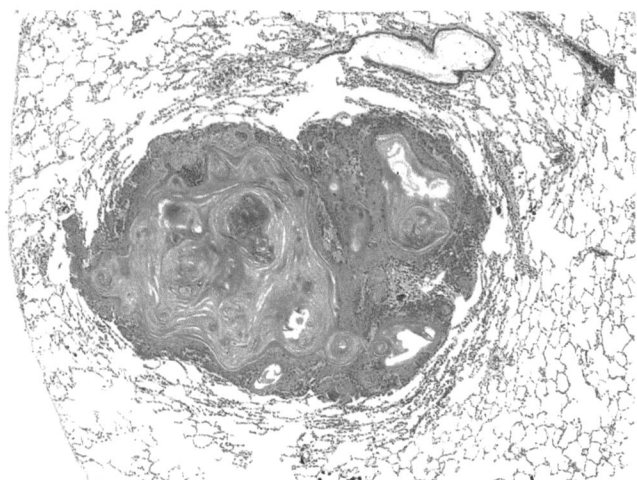

FIGURE 9.12 Lung – Cystic keratinizing epithelioma. Large keratin-filled spaces lined by squamous epithelium, which often lacks orderly maturation. *Figure reproduced from Haschek WM, Rousseaux CG, Wallig MA, editors:* Handbook of toxicologic pathology, *ed 2, 2002, Academic Press, Fig. 12, p 200, with permission.*

evidence of malignancy. They would diagnose a carcinoma based on histomorphologic appearance (e.g., anisocytosis, anisokaryosis, bizarre mitotic figures, hemorrhage, necrosis), without the requirement for invasion (Fig. 9.11) (Renne et al., 2009). The key in managing these equivocal findings is for the study pathologist to define, maintain, and then communicate within the report a clear diagnostic glossary. Such clear documentation will not only aid the study pathologist's interpretation but also will provide guidance to any peer review pathologist and regulatory reviewers what criteria should be used in evaluating the pathology raw data within the report.

Another controversial lesion in the lung involves the spectrum of squamous epithelium–lined cystic lesions that can occur in the alveolar parenchyma. Seen primarily in inhalation studies involving metals and fibers, these lesions have been diagnosed by various pathologists and expert groups as epithelial cysts, benign squamous tumors (which resemble keratoacanthomas morphologically), and squamous cell carcinomas (Fig. 9.12). Since the implications of diagnosing a cyst are quite different from those for a carcinoma, specific diagnostic criteria and nomenclature for distinguishing these lesions have been established (Boorman et al., 1996).

Another example is proliferation in the parathyroid gland that results in a focal enlargement, usually in only one of the glands. Diffuse bilateral enlargement of the parathyroid glands in older rats is often the hyperplastic response that is the result of secondary renal hyperparathyroidism as opposed to a primary neoplastic change of parathyroid tissue. For this reason, it is important that both parathyroid glands be examined grossly and microscopically. The differentiation between hyperplasia and neoplasia is more difficult if only one is sectioned and evaluated.

In the thyroid gland, there are several lesions that histologically appear to be related. Cysts, cystic hyperplasia, and follicular hyperplasia have all been used to diagnose similar lesions in the follicular epithelium (Brandli-Baiocco et al., 2018). The issue of whether a cyst should be considered a proliferative lesion is critical because proliferative and nonproliferative lesions have differing impacts on risk assessment when reviewed by regulatory agencies.

Sexual dimorphism is normal in a number of organs shared by males and females. It is important for pathologists to be aware of these differences, not only so that they have the ability to recognize normal sex-linked differences but, more importantly, so that they can detect any test article–related changes. For example, in male mice the epithelium lining Bowman's capsule in the kidney is cuboidal, while in females the epithelium is simple squamous (Figures 9.13 and 9.14). Sexual dimorphism is also present in the submandibular salivary gland and preputial/clitoral glands of rodents (Figures 9.15 and 9.16). The mammary gland in young rats undergoes age-related changes that could prove to be confusing (Cardy, 1991). Prior to puberty,

the immature mammary gland of females resembles those of postpubertal male rats. It is not until after estrogenic stimulation that the female mammary gland takes on its characteristic lobular appearance (Figures 9.17 and 9.18). Therefore, proper knowledge of the normal appearance of these tissues is necessary in order to detect abnormalities. It is important to remember that

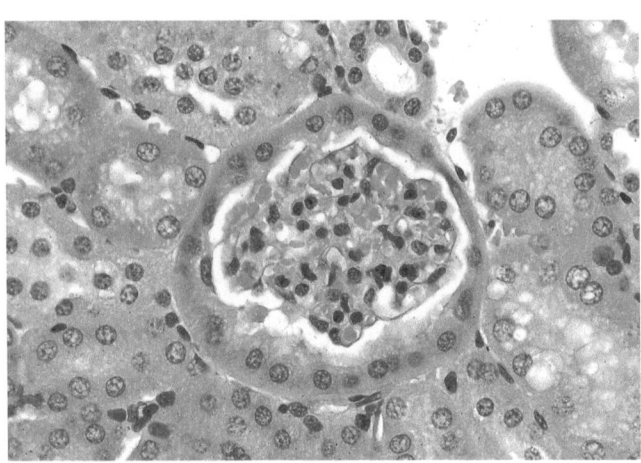

FIGURE 9.13 Male mouse – Kidney – Normal glomerulus. In males, parietal epithelial cells lining Bowman's capsule are cuboidal. *Figure reproduced from Haschek WM, Rousseaux CG, Wallig MA, editors:* Handbook of toxicologic pathology, *ed 2, 2002, Academic Press, Fig. 13, p 201, with permission.*

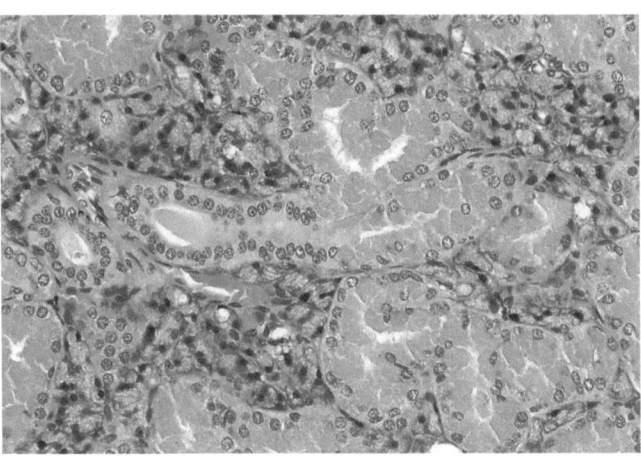

FIGURE 9.15 Male mouse – Submandibular salivary gland – Normal. Note prominent convoluted ducts lined by tall columnar cells with basally located nuclei, with numerous intracytoplasmic eosinophilic granules. *Figure reproduced from Haschek WM, Rousseaux CG, Wallig MA, editors:* Handbook of toxicologic pathology, *ed 2, 2002, Academic Press, Fig. 15, p 202, with permission.*

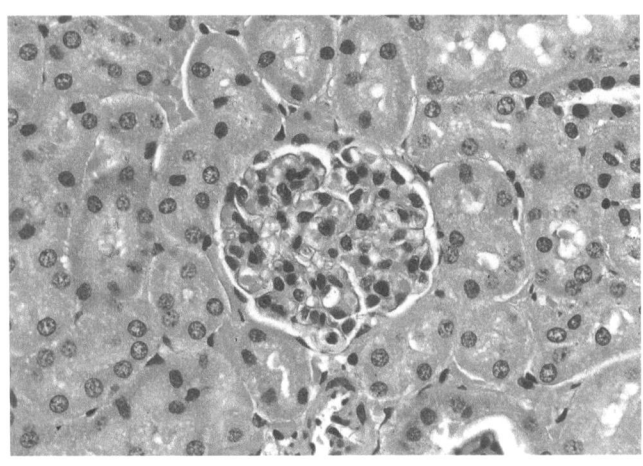

FIGURE 9.14 Female mouse – Kidney – Normal glomerulus. In females, parietal epithelial cells lining Bowman's capsule are flat. *Figure reproduced from Haschek WM, Rousseaux CG, Wallig MA, editors:* Handbook of toxicologic pathology, *ed 2, 2002, Academic Press, Fig. 14, p 201, with permission.*

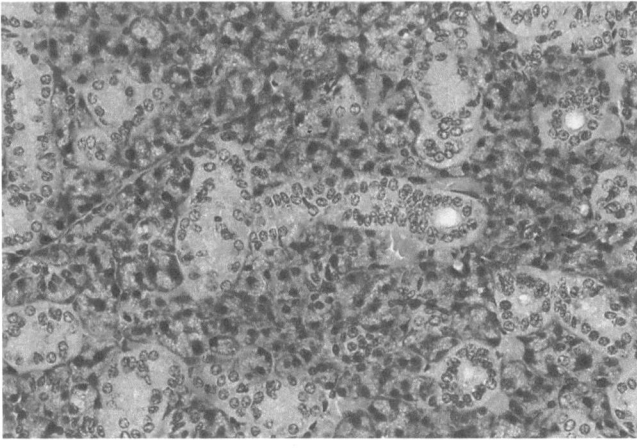

FIGURE 9.16 Female mouse – Submandibular salivary gland – Normal. Note smaller convoluted ducts lined by shorter columnar cells with centrally located nuclei, with fewer eosinophilic granules. *Figure reproduced from Haschek WM, Rousseaux CG, Wallig MA, editors:* Handbook of toxicologic pathology, *ed 2, 2002, Academic Press, Fig. 16, p 202, with permission.*

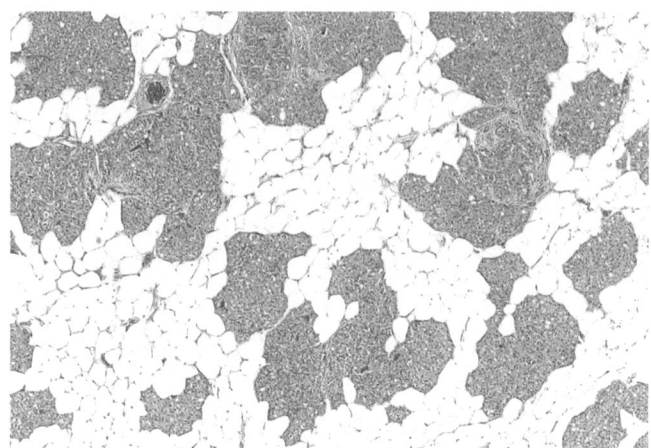

FIGURE 9.17 Male rat (sexually mature) – Mammary gland – Normal. Note the predominant lobuloalveolar pattern and lack of tubular or ductal development. *Figure reproduced from Haschek WM, Rousseaux CG, Wallig MA, editors:* Handbook of toxicologic pathology, *ed 2, 2002, Academic Press, Fig. 17, p 203, with permission.*

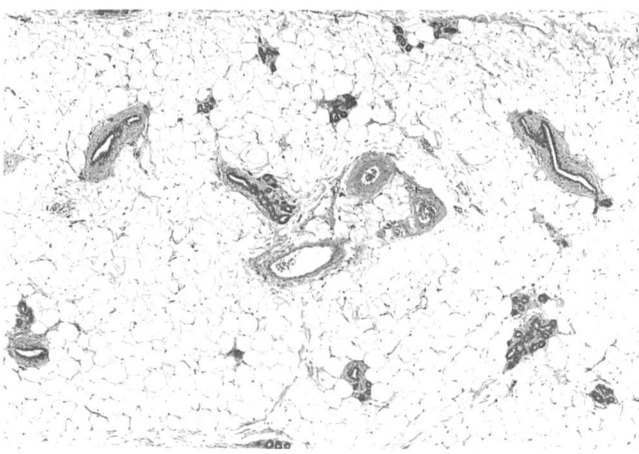

FIGURE 9.18 Female rat (sexually mature) – Mammary gland – Normal. Note the tubuloalveolar pattern. *Figure reproduced from Haschek WM, Rousseaux CG, Wallig MA, editors:* Handbook of toxicologic pathology, *ed 2, 2002, Academic Press, Fig. 18, p 203, with permission.*

exposure to androgenic or estrogenic compounds, such as the synthetic androgen oxymetholone, could result in changes in the normal appearance of these glands (Vidal, 2017).

A final topic that serves as an example of the way in which continuing growth of biomedical knowledge can lend to confusion in study interpretation is the changing preference in terminology with regard to cell death. In the past few years, basic researchers have adopted the term "apoptosis" to describe programmed cell death. However, the morphologic changes associated with apoptosis are often difficult to separate histologically from the classic diagnosis of "necrosis." While researchers have suggested the term "oncosis" to describe necrosis that involves cellular swelling, this term could be confused with a neoplastic process and so has not been generally accepted by pathologists. A special panel from the STP has issued recommendations for the nomenclature of necrosis (Levin et al., 1999). In this document, they recommend the use of the morphologic term "necrosis," with modifiers such as "apoptotic" or "oncotic" if it will help with the interpretation of a particular study, or aid in the characterization of the necrotic process present in the specific tissue being examined.

10. CONCLUSIONS

The goal of this chapter was to introduce the fundamental factors and components that critically influence the capable execution of regulatory toxicity studies with emphasis on anatomic pathology endpoints. It is essential that the toxicologic pathologists understand their role in the operational implementation of these studies despite not being directly responsible for performing many of its functions. The pathologist's job will be significantly influenced by the study director/toxicologist and the local IACUC and laboratory animal resources.

Many of the topics introduced in this chapter such as GLP guidelines, clinical pathology approaches, peer review, nomenclature considerations, and laboratory animal issues are discussed in much greater detail in other chapters, and thus have been cross-referenced to them. However, as the novice pathologist transitions into the regulatory environment of industrial toxicologic pathology, they are encouraged to become familiar with best practice recommendations (https://www.toxpath.org/best-practices. asp; Society of Toxicologic Pathology (STP)) and relevant regulations codified in the Federal Register, the Animal Welfare Act, and other regulatory documents (US EPA, 2002; FDA U.S. Food and Drug Administration, 2007; OECD Organisation for Economic Co-operation and Development, 2018).

REFERENCES

Abdo KM, Kari FW: The sensitivity of the NTP bioassay for carcinogen hazard evaluation can be modulated by dietary restriction, *Exp Toxic Pathol* 48:129–137, 1997.

Albrecht K: Microchip-induced tumors in laboratory rodents and dogs: a review of the literature 1990–2006. In *2010 IEEE international symposium on technology and society, Wollongong, NSW*, 2010, pp 337–349, 2010. https://doi.org/10.1109/ISTAS.2010.5514622.

Amacher DE, Schomaker SJ, Boldt SE, Mirsky M: The relationship among microsomal enzyme induction, liver weight, and histological change in rat toxicology studies, *Food Chem Toxicol* 44(4):528–537, April 2006.

American College of Veterinary Pathologists (ACVP): *Certifying Examination Candidate Handbook (website)*, 2020. https://cdn.ymaws.com/www.acvp.org/resource/resmgr/exam/candidate_handbook_03182020.pdf. (Accessed 10 June 2021).

American College of Veterinary Pathologists (ACVP): *2021 phase 1 certifying examination candidate handbook (website)*, 2020. https://cdn.ymaws.com/www.acvp.org/resource/resmgr/ACVP_Phase_I_Handbook_2021_-.pdf. (Accessed 10 June 2021).

American Veterinary Medical Association (AVMA): *AVMA guidelines for the euthanasia of animals*, Schaumberg, IL, 2020, AVMA, 2020.

Bailer SA, Zidell RH, Perry RW: Relationships between organ weight and body/brain weight in the rat: what is the best analytical endpoint? *Toxicol Pathol* 32:448–466, 2004.

Benavides A, Siches M, Llobera M: Circadian rhythms of lipoprotein lipase and hepatic lipase activities in intermediate metabolism of adult rat, *Am J Physiol-Reg I* 275(3):R811–R817, 1998.

Bolon B, Barale-Thomas E, Bradley A, Ettlin RA, Franchi CAS, George C, Giusti AM, Hall R, Jacobsen M, Konishi Y, Ledieu D, Morton D, Park JH, Scudamore CL, Tsuda H, Vijayasarathi SK, Wijnands MVW: International recommendations for training future toxicologic pathologists participating in regulatory-type, nonclinical toxicity studies, *Toxicol Pathol* 38(6):984–992, 2010.

Bolon B, Butt MT: Fixation and processing of central nervous system tissue. In Aminoff MJ, Daroff RB, editors: *Encyclopedia of Neurological Sciences*, 2nd Ed., San Diego, 2014, Academic Press (Elsevier), pp 312–316.

Bolon B, Garman R, Jensen K, Krinke G, Stuart B: An ad hoc working group of the STP Scientific and Regulatory Policy Committee: a 'best practices' approach to neuropathologic assessment in developmental neurotoxicity testing – for today, *Toxicol Pathol* 34:296–313, 2006.

Bolon B, Garman RH, Pardo ID, Jensen K, Sills RC, Roulois A, Radovsky A, Bradley A, Andrews-Jones L, Butt M, Gumprecht L: STP position paper: recommended practices for sampling and processing the nervous system (brain, spinal cord, nerve, and eye) during nonclinical general toxicity studies, *Toxicol Pathol* 41(7):1028–1048, 2013.

Bolon B, Krinke G, Butt MT, Rao DB, Pardo ID, Jortner BS, Garman RH, Jensen K, Andrews-Jones L, Morrison JP, Sharma AK, Thibodeau MS: STP position paper: recommended best practices for sampling, processing, and analysis of the peripheral nervous system (nerves and somatic and autonomic ganglia) during nonclinical toxicity studies, *Toxicol Pathol* 46(4):372–402, 2018.

Bolon B: Regulatory Forum opinion piece: effective brain trimming for regulatory-type nonclinical toxicity studies, *Toxicol Pathol* 46(2):115–120, 2018.

Boone L, Meyer D, Cusick P, Ennault D, Provencher Bollinger A, Everds N, Meador V, Elliott G, Honor D, Bounous D, Jordan H: Selection and interpretation of clinical pathology indicators of hepatic injury in preclinical studies, *Vet Clin Pathol* 34:182–188, 2005.

Boorman GA, Brockman M, Carlton WW, Davis JMG, Dungworth DL, Hahn FF, Mohr U, Richter Reichhelm R, Turosov VS, Wagner BM: Classification of cystic keratinizing squamous lesions of the ray lung: report of a workshop, *Toxicol Pathol* 24:564–572, 1996.

Brandli-Baiocco A, Balme E, Bruder M, Chandra S, Hellmann J, Hoenerhoff ML, Rosol TJ: Nonproliferative and proliferative lesions of the rat and mouse endocrine system, *Toxicol Pathol* 31(# Suppl):1S–95S, 2018.

Bregman CL, Adler RR, Morton DG, Regan KS, Yano BL: Recommended tissue list for histopathologic examination in repeat-dose toxicity and carcinogenicity studies: a proposal of the society of toxicologic pathology (STP), *Toxicol Pathol* 31:252–253, 2003.

Cardy RH: Sexual dimorphism of the normal rat mammary gland, *Vet Pathol* 28:139–145, 1991.

Carson FL, editor: *Histotechnology: a self-instructional text*, 2nd Ed., Chicago, 1997, ASCP Press.

Chlipala E, Bendzinski CM, Chu K, Johnson JI, Brous MA, Copeland K, Bolon B: Optical density-based image analysis method for the evaluation of hematoxylin and eosin staining precision, *J Histotechnol* 43:29–37, 2020.

Castelhano-Carlos MJ, Baumans V: The impact of light, noise, cage cleaning and in-house transport on welfare and stress of laboratory rats, *Lab Anim* 43(4):311–327, 2009.

Chapman K, Sewell F, Allais L, Delongeas J-L, Donald E, Festag M, Kervyn S, Ockert D, Nogues V, Palmer H, Popovic M, Roosen W, Schoenmakers A, Somers K, Stark C, Stei P, Robinson S: A global pharmaceutical company initiative: an evidence-based approach to define the upper limit of body weight loss in short term toxicity studies, *Regul Toxicol Pharmacol* 67(1):27–38, 2013.

Chatamra K, Daniel PM, Lam DK: The effects of fasting on core temperature, blood glucose and body and organ weights in rats, *Q J Exp Physiol* 69:541–545, 1984.

Committee for Proprietary Medicinal Products (CPMP): *Note for guidance on repeat dose toxicity testing*, 1999. Appendix A, https://www.ema.europa.eu/en/documents/scientific-guideline/note-guidance-repeated-dose-toxicity_en.pdf. (Accessed 10 June 2021).

Committee for Proprietary Medicinal Products (CPMP): *Note for guidance on carcinogenic potential*, 2000. Tissue List A, https://www.ema.europa.eu/en/documents/scientific-guideline/note-guidance-carcinogenic-potential_en.pdf. (Accessed 10 June 2021).

Coolidge BJ, Howard RM. *Animal Histology Procedures*, 2, 1979, National Institutes of Health, 1979.

Creasy D, Bube A, De Rink E, Kandori H, Kuwahara M, Masson R, Nolte T, Reams R, Regan K, Rehm S, Rogerson P, Whitney K: Proliferative and nonproliferative lesions of the rat and mouse male reproductive system, *Toxicol Pathol* 40: 40S–121S, 2012.

Crissman JW, Goodman DG, Hildebrandt PK, Maronpot RR, Prater DA, Riley JH, Seaman WJ, Thake DC: Best practices guideline: toxicologic histopathology, *Toxicol Pathol* 32:126–131, 2004.

De Vera Mudry MC, Kronenberg S, Komatsu S, Aguirre GD: Blinded by the light: retinal phototoxicity in the context of safety studies, *Toxicol Pathol* 41(6):813–825, 2013.

Diehl K-H, Hull R, Morton D, Pfister R, Rabemampianina Y, Smith D, Vidal J-M, van de Vorstenboch C: A good practice guide to the administration of substances and removal of blood, including routes and volumes, *J Appl Toxicol* 21:15–23, 2001.

Dillberger JE: Age-related pancreatic islet changes in Sprague-Dawley rats, *Toxicol Pathol* 22(1):48–55, 1994.

Dixon D, Yoshitomi K, Boorman GA, Maronpot RR: "Lipomatous" lesions of unknown cellular origin in the liver of B6C3F1 mice, *Vet Pathol* 31:173–182, 1994.

Elcock LE, Stuart BP, Wahle BS, Hoss HE, Crabb K, Millard DM, Mueller RE, Hastings TF, Lake SG: Tumors in long-term rat studies associated with microchip animal identification devices, *Exp Toxicol Pathol* 52(6):483–491, 2001.

Fossey S, Vahle J, Long P, Schelling S, Ernst H, Boyce RW, Leininger J: Nonproliferative and proliferative lesions of the rat and mouse skeletal tissues (bones, joints, and teeth), *Toxicol Pathol* 29(3 Suppl):49S–103S, 2016. https://doi.org/10.1293/tox.29.3S-2.

Frame SR, Hurtt ME, Green JW: Testicular maturation in prepubertal New Zealand white rabbits, *Vet Pathol* 31:541–545, 1994.

FDA (U.S. Food and Drug Administration): *Guidance for industry and other stakeholders: redbook 2000*, 2007. https://www.fda.gov/regulatory-information/search-fda-guidance-documents/guidance-industry-and-other-stakeholders-redbook-2000#TOC. (Accessed 10 June 2021).

FDA (U.S. Food and Drug Administration): *Guidance for industry. Drug induced liver injury: premarketing clinical evaluation*, 2009. http://www.fda.gov/Drugs/Guidance ComplianceRegulatoryInformation/Guidances/default.html. (Accessed 10 June 2021).

Fortin JS, Chlipala EA, Shaw DP, Bolon B: Methods optimization for routine sciatic nerve processing in general toxicity studies, *Toxicol Pathol* 48(1):19–29, 2020.

Gamble MR: Sound and its significance for laboratory animals, *Biol Rev* 57:395–421, 1982.

Garman RH: Evaluation of large-sized brains for neurotoxic endpoints, *Toxicol Pathol* 31:32–43, 2003.

Goedken MJ, Kerlin RL, Morton D: Spontaneous and age-related testicular findings in beagle dogs, *Toxicol Pathol* 36(3):465–471, 2008. https://doi.org/10.1177/0192623308315670.

González M: Dim light at night and constant darkness: two frequently used lighting conditions that jeopardize the health and well-being of laboratory rodents, *Front Neurol* 9: 609, 2018.

Greaves P, Chouinard L, Ernst H, Mecklenburg L, Pruimboom-Brees IM, Rinke M, Rittinghausen S, Thibault S, Von Erichsen J, Yoshida T: Proliferative and non-proliferative lesions of the rat and mouse soft tissue, skeletal muscle and mesothelium, *Toxicol Pathol* 26(3 Suppl):1S–26S, 2013.

Guo L, Johnson RS, Schuh JC: Biochemical characterization of endogenously formed eosinophilic crystals in the lungs of mice, *J Biol Chem* 275:8032–8037, 2000.

Halliwell WH: Submucosal mesenchymal tumors of the mouse urinary bladder, *Toxicol Pathol* 26:128–136, 1998.

Halpern WG, Ameri M, Bowman CJ, Elwell MR, Mirsky ML, Oliver J, Tomlinson L: Scientific and Regulatory Policy Committee points to consider review: inclusion of reproductive and pathology end points for assessment of reproductive and developmental toxicity in pharmaceutical drug development, *Toxicol Pathol* 44(6):789–809, 2016.

Hankenson FC, Marx JO, Gordon CJ, David JM: Effects of rodent thermoregulation on animal models in the research environment, *Comp Med* 68(6):425–438, 2018. https://doi.org/10.30802/AALAS-CM-18-000049.

Hart RW, Newmann DA, Robertson RT, editors: *Dietary restriction: implications for the design and interpretation of toxicity and carcinogenicity studies*, Washington, DC, 1995, ILSI Press.

Hoenerhoff MJ, Starost MF, Ward JM: Eosinophilic crystalline pneumonia as a major cause of death in 129S4/SvJae mice, *Vet Pathol* 43:682–688, 2006.

Hoffman JC: Light and reproduction in the rat: effects of photoperiod length on albino rats from two different breeders, *Biol Reprod* 2:255–261, 1970.

Howroyd PC, Peter B, de Rijk E: Review of sexual maturity in the minipig, *Toxicol Pathol* 44(4):607–611, 2016.

Ingram DK, de Cabo R: Calorie restriction in rodents: caveats to consider, *Ageing Res Rev* 39:15–28, 2017.

ICH (international council for harmonisation of technical requirements for pharmaceuticals for human use) S6(R1) guideline: preclinical safety evaluation of biotechnology-derived pharmaceuticals, 2011. https://database.ich.org/sites/default/files/S6_R1_Guideline_0.pdf. (Accessed 10 June 2021).

Jortner BS: The return of the dark neuron. A histological artifact complicating contemporary neurotoxicologic evaluation, *Neurotoxicology* 27(4):628–634, 2006.

Kanerva RL, Alden CL, Wyder WE: The effect of uniform exsanguination on absolute and relative organ weights and organ weight variation, *Toxicol Pathol* 10:43–44, 1982.

Keenan KP, Ballam GC, Soper KA, Laroque P, Coleman JB, Dixit R: Diet, caloric restriction, and the rodent bioassay, *Toxicol Sci* 52(Suppl):24–34, 1999.

Keenan KP, Coleman JB, McCoy CL, Hoe CM, Soper KA, Laroque P: Chronic nephropathy in ad libitum overfed Sprague-Dawley rats and its early attenuation by increasing degrees of dietary (caloric) restriction to control growth, *Toxicol Pathol* 28:788–798, 2000.

Keenan KP, Laroque P, Ballam GC, Soper KA, Dixit R, Mattson BA, Adams SP, Coleman JB: The effects of diet, ad libitum overfeeding, and moderate dietary restriction on rodent bioassay: the uncontrolled variable in safety assessment, *Toxicol Pathol* 24:757–768, 1996.

Kemi M, Keenan KP, McCoy C, Hoe CM, Soper KA, Ballam GC, vanZwieten MJ: The relative protective effects of moderate dietary restriction versus dietary modification on spontaneous cardiomyopathy in male Sprague-Dawley rats, *Toxicol Pathol* 28:285–296, 2000.

Kittel B, Ruehl-Fehlert C, Morawietz G, Klapwijk J, Elwell MR, Lenz B, O'Sullivan MG, Roth DR, Wadsworth PF: Revised guides for organ sampling and trimming in rats and mice – part 2. A joint publication of the RITA and NACAD groups, *Exp Toxic Pathol* 55:413–431, 2004.

Lasser KE, Allen PD, Woohandler SJ, Himmelstein DU, Wolfe SM, Bor DH: Timing of new black box warnings and withdrawals for prescription medications, *J Am Med Assoc* 287:2215–2220, 2002.

Latendresse JR, Warbrittion AR, Jonassen H, Creasy DM: Fixation of testes and eyes using a modified Davidson's fluid: comparison with Bouin's fluid and conventional Davidson's fluid, *Toxicol Pathol* 30(4):524–533, 2002.

Levin S, Bucci TJ, Cohen SM, Fix AS, Hardisty JF, LeGrand EK, Trump BF: The nomenclature of cell death: recommendations of an ad hoc committee of the Society of Toxicologic Pathologists, *Toxicol Pathol* 27:484–490, 1999.

Lewis DJ: Morphologic assessment of pathologic changes within the rat larynx, *Toxicol Pathol* 19:352–357, 1992.

Li X, Elwell MR, Ryan AM, Ochoa R: Morphogenesis of postmortem hepatocyte vacuolation and liver weight increases in Sprague-Dawley rats, *Toxicol Pathol* 31:682–688, 2003.

Long G: Recommendations to guide determining cause of death in toxicity studies, *Toxicol Pathol* 32:269–270, 2004.

Luna LG, editor: Agents and methods for specimen fixation. *Histopathologic methods and color Atlas of special stains and tissue artifacts*, Downers Grove, IL, 1992, Johnson Printers. Chapter 1.

Mann PC, Vahle J, Keenan CM, Baker JF, Bradley AE, Goodman DG, Harada T, Herbert R, Kaufmann W, Kellner R, Nolte T, Rittinghausen S, Tanaka T: International harmonization of toxicologic pathology nomenclature: an overview and review of basic principles, *Toxicol Pathol* 40(4 Suppl):7S–13S, 2012.

Matsuzawa T: Technical factors affecting clinical chemistry values in laboratory rats. In Matsuzawa T, Inouye H, editors: *Biological reference data on CD(SD)IGS rats -1999*, Tokyo, 1999, Best Printing Co. Ltd, pp 1–8.

McDowell E, Trump B: Histological fixatives for diagnostic light and electron microscopy, *Arch Pathol Lab Med* 100(8): 405–414, 1976.

McLarrin GM: Vacuoles in the fiber tracts of rat CNS tissues, *J Histotechnol* 5:171–173, 1982.

Mery S, Gross EA, Joyner DR, Godo M, Morgan KT: Nasal diagrams: a tool for recording the distribution of nasal lesions in rats and mice, *Toxicol Pathol* 22(4):353–372, 1994. https://doi.org/10.1177/019262339402200402.

Michael B, Yano B, Sellers RS, Perry R, Morton D, Roome N, Johnson JK, Schafer K: Evaluation of organ weights for rodent and non-rodent toxicity studies: a review of regulatory guidelines and a survey of current practices, *Toxicol Pathol* 35(5):742–750, 2007.

Minematsu S, Watanabe M, Tsuchiya N, Watanabe M, Amagaya S: Diurnal variations in blood chemical items in Sprague-Dawley rats, *Exp Anim* 44(3):223–232, 1995.

Morton D, Sellers RS, Barale-Thomas E, Bolon B, George C, Hardisty JF, Irizarry A, McKay JS, Odin M, Teranishi MF: Recommendations for pathology peer review, *Toxicol Pathol* 38(7):1118–1127, 2010.

Musigazi GU, De Vleeschauwer S, Sciot R, Verbeken E, Depreitere B: Brain perfusion fixation in male pigs using a safer closed system, *Lab Anim* 52(4):413–417, 2018.

National Research Council. *Guide for the Care and Use of Laboratory Animals*, 8th Ed., Washington, DC, 2011, National Academy Press, 2011 http://grants.nih.gov/grants/olaw/Guide-for-the-care-and-use-of-laboratory-animals.pdf.

Nemzek J, Bolgos G, Williams B, et al.: Differences in normal values for murine white blood cell counts and other hematological parameters based on sampling site, *Inflamm Res* 50:523–527, 2001.

Nold JB, Keenan KP, Nyska A, Cartwright ME: Society of Toxicologic Pathology position paper: diet as a variable in rodent toxicology and carcinogenicity studies, *Toxicol Pathol* 29:585–586, 2001.

OECD (Organisation for Economic Co-operation and Development): *Principles on good laboratory practice, OECD series on principles of good laboratory practice and compliance monitoring, No. 1*, Paris, 1998, OECD Publishing, 1998. https://www.oecd-ilibrary.org/environment/oecd-principles-on-good-laboratory-practice_9789264078536-en. (Accessed 19 August 2021).

OECD (Organisation for Economic Co-operation and Development): *Guidance document 116 on the conduct and design of chronic toxicity and carcinogenicity studies, supporting test guidelines 451, 452 and 453: second edition, OECD series on testing and assessment, No. 116*, Paris, 2014, OECD Publishing, 2014. https://www.oecd-ilibrary.org/environment/guidance-document-116-on-the-conduct-and-design-of-chronic-toxicity-and-carcinogenicity-studies-supporting-test-guidelines-451-452-and-453_9789264221475-en. (Accessed 19 August 2021).

OECD (Organisation for Economic Co-operation and Development): *Test No. 408: repeated dose 90-day oral toxicity study in rodents, OECD guidelines for the testing of chemicals, section 4*, Paris, 2018, OECD Publishing, 2018. https://www.oecd-ilibrary.org/environment/test-no-408-repeated-dose-90-day-oral-toxicity-study-in-rodents_9789264070707-en. (Accessed 19 August 2021).

Palazzi X. *The Beagle Brain in Stereotaxic Coordinates*, 2011, Springer Verlag, 2011.

Pandher K, Leach MW, Burns-Naas LA: Appropriate use of recovery groups in nonclinical toxicity studies: value in a science-driven case-by-case approach, *Vet Pathol* 49:357–361, 2012.

Pardo ID, Garman RH, Weber K, Bobrowski WF, Hardisty JF, Morton D: Technical guide for nervous system sampling of the cynomolgus monkey for general toxicity studies, *Toxicol Pathol* 40(4):624–636, 2012.

Parker GA, Picut CA, editors: *Atlas of histology of the juvenile rat*, New York, 2016, Academic Press/Elsevier.

Paxinos G, Watson C. *The Rat Brain in Stereotaxic Coordinates*, 6th Ed., 2007, Academic Press (Elsevier), 2007.

Paxinos G, Petrides M, Huang X-F, Toga AW. *The Rhesus Monkey Brain in Stereotaxic Coordinates*, 2nd Ed., San Diego, 2008, Academic Press (Elsevier), 2008.

Peirson SN, Brown LA, Pothecary CA, Benson LA, Fisk AS: Light and the laboratory mouse, *J Neurosci Methods* 300:26–36, 2018.

Pellizzon MA, Ricci MR: Choice of laboratory rodent diet may confound data interpretation and reproducibility, *Curr Dev Nutri* 4(4):nzaa031, 2020.

Perry R, Farris G, Bienvenu JG, Dean C, Foley G, Mahrt C, Short B: Society of Toxicologic Pathology position paper on best practices on recovery studies: the role of the anatomic pathologist, *Toxicol Pathol* 41:1159–1169, 2013.

Peter B, de Rijk E, Zeltner A, Emmen HH: Sexual maturation in the female Göttingen minipig, *Toxicol Pathol* 44(3):482–485, 2016.

Picut CA, Parker GA: Postnatal organ development as a complicating factor in juvenile toxicity studies in rats, *Toxicol Pathol* 45(1):248–252, 2017.

Picut CA, Remick AK: Impact of age on the male reproductive system from the pathologist's perspective, *Toxicol Pathol* 45(1):195–205, 2017.

Picut CA, Remick AK: *Pathology of juvenile animals. Toxicologic Pathology for Non-Pathologists*, 2nd Ed., New York, NY, 2019, Humana, pp 779–849, 2019.

Picut CA, Remick AK, DeRuk EPCT, Simons ML, Stump DG, Parker GA: Postnatal development of the testis in the rat: morphologic study and correlation of morphology to neuroendocrine parameters, *Toxicol Pathol* 43:326–342, 2015.

Rao DB, Little PB, Sills RC: Subsite awareness in neuropathology evaluation of National Toxicology Program (NTP) studies: a review of select neuroanatomical structures with their functional significance in rodents, *Toxicol Pathol* 42(3):487–509, 2014.

Rao GN: Diet and kidney diseases in rats, *Toxicol Pathol* 30(6):651–656, 2002.

Rao DB, Little PB, Malarkey DE, Herbert RA, Sills RC: Histopathological evaluation of the nervous system in National Toxicology Program rodent studies: a modified approach, *Toxicol Pathol* 39:463–470, 2011.

Renne R, Brix A, Harkema J, Herbert R, Kittel B, Lewis D, March T, Nagano K, Pino M, Rittinghausen S, Rosenbruch M, Tellier P, Wohrmann: Proliferative and nonproliferative lesions of the rat and mouse respiratory tract, *Toxicol Pathol* 37:5S–73S, 2009.

Renne RA, Gideon KM, Miller RA, Mellick PW, Grumbein SL: Histologic methods and interspecies variations in the laryngeal histology of F344/N rats and B6C3F1 mice, *Toxicol Pathol* 20:44–51, 1992.

Rothacker DL, Kanerva RL, Wyder WE, Alden CL, Maurer JK: Effects of variation of necropsy time and fasting on liver weights and liver components in rats, *Toxicol Pathol* 16:22–26, 1988.

Rubin RL: Mice housed at elevated vivarium temperatures display enhanced T-cell response and survival to *Francisella tularensis*, *Comp Med* 67(6):491–497, 2017.

Sagartz JW, Madarasz AJ, Forsell MA, Burger GT, Ayres PH, Coggins RE: Histologic sectioning of the rodent larynx for inhalation toxicity testing, *Toxicol Pathol* 20:118–121, 1992.

Schafer, Eighmy J, Fikes JD, Halpern WG, Hukkanen RR, Long GG, Francke S: Scientific and Regulatory Policy Committee points to consider: use of severity grades to characterize histopathologic changes, *Toxicol Pathol* 46(3):256–265, 2018.

Scheifele D, Bjornson G, Dimmick J: Rapid postmortem gut autolysis in infant rats: a potential problem for investigators, *Can J Vet Res* 51(3):404–406, 1987.

Sellers RS, Morton D, Michael B, Roome N, Johnson JK, Yano BL, Schafer K: Society of Toxicologic Pathology position paper: organ weight recommendations for toxicologic studies, *Toxicol Pathol* 35:751–755, 2007.

Sewell F, Chapman K, Baldrick P, Brewster D, Broadmeadow A, Brown P, Burns-Naas LA, Clarke J, Constan A, Couch J, Czupalla O, Danks A, DeGeorge J de Haan L, Hettinger K, Hill M, FestagM, Jacobs A, Jacobson-Kram D, Kopytek S, Lorenz H, Moesgaard SG, Moore E, Pasanen M, Perry R, Ragan I, Robinson S, Schmitt PM, Short B, Lima BS, Smith D, Sparrow S, van Bekkum Y, Jones D: Recommendations from a global cross-company data sharing initiative on the incorporation of recovery phase animals in safety assessment studies to support first-in-human clinical trials, *Reg Tox Pharm* 70(1):413–429, 2014.

Society of Toxicologic Pathology (STP): Best Practices & Points to Consider Papers (website). http://www.toxpath.org/best-oractices.asp. (Accessed 12 September 2020).

Sullivan DJ: The effect of exsanguination on organ weight of rats, *Toxicol Pathol* 13:229–231, 1985.

Suvarna SK, Layton C, Bancroft JD. *Bancroft's Theory and Practice of Histological Techniques*, 8th Ed., Oxford, 2019, Elsevier, 2019.

Taqi SA, Sami SA, Sami LB, Zaki SA: A review of artifacts in histopathology, *J Oral Maxillofac Pathol* 22(2):279, 2018.

The NTP interagency center for the evaluation of alternative toxicological methods (NICEATM)- interagency coordinating committee on the validation of alternative methods ICCVAM five Year plan (2008–2012): a plan to advance alternative test methods of high scientific quality to protect and advance the health of people, animals, and the environment, 2008. NIH Publication No. 08-6410.

Tomlinson L, Boone LI, Ramaiah L, Penraat KA, von Beust BR, Ameri M, Poitout-Belissent FM, Weingand K, Workman HC, Aulbach AD, Meyer DJ, Brown DE, MacNeill AL, Bolliger AP, Bounous DI: Best practices for veterinary toxicologic clinical pathology, with emphasis on the pharmaceutical and biotechnology industries, *Vet Clin Pathol* 42:252–269, 2013.

Tomlinson L, Ramaiah L, Tripathi NK, Barlow VG, Vitsky A, Poitout-Belissent FM, Bounous DI, Ennulat D: STP best practices for evaluating clinical pathology in pharmaceutical recovery studies, *Toxicol Pathol* 44(2):163–172, 2016.

Uriah LC, Maronpot RR: Normal histology of the nasal cavity and application of special techniques, *Environ Health Perspect* 85:187–208, 1990.

US EPA: *Good laboratory practice standards, 40 CFR§ 160.1-195*, 1998a. https://www.govinfo.gov/app/details/CFR-1999-title40-vol16/CFR-1999-title40-vol16-part160. (Accessed 19 August 2021).

US EPA: *Good laboratory practice standards, 40 CFR§ 792.1-195*, 1998b. https://www.govinfo.gov/app/details/CFR-2011-title40-vol32/CFR-2011-title40-vol32-part792. (Accessed 19 August 2021).

US FDA: *Good laboratory practice for nonclinical laboratory studies, 21 CFR § 58.1-219*, 2002. https://www.accessdata.fda.gov/scripts/cdrh/cfdocs/cfcfr/CFRSearch.cfm?CFR Part=58. (Accessed 19 August 2021).

Vidal JD: The impact of age on the female reproductive system: a pathologist's perspective, *Toxicol Pathol* 45(1):206–215, 2017.

Ward JM: Pulmonary pathology of the motheaten mouse, *Vet Pathol* 15:170–178, 1978.

Wheeler A: *Directive to prioritize efforts to reduce animal testing [at EPA]*, 2019. Retrieved from: https://www.epa.gov/sites/production/files/2019-09/documents/image2019-09-09-231249.pdf. (Accessed 10 June 2021).

Wilson NH, Hardisty JF, Hayes JR: Short-term, subchronic, and chronic toxicology studies. In Wallace Hayes A, editor: *Principles and methods of toxicology*, 5th Ed., 2008, pp 1223–1264.

World Health Organization: Rules and guidelines for mortality and morbidity coding. In *International statistical classification of diseases and related health problems. ICD-10*, Geneva, 1993, World Health Organization.

Young JT: Histopathologic examination of the rat nasal cavity, *Fundam Appl Toxicol* 1:309–312, 1981.

Young JK, Hall RL, O'Brien P, Strauss V, Vahle JL: Best practices for clinical pathology testing in carcinogenicity studies, *Toxicol Pathol* 39(2):429–434, 2011.

CHAPTER

10

Clinical Pathology in Nonclinical Toxicity Testing

A. Eric Schultze¹, Daniela Ennulat², Adam D. Aulbach³

¹Eli Lilly and Company, Indianapolis, IN, United States, ²GlaxoSmithKline, Collegeville, PA, United States, ³Inotiv, Maryland Heights, MO, United States

OUTLINE

1. Introduction 295
1.1. Value of Clinical Pathology Testing 295
1.2. The Role of a High-Quality Clinical Pathology Laboratory in Toxicity Testing 296
1.3. Samples Submitted to the Clinical Pathology Laboratory 302
1.4. Recommended Test Parameters 303
1.5. Kinetics 304
1.6. Controls 305

2. Clinical Pathology Parameters Commonly Included in Protocols for General Toxicity Studies 305
2.1. Hematology 305
2.2. Hemostasis 307
2.3. Clinical Chemistry 310
2.4. Urinalysis 315
2.5. Bone Marrow Evaluation 317

2.6. Flow Cytometry 318

3. Nonstandard Biomarkers 318
3.1. Introduction 318
3.2. Biomarker Assay Kits 318
3.3. Fit-for-Purpose (Analytical) Validation 319
3.4. Biologic Validation 319
3.5. Biomarker Application in Nonclinical Studies 319
3.6. Hormones 319
3.7. Acute Phase Proteins 321
3.8. Novel Renal Biomarkers 321
3.9. New Liver Biomarkers 325
3.10. Heart Biomarkers 327
3.11. Drug-induced Vascular Injury Biomarkers 329

4. Conclusions 330

References 330

1. INTRODUCTION

1.1. Value of Clinical Pathology Testing

Clinical pathology testing is a key component of nonclinical safety studies that evaluate the potential toxicity of test articles including therapeutic agents (new chemical entities and biologics), pesticides, and industrial chemicals to which humans and/or animals may be exposed. Clinical pathology data are used to detect treatment-related effects; monitor the onset, temporal progression, and reversibility of these effects; and characterize the dose response and severity of effect. For nonrodent studies, clinical pathology data are often one of the components used to assess animal health prior to entry onto the study. Changes in clinical pathology parameters may help to distinguish whether

Haschek and Rousseaux's Handbook of Toxicologic Pathology, Fourth Edition.
https://doi.org/10.1016/B978-0-12-821044-4.00017-0

effects are due to exaggerated pharmacology, metabolic adaptation, or overt toxicity. Target organ effects indicated by clinical pathology alterations can be compared across laboratory animal species and, when combined with other data and mechanistic insights, the importance and relevance of findings to humans can be assessed.

Regulatory guidelines for inclusion of hematologic, clinical chemistry, hemostasis, and/or urinalysis testing in nonclinical safety and/or efficacy assessment studies have been reviewed by several investigators (Hall, 1992, 2013; Tomlinson et al., 2013, Tomlinson et al., 2016; Young et al., 2011). Additional guidance regarding inclusion of hematologic analysis, clinical chemistry, and to a lesser extent hemostasis evaluation and urinalysis in studies for test article evaluation in the biopharmaceutical, biotechnology, and agrochemical industries have been provided by global regulatory agencies including the European Medicines Agency (EMA European Medicines Agency, 2010, EMA European Medicines Agency, 2020), Japanese Ministry of Health, Labour and Welfare (JMHLW, 1989, 1993, 1999, 2020), Organisation for Economic Co-operation and Development (OECD, 2008, 2020), United States (US) Environmental Protection Agency (EPA U.S. Environmental Protection Agency, 2001), and the US Food and Drug Administration (FDA U.S. Food and Drug Administration Center for Devices and Radiological Health, 1999, FDA U.S. Food and Drug Administration, 2003). These guidance documents are not comprehensive in study type or species, and they lack uniformity with respect to recommended clinical pathology testing. More recently, expert working groups of the Division of Animal Clinical Chemistry (DACC), Society of Toxicologic Pathology (STP), and the American Society for Veterinary Clinical Pathology (ASVCP) have produced "best practice" articles that offer specific recommendations for the use of clinical pathology testing in nonclinical safety studies (Weingand et al., 1992; Tomlinson et al., 2013, Tomlinson et al., 2016). Some organ- or study-specific recommendations also are provided in scientific literature. For example, recent articles provide a summary of regulatory guidelines as these relate to hematologic analysis and bone marrow examinations (Reagan et al., 2011a,b), hepatobiliary toxicity (Boone et al., 2005), and

carcinogenicity studies (Young et al., 2011) in nonclinical safety assessment. These societal "best practice" recommendations are consistent with existing regulatory guidance and thus are extremely helpful in directing the design of clinical pathology sampling and analysis in nonclinical toxicity studies.

Clinical pathology and biomarker research are fields that are rich in acronyms and abbreviations for various tests, clinical syndromes, and regulatory and scientific organizations. Acronyms and abbreviations used in this chapter are listed in Table 10.1.

1.2. The Role of a High-Quality Clinical Pathology Laboratory in Toxicity Testing

Essential Services

Clinical pathology testing in nonclinical toxicity studies encompasses hematology, hemostasis, clinical chemistry, and urinalysis as the core elements. The scope of testing is evolving constantly to include new technologies as well as additional test parameters and novel biomarkers. Despite the rapid advances in laboratory instrumentation and biomarker development, the core set of clinical pathology tests for nonclinical safety studies typically is limited to the four standard test panels for nonclinical safety studies.

Hematology: Ethylenediaminetetraacetic acid (EDTA)–anticoagulated blood for determination of a complete blood count (CBC) is the most frequently submitted sample for hematological analysis in all species used in toxicity testing. The CBC provides rapid, inexpensive, and noninvasive assessment of the erythron (red blood cells [RBCs]), leukon (white blood cells [WBCs]), and thrombon (platelets) (Table 10.2). A freshly made and stained blood smear from each animal is used to confirm cell counts and to evaluate blood cell morphology. These smears may be made by investigators at the time of phlebotomy or, provided that the blood samples are delivered to the clinical pathology laboratory within 1–2 h of collection, they can be made in the laboratory at the time of specimen processing.

Bone marrow cytologic smears, prepared at necropsy for each animal, are also submitted routinely for staining and potential future evaluation in toxicity studies. Although these

TABLE 10.1 Key Acronyms and Abbreviations

Acronym/Abbreviation	Meaning
5′NT	5′nucleotidase
α	Alpha
α-GST	Alpha glutathione *S*-transferase
AA	Arachidonic acid
A/G	Albumin/globulin ratio
ADP	Adenosine 5′-diphosphate
AGP	α-1 acid glycoprotein 1
ALP	Alkaline phosphatase (total activity)
ALT	Alanine aminotransferase
ANG-2	Angiopoietin-2
ANP	Atrial natriuretic peptide
APP	Acute phase protein
APTT	Activated partial thromboplastin time
ASCP	American Society for Clinical Pathology
AST	Aspartate aminotransferase
ASVCP	American Society for Veterinary Clinical Pathology
B-ALP	Bone alkaline phosphatase isozyme
BNP	Brain natriuretic peptide
BSEP	Bile salt export pump
BUN	Blood urea nitrogen
CAP	College of American Pathologists
CBC	Complete blood count
CHCM	Corpuscular hemoglobin concentration mean
CK	Creatine kinase

TABLE 10.1 Key Acronyms and Abbreviations—cont'd

Acronym/Abbreviation	Meaning
CRP	C-reactive protein
cTn	Cardiac troponin
cTnC	Cardiac troponin C
cTnI	Cardiac troponin I
cTnT	Cardiac troponin T
D-dimer	A specific, cross-linked fibrin degradation product
DIKI	Drug-induced kidney injury
DILI	Drug-induced liver injury
DIVI	Drug-induced vascular injury
EC	Endothelial cell
EDTA	Ethylenediaminetetraacetic acid
EMA	European Medicines Agency
EPA	US Environmental Protection Agency
Fabp3	Fatty acid binding protein 3
FDA	US Food and Drug Administration
FDP	Fibrinogen/fibrin degradation product
FSH	Follicle-stimulating hormone
GGT	Gamma-glutamyl transferase
GLDH	Glutamate dehydrogenase
GLP	Good laboratory practice
Hct	Hematocrit
HDW	Hemoglobin distribution width
HESI	Health and Environmental Sciences Institute
Hgb	Hemoglobin
I-ALP	Intestinal alkaline phosphatase isozyme

(*Continued*)

TABLE 10.1   Key Acronyms and Abbreviations—cont'd

Acronym/ Abbreviation	Meaning
IVD	In vitro diagnostic assay
JMHLW	Japanese Ministry of Health, Labour and Welfare
K18	Keratin 18
KIM-1	Kidney injury molecule-1
L-ALP	Liver alkaline phosphatase isozyme
LAP	Leucine aminopeptidase
LDH	Lactate dehydrogenase
LH	Luteinizing hormone
MCH	Mean corpuscular hemoglobin
MCHC	Mean corpuscular hemoglobin concentration
MCSFR	Macrophage colony-stimulating factor receptor
MCV	Mean corpuscular volume
M:E	Myeloid to erythroid ratio
miR-122	microRNA-122
MPV	Mean platelet volume
Myl3	Myosin light chain 3
NAG	N-acetyl-/β-glucosaminidase
NGAL	Neutrophil gelatinase–associated lipocalin
NHP	Nonhuman primate
NO	Total nitric oxide
NT-proANP	Amino cleavage equivalent of ANP
NT-proBNP	Amino cleavage equivalent of BNP
OECD	Organisation for Economic Co-operation and development

TABLE 10.1   Key Acronyms and Abbreviations—cont'd

Acronym/ Abbreviation	Meaning
OPN	Osteopontin
P5P	Cofactor pyridoxal 5' phosphate, the active form of vitamin B6
PAF	platelet activating factor
PDE3i	a phosphodiesterase inhibitor
PDW	platelet distribution width
PSTC	Predictive Safety Testing Consortium
PT	Prothrombin time
RBC	Red blood cell (erythrocyte)
RDW	Red cell distribution width
RPA-1	Renal papillary antigen-1
RUO	Research use only assay
sCr	Serum creatinine
SDH	Sorbitol dehydrogenase
SOP	Standard operating procedure
T3	Triiodothyronine
T4	Thyroxin
TBA	Total bile acids
TIMP-1	Tissue inhibitor of metalloproteinase-1
TSH	Thyroid-stimulating hormone
US	United States
VEGF-α	Vascular endothelial growth factor-α
WBC	White blood cell (leukocyte)

TABLE 10.2 Routine Clinical Pathology Testing Parameters in Nonclinical Toxicity Studies

Hematology	Hemostasis	Clinical chemistry	
Erythrocyte (red blood cell [RBC]) count	Activated partial thromboplastin time (APTT)	Sodium	
Hematocrit (Hct)	Prothrombin time (PT)	Chloride	
Hemoglobin (Hgb)	Fibrinogen concentration[b]	Potassium	
Mean corpuscular volume (MCV)		Phosphorus	
Mean corpuscular hemoglobin concentration (MCHC)		Calcium	
Mean corpuscular hemoglobin (MCH)		Total protein	
Reticulocyte count		Albumin	
Platelet count		Globulin	
Leukocyte (white blood cell [WBC], total and differential[a]) counts		Albumin/ globulin (A/G) ratio	
Collect and archive blood and bone marrow smears		Urea nitrogen (BUN)	
		Serum creatinine (sCr)	
		Triglyceride	
		Total cholesterol	
		Glucose	
		At least two hepatocellular markers	Alanine aminotransferase (ALT)
			Aspartate aminotransferase (AST)
			Sorbitol dehydrogenase (SDH[c]) or glutamate dehydrogenase (GLDH[c])
		At least two hepatobiliary markers	Alkaline phosphatase (ALP)
			Total bilirubin
			Gamma-glutamyl transferase (GGT[c])
			Bile acids

[a] *Neutrophils, lymphocytes, monocytes, eosinophils, basophils, large unclassified cells.*
[b] *Not required.*
[c] *Recommended in pigs and guinea pigs.*
Modified from Weingand et al., 1992, 1996; Tomlinson et al., 2013.

smears are collected in most studies, they are used infrequently in test article evaluation. Their use is reserved for studies in which the CBC combined with bone marrow histopathology is insufficient to explain the cause(s) for unexpected nonregenerative decreases in erythroid mass, neutropenia, and/or thrombocytopenia. They may also be used less frequently to investigate unexplained test article–induced increases in various blood cell lines and certain types of morphologic changes in blood cells (Hall, 2013; Reagan et al., 2011a,b).

Hemostasis: Citrated blood is the sample submitted most frequently for hemostasis evaluation. Citrated plasma is used for determining the prothrombin time (PT)—a rapid screen of the extrinsic and common pathways of coagulation; activated partial thromboplastin time (APTT)—a rapid screen of the intrinsic and common pathways of coagulation; and fibrinogen concentration—a measurement of the plasma protein precursor to fibrin (Table 10.2).

Clinical Chemistry: A variety of fluids may be submitted for biochemical analysis: serum, plasma, urine, and less frequently cerebrospinal fluid, synovial fluid, organ lavage fluids, semen, body effusions, and cell culture supernatants. Of these fluids, serum (the supernatant remaining after blood has been allowed to clot) followed by plasma (the supernatant following centrifugation of anticoagulated blood) is analyzed most frequently in clinical pathology laboratories in the United States. Specific tests may be requested individually, or a panel of tests may be selected to screen multiple organ systems (Table 10.2). These standardized panels are commonly used for safety assessment studies. A typical screening panel may include tests to evaluate renal function, liver injury, and electrolyte status as well as lipid, carbohydrate, and protein metabolism. The exact number of tests per panel may vary with the individual clinical pathology laboratory and institution as well as the sample size. If the amount of serum available for analysis is limited due to animal size, investigators may opt to modify the standard panel or select an organ-specific panel (such as a liver screen that includes total protein, albumin, and total bilirubin concentrations as well as the activities of the hepatobiliary enzymes: alanine aminotransferase (ALT), aspartate aminotransferase (AST), alkaline phosphatase (ALP), and/or gamma-glutamyl transferase (GGT)).

Urinalysis: Aliquots of fresh urine are submitted for complete urinalysis. The full evaluation includes assessment of physical parameters of urine (e.g., volume, color, clarity, and specific gravity); reagent stick (semiquantitative) biochemistry determinations (pH, protein, glucose, bilirubin, ketones, blood, urobilinogen) or quantitation of specific analytes on automated instrumentation; and microscopic examination of the sediment to observe cells, crystals, casts, and infectious agents. Urine may be submitted and analyzed within 4 h of collection or may be refrigerated for up to 24 h prior to analysis. It is essential for appropriate data interpretation that investigators specify the method of urine collection (voided midstream catch, cage pan, catheterization, cystocentesis, or metabolism cage) when submitting urine for analysis since collection methods can influence proper interpretation of urinalysis results. For certain renal toxicity/physiology studies, urine may be analyzed quantitatively to determine the concentrations of albumin, protein, glucose, sodium, potassium, chloride, calcium, phosphate, and creatinine. True quantitative studies of urine proteins, creatinine, and electrolytes, often referred to as "renal physiology studies," may require timed urine collection via metabolism cages, and values may be reported as urine analyte concentration and/or analyte concentration normalized to urine creatinine concentration.

Instrumentation

A detailed description of all instrumentation utilized in the clinical pathology laboratory is beyond the scope of this chapter. Excellent, comprehensive laboratory instrument reviews are provided by the College of American Pathologists (CAP, 2020). The ASVCP publishes numerous instrument validation and methods comparison studies in the journal *Veterinary Clinical Pathology* (ASVCP, 2020). Several reference textbooks review instrument methodology and the challenges of analyzing animal samples (Stockham & Scott, 2008; Weiss and Wardrop, 2010; Burtis et al., 2006). There are some important concepts that are common to laboratory instruments, and investigators should be aware of these when pursuing services from a clinical pathology laboratory. These guiding principles are covered briefly here.

The instrument for measurement of the CBC should be automated and accommodate high volumes of samples daily. Given the small sizes of laboratory mice and rats and the limited blood volumes that may be collected from these species, the hematology instrument should be capable of accurately analyzing a small EDTA blood sample (approximately 250 μL). Some newer automated hematology instruments that are under evaluation currently and not yet in widespread use have smaller sample volume requirements (approximately 125 μL) and may be very helpful for analysis of mouse blood samples. The instrument intended for animal hematologic analysis should be equipped with multispecies software to accommodate the laboratory animals that are being studied at that institution. The range of nonclinical test species most often includes mice, rats, dogs, rabbits, pigs, and nonhuman primates (NHPs); however, other species are also occasionally utilized such as guinea pigs, hamsters, gerbils, and/or cats. It is important to utilize appropriate instrumentation and optimize it accordingly in order to accurately analyze blood samples from a variety of laboratory animal species. An automated blood smear stainer also should be available for routine use. These instruments should provide an acceptable Romanowsky stain, such as modified Wright stain, Wright stain, or Wright–Giemsa stain, to highlight cytologic features of various cell types. This instrument also may be used to stain cytologic preparations of bone marrow and other body fluids, tissue aspirates, or impression smears. Manual staining of blood smears is a time-consuming and challenging task that may lead to much stain variation and so should be avoided.

Instruments dedicated to measurement of hemostasis assays are sometimes called "coagulometers." These instruments vary markedly in size and complexity. In the modern clinical pathology laboratory, these instruments are usually semi- or fully automated, accommodate high volumes of samples daily, and employ physical method, optical end points (turbidometry or nephelometry), or a combination of these methods to detect conversion of fibrinogen to fibrin. Most hemostasis assays are simple clotting or chromogenic substrate assays. A limiting factor in hemostasis testing in animals is the volume of the citrated plasma sample required for completion of a panel of the more commonly used assays (PT, APTT, and fibrinogen concentration)—usually approximately 400 μL minimum. Manual assays (tilt tube method) that use visual inspection for clot detection are used rarely today.

In the clinical chemistry section of the laboratory, the main instrument for biochemical analysis should accommodate large numbers of samples daily. This instrument should be equipped with reagents and assays to measure the 20–30 more common analytes (Table 10.2) of biochemical panels and should have open channels that can be programmed to accommodate unique assays (e.g., novel biomarkers) developed by the laboratory staff. Ideally, the sample volume requirement for the entire clinical chemistry panel should be small ($\leq$250 μL serum or plasma, which equates to approximately 500 μL of whole blood) to accommodate the limited blood volume of rodents.

Urine specific gravity should be measured by refractometry as the urine reagent sticks have proven unsatisfactory for measurement of urine specific gravity in animals. The refractometer may be a hand-held device or might be incorporated into a large bench-top instrument that is used to evaluate the semiquantitative urine reagent stick chemistry determinations.

All clinical pathology laboratory instruments should have an appropriate maintenance log and a standard operating procedure (SOP). Competency of laboratory personnel to operate instruments should be reassessed according to institutional guidelines on a regular basis. Every clinical pathology laboratory should have a quality assurance program to ensure the proper operation of each instrument, the appropriate use of assay reagents, and the correct actions of the instrument operator to generate accurate and precise data. Readers are referred to summaries in textbooks (Stockham & Scott, 2008; Weiss and Wardrop, 2010; Burtis et al., 2006) and the numerous publications and guidelines produced by the Quality Assurance and Laboratory Standards Committee of the ASVCP (ASVCP, 2020) for details on these important programs.

Laboratory Staffing

Clinical pathology laboratories may vary in size and number of employees, depending on the management objectives for individual institutions. In some organizations, the clinical pathology laboratory focuses on services in hematology, hemostasis, clinical chemistry, and urinalysis in laboratory animals only. In other institutions, the clinical pathology laboratory may be involved in active biomarker research, microbiological testing, development and validation of emerging molecular pathology techniques, and/or processing samples for test article absorption and metabolism determinations. Many of the Good Laboratory Practice (GLP)–compliant clinical pathology laboratories in biopharmaceutical research, contract research organizations, and the chemical industry are restricted to analysis of animal samples. Infrequently, institutions will have both human (where the GLP-equivalent standard is Clinical Laboratory Improvement Amendments [CLIA] compliance) and animal samples analyzed within the same clinical pathology laboratory. The common denominators for these laboratories should be high-quality analysis of samples in a timely manner.

The job titles for laboratory personnel vary widely among companies and organizations. Position titles such as research associate, research specialist, technologist, and technician often lack universally accepted definitions for education, training, skill level, and duties. These titles may confuse investigators and can be defined differently at various institutions. Since high-quality sample analysis depends on appropriate education and training of laboratory employees, it is desirable for clinical pathology laboratory employees to have earned certification in clinical pathology testing by a professional society of pathology such as the American Society for Clinical Pathology (ASCP). Individuals credentialed by the ASCP as Medical Laboratory Technician or Medical Laboratory Scientist [formerly known as Clinical Laboratory Scientist or Medical Technologist] are highly valued clinical pathology professionals. Many of these individuals, while originally educated in hospital- or university-based clinical pathology training programs focused on human sample testing, have completed additional years of training in a veterinary clinical pathology laboratory to familiarize themselves with the myriad species differences in hematology, cytology, clinical chemistry, hemostasis, and urinalysis. Clinical pathology laboratory personnel should be fluent in operation of the latest automated instruments for hematology, hemostasis, clinical chemistry, and urinalysis as well as have skills in manual techniques and procedures such as creation of blood and bone marrow smears, production of buffy coat preparations, analysis of body fluids, and performance of manual "quick" stains on cytologic specimens. Lastly, it is desirable that a veterinary clinical pathology laboratory have a board-certified veterinary clinical pathologist as the supervisor or scientific liaison to advise on challenging issues such as cellular identification in hematology or cytology, unique assay and instrument validation procedures, study designs, and data interpretation as well as to provide continuing education opportunities for laboratory employees (Schultze et al., 2008a; Schultze, 2011; Schultze and Irizarry, 2017). Commonly, clinical pathologists in animal facilities are veterinary pathologists with certification as a diplomate of the American College of Veterinary Pathologists (ACVP) or European College of Veterinary Clinical Pathology (ECVCP). The practice in some nonclinical facilities of having clinical pathology data evaluated solely by the toxicologist, the study director, or by the anatomic pathologist who is performing the histopathologic evaluation may be suitable in cases where few or obvious clinical pathology alterations are found, but unusual or challenging clinical pathology changes generally should be analyzed or reviewed by a veterinary clinical pathologist.

1.3. Samples Submitted to the Clinical Pathology Laboratory

Types of Samples and Identification

All specimens delivered to the clinical pathology laboratory should be properly labeled. An ideal specimen label contains the following information: study number, unique animal identifier, date the sample was collected, and species; in some institutions, a unique computer tracking bar code may be included to speed the analysis (by reducing the need for direct entry of the unique animal identifiers for all subjects of large studies). Upon receipt in the clinical pathology laboratory, all specimens from a study should be reviewed by laboratory personnel and matched to the study protocol. The number of samples is reviewed, and any missing samples should be noted immediately and recorded in the written and/or computer record for the study.

Quality of Samples—Volume, Hemolysis, Lipemia, and Icterus

Ideally, blood samples submitted to the clinical pathology laboratory for hematologic, hemostasis, and clinical chemistry analysis are obtained from rats, dogs, and NHPs fasted overnight. Fasting improves specimen quality by reducing variability in glucose, triglyceride, and some lipid concentrations compared to those analyte values obtained from nonfasted animals. Fasting also reduces the occurrence of lipemia, which may interfere with some test methods in hematology, hemostasis, and clinical chemistry. However, fasting of mice for longer than 4 h in preparation for clinical pathology sampling typically is not recommended since fasted mice also may decrease water consumption and become dehydrated, which can impact several clinical pathology parameters. Urine for urinalysis may be obtained from fasted or nonfasted animals.

Body fluid specimens (anticoagulated blood, serum, plasma, urine) should be evaluated for adequacy of sample volume. Any sample with inadequate volume to complete the tests listed in the study protocol should be recorded.

Anticoagulated blood samples (EDTA, citrate, and heparin) should be gently rocked back and forth and evaluated for clotting. A wooden applicator stick should be inserted and gently stirred in the anticoagulated samples to check for microclots. Any anticoagulated blood sample with gross or microclots should be rejected and not analyzed since clotting will alter some parameters by consuming proteins, causing release of some cellular constituents, and removing cells from the sample. Clotted samples also may potentially disable a hematology analyzer if large cellular clumps occlude the fluid mechanics of the instrument.

Samples of whole blood that are processed to serum and anticoagulated blood samples processed to plasma should be evaluated for the presence of hemolysis, lipemia, and icterus. If present, the magnitude of hemolysis, lipemia, or icterus should be assessed objectively by visually matching to a color chart or by biochemical determination using the chemistry analyzer. Any sample quality observations should be recorded and reported along with the study analyte data to the clinical pathologist to assist in data interpretation. Laboratory personnel should contact the study director to discuss any clotted samples or samples with an inadequate volume for analysis. Collection of another blood sample may be possible for certain prestudy or interim time points from animals with larger blood volumes (e.g., dogs, NHPs, and pigs). Body fluid samples from mice or rats are seldom redrawn as they are usually obtained at the time of necropsy.

If it is impossible to obtain adequate sample volume to complete all the tests listed in the study protocol, the study director should be asked to provide a list of prioritized tests that can be completed using the sample submitted to the laboratory. It is most expedient if the prioritized list of testing is established and communicated in advance in the study protocol and/or a facility SOP to avoid delays if this situation arises as an urgent need for a critical study time point.

1.4. Recommended Test Parameters

In 1996, a joint scientific committee for International Harmonization of Clinical Pathology Testing, composed of representatives from 10 scientific organizations, published minimum recommendations for clinical pathology testing of laboratory animals used in regulated safety assessment/toxicity studies (Weingand et al., 1996). These standards have been widely adopted and accepted by regulatory agencies globally. The list of hematology, hemostasis, clinical chemistry, and urinalysis analytes identified originally has essentially remained as "core" tests that should be included in clinical pathology protocols for nonclinical toxicity studies and has been updated infrequently (Table 10.2). Some of the more important recommendations from the joint scientific committee were the following: (1) clinical pathology testing (hematology, chemistry, and urinalysis) should be conducted at termination and following the recovery interval (when applicable) in rodent and nonrodent studies; (2) clinical pathology testing should be conducted at predose and at a minimum of one interim interval in nonrodent studies to help mitigate potential interpretive challenges due to small group sizes and inter-animal variation; (3) testing should occur within the first 7 days of dosing in nonrodent studies of less than 6 weeks duration; and (4) predose testing is not recommended in rodent studies, and interim evaluation in chronic rodent studies is not considered necessary if clinical pathology data were evaluated in prior studies of shorter duration (see following section on kinetics for additional information on sampling frequency). An exception to this recommendation for rodents is that clinical pathology analysis may be appropriate if the chronic study is conducted at higher dose levels or uses a different dosing regimen. Although the harmonization recommendation states that reticulocyte counts are not routinely necessary, automated instrumentation has made this evaluation standard today and reticulocyte counts generally should be included as part of a standard hematology evaluation in animal studies.

Additional clinical pathology parameters to those identified in Table 10.2 should be added to study protocols as necessary to optimize achievement of study objectives for a specific test article. Investigators should consider the projected potential changes in clinical pathology analytes based on awareness of the chemical structure, pharmacologic and biological properties, and pathologic findings in past studies with the test article or related agents. Importantly, it is necessary to know that changes in clinical pathology parameters are, in fact, real consequences of test article exposure and do not represent interference with assay performance or any other artifactual influence.

The selection of clinical pathology analytes and timing of sample collection for analyte determination should always be considered on case-by-case basis for nonstandard rodent and nonrodent studies. For example, studies of very short duration (several hours to 2 days) may benefit from inclusion of different clinical pathology analytes and sampling times compared to a study of longer duration (3 months or longer). The evolution of technology within the clinical pathology laboratory has provided an opportunity to develop a variety of exploratory biomarkers that may require unique sampling times for optimal interpretation.

1.5. Kinetics

Understanding the expected rates of change in clinical pathology analytes over time in response to normal physiologic stimuli and pathologic conditions is necessary to ensure that the timing of sample collection and clinical pathology parameter selection are appropriate to detect a test article–related effect. The kinetics of each parameter should be considered unique and may vary by species. When possible, a series of related analytes collected over time can provide more information than a single analyte determination at one time point. For example, if myocardial injury occurs in a dog following a single test article administration, increased serum myoglobin and cardiac troponin (cTn) concentrations can be observed within 2 h of test article administration. An increase in creatine kinase (CK) activity may follow shortly (within 2–4 h after the myocardial injury), and an increase in AST activity may occur later at a time when myoglobin and cTn concentrations and CK activity may already have returned to baseline or control values. Alternatively, a test article that hinders normal erythropoiesis may not result in a decreased erythrocyte count, hemoglobin (Hgb) concentration, or hematocrit (Hct) values for at least 2 weeks after exposure in a dog due to the bone marrow reserve and life span of erythrocytes in that species (100–120 days).

Knowledge of many kinetic parameters including enzyme half-life; the production times, tissue transit times, and life span of specific blood cell types; and effects of various physiologic and pathologic stimuli on clinical pathology parameters is valuable for study design. For example, for test articles that are anticipated or proven to alter glucose concentration, an analyte that can increase [stress (corticosteroid or epinephrine effect) or glucagon] or decrease [insulin] concentrations rapidly, customized study phlebotomy times and more frequent blood draws might be needed during a 24–48 h study to demonstrate the rapid concentration changes possible with this analyte. Investigators of test articles that are expected to affect neutrophil or platelet numbers might need to measure CBCs at multiple time points in order to gain an understanding of the kinetics between test article administration and expected hematopoietic regenerative response. Test article–induced liver injury could warrant inclusion of a panel of liver enzymes with different serum activity half-lives in order to characterize the onset and recovery a from a single test article–induced liver insult. By virtue of their unique education and training, veterinary clinical pathologists are well suited to incorporate study-specific sampling intervals in study designs.

1.6. Controls

Concurrent vehicle control animals should be included as part of the study design for small animal (mice, rats, guinea pigs, hamsters, gerbils) safety assessment studies and should be matched for vendor, stock/strain, age, and sex to the test article–treated animals. In regulatory studies of large nonrodents (including dogs, pigs, and NHPs), in which blood may be collected for toxicokinetic or pharmacokinetic testing, samples collected from control animals must be the same volume and acquired on the same schedule as test article–treated animals to avoid misinterpreting procedural effects as test article effects. In order to reduce the number of large animals used in certain types of research (screening, pilot toxicity, and/or investigative studies), some study designs may not have a separate vehicle control group. In such situations, it is important that all test animals have blood drawn at least twice prestudy to evaluate clinical pathology parameters and determine approximate baseline values so that clinical pathology analytes posttest article administration can be compared to a larger database of prestudy values for determination of test article–related effects. Evaluation of clinical pathology parameters at least two times prestudy is also advantageous in repeat-dose toxicity testing in nonrodent studies in which a concurrent vehicle control group is used. Finally, clinical pathology results need to be reported in accordance with laboratory quality control procedures. General principles for consideration in designing the clinical pathology component of nonclinical toxicity studies are highlighted in Table 10.3.

TABLE 10.3 Considerations in the Design of the Clinical Pathology Component of a Nonclinical Toxicity Study

- Study objectives
- Scientific criteria
- Endpoints
- Study type (acute, subacute, subchronic, chronic, carcinogenicity)
- Species
- Test article characteristics
- Regulatory guidelines
- Practical aspects
- Appropriate controls

Table reproduced from Haschek WM, Rousseaux CG, Wallig MA, editors: Handbook of Toxicologic Pathology, *ed 2, 2002, Academic Press, Table V, p. 142, with permission.*

2. CLINICAL PATHOLOGY PARAMETERS COMMONLY INCLUDED IN PROTOCOLS FOR GENERAL TOXICITY STUDIES

2.1. Hematology

The broad functions of the hematologic system are to provide oxygen to cells in tissues via Hgb in erythrocytes, host defense and immunologic surveillance by leukocytes, and hemostasis by platelets. Potential hematologic effects of test agents are identified primarily by evaluation of the CBC comprised of the erythrogram, leukogram, and thrombogram.

Testing for hematology endpoints in nonclinical safety studies is aimed at identifying toxicity of the hematologic and lymphoid systems as well as aiding in the characterization of inflammation and immunotoxicity. Minimum testing recommendations for routine hematology evaluation in repeat-dose toxicity studies include an erythrocyte (red blood cell [RBC]) count; Hgb concentration; Hct; mean corpuscular volume (MCV); mean corpuscular hemoglobin concentration (MCHC); mean corpuscular hemoglobin (MCH); reticulocyte count; leukocyte (white blood cell [WBC]) count with absolute differential counts of multiple leukocyte classes (neutrophils, lymphocytes, monocytes, eosinophils, and basophils); platelet count; and preparation of blood and bone marrow smears (Table 10.2) (Tomlinson et al., 2013; Weingand et al., 1996).

Additional specialized parameters may be added to the standard panels based on study objectives, design, duration, test material, animal species, biological activity of the test article, and regulatory requirements. Platform and reagent accessibility may also influence test selection.

In some studies, cytological evaluation of blood and/or bone marrow smears may be necessary to confirm or complete the characterization of automated cell count data. While not required in regulatory guidelines, microscopic evaluation of hematologic cells is important to verify automated data, particularly in instances of abnormal values flagged by the instrument. Microscopic evaluation of blood smears is also important to identify platelet clumps, immature cells, and to assess cellular morphology, all which aid in the overall hematology assessment.

Erythrogram

The erythrogram is comprised of several erythroid measurements including RBC count, Hgb, Hct, and reticulocyte count as well as several erythrocyte indices (e.g., MCV, MCH, MCHC, red cell distribution width (RDW), corpuscular hemoglobin concentration mean (CHCM), and/or hemoglobin distribution width (HDW). The RBC count, Hgb, and Hct are often collectively referred to as "red cell mass" parameters. Erythrocyte indices are a collection of instrument-based calculations generated from direct measurements of various characteristics (i.e., size, density) of RBC populations. Although erythrocyte indices can sometimes be used to provide additional supportive or mechanistic information, they most often are limited in their interpretive value and largely reflect expected changes associated with RBC turnover (regeneration and kinetics). MCV is a measure of RBC size, while RDW relates to the degree of size variability overall in the RBC population; changes to these parameters can be used to help characterize erythropoietic activity of the bone marrow (see *Interpretation and Reporting of Clinical Pathology Results in Non-clinical Toxicity Testing* Vol 2, Chap 14). MCH, MCHC, CHCM, and HDW are indices related to Hgb content and the overall degree of variability of Hgb content with the RBC population. Unlike most of the erythrocyte indices including MCHC, CHCM is a direct measure of Hgb content

within RBCs which can be used in conjunction with other markers to help characterize certain hematologic abnormalities.

Enumeration of reticulocytes is an important aspect of an erythrogram as reticulocytes are anucleate but immature RBCs. Reticulocyte counts are an indicator of bone marrow regeneration and overall erythropoietic activity. Reticulocytes correspond to polychromatophilic erythrocytes on blood smear evaluation, and assessment should be made based on absolute rather than relative reticulocyte counts. Nucleated RBCs should also be enumerated by counting the number per 100 WBCs, which is typically done by the automated hematology analyzer and incorporated into cell count results.

Leukogram

The leukogram is comprised of the total leukocyte (WBC) count and differential leukocyte (relative and absolute) counts, which include neutrophils, lymphocytes, monocytes, eosinophils, basophils, and large unstained (or unclassified) cells (LUC, which are large peroxidase-negative cells that cannot be further categorized). Interpretation of leukocyte responses should be made based on absolute rather than relative percentage counts, even if the laboratory includes both absolute and relative percent differential counts in the report. Changes in the number of individual leukocyte types in blood reflect the balance of cell production and release to the blood, margination (adhesion to endothelial cells [ECs]), migration to tissues, and destruction/consumption. Microscopic evaluation of blood smears can reveal important morphologic alterations to leukocytes that can further aid in the characterization of pathologic processes, particularly those involving inflammation.

Thrombogram

The thrombogram is composed of tests that evaluate platelets or circulating platelet mass. The key components of the thrombogram are a count of platelet number and various calculated platelet indices; these parameters are core components of hemostasis testing in all nonclinical species. The numbers of platelets in circulation vary considerably by species and reflect a balance of production, destruction, consumption, and redistribution to tissues such as the spleen (Weiss and Wardrop, 2010). While the platelet count is the most frequently reported parameter in the thrombogram, other parameters may be measured by the analyzer, but not always reported, depending on the study protocol.

More recently developed measurements of platelets are available from some types of automated cell counting instruments. These new techniques include the following: thrombocrit, large platelets, mean platelet volume (MPV), and platelet distribution width (PDW). The thrombocrit (or plateletcrit) is the percentage of blood volume occupied by platelets and is an assessment of circulating platelet mass. MPV is the average volume of all the particles in a blood sample that are counted as individual platelets. PDW is a measurement of platelet anisocytosis (size differences) calculated from the distribution of individual platelet volumes. These biomarkers may provide additional data regarding platelet numbers and bone marrow response to treatment in some specialized studies, especially those in which serial determinations occur in a longitudinal fashion (Moritz & Becker, 2010; Jordan et al., 2014).

Additional biomarkers used to assess platelets qualitatively are available from certain automated cell counters and can be measured during routine CBCs. Mean platelet component and platelet component distribution width are two biomarkers that change in association with platelet activation and have proven helpful in some safety assessment studies in rodents, dogs, and NHPs.

2.2. Hemostasis

Hemostasis is the physiological process that stops bleeding at the site of vascular injury while maintaining normal blood flow elsewhere in the circulation. The hemostatic system is composed of the vasculature, platelets, and soluble coagulation and fibrinolytic factors. Blood loss is stopped by the formation of a hemostatic plug. The hemostatic process can be divided into three phases: primary hemostasis, secondary hemostasis, and fibrinolysis (Smith, 2010; Gale, 2011). These phases and the tests used to evaluate the processes are discussed in sections below.

Hemostasis Screening

Historically, screening of the hemostatic system in safety assessment studies has been focused on the identification of potential bleeding liabilities. For most studies, platelet counts, APTT, PT, and less frequently fibrinogen concentration are included in protocols as markers of hemostasis in rats, dogs, and NHPs. Results of these tests are correlated with clinical observations and macroscopic and microscopic tissue examination to assess hemostatic liabilities. An appropriate battery of other, more specialized hemostasis tests (e.g., fibrinogen/fibrin degradation products [FDPs], specific factor assays, measures of fibrinolysis, antithrombin activity, thrombin generation tests, thromboelastography and other viscoelastic assays, and overall hemostasis potential) can provide significant additional information for safety assessment of test agents (Brooks et al., 2017a; Lubas, Caldin, Wiinberg, & Kristensen, 2010; Smith, 2010). It is important to select the relevant tests in accordance with the characteristics of the test agent or toxicological events (Criswell, 2010).

Samples for Hemostasis Screening

Platelet counts and platelet biomarkers may be obtained from EDTA-anticoagulated blood when the CBC is measured on certain automated hematology analyzers. Most coagulation tests, such as the APTT, PT, and fibrinogen concentration, require platelet-poor plasma obtained from blood collected in citrate. However, many platelet function tests, such as adhesion and aggregation studies, require platelet-rich plasma obtained from citrated blood and therefore are not routine endpoints in toxicity studies.

Blood sample quality is essential for successful hemostasis testing. Blood samples should be collected from high-flow, large-caliber vessels such as the jugular vein, abdominal aorta, and/or vena cava in rats. Blood obtained by techniques that cause tissue trauma and platelet activation during sampling, such as periorbital sinus collection in rats, is unsatisfactory for hemostasis evaluations. Due to blood volume limitations, mice are rarely used for hemostasis assessment in safety assessment studies. In dogs, the jugular vein and less frequently the cephalic and/or saphenous veins are used for blood collection for hemostasis testing. In NHPs, blood is usually collected from the femoral vein. It is important to fill the blood collection tube properly and maintain a 9:1 ratio of blood:citrate anticoagulant. Vacuum blood tubes with citrate anticoagulant that are underfilled (too little blood) may result in artifactually prolonged APTT and PT. Vacuum blood tubes with citrate anticoagulant that are overfilled with blood (too little citrate) may result in clotted samples and potentially yield falsely shortened APTT and PT. The citrate-anticoagulated blood sample for hemostasis testing should be held at ambient temperature for delivery to the clinical pathology laboratory within 1 h and must be free of clots or hemolysis resulting from improper collection to be useful for coagulation testing (Lubas, Caldin, Wiinberg, & Kristensen, 2010; Adcock Funk et al., 2012).

Primary Hemostasis—Platelets Adhere and Aggregate

Primary hemostasis is the initial platelet response to vascular injury and consists of platelet adhesion/aggregation and activation at the site of vascular injury. Many drugs are known to affect platelet function (e.g., nonsteroidal antiinflammatory agents, β-lactam–containing antibiotics, cardiovascular drugs such as β-blockers and calcium channel blockers, psychotropic drugs, antihistamines, and some chemotherapeutic agents). Some drugs are designed to inhibit platelet function; most of these are platelet receptor antagonists (Gale, 2011).

Platelets may be assessed quantitatively (counts) or qualitatively (function). Commonly used quantitative tests for platelets consist of automated platelet counts, performed routinely as part of the CBC, and microscopic assessment of platelet numbers and platelet morphology in blood smears.

Historically, tests of platelet function are done less frequently due to the larger blood volume requirements for certain tests, lack of stability of the specimen that necessitates immediate analysis, and/or complicated test procedures that may not fit well into a safety assessment study. Tests to evaluate platelet function such as adhesion (measured indirectly as platelet aggregation ex vivo by collagen or adenosine 5′-diphosphate [ADP] or by measurement of von Willebrand

factor); platelet release reactions (e.g., release of ADP, serotonin, adenosine triphosphate); or clot retraction are not routinely conducted in animal toxicity testing but can be performed as warranted. Platelet aggregation testing assesses the aggregation response of platelets prepared in platelet-rich plasma, to various agents. There are marked species differences in platelet aggregation. In designing a study, it is imperative to know the characteristics of platelet aggregation in different laboratory animals. Although a complete review of this topic is beyond the scope of this chapter, a few pertinent characteristics are described below.

Critical components in platelet function testing are proper sample collection, without activation of platelets or evidence of clotting on blood smears, and selection of the appropriate agonist for the species. Rat platelets do not respond to arachidonic acid (AA) with sodium citrate as an anticoagulant; however, they do respond if heparin is used. Also, rat platelets do not respond to platelet-activating factor (PAF) since they do not have the receptor for PAF. Differences in platelet aggregation have been reported in Sprague–Dawley rat substocks from different breeders. There are large differences in dog platelet aggregation in response to AA and other agonists, attributed due to genetic differences in signaling through the thromboxane A_2 receptor. Preparation of platelet-rich plasma in cynomolgus monkeys is problematic because the specific gravity of their platelets is close to that of other blood cells. Therefore, the yield of platelets for testing may be low and will vary among individuals. Centrifugation conditions may need to be adjusted for each individual NHP. Guinea pig platelets are relatively close to human platelets in terms of reactivity and respond well to collagen, ADP, AA, and PAF (Johnson et al., 1993; Baker and Brassard, 2011).

Secondary Hemostasis—Clotting, Soluble Factors Generate Insoluble Fibrin

Secondary hemostasis refers to processes leading to the generation of insoluble fibrin from soluble factors in plasma to help anchor the primary platelet plug in place. The classic concept of secondary hemostasis, that thrombin generation by soluble coagulation factors leads to fibrin formation by a cascade of proteolytic reactions via a scheme encompassing intrinsic, extrinsic, and common pathways, has been superseded by a new cell-based model that consists of initiation, amplification, and propagation (Smith, 2010). The APTT (a measure of the intrinsic and common pathways) and the PT (a measure of the extrinsic and common pathways) are the core coagulation tests employed in safety assessment studies to identify potential liabilities for hemorrhage. Fibrinogen, a glycoprotein synthesized in the liver and found in alpha (α) granules of platelets, plays a central role in hemostasis by forming a cross-linking meshwork of fibrin when cleaved by thrombin. Plasma fibrinogen concentration (measured by thrombin time, also called the thrombin clotting time) is occasionally included in study protocols along with APTT and PT as a measure of the blood coagulation process. Very rarely, mixing studies of fresh plasma from a healthy animal and the plasma of the bleeding animal may be undertaken or specific factor assays may be requested to better explain conditions characterized by hemorrhage and prolongation of the PT and/or APTT. If needed, these infrequently requested tests are best performed by an experienced hemostasis reference laboratory (Gale, 2011).

Fibrinogen is also an APP that is increased in blood during systemic inflammation. When the APTT or PT is prolonged without a concurrent decrease in fibrinogen concentration and in the absence of obvious mechanisms for clinically relevant prolongation in APTT and/or PT (e.g., disseminated intravascular coagulation, decreased absorption of vitamin K, vitamin K antagonism, or liver failure), further investigation to evaluate specific coagulation factors may identify the target of the test agent effect. Although the liver synthesizes almost all clotting factors, the large hepatic functional reserve means that severe liver injury generally is required before coagulation times are affected (Gale, 2011).

Fibrinolysis—Clot Dissolution

Fibrinolysis is the physiologic process in which thrombi within the vasculature are proteolytically degraded to restore blood circulation. The zymogen (plasminogen) is converted to the active enzyme (plasmin) by plasminogen activators [tissue plasminogen activator or urokinase], and once activated, it will digest thrombi until inactivated by circulating inhibitory proteins (e.g., α2-macroglobulin or α2-antiplasmin). The cleaving action of plasmin upon fibrin within the thrombi results in generation of FDPs and D-dimers (the terminal FDP produced when factor XIII cross-links fibrin monomers to form fibrin). Determination of FDPs and D-dimers in plasma may be selectively included in protocols to assess fibrinolysis. Plasminogen/plasmin activities can be determined to assess plasminogen activation. Increased concentrations of FDPs and D-dimers are markers of systemic fibrinolytic states and disseminated intravascular coagulation.

Hypercoagulable and Prothrombotic States

Concerns associated with hypercoagulability and/or development of thromboembolic events have caused research on new test articles in development to be stopped and some drugs that have been approved previously for human use to be removed from the market due to cardiovascular safety liabilities. The Cardiovascular Biomarkers Working Group of the Health and Environmental Sciences Institute (HESI) produced a survey asking scientists to identify specific gaps in hemostasis testing in nonclinical and clinical development (Schultze et al., 2013). A need for better harmonization of hemostasis testing between nonclinical and clinical development scientists and a critical lack of tests to identify hypercoagulable and prothrombotic states in laboratory animals and people were identified as major concerns. Factors such as small blood volumes, especially in rodents; a lack of immunological reagents used in hemostasis testing that will cross-react with laboratory animal species; limited availability of certain types of hemostasis analyzers; and few reference laboratories that specialize in animal hemostasis testing were identified as hurdles to improved nonclinical testing for hypercoagulable and prothrombotic states. Recent studies from the HESI Cardiovascular Biomarkers Working Group and associated investigators have identified several tests of hemostasis that provide improved ability to detect hypercoagulable states in rats (Brooks et al., 2017a,b). Thrombin generation tests, antithrombin, thrombin–antithrombin complexes, viscoelastic assays, and fibrinolytic pathway assays such as overall hemostasis potential can be performed using citrated plasma, like that obtained for routine PT and APTT determinations. These assays require moderate amounts of plasma (0.5–1.0 mL). When combined with plasminogen/plasmin activity and FDPs and/or D-dimer testing, these tests may help determine if hypercoagulable or prothrombotic conditions exist in the blood and provide insight regarding whether the altered hemostatic balance occurred due to excessive clotting activity or decreased fibrinolytic activity.

2.3. Clinical Chemistry

Glucose, Cholesterol, and Triglycerides

In animal toxicity studies, changes in glucose, cholesterol, or triglyceride concentrations generally reflect metabolic events rather than direct target organ toxicities. These changes can be due to minor physiologic (i.e., nontoxic) effects such as postprandial increases in serum glucose or triglyceride concentrations, so measurement of these parameters is best performed on fasted samples. Glucose or lipid changes can also be primary manifestations of an intended pharmacology (e.g., decreased serum glucose concentration following insulin administration), secondary effects indirectly related to test article administration (e.g., stress-induced hyperglycemia), or preanalytical changes due to experimental procedures (e.g., artifactual hypoglycemia due to delayed sample processing and in vitro consumption of glucose by erythrocytes). Interpretation of changes in glucose, cholesterol, or triglyceride concentrations requires knowledge of clinical status, food consumption, experimental design, associated pathology findings, and, in some cases, pharmacology of the test article.

Serum glucose concentration is determined by the interplay between intestinal absorption, hepatic production, and tissue utilization. Circulating glucose levels are tightly regulated by pancreatic hormones such as insulin, which lowers serum glucose by increasing tissue uptake of glucose, and glucagon, which increases serum glucose concentration by stimulation of hepatic gluconeogenesis and glycogenolysis. Other hormones that can increase serum glucose concentrations include glucocorticoids, which stimulate hepatic gluconeogenesis and decrease glycogenolysis, and catecholamines and growth hormone, which increase glycogenolysis.

Circulating lipids in mammalian plasma or serum include sterols (primarily cholesterol and associated esters, steroid hormones, and bile salts); acylglycerols (such as mono-, di-, or triglycerides); fatty acids; phospholipids (such as phosphatidylcholine, the most abundant circulating phospholipid); and sphingolipids. Of these, serum or plasma cholesterol and triglyceride concentrations are most commonly evaluated in toxicologic clinical pathology.

Cholesterol and triglycerides are derived from dietary intake and endogenous synthesis. The liver is the primary site of cholesterol and triglyceride synthesis, but essentially all tissues can synthesize cholesterol, particularly intestinal epithelium, gonads, adrenal gland, and placenta. The liver is the primary route of cholesterol excretion. Due to their hydrophobicity, triglycerides and cholesterol circulate as chylomicrons or lipoprotein complexes of differing densities.

There are species differences in both cholesterol transport and metabolism. For example, low-density lipoprotein cholesterol is the predominant circulating form in humans and NHPs, while high-density lipoprotein cholesterol is the major form in rodents and dogs. Cholesterol is not catabolized within mammalian cells—rather it is eliminated in bile conjugated to taurine or glycine, or to a lesser extent excreted as free cholesterol. Bile acid synthesis and cholesterol excretion also differ between humans and rodents (Chiang, 2013). In mice and rats, the predominant bile acid (muricholic acid) is hydrophilic, whereas in humans the predominant bile acid (chenodeoxycholic acid) is hydrophobic. These differences impact bile flow, a major determinant of cholesterol excretion. For example, in the rat, the absence of a gall bladder and the greater hydrophilicity of bile salts lead to larger biliary water content and greater choleresis (bile flow) than other species including humans. Total cholesterol rather than cholesterol subfraction concentrations is normally measured in animal toxicity studies. These species differences in lipid metabolism and transport limit the translatability of animal results for human safety risk assessment.

Blood Urea Nitrogen and Serum Creatinine

Renal injury is typically monitored in nonclinical studies by blood urea nitrogen (urea or BUN), serum creatinine (sCr), and urinalysis. Urea and sCr are considered renal functional indicators and are used as surrogates for glomerular filtration. Urea is derived from protein catabolism by conversion of ammonia to urea by the hepatic urea cycle, and it passively crosses membranes and equilibrates throughout the total body water compartment. Urea concentration tends to underestimate glomerular filtration because of its distribution between the intravascular and extravascular space and because of tubular resorption, especially with low urine flow rates. Urea can be highly variable and is influenced by diet, protein turnover, and hydration status.

Creatinine is a product of muscle metabolism, and although it is also influenced by diet and skeletal muscle mass, sCr tends to be less variable or vulnerable to preanalytic effects than urea. Although routinely included in the chemistry panel on nonclinical studies, urea and sCr are relatively insensitive. Specifically, values for these two analytes are only increased in humans when more than half of renal function is lost (Bonventre et al., 2010; Ferguson et al., 2008), or in animal species when more than 75% of renal functional mass is lost (Hall, 2013).

Total Protein, Albumin, and Albumin/Globulin Ratio

Total serum protein concentration includes all plasma proteins except those consumed during clot formation, mainly fibrinogen and some other clotting factors. Albumin and globulins are the main plasma protein fractions. Albumin is synthesized by the liver and generally accounts for up to 60% of total serum protein concentration. Albumin serves many functions including providing approximately 75% of plasma colloid osmotic pressure (or oncotic pressure), serving as a carrier protein for plasma constituents that are not transported by specific carrier proteins, or as a nutritive reservoir for peripheral tissues. There is a direct correlation between body size and albumin turnover (e.g., plasma albumin half-life is 2 days in mice and 8 days in dogs). Albumin is a negative APP, decreasing during inflammation due to increased catabolism, decreased synthesis, hemodilution, and/or extravascular loss. Albumin is often considered as an indicator of liver function. However, hypoalbuminemia due to hepatic insufficiency is extremely rare in animal studies.

In addition to immunoglobulins, the globulin fraction includes carrier proteins, clotting factors, APPs, and enzymes. Most globulins other than immunoglobulins are synthesized by the liver. The globulin fraction is calculated by subtraction of albumin concentration from the total protein concentration, and the albumin/globulin ratio is often assessed to evaluate relative changes in these two fractions.

Calcium and Phosphorus

Serum calcium and inorganic phosphorus concentrations reflect the balance between intestinal absorption, bone formation or resorption and urine excretion, and are tightly regulated by parathyroid hormone, calcitonin, vitamin D, and/or fibroblast growth factor 23 (FGF 23). About 99% of total body calcium is present in bone, while the rest is present within intra- and extracellular compartments. About 40% of serum calcium is bound to protein (primarily albumin), 10% is bound to anions such as citrate or phosphate, and 50% of serum calcium is free. Free or ionized calcium is the biologically active form and plays a role in a many processes including cell signaling, neuromuscular function, bone formation and coagulation. Total calcium concentration is normally measured in animal safety studies, and in the absence of a pharmacologically mediated effect, minor changes in serum total calcium concentration largely follow changes in albumin concentrations and generally do not reflect a biologically important change. Where needed, ionized calcium concentration can be measured to more fully assess calcium changes.

Like calcium, inorganic phosphorus is primarily found in bone (~85%, as hydroxyapatite). Most of the nonbone phosphorus is present within cells as intracellular mono- and dihydrogen phosphate anions, with lesser amounts in serum or plasma. Nonbone inorganic phosphorus is involved in both intra- and extracellular buffering. It also plays a pivotal role in energy metabolism and is an essential component of cellular organelles and metabolic systems.

Sodium, Chloride, and Potassium (Electrolytes)

Electrolyte concentrations are determined by intake, excretion (mainly alimentary and renal), and shifts between intra- and extracellular fluid compartments. Sodium is the major cation in serum or plasma, and its concentration largely determines plasma osmolality and extracellular fluid volume. Potassium is the major intracellular cation and is maintained within narrow limits because of its critical role in neuromuscular and cardiac excitability. Chloride is the major anion in serum. Serum chloride concentration is influenced by extracellular concentrations of sodium and bicarbonate. Therefore, interpretation of serum chloride concentration may require knowledge of both serum sodium concentration and acid–base status.

Unlike sodium concentration, serum potassium concentration is a poor indicator of total body potassium because it is localized predominantly in the intracellular fluid and will shift between intra- and extracellular compartments in response to changes in acid–base balance. For example, increased serum potassium concentration may occur with acidosis due to exchange of extracellular fluid hydrogen ions for intracellular potassium ions, and decreased serum potassium concentration may arise from alkalosis. Electrolyte concentrations must be interpreted with knowledge of hydration status and consideration of the extracellular fluid volume. While reference intervals for sodium, potassium, and chloride can be broad, the range of values among animals in a well-controlled animal toxicity study is generally quite narrow. However, small, statistically significant differences in electrolyte concentrations between treatment groups and controls are often not biologically important.

Enzymes

Serum enzyme activities are commonly measured in clinical and nonclinical safety evaluation. Enzymes in serum are typically of cellular origin; can have varied specificity for tissues, cell types, or subcellular organelles; and have species differences in both circulating half-lives and tissue expression. The magnitude of increase in serum enzyme activity is determined largely by the severity of injury and the concentration gradient between the tissue and serum. The time course of serum enzyme changes is determined by subcellular localization, clearance rate, and level of expression (e.g., constitutively expressed or induced with injury).

Serum enzyme activity increases are typically associated with lethal cellular injury, but increased serum activity can result from sublethal or reversible cellular injury through cytoplasmic blebbing (Solter, 2005). Decreases in serum enzyme activity are generally not biologically important and can arise due to preanalytic variables (e.g., storage stability or sample handling), assay methodology, or decreased functional tissue mass; however, test article–related decreases in liver enzyme activities are occasionally seen. The diagnostic utility of a serum enzyme activity value thus depends on factors including tissue specificity, cellular and/or subcellular location, serum half-life, in vitro stability, and accuracy of the measurement.

Alanine Aminotransferase and Aspartate Aminotransferase

Alanine aminotransferase (ALT) and aspartate aminotransferase (AST) have been used as markers of hepatocellular injury since the 1950s (Karmen et al., 1955). Although often referred to as "liver function tests," ALT and AST are not indicators of liver function but rather indicators of hepatocellular degeneration or necrosis. While neither enzyme is liver-specific, ALT is predominantly localized in liver, with lower levels of activity in cardiac and skeletal muscle. AST is primarily localized in heart, skeletal muscle, and, to a lesser extent, liver (Clampitt and Hart, 1978). In common laboratory animals, pigs and guinea pigs are the exception to this tissue distribution as they possess low levels of hepatic aminotransferases; as a result, glutamate dehydrogenase (GLDH) and sorbitol dehydrogenase (SDH) are suggested markers of hepatocellular injury in these two species (Tomlinson et al., 2013). Both ALT and AST are cytosolic and mitochondrial, although ALT is predominantly cytosolic, and both are primarily localized in periportal rather than centrilobular regions of the liver.

ALT is an enzyme in the alanine–glucose cycle that catalyzes the reversible transfer of an amino group from alanine to α-ketoglutarate to form pyruvate and glutamate. ALT exists as two isoforms that are relatively well conserved with similar tissue distribution across species: ALT1 primarily localizes to kidney, liver, fat, and heart, while ALT2 is mainly localized in skeletal muscle and fat. Although immunoassays for specific ALT isoforms exist, to date they have not yet demonstrated improved specificity. Instead, total serum ALT activity is most commonly measured as a hepatocellular injury marker in nonclinical toxicity studies. Serum half-life for ALT is less than 8 h in rats and about 60 h in dogs and monkeys.

AST reversibly catalyzes the deamination of aspartate and α-ketoglutarate to form oxaloacetate and pyruvate. AST is involved in glycolysis and electron transport and plays a pivotal role in the maintenance of intracellular NAD^+/ NADH balance and in the malate–aspartate shuttle. AST is present in almost all tissues, although hepatocytes and skeletal muscle are the main sources of serum AST. Serum half-life of AST is generally shorter than ALT (e.g., less than 1 day for AST vs. 45–60 h for ALT in the dog).

One major factor affecting measurement of both ALT and AST activities is inclusion of the cofactor pyridoxal 5′ phosphate (P5P), the active form of vitamin B6, in the activity assay. Because decreased aminotransferase activity can occur with insufficient P5P, it is recommended that P5P be incorporated into aminotransferase assays to ensure that all potential activity present in a sample is detected (Tarrant et al., 2013).

Glutamate Dehydrogenase

GLDH is a mitochondrial enzyme involved in amino acid oxidation and ureagenesis. GLDH is primarily present in liver with minimal or trace expression in other organs including kidney, brain, skeletal muscle, small intestine, salivary gland, and leukocytes. Serum GLDH is thus considered to be liver-specific. In contrast with ALT, GLDH is present at highest concentrations in centrilobular hepatocytes and is not affected by skeletal muscle injury or inducible by corticosteroids (Schmidt and Schmidt, 1988). GLDH has a large dynamic range and its half-life is comparable to that of ALT in the rat (~5 h) but is shorter than ALT in the dog (16 vs. 45–50 h). In the rat, biological variability of GLDH increases with age, reducing the diagnostic utility of

GLDH in rats older than 3 months (York, 2013). GLDH is recommended as a hepatocellular injury marker in species such as pig and guinea pig that lack high levels of ALT expression in liver.

Sorbitol Dehydrogenase

SDH is a cytosolic enzyme that converts sorbitol into glucose and is present predominantly in the liver with only small amounts in other tissues. SDH is generally regarded as liver-specific and is sometimes included in clinical chemistry panels in animal studies, particularly in species with low hepatic ALT; however, SDH has a short half-life and is extremely labile, limiting its utility. Measurement of SDH (and/or GLDH) is useful when additional indicators of hepatic injury are desired or in species where ALT activity is either low or nonspecific.

Alkaline Phosphatase

ALP catalyzes the hydrolysis of organic phosphate esters, optimally at alkaline pH. Many tissues have ALP activity, but few tissues release enough ALP to affect serum activity. Key sources of ALP include epithelia (primarily the lumenal aspect of epithelial membranes) and skeletal tissue (bone, chondrocytes in biologically active regions, osteoblasts, and osteoid) (Miao and Scutt, 2002). In humans, there are four ALP isoenzymes: tissue-nonspecific ALP (which includes liver, bone, and kidney isoforms); intestinal (I-ALP); placental; and a germ cell isoenzyme found in testis and thymus. NHPs express all the human ALP isoenzymes except for the germ cell isoenzyme. Other animal species have tissue-nonspecific and I-ALP isoenzymes except for the dog, which has a unique corticosteroid-inducible isoenzyme produced in response to high levels of exogenous or endogenous corticosteroids. Post-translational modification of the tissue-nonspecific isoenzyme by addition of carbohydrate and lipid side chains creates different isoforms: L-ALP (liver, hepatocytes, and biliary epithelium); B-ALP (bone, osteoblasts); and kidney-ALP. Serum ALP activity is determined by age and circulating half-life. B-ALP is the predominant form in young animals and decreases with maturity, whereas L-ALP generally predominates in mature animals. Increases in serum L-ALP activity are usually due to hepatobiliary injury, although drugs metabolized in the liver (such as phenobarbital and phenytoin) may induce L-ALP in the dog. In the dog, serum half-life for L-ALP and B-ALP is about 3 days, whereas I-ALP is short-lived and contributes little to total ALP activity. I-ALP is the predominant isoenzyme in rodents, and activity can be increased in response to feeding or decreased with fasting/inanition. Total ALP activity is generally measured in animal studies. Although of questionable value for routine use, electrophoretic separation of liver, bone, and intestinal isoenzymes in serum can aid in the interpretation of increased serum ALP activity.

Gamma-Glutamyl Transferase

GGT is involved in amino acid transport as part of the γ-glutamyl cycle, most notably catalyzing the transfer of a γ-glutamyl group to peptides such as glutathione. GGT is present in the cell membranes of many tissues, with greatest activity in kidney (proximal tubule brush border), biliary epithelia, hepatocyte membranes bordering bile canaliculi, pancreas, mammary gland, spleen, lung, intestine, and even ciliary body in the eye. Although GGT is most highly expressed in the kidney, particularly in the rat, increased GGT activity in serum indicates hepatobiliary toxicity, particularly cholestasis. Unlike ALP, GGT activity does not change with bone disease or growth. In rodents, serum GGT activity is generally low or even undetectable in normal animals, and liver GGT has a short circulating half-life of as little as 30 min depending on level of sialylation (Huseby et al., 1992). Like ALP, increased plasma GGT activity in cholestasis may be due to stimulation of hepatic synthesis and release by increased bile acids or other biliary constituents during cholestasis. GGT activity is generally considered to be a less sensitive yet more specific indicator of cholestasis than ALP activity. Like ALP activity, certain drugs and steroids may induce GGT activity, particularly in the rat.

Creatine Kinase

CK exists as four major isoenzymes: CK-1 predominates in brain, CK-2 and CK-3 in cardiac and skeletal muscle, and CK-Mt in mitochondria of various tissues. Most serum CK originates from skeletal muscle. CK has a relatively short half-life (about 2–4 h) in all species, and activity

rapidly returns to normal following cessation of muscle degeneration or necrosis. Consequently, skeletal muscle injury is assessed using a weight-of-evidence approach by evaluating total CK activity with AST and ALT activities, and, in some species, skeletal troponin (Tn) I concentration.

5′Nucleotidase, Leucine Aminopeptidase, and Lactate Dehydrogenase

Enzymes such as 5′nucleotidase (5′NT), leucine aminopeptidase (LAP), and lactate dehydrogenase (LDH) are used infrequently in nonclinical safety assessment. 5′NT catalyzes the hydrolysis of nucleotides and is found in many tissues including liver, where it is located on the bile canalicular and sinusoidal aspects of hepatocellular epithelial membranes. Serum 5′NT activity is considered to be liver specific. LAP is a proteolytic enzyme that hydrolyzes amino acids, particularly leucine from the N-terminus of proteins and polypeptides. At least in humans, it is widely distributed in tissues; however, activity is highest in liver, where it is located mainly in biliary epithelium. LAP and 5′NT are used rarely in nonclinical or human clinical laboratory medicine and do not appear to confer any advantages over ALP or GGT as indicators of hepatobiliary pathology.

LDH isoenzymes are tetramers of either H or M subunits. All tissues contain various amounts of the five LDH isoenzymes, but skeletal muscle, liver, and RBCs are the main sources of serum LDH activity. The liver isoenzyme is a less sensitive indicator of hepatotoxicity than the aminotransferases, and due to lack of specificity, LDH is rarely included in nonclinical safety studies.

Bilirubin

Most bilirubin is derived from the degradation of heme from senescent erythrocytes by macrophages in spleen, liver, or bone marrow. Small amounts of bilirubin also are formed from degradation of other heme-containing proteins including myoglobin, various cytochromes, and catalase. Bilirubin is soluble in lipid but virtually insoluble in water; as a result, it is transported in the blood bound to albumin or conjugated with glucuronides. There are three forms of bilirubin: unconjugated, conjugated, and bilirubin-delta. Unconjugated bilirubin, which is noncovalently bound to albumin, is the main circulating form in plasma. Conjugated bilirubin is formed within hepatocytes by microsomal glucuronyl transferase–catalyzed conjugation with glucuronic acid to form bilirubin mono- and diglucuronides. Glucuronide conjugates are largely secreted by active transport into bile canaliculi by multidrug resistance–associated protein 2, with small amounts of conjugated bilirubin escaping into the plasma at the glomerulus that are resorbed in the proximal tubule. Bilirubin-delta, also known as biliprotein, is covalently or irreversibly bound to albumin and has a circulating half-life equivalent to that of albumin.

Direct and indirect bilirubin are differentiated by the van den Bergh method. In this technique, direct bilirubin in serum reacts quickly with diazotized sulfanilic acid, while total bilirubin is measured following addition of an alcohol as accelerator. Direct bilirubin is an estimate of conjugated bilirubin. Indirect or unconjugated bilirubin is the calculated difference between total and direct bilirubin concentrations. Conjugated hyperbilirubinemia is generally due to impaired bilirubin secretion or cholestasis, while unconjugated hyperbilirubinemia is usually the result of a hemolytic or hemorrhagic episode that overwhelms the uptake and conjugation capacity of the liver. Total bilirubin concentration is routinely measured in toxicity studies, with determination of conjugated (direct) bilirubin only if there is a large increase in total bilirubin concentration in the absence of evidence of hemolysis or cholestasis.

Bile Acids

While bilirubin is derived from the degradation of heme proteins, bile acids are a major product of hepatic cholesterol degradation. Within hepatocytes, cholesterol is degraded to primary bile acids such as cholic or chenodeoxycholic acid and then conjugated with taurine or glycine. Conjugated bile acids are then secreted into the biliary system and transported to the duodenum where they facilitate fat absorption. Primary bile acids can be reabsorbed in the ileum or progress into the large intestine where they are deconjugated and dehydroxylated by colonic bacteria to form the secondary bile acids deoxycholic or lithocholic acid. Primary and secondary bile acids are largely recycled by absorption into portal blood as part of the enterohepatic circulation. The enterohepatic circulation is very active;

for example, at steady state, the entire bile acid pool completes the cycle approximately 10 times a day in the dog (Hofmann, 1966). As a result, only very minimal amounts of bile acids are excreted in feces.

In health, most bile acids are present within the enterohepatic circulation with only low concentrations in peripheral blood. Serum total bile acid (TBA) concentration is generally considered less sensitive for the evaluation of hepatocellular injury and cholestasis than are enzyme activities and bilirubin. However, inhibition of the bile salt export pump (BSEP) is a known risk factor for hepatotoxicity, and in vitro profiling of test articles for BSEP inhibition can trigger TBA measurement in nonclinical studies.

2.4. Urinalysis

Standard Urinalysis

Urinalysis is commonly included in nonclinical toxicity study protocols and is used to assess kidney function, urinary tract health, and other metabolic disturbances in laboratory animal species. Although standard urinalysis endpoints are a regulatory requirement, routine urinalysis screening as performed in most toxicity studies is an imprecise tool as common assays are largely qualitative or semiquantitative. Routine urinalysis can be used effectively to screen for overt changes such as hematuria, pyuria, glucosuria, bilirubinuria, presence of casts, or abnormal crystalluria as well as providing general information regarding hydration and concentrating ability.

Components of urinalysis may vary slightly among laboratories. However, urinalysis panels usually contain the following: physical examination (volume, color, clarity, and specific gravity or osmolality); chemical examination by reagent strip methods (e.g., pH, protein, glucose, ketones, heme [occult blood], bilirubin, urobilinogen, and also potentially nitrite and leukocyte esterase); and microscopic examination of unstained or stained sediment to identify erythrocytes, leukocytes, bacteria, casts, crystals, epithelial cells, and other nondissolved materials (Table 10.4).

As opposed to quantitative measurement of urinary components which can be expensive and often unnecessary, reagent strip methods

TABLE 10.4 Routine Urinalysis Testing Parameters in Nonclinical Toxicity Studies

Physiochemical	Biochemical	Microscopic[a]
Volume	Protein	Sediment examination for:
Color	Glucose	
Clarity	Bilirubin	Crystals
Specific gravity	Occult blood	Casts
pH	Ketones	Blood cells (erythrocytes and leukocytes)
	Urobilinogen	
		Epithelial/malignant cells
		Infectious agents

[a] Not required.

Modified from Weingand K, Bloom J, Carakostas M, Hall R, Helfrich M, Latimer K, Levine B, Neptun D, Rebar A, Stitzel K, Troup C: Clinical pathology testing recommendations for nonclinical toxicity and safety studies, Toxicol Pathol 20:539–543, 1992; Weingand K, Brown G, Hall R, Davies D, Gossett K, Neptun D, Waner T, Matsuzawa T, Salemink P, Froelke W, Provost JP, Dal Negro G, Batchelor J, Nomura M, Groetsch H, Boink A, Kimball J, Woodman D, York M, Fabianson-Johnson E, Lupart M, Melloni E: Harmonization of animal clinical pathology testing in toxicity and safety studies. The joint scientific committee for international harmonization of clinical pathology testing, Fundam Appl Toxicol 29(2): 198–201, 1996; Tomlinson L, Boone LI, Ramaiah L, Penraat KA, von Beust BR, Ameri M, Poitout-Belissent FM, Weingand K, Workman HC, Aulbach AD, Meyer DJ, Brown DE, MacNeill AL, Bolliger AP, Bounous DI: Best practices for veterinary toxicologic clinical pathology, with emphasis on the pharmaceutical and biotechnology industries, Vet Clin Pathol 42(3):252–269, 2013.

(i.e., urine dipstick) are inexpensive semiquantitative screening assays used to detect relative amounts of protein, glucose, ketones, occult blood, and other biochemical constituents. Brief description of commonly utilized reagent strip assays is described below.

pH: Urine pH reflects renal regulation of blood bicarbonate and hydrogen ion concentrations and helps to characterize overall acid–base status. Urine pH is affected by diet, with high-protein/meat-based diets contributing to a low urine pH, and vegetable-based diets contributing to a high urine pH. In addition, urine pH will increase if samples are left standing for a prolonged period of time before analysis, as bacteria will convert urea to ammonia.

Protein: The protein reagent pad is most sensitive to albumin and should be interpreted while considering urine volume and specific gravity, as a small degree of proteinuria is of greater concern in dilute urine than in highly concentrated urine.

Occult Blood: The blood reagent pad detects Hgb, myoglobin, intact erythrocytes and methemoglobin with equal sensitivity. Urine sediment exam and other ancillary tests (blood smear examination, hematology data, and CK measurement) may help differentiate the origin of a positive reaction.

Glucose: The renal threshold of the proximal tubules varies by species and is above 180 mg/dL in humans and dogs and above 280 mg/dL in cats. Glucosuria in the absence of elevated blood glucose concentrations may indicate proximal tubule injury or dysfunction.

Ketones: Ketones are not normally detected in the urine. Their presence in urine (i.e., ketonuria) is typically a consequence of negative energy balance, with a shift from carbohydrates to lipids for energy production.

Bilirubin: A small amount of bilirubin can occur in the urine of dogs (particularly males), but otherwise is not normally detected. The presence of bilirubin in the urine may occur secondary to hemolysis or hepatobiliary disease.

Urobilinogen: A positive urobilinogen reaction indicates a patent bile duct, and increased concentrations may be seen secondary to hemolysis or decreased liver function.

Nitrites: The nitrite reagent pad is used to screen for bacteria (nitrate reducing) but is unreliable in animal urine.

Leukocytes: The leukocyte reagent pad detects leukocyte esterase and is used in humans to detect leukocytes in the urine but is unreliable in animal urine.

Whether conduct of urine sediment examination is warranted for all test article–treated and control groups in studies is frequently questioned, and sediment evaluations are not a regulatory requirement. Determining whether or not to incorporate this endpoint is best decided on a case-by-case basis according to study objectives, experience in previous studies, and characteristics of the test article.

It is recommended that timed urine collections (e.g., overnight or 16 h) and urinalysis be conducted at a time interval(s) that matches hematology and clinical chemistry evaluations. Testing should be done on fresh urine (less than 1 h from collection if possible) that is uncontaminated. Delay in performing urinalysis results in the potential for deterioration of cellular components, in vitro crystal formation/dissolution, and bacterial overgrowth (Osborne & Stevens, 1999).

Quantitative Urinalysis

Although not included among core requirements, several urine chemistry tests have been used to enhance the detection of early kidney injury in nonclinical toxicity studies. Unlike most standard urinalysis endpoints that are qualitative or semiquantitative, quantitative urinalysis describes the method of characterizing the amount of a substance(s) excreted by kidneys when measured over a defined time period. Measurements of urine protein, albumin, glucose, creatinine, and other renal biomarkers (e.g., N-acetyl-β-D-glucosaminidase [NAG], kidney injury molecule-1 [KIM-1], and neutrophil gelatinase–associated lipocalin [NGAL]) (also see "Renal Biomarkers" section below) are incorporated into some study protocols when conducting mechanistic investigations of renal toxicity (Dieterle et al., 2010; Ennulat, Ringenberg, & Frazier, 2018) and can provide meaningful information related to renal injury/function. Fractional excretion of electrolytes (e.g., sodium, chloride, potassium) is included in some nonclinical toxicity studies to aid in characterizing alterations in renal electrolyte excretion. However, these data often have a high degree of inter-animal (differences among individuals of a population) and intra-animal (degree of normal physiologic variation within a single individual) variability and have numerous extrarenal influences (e.g., hydration, diet, fasting) to consider when interpreting results.

Because quantitative analytes in urine are often impacted by overall urine concentration, it is imperative that all urine chemistry tests be normalized to urine concentration and/or volume over time. As a result, these endpoints should be expressed as a function of rate of excretion relative to the clearance of creatinine (x/creatinine ratio) or rate over a defined collection period (x/16 h).

2.5. Bone Marrow Evaluation

Bone marrow histopathology and cytology are routinely assessed on definitive nonclinical studies. Histopathologic evaluation of bone marrow provides assessment of overall hematopoietic cellularity, maturation and cellularity of megakaryocytes, relative proportions and maturation of erythroid and granulocytic series, and marrow stromal architecture. Cytologic evaluation of bone marrow is a second-tier assessment sometimes used to characterize changes in hematopoietic cellularity observed by histopathology, to differentiate early hematopoietic precursors, or to assess maturation progression of hematopoietic lineages. Bone marrow flow cytometry also can be used to evaluate marrow hematopoiesis, but it should be used in conjunction with cytologic evaluation, particularly if hematopoietic cell morphology changes are suspected based on changes in peripheral blood. Bone marrow histopathologic and cytologic findings must be interpreted in the context of other study findings, most notably hematology changes observed in the peripheral blood as well as endpoints including food consumption and body weight changes, toxicokinetics, and dose response.

Cytologic evaluation of bone marrow smears is not recommended as a routine endpoint, although smears stained with Romanowsky stains are often prepared to allow for retrospective evaluation as necessary. Because hematopoietic cells are labile, bone marrow smears should ideally be the first sample collected at necropsy to preserve cytologic detail. Qualitative and often quantitative microscopic evaluations are sometimes performed to assess morphology and relative number and maturation of the different hematopoietic cell lines. The most common and simplest quantitative cytologic evaluation of marrow cells is the myeloid:erythroid (M:E) ratio, which includes all maturation stages of myeloid versus nucleated erythroid cells. However, the M:E ratio adds little value over peripheral blood cell counts and bone marrow histopathology as it reflects nothing more than the relative proportion of myeloid and erythroid lineages. A more labor-intensive and informative evaluation is the bone marrow differential cell count (typically of 300–500 nucleated cells) which provides information on both the relative proportion and maturation status of hematopoietic cells and thus mechanistic information (Reagan et al., 2011a,b; Hall and Everds, 2014).

The decision on whether to evaluate cytologic smears should be done on a case-by-case basis.

Bone marrow smear evaluation may be justified when there are unexplained peripheral blood changes in a particular cell lineage since histopathology is unable to reliably discriminate cell types and cytomorphologic changes of hematopoietic precursors. Evaluation of bone marrow smears also may be necessary to determine whether alterations in bone marrow cellularity are due to erythroid versus lymphoid cells, particularly in rodents which have more lymphocytes in bone marrow than nonrodents. Cytologic evaluation may not be needed when there are known effects on food consumption or body weight, particularly in rats (Levin et al., 1993), or for biopharmaceutical effects that occur at very high doses or exposure multiples. Bone marrow cytology is also not needed to characterize changes in peripheral blood and bone marrow histopathology that are adaptive or regenerative, or for decreased peripheral lymphocyte counts regardless of species since lymphocytes recirculate extensively between the lymphoid tissues and peripheral blood. Third-tier mechanistic studies including in vitro clonogenic assays and electron microscopy are infrequently used to characterize effects on the hematopoietic system.

2.6. Flow Cytometry

Over the past decade, the use of flow cytometry evaluation has steadily increased in nonclinical toxicity studies. This trend has largely been driven by the increasing availability of instrumentation and improved technical capability of laboratories, but also can be attributed to increased numbers of immunomodulating test articles requiring more thorough assessment of the immune and lymphoid systems. Standard flow cytometry is used most often in nonclinical toxicity studies to characterize lymphocyte subpopulations (e.g., T-cells, B-cells, helper T-cells, cytotoxic T-cells) in peripheral blood or quantify bone marrow hematopoietic subpopulations (granulocytic vs. erythroid cells; maturing vs. proliferating pools). Flow cytometric analysis of bone marrow is still relatively uncommon as light microscopy continues to be the gold standard for screening. However, lymphocyte subtyping analysis by flow cytometry has become a core expectation of contemporary immunotoxicology testing paradigms and often overlaps with the hematology assessment (see *Special Techniques in Toxicologic Pathology* Vol 1, Chap 11).

3. NONSTANDARD BIOMARKERS

3.1. Introduction

Biomarkers are playing an increasingly important role in pharmaceutical development and are receiving increased attention from both regulators and industry. Unlike traditional clinical pathology and other well-established testing methods, commercially available first-to-market biomarker kits often use ligand-based (immunoassay) testing methods and reagents that vary greatly in their quality, performance, and overall value. Despite the availability of a multitude of commercial kits from numerous vendors, the extent of assay characterization and critical reagent performance of these assays is often insufficient to support their use, especially as a routine element of conventional animal toxicity studies undertaken for safety assessment. Commercial biomarker kits and their associated reagents are not consistently regulated, monitored, or standardized. These factors result in inconsistent and sometimes improper use and application of biomarkers across different organizations/laboratories and emphasize the importance of stringent validation and assay characterization practices.

3.2. Biomarker Assay Kits

Two main categories of commercial biomarker kits are used in drug development and research purposes. These include in vitro diagnostic assays (IVD) and "Research Use Only" (RUO) assays. IVD assays make up a large majority of the traditional clinical pathology assays as well as several of the newer biomarker kits. These assays have been approved by the FDA (defined in 21 CFR 809.33) for an intended use in human clinical diagnosis or patient care and undergo intensive monitoring and regulation of material manufacture, distribution, and use in clinical laboratories (Khan et al., 2015). For these reasons, traditional clinical pathology assays and IVD biomarker tests are better characterized, standardized from laboratory to laboratory, and generally have better performance characteristics than novel first-to-market biomarker assays. Conversely, most commercially available novel biomarker kits used in nonclinical laboratories fall under the RUO category. Assays that are labeled as RUO are exempt from regulatory requirements and approvals that would be needed for clinical diagnosis or patient management. Since there are no rigorous requirements or guidelines for the RUO label, the extent of manufacturing quality compliance, assay characterization, and documentation vary considerably across different vendors and from assay to assay. Hence, most novel biomarker assays are not standardized among laboratories and require a robust performance characterization and validation prior to use for other than discovery research purposes.

3.3. Fit-for-Purpose (Analytical) Validation

The fit-for-purpose paradigm has been in use for over a decade and was initially described in 2006 with an intention to provide a framework for the validation and performance characterization of ligand-binding (immunoassay) biomarker kits (Lee et al., 2006). The core principle of the fit-for-purpose approach involves executing a performance characterization/validation equal in robustness to the intended use of the data being generated. Briefly, the key elements included in a fit-for-purpose validation/performance characterization include preparation of a validation plan; testing of dynamic range, precision, and accuracy; establishment of quality control and normal baseline ranges in species-specific sample material (e.g., serum/plasma/urine); and assessments of short- and long-term stability.

3.4. Biologic Validation

As critical as it is to verify sound analytical performance of a method, it is just as important to verify the biologic activity of any given biomarker. Biologic validations test the applicability of a proposed biomarker in a biologic setting. Is the biomarker giving you the expected response in relation to a known stimulus? Although it is neither necessary nor productive to use animals to generate positive control data in every case due to cost, animal welfare concerns, and availability of published method reports, in circumstances where the assay is relatively novel or unproven, it may be necessary to generate positive controls in vivo to substantiate the utility of the biomarker in a real-world setting. Biologic validation exercises also often incorporate traditional clinical pathology and/or anatomic pathology assessments in order to gain a better understanding of biomarker signals in relation to standard toxicity endpoints.

3.5. Biomarker Application in Nonclinical Studies

Inherent to the use of biomarker assays in animal toxicity studies is an understanding of what constitutes a definitive signal. Biomarker assays generally have much higher background variability than traditional clinical pathology tests. Thus, it remains crucial for the interpreting scientist to understand the inherent variation of the specific assay/reagent set based on the analytical validation data for a given species as well as the inter- and intra-animal variability over time and within a population. Once a definitive signal has been identified, a thorough understanding of what a signal represents in biological terms is fundamental to accurate hazard identification. For example, some cardiac biomarkers are indicators of direct cardiac myocyte injury (cTns), while others are indicators of a functional defect (natriuretic peptides). The renal biomarker NGAL is an indicator of renal tubular injury but can also be seen in cases of systemic and urinary tract inflammation (Han, Li, Liu, & Cong, 2012).

3.6. Hormones

Hormone concentrations are not routinely measured in animal toxicity studies, although serum hormone data are sometimes requested by regulatory agencies or are needed to provide context for study findings. For example, measurement of hormone levels may be useful for characterizing the mode of action of a test article, informing the safety risk assessment, or providing a translatable marker for monitoring potential clinical toxicities. Hormone concentrations can be highly variable and are influenced by factors such as pulsatility or pattern of secretion, diurnal or circadian rhythm, feeding status, sex, stage of the reproductive cycle, and even study duration. As a result, hormone assessment is ideally used in dedicated investigative (i.e., hypothesis-driven) studies. Addition of serum hormones as a terminal endpoint to other clinical pathology parameters on conventional nonclinical studies is generally not recommended.

Hormones, particularly reproductive hormones, should always be evaluated in the context of histopathologic findings, organ weight changes in hormone-responsive tissues, and target organ pharmacology (Stanislaus et al., 2012; Chapin and Creasy, 2012; Andersson, Rehm, Stanislaus, & Wood, 2013). Hormones most commonly assessed in association with morphologic changes in animal studies include male (testosterone, follicle-stimulating hormone [FSH], luteinizing hormone [LH]) and female (estrogen, progesterone) reproductive hormones; thyroid hormones including triiodothyronine (T3), thyroxin (T4), and thyroid-stimulating hormone (TSH); hormones of the hypothalamic–pituitary–thyroid (thyrotropin-releasing hormone [TRH] and TSH) and hypothalamic–pituitary–adrenal (corticotropin-releasing hormone [CRH], adrenocorticotropic hormone [ACTH], cortisol) axes; and markers of endocrine homeostasis (insulin and glucagon). Other less commonly measured hormones in animal studies include prolactin, natriuretic peptides, oxytocin, vasopressin, growth hormone and associated growth hormone axis hormones, eicosanoids, and pharmacodynamic hormone markers such as adiponectin.

General considerations for evaluation of hormones in animals include species relevance with respect to human risk assessment, biologic context, target organ histopathology, sampling regimen, experimental design, and species differences. For example, cortisol is the most abundant adrenal glucocorticoid in humans and dogs, corticosterone is the primary glucocorticoid in rodents, and rabbits produce both cortisol and corticosterone. Understanding these types of species differences is important in determining the appropriate hormones to measure. Interpretation of hormone concentrations should always include the assumption that a change in serum concentration for a given hormone may not necessarily reflect a primary disorder of the respective endocrine organ per se. For example, decreased free T4 concentrations can be the result of nonthyroid diseases including

hyperadrenocorticism, systemic inflammation, or treatment with agents such as prednisolone, sulfonamides, or phenobarbital.

Measurement of functionally related rather than individual hormone levels is critical because individual hormones are interdependent components of complex and tightly regulated hormonal axes that are generally controlled by the hypothalamus and pituitary gland. For example, T3, T4, and TSH are often measured together in rat studies where increased thyroid weight and thyroid follicular cell hypertrophy or hyperplasia were noted to confirm that these findings are caused by induction in liver of drug-metabolizing enzymes. Specifically, induction of T4-uridine diphosphate–glucuronyl transferase (UDPGT) would be expected to cause decreases in serum T4 and T3 levels and a compensatory increase in TSH (Curran and DeGroot, 1991). Many hormones circulate bound to carrier proteins, but species differences in both the carrier protein or its quantity or binding affinity may influence hormone turnover and data interpretation. For example, T3 and T4 circulate bound to the high-affinity thyroglobulin and the lesser affinity albumin in humans, NHP and dogs, while rodent T3 and T4 only bind albumin. Because albumin has lower binding affinity for thyroid hormones, rodent thyroid hormones have larger free circulating fractions and shorter circulating half-lives (e.g., T4 half-life is ≤24 h in rat vs. 5–9 days in human). As a result, rodent thyroid glands are more active and more sensitive to TSH overstimulation than human thyroid glands. Because of these species-specific differences in thyroid physiology, changes in the rat thyroid gland morphology and activity associated with induction of hepatic drug-metabolizing enzymes are of limited relevance for human safety.

Most hormones are secreted in a diurnal or pulsatile rhythm which can be influenced by environmental or feeding effects, leading to large variability that can make interpretation of endocrine data challenging, particularly if samples are collected at a single time point. Species differences in hormone pulsatility exist, but in general, release of hormones such as LH, FSH, and testosterone is pulsatile (except for LH and testosterone in rats), while T3 and T4 are not pulsatile (Stanislaus et al., 2012; Andersson, Rehm, Stanislaus, & Wood, 2013).

Investigators use several techniques to address variability in hormone concentrations. These include power analyses to determine the appropriate sample size needed to detect a meaningful change based on the inherent variability of that parameter, measurement of serial samples with calculation of an area under the curve unique for each animal based on as few as six time points per animal (Stanislaus et al., 2012), and, in the case of female reproductive hormones, sampling based on the stage of the estrus cycle as determined by vaginal smear cytology. Such experimental designs can require large group sizes. Other considerations related to sampling and study design include use of baseline measurements and longitudinal sampling over time, particularly in nonrodent species where group sizes are small and blood sample volume is less limiting relative to rodents, and collection of samples at the same time of day, all of which can create logistical challenges in large studies. Most importantly for hormone evaluation, minimizing stress associated with blood collection by limiting transport prior to sampling, separating housing or treatment areas from necropsy rooms, and use of decapitation or short duration anesthetics for euthanasia are advised to reduce the effects of stress on hormone concentrations.

3.7. Acute Phase Proteins

APPs are circulating blood proteins primarily synthesized in the liver in response to upstream inflammatory signals. APPs are used in context with other markers of inflammation to identify subtle inflammatory/immune signals. APPs can either be positive APPs, which increase with inflammation (e.g., fibrinogen, C-reactive protein [CRP], haptoglobin, serum amyloid A or P), or negative APPs (e.g., albumin), which decrease with inflammation. APPs have species-specific differences in expression patterns and can be classified as either a major (increase 10–100×) or minor (increase 2–10×) APP in any given species depending on the magnitude of change in response to an inflammatory stimulus (Table 10.5). It is critical to understand which APP is most appropriate for the test species in order to avoid mischaracterization of test article liabilities. For example, in the NHP, CRP is a major APP with pronounced increases in response to inflammatory stimuli, while in

rodents the CRP response will be comparatively minor or nonexistent (Cray et al., 2009). Results from APP biomarkers should always be interpreted in context with other inflammatory biomarkers (e.g., hematology, serum cytokine concentrations, etc.). APP assays are widely available on both automated clinical chemistry analyzers and as single or multiplex enzyme-linked immunosorbent assay platforms.

3.8. Novel Renal Biomarkers

Collaborations in consortia among industry, academia, and regulatory agencies have led to the qualification of or regulatory support for use of several novel and traditional urinary proteins for evaluation of acute drug-induced kidney injury (DIKI) in rats (FDA, 2020a,b). Many of these biomarkers have also been evaluated in humans (Brott et al., 2014, 2015) and, in a few cases, in nonrodent species in single toxicant experimental studies. However, formal regulatory qualification of urinary biomarkers across a wide range of toxicants in nonrodents has not been done.

Urinary markers recently qualified in rats, such as urine albumin, protein, NAG, α-glutathione S-transferase (α-GST), and glucose have been in use for decades. Other novel urinary protein markers such as KIM-1, lipocalin-2 (or NGAL), and clusterin were recently identified using genomics (Han et al., 2002; Thompson et al., 2004). Most urine markers are functionally and biologically conserved across species. They include proteins such as albumin or cystatin C that enter the urine passively by glomerular filtration, constitutively expressed proteins such as NAG or α-GST that enter urine following tubular injury, and inducible proteins such as KIM-1, NGAL, or clusterin that are upregulated in various regions of the nephron with renal injury.

Because of the biology unique to each marker, urinary marker changes can be used to characterize the location, timing, and extent of DIKI based on the pattern of marker changes. For example, KIM-1 is upregulated in proximal tubule epithelium in response to injury and will appear in urine later than a constitutively expressed proximal tubule injury marker such as NAG, which is rapidly released upon tubular injury. Segment-specific functional and structural injury markers are generally available for

TABLE 10.5   Positive Acute Phase Proteins (APPs) in Various Laboratory Animal
Species

Species	Major APP	Minor APP
Rat	α1-acid glycoprotein α2-macroglobulin	C-reactive protein Fibrinogen Haptoglobin
Mouse	Haptoglobin Serum amyloid A Serum amyloid P	C-reactive protein Fibrinogen
Nonhuman primate	C-reactive protein	α2-macroglobulin Fibrinogen Serum amyloid A
Dog	C-reactive protein Serum amyloid A	α1-acid glycoprotein ceruloplasmin Haptoglobin
Pig	Haptoglobin Serum amyloid A Major acute phase protein	α1-acid glycoprotein
Rabbit	Haptoglobin Serum amyloid A	α1-acid glycoprotein C-reactive protein Fibrinogen

Adapted from Cray et al., 2009.

common laboratory animal species for the evaluation of injury to proximal tubules, which are the predominant site of renal injury in DIKI. The exception to this is renal papillary antigen-1 (RPA-1), a marker of collecting duct injury that is only available for rat (Harpur et al., 2011). Traditional markers of proximal tubular injury or functional loss such as urine NAG, albumin, protein or glucose excretion can be used in all animal species and essentially perform as well as the newer markers. A subset of the urinary markers most commonly used in nonclinical studies, their localization, function or biology, and species applicability is detailed in Table 10.6.

While many of these markers monitor similar types of renal function or injury, they are often evaluated together because of differences in marker biology, qualification status, assay availability, or storage stability. For example, low-molecular weight markers such as β2-microglobulin, retinol-binding protein, or cystatin C freely pass the glomerular filtration barrier, and their presence in urine suggests impaired or saturated tubular absorption. In contrast, intermediate- or high-molecular weight proteinuria (albuminuria or proteinuria) may indicate concomitant glomerular and tubular disease. Urinary proteins such as KIM-1 or RPA-1 can localize renal injury to the proximal or distal (collecting duct) nephron, respectively, and can be upregulated in response to renal injury (KIM-1) or constitutively expressed (RPA-1). In contrast, clusterin and NGAL can be upregulated throughout the nephron with nephrotoxic injury. It should be noted that while KIM-1 performs well in the rat, it has not been useful in the dog despite use of dog-specific assays (Wagoner et al., 2017). NGAL and clusterin have been demonstrated to be effective in rat, dog, NHP, and minipig (Waggoner et al., 2017; Gautier et al., 2016; Phillips et al., 2016).

In summary, the properties of numerous urinary biomarkers and their potential value as noninvasive indicators of renal injury have been extensively investigated in rats. Translation of a number of these markers to other animal species and the human clinical setting is ongoing.

TABLE 10.6 Selected Urinary Biomarkers in Nonclinical Safety Studies with Regulatory Qualification Status (rat) and Assay Availability (dog, nonhuman primate (NHP) and minipig)

Urinary Marker	Regulatory Status (rat)	General Comments	Dog	NHP	Minipig
PROXIMAL TUBULE–SPECIFIC INJURY MARKERS					
KIM-1	Q	Upregulated with proximal tubular injury, functions in tubular repair as epithelial scavenger receptor for phosphatidylserine-mediated phagocytosis. Chronic upregulation associated with interstitial fibrosis in mice. Does not perform as well in humans or nonrodent species as in rat. Limited usefulness in dog regardless of canine-specific assay used.	X	X	
NAG	Q	Lysosomal enzyme that enters urine with proximal tubular injury. Automated measurement. Inhibited by endogenous urea, poor storage stability.	X	X	X
α-GST	NQ	Proximal tubular brush border enzyme involved in xenobiotic metabolism, also serum liver injury marker, so must be interpreted with other clinical chemistry and liver histopathology findings, poor urine stability.			
Glucose	n/a	Sensitive marker of impaired renal function since proximal tubule is site of >90% urinary glucose absorption. Must be interpreted with serum/plasma glucose concentration.	X	X	X
INTERMEDIATE TO HMW MARKERS OF GLOMERULAR/ TUBULAR DAMAGE					
Albumin	Q	Urinary albumin excretion is highly specific for renal injury, but immunoassays underestimate severity of renal injury due to proximal tubular resorption/excretion of variably sized nonimmunoreactive albumin fragments	X	X	X

(Continued)

TABLE 10.6 Selected Urinary Biomarkers in Nonclinical Safety Studies with Regulatory Qualification Status (rat) and Assay Availability (dog, nonhuman primate (NHP) and minipig)—cont'd

Urinary Marker	Regulatory Status (rat)	General Comments	Dog	NHP	Minipig
Protein	Q	Less specific for renal injury than urinary albumin because of potential extrarenal contamination	X	X	X
LMW MARKERS OF PROXIMAL TUBULAR INJURY WITH NORMAL GLOMERULAR FUNCTION					
β2-microglobulin	Q	Qualified in rat, demonstrated utility in the clinic, but poor stability at room temperature and in acid urine			
Cystatin C	Q	Comparable to other LMW markers including β2m, α1m, and RBP; therefore, can be substituted for species-specific assays. Demonstrated utility in clinic.	X	X	
α1-microglobulin	n/a	Comparable to other LMW markers. May be increased with inflammation. Demonstrated utility in human AKI as well as chronic interstitial nephritis.		X	
GENERAL RENAL INJURY MARKERS					
Lipocalin-2 (NGAL)	LOS	25 kD transport protein originally found in neutrophil-specific granules, induced with injury in many epithelia, in kidney primarily in distal nephron. Urinary NGAL is an early renal injury marker with a large dynamic range in many species and has excellent predictivity of AKI in a variety of clinical settings. Serum increases due to systemic inflammation or sepsis can cause increased urine levels in the absence of renal injury.	X		X
Clusterin	Q	Inducible antiapoptotic protein secreted by all nucleated cells, upregulated throughout kidney with renal injury. Clinical utility to be determined.	X	X	

TABLE 10.6 Selected Urinary Biomarkers in Nonclinical Safety Studies with Regulatory Qualification Status (rat) and Assay Availability (dog, nonhuman primate (NHP) and minipig)—cont'd

Urinary Marker	Regulatory Status (rat)	General Comments	Dog	NHP	Minipig
Osteopontin (OPN)	LOS	Extracellular matrix phosphoprotein produced in bone and epithelia, in kidney upregulated primarily distal thick ascending limb and distal tubule. Clinical utility to be determined.		X	
OTHER DISTAL NEPHRON MARKERS					
Calbindin D28	n/a	Ca-binding protein in distal tubule and early collecting duct of most species		X	
RPA-1	Q	Constitutive HMW glycoprotein in rat collecting duct—no human ortholog, not available for other animal species			

α1m, α1-microglobulin; *α-GST*, α Glutathione S-Transferase; *β2m*, β2-microglobulin; *AKI*, acute kidney injury; *HMW*, high molecular weight; *KIM-1*, Kidney injury molecule-1; *LMW*, low molecular weight; *LOS*, Letter of Support (regulatory support for the potential value of a candidate marker encouraging further evaluation); *n/a*, not applicable; *NAG*, N-acetyl-β-D-glucosaminidase; *NGAL*, neutrophil gelatinase–associated lipocalin; *NQ*, not qualified; *Q*, qualified (i.e., regulatory acceptance for reliability of interpretation and applicability within a specific context of use); *RBP*, retinol-binding protein; *RPA-1*, Renal papillary antigen-1.

These markers can provide insight into the location, severity and duration of nephrotoxic injury. However, inclusion of novel urinary biomarkers in toxicity studies slated for regulatory review requires careful selection of the most relevant analyte(s) on a case-by-case basis.

3.9. New Liver Biomarkers

Drug-induced liver injury (DILI) is the most common cause of safety-related attrition in drug development (Kaplowitz, 2005). Hepatobiliary markers in current use to monitor hepatotoxicity, such as ALT, AST, GGT, and ALP, have been used for decades. These markers generally lack sensitivity, specificity, or predictivity for liver injury and provide limited mechanistic insight. As a result, candidate novel markers of liver injury are being explored, primarily in clinical settings or biomarker consortia (Church et al., 2019; Fu et al., 2020), with limited evaluation in animal models or metaanalyses of nonclinical studies (Bailey et al., 2019). Some of the most promising markers are briefly discussed below and summarized in Table 10.7.

Several clinical DILI markers have recently received regulatory letters of support. These include microRNA-122 (miR-122), GLDH, osteopontin (OPN), macrophage colony-stimulating factor receptor (MCSFR), and keratin 18 (K18) (Church et al., 2019).

MicroRNAs such as the liver-specific miR-122 offer advantages over protein or enzymatic markers. They are readily translatable across species because of sequence conservation and are stable in samples during long-term storage. Increases in miR-122 with liver injury generally precede changes in traditional hepatobiliary markers in rats, dogs, and humans. However, miR-122 also appears to be actively released under physiologic conditions in the absence of liver injury.

As mentioned earlier, GLDH has been used in nonclinical studies for decades, and as an activity assay is applicable across species. GLDH has a larger dynamic range and lower variability

TABLE 10.7 Selected Investigative Clinical Drug-induced Liver Injury (DILI) Markers

Hepatobiliary marker	Mechanism	General comments	Species assay availability[a]
miR-122	Necrosis	Liver-specific miRNA with role in lipid metabolism, hepatocyte differentiation, and hepatitis C infection. Increases demonstrated in rodent and dog and with human liver injury. Large inter- and intra-subject variability in humans.	R, D, NHP
GLDH	Necrosis	Improved specificity for liver over ALT, low inter- and intra-subject variability, shorter elimination half-life than ALT, should be interpreted in concert with other hepatobiliary markers	R, M, D, NHP, MP
K18/ccK18	Necrosis/apoptosis	Intermediate filament found in all single-layer epithelia, in liver in hepatocytes, and biliary epithelium. Full-length peptide released passively with hepatocellular necrosis, while caspase-cleaved K18 enters circulation during hepatocyte apoptosis.	R
Osteopontin	Necrosis inflammation	Protein found in many tissues, in liver involved in cancer cell metastasis, and inflammatory cell migration.	R, M, D, NHP
MCSFR1	Inflammation	Macrophage receptor for CSF-1 shed by activated macrophages during liver injury	R

[a] Many of these assays are not validated for a given species and none have undergone regulatory qualification in animals. ALT, alanine aminotransferase; ccK18, caspase-cleaved K18; CSF-1, colony-stimulating factor-1; D, dog; GLDH, glutamate dehydrogenase; K18, total keratin 18; M, mouse; miR-122, microRNA 122; MCSFR1, macrophage colony-stimulating factor receptor 1; MP, minipig; NHP, nonhuman primate; R, rat.

than miR-122 in healthy human volunteers, and it has been prioritized in clinical qualification efforts by the Predictive Safety Testing Consortium (PSTC) (Church et al., 2019).

OPN, a phosphoprotein secreted by many cells including macrophages, ECs, and kidney, acts as a proinflammatory mediator in liver. Increased serum OPN in humans with severe liver disease has been predictive of a poor prognosis or the need for transplant in patients with DILI or other liver diseases (Church et al., 2019; Roth et al., 2020). Urinary OPN was recently qualified as a general renal injury biomarker in the rat (Phillips et al., 2016).

MCSFR is shed from activated macrophages including Kupffer cells, the largest population

of tissue-resident macrophages in the body. This marker has shown promise as a prognostic marker for identification of idiosyncratic DILI.

K18 is a type I intermediate filament found in essentially all single-layer epithelia. In liver, it is highly expressed in hepatocytes and cholangiocytes. K18 and its caspase-cleaved form ccK18 are potential markers of hepatocellular necrosis and apoptosis, respectively. Since necrosis is considered a more severe manifestation of liver injury, use of an apoptotic index based on the ratio of ccK18 to K18 may add value in patients as a predictor of risk of death or need for liver transplant (Church et al., 2019; Fu et al., 2020; Roth et al., 2020).

Other candidate DILI markers evaluated by international collaborations in healthy subjects and DILI patients include α-fetoprotein, arginase, fatty acid binding protein 1, α-GST, high mobility group box 1 and paraoxonase 1 (Church et al., 2019; Fu et al., 2020). Some of these markers have also been evaluated in nonclinical studies in various species.

3.10. Heart Biomarkers

The need for noninvasive, specific, and sensitive biomarkers for the evaluation of cardiac injury has been long standing in both human clinical and laboratory animal safety testing. cTns are established plasma or serum biomarkers that have essentially supplanted the use of serum LDH and CK activities and their isoenzymes (LD_1, LD_2; CK-MM) or myoglobin concentration analyses for determination of myocardial (nonischemic and ischemic) injury. Effective use of LDH and CK activities is limited due to lack of tissue specificity and sensitivity as well as the time required for analysis of isoenzymes. Activity of the isoenzymes that are more cardio-specific is relatively low compared to the total enzyme activity, thus rendering low sensitivity as cardiac injury biomarkers. Myoglobin is smaller than the enzymes and so may be released earlier, but it has a very short half-life. However, myoglobin lacks tissue specificity and is increased with both cardiac and skeletal muscle injury.

Cardiac Troponins

cTns are globular contractile proteins found in cardiac muscle that form a complex which regulates the actin–myosin interaction required for myocyte contraction. They are released from myocardium in proportion to the degree of tissue injury and disruption of cardiomyocyte membranes. There are three different cTns: cTnT, cTnI, and cTnC. The cTn complex binds to the the thin actin myofilament via tropomyosin (cTnT) and mediates both calcium activation (cTnC) and inhibition (cTnI) of thick and thin myoflilment sliding to produce contraction. cTns are found in two distinct pools within cardiac muscle cells: cytoplasm (~5%) and the sarcomere (~95%). The cytoplasmic pool is believed to be released more quickly and with substantially less injury than the sarcomeric pool (Walker, 2006; Reagan, 2010).

cTns I and T (cTnI and cTnT) have high sensitivity and specificity for damage to cardiac muscle from various causes in humans and across a wide range of animal species. These can be effectively used in mice, rats, rabbits, dogs, pigs, and NHPs. cTn is recognized as a translational safety biomarker for cardiotoxic injury, and cTnI and/or cTnT are included in many nonclinical safety studies and human clinical trials (O'Brien, 2008; Berridge et al., 2009). There is a need to use appropriate blood collection methods for cTn determinations that avoid cardiac injury due to cardiac puncture or cardiac ischemia associated with blood collection postmortem or during euthanasia using carbon dioxide.

Representatives from the Cardiovascular Biomarker Working Group of the HESI Cardiac Safety Committee evaluated commercially available immunoassays for measurement of cTn in people (Apple et al., 2008). There were numerous differences in cross-reactivity for antibodies used in these assays, assay precision, and dynamic range. Not all the assays performed equally well in rats, dogs, and NHPs. Readers are encouraged to review this article prior to selecting an assay to validate for their use in safety assessment studies. The newer ultrasensitive or high-sensitivity assays detect cTn in the low pg/mL range, thus increasing the sensitivity and precision of detection of baseline cTn concentrations in healthy, resting control populations at levels that were previously undetectable using earlier generation commercial assays. This increased sensitivity potentially increases the ability to detect test article–induced myocardial injury. An additional benefit of some of the ultrasensitive assays is a smaller sample volume requirement that makes the assays easier to use in rodents (Schultze et al., 2008b, 2009).

Inclusion of cardiac biomarkers in safety assessment studies of traditional length and design may necessitate adjusting phlebotomy times in order to increase the probability of detecting the unique biomarker at times of maximal change. cTn concentration may increase in serum within hours after a single toxicant-induced cardiac insult and then return to baseline values within 24–48 h in rats, dogs, and NHPs. Therefore, optimal design of a phlebotomy plan for the initial characterization of a test article with suspected or known cardiac liability that results in cardiac myocyte degeneration/necrosis would include multiple cTn determinations spread equally throughout the length of a longitudinal study. If reversibility is planned as part the study, cTn should also be measured at the end of the recovery period to evaluate success of the reversal of any cardiac lesions or onset of delayed cardiotoxicity. Determination of a single cTn concentration at study termination is considered insufficient characterization to provide an assurance of safety and may miss important but subtle and transient increases in cTn concentrations. The time interval between cTn measurements may vary among studies of different lengths, and there is no single phlebotomy schedule that fits every type of safety assessment study. It may not be possible, due to blood volume limitations or other animal handling restrictions, to obtain a complete set of cTn measurements in every study of a new test article under evaluation. In those instances in which the blood sampling opportunities are limited, the minimum of cTn measurement should consist of collection of three samples obtained during the dosing phase of the study: (1) very early (usually within 2–8 h of test article administration to detect potential acute cardiac myocyte injury), (2) a midstudy blood sample to evaluate the potential effects of repeated test article administration or the possibility for delayed onset of cardiac injury, and (3) at study termination (necropsy) to correlate cTn concentrations and histopathologic evidence of cardiac microscopic alterations. If a recovery phase is included in the study, cTn should be measured again at the end of the reversibility phase.

Atrial and Brain Natriuretic Peptides

Biomarkers for chronic and/or functional cardiac injury that will translate from nonclinical to clinical testing are of primary interest to toxicologists and pathologists. The natriuretic peptides regulate blood pressure, blood volume, and cardiac growth. Atrial and brain natriuretic peptides (ANP and BNP, respectively) are structurally related hormones secreted from the heart as prohormones in response to increased atrial or ventricular wall tension (Engle and Watson, 2016; Dunn et al., 2017).

ANP is synthesized and stored by myocytes in the cardiac atria. BNP, originally identified in porcine brain extracts, is primarily synthesized and secreted by myocytes in the ventricular myocardium in proportion to end-diastolic pressure and ventricular volume/stretch. The measurement of plasma BNP concentration was introduced to the clinical laboratory as a test to identify congestive heart failure and related cardiac indications in humans (Dunn et al., 2017).

Both ANP and BNP have relatively short half-lives. The amino cleavage equivalents of ANP and BNP are NT-proANP and NT-proBNP, respectively. NT-proANP and NT-proBNP are superior markers of decreased cardiac function compared to ANP and BNP due to their better stability and the availability of more sensitive and robust assays. ANP and NT-proANP are conserved across species and are good translational biomarkers for decreased cardiac function secondary to increased plasma volume, increased cardiac stretch due to heart failure, and certain types of cardiac hypertrophy in laboratory animals. Increases in ANP concentration secondary to hemodynamic alterations are generally sustained longer than increases in BNP concentration. There are numerous commercial assays available for analysis of the ANP and NT-proANP in rodents. In contrast, BNP and NT-proBNP are not well conserved across species lines, and the number of assays available for use with rodents is limited (Dunn et al., 2017; Vinken et al., 2016).

Fatty Acid Binding Protein and Myosin Light Chain 1

Other markers of cardiac injury that have been investigated in experimental animal models include fatty acid binding protein 3 (Fabp3) and myosin light chain 1 (also known as Myl3) (Schultze et al., 2011; Pritt et al., 2008). The concentration of Fabp3 in serum or plasma increases following cardiac damage and is reported to have a kinetic profile somewhat similar to cTnI. However, Fabp3 is a less specific marker of cardiotoxicity due to the presence of the protein in other tissues, including skeletal muscle, brain, and kidney.

My13 is an isoform of one of the subunits of myosin expressed in ventricular and slow-twitch skeletal muscles. My13 has an extended kinetic profile compared with cTns, thus providing a longer period for detection of cardiac injury. However, Myl3 is also not a specific marker for cardiac injury and can be affected by concurrent skeletal muscle injury (Schultze et al., 2011; Pritt et al., 2008). In a direct comparison study, neither Fabp3 nor Myl3 was as sensitive as cTnI in detection of acute cardiac injury in several stocks of rats treated with isoproterenol (Schultze et al., 2011). Detection of onset and progression as well as reversibility of cardiac damage may be optimized by use of an integrated panel of conventional and investigative cardiovascular biomarkers in longitudinal studies.

3.11. Drug-induced Vascular Injury Biomarkers

Biomarkers of Endothelial Cell Activation and Injury

Drug-induced vascular injury (DIVI) refers to any of a variety of pathologic processes leading to or resulting in injury to blood vessels. It is a significant cause of drug attrition as drug companies are often unable to proceed into the clinic following identification of a DIVI liability in nonclinical studies. The characterization of

DIVI in animal species generally relies on biomarkers related to the release of EC adhesion molecules, EC activation markers, and/or nonspecific acute phase inflammatory proteins (Weaver et al., 2008; Mikaelian et al., 2014). Although a long list of potential biomarkers can be gathered from a literature search, more recent evidence suggests that most markers will not apply equally to all animal species and/or types of injury. This list becomes even shorter when one considers the lack of species-specific assays for all DIVI biomarkers.

Biomarkers of EC injury make up a significant portion of DIVI biomarkers described in the literature. Common examples include the vascular cell adhesion molecules, intracellular adhesion molecules, and integrins/selectins as well as signaling molecules involved in vascular regeneration and repair. Though these families of molecules have many members, only a select few have been deemed to be useful for characterization of DIVI in the rat by the Vascular Injury Working Group of the PSTC (Table 10.8).

TABLE 10.8 Selected Investigative Drug-induced Vascular Injury (DIVI) Biomarkers in the Rat

Biomarker	Mechanism	General Comments
Angiopoietin-2 (ANG-2)	Endothelial cells	Increases in angiogenesis following vascular injury
Vascular endothelial growth factor (VEGF)	Endothelial cells	Increases in angiogenesis following vascular injury
Endothelin-1	Endothelial cells	Produced by activated ECs in response to nitric oxide; facilitates vasoconstriction and proliferation of VSMC
E-selectin	Endothelial cells	Associated with leukocyte adhesion and rolling; surface upregulation in EC activation
Tissue inhibitor of metalloproteinase-1 (TIMP-1)	Inflammation	Modulator of NGAL/lipocalin-2; positive acute phase protein
Neutrophil gelatinase—associated lipocalin (NGAL)/lipocalin-2	Inflammation	Produced by activated neutrophils in response to inflammation
α-1-Acid glycoprotein (α-1-AGP)	Inflammation	Major positive acute phase protein in the rat
Nitric oxide (NO)	Inflammation	Produced by ECs in response to injury/inflammation

ECs, endothelial cells; *VSMC*, vascular smooth muscle cell.
Adapted from Mikaelian I, Cameron M, Dalmas D, Enerson B, Gonzalez R, Guionaud S, Hoffman P, King N, Lawton M, Scicchitano M, Smith H, Thomas R, Weaver J, Zabka T, and The Vascular Injury Working Group of the Predictive Safety Testing Consortium: Nonclinical safety biomarkers of drug-induced vascular injury: current status and blueprint for the future, Toxicol Pathol 42:1533–1601, 2014.

Candidate biomarkers from this group include angiopoietin-2, endothelin-1, E-selectin, thrombospondin-1, and vascular endothelial growth factor-α (Mikaelian et al., 2014). Following administration of a known vascular toxicant (PDE3i, a phosphodiesterase inhibitor), positive signals in these circulating EC biomarkers were modest (2- to 5-fold) and tended to be most pronounced at 24–72 h postinjury. Notably, most of these biomarkers exhibited increases following injury, but E-selectin showed a decrease from baseline following injury.

Biomarkers of Inflammation

The second main category of biomarkers that is helpful in characterizing DIVI are those involved in inflammation. Although these markers are extremely sensitive indicators, they lack the specificity to localize injury to the vasculature and require the concurrent use of EC-specific markers to be useful in DIVI identification. The proinflammatory markers found to be useful included tissue inhibitor of metalloproteinase-1, lipocalin-2, KC/GRO (C-X-C motif chemokine ligand 1), α-1 acid glycoprotein 1, and total nitric oxide. These markers tended to give more robust positive signals following PDE3i administration (up to 200-fold) and were observed earlier (as soon as 1–4 h) relative to biomarkers of EC activation/injury.

4. CONCLUSIONS

Hematologic analysis, clinical chemistry testing, hemostasis evaluation, and urinalysis are staples for nearly all nonclinical toxicity studies (GLP and non-GLP). Special or nonstandard tests including hormones, APPs, and biomarkers are incorporated into animal safety studies when needed to answer specific questions. Results of clinical pathology testing are used by scientists and regulatory authorities to inform the risk assessment of a given test article. In the pharmaceutical setting, these data may be used to develop safety monitoring strategies for future animal and human trials.

It is essential that the clinical pathology component of any nonclinical toxicity study is designed to optimize the opportunity to achieve the specific study objectives. The fundamental characteristics of clinical pathology parameters and novel biomarkers included in the study need to be understood, and validated assays for the species of interest must be used so that results can be interpreted with confidence. Test article–related changes in clinical pathology parameters and biomarkers should be correlated with effects on anatomic pathology and/or live phase observations in order to help to identify safety concerns, underlying mechanisms of injury, or distinguish whether effects are due to exaggerated pharmacology, metabolic adaptation, or overt toxicity.

REFERENCES

Adcock Funk DM, Lippi G, Favaloro EJ: Quality standards for sample processing, transportation, and storage in hemostasis testing, *Semin Thromb Hemost* 38(6):576–585, 2012. https://doi.org/10.1055/s-0032-1319768. Epub June 1, 2012.

ASCVP (American Society for Veterinary Clinical Pathology). https://www.asvcp.org/default.aspx. (Accessed 20 June 2021).

Andersson H, Rehm S, Stanislaus D, Wood CE: Scientific and Regulatory Policy Committee (SRPC) paper: assessment of circulating hormones in nonclinical toxicity studies III. female reproductive hormones, *Toxicol Pathol* 41(6):921–934, 2013.

Apple FS, Murakami MM, Ler R, Walker D, York M: For the HESI Technical Committee of Biomarkers Working Group on Cardiac Troponins: analytic characteristic of commercial cardiac troponin I and T immunoassays in serum from rats, dogs, and monkeys with induced acute myocardial injury, *Clin Chem* 54:1982–1989, 2008.

Bailey WJ, Barnum JE, Erdos Z, LaFranco-Scheuch L, Lane P, Vlasakova K, Sistare FD, Glaab WE: A performance evaluation of liver and skeletal muscle-specific miRNAs in rat plasma to detect drug-induced injury, *Toxicol Sci* 168(1): 110–125, 2019.

Baker DC, Brassard J: Review of continuing education course on hemostasis, *Toxicol Pathol* 39:281–288, 2011.

Berridge BR, Pettit S, Walker DB, Jaffe AS, Schultze AE, Herman E, Reagan WJ, Lipshultz SE, Apple FS, York MJ: A translational approach to detecting drug-induced cardiac injury with cardiac troponins: consensus and recommendations from the cardiac Troponins Biomarker Working Group of the Health and Environmental Sciences Institute, *Am Heart J* 158:21–29, 2009.

Bonventre JV, Vaidya VS, Schmouder R, Feig P, Dieterle F: Next-generation biomarkers for detecting kidney toxicity, *Nat Biotechnol* 28(5):436–440, 2010.

Boone L, Meyer D, Cusick P, Ennulat D, Provencher Bolliger A, Everds N, Meador V, Elliott G, Honor D, Bounous D, Jordan H: Selection and interpretation of clinical pathology indicators of hepatic injury in preclinical studies, *Vet Clin Pathol* 34:182–188, 2005.

Brooks MB, Stablein AP, Schneider A, Johnson L, Schultze AE: Preanalytic processing of rat plasma influences thrombin generation and fibrinolysis assays, *Vet Clin Pathol* 46(3): 496–507, 2017a.

Brooks MB, Turk JR, Guerrero A, Narayanan PK, Nolan JP, Besteman EG, Wilson DW, Thomas RA, Fishman CE, Thompson KL, Ellinger-Ziegelbaurer H, Pierson JB, Paulman A, Chiang AY, Schultze AE: Non-lethal endotoxin injection: a rat model of hypercoagulability, *PLoS One* 12(1): e0169976, 2017b [Electronic Resource].

Brott DA, Adler SH, Arani R, Lovick SC, Pinches M, Furlong ST: Characterization of renal biomarkers for use in clinical trials: biomarker evaluation in healthy volunteers, *Drug Des Dev Ther* 8:227–237, 2014.

Brott DA, Furlong ST, Adler SH, Hainer JW, Arani RB, Pinches M, Rossing P, Chaturvedi N: DIRECT programme steering committee: characterization of renal biomarkers for use in clinical trials: effect of preanalytical processing and qualification using samples from subjects with diabetes, *Drug Des Dev Ther* 9:3191–3198, 2015.

Burtis CA, Ashwood ER, Bruns DE, editors: *Tietz textbook of clinical chemistry and molecular diagnostics*, 4, St. Louis, MO, 2006, Elsevier Saunders, pp 1–2412.

Chapin RE, Creasy DM: Assessment of circulating hormones in regulatory toxicity studies II. Male reproductive hormones, *Toxicol Pathol* 40(7):1063–1078, 2012.

Chiang JY: Bile acid metabolism and signaling, *Comp Physiol* 3(3):1191–1212, 2013. https://doi.org/10.1002/cphy.c120023. (Accessed 20 June 2021).

Church RJ, Kullak-Ublick GA, Aubrecht J, Bonkovsky HL, Chalasani N, Fontana RJ, Goepfert JC, Hackman F, King NMP, Kirby S, Kirby P, Marcinak J, Ormarsdottir S, Schomaker SJ, Schuppe-Koistinen I, Wolenski F, Arber N, Merz M, Sauer JM, Andrade RJ, van Bömmel F, Poynard T, Watkins PB: Candidate biomarkers for the diagnosis and prognosis of drug-induced liver injury: an international collaborative effort, *Hepatology* 69(2):760–773, 2019.

Clampitt RB, Hart RJ: The tissue activities of some diagnostic enzymes in ten mammalian species, *J Comp Pathol* 88(4): 607–621, 1978.

CAP (College of American Pathologists): CAP Today. http://digital.olivesoftware.com/Olive/ODN/CAPTODAY/?olv-cache-ver=20200710083345. (Accessed 20 June 2021).

Cray C, Zaias J, Altman N: Acute phase response in animals: a review, *Comp Med* 59(6):517–526, 2009.

Criswell KA: Preclinical evaluation of compound-related alterations in hemostasis. In Weiss DJ, Wardrop KJ, editors: *Schalm's veterinary hematology*, 6, Ames, Iowa, 2010, Wiley-Blackwell, pp 92–97.

Curran PG, DeGroot LJ: The effect of hepatic enzyme-inducing drugs on thyroid hormones and the thyroid gland, *Endocr Rev* 12(2):135–150, 1991.

Dieterle F, Perentes E, Cordier A, Roth D, Verdes P, Grenet O, Pantano S, Moulin P, Wahl D, Mahl A, End P, Staedtler F, Legay F, Carl K, Laurie D, Chibout S, Vonderscher J, Maurer G: Urinary clusterin, cystatin C, β2-microglobulin and total protein as markers to detect drug-induced kidney injury, *Nat Biotech* 28(5):463–468, 2010.

Dunn ME, Manfredi TG, Agostinucci K, Engle SK, Powe J, King NM, Rodriguez LA, Gropp KE, Gallacher M, Vetter FJ, More V, Shimpi P, Serra D, Colton HM: Cardiac Hypertrophy Working Group of the Predictive Safety Testing Consortium: serum natriuretic peptides as differential biomarkers allowing for the distinction between physiologic and pathologic left ventricular hypertrophy, *Toxicol Pathol* 45(2):344–352, 2017.

EMA (European Medicines Agency): *Guide on repeated dose toxicity, 2010*. https://www.ema.europa.eu/en/documents/scientific-guideline/guideline-repeated-dose-toxicity-revision-1_en.pdf. (Accessed 20 June 2021).

EMA (European Medicines Agency): *Scientific guidelines non-clinical: toxicology, 2020*. https://www.ema.europa.eu/en/human-regulatory/research-development/scientific-guidelines/non-clinical/non-clinical-toxicology. (Accessed 20 June 2021).

Engle SK, Watson DE: Natriuretic peptides as cardiovascular safety biomarkers in rats: comparison with blood pressure, heart rate, and heart weight, *Toxicol Sci* 149(2):458–472, 2016. https://doi.org/10.1093/toxsci/kfv240.Epub2015Nov25.

Ennulat D, Ringenberg M, Frazier K: Toxicologic Pathology Forum opinion paper: recommendations for a tiered approach to nonclinical mechanistic nephrotoxicity evaluation, *Toxicol Pathol* 46(6):636–646, 2018.

EPA (U.S. Environmental Protection Agency): *OCSPP harmonized test guidelines series 870- health effects test guidelines, 40CFR Part 261*, Washington, DC, 2001, US Government Printing Office. https://www.epa.gov/test-guidelines-pesticides-and-toxic-substances/series-870-health-effects-test-guidelines. (Accessed 20 June 2021).

FDA (U.S. Food and Drug Administration): List of qualified biomarkers. https://www.fda.gov/Drugs/DevelopmentApprovalProcess/DrugDevelopmentToolsQualificationProgram/BiomarkerQualificationProgram/ucm535383.htm. (Accessed 20 June 2021).

FDA (U.S. Food and Drug Administration): *Guidance for industry and other stakeholders. Toxicological principles for the safety assessment of food ingredients. Redbook 2000: IV.B.1 general guidelines for designing and conducting toxicity studies, 40CFR Part 261*, Washington, DC, 2003, US Government Printing Office. https://www.fda.gov/regulatory-information/search-fda-guidance-documents/guidance-industry-and-other-stakeholders-redbook-2000. (Accessed 20 June 2021).

FDA (U.S. Food and Drug Administration): FDA issued letters of support. https://www.fda.gov/Drugs/DevelopmentApprovalProcess/DrugDevelopmentToolsQualificationProgram/BiomarkerQualificationProgram/ucm602478.htm#FDA_issued_Letters_of_Support. (Accessed 20 June 2021).

FDA (U.S. Food and Drug Administration Center for Devices and Radiological Health): *United States department of health and human services: guidance for industry and FDA reviewers: immunotoxicity testing guidance, 40CFR Part 261*, Washington, DC, 1999, US Government Printing Office. https://www.fda.

gov/regulatory-information/search-fda-guidance-document s/immunotoxicity-testing-guidance. (Accessed 20 June 2021).

Ferguson MA, Vaidya VS, Bonventre JV: Biomarkers of nephrotoxic acute kidney injury, *Toxicology* 245(3):182–193, 2008.

Fu S, Wu D, Jiang W, Li J, Long J, Jia C, Zhou T: Molecular biomarkers in drug-induced liver injury: challenges and future perspectives, *Front Pharmacol* (10):1667, 2020.

Gale AJ: Continuing education course #2: current understanding of hemostasis, *Toxicol Pathol* 39:273–280, 2011.

Gautier JC, Zhou X, Yang Y, Gury T, Qu Z, Palazzi X, Leonard J-F, Slaoui M, Veeranagouda Y, Guizin I, Blitier E, Fliali-Ansary A, van den Berg BHJ, Poetz O, Joos T, Zhang T, Wang J, Detilleux P, Li B: Evaluation of novel biomarkers of nephrotoxicity in Cynomolgus monkeys treated with gentamicin, *Tox Appl Pharm* 303:1–10, 2016.

Hall RL: Clinical pathology for preclinical safety assessment: current global guidelines, *Toxicol Pathol* 20:472–476, 1992.

Hall RL: Principles of clinical pathology. In Sahota PS, et al., editors: *Toxicologic pathology: nonclinical safety assessment*, Boca Raton, FL, 2013, CRC Press Taylor & Francis Group, pp 133–174.

Hall R, Everds N: Principles of clinical pathology for toxicology studies. In Hayes AW, Kruger CL, editors: *Hayes' principles and methods of toxicology*, 6, London, 2014, CRC Press Taylor & Francis Group, pp 1305--1344.

Han M, Li Y, Liu M, Cong B: Renal neutrophil gelatinase associated lipocalin expression in lipopolysaccharide-induced acute kidney injury in the rat, *BMC Nephrol* 13(1): 25, 2012.

Han WK, Bailly V, Abichandani R, Thadhani R, Bonventre JV: Kidney Injury Molecule-1 (KIM-1): a novel biomarker for human renal proximal tubule injury, *Kidney Int* 62(1):237–244, 2002.

Harpur E, Ennulat D, Hoffman D, Betton G, Gautier JC, Riefke B, Bounous D, Schuster K, Beushausen S, Guffroy M, Shaw M, Lock E, Pettit S: HESI committee on biomarkers of nephrotoxicity: biological qualification of biomarkers of chemical-induced renal toxicity in two strains of male rat, *Toxicol Sci* 122(2):235–252, 2011.

Hofmann AF: A physiochemical approach to the intraluminal phase of fat absorption, *Gastroenterology* 50:56–64, 1966.

Huseby NE, Kindberg GM, Grostad M, Berg T: Clearance of purified human liver γ-glutamyltransferase after intravenous injection in the rat, *Clin Chim Acta* 205(3):197–3203, 1992.

JMHLW (Japanese Ministry of Health, Labour and Welfare): *Guidelines for toxicity studies for manufacturing (importing) approval application of drugs. Notification No. 24 of the first evaluation and registration division*, Pharmaceutical Affairs Bureau.

JMHLW (Japanese Ministry of Health, Labour and Welfare): *Partial revisions of the guidelines for repeated dose toxicity studies. Notification No. 655 of the evaluation and licensing division*, Pharmaceutical Affairs Bureau (ICH S4).

JMHLW (Japanese Ministry of Health, Labour and Welfare): *Revisions of the guidelines for single and repeated dose toxicity*

studies. Notification No. 88 of the evaluation and licensing division, Pharmaceutical Affairs Bureau (ICH S4).

JMHLW (Japanese Ministry of Health, Labour, and Welfare). https://www.mhlw.go.jp/english/. (Accessed 20 June 2021).

Johnson GJ, Leis LA, Dunlop PC: Thromboxane-insensitive dog platelets have impaired activation of phospholipase C due to receptor-linked G protein dysfunction, *J Clin Invest* 92(5):2469–2479, 1993. https://doi.org/10.1172/JCI116855. (Accessed 20 June 2021).

Jordan HL, Register TC, Tripathi NK, Bolliger AP, Everds N, Zelmanovic D, Poitout F, Bounous DI, Wescott D, Ramaiah SK: Nontraditional applications in clinical pathology, *Toxicol Pathol* 42(7):1058–1068, 2014.

Kaplowitz N: Idiosyncratic drug hepatotoxicity, *Nat Rev Drug Discov* 4:489–499, 2005.

Karmen A, Wroblewski F, Ladue JS: Transaminase activity in human blood, *J Clin Invest* 34(1):126–131, 1955.

Khan M, Bowsher RR, Cameron M, Devanarayan V, Keller S, King L, Lee J, Morimoto A, Rhyne P, Stephen L, Wu L, Wyant T, Lachno DR: Recommendations for adaptation and validation of commercial kits for biomarker quantification in drug development, *Bioanalysis* 7(2):229–242, 2015.

Lee J, Devanarayan V, Barrett YC, Weiner R, Allinson J, Fountain S, Keller S, Weinryb I, Green M, Duan L, Rogers JA, Millham R, O'Brien PJ, Sailstad J, Khan M, Ray C, Wagner JA: Fit-for-purpose method development and validation for successful biomarker measurement, *Pharm Res* 23(2):312–328, 2006.

Levin S, Semler D, Ruben Z: Effects of two weeks of feed restriction on some common toxicologic parameters in Sprague-Dawley rats, *Toxicol Pathol* 21(1):1–14, 1993.

Lubas G, Caldin M, Wiinberg B, Kristensen A: Laboratory testing of coagulation disorders. In Weiss DJ, Wardrop KJ, editors: *Schalm's veterinary hematology*, 6, Ames, Iowa, 2010, Wiley-Blackwell, pp 1082–1100.

Miao D, Scutt A: Histochemical localization of alkaline phosphatase activity in decalcified bone and cartilage, *J Histochem Cytochem* 50(3):333–340, 2002.

Mikaelian I, Cameron M, Dalmas D, Enerson B, Gonzalez R, Guionaud S, Hoffman P, King N, Lawton M, Scicchitano M, Smith H, Thomas R, Weaver J, Zabka T, The Vascular Injury Working Group of the Predictive Safety Testing Consortium: Nonclinical safety biomarkers of drug-induced vascular injury: current status and blueprint for the future, *Toxicol Pathol* 42:1533–1601, 2014.

Moritz A, Becker M: Automated hematology systems. In Weiss DJ, Wardrop KJ, editors: *Schalm's veterinary hematology*, 6, Ames, Iowa, 2010, Wiley-Blackwell, pp 1054–1066.

O'Brien PJ: Cardiac troponin is the most effective translational safety biomarker for myocardial injury in cardiotoxicity, *Toxicology* 245:206–218, 2008.

OECD (Organisation for Economic Co-operation and Development): guidelines for the testing of chemicals, Section 4. https://www.oecd-ilibrary.org/environment/oecd-guidelines-for-the-testing-of-chemicals-section-4-health-effects_20745788?page=1. (Accessed 20 June 2021).

OECD (Organisation for Economic Co-operation and Development): *Guideline for the testing of chemicals in chronic toxicity studies, 40CFR Part 261*, Washington, DC, 2008, U.S. Government Printing Office.

Osborne C, Stevens JB. *Urinalysis: A Clinical Guide to Compassionate Patient Care*, Leverkusen Germany, 1999, Bayer Corporation and Bayer AG Business Group Animal Health.

Phillips JA, Holder DJ, Ennulat D, Gautier JC, Sauer JM, Yang Y, Walker EG: Rat urinary osteopontin and neutrophil gelatinase-associated lipocalin improve certainty of detecting drug-induced kidney injury, *Toxicol Sci* 151(2):214–223, 2016.

Pritt ML, Hall DG, Recknor J, Credille KM, Brown DD, Yumibe NP, Schultze AE, Watson DE: Fabp3 as a biomarker of skeletal muscle toxicity in the rat: comparison with conventional biomarkers, *Toxicol Sci* 103:382–396, 2008.

Reagan WJ: Troponin as a biomarker of cardiac toxicity: past, present, and future, *Toxicol Pathol* 38(7):1134–1137, 2010.

Reagan WJ, Irizarry-Rovira A, Poitout-Belissent F, Bolliger AP, Ramaiah SK, Travlos G, Walker D, Bounous D, Walter G: Bone Marrow Working Group of ASVCP/STP: best practices for evaluation of bone marrow in nonclinical toxicity studies, *Toxicol Pathol* 39(2):435–448, 2011a.

Reagan WJ, Irizarry-Rovira A, Poitout-Belissent F, Bolliger AP, Ramaiah SK, Travlos G, Walker D, Bounous D, Walter G: Bone Marrow Working Group of ASVCP/STP: best practices for evaluation of bone marrow in nonclinical studies, *Vet Clin Pathol* 40(2):119–134, 2011b.

Roth SE, Avigan MI, Bourdet D, Brott D, Church R, Dash A, Keller D, Sherratt P, Watkins PB, Westcott-Baker L, Lentini S, Merz M, Ramaiah L, Ramaiah SK, Stanley AM, Marcinak J: Next-generation DILI biomarkers: prioritization of biomarkers for qualification and best practices for biospecimen collection in drug development, *Clin Pharmacol Ther* 107(2):333–346, 2020.

Schmidt ES, Schmidt FW: Glutamate dehydrogenase: biochemical and clinical aspects of an interesting enzyme, *Clin Chim Acta* 173(1):43–55, 1988.

Schultze AE: Veterinary clinical pathologists impact science and the biopharmaceutical industry, *Vet Clin Pathol* 40:117–118, 2011.

Schultze AE, Bounous DI, Provencher Bolliger A: Veterinary clinical pathologists in the biopharmaceutical industry, *Vet Clin Pathol* 37:146–158, 2008a.

Schultze AE, Carpenter KH, Wians FH, Agee SJ, Minyard J, Lu QA, Todd J, Konrad RJ: Longitudinal studies of cardiac troponin-I concentrations in serum from male Sprague Dawley rats: baseline reference ranges and effects of handling and placebo dosing on biological variability, *Toxicol Pathol* 37:754–760, 2009.

Schultze AE, Irizarry A: Recognizing and reducing analytical errors and sources of variation in clinical pathology data in safety assessment studies, *Toxicol Pathol* 45(2):281–287, 2017.

Schultze AE, Konrad RJ, Credille KM, Lu QA, Todd J: Ultra-sensitive cross species measurement of cardiac troponin-I

using the erenna immunoassay system, *Toxicol Pathol* 36:777–782, 2008b.

Schultze AE, Main BW, Hall DG, Hoffman WP, Lee H-YC, Ackermann BL, Pritt ML, Smith HW: A comparison of mortality and cardiac biomarker response between three outbred stocks of Sprague Dawley rats treated with isoproterenol, *Toxicol Pathol* 39:576–588, 2011.

Schultze AE, Walker DB, Turk JR, Tarrant JM, Brooks MB, Pettit SD: Current practices in preclinical drug development: gaps in hemostasis testing to assess risk of thromboembolic injury, *Toxicol Pathol* 41(3):445–453, 2013.

Smith SA: Overview of hemostasis. In Weiss DJ, Wardrop KJ, editors: *Schalm's veterinary hematology*, 6, Ames, Iowa, 2010, Wiley-Blackwell, pp 635–653.

Solter PF: Clinical pathology approaches to hepatic injury, *Toxicol Pathol* 33(1):9–16, 2005.

Stanislaus D, Andersson H, Chapin R, Creasy D, Ferguson D, Gilbert M, Wood CE: Society of Toxicologic Pathology position paper: review series: assessment of circulating hormones in nonclinical toxicity studies: general concepts and considerations, *Toxicol Pathol* 40(6):943–950, 2012.

Stockham SL, Scott MA. *Fundamentals of Veterinary Clinical Pathology*, 2, Ames, Iowa, 2008, Blackwell Publishing, pp 1–908.

Tarrant J, Meyer D, Katavolos P: Use of optimized aminotransferase methods in regulated preclinical studies, *Vet Clin Pathol* 42:535–538, 2013.

Thompson KL, Afshari CA, Amin RP, Bertram TA, Car B, Cunningham M, Kind C, Kramer JA, Lawton M, Mirsky M, Naciff JM, Oreffo V, Pine PS, Sistare FD: Identification of platform-independent gene expression markers of cisplatin nephrotoxicity, *Environ Health Perspect* 112(4):488–494, 2004.

Tomlinson L, Boone LI, Ramaiah L, Penraat KA, von Beust BR, Ameri M, Poitout-Belissent FM, Weingand K, Workman HC, Aulbach AD, Meyer DJ, Brown DE, MacNeill AL, Bolliger AP, Bounous DI: Best practices for veterinary toxicologic clinical pathology, with emphasis on the pharmaceutical and biotechnology industries, *Vet Clin Pathol* 42(3):252–269, 2013.

Tomlinson L, Ramaiah L, Tripathi NK, Barlow VG, Vitsky A, Poitout-Belissent FM, Ennulat D: STP best practices for evaluating clinical pathology in pharmaceutical recovery studies, *Toxicol Pathol* 44(2):163–172, 2016. https://doi.org/10.1177/0192623315624165. (Accessed 20 June 2021).

Vinken P, Reagan WJ, Rodriguez LA, Buck WR, Lai-Zhang J, Goeminne N, Barbacci G, Liu R, King NM, Engle SK, Colton H: Cross-laboratory analytical validation of the cardiac biomarker NT-proANP in rat, *J Pharmacol Toxicol Methods* 77:58–65, 2016. https://doi.org/10.1016/j.vascn.2015.10.002. Epub 2015 Oct 26.

Wagoner MP, Yang Y, McDuffie JE, Klapczynski M, Buck W, Cheatham L, Eisinger D, Sace F, Lynch KM, Sonee M, Ma JY, Chen Y, Marshall K, Damour M, Stephen L, Dragan YP, Fikes J, Snook S, Kinter LB: Evaluation of temporal changes in urine-based metabolomic and kidney injury markers to detect compound induced acute kidney tubular toxicity in Beagle dogs, *Curr Top Med Chem* 17(24): 2767–2780, 2017.

Walker DB: Serum chemical biomarkers of cardiac injury for nonclinical safety testing, *Toxicol Pathol* 34:94–104, 2006.

Weaver J, Snyder R, Knapton A, Herman E, Honchel R, Miller T, Espandiari P, Smith R, Gu Y, Goodsaid F, Rosenblum I, Sistare F, Zhang J, Hanig J: Biomarkers in peripheral blood associated with vascular injury in Sprague-Dawley rats treated with the phosphodiesterase IV inhibitors SCH 351591 or SCH 534385, *Toxicol Pathol* 36: 840–849, 2008.

Weingand K, Bloom J, Carakostas M, Hall R, Helfrich M, Latimer K, Levine B, Neptun D, Rebar A, Stitzel K, Troup C: Clinical pathology testing recommendations for nonclinical toxicity and safety studies, *Toxicol Pathol* 20: 539–543, 1992.

Weingand K, Brown G, Hall R, Davies D, Gossett K, Neptun D, Melloni E: Harmonization of animal clinical pathology testing in toxicity and safety studies. The Joint Scientific Committee for International Harmonization of Clinical Pathology Testing, *Fundam Appl Toxicol* 29(2):198–201, 1996.

Weiss DJ, Wardrop KJ, editors: *Schalm's veterinary hematology,* 6, Ames, Iowa, 2010, Wiley-Blackwell, pp 1–1206.

York MJ: Clinical pathology. In Faqi OS, editor: *A comprehensive guide to toxicology in preclinical drug development*, San Diego, CA, 2013, Academic Press, pp 167–211.

Young JK, Hall RL, O'Brien P, Volker S, Vahle JL: Best practices for clinical pathology testing in carcinogenicity studies, *Toxicol Pathol* 39:429–434, 2011.

Special Techniques in Toxicologic Pathology

Shari A. Price[1],[*], Kevin McDorman[1], Curtis Chan[2], Jennifer Rojko[1],[+],
James T. Raymond[1], Danielle Brown[3], Na Li[4], Christina Satterwhite[2],
Tracey Papenfuss[5], James Morrison[6]

[1]Charles River Laboratories, Preclinical Services, Frederick, MD, United States, [2]Charles River Laboratories, Preclinical Services, Reno, NV, United States, [3]Charles River Laboratories, Preclinical Services, Durham, NC, United States, [4]Charles River Laboratories, Preclinical Services, Morrisville, NC, United States, [5]Charles River Laboratories, Preclinical Services, Ashland, OH, United States, [6]Charles River Laboratories, Preclinical Services, Shrewsbury, MA, United States

O U T L I N E

1. Introduction	336
2. Immunohistochemistry	337
2.1. Introduction	337
2.2. Applications of Immunohistochemistry in Toxicologic Pathology	338
2.3. Technical Considerations for Immunohistochemistry	352
2.4. Conclusion	356
3. Enzyme Histochemistry	356
3.1. Introduction	356
3.2. Applications of Enzyme Histochemistry in Toxicologic Pathology	357
3.3. Technical Considerations for Enzyme Histochemistry	357
3.4. Conclusions	358
4. In Situ Hybridization	358
4.1. Introduction	358
4.2. Applications of In Situ Hybridization in Toxicologic Pathology	358
4.3. Technical Considerations for In Situ Hybridization	361
4.4. Conclusions	364
5. Flow Cytometry	365
5.1. Introduction	365
5.2. Applications of Flow Cytometry in Toxicologic Pathology	369
5.3. Advantages and Limitations of Flow Cytometry	373
5.4. Conclusions	374
6. Laser Capture Microdissection	374
6.1. Introduction	374
6.2. Applications of Laser Capture Microdissection in Toxicologic Pathology	375
6.3. Technical Considerations for Laser Capture Microdissection	375
6.4. Limitations	377
6.5. Conclusions	377
7. Confocal Microscopy	377
7.1. Introduction	377
7.2. Applications of Confocal Microscopy in Toxicologic Pathology	377
7.3. Technical Considerations for Confocal Microscopy	378
7.4. Limitations	380
7.5. Conclusions	380
8. Electron Microscopy	380
8.1. Introduction	380

[*]Lead/Contributing author.

[+]Retired.

8.2. *Applications of Electron Microscopy in Toxicologic Pathology*   380

8.3. *Technical Considerations for Electron Microscopy* 381

8.4. *Limitations*   382

8.5. *Conclusions*   382

9. **Stereology**   382

10. **Digital Pathology**   384

11. **Conclusions**   384

Glossary   384

References   385

1. INTRODUCTION

Advances in cell and molecular biology have engendered a wide range of techniques to investigate mechanisms of disease or toxicity that can be used to augment traditional morphologic tools used in toxicity testing. In the team-oriented scientific world of today, pathologists should be familiar with the technical basis and utility of these varied techniques, some of which are slide based and others that are solution (fluid) based.

In solution-based assays, tissue is homogenized and DNA, RNA, or protein is extracted for analysis in a test tube. In contrast, slide-based methods such as immunohistochemistry (IHC), in situ hybridization (ISH), and laser capture microdissection (LCM) retain tissue architecture and provide spatial localization of alterations in DNA, RNA, or protein at the cellular level. Slide-based techniques typically reside in the pathology laboratory and require the interpretation of the slide by a trained and experienced pathologist. While solution (fluid)-based assays may not require the morphologic training of a pathologist, the accurate interpretation of these data also should be made by individuals with appropriate training and expertise—and this can include molecular pathologists.

The application of special pathology techniques in the field of toxicology and risk assessment has experienced dramatic changes over the past decade (see *Risk Assessment*, Vol 2, Chap 16). Techniques once considered "special" techniques have become common and in some cases "expected" depending on the chemical/molecular structure or therapeutic type, therapeutic modality, anticipated tissue response, and needs of the project team. This chapter focuses on the more common special techniques that a toxicologic pathologist may utilize, although it is by no means a comprehensive list of all possible special methodologies. Techniques discussed in this chapter include IHC, enzyme histochemistry (EHC), ISH, flow cytometry, LCM, confocal microscopy (CM), electron microscopy (EM), and stereology. Digital pathology will be briefly reviewed, but more detail on this topic can be found in *Digital Pathology and Tissue Image Analysis*, Vol 1, Chap 12.

Careful evaluation of therapeutic candidates to fully understand their impact on biological systems requires a mechanistic understanding that often is deeper than that provided by classical light microscopic examination alone. Therapeutic candidates are becoming more complex (e.g., monoclonal antibodies linked to cytotoxic agents, chemical combinations or mixtures, cell-based therapies, gene therapies, etc.), and special techniques for fully evaluating these complex therapies also have increased in complexity and sophistication.

The development of specialized equipment to support these techniques has lagged behind with the exceptions of flow cytometry, multiplex IHC, and digital pathology. Notably, digital pathology has seen rapid development in application and use within toxicologic pathology. In contrast, IHC, ISH, LCM, and CM tools and methods have not changed dramatically, but rather the use and expectation for the application of these techniques has shifted. Previously, methods to determine expression levels and subcellular localization or activity directly in tissue (e.g., IHC, ISH, and EM) were considered to add clarity to a safety assessment but were not considered to be a critical component in characterizing the nonclinical safety profile. This philosophy and practice has changed for certain types of test articles (e.g., immunomodulatory molecules that deplete certain populations of immune cells). Currently, IHC and flow cytometry are critical in the evaluation of these types of test articles for both general toxicity studies and special immunotoxicity studies.

Toxicologic pathology and other risk assessment follow guidance provided by international regulatory agencies, particularly agency requests for information regarding mode of action or mechanistic understanding of new therapeutic modalities, chemicals, and devices. Specific agency requests for specialized techniques (e.g., IHC) are an indicator that these methods are becoming more accepted and, in some instances, are more of a routine expectation for a comprehensive risk assessment. This arena is a rapidly evolving field, and readers are encouraged to supplement their reading through the provided references and recent literature.

2. IMMUNOHISTOCHEMISTRY

2.1. Introduction

While microscopic examination of hematoxylin and eosin (H&E)–stained tissues remains the gold standard for the evaluation of toxicologic effects on animal tissues following administration of pharmaceuticals, biotherapeutics, and potential toxicants, IHC often has great value in conjunction with H&E in better characterizing potential hazards posed by novel test articles. IHC uses the precise antigen specificity of antibody reagents to localize target molecules in tissue sections. Antibodies can be produced to specifically recognize billions of different antigens and can be engineered to recognize almost any molecule of interest. In IHC, an antibody that has specificity for a target molecule of interest is applied to a tissue section and binds to its target molecule. This bound antibody can then be detected through a number of different techniques.

Antibodies can be labeled in various ways. Fluorescent dyes (e.g., Alexa Fluor or fluorescein-isothiocyante [FITC]) emit light photons that can be detected directly without the need for building a longer immunobridge. Immuno-tags (e.g., biotin, digoxigenin, fluorescent dyes, and hemagglutinin [HA]) serve as anchors for high-affinity binding of other reagents needed to build the immunobridge. Reporter enzymes (e.g., horseradish peroxidase [HRP] or alkaline phosphatase [AP]) conjugated to antibodies can convert

noncolored chromogens to produce a visible colored precipitate at the site of antibody binding. The choice of antibody label will depend on the desired manner of visualization (chromogenic or immunofluorescent) and the level of signal amplification needed for sufficient visualization. Considerations in making this choice include signal persistence (chromogenic products last longer than fluorescent signals, which have implications for retention of study materials required under Good Laboratory Practice [GLP]); available instrumentation; endogenous pigment or autofluorescence which might hamper interpretation; and signal sensitivity.

Often, the primary antibody itself (whether acting as the test article or the first link in the immunobridge for detecting a tissue antigen) serves as the target for a secondary antibody, which has specificity for the primary antibody (Fc region, heavy and light chains, or light chain only). The addition of the secondary antibody amplifies the signal and also allows the same detection reagents to be used for different primary antibodies. The development of IHC amplification procedures such as Avidin–Biotin Complex (ABC), Catalyzed Reporter Deposition (CARD), and tyramide signal amplification (TSA) has also greatly increased the sensitivity and utility of IHC as now even very rare antigens can theoretically be detected (Key, 2006).

IHC can be used to visualize changes that are not apparent with routine H&E staining. This can greatly expand the amount of information obtained from a toxicity study. For example, IHC can be used to detect the administered test article and its metabolites and may aid in determining the spatial and temporal distribution of the material in the body. Additionally, various substances may be either increased or decreased in tissue in response to administration of a test article, and IHC may be useful to detect such changes. Thus, the mechanisms of action and toxicity of the test article may be elucidated. In addition, specific cell populations affected by administration of a therapeutic candidate can be identified using specific IHC markers individually or in combination. These are just three examples of the value of IHC in toxicologic pathology.

The applications of IHC in toxicologic pathology are seemingly limitless given the myriad product candidates that are tested and the large number of questions that must be answered about each. The following section focuses on various ways IHC can be utilized, using specific examples and including discussions of cell proliferation markers, markers of apoptosis, biodistribution and immune complex evaluations, and tissue cross-reactivity (TCR) studies. The technical considerations of IHC in toxicologic pathology also are covered, as well as suggestions for study planning and tissue collection and fixation.

2.2. Applications of Immunohistochemistry in Toxicologic Pathology

Tissue Cross-Reactivity Studies

TCR studies are nonclinical safety studies conducted to assess the potential for off-target reactivity of therapeutic monoclonal antibody (mAb) and antibody-based therapeutics (see *Protein Pharmaceutical Agents,* Vol 2, Chap 6). The conduct and applicability of TCR studies is addressed in the scientific literature as well as in various TCR guidelines published by the US Food and Drug Administration (FDA), European Medicines Agency (EMA), and the International Council on Harmonisation (ICH) (EMA, 2016; FDA, 1997; ICH, 2012). Current industry best practices recommendations indicate that TCR should be performed on human tissues with inclusion of animal tissues if human TCR findings are present (Leach et al., 2010). It should be noted that for therapeutic candidates with no mammalian targets such as antiinfectious agents, TCR or other appropriate assessment of off-target binding might be one of the key components of a preclinical safety assessment package.

TCR performed on animal tissue is no longer considered the primary screen for species selection for toxicity and safety testing of therapeutic mAb therapeutics (ICH, 2012; Leach et al., 2010). Rather, TCR performed on tissues from toxicology models is useful and often included as part of the larger data package to support selection of a particular species for toxicity testing if the patterns of on- and/or off-target IHC labeling (synonym: IHC staining) are similar to that observed in human tissues and to investigate unexpected or nonpharmacologic toxicity findings in safety studies. In nonclinical toxicity studies in animals, cross-reactivity of the mAb or mAb-based test article with an unexpected tissue in combination with histopathological lesions in that tissue is strong evidence of an adverse result due to unexpected binding of the test article. If the human TCR studies also show a similar distribution of cross-reactivity, additional safety assessments may be needed prior to clinical trials or additional clinical safety monitoring may be warranted. TCR findings should always be interpreted in the context of the entire Investigational New Drug-enabling data package, and a weight-of-evidence approach should be taken in defining whether IHC labeling is linked to the expected expression of the antigen ("on target"), serves as evidence for unexpected antigen localization and potential off-target test article binding, or is spurious (Leach et al., 2010).

It is noteworthy that while the technology exists to test other types of therapeutics (such as ligand-binding fusion proteins or even small molecules designed to bind ligands) for binding specificity, human TCR studies are not recommended by the FDA or industry for these non-antibody test articles on a routine basis. In general, TCR studies are required or recommended when the test article includes a complementarity-determining region (CDR) (ICH, 2012). For test articles that do not contain a CDR, other methods are available that can be used to assess on- or off-target binding and biodistribution (e.g., qualitative whole body autoradiography).

In addition, an ICH S9 Q&A document states that TCR studies are not needed for test articles directed to oncology indications unless there is a specific cause for concern or there is no pharmacologically relevant species for toxicity studies (ICH, 2016). It should be noted that, as of 2016, there have been no truly tumor-specific antibody or antibody-based tumor therapies available (Klebanoff et al., 2016). Given the powerful pharmacologic nature and already precedented adverse effects associated with some of the newer antibody and antibody-based test articles, particularly multispecific molecules and cell-based therapies, some level of risk is indeed inherent in these materials (Bonifant et al., 2016; Sun et al., 2018). Moreover, for newer multispecific molecules and cell-based therapies, no adequate animal models exist, so TCR testing might still be necessary in these cases.

In a typical TCR study, the mAb or mAb-based therapeutic is applied at two IHC staining concentrations to cryosections of approximately 37 human tissues from at least three unrelated adult donors. Embryonic or fetal human tissues may be included as well for test articles that might be given to infants or women of child-bearing potential. Flash-frozen tissues are preferred for TCR studies as no modification in antigen structure will have been imparted by prior fixation. Ideally, the test article should be assessed in the form it is to be used clinically, but this may not be feasible technically, particularly for chimeric antigen receptor T-cells (CAR-Ts) where a version of the chimeric antigen receptor can be used as a surrogate for the cell-based therapeutic. Positive and negative control slides or cryosections are essential to ensure sensitive and reproducible staining. Such controls might include intact adult tissues, cell lines expressing or not expressing the target of interest, stem cells, or embryonic or fetal tissue that do or do not express the target of interest, or purified target or irrelevant antigens spotted onto and cross-linked to ultraviolet (UV)-activatable resin-coated slides. Other staining controls applied to donor samples include replicate sections stained with species, isotype, and concentration-matched negative control antibody and assay control (omitting the primary antibody) slides (Hall et al., 2008; Leach et al., 2010).

FDA guidance suggests that a positive control antibody against an antigen present on many tissues should be used as a tissue suitability and tissue validation control (FDA, 1997; Leach et al., 2010). The tissue suitability controls most commonly used include staining for β2-microglobulin (a ubiquitous antigen expressed on endothelium, many epithelia, and hematopoietic and lymphoid cells) (Figure 11.1); von Willebrand Factor; CD31 (an antigen expressed on endothelium and platelets); or transferrin receptor (a membrane protein on some endothelial, epithelial, endocrine, and Kupffer cells). In some cases, the use of antigen or positive control antibody blocking studies may be useful (Hall et al., 2008; Leach et al., 2010).

TCR slides are interpreted by a pathologist to identify the types and locations of each mAb (i.e., test article)-stained cellular and/or extracellular element. Particular attention is paid to "unexpected" staining (i.e., staining not predicted by known locations of the epitope recognized by the mAb) (Hall et al., 2008; Leach et al., 2010). For example, the T10B9 series of anti-CD3 (T-lymphocyte) monoclonal antibodies recognizes its target CD3 epitope in human tissues, especially T-cell-rich regions of lymphoid

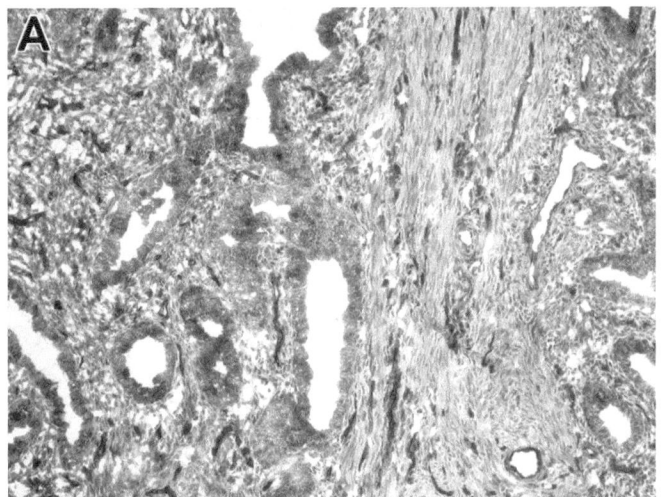 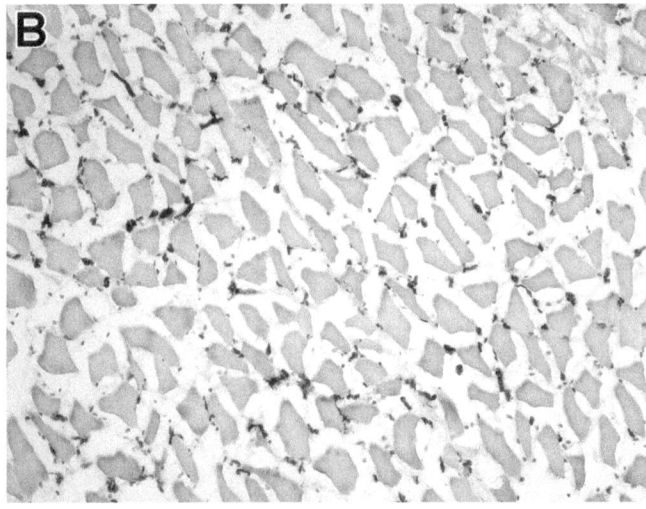

FIGURE 11.1 Human tissues stained for β2-microglobulin, a broadly expressed marker in normal human tissues that can serve as a marker for tissue validation (i.e., antigenic preservation) in tissue cross-reactivity (TCR) studies. Positive staining indicates that epitopes were sufficiently intact that they could be labeled using standard immunohistochemical (IHC) methods. β2-microglobulin staining is prominent in mononuclear cells, most epithelial cell types, and endothelium. (A) Human uterus—note positive staining of endometrial epithelium, endothelium, and endometrial stromal cells. (B) Human skeletal muscle—note positive staining of endothelium and scattered mononuclear cells between nonlabeled (negative) myocytes.

organs. It does not react with nonhuman primate (NHP) CD3 but does cross-react with an off-target, cytoplasmic filaments in human and NHP epithelial cells. This off-target cytoplasmic staining is not associated with toxic effects in safety studies (Waid et al., 1989).

Technical difficulties may arise during the conduct and interpretation of TCR studies. Since many therapeutic mAbs are fully human or "humanized" (chimeras of animal-derived variable regions and human-derived Fc domains with or without additional mutations to match human antibody protein sequences) proteins, TCR assays need to minimize background staining that may occur due to binding of the secondary antibody (which is antihuman) to human antibodies present within the human donor tissues being tested. Current best practices include labeling of the antibody with a protein tag (e.g., biotin or digoxigenin) or a fluorophore (e.g., FITC or AlexaFluor, which can be used as epitope tags for enzyme-conjugated detection antibody binding) or indirect labeling with a biotinylated secondary antibody via

a precomplexing approach (Fung et al., 1992; Hall et al., 2008; Hierck et al., 1994; Leach et al., 2010; Tuson et al., 1990) (Figure 11.2). Other technical difficulties arise when the epitope of interest is only expressed at low levels or undergoes a conformational alteration during freezing, storage, thawing, and/or a brief exposure to the tissue fixative during IHC staining (Hall et al., 2008; Leach et al., 2010).

Another challenge related to TCR studies lies in interpreting the pattern of staining observed. If a therapeutic mAb or mAb-based test article binds to unexpected tissues, it does not necessarily indicate whether the antibody will specifically bind to and adversely affect that tissue. Binding to membranes is considered to have greater potential toxicologic significance than binding to intracellular components as such sites in intact cells are considered to be less accessible to therapeutic mAbs in vivo. ICH S6(R1) indicates that binding to areas not typically accessible to the antibody in vivo (e.g., cytoplasm) is generally not relevant (Edwards and Sklar, 2015; Hall et al., 2008; ICH, 2012).

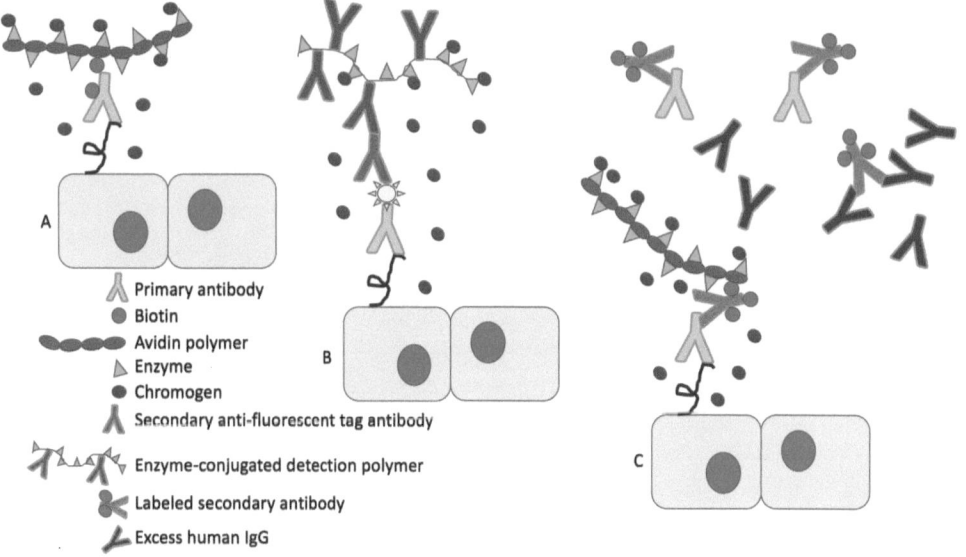

FIGURE 11.2   Schematic diagrams for immunohistochemical (IHC) labeling methods used for staining human tissues with fully human, humanized, or chimeric primary antibodies. (A) Direct avidin–biotin complex method. Target binding of the biotinylated primary antibody is detected with enzyme-conjugated avidin polymers and subsequent precipitation of colored chromogen. (B) Indirect tertiary staining method. Target binding of a fluorescent-tagged primary antibody is detected using a mouse or rabbit antifluorescent tag secondary antibody followed by an enzyme-conjugated antimouse or antirabbit polymer and subsequent precipitation of colored chromogen. (C) Precomplex staining method. The unlabeled primary antibody is first precomplexed with labeled secondary antibody (biotinylated secondary antibody shown here). Unbound secondary antibody is "mopped up" by addition of excess human IgG and precomplexes are then incubated with tissue sections. Target binding of primary: secondary antibody complexes is detected with enzyme-conjugated avidin polymers and subsequent precipitation of colored chromogen.

Furthermore, when mAb or mAb-based test articles cross-react with many nontarget tissues, the safety risk is not necessarily enhanced. However, in these cases, high levels of off-target binding might require further characterization and interpretation in light of the entire toxicity testing package. In addition, the potential for adverse events often does not relate well to the relative degree of cross-reactivity or abundance of off-target antigen as assessed by IHC. However, in other cases, TCR results have provided valuable information regarding potential sites of toxicity, in particular by identifying tissues that should receive close monitoring in human clinical trials. Greater than 20 case studies have been identified and described where TCR results either confounded, were inessential to, or greatly clarified the risk assessment of mAb drugs (Leach et al., 2010).

In some cases, a drug-related adverse event may occur in a tissue with apparently very little antigen, while tissues with abundant antigen may be spared. This has been observed with some toxin-conjugated antibodies (i.e., immunotoxins, a special category of antibody–drug conjugates). In these cases, the addition of the toxin to the therapeutic mAb may alter the biodistribution, uptake, transcellular transport, and clearance of the test article (see below). Other factors that can affect the safety profile include antibody class, which may relate to an antibody's ability to fix complement or elicit antibody-dependent cell cytotoxicity events, manufacturing-related variations in glycosylation and alterations of structure (often by virtue of the effect on pharmacokinetics [PK] or on organ of excretion), and conjugations (Hall et al., 2008). Overall, toxin-conjugated antibodies have much poorer safety records than plain antibodies.

There are now several array-based technologies also available for assessment of cross-reactivity of antibodies and antibody-based test articles (Freeth and Soden, 2020; Huston-Paterson, 2016). In general, these technologies involve screening cells transfected with vectors designed to overexpress various membrane-bound proteins. The potential benefits of such technologies include the speed and throughput of the in vitro assay, ability to rapidly screen a variety of constructs, ability to identify the protein that is being bound, and potentially lower cost than conventional TCR studies.

However, these technologies are still relatively new and have a few drawbacks including no tissue, cellular, or histologic context; incomplete representation of the membrane proteome; no representation of soluble or secreted proteins; no representation of proteomes from species of interest for toxicity studies; no representation of isoforms; and no context of other intramembrane proteins which might interact with the protein of interest.

Test Article Biodistribution

The most direct application of IHC in the evaluation of an administered test article is in detecting the test article and its metabolites. This detection allows one to determine the spatial distribution of the test article and to specifically localize it to certain cell types or extracellular sites. Distribution to unexpected (off-target) organs also may be detected. The ability to specifically visualize the test article in cellular, subcellular, or extracellular sites is an advantage over other methods to determine the amount but not the precise anatomic distribution, including measurement of test article levels in plasma or digested tissue.

USE OF IMMUNOHISTOCHEMISTRY FOR BIODISTRIBUTION OF CELL OR GENE THERAPIES

IHC can be a powerful tool for spatial localization of cell and gene therapy candidates and provide useful information regarding their safety and activity in vivo. Careful planning during study design is important to ensure that tissues are collected and processed appropriately for these analyses and that the staining method itself is suited to the species and tissues to be stained.

For cell-based therapies such as CAR-T or other modified cells, IHC can be used to localize the therapeutic cells in tissues after administration in toxicity/safety study models to determine their biodistribution and persistence over time (see *Stem Cells and Regenerative Medicine*, Vol 2, Chap 10). A variety of human-specific markers such as major histocompatibility complex proteins (HLA-ABC) or feature-specific molecules expressed in human mitochondria, stem cells (STEM121), and nuclei (HuNu, Ku80) are available that can facilitate localization of engrafted human cells in animal tissues (Figure 11.3). These analyses can be helpful in determining intratumor versus systemic

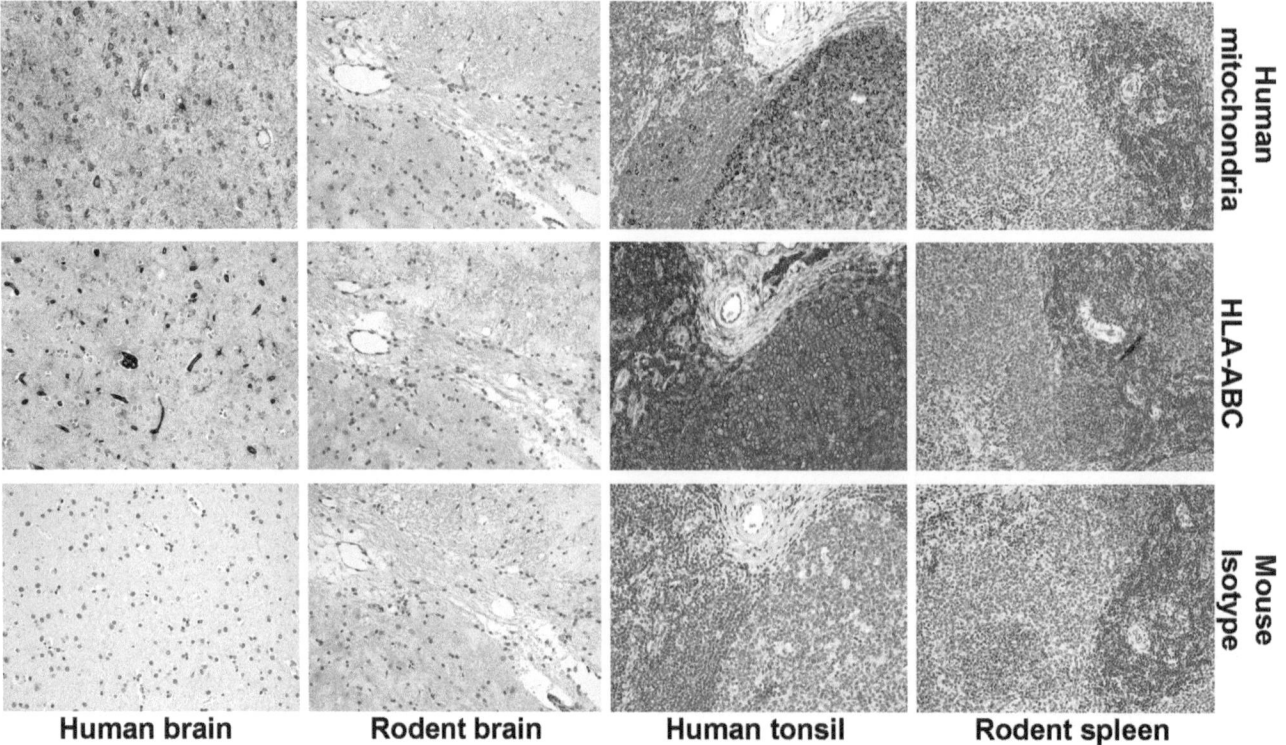

FIGURE 11.3   Examples of markers that can be used to localize human cell therapy test articles in nonclinical toxicity study test tissues. The chosen marker should be one that is specific for human and does not cross-react with the corresponding protein (or other proteins) in the animal species of interest. Note that staining for human mitochondria (mouse antihuman mitochondria clone 113-1) (top row) and HLA-ABC (middle row) are only observed in human brain and tonsil and not in rodent brain or spleen. No staining is observed with mouse isotype control in any of the tissues (bottom row).

localization of the cell-based therapeutic candidate over time. This tissue context cannot be demonstrated for cell-based therapies by simple quantification using polymerase chain reaction (PCR)–based biodistribution. In addition, other IHC stains including Ki67 and proliferating cell nuclear antigen (PCNA) can be applied to facilitate evaluation of proliferation and tumorigenicity of cell therapies.

For gene therapy, IHC can be used for assessing the biodistribution of the test article (see *Gene Therapy and Genome Editing*, Vol 2, Chap 8). It is important that a suitable marker for the therapeutic protein is available and/or that there is an antibody available that is specific for the human-derived test article that does not cross-react with any endogenous animal protein. Protein tags (i.e., artificial nonendogenous antigens) such as human influenza HA or FLAG-tag that can easily be detected with IHC methods can be used as a marker for the test article. These data provide tissue, cellular, and subcellular context

for the expression of the gene therapy candidate and can complement PCR-based quantitative biodistribution data. In addition, other IHC stains can be used to characterize downstream changes in protein expression or tissue effects. For example, in a mouse model of mucopolysaccharidosis Type IIID, IHC for glial fibrillary acidic protein (GFAP) has been used to demonstrate reduction in astrocytic activation after delivery of adeno-associated virus 9 (AAV9) vectors expressing N-acetylglucosamine 6-sulfatase (Roca et al., 2017). Similarly, in a mouse model of Alzheimer's disease, immunohistochemistry for GFAP has been used to demonstrate neuroinflammation in animals that received AAV vectors designed to express antibodies directed against β-amyloid. The observed neuroinflammation was attributed to presence of the expressed antibodies in the tissues (Elmer et al., 2019). Having a sensitive and specific staining method for such analyses is critical to their utility for assessing safety and functionality of cell and gene therapies.

USE OF IMMUNOHISTOCHEMISTRY FOR BIODISTRIBUTION OF SMALL OR LARGE MOLECULE THERAPIES

IHC can be used to assess the biodistribution of large or small molecules as well as cell and gene therapies in dosed animals. Unlike TCR studies, which are required for CDR-containing biotherapeutics to characterize potential off-target binding, biodistribution studies are not a standard component of a safety program but rather are performed on a case-by-case basis. These studies can provide valuable information about the distribution, persistence, association with observed lesions, or association with other tissue-based markers of effect of a therapeutic candidate in dosed tissues.

For large and small molecule therapies, the ideal IHC test article biodistribution study has the following characteristics (Rojko, 2008):

a. Provides sensitive, specific, and robust demonstration of the test article in paraffin sections (usually replicate sections from tissues obtained during a toxicity or efficacy study);

b. Demonstrates if the test article binds to expected **target** sites after in vivo dosing to test species;

c. Demonstrates if the test article binds to unexpected or undesired **off-target** sites after in vivo dosing to test species;

d. Can be used to compare test article distribution produced by different dosing routes;

e. May be employed to evaluate temporal shifts in test article distribution;

f. Demonstrates if the test article is associated with histopathologic findings; and

g. Demonstrates if the test article is associated with immune complex formation and deposition in vivo.

Sensitive and specific test article demonstration is easiest when the test article is antigenically distinct from any endogenous molecule found in the test species tissue and when a commercially available antibody is available with specificity for the test article, and this detection antibody and the staining method have been qualified. For example, IHC can localize microcystin-LR in mouse liver after intraperitoneal injection and associate distribution of this toxin with the temporal onset of hemorrhage and apoptosis affecting hepatocytes (Guzman and Solter, 2002). Similarly, a commercially available antiantibiotic antibody has been utilized to localize accumulation of the test article in activated lung macrophages (Yoshida et al., 1998).

Biodistribution studies are more difficult when the biomolecule test article is closely related to an endogenous protein. For example, when the test articles is a human enzyme administered to a heterologous species, that species may have an endogenous enzyme that is closely related to the administered human protein. Thus, even when an antienzyme antibody is available, it might detect both the administered human-derived test article and the endogenous animal enzyme in tissue.

Another example is the IHC evaluation of paraffin sections from animals administered human monoclonal IgG antibodies (mAbs), particularly when the test species of choice is an NHP. Sensitive and specific detection of the human mAb against the cross-reactive background of monkey IgG can be accomplished but only following extensive cross-adsorption of the antihuman IgG antibody (Lewis, 2018). Additionally, the exogenous human mAb becomes incorporated into the endogenous monkey IgG pool and is transported, taken up, and cleared according to the physiologic processes that govern IgG biodistribution (e.g., FcR-mediated clearance, etc.). Thus, in order to localize the human mAb (human IgG), one must also use extensively cross-adsorbed, anti-monkey IgG antibodies to identify the patterns of monkey IgG staining (Figure 11.4). These patterns are then "subtracted" from the patterns of human mAb staining to identify potential sites of target or off-target binding of the test article (Rojko, 2008; Rojko et al., 2014).

IHC may also allow evaluation of the temporal differences in distribution of the test article, including the determination of shifts between organ compartments and the total time of duration of the agent in certain tissues (see *Principles of Pharmacokinetics and Toxicokinetics*, Vol 1, Chap 5). Antisense oligonucleotide (ASO) test articles have been monitored in this manner using IHC, sometimes in combination with ISH (Goebl et al., 2007; Monteith et al., 1999). When ASO test articles are administered to an animal, basophilic granular material can be seen in the kidneys, liver, and lymph nodes on H&E-stained sections, particularly when higher

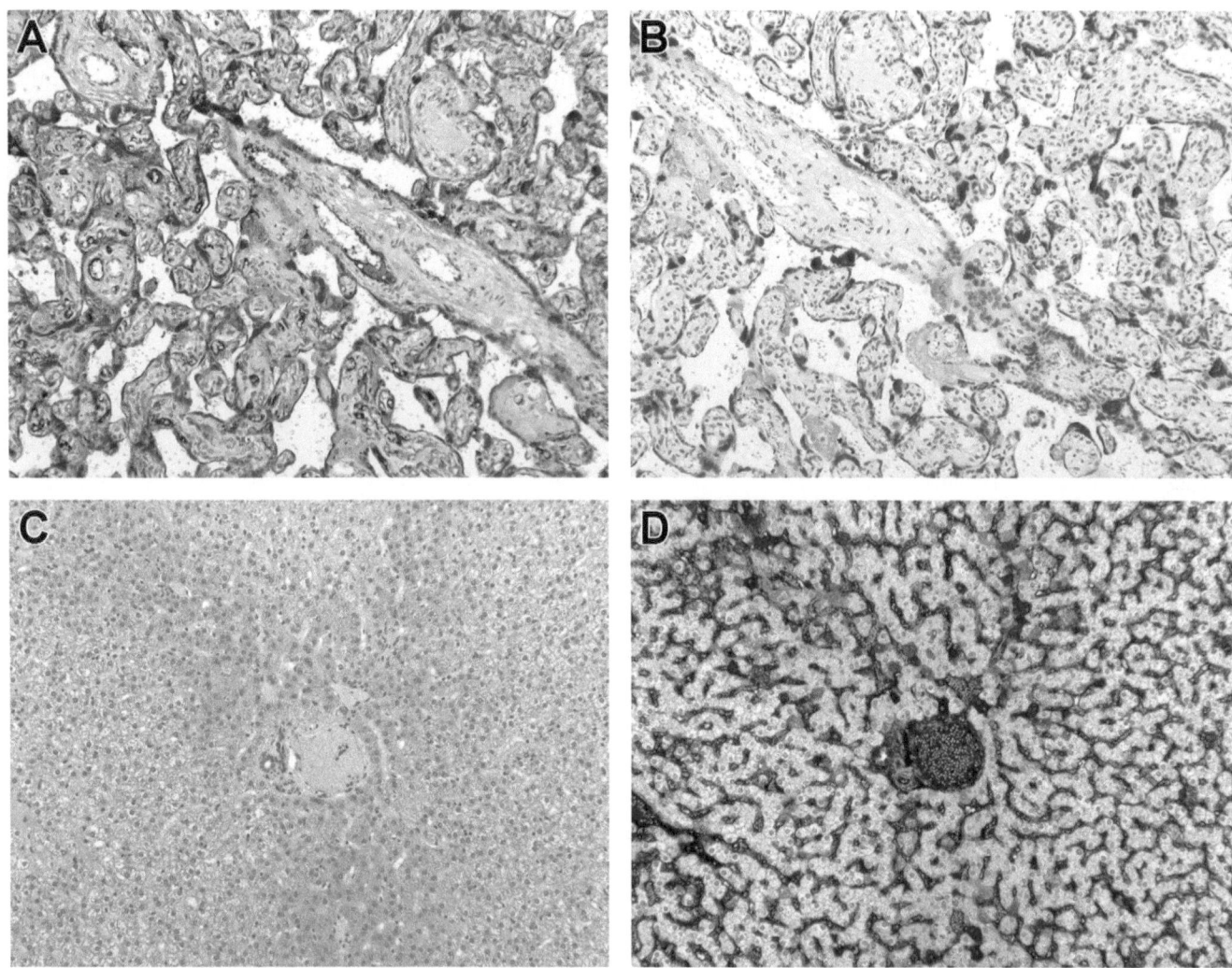

FIGURE 11.4   Example of controls used for evaluation of biodistribution of fully human, humanized, or chimeric antibody–based test articles in nonhuman primate tissues. Demonstration of lack of reactivity of monkey-adsorbed, goat antihuman IgG and human-adsorbed, goat antimonkey IgG with endogenous IgG in monkey and human tissue, respectively, permits localization of human antibody–based test articles in nonhuman primate tissues. (A) Human placenta stained with monkey-adsorbed goat antihuman IgG to show specific (positive) labeling. (B) Human placenta stained with human-adsorbed goat antimonkey IgG that demonstrates no labeling. (C) Cynomolgus monkey liver stained with monkey-adsorbed goat antihuman IgG to show no labeling. (D) Cynomolgus monkey liver stained with human-adsorbed goat antimonkey IgG to demonstrate extensive positive labeling.

doses are given (Farman and Kornbrust, 2003) (see *Nucleic Acid Pharmaceutical Agents*, Vol 2, Chap 6). Using an antibody directed toward the antisense test article demonstrated that these granules represent either the oligonucleotide itself or its metabolite. When new antisense test articles are developed, IHC can be used to evaluate their distribution. This method is particularly useful when tissue concentrations are not high enough to visualize the granule accumulation using standard H&E staining. Small interfering RNA test articles can be localized in tissues using fluorescent dye tags. Localization of these test articles can be further characterized using IHC and colocalization for other cell-specific markers (Aleku et al., 2008; Shi et al., 2011).

A potential caveat to using IHC to detect administered test articles in tissues is that in some cases the method may not be sensitive enough to detect low levels of the test article. For example, IHC may not detect the small amounts of mAb that reach other tissues via the systemic circulation following intravitreal exposure. Combining IHC with other, more sensitive methods such as ELISA to measure administered mAb in serum or using amplification techniques in the IHC protocol (e.g., ABC, CARD, and TSA) could resolve such problems.

Lesion Identification and Characterization

When a morphological alteration is identified by routine H&E evaluation in a nonclinical safety study, it may be important to further characterize that alteration. Characterization should always be designed on a case-by-case basis using a focused approach. IHC staining should only be done on slides from a safety study when the question to be answered is well defined and the appropriate methods development, qualification, and/or validation have been performed to ensure interpretable and reproducible data.

Depending upon the histopathologic alteration, IHC staining can provide valuable information regarding many aspects of the lesion pathogenesis. For example, IHC markers may be employed to identify the cell type, determine the lineages and/or functional states of responding cells (especially resident or infiltrating immune elements), assess the relative abundance of intracellular proteins such as hormones, provide evidence of cell death or proliferation, localize test article, and detect the presence of immune complexes. These data can add context and aid in risk assessment of observed tissue changes.

Finally, IHC staining using panels of antibodies can be useful in determining the histogenesis of a tumor. Use of marker panels expected to be expressed or not expressed in a given tissue can be useful in determining the origin of an observed mass and can offset the pathologist's internal bias (Painter et al., 2010). Epithelial cell markers (e.g., cytokeratins) as well as markers for mesenchymal cells (e.g., vimentin) and hematopoietic cells (e.g., CD45) should be included in such a staining panel (Painter et al., 2010). For example, in a U.S. National Toxicology Program (NTP) study, mouse uterine cervical granular cell tumors examined using IHC with a panel of antibodies were found to be positive for smooth muscle actin and desmin and negative for S-100 and other neural markers, suggesting myogenic rather than neural origin (Painter et al., 2010).

Evaluation of Responses to Test Article Administration

IHC is also valuable for evaluating alterations in host response to target organs following administration of a test article. In this respect, it can generate much information about the mechanisms of action and toxicity of an agent.

BIOMARKERS OF EXPOSURE AND EFFECT

EVALUATION OF LEUKOCYTE CD MARKERS OR OTHER SURFACE MARKERS (E.G., CHEMOKINE RECEPTORS) IN RESPONSE TO IMMUNE-MODULATING AGENTS

Current international guidelines include IHC as a potentially useful method to evaluate the immunotoxicity of a test article in nonclinical and clinical studies (ICH, 2006). In current toxicologic practice, IHC is used to evaluate changes in leukocyte cluster of differentiation (CD) antigens or other cell type–specific surface markers in response to the administration of agents that modulate the immune system. These types of changes might be difficult to observe with evaluation of H&E-stained sections alone as changes in numbers of some cell types after treatment might be subtle, especially for some immune-modulating test articles.

Flow cytometry provides a sensitive and specific monitor of CD, cytokine, and chemokine receptors on peripheral blood cells or ex vivo tissue suspensions but provides limited information regarding distribution of these markers with respect to tissue architecture. IHC staining for different CD antigens in lymphoid or nonlymphoid tissues can illustrate normal architecture (Figure 11.5) or can provide vital information regarding toxicologic or pharmacologic alterations. For example, IHC staining was used as part of the weight-of-evidence approach to demonstrate potential efficacy of combination therapy with the B-cell immunomodulators atacicept and rituximab in monkeys (Ponce, 2009).

When IHC labeling is used as a predictor of efficacy in nonclinical studies, a similar IHC assay also may be useful as a predictor of responsiveness in clinical trials, especially when the marker can be used as a selection criterion for clinical trial entry. The number of CD antigens and the availability of antibodies directed against them is constantly growing, and investigators should thoroughly review whether the CD

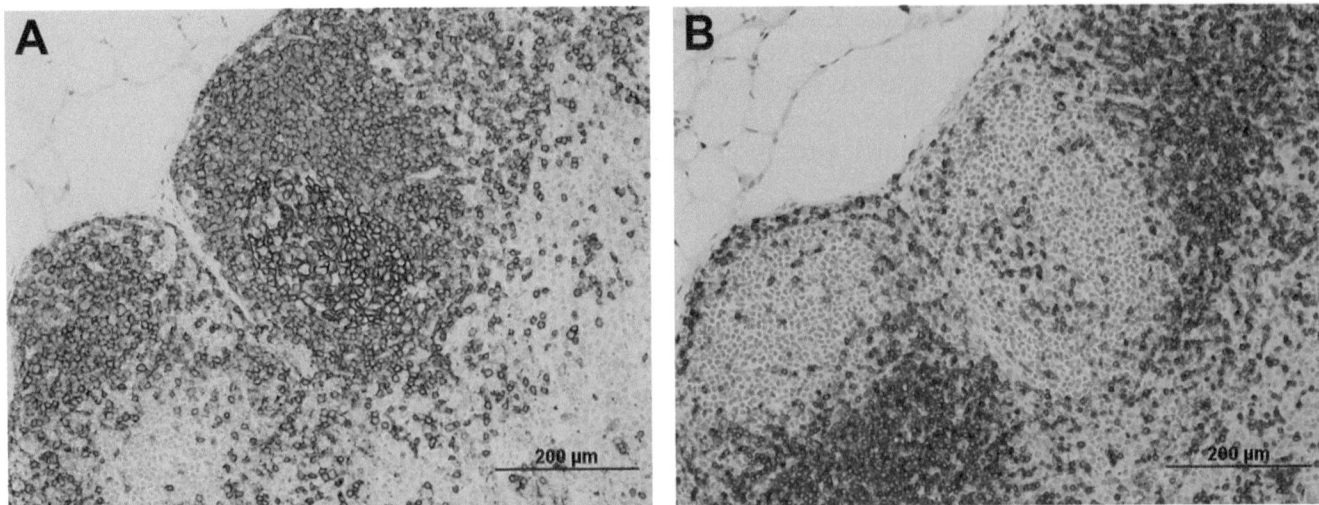

FIGURE 11.5   Rhesus monkey axillary lymph node stained by immunohistochemistry for lymphocyte markers (CD markers). The dark-stained regions consist of cells positive for the antibody marker. (A) Immunohistochemistry with an anti-CD20 antibody (Pan–B-lymphocyte marker) identifies B-cell specific regions (Original magnification 20X). (B) Immunohistochemistry with an anti-CD2 antibody (Pan–T-lymphocyte marker) identifies T-cell specific regions (Original magnification 20X). *Figure reproduced from the Haschek WM, Rousseaux CG, Wallig MA, editors:* Handbook of toxicologic pathology, *ed 3, 2013, Elsevier, Fig. 7.1, with permission.*

antigen in which they are interested is appropriate for the question being asked as well as for the test species (and ultimately for translation to support the human clinical trials indication) under consideration (Knapp, 1989; Schlossman, 1995).

If the test article targets a certain CD or chemokine receptor molecule, changes in the presence of that marker on cells may be evaluated by IHC (Ponce, 2009). On numerous occasions in our experience, no apparent changes were present in lymphoid tissues based on evaluation of H&E-stained sections, whereas changes in the numbers and/or distribution of various leukocytes were obvious using IHC evaluation of CD markers. However, because subtle differences in cell numbers may not be detectable by conventional semiquantitative evaluation of IHC-stained sections, quantification of cell numbers may be better approached by flow cytometry on peripheral blood cells or cells isolated from lymphoid organs or by digital image analysis of sections containing chromogenic or immunofluorescent signals for specific cell types.

Evaluation of CD markers not only has value in adult animals but also can give information about the effects of a test article on the developing immune system. In our experience, IHC evaluation of CD marker expression has illustrated on numerous occasions that there may be obvious effects on the numbers and distribution of various cell types without the presence of clinically detectable immunosuppression (including the lack of detectable opportunistic infections, a hallmark of clinical immunosuppression). This is often useful information for the developers of immunomodulatory compounds since it demonstrates that their therapeutic candidate has a desired, but not overwhelming, effect on regulating the function of the immune system.

One limitation of using IHC to evaluate changes in CD, cytokine, and chemokine receptor molecule expression is that it detects changes in numbers of cells and their distribution but does not generally give any information about cellular function. The exception to this is the use of antibodies against CD markers found on activated cells of various types where IHC effectively detects activated cells expressing activation state-specific markers (Knapp, 1989; Schlossman, 1995). A limitation of this approach is that many activation markers are expressed on multiple immune cell types; therefore, multiplex IHC labeling with fluorescently labeled antibodies is often used to detect subsets of activated cells. Commercial antibody suppliers are often very helpful in choosing appropriate activation markers via their catalogs and technical service representatives. Other methods including flow cytometry and functional assays that more specifically evaluate immune cell function can be combined with IHC to provide an overall functional assessment so that effects on the immune system are not missed if assays are used in isolation.

EVALUATION OF CHANGES IN COMMON TARGET ORGANS

Pharmaceutical and biopharmaceutical agents can affect target organs in different ways, and IHC can be used to study physiologically similar events in most organs. Thus, it is possible to compare changes in the kidney and liver in the distribution of organ-specific enzymes, cell type–specific markers, and the composition of cellular infiltrates by using IHC.

The liver is commonly affected by a wide variety of pharmaceutical and biopharmaceutical agents and toxicants by virtue of its roles in metabolism and detoxification. As a result, many substances in the liver may be altered depending on the mixture of potentially toxic entities that are presented for processing. Many of these substances can be detected by IHC, making this a useful method for evaluation of effects on the liver. Various hepatocellular enzymes or microsomal constituents may be evaluated by IHC, and thus changes in these parameters can be monitored. For example, IHC has been used to demonstrate reductions in cytochrome P450 enzymes in rats treated with Kava extracts (Clayton et al., 2007). In another study, immunohistochemistry was used to demonstrate hepatotoxicity by reductions in expression of cytochrome P450 enzymes in rats treated with triptolide (Lu et al., 2017). Antibodies are available to demonstrate various cell types within the liver, easing the structural evaluation of functional changes (e.g., hypertrophy and hyperplasia) of such cell populations. Certain molecules (exogenous or endogenous) may stimulate leukocyte accumulation in the liver, either without (i.e., infiltration) or with (i.e., inflammation) damage to the liver parenchyma and upregulation of cell adhesion molecules. These changes can often be detected using IHC. Finally, preneoplastic and neoplastic changes in the liver may be evaluated by detecting changes in expression of growth factors, markers of cell proliferation (e.g., Ki-67, PCNA) and cell apoptosis (e.g., cleaved caspase 3 [CC3]), and the protein products of oncogenes (e.g., c-met). A comprehensive review on the use of IHC in the evaluation of the liver is available (Hall and Rojko, 1996; Xi Yang et al., 2014). The liver has been used as an example of IHC utility in evaluating functional parameters and disease progression since this organ is so commonly affected by pharmaceutical and other bioactive agents. A similar approach using IHC may be employed profitably in other common target organs.

IMMUNE COMPLEX AND COMPLEMENT DEPOSITION

Some pharmaceutical agents or toxic compounds, particularly biotherapeutics, may incite an immune response when recognized by the body's immune system as foreign. Such reactions may lead to deposition of immune complexes and complement proteins in various organs, particularly in blood vessels and renal glomeruli. This process can occur when a human or humanized biotherapeutic such as a mAb is administered to a relevant animal species as part of the regulatory-directed safety assessment. When an immune complex pathogenesis is suspected based on clinical presentation (e.g., infusion reaction, protein losing nephropathy); clinical pathology findings (e.g., hypoalbuminemia, acute phase response); and/or microscopic features (membranoproliferative glomerulonephritis, vasculitis), it usually is preferable to assess immune complex deposition by performing retrospective IHC analysis on replicate paraffin sections rather than cryosections. Frozen tissues may not be available, the sensitivity of detection is generally considered equivalent in paraffin and frozen sections, and the paraffin sections provide the advantages of improved morphology and correlation with histopathologic lesions. A typical panel of immune complex markers might include IHC staining for one or more immunoglobulin (IgG, IgM, and/or IgA) classes or early or late markers of complement activation (e.g., complement factor C3 or soluble membrane attack complex sC5b-9 [also called sMAC]) (Chowdhury et al., 2005; Rojko, 2008; Rojko et al., 2014; Yamashina et al., 1989).

Furthermore, current IHC methods allow testing for deposition of immune complex components, including the concurrent presence of the test article, in serial sections. Combined test article biodistribution and immune complex studies have proven useful to understand the role of drug–antidrug immune complexes in animals on toxicity studies that experience infusion reactions and leukocyte sequestration in lung, liver or other tissues as well as in vascular or glomerular inflammatory alterations (Rojko, 2008; Rojko et al., 2014). The IHC demonstration that a histopathologic alteration associated with a test article noted during a toxicity study was due the biologic response of the test species to a foreign antigen (i.e., immune response of an animal to human IgG) and was not a direct pharmacologic/toxicologic effect of the test article is generally interpreted to mean that the effects in animals are less likely to occur in the treated human population (Frazier et al., 2015; Rojko et al., 2014).

ENDOCRINE EFFECTS

In 2009, the Endocrine Society published a review article expressing concern that certain naturally occurring compounds, therapeutics, and environmental contaminants likely disrupt the function of the endocrine system. The U.S. Environmental Protection Agency (EPA) has issued guidelines for Tier 1 (in vitro) and Tier 2 (in vivo) screening of endocrine disruptors (http://www.epa.gov/endo/). Although Tier two screening does not specify IHC evaluation for endocrine disruptors, IHC has been a classical adjunct to toxicity or experimental studies in which the test article targets the endocrine system (e.g., drugs for diabetes or targeting the hypothalamic-pituitary-adrenal or hypothalamic-pituitary-thyroid axes in rodents or NHPs at different stages of fetal or postnatal development). Furthermore, many antibodies suitable for use in common animal test species and humans are already available against hormones, their receptors, or other critical components of endocrine or neuroendocrine axes. Additional information can be found in (see *Endocrine Disruptors*, Vol 2, Chap 29).

IHC has proven valuable in elucidating the pathogenesis of some endocrine disruptors, including those with neuroendocrine effects in sexually dimorphic areas of the brain. For example, IHC has demonstrated alterations in calbindin in the preoptic area of rabbit hypothalamus following exposure to the antiandrogenic fungicide vinclozolin, which disrupts male sexual behavior (Bisenius et al., 2006; Bogdanffy, 1990). IHC also has contributed to the understanding of how vinclozolin, polychlorinated biphenyls (PCBs), and synthetic estrogens perturb sexually dimorphic regions of the developing rat hypothalamus (Dickerson et al., 2011a). Translation of this IHC-derived information to human health risk assessment has been assisted by other IHC studies which show species, gender, and age-related differences in distribution of estrogen, progesterone, and androgen receptors; calbindin protein; and gonadotropin-releasing hormone neurons and nerve terminals in different hypothalamic regions (Dudas and Merchenthaler, 2006; Fernández-Guasti et al., 2000; Kruijver et al., 2003; Scott et al., 2004). IHC also has been useful in monitoring neuroendocrine alterations affecting puberty and reproduction associated with environmental endocrine disrupters (e.g., heavy metals and PCBs) following experimental or environmental exposure (Dickerson et al., 2011b; Iavicoli et al., 2009). IHC using a variety of markers can also be useful in identifying hyperplastic and neoplastic lesions of the endocrine system. The panels of markers might include those that identify and/or illustrate neuroendocrine differentiation, epithelial origin, proliferation, and site of origin (Duan and Mete, 2016).

BIOTRANSFORMATION ENZYMES

Drug metabolizing enzymes, particularly the cytochrome P450 enzymes, are very important in the detoxification of many chemicals (see *Biochemical and Molecular Basis of Toxicity*, Vol 1, Chap 2). Evaluation of changes in these enzymes by IHC may help elucidate mechanisms of toxicity of certain toxicants. As a specific example, a variety of cytochromes P450 have been localized to specific cell types in the nasal cavity, helping to explain the mechanisms of toxicity of numerous inhaled and systemic toxicants that affect this region. Diversity in enzyme distribution among species has helped to explain species differences in response to formaldehyde, a nasal carcinogen (Anderson et al., 1989; Cui et al., 2000).

MECHANISMS OF TUMOR FORMATION

Carcinogenicity of exogenous compounds may occur via either genotoxic or epigenetic mechanisms. IHC is useful to investigate mechanisms of tumor formation by a wide variety of toxicants (see *Carcinogenesis: Mechanisms and Evaluation*, Vol 1, Chap 8). Some IHC techniques are suitable for mechanistic exploration whether the agent acts by a genotoxic or epigenetic mechanism. IHC detection of cell type-specific markers known to be produced by initiated or transformed cells is a useful method to evaluate the potential carcinogenicity of a toxicant. In a medium-term liver carcinogenesis model in rat, increased expression by IHC of the placental form of glutathione S-transferase (also termed GST-7-7) provides putative evidence of initiated hepatocytes (Moore et al., 1999). As noted above, species-agnostic IHC methods to detect apoptotic cells (CC3) or proliferating (5-bromo-2'-deoxyuridine [BrdU]), Ki-67, PCNA) cells provide important means for evaluating tumor viability and aggressiveness (Mitić and McKay, 2005). Many tumor cell type–specific markers are available to aid in the identification and characterization of organ-limited or multisystemic neoplasms (Kolenda-Roberts et al., 2013; Painter et al., 2010; Rehg et al., 2012). The importance of IHC as a tool for such investigations is clear, but a detailed review of this topic is beyond the scope of this chapter.

With respect to genotoxic mechanisms, IHC can be employed to examine specific forms of DNA damage and mechanisms of genotoxicity. For example, IHC can detect DNA adducts resulting from interaction of toxic metabolites with particular nucleotides at appreciable levels (Ewa and Danuta, 2017; Poirier et al., 2000). IHC using antibodies recognizing γH2AX, a marker for DNA double strand breaks, was used as an early marker for genotoxicity in the urinary bladders of rats treated with N-butyl-N-(4-hydroxybutyl)-nitrosamine (Toyoda et al., 2013). In addition, various IHC markers have been used to demonstrate the genotoxic mode of action of fine dust particles in rat lungs (Rittinghausen et al., 2013).

In recent years, the tremendous importance of epigenetic mechanisms of tumor formation has become clear. Extensive research has determined that mutations in genes that limit DNA damage (i.e., tumor suppressor genes such as *Trp53* ["p53"]) or promote increased tumor cell survival (e.g., proto-oncogenes like *k-ras*) are very important in the formation and progression of various types of neoplasms in both animals

and humans. For example, when engineered or carcinogen-induced mutations in the *Trp53* gene ablate its tumor suppressor function, the mutant p53 protein becomes easier to detect with IHC because it becomes localized to the nucleus and is much more stable than normal ("wild type") p53 protein. Importantly, p53 mutations are important in some tumor types but not others (Belinsky et al., 1997; Lee et al., 1999; Okudela et al., 1999). The same differential involvement also exists for oncogenes, where activating mutations detected by IHC are concentrated in some tumor types but appear to be inconsequential in others.

Cell Proliferation Studies and Evaluation of Cell Cycle–Related Proteins

IHC evaluation of cell proliferation is commonly performed, particularly for agents known or suspected to cause changes in cell proliferation rates or neoplasia. Numerous methods are available to perform these studies, each of which has advantages and disadvantages (Hall and Woods, 1990). They all have an advantage over simple evaluation of the numbers of mitotic figures in routinely stained H&E sections because the IHC-stained cells are easier to see and count, and for some markers cells are detectable in various stages of replication in addition to mitosis. Originally, tritiated thymidine was used to evaluate cell proliferation, but this method has mostly been replaced by nonradioactive methods. For example, BrdU, a thymidine analog, is incorporated into cellular DNA in the S (synthesis) phase of the cell cycle and can be detected by IHC using antibodies to BrdU resulting in an accurate and reliable technique for assessing cell proliferation. However, BrdU must be administered to test animals either by injection 1 to 2 hours prior to necropsy, by means of subcutaneously implanted minipumps, or by administration in the drinking water. As such, BrdU is not the ideal method, particularly in the context of toxicity studies, where there is often a preference to avoid techniques that require administration of an agent to the animals during the course of the study.

More popular methods for IHC evaluation of cell proliferation, especially for toxicity studies, include staining for PCNA, Ki67, and phosphohistone H3 (PhH3). PCNA and Ki67 staining offer advantages compared to BrdU staining since these techniques do not require prior injections and can often be performed retrospectively on formalin-fixed, paraffin-embedded tissue. Furthermore, BrdU stains only detect cells in S phase, while PCNA and Ki67 detect cells in all stages of the replicative portion of the cell cycle (G1 + S + G2 + M). Some investigators believe that PCNA-positive cells can be separated according to each of these stages based on characteristic differences in the pattern of nuclear staining. Studies using characteristic differences in nuclear staining of PCNA to compare S phase labeling of PCNA to that of BrdU have found that the labeling indices are similar for the two methods and that the methods are equally useful for evaluating cell proliferation. Histone H3 (PhH3) is a nuclear protein that is a component of chromatin. Its phosphorylation is a key event in chromatin condensation during mitosis and meiosis, and thus, it can serve as a useful marker of mitotic cells (Lee et al., 2014). PhH3 has been used as an early marker of carcinogens inducing cell proliferation in a number of tissues in rats treated with carcinogens targeting different organs (Yafune et al., 2013). In another study, PhH3 was used to demonstrate the role of p53 in microcystin-LR tumor promotion in mice (Clark et al., 2008). One method may be preferred over the other depending on the specific situation (Eldridge and Goldsworthy, 1996; Foley et al., 1991; Mundle et al., 1994; Roberts et al., 1997).

Examples of the use of cell proliferation markers in toxicologic pathology abound in the literature and it should not be difficult to find information appropriate for a desired situation. Experts in this field caution that with regard to evaluating cell proliferation in an attempt to assess for a potential carcinogenic effect, an increase in cell proliferation does not necessarily indicate that such proliferation will lead to neoplasia. For example, a specific study in which both proliferation and apoptosis were evaluated for two different agents determined that the relative balance of the two different processes might be important in determining why carcinogenesis occurs with some nongenotoxic agents and not others (Ghanayem et al., 1997). It should be noted that a single assessment for cell proliferation might not be sufficient for prediction of tumor outcome; rather, understanding the extent of cell proliferation over the entire course of the disease via assessment at multiple time points might provide more valuable information in this regard.

IHC also is used to evaluate changes in other molecules involved in cell cycle control, particularly caspases, cyclins, and cyclin-dependent kinases. Numerous antibodies are available commercially for these molecules. Various investigators have used IHC to evaluate changes in these cell cycle–related proteins in response to administration of various toxicants. The application of digital pathology techniques (see *Digital Pathology and Tissue Image Analysis*, Vol 1, Chap 12) should provide the ability to rapidly gather more quantitative cell proliferation data (Lee et al., 1999; Wang et al., 1998).

Evaluation of Apoptosis and Necrosis

Apoptosis, or programmed cell death (PCD), is an active cell process that plays a critical role in a number of normal physiological events, including embryonic modeling, organization of the central nervous system, metamorphosis, etc (Bursch et al., 1992). PCD has received widespread attention as a crucial component of a number of pathologic processes, including neoplasia and other disturbances in growth, inflammation, and immune responses (Corcoran et al., 1994; Elmore, 2007). The best-defined biochemical alteration in cells undergoing PCD is generation of an endonuclease that cleaves nuclear DNA at the regions between the nucleosomes. This cleavage yields characteristic DNA fragments with sizes that are multiples of approximately 180–200 base pairs. Gel electrophoresis of DNA extracted from apoptotic cells shows a characteristic "DNA ladder" that is diagnostic for PCD. Morphologic criteria for PCD are also very specific at the ultrastructural level. Apoptotic cells are characterized by the shrinkage of the cytoplasm and nuclear chromatin condensation. The cellular shrinkage results in apoptotic bodies, which are typically phagocytosed by macrophages or other surrounding cells (Elmore et al., 2016; Huppertz et al., 1999).

Although the morphologic criteria of PCD are well defined, apoptotic cells can be very difficult to recognize or confused with other cellular changes in standard histologic sections. This difficulty stems from both their relative rarity in most tissues and their transience—commonly a few hours only. Two methods have been described that utilize the presence of DNA breaks to label single cells undergoing PCD. One method uses DNA polymerase I (Pol 1), and is called either in situ nick translation (ISNT) or in situ end labeling (ISEL) in the literature, where "in situ" reflects the location where the method is employed (i.e., in a tissue section), "nick translation" indicates that the method leads to extension (by translation) from a site of DNA strand breakage, and "end labeling" denotes that the extension occurs at the broken end (Gold et al., 1993; Mainwaring et al., 1998). The second method uses terminal deoxynucleotidyl transferase (TdT) and has been called either the tailing reaction or TdT-mediated bio-dUTP nick end-labeling (TUNEL) (Sanders, 1997). While these methods involve a combination of molecular biology and IHC techniques, they will be covered here in order to include them in a discussion of IHC techniques used to evaluate various stages of the apoptotic pathway.

ISEL or ISNT relies on the ability of DNA Pol 1 to add labeled nucleotides to the 3'-hydroxyl end of a DNA strand in the presence of a template, thereby extending the strand in a 5' to 3' direction. It is hypothesized that ISEL probably detects the 3' recessed DNA fragments formed in apoptosis. Because DNA Pol 1 is primer- and template dependent, it cannot label the blunt-ended or 5' recessed DNA fragments that may also occur in PCD. DNA Pol 1 also has an exonuclease activity that, starting at the site of a single-strand break, may remove unlabeled nucleotides ahead of the enzyme, allowing their replacement by labeled nucleotides (Aschoff et al., 1996; Kressel and Groscurth, 1994). Many vendors now offer the large subunit of DNA Pol 1, known as the Klenow fragment, for use in molecular biology and related applications. The Klenow fragment lacks any 3' to 5' exonuclease activity while retaining the primer extension and proofreading capabilities of DNA Pol 1, and has also been used with success in the ISEL procedure (Woolveridge et al., 1999; Wu and Liu, 2000).

The TUNEL method is based on the specific binding of terminal TdT to 3'-OH ends of DNA, with subsequent incorporation of labeled deoxyuridine at the sites of DNA breaks. Biotin and digoxigenin are the common choices for labels. Because TdT is template independent, it can label blunt-ended, 3'-recessed or 5'-recessed DNA fragments at the hydroxylated 3' ends (Gold et al., 1993; Migheli et al., 1995; Sanders and Wride, 1996).

These methods have become very popular, and commercial kits are available to specifically label apoptotic cells. However, controversy has arisen regarding the specificity of these enzymatic reactions. Both methods rely on the enzymatic detection of DNA fragments in tissue sections. Although DNA fragmentation is a key feature of PCD, DNA fragmentation also occurs in necrosis, albeit at a later stage in the death of the cell. Some groups suggest that these methods do not reliably detect apoptotic cells in tissue sections, and in particular are unable to differentiate apoptotic from necrotic cells, or even from early postmortem autolysis. Other authors emphasize the value of these methods but caution that they must be used in conjunction with the morphologic assessment of the labeled cell in order to distinguish necrosis from PCD (Arends and Wyllie, 1991; Charriaut-Marlangue and Ben-Ari, 1995; Elmore et al., 2016; Grasl-Kraupp et al., 1995).

Many antibodies and methods are now available for detecting earlier changes in the apoptotic pathway by IHC (Arends and Wyllie, 1991). Some IHC markers for apoptosis include CC3, cleaved cytokeratin 18, phosphorylated histone H2AX, and cleaved lamin-A (Holubec et al., 2005). Some of these are more specific than the TUNEL assay, although all have their limitations. CC3 is frequently used as a marker for apoptotic cells. The epitope recognized by antibodies directed against CC3 is not present in healthy (i.e., nondegenerating) cells and is similar across species, making this an attractive marker for apoptotic cells (Gown and Willingham, 2002). However, using multiple methods in combination may provide more valuable information than using any single method alone. In our experience, use of CC9 and CC3 provides useful information about early and later events in the apoptotic cascade, respectively (Elmore, 2007; Elmore et al., 2016). Additionally, the application of digital pathology methods to apoptosis studies may facilitate the acquisition of more quantitative data and improve intergroup comparability in toxicity studies.

Necrosis is cell death usually resulting from acute cell injury and is characterized by loss of cell and organelle membrane integrity which leads to cell swelling, release of proteolytic enzymes, and ultimately cell death. The subsequent leakage of cellular components generally results in inflammation (Elmore et al., 2016). Necrosis is most often diagnosed by evaluation of H&E-stained slides and is generally characterized by loss of cellular detail, often associated with cellular debris and inflammation. Other changes associated with necrosis include cell swelling, nuclear swelling, karyolysis, karyorrhexis, nuclear pyknosis, pale eosinophilic cytoplasm, and cytoplasmic vacuoles (Elmore et al., 2016).

In some cases, apoptosis and necrosis can be difficult to distinguish. In these cases, transmission electron microscopy (TEM) is considered the "gold standard" for differentiation of these processes (Krysko et al., 2008). Other methods used for confirmation of necrosis include measurement of enzyme release into serum (e.g., beta-glucuronidase for hepatic necrosis and creatine kinase for myocardial necrosis) (Ohta, 1991; Ruzgar et al., 2006); exclusion dyes (e.g., propidium iodide, ethidium homodimer III) (Honda et al., 2000), or other methods such as flow cytometry and western blotting (Krysko et al., 2008). There are commercially available kits that use dyes to distinguish apoptotic cells from necrotic cells in suspension or adherent cells, but these kits cannot be used on whole tissue sections.

Use of IHC or exclusion dyes to detect necrosis in whole tissue can be difficult or impossible. IHC on tissue sections with necrotic areas can be difficult to interpret since antibodies often bind nonspecifically to necrotic tissue. In addition, there is no one marker that is truly a specific marker of necrosis. Use of exclusion dyes on tissue sections is also not possible since the nuclear membrane is cut during histological sectioning, thereby exposing nuclear DNA. However, exclusion dyes have been reported to detect necrosis in renal tissue after perfusion of the whole organ with an exclusion dye (Edwards et al., 2007). In addition, there are reports where IHC has been used successfully for elucidation of necrosis in tissue sections in conjunction with other markers for apoptosis and etosis (i.e., leukocyte death leading to release of an extracellular trap lattice composed of DNA, histones, and cytoplasmic proteins) (Pertiwi

et al., 2019). However, if IHC is being considered for detection of necrosis in tissue sections, careful method development is necessary to ensure that any observed binding is not due to nonspecific "sticking" of the antibody reagents to necrotic material.

Evaluation of Infectious Disease Agents

Immunohistochemistry using antibodies against various infectious agents is commonly performed in diagnostic pathology and can be useful in toxicologic pathology (see *Basic Approaches in Anatomic Toxicologic Pathology*, Vol 1, Chap 9). If immunomodulatory compounds are administered, it is possible that increased susceptibility to infectious agents may occur in the test species due to immunosuppression, and such agents may be detected using IHC. Evaluation of background infectious diseases in a research animal colony also may be undertaken in some instances. Animal models of infectious disease are used frequently to evaluate the efficacy of potential antiinfective test articles, and IHC for the particular infectious agent may help evaluate responses to therapy. Finally, viral vectors often are used to deliver therapeutic genes, and IHC may be used to detect the presence of the viral capsid proteins in the vector to ensure delivery to the target organ (though ISH for the transgene sequence is often used for this purpose as well) (Porter et al., 1990).

2.3. Technical Considerations for Immunohistochemistry

Availability of Antibodies

A significant problem facing investigators wishing to use IHC to detect target molecules is the availability of antibodies specific for the molecule. Proprietary mAb or mAb-based test articles generally will not have commercially available antibody reagents to enable IHC, so the antibodies needed for IHC will have to be specially generated for this purpose by the institution. In addition, even if antibodies to the target molecule are available commercially, they may not work in IHC but only in homogenized tissues (e.g., western blots). Commercial antibody vendors will generally have information regarding the applicability of their reagents to IHC and the ability of their products to detect related antigens from various species (animal and human); for specially generated antibodies designed to detect a novel test article, this information will have to be worked out experimentally. Commercial antibody reagents for IHC may have cross-reactivity with off-target antigens that may complicate interpretation.

Due to the widespread use of rodents in research, large numbers of antibody reagents specific for rodents have become available commercially. This is good news for those investigators using rodents in their studies and has been important in understanding many biologic responses (e.g., rat pituitary cell type determination). Some antihuman antibodies may cross-react with one or more animal species, but in the absence of such information, trial and error testing must be performed to determine the level of cross-reactivity across species. Many antihuman antibodies will cross-react with NHP tissue because of the close relationship between these species. If long-term studies with a critical test article are planned, a company may decide to synthesize (or have synthesized) a custom antibody reagent for the specific purpose of developing an IHC technique.

For some molecules, myriad antibodies are available, and the investigator must choose between a mAb (directed against a single epitope of the antigen) made in one species and a polyclonal antibody (directed against multiple epitopes of an antigen) made in a different species. There is no general rule of thumb regarding which type of antibody performs the best in IHC, and the choice of antibody must often be made empirically by testing several. In addition, some commercially available antibodies will only work in frozen tissues. Therefore, it is important to plan ahead with respect to tissue collection and fixation conditions if it is at all possible that IHC will be performed.

Tissue Collection and Fixation for Immunohistochemistry

Sampling of desired tissues should be considered before a toxicity study is even designed in order to have adequate tissue samples for both standard histological examination and IHC. For larger species, a particular tissue usually can be split into two parts, or in the case of lymph nodes, two or more of a specific type of node may be collected, if the fixation for routine

processing and IHC requires different conditions. However, due to the small size of rodents and fetuses, it is not always possible to split tissues. Therefore, additional animals may need to be added to the study, with some dedicated to IHC and the others to routine histology.

It may be desirable in larger institutions that perform IHC on an extensive scale to establish banks of appropriately collected and fixed tissues (both frozen and paraffin embedded) from normal animals. In this way, suitable control tissue is always available in the event that the cross-reactivity of a commercially available antibody reagent needs to be tested or for small pilot experiments in which concurrent control animals may not have been included in the study.

Target molecules in tissue sections need to be immobilized prior to the IHC because of the possibility of postmortem antigen diffusion. Target immobilization is usually accomplished through fixation (as in the case of formalin-fixed, paraffin-embedded tissue). The choice of fixative may impact the ability of the antibody reagent to bind to its target as not all epitopes or antigens survive all fixation procedures.

Some antibody reagents will only bind to their intended target in fresh frozen tissues, while others might be used successfully in both frozen or fixed tissues (Janardhan et al., 2018). If fixation may be used, overfixation should be avoided, which typically is accomplished by limiting the time spent in fixative and/or by using coagulating fixatives (also termed denaturing or precipitating fixatives, e.g., acetone, ethanol) rather than cross-linking (e.g., aldehydes) fixatives (Key, 2006). As mentioned above, it is important to plan ahead during the study design phase to ensure that tissues will have been collected and processed appropriately for any potential IHC staining that might be needed to interpret any histopathologic findings.

For tissues that have been fixed in neutral buffered 10% formalin (NBF, commercial formulations of which contain about 4% formaldehyde mixed with approximately 1% methanol as a stabilizing agent) or methanol-free 4% formaldehyde (known colloquially as 4% paraformaldehyde [PFA] since it is made from PFA pellets or powder), IHC may be problematic, depending on the antibody and depending on the length of time the tissues have been in fixative. It is most desirable that tissues only be fixed in aldehydes for no more than 24–48 h and then transferred to 70% ethanol if IHC is to be performed. Lengthy fixation in formaldehyde-based fixatives may destroy any hopes of performing IHC using many antibodies due to overcross-linking of protein. For many antibodies, retrieval of antigen in formalin-fixed, paraffin-embedded tissue may be necessary, using any of a variety of methods including enzymatic digestion and heat (Bohle et al., 1997; Cattoretti et al., 1993; Janardhan et al., 2018; Shi et al., 1997). Delicate antigens may be detected only if fixation occurs after acquisition of frozen sections. In such cases, sections are immersed in fixative (typically acetone, NBF, or other suitable fixative as determined during method development) for a few seconds up to several minutes.

Controls

Anyone who has performed IHC is aware that there are many potential pitfalls to accurate performance of the assays and interpretation of the results. Proper controls are always essential to the correct interpretation of the data. At a minimum, a serial section of tissue should be stained with an isotype-matched control antibody (for monoclonal antibodies) or pre- or nonimmune serum (for polyclonal antibodies) to demonstrate specificity of the primary antibody. In some cases, the IHC reagents may be the cause of nonspecific background staining. In this case, staining a series of sections where a different component of the IHC reaction is withheld would be useful in identifying the problematic reagent (Janardhan et al., 2018).

Knowledge of the expected staining results based on prior studies and a thorough understanding of the target protein is helpful (Janardhan et al., 2018). Expression patterns in various tissues gained by western blotting may be helpful in defining the list of expected binding sites for novel antibodies. Otherwise, trial and error and thorough investigation of the reasons for unexpected staining are often necessary to ensure accuracy.

Bright-Field Versus Immunofluorescence Microscopy for Immunohistochemistry

The choice of bright-field versus immunofluorescent microscopy for IHC can be made based on user preference or may be dependent on the staining method used. Multiplex IHC often is conducted more readily using immunofluorescence, for several reasons. First, distinct primary antibodies, each labeled with a different fluorophore having a unique emission spectrum from the other dyes, can be applied simultaneously. In contrast, for multiplex IHC using chromogenic methods, more care must be taken since the immunobridges to detect different antigens need to be built sequentially. Second, immunofluorescence might be the method of choice if there is interference from endogenous pigment (e.g., lipofuscin) or molecules used to label IHC reagents (e.g., biotin) in a chromogenic method. Third, in some instances, immunofluorescent staining is more sensitive than chromogenic staining and thus may better detect proteins expressed at very low levels. However, potential disadvantages of immunofluorescence methods include tissue autofluorescence (e.g., collagen and erythrocytes) and lack of fine tissue/cellular detail since the immunofluorescence method is dark field and other cellular/tissue structures are not readily visible with counterstain, thus limiting tissue or histologic context. Further, fluorescent staining is not permanent, so optimally whole-slide images (WSIs) would need to be prepared for long-term retention of fluorescent staining data. Consideration for long-term storage of large data files for high-resolution images would be necessary in these cases. In these instances, chromogenic IHC, where the colored product is more stable over time, might be the preferred method for long-term retention of the study materials needed to reproduce the data set.

Multiplex Labeling and Combination Techniques in Immunohistochemistry

Multiplex IHC, the staining of a single sample using multiple primary antibody reagents detecting distinct antigens, is an effective method to characterize the spatial distribution and coexpression of more than one biomarker in cells and tissues. The technique is becoming increasingly important as it enables the simultaneous collection of data for expanded lists of protein targets that have emerged to improve disease profiling or guide treatment while preserving limited sample material.

Multiplex labeling can be performed either using fluorescent or bright-field chromogenic techniques. Chromogenic immunohistochemistry labeling typically makes use of different enzymes (e.g., HRP, AP) and different soluble noncolored dyes that can be converted to colored precipitating products (Figure 11.6). The chromogenic double labeling technique is extremely useful in toxicologic pathology to determine the spatial location of an administered test article and a substance changed as a result of exposure to the test article, or to look for activated leukocytes infiltrating into tissue as a result of treatment with a certain test article or in response to a particular lesion (e.g., a tumor). However, study of biomarker colocalization is limited as commonly available chromogenic dyes used for IHC have poorly separated spectra features, which makes it challenging to unambiguously differentiate these dyes when they overlap.

In contrast, immunofluorescence labeling circumvents this limitation as fluorophores with disparate emission peaks can be separately imaged using fluorescence filters with restricted bandwidths so that binding of each labeled antibody can be interpreted in isolation, or paired antibodies can be assessed in any combination. Traditionally, immunofluorescence multiplex staining is performed with primary antibodies directly conjugated with fluorophores. However, it is cost inefficient to conjugate multiple primary antibodies, and sensitivity is often poor with low expression antigens. There are now commercially available and easy-to-use tyramide-based reagents that permit the staining of seven or more targets on a single tissue section (e.g., Opal multiplex assay, TSA kits) regardless of the species of the primary antibody host. Such techniques have also been applied successfully for the multiplex of ISH and immunofluorescence labeling (Dixon et al., 2015; Tan et al., 2020).

Quantitative Analysis in Immunohisotchemistry

A major limitation of IHC is that it has historically been more qualitative and not quantitative, demonstrating the presence but not the amount of the antigen. An exception to this is in studies where numbers of positively stained nuclei or cells (i.e., discrete objects) may be counted. Specific applications of quantitative IHC analysis in toxicologic pathology include cell proliferation assays and distinguishing the presence of human cells (cell-based therapies) in animal tissues. In most instances, however, a qualitative evaluation of changes in staining patterns and intensity has been sufficient to provide valuable information to the researcher. Digital pathology and computerized image analysis are rapidly evolving methodologies with the ability to objectively quantify IHC data through the use of algorithms (see *Digital Pathology and Tissue Image Analysis*, Vol 1, Chap 12). An important concept in IHC

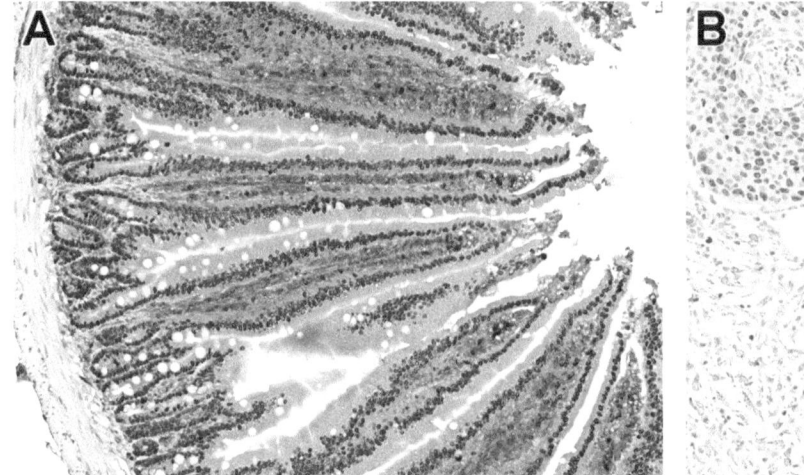
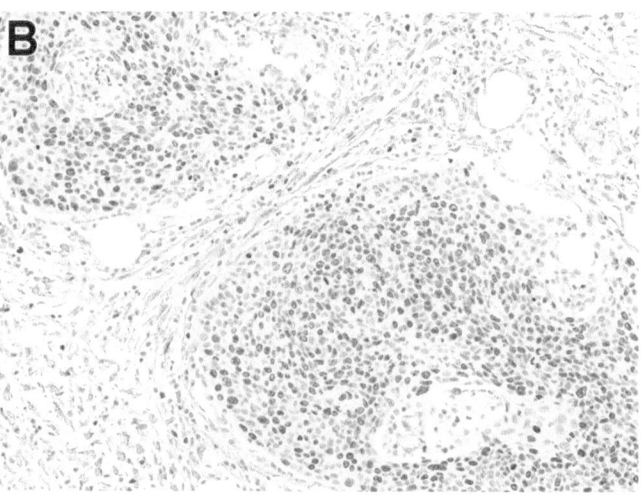

FIGURE 11.6   Examples of chromogenic multiplex staining. (A) BrdU and CD31. Dividing cell nuclei stained with BrdU marked with brown chromogen and endothelial cells expressing CD31 are marked with red chromogen. (B) Ki67 and smooth muscle actin (SMA). Dividing cell nuclei stained with Ki67 marked with purple chromogen and smooth myocytes stained with anti-SMA marked with yellow chromogen.

quantification of protein expression by digital image analysis is that true quantification cannot be done by counting positive pixels and their intensities. Instead, the algorithm must be calibrated to a known standard (e.g., cell pellets or tissues with known levels of protein expression) processed using the same IHC conditions and at the same time as the test samples.

When performing any type of quantitation, whether through manual counting or through the use of image analysis, it is important to design the study appropriately and understand when bias may be introduced into the quantitative methods. For example, manual counting of positively labeled cells in a certain number of "randomly chosen" fields of view contains significant inherent user bias, as the eye will always be drawn to fields with higher positivity. Care must be taken when choosing fields of view to count since bias related to sampling and processing of the tissue as well as geometrical features of the objects being counted may affect the accuracy of data acquired by image analysis. It is important to capture samples that are truly representative to minimize sampling bias, and unbiased sampling is the proper way to accomplish this task. It is also important to take tissue shrinkage, particularly when paraffin is used, into account when determining the density of positive cells within the tissue as packing density increases with increased tissue shrinkage. Finally, geometrical bias of the objects of interest can be important, particularly for larger objects that are irregularly shaped. Additional explanations of bias are given below in Section 9 (Stereology).

Regardless of whether the endpoints are qualitative or quantitative in nature, it is important to have an adequate sample size to ensure statistical power and suitably cover the range of normal staining in control animals. At least 5 animals/sex/groups are needed to come to any reasonable conclusion about the results with certainty, and 10 sex/groups are preferable to ensure adequate statistical power. Because quantitative analysis is more sensitive than qualitative evaluation, results may be more reliable if fewer samples per group are present for evaluation. In addition, the interpretation of TCR studies is primarily descriptive with no statistical analysis performed, so fewer donors (usually three) per tissue are generally included in those studies.

It is also important to consider staining variation within the tissue, particularly if the tissue is heterogeneous (i.e., staining for islets of Langerhans in the pancreas or staining for a particular neuron type in the brain). In these instances, it is imperative to capture several sections of the region of interest for evaluation, such as samples through the head, body, and tail of the pancreas.

2.4. Conclusion

In summary, IHC has many important applications in toxicologic pathology, in answering the many questions that arise in the development and overall safety assessment of pharmaceutical and biological agents for therapeutic purposes. The examples of its uses in this field are almost endless in the literature, and it is often very easily applied to novel questions that arise with new compounds. Although IHC is primarily qualitative, innovations in digital pathology analytical techniques may allow capture of more quantitative data in the future.

3. ENZYME HISTOCHEMISTRY

3.1. Introduction

EHC is a method that provides functional information about enzymes or pathways of interest in the context of their location in an intact cell or tissue. These methods generally involve the application of a colorless enzyme substrate to organ pieces ("whole mounts") or tissue sections and subsequent visualization of the colored metabolite as an insoluble dye product deposited at sites where the enzyme of interest is active (Meier-Ruge and Bruder, 2008; Vinod Sargaiyan, 2014). These techniques are usually fairly simple and can provide contextual information about changes in enzymatic function and other downstream tissue effects where quantitative biochemical measurements of enzyme activity cannot.

EHC was originally developed in the 1950's (Pearse, 1960) and rapidly became an important method in diagnostic pathology (Meier-Ruge and Bruder, 2008). Methods for a large number of enzymes of interest have been developed and widely used in diagnostic pathology (Meier-Ruge and Bruder, 2008). Immunohistochemistry, discussed in detail above and developed in the 1970s, later largely replaced EHC. However, EHC can provide spatial/tissue context information about an enzyme's activity where IHC only provides spatial information regarding its presence or level of expression in tissue. Changes in enzyme function often can be detected before histologic changes are observed. Thus, EHC can provide valuable information in the toxicologic pathology setting about dose-dependent and/or time-related changes cellular/tissue due after test article administration in a variety of species.

3.2. Applications of Enzyme Histochemistry in Toxicologic Pathology

EHC can be a useful tool in toxicologic pathology for demonstration of dose- or time-dependent cellular/tissue changes after administration of a test article. Subtle changes in enzyme activity can be observed before any histologic changes are apparent in tissues. In addition, morphology can be paired with EHC to provide information on cellular changes as they correlate to enzyme activity (Meier-Ruge and Bruder, 2008). For example, EHC was used in a cat model to elucidate the cause of the side effect of night blindness and retinal pigmentation in clinical trials with a tranquilizer (Meier-Ruge, 1969). In a primate model, EHC for acid phosphatase paired with morphometry facilitated understanding of the time-dependent increase in infarct size (Meier-Ruge et al., 1992). EHC can also provide contextual information about changes in enzymatic function and other downstream tissue effects. For example, EHC for AP and nonspecific esterase have been used as an effective early biomarker of cellular injury in the skin of Yorkshire pigs after topical exposure to jet fuel mixtures (Rhyne et al., 2002). In rats, EHC for hexosaminidase has been used to show differences in morphology and composition of aberrant crypt foci induced by either dextran sulfate, a nongenotoxic compound, or azoxymethane, a known genotoxin (Whiteley et al., 1996). EHC can also be a powerful tool for assessment of transgene expression and thus characterization of transgenic animal models. In a transgenic rodent model, whole mount beta-galactosidase activity (which can be added as a component of engineered genes but also is expressed endogenously in cells of many tissues as well as many intestinal bacteria) was evaluated during high-throughput necropsies and was shown to be useful for many but not all organs (Bolon, 2008). Other techniques including IHC and ISH are now more commonly used to characterize transgene expression in tissues.

3.3. Technical Considerations for Enzyme Histochemistry

EHC methods are usually fairly simple and have been extensively described (Meier-Ruge et al., 1971; Meier-Ruge and Bruder, 2005; 2008; Pearse, 1960; Schiebler, 1979). These methods most often involve application of the enzyme substrate to the tissue piece (whole mount) or tissue section followed by visualization of the resultant metabolite. The vast majority of these stains are performed on cryosections since extensive cross-linking associated with conventional aldehyde fixation often leads to permanent enzyme deactivation after just a few hours (Meier-Ruge and Bruder, 2008). EHC has been performed on fixed sections with variable results obtained under different fixation conditions (Bolon, 2008). Further, tissues to be used for EHC should be frozen using dry ice in a −80 degrees freezer or isopentane in a −25 degrees freezer rather than flash freezing in liquid nitrogen, which can cause severe tissue cracking. This compromise of tissue morphology can hamper interpretation of localization and tissue context for any observed signal (Meier-Ruge and Bruder, 2008). Tissues can be stored at −25 degrees until analysis (Meier-Ruge and Bruder, 2008). In addition, thicker sections (15 μm) are recommended to overcome the minimal enzyme activity threshold for the enzymatic starting reaction (Meier-Ruge and Bruder, 2005). Finally, a positive control section (a tissue with relevant cell types known to possess enzymatic activity) should be included for all experiments to ensure that the enzymatic staining method has worked consistently. Therefore, careful experimental planning is necessary to ensure that tissues are collected and processed in a manner suitable for EHC.

3.4. Conclusions

EHC can provide a useful tool for demonstration of changes in enzyme function and thus elucidate pathobiology of tissue/cellular processes after administration of a test article. Its ability to demonstrate changes in enzyme function in situ before observable changes on H&E or IHC makes these methods a valuable complement to other special techniques in toxicologic pathology.

4. IN SITU HYBRIDIZATION

4.1. Introduction

ISH is a uniquely sensitive method that allows localization of gene expression in tissues at the cellular or subcellular level. Similar to IHC techniques, which were developed through the application of immunologic methods and reagents to investigate pathology endpoints, ISH was developed by applying molecular biology techniques to address mechanistic questions. ISH was first described in 1969 and has primarily found applications in both basic and clinical research. Recently, ISH has become an increasingly valuable technique in the arsenal of the toxicologic pathologist (Gall and Pardue, 1969; Gillett and Chan, 1999; Goebl et al., 2007; Mikaelian et al., 2014).

ISH is based on the principle that nucleic acid probes that are complementary to the sequence of a target gene will specifically hybridize (bind) to the target gene (DNA) or the gene transcripts (RNA) in expressing cells in tissue. These probes initially consisted of labeled RNA or DNA molecules generated in the same manner as probes prepared for molecular techniques such as Southern blots (for DNA) or Northern blots (for RNA) (Gall and Pardue, 1969). In more recent years, alternative forms of nucleic acid probes such as locked nucleic acid (LNA) and peptide nucleic acid (PNA) probes have been developed as an alternative to the more common probe forms in order to improve hybridization efficiency and the speed of the assay (Kubota et al., 2006; Paulasova and Pellestor, 2004). Regardless of the type (RNA, DNA, LNA, or PNA), the probes need to be labeled with either radioisotopic (e.g., ^{33}P or ^{35}S) or nonradioisotopic (e.g., biotin or digoxigenin) labels

to allow visualization within the specimen of interest (Figure 11.7).

Molecular biology techniques such as Southern blots, Northern blots, PCR, and reverse transcription PCR that use homogenized tissues provide information on gene expression at the whole tissue level. These techniques require that DNA or RNA be extracted; however, once the tissue has been homogenized and the nucleic acids extracted, any information regarding spatial localization to particular cells or structures is lost. ISH is valuable in that it both preserves the tissue morphology and cellular location of the target gene while also providing quantitative information on the level of gene expression. ISH has also been used extensively in cytogenetics to identify chromosomes, chromosomal rearrangements, and gene amplification.

4.2. Applications of In Situ Hybridization in Toxicologic Pathology

ISH has primarily been used as a research tool in molecular biology and pathology laboratories and has more recently found acceptance in the clinical arena as a biomarker of gene amplification. Until recently, the use of ISH in toxicologic pathology has been limited to addressing specific questions encountered in very early discovery research studies and evaluation of efficacy in animal models. While useful in those environments, this technique also has broad applications in biopharmaceutical development, particularly for some biologic products such as gene therapies and ASOs.

ISH in Discovery Research

In early discovery research, ISH has been used to localize sites at which novel genes are expressed for which the function of the encoded protein product may not be known. Determining the cell type in which a gene is expressed can provide an insight into the potential function of the protein. For example, localization of a newly cloned guanylyl cyclase receptor to the photoreceptor layer of the eye provided an indication that this gene may function in phototransduction (Shyjan et al., 1992). Expression of guanylin mRNA has been determined by ISH to be restricted to the intestine and helped confirm that guanylin was an endogenous activator of an intestine-specific receptor guanylyl cyclase

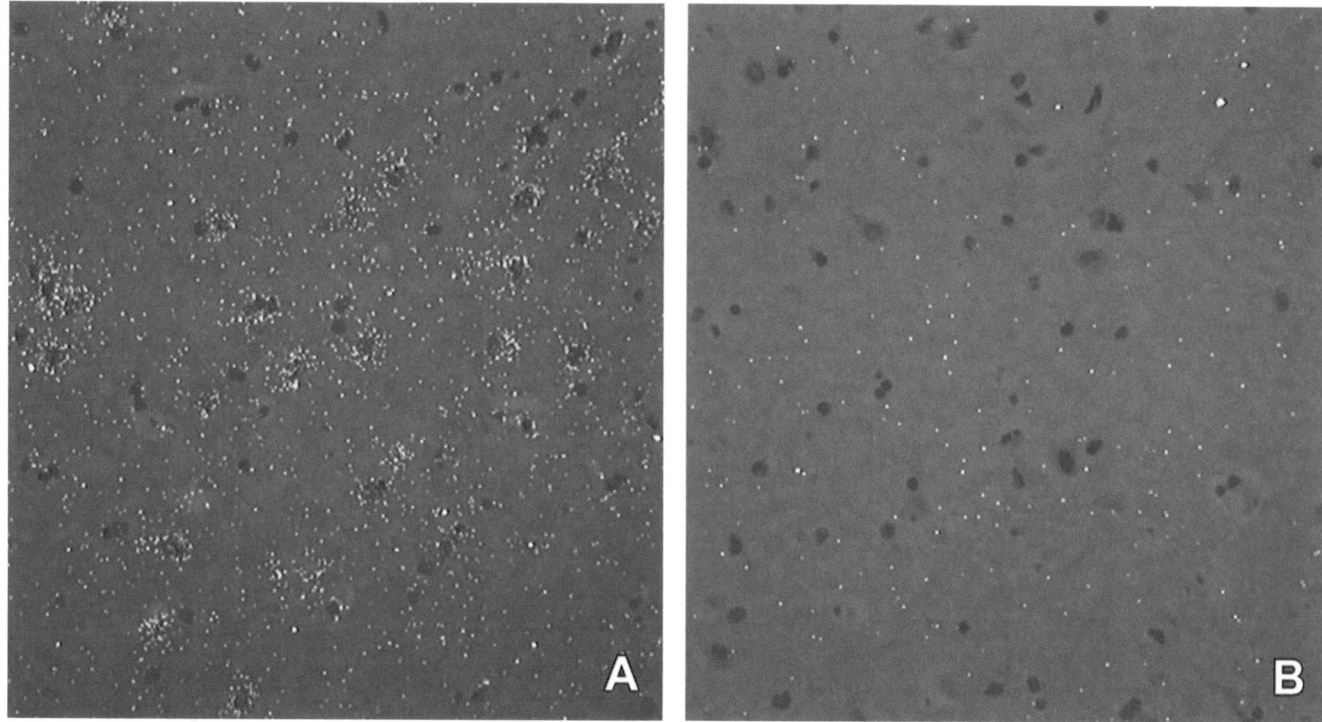

FIGURE 11.7   Section of rhesus monkey brain probed by in situ hybridization with ^{33}P-labeled human β-actin RNA probes (riboprobes). Clusters of silver grains indicate hybridization of the probe to target mRNA. (A) Human β-actin antisense RNA probe hybridizes to cells in rhesus monkey brain expressing β-actin mRNA (Original magnification 200X). (B) Human β-actin sense RNA probe (control) does not hybridize to cells in rhesus monkey brain. Only minimal background signal is present (Original magnification 200X). *Figure reproduced from the Haschek WM, Rousseaux CG, Wallig MA, editors:* Handbook of toxicologic pathology, *ed 3, 2013, Elsevier, Chapter 10, Fig. 2, p. 192, with permission.*

through which an *Escherichia coli*–derived enterotoxin worked (de Sauvage et al., 1992). Leptin, the product of the *ob* gene, is secreted by fat cells and is involved in body weight regulation. ISH has been used to demonstrate that expression of a form of the leptin receptor is expressed in the hypothalamus (Luoh et al., 1997). B1 bradykinin receptor mRNA has been localized with ISH in the primate nervous system to better understand its purported role in processes such as pain and nociception (Shughrue et al., 2003). Lymphotoxin-β and lymphotoxin-β receptor mRNA expression were examined by ISH in developing mouse embryos to provide insight into the role of the lymphotoxin system on the development of immune organs (Browning and French, 2002). The expression of endocrine gland–derived VEGF (EG-VEGF) mRNA expression has been examined by ISH in human prenatal and adult testis and in testicular tumors with findings suggesting that EG-VEGF may have a role in

angiogenesis both during the early endocrine development of the testis as well as in adult testis (Samson et al., 2004).

Study of Changes in Gene Expression in Animal Models to Assess Responses to Pharmacologic or Environmental Agents

Although ISH has been traditionally thought of as a tool for early discovery research, toxicologic pathologists are increasingly using ISH as a tool for monitoring gene expression following test article administration. For example, in carcinogenicity testing, ISH for connexin 32 in liver samples of treated rats has been used to determine if the compound might promote the formation of liver tumors. Though the connexin genes are not oncogenes or tumor suppressor genes, they are integral to cell signaling and have been implicated in abnormal growth (Shoda et al., 1999). ISH has been used to demonstrate that renin mRNA expression was increased in the kidneys of rats treated with the angiotensin II antagonist, ZENECA ZD8731 (Doughty et al., 1995).

In environmental toxicology, ISH has been used to assess changes in the expression of genes associated with lung extracellular matrix (ECM) proteins such as collagen I and III, elastin, fibronectin, and interstitial collagenase. The deposition of some of these ECM proteins is increased in the lungs of animals following chronic ozone exposure (Parks and Roby, 1994). Osteopontin has been shown to play a role in several inflammatory diseases and its expression has been localized by ISH in the livers of a rat model of alcoholic steatohepatitis (Banerjee et al., 2006, 2009). Clusterin mRNA expression by ISH has been proposed as a potential biomarker of nephrotoxicity in a rat model of unilateral ureteral obstruction (Ishii et al., 2007). In rat models of Parkinson's disease and L-DOPA–induced dyskinesia, ISH has been used to study changes in mRNA levels of α(2A) and α(2C) adrenoceptors (Alachkar et al., 2012).

ISH in the Study of Genetically Engineered Animals

The study of transgenic and gene-targeted (knockout, knockdown, and knockin) animals in biomedical research has provided a means to understand the function and interaction of specific genes in vivo. Animal models often provide the best means of studying diseases since they behave similarly in some or many respects to humans in many cases. ISH has been particularly valuable in the study of gene-altered animal models in characterizing tissue-specific transgene expression. In v-Ha-ras oncogene-transgenic mice, ISH has been used to verify expression of v-Ha-ras mRNA in both normal and neoplastic cells (Delker et al., 1999). Upregulation of IL-17Rh1, a receptor homolog for interleukin 17E (IL-17E), was confirmed by ISH in transgenic mice overexpressing human IL-17E resulting in eosinophilia, B-lymphocyte hyperplasia, and altered antibody production (Kim et al., 2002). Transgenic overexpression of Anks6 causes polycystic kidney disease in rats, and ISH was used to determine that the first 10 days of age was the time period during which transgene expression initiated cystic growth (Neudecker et al., 2010).

Gene knock-out animals provide an opportunity to study the effects of gene deletion in vivo. ISH was used to characterize the effects of estrogen receptor-α–dependent processes in estrogen receptor-α knock-out (ERKO) mice. ISH of ovaries from ERKO mice shows a high level of luteinizing hormone receptor (LHR) mRNA expression in the granulosa and thecal layers of antral follicles indicating that ER-α action was not a prerequisite for LHR gene expression (Schomberg et al., 1999).

Gene knock-out animals can be used as models of human diseases. ISH was used to help determine the mechanism in the development of myasthenia gravis in interferon-γ (IFN-γ) receptor–deficient mice. Lymphoid cells from these animals were examined by ISH for changes in the expression of various cytokine mRNAs including IFN-γ. Upregulation of IFN-γ mRNA expression is believed to contribute to the susceptibility to myasthenia gravis in these mice (Zhang et al., 1999). TNF-like weak inducer of apoptosis (TWEAK) has been shown to selectively stimulate the proliferation of a hepatic progenitor cell population known as oval cells through the expression of the TWEAK receptor (Fn14) mRNA using ISH (Jakubowski et al., 2005).

Comparing Gene Expression Across Species

ISH also can be used to explore mechanisms of disease in both animal models and humans. Because regions of gene sequences are often conserved across species, it often is possible to design ISH reagents that can be used to examine gene expression in both animal models of a disease and samples from human patients with the disease. For example, due to the homology between mouse (flk-1) and human (KDR) growth factor receptors, it was possible to use the same probe to study expression in human colorectal liver metastases and a mouse model of colorectal liver metastases (Warren et al., 1995). Such evaluation of multiple species is often not possible using IHC because of the lack of cross-reactivity of antibody reagents across species. Even when the gene sequence homology between species is not high enough to allow the use of the same reagents, ISH can still provide valuable information. For example, ISH using probes specific for cyclooxygenase 1 (COX-1) or COX-2 was able to demonstrate the differential expression of these isoforms in the kidneys of rats based on differences in localization of ISH probe binding (Khan et al., 1998).

ISH in the Evaluation of Gene Therapy and Antisense Therapeutics

The emergence of gene therapy products and ASOs as therapies has highlighted the utility of ISH later in the product development pathway. Because ISH allows cellular localization of gene expression, questions regarding the safety and efficacy of these products can be answered at a cellular level. For example, in the case of gene therapy, ISH has been used numerous times to localize the vector, indicate if the transgene has entered the targeted host cells, and confirm whether transgene transcription to produce the associated mRNA has occurred. In addition, in some tissues or cell types, ISH can determine if observed lesions are occurring at the site of cellular transduction, or are spatially unrelated to the presence of the transferred DNA. ISH can also reveal whether transduction and gene expression is occurring in germ line cells in the testes or ovaries (Sterman et al., 1998; Verdier and Descotes, 1999; Xiao et al., 1998). ISH was used to confirm the successful delivery of genes across the blood–brain barrier (BBB) by intravenously injected AAV9 to neonatal neurons and adult astrocytes of mouse brain and spinal cord (Foust et al., 2009). AAV9-mediated gene therapy across the BBB following intravenous injection was further confirmed by ISH in a study in cynomolgus macaques (Mattar et al., 2013).

Following administration of ASOs, ISH can be used to evaluate the relative level of target mRNA in the cells of interest, both before and after ASO administration (Goebl et al., 2007). Just as the advent of mAbs and other proteins as potential therapeutics has broadened the application of IHC during efficacy and safety testing, it is likely that the development of DNA- and RNA-based therapies will increase the usefulness of ISH in safety assessment.

4.3. Technical Considerations for In Situ Hybridization

A review of the literature reveals a plethora of ISH techniques, using a variety of probe types, different labeling methods, etc. The truth that emerges from this survey is that, similar to IHC, there is probably not a single "best" method for ISH. Though some protocols work over a broad range of conditions, in general, experimental conditions must be customized for each target and tissue and, as always, appropriate controls must be run for the proper interpretation of the data.

Selection of Probe Type

The first technical consideration for ISH is the type of probe to use. There are three main types of probes that are used in ISH: DNA (single or double stranded of variable length), RNA (riboprobes of variable length), or oligonucleotides (short synthetic DNA or RNA sequences). Of these options, riboprobes and oligonucleotides are the most commonly used, and each probe type has distinct advantages and disadvantages (Kumar, 2010).

DNA probes, created by DNA purification and labeled using nick translation or random priming, were originally used for ISH. However, use of DNA probes was limited by availability of DNA for probes and low sensitivity. With the advent of molecular cloning and DNA synthesis technology which simplified probe creation, other probe types such as oligonucleotide probes became more commonly used for ISH (Brown, 1998).

The advantages of riboprobes are that they probably offer the greatest sensitivity in detecting gene targets because of their length (typically 100–500 bp), their ability to be labeled to a high specific activity, and the greater stability of the DNA–RNA hybrids that are formed. In addition, sense riboprobes that are complementary to the antisense riboprobes and identical to the target gene can be used as negative control reagents on serial tissue sections to identify areas of nonspecific tissue probe binding. Riboprobes also have the advantage that RNAse can be used in a posthybridization wash to degrade unbound RNA thereby decreasing the background (Brown, 1998; Kind, 2000; Kumar, 2010).

One disadvantage of riboprobes is that RNA is quite labile. Therefore, precautions must be used to ensure that the procedure (reagents and reactor vessels) is RNAse free so that the riboprobe is not degraded during the preparation of the probe or during the hybridization process. Another disadvantage of RNA probes is that they require some level of molecular biology skill to produce them (Altar, 1989; Kumar, 2010). Riboprobes are generated by in vitro transcription from DNA templates containing RNA polymerase promoter sequences. Riboprobe templates can be created by either subcloning the gene of interest into a plasmid ribovector, or alternatively, PCR techniques can be used to attach RNA polymerase recognition sites to the sequence of interest for subsequent in vitro transcription.

Oligonucleotide probes ("oligos") are gaining popularity for use in ISH. Typically, these are 20–50 nucleotide oligomers that are designed to specifically hybridize to target sequences. Many organizations already have in-house facilities that are able to synthesize oligonucleotides. Alternatively, oligonucleotides can be purchased at modest cost from a number of commercial synthesis firms. Most synthesis laboratories can attach labels to the oligo probes at the time of synthesis, or alternatively, "kits" are available to label them prior to hybridization. Thus, oligo probes are often easier for nonmolecular biologists to obtain and use. The main disadvantage of oligo probes is that they are much less sensitive than riboprobes due to their small size. They generally require a relatively high copy number of mRNA in the tissue in order to detect a signal (Kumar, 2010; Lewis et al., 1985).

Selection of Probe Label

The other major technical consideration with ISH is the choice of probe label. There are two primary types: radioisotopic and nonisotopic. ISH was initially performed using radioisotopic labels, and this is still the method of choice in many research laboratories. Types of radioisotopic labels are shown in Table 11.1.

The choice of label is a compromise between better cellular resolution, which requires relatively weak β-emitters, and short exposure times, which are achieved by more energetic isotopes. At this time, medium energy β-emitters such as ^{35}S and increasingly ^{33}P are the radioisotopes of choice in most laboratories using radioactivity. While both of these isotopes offer similar half-lives and tissue resolution (10–20 μm), there are practical and technical differences that influence label selection. For example, ^{33}P is generally more expensive than ^{35}S but is often is preferred for ISH, for two reasons. First, ^{33}P produces less nonspecific background hybridization than ^{35}S (McLaughlin and Margolskee, 1993). Second, ^{33}P is amenable to convenient end-labeling methods, while ^{35}S is not (Carter et al., 2010). Most, though not all, investigators feel that ISH with radioisotopic-labeled probes is more sensitive in detecting low-level gene expression as compared to ISH with nonisotopic–labeled probes. Though isotopically labeled probes are generally more sensitive than nonisotopic probes, they require relatively long incubation times (sometimes weeks) and have poorer cellular resolution owing to the pattern of radioactive emissions (Frantz et al., 2001; Ky and Shughrue, 2002; Moorman et al., 1993).

Protocols are available for ISH using isotopic-labeled probes that have been optimized and standardized for use on a variety of tissues and different probe sequences. This has not been possible for nonisotopic–labeled probes, where the protocol must be optimized for each new probe and tissue, similar to that required for antibodies in IHC. Nevertheless, ISH with nonisotopic labeled probes will probably be the method of choice for many laboratories in the future as there are distinct advantages to working with nonisotopic labels, chief among them being not having to deal with the extra precautions associated with using and safely disposing of radioactive reagents and solutions. Nonisotopic labels for ISH probes are similar to those used in IHC (Table 11.2).

TABLE 11.1 β-emitting Isotopes for In Situ Hybridization

Isotope	$T_{1/2}$	Max Energy (MeV)	Resolution	Exposure Time
^{3}H	12.35 years	0.018	High	Long
^{35}S	87.4 days	0.167	Moderate	Intermediate
^{33}P	28 days	0.250	Moderate	Intermediate
^{32}P	14.29 days	1.710	Poor	Short

H, Hydrogen; *P*, Phosphorus; *S*, Sulfur;

TABLE 11.2 Commonly Used Nonisotopic Labeling Techniques for In Situ Hybridization

Direct
    Fluorochromes (FITC, Texas
        Red, Phycoerythrin)
    Enzymes (Horseradish
        Peroxidase, Alkaline
        Phosphatase)

Indirect
    Antibodies
        DNA−RNA
        RNA−RNA
    Biotin
    Digoxigenin
    BrdU

The most common nonisotopic labels for nucleotides at this time are biotin and digoxigenin, which then can be detected through a secondary detection system. Direct labeling, such as with a fluorescent tag, does not usually provide a signal with sufficient strength for direct visualization. The choice of nonisotopic label is usually determined by the commercial availability of labeled nucleotides and the availability of sensitive detection systems to detect them. In addition to the benefit of not having to work with radioactivity, the use of nonisotopic probes allows for markedly shorter detection times (hours instead of weeks), lowers reagent costs, better cellular resolution, and increased shelf life of the reagents (since nonisotopic labels do not decay like isotopic labels). In addition, new amplification strategies are being introduced that may markedly increase the sensitivity of nonisotopic techniques. Tyramide amplification, for example, uses the deposition of haptenized tyramide molecules in the vicinity of hybridized probes catalyzed by HRP to greatly amplify the signal produced by digoxigenin- or biotin-labeled nucleotides (Holm et al., 1992; Pacchioni et al., 1992; Rihn et al., 1995; Speel et al., 1998, 1999, 2006).

Fixation

For ISH, the choice of tissue fixative should balance accessibility of the probe to the target DNA or RNA, maximal retention of target DNA or RNA, and morphological details of the tissue (Hofler, 1990; Kumar, 2010; Valentino, 1987). Precipitating fixatives such as acetic acid–alcohol mixtures might allow the best penetration of probe but might also permit the greatest loss of RNA target and offer less crisp cytoarchitectural detail (Kumar, 2010). Cross-linking fixatives such as aldehydes and acrolein might yield the best retention of DNA or RNA targets and provide improved structural preservation but might limit probe penetration likely due to steric hindrance of cross-linked proteins near or around the DNA or RNA targets. Pretreatments with detergents or proteases can reduce this problem but also might result in loss of probe target (Kumar, 2010). Use of 4% PFA appears to provide a reasonable balance between probe penetration and DNA/RNA target retention. ISH also can be performed on snap-frozen tissues that are subsequently fixed briefly with PFA after sectioning, but tissue morphology is often compromised in this situation (Kumar, 2010).

Controls for In Situ Hybridization

Appropriate reagent and tissue controls are necessary to demonstrate the sensitivity and specificity of an ISH method. Positive and negative control tissues (or cell pellets) should be included in a manner analogous to that described above for IHC. A positive control tissue will express the nucleic acid target of interest and can be used to demonstrate that the ISH assay is working and is sensitive and reproducible. A negative control tissue will not express the target of interest and can be used to demonstrate the specificity of the assay. For ISH, these positive and negative controls can be expressing- or nonexpressing cells within a tissue; however, in some cases, a true negative can be hard to identify in tissue sections. Alternatively, transfected and nontransfected cell lines can be used as positive and negative control "tissues," respectively (MacDonald et al., 2014).

Several options exist for control probes. Inclusion of an alternate (nonsense) sequence or sense probe (with a sequence that matches the gene of interest) will control for specificity (Kumar, 2010). Another control step for specificity involves hybridizing first with unlabeled antisense probe followed by labeled antisense probe. This step eliminates hybridization of labeled probe to target sequences leaving only background staining (Kumar, 2010). Tissue validation controls can also be performed using probes that recognize housekeeping genes to demonstrate that the DNA/RNA in the tissue sample has been sufficiently preserved to be recognized using standard ISH methods.

4.4. Conclusions

ISH is a powerful tool for studying gene expression and distribution at the cellular level. While there are a number of parallels and synergies between IHC and ISH—indeed the two techniques complement each other, as will be discussed—there is danger in overstating the similarities between the two techniques, because the reagent requirements and technical expertise for each is quite different. An understanding of the principles underpinning each method is essential to "troubleshooting" the procedures and interpreting the results.

Obviously, information regarding the gene and its protein product can be maximized if both IHC and ISH are performed. A variety of different patterns can be obtained if both IHC and ISH are applied to a given cell population (Table 11.3).

In recent years, dual detection methods have been developed where multiple genes or gene products can be detected in the same tissue section using a combination of IHC and ISH. Alternatively, these techniques can be used in serial sections from the same tissue block to determine the tissue distribution of the mRNA and their cognate protein. There are a number of instances where ISH and IHC will show differing patterns, depending upon the differing sites of protein manufacture versus storage or use, the degree of posttranslational processing, and intracellular degradation of the protein. An obvious example of such discrepancies is found in the peripheral nervous system where neurons house the genetic blueprint (nucleus) and protein fabrication apparatus (cytoplasm in the cell body) even if the proteins are deployed to far-distant nerve termini.

The decision to perform either IHC or ISH will often depend upon the availability of the reagents and the nature of the scientific question. Sometimes, antibodies will not be available to perform IHC for the protein product of interest. Usually, the gene sequence is known prior to

TABLE 11.3   Interpretation of ISH and IHC Results

ISH	IHC	Interpretation
+	+	- Detectable synthesis of mRNA - Synthesis and storage of protein[a]

+	−	- Detectable synthesis of mRNA
		- No detectable protein
		  - No storage of protein
		  - Rapid degradation of protein
		  - Below limit of detection

−	+	- No detectable mRNA
		  - Rapid degradation of mRNA
		  - Protein synthesized in a different cell
		  - Below limit of detection
		- Detectable protein
		  - Synthesis and storage of protein
		  - Uptake of protein

−	−	- No detectable mRNA
		  - Rapid degradation of mRNA
		  - Protein synthesized in a different cell
		  - Below limit of detection
		- No detectable protein
		  - No storage of protein
		  - Rapid degradation of protein
		  - Below limit of detection

[a] Note that a positive signal for in situ hybridization (ISH) might not be observed in the same subcellular location as a positive signal for immunohistochemistry (IHC). For example, for many molecules in the peripheral nerve system, a positive ISH result in ganglionic neurons corresponds to IHC staining observed in distant nerve terminals.

the availability of antibodies; thus, ISH may be the first procedure available to determine cellular localization for expression of a given gene. In some cases, knowledge of the location of the protein is more important than knowledge of the mRNA levels. In other instances, such as in endocrine tumors, the cells may be synthesizing a prohormone that is not detected by conventional antibodies but can be detected through ISH by nucleotide-based probes.

The obvious advantage of ISH as compared to PCR or Northern blots is that the mRNA can be localized to the cell, thus cytoarchitectural context to the observed binding. In some cases, ISH is likely to be more sensitive than Northern blots. For example, when a small proportion of the cell population is expressing mRNA at high levels, it is more easily detected by ISH than Northern blots. Conversely, when 100% of the cell population is expressing mRNA at low levels, it will be more easily detected by Northern blot than by ISH.

5. FLOW CYTOMETRY

5.1. Introduction

Flow cytometry is a powerful technology that allows for multiparameter assessments of numerous elements, including cells, subcellular components, transcription factors, microparticles, infectious agents, and numerous others. Since the development of flow cytometry, the parameters that can be assessed by this technique have expanded exponentially with the refinement of the technology, including increased numbers of assessments that can be evaluated with one sample and increased availability of reagents. This platform now is used widely in basic research, biopharmaceutical development (both nonclinical and clinical), and as a diagnostic tool. Flow cytometry can be utilized in all stages of biopharmaceutical development to measure cellular changes on the cell surface, in intracellular compartments, and in matrices.

Common Uses of Flow Cytometry in Nonclinical and Clinical Testing

The expansion over the last decade of biotechnology drugs such as proteins, peptides, bi- and trispecific antibodies, CAR-T cell therapies, antidrug antibodies, vaccines, and oligonucleotides along with an increasing number of small molecule therapeutics that target the immune system has led to an increased need for tools that can explore the biology of the immune system. Significant advances in flow cytometry have allowed this technique to support many immunotoxicologic endpoints established by the FDA (e.g., hypersensitivity, chronic inflammation, immunosuppression, immunomodulation, immunostimulation, and autoimmunity) (FDA, 1997, 2002, 2006, 2014, 2020). Flow cytometry can be used not just to evaluate the potential for an agent to alter immune system function but also can evaluate test article efficacy (e.g.,

the expansion of CAR-T cells engineered to target cancer cells). Predicting potential immunotoxicologic effects depends on several factors including understanding the therapeutic target, determining the mechanism of action of the test article, and the accrued nonclinical and clinical safety data relevant to the immune system. The scope of this brief discussion will be limited to flow cytometry applications and technology commonly used by toxicologic pathologists in nonclinical research.

Therapeutic development programs aim to reduce the time and cost required to bring a new product to market without impacting the quality of the safety and efficacy data obtained. Flow cytometry over the last several decades has become an instrumental technique in this quest due to its ability to simultaneously measure changes at the cellular level in protein expression, drug receptor occupancy for therapeutic candidates, activation and internalization of receptor-mediated signaling pathways, and functional cellular assessments.

The use of flow cytometry in the human clinical setting expanded after the 1980s with the rapid spread of human immunodeficiency virus and acquired immunodeficiency syndrome, investigations of which require the analysis of lymphocyte subsets (specifically T-cells) to monitor progression of this disease. Subtyping of hematologic malignancies using cell type–specific antibodies detected using flow cytometry has provided valuable information about the cell lineage(s) involved in forms of leukemia and lymphoma and has become the basis for treatment, prognosis, and monitoring of recurrence. Flow cytometry also can be used to measure the content of DNA in tumor cells as a marker of carcinoma (e.g., breast and prostate) recurrence in patients.

Historically, in the arena of therapeutic discovery and development, a primary consideration has been to determine whether therapies are directly toxic to the immune system and result in immunosuppression. While decreased cellularity in lymphoid organs as evident by microscopic evaluation of tissue sections suggests the likelihood of reduced leukocyte (especially lymphocyte) populations, the incorporation of flow cytometric analysis has significantly improved the quantification of these effects and has been instrumental in identifying

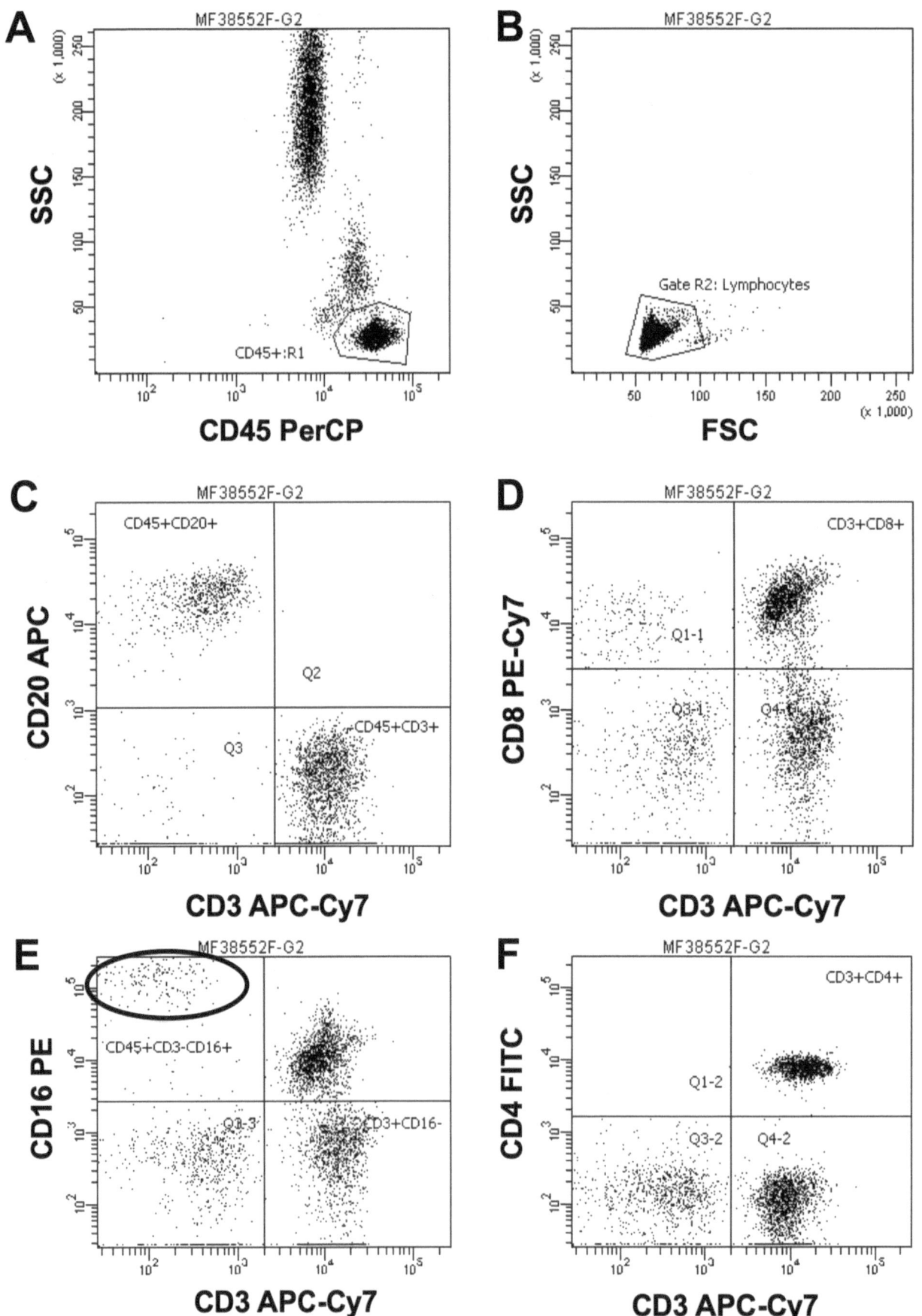

FIGURE 11.8 Calculating absolute counts of lymphocyte populations. Cells can be gated based on expression of a common leukocyte marker CD45 and granularity/complexity (side scatter; panel A) and/or cell size (forward

the affected immune cell populations. With the growing number of therapies that target or affect the immune system in multiple and often subtle ways, there is an increasing need to include endpoints besides immunosuppression and characterize the nature of the immunomodulation occurring with these agents when given alone or in combinations with other therapies (Danilenko and Wang, 2012; Edwards and Sklar, 2015; Lappin, 2010). Immunosafety is the field of assessing the impact of new therapies on the immune system and incorporates immunotoxicologic assays (both in vitro and flow cytometric), hematologic endpoints, and morphologic evaluation of immune organs. In particular, flow cytometry is an essential tool for immunophenotyping, in which immune cell populations and their immune responses are characterized based on the size, granularity (complexity), and expression of cell type–specific markers present on the cell surface or within the cell. The robust applications of immunophenotyping by flow cytometry have made this methodology extremely useful in safety assessment (Papenfuss, 2017; Wang and Lebrec, 2017). In addition to an ever-increasing set of immune cell subsets that can be identified by immunophenotyping, flow cytometry can be utilized to assess levels of biomarkers (e.g., CD membrane proteins, cytokines), the activation states of key molecules (e.g., enzymes, transcription factors), and numerous other applications (Baumgarth and Roederer, 2000; Edwards and Sklar, 2015; Gossett et al., 1999; Lappin, 2010; Ramanathan, 1997).

Basic Principles of Flow Cytometry

Flow cytometry is based on the examination of cells or other particles suspended in a hydrodynamically focused fluid stream that sorts individual objects (cells or particles) for examination (Shapiro, 2003). Suspended objects pass individually through the flow cell where they are exposed to a focused laser light source. The light emission that results from the diffraction of laser light by the objects is filtered and directed to a series of photodetectors where the light signal is converted to electronic signals that are digitized and displayed as object-related attributes. Each cell or particle type has a characteristic light scatter pattern that can be qualitatively and quantitatively evaluated. Many hematology analyzers currently in use incorporate this technology for counting erythrocytes, leukocyte classes, and platelets, converting light scatter properties of individualized blood cells (shape, size, and granularity) to information used in blood cell differential analysis. Fluorescence-activated cell sorting (FACS) is a specialized flow cytometry application that sorts heterogeneous mixtures of cells into bins by adding signal detection from fluorochrome-labeled reagents (antibodies, proteins, or nucleic acids) that selectively bind to certain cells or cell components. FACS can detect and localize cell surface, intracellular, soluble (cytokines), and drug or antidrug targets. The additional stratification supplied through the use of fluorescent probes results in enhanced analysis of cellular and functional attributes that cannot be observed with other classic toxicologic pathology techniques.

Gating is a fundamental approach to evaluating the immunophenotype of specific populations by flow cytometry. Gating involves identifying cell subpopulations based on deflection of laser light by specific cell features; in general, cells of a given subset are grouped together (within a particular quadrant or region) when visualized via a dot plot. Gating typically sorts first using forward scatter (FSC; cell size) and side scatter (SSC; granularity) to isolate the lymphocyte (or mononuclear) subsets from the granulocytes. The population of leukocytes can be separated on a dot plot based on the relative expression granularity (or complexity) and the expression of the common leukocyte antigen CD45 (Figure 11.8A). Note that cell populations

---

scatter; FSC) or SSC (panel B). Populations of each lymphocyte subset can then be shown in a dot plot and quadrant gating which can provide the percentage of lymphocytes possessing each cell marker (e.g. the percentage of CD45+/CD3−/CD16+ lymphocytes). The percentage of each gated population can then be multiplied by the total number of lymphocytes (as determined by conventional hematology or bead counts) to determine the number of cells per microliter for each lymphocyte population. *Figure modified from the Haschek WM, Rousseaux CG, Wallig MA, editors:* Handbook of toxicologic pathology, *ed 3, 2013, Elsevier, Fig. 7.3, with permission.*

can also be identified based simply on size (FSC) and granularity (Figure 11.8B), where lymphocytes are smaller in size and less granular and thus are visualized on the flow cytometry dot plot toward the bottom left quadrant (i.e., low SSC and low FSC). Note that since granulocytes are typically larger and have higher granularity than lymphocytes, they have higher SSC and FSC so would be toward the top right corner. In assessing the typical T, B, and NK cell lymphocyte panel, an initial gate is "drawn" around the population of interest by defining ranges for size and granularity characteristics (Figure 11.8A). From there, additional gating of subpopulations can be employed by establishing gates for other parameters so that the relative expression of lymphocyte-specific markers on CD45+ cells can be visualized by their fluorescent intensity. Marker combinations can be selected to identify specific populations or subpopulations that are double negative, single positive, and double positive. For example, the relative expression of CD20 and CD3 can identify CD45+CD20+ B cells compared to CD45+CD3+ T cells, subpopulations of CD45+CD3+CD8+ and CD45+CD3+CD4+ T cells, and CD45+CD3−CD16+ NK cells (Figure 11.8C–F). Data for subpopulations are usually reported as a percentage (%) of the parent population. Gating of well-defined markers such as the standard T, B, and NK cell panel typically are straightforward, and for a given study should be kept consistent for all animals, and across all time points evaluated for the same animal. As with any assays in safety assessment, immunophenotyping panels typically should be validated before use, and considerations for a GLP toxicity studies should at minimum include titration of the antibodies, checking for cross-reactivity with other antibodies, intra- and interassay precision, range of response, and stability assessments (in whole blood/tissue and processed tissue).

In addition to standard light scatter/fluorescence evaluation, flow cytometry principles also may be applied to sort cells or particles in tissue sections. This advance, termed laser scanning cytometry, is used to measure the fluorescence intensity or light loss (absorbance) of molecular targets within various cell compartments (usually the nucleus or cytoplasm) in tissue sections. This technique has been deployed in basic biomedical research but to date has been performed rarely in the nonclinical arena. For this reason, this technique will not be discussed further. Additional detail may be gained in selected reviews (Harnett, 2007; Pozarowski et al., 2013).

The use of multiple fluorescent probes in one sample, which has increased with technological enhancements to flow cytometers and increased availability of reagents, has expanded in recent years. Multicolor flow cytometry has expanded the number of markers an investigator can evaluate from a single sample. Today, instruments with multiple filters readily support experiments assessing 3 colors per study, but more complex instruments can deal with greater than 18 colors (Islam et al., 1995; Maecker et al., 2004; O'Hara et al., 2011; Shapiro, 2003). The ability to evaluate multiple endpoints in tandem should be tempered so that the resulting flow cytometric data are tailored to address a specific question of relevance to the overall interpretation of the collated pathology data.

Flow Cytometry in Animal Toxicity Studies

In nonclinical safety assessment, flow cytometry is primarily used to evaluate peripheral whole blood samples due to the ease of sampling, limited blood volume required to measure multiple parameters (typically 0.5–1.0 mL collected in sodium heparin or EDTA), commercial availability of immunophenotyping reagents and kit-based assays in multiple species (from rodent to human), and the capability to translate data across species for specific pharmacodynamic (PD) markers (e.g., CD3, CD4, CD8, CD45RA, CD19, and CD21 markers, which can be used to compare counts of T- and B-cells between species). Tissues samples taken by biopsy or at necropsy can be collected and processed using various homogenization techniques (enzymatic and/or mechanical) for evaluation of key cell populations by flow cytometry. The most commonly evaluated samples are tissues with relatively little stroma (which permits easier cell dispersal) and large numbers of hematopoietic and or immune cell elements, such as bone marrow, thymus, lymph nodes, and spleen.

Over the last several years, the biomedical industry has moved from simply identifying major cell classes by measuring cell surface markers such as T-lymphocyte, B-lymphocyte, and natural killer (NK) cell subsets to complex assessments of immune cell subpopulations based on their activation states (e.g., Th1, Th2, or Th17 lymphocytes) or function (e.g., cytotoxic or T-regulatory [Treg] lymphocytes). *Ex vivo* evaluation of cultured blood or lymphoid organ cells by flow cytometry may be employed to identify changes in the physical (cell phenotype) or functional (activity, proliferation, viability) attributes of cells that may be induced by addition of immune modifying agents or challenges (antigens). Prior to study start, flow cytometry also can be used to quantify target expression in study animals to ensure that all treatment groups contain animals with equivalent beginning complements of target-expressing cells. Other endpoints of interest that may be examined by flow cytometry include the effectiveness and timing of cellular/tissue repair as well as the initiation and evolution of neoplasia.

Flow cytometry is a technique that evaluates large numbers of cells in a short period of time across multiple time points within a study. The small sample sizes needed permit the analysis of cell populations during the predose, dosing, and recovery phases of nonclinical studies.

Flow cytometry is a powerful tool in toxicologic pathology when combined with more traditional methods of nonclinical immune system testing such as routine hematology and morphologic evaluation of bone marrow and lymphoid organs. In addition, many immunophenotyping markers used to identify changes in cells from test animals have counterparts that react with similar constituents on human cells; as such, the results from animal experiments translate fairly well to clinical evaluation of the same parameters in humans (Wang and Lebrec, 2017). For example, rituximab (Rituxan) is a marketed biotherapeutic that depletes B-lymphocytes as its primary mechanism of action. Flow cytometry was utilized as a tool during the development of rituximab to evaluate the PD effects of the test article on circulating and organ-specific B-cell numbers in both nonclinical and clinical development, while other toxicologic pathology endpoints including both evaluation of H&E- and IHC-stained sections highlighted that B-cells were depleted in the expected anatomic regions of lymphoid organs in situ (Vugmeyster et al., 2003). Rituxan is a classic example of the important role that flow cytometry can play in therapeutic development. Similarly, flow cytometry can play an important role in evaluating immuno-oncology agents, such as the relative efficacy of PCD protein 1 and programmed death-ligand 1 (PD-L1) inhibitors, or for other aspects of immunotherapy monitoring (Butterfield, 2018; De Sousa Linhares et al., 2019; Rusdi, 2019).

5.2. Applications of Flow Cytometry in Toxicologic Pathology

Flow cytometry is a useful tool in toxicologic pathology given its versatility which includes tasks such as cellular immunophenotyping, numerous functional assays, and receptor occupancy and binding assays. The advantages that flow cytometry has over other techniques, specifically the ability to evaluate samples acquired at several time points and the ability to assess multiple endpoints in one sample, increase the quantity of data that can be obtained, while the advanced software greatly enhances the efficiency and speed of data collection and automated analysis. These advantages have helped make flow cytometry instrumental in the therapeutic development process, and it can be a key method to reduce the time to get a therapeutic candidate to market.

Some potential applications of flow cytometry in toxicologic pathology are described in the following sections with comments regarding advantages and disadvantages of this technology over more traditional methods used in nonclinical safety evaluation studies.

Cell Immunophenotyping

Cell immunophenotyping is a standard endpoint for both small molecule and biotherapeutics that have the potential to modulate the immune system. Classical immunophenotyping is conducted on cells in peripheral blood collected prior to dose administration, during the dosing phase, and during the recovery period (if applicable to the study design) of a nonclinical toxicity study. In addition, organ-specific immunophenotyping can be conducted, typically on immune organs including the bone marrow, lymph nodes, spleen, and thymus. Immunophenotyping data are typically added in concert with hematological assessments, and most study designs collect samples for immunophenotyping and hematology at concurrent time points. Standard hematology parameters related to immunophenotyping will include absolute and differential white blood cell counts and often cytologic evaluation of a blood smear. Bone marrow smears often are collected, and a morphologic evaluation of these smears may be conducted to characterize the light microscopic features of the various marrow elements. Flow cytometry allows the analysis of cell populations and often selected cell subsets based on the expression of cell surface markers, shape and size, and granularity (complexity). Given that morphology and cellular marker expression may differ for individual cell populations, findings may differ between clinical pathology and immunophenotyping results. This is particularly true for monocytes given the wide array and subpopulations of monocytes that have differing antigenic and functional profiles. It is important to consider this potential disparity when evaluating findings and integrating multiple pathology data sets within a study.

An immunophenotyping panel often includes T, B, and NK cell markers (Table 11.4) although numerous other markers can be evaluated based on the cell type of interest. The cell surface markers that are examined most commonly are CD3+ (T-lymphocytes), CD3+/CD4+ (T-helper lymphocytes), CD3+/CD8+ (T-cytotoxic lymphocytes), and CD20+ (B-lymphocytes). The NK cell phenotype is species dependent and typically is characterized by the following cell surface markers: CD3-/CD56+/CD16+/CD159a+/NKp46+ for humans; CD3-/CD16+/CD159a+/NKp46+ for NHPs; CD3-/CD161a+/NKp46+ for rats; and NK1.1+/NKp46+ for mice (Veiga-Fernandes et al., 2010). Total monocyte counts can vary if comparing hematology counts on conventional analyzers and the CD14+ monocyte absolute counts via automated flow cytometry. The NHP monocyte populations have been categorized into three distinct phenotypes based on CD14 and CD16 expression: CD14+/CD16-, CD14+/CD16+, and CD14-/CD16+; these subpopulations correspond to classical, intermediate, and nonclassical monocytes in NHP peripheral blood (Sugimoto et al., 2015). However, when

evaluating any cells of the myelomonocytic lineage (e.g., monocytes, macrophages, dendritic cells, and granulocytes), it is important to recognize that the plasticity of these cells and the myriad potential markers for these elements that are expressed differentially based on functionality may make fluorochrome selection and data interpretation difficult.

As we obtain greater understanding of the immune system, the cell subpopulations that can be evaluated by flow cytometry expand as the reagents become available for the toxicology models used in nonclinical toxicology research (Cossarizza et al., 2017; McFarland, 2010; Wang and Lebrec, 2017). A great example is the Treg population. Tregs are a rare subset of lymphocytes that inhibit the activation and effector functions of other T-lymphocytes and have been shown to be integral cell components in modulating normal immune system function. Evaluation of Tregs as an added endpoint in nonclinical studies has become an increasingly common endpoint. The markers used to define Tregs in NHPs are CD3+/CD4+/CD25+/FoxP3+ (Dons et al., 2010). FoxP3 is an intracellular marker, so the procedures to define this population may take 8–10 h in the laboratory. Recently, a high-throughput 96-well microtiter plate-based assay has been developed to detect circulating Tregs in NHPs using a cell surface marker. Cell surface marker assays take far less time in the laboratory; therefore, the data derived from this plate-based method, in which CD3+/CD4+/CD25+/CD127+ (where CD127 is a surface marker) was shown to identify an equivalent population, will potentially decrease the time to perform (Clark et al., 2012).

There are numerous scientific and technical considerations for incorporating cytometry and immunophenotyping in a nonclinical study that are beyond the scope of this chapter. These factors include, but are not limited to, study design; sample collection; time points to be evaluated; practical considerations (e.g., blood volume, tissue availability and processing limitations, etc.); fluorochrome availability; instrument settings (compensation, gating parameters, validation, etc.); and the evaluation of results within the context of the compound, biology of the antibodies, and potential target cells of interest (der Strate et al., 2017; Green et al., 2016; O'Hara et al., 2011; Papenfuss, 2017; Shapiro, 2003; Wood et al., 2013). As

TABLE 11.4 Example of Immunophenotyping Panels

	Species			
	Nonhuman primate	Canine	Rat	Mice
Blood immunophenotyping (standard panel)	T-Cells (CD45/CD3/ CD4/CD8) B-Cells (CD45/ CD20) NK cells (CD16)	T-Cells (CD3/CD4/ CD8) B-cells (CD21)	T-Cells (CD3/CD4/ CD8) B-Cells (CD45RA) NK cells (CD161a)	T-Cells (CD3/CD4/ CD8) B-Cells (CD19) NK cells (NK1.1)
Spleen Immunophenotyping (standard panel)	—	—	T-Cells (CD3/CD4/ CD8 B-Cells (CD45RA) NK cells (CD161a)	T-Cells (CD3/CD4/ CD8) B-Cells (CD19) NK cells (NK1.1)
Thymus Immunophenotyping (standard panel)	—	Mature and immature T-cells (CD3/CD4/ CD8)[a]	Mature and immature T-cells (CD3/CD4/CD8)	Mature and immature T-cells (CD3/CD4/CD8)
Other panels	**Blood** B-Cells (CD3/CD19, CD45/CD3/CD20/ CD21 and CD45/ CD20/HLA-DR[a]) Activated/ Regulatory T-cells (CD45/CD4/CD25/ FoxP3 and CD45/ CD8/CD25/FoxP3) Activated T-cells (CD45/CD3/CD25/ CD69) Memory/Naive T-cells (CD3/ CD45RA/CD62L/ CD4[a] and CD3/ CD45RA/CD62L/ CD8[a]) Platelet activation (CD61/CD62P/ PAC1)	—	**Blood** Memory T-cells (CD4/CD45RC/ CD90) Regulatory T-cells (CD3/CD4/FoxP3/ CD25) **Spleen** Memory B-cells (IgD/IgM) Memory T-cells (CD4/CD45RC/ CD90) **Thymus** Regulatory T-cells (CD3/CD4/FoxP3/ CD25)	**Blood** Memory T-cells (CD4/CD62L/CD44 and CD8/CD44/ CD62L/Ly-6C) **Spleen** Memory T-cells (CD4/CD62L/CD44 and CD8/CD44/ CD62L/Ly-6C) Memory B-cells (CD3/NK1.1/F4/ 80/CD19/CD45/ B220)

[a] These panels are reported as relative percentages (absolute counts not included).

with any assay in a safety assessment study, ensuring validation of the assay and determining the parameters and guidelines involved in sample collection, data acquisition, and data interpretation are critical. The analysis of the results should involve scientists aware of not only the technical considerations related to flow cytometry but also the scientific ones defined in the study objective. It is particularly important to consider the impact of immune system biology and how a therapeutic may impact the phenotype or function. For example, an engineered biotherapeutic that has an Fc portion of the antibody that binds to the FcγRIII (CD16) receptor as parts of its mechanism of action will bind CD16 on NK cells. The net effect is that this biotherapeutic will block a fluorochrome directed against CD16, a marker for NK cells, and result in an apparent "depletion" of NK cells. Similarly, an alternative marker such as CD19 would be appropriate to monitor B lymphocytes for Rituxan, which binds to CD20 on the surface of B-lymphocytes. An understanding of the biology of both the therapeutic agent and immune cells is necessary to avoid misinterpretation of the data and to prompt the selection of a different NK (e.g., CD159a) or B (i.e., CD20)-lymphocyte marker in the study design.

Test article–related effects observed in the flow cytometry data should be substantiated by and integrated with hematology data and the overall results of other endpoints such as microscopic changes in lymphoid tissues, IHC findings, and any additional immune function assessments evaluated within the study.

Functional Assays in Flow Cytometry

Perhaps the most frequent application of flow cytometry in toxicologic pathology is in the functional assessment of the immune system. Typically, a tiered approach is taken to evaluate the toxicity and impact of a therapeutic on the immune system and provide a weight of evidence indicating immunotoxicity for regulatory agencies (Dean et al., 1979; FDA, 2006, 2020; Germolec et al., 2017; Huppertz et al., 1999).

In addition to immunophenotyping, immune function tests that can be added to standard toxicity studies include the T-cell–dependent antibody response (TDAR), cytokine evaluations, cytotoxic T-cell function, NK cytotoxicity (activity), macrophage/neutrophil functions, and host resistance assays. The TDAR is the primary immune function test that assesses multiple components involved in the development of a T-cell–dependent immune response that results in antibody development. Animals are immunized with a specific antigen such as keyhole limpet hemocyanin, and generation of antibodies is evaluated postimmunization. NK cell function via evaluation of cytotoxicity is a required assessment if the test article is known to impact the innate immune system, the NK cell response, or NK numbers. NK cells are cultured with prelabeled target cells, and the amount of target cell killing is determined. Cytokine assessments can evaluate serum levels of cytokines or intracellular cytokines, such as IFN-γ, via flow cytometry. Functional evaluation of other innate immune cell function (e.g., macrophage/neutrophil activity) can be evaluated as a stand-alone assay or in conjunction with functional evaluation of other immune cells. Other PD assessments might include antibody-dependent cell-mediated cytotoxicity, complement-dependent cytotoxicity, oxidative burst, phagocytosis, apoptosis, platelet activation and neutralizing antibody assays, and biomarker assessment. These functional assays can be performed to support a therapeutic development program either as in vitro assessments or as added endpoints to nonclinical toxicity studies.

In addition to applications in nonclinical safety assessment, immune function assays often can be translated for use in the clinic as both important biomarkers and/or prognostic indicators for both therapeutic response and disease outcome. For example, cytokine levels of IL-6 and IL-10 are prognostic indicators in patients with COVID-19 (where "CO" stands for corona, "VI" for virus, "D" for disease, and "19" for the outbreak year) and may identify at-risk patients and the impact of potential therapeutics on ameliorating coronavirus-related organ damage (Han et al., 2020; Schett et al., 2020). In safety assessment, functional assay evaluation and biomarkers may be useful to monitor the efficacy and immune system toxicity of the therapeutic candidates in patient populations.

Receptor Occupancy and Binding Assays

Biotherapeutics that target extracellular antigens may be evaluated for binding to the target receptor using flow cytometry. Receptor occupancy and binding measurements are becoming more common in nonclinical toxicity studies. In addition, binding assessments using cells that express the target of interest may be used to characterize multiple lots of drug to ensure that binding characteristics have not changed during the manufacturing process (i.e., from the engineering lots generated for early studies to the Good Manufacturing Practice–compliant lots that are utilized for GLP nonclinical studies and clinical trials.

Establishing the level of receptor occupancy on the cell surface can be used to provide PD biomarker data and, in conjunction with PK evaluations, help inform decisions on dose level and frequency (Liang et al., 2016). Typically, competing and noncompeting monoclonal antibodies are used to assess the amount of drug that is bound compared to the amount of drug that remains unbound. The information acquired in these assessments along with PK and efficacy data can aid in determining appropriate dose levels for nonclinical toxicity studies when performed on early in vivo PK studies.

5.3. Advantages and Limitations of Flow Cytometry

Flow cytometry is a powerful tool that can provide detailed information on immunophenotyping, functional assays, receptor occupancy, transcription factor activation, and numerous others immunotoxicologic parameters that help characterize the immunomodulation and immunotoxic effects of therapies in drug development. The ability to serially evaluate parameters over time in blood samples generates important information regarding the kinetics of a therapy's impact on the immune system. Additionally, the various assays that can be performed by flow cytometry or via other methodology can help in the interpretation of other immunophenotyping and immune function data sets and provide a "big picture" of the immune changes that may be present. A weight-of-evidence approach integrating these multiple data sets can provide detailed information on the cells and processes affected, the kinetics of this response, potential reversibility, utility of biomarkers to monitor the response, and numerous other parameters that evaluate safety and efficacy during drug development. Additionally, the continual development of new applications utilizing the power and flexibility of flow cytometry is a distinct advantage of this technology.

However, there are some limitations, both scientific and technical. By its very nature, flow cytometry is performed on a cell suspension. Although this is not an issue with most clinical pathology applications, it does result in a loss of tissue and organ structural information of various cellular populations that are present in anatomic pathology evaluation. The application of IHC to identify specific populations and subpopulations of immune cells (beyond their phenotypic characteristics recognizable on H&E-stained sections) can help identify the architectural arrangements in situ and, together with peripheral flow cytometry of blood, can provide a comprehensive assessment of immune system biology over time. Technical limitations also are factors that need to be taken into consideration when adding flow cytometry analysis to nonclinical toxicity studies including operator and instrument capabilities, instrument settings, maintenance, cleaning, quality control, and validation, study planning and design, sample collection and preparation, appropriate baseline measurements, controls, gating, and compensation, and data analysis and interpretation. Sample preparation is as important to the success of flow cytometry as proper experimental design and instrument operation. One important limitation that may be overlooked during study design is that preparation of tissue homogenates for flow cytometric evaluation on fixed tissues is difficult and rarely performed due to technical difficulties and time-intensive aspect of this approach (Bolon et al., 1990). This necessitates planning to allow for fresh tissues to be separated into subsamples at necropsy that can be analyzed in parallel by flow cytometry, histopathology, or other methodologies (e.g., molecular biology). Study design must also take into account the potential species-specific limitations including small sample size/volume for rodent studies and small group size for nonrodent studies. Samples for flow cytometry must be prepared appropriately since particulate matter or clotted samples can result in nonspecific results or nonspecific binding of antibodies. Additionally, flow cytometric samples and antibody reagents can be relatively labile, and exposure to heat, light, and/or vigorous agitation may change and lose (or gain) properties that are incorrectly "read" by the analyzer. Sample stability and integrity in relation to the analyte of interest should be evaluated so that samples submitted for labeling or labeled samples do not give rise to spurious results. Accurate interpretation of flow cytometry data relies not only on a skilled operator setting up controls, compensation, and gating parameters correctly but also requires an understanding of the mechanism of the therapeutic as well as an awareness of species-specific differences in the parameters being analyzed.

It is imperative that baseline flow cytometric measurements are taken prior to the dosing phase of the study. At least one, but more commonly more than one, predose sample is taken to provide baseline data and help address inherent biological variability with these measurements ideally separated at least 1 week apart. In addition, data for individual animals should be (1) evaluated over time for changes above or below that individual's baseline, (2) compared to the individual's hematological data, (3) compared to the control group means, and (4) analyzed statistically. The design of the experiment should be thoroughly considered to ensure that appropriate antibodies are used in the relevant species, that blood volumes are within the limits defined for collection, that evaluation of the markers of interest is conducted to determine whether or not the selected markers identify function or numbers of cells, and that stability of the analyte is addressed. It is rarely possible to add flow cytometry endpoints to a study after necropsy, so it is particularly important to incorporate flow cytometry (and other in vitro functional immune assays for immunotoxicologic evaluation) into the study design in advance to ensure appropriate resource scheduling. Flow cytometric processing methods, gating strategies for various markers, instrument operational parameters, and automated analytical software also should be qualified or validated prior to the study start.

5.4. Conclusions

Flow cytometry should be added to nonclinical study designs on a case-by-case basis considering the mechanism of action of the test article being evaluated, findings from traditional safety assessment methods such as hematology, microscopic evaluation of lymphoid tissues and Tier I immunosafety assays, stage of clinical development,

and intended therapeutic use. Flow cytometry is a multiparameter technique widely used in nonclinical toxicology and in the overall product development process. Flow cytometry can be used to evaluate multiple endpoints including peripheral blood and tissue cell subset percentage and number changes; functional changes (oxidative burst, phagocytosis, apoptosis, and NK cell function); measurement of drug; antidrug antibodies; and neutralizing antibodies. Methods should be appropriately conducted with controls, and qualification or validation should be performed if necessary to ensure that the data are of high quality. The instrument capabilities are continually expanding, and new techniques are being evaluated for use in nonclinical research. In the next 10 years as in the last, the use of flow in drug development will continue to evolve.

6. LASER CAPTURE MICRODISSECTION

6.1. Introduction

LCM was first described in 1996, and it has rapidly gained wide acceptance as an important tool in both diagnostic pathology and pathology research. A PubMed search on LCM in April 2020 yielded more than 5500 articles, and this number has grown steadily and consistently since the commercialization of the technology. Prior to the development of LCM, molecular analysis of cellular populations was limited to either the analysis of heterogeneous fragments of tissues containing mixed cell populations or the analysis of a thin tissue section on a glass slide using IHC or ISH. Analyzing microdissected and homogenized tissue fragments is a powerful approach that allows for the quantification of many different genes or proteins simultaneously, but it is limited in that the results represent an average of every cell contained in the sample and not the particular cell population(s) of interest. Such bulk analyses may mask important changes that are confined to a single cell subset. Assessment of cell populations in tissue sections on a slide has the advantage of using morphology to aid in the interpretation of the result, and therefore, a single cell type can be targeted, but historically these in situ molecular techniques have been limited by being technically challenging to perform (ISH) and/or having few high-quality, commercially available reagents (both IHC and ISH). LCM overcomes these deficiencies by using microscopic cell features to isolate nearly pure cellular populations that then can be subjected to molecular analysis (Datta et al., 2015; Liu et al., 2014; Mahalingam, 2018).

6.2. Applications of Laser Capture Microdissection in Toxicologic Pathology

LCM has been widely utilized in the various subspecialties of pathology, from medical diagnostic pathology to toxicologic pathology (Aguilar-Bravo and Sancho-Bru, 2019; Corgiat and Mueller, 2017; Gagner and Zagzag, 2018; Kato et al., 2018; Roy et al., 2020; Yamazaki et al., 2018). The ability to reliably isolate specific cell populations using LCM is particularly a powerful tool when coupled with any of the various "omic" approaches currently used in research and diagnostics (see *Toxicogenomics: A Primer for Toxicologic Pathologists*, Vol 1, Chap 15). The subsequent analysis of any of the major classes of biological macromolecules or cellular metabolites, such as DNA (mutation analysis—the "genome"), RNA (transcriptional profiling—the "transcriptome"), protein (expression analysis—the "proteome"), and/or metabolites (metabolic profiling—the "metabolome"), can be performed on the isolated sample depending on the scientific question, provided that appropriate modifications to the fixation and processing protocols are made (Frost et al., 2015; Liu et al., 2014).

Applications of LCM to toxicologic pathology are numerous. Researchers have utilized LCM in the analysis of proliferative lesions, various toxicities, and animal models of disease (Aguilar-Bravo and Sancho-Bru, 2019; Boone et al., 2018; Corgiat and Mueller, 2017; Gagner and Zagzag, 2018; Kato et al., 2018; Moto et al., 2006; Roberts et al., 2008; Wei et al., 2008). By analyzing the cellular responses to toxicant exposure or the particular disease state, important information is gleaned regarding the subcellular target of the toxicity, ultimately leading to a better understanding of the pathogenesis.

6.3. Technical Considerations for Laser Capture Microdissection

Two types of LCM systems have been developed and marketed commercially. The first involves several steps: placement of a thin thermoplastic film over the tissue section, morphological identification of the cell type of interest using a light microscope, brief (microsecond) firing of an infrared laser pulse to temporarily melt the polymer film so that it bonds with the underlying cells, and then removal of the bonded polymer and cell sample for subsequent analysis (Figure 11.9). This technology has been widely adopted and can be applied to paraffin-embedded or frozen tissue sections (Mahalingam, 2018). The width of the laser beam is generally 7–8 microns, so single cells can easily be identified and harvested.

An alternate system operates using similar principles. The distinguishing feature is that a UV laser is used to cut the cells of interest away from the remaining tissue section, rather than capturing it using a polymer. The laser is typically very narrow (only approximately 0.5 microns in diameter) so that very precise cuts can be made. The dissected tissue of interest then either falls into a collection tube via gravity or is catapulted into a tube cap (Datta et al., 2015). In addition to finding application in paraffin-embedded or frozen tissue sections, this system can be used with live cells. Furthermore, this platform has been more widely applied to protein and metabolic analyses to avoid the need for adhesive polymers, binding of which may have detrimental effects on the biomolecules associated with the plastic.

Regardless of the type of system employed, special fixation or tissue handling is necessary in order to optimize the results, depending on the type of analysis being performed. For example, DNA analysis can be performed after standard formalin fixation, even if quite prolonged, given the inherent stability of the macromolecule and its resistance to aldehyde cross-linking. However, the analysis of more labile molecules (e.g., RNA) or molecules that are more susceptible to cross-linking with aldehyde fixatives (e.g., proteins) requires dedicated solutions incorporating RNase inhibitors and/or rapid freezing at the time of necropsy. Numerous technical or methods manuscripts have been published describing

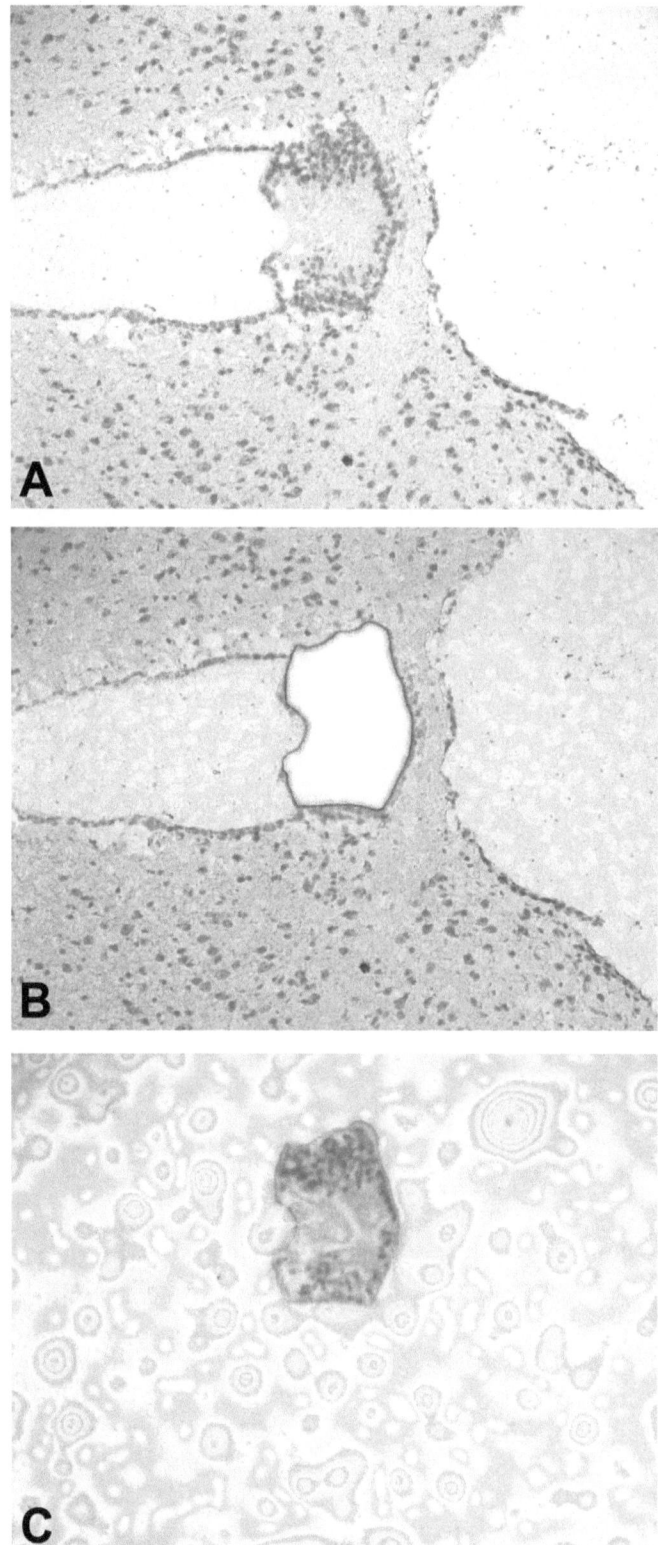

FIGURE 11.9   Example of laser capture microdissection (LCM). (A) High-magnification image of the sub-commissural organ (SCO) of the normal rat brain; (B) same section after the specific SCO excision by LCM; and (C) the excised SCO ready for subsequent analysis. The instrument used for the microdissection was an MMI CellCut. Frozen section, H&E stain.   *Figure reproduced from the Haschek WM, Rousseaux CG, Wallig MA, editors: Handbook of toxicologic pathology, ed 3, 2013, Elsevier, Fig. 7.4, with permission, from images provided by Julie Foley, Yu Wang and Ping Xu; National Institute of Environmental Health Sciences, National Institutes of Health, United States Department of Health and Human Services.*

these considerations (Datta et al., 2015; Liu et al., 2014; Mahalingam, 2018; Watanabe et al., 2015; Yamazaki et al., 2018).

6.4. Limitations

Depending on the type of analysis being performed subsequent to LCM, there are inherent difficulties which must be overcome for success. Most notably, the manner in which the tissue is handled before and during LCM is critically important. For DNA analysis, tissue handling is more flexible given the inherent stability of the molecule and its relative lack of reactivity with the aldehyde fixatives that are typically used for tissue fixation.

Formalin-fixed tissue allows for excellent DNA recovery and subsequent analysis from LCM samples, even from paraffin-embedded archival samples. Expression analysis of mRNA is more challenging and the results more variable. Flash-frozen samples are ideal for transcriptional profiling, but care must be exercised in tissue and sample handling to minimize RNase contamination leading to RNA degradation. Proteomic and metabolic analyses can utilize fixed or frozen tissue but, if fixed, the type of fixative must be chosen carefully. Denaturing fixatives (e.g., ethanol) are preferred over aldehyde fixatives since cross-linked protein adducts compromise subsequent molecular identification. Protein analysis and identification also typically require large samples given the inability to perform an amplification of the original molecules of interest. Advances in protocols for tissue preparation and handling, no matter what type of subsequent analysis is being performed, have progressed considerably and make it possible to achieve reasonable results under less than ideal conditions (Datta et al., 2015; Frost et al., 2015; Liu et al., 2014; Mahalingam, 2018).

6.5. Conclusions

Since its introduction in the mid-1990s, LCM has rapidly gained acceptance in all fields of pathology, including toxicologic pathology. Recent technological advances and improvements in tissue handling and sample amplification protocols continue to be made which make the systems easier to use and the results more consistent. LCM has become, and will continue to be, a very helpful tool to study molecular changes in individual cell types in the context of their original tissue.

7. CONFOCAL MICROSCOPY

7.1. Introduction

CM has been used to image biological samples for nearly four decades and has distinct advantages over alternate imaging techniques, particularly in research settings, including a dramatic increase in image resolution, the ability to optically section through thick pieces of tissue or living organisms, and the ability to record changes occurring at the cellular level in real time. Using this technique, investigators are not limited to viewing moments frozen in time as in standard tissue sections, but rather can view and record changes in dynamic systems in three dimensions (3D). The capabilities of CM have provided tremendous insights into basic biology, the pathogenesis of numerous diseases and toxicities, and the perturbations of cellular processes and pathways induced by pharmaceuticals.

7.2. Applications of Confocal Microscopy in Toxicologic Pathology

Since its introduction, CM has been broadly applied to biomedical research. The ability to optically section through a relatively thick piece of tissue allows for the visualization of cellular components or subcellular proteins in 3D without having to physically section (and then reassemble mentally or mathematically) the tissue, thus enabling the detailed study of cells and cellular processes in their native microenvironment (Amos and White, 2003; Bayguinov et al., 2018; Conchello and Lichtman, 2005; Jonkman and Brown, 2015). This ability is a particular advantage when studying anatomically complex tissues such as the central and peripheral nervous systems as well as rapidly evolving embryonic tissues. Researchers have applied CM to synaptic degeneration in inherited neurodegenerative diseases, corneal nerve fiber degeneration as a marker of peripheral neuropathies, and detailed studies of neurogenesis in specific brain regions (Chamaa et al., 2018; Martínez-Hernández et al., 2013; Martinez et al., 2015; Petropoulos et al., 2020; Vulovic et al., 2018), to cite a few examples.

The ability to view cellular processes in 3D in real time has enabled researchers to study critical cellular functions such as protein trafficking and to visualize, quantify, and record perturbations of these processes driven by various toxicants and therapeutics. Since the scanning and viewing processes are nondestructive, the technique can easily be applied to isolated live cells, tissues within living animals, and isolated organ fragments such as the cornea, skin, gastrointestinal epithelium, and even the brain (Pygall et al., 2007; Que et al., 2016; Tavakoli et al., 2008). For example, confocal laser endomicroscopy has been applied during gastrointestinal biopsy and even intraoperatively during brain surgery to better assess tumor margins. CM information at the time of biopsy or surgery enables clinical decisions to be made regarding the need for additional tissue biopsy or resection in an attempt to get clean margins, which can directly impact patient outcome (Belykh et al., 2018; Ragazzi et al., 2014, 2016).

CM also has become an increasingly important tool in therapeutic development, particularly during the discovery and early development phases or when investigating the mechanism of an unanticipated toxicity (Martinez et al., 2015; Pygall et al., 2007). These advances have been notably beneficial in the fields of ocular pharmacology (Furrer and Gurny, 2010; Petropoulos et al., 2020). Retinal and lenticular cytoskeletal alterations can be recorded directly using CM for potential use as a marker of drug-related ocular toxicity. In addition, sequential monitoring of infiltrating leukocytes in ocular tissue has demonstrated a diminished response following treatment with antiinflammatory agents. There are numerous additional published examples of CM applications within biological research, diagnostic pathology, and toxicologic pathology (Du Toit et al., 2013; Mantopoulos et al., 2010; Verdugo-Gazdik et al., 2006).

7.3. Technical Considerations for Confocal Microscopy

Conventional epifluorescence microscopes were first developed approximately a century ago and are suitable for many purposes in diagnostic and toxicologic pathology. These systems use a wide-spectrum fluorescent light source and illuminate an entire tissue section at once. The light excites a fluorochrome bound to the cell component or molecule of interest, which then emits a photon of a characteristic wavelength in all directions. The microscope objective collects the photons of emitted light for viewing by the observer. Although effective in many situations, images generated by epifluorescence represent features evident at a fixed moment in time and are of low resolution and blurred since the microscope objective collects light from all aspects of the tissue section simultaneously, including those areas from tissue planes that are out of focus (Jonkman and Brown, 2015; Wright and Wright, 2002).

In contrast, CM overcomes many of the shortcomings of classical epifluorescence microscopy. Instead of utilizing a wide-spectrum light source that illuminates the entire tissue section simultaneously, a confocal microscope utilizes a narrow-spectrum laser and a raster sampling approach to scan the entire section a small piece at a time. Each individual image in the raster pattern is a very tightly defined tissue region (a small cluster of pixels with distinct X and Y coordinates) at the surface or at some depth beneath the surface (which defines the Z coordinate); the small image size maintains all features at high resolution. A digital montage of all images then is reconstructed to provide a detailed high-resolution 3D view of the entire tissue sample (Figure 11.10). With recent technical advances in the speed with which samples can be scanned, digital computer storage, and image processing, CM also supports the generation of real-time, high-resolution videos of active cell processes such as the trafficking of cell components (Bayguinov et al., 2018; Conchello and Lichtman, 2005; Jonkman and Brown, 2015; Lichtman and Conchello, 2005; Murray, 2011).

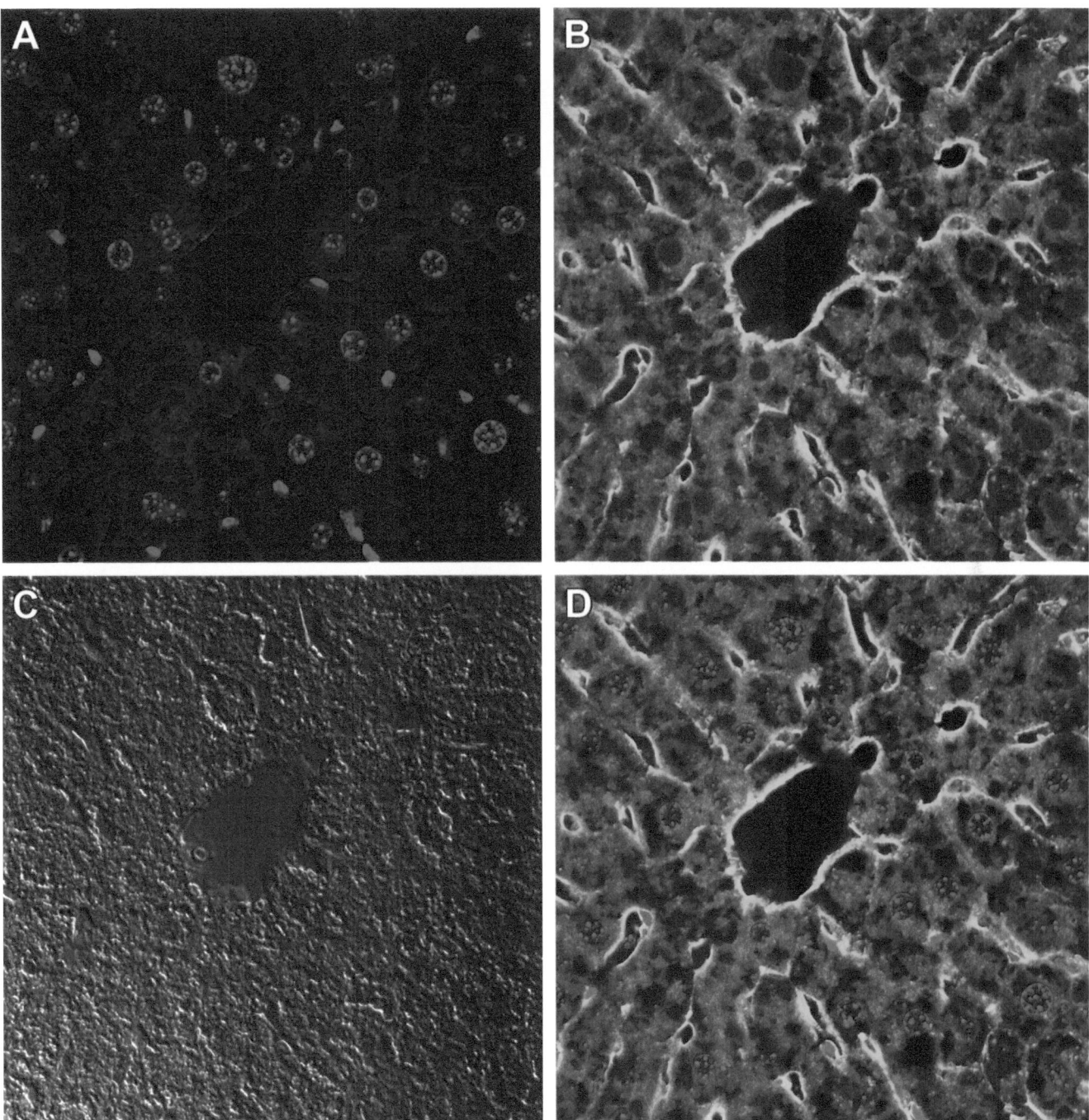

FIGURE 11.10 Example of confocal microscopy; liver from a mouse with diet-induced obesity after bromodi-chloromethane exposure. (A) Staining with 4′,6-diamidino-2-phenylindole (DAPI), a fluorescent stain that binds strongly to AT-rich regions in DNA and is commonly used to label nuclei. (B) Immunofluorescent staining for nitrotyrosine, a marker of free radical damage (fluorochrome = Alexa 488) showing increased labeling of the cell membrane indicative of lipid oxidation. (C) A gray-scale Differential Interference Contrast (DIC) image used to visualize the structure of the tissue. (D) Composite of images A and (B) *Figure reproduced from the Haschek WM, Rousseaux CG, Wallig MA, editors:* Handbook of toxicologic pathology, *ed 3, 2013, Elsevier, Fig. 7.3, with permission, from images provided by Dr. Saurabh Chatterjee and Jeff Tucker, National Institute of Environmental Health Sciences, National Institutes of Health, United States Department of Health and Human Services.*

7.4. Limitations

The principal limitation of CM is cost, not only for the initial equipment but also for ongoing maintenance and operation of this equipment. In order to fully realize the capabilities of the system, most institutions have dedicated personnel to oversee its operation, which allows the institution to maximize its utilization and ensure that features of the systems are fully exploited.

In contrast to epifluorescence systems, which have a lamp with a full emission spectrum including UV, confocal microscopes are limited by the available wavelength of their laser, which typically has a fairly narrow range. Whereas this can limit the fluorochrome choices available for labeling, the impact of this limitation has been lessened by the introduction of a wide variety of new fluorochromes.

7.5. Conclusions

CM has proven to be an immensely powerful technique with broad applications in biomedical research. The intrinsically high resolution and ability to visualize tissue features in 3D using CM have revolutionized fluorescence microscopy and dramatically furthered our understanding of dynamic biological processes and diseases.

8. ELECTRON MICROSCOPY

8.1. Introduction

The imaging of biological samples by TEM began in earnest in the 1940s and 1950s. The 40 years that followed were a golden era in which widespread use of the technology to explore a wide variety of biological tissues significantly increased our understanding of subcellular anatomy and morphology during health and disease (Cheville, 1983, 2009; Dykstra and Reuss, 2003; Ghadially, 1997, 1998; Ghiadially, 1985; Hayat, 2000; Lewis, 1998, 1999; Peters, 1991). The technology is ideal for visualizing cellular organelles and structures that are below the limits of resolution of light microscopy (magnifications routinely ranging from 500–80,000X). Modern advances have allowed TEM to be adapted for in situ molecular pathology analyses (e.g., IHC and ISH) and for evaluation of isolated nucleic acids and proteins. Related EM techniques have been used on occasion in toxicologic research to explore the surface features (i.e., scanning EM) or internal membrane organization (i.e., freeze fracture EM), but these tools are employed less often than TEM based on the nature of questions encountered during risk assessment and investigational toxicity experiments. Today, although its use has waned considerably since the 1980s in favor of other techniques and assays that provide dynamic microscopic and molecular information, TEM remains an indispensable technique and the gold standard for answering certain questions.

8.2. Applications of Electron Microscopy in Toxicologic Pathology

Although its use has waned, TEM is still employed consistently in the field of toxicologic pathology as reflected in a 2019 industry survey conducted by the Society of Toxicologic Pathology's Scientific and Regulatory Policy Committee (Keirstead et al., 2019). The most commonly cited reasons for performing TEM in product development were to characterize the ultrastructural morphology of a light microscopic finding (96%) and to investigate the pathogenesis or test a mechanistic hypothesis (65%). It is important to note that most respondents to the survey selected both reasons. Other less common reasons for TEM were in response to a regulatory request or to establish a threshold value (e.g., no observed effect level or no observed adverse effect level) of an ultrastructural finding. Common situations in the authors' experience in which TEM is employed are the characterization of vacuolation in various tissues related to drug-induced phospholipidosis (Nonoyama and Fukuda, 2008), brain or liver vacuolation after exposure to neurotoxicants or hepatotoxicants (Butler et al., 1987), or the assessment of renal glomerular changes related to cell or protein deposition (Hoane et al., 2016).

Although the low numbers of TEM studies performed per year might suggest that TEM is not particularly valuable, this technique retains a place of importance in the field of toxicologic pathology since there are certain situations in which alternative techniques do not provide comparable information. In addition, for pathologists, TEM is a natural extension of light microscopy evaluations, simply at higher magnifications to provide enhanced resolution.

8.3. Technical Considerations for Electron Microscopy

TEM is a technically complex technique requiring expensive equipment and highly trained technical personnel, factors which have historically been and remain obstacles to its use. A thorough discussion of the technical aspects is beyond the scope of this chapter, particularly the laboratory aspects of tissue processing, embedding, and imaging. Such details may be gleaned from several excellent references (Dykstra et al., 2002; Dykstra and Reuss, 2003; Hayat, 2000; Lewis, 1999; Russell, 1999). The paragraphs below will instead focus on aspects that the authors consider to be important knowledge for the toxicologic pathologist tasked with designing or interpreting a TEM study. While this section is focused on TEM, it should be noted that the fixation and processing techniques used for TEM are also used in the light microscopic evaluation of certain organs in order to obtain superior morphologic preservation. Perhaps the most obvious example of this adaptation is to stabilize myelin sheaths in the peripheral nervous system (Bolon et al., 2018; Jortner, 2011; Jortner et al., 2005).

When embarking on a TEM analysis, the single most important aspect influencing success is the quality of tissue fixation. Although it is possible to perform TEM on tissue fixed in commercially available formalin (containing methanol as a stabilizer)—and at times this is the only option—if an investigator considers TEM to be a possibility, there is considerable benefit to planning prospectively during study design so that tissue collection and fixation for TEM can be optimized. Tissue that is apparently well fixed when viewed using light microscopy may have considerable artifactual changes when viewed by TEM. Paraffin-embedded tissue may be deparaffinized and processed for TEM in extraordinary circumstances, but in general, this is not suitable for safety assessment.

Ideally, tissue slated for TEM should be selected and processed deliberately at the time of necropsy. The organ in question should be harvested as soon as possible to minimize any autolysis. Tissue blocks (about 1 mm^3) should be procured by placing an organ piece in a drop of fixative on a hard plastic surface and then mincing it using a very sharp blade. Employing dedicated and experienced necropsy personnel for this step is advised. Blocks typically are fixed at 4°C for 2–3 h, although longer fixation times may be used (e.g., overnight when processing many TEM samples from a large toxicity study). Very thin tissue slices are also acceptable.

Samples for TEM typically are fixed in mixtures of aldehydes. Glutaraldehyde (GLUT) is one key fixative since it provides improved molecular cross-linking and the other fixative usually is methanol-free formaldehyde (i.e., PFA). Combinations often used in toxicologic pathology include modified Karnovsky's solution (2% PFA and 2.5% GLUT) and McDowell–Trump's solution (4% PFA and 1.0% GLUT). Although perfusion fixation is ideal since it rapidly delivers fixatives deep into tissues, most TEM projects in toxicologic pathology are performed using immersion-fixed tissues; this reflects the fact that TEM specimens are only one sample type obtained at necropsy, and many of the other samples are dedicated to endpoints requiring fresh tissue for analysis. This immersion fixation step typically is performed at 4°C for a minimum of 2–24 h. Ensuring rapid immersion in the fixative at necropsy and limiting the tissue size and/or thickness are both critical to ensure adequate fixation. Since GLUT is a much larger molecule than formaldehyde, its diffusion into tissues is much more limited. Aldehyde fixatives are excellent for cross-linking proteins and nucleic acids but not lipids, and so after the initial fixation in the GLUT-containing fixative, samples are postfixed by immersion in osmium tetroxide (typically 1%) at 4°C for 1–2 h to stabilize lipid-rich structures like cell and organelle membranes.

Once fixed, tissue cubes typically are processed into epoxy resin (i.e., hard plastics like araldite, epon, or Spurr's). One-micron-thick sections are taken from each block, placed on glass slides, and stained with toluidine blue for light microscopic evaluation by the pathologist. Regions for further analysis are selected by the pathologist; the resin block is further trimmed using a diamond knife to produce 80- to 90-nm-thick "thin" sections that are applied to grids for staining, usually in lead citrate and/or uranyl acetate.

The operation of the microscope and capture of the images are typically performed by trained technical personnel, but it is beneficial for the pathologist to also review the entire section(s) in order to ensure that images for key regions of interest or ultrastructural lesions have been captured. Image magnifications should range from low to high to allow careful review of any changes by the evaluating pathologist. Digital images at the same magnifications should be taken from the control tissues as well as the treated tissues for subsequent evaluation by the pathologist.

8.4. Limitations

The principle limitation of TEM is the overall cost of either starting or maintaining a TEM facility. The initial cost for the microscope is high, and it has ongoing utility and maintenance costs and requires dedicated, trained personnel to process the samples and operate the microscope. The relatively small number of studies performed by each institution makes the economic argument for maintaining a TEM facility difficult to make, and as a result, most institutional facilities have closed.

In addition, the pathologist performing the evaluation ideally should have experience with TEM evaluations and interpretations, which is not easy to acquire now that many TEM facilities, even in academic institutions, have closed. Whereas the basic principles of ultrastructural anatomy and pathology can be learned from textbooks and the literature (Cheville, 1983, 2009; Cheville and Stasko, 2014; Dykstra et al., 2002; Dykstra and Reuss, 2003; Fagerland et al., 2012; Ghadially, 1997, 1998; Ghadially, 1985; Peters, 1991; Russell, 1999), training under the guidance of a more experienced pathologist is beneficial. As facilities have closed, TEM studies increasingly are outsourced to other facilities, often to contract research organizations or universities that have retained the internal expertise to perform not only the technical aspects but also the scientific interpretation.

Last, even with careful attention to fixation and processing, TEM is prone to artifacts, which makes the subsequent evaluation of the images

and interpretation challenging, and there is a constant risk of overinterpretation (Fagerland et al., 2012). As with any other piece of study data, it is important to always put any potential findings into context of the overall study.

8.5. Conclusions

TEM is a powerful investigative tool that can provide important study information that cannot be easily attained using other technologies. Although its use has declined in the last several decades, there are certain experimental situations in which the subcellular morphologic information it provides is invaluable. There are technical challenges that must be overcome for best results, but with thoughtful planning, a well-trained technical staff, and, ideally, an experienced pathologist, TEM has considerable and continued value to toxicologic pathology.

9. STEREOLOGY

Two-dimensional (2D) morphometry, such as image analysis of lengths or areas, can provide additional quantitative data on tissue sections. The results, however, are only applicable to the section that has been measured, and the results are expressed as densities or ratios. Furthermore, such measurements are accurate only if sections in which the features are to be measured are highly homologous in terms of the trimming plane (Garman et al., 2016). This type of analysis also contains many assumptions, which are sources of bias, or inaccuracy. Examples of bias in 2D morphometry and how these are minimized in stereology are detailed in several recent reviews (Boyce et al., 2010; D. L. Brown, 2017a).

In contrast, stereology provides absolute 3D estimates using strict sampling paradigms that both improve accuracy and minimize bias. The sampling principle utilized in stereology is termed Systematic Uniform Random Sampling (SURS). This principle ensures that every object of interest has an equal chance of being sampled. The tissue is measured, and a sampling interval (T) is determined that will result in 8–10 sections being sampled from the tissue or area of interest. The first section is captured at a random start between 0 and T, and sections are captured regularly thereafter at intervals of T. If the tissue is small, SURS can be completed at the microtomy stage. The entire tissue is processed and embedded, with the tissue measured prior to embedding (but after processing to capture shrinkage), and the sampling interval is chosen. The microtome is then calibrated to the desired section thickness (typically 3–5 μm), and the block is faced into until the appropriate depth (i.e., randomly chosen first section) is reached. Sections are captured and microtomy continues until the next sampling interval is reached. This continues until the tissue is sectioned exhaustively; therefore, it is important to capture several additional sections at each interval for backups or other analyses. For medium to large tissues, one or more subsampling steps are typically needed before the microtomy stage. How a tissue is sectioned unbiasedly depends on its size and shape. For examples of unbiased sectioning of different tissue types, the reader is directed to the third edition of this textbook (Gundersen et al., 2013). The same unbiased sampling principles are applicable to any tissue or any species.

The objects of interest are then counted or measured within the tissue sections using stereology software. If number is the desired endpoint, it is important to collect disectors at each sampling interval. There are two types of disectors: physical disectors and optical disectors. These are 3D "probes" (see other types of stereological "probes" below) that ensure objects are sampled according to their presence (number) rather than according to their size, shape, or orientation. Physical disectors consist of two consecutive sections (or two sections with a defined distance between them when counting larger objects such as glomeruli or alveoli) of average thickness (3–5 μm) captured at each sampling interval, whereas optical disectors are single thick sections (typically ≥ 30 μm) captured at each sampling interval. The main difference between the two types of disectors is how objects are counted within them. Physical disectors are typically digitized slides, and these virtual slides are imported into the stereology software system. The software samples fields of view according to SURS, and the user counts objects if they are present in one section but not the other one. In contrast, optical disectors are imaged using a live microscope under a high-magnification oil objective (typically 60–100x),

and objects are counted when they come into focus. For practical examples of the use of physical or optical disectors to obtain object number, the reader is referred to a recent review article (Brown, 2017b).

Other common endpoints for stereology are volume, surface area, and length, and these are analyzed using single sections captured at each sampling interval. All stereological endpoints can be obtained at any tissue level, from the whole tissue to subcellular organelles/inclusions. Volume is estimated simply using the Cavalieri method, where the volume of an object divided into segments is equal to the sum of the cross-sectional area of each segment multiplied by the distance between the segments, which in SURS is designated as T (Gundersen and Jensen, 1987). This cross-sectional area can be obtained through applying a stereologic "point probe" onto the section and counting the number of points that intersect the tissue or area of interest. The sum of points across all sections is multiplied by the cross-sectional area per point and the distance between the sections to estimate the total volume. Alternatively, WSI analysis can be performed to determine the total area of tissue or area of interest, and the sum across all slides can be multiplied by the distance between the sections. For details on estimating surface area and length, the reader is directed to the third edition of this textbook (Gundersen et al., 2013).

Stereology is employed selectively in safety assessment, serving more as an advanced technique to answer specific questions than as a primary screen. In the context of toxicologic pathology, if the pathologist can detect a change by qualitative evaluation, quantitative analysis such as stereology may not be indicated unless the change is a significant safety concern (i.e., for certain families of test articles such as anti-nerve growth factor compounds, which cause neuronal atrophy of sympathetic ganglia that cannot be detected qualitatively unless the cell changes are fairly marked). Stereology should also be considered when an investigator is interested in detecting small differences in quantity between groups, particularly for tissues that are heterogeneous (such as the brain) or dynamic (such as the lung). Indeed, if smaller differences between groups are important to detect, stereology may be essential to provide sufficient sensitivity; examples include if a low-intensity signal is detected by other methods, if the underlying mechanism is an important question, or if the class of agents has a known safety concern. Stereology is also employed in drug discovery and efficacy studies, particularly those involving animal models of disease. For detailed examples of cases in which stereology should be considered, the reader is directed to prior extensive reviews (Brown, 2017b; Gundersen et al., 2013).

10. DIGITAL PATHOLOGY

Digital pathology is an image-based information environment enabled by computer technology that allows for the management of information generated from a digitized slide (i.e., WSIs). Equipment speeds, scanning resolutions, and analytical software sophistication have improved and now provide a reasonable application platform for performing routine evaluations, non-GLP peer reviews, detailed morphologic characterization, and sensitive quantitation for elucidate changes in cell number, localization, or protein expression. Digital pathology provides unique and outstanding tools that not only save time compared to standard descriptive morphologic or morphometric approaches but also provide more quantifiable data relevant to risk assessment activities. Digital pathology is instrumental as a platform for enhancing special pathology techniques, in particular IHC, EHC, and ISH. A detailed discussion of digital pathology is outside the scope of this chapter, but more information is available in the chapter on (*Digital Pathology and Tissue Image Analysis*, Vol 1, Chap 12).

11. CONCLUSIONS

A wealth of special techniques are available that can provide valuable information about the function of or downstream effects induced by a test article or a toxicant of interest. These techniques include IHC, ISH, EHC, confocal microscopy, LCM, TEM, flow cytometry, stereology, and digital pathology as discussed in this chapter, to name a few of the most important. Used individually or in combination, these special techniques can facilitate a greater

understanding of the functionality, on- or off-target effects, and other downstream events that might occur after administration of a therapeutic candidate. For any of these techniques, careful experimental planning is critical to ensure proper sample procurement, handling, and preparation so that the most meaningful, accurate results can be obtained from such analyses. Performance of these techniques as well as evaluation and interpretation of the data they provide should be performed by well-trained personnel to ensure that the information obtained is suitable for predicting or understanding possible effects that might occur in later stages of product development (e.g., clinical trials) or following occupational or environmental exposures.

GLOSSARY

Adsorption – process of removing antibody by exposure to a specific antigen; to reduce cross-reactivity of detection antibodies with proteins of a given species, immunoglobulins from that species are incubated with the detection antibody to bind to and thus block binding ability of any cross-reactive antibody

Antigen – a molecule foreign to the body that evokes an immune response

Bias – deviation from objective reality in collected data that can lead to a false conclusion, based on conscious or unconscious selection of a sampling method that systematically favors some outcomes over others

Chimeric antibody – antibody comprising peptide derived from more than one species; many such antibodies have variable regions derived from mouse and the constant regions derived from human

Compensation – correction of signal overlap between channels of emission spectra for various fluorochromes

Chromogen – a noncolored chemical that can be enzymatically converted to a dye or colored substance

Epitope – a specific portion of an antigen against which an immune response is directed

Epitope tag – short protein sequences genetically fused to a larger protein and used for the purpose of antibody recognition for purification or detection in immune assays

Fluorochrome – a chemical that can be used as a label for detection because it absorbs high-energy (shorter wavelength) light and then emits lower-energy (longer wavelength) light

Humanized antibody – antibodies derived from nonhuman species that are genetically modified to have sequences more similar to naturally occurring human antibodies

Immunobridge – series of proteins/antibodies between the primary antibody bound to the target antigen and the ultimate detection compound in an immunohistochemistry assay

Morphometry – process of measuring in 2D the shape and/or dimensions of various structures in tissues

Qualification – demonstration that an established method will provide meaningful data for the conditions being evaluated

Raster pattern – a grid-like scan pattern where an area is assessed from side to side and top to bottom using narrow lines

Stereology – an unbiased quantitative method for 3D evaluation of an object using 2D sections

Systemic Uniform Random Sampling (SURS) – an unbiased sampling method for stereology requiring random sampling

Validation – a process for demonstrating specificity of binding, specificity of the assay, and reproducibility for an antibody in a given immuno-assay

REFERENCES

Aguilar-Bravo B, Sancho-Bru P: Laser capture microdissection: techniques and applications in liver diseases, *Hepatol Int* 13:138–147, 2019.

Alachkar A, Brotchie JM, Jones OT: Changes in the mRNA levels of α2A and α2C adrenergic receptors in rat models of Parkinson's disease and L-DOPA-induced dyskinesia, *J Mol Neurosci* 46:145–152, 2012.

Aleku M, Fisch G, Möpert K, et al.: Intracellular localization of lipoplexed siRNA in vascular endothelial cells of different mouse tissues, *Microvasc Res* 76:31–41, 2008.

Altar C: Gene probes. In Conn P, editor: *Methods in neurosciences*, 1989, Elsevier.

Amos WB, White JG: How the confocal laser scanning microscope entered biological research, *Biol Cell* 95:335–342, 2003.

Anderson LM, Ward JM, Park SS, et al.: Immunohistochemical localization of cytochromes P450 with polyclonal and monoclonal antibodies, *Pathol Immunopathol Res* 8:61–94, 1989.

Arends MJ, Wyllie AH: Apoptosis: mechanisms and roles in pathology, *Int Rev Exp Pathol* 32:223–254, 1991.

Aschoff A, Jantz M, Jirikowski GF: In-situ end labelling with bromodeoxyuridine–an advanced technique for the visualization of apoptotic cells in histological specimens, *Horm Metab Res* 28:311–314, 1996.

Banerjee A, Burghardt RC, Johnson GA, et al.: The temporal expression of osteopontin (SPP-1) in the rodent model of alcoholic steatohepatitis: a potential biomarker, *Toxicol Pathol* 34:373–384, 2006.

Banerjee A, Rose R, Johnson GA, et al.: The influence of estrogen on hepatobiliary osteopontin (SPP1) expression in a female rodent model of alcoholic steatohepatitis, *Toxicol Pathol* 37:492–501, 2009.

Baumgarth N, Roederer M: A practical approach to multicolor flow cytometry for immunophenotyping, *J Immunol Methods* 243:77–97, 2000.

Bayguinov PO, Oakley DM, Shih CC, et al.: Modern laser scanning confocal microscopy, *Curr Protoc Cytom* 85:e39, 2018.

Belinsky SA, Swafford DS, Finch GL, et al.: Alterations in the K-ras and p53 genes in rat lung tumors, *Environ Health Perspect* 105(Suppl 4):901–906, 1997.

Belykh E, Cavallo C, Gandhi S, et al.: Utilization of intraoperative confocal laser endomicroscopy in brain tumor surgery, *J Neurosurg Sci* 62:704–717, 2018.

Bisenius ES, Veeramachaneni DN, Sammonds GE, et al.: Sex differences and the development of the rabbit brain: effects of vinclozolin, *Biol Reprod* 75:469–476, 2006.

Bogdanffy MS: Biotransformation enzymes in the rodent nasal mucosa: the value of a histochemical approach, *Environ Health Perspect* 85:177–186, 1990.

Bohle RM, Bonczkowitz M, Altmannsberger HM, et al.: Immunohistochemical double staining of microwave enhanced and nonenhanced nuclear and cytoplasmic antigens, *Biotech Histochem* 72:10–15, 1997.

Bolon B: Whole mount enzyme histochemistry as a rapid screen at necropsy for expression of beta-galactosidase (LacZ)-bearing transgenes: considerations for separating specific LacZ activity from nonspecific (endogenous) galactosidase activity, *Toxicol Pathol* 36:265–276, 2008.

Bolon B, Calderwood Mays MB, Hall BJ: Characteristics of canine melanomas and comparison of histology and DNA ploidy to their biologic behavior, *Vet Pathol* 27:96–102, 1990.

Bolon B, Krinke G, Butt MT, et al.: STP position paper: recommended best practices for sampling, processing, and analysis of the peripheral nervous system (nerves and somatic and autonomic ganglia) during nonclinical toxicity studies, *Toxicol Pathol* 46:372–402, 2018.

Bonifant CL, Jackson HJ, Brentjens RJ, et al.: Toxicity and management in CAR T-cell therapy, *Mol Ther Oncolytics* 3: 16011, 2016.

Boone DR, Weisz HA, Sell SL, et al.: Laser capture microdissection in traumatic brain injury research: obtaining hippocampal subregions and pools of injured neurons for genomic analyses, *Methods Mol Biol* 1723:235–245, 2018.

Boyce RW, Dorph-Petersen KA, Lyck L, et al.: Design-based stereology: introduction to basic concepts and practical approaches for estimation of cell number, *Toxicol Pathol* 38: 1011–1025, 2010.

Brown C: In situ hybridization with riboprobes: an overview for veterinary pathologists, *Vet Pathol* 35:159–167, 1998.

Brown DL: Bias in image analysis and its solution: unbiased stereology, *J Toxicol Pathol* 30:183–191, 2017a.

Brown DL: Practical stereology applications for the pathologist, *Vet Pathol* 54:358–368, 2017b.

Browning JL, French LE: Visualization of lymphotoxin-beta and lymphotoxin-beta receptor expression in mouse embryos, *J Immunol* 168:5079–5087, 2002.

Bursch W, Oberhammer F, Schulte-Hermann R: Cell death by apoptosis and its protective role against disease, *Trends Pharmacol Sci* 13:245–251, 1992.

Butler WH, Ford GP, Newberne JW: A study of the effects of vigabatrin on the central nervous system and retina of Sprague Dawley and Lister-Hooded rats, *Toxicol Pathol* 15: 143–148, 1987.

Butterfield LH: The society for immunotherapy of cancer biomarkers task force recommendations review, *Semin Cancer Biol* 52:12–15, 2018.

Carter BS, Fletcher JS, Thompson RC: Analysis of messenger RNA expression by in situ hybridization using RNA probes synthesized via in vitro transcription, *Methods* 52: 322–331, 2010.

Cattoretti G, Pileri S, Parravicini C, et al.: Antigen unmasking on formalin-fixed, paraffin-embedded tissue sections, *J Pathol* 171:83–98, 1993.

Chamaa F, Bahmad HF, Makkawi AK, et al.: Nitrous oxide induces prominent cell proliferation in adult rat hippocampal dentate gyrus, *Front Cell Neurosci* 12:135, 2018.

Charriaut-Marlangue C, Ben-Ari Y: A cautionary note on the use of the TUNEL stain to determine apoptosis, *Neuroreport* 7:61–64, 1995.

Cheville N: *Cell pathology*, ed 2 Ames, Iowa, 1983, Iowa University Press.

Cheville N: *Ultrastructural pathology: the comparative cellular basis of disease*, Hoboken, NJ, 2009, Wiley-Blackwell.

Cheville NF, Stasko J: Techniques in electron microscopy of animal tissue, *Vet Pathol* 51:28–41, 2014.

Chowdhury AR, Ehara T, Higuchi M, et al.: Immunohistochemical detection of immunoglobulins and complements in formaldehyde-fixed and paraffin-embedded renal biopsy tissues; an adjunct for diagnosis of glomerulonephritis, *Nephrology* 10:298–304, 2005.

Clark SM, Narayanan PK, Fort MM: Determination of absolute counts of circulating regulatory T cells in cynomolgus macaques using an optimized flow cytometric method, *Toxicol Pathol* 40:107–112, 2012.

Clark SP, Ryan TP, Searfoss GH, et al.: Chronic microcystin exposure induces hepatocyte proliferation with increased expression of mitotic and cyclin-associated genes in P53-deficient mice, *Toxicol Pathol* 36:190–203, 2008.

Clayton NP, Yoshizawa K, Kissling GE, et al.: Immunohistochemical analysis of expressions of hepatic cytochrome P450 in F344 rats following oral treatment with kava extract, *Exp Toxicol Pathol* 58:223–236, 2007.

Conchello JA, Lichtman JW: Optical sectioning microscopy, *Nat Methods* 2:920–931, 2005.

Corcoran GB, Fix L, Jones DP, et al.: Apoptosis: molecular control point in toxicity, *Toxicol Appl Pharmacol* 128:169–181, 1994.

Corgiat BA, Mueller C: Using laser capture microdissection to isolate cortical laminae in nonhuman primate brain, *Methods Mol Biol* 1606:115–132, 2017.

Cossarizza A, Chang HD, Radbruch A, et al.: Guidelines for the use of flow cytometry and cell sorting in immunological studies, *Eur J Immunol* 47:1584–1797, 2017.

Cui L, Takahashi S, Tada M, et al.: Immunohistochemical detection of carcinogen-DNA adducts in normal human prostate tissues transplanted into the subcutis of athymic nude mice: results with 2-amino-1-methyl-6-phenylimidazo [4,5-b]pyridine (PhIP) and 3,2′-dimethyl-4-aminobiphenyl (DMAB) and relation to cytochrome P450s and N-acetyltransferase activity, *Jpn J Cancer Res* 91:52–58, 2000.

Danilenko DM, Wang H: The yin and yang of immunomodulatory biologics: assessing the delicate balance between benefit and risk, *Toxicol Pathol* 40:272–287, 2012.

Datta S, Malhotra L, Dickerson R, et al.: Laser capture microdissection: big data from small samples, *Histol Histopathol* 30:1255–1269, 2015.

de Sauvage FJ, Keshav S, Kuang WJ, et al.: Precursor structure, expression, and tissue distribution of human guanylin, *Proc Natl Acad Sci USA* 89:9089–9093, 1992.

De Sousa Linhares A, Battin C, Jutz S, et al.: Therapeutic PD-L1 antibodies are more effective than PD-1 antibodies in blocking PD-1/PD-L1 signaling, *Sci Rep* 9:11472, 2019.

Dean JH, Padarathsingh ML, Jerrells TR: Assessment of immunobiological effects induced by chemicals, drugs or food additives. I. Tier testing and screening approach, *Drug Chem Toxicol* 2:5–17, 1979.

Delker DA, Yano BL, Gollapudi BB: V-Ha-ras gene expression in liver and kidney of transgenic Tg.AC mice following chemically induced tissue injury, *Toxicol Sci* 50:90–97, 1999.

der Strate BV, Longdin R, Geerlings M, et al.: Best practices in performing flow cytometry in a regulated environment: feedback from experience within the European bioanalysis forum, *Bioanalysis* 9:1253–1264, 2017.

Dickerson SM, Cunningham SL, Gore AC: Prenatal PCBs disrupt early neuroendocrine development of the rat hypothalamus, *Toxicol Appl Pharmacol* 252:36–46, 2011a.

Dickerson SM, Cunningham SL, Patisaul HB, et al.: Endocrine disruption of brain sexual differentiation by developmental PCB exposure, *Endocrinology* 152:581–594, 2011b.

Dixon AR, Bathany C, Tsuei M, et al.: Recent developments in multiplexing techniques for immunohistochemistry, *Expert Rev Mol Diagn* 15:1171–1186, 2015.

Dons EM, Raimondi G, Cooper DK, et al.: Non-human primate regulatory T cells: current biology and implications for transplantation, *Transplantation* 90:811–816, 2010.

Doughty SE, Ferrier RK, Hillan KJ, et al.: The effects of ZENECA ZD8731, an angiotensin II antagonist, on renin expression by juxtaglomerular cells in the rat: comparison of protein and mRNA expression as detected by immunohistochemistry and in situ hybridization, *Toxicol Pathol* 23:256–261, 1995.

Du Toit LC, Govender T, Carmichael T, et al.: Design of an anti-inflammatory composite nanosystem and evaluation of its potential for ocular drug delivery, *J Pharm Sci* 102: 2780–2805, 2013.

Duan K, Mete O: Algorithmic approach to neuroendocrine tumors in targeted biopsies: practical applications of immunohistochemical markers, *Cancer Cytopathol* 124:871–884, 2016.

Dudas B, Merchenthaler I: Three-dimensional representation of the neurotransmitter systems of the human hypothalamus: inputs of the gonadotrophin hormone-releasing hormone neuronal system, *J Neuroendocrinol* 18:79–95, 2006.

Dykstra MJ, Mann PC, Elwell MR, et al.: Suggested standard operating procedures (SOPs) for the preparation of electron microscopy samples for toxicology/pathology studies in a GLP environment, *Toxicol Pathol* 30:735–743, 2002.

Dykstra MJ, Reuss LE: *Biological electron microscopy: theory, techniques, and troubleshooting*, 2003, Springer US.

Edwards BS, Sklar LA: Flow cytometry: impact on early drug discovery, *J Biomol Screen* 20:689–707, 2015.

Edwards JR, Diamantakos EA, Peuler JD, et al.: A novel method for the evaluation of proximal tubule epithelial cellular necrosis in the intact rat kidney using ethidium homodimer, *BMC Physiol* 7(1), 2007.

Eldridge SR, Goldsworthy SM: Cell proliferation rates in common cancer target tissues of B6C3F1 mice and F344 rats: effects of age, gender, and choice of marker, *Fundam Appl Toxicol* 32:159–167, 1996.

Elmer BM, Swanson KA, Bangari DS, et al.: Gene delivery of a modified antibody to Aβ reduces progression of murine Alzheimer's disease, *PLoS One* 14:e0226245, 2019.

Elmore S: Apoptosis: a review of programmed cell death, *Toxicol Pathol* 35:495–516, 2007.

Elmore SA, Dixon D, Hailey JR, et al.: Recommendations from the INHAND apoptosis/necrosis working group, *Toxicol Pathol* 44:173–188, 2016.

EMA: *Guideline on development, production, characterisation and specification for monoclonal antibodies and related products*, 2016. Published, https://www.ema.europa.eu/en/documents/scientific-guideline/guideline-development-production-ch aracterisation-specification-monoclonal-antibodies-related_en.pdf. (Accessed 10 December 2020).

Ewa B, Danuta M: Polycyclic aromatic hydrocarbons and PAH-related DNA adducts, *J Appl Genet* 58:321–330, 2017.

Fagerland JA, Wall HG, Pandher K, et al.: Ultrastructural analysis in preclinical safety evaluation, *Toxicol Pathol* 40: 391–402, 2012.

Farman CA, Kornbrust DJ: Oligodeoxynucleotide studies in primates: antisense and immune stimulatory indications, *Toxicol Pathol* 31(Suppl):119–122, 2003.

FDA: *Points to consider in the manufacture and testing of monoclonal antibody products for human use*, 1997. Published, https://www.fda.gov/regulatory-information/search-fda-guidance-documents/points-consider-manufacture-and-testing-monoclonal-antibody-products-human-use. (Accessed 10 December 2020).

FDA: *Immunotoxicology evaluation of investigational new drugs*, 2002. Published, https://www.fda.gov/regulatory-information/search-fda-guidance-documents/immunotoxicology-evaluation-investigational-new-drugs. (Accessed 10 December 2020).

FDA: *S8 immunotoxicity studies for human pharmaceuticals*, 2006. Published, https://www.fda.gov/regulatory-information/search-fda-guidance-documents/s8-immunotoxicity-stud ies-human-pharmaceuticals. (Accessed 10 December 2020).

FDA: *Flow cytometric devices; draft guidance for industry and Food and drug administration staff; availability*, 2014. Published, https://www.federalregister.gov/documents/2014/10/14/2014-24308/flow-cytometric-devices-draft-guidance-for-industry-and-food-and-drug-administration-staff. (Accessed 10 December 2020).

FDA: *Medical devices; exemption from premarket notification: class II devices; flow cytometer instruments; request for comments*, 2020. Published, https://www.federalregister.gov/documents/2020/07/22/2020-15256/medical-devices-exemptions-from-premarket-notification-class-ii-devices. (Accessed 10 December 2020).

Fernández-Guasti A, Kruijver FP, Fodor M, et al.: Sex differences in the distribution of androgen receptors in the human hypothalamus, *J Comp Neurol* 425:422–435, 2000.

Foley JF, Dietrich DR, Swenberg JA, et al.: Detection and evaluation of proliferating cell nuclear antigen (PCNA) in rat tissue by an improved immunohistochemical procedure, *J Histotechnol* 14:237–241, 1991.

Foust KD, Nurre E, Montgomery CL, et al.: Intravascular AAV9 preferentially targets neonatal neurons and adult astrocytes, *Nat Biotechnol* 27:59–65, 2009.

Frantz GD, Pham TQ, Peale Jr FV, et al.: Detection of novel gene expression in paraffin-embedded tissues by isotopic in situ hybridization in tissue microarrays, *J Pathol* 195:87–96, 2001.

Frazier KS, Engelhardt JA, Fant P, et al.: Scientific and regulatory policy committee points-to-consider paper*: drug-induced vascular injury associated with nonsmall molecule therapeutics in preclinical development: part I. Biotherapeutics, *Toxicol Pathol* 43:915–934, 2015.

Freeth J, Soden J: New advances in cell microarray technology to expand applications in target deconvolution and off-target screening, *SLAS Discov* 25:223–230, 2020.

Frost AR, Eltoum IE, Siegal GP, et al.: Laser microdissection, *Curr Protoc Mol Biol* 112:25a.21.21–25a.21.30, 2015.

Fung KM, Messing A, Lee VM, et al.: A novel modification of the avidin-biotin complex method for immunohistochemical studies of transgenic mice with murine monoclonal antibodies, *J Histochem Cytochem* 40:1319–1328, 1992.

Furrer P, Gurny R: Recent advances in confocal microscopy for studying drug delivery to the eye: concepts and pharmaceutical applications, *Eur J Pharm Biopharm* 74:33–40, 2010.

Gagner JP, Zagzag D: Probing glioblastoma tissue heterogeneity with laser capture microdissection, *Methods Mol Biol* 1741:209–220, 2018.

Gall JG, Pardue ML: Formation and detection of RNA-DNA hybrid molecules in cytological preparations, *Proc Natl Acad Sci USA* 63:378–383, 1969.

Garman RH, Li AA, Kaufmann W, et al.: Recommended methods for brain processing and quantitative analysis in rodent developmental neurotoxicity studies, *Toxicol Pathol* 44:14–42, 2016.

Germolec D, Luebke R, Rooney A, et al.: Immunotoxicology: a brief history, current status and strategies for future immunotoxicity assessment, *Curr Opin Toxicol* 5:55–59, 2017.

Ghadially F: *Ultrastructural pathology of the cell and matrix*, ed 4, Burlington, MA, 1997, Butterworth-Heinemann.

Ghadially F: *Diagnostic ultrastructural pathology: a self-evaluation and self-teaching*, ed 2, Lpndon, 1998, Hodder Arnold.

Ghanayem BI, Elwell MR, Eldridge SR: Effects of the carcinogen, acrylonitrile, on forestomach cell proliferation and apoptosis in the rat: comparison with methacrylonitrile, *Carcinogenesis* 18:675–680, 1997.

Ghiadially F: *Diagnostic electron microscopy of tumors*, Oxford, UK, 1985, Butterworth-Heinemann.

Gillett NA, Chan CM: Molecular pathology in the preclinical development of biopharmaceuticals, *Toxicol Pathol* 27:48–52, 1999.

Goebl N, Berridge B, Wroblewski VJ, et al.: Development of a sensitive and specific in situ hybridization technique for the cellular localization of antisense oligodeoxynucleotide drugs in tissue sections, *Toxicol Pathol* 35:541–548, 2007.

Gold R, Schmied M, Rothe G, et al.: Detection of DNA fragmentation in apoptosis: application of in situ nick translation to cell culture systems and tissue sections, *J Histochem Cytochem* 41:1023–1030, 1993.

Gossett KA, Narayanan PK, Williams DM, et al.: Flow cytometry in the preclinical development of biopharmaceuticals, *Toxicol Pathol* 27:32–37, 1999.

Gown AM, Willingham MC: Improved detection of apoptotic cells in archival paraffin sections: immunohistochemistry using antibodies to cleaved caspase 3, *J Histochem Cytochem* 50:449–454, 2002.

Grasl-Kraupp B, Ruttkay-Nedecky B, Koudelka H, et al.: In situ detection of fragmented DNA (TUNEL assay) fails to discriminate among apoptosis, necrosis, and autolytic cell death: a cautionary note, *Hepatology* 21:1465–1468, 1995.

Green CL, Stewart JJ, Högerkorp CM, et al.: Recommendations for the development and validation of flow cytometry-based receptor occupancy assays, *Cytometry B Clin Cytom* 90:141–149, 2016.

Gundersen HJ, Jensen EB: The efficiency of systematic sampling in stereology and its prediction, *J Microsc* 147:229–263, 1987.

Gundersen HJG, Mirabile R, Brown D, Boyce RW: Stereological principles and sampling procedures for toxicologic pathologists. In Haschek WMRC, Wallig MA, editors: *Handbook of toxicologic pathology*, San Diego, CA, 2013, Academic Press, pp 215–286.

Guzman RE, Solter PF: Characterization of sublethal microcystin-LR exposure in mice, *Vet Pathol* 39:17–26, 2002.

Hall PA, Woods AL: Immunohistochemical markers of cellular proliferation: achievements, problems and prospects, *Cell Tissue Kinet* 23:505–522, 1990.

Hall WP-SS, Wicks J, Rojko J: Tissue cross-reactivity studies for monoclonal antibodies: predictive value and use for selection of relevant animal species for toxicity testing. In Cavagnaro JA, editor: *Preclinical safety evaluation of biopharmaceuticals: a science-based approach to facilitating clinical trials*, Hoboken,NJ, 2008, Wiley-Interscience, pp 207–240.

Hall WC, Rojko JL: The use of immunohistochemistry for evaluating the liver, *Toxicol Pathol* 24:4–12, 1996.

Han H, Ma Q, Li C, et al.: Profiling serum cytokines in COVID-19 patients reveals IL-6 and IL-10 are disease severity predictors, *Emerg Microbes Infect* 9:1123–1130, 2020.

Harnett MM: Laser scanning cytometry: understanding the immune system in situ, *Nat Rev Immunol* 7:897–904, 2007.

Hayat: *Principles and techniques of electron microscopy: biological applications*, Boca Raton, FL, 2000, CRC Press.

Hierck BP, Iperen LV, Gittenberger-De Groot AC, et al.: Modified indirect immunodetection allows study of murine tissue with mouse monoclonal antibodies, *J Histochem Cytochem* 42:1499–1502, 1994.

Hoane JS, Johnson CL, Morrison JP, et al.: Comparison of renal amyloid and hyaline glomerulopathy in B6C3F1 mice: an NTP retrospective study, *Toxicol Pathol* 44:687–704, 2016.

Hofler H: Principles of in situ hybridization. In JO'D PJM, editor: *In situ hybriziation: principle and practice*, Oxford, UK, 1990, Oxford Univeristy Press.

Holm R, Karlsen F, Nesland JM: In situ hybridization with nonisotopic probes using different detection systems, *Mod Pathol* 5:315–319, 1992.

Holubec H, Payne CM, Bernstein H, et al.: Assessment of apoptosis by immunohistochemical markers compared to cellular morphology in ex vivo-stressed colonic mucosa, *J Histochem Cytochem* 53:229–235, 2005.

Honda O, Kuroda M, Joja I, et al.: Assessment of secondary necrosis of Jurkat cells using a new microscopic system and double staining method with annexin V and propidium iodide, *Int J Oncol* 16:283–288, 2000.

Huppertz B, Frank HG, Kaufmann P: The apoptosis cascade–morphological and immunohistochemical methods for its visualization, *Anat Embryol* 200:1–18, 1999.

Huston-Paterson DJ, Banik SSR, Doranz BJ: A high-throughput platform for identifying membrane protein antibody targets, *Genet Eng Biotechnol News* 36, 2016.

Iavicoli I, Fontana L, Bergamaschi A: The effects of metals as endocrine disruptors, *J Toxicol Environ Health B Crit Rev* 12:206–223, 2009.

CH: *S8 immunotoxicity studies for human pharmaceuticals*, 2006. Published, https://www.fda.gov/regulatory-information/search-fda-guidance-documents/s8-immunotoxicity-studies-human-pharmaceuticals. (Accessed 10 December 2020).

ICH: *S6(R1) preclinical safety evaluation of biotechnology-derived pharmaceuticals*, 2012. Published, https://www.fda.gov/regulatory-information/search-fda-guidance-documents/s6r1-preclinical-safety-evaluation-biotechnology-derived-pharmaceuticals. (Accessed 10 December 2020).

ICH: *S9 guideline on nonclinical evaluation for anticancer 5 pharmaceuticals - questions and answers*, 2016. Published, https://www.ema.europa.eu/en/documents/scientific-guideline/ich-s9-guideline-nonclinical-evaluation-anticancer-4-pharmaceuticals-questions-answers-step-2b_en.pdf. (Accessed 10 December 2020).

Ishii A, Sakai Y, Nakamura A: Molecular pathological evaluation of clusterin in a rat model of unilateral ureteral obstruction as a possible biomarker of nephrotoxicity, *Toxicol Pathol* 35:376–382, 2007.

Islam D, Lindberg AA, Christensson B: Peripheral blood cell preparation influences the level of expression of leukocyte cell surface markers as assessed with quantitative multi-color flow cytometry, *Cytometry* 22:128–134, 1995.

Jakubowski A, Ambrose C, Parr M, et al.: TWEAK induces liver progenitor cell proliferation, *J Clin Invest* 115:2330–2340, 2005.

Janardhan KS, Jensen H, Clayton NP, et al.: Immunohistochemistry in investigative and toxicologic pathology, *Toxicol Pathol* 46:488–510, 2018.

Jonkman J, Brown CM: Any way you slice it-A comparison of confocal microscopy techniques, *J Biomol Tech* 26:54–65, 2015.

Jortner B: High-definition microscopic analysis of the nervous system. In Butt BBM, editor: *Tundamental neuropathology of pathologists and Toxicologists: principles and techniques*, Hoboken, NJ, 2011, John Wiley and Sons, pp 203–208.

Jortner BS, Hancock SK, Hinckley J, et al.: Neuropathological studies of rats following multiple exposure to tri-ortho-tolyl phosphate, chlorpyrifos and stress, *Toxicol Pathol* 33:378–385, 2005.

Kato Y, Masago Y, Kondo C, et al.: Comparison of acute gene expression profiles of islet cells obtained via laser capture microdissection between alloxan- and streptozotocin-treated rats, *Toxicol Pathol* 46:660–670, 2018.

Keirstead ND, Janovitz EB, Meehan JT, et al.: Scientific and regulatory policy committee points to consider*: review of scientific and regulatory policy committee points to consider: review of current practices for ultrastructural pathology evaluations in support of nonclinical toxicology studies, *Toxicol Pathol* 47:461–468, 2019.

Key M: *Immunohistochemical staining methods carpenteria*, CA, 2006, Dako Corporation.

Khan KN, Venturini CM, Bunch RT, et al.: Interspecies differences in renal localization of cyclooxygenase isoforms: implications in nonsteroidal antiinflammatory drug-related nephrotoxicity, *Toxicol Pathol* 26:612–620, 1998.

Kim MR, Manoukian R, Yeh R, et al.: Transgenic over-expression of human IL-17E results in eosinophilia, B-lymphocyte hyperplasia, and altered antibody production, *Blood* 100:2330–2340, 2002.

Kind CN: The application of in-situ hybridisation and immuno-cytochemistry to problem resolution in drug development, *Toxicol Lett* 112–113:487–492, 2000.

Klebanoff CA, Rosenberg SA, Restifo NP: Prospects for gene-engineered T cell immunotherapy for solid cancers, *Nat Med* 22:26–36, 2016.

Knapp W: *Leucocyte typing IV: white cell differentiation antigens*, 1989, Oxford University Press.

Kolenda-Roberts HM, Harris N, Singletary E, et al.: Immunohistochemical characterization of spontaneous and acrylonitrile-induced brain tumors in the rat, *Toxicol Pathol* 41:98–108, 2013.

Kressel M, Groscurth P: Distinction of apoptotic and necrotic cell death by in situ labelling of fragmented DNA, *Cell Tissue Res* 278:549–556, 1994.

Kruijver FP, Balesar R, Espila AM, et al.: Estrogen-receptor-beta distribution in the human hypothalamus: similarities and differences with ER alpha distribution, *J Comp Neurol* 466:251–277, 2003.

Krysko DV, Vanden Berghe T, D'Herde K, et al.: Apoptosis and necrosis: detection, discrimination and phagocytosis, *Methods* 44:205–221, 2008.

Kubota K, Ohashi A, Imachi H, et al.: Improved in situ hybridization efficiency with locked-nucleic-acid-incorporated DNA probes, *Appl Environ Microbiol* 72:5311–5317, 2006.

Kumar A: In situ hybridization, *Int J Appl Biol Pharmaceut Technol* 1:418–430, 2010.

Ky B, Shughrue PJ: Methods to enhance signal using isotopic in situ hybridization, *J Histochem Cytochem* 50:1031–1037, 2002.

Lappin PB: Flow cytometry in preclinical drug development, *Methods Mol Biol* 598:303–321, 2010.

Leach MW, Halpern WG, Johnson CW, et al.: Use of tissue cross-reactivity studies in the development of antibody-based biopharmaceuticals: history, experience, methodology, and future directions, *Toxicol Pathol* 38:1138–1166, 2010.

Lee CC, Ichihara T, Yamamoto S, et al.: Reduced expression of the CDK inhibitor p27(KIP1) in rat two-stage bladder carcinogenesis and its association with expression profiles of p21(WAF1/Cip1) and p53, *Carcinogenesis* 20:1697–1708, 1999.

Lee LH, Yang H, Bigras G: Current breast cancer proliferative markers correlate variably based on decoupled duration of cell cycle phases, *Sci Rep* 4:5122, 2014.

Lewis AGP: *Biological specimen preparation for transmission electron microscopy,* Princeton, NJ, 1998, Princeton Univerisity Press.

Lewis Ga: *Biological specimen preparation for transmissio electron microscopy,* Princeton, NJ, 1999, Princeton University Press.

Lewis M: *Cross-adsorbed secondary antibodies and cross-reactivity,* 2018.

Lewis ME, Sherman TG, Watson SJ: In situ hybridization histochemistry with synthetic oligonucleotides: strategies and methods, *Peptides* 6(Suppl 2):75–87, 1985.

Liang M, Schwickart M, Schneider AK, et al.: Receptor occupancy assessment by flow cytometry as a pharmacodynamic biomarker in biopharmaceutical development, *Cytometry B Clin Cytom* 90:117–127, 2016.

Lichtman JW, Conchello JA: Fluorescence microscopy, *Nat Methods* 2:910–919, 2005.

Liu H, McDowell TL, Hanson NE, et al.: Laser capture microdissection for the investigative pathologist, *Vet Pathol* 51:257–269, 2014.

Lu Y, Xie T, Zhang Y, et al.: Triptolide Induces hepatotoxicity via inhibition of CYP450s in rat liver microsomes, *BMC Complement Altern Med* 17(15), 2017.

Luoh SM, Di Marco F, Levin N, et al.: Cloning and characterization of a human leptin receptor using a biologically active leptin immunoadhesin, *J Mol Endocrinol* 18:77–85, 1997.

MacDonald C, Finlay DB, Jabed A, et al.: Development of positive control tissue for in situ hybridisation using Alvetex scaffolds, *J Neurosci Methods* 238:70–77, 2014.

Maecker HT, Frey T, Nomura LE, et al.: Selecting fluorochrome conjugates for maximum sensitivity, *Cytometry A* 62:169–173, 2004.

Mahalingam M: Laser capture microdissection: insights into methods and applications, *Methods Mol Biol* 1723:1–17, 2018.

Mainwaring PN, Ellis PA, Detre S, et al.: Comparison of in situ methods to assess DNA cleavage in apoptotic cells in patients with breast cancer, *J Clin Pathol* 51:34–37, 1998.

Mantopoulos D, Cruzat A, Hamrah P: In vivo imaging of corneal inflammation: new tools for clinical practice and research, *Semin Ophthalmol* 25:178–185, 2010.

Martínez-Hernández R, Bernal S, Also-Rallo E, et al.: Synaptic defects in type I spinal muscular atrophy in human development, *J Pathol* 229:49–61, 2013.

Martinez NJ, Titus SA, Wagner AK, et al.: High-throughput fluorescence imaging approaches for drug discovery using in vitro and in vivo three-dimensional models, *Expert Opin Drug Discov* 10:1347–1361, 2015.

Mattar CN, Waddington SN, Biswas A, et al.: Systemic delivery of scAAV9 in fetal macaques facilitates neuronal transduction of the central and peripheral nervous systems, *Gene Ther* 20:69–83, 2013.

McFarland D, Harkins KR: Flow cytometry in preclinical toxicology/safety assessment. In Litwin V, Marder P, editors: *Flow cytometry in drug discovery and development,* Hoboken, New Jersey, 2010, Wiley, pp 123–150.

McLaughlin SK, Margolskee RF: 33P is preferable to 35S for labeling probes used in in situ hybridization, *Biotechniques* 15:506–511, 1993.

Meier-Ruge W: Drug induced retinopathy, *Ophthalmologica* 158(Suppl):561–573, 1969.

Meier-Ruge W, Bielser Jr W, Wiederhold KH, et al.: Incubation media for routine laboratory work on enzyme histotopochemistry, *Beitr Pathol* 144:409–431, 1971.

Meier-Ruge W, Bruder A, Theodore D: Histochemical and morphometric investigation of the pathogenesis of acute brain infarction in primates, *Acta Histochem Suppl* 42:59–70, 1992.

Meier-Ruge WA, Bruder E: Pathology of chronic constipation in pediatric and adult coloproctology, *Pathobiology* 72:1–102, 2005.

Meier-Ruge WA, Bruder E: Current concepts of enzyme histochemistry in modern pathology, *Pathobiology* 75:233–243, 2008.

Migheli A, Attanasio A, Schiffer D: Ultrastructural detection of DNA strand breaks in apoptotic neural cells by in situ end-labelling techniques, *J Pathol* 176:27–35, 1995.

Mikaelian I, Cameron M, Dalmas DA, et al.: Nonclinical safety biomarkers of drug-induced vascular injury: current status and blueprint for the future, *Toxicol Pathol* 42:635–657, 2014.

Mitić T, McKay JS: Immunohistochemical analysis of acetylation, proliferation, mitosis, and apoptosis in tumor xenografts following administration of a histone deacetylase inhibitor–a pilot study, *Toxicol Pathol* 33:792–799, 2005.

Monteith DK, Horner MJ, Gillett NA, et al.: Evaluation of the renal effects of an antisense phosphorothioate oligodeoxynucleotide in monkeys, *Toxicol Pathol* 27:307–317, 1999.

Moore MA, Tsuda H, Tamano S, et al.: Marriage of a medium-term liver model to surrogate markers–a practical approach for risk and benefit assessment, *Toxicol Pathol* 27:237–242, 1999.

Moorman AF, De Boer PA, Vermeulen JL, et al.: Practical aspects of radio-isotopic in situ hybridization on RNA, *Histochem J* 25:251–266, 1993.

Moto M, Okamura M, Muguruma M, et al.: Gene expression analysis on the dicyclanil-induced hepatocellular tumors in mice, *Toxicol Pathol* 34:744–751, 2006.

Mundle S, Iftikhar A, Shetty V, et al.: Novel in situ double labeling for simultaneous detection of proliferation and apoptosis, *J Histochem Cytochem* 42:1533–1537, 1994.

Murray JM: Methods for imaging thick specimens: confocal microscopy, deconvolution, and structured illumination, *Cold Spring Harb Protoc* 2011:1399–1437, 2011.

Neudecker S, Walz R, Menon K, et al.: Transgenic overexpression of Anks6(p.R823W) causes polycystic kidney disease in rats, *Am J Pathol* 177:3000–3009, 2010.

Nonoyama T, Fukuda R: Drug-induced phospholipidosis -pathological aspects and its prediction, *J Toxicol Pathol* 21: 9–24, 2008.

O'Hara DM, Xu Y, Liang Z, et al.: Recommendations for the validation of flow cytometric testing during drug development: II assays, *J Immunol Methods* 363:120–134, 2011.

Ohta H: Measurement of serum immunoreactive beta-glucuronidase: a possible serological marker for histological hepatic cell necrosis and to predict the histological progression of hepatitis, *Hokkaido Igaku Zasshi* 66:545–557, 1991.

Okudela K, Ito T, Mitsui H, et al.: The role of p53 in bleomycin-induced DNA damage in the lung. A comparative study with the small intestine, *Am J Pathol* 155:1341–1351, 1999.

Pacchioni D, Papotti M, Bonino F, et al.: Detection of cytomegalovirus by in situ hybridization using a digoxigenin-tailed oligonucleotide, *Liver* 12:257–261, 1992.

Painter JT, Clayton NP, Herbert RA: Useful immunohistochemical markers of tumor differentiation, *Toxicol Pathol* 38: 131–141, 2010.

Papenfuss: Flow cytometry and immunophenotyping in drug development. In Parker G, editor: *Immunopathology in toxicology and drug development*, 2017, Springer International.

Parks WC, Roby JD: Consequences of prolonged inhalation of ozone on F344/N rats: collaborative studies. Part IV: effects on expression of extracellular matrix genes, *Res Rep Health Eff Inst* 3–20:21–29, 1994. Discussion.

Paulasova P, Pellestor F: The peptide nucleic acids (PNAs): a new generation of probes for genetic and cytogenetic analyses, *Ann Genet* 47:349–358, 2004.

Pearse: Histochemistry: *Theoretical and applied London, England*, London, 1960, Royal Postgraduate Mcd. Sch. Univ.

Pertiwi KR, de Boer OJ, Gabriels P, et al.: Development of immunohistochemical triple staining method for the evaluation of different types of cell death in coronary thrombus, *J Phys Conf* 1241:012013, 2019.

Peters A, Palay SL, Webster HD: *The fine structure of the nervous system: neurons and their supporting cells*, ed 3, New York, 1991, Oxford University Press.

Petropoulos IN, Ponirakis G, Khan A, et al.: Corneal confocal microscopy: ready for prime time, *Clin Exp Optom* 103:265–277, 2020.

Poirier MC, Santella RM, Weston A: Carcinogen macromolecular adducts and their measurement, *Carcinogenesis* 21: 353–359, 2000.

Ponce R: Preclinical support for combination therapy in the treatment of autoimmunity with atacicept, *Toxicol Pathol* 37: 89–99, 2009.

Porter HJ, Heryet A, Quantrill AM, et al.: Combined non-isotopic in situ hybridisation and immunohistochemistry on routine paraffin wax embedded tissue: identification of cell type infected by human parvovirus and demonstration of cytomegalovirus DNA and antigen in renal infection, *J Clin Pathol* 43:129–132, 1990.

Pozarowski P, Holden E, Darzynkiewicz Z: Laser scanning cytometry: principles and applications-an update, *Methods Mol Biol* 931:187–212, 2013.

Pygall SR, Whetstone J, Timmins P, et al.: Pharmaceutical applications of confocal laser scanning microscopy: the physical characterisation of pharmaceutical systems, *Adv Drug Deliv Rev* 59:1434–1452, 2007.

Que SK, Grant-Kels JM, Rabinovitz HS, et al.: Application of handheld confocal microscopy for skin cancer diagnosis: advantages and limitations compared with the wide-probe confocal, *Dermatol Clin* 34:469–475, 2016.

Ragazzi M, Longo C, Piana S: Ex vivo (fluorescence) confocal microscopy in surgical pathology: state of the art, *Adv Anat Pathol* 23:159–169, 2016.

Ragazzi M, Piana S, Longo C, et al.: Fluorescence confocal microscopy for pathologists, *Mod Pathol* 27:460–471, 2014.

Ramanathan M: Flow cytometry applications in pharmacodynamics and drug delivery, *Pharm Res* 14:1106–1114, 1997.

Rehg JE, Bush D, Ward JM: The utility of immunohistochemistry for the identification of hematopoietic and lymphoid cells in normal tissues and interpretation of proliferative and inflammatory lesions of mice and rats, *Toxicol Pathol* 40:345–374, 2012.

Rhyne BN, Pirone JR, Riviere JE, et al.: The use of enzyme histochemistry in detecting cutaneous toxicity of three topically applied jet fuel mdttures, *Toxicol Mech Methods* 12: 17–34, 2002.

Rihn B, Bottin MC, Coulais C, et al.: Use of non-radioactive methods for the determination of the expression, the sequence and the copy-number of transgene in mice, *Cell Mol Biol (Noisy-le-grand)* 41:907–915, 1995.

Rittinghausen S, Bellmann B, Creutzenberg O, et al.: Evaluation of immunohistochemical markers to detect the genotoxic mode of action of fine and ultrafine dusts in rat lungs, *Toxicology* 303:177–186, 2013.

Roberts ES, Thomas RS, Dorman DC: Gene expression changes following acute hydrogen sulfide (H2S)-induced nasal respiratory epithelial injury, *Toxicol Pathol* 36:560–567, 2008.

Roberts RA, Nebert DW, Hickman JA, et al.: Perturbation of the mitosis/apoptosis balance: a fundamental mechanism in toxicology, *Fundam Appl Toxicol* 38:107–115, 1997.

Roca C, Motas S, Marcó S, et al.: Disease correction by AAV-mediated gene therapy in a new mouse model of mucopolysaccharidosis type IIID, *Hum Mol Genet* 26:1535–1551, 2017.

Rojko JP-SS: Physiologic IgG biodistribution, transport, and clearance: implications for monoclonal antibody products. In Cavagnaro JA, editor: *Preclinical safety evaluation of biopharmaceuticals: a science-based approach to facilitating clinical trials*, Hoboken NJ, 2008, Wiley-Interscience, pp 242–276.

Rojko JL, Evans MG, Price SA, et al.: Formation, clearance, deposition, pathogenicity, and identification of biopharmaceutical-related immune complexes: review and case studies, *Toxicol Pathol* 42:725–764, 2014.

Roy A, Deng M, Aldinger KA, et al.: Laser capture microdissection (LCM) of neonatal mouse forebrain for RNA isolation, *Bio Protoc* 10, 2020.

Rusdi NK: PJA: cancer immunotherapy and flow cytometry in immunotherapy monitoring, *Biomed Pharmacol J* 12, 2019.

Russell B: *Electron biology principles and techniques for biologists sudbury*, MA, 1999, Jones and Bartlett Learning.

Ruzgar O, Bilge AK, Bugra Z, et al.: The use of human heart-type fatty acid-binding protein as an early diagnostic biochemical marker of myocardial necrosis in patients with acute coronary syndrome, and its comparison with troponin-T and creatine kinase-myocardial band, *Heart Vessels* 21:309–314, 2006.

Samson M, Peale Jr FV, Frantz G, et al.: Human endocrine gland-derived vascular endothelial growth factor: expression early in development and in Leydig cell tumors suggests roles in normal and pathological testis angiogenesis, *J Clin Endocrinol Metab* 89:4078–4088, 2004.

Sanders EJ: Methods for detecting apoptotic cells in tissues, *Histol Histopathol* 12:1169–1177, 1997.

Sanders EJ, Wride MA: Ultrastructural identification of apoptotic nuclei using the TUNEL technique, *Histochem J* 28:275–281, 1996.

Schett G, Sticherling M, Neurath MF: COVID-19: risk for cytokine targeting in chronic inflammatory diseases? *Nat Rev Immunol* 20:271–272, 2020.

Schiebler ZLRGT: *Enzyme histochemistry: a laboratory manual Berlin Heidelberg*, 1979, Springer-Verlag.

Schlossman SF: *Leucocyte typing V: white cell differentiation antigens*, 1995, Oxford University Press.

Schomberg DW, Couse JF, Mukherjee A, et al.: Targeted disruption of the estrogen receptor-alpha gene in female mice: characterization of ovarian responses and phenotype in the adult, *Endocrinology* 140:2733–2744, 1999.

Scott CJ, Clarke IJ, Rao A, et al.: Sex differences in the distribution and abundance of androgen receptor mRNA-containing cells in the preoptic area and hypothalamus of the Ram and Ewe, *J Neuroendocrinol* 16:956–963, 2004.

Shapiro H: *Practical flow cytometry*, New York NY, 2003, Wiley-Liss, Inc.

Shi B, Keough E, Matter A, et al.: Biodistribution of small interfering RNA at the organ and cellular levels after lipid nanoparticle-mediated delivery, *J Histochem Cytochem* 59:727–740, 2011.

Shi SR, Cote RJ, Taylor CR: Antigen retrieval immunohistochemistry: past, present, and future, *J Histochem Cytochem* 45:327–343, 1997.

Shoda T, Onodera H, Takeda M, et al.: Liver tumor promoting effects of fenbendazole in rats, *Toxicol Pathol* 27:553–562, 1999.

Shughrue PJ, Ky B, Austin CP: Localization of B1 bradykinin receptor mRNA in the primate brain and spinal cord: an in situ hybridization study, *J Comp Neurol* 465:372–384, 2003.

Shyjan AW, de Sauvage FJ, Gillett NA, et al.: Molecular cloning of a retina-specific membrane guanylyl cyclase, *Neuron* 9:727–737, 1992.

Speel EJ, Hopman AH, Komminoth P: Amplification methods to increase the sensitivity of in situ hybridization: play card(s), *J Histochem Cytochem* 47:281–288, 1999.

Speel EJ, Hopman AH, Komminoth P: Tyramide signal amplification for DNA and mRNA in situ hybridization, *Methods Mol Biol* 326:33–60, 2006.

Speel EJ, Saremaslani P, Roth J, et al.: Improved mRNA in situ hybridization on formaldehyde-fixed and paraffin-embedded tissue using signal amplification with different haptenized tyramides, *Histochem Cell Biol* 110:571–577, 1998.

Sterman DH, Treat J, Litzky LA, et al.: Adenovirus-mediated herpes simplex virus thymidine kinase/ganciclovir gene therapy in patients with localized malignancy: results of a phase I clinical trial in malignant mesothelioma, *Hum Gene Ther* 9:1083–1092, 1998.

Sugimoto C, Hasegawa A, Saito Y, et al.: Differentiation kinetics of blood monocytes and dendritic cells in macaques: insights to understanding human myeloid cell development, *J Immunol* 195:1774–1781, 2015.

Sun S, Hao H, Yang G, et al.: Immunotherapy with CAR-modified T cells: toxicities and overcoming strategies, *J Immunol Res* 2018:2386187, 2018.

Tan WCC, Nerurkar SN, Cai HY, et al.: Overview of multiplex immunohistochemistry/immunofluorescence techniques in the era of cancer immunotherapy, *Cancer Commun (Lond)* 40:135–153, 2020.

Tavakoli M, Hossain P, Malik RA: Clinical applications of corneal confocal microscopy, *Clin Ophthalmol* 2:435–445, 2008.

Toyoda T, Akagi J, Cho YM, et al.: Detection of γ-H2AX, a biomarker for DNA double-strand breaks, in urinary bladders of N -butyl- N -(4-Hydroxybutyl)-Nitrosamine-Treated rats, *J Toxicol Pathol* 26:215–221, 2013.

Tuson JR, Pascoe EW, Jacob DA: A novel immunohistochemical technique for demonstration of specific binding of human monoclonal antibodies to human cryostat tissue sections, *J Histochem Cytochem* 38:923–926, 1990.

JTJeJBK V: Methodological considerations in the utilization of in situ hybridization. In Barchas KVJEJ, editor: *In situ hybridication: applications to neurobiology*, New York, 1987, Oxford University Press.

Veiga-Fernandes H, Kioussis D, Coles M: Natural killer receptors: the burden of a name, *J Exp Med* 207:269–272, 2010.

Verdier F, Descotes J: Preclinical safety evaluation of human gene therapy products, *Toxicol Sci* 47:9–15, 1999.

Verdugo-Gazdik ME, Simic D, Opsahl AC, et al.: Investigating cytoskeletal alterations as a potential marker of retinal and lens drug-related toxicity, *Assay Drug Dev Technol* 4:695–707, 2006.

Vinod Sargaiyan AB: Enzyme histochemistry: a review, *J Adv Med Dent Sci Res* 2:191–195, 2014.

Vugmeyster Y, Howell K, McKeever K, et al.: Differential in vivo effects of rituximab on two B-cell subsets in cynomolgus monkeys, *Int Immunopharmacol* 3:1477–1481, 2003.

Vulovic M, Divac N, Jakovcevski I: Confocal synaptology: synaptic rearrangements in neurodegenerative disorders and upon nervous system injury, *Front Neuroanat* 12:11, 2018.

Waid TH, Lucas BA, Amlot P, et al.: T10B9.1A-31 anti-T-cell monoclonal antibody: preclinical studies and clinical treatment of solid organ allograft rejection, *Am J Kidney Dis* 14:61–70, 1989.

Wang QS, Papanikolaou A, Sabourin CL, et al.: Altered expression of cyclin D1 and cyclin-dependent kinase 4 in azoxymethane-induced mouse colon tumorigenesis, *Carcinogenesis* 19:2001–2006, 1998.

Wang X, Lebrec H: Immunophenotyping: application to safety assessment, *Toxicol Pathol* 45:1004–1011, 2017.

Warren RS, Yuan H, Matli MR, et al.: Regulation by vascular endothelial growth factor of human colon cancer tumorigenesis in a mouse model of experimental liver metastasis, *J Clin Invest* 95:1789–1797, 1995.

Watanabe T, Kato A, Terashima H, et al.: The PFA-AMeX method achieves a good balance between the morphology of tissues and the quality of RNA content in DNA microarray analysis with laser-capture microdissection samples, *J Toxicol Pathol* 28:43–49, 2015.

Wei BR, Edwards JB, Hoover SB, et al.: Altered {beta}-catenin accumulation in hepatocellular carcinomas of diethylnitrosamine-exposed rhesus macaques, *Toxicol Pathol* 36:972–980, 2008.

Whiteley LO, Hudson Jr L, Pretlow TP: Aberrant crypt foci in the colonic mucosa of rats treated with a genotoxic and nongenotoxic colon carcinogen, *Toxicol Pathol* 24:681–689, 1996.

Wood B, Jevremovic D, Béné MC, et al.: Validation of cell-based fluorescence assays: practice guidelines from the ICSH and ICCS - part V - assay performance criteria, *Cytometry B Clin Cytom* 84:315–323, 2013.

Woolveridge I, de Boer-Brouwer M, Taylor MF, et al.: Apoptosis in the rat spermatogenic epithelium following androgen withdrawal: changes in apoptosis-related genes, *Biol Reprod* 60:461–470, 1999.

Wright SJ, Wright DJ: Introduction to confocal microscopy, *Methods Cell Biol* 70:1–85, 2002.

Wu A, Liu Y: Apoptotic cell death in rat brain following deltamethrin treatment, *Neurosci Lett* 279:85–88, 2000.

Xi Yang LKS, Shi Q, Salminen WF: Hepatic toxicity biomarkers. In Gupta R, editor: *Biomarkers in toxicology*, 2014, Academic Press, pp 241–259.

Xiao W, Berta SC, Lu MM, et al.: Adeno-associated virus as a vector for liver-directed gene therapy, *J Virol* 72:10222–10226, 1998.

Yafune A, Taniai E, Morita R, et al.: Aberrant activation of M phase proteins by cell proliferation-evoking carcinogens after 28-day administration in rats, *Toxicol Lett* 219:203–210, 2013.

Yamashina M, Takami T, Kanemura T, et al.: Immunohistochemical demonstration of complement components in formalin-fixed and paraffin-embedded renal tissues, *Lab Invest* 60:311–316, 1989.

Yamazaki M, Yabuki N, Suzuki Y, et al.: PAXgene-fixed paraffin-embedded sample is applicable to laser capture microdissection with well-balanced RNA quality and tissue morphology, *J Toxicol Pathol* 31:213–220, 2018.

Yoshida T, Makita Y, Tsutsumi T, et al.: Immunohistochemical localization of microcystin-LR in the liver of mice: a study on the pathogenesis of microcystin-LR-induced hepatotoxicity, *Toxicol Pathol* 26:411–418, 1998.

Zhang GX, Xiao BG, Bai XF, et al.: Mice with IFN-gamma receptor deficiency are less susceptible to experimental autoimmune myasthenia gravis, *J Immunol* 162:3775–3781, 1999.

Digital Pathology and Tissue Image Analysis

Famke Aeffner[1], Thomas Forest[2], Vanessa Schumacher[3], Mark Zarella[4],
Alys Bradley[5]

[1]Amgen Inc., Amgen Research, Translational Safety and Bioanalytical Sciences, South San Francisco, CA, United States,
[2]Merck & Co, Inc., West Point, PA, United States, [3]Roche Pharma Research and Early Development, Roche Innovation
Center Basel, F. Hoffmann-La Roche Ltd., Basel, Switzerland, [4]Johns Hopkins University, Department of Pathology,
Baltimore, MD, United States, [5]Charles River Laboratories Edinburgh Ltd., Tranent, Scotland, United Kingdom

OUTLINE

1. Introduction   395

2. Whole-Slide Imaging   396
    2.1. Scanning Modalities   396
    2.2. Scanning in Focus   397
    2.3. Scanning Capacity and Time   398
    2.4. Scanning Magnification   398
    2.5. Scanning Resolution   399
    2.6. Color Preservation   399
    2.7. Image Compression   400
    2.8. Pyramid Representation   401
    2.9. Digital Workflow   401

3. Tissue Image Analysis   406
    3.1. Visual and Cognitive Biases of Manual Slide
       Review   407
    3.2. Application Areas   407
    3.3. Impact of Preanalytical Variables on Image
       Analysis   409
    3.4. Manual versus Automated Image Annotations   409

3.5. The Basics of Quantitative Image Analysis   410
3.6. Nonquantitative Image Analysis   412
3.7. Available Tools   412
3.8. The Pathologist's Role in the Image Analysis
      Workflow   413
3.9. Computational Pathology   414
3.10. Introduction to Artificial Intelligence and
       Machine Learning in Tissue Image Analysis   414

4. Regulatory Considerations for Digital Pathology
   Evaluation   416

5. Related Topics   418
    5.1. Stereology   418
    5.2. 3D Reconstruction   419
    5.3. Other Imaging Modalities   419

6. Conclusion   419

References   420

1. INTRODUCTION

The age of digitalization has arrived in light microscopy. While the current practice of toxicologic pathology remains largely based on the light microscopic evaluation of stained tissue sections, it is no longer limited to it. Thanks to the availability of whole-slide imaging (WSI), histopathologic evaluation can now be accomplished via a computer screen (Farahani et al., 2015; Hamilton et al., 2014; Higgins, 2015). Substituting a computer monitor for a traditional microscope may seem at first to be a minor change. However, the digitization of glass slides

Haschek and Rousseaux's Handbook of Toxicologic Pathology, Fourth Edition.
https://doi.org/10.1016/B978-0-12-821044-4.00010-8

has opened up a host of options to interrogate tissue sections that were previously not possible. These new options include geographically remote viewing of slides for more convenient and expedient pathology peer review, simplification in obtaining rapid and even real-time consultations with specific subject matter experts, formation of pathology working groups with global membership, building electronic workflows that link whole-slide images to associated metadata stored in laboratory information management systems, integration of other relevant data (e.g., in vivo observations and macroscopic findings) directly to tissue sections, enhancing teaching and training capabilities, and applying image analysis algorithms to whole-slide images to extract quantitative data (Aeffner et al., 2018; Bertram and Klopfleisch, 2017; Malarkey et al., 2015). These assessments may include features previously not accessible or quantifiable. While WSI has been commercially available for over 20 years and is being rapidly adopted by the global pathology community, regulatory guidance on the use of digital pathology and related topics in toxicologic pathology is still evolving and currently incomplete.

This chapter introduces digital pathology, including basic principles and useful practices for WSI and tissue image analysis (Abels et al., 2019; Aeffner et al., 2018, 2019; Zarella et al., 2019), and explores potential future use in experimental and nonclinical toxicology. Additional related topics such as stereology and alternative imaging modalities are briefly introduced. General principles for consideration in use of WSI in regulated studies are included. A reference list provides helpful resources for suggested reading for those who wish to seek additional information on this rapidly growing discipline.

2. WHOLE-SLIDE IMAGING

WSI, first developed by Wetzel and Gilbertson in 1999, consists of the digitization of glass slides in their entirety (Ghaznavi et al., 2013). Slide scanners, much like conventional bright-field microscopes, usually consist of four main components: a light source, a slide stage or tray, objective lenses, and a high-resolution sensor for digital image capture (Bueno et al., 2014; Farahani et al., 2015; Pantanowitz et al., 2013). Scanning of cytology slides and other specimens (e.g., plant material) is possible (Farris et al., 2017; Wilbur, 2016). Similarly, microscope-mounted digital cameras enable some aspects of digital pathology in photomicrographs for a portion of a tissue section. However, this chapter is focused on the use of stand-alone whole-slide scanners for evaluating traditional histology sections of tissue mounted under coverslips.

2.1. Scanning Modalities

Whole-slide images can be created using bright-field (including polarized light), fluorescent, and multispectral imaging, and the scanner type should be paired with the appropriate slide staining technique (Aeffner et al., 2018; Farahani et al., 2015; Zarella et al., 2019). Commercially available scanners that accommodate several modalities are available. However, instruments with increased scanning modalities often trade-off increased imaging capability for other potentially desirable functionality such as a higher scanning speed and/or larger number of slides that can be loaded and scanned in a single batch. Therefore, it is important to consider the typical ranges of study types to be evaluated and the potential workflow in the laboratory when selecting a scanner.

Bright-field whole-slide scanning is similar to standard bright-field microscopy and represents the most common and cost-effective WSI approach. While most scanners are capable of creating bright-field images, some models are optimized for high scan throughput (by allowing for large batch sizes of thousands of slides or continuous slide feeding) and have enhanced features that enable minimal oversight of the instrument by laboratory personnel during the scan run. These enhanced features include automated tissue recognition and focusing, prioritization of specific slides in the batch, and skipping of slides that fail quality control (QC) without interrupting the overall scanning process. Such aspects permit round-the-clock scanning, which makes WSI cost effective in high-throughput workflows. Similarly, fluorescent whole-slide scanning emulates fluorescent microscopy and is used to digitize fluorescently labeled slides (i.e., fluorescent immunohistochemistry [IHC], fluorescent in situ hybridization [ISH]). Multispectral imaging captures information in separate spectral channels across the spectrum of light and can be used in both bright-field and fluorescent scanning (Feng et al., 2015; Ghaznavi et al., 2013; Indu et al., 2016; Mansfield, 2014). This form of imaging is particularly well suited in fluorescent applications to overcome issues due to tissue autofluorescence because the spectrum of each individual marker is separated (unmixed) (Ghaznavi et al., 2013; Indu et al., 2016). It also provides an opportunity to use bright-field multiplexing IHC, especially when there is colocalization of two or more IHC biomarkers. Fluorescent or multispectral scanners typically require more user interaction and provide low-throughput scanning, and therefore are more suited to laboratory workflows focused on in-depth characterization of a smaller number of specimens as is done in a special techniques laboratory or to support discovery research.

The two most common approaches for creating whole-slide scans are image capture by tile or by line scanning (Figure 12.1) (Aeffner et al., 2018).

After capture, the tiles or lines are digitally stitched together by software algorithms to create the virtual image of the entire scanned slide (Hamilton et al., 2014; Indu et al., 2016).

2.2. Scanning in Focus

Scanners apply focus to slides along the so-called z-axis, which is the tissue expanse (i.e., thickness) perpendicular to the x–y plane in which the tissue section and coverslip are arranged. Slides may contain tissue with slightly varying thickness or uneven cover-slipping, making it more challenging for the scanner to capture the entire section in focus in a single plane of the z-axis. Whole-slide scanners employ a variety of approaches to maintain focus across the slide, from focusing on every tile, focusing on a subset of tiles, or to distribute multiple focus points across the slide independent of tile positions (Figure 12.1) (Aeffner et al., 2018; Zarella, Bowman, & Aeffner, 2019). Increasing the number of focus points and strategically positioning them across the slide typically decreases the number of tiles with "out-of-focus" regions, but also increases scanning time due to repeated automatic focus adjustments. In an attempt to balance image quality with slide throughput, some scanners allow for the operator to specify

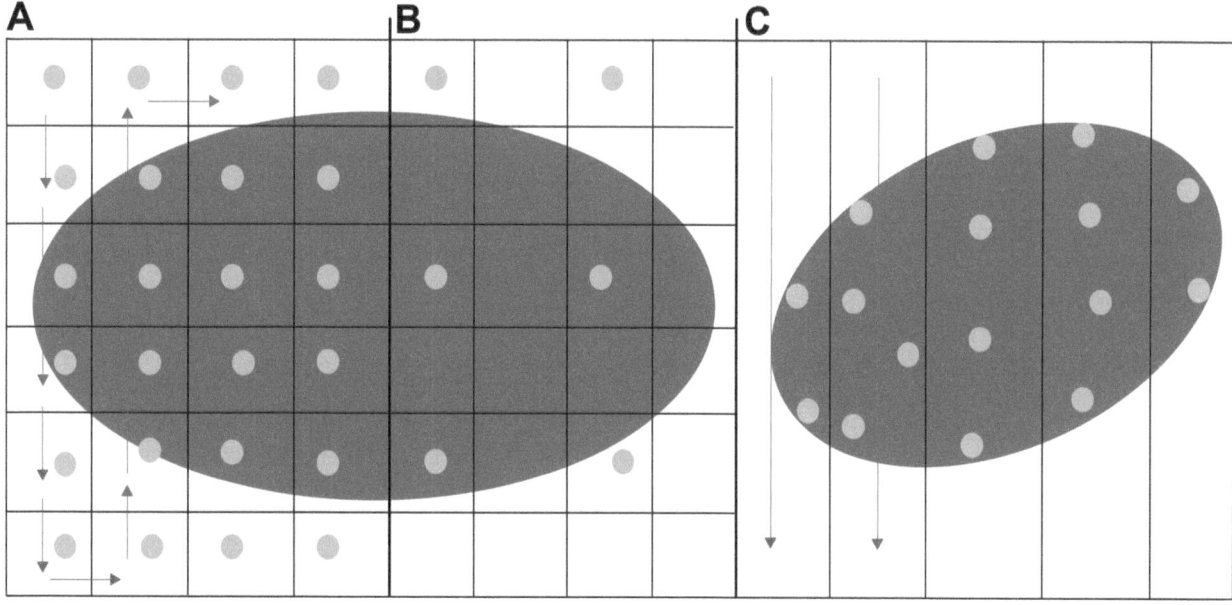

FIGURE 12.1 Scanning patterns. (A) Tile scanning of every tile. The *arrows* indicate direction of scanning. *Dots* within a tile indicate a focus point. (B) Tile scanning of every nth field. (C) Line scanning pattern. *Dots* indicate focus points of a focus map. *Figure reproduced from Aeffner F, Adissu HA, Boyle MC, et al.: Digital microscopy, image analysis, and virtual slide repository,* ILAR J: 59(1):66–79, 2018, with permission.

the number of focus points. Line scanning instruments typically approach focusing by use of focus maps (a method also used in some tile scanners). Focus maps are generated by placing a network of focus points (automatically or manually generated) across the tissue section, which often results in faster scan times. Similar to tile scanning, the trade-off consists of having a higher potential error rate (i.e., out-of-focus areas) (Indu et al., 2016; Montalto et al., 2011). Most recently, scanning technology has been developed that incorporates continuous automatic refocusing (Al-Janabi et al., 2012; Higgins, 2015).

2.3. Scanning Capacity and Time

Slide capacity is an important consideration when selecting a whole-slide scanner. Different models vary from holding just a single slide to automatically loading slide after slide from a preloaded unit holding up to thousands of slides arranged in one or more trays (Farahani et al., 2015; Indu et al., 2016; Zarella et al., 2019). Technological advances have reduced the cost of low-capacity (4- to 8-slide) instruments to a few thousand dollars. Some scanners can accommodate bigger specimens, such as whole tissue mounts and nonstandard glass slides holding large organ sections (e.g., bone, brain, eye) from nonrodents (Farahani et al., 2015).

Scan time is another key element that impacts the choice of slide scanner. As discussed above, the mechanical capabilities of scanners are critical determinants of the amount of time and effort required to create a whole-slide image. Scan time is also affected by the desired magnification, where the amount of time required for a scan increases with the desired magnification, size of the tissue section, number of imaging modalities used, and the number of planes collected along the z-axis (Bertram and Klopfleisch, 2017; Higgins, 2015). In addition, data transmission rates from the sensor to the image file being generated also can impact overall scanning speed.

2.4. Scanning Magnification

Scanners are typically capable of creating scans at various magnifications specified by the user, and the specific magnification choices may be workflow dependent. Most scanners are limited to one or two objective magnifications (20× and 40×), but some instruments include a wider range of objectives (1.25× or 2.5×, 5×, 10×, 20×, 40×, 63× [dry or oil], or 100× [oil]). Additionally, some scanners can perform both dry objective and oil immersion scanning. While pathologists often find 20× scans sufficient for routine hematoxylin and eosin (H&E) and IHC tissue section review in a research setting, many institutions with established fully digital workflows and appropriate information technology (IT) infrastructure are routinely scanning at 40×. Common reasoning for this routine use of 40× is that a 40× objective is the highest one usually available on a traditional light microscope used to screen tissue sections in anatomic toxicologic pathology, and therefore whole-slide images created using 40× have approximately equivalent resolution to the maximum resolution typically available by traditional microscopy. In addition, standard 40× scanning avoids the workflow disruptions that would result when rescanning selected slides at 40×. The trade-off for establishing this equivalence is that 40× whole-slide images may take approximately 4 times longer to scan than 20× images, and the resulting files are proportionally larger (Bertram and Klopfleisch, 2017; Cornish et al., 2012; Hamilton et al., 2014). For slides from Good Laboratory Practice (GLP)–compliant studies, regulatory guidance will need to be considered for the minimum scanning magnification when seeking to use whole-slide images to perform primary histopathologic evaluation or pathology peer reviews (FDA, 2016).

Higher scanning magnifications are required for certain applications. Digitization of ISH should always be performed with at least 40× magnification to resolve individual ISH dots that may be less than about 0.5 μm apart (Laurent et al., 2013). Even then, some dots will remain slightly out of focus. Specialized scanners that can accommodate higher magnifications are now available (60×/63× or 100×, under oil) and are used regularly for WSI of blood smears and other cytological preparations (Bertram and Klopfleisch, 2017; Bueno et al., 2014; Higgins, 2015).

2.5. Scanning Resolution

Resolution determines the minimum distance at which two distinct objects can be identified as separate objects. For a purely optical system, such as a light microscope, the resolution is determined by the numerical aperture of the objective. In a slide scanner, which combines optical and digital components, resolution is determined both by the numerical aperture of the objective and the number of pixels per unit area of the camera sensor (termed "pixel density") (Sellaro et al., 2013). If this sensor density creates a lower resolution than the objective's numerical aperture, not all information from the optical projection is gathered.

Vendors usually express the resolution of their scanners in units of μm per pixel. Color depth is expressed as the number of bits per pixel allocated to a channel, which in turn specifies the total number of distinct colors possible in the image. Typically, a 40× bright-field whole-slide scan has a resolution of about 0.25 μm per pixel and 24-bit color depth. This means that a 1 mm^2 area of a scanned section is equivalent to 384 million bits of information.

Lastly, the resolution of the monitor used to view the image can impact the effective resolution of the digital system. In addition, because in a digital pathology system the light path is not projected directly onto the observer's retina, perceived resolution of the viewed image is also limited by the observer's visual acuity, ambient light conditions, and distance from the monitor.

2.6. Color Preservation

One of the challenges of digital pathology is the preservation of color along the workflow (Clarke and Treanor, 2017). The color captured during scanning may not match the original slide, and the colors displayed on a monitor may not accurately reflect the colors captured during scanning.

Aside from general color variability introduced by preanalytical variables (e.g., fixation and histologic processing), the act of scanning itself may introduce color variation. Two different scanners may be used to digitize the same slide, but the precise colors rendered by each scanner are likely to be slightly different, especially if they have not been calibrated in the same manner. Similarly, displaying a single scanned image via different viewing software may result in visible color differences. The impact of monitors on variability in color displays is discussed in depth later in this chapter.

To control for color variability, it is recommended that a test slide should be scanned with each scanned batch of slides, or at least daily. The test slide should have multiple tissues (e.g., a tissue microarray [TMA] slide of the major organs) with different structures having a range of affinities for the dyes applied in staining to demonstrate the full array of expected colors in a routine study. Color variations can then be compared to the test slide. If the same test slide is run with the scan batches, any color artifacts should be obvious to the reader.

To mitigate the impact of color variability after the slide has been scanned, various color normalization algorithms can be applied to the whole-slide image (Zarella et al., 2017). These transform the colors of a series of images to align to a single standard or reference slide. While many of the tools have demonstrated a reduction in color variability among images by a significant margin, it is important to detect and assess any distortions in the image that may potentially be introduced during the color normalization process, such as incorrect color representation. Notably, regulatory guidance regarding color normalization tools is lacking, and therefore, it is not clear if these means are suited for usage in a regulated environment.

Color preservation can be achieved by color calibrating the entire digital workflow. For example, the International Color Consortium (ICC) has released an open, vendor-neutral color management protocol (with the most recent version available on the ICC website; www.color.org). Briefly, this protocol involves scanning a reference slide that contains known color attributes and then comparing those attributes to the color values produced by the scanner. Similarly, the colors displayed on a monitor can be compared to known color attributes of the reference slide as initially scanned (Shrestha and Hulsken, 2014; Yagi, 2011). In addition, tools are commercially available to perform color calibration of computer monitors. The landscape for color calibration is rapidly evolving.

Color preservation is a demanding aim, which is further complicated by the fact that there is variability in staining within a single laboratory, and among different laboratories (Chlipala et al., 2021). Especially when scans are intended for image analysis, setting thresholds for certain stain colors may be an important part of the pre-analytical work, and the quality of the final data can be greatly influenced by staining and color consistency. Likewise, manual review of whole-slide scans can be hampered by suboptimal color preservation along the digitization and display process.

2.7. Image Compression

Since WSI creates large file sizes, usually in proprietary formats, image compression is commonly used to facilitate file transfer and storage (Aeffner et al., 2018; Webster and Dunstan, 2014; Zarella et al., 2019). Many commercially available scanners compress images in JPEG (Joint Photographic Expert Group), JPEG 2000, or LZW (Lempel–Ziv–Welch) codecs (i.e., where a codec is a device or program that compresses data to enable faster transmission and decompresses received data), which can reduce file size. While smaller files save resources, such "lossy" compression algorithms (e.g., JPEG) should be used with caution as the loss of information that accompanies the compression is unrecoverable. For this reason, compressed files may not be suitable for pathology peer review purposes. Some scanners allow the user to determine the level of compression (on a quality factor scale of 0 to 1). The selection of this value balances image quality and file size. It is important to avoid application of successive rounds of JPEG compression to the same image file, as each round will result in further reduction of image quality, potentially introducing visible image artifacts such as an excessively grainy appearance, blockiness (particularly in homogeneous patches such as white space), and color distortions (Figure 12.2). The standard JPEG and JPEG2000 standards are compatible with Digital Imaging and Communications in Medicine (DICOM) standards for image storage (Tuominen and Isola, 2010).

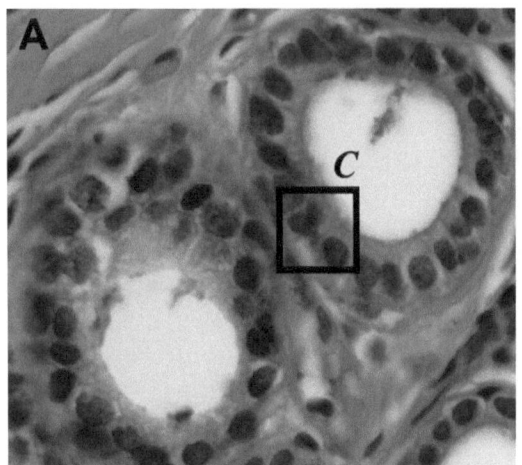
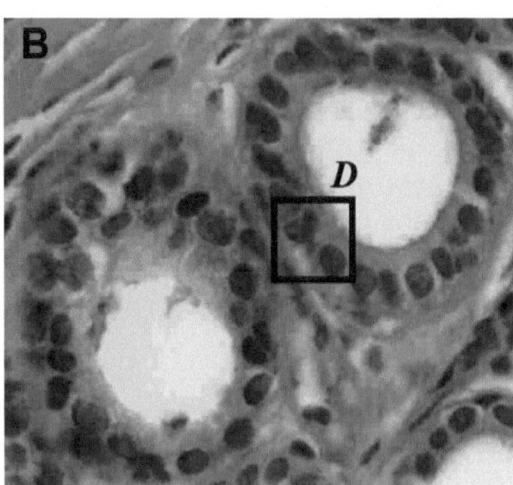
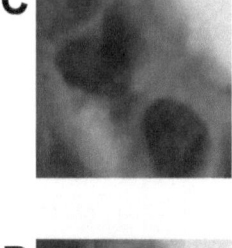
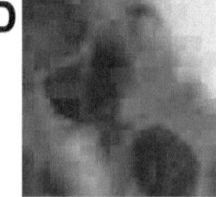

FIGURE 12.2   Image quality following JPEG compression. (A) Sample hematoxylin and eosin (H&E) image was compressed using a JPEG quality factor of 0.8, resulting in a reduction in file size by a factor of 15.9 (compared with the uncompressed image). (B) The sample was compressed using a JPEG quality factor of 0.1, with a compression ratio of 108.3, resulting in visible artifacts such as blurring and pixilation. (C and D) Magnified views of the fields of view indicated in (A and B), respectively, reveal substantial visible artifacts following compression (original magnification 20× [A through D]). *Figure reproduced from Zarella MD, Bowman D, Aeffner F, et al.: A practical guide to whole slide imaging: a white paper from the Digital Pathology Association,* Arch Pathol Lab Med *143:222–234, 2019, with permission.*

It has been shown that modest image compression in the range of 1:7 has no appreciable effect on the ability of skilled observers to perform qualitative and semiquantitative assessments of tissue sections and cells (Hamilton et al., 2014; Krupinski et al., 2012). However, fully quantitative assessments such as tissue image analysis and densitometric assessments may be sensitive to a loss of information caused even by visually imperceptible image compression (Hamilton et al., 2014; Krupinski et al., 2012). In addition to image compression, whole-slide scanners often reduce file sizes by excluding scanned regions of the slide that do not contain tissue.

2.8. Pyramid Representation

Although a variety of methods exist to reduce the file size, as described above, a single whole-slide scan file commonly exceeds the working capacity of the RAM (random access memory) in a typical office computer. Therefore, the whole-slide image in its entirety cannot be displayed at maximum resolution on commercially available monitors. The limitations of typically available computational power can therefore be managed by creating whole-slide images as "image pyramids" consisting of a base layer collected at high magnification, such as 40×, and multiple "down-sampled" layers stored, for example, at 10×, 2.5×, 1.25×, etc (Figure 12.3). The image pyramid approach makes use of available resources by displaying the down-sampled layer when the observer is viewing the image at low magnification and displaying a smaller field of view at high resolution when the observer wishes to view a portion of the specimen at high magnification. The more layers in the pyramid, the larger the file's size, but the more efficient the bandwidth usage during viewing. Some systems allow for the user to determine the number of image levels within the pyramid. Typically, there are three to four levels, balancing bandwidth requirements with overall file size.

Other information ("metadata") related to the image typically are embedded into the overall file. Examples of common metadata include image properties, scanner acquisition details, organization of the file, color profiles, subject-

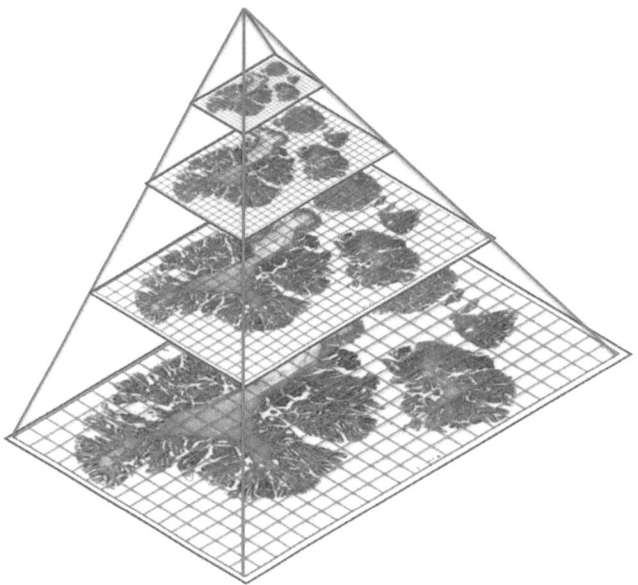

FIGURE 12.3 Digital slide images are represented as a tiled pyramidal structure to allow "on-demand" viewing of images online by serving image tiles at specific locations and at different resolutions. *Figure reproduced from Hamilton PW, Bankhead P, Wang Y, et al.: Digital pathology and image analysis in tissue biomarker research, Methods 70:59–73, 2014, with permission.*

specific data, an image of the slide label, and a low-resolution snapshot of the entire slide. These data typically add a small fraction to the overall file size.

2.9. Digital Workflow

When transforming a traditional histology laboratory to a digital workflow, it is crucial to understand that not only are appropriately trained staff and novel equipment needed but that also the overall workflow is extended by new steps for slide digitization and corresponding QC (Griffin and Treanor, 2017). Despite these additional steps, creating a fully digital pathology workflow ultimately can increase the efficiency and throughput of the laboratory (Hanna et al., 2019). In general, there may be a need for increased laboratory space and machinery, expanded staff expertise, new QC steps, software maintenance and IT infrastructure, and ergonomic end-user workstations.

The Impact of Preanalytical Variables on Whole-Slide Imaging

Every step along the workflow from initial tissue collection to final cover-slipping has an impact on the quality of the slide produced. With that, so-called "preanalytical variables" also greatly affect the overall quality of the whole-slide scan and the data that are generated from it (Aeffner et al., 2016; Shakeri et al., 2015; Webster and Dunstan, 2014). Examples of important preanalytical variables are as obvious as effects of improper physical handling of unfixed tissue in generating disrupted cellular morphology (e.g., crush artifacts), and as subtle as the influence of water bath temperature on the expansion or shrinkage of individual thin tissue sections. Pathologists are uniquely qualified to evaluate the impact of these preanalytical variables due to their knowledge of all aspects of this process.

Once tissues are processed, artifacts can be introduced during sectioning, including variability in section thickness, differences in tissue expansion, or shrinkage introduced during flotation on the water bath or slide backing. Histological artifacts such as tissue folds may not be preanalytical variables per se but can nevertheless significantly impact the data generated from affected slides. Rare folds can be manually or automatically excluded from analysis, but excessive tissue folding may require generating a new section/slide.

Differences in sample staining may be caused by variability in tissue sampling, handling, fixation timing, and processing, as these may vary study to study, laboratory to laboratory, and even tissue to tissue. Such differences may be visible for routine histological stains, such as H&E (Figure 12.4), and for common IHC applications (Aeffner et al., 2019; Chlipala et al., 2019, 2021). Digital analysis of scanned images may be used for evaluating staining reproducibility, which, for example, may facilitate development and validation of medical diagnostic kits based on cytological or histopathological evaluation.

As a general concept, the impact of some of the preanalytical variables can be minimized by standardizing laboratory workflows and tracking relevant aspects of tissue processing such as the staining protocol; time of staining (e.g., during the day or overnight, as room

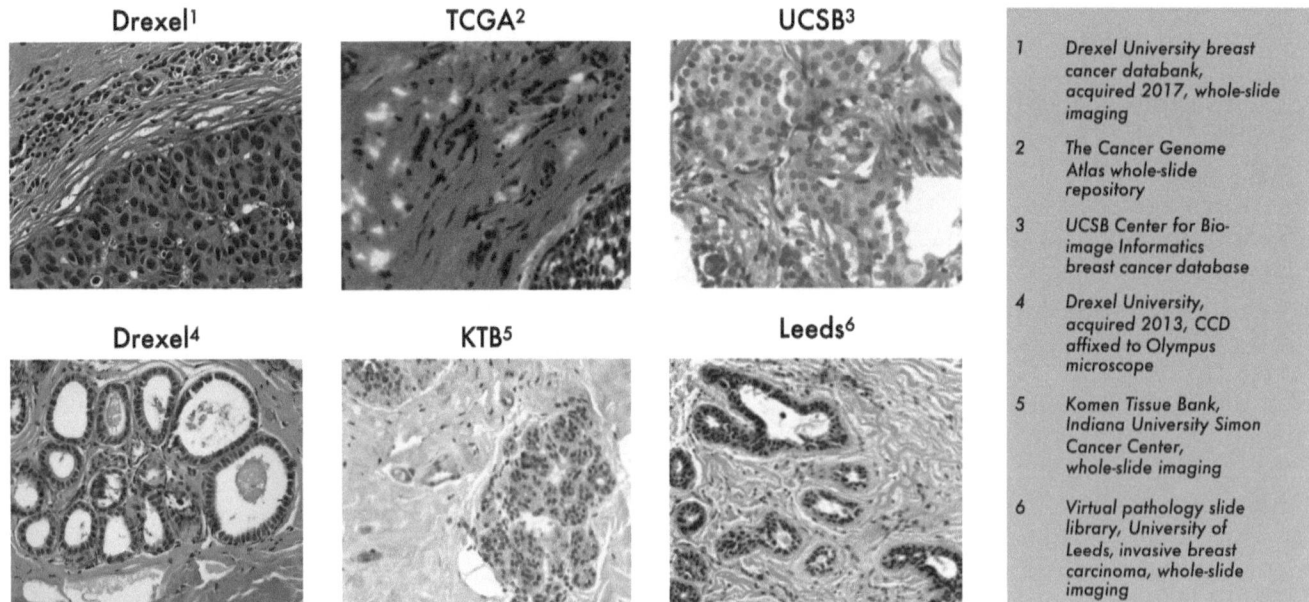

FIGURE 12.4 Sample hematoxylin and eosin (H&E) images obtained from six sources designated on the right depict different color attributes commonly encountered when viewing digital images of slides across laboratories or across imaging modalities. *Figure reproduced from Aeffner F, Zarella MD, Buchbinder N, et al.: Introduction to digital image analysis in whole-slide imaging: a white paper from the Digital Pathology Association,* J Pathol Inform *10:9, 2019, with permission.*

temperature and length of holding cycles affect the chemical reactions during staining); reagent batch/lot numbers (especially for antibodies); and the specific stainer used. Similarly, the use of automated staining platforms, and the uniform use of appropriate on-run (concurrent) assay controls can play an important role in creating consistent staining results (Aeffner et al., 2016; Dunstan et al., 2011). Lastly, proper staining protocol optimization and stain QC are important aspects of minimizing the impact of preanalytical variables on the quality of data obtained from analyzing whole-slide images.

Slide Viewing

Image viewing software may be installed on a local computer to view whole-slide images. Alternatively, some vendors support web-based viewing tools. Digital slides are typically viewed by navigating across the image in a 2-dimensional (2D) fashion in the x/y plane, using peripheral input devices (e.g., computer mouse, joystick, trackball). When multiple x/y planes are collected from the specimen and assembled into a stack in the z-plane, additional navigation is possible along the z-axis to adjust the fine focus (Bertram and Klopfleisch, 2017; Higgins, 2015).

Currently, most commercial slide scanners create images in proprietary scan file formats compatible with their accompanying viewing software. With the growing number of choices, many scanners may also be compatible now with third-party software. Open source libraries and viewers exist that can display a number of different file formats proprietary to different whole-slide scanners (e.g., the OpenSlide library [https://openslide.org/], Bio-Formats toolbox [https://www.openmicroscopy.org/bio-formats/]) (Goode et al., 2013; Moore et al., 2015).

While there has been a long-standing call to harmonize file formats, only recently have the first vendors adopted a DICOM-compatible file format, which allows for harmonization and standardization across WSI platforms. DICOM was previously established and successfully implemented worldwide in digital radiology (Kayser et al., 2008). Now efforts are ongoing to expand and widely adopt a similar standard in digital pathology, in part driven by the effort to seek regulatory acceptance for pathology data generated from digital scans of slides from nonclinical safety studies.

Slide Scan Storage, Retrieval, Databases, and Metadata

Storage of histology slides requires a significant amount of space. Such archives need to be constructed in a way that supports the enormous weight of accumulated glass slides. Furthermore, manual filing and retrieval of slides is time consuming, and both initial filing and refiling are error prone. Storage of glass slides is also finite as many sponsors opt to destroy the archived slides and blocks from non-GLP studies after a defined period. In contrast, whole-slide images do not take up physical space and are easily and rapidly accessed on demand through digital storage systems. Nevertheless, using current technology, physical slides must still be produced, and for some uses, physical slides must be retained per current regulatory guidance, resulting in the need to store both glass slides and whole-slide image files for extended periods.

Adequate and functional digital storage in a secure and searchable system is critical for creating a meaningful digital database. To enable this accessibility, a minimum of adequate specimen-specific metadata need to be retained in a standardized fashion. Establishing such digital storage databases should be accompanied by designing strategies to back up data and protect the database in worst-case scenarios (e.g., server failure).

The advantages and opportunities of accessing whole-slide images in searchable databases or repositories are manifold. In general, searching a digital database is less time consuming than retrieving physical slides. Compared to glass slides, digitized whole-slide images are stable in quality indefinitely in contrast to fading, breaking, or loss of cover slips, as is often encountered with glass slides. Remote access to digitized slides stored within such a database can be established, enabling extensive real-time collaborations beyond the physical location of the glass slide. This avoids the need for shipping glass slides, which can be time consuming, costly, and subject to potential damage and/or loss of materials. Specifically, in the context of non-human primate tissues, utilization of digital slides avoids the need for seeking CITES (Convention on International Trade in Endangered Species of Wild Fauna and Flora) permits for international shipping of physical slides. The CITES permit approval timeline is unpredictable and often can be lengthy.

The storage strategy for whole-slide images should be chosen based on their intended use. For scenarios where there are limited numbers of users, in the same physical location, and in the absence of a need to retain whole-slide images for the long term, local storage on a single computer or server may be sufficient. However, proper retention and archiving are usually an important part of the overall digital workflow, and various options for computer hardware, software, and data backup should be evaluated to create a fit-for-purpose solution for a given laboratory. These may include off-site storage, RAID (Redundant Array of Independent Disks) storage or equivalent, optical/tape, or some combination thereof. More commonly, access is granted to multiple users, working from different computers and potentially in different locations (at a single work site or geographically distant sites). In this case, network-based access and storage solutions are needed. One major decision involves choosing between cloud-based or on-premises network access and storage. Either option needs to be evaluated in the context of the organization's information systems policies, the source of the slide scans, and the speed of data streaming supported by internal and external network connections. Combination solutions that blend both local and cloud-based storage and access, or so-called "hub-and-spoke" models for multisite organizations, can be effective approaches. Finalization of an effective strategy that fits the organization's needs requires the input of various stakeholders, including IT, compliance, and informatics teams. Special considerations need to be given to storage, archival procedures, and data security within the regulatory environment. (For more information, see the "Regulatory Considerations for Digital Pathology Evaluation" section below.)

WSI also offers an opportunity to integrate scanned slides into a database system that expands the amount of information immediately accessible to the viewer. For example, a scanned slide can be linked to the other data generated from the same study subject (including in vivo, ex vivo, and postmortem data) or can be viewable alongside images of other slides that may have been acquired from the same subject (e.g., recuts, serial sections, other tissues, other stains, necropsy photos, other imaging modalities). Some image viewers that support simultaneous viewing of multiple images side by side enable users to easily navigate several slides in parallel to maintain the same field of view or allow for overlay of different serial sections. Similarly, some image viewers permit simultaneous inspection of images of the same organ from multiple animals, and a few will sequentially load scans of the same organ from multiple animals in random order to permit a "blinded" evaluation. Lastly, individual slides or entire studies can be linked to other relevant documents, such as a study protocol or final report, to facilitate a quick access to all materials pertaining to a given study (Higgins, 2015; Huisman et al., 2010; Wienert et al., 2009).

In addition, image management systems also include the ability to regulate overall database access (e.g., requiring unique usernames and passwords) and restrict the access of individual users to specific slides or studies. Some systems can facilitate audit trails. The choice and structure of a digital slide repository and how it is managed are crucial parts of establishing an effective digital pathology workflow. This includes maintaining backups of previous software versions to ensure that whole-slide images and data can be accessed years after their creation. The transition to more universal formats for whole-slide images over time should prevent image files from becoming obsolete.

The Role of the Pathologist in a Digital Workflow

Pathologist input should be central to all major steps along the digital pathology workflow (Aeffner et al., 2016). This input should begin with the study design and should continue through sample quality assessment, tissue staining approval, setting scan quality and analysis parameters, designing data capture protocols, and final data interpretation and reporting. While some QC checks can and should be delegated to qualified personnel, the QC process itself should be overseen by a pathologist (Aeffner et al., 2016).

In general, a pathologist must decide whether the tissue sections are of required quality and confirm that the target tissue is present in sufficient quantity for slides to be included in any evaluation. This review may happen prior to digitization (to reduce scan load), or after (e.g., when the protocol requires that all slides of a study need to be digitized, independent of quality). Such decisions often are made on a case-by-case basis depending on the size of the project, the laboratory's general workflow, standard operating procedures (SOPs), and relevant regulatory guidance.

For IHC and ISH, a sufficiently optimized staining protocol not only demonstrates the presence or absence of a biomarker but also provides the opportunity to answer more detailed questions. Common objectives include localizing the presence of the biomarker in subcompartments of cells, determining biomarker expression levels, and evaluating colocalization with other markers of interest. It is especially important that IHC-/ISH-stained specimens are checked by a pathologist to confirm that the staining occurs in the correct tissue and cellular compartment(s). In addition, for experiments involving assessment of staining intensity, it is vital to verify that staining intensity occurs within the appropriate dynamic range of the detector being used. Chromogenic IHC has a lower and nonlinear dynamic range compared to fluorescence IHC (Watanabe et al., 1996), which can make quantification of staining intensity challenging for chromogenic methods (Kim et al., 2016; Taylor and research, 2015). Detailed considerations on optimizing IHC or ISH assays are beyond the scope of this chapter. Please see sections on IHC and ISH in *Special Techniques in Toxicologic Pathology*, Vol 1, Chap 11 for more information.

Considerations for Designing a Pathologist's Digital Pathology Workstation

Currently, a pathologist's workstation likely includes a microscope, a computer with standard peripherals (e.g., mouse or trackball), and one or more conventional monitors. While sufficient for pathology workflows in which the materials to be evaluated are tissue sections mounted on glass slides, additional specialized equipment is needed for efficient and effective analysis when evaluating digitized images.

More ergonomic peripherals than the standard keyboard and mouse are readily available for viewing and annotating scanned images.

However, there is little guidance from regulatory agencies or in the published literature on how to best set up the digital pathology workspace.

Within the context of digital pathology, some thought should be given to the proper workstation arrangement to enable digital slide viewing. This design should include general ergonomics, such as the number of computer monitors, ambient light settings, room temperature, etc. A Swedish study in human medicine reported that pathologists themselves rated working at an ergonomically optimized workstation as an improvement over traditional microscope setups (Thorstenson et al., 2014). In addition, improved ergonomic pathologist workstations have been linked to increased productivity (Thorstenson et al., 2014).

While the quality of a whole-slide image depends on the quality of the physical slide being scanned, one should not underestimate the impact that an inadequate computer monitor may have on the quality of a displayed image (Al-Janabi et al., 2012; Clarke and Treanor, 2017; Neil and Demetris, 2014). It has been shown that failure of color preservation impacts the diagnostic performance of pathologists (Avanaki et al., 2015). Color differences can be introduced when the color gamut of the display does not match that of the scanner (i.e., when the monitor can display only a limited color range that is significantly reduced compared to the color range that the slide scanner camera can capture). In addition, there are vast differences in monitor quality and color calibration that are imparted during manufacturing, and a profound impact on viewing experience may occur when changing monitor settings. Lastly, it is important to remember that monitors fade, so that even high-end, color-calibrated monitors lose their ability to accurately display color over time (approximately after 2–3 years for existing equipment). The aging of monitors reduces color saturation and luminosity and impacts the ability to adequately display white light. These changes have been shown to increase the average time required for pathologists to score digital slides, and pathologists report a notable decrease in "ease of reading" when scans are evaluated on aged monitors (Avanaki et al., 2015). In addition, the percent agreement of diagnostic scores for slides shown on non-aged displays was about 20% higher than that of aged displays (Avanaki et al., 2015). The variability in displaying colors may be amplified if slides from the same study are displayed and evaluated on different monitors, even if viewed by the same pathologist.

In addition to color calibration and the number of monitors used, display size and resolution are important factors to consider in designing the workstation (Treanor et al., 2009; Vodovnik, 2016). As described above, if a monitor has a lower resolution than the whole-slide scan, there is a loss of detail at higher magnifications (Neil and Demetris, 2014; Zarella et al., 2019"). It has been described that larger monitors may improve viewer experience due to better navigation (i.e., turning one's head instead of relying on peripheral vision to provide image context, the former being more ergonomically desirable) (Randell et al., 2015). Viewing angle and screen refresh rate also are additional important factors to consider in monitor selection.

As such, a color-calibrated monitor with full high-definition display should be considered the ideal platform for properly assessing detailed whole-slide images (Neil and Demetris, 2014). Pathologists can purchase a monitor that was calibrated at the time of manufacture or utilize commercial products to calibrate monitors in an after-market setting (e.g., calibration software) (Linden et al., 2015). For GLP studies, color calibration procedures (including frequency of calibration) should be listed in relevant SOPs.

While viewing angle and surrounding light can influence perception of bright-field scanned images, it is paramount to have a more controlled and consistent viewing environment when evaluating fluorescent scans (e.g., ability to adjust and control ambient light). Reviewing fluorescent scans requires a consistent and dark viewing environment, with minimal screen glare.

When whole-slide images are not hosted directly on the computer on which they are viewed, internet bandwidth and latency can increase the time required for the view to come into focus when navigating across the slide, changing magnifications, or switching to a new slide. Larger medical centers with fully digital pathology workflows funnel extra bandwidth to pathologists' offices to minimize such image-loading latency.

An important aspect of an ergonomic setup of pathologists' workstations is the device used for slide navigation. The most commonly used tool remains the standard computer mouse, but it may not be the most appropriate and ergonomic tool. Electronic pens that can be used to trace areas of interest and impart layers of annotation to a scanned image when it is displayed on a tilting monitor are viewed by some as an effective means for navigating quickly and reliably through a scanned image. Currently, the input device selection appears to be largely based on personal preference. Some vendors have identified the need for improved navigation tools and have developed alternative devices that are entering the marketplace.

Increased screen time for pathologists involved in large-scale digital pathology studies can cause repetitive strain injuries, including eye strain. Pathologists viewing digitized images on a regular basis should work in an environment that provides regular breaks from the screen and are encouraged to practice the 20-20-20 rule: for every 20 min of screen work, take a 20-second break looking at an object 20 feet (6m) in the distance (Sheppard and Wolffsohn, 2018). In addition, the monitor should be placed approximately an arm's length (50–66 cm) away from the user's face, which aids in creating a more eye-friendly and ergonomic work environment.

Due to the rapid advancements in computer technology, it is challenging to provide a list of even the minimum recommendations for an adequate computer setup for evaluating whole-slide images. However, it is important to consider that the graphics card needs to be selected such that it can enable optimal monitor function. For such purposes, hardware of "gaming" quality should be considered as a logical starting point.

3. TISSUE IMAGE ANALYSIS

Toxicologic pathology is traditionally an observational discipline based on semiquantitative histopathologic evaluation, in which microscopic diagnoses based on extensive training in pathology are informed by personal experience. However, there is an increasing effort toward quantification to optimize the objectivity of the assessment when evaluating the spectrum of tissue findings, and digital tissue image analysis is suitable for supporting this purpose. Despite extensive training and experience, differences in diagnostic terminology and severity grading may be encountered between pathologists who have evaluated the same tissue sections independently, reflecting the descriptive and semiquantitative nature of the discipline. Image analysis aims to minimize diagnostic divergence by providing quantitative information using reproducible algorithms based on specific features within images (Aeffner et al., 2019).

Measurement of microscopic images dates back to the 17th century, when Antonie van Leeuwenhoek used sand grains and strands of his own hair to measure microscopic objects (Meijer et al., 1997). The wide commercial availability of whole-slide scanners has greatly facilitated the adoption of tissue-based image analysis, which may be applied only to an area of interest on a slide or to an entire whole-slide image. Analysis of entire whole-slide images may help to reduce bias as compared to manual selection of specific regions of interest (ROI) for analysis and has now become more common practice (Zarella et al., 2019). When conducted correctly, image analysis provides the pathologist with a powerful tool to complement the traditionally descriptive pathologic assessment with quantitative data. It allows for the identification and quantification of features not easily discernible by eye. The added value of image analysis for prognostic decision-making in medical diagnostic pathology in human medicine has led to the development of several diagnostic image analysis–based tests that have received 510k clearance from the U.S. Food and Drug Administration (FDA). The 510k clearance allows for marketing as a safe and effective medical device for clinical diagnostic practice. Image analysis is widely used in early research and clinical settings, and adoption in the field of toxicologic pathology (including for some aspects of GLP-compliant studies) is on the rise. The benefits of adding image analysis to a routine toxicologic pathology workflow include standardization of tissue measurement, automation, and improved transparency to reviewers.

3.1. Visual and Cognitive Biases of Manual Slide Review

The rich image-based information available on a histologic slide is usually evaluated by a pathologist, whose expertise is dependent on his or her training and past experience. However, readouts by a human observer may be influenced by inherent cognitive and/or visual biases. Image analysis tools can improve standardization and reproducibility and help to minimize inherent bias (Aeffner et al., 2017). Table 12.1 provides an overview of common visual biases and traps that may affect a pathologist's evaluation of slides and notes which biases may be reduced or minimized using traditional tissue image analysis algorithms.

3.2. Application Areas

Digital tissue image analysis can be applied to a variety of media including formalin-fixed, paraffin-embedded, or frozen 2D tissue sections, transmission electron micrographs, tissue whole mounts, three-dimensional (3D) confocal or light sheet microscopy, and cytological preparations (Aeffner et al., 2018). Staining techniques that can be assessed by image analysis include histochemical stains (including H&E) as well as IHC or ISH procedures utilizing either conventional chromogenic or fluorescent signals.

In toxicologic pathology, image analysis is useful in cases where area- and cell-based quantification may be especially difficult for a pathologist to reproducibly assess, or when a task is tedious and time consuming, and might be streamlined with the help of automation and appropriate QC. Traditionally, toxicologic pathology assessments are scored on either a nominal scale (qualitative: "Is a tissue change perceived, yes or no?") or ordinal scale (semiquantitative: "On a tiered scale, what is the score for an observed tissue change?"), neither of which is based on completely objective criteria (e.g., numerical values for staining intensity). To the extent that these scoring schemes are informed by the pathologist's prior experience, they may be prone to observer bias or visual limitations and may not be appropriate for statistical data interrogation. Furthermore, nominal and ordinal data are discontinuous,

TABLE 12.1 Overview of Visual and Cognitive Traps and Features

Name	Brief description	Effects mitigated by tissue image analysis
VISUAL TRAPS		
Illusion of size	Perception of an object's size is influenced by the context in which it is displayed as influenced by memory and other stimuli	Yes
Craik–O'Brien –Cornsweet illusion	Perception of brightness (or staining intensity) of an object or surface is solely determined by the brightness of its edge or interface and not the brightness of the entire surface	Yes
Checker shadow illusion	Perception of a surface's brightness is influenced by our knowledge of how it should appear, even if it is covered by a shadow, ignoring variations at the edges of shadows but recognizing those associated with sharp color changes at edges	Yes
Distinguishing colors and hues	Perception of colors and hues depends on their context, where more are recognized if presented as a gradient rather than in isolation	Yes
Lateral inhibition	Tendency for activated neurons to influence neighboring neurons in the visual pathway, yielding an increased ability to respond to edges of surfaces	Yes
Inattentional blindness	Phenomenon of failing to observe salient features or events when engaged in a different task	Maybe
COGNITIVE TRAPS		
Confirmation bias	Predisposition of people to seek information supportive of a favored hypothesis	Yes
Diagnostic drift	Situation in which scoring values vary slightly and in a consistent fashion during the course of a study	Yes
Anchoring (tunnel vision or fixation error)	Predisposition to rely too heavily on the first information presented (the so-called anchor)	No
Search satisfaction	Tendency to stop searching for a diagnosis once one event confirms an opinion, even if more events are available for evaluation	No
Context bias	Predisposition to consider a sample as "abnormal" when viewed in series with other samples showing a high disease prevalence but as "within normal limits" when the sample is interpreted as part of a sample series with lower disease prevalence	Yes
Avoidance of extreme ranges	Tendency to avoid extremes of ranges when assigning pathology scores	Yes
Number preference	Predisposition to assign numerical scores ending in 0 or 5	Yes
Gambler's fallacy	Inability to consider individual samples and endpoints (e.g., cytoplasmic vs. membrane staining) as events independent from previous and following slides or scoring events	Yes

Modified after Aeffner F, Wilson K, Martin NT, et al.: The gold standard paradox in digital image analysis: manual versus automated scoring as ground truth, Arch Pathol Lab Med *141(9):1267–1275, 2017.*

and thus inherently not quantitative. When appropriately utilized, image analysis can be used to generate continuous data, and the reliance on optical properties intrinsic in the sample typically yields a more reproducible readout.

In cases where manual measurements are used to quantify toxicity, such analyses are usually done in a subset of the structures to be measured, or in small fields of view. An example is calculation of axon G-ratios, a measurement of myelination in axons (Karumuthil-Melethil et al., 2016). Applying automated image analysis to this task can minimize interindividual influence on anchoring such measurements, which will improve accuracy and also enhance productivity by measuring the structural feature of interest throughout the whole tissue or cell population in a fraction of the time needed by a pathologist or technician to acquire such data manually.

A significant portion of tissue image analysis revolves around the interrogation of biomarker distribution via IHC or ISH. Chromogenic IHC analysis is a widespread method to assess the presence of a biomarker in the context of tissue structures. However, these assays are limited by a low dynamic range (i.e., little variation between light and dark staining) and nonlinear increase of staining intensity. These considerations are particularly important for chromogenic multiplex staining, where multiple biomarkers are assessed simultaneously (usually ranging from two to four colors, though new staining modalities with more color options are becoming available); in such cases, it may not be possible to fully separate the different colors at a given location due to their overlapping color spectra. Fluorescent imaging, therefore, is emerging as a tool for evaluating the distribution and relative expression of tissue-based biomarkers—particularly for multiplex assays. Each antibody is labeled with a fluorophore that emits photons when stimulated with light, and the wavelengths emitted by each fluorophore are detected separately by specific filters (channels), often without the need for color separation. Thus, multiplex fluorescence IHC slide scans lead to acquisition of multiple, entirely overlapping whole-slide images (one for each filter–wavelength pair). In some cases, there may be bleed-through or cross-talk between two channels, where spectral deconvolution may still be required to distinguish between

biomarkers (Hamilton et al., 2014). Please see sections on IHC and ISH in *Special Techniques in Toxicologic Pathology*, Vol 1, Chap 11 for more information.

TMAs consist of multiple aligned tissue cores from paraffin-embedded samples, which are commonly used to compare IHC or ISH biomarkers across several donors or tissues simultaneously, thereby saving time and resources in screening. TMAs are used in toxicologic pathology to identify potential target organs of toxicity, as color calibration reference and to assess the suitability of animal models based on protein expression. Their analysis can be greatly streamlined through image analysis to quantify staining in each individual tissue core, including specific features (e.g., cell membranes or nuclei) of each core.

A common challenge in tissue-based quantification is regional heterogeneity. Visualization of a biomarker by creating a spatial plot of cell data and color-coded dots based on the level of biomarker expression can be a useful feature. These can be used to generate a "heat map" for the pathologist to easily identify "hot spots" of high (or low) expression across whole tissue sections to facilitate interpretation.

In the realm of artificial intelligence (AI)–powered analysis tools (discussed later), augmented visualization is emerging. These tools convert quantitative tissue data into a visual overlay for the pathologist to aid in diagnosis and grading.

3.3. Impact of Preanalytical Variables on Image Analysis

The effect of preanalytical variables on whole-slide images has been discussed above. For tissue image analysis, the impact especially of staining optimization, quality, and consistency cannot be overstated. Please also see sections on IHC and ISH in *Special Techniques in Toxicologic Pathology*, Vol 1, Chap 11 for more information on proper reagent qualification and optimization.

3.4. Manual versus Automated Image Annotations

Image annotations, or image masking, of ROIs are usually applied to whole-slide images to focus the assessment on a particular area of the slide (e.g., an anatomical area of an organ or lesion). They can be used to specifically include one or more ROIs but can also be used to exclude specific areas of the slide from analysis by the algorithm (e.g., necrotic areas, tissue folds). ROIs can be manually or automatically annotated. Manual annotation involves drawing virtual lines or shapes on the digital image to mark an ROI for the algorithm. These annotations may be applied by the pathologist; alternatively, such annotation may be made by a technician or scientist with morphological training, in which case subsequent QC by a pathologist is advised. The annotation process may be facilitated by using a drawing tablet or similar device. Automated annotation features are available with many software packages to further facilitate this workflow step by rapidly applying an initial annotation layer to demarcate the ROI. The level of automation may vary from using basic image analysis techniques (i.e., edge detection of large objects) to AI-enabled recognition of tissue structures (e.g., renal glomeruli). As with manual annotations, automated annotations should be confirmed and, if necessary, adjusted by a pathologist prior to proceeding with the analysis.

3.5. The Basics of Quantitative Image Analysis

Quantitative image analysis encompasses the generation of any type of numerical value that quantifies an event present in a specimen (e.g., tissue section or cells). The most commonly used categories of measurements in toxicologic pathology scans are the following: area-based, cell-based, and object-based (Aeffner et al., 2016). Area-based measurements include quantification of the area of a certain morphological feature or stain. Cell-based measurements aim to identify and enumerate cells, which also enables subsequent assessment of subcellular compartments. Object-based algorithms may assess features present on tissue sections that may not be comprised of individual cells.

Area/Pixel-Based Measurements

Since the area of a given pixel in an image is known, algorithms can be used to determine the area of the feature being measured. Common outputs of area-based measurements include the size of a specific structure (e.g., tumor, focus of necrosis) or the dimensions covered by a stain (or particular extent of staining within a given range of intensity for that stain). It is important to note that the area measured within a tissue does not translate directly to an area of the tissue in situ as multiple preanalytical variables impact tissue deformation, resulting in either shrinkage or expansion of structures to unpredictable degrees. Nevertheless, area-based measurements may be powerful, and quickly obtained analytical endpoints often can be obtained with relatively little need for manually adjusting the automatically applied annotation.

Cell-Based Measurements

The cell is the basic unit of histopathology and in stained tissue sections is characterized by a prominent nucleus and variable visibility of other cellular compartments. Demarcating cells or subcellular structures is among the first and most important steps of many image analysis approaches. Segmentation is the spatial separation of an image into constituent parts that have some significance or utility. Therefore, cell segmentation generally refers to the process where pixels are grouped based on staining and/or intensity similarities to defined cellular structures such as the nucleus, nucleolus, plasma membrane, or cytoplasm. These features then aid in differentiating ("segmenting") individual cells from each other. Examples of common cell-based image analysis applications include evaluating terminal deoxynucleotidyl transferase dUTP nick end labeling distribution for apoptosis, Ki67 expression for proliferation (Figure 12.5), or IHC labeling of various tumor-associated antigens on neoplastic cells.

Once an algorithm has appropriately segmented the tissue's individual cells, their shapes and sizes may aid in the differentiation of specific cell types or categories (e.g., tumor cells vs. fibroblasts). In addition, their relationship (e.g., spatial relationship, orientation, arrangement) can be analyzed to identify structures that are comprised of cells (e.g., tumor nests, renal glomeruli, vessels). Once these structures are digitally detected, their cells can be grouped as a unit so that data can be generated and extracted on a per unit basis (e.g., the circumference or area of each individual vascular

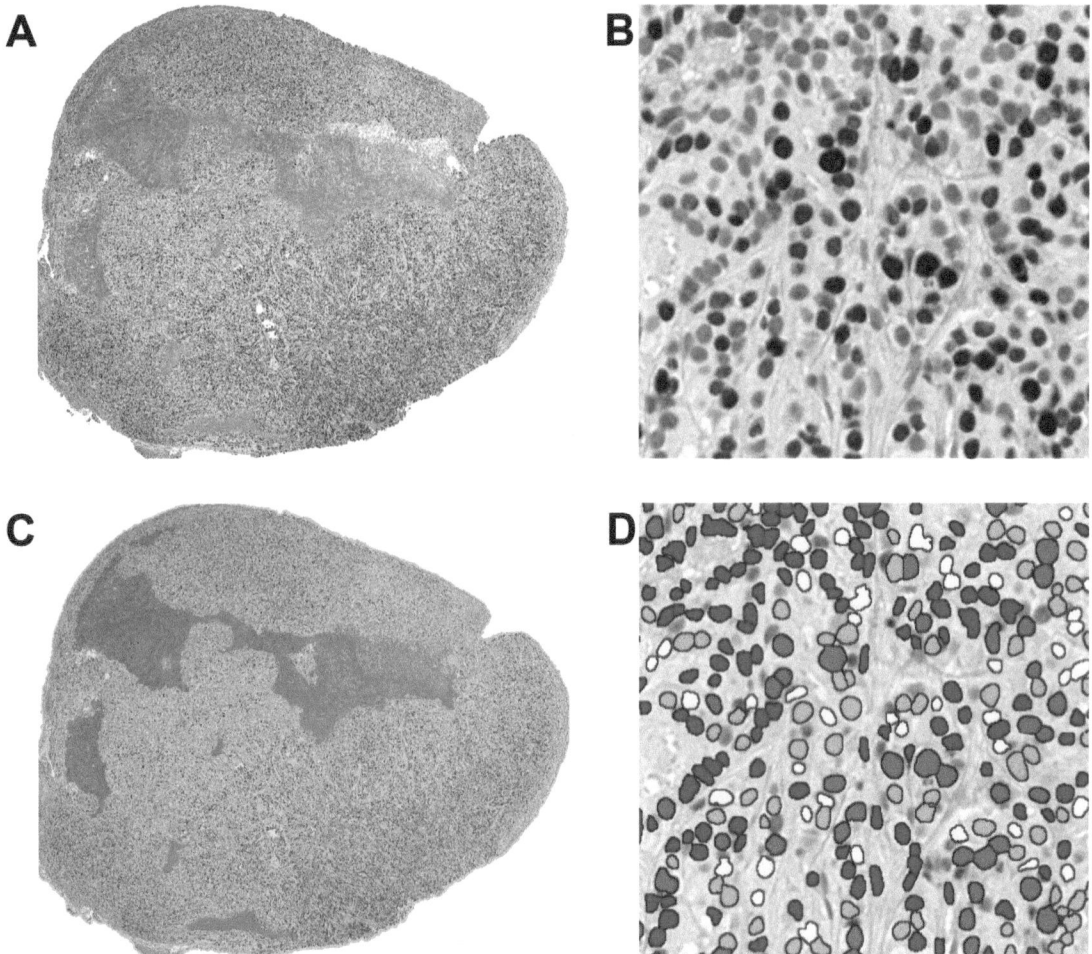

FIGURE 12.5   Digital analysis can evaluate subpopulations of cells expressing different features and variable stain intensities. (A) Mouse xenograft tumor sample stained with hematoxylin and anti-Ki67 IHC (chromogen = DAB). (B) Higher magnification image of the xenograft showing nuclei that are stained blue and Ki67+ cells that are brown. (C) An algorithm was developed to identify, classify, and label components [e.g., tumor (green), stroma (blue), necrosis (red), and glass (gray)]. (D) The algorithm parameters are fine-tuned with the pathologist's input to optimize the nuclear segmentation and to define staining intensity thresholds to categorize the expression into four bins: 0+ (blue), 1+ (yellow), 2+ (orange), and 3+ (red). *Figure reproduced from Aeffner F, Zarella MD, Buchbinder N, et al.: Introduction to digital image analysis in whole-slide imaging: a white paper from the Digital Pathology Association,* J Pathol Inform *10:9, 2019, with permission.*

profile in a tissue section). Similarly, cellular features per unit can be interrogated (e.g., the number of Ki67-positive cells per pancreatic islet). Finally, the spatial relationship between individual categories of cells, between cells and other structures (e.g., blood vessels or organ edges), or structures to each other can be interrogated. As an example, cell-based measurements are appropriate for evaluating the distance of a specific immune cell to the nearest tumor cell (Figure 12.6) or the closest vascular profile.

Object-Based Measurements

Not every feature on a slide that may need to be quantified is comprised of cells. For example, one application is to assess subcellular objects (e.g., ISH dots representing labeled genes on chromosomes). Alternatively, features that are independent of discrete cells may need to be evaluated (e.g., numbers and sizes of plaques in Alzheimer's disease models). Such features may be analyzed as discrete objects as long as their margins can be visualized or extrapolated.

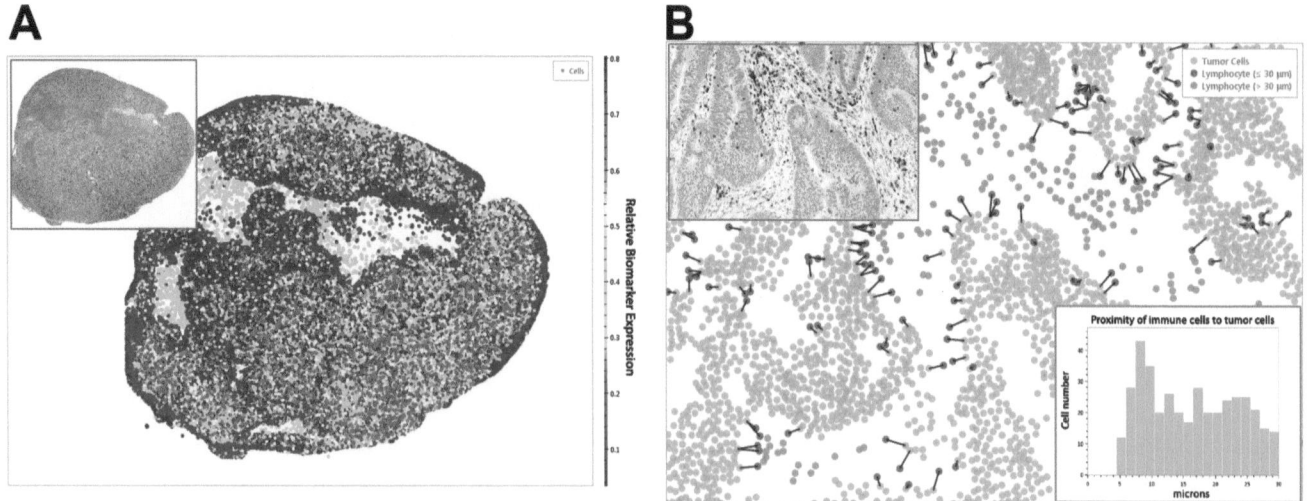

FIGURE 12.6   Digital pathology image analysis in spatial context reveals biomarker and cell heterogeneity. (A) The inset digital slide with a DAB-stained biomarker (brown) was analyzed. Cells identified in the analysis were plotted spatially as a dot plot and each cell "dot" color coded according to the optical density of DAB stain in that cell. Cells in "cooler" colors (blues and greens) have lower stain optical density compared to cells in "warmer" colors (yellow, orange, and red). (B) Tumor cells (blue) and immune cells (DAB positive) identified by image analysis were plotted spatially and analyzed to quantify immune cells within 30 μm of tumor cells (termed "proximal" immune cell). Tumor cells are colored blue, proximal immune cells are colored red, and nonproximal immune cells are green. The distance between tumor cells and proximal immune cells is recorded to create a histogram (inset, bottom right) and is connected by nearest neighbor lines in the dot plot. *Figure reproduced from Aeffner F, Zarella MD, Buchbinder N, et al.: Introduction to digital image analysis in whole-slide imaging: a white paper from the Digital Pathology Association,* J Pathol Inform *10:9, 2019, with permission.*

3.6. Nonquantitative Image Analysis

In some cases, a quantitative output is not useful or required when evaluating tissue. In these cases, pattern recognition is the preferred analytical endpoint. These algorithms may generate analysis markups that create an augmented viewing experience for the pathologist, highlighting areas of tissue where an abnormal event is more likely to be present (e.g., altered hepatic focus, area of necrosis, micrometastasis of neoplastic cells in the lymph node). The ability of an algorithm to accurately identify normal versus abnormal tissues is an active area of research, as generation of such tools may yield a significant improvement in the efficiency of evaluating tissue sections for toxicologic pathology studies.

3.7. Available Tools

A variety of commercial and open source software options are available to facilitate the analysis of whole-slide images. In addition, several service providers (i.e., contract research organizations) specialize in image analysis. Some are expert users of specific commercially available software packages, whereas others utilize their own proprietary software to build completely customized analysis tools for use by their client companies.

Commercially available software solutions have a graphical user interface (GUI) that enables the user to change parameters in the analytical algorithm without the need to be able to write computer code. These parameters can be used to "tune" an algorithm, meaning that they can be combined and tested on the use case images (i.e., images of tissues known to contain the features of interest to be analyzed) to develop an algorithm that meets the intended use criteria (Aeffner et al., 2019). Intuitive GUIs walk the user through the right progression of analytical steps to generate appropriate algorithms.

Broadly, there are three different types of image analysis platform tools: prebuilt application modules, development environments that enable a high degree of customization by the end user, or machine learning (ML)–based training modules. In general, there is a trade-off between the ease of use and flexibility.

Prebuilt applications have modules that are designed for a specific purpose and offer the end user a nearly ready-made solution, which may require no or only minimal fine-tuning of parameters. An example would be a cell detection measurement algorithm where the end user must only input the counterstain, color, and threshold of the stain that is being measured as well as the desired analysis output (e.g., the number of stain-positive cells). Another use case is measurement of multiple biomarkers in a single tissue section, known as multiplex analysis; this strategy is used frequently in basic biomedical research and especially in clinical immuno-oncology research. Basic prebuilt tools usually must be adapted for multiplex image analysis, typically requiring more input from the end user (e.g., color, threshold, and cellular locations of each biomarker). A benefit of this prebuilt module approach is that extensive training in image analysis principles is not required. These tools are particularly well suited for routine analyses such as area measurements and positive cell counts.

The second type of approach for image analysis algorithms is the development environment. Here, the user has more flexibility to build an algorithm by using a modular approach to combine different functions such as preprocessing, color separation, filtering, and postprocessing. Such an approach requires that the user possess more background knowledge of the principles of image analysis to ensure that the appropriate functions are applied in the correct order and with the optimal parameters. This strategy is well suited for more advanced analytical applications (e.g., less routinely assessed features or lesions, such as distinguishing regional variations in biomarker expression across a heterogeneous population of tumor cells). In both prebuilt applications and development environments, the algorithm can be saved and applied to another study set. In such cases, the pathologist is a team member who engages primarily in definition of scientific questions to be answered by the algorithm, analysis QC, and data interpretation but does not necessarily perform the algorithm tuning him/herself.

The third approach is an ML-based interface (see below for more on ML). In this approach, the end user gives inputs in the form of annotations that train the ML application. The trained algorithm can detect complex features without the need to manually input the image analysis filters (e.g., color, texture). Therefore, the software can learn to separate different features, which then are analyzed in a next step. An example would be to train the software to distinguish tumor cells and normal cells as distinct ROIs and recognize the interface between tumor foci and adjacent normal tissue, after which analysis of different cell types is performed in each of these defined regions.

3.8. The Pathologist's Role in the Image Analysis Workflow

The pathologist plays a crucial role along the entire image analysis workflow (Aeffner et al., 2016). Key tasks include ensuring appropriate study design, confirming the quality of specimen preparation to control for preanalytical variables (discussed above), performing the algorithm QC, and undertaking the data interpretation. The pathologist may fulfill any or all of these roles depending on the nature of the available tools, familiarity with image analysis principles, and the time available for performing this function relative to other pathologist-oriented tasks.

A pathologist must also be aware of the limitations of a particular assessment. For example, while biomarker expression may be calculated due to the linear relationship between fluorescent staining intensity and the amount of bound fluorophore-conjugated antibody, such calculations are not feasible for chromogenic IHC staining due to the nonlinear staining intensity of such enzyme-based detection methods. A multiplex staining assay that looks good for routine histopathologic evaluation by a pathologist may display a staining intensity that is too dark for image analysis and therefore may not provide optimal results in the color deconvolution steps of the image analysis workflow. Running image analysis and color deconvolution on a range of staining intensities on a subset of images can determine the optimal staining conditions for a study.

The pathologist's role in the QC of WSI is discussed above. Specifically, for image analysis, assessment of appropriate staining (localization, intensity, etc.) by a pathologist is paramount. Analysis of biomarker expression (via IHC or ISH) requires the pathologist to approve all adjustable algorithm parameters (e.g., threshold of staining intensity for a particular biomarker to be considered positive or number of ISH dots required per cell for it to be assigned a specific scoring category). Thresholds should be tested on a subset of slides for review by a pathologist prior to lockdown of parameters that are to be applied to all specimens of an entire study.

In general, algorithm development is an iterative process. The generation may start with an automated algorithm, but it usually requires several additional rounds of tuning, algorithm QC by a pathologist, and retuning based on the knowledge of why the previous algorithm failed to meet performance criteria. For any image analysis project, it is advisable to establish the desired performance criteria prior to beginning the process of algorithm tuning. For screening approaches, less stringent pass/fail criteria may be sufficient, whereas for other scenarios, a more stringent set of criteria may be needed to produce appropriate quantitative data for the endpoints of interest.

Once an algorithm meets the desired performance criteria, it may be applied to the test set of whole-slide images. A useful tool for pathologist evaluation of algorithm performance available in most image analysis software is to assess a visual representation of the image segmentation and classification known as the "markup" or the "segmentation overlay." The pathologist reviews the markup to assess if the algorithm performance meets the study-specific and predefined analysis criteria. In general, this review should include assessment regarding whether the correct structure or tissue compartment is analyzed, if cells and/or subcellular structures are adequately identified and enumerated, and if scoring parameters or staining thresholds are appropriately applied (Aeffner et al., 2016). Confirmation that the algorithm markup reflects adequate identification and analysis of desired tissue features provides confidence that the quantitative image analysis results are suitable for interpretation.

Data extraction should only commence after appropriate pathology review and approval.

In medical diagnostic practice and clinical trials, pathologist review of every individual algorithm is a requirement by regulatory agencies (e.g., FDA). This same "complete review" practice is not mandated for regulatory-type animal toxicity studies (whether GLP or non-GLP) used in product registration. Nevertheless, algorithm markup review of every slide by a pathologist prior to data extraction is a strongly advisable ("best") practice in the nonclinical regulatory setting and is also encouraged in the nonregulated environment.

3.9. Computational Pathology

Computational pathology is the field of extracting meaningful information by combining morphologic pathology images with other sources of raw data including metadata, clinical pathology, omics analyses, and other "big data" (Abels et al., 2019). This information may be presented as a data output, or—as in the case of Computer-Assisted Diagnosis—presented to the pathologist as an integrated assessment to the pathology expert for assisting in medical decision-making. This concept focuses on the core competency of pathology: leveraging and integrating diverse data sources and knowledge of disease mechanisms to create meaningful interpretations. Successful integration of computational endpoints into pathology assessments will require a shift to a strongly collaborative culture where computer scientists, imaging experts, and pathologists work as a multidisciplinary team. There is currently a trend toward the development of multidisciplinary educational programs that combine computational and biological training. The development of online platforms for sharing tissue-based image data is a global approach to enabling this cultural acceptance.

3.10. Introduction to Artificial Intelligence and Machine Learning in Tissue Image Analysis

AI is a branch of computer science focused on the simulation of intelligent behavior by computers. For histopathologic evaluation as applied in toxicologic pathology, AI shows promise as a potential means for screening large tissue sets for potential abnormalities. ML is considered a subset of AI in which an algorithm learns to make associations by being exposed to large representative data sets, and can be categorized as supervised, weakly supervised, or unsupervised (Figure 12.7) (Turner et al., 2019). In supervised ML, an algorithm is trained explicitly by associating an input data set with ground truth labels provided by the user, such as the identity of an image or cell. In contrast, unsupervised ML does not rely on a user-supplied ground truth for training and instead seeks to identify natural divisions in the data; an algorithm trained to cluster images by similar features is one example of this approach. Weakly supervised learning can be considered a special case of supervised ML in which the ground truth is known to be excessively noisy or is surmised from other data that are known; an

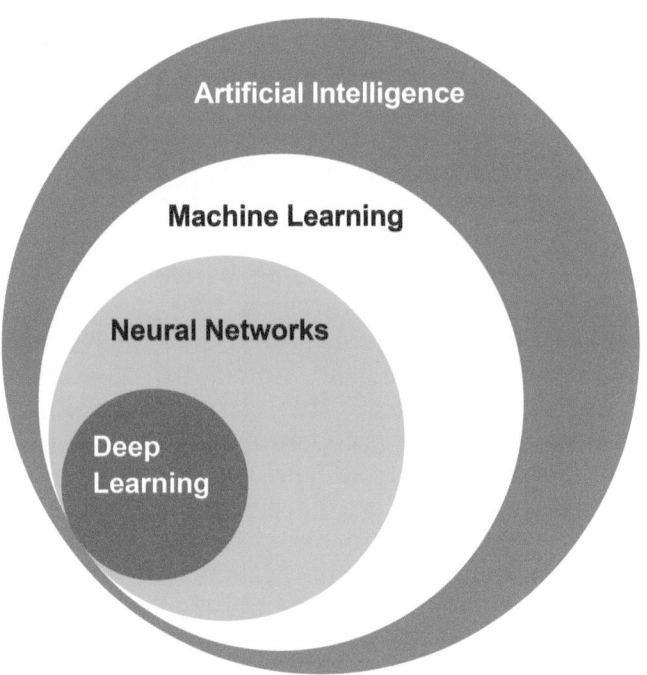

FIGURE 12.7 Overview of the relationships between Artificial Intelligence, Machine Learning, Neural Networks, and Deep Learning. *Figure reproduced from Turner OC, Aeffner F, Bangari DS, et al.: Society of Toxicologic Pathology Digital Pathology and Image Analysis Special Interest Group article*: Opinion on the application of artificial intelligence and machine learning to digital toxicologic pathology,* Toxicol Pathol 48:277–294, 2019, Figure 1, *p 279, with permission.*

example of this strategy is the use of a surrogate value as ground truth, or case-level ground truth applied to regions of a whole-slide image that were not explicitly annotated. ***Deep learning*** (DL) is a type of ML based on neural networks, best distinguished by not requiring explicit representation of image features prior to training. Rather, DL learns to identify features relevant for learning. ***Convolutional neural networks*** (CNNs) are among the most commonly used DL approaches. CNNs are based on the analysis of an image by a series of filters, typically followed by a pooling step (to reduce the number of parameters and amount of computation), rectification, and followed by another round of convolution and so on. Each layer of a deep network operates on the output of a previous layer. As more layers are added, the network is considered "deeper," which distinguishes DL from other neural network–based approaches. However, this also adds computational complexity.

One of the current challenges of ML in the context of toxicologic pathology is the availability and generation of ground truth data. In supervised learning, this may require time-consuming annotation. The number of organs assessed in a toxicity study and the variation in background findings across species, strains, ages, and sometimes sex further amplifies this challenge. A whole-slide image viewer or image analysis software with integrated annotation and collaboration tools may streamline this process sufficiently so that ML may be deployed for some toxicologic pathology endpoints in the future.

Appropriate training, testing, and QC'ing of AI-based image analysis approaches are rapidly evolving, and a detailed review is beyond the scope of this chapter. However, it is essential that trained algorithms are thoroughly evaluated using a separate validation data set. A specific challenge that DL algorithms impose is that the image features used by the algorithm to make a decision are not transparent to a human observer. Methods have been devised to improve transparency, which may include demonstrating to the viewer representative structures or regions of the slide that exemplify a particular decision. In the absence of specific regulatory guidance on QC practices for AI-based image analysis, it is incumbent on the user to provide the rationale and demonstrate the suitability of the QC process selected for a given study.

4. REGULATORY CONSIDERATIONS FOR DIGITAL PATHOLOGY EVALUATION

Currently, guidelines are sparse (OECD, 2020) for the primary evaluation or pathology peer review of whole-slide images from GLP-compliant animal toxicity studies. However, accounts have been published of such efforts for non-GLP studies in relation to use of whole-slide images in an ancillary role to traditional bright-field light microscopy, use in diagnostic settings, and some general regulatory considerations (Bertram and Klopfleisch, 2017; Bradley and Jocobsen, 2019; OECD, 2020; Fikes et al., 2015; Gauthier et al., 2019; FDA, 2016; Long et al., 2013; Pantanowitz et al., 2013; Tuomari et al., 2007; Vodovnik, 2016). Moreover, discussion is ongoing between members of societies of toxicology and regulatory authorities on points to consider and potential best practices for use of WSI. Therefore, further guidelines are likely to be proposed soon, and it is feasible at this time to describe some principles that will very likely pertain to use of whole-slide images for pathology peer review of GLP toxicity studies.

In general, the principles that apply to the conduct of histopathologic evaluation during GLP studies or substitution of methods in GLP studies will also apply to WSI. The system used must be qualified by demonstrating that it is not inferior to traditional bright-field light microscopy, it must be validated as fit for use as installed within the test facility, and it must be verified as functioning within specifications on a regular schedule described in an SOP. Evaluations conducted on noncompliant equipment or outside a test facility should be described as "GLP exceptions," for example, when the input of a specific subject matter expert is desired and use of GLP-compliant equipment is not feasible. Similar to other study activities, the intent to create whole-slide images should be identified in the study protocol or amendments, and the process used for scanning the glass slides should be described. Likewise, test facility

management is responsible for ensuring that users are adequately trained to use the system and that users can perform their assigned duties. Finally, data generated using a WSI system must conform to the "ALCOA" integrity standard whereby data can be demonstrated to be Attributable, Legible, Contemporaneous, Original, and Accurate.

While GLP principles generally apply to the use of WSI systems in regulated nonclinical toxicity studies, there are also some specific points to consider that are unique to current digital imaging technology. Because WSI systems contain multiple hardware and software subsystems and can be configured in various ways from components obtained from many sources, it can be useful to consider the quality of the system based on the entire "pixel pathway" from surface of the glass slide being scanned to the surface of the monitor being used to evaluate the resulting image (FDA, 2016). This perspective will facilitate design of tests to establish that the performance of a WSI system is comparable to traditional bright-field microscopy, thereby establishing diagnostic concordance of the two approaches. Using a diagnostic concordance approach to qualification, noninferiority of a WSI system configuration can be established through statistical comparison of diagnoses in which a group of suitably trained and experienced pathologists evaluate tissue sections on glass slides and corresponding whole-slide images of the sections, with the microscopic and WSI analyses separated by a suitable "washout" period. This type of proof-of-concept/end-user acceptance qualification need not be conducted for each installation of the system, but only on the generic configuration of the components using specimens relevant to the eventual use of the system. Although the GLP stakeholder community is still in the process of gaining experience with WSI system qualification, the standard of practice appears to be moving toward qualification specifications of some hardware components that are based on minimum technical attributes rather than on specific models for components of the pixel pathway. This approach would allow substitutions of some hardware components without a new qualification or validation effort in a qualified system, such as using different models of monitors or input peripherals that meet or exceed the performance characteristics of devices used in qualification tests.

Although specific guidance has yet to be established for validating WSI systems that have undergone vendor qualification to demonstrate diagnostic equivalency, validation of vendor-qualified WSI systems installed in test facilities may be based on demonstrating the representative nature of whole-slide images produced by the system in comparison to the parent glass slide for the test facility use cases. Using this approach, a suitable number of critical features particular to the work being conducted could be identified that are often challenging to identify on glass slides, and a comparison check conducted to validate that the same critical features appear in the whole-slide image generated by the system as configured (Williams and Treanor, 2019). Significant changes to the imaging system or use of the system for new purposes would necessitate a new validation effort. In addition to checking for the presence of critical microscopic features by visual inspection of the whole-slide image, regulatory guidance supports a validation assessment of several critical technical attributes of the system including color reproducibility, spatial resolution, focusing, whole-slide coverage, scan quality, image rendering latency, accessibility and proper function of the user interface (software viewer), and a hazard analysis of use-related failures (FDA, 2016). Because diagnostic equivalence with traditional light microscopy has not been established for many WSI systems, some organizations may elect to create this type of qualification in the validation package for their system as it is installed in their facility. Since establishing diagnostic equivalency has been typically performed by the resource-intensive means of statistically comparing the diagnostic performance of pathologists using whole-slide images and traditional light microscopy, it is advisable to carefully plan these undertakings with appropriate involvement of subject matter experts.

Similar to use of other types of validated equipment in GLP studies, periodic tests should be conducted to verify that the equipment is performing within specification, and preventive maintenance should be conducted on an appropriate schedule specified in an SOP. For example, light sources in WSI scanners and display monitors are components known to deteriorate over time, and therefore require ongoing testing to confirm that they are operating within specification. Performance verification standards for WSI systems used in GLP studies are a current topic of discussion. Using the aforementioned "pixel pathway" model for testing, one possible approach would be to establish that critical features relevant to the use case are identifiable using a TMA slide. Another approach would be to establish critical technical outputs at the surface of the monitor based on a standardized WSI scanner input (FDA, 2016). For example, a calibration slide etched with a micrometer scale and a calibration slide containing patches of known color could be scanned periodically and a comparison made at the surface of the monitor between the new WSI system and the whole-slide image of the calibration standards created during system validation to confirm that spatial resolution and color reproducibility have been maintained over time. Kinetic monitor performance characteristics such as image refresh rates might also be included to confirm image turnaround time. Whatever timing and details of the verification process may be specified in an SOP, it would remain the responsibility of the pathologist to establish that the overall output of the system for viewing images is fit for purpose, as is currently the case for traditional bright-field light microscopy.

Given the complexity of WSI systems, the opacity of computer files to direct human observation, and the potential for the introduction of untraceable changes in digitized data, robust digital audit and security measures will need to be incorporated into WSI systems used on GLP studies, particularly when images and image metadata move across institutional boundaries or are archived for extended periods (especially in the cloud). As part of this security system, any whole-slide image used as the basis for a diagnosis should be preserved in its original unaltered form, along with the related metadata and any relevant alterations or annotations applied to support the interpretation. Understanding the appropriate specifics of security measures needed to establish the *bona fides* of WSI used in GLP-compliant studies is a technical subject outside the competence of most end users of WSI systems, and therefore, experts on these topics should be involved in the process of choosing, installing, validating, and verifying WSI systems that will be used for toxicologic pathology applications. A topic of special interest in the current discussion is the suitability of computer cloud-based storage for archiving whole-slide images. This issue is of particular concern since input from GLP inspectors on implementing this practice differs depending on jurisdiction. Public third-party cloud storage has practical advantages because it typically exists outside the IT firewall of a sponsor or test facility, which facilitates collaboration across institutions or institutional locations, and because third-party archival cloud storage can be inexpensive. However, GLP regulations currently stipulate that archives must be identified in the study record with a specific geography. While this geographical requirement for archives facilitates the physical inspection of study materials, the advantages of third-party cloud computing are based in part on an absence of geographic permanence. The question of archiving GLP study materials in the public cloud extends beyond the storage of whole-slide images, and further discussion of this topic among GLP stakeholders is anticipated. Until the question has been fully addressed, public third-party cloud-based computer long-term storage of whole-slide images is acceptable for non-GLP use. Currently, whole-slide images from GLP studies can be archived in private cloud systems with defined geographies or on tangible media such as flash memory/external hard drives kept in a traditional physical GLP archive along with the rest of the study materials.

In GLP nonclinical toxicity studies, the glass slides are considered specimens because they are objects derived from the test system, and only the signed pathology report is considered to be the raw data. GLP specimens and raw data must be retained subject to schedules specific to the geographic location of the test facility and the regulatory use of the study report. In this context, whole-slide images and annotations used only for the purposes of refining the analytical algorithm or GLP pathology peer review may be viewed as supportive information not needing to be archived. While whole-slide images are not specimens and do not fit the current definition of pathology raw data, if they are used to establish a diagnosis then they are necessary to reconstruct the study and must be archived (Tuomari et al., 2007). Therefore, in the specific case where the study pathologist conducts a GLP histopathologic evaluation based on traditional light microscopy using glass slides, and the peer reviewer assesses whole-slide images before the study report is signed, then the whole-slide images may not need to be archived. However, in such cases, it may be prudent for the test facility to have a validated means established for archiving scans in the unlikely event that a diagnosis is identified that can only be seen on a whole-slide image. It is important to note that the discussion about the classification and retention requirements of whole-slide images continues to evolve. Therefore, the reader is advised to always consult the most recent regulatory guidance.

A final consideration specific to the use of WSI relates to the evolving nature of the technology and concerns about accessibility of archived whole-slide images. This issue is important since the systems and file protocols currently in use may not be in existence decades hence, especially given the current proliferation of vendor-specific file types. The proposed solution currently under discussion is a push for industry-wide adoption of the DICOM standard (discussed above) for WSI. Indeed, some vendors already are moving in this direction with their newest scanners. Consideration of DICOM compatibility should be included in assessments of WSI systems before purchase and validation to avoid the need to implement a retrofitting solution to preserve the functionality and GLP compliance of whole-slide image archives.

5. RELATED TOPICS

5.1. Stereology

While WSI enables digital image analysis of entire tissue sections, analysis of a single section is limited to 2D analysis of a 3D object. This approach has the potential of introducing bias of multiple sources into the generated data. To avoid this and appropriately sample the 3D space, the field of stereology utilizes stringent sampling methods (e.g., systematic uniform random sampling), aiming at generating absolute 3D numbers/values rather than density estimates and ratios. Advances in the field of digital image analysis have made stereological approaches more efficient, but it remains a time- and planning-intensive methodology that requires the skills of experienced stereologists. For an introduction to stereology, the reader may refer to *Special Techniques in Toxicologic Pathology,* Vol 1, Chap 11. A detailed consideration of digital image analysis as applied to stereology is beyond the scope of this chapter, but basic considerations may be obtained from other sources (Brown, 2017).

5.2. 3D Reconstruction

WSI of consecutive sections with subsequent registration of images from the 2D sections allows for digital 3D reconstruction of the sectioned tissue or organ. Multiple software solutions (commercial and open source) as well as service providers are available for this purpose. While digitization of the individual sections is an important first step, the introduction of tissue deformation and artifacts in the process of tissue harvest, fixation, processing, and sectioning may be substantial. These factors need to be addressed when digitally aligning individual sections to each other ("registration") in order to assemble an entire 3D structure to represent its shape. In the context of toxicologic pathology, 3D reconstruction may be of use when a lesion is challenging to capture in a single section, or its 3D appearance provides significant information related to the microscopic diagnosis or its interpretation. This may be the case when evaluating atherosclerotic plaques in vascular lesions, or when evaluating entire heart samples instead of individual section levels.

5.3. Other Imaging Modalities

The number of alternative or extended tissue imaging modalities is rapidly increasing. It includes, but is not limited to, light sheet fluorescence microscopy (LSFM), optical coherence tomography (OCT), confocal microscopy, Raman spectrography, and MUSE (microscopy with UV surface excitation). These methods all can be applied to routinely fixed tissues, and some also can be used on other kinds of specimens.

LSFM is a technique whereby tissues, organs, and even whole animals may be cleared and imaged by a sheet of light on each plane. These light sheet images can then be reconstructed into a volumetric image. A benefit of this technique is that it can also image living organisms or microphysiological systems, enabling a four-dimensional evaluation. To enable the light to pass through, the samples may be cleared using a variety of available chemical processes (e.g., Clear, Unobstructed Brain/Body Imaging Cocktails and Computational Analysis (CUBIC), 3D imaging of solvent-cleared organs). Samples can then be immunostained *en bloc* or even imaged as unstained tissues as many structures of toxicologic pathology significance can be visualized by tissue autofluorescence. Following LSFM, organs can be processed routinely for follow-up H&E and/or IHC evaluations in 2D sections.

OCT uses low-coherence light scattering to generate 2D and 3D images. Because it uses long wavelength light, it can penetrate deeper into tissue compared to confocal microscopy. Raman spectroscopy, in contrast, generates images by determining the vibrational modes of molecules via inelastic scattering of photons.

A detailed review of these and other alternative imaging modalities is beyond the scope of this chapter. The reader is encouraged to consult current review publications focusing on the individual imaging modality of interest.

6. CONCLUSION

In conclusion, the age of digitalization has arrived in toxicologic pathology, and these technological advances have revealed new possibilities that will impact all members of the pathology team. These include geographically remote viewing of slides, digital consults and pathology peer review, building of electronic workflows and digital databases linking WSI to associated metadata, applying image analysis algorithms to whole-slide scans to extract quantitative data previously not easily accessible, and enhancing teaching and training capabilities. While this technology has been commercially available for decades, regulatory guidance on the use of digital pathology and related topics in toxicologic pathology is evolving and is currently incomplete. This continues to be a rapidly evolving field in all aspects, including broad adoption, hardware updates, evolving software capabilities, and regulatory guidance and acceptance. Digital pathology applications will significantly shape how toxicologic pathologists perform their craft in the future.

REFERENCES

Abels E, Pantanowitz L, Aeffner F, et al.: Computational pathology definitions, best practices, and recommendations for regulatory guidance: a white paper from the digital pathology association, *J Pathol* 249:286–294, 2019.

Aeffner F, Adissu HA, Boyle MC, et al.: Digital microscopy, image analysis, and virtual slide repository, *ILAR J* 59(1): 66–79, 2018.

Aeffner F, Wilson K, Bolon B, et al.: Commentary: roles for pathologists in a high-throughput image analysis team, *Toxicol Pathol* 44:825–834, 2016.

Aeffner F, Wilson K, Martin NT, et al.: The gold standard paradox in digital image analysis: manual versus automated scoring as ground truth, *Arch Pathol Lab Med* 141(9): 1267–1275, 2017.

Aeffner F, Zarella MD, Buchbinder N, et al.: Introduction to digital image analysis in whole-slide imaging: a white paper from the Digital Pathology Association, *J Pathol Inform* 10(9), 2019.

Al-Janabi S, Huisman A, Van Diest PJ: Digital pathology: current status and future perspectives, *Histopathology* 61: 1–9, 2012.

Avanaki A.R., Espig K., Sawhney S., et al: 2015. Aging display's effect on interpretation of digital pathology slide, Proc SPIE 9420, Medical Imaging: Digital Pathology, 942006. https://doi.org/10.1117/12.2082315.

Bertram CA, Klopfleisch R: The pathologist 2.0: an update on digital pathology in veterinary medicine, *Vet Pathol* 54: 756–766, 2017.

Bradley A, Jacobsen M: Toxicologic pathology forum: opinion on considerations for the use of whole slide images in GLP pathology peer review, *Toxicol Pathol* 47:100–107, 2019.

Brown DL: Bias in image analysis and its solution: unbiased stereology, *J Toxicol Pathol* 30:183–191, 2017.

Bueno G, Deniz O, Fernandez-Carrobles Mdel M, et al.: An automated system for whole microscopic image acquisition and analysis, *Microsc Res Tech* 77:697–713, 2014.

Chlipala EA, Bendzinski CM, Dorner C, et al.: An image analysis solution for quantification and determination of immunohistochemistry staining reproducibility, *Appl Immunohistochem Mol Morphol* 28(6):428–436, 2019.

Chlipala EA, Butters M, Brous M, Fortin JS, Archuletta R, Copeland K, Bolon B: Impact of pre-analytical factors during histology processing on section suitability for digital image analysis, *Toxicol Pathol* 49(4):755–772, 2021.

Clarke EL, Treanor D: Colour in digital pathology: a review, *Histopathology* 70:153–163, 2017.

Cornish TC, Swapp RE, Kaplan KJ: Whole-slide imaging: routine pathologic diagnosis, *Adv Anat Pathol* 19:152–159, 2012.

Dunstan RW, Wharton Jr KA, Quigley C, et al.: The use of immunohistochemistry for biomarker assessment—can it compete with other technologies? *Toxicol Pathol* 39:988–1002, 2011.

FDA (U.S. Food and Drug Administration): *Technical performance assessment of digital pathology whole slide imaging devices*, 2016. https://www.fda.gov/regulatory-information/search-fda-guidance-documents/technical-performance-assessment-digital-pathology-whole-slide-imaging-devices. (Accessed 17 May 2021).

Farahani N, Parwani A, Pantanowitz L: Whole slide imaging in pathology: advantages, limitations, and emerging perspectives, *Pathol Lab Med Int* 23–33, 2015.

Farris AB, Cohen C, Rogers TE, et al.: Whole slide imaging for analytical anatomic pathology and telepathology: practical applications today, promises, and perils, *Arch Pathol Lab Med* 141:542–550, 2017.

Feng Z, Puri S, Moudgil T, et al.: Multispectral imaging of formalin-fixed tissue predicts ability to generate tumor-infiltrating lymphocytes from melanoma, *J Immunother Cancer* 3:47, 2015.

Fikes JD, Patrick DJ, Francke S, et al.: Scientific and regulatory policy committee review: review of the organisation for economic Co-operation and development (OECD) guidance on the GLP requirements for peer review of histopathology, *Toxicol Pathol* 43:907–914, 2015.

Gauthier BE, Gervais F, Hamm G, et al.: Toxicologic pathology forum: opinion on integrating innovative digital pathology tools in the regulatory framework, *Toxicol Pathol* 47:436–443, 2019.

Ghaznavi F, Evans A, Madabhushi A, et al.: Digital imaging in pathology: whole-slide imaging and beyond, *Annu Rev Pathol* 8:331–359, 2013.

Goode A, Gilbert B, Harkes J, et al.: OpenSlide: a vendor-neutral software foundation for digital pathology, *J Pathol Inform* 4:27, 2013.

Griffin J, Treanor D: Digital pathology in clinical use: where are we now and what is holding us back? *Histopathology* 70: 134–145, 2017.

Hamilton PW, Bankhead P, Wang Y, et al.: Digital pathology and image analysis in tissue biomarker research, *Methods* 70:59–73, 2014.

Hanna MG, Reuter VE, Samboy J, et al.: Implementation of digital pathology offers clinical and operational increase in efficiency and cost savings, 143:1545–1555, 2019.

Higgins C: Applications and challenges of digital pathology and whole slide imaging, *Biotech Histochem* 90:341–347, 2015.

Huisman A, Looijen A, van den Brink SM, et al.: Creation of a fully digital pathology slide archive by high-volume tissue slide scanning, *Hum Pathol* 41:751–757, 2010.

Indu M, Rathy R, Binu MP: "Slide less pathology": fairy tale or reality? *J Oral Maxillofac Pathol* 20:284–288, 2016.

Karumuthil-Melethil S, Marshall MS, Heindel C, et al.: Intrathecal administration of AAV/GALC vectors in 10–11-day-old twitcher mice improves survival and is enhanced by bone marrow transplant, *J Neurosci Res* 94:1138–1151, 2016.

Kayser K, Gortler J, Goldmann T, et al.: Image standards in tissue-based diagnosis (diagnostic surgical pathology), *Diagn Pathol* 3(17), 2008.

Kim S-W, Roh J, Park C-SJJ, et al.: Immunohistochemistry for pathologists: protocols, pitfalls, and tips, 50:411, 2016.

Krupinski EA, Johnson JP, Jaw S, et al.: Compressing pathology whole-slide images using a human and model observer evaluation, *J Pathol Inform* 3(17), 2012.

Laurent C, Guérin M, Frenois F-X, et al.: Whole-slide imaging is a robust alternative to traditional fluorescent microscopy for fluorescence in situ hybridization imaging using break-apart DNA probes, 44:1544–1555, 2013.

Linden MA, Sedgewick GJ, Ericson M: An innovative method for obtaining consistent images and quantification of histochemically stained specimens, *J Histochem Cytochem* 63:233–243, 2015.

Long RE, Smith A, Machotka SV, et al.: Scientific and Regulatory Policy Committee (SRPC) paper: validation of digital pathology systems in the regulated nonclinical environment, *Toxicol Pathol* 41:115–124, 2013.

Malarkey DE, Willson GA, Willson CJ, et al.: Utilizing whole slide images for pathology peer review and working groups, *Toxicol Pathol* 43:1149–1157, 2015.

Mansfield JR: Multispectral imaging: a review of its technical aspects and applications in anatomic pathology, *Vet Pathol* 51:185–210, 2014.

Meijer GA, Belien JA, van Diest PJ, et al.: Origins of … image analysis in clinical pathology, *J Clin Pathol* 50:365–370, 1997.

Montalto MC, McKay RR, Filkins RJ: Autofocus methods of whole slide imaging systems and the introduction of a second-generation independent dual sensor scanning method, *J Pathol Inform* 2:44, 2011.

Moore J, Linkert M, Blackburn C, et al.: OMERO and Bio-Formats 5: flexible access to large bioimaging datasets at scale. In *Medical imaging 2015: image processing*, 2015, International Society for Optics and Photonics.

Neil DA, Demetris AJ: Digital pathology services in acute surgical situations, *Br J Surg* 101:1185–1186, 2014.

OECD (Organisation for Economic Co-operation and Development): *Frequently asked questions - histopathology*, 2020. http://www.oecd.org/chemicalsafety/testing/glp-frequently-asked-questions.htm#Histopathology. (Accessed 17 May 2021).

Pantanowitz L, Sinard JH, Henricks WH, et al.: Validating whole slide imaging for diagnostic purposes in pathology: guideline from the College of American Pathologists Pathology and Laboratory Quality Center, *Arch Pathol Lab Med* 137:1710–1722, 2013.

Randell R, Ambepitiya T, Mello-Thoms C, et al.: Effect of display resolution on time to diagnosis with virtual pathology slides in a systematic search task, *J Digit Imaging* 28:68–76, 2015.

Sellaro TL, Filkins R, Hoffman C, et al.: Relationship between magnification and resolution in digital pathology systems, *J Pathol Inform* 4:21, 2013.

Shakeri SM, Hulsken B, van Vliet LJ, et al.: Optical quality assessment of whole slide imaging systems for digital pathology, *Opt Express* 23:1319–1336, 2015.

Sheppard AL, Wolffsohn JS: Digital eye strain: prevalence, measurement and amelioration, *BMJ Open Ophthalmol* 3: e000146, 2018.

Shrestha P, Hulsken BJJMI: Color accuracy and reproducibility in whole slide imaging scanners, 1:027501, 2014.

Taylor CRJC: Quantitative in situ proteomics; a proposed pathway for quantification of immunohistochemistry at the light-microscopic level, 360:109–120, 2015.

Thorstenson S, Molin J, Lundstrom C: Implementation of large-scale routine diagnostics using whole slide imaging in Sweden: digital pathology experiences 2006–2013, *J Pathol Inform* 5:14, 2014.

Treanor D, Jordan-Owers N, Hodrien J, et al.: Virtual reality powerwall versus conventional microscope for viewing pathology slides: an experimental comparison, *Histopathology* 55:294–300, 2009.

Tuomari DL, Kemp RK, Sellers R, et al.: Society of toxicologic pathology position paper on pathology image data: compliance with 21 CFR parts 58 and 11, *Toxicol Pathol* 35: 450–455, 2007.

Tuominen VJ, Isola J: Linking whole-slide microscope images with DICOM by using JPEG2000 interactive protocol, *J Digit Imaging* 23:454–462, 2010.

Turner OC, Aeffner F, Bangari DS, et al.: Society of Toxicologic Pathology Digital Pathology and Image Analysis Special Interest Group article: Opinion on the application of artificial intelligence and machine learning to digital toxicologic pathology, *Toxicol Pathol* 48(2):277–294, 2019.

Vodovnik A: Diagnostic time in digital pathology: a comparative study on 400 cases, *J Pathol Inform* 7(4), 2016.

Watanabe J, Asaka Y, Kanamura S: Relationship between immunostaining intensity and antigen content in sections, *J Histochem Cytochem* 44:1451–1458, 1996.

Webster JD, Dunstan RW: Whole-slide imaging and automated image analysis: considerations and opportunities in the practice of pathology, *Vet Pathol* 51:211–223, 2014.

Wienert S, Beil M, Saeger K, et al.: Integration and acceleration of virtual microscopy as the key to successful implementation into the routine diagnostic process, *Diagn Pathol* 4(3), 2009.

Wilbur DC: Digital pathology and its role in cytology education, *Cytopathology* 27:325–330, 2016.

Williams BJ, Treanor D: Practical guide to training and validation for primary diagnosis with digital pathology, *J Clin Pathol* 73(7):418–422, 2019.

Yagi Y: Color standardization and optimization in whole slide imaging. In *Diagnostic pathology*, 2011, Springer.

Zarella MD, Bowman D, Aeffner F, et al.: A practical guide to whole slide imaging: a white paper from the Digital Pathology Association, *Arch Pathol Lab Med* 143:222–234, 2019.

Zarella MD, Yeoh C, Breen DE, et al.: An alternative reference space for H&E color normalization, *PLoS One* 12:e0174489, 2017.

C H A P T E R

13

In Vivo Small Animal Imaging: A Comparison to Gross and Histopathologic Observations in Animal Models

Kathleen Gabrielson[1], Polina Sysa-Shah[2], Claire Lyons[3], Dmitri Artemov[4], Catherine A. Foss[4], Christopher T. Winkelmann[5], Sébastien Monette[6]

[1]Departments of Molecular and Comparative Pathobiology and Environmental Health and Engineering, School of Medicine and Bloomberg School of Public Health, Johns Hopkins University, Baltimore, MD, United States, [2]Department of Urology, School of Medicine, Johns Hopkins University, Baltimore, MD, United States, [3]Department of Molecular and Comparative Pathobiology, School of Medicine, Johns Hopkins University, Baltimore, MD, United States, [4]Department of Radiology and Radiological Sciences, School of Medicine, Johns Hopkins University, Baltimore, MD, United States, [5]Takeda Pharmaceutical Company Ltd., Cambridge, MA, United States, [6]Laboratory of Comparative Pathology, Memorial Sloan Kettering Cancer Center, The Rockefeller University, Weill Cornell Medicine, New York, NY, United States

O U T L I N E

1. Introduction — 424

2. Magnetic Resonance Imaging and Magnetic Resonance Microscopy — 426
2.1. Basic Principles of MRI/MRM — 426
2.2. Advantages — 428
2.3. Disadvantages — 429
2.4. Correlation of MRI or MRM to Gross or Histopathological Lesions — 429

3. Computed Tomography — 430
3.1. Basic Principles of CT — 430
3.2. Image Information — 432
3.3. Experimental Procedures — 433
3.4. Advantages — 433
3.5. Disadvantages — 433
3.6. CT Imaging in Preclinical Toxicology — 434

4. Radionuclide-based Imaging: PET and SPECT — 435
4.1. Basic Physics of PET — 435

4.2. Basic Physics of SPECT — 437
4.3. Comparative Utility of PET and SPECT — 437
4.4. Advantages — 437
4.5. Disadvantages — 438
4.6. Radionuclide-Based Imaging in Preclinical Toxicity Studies — 439

5. Optical Imaging — 442
5.1. Basic Principles of Bioluminescence Imaging — 442
5.2. Basic Principles of Fluorescence Imaging — 443
5.3. Advantages — 443
5.4. Disadvantages — 444
5.5. Optical Imaging in Preclinical Toxicity Studies — 447

6. Ultrasound — 450
6.1. Basic Physics — 450
6.2. Advantages — 451
6.3. Disadvantages — 452
6.4. Ultrasound Imaging in Preclinical Efficacy Studies — 452

7. Translational Application, Safety Assessment, and Drug Screening with In Vivo or Ex Vivo Imaging   453

Abbreviations for Imaging Modalities   453

References   453

1. INTRODUCTION

Few publications have compared noninvasive in vivo imaging to either gross findings or histopathology in rodent models. Many researchers are using either in vivo imaging or histology to test their hypotheses. In vivo imaging methods are ideal for longitudinal evaluations to follow disease progression or to probe different disease processes that histopathology does not address, but in most cases, imaging has been used in investigational toxicity studies rather than routine safety assessment. Evaluation of drugs for toxicity or efficacy typically uses gross pathology as an initial morphologic screening method followed by the gold standard, histopathology. Each of these methods has its own merits and, in most cases, can complement or validate each other. This chapter will focus on examples that utilize both imaging (in vivo or ex vivo) and postmortem pathologic analysis to compare and contrast the strengths and weaknesses of each morphological method.

Molecular in vivo imaging has emerged as an invaluable tool to probe biological processes and pathways in humans and animals. It is now possible to image antibodies or drugs within humans and rodents to detect the molecular distribution of these molecules and validate targets. This is a very important accomplishment as aberrant proteins can be imaged and, at the same time, enable the investigator to visualize a therapeutic at the cellular level. Molecular imaging methods that target disease biomarkers at early time points in principle can replace conventional survival studies which require large numbers of animals, thus serving as a refinement tool in biomedical research (see

Issues in Laboratory Animal Science That Impact Toxicologic Pathology, Vol 1, Chap 29). Since animals can serve as their own controls, longitudinal imaging studies can be designed with powerful statistical methods which require fewer animals to reliably measure toxicity or efficacy outcomes.

The imaging modalities reviewed in this chapter include magnetic resonance imaging (MRI), including magnetic resonance microscopy (MRM); nuclear imaging methods such as positron emission tomography (PET) and single-photon emission computed tomography (SPECT); computed tomography (CT); ultrasound; and optical imaging. Each of these modalities has the capability of assessing molecular expression, and all are currently used on a routine basis in human medicine. Table 13.1 compares and contrasts the important features of each modality as they apply to other small animal imaging options, and also provides a comparison of the imaging options with conventional pathology endpoints. The breadth of currently available imaging systems provides the opportunity to simultaneously elucidate anatomic, functional, and molecular expression within an animal model, permitting rapid translation of new knowledge regarding disease pathogenesis to the human clinical setting. This chapter will focus on the fundamentals of each of these in vivo imaging methods, in comparison to routine gross examination or histopathology, using a broad spectrum of applications in rodent models for human toxicities or diseases.

Miniaturized ("micro") versions of clinical imaging modalities (micro-CT, micro-MRI, micro-PET, micro-SPECT, etc.) have been developed for small laboratory animals (e.g., rodents and rabbits) and have significantly improved

TABLE 13.1 Comparison of the Small Animal Imaging Modalities

	MRI	CT	PET/SPECT	Optical	US	Histology
Modality physics	Magnetic field	X-ray	Radioactivity	Bioluminescence Fluorescence	Sound waves	Light Fluorescence
Noninvasive	√	√	√	√	√	
Longitudinal	√	√	√	√	√	
Reduction of animals	√	√	√	√	√	
Imaging time/animal	10–60 min	min	30–60 min	min	min	days
Spatial resolution	<0.05 mm	<0.05 mm	1–1.5 mm	1.0 mm	<0.03 mm	0.0002–0.001 mm
Sensitivity	µM-mM	nM-µM	pM-nM	pM	µM-mM	
Structure	√	√	√	√	√	√
Measure function	MR spectroscopy, fMRI	√	√	√	√	
Quantitative	√	√	√	√	√	√
Identify gene expression	√	√	√	√	√	√
Translational to humans	√	√	√	√	√	√
Cost	++++	+++	++++	+	+	+
Anesthesia	√	√	√	√	Not always	√

Modified from Haschek WM, Rousseaux CG, Wallig MA, editors: Haschek and Rousseaux's Handbook of Toxicologic Pathology, *ed 3, 2013, Academic Press, Table 9.1, p 289, with permission.*

since the early 1980s. Now these systems are commercially available throughout the world and optimized for small animal imaging in preclinical research. Figure 13.1 illustrates the number of publications using these imaging methods revealed by a PubMed search covering the last 30 years. The leading imaging method, optical imaging, is a broader term which includes several modalities, from more traditional bioluminescence and fluorescence imaging to newer applications, such as photoacoustic (optoacoustic) imaging and optical coherence tomography. Micro-CT continues to be one of the most popular methods in use today, probably due to its growing application in anatomical imaging for preclinical testing. This may be due to the recent development of micro-CT systems with sensitive X-ray detectors, cone beam reconstruction algorithms, new blood contrast agents (to enable dynamic preclinical imaging in soft tissue, tumors, fat distribution, and vessel morphology with improved spatial and temporal resolution), and the ability to process certain micro-CT specimens subsequently for routine histopathology analysis.

We have been frequently asked how the resolution of rodent in vivo imaging compares to the resolution of traditional histopathology methods and examination with standard bright-field microscopy. Spatial resolution is the

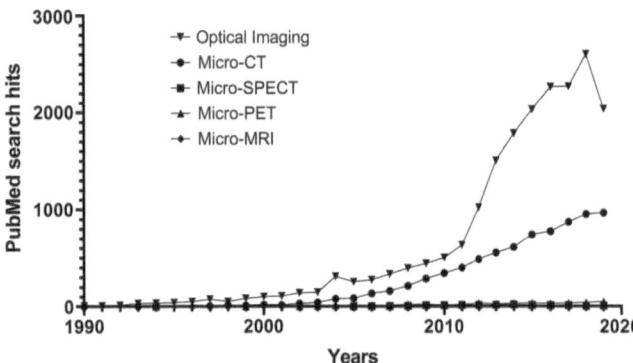

FIGURE 13.1 **PubMed citations for publications in which noninvasive imaging of laboratory rodents was a key feature, summarized for the last 30 years.** Miniaturized versions of human clinical imaging modalities, such as micro-CT, micro-MRI, micro-PET, micro-SPECT, optical imaging, and ultrasound (US), for small animals have been built and considerably improved since the early 1980s. Now these systems are commercially available and optimized for small animal imaging in preclinical research. Optical imaging citations are the most prevalent modalities compared to other imaging modalities as of April 2020.

distance needed between two objects to identify the objects as distinct entities. Diffraction of light limits the resolution of the bright-field (light) microscope to about 0.2 μm (or microns). Bright-field data can provide resolution of about 100 nm using appropriate mathematical algorithms. New superresolution microscopy techniques can further improve resolution to a single protein molecule. However, in the usual practical applications, most pathologists agree that we can discriminate two adjacent bacilli in a field (i.e., 1–2 microns apart) at 400× magnification. Resolutions of various imaging modalities (Table 13.1) are all substantially reduced relative to histopathology, ranging from 10 to 50 microns for micro-MRI, micro-CT, and ultrasound to a millimeter or more for optical imaging micro-PET and micro-SPECT. In vivo imaging technology has improved in spatial resolution over the last 20 years. In most cases, the physics of the in vivo imaging methods may prevent any further major improvements to resolution, emphasizing the need for histopathology to provide the most detailed morphological evaluations, a necessary part of rodent studies.

2. MAGNETIC RESONANCE IMAGING AND MAGNETIC RESONANCE MICROSCOPY

2.1. Basic Principles of MRI/MRM

Both MRI and MRM are based on the principles of nuclear magnetic resonance (NMR), a spectroscopic technique used by scientists to obtain structural information for molecules. NMR is a phenomenon of absorption and emission of energy in the radio frequency range of the electromagnetic spectrum by certain atomic nuclei when placed within a magnetic field. Clinical MRI uses magnetic resonance of hydrogen atoms to obtain detailed anatomical information in living tissue. High-field preclinical MRI/MRS can also use different nuclei such as ^{13}C, ^{29}Na, ^{31}P, ^{19}F, etc., to obtain unique biological information in animal models of human diseases.

An MRI scanner consists of the several key components. The first is a permanent magnet capable of producing a strong static magnetic field. Typically, superconductive magnets produce magnetic fields in the range from 1.5 to 3T (Tesla) for clinical imaging and up to 17.6T for preclinical MRI. The second constituent is a radiofrequency (RF) system consisting of transmitter(s) and receiver(s) that excites the nuclei in the sample and receives the emitted signal; an RF coil or arrangement of multiple RF coils is used to measure signals from the whole body or a sample region to be scanned. Finally, the scanner features a gradient system that includes three orthogonal controllable magnetic field gradients to encode the spatial information required to form an image. The strength of the magnetic field is one of the most crucial factors dictating image quality. Higher magnetic fields enhance signal-to-noise ratio (SNR), allowing higher spatial and temporal resolution with shorter scanning times for rodent models.

Many institutions have imaging core facilities with MRI equipment dedicated for small animal imaging, with higher magnetic field strengths ranging from 3 to 11 T. In comparison, clinical MRI facilities for human patients have significantly larger available diameter and provide a lesser resolution within a large field of view.

For animal imaging, just as in human imaging, specially designed RF coils are placed around the whole body or a specific region of the body that is to be scanned. The inherent isotropic three-dimensional (3D) nature of MRI allows detailed analysis of organs and retrospective studies through any arbitrary plane within the object, whereas individual two-dimensional (2D) planar images can also be recombined into 3D data sets for volumetric rendering. Moreover, MRI has the ability to obtain exquisite contrast between various types of tissue (e.g., gray vs. white matter in the brain) by exploiting the inherent differences in their tissue-specific properties, such as relaxation time, water/fat ratio, diffusion, spectral signatures, etc., by using specific MRI image acquisition modes ("pulse sequences"). The most widely used properties are the longitudinal relaxation time (T_1) and the transverse relaxation time (T_2). Depending on the pulse sequence, either T_1 or T_2 contrast can be emphasized in the image, producing MRI images with differential enhancement of contrasting soft tissues. When applied to excised tissue samples, these contrast enhancement methods have been coined "proton staining," as the unique proton contrasts provided by MRM enable direct examination of the state of water protons in tissues (Johnson et al., 1993).

One of the most important determinants of the SNR is the choice of the RF coil. High-quality coils are made up of multiple smaller coil elements (i.e., array coils). Superconductive RF coils can also improve SNR for micro-MR imaging. However, in spite of these instrument innovations, low signal sensitivity issues continue to be a hurdle for some rodent MRI studies.

The signal sensitivity and contrast can sometimes be improved by the use of contrast agents in MR imaging. The use of contrast agents based on gadolinium (Gd) or iron oxide particles can influence the relaxation times of water molecules in their immediate vicinity. Iron oxide nanoparticles have been used to track cell migration, angiogenesis, apoptosis, and gene expression in various organs. Targeted ("smart") contrast agents have been developed to focus particles to specific cell-surface receptors using conjugated antibodies or smaller high-affinity molecules, such as "affibodies." For example,

molecular imaging of HER2 can be undertaken successfully using a novel class of multiple modality imaging affibodies that include a Gd^{3+}-binding protein or iron oxide nanoparticles and near-infrared (NIR) fluorescent probe Cy5.5 (Gao et al., 2011; Qiao et al., 2011). The protein-based MRI contrast moiety (ProCA1) agent greatly enhanced the MR imaging, was specific for HER2, and required less Gd^{3+}, thus reducing the chances for nephrotoxicity (Qiao et al., 2011).

Diffusion-weighted MR imaging (DWI) is an MRI method that is capable of detecting the extent of apoptosis and potential edema without using a contrast agent. DWI may also be utilized to monitor changes in tissue volume and/or fluid content caused by cell swelling, tumor shrinkage, necrosis, hydrocephalus, and other processes that can occur in the course of therapy. In addition, diffusion tensor imaging can be used to image microstructure of white matter and other organs based on spatially anisotropic diffusion of water molecules along tissue fibers. Alternatively, apoptosis has been detected by MRI using contrast agents based on annexin V conjugated to nanocrystals of iron oxides, Gd-containing liposomes, or quantum dots (QDs) with a paramagnetic lipid coating. Cell death induced by domoic acid, carbonyl sulfide (COS), or acetaminophen can be easily detected by MRI (Nishie et al., 2019; Brown et al., 2012).

The images obtained with MRM are often correlated with gross or histopathologic findings. MRM shares the same physical principles as MRI. The delineation of high-resolution MRI and MRM is somewhat unclear, but does relate to the higher resolution provided by MRM. To obtain the higher resolution, MRM requires much stronger magnetic gradients, typically about 50- to 100-fold higher than those of most clinical imaging systems. MRM can be utilized to image both live and fixed tissues. Usually, the resolution of MRM images is less than 100 μm depending on the length of the scanning time. For example, image acquisition from a fixed adult mouse with a uniform resolution of 43 μm would take roughly 30 min. Further increase in the spatial resolution would require significant increase in the acquisition time to maintain the same SNR in images (theoretically proportional to the power 6 of the resolution increase ratio). MRM is a superb imaging modality for toxicity evaluation in the nervous system, as lesions revealed by imaging correlate well with those observed using light microscopy (Morgan et al., 2004; Ngen et al., 2016).

MRI/MRM has broad applications in studying rodent models of various neurologic injuries and disorders, including hydrocephalus, stroke (especially ischemic), head injury, brain tumors, and spinal cord injuries. MRI can be applied to optimize interventional treatment schedules, validate functional endpoints, or to select the most appropriate sites for tissue harvest and pathology sampling. Longitudinal studies using MRI to define the most appropriate time for tissue harvesting have the capacity to greatly reduce the number of animals required in research studies. In toxicological studies, routine evaluation by conventional histopathology is problematic due to the anatomical heterogeneity of the central nervous system (CNS) and PNS as well as the relatively limited number of planar (2D) sections that can be analyzed from any single subject (see *Nervous System,* Vol 3, Chap 9). In contrast, a comprehensive MRI or MRM study of the brain or spinal cord offers a complementary approach to histopathology by providing individual planar images of a lower resolution that can be combined into a 3D composite image that permits assessment of the entire nervous system as well as digital "dissection" of 2D planes at any angle. The MRI modality is especially well suited for neuroimaging because it can clearly distinguish gray and white matter, and thus can be used to quantitatively map brain regions—especially in the course of developmental neurobiology and aging experiments in rodents conducted in a longitudinal fashion (Chuang et al., 2011).

2.2. Advantages

Compared to CT, MRI provides much greater contrast and more detailed resolution between the soft tissues of the body, making it especially useful for imaging neurological, musculoskeletal, cardiovascular, and oncology models. Additionally, MRI, unlike CT, uses no ionizing radiation. MRM is nondestructive and takes advantage of a unique "proton staining" as define earlier. Both MRM and MRI data are

inherently 3D and digital. Thus a 2D section can be sliced along any plane. Since no distortion from dehydration or sectioning occurs in MRM, morphometric measurements are more accurate than those from traditional histologic preparations.

Movement of the subject during image acquisition can cause artifacts and confound the contrast needed for signal interpretation in MRI/MRM. Consequently, there has been a significant effort to reduce movement artifacts by developing improved animal handing and monitoring methods, as well as novel gated or navigator imaging pulse sequences. Gated sequences synchronize MRI acquisition with respiratory motions and cardiac cycle measured by a physiology monitoring system. Alternatively, navigator techniques monitor motion in real time using an additional pulse to selectively produce echo signals from the diaphragm region and to trigger image acquisition at the end of expiration or to retrospectively select out imaging data that were acquired at end of expiration (Huang et al., 2015). Increasingly sophisticated anesthetic delivery systems are able to provide physiological monitoring and supportive care for rodent species during imaging studies. These monitoring devices typically employ fiber optic technology, making them MRI compatible while monitoring respiratory rate, heart rate, body temperature, tidal volume, and electrocardiographic readings during image acquisition. Furthermore, spatial resolution can be significantly enhanced during MRI of rodents by cardiac gating and respiratory synchronization, thus decreasing the motion artifact while images are being acquired. Complete control of respiration requires intubation or tracheotomy and mechanical ventilation of the experimental animals; these procedures are not typically employed for rodents. Finally, cardiac (i.e., electrocardiographic) and thoracic motion information is processed by a scan management system to control timing of the MR sequence recording.

2.3. Disadvantages

As applied to small animals, MRM has two major weaknesses. The first is related to the "newness" of the method. The interpretation of MR images must be built upon experience from comparison of tissue sections from diseased organs to the images produced with MRM. For example, using MRM, some lesions cause a hypointense signal, while others produce hyperintense signals. Consequently, from our experience, there is a fairly steep learning curve to acquire the skills needed to interpret MR signals and correlate them with tissue damage that is observed with histopathology.

The second weakness is the accessibility and affordability of the modality. The equipment required is expensive, and the personnel required for development and operation of the facility are in short supply. It is our experience that to establish a high-field MRI/MRM facility, a minimum of $3 million in capital equipment with a one- to two-year lead time is needed to establish a functional center. Furthermore, the higher field strengths in MRI/MRM come with greater maintenance costs and raise increased safety concerns around the use of accessory equipment, as all devices housed in the vicinity of the magnet need to be devoid of magnetic ferrous components.

2.4. Correlation of MRI or MRM to Gross or Histopathological Lesions

Several studies have shown the potential for comparing MRM imaging to histology (Morgan et al., 2004; Ngen et al., 2016; Hanig et al., 2014; Liu et al., 2015; Ramot et al., 2017; Taketa et al., 2015; Tempel-Brami et al., 2015). One signature publication evaluates the utility of MRM in detecting and characterizing COS neurotoxicity in rats (Morgan et al., 2004). Male F344 rats were exposed to 400 ppm of COS for 4 weeks (6 h/day), anesthetized, and then imaged with MRM utilizing a Gd-based contrast dye. As shown in Figure 13.2, exposure to COS was associated with a hyperintense (bright) signal unilaterally in the parietal cortex, where the Gd was able to diffuse; this hyperintense focus corresponds to the region of malacia seen in the corresponding H&E-stained tissue section. Without contrast, hypointense MRM signals in the brain have been shown to correspond to foci of microgliosis with or without neuronal

loss, while hyperintense signals correspond to hemorrhage. Lesions with a hyperintense rim surrounding a hypointense center correspond to peripheral hemorrhage and hemosiderin-laden microgliosis surrounding necrotic cores. Complete evaluation of the entire brain using 3D digital MRM images acquired in vivo was critical for defining a strategy for trimming the brain for subsequent histopathological analysis. This capability is likely to be especially useful in future studies where the heterogeneous parenchyma of the brain will show site-specific toxic responses that might be missed using conventional brain sampling schemes for histopathology. Currently, standard histopathological sampling methods include seven coronal sections for evaluation with placement using brain gross external anatomical landmarks. In the rat neurotoxicity study, only three coronal sections were originally being collected for microscopic examination (i.e., the conventional method at that time) and MRM was able to uncover a previously unidentified region of the brain with lesions which likely would not have been discovered during the previous routine trimming and microscopic assessment.

Using MRI to image tissues in an anesthetized mouse can be useful to evaluate toxicity or to monitor tumor development and progression. For example, male mice have been evaluated for bladder tumors using dynamic MRI with a Magnevistcontrast agent. Transgenic mice expressing the Harvey Ras oncogene driven by the urothelial-specific uroplakin II promoter develop papillary tumors in the urinary bladder. The mice were scanned on a Bruker 4.7T MRI machine for 20–30 min to acquire T_1-weighted images. Figure 13.3 is a composite of images providing comparison of the MRI, gross, and histopathologic features of these lesions. Although MRI can demonstrate a tumor in the bladder cavity, it is difficult to appreciate that the tumor is a papilloma due to the lower resolution with MRI versus histopathological examination. Additionally, the MR image has a band artifact related to the contrast agent on the urine surface. Nonetheless, MRI can be used to screen live rodents for carcinogenic effects of toxicants to provide guidance for when and where to focus the microscopic evaluation.

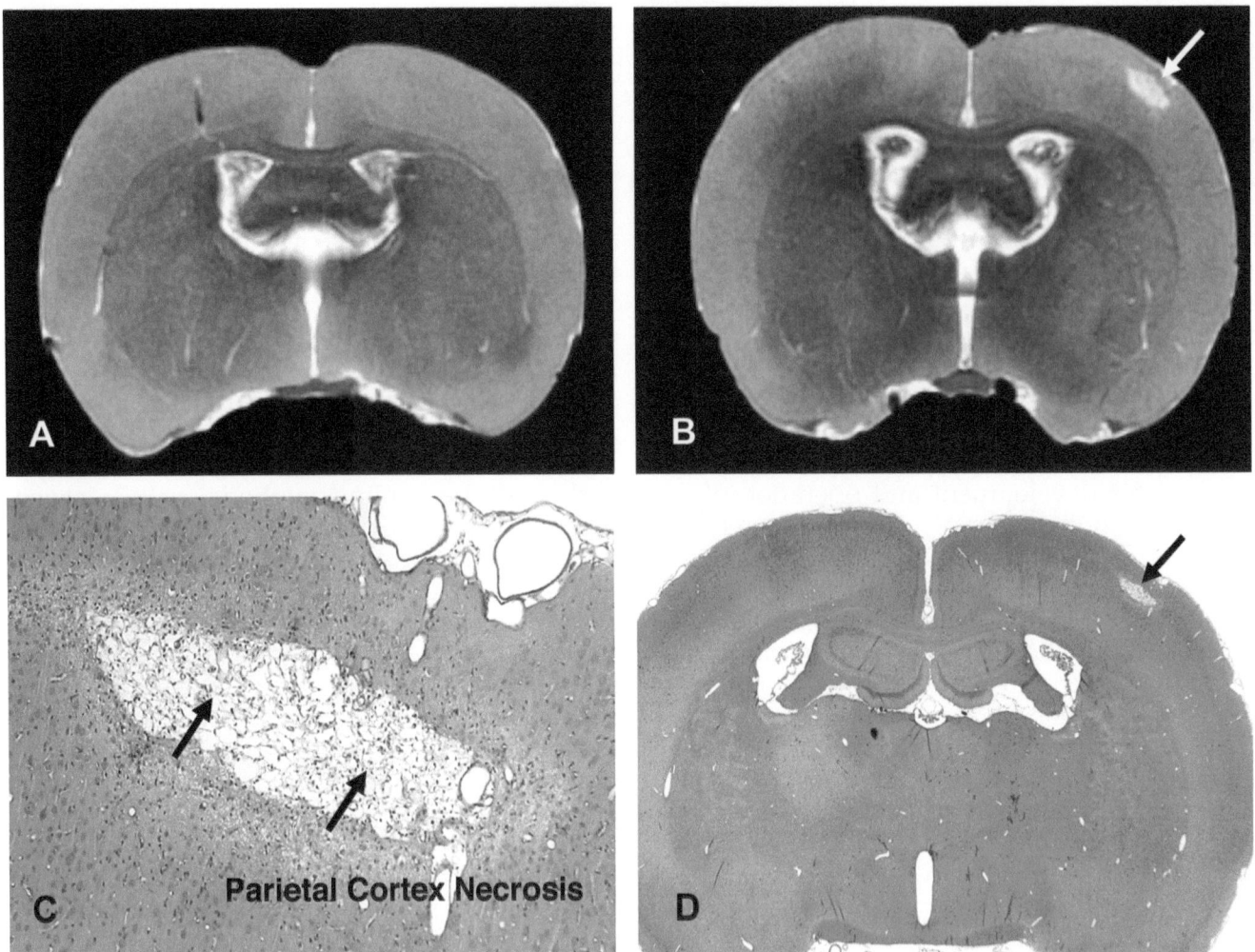

FIGURE 13.2 **Detection of chemically induced neurotoxic lesions in the frontal cortex of rats is well correlated when comparing the results of magnetic resonance microscopy (MRM) and conventional neuropathology methods.** Male Fischer 344 (F344) rats were exposed to carbonyl sulfide at 400 ppm for 4 weeks (6 h/day). MRM images from a control rat (A) and a treated rat (B) reveal cortical necrosis as a hyperintense (bright) unilateral signal (arrows) associated with the parietal cortex. (C) Comparable H&E-stained sections of the treated rat (C and D) showing malacia and necrosis in the parietal cortex; the magnification of panel (D) is comparable to that of the MRM image in panel (B). Since MRM is nondestructive and can rapidly evaluate the entire brain in three dimensions, MRM may give a more complete evaluation of the very heterogeneous brain, compared to the limited survey available using standard sectioning for conventional neuropathology. *Figure reproduced from Haschek WM, Rousseaux CG, Wallig MA, editors:* Haschek and Rousseaux's Handbook of Toxicologic Pathology, *ed 3, 2013, Academic Press, Figure 9.2, p 293, with permission.*

3. COMPUTED TOMOGRAPHY

3.1. Basic Principles of CT

X-ray CT can produce high-quality 3D anatomical images. CT is a mature imaging modality with the first human clinical system having been introduced in 1972 (Pan et al., 2008). More recently, numerous improvements and advancements in the field of CT imaging have allowed development of high-resolution preclinical CT systems for rodents and small specimens; these instruments have been dubbed "micro-CT" due to their spatial resolution in the micrometer scale (typically in the 50–100 μm range for in vivo scans or down to ~100 nm for specimens). The detailed anatomical images produced by CT and micro-CT systems allow

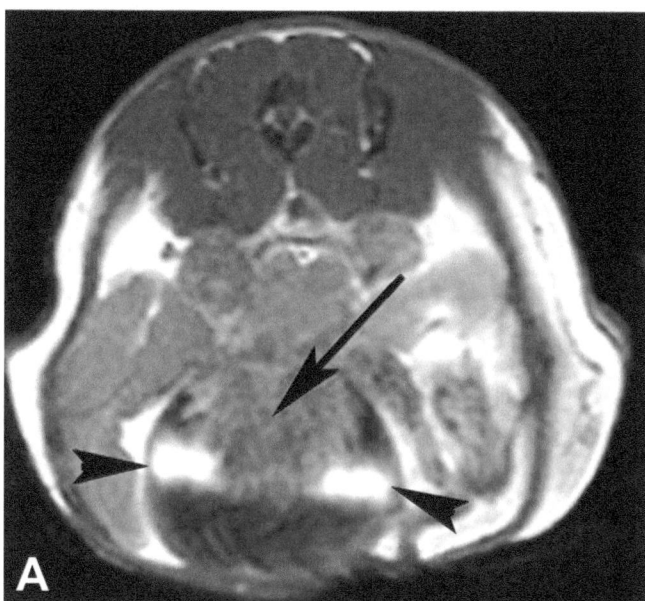

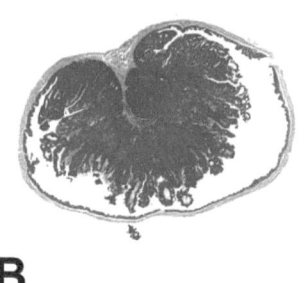

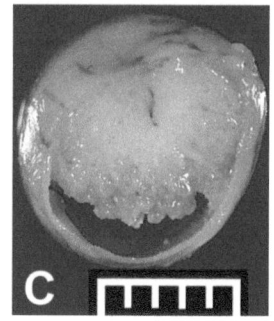

FIGURE 13.3 **Magnetic resonance imaging (MRI), gross appearance, and histopathologic sections offer coordinated views of a murine urinary bladder tumor model.** Transgenic mice expressing the HaRas oncogene driven by the uroplakinII (UPII) urothelial-specific promoter develop superficial, noninvasive, papillary tumors of the urinary bladder. Anesthetized mice were scanned on a Bruker 4.7T MRI machine for 20–30 min to acquire a T_1-weighted image (A). Contrast agent (Magnevist, dilution of 1:5) was used to improve the ability to visualize the bladder tumors with MRI. Although MRI can demonstrate a tumor in the urinary bladder lumen (*arrow*), it is difficult to identify the tumor as a papilloma due to the lower resolution provided by MRI versus conventional macroscopic (B) and microscopic (C) preparations. A band artifact (arrowheads) visible in the MR image is related to accumulation of contrast agent on the surface of the retained urine. *Figure modified from Haschek WM, Rousseaux CG, Wallig MA, editors:* Haschek and Rousseaux's Handbook of Toxicologic Pathology, *ed 3, 2013, Academic Press, Figure 9.3, p 294, with permission.*

this technology to be applied to toxicology studies to provide unique anatomical and/or functional information.

A complete discussion of CT physics and image production is beyond the scope of this chapter, and the reader is directed to several references for additional information (Badea et al., 2008; Krishnamurthi et al., 2005; Ritman, 2004). In general, the production of CT images includes two major steps: acquisition and reconstruction. For image acquisition, an X-ray source is mounted opposite an X-ray detector, and the pair is rotated around a subject positioned in the center. In some micro-CT systems, the X-ray source and detector are stationary and the specimen is rotated. As the X-rays pass through the subject, the radiation is differentially absorbed or scattered depending on the material properties of the different tissues in the path. The attenuated X-rays then leave the subject and strike the detector, after which the incident radiation is detected at a single angular position. This radiation detection at a single position is termed a projection and can be thought of as being similar to a planar radiograph. The X-ray source and detector are then rotated to collect additional projections around the subject (usually several hundreds of projections collected in an arc ranging from 180 to 360 degrees). The CT projections are then converted into tomographic 3D image slices taken through the subject in a process termed reconstruction. This mathematical process takes 2D image elements (pixels) from the projections and then "back-projects" them to form reconstructed 3D image elements (voxels) in the CT image space. Reconstruction is computationally expensive, so methods have been developed to perform these calculations on CPU (central processing unit)-based computer clusters, or more recently, on GPU (graphics processing unit)-based systems to substantially reduce reconstruction times. During the reconstruction process, various image filters can be applied to the input projection data and/or the output image slice data to improve image quality. The output image slices may also be scaled to CT units, termed Hounsfield units (HU), that are typical of clinical CT systems. The HU scale is linear and is defined with air having a density value equal to −1000 HU and water being equal to 0 HU. After reconstruction, the CT images can then be viewed and analyzed by any number of image analysis software programs.

3.2. Image Information

A powerful aspect of the CT platform is that the resultant image data are quantitative both in regard to voxel intensity scaling and for defined voxel dimension. Combined with relatively high spatial resolution compared to other imaging modalities, these CT image attributes can be exploited to obtain unique data. For example, the 3D image can be used to obtain quantitative spatial information, such as measurements of length, width, and volume. The very high spatial resolutions permit "virtual histology" evaluations to be performed by micro-CT for such tiny objects as biopsy specimens and mouse embryos (Cnudde et al., 2008; Metscher, 2009a, b; Albers et al., 2018). Given the linear nature of CT image voxel intensity scaling, the image voxel values can be calibrated using density phantoms within the field of view of the scan as scales for quantifying chemical composition of certain structures. For example, rods of known hydroxyapatite concentration can be used to derive a calibration equation to convert voxel values from HU to units of bone mineral density (e.g., mg hydroxyapatite/cm^3). The exquisite detail offered by micro-CT permits the structural analysis of complex features, such as bone microarchitectural parameters in safety toxicology studies (Vahle et al., 2002). In addition, micro-CT measurements of anatomical parameters at the organ level can be employed to obtain functional data, such as ejection fraction, stroke volume, and cardiac output for the heart and lung ventilation (Badea et al., 2004, 2005, 2006, 2007). Dynamic CT has been used to measure renal parameters relevant to parenchymal (e.g., glomerular filtration rate, fractional tubular volumes, and urine formation rates) and vascular (renal blood flow) functions (Chang et al., 2011). One group has even correlated CT imaging findings to gene expression in liver cancer where a set of distinctive CT features or "traits" specific for individual hepatocellular carcinomas were identified (Segal et al., 2007). The traits were further filtered based

on their frequency, prominence, interobserver agreement between two radiologists, and independence. A module network algorithm was employed to identify associations between filtered trait combinations and expression levels of over 6000 genes as determined by microarray analysis.

Techniques on the cutting edge of CT technology include dynamic contrast, dual energy, and phase-contrast imaging. With dynamic contrast CT, multiple short (1–3 s) scans are acquired over a longer time frame (minutes) while a contrast agent is injected slowly into the subject. As the contrast agent enters the region of interest (ROI) (e.g., a tumor), various functional parameters can be extracted from the dynamic CT data set, such as regional blood flow and volume, mean transit time, and microvessel permeability surface area product (Cao et al., 2009; Kan et al., 2005; Purdie et al., 2001). For dual energy CT, image data sets are acquired at two different energy levels(Petersilka et al., 2008). Since materials (e.g., bone vs. contrast agent) absorb radiation at different amounts along the X-ray energy spectrum, these material properties can be exploited to visually remove tissue from an image data set (e.g., remove the voxels corresponding to bone, but leave the voxels corresponding to contrast agent) (Granton et al., 2008; Tran et al., 2009). Dual energy imaging can also be used to improve temporal resolution in cardiac imaging. For phase-contrast CT, the X-ray radiation passes through the subject and then forms interference patterns based on the phase discrepancy produced by various tissues (Momose, 2002; Momose et al., 1996, 2000; Takeda et al., 2000). These interference patterns have been shown to highlight soft tissue structures much better than typical CT images; however this type of CT technology is not widely available at present.

3.3. Experimental Procedures

Contrast resolution refers to the ability of an imaging modality to discern between objects of similar contrast, or gray value. In CT, similar to conventional radiographs, the image is usually scaled so that air is close to black in color, bone is visualized as white, and soft tissues adopt various shades of gray. Given the biologic contrast provided by bone and lung (air),

CT imaging provides excellent information on the skeleton and lung without the need for externally administered contrast agents (Campbell and Sophocleous, 2014; Vasquez et al., 2008). Since most soft tissue structures have a high water content, the contrast between most of these tissues is minimal (e.g., kidney vs. liver). To be able to differentiate soft tissue structures, contrast agents and protocols have been developed to selectively highlight various organs and systems (Ford et al., 2006; Herman, 2004; Johnson et al., 2005; Lam et al., 2007; Willekens et al., 2009). For example, iodine-based contrast agents are routinely given by intravascular injection to highlight the vessels and heart. Some of these agents are filtered and excreted by the kidneys, which then allows the kidneys to be easily visualized (Almajdub et al., 2008). In addition, lipid nanoparticle–based contrast agents have been developed that are taken up by hepatocytes to emphasize the liver (Graham et al., 2008a, b; Suckow and Stout, 2008). Inflation with ambient air has been used as a technique to provide negative contrast for CT-based virtual colonoscopy in mouse tumor models, while barium contrast agents have been employed as positive contrast agents to monitor for the development of tumors and inflammation in the colon in mouse models (Fredin et al., 2008; Pickhardt et al., 2005; Sodir et al., 2006). Another ex vivo technique to increase soft tissue contrast is to perfuse organs of interest with contrast-permeated silicone to form vascular casts. These casts can then be used to obtain high quality micro-CT images, while subsequent digestion of the tissue around the casts permits the direct observation of the vessel networks.

An essential experimental consideration for CT is reducing image blurring due to respiration and/or heart movement (Badea et al., 2005, 2007; Johnson et al., 2008; Johnson, 2007; Walters et al., 2004). Gating refers to the collection of image projections at defined positions within the respiratory and/or cardiac cycle (e.g., collecting projections only during peak inspiration) so that the moving organs appear stationary. This procedure can be accomplished by the use of a small pillow under the subject to detect respiratory frequency and electrocardiographic electrodes to provide cardiac cycle information. Software can then be used to trigger the CT acquisition only when the subject is in the correct phase of the respiratory and/or cardiac cycles. Although gating increases image acquisition times, it results in images with much higher quality.

3.4. Advantages

X-ray CT has several advantages when compared to other imaging modalities. CT is quantitative with high spatial resolution that allows for accurate measurement of many anatomical features. Under certain circumstances, CT also can provide additional functional information. It has relatively fast image acquisition times (as low as a few seconds) allowing for high-throughput studies. In addition, CT imaging is a mature technology that can be translated directly to human clinical medicine. Another exciting advantage of CT imaging (and other imaging modalities) is the potential for automated analysis of image data sets (Baiker et al., 2010; Dogdas et al., 2015; Dullin et al., 2007; Olafsdottir et al., 2007).

3.5. Disadvantages

However, CT also has several disadvantages and challenges. A major concern with CT imaging is radiation dose. For short-term applications, the cumulative dose is unlikely to be a factor, but repeated exposures during the course of longitudinal studies can be substantial. Many factors affect the amount of radiation dose delivered to a subject during a CT scan, including the X-ray source voltage and current, number of projections taken, and the exposure time for each projection. Radiation effects on bone architecture appear to be minimal, but the potential effect of radiation dose on the study outcome still should be considered when designing an experiment (Klinck et al., 2008). Detrimental effects from radiation exposure (see *Radiation and Physical Agents*, Vol 2, Chap 32) in study animals and personnel can be minimized by including appropriate control groups, reducing the number of scan acquisitions over time, and using the lowest spatial resolution that is necessary to achieve the study objectives. Another disadvantage of CT is that data generated by this modality do not provide adequate delineation between adjacent soft tissue structures. This limitation can sometimes be overcome through the use of appropriate contrast agents. A final challenge of the CT modality is the large amount of data it generates. A single CT data set can range from a few megabytes to more than 10 gigabytes depending on the size of the volume of interest and the voxel dimensions. Highly utilized micro-CT systems can easily generate terabytes of data per year. Dedicated image storage systems are typically required to store and manage these data sets, and specialized hardware and software typically is needed to visualize and process CT imaging data.

3.6. CT Imaging in Preclinical Toxicology

Fetal Evaluation

According to regulatory guidelines, pharmaceutical candidates are required to be tested for their ability to induce fetal abnormalities when administered to pregnant animals (Solomon et al., 2016). Visual gross examination of external fetal features, internal organs, and skeletal elements (after staining with Alizarin red) is commonly performed in support of embryo–fetal developmental safety assessment studies. Micro-CT has been developed as a high-throughput modality to evaluate fetal skeletal anatomy in rodents and rabbits (French et al., 2010; Guldberg et al., 2004; Liang et al., 2009; Oest et al., 2008). Also, methods using iodine stains have been devised to allow for CT evaluation of soft tissues.

Micro-CT imaging has been evaluated as a method in developmental toxicology to replace Alizarin red staining in the assessment of rat and rabbit fetal skeletons. Procedures have been developed to enable high-throughput ex vivo imaging of numerous fetal specimens, including fabrication of specimen holders to allow for simultaneous image acquisition from multiple fetuses (up to 20 rat fetuses per scan) and robust processing techniques for image reconstruction and cropping of individual fetuses from scans of entire litters (Winkelmann and Wise, 2009). The micro-CT method has been validated by performing several positive-control studies in rats and rabbits using known skeletal teratogens in which head-to-head comparisons were performed between imaging and skeletal staining outcomes; the model agents were boric

acid, hydroxyurea, and retinoic acid. These studies have shown that CT imaging results are equivalent to staining data at identifying the no-effect and low-effect levels of these chemicals (Wise and Winkelmann, 2009a, b; Wise et al., 2010). In addition, specific skeletal abnormalities such as fused ribs (Figure 13.4) were robustly observed by both imaging and staining. Due to spatial resolution limitations inherent in imaging technology, the smallest and least ossified skeletal elements are sometimes not detected by CT imaging. Additional work has included automating skeletal image evaluation to reduce the resources needed to perform and analyze these studies as well as to decrease interobserver variability in reporting skeletal findings (Wise et al., 2013).

MICRO-CT MICROSCOPY

CT is a very useful technique for evaluating microscopic features of disease. The utility of this technique is particularly good for detecting lesions in tissues with high contrast, such as lung (normal airways are radiolucent [black]) and bone (normal cortical bone is radioopaque [bright white]). For example, female F344 rats given a tracheal instillation of bleomycin solution (3 mg/kg) and imaged by micro-CT 1 week later had increased opacity of the pulmonary parenchyma (Johnson, 2007). The areas of opacity in the CT image corresponded with a peribronchiolar inflammatory infiltrate seen in H&E-stained lung sections (Figure 13.5). The noninvasive CT method can detect very subtle pulmonary parenchymal changes, and can be used to follow these findings as they evolve in the same animal.

4. RADIONUCLIDE-BASED IMAGING: PET AND SPECT

4.1. Basic Physics of PET

PET is based on the principle of electron–positron annihilation. The collision of a positron (positive electron) with an ordinary (negative) electron results in the generation of two 511 keV annihilation photons at an angle that approximates 180 degree, which can be detected by the appropriate apparatus. When PET tracers labeled with positron-emitting radioisotopes are injected into a subject, the decay of the

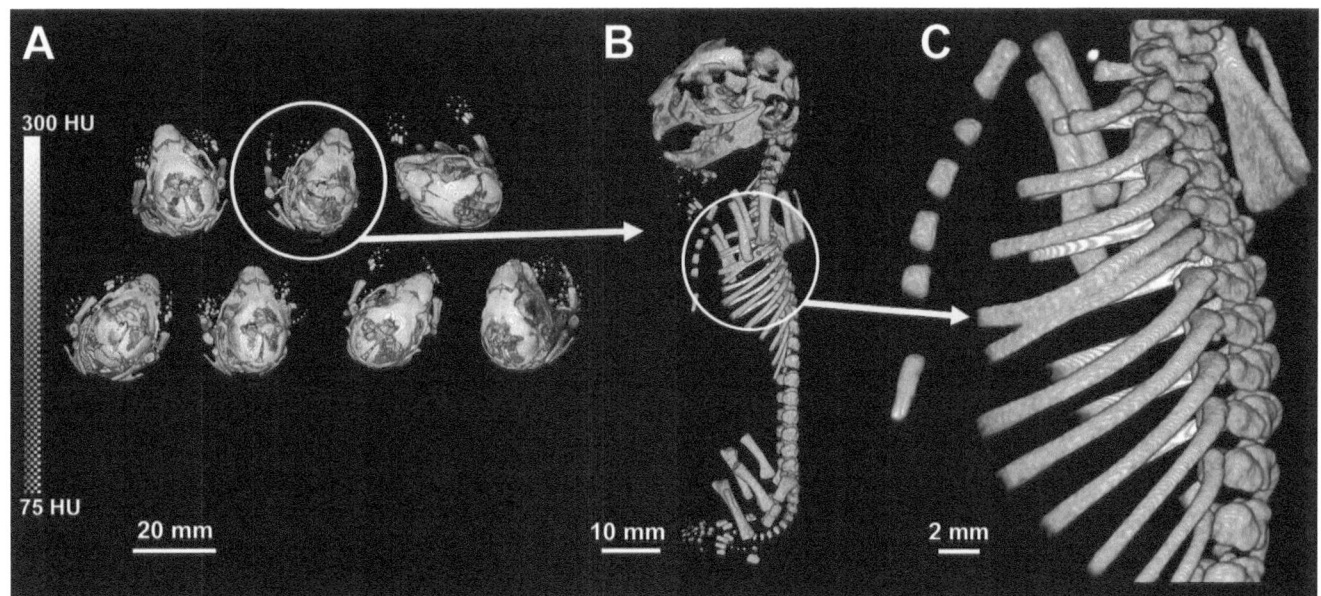

FIGURE 13.4 **Microcomputed tomography (micro-CT) image of a fused rib in a near-term rabbit fetus exposed to a teratogenic compound.** (A) Volume rendering of micro-CT images of an entire rabbit litter (7 fetuses). The fetus in the center of the top row (*yellow circle*) was then cropped digitally and displayed at higher magnification. (B) Volume rendering of this fetus, which allowed demonstration of a fused rib (*yellow circle*). (C) A magnified view showing fusion of the fourth and fifth ribs (*yellow arrow*). A Hounsfield unit (HU) scale bar is present at the left of the figure, displaying the radiodensity of the cartilage and bone structures from lower (75 HU) to higher (300 HU) values conveyed over a range of colors. *Figure reproduced from Haschek WM, Rousseaux CG, Wallig MA, editors: Haschek and Rousseaux's Handbook of Toxicologic Pathology, ed 3, 2013, Academic Press, Figure 9.4, p. 297, with permission.*

radioisotope produces positrons, which travel in space in a random fashion until they collide with an electron of similar energy. The coincidence of their arrival at opposed detectors marks the recorded event, and various reconstruction algorithms can be employed to generate a tomographic image, such as the 3D-ordered subsets implementations (OSEM) algorithm, which converts detected photons into a 3D image (Ortuno et al., 2006). PET cameras have detectors arranged in a circle around the subject. The stimulation of two detectors (at 180 degree) reveals the location of the annihilation event and thus the position of the radioactive molecule or tracer at that point in time; the assembly of many such signals in a single plane will produce a 2D image of a slice through the subject (i.e., tomography) while assembly of the slices produced a 3D dataset. The most frequently used radioisotopes for PET imaging include [^{11}C] (with a half-life [$t_{1/2}$] of 20.4 min), [^{18}F] ($t_{1/2}$, 110 min), [^{124}I] ($t_{1/2}$, 4.18 days), [^{64}Cu] ($t_{1/2}$, 12.7 h), and [^{89}Zr] ($t_{1/2}$, 78.4 h).

In cancer imaging, [^{18}F]-fluorodeoxyglucose ([^{18}F]-FDG) is one of the most commonly used PET imaging tracers (Miele et al., 2008). This agent is widely used for both the detection of tumor cells and monitoring efficacy of antineoplastic therapeutics in the preclinical and clinical settings. [^{18}F]-FDG is a glucose analog and thus is actively transported into cells by glucose transport proteins (GLUT). Once inside cells, [^{18}F]-FDG is phosphorylated by hexokinase, which is the first enzyme involved in glycolysis. Phosphorylated [^{18}F]-FDG cannot continue along the glycolytic cycle and becomes trapped inside the cells as [^{18}F]-FDG-6-phosphate, whose accumulated radioactivity is detected by PET. Tumor cells have increased glucose metabolism (known as the Warburg effect) (Miele et al., 2008; Serkova and Eckhardt, 2016) and are also known to have upregulated GLUT expression, demonstrating the utility of FDG-PET for cancer diagnosis. However, host cells in stromal compartments also display increased glucose metabolism; therefore, FDG-PET cannot always

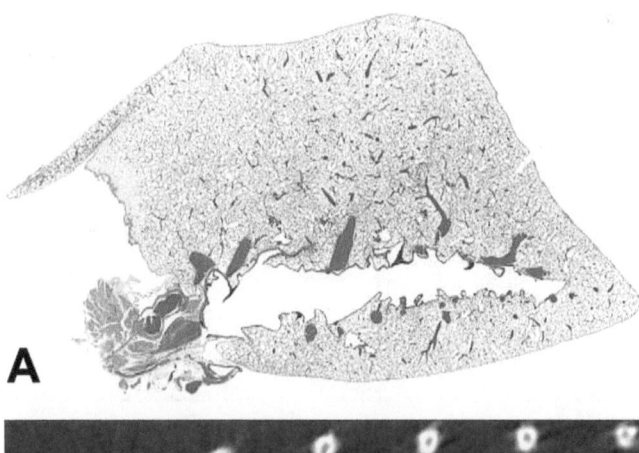

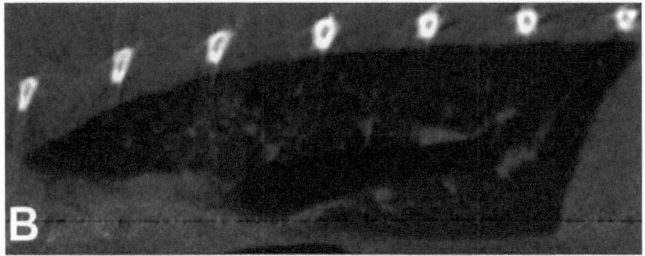

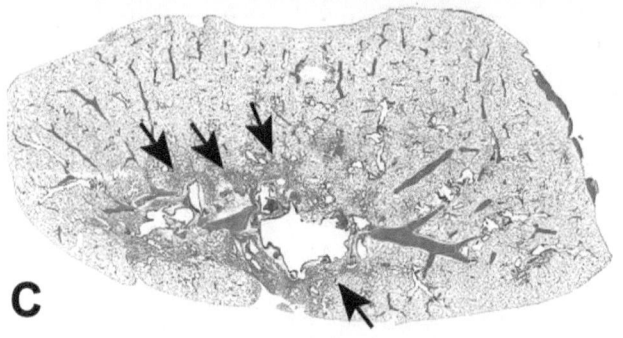

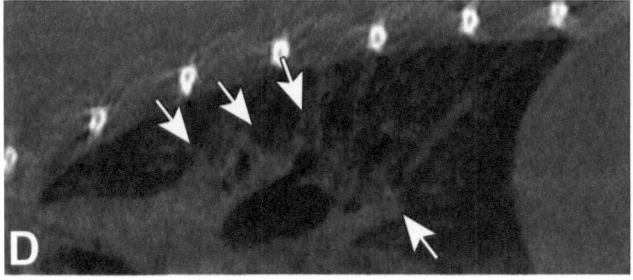

FIGURE 13.5 **Comparison of detection sensitivity for bleomycin-induced pulmonary inflammation between microcomputed tomography (micro-CT) and conventional histopathology.** Histopathologic (A) and micro-CT (B) representations of a saline-treated control lung demonstrate normal morphology of the lung parenchyma, while histopathologic (C) and micro-CT (D) images of a bleomycin-treated lung exhibited substantial peribronchiolar infiltrates (*black arrows* (C); *white arrows* (areas of opacity) (D)). Female Fischer 344 (F344) rats were treated by tracheal instillation with bleomycin (3 mg/kg) and evaluated 1 week later. The noninvasive micro-CT method can detect subtle pulmonary inflammation, although microscopic

distinguish between tumor and associated or stand-alone inflammation.

This imaging modality has been employed in the examination of the CNS. The majority of animal and human ligand activation studies have been performed in the dopaminergic (DA) system to evaluate binding saturation of new neuroleptics (i.e., for understanding novel drug efficacy) even though ligands are available for most major neurotransmitter systems. In the DA system, many of these studies have used [11C]-raclopride, a compound that competes with endogenous dopamine (Ikoma et al., 2008). The high affinity of [11C]-raclopride for dopamine $D_{2/3}$ receptors makes it very useful for monitoring the effects of potential drug candidates on DA neurons that may be therapeutic for certain neurodegenerative and neuropsychiatric diseases. Since CNS diseases represent one of the final frontiers of medicine with few new treatments and a tissue compartment refractory to biopsy, PET imaging represents an ideal tool to examine altered biochemical states within individuals during an episode of illness and during remission. Additionally, the use of PET to verify drug delivery across the blood–brain barrier and target engagement within the affected subregions and/or lesions is paramount to the development of new diagnostics. It can also enhance understanding of CNS pathologies at the molecular level that currently are defined by subjective symptoms or behavioral scores (Slough et al., 2016). Because pharmacotherapies target biochemistry and, secondarily, physiological processes such as blood pressure and electrolyte balance, PET and SPECT are the ideal tools to reveal and quantitate pathological biochemical changes to direct diagnosis and therapeutic regimen in affected individuals. These changes noted by imaging can and should be correlated to gross pathologies noted in anatomy, physiology, and behavior so that clinicians can understand the relationships between what they observe and the true diagnosis.

examination of H&E-stained formalin-fixed tissue sections is necessary to define the cellular nature of the CT lesion. *Figure reproduced from Haschek WM, Rousseaux CG, Wallig MA, editors:* Haschek and Rousseaux's Handbook of Toxicologic Pathology, *ed 3, 2013, Academic Press, Figure 9.5, p. 298, with permission.*

4.2. Basic Physics of SPECT

SPECT takes advantage of isotopes that decay by gamma emission and/or electron capture (Khalil et al., 2011). Some radionuclide nuclei that are rich in protons are able to capture an orbiting electron, resulting in the generation of a neutron. The daughter nucleus formed by electron capture often remains in an excited or metastable state, subsequently achieving a ground state and producing a single gamma photon in the process. The most widely used radioisotopes for SPECT imaging include $[^{125}I]$ ($t_{1/2}$, 59.4 days), $[^{111}In]$ ($t_{1/2}$, 2.83 days), $[^{123}I]$ ($t_{1/2}$, 13.2 h), and $[^{99}Tc]$ ($t_{1/2}$, 6.01 h).

Since gamma rays are directly emitted from the site of decay, theoretically there is no limit on spatial resolution for SPECT. However, the emission of a single photon in SPECT means that the instrumentation must be different from that of PET. SPECT requires the use of a collimator instead of coincidence detection as is practiced in PET. A collimator is a lead block containing one or more tiny holes that is placed between the subject and the radiation detector. The holes are designed to permit only photons of parallel trajectory to pass through the collimator to reach the detector. The origin of the detected photon can be linearly extrapolated from the knowledge of the orientation of the holes in the collimator. In contrast to parallel photons, nonparallel gamma rays are not detected because they deviate slightly and become absorbed by the lead. As many potentially informative photons are filtered out by collimation, SPECT detection is about 1000 times less efficient than PET coincidence detection but has higher resolution in preclinical settings (Khalil et al., 2011; Bernsen et al., 2014; Chatziioannou, 2005).

4.3. Comparative Utility of PET and SPECT

Because SPECT photons must be collimated for detection, the SPECT technique is considered to be the less sensitive modality compared with PET. In general, SPECT permits clearer imaging of non-CNS biological processes because of a longer physical $t_{1/2}$ of the SPECT tracers, has more readily available tracers, and employs less expensive equipment. Although less sensitive than PET, advances in collimator design and radiation detection have made SPECT sensitive enough for use in nearly all of the same applications. Because the nuclides used to label SPECT radiotracers are either relatively high molecular weight or require a chelator to attach them to the probe ($[^{111}In]$ and $[^{99m}Tc]$), the probes then are unsuitable for the CNS except in cases where the blood–brain barrier has been disrupted as in the case of grade IV glioma, meningitis, or encephalitis (Bernsen et al., 2014). Alternatively, probes that were produced for PET using $[^{11}C]$, $[^{18}F]$, and sometimes $[^{124}I]$ can be repurposed for use with SPECT, and are typically small enough and uncharged and may then be suitable to probe targets in an otherwise healthy CNS (Franc et al., 2008).

4.4. Advantages

The biggest advantage of preclinical radionuclide-based imaging is its potential for translation to the clinic. PET employs physiologic tracers; chelation chemistry (binding metals to other compounds) methods are not required. The tracers for PET and SPECT can be identical to the drug candidate to be tested, and the methods lend themselves easily to quantification (Franc et al., 2008). Information acquired from radionuclide-based imaging can be directly applicable to clinical use for patients through dosimetric analysis. Another advantage of radionuclide-based imaging is its extraordinarily high sensitivity (10^{-9} to 10^{-12} M), which results from its great depth of tissue penetration (Lu and Yuan, 2015). Accordingly, the detection of radioactivity at the surface can reveal the metabolic function from internal organs.

Before analyzing PET or SPECT data, investigators overlay the radionuclide imaging information with MRI or CT images to obtain the precise anatomical location of the radioactivity (Bernsen et al., 2014; Franc et al., 2008; Judenhofer et al., 2007). The MRI and CT images impart structural relevance to the functional/molecular imaging data acquired by SPECT and PET in the ROIs. Anatomical details of ROIs are defined by using CT or MR images before examining the PET data to permit unbiased assessment of how an independent variable (e.g., drug treatment) affected PET measurements in specific regions of an organ. For example, for studies using radiolabeled ligands, the analysis of the PET data follows a three-compartment model: radioactivity in the blood, in the extracellular space, and bound to the ligand's receptor (Nader and Czoty, 2008). Rates of movement of the tracer between compartments are analyzed by sequential PET images acquired over minutes to hours to days, depending on the kinetics of the tracer-labeled ligands and $t_{1/2}$ of the chosen radionuclide. These images are used to generate a distribution volume (DV) in the ROI, which serves as a measure of the percent of the injected dose of radioactive substance in the ROI across time. To quantify and compare PET data after some manipulation, the DV for one ROI is studied in relation to a control region that contains relatively few receptors that have bound the labeled ligand. The ratio of these DVs constitutes the distribution volume ratio, which is the primary dependent variable in most PET imaging studies (Krueger et al., 2020). See *Experimental Design and Statistical Analysis for Toxicologic Pathologists*, Vol 1, Chap 16 for a more comprehensive consideration of independent and dependent variables in biomedical study designs.

Growing interest and recent advances have brought dual-modal imaging systems (i.e., functional imaging with SPECT or PET combined with anatomical imaging like CT or MRI) into routine use in human clinical medicine and animal-based experimentation (Bernsen et al., 2014; Franc et al., 2008; Judenhofer et al., 2007). Indeed, trimodal imaging systems that merge PET, SPECT, and CT data are now commercially available for preclinical research. Efforts to combine optical imaging modalities (e.g., bioluminescence) with other modalities, including PET and SPECT, are underway (van der Have et al., 2009). Multimodal imaging systems enable investigators to acquire imaging data sets more conveniently without moving the subject, which can interrupt perfect coregistration of functional and anatomical images.

Multitracer (dual tracer) PET methods (not to be confused with dual-modal or multimodal methods, such as PET/SPECT or PET/MR) are being developed for use in human diagnostics (Kadrmas and Hoffman, 2013). Only a few studies have been published on multitracer PET applications in nonhuman primates, dogs,

and rats (Nader and Czoty, 2008; Kadrmas and Hoffman, 2013; Black et al., 2009; Casteels et al., 2006; Figueiras et al., 2011). With new cylindrical multipinhole collimators now available for preclinical and soon for clinical imaging, simultaneous multinuclide imaging is now available, allowing an investigator to inject multiple and differently labeled radiotracers for simultaneous imaging obtaining context with a primary target probe. At this time, this technology is exclusively offered by MILabs (Utrecht, Netherlands). Since each nuclide decays with a conserved energy, nuclide decays can be distinguished and reconstructed separately then displayed together. This allows for the probing of activities such as drug docking and selected host responses.

4.5. Disadvantages

Imaging results for PET and SPECT in preclinical applications should be validated by histopathology to confirm target specificity, pharmacological properties, and cytotoxicity of imaging agents. However, histopathologic processing and analysis of tissues permeated with radionuclides is complicated by the presence of residual radioisotopes. Concerns about contamination with radioactivity are particularly serious in cases involving isotopes with a long $t_{1/2}$. If an institution does not have histology core facilities or equipment designated for samples that are contaminated with radioactive materials, investigators should not process fixed tissue specimens until radioisotopes decay (10 half-lives). The emerging protocol for verification of the final disposition of a new radiotracer is to fluorescently label the probe, if feasible, and conduct imaging of the whole animal to assess the amount of fluorescence followed by examination of tissues using immunofluorescence microscopy. If adding a fluorophore is chemically or biochemically unfavorable, whole-body autoradiography is carried out where whole coronal sections are made on a microtome and exposed to film. The frozen or thawed slices are then also available for gross pathological examination to confirm or refute specific binding of the radiotracer to relevant sites of pathology.

General safety concerns about contamination with radioactive materials make PET- or SPECT-based imaging studies more complicated and will require a greater institutional investment in capital resources and ongoing material costs. In most vivariums, animals injected with radiotracers must be housed in a specially designed space and cannot be housed with other animals in the same area. In addition, any waste from animal husbandry (e.g., disposable cages and soiled bedding), imaging procedures, and animal carcasses must be collected and stored separately until radioisotopes decay after 10 half-lives. Furthermore, radioisotope $t_{1/2}$ is important for orchestrating the study design beginning from the isotope production, synthesis, and transportation of the radiotracer, delivery to the patient, and conduct of the study itself—which in total should not take more than two half-lives of the radioisotope. Thus, a radioisotope with a short $t_{1/2}$ cannot be shipped from a distant location so one or more cyclotrons must be maintained on site. Radionuclide-based imaging modalities also necessitate many specialized personnel, such as radiochemists who can produce tracers and medical physicists who can conduct data reconstruction. PET or SPECT imaging takes a longer time per subject compared to CT or optical imaging, with one scan of an animal typically taking from 10 to 90 min. The size of data set is large, ranging from a few hundred megabytes to a few gigabytes for a single data set that includes both CT and SPECT images. Thus, servers with ample storage capacity should be prepared in advance.

4.6. Radionuclide-Based Imaging in Preclinical Toxicity Studies

One application of radionuclide-based functional imaging is to determine the distribution of reporter gene products to detect cancer metastases. For example, herpes simplex virus type 1 thymidine kinase (HSV1-TK) has been widely used as a reporter gene whose expression can be regulated by the progression-elevated gene-3 (PEG-3) promoter, which has specificity for many types of cancer (Bhang et al., 2011). 2-Fluoro-2-deoxy-1-D-arabinofuranosyl-5-iodo-uracil (FIAU) is a specific substrate for HSV1-TK. The working mechanism of HSV1-TK and FIAU is somewhat analogous to that of hexokinase and FDG, except that hexokinase is an endogenously expressed enzyme, while HSV1-TK must be exogenously expressed as a "beacon" reporter. Once a pyrimidine analog FIAU enters a cell and becomes phosphorylated by HSV1-

TK, the negative charge of the phosphate group prevents FIAU from escaping across the cell membrane so that FIAU monophosphate will accumulate in the cytoplasm. By labeling FIAU with a gamma ray emitter like $[^{125}I]$ or a positron emitter such as $[^{124}I]$, the localization and quantity of $[^{125}I]$-FIAU or $[^{124}I]$-FIAU can be detected by external imaging devices such as SPECT and PET, respectively. When mice with human melanoma xenografts are intravenously administered a plasmid construct expressing HSV1-TK under the control of the PEG-3 promoter, HSV1-TK expression occurs preferentially within cancer cells (Figure 13.6A). Since $[^{125}I]$ has a long $t_{1/2}$ of 59 days, the tissue samples from this animal could not be used for histologic analysis because of the contamination and safety issues discussed above. However, large masses still can be confirmed by gross evaluation (Figure 13.6B). As with imaging-based diagnosis in human patients, the locations of gamma ray-emitting masses can be predicted based on the tomographic SPECT-CT images. Another commonly employed reporter gene for radionuclide imaging is the sodium iodide symporter.

Another application for SPECT imaging has been to identify cell death within tissues. For instance, technetium 99m–Hydrazinonicotinamide (HYNIC)–annexin V has been demonstrated by SPECT as a sensitive tool for detecting dead cells in vivo in the heart (Gabrielson et al., 2008). Female Sprague–Dawley rats treated with doxorubicin (2.5 mg/kg once a week for 6 weeks) were injected intravenously with ^{99m}Tc-HYNIC-Annexin V (Gabrielson et al., 2008). The annexin V molecule naturally binds to exposed phosphatidylserine on membranes from dying cells. A SPECT image from a control rat (upper body, Figure 13.7A) contains much less tracer-labeled annexin V than in tissue in a corresponding SPECT image from a doxorubicin-treated rat (Figure 13.7B). Corresponding terminal deoxynucleotidyl transferase dUTP nick end labeling images of heart from control and doxorubicin-treated rats are provided to demonstrate a comparable change shown with SPECT imaging. Importantly, SPECT imaging was able to detect a dose response in myocardial cell death using this model.

Similarly, PET imaging can be employed to evaluate the amount of cell proliferation in neoplasms. For example, 3'-deoxy-3'-[^{18}F]-fluorothymidine is a thymidine analog that is incorporated into the nucleus during DNA synthesis. Following

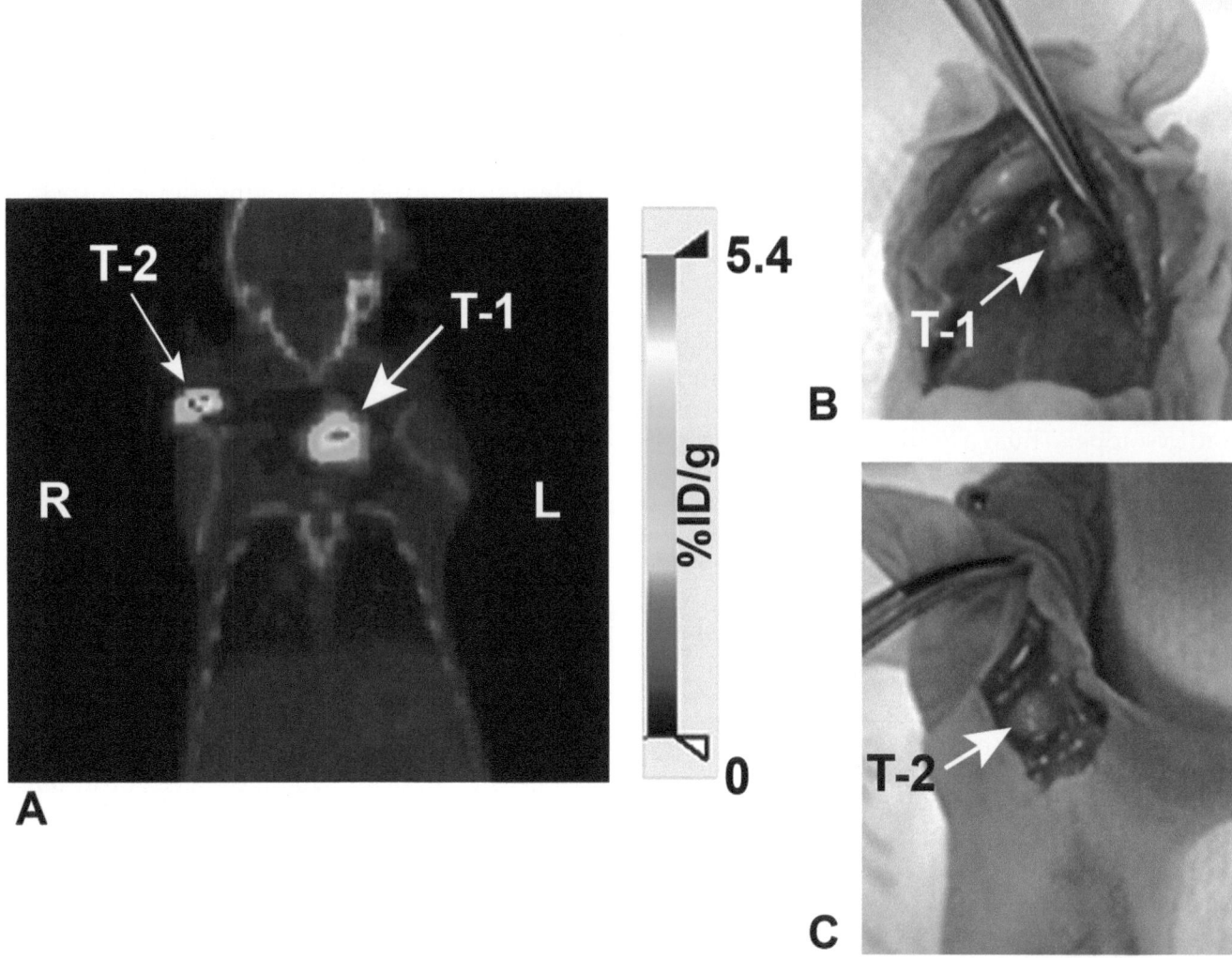

FIGURE 13.6 **Detection and localization of metastases using combined functional and structural imaging in a mouse model of human melanoma.** (A) A coronal view of the coregistered single-photon emission computed tomography (SPECT (functional [colored foci]) and CT [structural grayscale contours]) images. The combined image was obtained at 48 h after intravenous administration of [^{125}I]-FIAU [2′-fluoro-2′-deoxy-β-d-5-[^{125}I]-iodouracil-arabinofuranoside], which was 94 h after injection of the HSV1-TK (herpes simplex virus type 1 thymidine kinase) expression plasmid construct under the control of the cancer-specific progression-elevated gene-3 (PEG-3) promoter. Two metastases were located based on the SPECT-CT image (**T-1** and **T-2**). The radiotracer uptake in tissues is expressed in %ID/g (percentage of injected dose per gram), color-coded from dark blue (lowest) to red (highest). (B) Gross image of the masses that were located based on the SPECT-CT image. Necropsy revealed two tumors under the brown fat (**T-1**) (B) and presumably in the salivary gland (**T-2**) (C), the locations of which correlated with the SPECT-CT image (A). *Figure reproduced from Haschek WM, Rousseaux CG, Wallig MA, editors:* Haschek and Rousseaux's Handbook of Toxicologic Pathology, *ed 3, 2013, Academic Press, Figure 9.6, p 302, with permission.*

intravenous administration of this [^{18}F]-labeled tracer, PET-CT images reveal extensive metastases in a mouse model of prostate cancer. The presence of the metastatic masses was confirmed at the predicted location (regional lymph node) by gross examination, and subsequent microscopic assessment of H&E-stained tissue sections demonstrated the presence of prostatic cancer cells in the affected axillary lymph nodes (Peck et al., 2015; McKinley et al., 2013).

Radionuclide-based imaging signals can be successfully captured using specific cellular proteins to understand disease-related pathways. For instance, a small molecule-based PET imaging agent for cancer diagnosis has been developed that uses the C-X-C chemokine receptor type 4

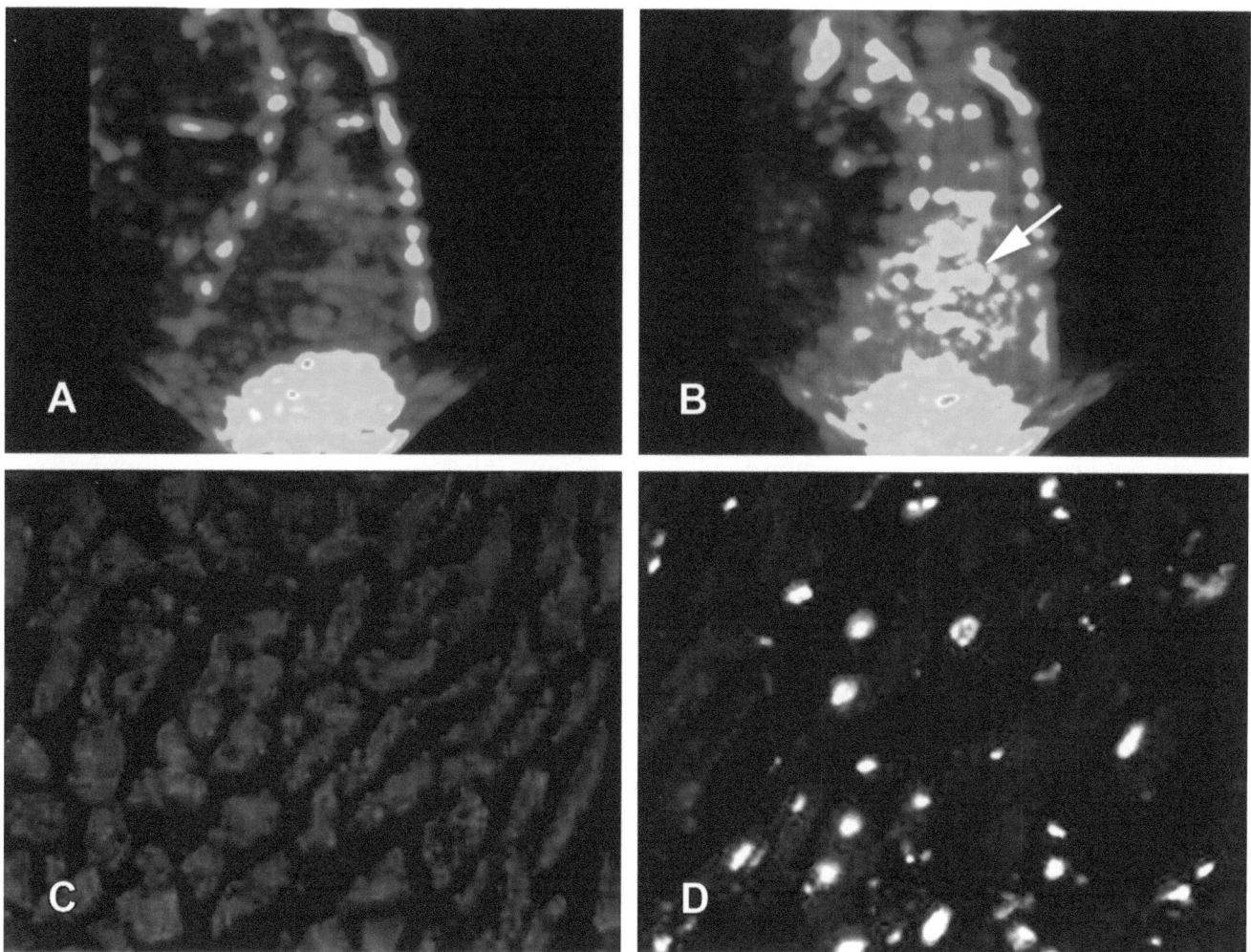

FIGURE 13.7 **Single-photon emission computed tomography (SPECT) imaging of cell death in the rat heart.**
Female Sprague–Dawley rats were treated with doxorubicin at 2.5 mg/kg once a week for 6 weeks. Rats were
injected with ^{99m}Tc-HYNIC-Annexin V; annexin binds to newly exposed phosphatidylserine (a cell membrane
component that is normally hidden in the membrane interior) on dying cells. Relative to a SPECT image of the
thorax of a control rat (A), SPECT images from a doxorubicin-treated rat show increased uptake of radiolabeled
annexin (*arrow*) in the heart (B). The extent of cardiac cell death in TUNEL (terminal deoxynucleotidyl transferase
dUTP nick end labeling)-labeled myocardial sections from control (C) and doxorubicin-treated (D) rats correlated
well with the SPECT data, indicating that SPECT imaging is a useful noninvasive means of identifying cell death
in vivo. *Figure reproduced from Haschek WM, Rousseaux CG, Wallig MA, editors:* Haschek and Rousseaux's Handbook
of Toxicologic Pathology, *ed 3, 2013, Academic Press, Figure 9.7, p. 303, with permission.*

(CXCR4) as a target molecule (De Silva et al., 2011). A ^{64}Cu-labeled version of AMD3465, a monocyclam analog and well-characterized CXCR4 inhibitor, binds specifically to colon cancer xenografts when delivered intravenously into mice. The target-specific binding of [^{64}Cu]-AMD3465 was proven by PET imaging through the coadministration of [^{64}Cu]-AMD3465 with nonradiolabeled AMD3465 to demonstrate competition-dependent binding of the labeled tracer. Following the PET scan, tumors were extracted and confirmed for CXCR4 expression by immunohistochemistry. The relatively short $t_{1/2}$ of [^{64}Cu] allowed processing and histological analysis of the tumor samples from the animals that were also used for the PET imaging, which is the ideal situation when validating such innovative imaging techniques.

5. OPTICAL IMAGING

Rapid advances in optical probes and detection systems as well as genetic engineering have expanded the potential applications of optical imaging for preclinical drug efficacy and toxicity studies. Optical imaging depends on the detection of emitted light in the visible and NIR regions of the electromagnetic spectrum from a ROI. As such, the success of this technology depends on the ability to detect light from tissues of variable thickness and opacity. Light detection in this context depends on highly sensitive charged-couple device (CCD) detectors that are cryo-cooled to minimize noise. Light detectors are composed of thermally generated electrons that flow through a photosensitive device independently of photons that are entering it, hence allowing detection of very low intensity light signal (Moomaw, 2013). Well-established and commonly used optical imaging modalities include bioluminescent and fluorescent imaging methods. In the context of preclinical studies, optical imaging is accelerating pharmaceutical discovery and development through applications that include directly tracking molecular targets, following drug distribution longitudinally, and quantifying the therapeutic effect on the cellular or subcellular target. Moreover, advances in nanobiotechnology have opened the door for examining the molecular aspects of many basic biological questions (e.g., cellular interactions in immunology); numerous disease processes (e.g., cancer and infection); and the interactions of xenobiotics (e.g., drug pharmacokinetics and physiological effects) in the whole animal (Alves et al., 2017).

5.1. Basic Principles of Bioluminescence Imaging

Bioluminescence is a naturally occurring form of chemiluminescence occurring in living organisms, where a chemical reaction releases energy in the form of light. The basis of noninvasive in vivo bioluminescent imaging is detection by a CCD camera of light output occurring deep in tissues as a luciferin substrate is acted upon by a luciferase enzyme reporter (Alves et al., 2017). Luciferase derived from the North American firefly (*Photinus pyralis*) is most commonly used for bioluminescent imaging as it is retained in the cytoplasm of cells expressing the enzyme. Other forms of luciferase that have been cloned and used for imaging include those from the sea pansy (*Renilla reniformis*, also cytoplasmic) and the copepod marine organism *Gaussia princeps* (secreted into body fluids). Firefly luciferase catalyzes the oxidation of its substrate D-luciferin into oxyluciferin using adenosine triphosphate (ATP) as a cosubstrate. This oxidization reaction results in emission of photons at wavelengths of 530–640 nm with a peak at 562 nm. *Renilla* and *Gaussia* luciferases oxidize coelenterazine in an ATP-independent manner leading to light emission peaking at about 480 nm (Hastings, 1996). As bioluminescent signal from a luciferase can only occur as the result of an oxidation reaction with its substrate, there is no background signal generated by the substrate itself. Therefore, the high target-to-background ratio is one of the strengths of luciferase-based in vivo bioluminescence imaging.

Luciferase reporters do not occur as endogenous proteins in vertebrates, so their genes must be introduced into target cells or organs. Necessary strategies for this purpose include the direct delivery of reporter genes through the use of viral or nonviral vectors or transient or stable transfection of cultured cells in vitro with reporter expression vectors followed by implantation of the reporter-expressing cells into animals. Another approach is through generation of transgenic animals expressing reporter genes under the control of a ubiquitous or tissue-specific promoter (Herschman, 2004). The substrate must be administered shortly before imaging. The kinetics of bioluminescence is affected by the route of administration (e.g., intraperitoneal, subcutaneous, or intravenous), the organ or lesion being imaged, and the type of luciferase used.

5.2. Basic Principles of Fluorescence Imaging

The excitation of a fluorophore with one wavelength of light induces fluorescence, which is the emission of light with a longer wavelength and therefore lower energy. As with bioluminescence, fluorescence emissions are also collected by CCD cameras, with the difference that the later requires illumination of the subject during imaging. Unlike bioluminescence imaging, which does not require specific filter sets, investigators engaged in fluorescence imaging must choose filter sets optimized for the excitation and emission spectra of each fluorophore. For this reason, most fluorescence imaging systems contain prepaired excitation and emission filter sets for commonly used fluorophores.

Fluorophores may be naturally occurring or synthesized molecules and include organic dyes and QDs specifically generated to label cells or proteins through direct binding and fluorescent proteins (FPs) such as green fluorescent protein (GFP) and red fluorescent protein (RFP) expressed by genetic engineering or viral or nonviral transfection. After their discovery, wild-type FPs occurring naturally in living organisms, such as the GFP from the jellyfish *Aequorea victoria*, and the RFP DsRed from sea anemones *Discosoma* spp., were originally used for biomedical imaging. Several improved variants of these FPs have since been developed by mutagenesis and now span the entire visible light spectrum (Day and Davidson, 2009). Classic examples of organic fluorescent dyes for use in vivo include FITC (fluorescein isothiocyanate), TRITC (tetramethylrhodamine), and BODIPY (4,4-difluoro-4-bora-3a,4a-diaza-s-indacene) probes (Alves et al., 2017). Organic probes with various excitation and emission spectra are commercially available that can be conjugated to a compound of interest, such as novel therapeutic molecules or imaging agents. One of the most extensively studied nanoparticle-based optical imaging agents is the semiconductor QD (Alves et al., 2017). The use of QDs with sharp emission spectra has become an important means of reducing emission wavelength overlap, thereby allowing the simultaneous acquisition of images for multiple molecular targets labeled using different emission wavelengths (i.e., multiplexing). The QD reagents are synthetic nanocrystals with a variety of metalloid–crystalline complex cores (e.g., zinc–selenium, ZnSe; cadmium–selenium, CdSe; and zinc–sulfide, ZnS) that can be attached to small molecules (nucleic acids, peptides, and proteins). Several factors make QD useful biologic labels, especially their hydrophilic and photostable properties. However, noncoated semiconductor nanocrystals also have demonstrated toxicities and bioincompatibilities that preclude their current use in toxicity studies. Current work with QD is geared toward reducing their toxicity and bioreactivity, for example, by encapsulation in phospholipid micelles (Dubertret et al., 2002).

5.3. Advantages

Compared to other modalities, optical imaging is generally a less expensive and more convenient method, assuming that the location of the target tissues is amenable to the technique (Gabrielson et al., 2018). Software involved with the operation of optical imaging equipment and analysis of data is user friendly. Procedures for operating the equipment are straightforward; in most cases, researchers can perform both bioluminescence and fluorescence imaging without help from staff members with special expertise. In addition, unlike PET or SPECT imaging, the initial data files acquired from optical imaging do not need complex postprocessing and can be analyzed by users immediately after acquisition. The size of the data file is usually significantly smaller than data sets from other imaging modalities. Therefore, data storage space is not a concern for optical imaging. Another significant advantage of optical imaging modalities is the high speed of data acquisition. Even though the acquisition time is determined by the light intensity, data acquisition normally takes between 5 s and 5 min per optical image. This feature enables investigators to apply these modalities to achieving objectives such as serially monitoring the pharmacokinetics of novel imaging or therapeutic agents, following dynamic molecular interactions, or tracking the movement of reporter-tagged cells at multiple time points within a narrow window (Alves et al., 2017). Therefore, optical imaging is useful for high-throughput in vivo screening studies because of its relatively low cost, short data acquisition time, and turn-key user-friendliness.

Recently, small animal imaging has become more frequently used for pharmacological or toxicological testing of novel imaging agents or therapeutics (Maronpot et al., 2017). In these preclinical studies, imaging results must be validated by histopathologic analysis to confirm target specificity, pharmacokinetic or pharmacodynamic properties, and cytotoxicity of the molecules. Unlike radionuclide-based imaging methods, the optical imaging methods are free from radiation hazards, which make not only the in vivo imaging procedure safer but also the subsequent necropsy and histologic preparation. Therefore, optical imaging is a preferred choice for proof of principle studies that can be performed before functional modalities using radionuclide-based imaging are undertaken. Additionally, investigators should consider only the physiological $t_{1/2}$ of the fluorescent probe–labeled molecules and not the physical $t_{1/2}$ when designing imaging studies which makes optical imaging a more attractive option for recurring and longitudinal studies. For example, bioluminescence imaging based on the enzymatic activity of firefly luciferase can be performed every 2 to 3 h since D-luciferin is nontoxic at the standard concentration (i.e., 150 mg/kg body weight or less), while the fast kinetics of bioluminescent signals leads to a return to background levels within 2 h after dosing in most cases. On the other hand, in vivo fluorescence imaging using FPs does not require the administration of any substrates or tracers, which makes the procedure even simpler.

Many of the optical modalities that were primarily developed for in vivo imaging are also amenable to macroscopic and microscopic postmortem imaging, which makes them particularly useful for correlation of in vivo data with anatomic pathology findings (Gabrielson et al., 2018). With appropriate illumination and equipment, fluorescence can be observed macroscopically during necropsy and can guide the prosector in finding lesions not otherwise visible with the naked eye, such as small metastases in lymph nodes. Similarly for bioluminescence, if animals are euthanized shortly after luciferin administration, dissected organs can be imaged and signal quantified at the level of individual organs. Such postmortem macroscopic imaging provides improved resolution relative to in vivo imaging of the whole animal and can be useful in guiding sampling for histology. Microscopic examination can then provide signal detection at the tissue and cellular level, providing further improvement in resolution and correlation with histopathologic findings. This can be accomplished through application of immunohistochemistry using antibodies for luciferase (Figure 13.8) or FPs on formalin-fixed paraffin-embedded tissue sections, or direct observation of fluorescence in frozen sections (most fluorescent molecules do not retain their light emitting properties after processing and paraffin embedding). Therefore, it is possible to harness optical modalities at all stages of an animal study (in vivo, gross necropsy, histopathology), with increasing resolution at each stage, making these methods particularly useful.

5.4. Disadvantages

The most significant challenge for in vivo optical imaging is the limited tissue penetration of the signal. As photons are absorbed and scattered by tissues, the intensity and spatial resolution are significantly affected, and this becomes more problematic when attempting to detect signal located deep within the body. Generally, light of higher wavelengths penetrates better through tissues. Therefore, the wide emission spectrum of firefly luciferase, which includes light above 600 nm, allows imaging of internal organs in mice. For the same reason, NIR probes are the preferred fluorescence modality when deep tissue imaging is required, while probes emitting light at shorter wavelengths, such as GFP, are used for imaging of relatively superficial structures. Even if light can travel through the required depth of tissue, light scattering between the emission site and the surface of the animal often results in poor resolution, often in the order of several millimeters for bioluminescence in internal organs. Therefore, the positioning of the subject is very important to detect the maximal signal; the source of light output must be as close as possible to the imaged surface of the animal. Another disadvantage of most optical modalities is that they are not used clinically, and therefore, their use in small animal models usually cannot be directly translated to application in patients. Bioluminescence imaging is not possible in humans due to the need for expression of a luciferase transgene. Fluorescence imaging with various targeted probes has been shown to have some useful clinical applications, but those are mostly limited to intraoperative imaging (Pogue et al., 2018) (Figure 13.9) due to the

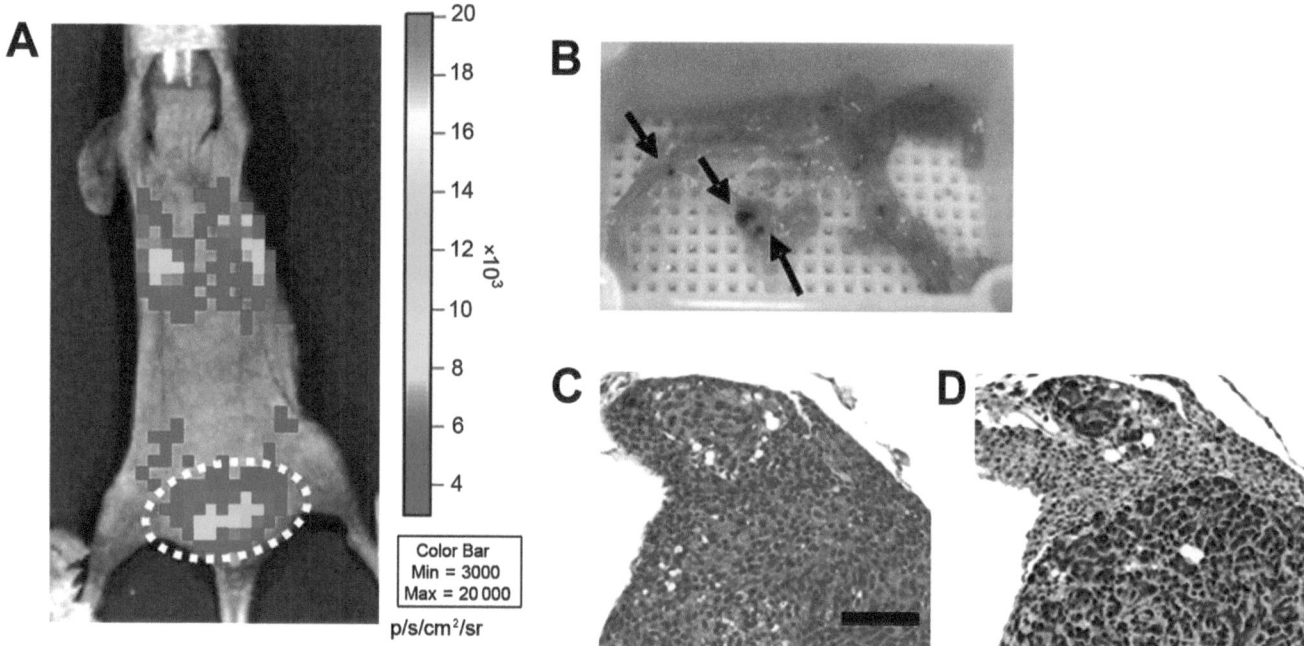

FIGURE 13.8 **Correlation between progression-elevated gene-3 (PEG-3) gene promoter-driven firefly luciferase (Luc) expression and metastatic sites shown by histopathological analysis in a mouse model of metastatic melanoma.** (A) Bioluminescent image (ventral view) acquired 48 h after the delivery of the Luc expression plasmid construct under the control of the cancer-specific PEG-3 promoter. The bioluminescent image is superimposed on a photograph of a mouse, using a scale in photons per second per square centimeter per steradian (p/sec/cm^2/sr) ranging from the lowest (dark blue) to the highest (red) values. (B) Melanoma-associated melanin pigmentation was observed in the abdominal inguinal adipose tissues by macroscopic examination (*black arrows*). (C) Hematoxylin and eosin (H&E) and (D) anti-Luc immunohistochemical staining of the formalin-fixed, paraffin-embedded (FFPE) tissues collected from the animal shown in (A). Organs tentatively associated with Luc expression (A, *circle*) were harvested for histological analysis. H&E staining confirmed metastatic foci of melanoma cells in the abdominal inguinal adipose tissues adjacent to the urinary bladder (C). Immunostaining of serial sections with rabbit anti-Luc antibody (D) shows precise correlation between the localization of microscopic metastasis and Luc expression. Scale bars, 100 μm. *Figure reproduced from Haschek WM, Rousseaux CG, Wallig MA, editors:* Haschek and Rousseaux's Handbook of Toxicologic Pathology, *ed 3, 2013, Academic Press, Figure 9.8, p 307, with permission.*

intrinsically poor depth of penetration of the signal. For the same reason, optical modalities have limited applications in large animal models and are mostly used in rodents.

Another limitation of optical imaging is the availability of reagents. Many classes of fluorophores have limited application in multiplex imaging because their emission wavelengths overlap. This disadvantage can be addressed by using fluorophores with narrow emission wavelengths and selection of optimal image acquisition methods.

For small animal fluorescence imaging, autofluorescence is a major hurdle that significantly affects the sensitivity of detection and the target to background ratio (Leblond et al., 2010).

Autofluorescence is caused by many elements, including hemoglobin (Hb) in erythrocytes and fur, and chlorophyll contained in plant fragments within standard rodent feed. Autofluorescence occurs over a wide range of wavelengths, but the degree to which it interferes can be adjusted by selecting the proper spectrum in which to detect genuine signals. For instance, autofluorescence of Hb decreases significantly at wavelengths >600 nm (i.e., within the NIR range), so the use of an imaging probe that emits in this range is desirable. In addition, autofluorescence can be reduced significantly by feeding animals with alfalfa-free diet instead of standard feed for at least 10 days prior to starting any imaging studies.

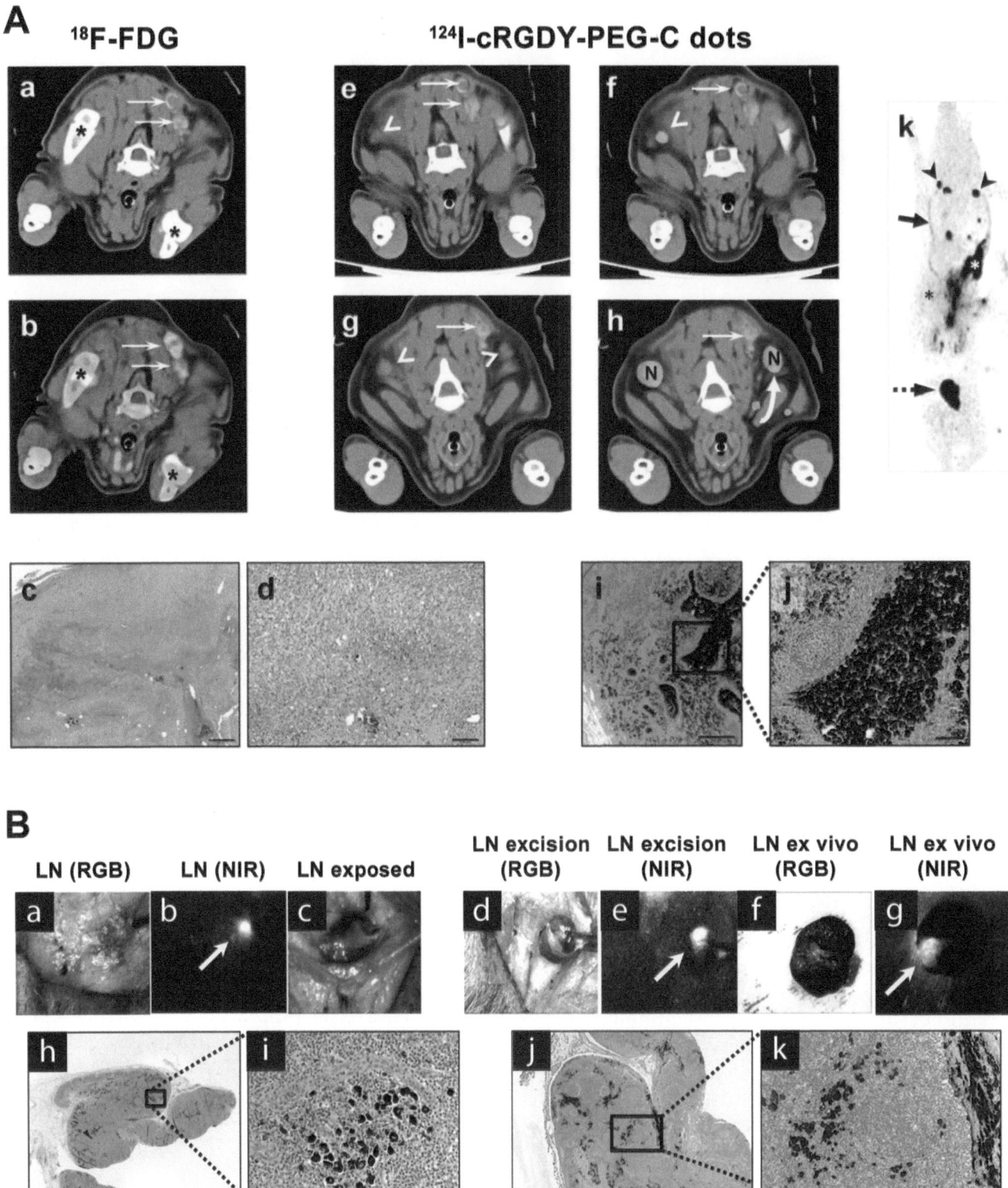

FIGURE 13.9 **Swine model of melanoma PET and optical imaging with pathology validation.** (A) In a Sinclair swine model of melanoma, a novel targeted nanoparticle PET tracer, ^{124}I-cRGDY-PEG-C-dots, was compared to a conventional nontargeted tracer, ^{18}F-FDG. The former uses cRGDY peptide for targeting of integrin expressing tumors, while ^{18}F-FDG relies on the detection of enhanced glucose metabolism, a process which occurs in neoplastic tissue but may also detect other processes such as inflammation. (a, CT; b, fused PET-CT) On fused

5.5. Optical Imaging in Preclinical Toxicity Studies

The strengths of bioluminescence imaging, such as affordability, simple data acquisition and processing, and the lack of safety concern, make optical imaging techniques a preferred proof-of-principle technique for use prior to more complex radionuclide-based imaging modalities, such as PET and SPEC. As shown in Figure 13.8A, the PEG-3 gene promoter was used to drive preferential expression of the luciferase reporter gene in cancer cells in a mouse model bearing melanoma metastases, and the light-emitting metastatic foci could be reliably defined using bioluminescence imaging (Bhang et al., 2011). Because tomography images cannot be acquired using bioluminescent signals, optical imaging is followed by organ harvesting of the labeled regions (e.g., the abdominal inguinal adipose tissues marked with a circle in Figure 13.8A). Subsequent evaluation of H&E-stained tissue sections created from the light-emitting foci confirmed the presence of metastatic nodules of melanoma cells observed grossly (Figure 13.8B and C), and immunostaining of serial sections with an antibody specific for firefly luciferase showed precise correlation between localization of the microscopic metastases and the cell clusters expressing luciferase (Figure 13.8D). The excellent correlation between firefly luciferase expression (as indicated by light emission on optical imaging) and locations of metastatic sites (shown by gross and microscopic examination) provided confidence that follow-on radionuclide-based imaging studies might be expected to provide relevant functional information on the progression of disease in this cancer model.

Similar correlations may be defined using fluorescence imaging and may be applicable to investigation of nonneoplastic diseases. For example, upregulation of the folate receptor is observed on the surface of activated macrophages involved in inflammatory joint diseases. Receptor-mediated folate endocytosis has been harnessed as a means of driving NIR fluorochrome–conjugated folate (NIR2-folate) uptake into synovial cells as an imaging agent for arthritis (Chen et al., 2005). Syngeneic C57BL/6 mice that receive serum from adult transgenic KRN mice with arthritis accumulate NIR2-folate at a proximal interphalangeal joint as detected by in vivo fluorescence imaging. The labeled joint was later shown to exhibit macroscopic evidence of discoloration and swelling that correlated with inflammatory cell infiltration in H&E-stained sections.

Other modalities of optical imaging include optical coherence tomography, photoacoustic imaging (PAI), multiphoton microscopy, Raman spectroscopy, and hybrid methods such as laser speckle and fluorescence and bioluminescence imaging.

PAI employs the photoacoustic effect, which is based on light to sound conversion. This imaging modality has gained particular attention in preclinical studies, with over 2000 PubMed search hits to date. A photoacoustic wave is generated when a short-pulsed light (nanoseconds) illuminates a biological sample and thermoelastic expansion of the optically

---

^{18}F-FDG PET-CT images, hypermetabolic foci were detected in calcified lymph nodes in the neck (*yellow arrows*) and bone marrow (*black asterisks*), and histopathology revealed chronic lymphadenitis with calcification, but no evidence of neoplasia (c, d). Bone marrow uptake was attributed to high hematopoietic activity. In the same animal, after injection of targeted tracer [124]I-cRGDY-PEG-C-dots (e, g, CT; f, h, fused PET-CT), no activity was detected in the calcified nodes (*yellow arrows*) or bone marrow, but PET-avid enlarged nodes were detected (N and *arrowheads*) as well as lymphatic drainage (*white curved arrow*), and these nodes were confirmed to contained metastatic melanoma on histopathology (i, j). Single frame from a three-dimensional (3D) PET image reconstruction shows multiple bilateral metastatic nodes (*arrowheads*) and lymphatic channels (solid arrow) draining injection site (*white asterisk*) (k). Bladder activity is seen (*dashed arrow*). (B) The [124]I-cRGDY-PEG-C-dots also contained Cy5.5, a near-infrared (NIR) organic dye, which was correlated with bright-field macroscopic images (RGB), allowing real-time intraoperative visualization of sentinel lymph node (a to g). Histopathology confirmed a correlation between the optical signal and presence of metastatic melanoma cells within lymph nodes (h, i, H&E, j, k, immunohistochemistry for HMB45 melanocyte marker). *Figure reproduced from Bradbury et al., Integr Biol (Camb). 2013, Figures 6 and 7 with permission Bradbury MS, et al.: Clinically-translated silica nanoparticles as dual-modality cancer-targeted probes for image-guided surgery and interventions, Integr Biol (Camb) 5(1):74–86, 2013.*

absorbing target occurs (Needles et al., 2013). The resulting wave can be further detected by an ultrasound transducer.

PAI combines the advantages of both optical and ultrasound imaging without ionizing radiation or tissue damage: good contrast and multiplexing capabilities characteristic of optical imaging methods complement high spatial and temporal resolution of ultrasound. PAI systems come in different designs, offering resolution from whole organs to organelles. Generally, two configurations are most frequently used: photoacoustic tomography (particularly multispectral optoacoustic tomography or functional photoacoustic tomography) and photoacoustic microscopy (Attia et al., 2019). PAI uses many of the intrinsic optical absorbers occurring in living organisms, the most common chromophores being Hb, lipid, melanin, and water. Detection of Hb is useful in studies of hypoxia, ischemia, or hypoxemia, since PAI can differentiate between Hb and oxyhemoglobin, allowing measurements of the oxygen saturation (Needles et al., 2013; Attia et al., 2019). Imaging of lipids is useful in atherosclerosis studies, while epidermal melanin imaging aids in melanoma, dermatological, and hair follicle studies. Since all these chromophores possess their own absorption spectra, PAI at various wavelengths permits their relative quantification. If the differences in optical absorption are insufficient, extrinsic contrast agents can be employed. Organic dye–based photoacoustic agents are common exogenous chromophores with high extinction coefficients and low quantum yields in NIR-I (650–950 nm) or NIR-II (1000–1700 nm) biological windows. Organic probes such as porphyrin, indocyanine green, methylene blue, and aza-BODIPY have been used in PAI (Fu et al., 2018). In addition, usage of nanoparticle-based PAI contrast agents (gold nanomaterials and polymeric nanoparticles) has gained attention as another prospective PAI application.

Raman spectroscopy is an emerging optical modality that presents significant advantages and opportunities. When matter is illuminated, most of the light is elastically scattered and retains its energy and wavelength (Rayleigh scattering), but a smaller fraction of the light is inelastically scattered with a lower energy and longer wavelength, a phenomenon termed Raman scattering. Because materials of different molecular composition inelastically scatter light differently, they have distinct spectra of inelastically scattered light, terms Raman "fingerprints" (Andreou et al., 2015). Raman spectroscopy is performed by illuminating a specimen and using a scattered light detector to characterize its Raman spectrum. Raman spectroscopy can be performed on cells and tissues without the use of probes, revealing their molecular composition as endogenous proteins and lipids produce distinct signatures, but it can also make use of probes which can be designed to target biological structures or functions. As the Raman effect is a very weak phenomenon in natural materials, because a very small proportion of light is inelastically scattered, nanoparticles have been designed to enhance the intensity of the Raman phenomenon by several orders of magnitude, a strategy called surface-enhanced Raman Scattering (SERS), thereby increasing sensitivity of this imaging modality. In an example of Raman spectroscopy imaging in Figure 13.10, surface-enhanced resonance Raman scattering (an improvement of SERS in which the signal is amplified by resonance between the probe and incident detection laser) nanoparticles were used to detect pancreatic tumors during surgery in a mouse model. Precise correlation of imaging, macroscopic, and microscopic pathologic findings, as well as immunohistochemistry for the nanoparticles, validated the accuracy of the imaging method, which detected not only advanced neoplasms but also early preneoplastic lesions (Harmsen et al., 2015).

6. ULTRASOUND

6.1. Basic Physics

Ultrasound imaging utilizes the interaction of sound waves with living tissue to produce an image. These sound waves are not detected by the human ear as they occur at frequencies of more than 20,000 cycles/sec (Hz); for rodent imaging, ultrasound machines use transducers ranging from frequencies of 2 to 15 MHz. Ultrasound biomicroscopy systems (e.g., VisualSonics units) use frequencies up to 100 MHz to increase

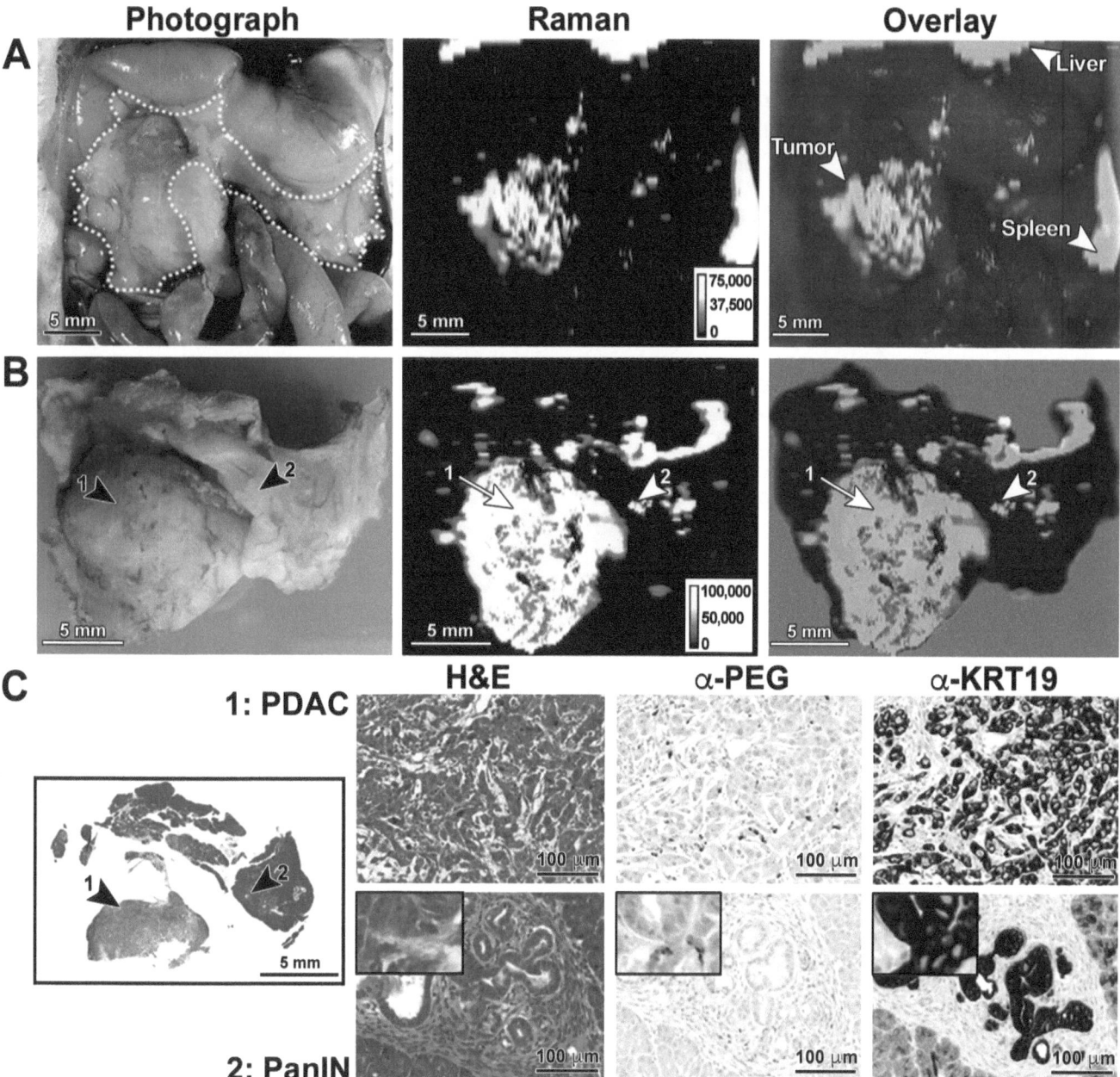

FIGURE 13.10 **Surface-enhanced resonance Raman scattering (SERRS) nanoparticles detect pancreatic tumors at surgery in real time.** Surface-enhanced resonance Raman scattering (SERRS) nanoparticles, designed for resonance in the near-infrared window, and conjugated with polyethylene glycol (PEG), were administered to mice with pancreatic ductal neoplasia as a proof of concept of their use as an intraoperative imaging agent. Imaging of the pancreas in situ (A) and ex vivo (B) revealed diffuse signal in a grossly visible tumor (*arrows 1*), and in multiple small foci in grossly normal pancreatic parenchyma (*arrows 2*), which corresponded to a pancreatic ductal adenocarcinoma and microscopic pancreatic intraepithelial neoplasia, respectively, therefore confirming their high sensitivity for the detection of malignant and premalignant lesions. (C) Immunohistochemistry for PEG was used to detect nanoparticles and for cytokeratin 19 (KRT19) to enhance visualization of proliferative ductal lesions. *Figure reproduced from Figure 13.5 with permission Harmsen S., et al.: Surface-enhanced resonance Raman scattering nanostars for high-precision cancer imaging, Sci Transl Med 7(271):271ra7, 2015.*

structural detail, ultimately providing images with spatial resolutions down to 30 microns (Greco et al., 2012).

Sound waves are transmitted through tissue relative to the acoustic impedance, which depends on the transmission velocity and the tissue density. If two tissues located next to each other have a distinct difference in tissue density, such as myocardium (i.e., a thick wall of cardiac muscle) and the left ventricle (i.e., a chamber filled with blood), there is a significant acoustic impedance mismatch at the interface between these features that causes sound waves to be reflected back to the transducer differently. In general, areas with more dense tissue, such as myocardium, will produce more reflected sound waves and a brighter image. In contrast, fewer sound waves are returned by the ventricular blood, thereby creating the black image of the chamber. Due to these properties, ultrasound is well suited for soft tissue imaging where closely apposed structures often possess different acoustic properties (Coatney, 2001).

The basic components of the ultrasound system include the CPU (or computer), a sound transducer, a monitor, and a storage unit for images. Images (static representations) and movies (dynamic views) usually are acquired and transferred to 640 MB magneto-optical diskettes for storage; a typical cardiac study requires approximately 1.5 MB for a 2D and M-mode ultrasound of the left ventricle. The CPU provides the software for analyzing and obtaining measurements from images. Systems with high frame rates are necessary to image conscious rodent hearts as their cardiac rates often approach 500–600 beats/min. Conventional ultrasound units (i.e., adapted to large animals and humans with slowly beating hearts) and high-resolution ultrasound biomicroscopy systems (i.e., VisualSonics rodent imaging units) may be upgraded when necessary. The high-resolution rodent units have applications that span a range from cardiac evaluation to cancer and development studies.

The transducer is the device that produces pulses of sound and then receives the reflected sound waves. Sounds are generated in the transducer by piezoelectric crystals that vibrate when exposed to electrical currents. Sound waves are focused into a beam and transmitted into the tissue as the transducer is held in contact with the surface of the body. Warm gel is placed on the skin to reduce artifacts created at the air: tissue interface; fur is commonly shaved to further improve contact between the transducer and body surface. The returning sound waves interact with the transducer crystals to produce a small current that is then processed by the CPU to produce an image. Transducers can be handheld or fixed on a grid system. The grid systems are important when conducting delicate in utero ultrasound-assisted injection, such as injections into the lateral ventricle of a mouse fetus (Pierfelice and Gaiano, 2010).

There are multiple modes for tissue imaging with ultrasound. The most common imaging format is the B-mode, in which the image is displayed on the monitor as a gray scale, 2D image of the target organ moving in real time. The real-time image provides information on motion, function, appearance, and size of a target tissue over time. In the heart, the 2D image is initially used to locate a valve or blood vessel. Another analytical variant is the Doppler mode, which is used to measure the velocity of blood. Doppler images represent a color-enhanced map where the flow velocity and direction of fluid movement are superimposed on a 2D image (Figure 13.11). This method can be used to evaluate cardiac valve competency and regurgitation or to assess vessel patency or turbulence. A third option is the M-mode, which is generated when a focused ultrasound beam ("ice-pick view") is transmitted through the heart or other target organ and the resulting image is displayed over time. The M-mode image is used to measure the left ventricular (LV) wall thickness and LV chamber dimensions at systole (i.e., during ventricular contraction) and diastole (i.e., ventricular dilation). Measurements of these chamber dimensions in M-mode permit ejection fraction or fraction shortening calculations to acquire functional data with respect to cardiac contractility (Coatney, 2001; Ram et al., 2011).

Contrast-enhanced ultrasound imaging is another advance that can facilitate visualization of the vascular system, detect targets such as endothelial gene expression, or deliver agents to the vascular bed. Microbubbles filled with inert gas are used to increase the contrast in the blood and the SNR between the blood and adjacent tissues (Denbeigh et al., 2014, 2015;

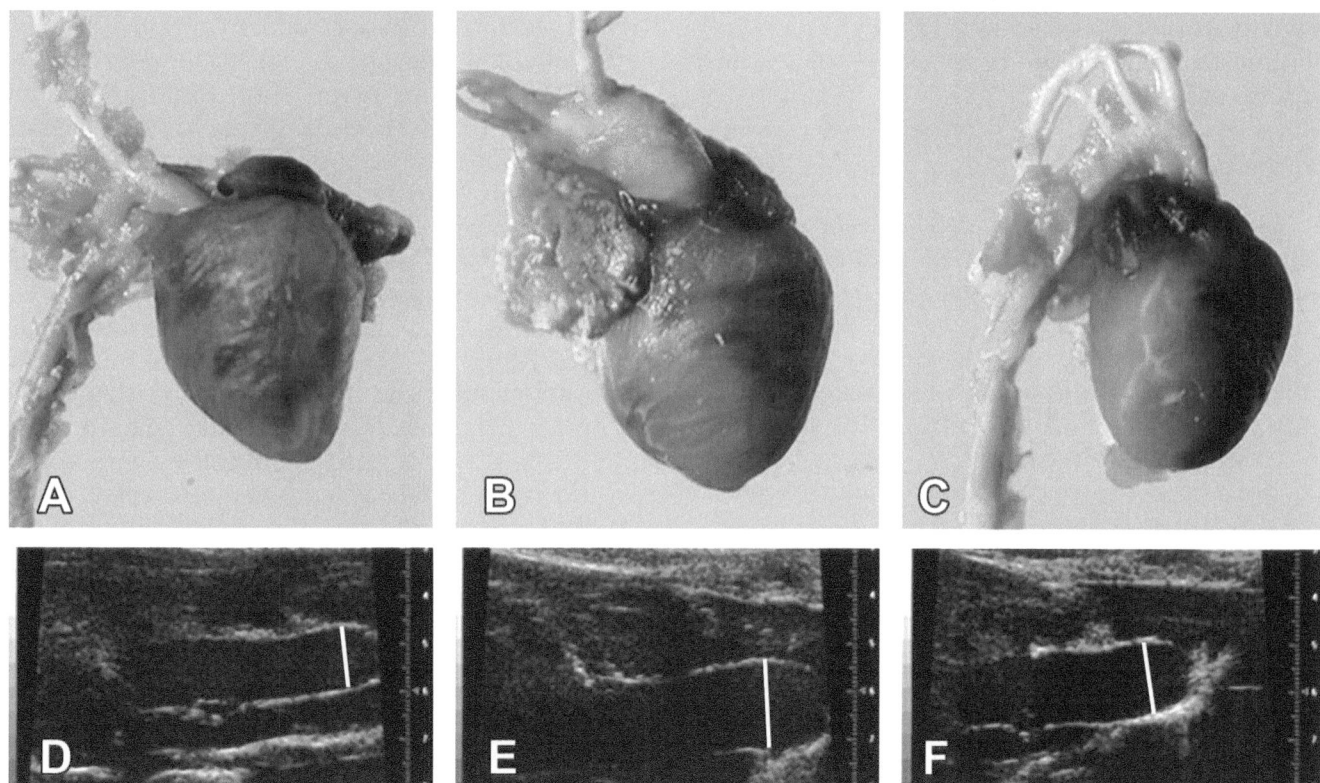

FIGURE 13.11   **Comparison of gross pathology to two-dimensional (2D) ultrasound (US) imaging in a mouse model of Marfan's disease.** Gross pathology and US images of hearts from wild-type mice (A, D) compared to fibrillin-1 (Fbn1) C1039G/+ animals that were untreated (B, E) or that had received Losartan (C, F). Losartan inhibits aortic dilation that develops secondary to the Fbn1 mutation–induced increase in transforming growth factor-beta (TGF-β) signaling. The white bars in the US images span the diameter of the aortic root. *Figure reproduced from Haschek WM, Rousseaux CG, Wallig MA, editors:* Haschek and Rousseaux's Handbook of Toxicologic Pathology, *ed 3, 2013, Academic Press, Figure 9.9, p 309, with permission.*

Kiessling et al., 2012). Additionally, bubbles can be loaded with recombinant material, such as DNA, to carry a payload to target vascular beds. The payload is released for uptake when the bubbles are ruptured using high-energy sound waves (Kiessling et al., 2012).

6.2. Advantages

In general, ultrasound is the only imaging method for use in laboratory animals that does not require anesthesia to acquire an image, although novel methodologies are becoming available for MRI and nuclear imaging applications. An experienced sonographer can pick up a mouse prepared for examination (i.e., gel has been applied and the animal has undergone suitable prior acclimatization to handling and the ultrasound procedure), apply the transducer in the correct body location and at the proper angle, and in seconds locate and acquire an image of the target organ with B-mode or 2D imaging. Routine imaging of conscious mice greatly reduces the amount of time and effort required to perform an experiment. From personal experience, it is possible to screen 40 mouse aortas in an hour, or perform 10 rat echocardiograms in an hour, which serves as an effective demonstration of the high-throughput capabilities of this imaging method.

Since sound waves are not considered harmful compared to ionizing radiation or radioactivity, mice can be imaged longitudinally for months to evaluate a novel drug treatment without safety concerns. This capability reduces the number of mice needed for each time point, as animals can serve as their own baseline controls and undergo serial evaluation. Before ultrasound evaluation was possible, mice necessarily would have to be euthanized at each time point to perform progressive studies.

6.3. Disadvantages

Specialized ultrasound biomicroscopy systems have been developed with a sufficiently high resolution (30 microns) to permit guided injections into structures as small as the ventricles of the brain in mouse embryos. However, the resolution is too limited to discern details at the cellular level. More importantly, specialized ultrasound biomicroscopy systems have limited penetration; therefore, deep structures cannot be effectively imaged.

The high throughput feature of this technique does require a sonographer with extensive animal handing experience and proficiency with the equipment and its capabilities. This skill can be learned with practice on anesthetized animals but must be relearned on conscious animals in order to attain the highest speeds. The majority of sonographers do use anesthesia due to the risk of transducer damage when examining conscious rodents. Transducers can cost $10,000 to $20,000, so considerable care must be taken to prevent damage.

6.4. Ultrasound Imaging in Preclinical Efficacy Studies

Ultrasound imaging of a mouse model of Marfan's disease is one of the best examples of how longitudinal in vivo imaging can drive investigations related to disease mechanisms and ultimately lead to development of a novel drug treatment for human conditions. Marfan's disease is caused by a mutation in the fibrillin-1 (*Fbn1*) gene which manifests as an enlarged aorta that frequently will rupture if not treated. Aortic dilation and aneurysms can be blocked in mutant mice by antibodies that downregulate expression of transforming growth factor-beta (TGF-β); the success of this regimen was shown by serial ultrasound assessments (Ng et al., 2004). Subsequent studies found that Losartan (an angiotensin II receptor antagonist) [COZAAR; Merck & Co] was also successful in blocking the development of aortic dilation and aneurysms in mice, supporting application of this agent in human clinical trials in children

with Marfan's disease which showed similar efficacy of Losartan to previous beta-blocker treatments and an increase in protection against aortic root dilation when given in combination therapy (Habashi et al., 2006; Lacro et al., 2014; Chiu et al., 2013). Figure 13.11 demonstrates the appearance of the normal wild-type mouse aorta compared to the macroscopic pathology observed in aortas of mutant mice (Fbn1 C1039G/+) with and without Losartan treatment. Roughly 700 ultrasound scans were completed on hundreds of mice for this study over 4–6 months. If longitudinal imaging had not been possible, gross pathology evaluation would have had to have been performed on 8–10 times as many mice to reveal the finding that Losartan was effective in blocking aortic dilation. It seems unlikely that such a costly study would have been possible in the absence of ultrasound capabilities. For more information on animal number optimization in preclinical studies, see *Issues in Laboratory Animal Science That Impact Toxicologic Pathology*, Vol 1, Chap 29.

Ultrasound is also very useful in monitoring the development of ventricular hypertrophy and assessing the pathways that can modulate or prevent this change. Surgically induced trans-aortic constriction (TAC) uses a ligature about the aortic arch to induce pressure overload in the left ventricle, which will create cardiac hypertrophy over time. Serial M-mode images of heart may be generated over the course of a 4–6 week study to document the progressive remodeling that occurs in the heart. The phosphodiesterase inhibitor sildenafil has been shown to block the development of ventricular hypertrophy when given to mice with TAC, an effect which can be easily and effectively followed using ultrasound imaging (Nagayama et al., 2009). In such studies, ultrasound imaging is used to capture a 2D image of the heart, after which the scan is switched to M-mode to capture images that can be used for measurements (e.g., ventricular wall thickness and chamber diameter) to probe functional parameters. The structural changes evident by ultrasound compare well to those revealed by histopathology.

Other applications for ultrasound using B-mode or 2D imaging include longitudinal evaluation of tumor xenografts under treatment with various molecule-specific inhibitors (Zlitni et al., 2017) and examination of pregnant mice to define placental and developmental defects (Flores et al., 2014). Many of the cases in which ultrasound imaging is used as a modality for probing mouse disease models can be translated for use in developing new treatments or monitoring patient progress during clinical trials.

7. TRANSLATIONAL APPLICATION, SAFETY ASSESSMENT, AND DRUG SCREENING WITH IN VIVO OR EX VIVO IMAGING

The high and ever-improving resolution of preclinical imaging modalities has the capacity to enable investigators to detect abnormalities at light microscopic levels (e.g., MRM). Nevertheless, bright-field microscopy still provides superior resolution of fine tissue and cellular detail. The various imaging modalities described here offer other advantages, however, such as functional, physiologic, and/or metabolic data acquired in the context of anatomic distribution, which may provide additional information to complement histopathologic evaluation and yield information that may serve as better biomarkers of efficacy and/or safety than standard microscopic tissue analysis.

To date, the main roles of noninvasive imaging in preclinical studies are for phenotyping transgenic animals developed as disease models, target validation using targeted probes, and testing compounds in rodent models of disease. The use of imaging to characterize animal models of human disease in drug discovery may facilitate the translation of novel methods and technological breakthroughs more rapidly from preclinical studies to clinical drug research and development programs. For example, in recent years, the most common imaging method for drug safety evaluation has been MRM for neurotoxicity evaluation (Taketa et al., 2015; Wang Yan, 2008). Recently, new developments in micro-CT have allowed rat and rabbit fetal skeletal morphology to be assessed rapidly and reliably for developmental toxicity studies (Solomon et al., 2016). We look forward to the future when a combination of histopathology and in vivo or ex vivo imaging will be used together to screen new drugs more rapidly and effectively, with a more mechanistic focus, when investigating potential toxicity or treatment efficacy.

ABBREVIATIONS FOR IMAGING MODALITIES

micro-CT microcomputed tomography
micro-MRI magnetic resonance imaging
micro-PET positron emission tomography
micro-SPECT single-photon emission computed tomography
MRM magnetic resonance microscopy

Acknowledgments

The authors are grateful for figure contributions for this chapter. We would like to thank Dr. Robert Maronpot and Dr. Robert Sills of NIEHS, Dr. Alan Johnson of the Duke University Center for In vivo Microscopy, Dr. Marty Pomper, Dr. Hal Dietz, and Dr. Jennifer Habashi of Johns Hopkins University, School of Medicine. From Baylor University, we would like to thanks Dr. Roger Price and Dr. Anita Sabichi. We would also like to thank Merck Research Laboratories for a review of the manuscript.

REFERENCES

Albers J, et al.: X-ray-Based 3D virtual histology-adding the next dimension to histological analysis, *Mol Imaging Biol* 20(5):732–741, 2018.

Almajdub M, et al.: Kidney volume quantification using contrast-enhanced in vivo X-ray micro-CT in mice, *Contrast Media Mol Imaging* 3(3):120–126, 2008.

Alves F BJ, Cimalla P, Hilger I, Hofmann M, Jaedicke V, Koch E, Licha K, Rademakers T, Razansky D, Zandvoort MA: Optical imaging, chapter 16. In Kiessling F, et al., editors: *Small animal imaging*, 2nd Edition, Springer, pp 403–490.

Andreou C, Kishore SA, Kircher MF: Surface-enhanced Raman spectroscopy: a new modality for cancer imaging, *J Nucl Med* 56(9):1295–1299, 2015.

Attia ABE, et al.: A review of clinical photoacoustic imaging: current and future trends, *Photoacoustics* 16:100144, 2019.

Badea CT, et al.: 4-D micro-CT of the mouse heart, *Mol Imaging* 4(2):110–116, 2005.

Badea CT, et al.: Imaging methods for morphological and functional phenotyping of the rodent heart, *Toxicol Pathol* 34(1):111–117, 2006.

Badea CT, et al.: Cardiac micro-computed tomography for morphological and functional phenotyping of muscle LIM protein null mice, *Mol Imaging* 6(4):261–268, 2007.

Badea CT, et al.: In vivo small-animal imaging using micro-CT and digital subtraction angiography, *Phys Med Biol* 53(19): R319–R350, 2008.

Badea C, Hedlund LW, Johnson GA: Micro-CT with respiratory and cardiac gating, *Med Phys* 31(12):3324–3329, 2004.

Baiker M, et al.: Atlas-based whole-body segmentation of mice from low-contrast Micro-CT data, *Med Image Anal* 14(6): 723–737, 2010.

Bernsen MR, et al.: The role of preclinical SPECT in oncological and neurological research in combination with either

CT or MRI, *Eur J Nucl Med Mol Imaging* 41(Suppl 1):S36–S49, 2014.

Bhang HE, et al.: Tumor-specific imaging through progression elevated gene-3 promoter-driven gene expression, *Nat Med* 17(1):123–129, 2011.

Black NF, McJames S, Kadrmas DJ: Rapid multi-tracer PET tumor imaging with F-FDG and secondary shorter-lived tracers, *IEEE Trans Nucl Sci* 56(5):2750–2758, 2009.

Bradbury MS, et al.: Clinically-translated silica nanoparticles as dual-modality cancer-targeted probes for image-guided surgery and interventions, *Integr Biol (Camb)* 5(1):74–86, 2013.

Brown AT, et al.: Correlation of MRI findings to histology of acetaminophen toxicity in the mouse, *Magn Reson Imaging* 30(2):283–289, 2012.

Campbell GM, Sophocleous A: Quantitative analysis of bone and soft tissue by micro-computed tomography: applications to ex vivo and in vivo studies, *Bonekey Rep* 3:564, 2014.

Cao M, et al.: Developing DCE-CT to quantify intra-tumor heterogeneity in breast tumors with differing angiogenic phenotype, *IEEE Trans Med Imaging* 28(6):861–871, 2009.

Casteels C, et al.: Construction and evaluation of multitracer small-animal PET probabilistic atlases for voxel-based functional mapping of the rat brain, *J Nucl Med* 47(11):1858–1866, 2006.

Chang J, et al.: Evaluation of glomerular filtration rate by use of dynamic computed tomography and Patlak analysis in clinically normal cats, *Am J Vet Res* 72(9):1276–1282, 2011.

Chatziioannou AF: Instrumentation for molecular imaging in preclinical research: micro-PET and Micro-SPECT, *Proc Am Thorac Soc* 2(6):533–536, 2005, 510-11.

Chen WT, et al.: Arthritis imaging using a near-infrared fluorescence folate-targeted probe, *Arthritis Res Ther* 7(2):R310–R317, 2005.

Chiu H, Wu M, Wang J, Lu C, Chiu S, Chen C, Hu F: Losartan added to β-blockade therapy for aortic root dilation in Marfan syndrome: a randomized, open-label pilot study, *Mayo Clin Proc* 88(3):271–276, 2013.

Chuang N, et al.: An MRI-based atlas and database of the developing mouse brain, *Neuroimage* 54(1):80–89, 2011.

Cnudde V, et al.: Virtual histology by means of high-resolution X-ray CT, *J Microsc* 232(3):476–485, 2008.

Coatney RW: Ultrasound imaging: principles and applications in rodent research, *ILAR J* 42(3):233–247, 2001.

Day RN, Davidson MW: The fluorescent protein palette: tools for cellular imaging, *Chem Soc Rev* 38(10):2887–2921, 2009.

De Silva RA, et al.: Imaging CXCR4 expression in human cancer xenografts: evaluation of monocyclam 64Cu-AMD3465, *J Nucl Med* 52(6):986–993, 2011.

Denbeigh JM, et al.: VEGFR2-targeted molecular imaging in the mouse embryo: an alternative to the tumor model, *Ultrasound Med Biol* 40(2):389–399, 2014.

Denbeigh JM, et al.: Contrast imaging in mouse embryos using high-frequency ultrasound, *J Vis Exp* 97, 2015.

Dogdas B, et al.: Characterization of bone abnormalities from micro-CT images for evaluating drug toxicity in developmental and reproductive toxicology (DART) studies. In *12th international symposium on biomedical imaging*, 2015, pp 671–674.

Dubertret B, et al.: In vivo imaging of quantum dots encapsulated in phospholipid micelles, *Science* 298(5599):1759–1762, 2002.

Dullin C, et al.: Semi-automatic classification of skeletal morphology in genetically altered mice using flat-panel volume computed tomography, *PLoS Genet* 3(7):e118, 2007.

Figueiras FP, et al.: Simultaneous dual-tracer PET imaging of the rat brain and its application in the study of cerebral ischemia, *Mol Imaging Biol* 13(3):500–510, 2011.

Flores LE, et al.: Early detection and staging of spontaneous embryo resorption by ultrasound biomicroscopy in murine pregnancy, *Reprod Biol Endocrinol* 12:38, 2014.

Ford NL, et al.: Time-course characterization of the computed tomography contrast enhancement of an iodinated blood-pool contrast agent in mice using a volumetric flat-panel equipped computed tomography scanner, *Invest Radiol* 41(4):384–390, 2006.

Franc BL, et al.: Small-animal SPECT and SPECT/CT: important tools for preclinical investigation, *J Nucl Med* 49(10):1651–1663, 2008.

Fredin MF, et al.: Predicting and monitoring colitis development in mice by micro-computed tomography, *Inflamm Bowel Dis* 14(4):491–499, 2008.

French J, et al.: Use of magnetic resonance imaging (MRI) and micro-computed tomography (micro-CT) in the morphological examination of rat and rabbit fetuses from embryofetal development studies, *Reprod Toxicol* 30(2):292–300, 2010.

Gabrielson KL, et al.: Detection of dose response in chronic doxorubicin-mediated cell death with cardiac technetium 99m annexin V single-photon emission computed tomography, *Mol Imaging* 7(3):132–138, 2008.

Fu Q, Zhu R, Song J, Yang H, Chen X: Photoacoustic imaging: contrast agents and their biomedical applications, *Adv Mater* 31(6):e1805875.3, 2018.

Gabrielson K, et al.: In vivo imaging with confirmation by histopathology for increased rigor and reproducibility in translational research: a review of examples, options, and resources, *ILAR J* 59(1):80–98, 2018.

Gao J, et al.: Affibody-based nanoprobes for HER2-expressing cell and tumor imaging, *Biomaterials* 32(8):2141–2148, 2011.

Graham KC, et al.: Contrast-enhanced microcomputed tomography using intraperitoneal contrast injection for the assessment of tumor-burden in liver metastasis models, *Invest Radiol* 43(7):488–495, 2008a.

Graham KC, et al.: Noninvasive quantification of tumor volume in preclinical liver metastasis models using contrast-enhanced x-ray computed tomography, *Invest Radiol* 43(2):92–99, 2008b.

Granton PV, et al.: Implementation of dual- and triple-energy cone-beam micro-CT for postreconstruction material decomposition, *Med Phys* 35(11):5030–5042, 2008.

Greco A, et al.: Ultrasound biomicroscopy in small animal research: applications in molecular and preclinical imaging, *J Biomed Biotechnol* 2012:519238, 2012.

Guldberg RE, et al.: Microcomputed tomography imaging of skeletal development and growth, *Birth Defects Res C Embryo Today* 72(3):250–259, 2004.

Habashi JP, et al.: Losartan, an AT1 antagonist, prevents aortic aneurysm in a mouse model of Marfan syndrome, *Science* 312(5770):117–121, 2006.

Hanig J, et al.: The use of MRI to assist the section selections for classical pathology assessment of neurotoxicity, *Regul Toxicol Pharmacol* 70(3):641–647, 2014.

Harmsen S, et al.: Surface-enhanced resonance Raman scattering nanostars for high-precision cancer imaging, *Sci Transl Med* 7(271):271ra7, 2015.

Hastings JW: Chemistries and colors of bioluminescent reactions: a review, *Gene* 173(1 Spec No):5–11, 1996.

Herman S: Computed tomography contrast enhancement principles and the use of high-concentration contrast media, *J Comput Assist Tomogr* 28(Suppl 1):S7–S11, 2004.

Herschman HR: Noninvasive imaging of reporter gene expression in living subjects, *Adv Cancer Res* 92:29–80, 2004.

Huang SY, et al.: Body MR imaging: artifacts, k-space, and solutions, *Radiographics* 35(5):1439–1460, 2015.

Ikoma Y, et al.: Error analysis for PET measurement of dopamine D2 receptor occupancy by antipsychotics with [11C]raclopride and [11C]FLB 457, *Neuroimage* 42(4):1285–1294, 2008.

Johnson GA, et al.: Histology by magnetic resonance microscopy, *Magn Reson Q* 9(1):1–30, 1993.

Johnson EM, et al.: Intraperitoneal administration of an iodine-based contrast agent to improve abdominal microcomputed tomography imaging in mice, *Contemp Top Lab Anim Sci* 44(6):20–27, 2005.

Johnson EM, et al.: A new method for respiratory gating during microcomputed tomography of lung in mice, *J Am Assoc Lab Anim Sci* 47(4):46–56, 2008.

Johnson KA: Imaging techniques for small animal imaging models of pulmonary disease: micro-CT, *Toxicol Pathol* 35(1):59–64, 2007.

Judenhofer MS, et al.: PET/MR images acquired with a compact MR-compatible PET detector in a 7-T magnet, *Radiology* 244(3):807–814, 2007.

Kadrmas DJ, Hoffman JM: Methodology for quantitative rapid multi-tracer PET tumor characterizations, *Theranostics* 3(10):757–773, 2013.

Kan Z, et al.: Functional CT for quantifying tumor perfusion in antiangiogenic therapy in a rat model, *Radiology* 237(1):151–158, 2005.

Khalil MM, et al.: Molecular SPECT imaging: an overview, *Int J Mol Imaging* 2011:796025, 2011.

Kiessling F, et al.: Ultrasound microbubbles for molecular diagnosis, therapy, and theranostics, *J Nucl Med* 53(3):345–348, 2012.

Klinck RJ, Campbell GM, Boyd SK: Radiation effects on bone architecture in mice and rats resulting from in vivo micro-computed tomography scanning, *Med Eng Phys* 30(7):888–895, 2008.

Krishnamurthi G, et al.: Functional imaging in small animals using X-ray computed tomography–study of physiologic measurement reproducibility, *IEEE Trans Med Imaging* 24(7):832–843, 2005.

Krueger M, Calaminus C, Schmitt J, Pichler B: Circadian rhythm impacts preclinical FDG-PET quantification in the brain, but not in xenograft tumors, *Sci Rep* 10, 2020.

Lacro RV, et al.: Atenolol versus losartan in children and young adults with Marfan's syndrome, *N Engl J Med* 371(22):2061–2071, 2014.

Lam WW, et al.: Micro-CT imaging of rat lung ventilation using continuous image acquisition during xenon gas contrast enhancement, *J Appl Physiol* 103(5):1848–1856, 2007.

Leblond F, et al.: Pre-clinical whole-body fluorescence imaging: review of instruments, methods and applications, *J Photochem Photobiol B* 98(1):77–94, 2010.

Liang C, et al.: Gestational high saturated fat diet alters C57BL/6 mouse perinatal skeletal formation, *Birth Defects Res B Dev Reprod Toxicol* 86(5):362–369, 2009.

Liu Y, et al.: Mammalian models of chemically induced primary malignancies exploitable for imaging-based preclinical theragnostic research, *Quant Imaging Med Surg* 5(5):708–729, 2015.

Lu FM, Yuan Z: PET/SPECT molecular imaging in clinical neuroscience: recent advances in the investigation of CNS diseases, *Quant Imaging Med Surg* 5(3):433–447, 2015.

Maronpot RR, et al.: Regulatory forum opinion piece*: imaging applications in toxicologic pathology-recommendations for use in regulated nonclinical toxicity studies, *Toxicol Pathol* 45(4):444–471, 2017.

McKinley ET, et al.: Limits of [18F]-FLT PET as a biomarker of proliferation in oncology, *PLoS One* 8(3):e58938, 2013.

Metscher BD: MicroCT for comparative morphology: simple staining methods allow high-contrast 3D imaging of diverse non-mineralized animal tissues, *BMC Physiol* 9:11, 2009a.

Metscher BD: MicroCT for developmental biology: a versatile tool for high-contrast 3D imaging at histological resolutions, *Dev Dyn* 238(3):632–640, 2009b.

Miele E, et al.: Positron Emission Tomography (PET) radiotracers in oncology–utility of 18F-Fluoro-deoxy-glucose (FDG)-PET in the management of patients with non-small-cell lung cancer (NSCLC), *J Exp Clin Cancer Res* 27:52, 2008.

Momose A, et al.: Phase-contrast X-ray computed tomography for observing biological soft tissues, *Nat Med* 2(4):473–475, 1996.

Momose A, Takeda T, Itai Y: Blood vessels: depiction at phase-contrast X-ray imaging without contrast agents in the mouse and rat-feasibility study, *Radiology* 217(2):593–596, 2000.

Momose A: Phase-contrast X-ray imaging based on interferometry, *J Synchrotron Radiat* 9(Pt 3):136–142, 2002.

Moomaw B: Camera technologies for low light imaging: overview and relative advantages, *Methods Cell Biol* 114: 243–283, 2013.

Morgan DL, et al.: Neurotoxicity of carbonyl sulfide in F344 rats following inhalation exposure for up to 12 weeks, *Toxicol Appl Pharmacol* 200(2):131–145, 2004.

Nader MA, Czoty PW: Brain imaging in nonhuman primates: insights into drug addiction, *ILAR J* 49(1):89–102, 2008.

Nagayama T, et al.: Pressure-overload magnitude-dependence of the anti-hypertrophic efficacy of PDE5A inhibition, *J Mol Cell Cardiol* 46(4):560–567, 2009.

Needles A, et al.: Development and initial application of a fully integrated photoacoustic micro-ultrasound system, *IEEE Trans Ultrason Ferroelectr Freq Control* 60(5):888–897, 2013.

Ng CM, et al.: TGF-beta-dependent pathogenesis of mitral valve prolapse in a mouse model of Marfan syndrome, *J Clin Invest* 114(11):1586–1592, 2004.

Ngen EJ, et al.: A preclinical murine model for the early detection of radiation-induced brain injury using magnetic resonance imaging and behavioral tests for learning and memory: with applications for the evaluation of possible stem cell imaging agents and therapies, *J Neuro Oncol* 128(2):225–233, 2016.

Nishie A, et al.: In vitro and in vivo detection of drug-induced apoptosis using annexin V-conjugated ultrasmall superparamagnetic iron oxide (USPIO): a pilot study, *Magn Reson Med Sci* 18(2):142–149, 2019.

Oest ME, et al.: Micro-CT evaluation of murine fetal skeletal development yields greater morphometric precision over traditional clear-staining methods, *Birth Defects Res B Dev Reprod Toxicol* 83(6):582–589, 2008.

Olafsdottir H, et al.: Computational mouse atlases and their application to automatic assessment of craniofacial dysmorphology caused by the Crouzon mutation Fgfr2(C342Y), *J Anat* 211(1):37–52, 2007.

Ortuno J, Guerra-Gutierrez P, Rubio J, Kontaxakis G, Santos A: 3D-OSEM iterative image reconstruction for high-resolution PET using precalculated system matrix, *Nucl Instrum Methods Phys Res*, 2006.

Pan X, et al.: Anniversary paper. Development of x-ray computed tomography: the role of medical physics and AAPM from the 1970s to present, *Med Phys* 35(8):3728–3739, 2008.

Peck M, et al.: Applications of PET imaging with the proliferation marker [18F]-FLT, *Q J Nucl Med Mol Imaging* 59(1): 95–104, 2015.

Petersilka M, et al.: Technical principles of dual source CT, *Eur J Radiol* 68(3):362–368, 2008.

Pickhardt PJ, et al.: Microcomputed tomography colonography for polyp detection in an in vivo mouse tumor model, *Proc Natl Acad Sci USA* 102(9):3419–3422, 2005.

Pierfelice TJ, Gaiano N: Ultrasound-guided microinjection into the mouse forebrain in utero at E9.5, *J Vis Exp* (45).

Pogue BW, et al.: Perspective review of what is needed for molecular-specific fluorescence-guided surgery, *J Biomed Opt* 23(10):1–9, 2018.

Purdie TG, Henderson E, Lee TY: Functional CT imaging of angiogenesis in rabbit VX2 soft-tissue tumour, *Phys Med Biol* 46(12):3161–3175, 2001.

Qiao J, et al.: HER2 targeted molecular MR imaging using a de novo designed protein contrast agent, *PLoS One* 6(3): e18103, 2011.

Ram R, et al.: New approaches in small animal echocardiography: imaging the sounds of silence, *Am J Physiol Heart Circ Physiol* 301(5):H1765–H1780, 2011.

Ramot Y, et al.: Compact MRI for the detection of teratoma development following intrathecal human embryonic stem cell injection in NOD-SCID mice, *Neurotoxicology* 59:27–32, 2017.

Ritman EL: Micro-computed tomography-current status and developments, *Annu Rev Biomed Eng* 6:185–208, 2004.

Segal E, et al.: Decoding global gene expression programs in liver cancer by noninvasive imaging, *Nat Biotechnol* 25(6): 675–680, 2007.

Serkova NJ, Eckhardt SG: Metabolic imaging to assess treatment response to cytotoxic and cytostatic agents, *Front Oncol* 6:152, 2016.

Slough C, Masters S, Hurley R, Taber K: Clinical positron emission tomography (PET) neuroimaging: advantages and limitations as a diagnostic tool, *J Neuropsychiatry Clin Neurosci*, 2016:A4–A71, 2016.

Sodir NM, et al.: Smad3 deficiency promotes tumorigenesis in the distal colon of ApcMin/+ mice, *Cancer Res* 66(17):8430–8438, 2006.

Solomon HM, et al.: Micro-CT imaging: developing criteria for examining fetal skeletons in regulatory developmental toxicology studies - a workshop report, *Regul Toxicol Pharmacol* 77:100–108, 2016.

Suckow CE, Stout DB: MicroCT liver contrast agent enhancement over time, dose, and mouse strain, *Mol Imaging Biol* 10(2):114–120, 2008.

Takeda T, et al.: New types of X-ray computed tomography (CT) with synchrotron radiation: fluorescent X-ray CT and phase-contrast X-ray CT using interferometer, *Cell Mol Biol (Noisy-le-grand)* 46(6):1077–1088, 2000.

Taketa Y, et al.: Application of a compact magnetic resonance imaging system for toxicologic pathology: evaluation of lithium-pilocarpine-induced rat brain lesions, *J Toxicol Pathol* 28(4):217–224, 2015.

Tempel-Brami C, et al.: Practical applications of in vivo and ex vivo MRI in toxicologic pathology using a novel high-performance compact MRI system, *Toxicol Pathol* 43(5): 633–650, 2015.

Tran DN, et al.: Dual-energy CT discrimination of iodine and calcium: experimental results and implications for lower extremity CT angiography, *Acad Radiol* 16(2):160–171, 2009.

Vahle JL, et al.: Skeletal changes in rats given daily subcutaneous injections of recombinant human parathyroid hormone (1-34) for 2 years and relevance to human safety, *Toxicol Pathol* 30(3):312–321, 2002.

van der Have F, et al.: U-SPECT-II: an ultra-high-resolution device for molecular small-animal imaging, *J Nucl Med* 50(4):599–605, 2009.

Vasquez SX, et al.: Optimization of volumetric computed tomography for skeletal analysis of model genetic organisms, *Anat Rec* 291(5):475–487, 2008.

Walters EB, et al.: Improved method of in vivo respiratory-gated micro-CT imaging, *Phys Med Biol* 49(17):4163–4172, 2004.

Wang YX, Yan SX: Biomedical imaging in the safety evaluation of new drugs, *Lab Anim* 42(4):433–441, 2008.

Willekens I, et al.: Time-course of contrast enhancement in spleen and liver with Exia 160, Fenestra LC, and VC, *Mol Imaging Biol* 11(2):128–135, 2009.

Winkelmann CT, Wise LD: High-throughput micro-computed tomography imaging as a method to evaluate rat and rabbit fetal skeletal abnormalities for developmental toxicity studies, *J Pharmacol Toxicol Methods* 59(3):156–165, 2009.

Wise LD, et al.: Micro-computed tomography imaging and analysis in developmental biology and toxicology, *Birth Defects Res C Embryo Today* 99(2):71–82, 2013.

Wise LD, Winkelmann CT: Evaluation of hydroxyurea-induced fetal skeletal changes in Dutch belted rabbits by micro-computed tomography and alizarin red staining, *Birth Defects Res B Dev Reprod Toxicol* 86(3):220–226, 2009a.

Wise LD, Winkelmann CT: Micro-computed tomography and alizarin red evaluations of boric acid-induced fetal skeletal changes in Sprague-Dawley rats, *Birth Defects Res B Dev Reprod Toxicol* 86(3):214–219, 2009b.

Wise LD, Xue D, Winkelmann CT: Micro-computed tomographic evaluation of fetal skeletal changes induced by all-trans-retinoic acid in rats and rabbits, *Birth Defects Res B Dev Reprod Toxicol* 89(5):408–417, 2010.

Zlitni A, et al.: Development of prostate specific membrane antigen targeted ultrasound microbubbles using bio-orthogonal chemistry, *PLoS One* 12(5):e0176958, 2017.

CHAPTER

14

Biomarkers: Discovery, Qualification, and Application

Myrtle A. Davis[1], Sandy Eldridge[2], Calvert Louden[3]

[1]Discovery Toxicology, Pharmaceutical Candidate Optimization, Bristol Myers Squib, Princeton, NJ, United States, [2]Toxicology and Pharmacology Branch, Division of Cancer Treatment and Diagnosis, National Cancer Institute, NIH, Bethesda, MD, United States, [3]Tox-Path-LAM, Janssen Pharmaceuticals R&D, Raritan, NJ, United States

OUTLINE

1. Introduction   459
   1.1. Biomarker versus Surrogate   460
   1.2. Qualification versus Validation   460

2. Categories of Biomarkers   460
   2.1. Biomarkers of Tissue Injury/Damage   460
   2.2. Biomarkers of Altered Organ Function   468
   2.3. Mechanistic Biomarkers   469
   2.4. Biomarkers of Environmental Exposure   472
   2.5. Drug Response or Pharmacodynamic Biomarkers (See "Principles of Pharmacodynamics and Toxicodynamics, Vol 1, Chap 5)   473
   2.6. Predictive Biomarkers   474
   2.7. Patient/Clinical Trial Subject Selection   475
   2.8. Surrogate Endpoint   476
   2.9. Pharmacogenomic Biomarkers   478
   2.10. Prognostic Biomarkers   478

3. Strategies for Discovery of Biomarkers   481

   3.1. Discovery and Application of Panels of Biomarkers   483

4. Methods for Biomarker Measurement and Quantitation   483
   4.1. Genomics   485
   4.2. Proteomics   485
   4.3. Metabolomics   485
   4.4. Histocytomics   486
   4.5. Antibody-Based Detection Systems   486
   4.6. Multiplexed Assays   486
   4.7. Morphology-Based Methods   486

5. Qualification of Biomarkers: Major Considerations   488

References   489

1. INTRODUCTION

Biomarker discovery has rapidly progressed from a classical empirical approach to a high-priority, technology-supported research activity. According to the Food and Drug Administration's (FDA) Biomarkers, EndpointS and other Tools glossary (https://www.ncbi.nlm.nih.gov/books/NBK326791/), a biomarker is a defined characteristic that is measured as an indicator of normal biological processes, pathogenic processes, or responses to an exposure or intervention, including therapeutic interventions. Within this characterization, the types of measurements and observations that are included in the various categories of biomarkers are extremely broad in both technical attributes and application. Molecular, histologic, radiographic, or physiologic characteristics are types of biomarkers. In practice, many bioassay results

Haschek and Rousseaux's Handbook of Toxicologic Pathology, Fourth Edition.
https://doi.org/10.1016/B978-0-12-821044-4.00026-1

459

that are now included in various biomarker categories were developed by clinical pathologists long before the terminology was used to describe them as such. In fact, clinical signs, hematology, clinical chemistry, and histopathology all fit within the definition of "biomarkers" in the hands of the toxicologic pathologist. One could argue that successful identification, interpretation, and application of many biomarkers are partially dependent upon the body of knowledge that has been obtained via histopathological evaluations. Histopathological interpretation is a critical standard that is often paired with development of safety biomarkers. Therefore, the toxicologic pathologist will continue to play a key role in providing the context, interpretation, and qualification of biomarkers.

1.1. Biomarker versus Surrogate

It is important to distinguish the term biomarker from that of surrogate endpoint or surrogate marker. **Surrogate endpoints** are considered a subset of biomarkers that serve as an indirect measure of clinical benefit. The benefit ascribed to the response of a surrogate endpoint can be used to support a traditional or accelerated approval of drug. Although all surrogate endpoints may be considered biomarkers, it is clear that only a few biomarkers will meet the rigorous scientific and regulatory requirements to achieve inclusion in this distinct subset. Since the term "surrogate" literally means "to substitute for," the use of the term "surrogate marker" is discouraged. Readers are referred to the FDA's downloadable Table of Surrogate Endpoints for a complete listing that of clinical endpoints that is updated every 6 months (https://www.fda.gov/drugs/development-resources/table-surrogate-endpoints-were-basis-drug-approval-or-licensure#top).

1.2. Qualification versus Validation

Another key concept to introduce is the distinction between the term *qualification* and *validation*. The FDA describes biomarker qualification and validation as two distinct processes (FDA, 2018). We define qualification as the measure of the evidence that will support the intended use

or purpose for the biomarker. With this definition for qualification, a fit-for-purpose approach to biomarker qualification can be used. We use of the term "validation" to mean analytical validation, which is a measure of the performance characteristics of an assay that ensure that the assay is reliable, reproducible, and adequately sensitive for the intended use.

2. CATEGORIES OF BIOMARKERS

Using the intended purpose of the biomarker as the defining characteristic, biomarkers may be broken into subsets as is provided in Table 14.1. The narrative within this section will use specific examples (within text boxes) to illustrate the discovery process, qualification, and expectations for use and, if applicable, regulatory requirements that the biomarker would need to meet.

2.1. Biomarkers of Tissue Injury/Damage

It was first recognized in the 1950s that cellular, tissue, and organ injury, as a result of toxic or pathological insults, resulted in the movement of cellular constituents, such as cytoplasmic enzymes, into blood or urine because of altered structural integrity of affected cells, tissues, and organs. Traditional markers of cell and tissue integrity and function such as serum transaminases (liver), creatine kinases (heart and muscle), lipases (pancreas), blood urea nitrogen (BUN, kidney), and urinary albumin (kidney) have been successfully exploited to monitor organ damage. These biomarkers have become an indispensable element of clinical pathology, toxicological assessment, and clinical practice. The utility of these markers has stood the test of time, and most of those currently used in regulatory practice have been in use for almost 50 years. However, changes in biofluids without histopathologic evidence of cellular damage may lead to inaccurate conclusions; therefore, histopathology remains the cornerstone and "gold standard" confirmatory test for organ damage.

In drug discovery as well as toxicology, the use of mechanistic models and nonhistopathologic markers is relevant to both safety and efficacy;

TABLE 14.1   Categories of Biomarkers According to Intended Purpose.

Biomarker purpose (category)	Expectation	Example
Patient/clinical trial subject selection	Predict a response to a molecularly targeted agent; has the potential to enrich clinical trials such that the patient pool includes patients more likely to benefit. For this purpose, the use of biomarkers intended to be prognostic or predictive biomarkers may be employed. This category is largely populated by genomic biomarkers	EGFR mutations in NSCLC are strongly associated with sensitivity to gefitinib and erlotinib and a higher rate of clinical benefit to treatment with EGFR tyrosine kinase inhibitors was demonstrated in patients with EGFR mutations than in those without such mutations
Pharmacogenomic/ Genomic	A measurable DNA and/or RNA characteristic that indicates normal biologic processes, pathogenic processes, and/or response to therapeutic or other interventions	Dihydropyrimidine dehydrogenase (DPD) is used to predict responsiveness to capecitabine. High levels of DPD relative to TP associated with poor response or outcome in capecitabine-treated patients
Surrogate endpoint	Used as a substitute for a direct measure of a clinical efficacy or toxicologic endpoint.	Disease-free survival is considered a surrogate endpoint for overall survival in anticancer therapy trials
Prognostic	Used to predict the natural course of the disease/effect and to distinguish the outcome	Elevated CA125 antigen in adenosarcomas of the ovary; CA 125 half-life < or = 20 days versus > 20 days provides an independent prognostic factor for patient survival in stage III–IV patients early in the course of therapy; must be FDA approved
Disease state or pathological process	Indicates the existence of pathological changes in tissue or organs or occurrence of abnormal cells or tissue function. Biomarkers intended for tissue injury may also be used for this purpose	Aspartate aminotransferase to platelet ratio index (APRI) for liver fibrosis
Mechanistic	Linked directly to the modulation of a specific target or signaling pathway	Adipsin is used as a biomarker for disruption of NOTCH-1 signaling and induction of goblet cell proliferation in the small intestine. Pharmacological inhibition of γ-secretase is one means to disrupt NOTCH-1 processing
Exposure	Indicators of absorbed or target dose (including an absorbed pollutant, its metabolite(s), or products resulting from interaction with endogenous substances), which are measured in a body tissue, fluid, or excreta.	Urinary dialkylphosphate (and other metabolites) is used to indicate exposure to organophosphates; guidelines for the interpretation of these biomarkers of exposure have not been established

(Continued)

TABLE 14.1   Categories of Biomarkers According to Intended Purpose.—cont'd

Biomarker purpose (category)	Expectation	Example
Dose optimization	Used to measure responses linked to variable exposure or metabolism; includes many pharmacogenomic biomarkers	Variability in the anticoagulation response (INR) has been linked to the genetic variants of CYP2C9 and VKORC1. Knowledge of the polymorphisms in these genes in addition to other clinical and patient considerations, such as age and BMI, helped in selecting the optimal initial dose of warfarin to be prescribed, achieving a target INR more efficiently and lowering the risk of bleeding adverse events. The US label of warfarin (Coumadin®) was updated with this information
Drug response or pharmacodynamic (PD)	Measure of a specific biological response that occurs after receiving a drug	Plasma vascular endothelial growth factor (VEGF)-C, and soluble VEGF receptor-3 as measures of response to tyrosine kinase inhibitors targeting vascular endothelial growth factor receptors
Toxicity	Measure of a specific toxicologic response (e.g., cellular response, organ/tissue response, or physiologic response that is considered a signal of an adverse response). Biomarkers intended for tissue injury may also be used for this purpose. May include subsets of pharmacogenomic markers	Transmembrane tubular protein kidney injury molecule-1 (Kim-1) is markedly induced in response to renal tubular injury; cystatin C to monitor generalized decreases in renal function; serum cardiac troponin I for myocardial necrosis
Predictive	Baseline characteristics that can indicate the likelihood a specific response will occur to a given treatment.	Use of mutation of the KRAS oncogene as a negative predictive biomarker to identify patients with metastatic colorectal cancer who do not benefit from EGFR-I therapy; PTEN loss in metastases may be predictive of resistance to cetuximab
Tissue injury or damage	A measure that is abundant preferentially (or exclusively) produced in the tissue of interest, be typically present at low concentrations in the blood and other body fluids when there is no tissue injury, increase upon tissue injury, and released into the systemic circulation or other body fluid, where it can be detected and measured	Aspartate transaminase (AST) and alanine transaminase (ALT) are among the first biomarkers of tissue injury; enzymes that are released into the circulation after injury to the liver or muscle
Organ function	Measure of a shift from normal to abnormal organ physiology or organ dysfunction	A change in glomerular filtration rate measured by a clearance method (e.g., radiolabeled-tracer plasma or urinary clearance)

however, the challenges for toxicology (safety) are significant because there are often multiple mechanisms of toxicity in play and multiple pathologic changes observed. Consequently, in toxicology studies, the "gold standard" remains histopathology, which emphasizes morphologic changes and response of cells and tissues to injury. In toxicology studies, histopathology is used to identify and characterize the nature of the morphologic changes seen within the phenotypically altered cells that are the target of toxicity. The histologic evaluation plays an important role in forming the basis for initiation and development of biomarker strategies for translation medicine and for the current industry and regulatory focus to predict, identify, and manage target organ toxicity in humans. Ideally, biological markers of toxicity should be cellular products of the phenotypically altered cells that are damaged within the specific tissue and/or organ. Because the nature and character of the histopathology observations can be quite diverse, minimal tissue damage/injury does not necessarily reflect major disturbances in organ function or specific mode of action responsible for the toxicity. Furthermore, a concerted effort to identify mechanistically linked biomarkers using histopathology observations is questionable because identification and use of biological markers that truly reflect mechanism(s) of toxicity is rare. Rather, the currently used biomarkers are "reporters" of cell and/or tissue injury and have gained acceptance through use over many years. This explains why most biomarkers used in toxicity testing are diagnostic and reflect damage already done, rather than being predictive or mechanistic. In recent years, there are only a few limited examples of newly introduced novel biomarkers that have been identified and qualified preclinically and later translated further for use in clinical evaluation. Given these constraints, in the process of identification and qualification of injury biomarkers, histopathology still plays a crucial role because it links structural morphological changes with alterations in biofluids organ physiology and function that reflect the status of cellular and tissue integrity.

Examples of Organ-specific Biomarkers of Tissue Injury

BIOMARKERS OF LIVER INJURY

(See also *Liver and Gallbladder*, Vol 3, Chap 2; *Clinical Pathology in Nonclinical Toxicity Testing*, Vol 1, Chap 18; *and Interpretation and Reporting of Clinical Pathology Results in Nonclinical Toxicity Testing*, Vol 2, Chap 14.)

Despite the known drawbacks of tissue injury biomarkers, additional biomarkers of liver injury, including hepatocellular toxicity and biliary effects, are being explored using comparative biomarker discovery efforts and "omics" methods (Adler et al., 2010; Fu et al., 2020; Meunier and Larrey, 2019). Novel promising biomarkers include glutamate dehydrogenase, keratin 18, sorbitol dehydrogenase, glutathione S-transferase, bile acids, cytochrome P450, osteopontin (OPN), high-mobility group box-1 protein, fatty acid–binding protein 1, cadherin 5, miR-122, genetic testing, and omics technologies, among others.

Drug-induced hepatocellular injury biomarkers considered most likely to be qualified in the near future for preclinical, clinical, and translational applications include the following enzymatic or immunoassay multiplexes: arginase I, glutamate dehydrogenase, glutathione S-transferase *alpha*, 4-hydroxyphenylpyruvate dioxygenase, malate dehydrogenase, paraoxonase, purine nucleoside phosphorylase, serum F protein, and sorbitol dehydrogenase. These biomarkers show utility based on receiver operating characteristic (ROC) curves performed to correlate biomarker measurements to histopathology findings. However, these biomarkers have not yet been adequately qualified for use in preclinical and early clinical development. Furthermore, large qualification studies and robust assay development are required to determine a biomarker combination that provides additional information relative to alanine aminotransferase (ALT). For example, the performance of new biomarkers in the qualification paradigm might define beneficial activities to aid in interpretation of subtle elevations in ALT. Added cost, increased statistical complexity and data analysis, use of multiple platforms, and greater complexity of qualification and validation efforts are some of the disadvantages of a multimarker strategy, but these potential downsides must be weighed against the cost associated with unanticipated toxicity and more effective safety monitoring for patients.

Comparative pan-genomic approaches are being used in rats to identify biomarkers capable of distinguishing pairs of drugs that are structurally and pharmacologically similar, but where one compound is capable of AIHI and the other drug is not. Another path to identifying potential

---

A CLASSIC: ALANINE AMINOTRANSFERASE (FDA, 2009)

ALT is the classic example of a liver-specific biomarker and extensively qualified measure of hepatocellular injury. A colorimetric assay for ALT was first described by Wroblewski and Cabaud in 1957 when they compared values in healthy individuals to patients with pathologic processes, including infectious hepatitis. Over the next few years, the clinical significance of elevated ALT activity in hepatic disease was established. Although ALT represents a clinical chemistry gold standard for detection of liver injury for both preclinical and clinical utility, guidelines for interpretation are still evolving. Current guidelines for the interpretation of biomarkers of hepatotoxicity in preclinical studies recommend that increases in ALT activity that correlate with histopathologic lesions should be considered adverse. However, the guidelines do not provide guidance regarding the interpretation of elevated ALT in the absence of correlative histopathologic changes. Therefore, the combined use of several serum biomarkers for hepatotoxicity is expected to add interpretive value. A correlation between histopathology and biomarker response serves as the principle standard for biomarker qualification. Since liver histopathology is not as readily attainable in a human clinical trial setting, translatable and analytically validated biomarkers to be compared with a standard measure like ALT are required. Investigations are focused on identifying biomarkers for evaluation of liver injury and integration of multiple analyte measurements to enhance the utility of ALT as a standard. The most promising biomarkers will be able to bridge preclinical toxicity testing and monitor drug-induced liver injury in the clinical setting.

A major type of liver injury of concern is acute idiosyncratic hepatocellular injury (AIHI). The event is termed "idiosyncratic" because the vast majority of treated patients are able to take the drug safely at the recommended dose range, and it is not possible to identify or predict patient susceptibility to AIHI. If a drug treatment is associated with recurrent bouts of AIHI, progressive loss of hepatocytes can lead to irreversible liver dysfunction and, in some cases, mortality. Thus, discovery and development of biomarkers that measure the potential to cause idiosyncratic liver injury or identify individual susceptibility to a drug with established AIHI potential is an area of active research and investigation.

Candidate biomarkers for AIHI are being identified from many paths of investigation.

biomarkers for AIHI is studies focused on an assessment of patients who have experienced AIHI. The Severe Adverse Event Consortium began whole-genome single nucleotide polymorphism analysis on germ-line DNA obtained from patients who have experienced varying degrees of drug-induced liver injury, including AIHI. Several efforts are also underway in which various "omics" technologies are used to analyze blood and urine samples from large cohorts of subjects. Additionally, large postmarketing adverse events databases are being mined to elucidate drug/environment susceptibility factors. These efforts could lead to testable hypotheses or be used to provide supportive data for genetic associations observed in these networks. Studying differences in hepatotoxicity susceptibility across panels of inbred strains of mice and quantitative trait loci mapping is also a promising approach to generating hypotheses that would be testable in relatively small numbers of human subjects.

BIOMARKERS OF VASCULAR TOXICITY (BROTT ET AL., 2005A, B; LOUDEN ET AL., 2006)

(See also *Cardiovascular System*, Vol 4, Chap 1.) Clinical development of novel life-saving therapies is often hindered because the nonclinical safety profiles of candidate drugs are associated with occult pathological changes that are not detected by noninvasive, routine clinical monitoring. In nonclinical safety studies, drug-induced vascular injury is an example of such a profile, because there are no biochemical markers for monitoring this lesion clinically and our understanding of the pathophysiology is limited. This type of vascular toxicity is most often associated with candidate drugs that are pharmacologically active in the vascular bed. In addition, immune complex vasculitis can be induced in animal studies of biotherapeutics, and while the relevance of these to humans is uncertain, there is often a need to monitor for vascular injury in clinical trials for these programs. There are a number of drugs from different pharmacologic classes and chemical structures that have been approved for human use but known to cause occult mesenteric or coronary arterial vascular lesions in animal studies.

At high doses in dogs, structurally and pharmacologically diverse vasoactive agents induce a distinctive morphologic coronary arterial pathology. Generally, drug-induced cardiovascular toxicity is regional, with some predilection for the right side of the heart, particularly the right extramural coronary arteries. Macroscopically, hemorrhagic areas are seen in the right atrium with petechial hemorrhages or short, linear, hemorrhagic streaks overlying or adjacent to the right branches of extramural coronary arteries. Similar small areas of hemorrhage are also seen infrequently in the left atrium. The ventricles are usually not affected. Whereas this change is a consistent feature of potential vascular toxicity in dogs and might serve as a biomarker for

vascular toxicity, the challenge remains to identify, qualify, and validate a preclinical marker in humans that will bridge the gap between the biomarker used in dogs and the marker(s) of toxicity in preclinical studies.

BIOCHEMICAL MARKERS OF DRUG-INDUCED VASCULAR INJURY (KERNS ET AL., 2005) von Willebrand Factor (vWF) and its propeptide (vWFpp) have been studied as potential markers of endothelial cell (EC) perturbation and drug-induced vascular injury. Release of vWF and vWFpp into circulation is controlled by well-defined constitutive and regulated pathways as well as biochemical processes. In models of drug-induced vascular injury, plasma vWF was evaluated as a potential marker of vascular injury in the rat and dog. Minor increases in plasma vWF have been observed following administration of a potassium channel opener drug and also fenoldopam. This observation in conjunction with other reports raises the possibility that the transient 2- to 6-h increase in circulating plasma vWF could be a reporter of endothelial activation/perturbation prior to morphologic evidence of vascular damage because levels had returned to baseline when vascular injury was confirmed histologically. Studies in the dog have indicated that minimal lesions induced by a potassium channel opener drug do not result in increased vWF levels. Therefore, vWF is not a suitable marker for use in nonclinical safety studies to monitor progressive vascular damage. However, it has been suggested that measurement and analysis of the vWF:vWFpp ratio in humans, dogs, and baboons allows discrimination between chronic and acute phases of EC perturbation, activation, and injury. There is also experimental evidence which suggests that measurement of plasma vWFpp levels may be a useful biochemical marker of *regional* drug-induced vascular injury because vWFpp is found in low levels in plasma, it has a short terminal half-life, it does not bind to the vascular wall subendothelial collagen, and its major source is ECs. Based on these properties, transient physiological increases in vWFpp can be differentiated from pathological increases that would lead to a sustained elevation.

SEEKING SITE-SPECIFIC AND SELECTIVE BIOMARKERS OF DRUG-INDUCED VASCULAR INJURY (BROTT ET AL., 2005B; GREAVES, 1998; ISAACS ET AL., 1989; LOUDEN ET AL., 2006; MESFIN ET AL., 1989; METZ ET AL., 1991)

Microscopically, vasodilators and/or positive inotropic agents such as minoxidil, hydralazine, phosphodiesterase inhibitors, and endothelin receptor antagonist (ETRA) are associated with this unique coronary arterial lesion, characterized by acute segmental changes of medial necrosis and hemorrhage that can develop as early as 12–24 h following intravenous administration and between 3 and 7 days with oral dosing. Medial hemorrhage can be transmural and/or circumferential, with well-preserved extravasated red blood cells and perivascular edema. Vascular lesions are seen primarily in muscular branches of the coronary arteries, in coronary arterioles and possibly capillaries. Subepicardial branches of the right coronary arteries composed of five to eight cell-layer thickness were most frequently affected and mural branches of the right and left coronary arteries were affected less frequently. Terminal arterioles and capillaries, particularly those in the outer third of the right atrial wall, were quite prominent due to enlargement related to swelling and/or activation of ECs. Chronic lesions are intimal proliferation, smooth muscle cell (SMC) hyperplasia with deposition of mucinous ground substance, and adventitial fibroplasia. Also present are varying degrees of a mixed mononuclear inflammatory cell infiltrate.

In the dog, understanding drug-induced vascular injury pathophysiology and potential mode of action has been aided by data describing a relationship between predisposed toxicity site(s) and the distribution, density, type, and ratio of vasoactive endothelin receptors in the heart and coronary arteries. Additionally, the composite analysis of receptor subtype profiles, mRNA expression, and regional blood flow measurements clearly supported the hypothesis that a disproportionate receptor distribution was responsible in the initial studies for the marked functional differences in regional blood flow at the affected sites of injury, the right atrium and right coronary arteries. Collectively, these data strongly suggest that exaggerated pharmacology is the basis for selective, site-specific, mesenteric, or coronary arterial damage in rats and dogs caused by these drugs (Louden et al., 2006; Louden and Morgan, 2001). Concomitantly, there is loss of regulation and control of key biochemical pathways in ECs and SMC, breakdown in cell-to-cell communications, and, ultimately, arterial wall damage. Therefore, both physiological and biochemical markers of endothelial and SMCs should be evaluated to identify and develop translational markers of vascular toxicity.

BIOMARKERS OF RENAL INJURY (PINCHES ET AL., 2012)

(See also *Kidney*, Vol 4, Chap 2; *Clinical Pathology in Nonclinical Toxicity Testing*, Vol 1, Chap 10; *Interpretation of Clinical Pathology Results in Nonclinical Toxicity Testing*, Vol 2, Chap 14.)

In 2010, the FDA issued the first formal biomarker qualification decision about novel safety biomarkers of drug-induced kidney injury for preclinical drug development. The ILSI Health and Environmental Sciences Institute (HESI) evaluated four urinary biomarkers of nephrotoxicity (α-glutathione S-transferase, μ-glutathione S-transferase, renal papillary antigen [RPA-1], and clusterin) and compared their performance against traditional measurements indicative of renal injury in male Sprague–Dawley and Wistar rats. In this biomarker discovery effort, compounds that cause injury to specific anatomical regions of the nephron and corresponding biomarker values to defined histopathologic lesions were used to generate a histopathological "gold standard" to assess

biomarker performance. Immunohistochemistry (IHC) was applied to confirm the location of regional lesions. The discriminatory accuracy of each biomarker was assessed using ROC curve methods. Immunolocalization of RPA-1 in gentamycin-treated rats demonstrated that RPA-1 is increased in the cytoplasm of intact injured collecting duct epithelial cells and in necrotic cells within the proximal tubular epithelium. It is also detected in the urine using immuno-based assays. Based on the review of the data submitted by an ad hoc appointed Biomarkers Qualification Team, RPA-1 and clusterin were qualified for use in Good Laboratory Practice preclinical toxicology studies, but not for routine monitoring of drug-induced nephrotoxicity in the clinical setting. RPA-1 represented a novel biomarker not previously qualified for this purpose.

Over the course of several months in 2007, the C-Path Predictive Safety Testing Consortium (PSTC) submitted data to the FDA/EMEA supporting claims for additional renal toxicity biomarkers. The newly proposed biomarkers included urinary albumin, β2-microglobulin, cystatin C, kidney injury molecule (Kim-1), total protein, and urinary trefoil factor 3. Performance of each biomarker was compared to accepted standards of BUN and serum creatinine by comparing the area under the curve (AUC) of the ROC analysis for each biomarker. Similar to the HESI studies discussed in the previous paragraph, histopathology was the standard used to qualify biomarker measurements. Although an ad hoc panel of reviewers concluded that the panel of proposed biomarkers is acceptable for nonclinical drug development, they noted several limitations of the data set, including lack of a clear correlation between the biomarkers and the temporal pathogenesis of the renal lesions (as determined by histopathology) and a lack of correlation between reversibility and recovery of kidney function. The panel concluded that use of these biomarkers to predict or **monitor** renal toxicity was insufficiently demonstrated. The panel did, however, consider the group biomarkers acceptable for the **detection** of acute drug-induced nephrotoxicity in preclinical drug development. Hence, the biomarker review panel did recognize the potential of these biomarkers to be qualified for use as clinical markers of acute drug-induced renal injury. Albumin, β2-microglobulin, cystatin C, Kim-1, total protein, urinary clusterin, and urinary trefoil factor 3 thus provide additional and complementary information to BUN and serum creatinine to correlate the histopathology, which is considered the gold standard.

REGION-SPECIFIC KIDNEY DAMAGE The use of renal injury biomarkers to define the specific region of the kidney subject to injury is promising. A marker that is strongly induced in proximal tubular injury is urinary Kim-1. Kim-1 has been cloned by representational difference analysis, a polymerase chain reaction–based technique, which was conducted to compare gene expression in normal versus postischemic rat kidney, to identify genes that were upregulated with renal ischemia. Researchers demonstrated that the ectodomain of Kim-1 is shed from cells in vitro and in vivo into the urine in rodents as well as humans after proximal tubular

kidney injury. Thus, urinary Kim-1 serves as a translational biomarker in preclinical and clinical studies and is a diagnostic indicator of kidney injury that is detected earlier and with greater specificity compared to conventional biomarkers (e.g., serum creatinine, BUN, glycosuria, increased proteinuria or increased urinary N-acetyl-β-D-glucosaminidase, γ-glutamyltransferase , alkaline phosphatase levels). Initially, an enzyme-linked immunosorbent assay (ELISA) was developed to measure Kim-1 in rodent and human urine samples. More recent technological advances facilitated the development of a high-throughput microbead-based assay to quantify Kim-1 in rat urine that is more sensitive, has a greater dynamic range, and requires less urine volume and reagents than the conventional ELISA. Kim-1 has been shown to clearly outperform serum creatinine as a marker for tubular injury in rats in terms of sensitivity and specificity.

BIOMARKERS FOR REVERSIBILITY OF KIDNEY DAMAGE Based on recommendations resulting from the FDA's biomarker qualification process, a study was recently reported in which reversibility and comparative injury data for several candidate urinary biomarkers of kidney injury were evaluated. The nephrotoxin gentamicin was given to rats once on each of 3 days and the animals were humanely euthanized at various time points. Between days 1 and 3, all biomarkers except albumin were elevated, peaked at day 7, and returned to control levels by day 10 (μ- and α-glutathione S-transferases, and RPA-1) or by day 15 in the case of Kim-1, lipocalin-2, OPN, and clusterin. All biomarkers performed better during injury than during recovery except OPN, which performed equally well at both time periods. During the evolution of injury, Kim-1, RPA-1, and clusterin correlated best with histopathologic lesions that included necrosis, apoptosis, and regeneration. During the recovery period, Kim-1, OPN, and BUN were the best markers of injury resolution based on correlation with histopathology. RPA-1 was the best indicator of tubular and/or collecting duct regeneration, especially during recovery.

BIOMARKERS OF CARDIAC INJURY (WANG ET AL., 2020)

(See also *Cardiovascular System*, Vol 4, Chap 1; *Clinical Pathology in Nonclinical Toxicity Testing,*

Vol 1, Chap 10; *and Interpretation of Clinical Pathology Results in Nonclinical Toxicicity Testing*, Vol 2, Chap 14.)

Historically, lactate dehydrogenase, myoglobin, and creatinine kinase isoenzyme analyses have been used as a measure of ischemia-induced cardiac injury. These serum-based myocardial markers have limited cardiac specificity and relatively short serum half-lives. Cardiac troponins (cTns) T and I are more recent additions to the list of biomarkers of cardiac injury recommended for assessing injury associated with myocardial ischemia and drug-induced cardiac toxicity.

Troponins are a complex of three proteins that regulate the calcium-mediated interaction of actin and myosin. Separate genes encode each cTn isoform. The isoform for cTnC is common to all types of muscle, whereas those for cTnI and cTnT are considered cTns. To date, the cardiac isoform of cTnI has not been found outside of cardiac tissue, whereas isoforms of cTnT exist in skeletal muscle as well as cardiac tissue.

cTnI and cTnT are released from the cytoskeleton during myocardial infarction, cardiac myocyte injury, or other cardiovascular conditions, with increased levels detected in blood. The American College of Cardiology and the European Society of Cardiology declared cTns the biomarker of choice for acute myocardial infarction in 2000. According to the "gold standard," analytical assays for cTns should include free cTnI, the I–C binary complex, the T–I–C ternary complex, and oxidized, reduced, and phosphorylated isoforms of the three cTnI forms; however, epitopes located on the stable part of the cTnI molecule should be a priority. Currently, cTns are the markers of choice for detection of clinical cardiotoxicity and cardiac ischemic necrosis based on their cardiac specificity and their longer serum half-life. Furthermore, cTnI and T have been promoted as the gold standard biomarkers of drug-induced cardiac toxicity in the preclinical setting as well. In fact, cTns are now routinely included in nonclinical safety studies (Babuin and Jaffe, 2005; Walker, 2006).

2.2. Biomarkers of Altered Organ Function

Functional biomarkers are expected to monitor specific changes in function associated with pathological events at the cellular, tissue, or systemic level (e.g., changes in biological function, diagnostic/disease state). A molecular biomarker is an entity whose release, abundance, and/or modification state is altered as a result of injury or disease and can be used to aid diagnosis.

THE DISCOVERY AND QUALIFICATION OF CYSTATIN C: A MEASURE OF GLOMERULAR FUNCTION (DHARNIDHARKA ET AL., 2002; DIETERLE ET AL., 2010; GRUBB ET AL., 1985; SIMONSEN ET AL., 1985)

The use of serum cystatin C as a measure of glomerular filtration rate was first proposed in 1985. Since then, numerous studies have been conducted to qualify cystatin C as a biomarker of glomerular function. Most of the studies have been comparative biomarker analyses comparing cystatin C to other standard references in healthy subjects compared to patients with impaired glomerular function. Cystatin C is an endogenous inhibitor of cysteine proteinases that is freely filtered by the glomeruli and reabsorbed from ultrafiltrate by the tubules, where it is almost completely catabolized, with the remainder eliminated in urine (similar to β2-microglobulin). Increased urinary cystatin C concentrations allow the detection of a direct impairment of the tubular protein reabsorption complex or an indirect impairment caused by a tubular protein overload due to glomerular alterations and injury in various nephropathies. Mean urinary cystatin C concentrations in patients with kidney tubular disease are elevated compared to healthy patients or patients with glomerular disease. Thus, increased urinary cystatin C reflects a direct or indirect functional renal tubular impairment independent of glomerular filtration rate. However, the concentration of serum cystatin C is mainly determined by the glomerular filtration rate. Serum cystatin C as an endogenous marker of glomerular filtration rate and kidney function is superior to serum creatinine because cystatin C is less dependent on extrarenal factors than creatinine and is completely cleared by the glomerulus, in contrast to creatinine, which is also cleared by tubular secretion. Metaanalysis of combined clinical studies done to qualify the performance of cystatin C as a marker of glomerular function confirms the superiority of cystatin C over creatinine with respect to glomerular filtration rate measurements, by both superior correlation coefficients and greater ROC plot AUC values.

Functional Markers of Vascular Toxicity: Heart Rate and Mean Arterial Pressure (Pugsley et al., 2008)

In nonclinical safety studies, vascular toxicity is associated with structurally and pharmacologically diverse agents. In the dog, this toxicity is oftentimes associated with profound cardiovascular hemodynamics changes in mean arterial pressure (MAP) and heart rate (HR). These parameters have been used as biomarkers to monitor potential vascular toxicity in humans at therapeutic doses. Minoxidil, a potent antihypertensive agent, causes profound decreases in MAP with compensatory increase in HR and vascular lesions in nonclinical studies in the dog. Similar findings have been reported with hydralazine. However, experiences with ETRAs, a novel class of vasoactive agents, suggest that profound hemodynamic changes in MAP and HR are not a prerequisite for development of coronary arterial lesions in the dog. For ETRAs, the lack of concordance with HR and MAP suggests that extrapolation of the potential risk to the human population can only be made on the basis that the dog is a very sensitive species. This species sensitivity response is supported by data in monkeys administered an ETRA that required higher systemic exposure and longer duration of treatment to develop less severe coronary arterial lesions.

In the dog, drug-induced vascular injury is associated with vasodilatation and increased blood flow, and these changes precede arterial damage. Increased regional coronary blood flow has been reported with minoxidil, hydralazine, SB209670, and adenosine agonists. In the rat, mesenteric arterial damage and increase in mesenteric arterial blood flow was associated with administration of minoxidil, fenoldopam, and SK&F 95654. In dogs and humans, exercise can cause an increase in coronary blood flow, and this suggests that physiological regulation plays a critical role in maintaining vascular integrity. In humans, because of the relationship between vasodilatation and blood flow, flow-mediated dilatation can be used to determine and measure regional blood flow drug-related effects.

Circulating micro-RNA as Biomarkers of Tissue Injury (Howell et al., 2018; Iguchi et al., 2017, 2018; Kagawa et al., 2018; Laterza et al., 2009)

Micro-RNAs (miRNAs) are small noncoding RNAs that regulate posttranscriptional gene expression by repressing or degrading target mRNA. Several research efforts have focused on exploring their potential to serve as tissue-specific biomarkers. Data supporting the potential

for miRNAs to be used in this way are compelling as are the qualities miRNA that make them ideal. miRNAs are stable in body fluids and can withstand freezing and thawing and extended storage at room temperature. Importantly, miRNA may originate from tissues and particular cells within the tissue in which they are highly and specifically expressed. This quality lends itself to miRNA being used to distinguish between the type of cellular injury and subsequent pathology within a tissue. Last, miRNA also have a particular advantage for nonclinical to clinical translation because of the conservation of sequences for most miRNAs between animal species and humans. There are numerous clinical and nonclinical studies that have explored miRNAs as biomarkers of tissue injury. Examples of tissue specific miRNA are provided in the following table (Table 14.2).

TABLE 14.2 Categories of Biomarkers According to Intended Purpose

Tissue/Cell type	miRNA
Brain	miR-9, miR-124—3p
Bone marrow	miR-223
Heart/skeletal muscle	miR-1, miR-133a, miR-208a, miR499a, miR126
Liver hepatocytes	miR-122a, miR122-5p, miR192-5p,
Liver sinusoidal endothelial	miR-511-3p
Lung	miR126
Pancreas	miR-216
Pituitary	miR-7
Peripheral nerves	miRNAs -199a-3p, miRNA-146, miRNA-499a
Skeletal muscle	miR-206
Testis	miR-204, miR-34b-5p. miR34c-5p, miR-449a, miR-202—5p, miR-508—3p
Thyroid	miR-144

2.3. Mechanistic Biomarkers

A mechanistic biomarker is expected to provide a measurable index of the pathogenesis and/or mechanism of action leading to the drug-induced effects. As one might imagine, this category of biomarkers as applied to mechanism of toxicity can be highly useful in developing approaches to

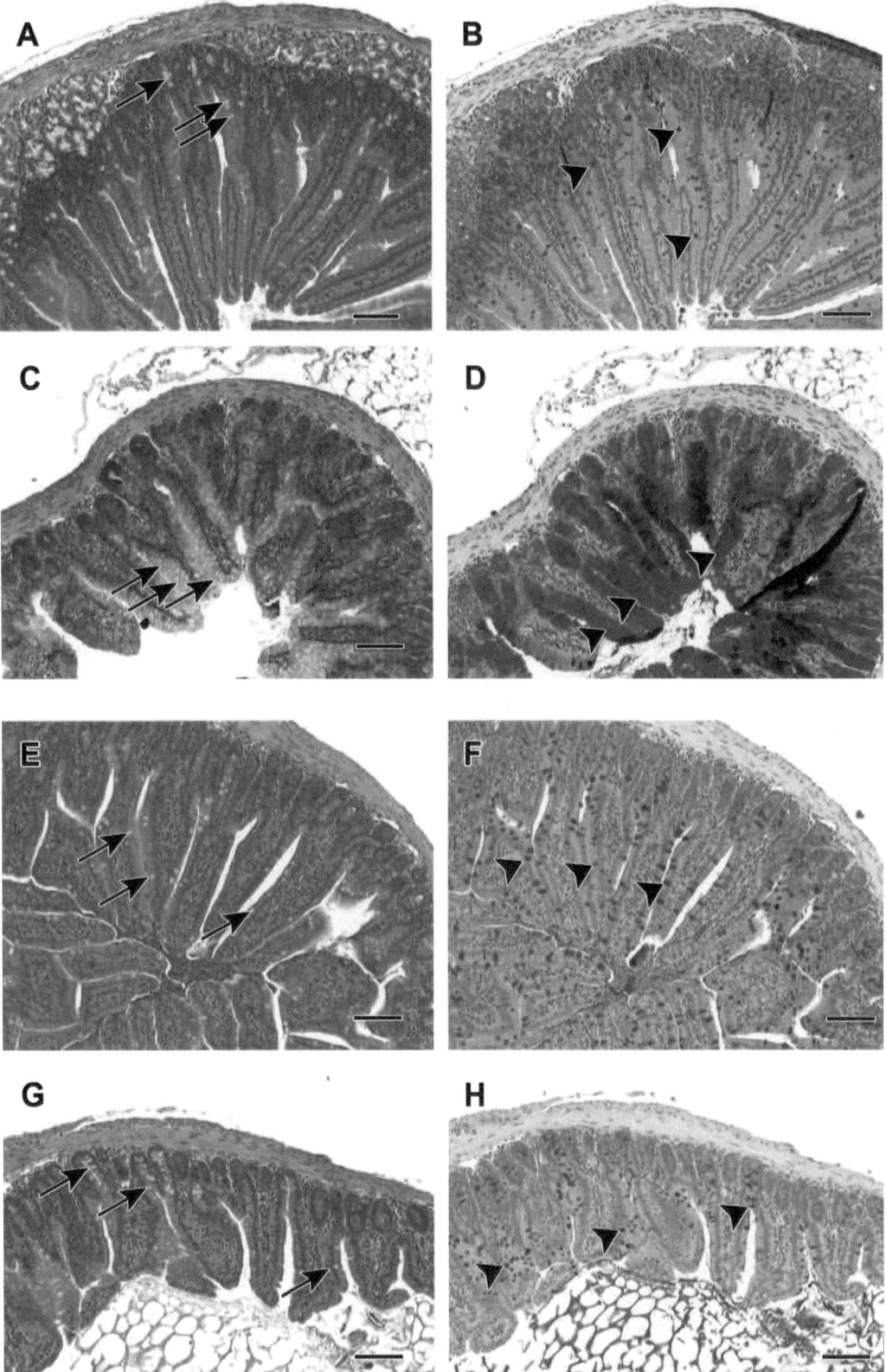

FIGURE 14.1 Photomicrographs of ileum sections (10× magnification) from mice treated 7 days × bid with gamma-secretase inhibitors noted below. Selected sections represent the range of goblet cell hyperplasia observed in this study. In H&E-stained sections (A, C, E, and G), goblet cells appear as cells with clear or foamy cytoplasm (*arrows*); in PAS-stained sections (B, D, F, and H), they appear as dark-stained cells (*arrow heads*). A normal

THE DISCOVERY AND APPLICATION OF A MECHANISTIC BIOMARKER: ADIPSIN (SEARFOSS ET AL., 2003)

Several important correlations led to the discovery and qualification of adipsin as a mechanistic biomarker for intestinal injury. The small intestine relies upon continuous cycles of rapid maturation, transport, and cell loss by a small population of stem cells in the intestinal crypts (giving rise to goblet cells, enterocytes, Paneth cells, and enteroendocrine cells) to maintain tissue homeostasis and populations of differentiated cells. This feature makes the small intestine (and bone marrow) particularly susceptible to toxicants which affect cell differentiation and proliferation. Understanding the process by which dividing intestinal epithelial stem cells in the crypt produces differentiated cell populations was critical to identification of adipsin as a mechanistic biomarker for disruption of NOTCH-1 signaling and subsequent induction of goblet cell proliferation in the small intestine.

Notch-1 signaling disruption and Hairy and Enhancer of Split homolog-1 (Hes-1) knock-out studies have shown that the Notch-1/Hes-1 pathway plays a critical role in the differentiation processes of the gastrointestinal tract and regulates whether cells adopt an exocrine/secretory (goblet cell, enteroendocrine cell, Paneth cell) fate or an absorptive (enterocyte) phenotype. When Notch-1 binds ligand (Delta, Serrate, or Jagged) on the surface of an adjacent cell, it stimulates a cleavage of the Notch-1 protein within the plasma membrane by an aspartyl protease, similar or identical to the γ-secretase activity implicated in Alzheimer's disease or in the pathogenesis of certain cancers. Cleavage of Notch-1 releases the Notch intracellular domain that translocates to the nucleus, and it associates with the transcriptional activator protein RBP-Jk (CSL/CBF/Su(H)/Lag-1) to stimulate the expression of target genes, most notably Hes-1. Disruption of this Notch-1 processing by γ-secretase inhibitors that function

to inhibit Notch-1 intramembrane cleavage mirrors differentiation effects seen in Hes-1 knock-out studies. High doses of an experimental γ-secretase inhibitor administered to Fischer 344 rats by George Searfoss and colleagues produced gastrointestinal changes similar to those described in Hes-1 knock-out mice, including an increased number of goblet cells (Fig. 14.1) and elevated mRNA levels for a number of enteroendocrine-specificgene products. Through gene expression analysis, they showed that the secreted adipocyte-specific protein, adipsin, had elevated mRNA levels and flagged it as a potential marker for Notch/Hes-1 signaling disruption effects in the gastrointestinal tract of rats. Subsequently, levels of the adipsin protein were found to be dramatically upregulated in the intestinal contents and feces of treated rats and could be monitored noninvasively. Histochemical staining revealed that adipsin was produced by cells present in the crypt region of the intestinal epithelium and that adipsin labeling was greater in treated rats. These investigators also provided critical mechanistic evidence for adipsin gastrointestinal expression by showing that adipsin expression can be repressed by Hes-1, and reduction of Hes-1 levels by an experimental γ-secretase inhibitor released Hes-1 repression of adipsin, thus allowing for its transcriptional upregulation. The connectivity between cell and molecular biology of the normal tissue, the pathological observation of cellular proliferation and differentiated phenotype and use of toxicogenomic approaches, and mechanistic validation is an elegant example of how mechanistic biomarkers can be elucidated. The biomarker was subsequently applied to several drug development programs for γ-secretase inhibitors.

population of goblet cells was observed in all vehicle control mice (A, B). All positive control LY411575 treated mice had a moderate increase in goblet cells (C, D). There was no apparent dose-related increase in goblet cells across ELN475516 treated groups among all mice in these groups, 21 had no increase in goblet cells, and 8 had a questionable increase (illustrated by a single animal from 100-mg/kg dose group, G, H). A single mouse from the 600-mg/kg dose group had a mild increase in goblet cells, which is shown for comparison purposes (panels E and F). Scale bar = 100 μm. *Reproduced from Basi GS, Hemphill S, Brigham EF, et al.: Amyloid precursor protein selective gamma-secretase inhibitors for treatment of Alzheimer's disease, Alz Res Therapy 2:36(2010) (©2010 Basi et al.; licensee BioMed Central Ltd), with permission. This is an open access article distributed under the terms of the Creative Commons Attribution License (http://creativecommons.org/licenses/by/2.0), which permits unrestricted use, distribution, and reproduction in any medium, provided the original work is properly cited).*

mitigate toxicity, but their use and validation require rigorous scientific investigations aimed at elucidating this mechanism of action.

Table 14.3 (FDA, 2020a) is a partial listing of qualified biomarkers of injury that are currently being or will be used. There is no doubt that there are others "in the pipeline," close to or ready to be fully qualified and validated for use.

2.4. Biomarkers of Environmental Exposure (Espín-Pérez et al., 2014)

Biomarkers of exposure to xenobiotics are particularly useful in toxicology and risk assessment, because they are indicators of internal dose or chemical exposure. For certain chemicals, state or federal regulations require regular

TABLE 14.3   Examples of Discovered Commonly Used Biomarkers

Biomarker	Associated tissue	Source	Matrix	Biomarker type/Measurement
Kim-1	Kidney	Urine	Protein	Proximal tubular injury
Albumin	Kidney	Urine	Protein	Glomerular permeability
Cystatin C	Kidney	Serum, urine	Protein	Glomerular filtration rate and tubular reabsorption
Clusterin	Kidney	Urine	Protein	Proximal tubular injury
β2-microglobulin	Kidney	Urine	Protein	Glomerular injury and tubular reabsorption
Trefoil factor 3	Kidney	Urine	Protein	Proximal tubular injury
Total protein	Kidney	Urine	Protein	Glomerular injury and tubular reabsorption
ALT1	Liver	Serum	Protein	Necrosis
SDH	Liver	Serum	Protein	Necrosis
GLDH	Liver	Serum	Protein	Necrosis
PNP	Liver	Serum	Protein	Necrosis
MDH	Liver	Serum	Protein	Necrosis
PON1	Liver	Serum	Protein	Necrosis
α-GST	Liver	Serum	Protein	Necrosis
Serum protein F	Liver	Serum	Protein	Necrosis
Arginase I	Liver	Serum	Protein	Necrosis
Thiostatin	Liver	Serum, urine	Protein	Necrosis
Troponin I and T	Heart	Plasma	Protein	Acute myocardial infarction
Cytokines	Multiple	Blood	Protein	Immunotoxicity
Histopathology	Vascular	Organs	Tissue	Drug-induced vascular injury
BRAF mutation	Melanoma	Blood	DNA	Predictive/sensitivity to drug treatment
CYP genes	Multiple organs	Blood	DNA	Metabolism

ALT1, alanine aminotransferase isoform 1; BRAF, serine/threonine protein kinase B-raf proto-oncogene; CYP, cytochrome P450 family of metabolizing enzymes; GI, gastrointestinal; GLDH, glutamate dehydrogenase; α-GST, alpha glutathione S-transferase; Kim-1, kidney injury molecule-1; MDH, malate dehydrogenase; PNP, purine nucleoside phosphorylase; PON1, paraoxonase-1; SDH, sorbitol dehydrogenase.

biomonitoring of individuals who may be at risk of exposure, and biomarkers of exposure are critical to this monitoring effort. Biomarkers of exposure must provide measurable indices of exposure but are not expected to indicate an adverse physiologic or pathologic effect. Biomarkers primarily used for assessment of exposure are most often endpoints in the continuum of events ranging from external dose to absorbed dose. Many exposure biomarkers are limited to direct measures of the chemical to which the individual has been exposed and only provide an estimate of absorbed dose proximal to the time of exposure. In many cases, it is difficult to find measures of exposure that serve as measures of internal dose for exposures that may have occurred months or years prior to the measurement. Only in a few cases is there a measurable continuum from exposure to disease causation.

The use of urinary carcinogens and their metabolites as biomarkers for investigating the links between tobacco and cancer serves as an excellent example that has been comprehensively reviewed (Yuan et al., 2014). Exposure to benzene is also monitored via several biomarkers, including urine trans,transmuconic acid. These metabolites are known to be involved in bone marrow leukemogenesis and the causal association between benzene exposure and leukemogenesis, and thus the carcinogenic potential of benzene exposure has been made (McHale et al., 2012).

The contribution of toxicological pathology in discovery and elucidation of exposure biomarkers is considered essential for many reasons. For example, it is now clear that the histological biomarkers seen at the end of most 6- or 12-month toxicology studies in rats can predict the outcome of a 2-year carcinogenicity study. The histological outcome combined with measure of exposure markers can provide the basis for the continuum from exposure to disease. Moreover, the link between exposure and early onset of disease can be made through the careful assessment of "predisease" pathological change as determined through histopathological assessment. The translation from these studies to human risk assessment has been the underpinning for the qualification of exposure biomarkers. Combined interpretation of results from histopathology, molecular techniques, and

analytical measurements of exposure will continue to be a powerful strategy in the future of environmental risk assessment.

2.5. Drug Response or Pharmacodynamic Biomarkers (See "Principles of Pharmacodynamics and Toxicodynamics, Vol 1, Chap 5)

Biomarkers that are drug responsive, known as pharmacodynamic (PD) biomarkers, are considered to be key to the modern era of drug discovery and development. It is commonly argued that PD markers provide the critical translational measures that link, in a quantitative manner, the interactions between drug (or combinations of drugs), pharmacological targets, (semi) mechanistic modeling across species, physiological pathways, and, ultimately, integrated disease systems (Campion et al., 2013). In this context, PD biomarkers have also been referred to as therapeutic biomarkers and can, in most cases, be considered synonymous. Therapeutic biomarkers are a subcategory of biomarkers that may be unique to a drug or therapeutic strategy that are used to measure whether the drug is reaching the target and causing its intended biologic effect on the target. A PD therapeutic biomarker thereby becomes a surrogate marker of drug activity if its presence or modulation is determined to correlate with a clinical response.

The expectations for a PD biomarker are different from those of the patient selection marker (although a PD marker may become validated for use as a patient selection biomarker). In general, the PD biomarker is expected to determine whether the drug inhibits the targeted pathway and is a measure of optimal effects of the test substance on the target at a tolerable and optimal biologic dose of the test substance. The ideal PD biomarker would be truly useful at all stages of drug development and clinical treatment, and could be used to

1. monitor dose-dependent effects of the drug on the target or target pathway;
2. provide a functional measure of the critical disease pathway or tissue type in which the targeted pathway is present and active.

The PD Biomarker and Dose Optimization

The connection between the PD response and the pharmacokinetics of a drug creates a natural role for the PD marker in dose selection. This approach could potentially be used to provide an accurate assessment of drug target modulation in early trials and the exposures or dose required for such. The recognition that it may be inappropriate to use a maximally tolerated

Predictive biomarker qualification is extremely complex, and exceptionally high standards of evidence are required. There is a growing interest in how responses to drugs differ among individuals or subsets, and there are a small number of predictive biomarkers that have found utility in answering the question "Will this drug work for this patient?" or "Will this drug cause an adverse effect in this patient?"

OLD DRUG, ESTABLISHED BIOMARKER, MODERN USE: ASPIRIN, SERUM THROMBOXANE B2, AND TYPE 2 DIABETES MELLITUS PATIENTS WITH CORONARY ARTERY DISEASE (CAPODANNO ET AL., 2011)

Patients with type 2 diabetes mellitus (T2DM) were shown to have reduced aspirin-induced PD responses. It was hypothesized that this may have been due to increased platelet turnover, resulting in an increased proportion of nonaspirin−inhibited platelets during the daily dosing interval. If true, this acquired condition may lead to a considerable proportion of circulating platelets with uninhibited cyclooxygenase-1 activity which in turn would continue to generate high levels of serum thromboxane. This would promote activation of circulating platelets (acetylated and nonacetylated) via thromboxane receptors (TP) on the platelet surface. Hence, a study was conducted to determine if an increase in the frequency of drug administration (twice daily [bid] vs. once daily [od]) would provide more effective platelet inhibition in T2DM patients. The PD marker for platelet inhibition used in the study was

serum thromboxane B2 (TXB2), an eicosanoid and well-established (qualified) measure of platelet production. With a twice-daily, low-dose aspirin administration, greater platelet inhibition than once-daily administration was achieved, as assessed by aspirin-sensitive assays, and an identified dose-dependent effect on serum TXB2 levels ($P = .003$). The clinical implication of a modified aspirin regimen tailored to T2DM patients is now undergoing further investigation. In another recent Phase 1 clinical trial, serum TXB2 levels were used to determine if concomitant multiple-dose administration of an investigational drug, PN 400, interferes with the platelet inhibitory effects of enteric-coated low-dose aspirin (81 mg). These and several other trials using this PD biomarker illustrate the long-term utility of a qualified PD marker to future drug development opportunities and new therapeutic indications.

---

dose in later phase development because target pathway modulation or PD response is maximized at a much lower exposure clearly illustrates the need to use the PD biomarker as a dose selection marker. The ability to monitor the effects of pathway inhibition in vivo and determine the most effective exposure and dosing schedule is a critical advantage for a clinical program that achieves early qualification of a PD marker and validation of an appropriate assay for measurement.

2.6. Predictive Biomarkers

Predictive biomarkers are used to assess the likelihood that a biological response *will* occur.

The use of preclinical models to qualify candidate predictive biomarkers is a promising means to obtain in vivo qualification data for translation to clinical trials or human studies. Preclinical retrospective studies using an existing predictive marker can be effectively used to validate the animal model for new predictive biomarker discovery (when a predictive marker exists) or to predict the likelihood that a treatment will have the desired effect on disease or an undesirable adverse effect. For example, clinically relevant orthotopic animal models are frequently used to investigate tumor biomarkers. In one such study, investigators used multimodality imaging with correlative histopathology to demonstrate the utility and accuracy of the mouse model in investigating tumor biomarkers—serum soluble mesothelin–related peptide (SMRP) and OPN (Servais et al., 2011). A percentage change in SMRP level was shown to be an accurate biomarker of tumor progression and therapeutic response—a finding consistent with clinical studies.

populations at risk through predictive toxicity biomarkers) (Jones et al., 2012). It is apparent that increased understanding of mechanisms of toxicity will contribute greatly to identification and qualification of many promising biomarkers that predict toxicity.

RECEIVER OPERATING CHARACTERISTIC CURVE (HANLEY AND MCNEIL, 1982; PARK ET AL., 2004)

Historically, ROC curves have been used by the diagnostic imaging community concerned with the content of information generated by a variety of imaging systems. The ROC curve is defined as a plot of test sensitivity (y coordinate) versus specificity (x coordinate) and used to evaluate the performance of diagnostic tests. Sensitivity is defined as the number of true positive decisions/the total number of true positive plus false-negative cases. Specificity is defined as the number of true negative decisions/ the number of true negative cases plus false-positive cases. These two determinations constitute the basic measures of performance of diagnostic tests. ROC curves are applied to correlate biomarker and histopathology findings for evaluating the biological performance of a biomarker in the preclinical setting. To understand the biological performance of a biomarker in the preclinical setting, statistical criteria are used to compare biomarker

changes with histopathologic change, which is considered the gold standard. Novel biomarkers can also be correlated directly to traditional biomarkers in order to compare performance characteristics. The area under the ROC curve (AUCROC) indicates the biomarker performance across the entire curve, where a biomarker can perform no worse than chance alone (0.5) and a perfect correlation with histopathology or other qualified biomarker is a value of 1.0. The AUCROC is a commonly used index of diagnostic accuracy that is utilized to compare the performance of biomarkers. The performance of numerous biomarkers can be determined and compared with one another on the same plot relative to the reference standard such as histopathology. An AUCROC greater than 0.75 is an indication of good biomarker performance, and a value greater than 0.9 is considered excellent.

The use of biomarkers to predict toxicity has been plagued by an unrealistic expectation for a predictive accuracy of almost 100%, with virtually no false-negative or false-positive results tolerated and 100% sensitivity and specificity. (Sensitivity is defined as the probability that a subject at risk will be correctly identified, and specificity is the probability that a subject who is NOT at risk will be correctly identified). Many have proposed a less restrictive way to evaluate the predictive value of a putative biomarker. Instead, the use of the predictive marker might be to place the value of the biomarker's prediction on its ability to reduce uncertainty. In this context, the sensitivity of the biomarker (and the assay) would usually be directly related to incidence; therefore, for an incidence rate of 0.03%, a biomarker and diagnostic test may be expected to have a sensitivity of 90% or more to be "acceptable" (as is suggested by published analyses of what would be required to effectively exclude

2.7. Patient/Clinical Trial Subject Selection

The use of biomarkers in early clinical trials is an important paradigm shift in the design and interpretation of the data derived from Phase 1 and Phase 2 clinical trials. The discovery and ultimate use of scientifically qualified biomarkers (and analytically validated assays) in rationally designed clinical hypothesis testing is a goal that is now set out early in drug discovery for most therapeutic areas. It is expected that an early focus on biomarker discovery and qualification during the preclinical phase will facilitate the use of biomarkers in clinical trials and allow the qualification process to continue seamlessly from the preclinical to the clinical setting. The success of a biomarker-driven program requires early application of the qualification criteria in the preclinical setting and extensive collaboration among many scientific disciplines. Most biomarker efforts depend heavily on a bridge between animal and human data via proof of mechanism or other gross, histological, or ultrastructural observations, creating an indispensable role for the pathologist in this effort.

A biomarker that is intended for patient selection must be qualified by a unique and rigorous set of criteria. Misleading results are an undesirable outcome for biomarkers in any category, but the patient selection biomarker has a particularly heavy influence on critical clinical decisions. Because of this role, any misinterpretation associ-

defined feature are not included (by chance) in an unselected population trial to allow a reasonably powered retrospective analysis. The inclusion of a biomarker in a clinical trial for the intent of patient selection is regulated by the FDA/EMEA and to an extent the institutional review boards that approve the research plan and clinical trial design. The uses of a biomarker for decision-making, dose finding, secondary/tertiary claims, or as supporting evidence (along with primary clinical evidence) are all uses covered by published guidance documents (Table 14.4).

THE DISCOVERY AND APPLICATION OF A BIOMARKER FOR PATIENT SELECTION: GENETIC MUTATION BRAF V600E (CHENG ET AL., 2018)

The role of consistent activating mutations in tyrosine kinases in human cancer has been and continues to be a stimulus for the development of tyrosine kinase inhibitor drugs, but when "kinome" exon sequencing efforts were applied, consistent activating mutations in serine/threonine kinases were uncovered. In particular, an activating V600E mutation in BRAF, a gene encoding for the serine/threonine kinase B-raf, was revealed to be present in a high proportion of human melanomas, providing an opportunity for development of selective small molecule inhibitors of V600E BRAF. The presence of a BRAF gene mutation in over 50% of melanoma patients and 10% in other cancers was discovered in 2002. Within several years after discovery of the gene mutation, a potent and selective inhibitor of active BRAF (PLX 4032) had been discovered, using a scaffold-based discovery approach. The IND for the

product, vemurafenib, was filed in 2006, with Phase 1 clinical trials started the same year. Encouraging results from Phase 1 trials resulted in start of Phase 2 trial in September 2009 and Phase 3 trials in January 2010. On August 17, 2011, the FDA approved Zelboraf (vemurafenib) to treat patients with late-stage (metastatic) or nonresectable melanoma. A diagnostic test for the genetic mutation was also approved. Several signal transduction pathways have been found to be constitutively active or mutated in other subsets of melanoma tumors that are potentially targetable with new agents. Effective use of data from molecular analysis of patient-derived tumor (or diseased tissue) used to assign the most appropriate therapeutic modality for each individual patient will continue to be explored with the codevelopment of therapeutic modalities and diagnostic kits to maximize therapeutic benefit.

---

ated with use of the biomarker can have particularly serious consequences. For example, the primary goal for this type of marker is the identification of subgroups of patient populations that will likely experience benefit from a particular treatment or treatment regimen. Inability to define these populations can lead to a significant number of patients receiving ineffective treatment and a lack of statistical power to determine benefit, particularly when enough patients with the

2.8. Surrogate Endpoint

A surrogate endpoint is expected to predict clinical outcome (benefit or harm, or lack of benefit or harm) based on epidemiologic, therapeutic, pathophysiologic, or other scientific evidence. For example, a surrogate endpoint for efficacy may be used to assess whether a drug has a clinically significant effect, and a surrogate endpoint for safety is expected to predict a safety

TABLE 14.4   Regulatory Guidance Documents Pertaining to Biomarkers

Document	Link
Biomarker qualification: Evidentiary framework — Draft guidance, December 2018	https://www.fda.gov/regulatory-information/search-fda-guidance-documents/biomarker-qualification-evidentiary-framework
Qualification process for drug development tools guidance — December 2019	https://www.fda.gov/regulatory-information/search-fda-guidance-documents/qualification-process-drug-development-tools-guidance-industry-and-fda-staff
CDER biomarker qualification program — current as of April 2018	https://www.fda.gov/drugs/drug-development-tool-ddt-qualification-programs/cder-biomarker-qualification-program
Considerations for use of histopathology and its associated methodologies to support biomarker qualification — May 2016	https://www.fda.gov/drugs/cder-biomarker-qualification-program/biomarker-guidances-and-reference-materials#guidance
Developing and labeling in vitro companion diagnostic Devices for a specific group or class of oncology therapeutic products — Draft guidance, December 2018	https://www.fda.gov/regulatory-information/search-fda-guidance-documents/developing-and-labeling-vitro-companion-diagnostic-devices-specific-group-or-class-oncology
Principles for codevelopment of an in vitro companion diagnostic Device with a therapeutic product — Draft guidance, July 2016	https://www.fda.gov/regulatory-information/search-fda-guidance-documents/principles-codevelopment-vitro-companion-diagnostic-device-therapeutic-product
E16 biomarkers related to drug or biotechnology product development: Context, structure, and format of qualification submissions — current as of August 2018	https://www.fda.gov/regulatory-information/search-fda-guidance-documents/e16-biomarkers-related-drug-or-biotechnology-product-development-context-structure-and-format
Use of public human genetic variant databases to support clinical validity for genetic and genomic-based in vitro diagnostics guidance — April 2018	https://www.fda.gov/regulatory-information/search-fda-guidance-documents/use-public-human-genetic-variant-databases-support-clinical-validity-genetic-and-genomic-based-vitro
Considerations for design, development, and analytical validation of next generation sequencing (NGS)—Based in vitro diagnostics (IVDs) intended to aid in the diagnosis of suspected germline diseases guidance — April 2018	https://www.fda.gov/regulatory-information/search-fda-guidance-documents/considerations-design-development-and-analytical-validation-next-generation-sequencing-ngs-based
Investigational in vitro diagnostics in oncology trials: Streamlined submission process for study risk determination — October 2019	https://www.fda.gov/regulatory-information/search-fda-guidance-documents/investigational-vitro-diagnostics-oncology-trials-streamlined-submission-process-study-risk
Developing targeted therapies in low-frequency molecular subsets of a disease — October 2018	https://www.fda.gov/regulatory-information/search-fda-guidance-documents/developing-targeted-therapies-low-frequency-molecular-subsets-disease
Bioanalytical method validation guidance for industry — May 2018	https://www.fda.gov/regulatory-information/search-fda-guidance-documents/bioanalytical-method-validation-guidance-industry

profile. There are several well-known examples of surrogate endpoints for efficacy, such as progression-free survival in colorectal cancer. An accepted and complex panel of surrogate endpoints for insulin resistance includes fasting insulin, fasting glucose, homeostatic model assessment of insulin resistance, and the insulin sensitivity index. Another prominent example is the use of blood cholesterol as a surrogate for risk of cardiovascular disease and stroke.

Perhaps due to the complexity of the burden of proof in a clinical trial, only a few biomarkers will likely achieve surrogate endpoint status. The use of surrogate endpoints in a clinical trial requires specification of the clinical endpoints that are being substituted, the class of therapeutic intervention being applied, and characteristics of population and disease state in which the substitution is being made. Furthermore, FDA approval for the use of a surrogate endpoint to establish therapeutic efficacy in registration trials may be predicated on obtaining additional clinical evidence to verify and describe clinical benefit, especially when there is uncertainty about the relation of the surrogate endpoint to clinical benefit or uncertainty about the relationship between the observed clinical benefit and ultimate outcome. Even with this high level of scrutiny, surrogate endpoints can still fail to serve as valid substitutes for other sources of data that may provide more direct evidence for a primary outcome. For example, many have acknowledged that lowering blood cholesterol levels in humans cannot always protect against cardiovascular disease. Thus, simply stating that lowering cholesterol will protect against cardiovascular disease may need to be proven. The biggest hurdle facing this biomarker subset is accumulating data to show that a surrogate is **causally related to disease outcome**, rather than being merely a correlate. Those points being taken, regulatory agencies such as the FDA may on occasion allow sponsors to bypass long-term safety studies and conditionally approve a drug based on small studies using a surrogate marker, on the basis that future studies will be done to more fully establish its clinical efficacy and safety.

2.9. Pharmacogenomic Biomarkers

A pharmacogenomic biomarker can be as a measurable DNA and/or RNA characteristic that is an indicator of normal biologic processes, pathogenic processes, and/or response to therapeutic or other interventions. A partial list of biomarkers that have been approved for use as pharmacogenomic markers can be found in Table 14.5. A complete listing may be found at the FDA website (FDA, 2020b). The pharmacogenomic marker serves to identify responders and nonresponders to medications, avoid adverse events, predict unique variations in drug metabolism (or drug–drug interactions), and optimize drug dose. This list has grown over 10-fold since 2013. Of interest, the type of approval given to pembrolizumab (Keytruda), larotrectinib (Vitrakvi), and entrectinib (Rozlytrek) represents use of a specific genetic defect to define the clinical use for a drug. FDA granted approval to treat solid tumors based on evidence of these tumors harboring microsatellite instability-high or being mismatch repair deficient. Keytruda (pembrolizumab) was approved to treat any solid tumors with these genetic features. FDA approval was also granted to Vitrakvi (larotrectinib) and Rozlytrek (entrectinib) for the treatment of solid tumors that have a neurotrophic receptor tyrosine kinase gene fusion.

2.10. Prognostic Biomarkers

Prognostic biomarkers are often defined as measurements used in the course of clinical diagnosis that serve to monitor about patient outcomes. In most cases, large multicenter retrospective and prospective studies in patients are required to determine if the biomarker can be of value in monitoring and to provide information about the state of the disease. Alternatively, studies using archived tissues, when conducted under ideal conditions and when independently confirmed, also can provide a sufficient level of evidence to support the biomarker for a prognostic purpose.

THE LIFE OF A CANDIDATE PROGNOSTIC MARKER: YKL-40 (JOHANSEN ET AL., 2006; SCHULTZ AND JOHANSEN, 2010)

YKL-40 is a member of the "mammalian chitinase—like proteins," that is expressed and secreted by several types of solid tumors. YKL-40 exhibits growth factor activity for cells involved in tissue remodeling processes. YKL-40 may have a role in cancer cell proliferation, survival, and invasiveness, in the inflammatory process around the tumor, angiogenesis, and remodeling of the extracellular matrix. YKL-40 is neither organ- nor tumor specific. In fact, the protein was discovered in a search for new bone proteins and was identified as a protein secreted in vitro in large amounts by the human osteosarcoma cell line MG63. Moderate to significant elevated serum concentrations of YKL-40 have been found in a variety of diseases characterized by inflammation and remodeling of the extracellular matrix such as active rheumatoid arthritis, osteoarthritis, bacterial pneumonia, and liver fibrosis. Increased serum levels of YKL-40 are correlated with an unfavorable prognosis for patients with recurrent breast cancer or with colorectal cancer. Elevated serum YKL-40 during postoperative follow-up appeared to be a negative predictor of survival. To validate these claims, several clinical studies have been conducted including a study to examine relationships between survival, serum CA-125, and plasma YKL-40, as measured in pretherapeutic samples from patients presenting with recurring ovarian cancer. The study included 73 women (mean age 55, range 25—76 years) with recurrent ovarian cancer. Blood was obtained at the time of diagnosis of the recurrence and before initiation of second-line chemotherapy. Although the study demonstrated that an elevated plasma level of YKL-40 was associated with high risk of short survival in patients with recurrent ovarian cancer, the mechanism by which plasma YKL-40 reflects disease status is unknown. To date, YKL-40 has not been approved for use as a prognostic indicator. Therefore, the elucidation of YKL-40 function will be an important objective of future studies in order to gain approval for use as a prognostic indicator.

TABLE 14.5 Biomarkers Approved for Pharmacogenomic Indications

Biomarker	Biomarker full name	Biomarker activity	Indication of biomarker
ALK	Anaplastic lymphoma receptor tyrosine kinase	Novel receptor tyrosine kinase having a putative transmembrane domain and an extracellular domain; these sequences are absent in the product of the transforming ALK gene rearrangement	Identify patients with an ALK rearrangement for clinical benefit
BCR-ABL1	Philadelphia chromosome	The BCR-ABL1 fusion gene and protein encoded by the philadelphia chromosome affects multiple signaling pathways that directly affect apoptotic potential, cell division rates, and different stages of the cell cycle to achieve unchecked proliferation	The presence of this translocation is required for diagnosis of chronic myeloid leukemia
BRAF	v-raf murine sarcoma viral oncogene homolog B1	Mutated BRAF is an oncogene associated with many different human cancers; activates RAF-ERK signal transduction pathways	Identify patients with genetic mutation for clinical benefit

(Continued)

TABLE 14.5   Biomarkers Approved for Pharmacogenomic Indications—cont'd

Biomarker	Biomarker full name	Biomarker activity	Indication of biomarker
BRCA	*BRCA1* and *BRCA2* are human genes that produce tumor suppressor proteins	Inherited mutations in *BRCA1* and *BRCA2* increase the risk of breast and ovarian cancer	Identify patients at risk for breast and ovarian cancer
CD274 (PD-L1)	Programmed cell death ligand	Upregulation of PD-L1 allows tumors to evade host immune system	Identify patients whose cancer is susceptible to treatment with PD-L1 inhibitors
C-kit	v-kit Hardy–Zuckerman 4 feline sarcoma viral oncogene homolog	Cytokine receptor expressed on the surface of hematopoietic stem cells; signaling through c-kit plays a role in cell survival, proliferation, and differentiation	Identify patients with c-kit mutations for clinical benefit
EGFR	Epidermal growth factor receptor	Autophosphorylation of EGFR dimer elicits several downstream signal transduction pathway cascades leading to DNA synthesis and cell proliferation	Identify patients with EGFR mutations for clinical benefit
ERBB2 (HER2)	Receptor tyrosine kinase human epidermal growth factor receptor 2	Amplification of HER2 associated with poor prognosis and increased disease recurrence	HER2 is the target of the monoclonal antibody trastuzumab (marketed as Herceptin)
ER	Estrogen receptor	DNA-binding transcription factor	ER status used to determine sensitivity of breast cancer to drug treatment
G6PD	Glucose-6-phosphate dehydrogenase	Metabolic enzyme involved in the pentose phosphate pathway, particularly important in red blood cell metabolism; G6PD deficiency is the most common human enzyme defect	Identify patients with G6PD deficiency; risk of toxicity
HLA-B	Major histocompatibility complex, class I, B	HLA-B is part of a family of genes called the human leukocyte antigen (HLA) complex that plays a critical role in the immune system	Identify individuals who have HLA-B and are at risk for toxicity to certain compounds
IL28B	Interleukin 28B (interferon, lambda 3)	IL-28 is a cytokine that plays a role in the adaptive immune response	Identify patients with a single nucleotide polymorphism (SNP) near the IL28B gene for prediction of clinical response

(Continued)

TABLE 14.5 Biomarkers Approved for Pharmacogenomic Indications—cont'd

Biomarker	Biomarker full name	Biomarker activity	Indication of biomarker
KRAS	v-Ki-ras2 Kirsten rat sarcoma viral oncogene homolog	KRAS protein is a GTPase and is an early player in many signal transduction pathways	Identify patients with KRAS mutation for poor clinical response rate
LDLR	Low-density lipoprotein receptor	Cell-surface receptor that mediates the endocytosis of cholesterol-rich LDL	Identify patients with LDLR polymorphisms for risk of disease
MSI-H; dMMR	Microsatellite instability-high; mismatch repair deficient	DNA repair pathway that plays a key role in maintaining genomic stability	Any solid tumor with specific genetic feature (biomarker)
NAT1; NAT2	N-acetyl-transferase 1 (arylamine N-acetyltransferase); N-acetyl-transferase 2 (arylamine N-acetyltransferase)	Responsible for N-acetylation of certain arylamine drugs such as p-aminosalicylic acid; polymorphisms associated with slow inactivator and rapid inactivator phenotypes	Identify variants that may lead to changes in drug exposure with risk of toxicity
PDGFRB	Platelet-derived growth factor receptor, beta polypeptide	Cell-surface tyrosine kinase receptor important for regulating cell proliferation, cellular differentiation, cell growth, development, and many diseases including cancer	Identify therapeutic target for anticancer drugs for clinical benefit
RAS	Retroviral proto-oncogene	Ras proteins are founding members of a large superfamily of small GTPases that regulate all key cellular processes	Ras point mutations are the single most common abnormality of human proto-oncogenes and are targets for cancer therapies

3. STRATEGIES FOR DISCOVERY OF BIOMARKERS

Biomarkers contribute to rational drug discovery and development. Although biomarkers have been used in drug development and to assess treatment of disease for a long time, the identification of new, predictive safety, and efficacy biomarkers is expected to reduce the time and cost of drug development. The use of novel biomarkers can further facilitate decision-making from discovery through preclinical development and into clinical trials. Rapid advances in genomics and proteomics have increased the discovery of new biomarkers and their value in drug development and treatment of disease. Discovery of novel biomarkers is challenging, and acceptance by the scientific and regulatory communities is often a long and arduous process. Various "omics" platforms have been applied to rapidly identify novel protein biomarkers in various biological matrices from cell cultures (lysates, supernatants) to preclinical samples (animal tissue, biological fluids, tumor xenografts) to human clinical samples (tissue, biological fluids). A number of strategies have been successfully applied to biomarker discovery. A common strategy is shown in Fig. 14.2.

Using this approach, analytical techniques are applied to compare molecular, structural, and functional differences between the sample groups without necessarily assigning relative importance to the changes. However, discovery of differentially identified measurements that distinguish the two sample groups becomes potential biomarkers for hypothesis-driven biomarker qualification. The stages of biomarker discovery and development using a comparative strategy can be divided into three main phases that address each of the key steps of the process: discovery, qualification, and verification (Fig. 14.3) (Kraus, 2018).

In the initial stage of discovery, the objective is to establish the purpose for the biomarker, which includes the clinical question being asked. A robust experimental design of the comparative studies is critical, including, but not limited to, types and number of samples, time points

examined, compound and dose selection, technology platforms to be used, and endpoint measurements. Samples must be carefully chosen and in sufficient numbers to produce statistical significance. Those biomarkers that show significant disease-, group-, or time-dependent differences are selected as candidate biomarkers.

Once candidate biomarkers are identified and prioritized, the purpose of the qualification stage is to link a biomarker to a preclinical or clinical endpoint or to a biological process using a fit-for-purpose process. Biomarkers must be sensitive for tissue-specific lesions and specific in terms of being differentially detected in comparative test systems, such as treated animals with drug-induced injured tissues compared to untreated animals. Confirmation of specificity of novel biomarkers is frequently the role of the toxicology pathologist and is often achieved by applying more traditional toxicologic pathology tools. IHC is a good method for localizing the differentially expressed protein(s) to a specific

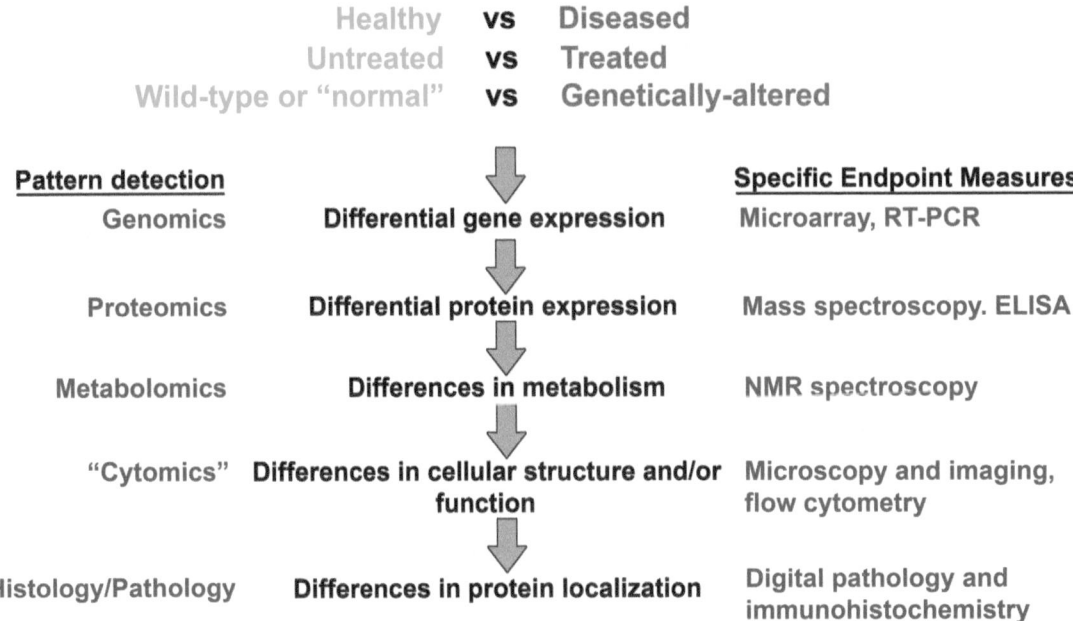

FIGURE 14.2 Strategy for biomarker discovery that involves comparing patterns of biological responses between different populations of samples. Various platforms and endpoints may be employed and measured.

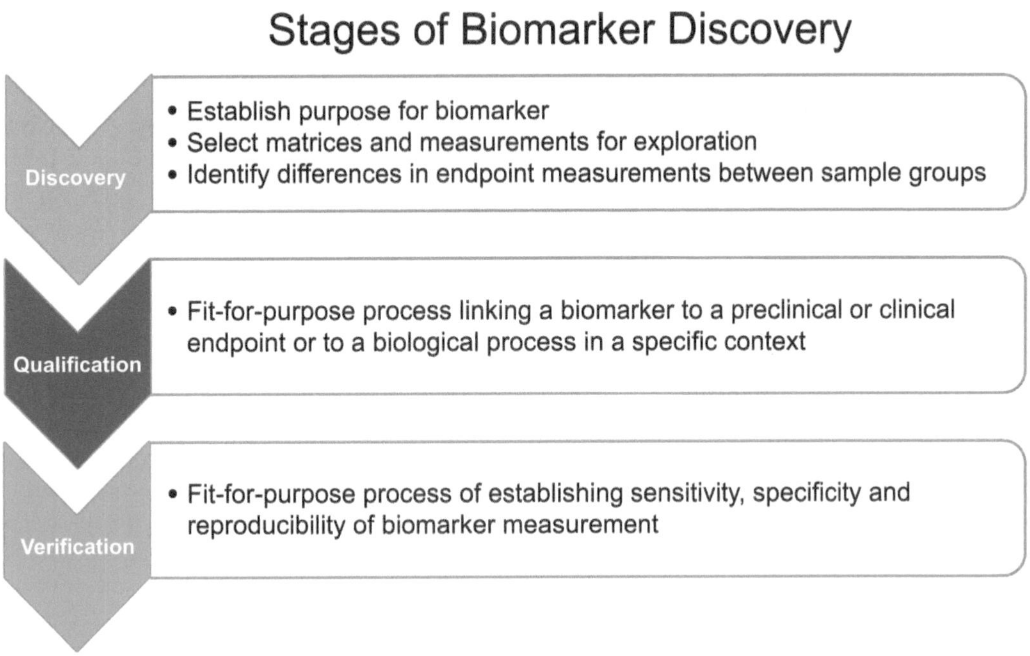

Stages of Biomarker Discovery

FIGURE 14.3 Stages of biomarker discovery.

region of the tissue so that site specificity of the biomarker(s) may be better characterized and qualified.

Verification is the fit-for-purpose process of measuring performance characteristics, and determining the range of conditions in which the assay will perform reproducibly and accurately, whereas validation is a regulated procedure to prove suitability of an analytical assay for intended use that involves demonstration of accuracy, precision, limits of quantification, and stability of an analyte in a matrix.

3.1. Discovery and Application of Panels of Biomarkers

Although a single biomarker is attractive, as the verification stage of biomarker discovery/ development is more achievable in terms of establishing sensitivity, specificity, and reproducibility, it is unlikely that a sole biomarker would be considered definitive. It is more likely that a combination of markers would be required to identify meaningful biomarkers and discover the appropriate weight of evidence applied to each to generate a final algorithmic conclusion. Given that "omics" technologies enable the

identification and assessment of thousands of genes and proteins, sophisticated technology platforms and biostatistical approaches are rapidly evolving and greatly contributing to biomarker discovery and application. The advent of "omics" disciplines has facilitated the discovery of novel biomarkers that may be measured in a variety of matrices, including DNA, RNA, and protein from biological fluids, cells, tissues, and organs.

4. METHODS FOR BIOMARKER MEASUREMENT AND QUANTITATION

Examples of methods used to measure biomarkers are presented in Table 14.6. The development and application of technologies and platforms that are used to assess differentially expressed genes, proteins, and cellular responses represent an evolving discipline by which new technologies are introduced and applied to biomarker discovery and measurement. With this in mind, only a few key technology platforms will be discussed as they are currently applied.

DISCOVERY OF THIOSTATIN AS A CANDIDATE BIOMARKER FOR DRUG-INDUCED HEPATIC INJURY (ADLER ET AL., 2010)

A good example of a discovery strategy that combined "omics" technologies with conventional clinical chemistry methods and ultimately immunohistochemical assessment is represented by the discovery of serum thiostatin, a candidate biomarker better for drug-induced hepatobiliary injury. The goal was to link onset of histopathologic change with biomarkers detected in serum/urine and their expression/localization in the liver, thus providing phenotypic anchoring to both the target organ and toxicity. In this study, genomics, transcriptomics, proteomics, and metabolomics responses to drug candidates that had failed during preclinical development due to hepatotoxicity and/or nephrotoxicity were extensively characterized to obtain mechanistic insight and identify potential biomarkers of organ-specific toxicity. Based on analysis of the extensive integrated "omics" profiles, paraoxonase (PON1), clusterin, neutrophil gelatinase–associated lipocalin (NGAL), and thiostatin were selected and compared to conventional clinical chemistry parameters, i.e., ALT and aspartate transaminase (AST). Rats were treated with drug candidates that had previously failed during development at two-dose levels for 1, 3, and 14 days. The biomarkers mined from the "omics" responses were measured in serum and urine by ELISA. These results were supplemented by confirmatory qRT-PCR performed on total RNA isolated from frozen livers and kidneys. Finally, immunohistochemical staining of liver and kidney tissue sections was used to localize the protein biomarkers to specific sites of injury, thus providing phenotypic anchoring in terms of histopathologic changes that correlated well with the increase in serum/urine markers accompanied by a corresponding increase in mRNA of the biomarkers. ROC analyses were applied to determine the ability of the biomarker candidates to discriminate animals without microscopic evidence of liver injury from those with histopathological lesions. Moreover, the results from this study were able to distinguish tissue specificity and demonstrate a dose response as well as a temporal response. Taken together, the results of this study demonstrated serum thiostatin to perform better than PON1, clusterin, or NGAL, as well as the traditional biomarkers of hepatic toxicity, ALT, and AST.

TABLE 14.6   Methods of Biomarker Measurement

Measurement	Matrix	Analytical technique	"Omics" discipline (pattern Detection)
Genome	DNA	DNA sequencing	Genomics
Gene expression	RNA, miRNA	Microarrays, RT-PCR	Transcriptomics
Protein characterization	Protein	Electrophoresis and mass spectrometry	Proteomics
Protein expression	Cell/tissue lysates, biological fluids	ELISA, Western	Proteomics
Metabolic profiling	Metabolites	NMR spectroscopy	Metabolomics
Structural and functional analysis	Cells	Microscopy and imaging, flow cytometry	"Histocytomics"
Phenotypic anchoring	Tissues	Digital pathology and immunohistochemistry	Histology/pathology

DNA, deoxyribonucleic acid; ELISA, enzyme-linked immunosorbent assay; miRNA, micro-RNA; NMR, nuclear magnetic resonance; RNA, ribonucleic acid; RT-PCR, reverse transcriptase–polymerase chain reaction.

4.1. Genomics

"Closed" genomic systems generally use microarray-type formats that are based on predefined sets of genes selected to address a specific hypothesis, to characterize a certain tissue, or to profile an entire genome. Microarrays are typically based on cDNA clones, PCR-amplified cDNA fragments, or chemically synthesized oligonucleotides that are affixed to a solid support material, such as a glass slide or nylon membrane. Depending on the specific platform, absolute or differential expression levels of the genes represented on the arrays are then calculated and used for statistical analysis. Alternatively, "open" gene expression-profiling systems do not begin with a preselected set of genes. Instead, the differences between two populations of RNA are determined directly, generally using some combination of RT-PCR, gel electrophoresis, and DNA sequencing. Examples include SAGE (Serial Analysis of Gene Expression), differential display, and subtractive hybridization.

Several representative types of biomarkers identified using comparative biomarkers discovery approaches and applying various "omics" pattern detection analytical methods are listed in Table 14.6. The list will continue to expand with increased understanding of the biology, advances in technology, and improvements in data mining. Clearly, the application of "omics" disciplines is advancing the discovery of biomarkers at an unprecedented pace.

4.2. Proteomics

Proteomics technologies are broadly characterized as tools designed to examine the expression of proteins in a given set of samples. Types of information derived from proteomics technologies include protein identity, quantity, interactions, structure, and posttranslational modification. The nature of the proteome presents a series of challenges, most importantly protein heterogeneity, that limit the ability of any single technology to completely assay and characterize it. Proteins are complex molecules, often with posttranslational modifications, such as glycosylation, lipidation, or phosphorylation. These can have dramatic effects on how the proteins behave in biochemical assays. A second challenge of the proteome is the extraordinarily wide dynamic range of protein expression, resulting in detection limitations. A third challenge of the proteome is the absence of a method of direct amplification. Whereas the polymerase chain reaction can amplify DNA and RNA, no such technique exists for proteins (although there are promising approaches in development). With advances in technological approaches and platforms, these challenges are being met and are providing powerful tools to discover biomarkers and understand fundamental mechanisms.

Most proteomic techniques are broadly aimed at expression profiling, although there have been recent advances in additional applications, such as detecting posttranslational modifications, for example, phosphorylation. All proteomics technologies consist of some permutation of separation followed by detection. Classically, two-dimensional gel electrophoresis has been used to assay the proteome. Protein samples are first separated based on pI using an isoelectric focusing gradient. Proteins are then further separated in a second dimension based on their migration in an electric field, which generally correlates to their molecular weight. Detection is achieved using any of a myriad of agents, including silver staining and fluorescent dyes. Individual spots on the gels can be excised, digested with trypsin, and tryptic fragment fingerprint matched against a database. Mass spectrometry can be performed and matched against the theoretical mass spectra of peptide sequences to provide definitive identification.

4.3. Metabolomics

The metabolome refers to the complete set of small-molecule metabolites (such as metabolic intermediates, hormones, other signaling molecules, and secondary metabolites) to be found within a biological sample. Metabolomics combines the techniques of high-resolution nuclear magnetic resonance spectroscopy and pattern recognition technology to rapidly generate differential metabolic fingerprints. For more in-depth information, see *Toxicogenomics: A Primer for Toxicologic Pathologists* [**Vol 1, Chap 15**].

4.4. Histocytomics

Quantitative and functional information may be obtained by analyzing accessible circulating cells. Circulating cells present in the blood may exhibit differential phenotypes between two populations such as those exemplified in Fig. 14.2. Flow cytometry has wide application in the study of circulating cells, which may be collected by minimally invasive means. It permits rapid simultaneous acquisition of multiple parameters, which are valuable for analyzing diverse functional or quantitative changes in individual cells. Advances in flow cytometry technology allow analysis of extremely large numbers of cells, leading to subsequent identification of even rare cells such as circulating tumor cells.

4.5. Antibody-Based Detection Systems

Quantitative antibody-based assays are the current method of choice for quantitative measurement of biomarkers (Table 14.7). The format used most often as a conventional biomarker assay is the two-step sandwich colorimetric ELISA format. Improvement in the affinity of the capture and signal antibodies, plus the use of detection systems such as fluorescence, including infrared, chemiluminescence, and electrochemiluminescence, has enabled assay manufacturers to produce platforms that require reduced specimen volumes and have wider dynamic ranges and higher throughput.

4.6. Multiplexed Assays

Multiplexing can accelerate biomarker discovery in both drug development and clinical applications. In a multiplexed assay, many different biomarkers may be measured simultaneously in one sample. Common multiplex platforms are flow cytometry–based assays with fluorescent microspheres and capture antibody–spotted plate-based assays. By combining multiple different antigen–antibody reactions into one assay, assay factors such as incubation time, buffers, and specimen dilution are inevitably compromised to accommodate measurement of all the analytes together. Such compromises may result in reduced sensitivity and/or dynamic range for some markers and

variation between different multiplexes. Given the numerous platforms and vendors actively engaged in the evolution of quantitative, immuno-based assays, the speed at which advances are being made equates with advances from "omics" technologies.

4.7. Morphology-Based Methods

Morphology-based approaches that combine anatomic/toxicologic pathology with IHC are used to define the expression and characterize the location of biomarker proteins. However, tissue-based IHC as a platform for biomarkers has been challenged by more quantitative molecular assays with reference standards, but lacking in morphologic context. Historically, IHC assays were not truly quantitative or on a par with nonmorphologic assays. A major step in transforming anatomic/toxicologic pathology from a discipline that is descriptive to one that is quantitative has been advances in digital microscopy, a comprehensive integration of digital imaging and light microscopy. To meet the challenges of the postgenomic era, a new concept of high-content pathology was created for integrating automated high-throughput digital whole-slide imaging, quantitative image analysis, high-content cell/tissue screening, and pathology informatics in order to provide multiplexed and data-rich information. New digital pathology applications that provide whole-slide imaging and automated quantitative analysis are transforming the integral role of the toxicological pathologist in drug discovery and development, including biomarker discovery efforts.

One of the biggest challenges to obtaining accurate image analysis results is the segregation of target tissue (region of interest) from other tissues on a slide. Conventionally, a limited sample of representative images that contained only the target tissue was captured with a microscope-fitted camera, and evaluations and/or image analysis was performed on these selected areas. The use of whole-slide imaging enables orders of magnitude more tissue to be analyzed because the image analysis can be conducted across the entire tissue present on the slide. Furthermore, with emerging automated pattern recognition software as a preprocessing utility to segregate target and nontarget tissue during analysis, an individual tissue type can then be

TABLE 14.7 Antibody-Based Technologies for Biomarker Measurements

Technique	Basis of assay	Platform	Measurement
Enzyme-linked immunosorbent assay (ELISA)	Ligand-binding assay	96-Well plate	Target protein concentration
Western blot	Protein immunoblot	Gel electrophoresis; nitrocellulose membrane	Molecular weight and relative amount of target protein
Immunoprecipitation	Antibody capture and immobilization	Solid state antibody-coated beads	Isolate protein complexes, DNA-binding proteins, RNA-binding proteins
Flow cytometry	Hydrodynamic focusing of particles with detection of fluorescent emission	Flow cytometer	Physical and biochemical properties of individual particles
Fluorescence-activated cell sorting (FACS)	Hydrodynamic focusing and separation of particles based on preselected fluorescent emission characteristics	FACS machine	Physical and biochemical properties of individual particles
Immunohistochemistry (IHC)	Labeled antibody reagents	Tissue based	Localization of target antigens
Enzyme-linked immunospot	Ligand-binding assay	96-Well plate	Number and percentage of cells secreting the target protein (e.g., cytokines)
Aptamer-based proteomics	Transforms a signature of protein concentrations into a corresponding signature of DNA aptamer concentrations, which is quantified on a DNA microarray	96-Well plate; DNA microarray	Quantified protein signature

selected for subsequent image analysis, without the pathologist making tedious region-of-interest drawings on the image. Histology pattern recognition is a powerful utility capable of identifying and categorizing specific histologic tissue types, thus enabling subsequent analysis of target regions by standard image analysis tools. The ability to digitize entire tissue specimens on slides and subsequently perform morphometric analysis on the images is a valuable tool being applied to biomarker discovery efforts. Anatomic imaging has promising application to biomarkers and is discussed in detail in *In Vivo Small Animal Imaging: A Comparison with Gross and Histopathologic Observations in Animal Models* [**Vol 1, Chap 13**].

5. QUALIFICATION OF BIOMARKERS: MAJOR CONSIDERATIONS

The Biomarkers Definitions Working Group published consensus definitions used for the discussion of biomarkers in 2001 that included validation and qualification as key terms used in the context of biomarkers. Validation was defined as "The fit-for-purpose process of assessing the assay and its measurement performance characteristics, determining the range of conditions under which the assay will give reproducible and accurate data." Qualification was defined as "The fit-for-purpose evidentiary process of linking a biomarker with biological processes and clinical endpoints." Currently, there are no clear regulatory guidelines on the requirements for novel biomarker assay validation; neither is there a consistent approach for qualifying biomarkers for regulatory use. However, there has been considerable coordination among industry, regulatory agencies, NIH, and academia to develop consensus practices for novel biomarker discovery, validation, and qualification, and reviews on the topic have been published.

Certain principles and considerations are applicable regardless of the approach taken for biomarker qualification. One core principle for the qualification process is that a biomarker must be developed in a specific "fit-for-purpose" context and in an iterative and progressive framework. For this reason, a biomarker qualification plan can be very helpful. Most qualification plans focus on identifying what types of evidence are required to link a biomarker with disease/toxicity biology or other physiological endpoints. For each biomarker effort, it is helpful if the objectives (or intended use for the biomarker) and potential issues are also identified in the qualification plan. For example, a biomarker intended to fulfill an exploratory objective in a preclinical or Phase 1 study would not necessarily need to meet the same qualification objectives as a biomarker being used for decision-making in a clinical study.

Biomarkers used in drug development may be categorized into three general classes of qualification, each one with increasing evidentiary requirements: (1) *exploration biomarkers* are research and development tools applied to the preclinical setting without evidence necessarily linking the biomarker to clinical outcomes in humans; (2) *demonstration biomarkers* have been qualified in terms of preclinical sensitivity and specificity, and have been linked with clinical outcomes, but have not been reproducibly demonstrated in clinical studies; and (3) *characterization biomarkers* have demonstrated adequate preclinical sensitivity and specificity, and are reproducibly linked with clinical outcomes. The progression of qualification leads to increased utility of a biomarker in decision-making and regulatory application.

Typically, a biomarker qualification process is based on strength-of-evidence criteria applied during the evaluation of a biomarker(s). For example, the C-Path PSTC considered several criteria during the process of evaluating biomarkers of drug-induced renal toxicity for use in early drug development. Although the criteria listed in the Strength-of-Evidence Biomarker Qualification box provide a framework for biomarkers associated with toxicity, they can be applied to biomarker qualification in general.

Method validation and biomarker qualification are linked due to the graded nature of the validation and qualification processes and close interaction between method validation and biomarker qualification, with both of these activities dependent on overall purpose. For example, repurposing a biomarker that is already being utilized for another purpose and qualified can be more readily tested for a new application. Having a validated assay will facilitate a much more rapid generation of data that can be used to qualify the biomarker for the new intended purpose.

This chapter is an introduction to the extensively reviewed and expansive topic of biomarker discovery and application. It is expected that

STRENGTH-OF-EVIDENCE BIOMARKER QUALIFICATION (AMUR ET AL., 2015)

1. Demonstrate dose response and temporal relationships between biomarker changes, onset of injury, and severity of injury that correspond to progression of the injury.
2. Identify a strong association between magnitude of biomarker changes and biological outcome; that is, identification of a biomarker threshold or quantitative changes that indicate reversibility of injury.
3. Provide adequate tissue specificity to ensure that the biomarker does not reflect injury to other organs or

activation of physiological processes in the target organ unrelated to injury.
4. Define molecular, biochemical, genetic, immunological, or physiological associations that link the biomarker to the organ, pathophysiology of injury, or mechanism of toxicity.
5. Provide experimental evidence connecting the molecular mechanism of the biomarker response with biological outcome.

the selected citations will provide detailed content and comprehensive background on the key concepts that have been introduced in this chapter.

REFERENCES

Adler M, Hoffmann D, Ellinger-Ziegelbauer H, et al.: Assessment of candidate biomarkers of drug-induced hepatobiliary injury in preclinical toxicity studies, *Toxicol Lett* 196:1–11, 2010.

Amur S, LaVange L, Zineh I, et al.: Biomarker qualification: toward a multiple stakeholder framework for biomarker development, regulatory acceptance, and utilization, *Clin Pharmacol Ther* 98:34–46, 2015.

Babuin L, Jaffe AS: Troponin: the biomarker of choice for the detection of cardiac injury, *CMAJ* 173:1191–1202, 2005.

Basi GS, Hemphill S, Brigham EF, et al.: Amyloid precursor protein selective gamma-secretase inhibitors for treatment of Alzheimer's disease, *Alz Res Therapy* 2:36, 2010.

Brott DA, Jones HB, Gould S, et al.: Current status and future directions for diagnostic markers of drug-induced vascular injury, *Cancer Biomark* 1:15–28, 2005a.

Brott D, Gould S, Jones H, et al.: Biomarkers of drug-induced vascular injury, *Toxicol Appl Pharmacol* 207:441–445, 2005b.

Campion S, Aubrecht J, Kim B, et al.: The current status of biomarkers for predicting toxicity, *Expert Opin Drug Metabol Toxicol* 9:1391–1408, 2013.

Capodanno D, Patel A, Dharmashankar K, et al.: Pharmacodynamic effects of different aspirin dosing regimens in type 2 diabetes mellitus patients with coronary artery disease, *Circ Cardiovasc Interv* 4:180–187, 2011.

Cheng L, Lopez-Beltran A, Massari F, et al.: Molecular testing for BRAF mutations to inform melanoma treatment decisions: a move toward precision medicine, *Mod Pathol* 31:24–38, 2018.

Dharnidharka VR, Kwon C, Stevens G: Serum cystatin C is superior to serum creatinine as a marker of kidney function: a meta-analysis, *Am J Kidney Dis* 40:221–226, 2002.

Dieterle F, Perentes E, Cordier A, et al.: Urinary clusterin, cystatin C, beta2-microglobulin and total protein as markers to detect drug-induced kidney injury, *Nat Biotechnol* 28:463–469, 2010.

Espín-Pérez A, Krauskopf J, Theo M, de Kok, et al.: 'OMICS-based' biomarkers for environmental Health studies, *Curr Environment Health Rep* 1:353–362, 2014.

FDA: *Guidance for industry drug-induced liver injury: premarketing clinical evaluation*, 2009, US Food and Drug Administration. https://www.fda.gov/regulatory-information/search-fda-guidance-documents/drug-induced-liver-injury-premarketing-clinical-evaluation.

FDA: *Biomarker qualification: evidentiary framework – draft guidance*, 2018. https://www.fda.gov/regulatory-information/search-fda-guidance-documents/biomarker-qualification-evidentiary-framework.

FDA: *List of qualified biomarkers*, 2020a, US Food and Drug Administration. https://www.fda.gov/drugs/cder-biomarker-qualification-program/list-qualified-biomarkers.

FDA: *Table of pharmacogenomic biomarkers in drug labeling*, 2020b, US Food and Drug Administration. https://www.fda.gov/drugs/science-and-research-drugs/table-pharmacogenomic-biomarkers-drug-labeling.

Fu S, Wu D, Jiang W, et al.: Molecular biomarkers in drug-induced liver injury: challenges and future perspectives, *Front Pharmacol* 10:1667, 2020.

Greaves P: Patterns of drug-induced cardiovascular pathology in the beagle dog: relevance for humans, *Exp Toxicol Pathol* 50:283–293, 1998.

Grubb A, Simonsen O, Sturfelt G, et al.: Serum concentration of cystatin C, factor D and beta 2-microglobulin as a measure of glomerular filtration rate, *Acta Med Scand* 218:499–503, 1985.

Hanley JA, McNeil BJ: The meaning and use of the area under a receiver operating characteristic (ROC) curve, *Radiology* 143:29–36, 1982.

Howell LS, Ireland L, Park BK, et al.: MiR-122 and other microRNAs as potential circulating biomarkers of drug-induced liver injury, *Expert Rev Mol Diagn* 18:47–54, 2018.

Iguchi T, Niino N, Tamai S, et al.: Comprehensive analysis of circulating microRNA specific to the liver, heart, and skeletal muscle of cynomolgus monkeys, *Int J Toxicol* 36: 220–228, 2017.

Iguchi T, Sakurai K, Tamai S, et al.: Circulating liver-specific microRNAs in cynomolgus monkeys, *J Toxicol Pathol* 31: 3–13, 2018.

Isaacs KR, Joseph EC, Betton GR: Coronary vascular lesions in dogs treated with phosphodiesterase III inhibitors, *Toxicol Pathol* 17:153–163, 1989.

Johansen JS, Jensen BV, Roslind A, et al.: Serum YKL-40, a new prognostic biomarker in cancer patients? *Cancer Epidemiol Biomarkers Prev* 15:194–202, 2006.

Jones B, Smith DA, Schmid EF: Are predictive biomarkers of toxicity worth having? An economic model, *Xenobiotica* 42: 4–10, 2012.

Kagawa T, Shirai Y, Oda S, et al.: Identification of specific MicroRNA biomarkers in early stages of hepatocellular injury, cholestasis, and steatosis in rats, *Toxicol Sci* 166:228–239, 2018.

Kerns W, Schwartz L, Blanchard K, et al.: Drug-induced vascular injury—a quest for biomarkers, *Toxicol Appl Pharmacol* 203:62–87, 2005.

Kraus VB: Biomarkers as drug development tools: discovery, validation, qualification and use, *Nat Rev Rheumatol* 14:354–362, 2018.

Laterza OF, Lim L, Garrett-Engele PW, et al.: Plasma MicroRNAs as sensitive and specific biomarkers of tissue injury, *Clin Chem* 55:1977–1983, 2009.

Louden C, Brott D, Katein A, et al.: Biomarkers and mechanisms of drug-induced vascular injury in non-rodents, *Toxicol Pathol* 34:19–26, 2006.

Louden C, Morgan DG: Pathology and pathophysiology of drug-induced arterial injury in laboratory animals and its implications on the evaluation of novel chemical entities for human clinical trials, *Pharmacol Toxicol* 89:158–170, 2001.

McHale CM, Zhang L, Smith MT: Current understanding of the mechanism of benzene-induced leukemia in humans: implications for risk assessment, *Carcinogenesis* 33:240–252, 2012.

Mesfin GM, Piper RC, DuCharme DW, et al.: Pathogenesis of cardiovascular alterations in dogs treated with minoxidil, *Toxicol Pathol* 17:164–181, 1989.

Metz AL, Dominick MA, Suchanek G, et al.: Acute cardiovascular toxicity induced by an adenosine agonist-antihypertensive in beagles, *Toxicol Pathol* 19:98–107, 1991.

Meunier L, Larrey D: Drug-induced liver injury: biomarkers, requirements, candidates, and validation, *Front Pharmacol* 10:1482, 2019.

Park SH, Goo JM, Jo CH: Receiver operating characteristic (ROC) curve: practical review for radiologists, *Korean J Radiol* 5:11–18, 2004.

Pinches MD, Betts CJ, Bickerton SJ, et al.: Evaluation of novel urinary renal biomarkers: biological variation and reference change values, *Toxicol Pathol* 40:541–549, 2012.

Pugsley MK, Authier S, Curtis MJ: Principles of safety pharmacology, *Br J Pharmacol* 154:1382–1399, 2008.

Schultz NA, Johansen JS: YKL-40-A protein in the field of translational medicine: a role as a biomarker in cancer patients? *Cancers* 2:1453–1491, 2010.

Searfoss GH, Jordan WH, Calligaro DO, et al.: Adipsin, a biomarker of gastrointestinal toxicity mediated by a functional γ-secretase inhibitor, *J Biol Chem* 278:46107–46116, 2003.

Servais EL, Suzuki K, Colovos C, Rodriguez L, Sima C, Fleisher M, Adusumilli PS, et al.: An in vivo platform for tumor biomarker assessment, *PLoS One* 6(10):1–6, 2011. https://doi.org/10.1371/journal.pone.0026722.

Simonsen O, Grubb A, Thysell H: The blood serum concentration of cystatin C (gamma-trace) as a measure of the glomerular filtration rate, *Scand J Clin Lab Invest* 45:97–101, 1985.

Walker DB: Serum chemical biomarkers of cardiac injury for nonclinical safety testing, *Toxicol Pathol* 34:94–104, 2006.

Wang X-Y, Zhang F, Zhang C, et al.: The biomarkers for acute myocardial infarction and heart failure, *BioMed Res Int* 2020:2018035, 2020.

Yuan J-M, Butler LM, Stepanov I, et al.: Urinary tobacco smoke-constituent biomarkers for assessing risk of lung cancer, *Canc Res* 74:401–411, 2014.

CHAPTER

15

Toxicogenomics: A Primer for Toxicologic Pathologists

Arun R. Pandiri[1], Pierre R. Bushel[2], Eric A. Blomme[3]

[1]Molecular Pathology Group, Comparative and Molecular Pathogenesis Branch, Division of the National Toxicology Program, National Institute of Environmental Health Sciences, Durham, NC, United States, [2]Biostatistics & Computational Biology Branch, National Institute of Environmental Health Sciences, Durham, NC, United States, [3]AbbVie, Chicago, IL, United States

OUTLINE

1. Introduction	491		6.2. Collection and Processing of the -Omics Samples	503
2. Basics of Toxicogenomics	492		6.3. Extraction of Biomolecules	504
			6.4. Controls for -Omics Assays	505
3. Overview of Toxicogenomic Technologies	493		6.5. Study Designs and Statistical Considerations	507
3.1. Nucleic Acid-Based -Omics Platforms	493		6.6. Software Tools and Databases	509
3.2. Microarray Technologies	495		6.7. Data Analysis and Interpretation	509
3.3. Next-Generation Sequencing Technologies	496			
3.4. Protein- and Metabolome-Based -Omics Platforms	497		7. Applications of Toxicogenomics	519
3.5. Proteomics Technologies	497		7.1. Predictive Toxicology	519
3.6. Metabolomics Technologies	500		7.2. Mechanistic Toxicology	527
			7.3. Carcinogenicity Assessment	529
4. Key Considerations for Conducting Toxicogenomic Studies	500		8. Regulatory Considerations	534
5. Goals and Applications of Toxicogenomic Studies	501		9. Conclusions	536
			Glossary	537
6. Sample Considerations	502		References	538
6.1. Study Planning for -Omics Endpoints	502			

1. INTRODUCTION

Toxicologic pathologists evaluate and integrate data in nonclinical and environmental toxicity studies from multiple sources (e.g., clinical signs, clinical pathology, gross, and microscopic pathology data). Traditional pathology assays have been developed over a couple of centuries and have become well established with but incremental technological advances (van den Tweel and Taylor, 2010). The acquisition and interpretation of pathology data are relatively standardized, resulting in reasonable confidence that the underlying biological alterations and the translational relevance are well understood and that these assays can be appropriately utilized for hazard identification and characterization as well as risk assessment (Foster et al., 2013).

Haschek and Rousseaux's Handbook of Toxicologic Pathology, Fourth Edition.
https://doi.org/10.1016/B978-0-12-821044-4.00028-5

491

With the advent and continuing evolution of innovative research technologies, the number of biological endpoints that can be reliably measured from individual subjects in these toxicity studies has increased exponentially. Traditional pathology endpoints (e.g., macroscopic and microscopic assessments, organ weights, clinical pathology analysis) reflect numerous underlying molecular processes (see *Morphologic Manifestations of Toxic Cell Injury*, Vol 1, Chap 6). Technological advances enable the rapid measurement of alterations in DNA, RNA, proteins, lipids, metabolites, and epigenetic markers (i.e., chemical modifications [like methylation] or associated proteins [like histones] that control DNA transcription), thereby providing a basis to understand the molecular mechanisms that lead to a phenotype as measured by traditional pathology assays. This ability to simultaneously measure hundreds of thousands of molecular variables and, more importantly, enhance interpretation of the underlying biological processes represents a unique opportunity to substantially advance the field of toxicologic pathology and associated disciplines (Foster et al., 2013).

2. BASICS OF TOXICOGENOMICS

Approaches that are typically grouped under the broad field of toxicogenomics include several "-omics" disciplines such as genomics, transcriptomics, proteomics, metabolomics, and epigenomics (also referred to as epigenetics). These technologies enable a systems biology approach where toxicogenomics data are integrated with traditional assay endpoints to generate a comprehensive understanding of toxic and carcinogenic mechanisms. Toxicologic pathologists are key contributors to a successful "systems toxicology" approach given that their knowledge and experience with traditional toxicology endpoints provide the necessary insight for the biological interpretation of toxicogenomics data. This approach is also referred to as "phenotype anchoring" where the morphologic endpoints are linked to molecular alterations detected by -omics technologies. Phenotypic anchoring provides confidence that molecular changes are biologically meaningful and also validates the appropriate development of bioinformatics methods. In addition, toxicogenomics is being used in predictive toxicology where chemicals are evaluated using molecular signatures that

were previously defined during in vitro and/or in vivo studies. These molecular signatures are explored based on prototype compounds or test conditions.

Toxicogenomics is a multidisciplinary area that requires expertise in traditional toxicology, pathology, molecular biology, and bioinformatics. As a result, it is important to at least understand the basics of each of these disciplines to optimally apply -omics technologies to toxicity investigations. Toxicogenomics technologies assess increasingly complex biological parameters by evaluating molecules ranging from DNA to metabolites (i.e., small [< 1.5 kDa] molecules that represent substrates, intermediates, and products of metabolism) within cells, biofluids, tissues, or organs (Figure 15.1).

The genetic material of all organisms is captured in the genome (i.e., the DNA). Examining the DNA (i.e., genomics) provides information regarding "what can happen" in an organism since DNA is relatively static across all tissues in an organism. In contrast, RNA expression is dynamic and may be altered in a tissue-specific manner under various physiological conditions and in response to exposure to xenobiotics. DNA is transcribed to generate RNA (e.g., messenger RNA [mRNA] and several types of noncoding RNAs [ncRNAs]), and examination of these transcripts (i.e., transcriptomics) provides information about "what might happen" when physiological homeostasis is altered. Translation of mRNA results in formation of proteins, and examination of the complement of proteins (i.e., proteomics) provides information regarding "what is happening" at the moment. Proteins can undergo posttranslational modifications and alteration by enzymatic reactions, resulting in the formation of metabolites; examination of the metabolites (i.e., metabolomics) gives an idea regarding "what already happened." Epigenomics involves examination of heritable phenotypes that occur without altering the DNA sequence. Epigenetic alterations may be mediated through changes in chromatin packaging, histone modification, DNA methylation, imprinted genes, and ncRNAs (Jeffries, 2020; van den Tweel and Taylor, 2010; Zhang et al., 2020).

All of these omics technologies can be applied to promote greater understanding of nonclinical study findings. However, transcriptomics largely dominates the field for various pragmatic reasons. First, it is relatively simple and inexpensive to

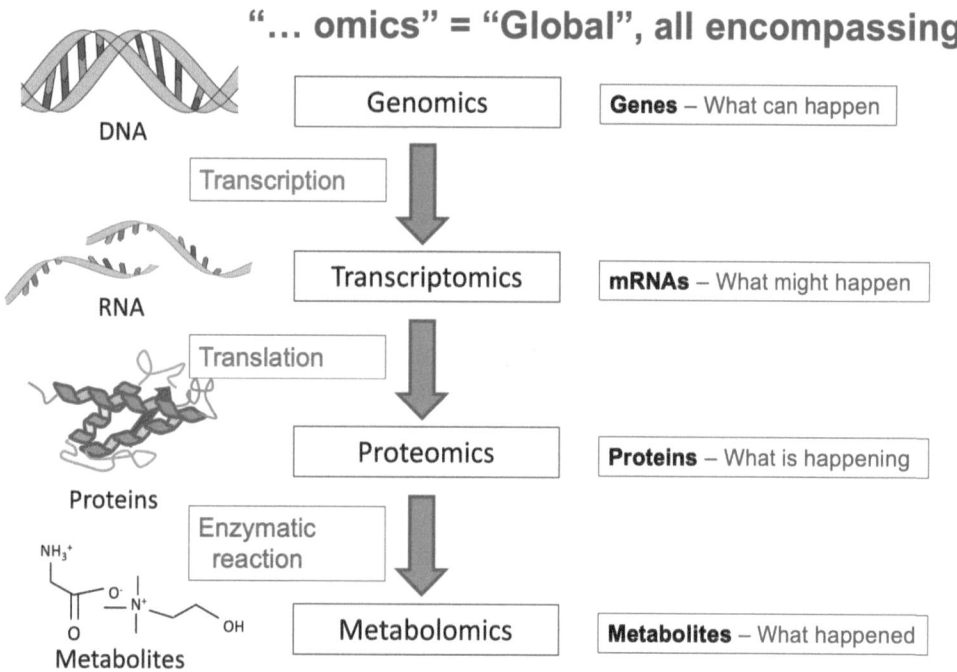

"… omics" = "Global", all encompassing

FIGURE 15.1   An overview of the molecules (e.g., DNA, RNA, proteins, and metabolites) in the central dogma and the corresponding toxicogenomics approaches (e.g., genomics, transcriptomics, proteomics, and metabolomics) to examine the biological program directed by these molecules. *Courtesy of Dr. Rick Paules, U.S. National Toxicology Program (NTP), National Institute of Environmental Health Sciences (NIEHS).*

capture the whole transcriptome compared to the whole genome since the size of the transcriptome in any given tissue or organ is approximately 5% of the genome. Second, capturing the entire proteome and metabolome is technologically challenging compared to capturing the entire transcriptome due to the massive dynamic range (i.e., abundance and size) of proteins and metabolites as well as the lack of inexpensive and high-throughput bioanalytical platforms (Zubarev, 2013). For a given sample, the dynamic range of proteins and metabolites can be in the order of billions, while that of transcripts is only in the range of 10–100s. Third, the transcriptome provides a snapshot at a point in time that offers an insight into "what might happen" (i.e., helps in generating hypotheses regarding the possible molecular alterations underlying the phenotype). These hypotheses can be tested at the protein ("what is happening") and/or metabolomic ("what already happened") levels. In most cases, the transcriptome provides sufficient actionable data in toxicity studies, so further investigations frequently are not pursued. As a result, this chapter will mainly focus on the principles of transcriptomics. However, these same concepts can be applied to other -omics technologies.

3. OVERVIEW OF TOXICOGENOMIC TECHNOLOGIES

Toxicogenomics may be broadly classified into nucleic acid-based approaches such as genomics, transcriptomics, and epigenomics and nonnucleic acid-based approaches such as proteomics and metabolomics. The following section provides brief overviews of the key -omics technologies commonly applied in animal toxicity studies. In general, genomics, transcriptomics, and epigenomics utilize similar technologies, such as microarrays or sequencing, while proteomics and metabolomics employ nuclear magnetic resonance (NMR) spectroscopy and mass spectroscopy (MS) methods.

3.1. Nucleic Acid-Based -Omics Platforms

Genomics refers to the systematic examination of the DNA sequences of the whole genome or part of the genome. However, genomics is also used as an umbrella term to refer to all genome-wide -omics approaches. Genomics may be conducted using array-based technologies such as single-nucleotide polymorphism (SNP) arrays and comparative genomic hybridization

(CGH) arrays or sequencing-based technologies such as whole-genome sequencing (WGS), whole-exome sequencing (WES), or targeted gene panels (McCombie et al., 2019; NRC, 2007). The array-based chips as well as targeted sequencing panels are efficient tools for screening cell or animal populations for known target genes (representing specific sequences of shorter-length DNA), whereas the sequencing-based approaches, especially the WGS, allow for discovery of new genomic biomarkers. Sequencing of DNA from the entire genome (WGS) is becoming more accessible as a research tool with reduction in sequencing costs but is still quite challenging in terms of data acquisition, analysis, and interpretation. However, more targeted genomic sequencing approaches such as WES or sequencing a panel of gene targets designed to evaluate a specific aspect of biology are increasingly being used in toxicogenomics and cancer research (Garcia et al., 2017; Levy and Myers, 2016; Mardis, 2019). Genomics has been used in the field of toxicology in fewer instances compared to transcriptomics.

Transcriptomics refers to the systematic examination of the products of gene transcription. The molecules that can be measured include fully processed mRNA coding for proteins; splice variants (versions of mRNA where exons have been deleted or added during transcription to produce proteins with different functions); mRNA variants with SNPs; and various RNAs that do not code for proteins but instead serve to regulate the expression of mRNAs such as microRNAs (miRNAs) or long ncRNAs (lncRNAs). In general, most toxicogenomics data are focused on assessment of mRNA expression because it is easier to interpret the data and also inexpensive to capture these data. The bulk of the transcriptomic data in the literature as well as in commercial or public databases consists of microarray data. However, with the advent of next-generation sequencing (NGS) technology such as RNA-sequencing (RNA-Seq), ncRNAs are also included in some toxicogenomics assessments.

Epigenomics refers to the systematic examination of the reversible modifications of DNA structure and conformation that affect gene expression without altering the DNA sequence. Epigenetic alterations may be mediated through alterations in chromatin packaging, histone modification, DNA methylation, imprinted genes, and ncRNAs (Chung and Herceg, 2020; Darwiche, 2020). Chromatin packaging determines the accessibility of transcription factors to DNA for downstream signaling. Chromatin is a tightly coiled nucleoprotein complex composed of DNA wrapped around histone proteins. Chromatin packaging may be altered by posttranslational modifications of the histone proteins by acetylation, methylation, phosphorylation, ubiquitination, SUMOylation (addition of small ubiquitin-like modifiers), and ADP-ribosylation. In general, histone acetylation decreases affinity of histone proteins for DNA and causes relaxation of chromatin packaging, leading to increased transcriptional activation. Methylation status of the cytosines in CpG dinucleotides within the promoter regions of protein-coding genes influences gene expression; hypermethylation of the promoter typically represses gene expression. Similarly, other histone modifications can increase DNA access either singly or in combination with other proteins and influence gene regulation.

ncRNAs constitute another major regulator of the epigenome. These transcripts are not translated into proteins but instead regulate gene expression at the transcriptional and posttranscriptional levels, typically acting to silence genes. They include small ncRNAs (19–31 nucleotides) such as miRNAs and piRNAs (PIWI [P-element-Induced WImpy testis]-interacting RNA), midsize ncRNAs (~20–200 nucleotides) such as SnoRNAs (small nucleolar RNA), and the lncRNA (>200 nucleotides) (Hombach and Kretz, 2016; Slack and Chinnaiyan, 2019). In toxicogenomics, the focus has been mainly on miRNAs and to a lesser extent on lncRNAs (Huang et al., 2018; Marrone et al., 2014). MiRNAs primarily function as negative regulators of gene expression at the posttranscriptional level. lncRNAs interact with DNA, RNA, and protein molecules and regulate gene expression and protein synthesis in various ways. For example, lncRNAs act as molecular scaffolds to modify chromatin complexes and interfere with the transcriptional machinery; modulate RNA processing events such as splicing, translation, and degradation; and regulate miRNA (Grixti and Ayers, 2020; Peschansky and Wahlestedt, 2014). Both miRNA and lncRNA are expressed in a tissue-specific manner, but in contrast to miRNAs, lncRNAs are not conserved across species (Bushel et al., 2020). Both miRNAs and lncRNAs can serve as sensitive biomarkers of toxicity (Balasubramanian et al., 2020; Dempsey and Cui, 2017; Guo et al., 2020; Machtinger et al., 2018). Each of these ncRNAs not only regulates normal cellular homeostasis but also exhibits altered expression in various toxicities and spontaneous and agent-induced cancers (Anastasiadou et al., 2018; Slack and Chinnaiyan, 2019; Wang et al., 2019). Several -omics technologies, such as array-based platforms (e.g., whole-genome arrays, miRNA arrays, and methylation arrays) and NGS-based approaches (e.g., chromatin immunoprecipitation sequencing [Chip-Seq], DNase I hypersensitive sites sequencing, assay for transposable accessible chromatin sequencing, whole-genome bisulfite sequencing, and RNA-Seq), are used to study epigenomics in various in vitro and in vivo biological systems.

Technologies that can comprehensively examine the genome (DNA), transcriptome (RNA), and the epigenome primarily employ microarrays or NGS. Early toxicogenomics investigations used microarrays, a technology that initiated and drove this discipline (Nuwaysir et al., 1999). Since then, microarray technologies as well as data analysis methods have been refined and standardized, and have contributed to the bulk of the existing toxicogenomics (transcriptomic mainly) data in the literature. Due to decrease in sequencing costs and also innovations in sequencing technology, NGS approaches are being increasingly used in toxicogenomics studies. Compared to microarrays, NGS technologies such as RNA-Seq are superior due to the higher dynamic range in quantification, absolute quantification of gene expression changes, low background signal, and potential for discovering novel transcripts and isoforms. Currently, both microarray and NGS technologies are comparable in terms of reagent and assay costs; however, the costs associated with data analysis and storage are still higher with NGS approaches because the data analysis methods for microarrays are standardized, while those of NGS methods are still in various stages of development. Most of the legacy transcriptomic data are based on microarrays and are deposited in easily accessible databases such as Gene Expression Omnibus (GEO, https://www.ncbi.nlm.nih.gov/geo/), DrugMatrix (https://ntp.niehs.nih.gov/data/drugmatrix/), TG-GATES (https://toxico.nibiohn.go.jp/english/), and the Comparative Toxicogenomics Database (https://ctdbase.org) where they serve as critical reference for new toxicogenomic data analysis and interpretation (Calvier and Bousquet, 2020; Davis et al., 2019; Ganter et al., 2006; Igarashi et al., 2015). In contrast, transcriptomic databases with RNA-Seq data are still in their infancy, which limits toxicogenomic data interpretation and metaanalysis (Rao et al., 2018). Overall, if the goal is to examine the gene expression of tissues after test article exposure and then compare expression to the legacy transcriptomic data, microarray platforms are probably more appropriate. However, if the purpose is to discover novel transcripts, alternative splicing isoforms, fusion transcripts, and/or ncRNAs, along with generating the whole-genome transcriptomic data, then NGS technologies are preferred.

In addition to the above platforms, more cost-effective, high-throughput transcriptomic platforms have been developed that are based on landmark transcriptomic biomarkers which can capture significant changes in biology using a small subset of the transcriptome. These platforms include the S1500+, which is based on TempO-Seq technology (Mav et al., 2018); L1000, which is based on Luminex technology (Subramanian et al., 2017); or variations on these approaches (Haider et al., 2018). These platforms are being used increasingly to screen chemical libraries that contain appropriate reference compounds (usually small molecules, but biomolecules may be used) (Gwinn et al., 2020; Ramaiahgari et al., 2019).

3.2. Microarray Technologies

Various microarray platforms can be used in toxicity and carcinogenicity assessment depending on the objective. Microarrays (often termed "genechips" from Affymetrix) typically are used to assess various nucleic acids such as RNA for gene expression analysis, DNA for SNP genotyping, DNA for CGH to identify gene structural differences and copy number variants, and DNA/RNA bound to a particular protein that is immunoprecipitated (ChIP) for the analysis of epigenetic effects/gene regulation ("ChIP-on-chip" studies). The principles of microarray studies are very similar across various applications (Jaksik et al., 2015).

A DNA microarray chip is a collection of pre-designed oligonucleotide (nt) probes with known sequences (~25 nt per spot in Affymetrix, 60 nt in Agilent) attached to a glass surface in a two-dimensional grid where each spot is assigned specific coordinates. A typical protocol for gene expression analysis, demonstrated here using an RNA-based example, includes the following steps. (1) High-quality RNA (with an RNA integrity number [RIN] of >7 assessed using an Agilent Bioanalyzer) extracted from cells or tissues is reverse- ranscribed using reverse transcriptase PCR (RT-PCR) into complementary DNA (cDNA). This cDNA represents the targets. (2) The resulting cDNA is amplified by in vitro transcription in the presence of biotinylated ribonucleotides to generate labeled complementary RNA (cRNA). (3) These biotinylated cRNA targets are hybridized to the antisense oligonucleotide (DNA) probes arrayed on the glass surface. (4) After hybridization, the arrays are stained with streptavidin-phycoerythrin (where streptavidin binds to the biotin in the cRNA and phycoerythrin is a fluorophore). (5) The fluorescent signals are captured with a scanner and a differential gene expression list is generated based on the comparison of groups identified in the experimental design.

Microarray experiments typically have one of two designs. In the case of a single-color microarray, the test and control samples are hybridized to separate chips containing an identical gene array, and the differential gene expression levels for the two samples are evaluated by comparing the fluorescent signals from two chips. In the case of a dual-color microarray, the test and control samples are labeled with different fluorescent probes (e.g., Cy3 and Cy5) and then hybridized simultaneously to the same chip so that the differential gene expression is obtained from a single chip. Due to the complicated experimental designs associated with dual-color microarrays, single-color microarrays have been and remain more popular. In addition, single-color microarrays are more efficient because they permit comparison of data from each chip (since it is one sample per chip), which is not possible in dual-color microarray since the experiment has to be repeated if new comparisons are needed between samples. Hence, single-color microarray enables comparison of each individual experimental sample and also both allows more efficient comparison of new data with findings from other microarray experiments and better supports metaanalyses. Much of the published microarray data are based on single-color microarray experiments. Some of the major vendors of microarrays used in animal toxicity studies include Affymetrix, Agilent, and Illumina.

3.3. Next-Generation Sequencing Technologies

Sequencing is the process by which the order ("sequence") of nucleotides is determined in DNA or RNA fragments. The technologies used for sequencing of genomic material have evolved from the low-throughput Sanger sequencing-based methods to NGS methods that use highly parallel protocols (McCombie et al., 2019; Slatko et al., 2018). The principles of NGS are very similar for genomic, transcriptomic, and epigenomic endpoints. In order, activities include library construction, sequencing, assembly, alignment, variant calling, and sometimes other downstream purpose-driven analyses. The basic premise of library construction includes harvesting total DNA (or total RNA that is converted to cDNA) from a tissue sample followed by fragmentation into small pieces of a certain size (typically 100–5000 bp) using physical forces (sonication) and/or enzymes (Head et al., 2014). Next, sequencing adapters are attached to the uniformly sized fragments on both their 3′ and 5′ ends. These adapters not only help in immobilizing the DNA fragments onto a solid surface (e.g., beads or a glass surface) but also contain priming sites to permit clonal amplification of the molecules (DNA fragments) attached to the adapter. Sequencing priming sites may be present in one or both of the adapters to conduct single-end or paired-end sequencing, respectively. Generally, paired-end sequencing is preferred for long genomic DNA fragments, such as de novo genome assemblies, while single-end sequencing is preferred for small fragments such as small RNA-Seq or ChIP-Seq. For some libraries, up to 96 unique indices (with molecular barcodes comprised of unique nucleotide sequences) are added within the adapters of each sample to enable multiplexing of samples within a single sequencing run. There are several NGS platforms such as the Roche 454, Illumina/Solexa, SoliD, Ion Torrent and PacBio sequencers, and each of these instruments has their pros and cons (Goodwin et al., 2016; van Dijk et al., 2014). Currently, Illumina is the industry leader due to their sequencing and cost efficiencies as well as their higher throughput, so most NGS data are being generated on Illumina sequencers.

For RNA-Seq studies, some additional principles should be considered that are specific to library preparation using RNA samples (Head et al., 2014). The total RNA isolated from any tissue comprises 80% ribosomal RNA (rRNA), 15% transfer RNA (tRNA), and 5% mRNA. Transcriptomic studies are mainly focused on biologically relevant protein-coding mRNA, so RNA-Seq library preparation is focused on selectively concentrating the mRNA population. This is accomplished by enriching transcripts with polyA tails or depleting rRNA (e.g., utilizing Ribo-zero kits). Since some mRNAs lack polyA tails, the rRNA depletion method that enriches mRNA both with and without polyA tails is usually preferred. The purified mRNA is enzymatically fragmented into 200–400 bp length, after which RT-PCR is used to convert RNA into cDNA. The cDNA is then included in the NGS workflow as described above. Care must be taken when constructing RNA libraries to maintain an RNase-free environment.

The NGS workflow is significantly different from that used with microarrays. Therefore, several decisions must be made during development of the experimental design. A detailed discussion of these factors is beyond the scope of this chapter, but some of the key considerations are given below in Table 15.1.

3.4. Protein- and Metabolome-Based -Omics Platforms

Proteomics is broadly defined as "the effort to establish the identities, quantities, structures, and biochemical and cellular functions of all proteins in an organism, organ, or organelle, and how these properties vary in space, time, or physiological state" (Kenyon et al., 2002). The field of protein sequencing had a head start (1950s) compared to RNA and DNA sequencing (1960s), but the technical limitations associated with proteins have hampered the field of

proteomics compared to genomics (Timp and Timp, 2020). Some of these technical limitations include a wide dynamic range in abundance and size, difficulties in physical handling, extensive posttranslational modifications, and the tendency to form insoluble complexes as well as preenzymatic, enzymatic, and nonenzymatic alterations that disrupt the actual protein structure. Less than 40% of the protein spectrum can be explained by mRNA transcript levels. In addition, proteins are in a constant state of flux associated with the phases of translation, maturation (three-dimensional folding and posttranslational modifications), regulation, and termination (Bereman, 2018). There are an estimated 300,000 proteins considering only splice variants and immediate posttranslational modifications (Kenyon et al., 2002). The proteome has a massive dynamic range in abundance (12 orders of magnitude), so MS approaches require a million to a billion copies of a protein molecule for detection even when combined advanced analytical techniques such as depletion of abundant proteins and enrichment of particular proteins of interest are used (Timp and Timp, 2020). In spite of these limitations, significant progress in bioanalytical technologies and bioinformatics approaches has been made in the proteomics arena in recent years, so proteomics is being used more frequently in toxicogenomic studies.

3.5. Proteomics Technologies

Proteins can be studied using antibodies (protein arrays), two-dimensional gel electrophoresis (2D-GE) or 2D differential gel electrophoresis (2D-DIGE), NMR spectroscopy, and MS (Altelaar et al., 2013; Angel et al., 2012).

Protein arrays are limited in their application since antibodies are required against particular peptide targets but usually are not available for novel peptides. As a result, protein arrays are mainly used as screening tools.

2D-GE and 2D-DIGE approaches separate proteins based on their differences in charge (by isoelectric focusing) and size (as migration within the gel depends on molecular mass). For 2D-GE, proteins are visualized after staining with Coomassie blue. The 2D-DIGE method uses fluorescent probes (e.g., Cy2, Cy3, Cy5) to label the proteins from reference and test samples to compare their electrophoretic

TABLE 15.1   Next-Generation Sequencing

Next-generation sequencing (NGS) technologies are increasingly used for toxicogenomics projects. Each new omics technology comes with its own technical jargon, and it is important to understand such terms in order to interpret the data.

The RNA/DNA samples are submitted to a sequencing core laboratory to obtain the transcriptomic/genomic data. In a typical microarray experiment, relatively few decisions need to be made by the investigator prior to sample submission; the key decisions are the desired platform (Affymetrix, Agilent, or other) and the type of the gene chip for the desired molecular endpoints. However, in an NGS experiment, several issues need to be considered before samples are submitted to the core laboratory. Before starting the study, it is recommended to review the relevant literature, refer to educational resources and tutorials (from Illumina (https://www.illumina.com/science/techno logy/next-generation-sequencing/beginners.html) and Genohub (https://genohub.com/next-generation-sequenc ing-guide/#top)), and often to consult with expert technical staff at the core laboratory. Here, we will discuss a few practical issues to be considered in planning a sequencing analysis.

1. What is a sequencing read/cycle? Do I need a single-end read or paired-end reads?

Sequencing instruments "read" or detect the order of the nucleotides in a DNA fragment from one end to the other in a single-end read assay, while in a paired-end assay, it reads from one end to the other and then reads the fragment again from the opposite end. Obviously, single-end reads are faster and cheaper and thus are typically used for general profiling studies such as RNA-Seq and small RNA-Seq. Paired-end reads give double the sequencing data at less than double the sequencing costs while providing additional confidence in the inferred nucleotide sequence. Paired-end reads give additional positional information in the genome and thus are preferred for de novo genome assemblies as well as to study structural rearrangements such as deletions, insertions, and inversions. Paired-end reads can also be used to examine splice variants, SNPs, and epigenetic modifications.

2. What read length and how many reads do I need?

A read length refers to the number of base pairs (bp) that can be analyzed at a time. Since each base is read in one cycle, the read length also corresponds to the number of cycles. Typically, read lengths or cycles of 50–75 are used for RNA-Seq applications and 150–300 are used in DNA-seq applications on Illumina sequencing machines. However, other sequencers such as those from PacBio can read up to 1500 bp. Currently, Illumina sequencing is the dominant player in the field. Read lengths of 75 bp with paired-end reads (2×75) for transcriptome analysis and 50 bp using single-end reads (1×50) for small RNA sequencing are typical. Likewise, read lengths of 2×150 bp for whole-genome or whole-exome sequencing and 2×150 bp or larger for de novo sequencing read lengths are preferred.

3. What read depth or coverage do I need?

Read depth refers to the total number of times a single base is read during a sequencing run. Coverage describes the reads for the novel sequence in the context of the reference sequence (i.e., whole genome or a targeted region). During sequencing, library fragments are read randomly and independently. As a result, some fragments are read (or "covered") a greater (or lesser) number of times than others (i.e., the coverage is not uniform for all portions of a long sequence). If the sequencing reads align to only 90% of the target reference, then the coverage is 90%. Higher coverage provides greater confidence that all the fragments that overlap the entire target region are represented (or "covered") adequately in the data. Ideally, uniform sequence coverage can be confirmed by the demonstration that the data produce a Poisson-like distribution with a small standard deviation and a low interquartile range. Depending on the goals of the experiment, the recommended coverage or read depth varies. With whole-genome sequencing, whole-exome sequencing, Chip-Seq, and targeted sequencing, coverage of ~20×, 100×, 40×, and >500× is recommended, respectively. For RNA-Seq studies, read depth is typically used instead of coverage; depending on the goals of the RNA-Seq study, the read depths may range from 5 million (M) to 100M reads (e.g., 20M for typical gene expression profiling, 60M or higher to obtain information on alternative splicing, and about 5M for small RNA-Seq). Sequencing capacities of different sequencers vary and, as a result, multiple samples can be pooled (i.e., with unique molecular identifier [UMI] adapters for each sample) and run in a single lane (multiplexed) to take advantage of the sequencing capacity of the instrument. Coverage calculators are also provided by vendors and other sources to calculate how many samples may be pooled together for a given run depending on the instrument and the type of sequencing kit being used (https://support.illumina.com/downloads/sequencing_coverage_calculator.html).

spectra when both are run on the same gel simultaneously. The individual protein spots on the 2D-GE and 2D-DIGE subsequently can be extracted and subjected to MS to further characterize the proteins.

NMR spectroscopy measures the characteristic frequency changes of the electromagnetic signals produced by the charged atomic nuclei in a molecule when placed in a strong magnetic field and pulsed with varying radiofrequencies (RFs). The frequencies at which the atomic nuclei resonate (i.e., match the frequencies of the RF pulses) produce an exclusive NMR spectrum for that sample (i.e., a unique pattern of resonance peaks at different frequencies). NMR spectra are widely used for measuring small molecules, and identification of proteins is usually limited to proteins smaller than 35 kDa.

MS measures the mass-to-charge ratio (m/z) of ionized molecules moving through electric and magnetic fields. Typically, samples for MS are bombarded with electrons to fragment and ionize them. As the ionized peptide fragments migrate through the electric fields at certain speeds based on their m/z and travel through the magnetic fields in specific paths (straight or deviated since ions with a higher m/z deviate less than ions with lower m/z charge in the magnetic field), a detector captures the mass spectrum. The resulting mass spectrum provides an idea on the structure of the sample in terms of its elemental composition while the isotopic makeup of the fragmented constituents is generally confirmed by comparing to a database of known molecules. Technologies based on MS have a limited dynamic range of detection (5 orders of magnitude). There are many variations in MS depending on the type of sample (e.g., solid, liquid, gas, complexity of the protein molecule, mixtures), ionizer, mass analyzer, and detector. Discussion on the variations of MS is beyond the scope of this chapter, but further information can be found elsewhere (Angel et al., 2012).

Proteomics using MS may be categorized into bottom-up (BU-MS) or top-down (TD-MS) approaches. Due to the scale and throughput for protein identification, BU-MS proteomics has dominated the field (Bereman, 2018; Timp and Timp, 2020). For more technical details on proteomics and potential future technologies, please refer to Timp and Timp (2020).

The BU-MS approach (also called "shotgun" proteomics) is used in global protein identification as well as to systematically profile the dynamic proteome. The proteins are digested by trypsin into smaller peptides (0.8–3 kDa). The "tryptic peptides" are analyzed by electrospray ionization or matrix-assisted laser desorption/ionization, both of which ionize peptides in a gas phase, analyze their masses, and then fragment the ions to recover information about their sequence from MS. Alternatively, liquid chromatography–MS (LC-MS) can be used to separate molecules before they are ionized and subjected to MS. The resulting peptide information is not a sequence but more like a fingerprint that is compared to a database using search engines like Mascot (http://www.matrixscience.com/) or Comet (http://comet-ms.sourceforge.net/) to identify the protein (Timp and Timp, 2020). The sensitivity of the BU-MS approach is compromised by the number of spectra required to accurately identify the protein sequence. It is estimated that about 60% of spectra are unresolved and do not provide a complete identification for the protein.

The TD-MS approach is advantageous to identify protein isoforms, sequence variants, and posttranslational modification. In the TD-MS approach, intact protein ions are introduced into the gas phase by electrospray ionization and fragmented by collision-induced or electron transfer dissociation in the mass spectrometer. The masses of both the proteins and fragment ions provide a picture of the protein structure and its modifications. However, the TD-MS approach is limited to larger proteins (50–70 kDa) and is complicated by the fact that the fragmentation efficacy of the intact proteins decreases as the molecular weight and the complexity of the tertiary protein structure increases. Therefore, the TD-MS approach mainly focuses on proteins <70 kDa, and only a few projects focus on larger proteins >100 kDa.

Metabolomics is the systematic study of small molecule by-products in cells, tissues, or biofluids (Bujak et al., 2015; Cui et al., 2018; Wishart, 2016, 2019). These small molecules are 50–2000 kDa and include sugars, nucleotides, peptides, amino acids, and lipids of either endogenous or exogenous origin. Endogenous metabolites are produced by the cell or organism during normal physiological processes. The endogenous metabolome is considered to have 3000–5000 metabolites. The animal's microbiome is another significant contributor to the metabolome and contributes to more than 6700 unique metabolites (Karu et al., 2018). The exogenous metabolome is much larger and depends on various sources such as foods, drugs (e.g., therapeutic or recreational), chemicals (e.g., agricultural and occupational), several environmental attributes (e.g., air and water pollution), and lifestyle factors (e.g., alcohol- or caffeine-containing beverages, smoking). Most metabolites regardless of source are a direct reflection of the underlying biological functions of the organism and are usually conserved across species; hence, they serve as a valuable source of biomarkers for exposure and/or disease. In addition, the examination of metabolites in body fluids collected noninvasively and repeatedly enables longitudinal human epidemiological and animal studies. As a result, metabolomics is considered an ideal technology for exposome research, where the exogenous compounds as well as the consequent endogenous metabolites are queried simultaneously to gain a better understanding of the exposure and its consequences on the biological system (Walker et al., 2019). Consequently, metabolomics may provide greater confidence when interpreting the underlying biology responsible for homeostatic processes in health. In general, metabolomics may be used for early detection and interventions, disease diagnosis, prognosis and monitoring, identification of exposures and their impact on the organism, and target identification of therapeutics and toxicants.

3.6. Metabolomics Technologies

As discussed earlier, unlike DNA, RNA, and protein, the metabolome is the ultimate measurable endpoint of the organism's interaction with the environment because it measures "what already happened." Many technologies related to liquid (LC) or gas (GC) chromatography coupled to MS as well as NMR spectroscopy are used to identify and quantify metabolites in biological samples. The MS methods are generally coupled with LC or GC to achieve separation of the molecules within the sample before entering the MS detector. LC-MS is particularly useful to detect lipids, fatty acids, and peptides, while GC-MS is useful to detect small molecules (<500 Da) and highly volatile compounds such as esters, amines, and ketones. The MS approaches are very sensitive and have higher throughput and lower cost than NMR-based methods. However, NMR methods have several other advantages as they do not require separation of the analytes, do not destroy the sample, require little to no molecular separation prior to entering the detector cell, and handle complex mixtures. For comprehensive insight into the metabolome, both the MS and NMR methods may be considered depending on the study objectives, but in general, MS methods are more widely used.

4. KEY CONSIDERATIONS FOR CONDUCTING TOXICOGENOMIC STUDIES

This section highlights the key technical issues and methods that must be addressed to design, conduct, analyze, and interpret toxicogenomic studies. Specific topics will include study goals and design, sample considerations, toxicogenomic software tools and databases, data analysis and interpretation, biological or technical validation, and study reporting.

As described elsewhere in this chapter, toxicogenomics may be used for hypothesis generation, mechanistic investigations, and prediction of the apical endpoints of likely regulatory significance. This "begin with the end in mind" approach acknowledges several potentially very significant contributions of the toxicologic pathologist to various aspects of toxicogenomics projects. In particular, pathologists are well suited to assist with study design, sample acquisition, and biological interpretation of data. Since toxicologic pathologists have expertise in interpreting the traditional biological endpoints such as clinical signs as well as clinical pathology values and anatomic pathology findings, they can integrate these data with the toxicogenomics data using a systems biology approach and understand the translational relevance of the experimental models. In fact, toxicogenomics studies have proven useful in translating findings in traditional animal-based toxicity assessments especially in the pharmaceutical and agrochemical industry (Vahle et al., 2018). Involvement of toxicologic pathologists during study design contributes to a successful toxicogenomics project as they will ensure that appropriate biological responses (apical endpoints) are benchmarked and anchored to the toxicogenomics data. The toxicologic pathologist will advise on the appropriate tissue sampling approaches, such as the type or subsite of the organ, method of collection, time of collection, storage prior to processing, and relevant -omics analysis. In addition, the toxicologic pathologist can serve an important role in data interpretation. For example, clusters of genes may be identified by software designed to detect unsupervised hierarchical clustering, but the expert judgment of the toxicologic pathologist or toxicologist is necessary to determine if these clusters are mechanistically related to the phenotypic changes being investigated or if they simply reflect the technical or biological variability inherent to any life-science study.

5. GOALS AND APPLICATIONS OF TOXICOGENOMIC STUDIES

Toxicogenomics aims to understand the adverse effects of intentional (therapeutic or recreational substances) or unintentional (environmental) exposures on human or animal health and the environment (National Research Council, 2007). In practical terms, the goals of toxicogenomics studies can be more specific. One set of related purposes is to improve understanding of the mode of action (MOA) and key molecular events of a xenobiotic-induced phenotype in animal or in vitro models, thereby determining the translational relevance or a cross-species extrapolation of a mechanism of action observed in an experimental model. A second series of linked objectives includes (1) deriving points of departure via benchmark dosing (BMD) for regulatory assessment, (2) discovering gene signatures or biomarkers that can predict toxicity or a phenotype without running expensive and time-consuming studies such as the rodent cancer bioassays, (3) screening compounds or groups of compounds

for hazard identification, and (4) monitoring xenobiotic exposure in human populations and the environment. Application of toxicogenomics methods also has the goal of better discerning interindividual and life-stage susceptibility to chemical hazards. Toxicogenomics is also being used in risk assessment, mainly as a tool for providing adjunct data to toxicity or carcinogenicity studies outlined in regulatory guidance documents to support MOA experiments and contribute to a weight-of-evidence approach.

These goals may be accomplished by the following three broad categories of toxicogenomics experiments: class discovery, class comparison, and class prediction (National Research Council, 2007). *Class discovery* takes an unbiased approach and attempts to identify patterns in a dataset with a defined similar biological endpoint. This is accomplished by using unsupervised data analysis methods based on some measure of similarity between the samples in a dataset. For example, hepatic gene expression data from various mouse hepatotoxicants can identify a common mechanism of action for all the samples in a dataset (e.g., cytotoxicity) or identify subclasses of hepatotoxicants with unique modes of action (e.g., receptor-mediated toxicity). *Class comparison* examines the gene expression profiles of different experimental groups (such as a control group and various treatment groups) to identify gene expression profiles (i.e., gene signatures) that effectively distinguish the different groups from each other. For example, gene expression data from exposure to various xenobiotics could help distinguish toxic from nontoxic agents or discriminate pathways indicative of particular disease processes (e.g., cytotoxicity vs. inflammation vs. neoplasia). This is accomplished by supervised data analysis methods to distinguish different treated groups from control animals. This approach will allow identification of gene signatures that are specific to each treatment which then can be further validated in mechanistic studies or serve as a starting point to classify new test articles based on the gene signatures specific to various process-related phenotypes. *Class prediction* attempts to predict the biological effect of an unknown test article based on the gene expression profiles that have been identified in the class comparison studies. The principle of class prediction relies on the assumption that test articles with similar mechanisms of toxicity will have similar gene expression profiles. In order to gain confidence with the prediction models, the training sets (i.e., gene expression -omics data sets obtained from known chemicals) have to be comprehensive and of high quality. Mathematical algorithms are used to generate a gene signature specific to a mechanism of toxicity, and these gene expression signatures will be used to predict the potential toxicity of the novel test article. These predicted phenotypes might still need follow-up investigations to confirm that the MOA predicted by the algorithms based on machine learning actually is relevant to the cell type or organism in question.

6. SAMPLE CONSIDERATIONS

The various -omics technologies use biomolecules such as DNA, RNA, and protein from many organs, body fluids, or cell cultures. The biological samples often are in different states of preservation, though less so for toxicity studies performed in accordance with existing regulatory guidelines and industrial best practice recommendations. The initial sample quality and quantity determines the toxicogenomic technology that may be used and ultimately defines the quality of the -omics data. Hence, improving the quality of sample collection and processing is essential to the success of a toxicogenomics project.

6.1. Study Planning for -Omics Endpoints

Ideally, the required sample type and biomolecule for the toxicogenomics experiment is determined during the experimental design phase. Early availability of this information aids the sampling team to properly prepare the tissue or fluid collection instruments and necessary sample preservation media. However, this may not always be the case, since toxicogenomics analysis may be implemented after the animal studies have been completed based on findings from routine toxicity or carcinogenicity studies. In these instances, the only samples that often are available are formalin-fixed "wet" tissue or blocks of formalin-fixed paraffin-embedded (FFPE) tissues. Such preservation methods impact the integrity of biomolecules in various cells and tissues (especially RNA), and this

tissue condition limits the types of toxicogenomics analysis that may be performed. Therefore, it is important to include a sample collection strategy in conventional animal studies especially if a toxicogenomics evaluation is a potential consideration in the future. Indeed, it may be resource appropriate to appropriately collect and store tissue samples "just in case" to avoid repeating a study, especially for studies of long duration and/or in nonrodents.

The toxicologic pathologist typically ensures that the sample collection and preservation strategy is adequate for toxicogenomics studies. This oversight may or may not be done in consultation with the staff who will implement any -omics technology; entry-level practitioners typically should work with a molecular biologist and/or experienced molecular pathologist to optimize the sampling and archiving procedures since the preanalytical variables dictate optimal tissue collection, processing, and storage that are integral factors to the success of a toxicogenomics study. These practices should be standardized and consistently followed during collection of all samples that will be subjected to toxicogenomics analysis in order to maintain appropriate historical controls. Institutions should consider developing standard operating procedures to maximize the likelihood that sample acquisition and handling will permit subsequent -omics analysis.

The study design phase and preparation of the study protocol are the initial points at which consideration should be given to the potential need for toxicogenomics endpoints. Useful sections in the study protocol might include a list of clinical observations that would trigger collection of tissues for -omics analyses and a detailed necropsy plan describing sampling and retention of -omics samples. Key elements of the necropsy plan should include the organs (or subsites within the organs) to be collected, the order and speed of sample collection, the quantity of tissue to harvest, the quality of that tissue (and how to assess that quality), target biomolecules for the toxicogenomic studies, any special harvesting conditions (e.g., extra instruments and RNase-free solutions for RNA preservation), and processing conditions for the samples. In particular, the tissue preservation procedures should encompass a range of details including the choice of tissue fixative, fixation temperature, duration of fixation, need for special fixatives, collection of frozen tissue (including how to freeze it and at what temperature to hold it), sample labeling, storage, and transportation. The individual animal necropsy record should be used to record all the above information and any deviation from the necropsy protocol. These preanalytical processes for sample collection should be defined, documented, and verified in the study protocol prior to the start of the study (see *Basic Approaches to Anatomic Toxicologic Pathology*, Vol 1, Chap 9 and *Practices to Optimize Generation, Interpretation, and Reporting of Pathology Data from Toxicity Studies*, Vol 1, Chap 28). Details of the sample collection defined above as well as the chain of custody of the samples should be recorded at every step, and any deviations from the protocol should be documented.

6.2. Collection and Processing of the -Omics Samples

Since -omics studies are highly sensitive in order to detect subtle effects, extra consideration regarding the fasting status, circadian rhythms, and accurate subsite tissue collection is essential (Morgan et al., 2005). For example, if liver tissue is being collected, a similar region of the same liver lobe should be collected from all animals (including controls) to minimize potential confounding factors in the interpretation of differences in gene expression related to normal biological variation (Irwin et al., 2004, 2005). Similarly, if the brain is being collected, the specific subsites (i.e., cell populations) for collection should be defined in the necropsy plan and collected appropriately. The order of collection of tissues and subsites should be clearly defined in the necropsy plan as some tissues such as bone marrow, gastrointestinal tract, and pancreas are more prone to degradation due to high levels of endogenous proteases and RNases, and thus should be harvested expeditiously. The order in which animals are necropsied should be randomized across control and treatment groups to prevent batch effects (i.e., artifacts leading to biased data associated with the order in which tissues/animals are processed). The labeling of tissue containers should be consistent and informative.

Obviously, freshly collected tissues are preferred for extracting biomolecules with the highest molecular and structural integrity.

However, snap-freezing in liquid nitrogen or isopentane cooled to $-80°C$ is the optimal method of tissue preservation for maintaining the biomolecules in a near native state when fresh samples cannot be processed and analyzed immediately. This rapid freezing will ensure extraction of high-quality DNA, RNA, and protein by halting enzyme activity that begins immediately after blood flow ceases. While RNA and protein are denatured after standard tissue fixation methods (e.g., immersion or perfusion with aldehyde-based fixatives), DNA is relatively stable and can be extracted from optimally fixed tissues. In general toxicity studies, tissues are collected mainly for histopathology and as a result are fixed in neutral buffered 10% formalin solution. Tissues fixed in formalin for greater than 48 h will result in extensive protein cross-linking and contribute to excessive DNA fragmentation. In order to use the DNA for NGS studies, formalin fixation of the tissues should be limited to 24–48 h; the samples may be transferred into ethanol for up to 30 days if they cannot be processed immediately into paraffin blocks.

If both the morphological examination and multiple -omics assessments are planned in advance (i.e., prior to the day of necropsy) to be a consideration, then tissues may be collected in OCT (optimal cutting temperature) compound and frozen while placed over liquid nitrogen, immersed in isopentane cooled to $-80°C$, or processed with a more efficient method such as PrestoCHILL (Milestone Medical, Kalamazoo, MI). Tissues in OCT are rapidly frozen (~60 s) using PrestoCHILL compared to liquid nitrogen vapors (~5–10 min), and have minimal artifacts associated with ice crystal formation. If morphological examination is not a consideration, the fresh tissue may be cut into 5 mm cubes and collected in screwcap cryovials to be snap-frozen in liquid nitrogen. In the absence of facilities to freeze the tissues, specialized fixatives such as RNAlater or PAXgene may be used to stabilize the nucleic acids, after which the tissues may be routinely processed and embedded in paraffin. The -omics samples may be immersed in these special fixatives and stored for a week at room temperature or a month at 4°C. The cellular morphology in tissues immersed in these specialized fixatives does show alterations (e.g., hyperchromatic tinctorial changes in nuclear and cytoplasmic morphology) compared to standard formalin fixation, but there is sufficient tissue quality to enable microscopic examination. While tissues fixed in RNAlater or PAXgene are perfect for in situ hybridization, immunohistochemical (IHC) identification of some proteins is not consistent as certain protein epitopes may be differentially altered with these fixatives (Suhovskih et al., 2019).

In addition to the fresh or frozen tissue collection described above, sample collection for metabolomics usually includes body fluids such as blood, plasma, serum, urine, feces, and/or saliva. Extreme care is required during sample collection in order to control the introduction of contaminants into the sample (Kurien et al., 2004). Ideally, fluid samples are collected fresh on dry ice and frozen at −70°C within an hour. Some chemicals such as anticoagulants may be added to blood samples, or antimicrobial agents such as sodium azide may be added to stabilize urine samples. After collection, biomolecules are extracted from the tissue homogenate or biological fluids using organic solvents and then lyophilized (freeze dried) before reconstituting in another solvent compatible with the appropriate analytical method.

6.3. Extraction of Biomolecules

Germline DNA is relatively stable over time in a tissue compared to RNA and proteins. Hence, it is critical to keep preanalytical variables such as the time required for collection, circadian rhythm, nutrition (fasting) status, and subsite of the sampled organ consistent across all experimental groups. Ideally, tissue sections for histopathologic evaluation should be made adjacent to the cut surface of the tissue sampled for -omics analysis in order to enable correlation of molecular and microscopic changes in the tissues selected for extraction of biomolecules. This is especially important for tumors containing both neoplastic and stromal tissues admixed with normal parenchymal tissues. In cases where a particular cell population or histologic tissue type is the focus of the investigation, then approaches such as laser capture microdissection (LCM) are essential (see *Special Techniques in Toxicologic Pathology*, Vol 1, Chap 11). It is important when preparing to collect samples to have an idea regarding the quantity and quality of the estimated starting material needed for the specific toxicogenomic assay. This will help in estimating the starting amount of tissue that is needed to obtain the necessary amount of the biomolecule of interest. If using LCM to collect tissue, then transcriptomic assays with low-input kits (i.e., made for use with very small specimens or low amounts of recovered biomolecules) are recommended. In general, each diploid cell in common test species and humans contains about 6 pg of DNA, and on average, each mg of tissue yields about 1 µg of DNA. The DNA and RNA yields from proliferating tumor cells are slightly higher than with normal cells. The RNA yields are a bit harder to predict as they vary based on the cell type, but RNA quantities per cell range from 10 to 30 pg. As discussed earlier, the majority of the total RNA consists of rRNA (~80%) and tRNA (~15%), and mRNA generated by gene transcription accounts for only 1%–5% depending on the cell type and its physiological state. In general, a single mammalian cell contains about 360,000 mRNA molecules made up of 12,000 different transcripts with a typical length of around 2 kb. Rare low-abundance mRNAs may account for only 0.01% of the mRNA (5–15 molecules/cell) but nevertheless may play a significant role in determining cell function during health and disease.

Since DNA is relatively stable, it can be extracted from promptly (and properly) fixed and paraffin-embedded tissues. Prompt fixation entails addition of the tissue to the fixative solution within minutes of death (ideally 5 min or fewer for metabolically active organs like gastrointestinal tract and pancreas). Proper fixation entails immersion in neutral buffered 10% formalin at 4°C (ideally) to halt autolytic digestion of biomolecules as soon as possible (Berrino et al., 2020; Jones et al., 2019). Ideally, alcohol-based coagulative fixatives such as methacarn and RCL2 should be considered for molecular pathology studies since they degrade nucleic acids less than cross-linking fixatives such as formalin (Delfour et al., 2006). If the tissues are fixed for long durations (weeks) in formalin before processing as in most rodent cancer bioassays, the quality of DNA is severely degraded. In most of the publications that report successful DNA extraction and NGS data generation from FFPE tissues, investigators utilized samples that had been fixed in formalin for 24–72 h (Gao et al., 2020; Merrick et al., 2012).

Thus, the critical point in achieving a successful -omics analysis of FFPE tissues is the duration of fixation rather than the age of the tissue (i.e., the length of time in the paraffin block).

Prior to -omics analysis, the suitability of the isolated biomolecules needs to be confirmed. The common quality metrics used in nucleic acid extraction include spectrometric, fluorometric, and electrophoretic methods. Spectrometric methods quantify nucleic acid concentrations by measuring the absorbance of ultraviolet light at 260 nm. Absorbance at other wavelengths indicates the presence of other materials in the nucleic acid preparation; a peak at 280 nm indicates substantial protein contamination, and one at 230 nm indicates organic contaminants from the extraction process. In neutral buffered solutions, a 260/280 ratio of ~1.8 indicates pure dsDNA, while a ratio of ~2.1 indicates pure RNA. Acidic solutions underestimate and basic solutions overestimate the 260/280 ratios by 0.2–0.3. While the spectrometric methods provide an idea about the relative purity of the nucleic acids and potential contaminants, they frequently overestimate the concentrations of the nucleic acids by up to fivefold especially when the concentration of the nucleic acids is lower than 20 ng/μL. To accurately measure lower concentrations, fluorometric methods such as Qubit are used that feature specialized dyes which selectively bind to dsDNA, ssDNA, or RNA. The electrophoretic methods provide information on the fragment size distribution of the nucleic acids within the sample. This is especially important for nucleic acid samples extracted from suboptimal samples such as FFPE tissue. Agilent's Tapestation or Bioanalyzer provides a DNA integrity number (DIN) or RIN, respectively, based on the electrophoretic traces. A DIN value > 3 and a RIN >7 is needed for a successful library preparation for NGS studies. In addition to the DIN and RIN, it is also important to examine the respective electropherogram traces to determine the overall size distribution (i.e., to confirm sample quality) of the starting nucleic acids as well as the NGS libraries. For RNA samples especially, those extracted from FFPE tissue, a DV_{200} value provides a percentage of nucleotides longer than 200 bp, and this value should be 30% or greater to confirm high sample quality and ensure a successful RNA library construction.

6.4. Controls for -Omics Assays

By definition, controls are designed to eliminate experimental errors and biases by minimizing the extraneous variables other than the independent variable under study. The controls in an experiment ideally should include technical controls as well as biological controls. Technical controls help in building the confidence in an assay, while biological controls help in avoiding interference from irrelevant variables unrelated to the biology of the toxicity or disease. Toxicogenomics approaches are incredibly sensitive by design in order to detect subtle molecular alterations. Without appropriate technical and biological controls as well as robust statistical methods, there is an increased likelihood of false-positive signals. Statistical considerations for -omics technologies will be covered in detail in the data analysis section of this chapter, but additional information can be found in *Experimental Design and Statistical Analysis for Toxicologic Pathologists*, Vol 1, Chap 16.

Several technical controls are incorporated into the -omics platforms. For example, both internal and external technical controls are included in the design of gene arrays to help troubleshoot a failed microarray experiment. The internal controls include probes for one or more housekeeping genes (i.e., genes expressed in all viable cells of a given specimen) and RNA degradation controls. The external ("spike in") controls include polyA + tailed *Bacillus subtilis* transcripts (to test the adequacy of RNA synthesis, amplification, and biotin labeling) and biotin-labeled *Escherichia coli* transcripts (to test for appropriate hybridization of the material in the sample with the probe). Comparing the relative intensities of the signals from the internal and external spike ins with the biological samples provides a metric on the performance of the assay (Lippa et al., 2010). Similar technical controls also may be considered in NGS platforms to assess the efficiency of each step in the assay. In some cases, the same biological sample (RNA or DNA) is aliquoted and run as replicates as a confirmation control to demonstrate confidence in the reproducibility of the assay.

Proper biological controls are very important to produce data that can be interpreted with a high degree of confidence. Biological controls are tissues, particular regions of tissues, or purified cell populations. These samples may include positive controls (having the molecule of interest), negative controls (lacking the molecule), sham-procedure or chamber (inhalation) controls, and vehicle controls. Ideally, effects related to differences in species, strain/breed, age, sex, metabolic status, health condition, fasting status, physical activity, and circadian rhythms also should also be controlled. In toxicity studies with -omics endpoints, these latter factors generally are handled by including relevant concurrent control groups in the experimental design. The critical nature of such controls is illustrated by examples of reproducible, wide-scale, poorly controlled toxicogenomic effects across many experimental variables (see Table 15.2).

TABLE 15.2 Variation in Experimental Factors and Their Impact on mRNA Transcripts in Rodent Liver[a]

Factor	Approximate number of transcripts affected	Example analytes	Functional role
Sex	~100 by > 5× difference compared to controls	Cyp3A (cytochrome P450 3A, higher in males)	Xenobiotic metabolism
		A1bg (alpha-1-B glycoprotein, higher in females)	Glycoprotein of unknown function whose expression in mice is controlled by growth hormone. Urinary protein levels of A1bg are a potential clinical marker of steroid-resistant nephrotic syndrome
Time of day	Hundreds	P21	Regulates cell cycle, increased hepatic expression in response to DNA damage, and transcription controlled by clock genes
		ARNTL (aryl hydrocarbon receptor nuclear translocator like)	Participates in creating circadian rhythms—regulates P21. Pattern of expression of ARNTL is reported to change in cancer and diabetes
Fasting	Hundreds	Cholesterol metabolism (transcripts downregulated)	Cholesterol biosynthesis
		Lipid metabolism (transcripts upregulated)	Fatty acid metabolism including β-oxidation
Acute phase response	Thousands	Cholesterol metabolism (transcripts downregulated)	Cholesterol biosynthesis
		Lipid metabolism (transcripts downregulated)	Fatty acid metabolism including β-oxidation
Enzyme induction	Thousands	CYP450 (cytochrome) oxidoreductases (transcripts upregulated)	Transfers electrons from NADPH (reduced nicotinamide adenine dinucleotide phosphate) to microsomal P450 enzymes
		Glutathione transferase (Yc2) (transcript upregulated)	Conjugation of glutathione (GSH) to toxicants; decreased expression during fasting and in acute phase response

[a] *Table modified from* Haschek and Rousseaux's Handbook of Toxicologic Pathology, *3rd ed., W. M. Haschek, C. G. Rousseaux and M. A. Wallig, eds. (2013), Academic Press, Table AD3, p 393, with permission.*

Another important design consideration is the collection of ancillary tissues for toxicogenomics studies. For example, collection of tissue adjacent to a lesion of interest that is sampled for -omics analysis may be important to understand the biology related to test article exposure. Histologically, normal tissue may be used to tease out the effects associated with exposure where a lesion has not developed, as in the case of a tumor and histologically normal tissue from the same organ. Affected tissue from within the lesion is essential for linking exposure and any molecular changes demonstrated by -omics to structural changes indicative of particular disease mechanisms. When comparing toxicogenomic data across different studies and organs, it is important to match the ages of control and treated animals as well as the sites from which organs are sampled since coding and noncoding transcript expression as well as epigenomic alterations such as DNA methylation are both age dependent and tissue specific. When considering whole-genome, whole-exome, or targeted sequencing of DNA samples, it is essential to compare results from the affected tissue to genomic data from a different organ within the same animal without the lesion or condition of interest. These genomic data from the normal tissue will serve as a reference baseline for genomic alterations resulting from test article exposure. Normally, a skin sample (tail snip or ear punch) is an adequate genomic control in rodent models, while leukocytes (nucleated cells) isolated from blood samples are a common genomic control in molecular epidemiological studies.

6.5. Study Designs and Statistical Considerations

The principles of good study design are arguably more important for investigations with toxicogenomic endpoints than with traditional toxicity studies due to the cost of -omics assays, likelihood that small systematic errors in the experimentation processes will multiply across numerous analytes, the limited understanding of toxicogenomic background levels or unpredictable random error, and the inability to undertake a thorough, direct examination of the raw -omics data given the large number of data points. One way of addressing this issue from a qualitative perspective is to visualize -omics data using various "heat map" options. In such preparations, a 2D display is constructed where columns represent a group or animal, a laddered stack of rows represent genes, and the expression of each gene relative to a reference value is shown as a distinct color. Inspection of such heat map "clustergrams" often permits identification of global gene expression patterns that are associated with a particular physiological or treatment status. Heat maps will be explained in greater detail below.

Statistical analysis based on hypothesis testing is an essential tool for analyzing toxicogenomic data sets to manage the large quantities of data. Common options for evaluating toxicogenomic data include calculating means (with standard deviations as needed), t-tests, parametric or nonparametric analysis of variance (ANOVA), and multiple comparison tests (see *Experimental Design and Statistical Analysis for Toxicologic Pathologists*, Vol 1, Chap 16). Multiple comparisons are especially important in toxicogenomics, where tens of thousands of analytes are each tested for significance by a t-test or ANOVA. One of the consequences of the multiple comparisons approach is the possibility of false positives that may occur solely due to the numerous statistical tests performed to determine significance. For example, if one performs 20 t-tests with a significance level of 0.05, the probability of observing at least one significant result by chance is approximately equal to 0.64, even if all of the tests are actually not significant. This is controlled by testing for false discovery rates that estimate the percentage of a list of analytes that are false positives.

To maximize the possibility of having reliable and interpretable results from a toxicogenomic experiment, an important consideration well before commencing the study is to decide on the extent of replication to incorporate in the design. Replication is desirable in order to optimize the power of the analysis, which is necessary to observe an effect of a specific size in the response to a test article. Selecting the degree of replication is often a challenging task and requires input from statisticians, bioinformaticians, or data scientists who are knowledgeable about the important considerations to sufficiently power a genomic experiment (see *Experimental Design and Statistical*

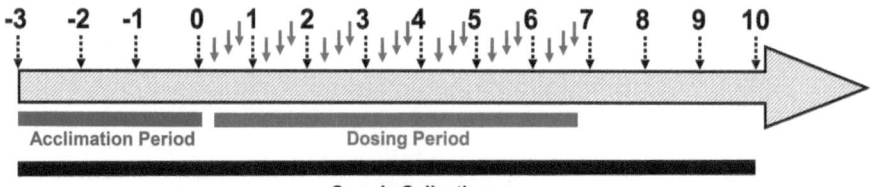

FIGURE 15.2 Design for a time course -omics study for repeated dosing (red arrows). Numbers are the days relative to the start of dosing.

Analysis for Toxicologic Pathologists, Vol 1, Chap 16). Understandably, the investigator typically has a primary interest in the design of the study so that sufficient experimental factors are modeled broadly enough to capture changes in a reasonable and realistic aspect of the biological test system. On the other hand, the data analyst might warrant that more samples should be incorporated to increase biological replication. Both viewpoints are certainly valid and should be valued. While replication is desirable, limited resources for any given study often will require a decision to be made in terms of where in the study design to invest the resources and that it does not interfere with the primary objective(s) of the toxicity study. For toxicogenomic studies, the de facto replication per factor level in a study design is at least three biological replicates (i.e., liver samples from three rats). This repetition ensures that the estimation of the variance is reliable when analyzed statistically using common tests (e.g., a one-way ANOVA with two factors and contrast or alternatively analysis with a Student's t-test).

As toxicogenomic experiments evolve toward increasingly complex study designs, more sophisticated analytical models are needed to reliably capture the underlying molecular alterations. For example, a time course study in rodents to evaluate gene expression responses to a test article to identify early (before apical endpoints) transcriptomic indicators of an adverse effect provides a good example of a more complex toxicogenomic experiment. The experimental factors that must be considered in the study design include replication of the samples, dosing regimen, inclusion of an acclimatization period, and eliminating factors such as batch effect when designing data collection processes. General statistical models (e.g., ANOVA, t-test) would not be appropriate for this complex design. The dosing aspect requires an account for the time series and the linear model can be in two parts: one for the acclimatization period and the other for the dosing period (Figure 15.2). In fact, the batch effect can confound the results if it is not properly corrected prior to analysis. Again, it is extremely important for toxicologists and pathologists to consult with statisticians, bioinformaticians, or data scientists to assist with the modeling and analysis of data especially when the study design is complex in nature.

An additional consideration for an appropriate toxicogenomic study design is the relationship between toxicogenomic and traditional toxicologic pathology endpoints in study conduct, sample collection, and data analysis. For a traditional Good Laboratory Practice (GLP)–compliant general toxicity study (i.e., for safety screening) in which toxicogenomic endpoints also will be assessed, the study design (e.g., time of collection, sequence of work and work load at necropsy, fasting prior to collection, sample availability) should emphasize successful collection of samples to fulfill the traditional endpoints if they conflict with the ideal toxicogenomic collection procedures (e.g., if a limited number of animals are available and/or if sample quantity is limiting). Nonetheless, though it adds to the complexity of study conduct, evaluation of traditional pathology endpoints and toxicogenomic endpoints in the same animal provides an opportunity to correlate individual responses, increasing the possibility of discerning toxicogenomic signals that may be secondary to, or diagnostic of, test article–related pathological effects versus molecular signals that may precede microscopically detectable alterations. In general, pathologists and toxicologists provide a pragmatic perspective for study design that is unlikely to be offered by professionals approaching the study design problem from more purely bioinformatic, statistical, or molecular biology perspectives (see *Basic Approaches to Anatomic Toxicologic Pathology*, Vol 1, Chap 9 and *Practices to Optimize Generation, Interpretation, and Reporting of Pathology Data from Toxicity Studies*, Vol 1, Chap 28).

6.6. Software Tools and Databases

To perform toxicogenomic analyses, intricate software programs are required to store, view, and manipulate these complicated data sets (see Table 15.3). Both commercial and free versions of analytical software are available for -omics. While such software programs are essential when conducting toxicogenomic analysis, the intellectual resources required to install, maintain, and become proficient in their use are frequently beyond what might be useful to a typical toxicologic pathologist who supports toxicogenomic studies as a sideline activity. This consideration should be kept in mind as resources are being allocated so that technical staff who are the regular gatekeepers for toxicogenomic databases have appropriate training and expertise, either through internal sources or through the software vendor. Such -omics expertise should be available to the pathologist when needed, and the responsible staff should be able to maintain the software and -omics database as well as deal effectively with new technological advances.

Beyond the software packages, various online toxicogenomic databases are available to the public (also listed in Table 15.3). These repositories provide direct access to findings acquired for many genetically engineered animal models and toxicity studies with various test articles including chemicals across multiple organ systems. In particular, such archives often allow access to entire sets of historical toxicogenomic data for which summaries have been reported in the scientific literature, but for which a comprehensive interpretation was impossible to capture within a single scientific paper or even a series of related manuscripts. For instance, the Chemical Effects in Biological Systems database (https://manticore.niehs.nih.gov/cebssearch/) allows for conducting queries to identify organs with site-specific neoplasia from rodents exposed to chemicals that produced clear or some evidence of carcinogenicity based on the U.S. National Toxicology Program's (NTP) criteria for carcinogenicity in rodents (Lea et al., 2017) (Figure 15.3).

Computer programming advances such as integrated development environments coupled with software development platforms and cloud computing for genomic data analysis empower novice analysts to string complex and intense analyses of -omics data together in a unified workflow. For example, a Galaxy (web-based platform for data-intensive biomedical research, https://usegalaxy.org/) workflow joined together to download and filter RNA-Seq aligned sequence reads (where a "read" is an output from a genome sequencer containing a string of nucleotide sequences) in binary alignment map format works to assign and count the sequence reads on gene features and then perform quality control on the data (Figure 15.4). Years ago, data analysts would need a bioinformatician trained in RNA-Seq analysis to acquire, store, and process the data. With these advanced, user-friendly, and integrated tools, the reasonably educated and patient scientist can perform sophisticated analyses with limited experience and minimal outside technical support. However, it is prudent to consult trained bioinformaticians to assure that optimal parameter settings are being used.

6.7. Data Analysis and Interpretation

To employ traditional statistical tests (e.g., ANOVA) in an effective manner, toxicogenomic data typically require preprocessing. This manipulation increases the accuracy of estimates of the mean values of treatment groups given that the raw -omics data are often expressed as relative values (e.g., to a baseline representing the midrange measured in healthy control tissues) rather than absolute values (as with MS data). These relative values (the "signal") may be confounded by multiple sources of incompletely controlled variation in the normal dynamic range of molecular expression ("noise") or the readout may vary according to how much data are collected for a given sample (i.e., read depth in RNA-Seq). A full description of these complex preprocessing techniques is beyond the scope of this chapter, but details may be explored in other sources (Li, 2020; Raghavachari and Garcia-Reyero, 2018; Wang, 2016; Wei, 2019). Standard methods typically

TABLE 15.3 Toxicogenomic Analysis Software and Databases[a]

Type of tool	Reference/source
MICROARRAY ANALYSIS SOFTWARE	
Commercial	
GeneSpring	http://www.genespring.com
Qiagen Digital insights	https://digitalinsights.qiagen.com/
Partek	http://www.partek.com/software
Genedata expressionist	http://www.genedata.com/
Free	
ArrayTrack	https://www.fda.gov/science-research/bioinformatics-tools/arraytracktm-hca-pca-standalone-package-powerful-data-exploring-tools
BioConductor	http://bioconductor.org/
dChip	https://sites.google.com/site/dchipsoft/
TM4	http://mev.tm4.org/#/welcome
Galaxy	https://usegalaxy.org/
PATHWAY/ONTOLOGY ANALYSIS	
Commercial	
Ingenuity pathway analysis tool	https://digitalinsights.qiagen.com/
GeneGo	https://portal.genego.com/
Free	
WikiPathways	http://pathvisio.org/, http://www.wikipathways.org
Geneontology	http://geneontology.org
GeneTrail	http://genetrail.bioinf.uni-sb.de/
GSEA	http://www.broad.mit.edu/gsea/
Cytoscape	http://www.cytoscape.org/
PUBLIC DATABASES	
Transcriptomics	
Gene expression omnibus (GEO)	http://www.ncbi.nlm.nih.gov/geo/
ArrayExpress at EBI	http://www.ebi.ac.uk/arrayexpress/
ArrayTrack	https://www.fda.gov/science-research/bioinformatics-tools/arraytracktm-hca-pca-standalone-package-powerful-data-exploring-tools
Comparative toxicogenomics database (transcripts, protein, chemicals)	http://ctd.mdibl.org/
TG-GATEs—from toxicogenomics project in Japan (Japanese)	https://toxico.nibiohn.go.jp/english/
Chemical effects in biological systems	https://cebs.niehs.nih.gov/cebs/

(Continued)

TABLE 15.3 Toxicogenomic Analysis Software and Databases[a]—cont'd

Type of tool	Reference/source
Drug matrix	https://ntp.niehs.nih.gov/data/drugmatrix/index.html
Metabolomics	
National institute of standards and technology	https://www.nist.gov/srd/search-srd
Golm metabolome database	http://gmd.mpimp-golm.mpg.de/
Human metabolome database	http://www.hmdb.ca
Genotypes and phenotypes	
dbGaP	http://www.ncbi.nlm.nih.gov/gap

[a] *Table modified from* Haschek and Rousseaux's Handbook of Toxicologic Pathology, *3rd ed., W. M. Haschek, C. G. Rousseaux and M. A. Wallig, eds. (2013), Academic Press, Table AD6, p. 396, with permission.*

	Publication No.	CASRN	Test Article Name	Species	Sex	Route	Organ	Level of Evidence	Tumor Type/Incidence
	TR-000 (143-50-0)	143-50-0	Chlordecone (kepone)	Mice	Female	Dosed-Feed	Liver	Positive	CARCINOMA; HYPERPLASIA
	TR-000 (143-50-0)	143-50-0	Chlordecone (kepone)	Mice	Male	Dosed-Feed	Liver	Positive	CARCINOMA; HYPERPLASIA
	TR-000 (143-50-0)	143-50-0	Chlordecone (kepone)	Rats	Female	Dosed-Feed	Liver	Positive	CARCINOMA; HYPERPLASIA
	TR-000 (143-50-0)	143-50-0	Chlordecone (kepone)	Rats	Male	Dosed-Feed	Liver	Positive	CARCINOMA; HYPERPLASIA
	TR-000 (67-66-3)	67-66-3	Chloroform	Mice	Female	Gavage	Liver	Positive	CARCINOMA
	TR-000 (67-66-3)	67-66-3	Chloroform	Mice	Male	Gavage	Liver	Positive	CARCINOMA
	TR-002	79-01-6	Trichloroethylene	Mice	Female	Gavage	Liver	Positive	(CARCINOMA)
	TR-002	79-01-6	Trichloroethylene	Mice	Male	Gavage	Liver	Positive	(CARCINOMA)

FIGURE 15.3 Test articles manifesting neoplasia as stored in the Chemical Effects in Biological Systems (CEBS) database.

employed to increase the precision and accuracy of microarray data include the use of error models, local and regional background subtraction, variance stabilization, normalization, and log transformation to achieve a normal distribution. For example, for bulk RNA-Seq data or TempO-Seq data, sequence reads are trimmed away from the adapter oligos, filtered to remove low-quality reads and those with low complexity, and then aligned to a reference genome. Subsequently, sequence read counts are quantified by a transcriptome gene model and then log transformed to produce a normally distributed data set. Automated preprocessing may yield values for individual analytes induced by the treatment that upon manual review do not appear to be quantitatively consistent across individual animals, among group means, and with respect to the fold change in amount (vs. matched controls or reference values). Such discrepancies are due to error propagation (due to any errors from sequencing, reference genome versions, contaminants, in silico errors related to many systematic experimental errors carried through the entire analysis or other transformations, where additional parameters are acting behind the scenes). For example, group mean and p-value estimates calculated for one tissue and sex may be slightly altered if data from the other sex and additional

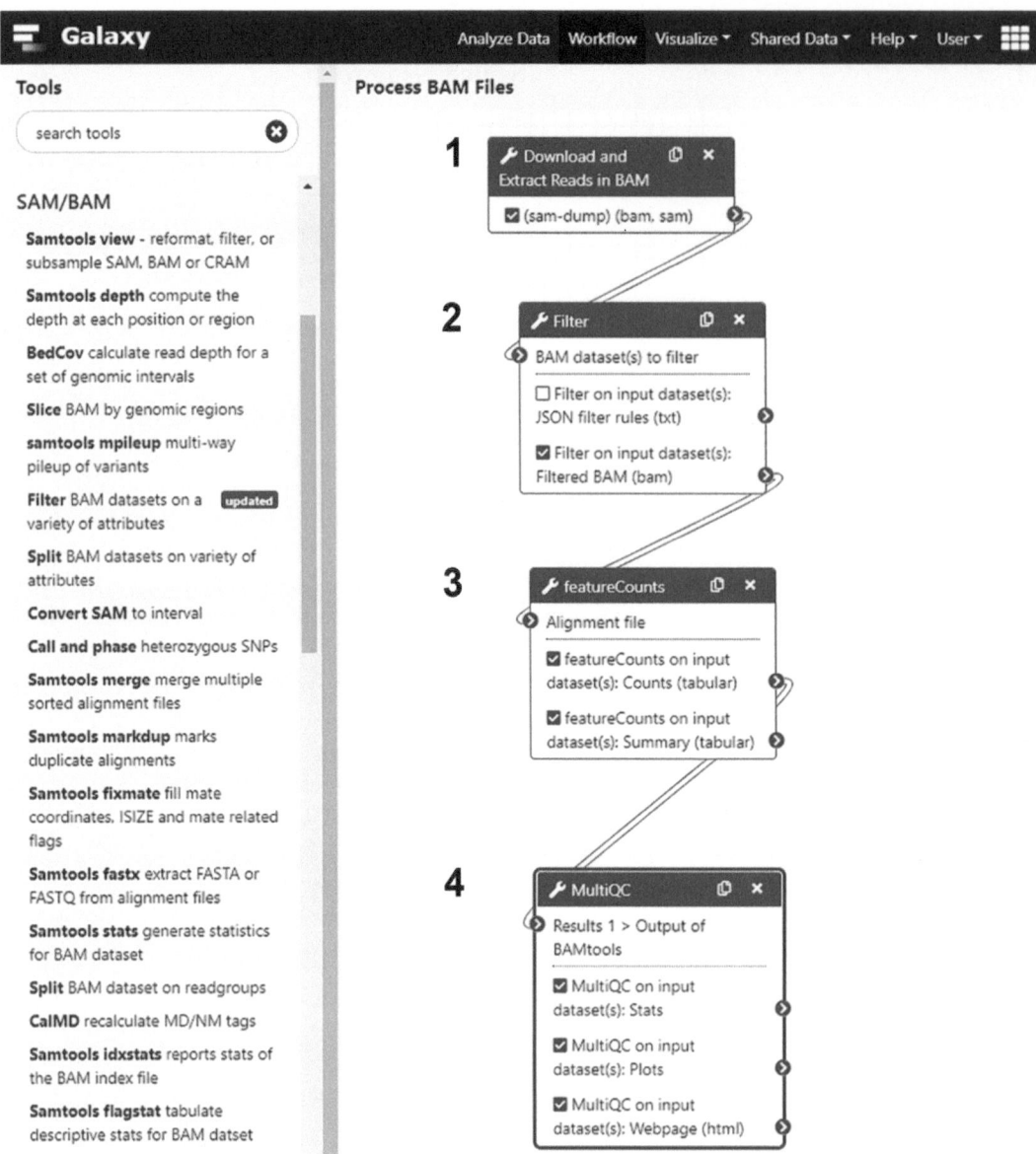

FIGURE 15.4   Galaxy workflow to automatically process binary alignment map (BAM)–formatted files, where BAM files are the compressed binary version of Sequence Alignment/Map (SAM) files representing aligned sequences from an -omics analysis. Step 1: Sequencing reads that were aligned to a gene model are downloaded as BAM files. Step 2: The BAM files are then automatically filtered based on quality attributes (e.g., sequence quality). Step 3: The BAM files are processed to count the number of sequence reads assigned to a given gene model feature. Step 4: Summary statistics are performed on the processed data, graphs generated, and quality control results reported in an HTML web page document.

tissues are incorporated in the analysis since noise and variance or dispersion (in RNA-Seq and TempO-Seq count data) estimates may draw on the entire data set to improve accuracy. Standardized preprocessing methods embedded in software algorithms yield highly reproducible results that can be verified qualitatively by more traditional techniques, like RT-PCR or LC-MS using quantitative standards, targeting a few analytes at a time.

Beyond traditional statistical methods and data preprocessing, toxicogenomics relies on multiple alternative analytical methods that likely will be unfamiliar to most toxicologic pathologists. These methods arose from the need to analyze large quantities of data to select signals requiring further investigation. To explain some commonly used alternative methods that are typically applied to toxicogenomic data, a conventional clinical pathology data set collected from a general toxicity study conducted in nonhuman primates will be used as an illustration. In this toxicity study (Figure 15.5), $n=5$ monkeys/sex/group received daily oral doses of either vehicle or a low or high dose of a test article for 1 month. At the high dose, conventional clinical pathology analysis demonstrated that red blood cell (RBC) parameters were decreased, clotting times were increased, and total bilirubin (TBIL) was elevated. In addition, serum gamma-glutamyl transferase (GGT) activity was decreased, suggesting the presence of altered thyroid hormone homeostasis. For the alternative -omics-like analytical approach, 11 traditional clinical pathology parameters (6 serum chemistry analytes, 2 clotting endpoints, and 3 hematology parameters) were analyzed for 30 animals (10 per group), thereby providing a total data set of 330 points. This data set is small enough to be viewed directly in tabular form without the use of visualization techniques, but the implications may be grasped quickly using graphic plots and heat maps as well (Figure 15.5). In contrast, it is impossible to productively navigate a full toxicogenomic data set for 30 animals using direct inspection of data tables due to the exponentially larger number of data points (e.g., 25,000 mRNAs per tissue). Unlike clinical pathology data, the viewing of toxicogenomic data is often limited to drug-related changes in treatment groups due to the sheer complexity of the data set.

A common dimension reduction method for an initial evaluation of a toxicogenomic data set is principal component analysis (PCA), a simple linear transformation technique that is illustrated graphically in Figure 15.5A for the 11 clinical pathology parameters in 30 animals. In this method, the original data are (1) projected in a new data space; however, the axes (principal components) are orthogonal to each other and (2) the newly formed axes are ordered in a sequentially reduced fashion in terms of their weights. In other words, any given principal component captures more variability than the one that immediately follows it. Hence, the multidimensional data from each sample are plotted along axes that represent the directions

of maximum variation. For instance, if RBC parameters exhibit the greatest change, then a weighted sum of these analytes would be the first principal component in the initial analysis. Subsequent principal components are chosen from the weighted sums of the parameters that capture the next highest amounts of variation in the data, thereby ensuring a unique graphical projection of the complex 11-dimensional data in a simplified 2D or 3D representation. In this fashion, the PCA technique visually captures the majority of variation in the assessment.

Though the principal component directions have genuine meaning (the weightings of the assays involve magnitude and correlation relationships), typically the weights are not evaluated in a formal sense using mathematics when analyzing -omics data. Rather, the graphical location of samples plotted in this abstract space of maximal change is assessed visually in a qualitative fashion. For instance, if a biological replicate does not group closely together in 2D or 3D space, then the sample may be an outlier that needs to be discarded or regenerated/reanalyzed before further consideration of the data set. In addition, if samples are separated in the dimensional space by some technical factor (e.g., mRNA preparation date, necropsy order, etc.), then the data may exhibit a batch effect which needs to be accounted for (if possible) before further analysis. If the data from the control (vehicle or other control) and test article–dosed groups appear in different regions of the graph (as they do in Figure 15.5A), then there is reasonable evidence of a test article–related change that can be distinguished using the major principal components. Thus, rapid inspection of the qualitative PCA graph identifies whether or not further statistical analysis is likely to be fruitful: Are there extreme outliers suggesting problems in study conduct? Is there a clear pattern of dose-related change indicative of a genuine test article–related effect? Is there evidence of a significant differential response to the test article based on age or sex? In the current example (Figure 15.5A), the data for the two sexes separate along principal component 2 due to sex-related differences in clinical pathology parameters reflective of established sex-specific reference intervals (e.g., lower values for hematocrit [HCT], GGT activity, and activated partial thromboplastin time in females than in males).

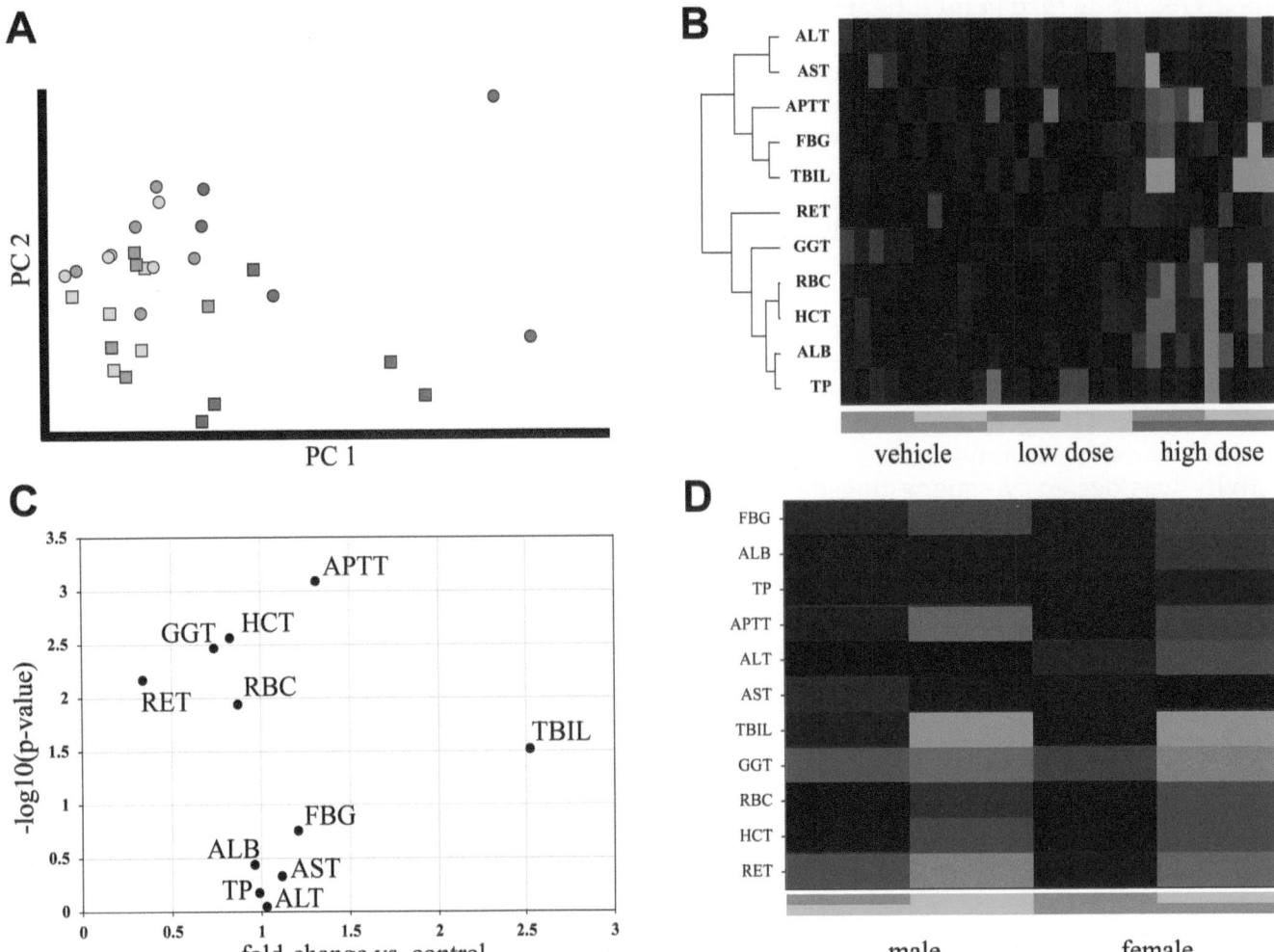

FIGURE 15.5   Toxicogenomic analysis representations of traditional clinical pathology parameters showing data display options commonly used for toxicogenomics data. (A) Principal component analysis (PCA) of changes in 11 clinical pathology parameters following exposure to a model test article, measured across 5 monkeys/sex/group. This conventional two-dimensional PCA representation shows all animals plotted versus the two greatest (arbitrarily chosen) principal components: PC1 (the direction of maximal change, x-axis) and PC2 (which specifies the second highest direction of variation in the data, y-axis); squares represent males, circles represent females; vehicle shows as blue, low dose as orange, and high dose as red. The position of individuals differs by dose along PC1 regardless of sex, indicating that some pattern of clinical pathology changes is dependent on dose. The position of the females and males differs along principal PC2 across all dose groups, indicating a sex-based difference in some clinical pathology analytes. The graphic does not indicate the parameters PC1 and PC2 that underlie either change, but subsequent analysis can reveal the causes. For instance, multiway analysis of variance (ANOVA) indicated sex-associated variations in hematocrit (HCT), serum gamma-glutamyl transferase (GGT) activity, and activated partial thromboplastin time (APTT). (B) Heat map representation of clinical pathology parameters across all individuals in the study (sex is shown in the color bar nearest the bottom of the heat map, with blue for males and green for females), where pink denotes higher and blue denotes lower values than the mean for that parameter, while brighter colors indicate a greater degree and darker colors a lesser degree of change. Prolongation of APTT and reduction in red blood cell parameters in some high-dose animals, predominantly male, is apparent. The dendrogram, or family tree, to the left of the map graphically conveys the Pearson correlation among the various analytes used to derive the plot. The dendrogram has two separate clusters of clinical analytes driven particularly by the high-dose treatment. Additional analyte abbreviations: albumin (ALB), alanine aminotransferase (ALT), aspartate aminotransferase (AST), total protein (TP), and fibrinogen (FBG); the changes are not necessarily significant by ANOVA. (C) Volcano plot across the parameters of the ANOVA P-values for high-dose males versus

A heat map clustergram, as shown in Figure 15.5B, provides another common means for providing a simple visual overview of toxicogenomic data sets. Clustering is a 2D similarity representation of vectors for data values of features (e.g., genes, proteins, etc.) grouped to demonstrate closeness to each other. Data may be arranged in a dendrogram (family tree) using a merging algorithm in whatever orientation and level of summarization is most helpful (e.g., genes in rows and dose groups in columns, or individual animals in rows and genes in columns). Signal intensity or another type of data relative to the mean across all animals or relative to the control group or reference value (all choices that may be selected in commercial software) is expressed in terms of color and brightness in the heat map. Values higher or lower than the mean across all animals (or vs. the control group or reference value) are represented by graded shades of two different colors; the choice of colors is arbitrary, but many contemporary publications have heat maps that employ red to designate higher/upregulated measurements and fluorescent green to represent lower/downregulated measurements. Some software tools use other color choices that permit color-blind viewers to discriminate values (as in the heat maps of Figure 15.5). The graphic provides a rapid and easy indication regarding which biological features are varying with treatment, though with all the potential choices, interpretation of the visualization requires knowing what choices have been used in the construction of the heat map. This presentation also shows that some high-dose animals have multiple clinical pathology parameters above and below their mean values (columns with brighter pink and blue, respectively; Figure 15.5B). Combined with hierarchical clustering (family tree of Figure 15.5B), an iterative computing of the similarity of biological features across individuals or groups rendered as a heat map can quickly identify similarities that may be important. In this case, the family tree identifies higher similarity across animals between biological feature values of RBC and HCT and also fibrinogen (FBG) and TBIL, illustrating that high correlation may be due to a mechanistic relationship (RBC and HCT) or may simply be an association present in the particular study.

In Figure 15.5C, the statistical significance and magnitude of changes in the high-dose males versus controls is represented as a volcano plot. Such plots are used to simultaneously convey the extent of change versus control (x-axis) and the statistical significance of this change (as in ANOVA-derived P-value; y-axis). Some assays with variation in Figure 15.5B did not reach significance by ANOVA (e.g., alanine aminotransferase [ALT], FBG). Figure 15.5D is a heat map of the same-sex fold change in group mean values versus control values for the 11 parameters, with larger positive fold changes appearing to be brighter pink and the larger negative fold changes appearing brighter blue.

Each of these commonly used analyses and representations provides a different view of a large multifactorial (i.e., toxicogenomic) data set and can contribute to answering different questions more rapidly and accurately. Examples of their utility include the following kinds of assessments:

1. Is there a test article- or dose-related change that is relatively consistent across individuals and sexes? PCA and heat maps (Figure 15.5) address this issue.
2. Which parameters are changing together, and which are consistently changed across animals? Heat maps (Figure 15.5B and D) combined with hierarchical clustering (Figure 15.5B) and the volcano plot (Figure 15.5C) across assays and individuals evaluate this possibility.

control. The y-axis is -$\log_{10}$ ANOVA P-value, while the x-axis is the fold change versus control males. Significant ($P<.05$ [equivalent to > 1.3 on (A)$\log_{10} P$ value scale on the y-axis]) increases in total bilirubin (TBIL) and APTT as well as decreases (mostly $P<.01$) in red blood cell count (RBC), reticulocyte count (RET), HCT, and GGT occurred in the high-dose males. (D) Graphic depiction of the group-mean fold change in treated animals (dose is indicated by the color bar nearest the bottom of the heat map, with blue for low dose and green for high dose) versus the values from the same-sex control across the 11 parameters. Pink denotes higher and blue lower fold changes (and brighter colors indicate a greater degree and darker colors a lesser degree of change); the changes are not necessarily significant by ANOVA. *Figure modified from Haschek WM, Rousseaux CG, Wallig MA, editors.* Haschek and Rousseaux's Handbook of Toxicologic Pathology, *ed 3, 2013, Academic Press Figure 11.3, p. 366, with permission.*

3. Which parameters meet statistical significance and have large fold changes versus control in the group means of treated animals? Volcano plots (Figure 15.5C) handle this topic.
4. Which parameters have large fold changes versus control in the group mean, and which assays or dose groups have the most correlated changes? This point is addressed by heat maps showing fold changes across various factors (e.g., sex) of treated versus control animals (Figure 15.5D) with hierarchical clustering of assays and dose groups.

In addition to the approaches illustrated in Figure 15.5, toxicogenomic analysis also commonly relies on approaches that leverage the experimental design in the analysis. For instance, Extracting Patterns and Identifying coexpressed Genes (EPIG) is a tool for analysis of microarray gene expression data using signal-to-noise, magnitude of fold change, and correlation of gene expression profiles across the toxicogenomic experimental factors or exposures to (1) identify all the significant coexpressed patterns in the data and then (2) cluster the gene expression profiles to the patterns (Chou et al., 2007). Figure 15.6A illustrates an EPIG analysis of gene expression patterns from the bone marrow of rats exposed to topotecan, oxaliplatin, their respective control vehicles, or a combination of the treatments for 24 h. The control samples are used as reference specimens to the test article–treated samples, and as such, the log2 ratio (e.g., a proportional change where +1 or −1 ratio means a doubling or halving of the original value) of the samples relative to the average of their respective controls is approximately 0. The order that the vehicles are given alone has no impact on the gene expression. When a control vehicle is given in combination with either topotecan or oxaliplatin individually, the gene expression decreases. However, when the agents are given in combination, the expression of the genes decreases relative to the reductions when the agents are given individually regardless of the order in which the two agents are administered. A version of EPIG for RNA-Seq data (EPIG-Seq) uses the sequence read counts and dispersion in the data to identify coexpressed genes (Li and Bushel, 2016).

In using gene expression data for BMD analysis, BMDExpress (Kuo et al., 2016; Yang et al., 2007) defines subsets of genes that demonstrate a significant dose–response behavior via ANOVA, after which they are fitted using a selection of statistical models to find the one which best describes the data with the least amount of complexity while bracketing the BMD. Figure 15.6B depicts an enhanced BMD analysis platform (BMDExpress2) that incorporates biological processes/pathways enrichment analysis of the genes exhibiting a significant dose–response behavior to optimize the fit of the statistical models to gene expression data used to identify the BMD (Phillips et al., 2019).

Signature analysis of variants in DNA is a means to identify somatic mutations derived by exposure to carcinogens or other mutagens. DNA sequencing of the exome or whole genome of tissue samples permits alignment of the sequence reads to a respective genome similar to the initial step in RNA-Seq analysis. However, the analysis encompasses tallying, at various loci of the genome, the number of variations in the sequence reads that differ from the reference base and are not either known SNPs, germline variants, or incidental substitutions also found in matched control samples. These single-nucleotide variants (SNVs) are then compiled into counts representative of 96 possible single-base substitution mutation types (constituted by the *six* known base substitutions C > A, C > G, C > T, T > A, T > C, and T > G that occur in the context of the *four* 5′ bases and *four* 3′ bases flanking the SNV for each codon, i.e., six substitutions x four 5′ bases x four 3′ bases = 96) in the form of a mutation spectrum. The same analysis can be performed for doublet-base substitutions and insertions/deletions (indels, which are gains or losses of multiple base pairs ranging from a few to several thousand in length). If the mutation spectra counts are not sparse (i.e., there are not many of the mutation types with zero counts or very low counts), then the data can be deconvoluted mathematically (Alexandrov et al., 2020) to decipher mutational signatures associated with a given test article exposure (Figure 15.7). These signatures then can be compared to a relevant repository, such as the human Catalogue Of Somatic Mutations In Cancer database (Bamford et al., 2004; Forbes et al., 2008; Tate et al., 2019), in order to infer their potential contributions to the etiology of chemically induced cancer.

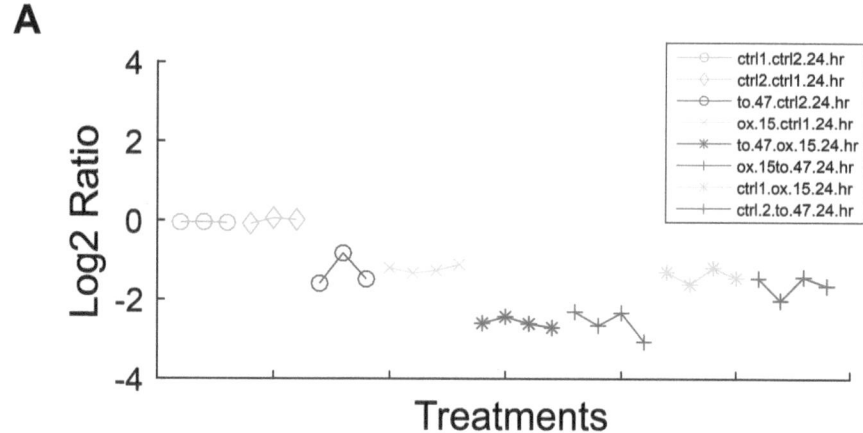

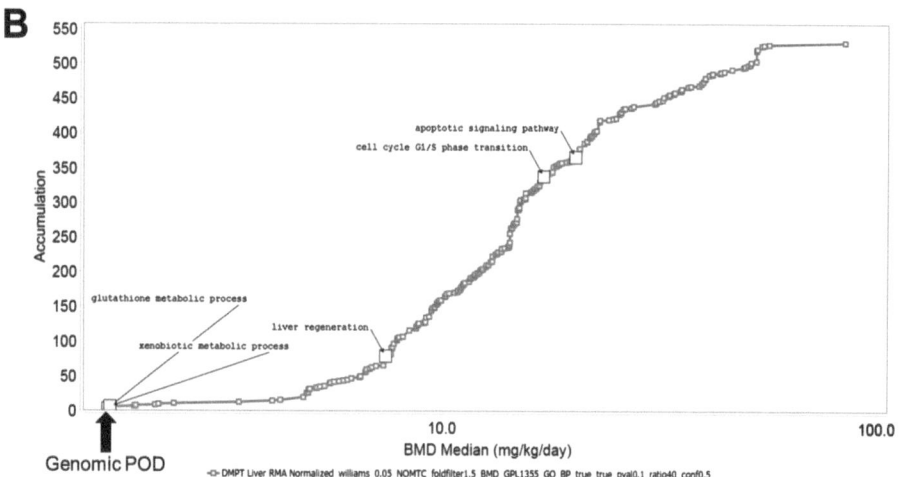

FIGURE 15.6   1 Gene expression patterns related to exposure to single or combinations of drugs. (A) Rats were exposed and mRNA from the bone marrow was analyzed for gene expression changes. Expression pattern of genes coexpressed in response to exposure for 24 h to either 47 mg/kg topotecan (to), 15 mg/kg oxaliplatin (ox), their respective control vehicles (ctrl1, ctrl2), or combination of the treatments (ox, to). The x-axis represents the samples from the treatments (three or four replicates), and the y-axis the log2 ratio of the treated values compared to the average of the matched controls. (B) Accumulation plot of the benchmark dose (BMD) estimation from the livers of rats exposed to N,N-dimethyl-p-toluidine (five replicates per dose level). The x-axis is the median dose (mg/kg/day) and represents the range of the BMD exposure concentrations examined. The y-axis represents benchmark concentration accumulation (integer accumulation for each BMD), and genomic point of departure (POD). The goodness of a fit of the data along a trend related to the dosing in combination with a 1.5-fold change was used to identify responsive genes. The microarray expression data for each gene normalized by the robust multichip average (RMA) method was fit to a suite of parametric (data meeting certain statistical assumptions) dose–response models. The best fit models were then filtered for goodness of fit and the genes collapsed into the Gene Ontology (GO) biological process (BP) terms. The yellow boxes denote the GO BPs enriched significantly by subsets of genes exhibiting a dose–response behavior induced by the exposures. "Active" GO BP terms shown on the plot were required to be populated by at least three genes, and the annotated genes in a category populated at $\geq$ 5%.

Other analytical approaches use supervision by the data analyst to enable classification of results relative to prior knowledge or external data. In pathway analysis, a list of analytes meeting a criterion of interest (perhaps a specific ANOVA-derived p-value as calculated across dose groups) is scored with respect to the probability that a randomly generated analyte list of the same length would contain as many or more members of a given biochemical or other canonical pathway. For instance, in the clinical pathology example above, if hemoglobin

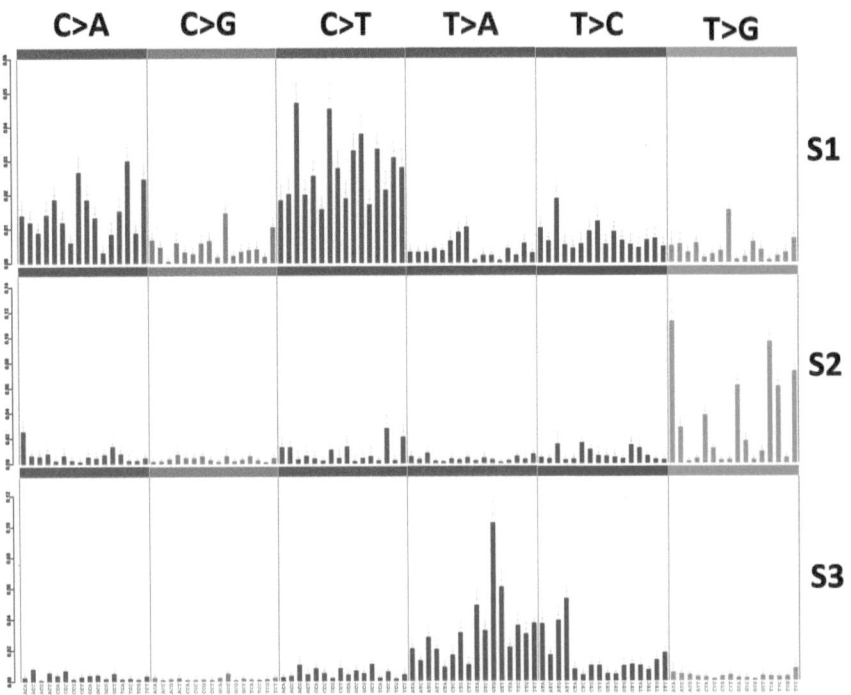

FIGURE 15.7   Mutational Signatures. The *x*-axis is the 96 possible mutation types and the y-axis is proportion. The colors represent the mutations from one base to another base substitution (C>A, C> G, C> T, T>A, T>C, and T>G). S1, S2, and S3 are the signatures derived from the mutations.

content, HCT, counts of RBC and reticulocyte numbers, and the RBC distribution width (RDW) all changed relative to control values in the absence of any other clinical pathology changes, a pathway analysis would indicate that there was a statistically significant enrichment for members of the "RBC" pathway. Such a statistical statement must be cross-checked against biological plausibility. For example, an increased HCT, increased reticulocyte numbers, and decreased RDW represent a virtually impossible biological combination, but it would still be viewed as a significant "pathway score" if the statistical analysis identified this pattern of multiple changes in RBC parameters. The software techniques automatically score the list regardless of magnitude and direction. In pathway analysis, the pathway being scored may not be a good fit to the data (e.g., members of a protein complex or of a biochemical pathway may not be transcriptionally regulated in a coordinated fashion in response to test article treatments or a particular disease state). Thus, biological plausibility of an explanation or mapped pathway still depends on review by a toxicologic pathologist or other biologist.

Another approach to classifying toxicogenomic data relative to prior knowledge is to generate and score data with multidimensional classifiers. These highly sophisticated approaches typically are pursued by statisticians, data scientists, or bioinformaticians. Using them, toxicogenomic responses associated with distinct test articles or well-characterized agent classes (e.g., mycotoxins as a class vs. other toxicant types) are processed to derive parameters (e.g., weights) that classify future data sets as belonging to one of the known classes. The weights derived by the classification methods generally have no clear meaning for any individual analyte as there may be tens or hundreds of weights acting together to place data within or outside of a given class. The computational methods for deriving classifiers strive to avoid bias and overfitting (i.e., matching the existing data well, but unable to be extrapolated to classify new data) by the use of diverse data sets to build the classes coupled with separate data sets to train and test the classifying algorithms. However, overfitting is a major issue for multidimensional classifiers that have not been tested across many laboratories and in potentially confounding situations (e.g., data from different sequencers, data from samples using different library preparation methods, batch effects due to processing site, etc.). Experience suggests that initial enthusiasm for a new, solidly performing multidimensional classifier, also known as a gene or metabolite "signature," is likely to fade upon wider use, just as the robust safety margins in short-duration early exploratory toxicity studies may narrow in pivotal longer duration studies or promising Phase 2a human clinical data are often followed by more modest Phase 3 findings.

In toxicogenomic publications or presentations, typically only a subset of the types of analyses as illustrated in Figure 15.5 are presented to concisely develop an argument. However, in practice, multiple analytical approaches create a more robust understanding of toxicogenomic data sets. To extend the clinical pathology example above, the analysis of a hepatic transcriptomic study in a mouse model of endotoxemia (cecal ligation and puncture) will be helpful to illustrate the value of multiple/ensemble data views when interpreting -omics data. In this animal model, hepatic transcript abundance in controls versus surgically manipulated wild-type (WT) mice and gene-targeted mice lacking a receptor involved in inflammatory signaling (gp130, the signal-transducing component of the interleukin [IL]-6 receptor) were generated. These microarray data are publicly available in the GEO data repository (https://www.ncbi.nlm.nih.gov/geo/) under the accession number GSE22009 (https://www.ncbi.nlm.nih.gov/geo/query/acc.cgi?acc=GSE22009). Some summary statistics of the transcriptomic data are provided in Table 15.4, more detailed data are given in Tables 15.5 and 15.6, and some graphical views of the study findings are shown in Figures 15.8–15.13. These graphical views are based on data analyses commonly performed in toxicogenomic studies. The exact quantitative values for the analyses of Table 15.4 will vary depending on the software analysis procedures used, but qualitative relationships will remain. The table also shows how different tests still may provide reinforced views of the data set, as with the Pearson correlation results across samples from individual animals versus ANOVA and t-test findings across group mean values for treatment groups. As illustrated in the multiple views of the data for this study,

there is a greater treatment-related change in gp130 knock-out animals versus WT mice, and the difference in response involves inflammatory genes and pathways, including genes directly downstream of the disrupted IL-6 receptor.

7. APPLICATIONS OF TOXICOGENOMICS

It is unclear how often pharmaceutical and chemical industries use toxicogenomics to characterize new entities. There have been regular publications in the scientific literature reporting interesting applications and results of toxicogenomics technologies in these settings, but often they have been in the form of review articles from academic authors or regulators and not new data originating from these industries. A recent cross-institutional survey regarding the application of and objectives for -omics technologies in the pharmaceutical industry (Vahle et al., 2018) indicated that toxicogenomics currently is used mostly in the context of non-GLP screening or exploratory rodent toxicity studies that are conducted during the lead identification and optimization stages of drug discovery. The value of a toxicogenomics component in these early studies is to provide a mechanistic understanding of toxicity and/or to predict future toxic effects. Additional applications include biomarker identification and assessing target engagement. These non-GLP studies are intended mainly to evaluate the suitability from a toxicology perspective of a test article and/or to generate dose range-finding data that then can be used to design robust GLP studies. These two aspects and the more specific application for carcinogenesis assessment are discussed below in more depth.

7.1. Predictive Toxicology

Predictive toxicology will be used here to cover the use of -omics tools and markers to predict the future occurrence of a toxic event as opposed to the use of animal models to predict toxicity in humans. In that context, since changes in tissue transcriptomes following exposure to a test article are very sensitive and most often happen before morphological and functional

TABLE 15.4   Summary Statistics for Hepatic Toxicogenomic Data Acquired Using a Cecal Ligation and Puncture Model in Wild Type and gp130 Knockout Mice[a,b]

Parameter	Value (across 45,000 analytes)
% Analytes expressed above background at $P<.01$ in individual samples (based on noise estimates for the array technology)	42%—46%
% Analytes expressed above background at $P<.01$ in groups (based on $n=3$ replicates per group and technology specific noise parameters)	77%—78% (replicates increase detection of low abundance analytes)
Pearson correlation of analyte abundance across controls—both genotypes	98% (similarity higher in controls)
Pearson correlation of analyte abundance across treated—within genotypes	96%—98%
Pearson correlation of analyte abundance across treated—across genotypes	95%—96%
Pearson correlation of analyte abundance—treated versus control for wild type	93%—94%
Pearson correlation of analyte abundance—treated versus control for knockout	95%—97%
% Analytes with significantly altered abundance at t-test $P<.01$—control versus treated for wild type	21%
% Analytes with significantly altered abundance at t-test $P<.01$—control versus treated for knockout	13%
% Analytes with significantly altered abundance at t-test $P<.01$—wild type control versus knock-out control	0.5% (insignificant effect of genotype in controls)
% Analytes with significantly altered abundance at ANOVA $P<.01$ for treatment	25%
% Analytes with significantly altered abundance at ANOVA $P<.01$ for treatment, using Benjamini—Hochberg false discovery rate multiple comparisons correction	16% (fewer analytes pass multiple comparisons test)

[a] Multiple traditional analysis methods provide logically consistent results indicating how use of multiple approaches builds understanding of a large toxicogenomic data set.
[b] Table modified from Haschek and Rousseaux's Handbook of Toxicologic Pathology, 3rd ed., W. M. Haschek, C. G. Rousseaux and M. A. Wallig, eds. (2013), Academic Press, Table 11.4, p 368, with permission.

effects indicative of toxicity, genome-wide expression profiling offers a unique opportunity to identify new gene-based markers (i.e., predictive gene expression signatures or classifiers) that can be used to foretell the long-term effects of new chemical entities (NCEs). These gene-based biomarkers are not designed to replace, but rather to complement the battery of other endpoints (e.g., hematology, serum [or plasma] chemistry, and histopathology) already used routinely in toxicity studies. Several research groups have provided evidence that gene expression–based classifiers have predictive value, at least for some toxic changes and some tissues.

The liver is one of the target organs most susceptible to chemical insults. The two key reasons are (1) its central role in metabolism and detoxification as well as (2) its high exposure to xenobiotics after oral intake (Weaver et al., 2020). Consequently, liver toxicity is a common finding in nonclinical toxicity studies, and drug-induced liver injury (DILI) is a major cause of nonclinical and clinical attrition, market withdrawal, and product labels with a "black box" warning regarding the potential for serious adverse effects (Kaplowitz, 2004). The liver is also a relatively homogenous tissue, which makes gene expression profiling experiments more reproducible and facilitates identification

TABLE 15.5 Comparison of gp130 Knockout and Surgically Manipulated Wild Type Versus Controls[b] for the Hepatic Abundance of Five mRNA Transcripts in a Mouse Cecal Ligation and Puncture Model[a]

| Analyte | Protein class[d] | gp130 knockout | | Wildtype | Affymetrix |
		Fold-change	P-value	Fold-change	Probeset ID[c]
Alpha-2-macroglobulin (A2m)	Protease inhibitor	−1.4	0.6	100	1434719_at
Lipocalin 2 (Lcn2)	Transfer/carrier protein	60	0	46	1427747_a_at
RIKEN cDNA D730039F16 gene	N/A	−7.4	0	−23	1425746_at
CYP450, family 7, subfamily A, polypeptide 1 (Cyp7a1)	Oxygenase	−2.3	0.12	−65	1422100_at
Glucokinase (Gck)	Protein kinase	−1.3	0.01	−100	1419146_a_at

[a] *Table modified from* Haschek and Rousseaux's Handbook of Toxicologic Pathology, *3rd ed., W. M. Haschek, C. G. Rousseaux and M. A. Wallig, eds. (2013), Academic Press, Table 11.5, p. 369, with permission.*
[b] *Controls are mouse genotypes without cecal ligation and puncture (CLP) treatment.*
[c] *NetAffx database: https://www.affymetrix.com/analysis/index.affx.*
[d] *Protein class annotation obtained from the Panther Classification System v15.0: http://pantherdb.org/.*
Values based on $n = 3$ per group.
The P-values for all transcripts in wild type were <.01.
N/A: None available.

TABLE 15.6 Gene Ontology Analysis for Transcripts That Changed During a Mouse Cecal Ligation and Puncture Model[a]

| Primary gene ontology (GO) term name | # of analytes in category | Wildtype | | gp130 knockout | |
		# Analytes changing	P-value for category	# Analytes changing	P-value for category
Inflammatory response	197	12	3.21E-17	5	3.79E-07
Immune response	487	12	1.55E-12	3	0.0058
Extracellular region	684	12	7.86E-11	6	1.12E-05
Chemokine activity	58	6	1.48E-10	2	0.0009
Cytokine activity	248	7	3.73E-08	2	0.015

[a] *Table modified from* Haschek and Rousseaux's Handbook of Toxicologic Pathology, *3rd ed. W. M. Haschek, C. G. Rousseaux and M. A. Wallig, eds. (2013) Academic Press, Table 11.6, p. 369, with permission.*
The number of analytes changing was based on transcripts that were strongly altered (fold-change >20) versus wild-type controls without cecal ligation and puncture (CLP) at t-test $P<.01$.

and interpretation of test article–related gene expression changes. For these reasons, early "proof of concept" and later predictive toxicology applications of toxicogenomic technologies have focused mainly on the liver. Likewise, as will be discussed later, the liver has been the most studied tissue to predict carcinogenicity using transcriptomics due to the relatively common ability of novel test articles to induce tumors in this organ during rodent bioassays.

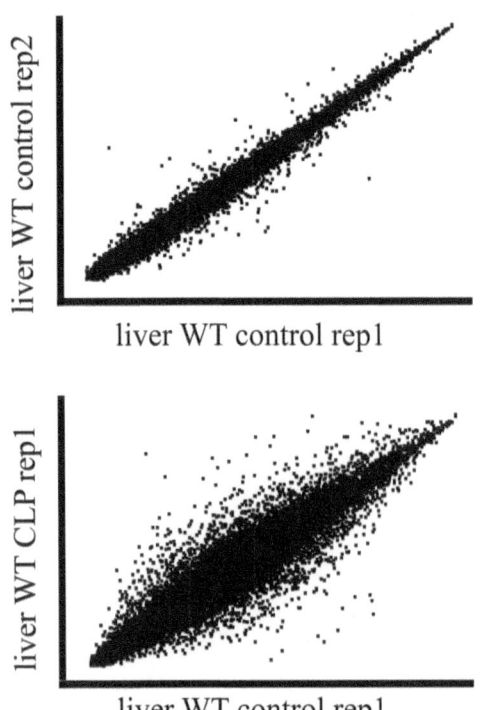

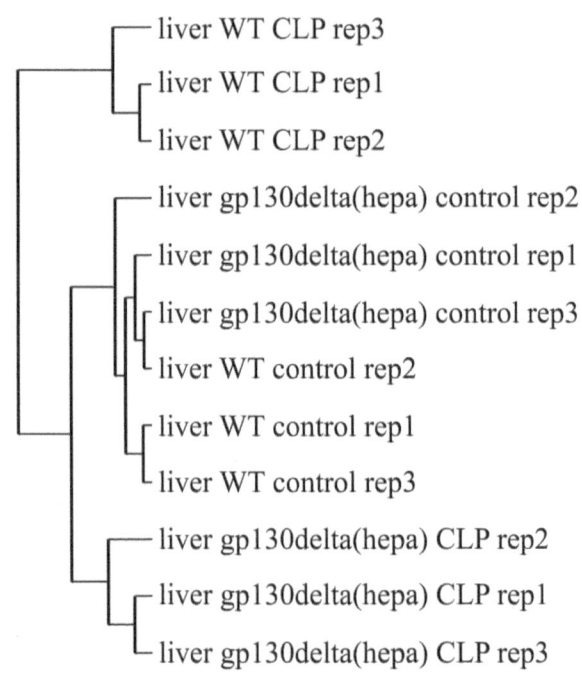

FIGURE 15.9   Hierarchical clustering of hepatic mRNA transcriptional profiles from wild-type mice and hepatocyte-specific gp130-delta knock-out mice (hepa) for both untreated controls and following treatment with cecal ligation and puncture (CLP). The data set was obtained using 12 samples, n = 3 mice per group, and correlating across 45,000 analytes. Controls of both genotypes cluster together closely in the center of the cladogram (family tree), indicating that the gene knockout did not significantly alter the overall pattern of transcript abundance. The response in the treated wild-type animals clusters further from the controls than does the response in the treated knockouts, indicating that loss of the gp130 gene decreased the molecular response to cecal ligation and puncture. Rep = replicates, animals with the same genotype in the same treatment group. Microarray data used in this analysis are publicly available in the Gene Expression Omnibus (GEO) data repository, http://www.ncbi.nlm.nih.gov/geo/under accession GSE22009. *Figure modified from Haschek WM, Rousseaux CG, Wallig MA, editors.* Haschek and Rousseaux's Handbook of Toxicologic Pathology, *ed 3, 2013, Academic Press, Figure 11.5, p. 370, with permission.*

FIGURE 15.8   Log of hepatic analyte abundance across 45,000 mRNA transcripts in 8- to 12-week-old male mice: two wild-type control individuals (top) versus one wild-type control animal and one wild-type animal with cecal ligation and puncture (bottom). The narrower range of the expression pattern for the top panel clearly demonstrates that the similarity of transcript abundance is higher in animals from a common treatment group. The comparison of control and treated individuals (bottom) shows that the treatment affects a multiplicity of transcripts. Data are publicly available in the Gene Expression Omnibus (GEO) data repository, http://www.ncbi.nlm.nih.gov/geo/under accession GSE22009. *Figure modified from Haschek WM, Rousseaux CG, Wallig MA, editors.* Haschek and Rousseaux's Handbook of Toxicologic Pathology, *ed 3, 2013, Academic Press, Figure 11.4, p. 370, with permission.*

Several independent groups have shown that predictive gene expression classifiers can be developed for the liver. For example, a neural network–based algorithm to predict hepatotoxicity in rats developed in one author's laboratory (Semizarov and Blomme, 2008) was built using liver mRNA profiles from 3-day rat studies evaluating 50 prototypical hepatotoxic and nonhepatotoxic agents at two dose levels: a high dose expected (based on proprietary and/or literature data) to induce hepatotoxicity after at least

1 week of daily treatment and a lower, nonhepatotoxic dose. The quantitative algorithm classified test articles according to the probability that they would induce hepatotoxicity in rats upon continued dosing. In a forward validation exercise using an independent testing set of agents, the algorithm classified correctly 89% of

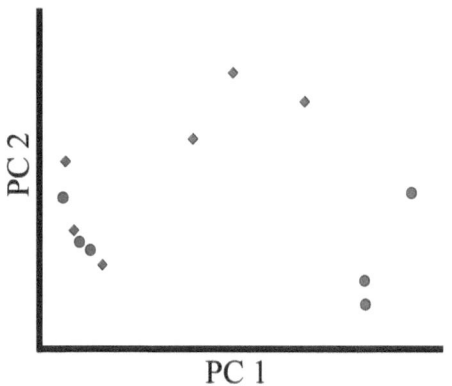

FIGURE 15.10 Principal component analysis (PCA) of each individual microarray in the mouse cecal ligation and puncture (CLP) study shown in Figure 9 (circles are wild type, diamonds are gp130 knockouts; blue are controls, red are treated; and $n = 3$ hepatic transcriptional profiles per treatment and genotype). The array for each animal is shown as a single point (summarizing all of the changes in 45,000 analytes) plotted along axes representing the two arbitrarily chosen principal components (PC) where the data vary most significantly. Controls of both genotypes cluster together, while CLP groups of each genotype cluster separately and with higher variance than is evident in controls. For CLP data, wild-type animals fall further from controls along PC1 (the direction of maximum change) than do the knockouts, indicating that loss of gp130 attenuates the CLP response. Microarray data used in this analysis are publicly available in the Gene Expression Omnibus (GEO) data repository, http://www.ncbi.nlm.nih.gov/geo/ under accession GSE22009. *Figure modified from Haschek WM, Rousseaux CG, Wallig MA, editors.* Haschek and Rousseaux's Handbook of Toxicologic Pathology, *ed 3, 2013, Academic Press, Figure 11.6, p. 371, with permission.*

the test articles. Furthermore, an additional validation evaluated 52 proprietary chemical entities for which data were available from short-term (3–5 days) and long-term (>2 weeks) rat studies. The model produced correct predictions for 50 entities (89% sensitivity, 98% specificity, and 96% predictive accuracy). Studies from other research groups using alternative experimental approaches have reported comparable results (Dai et al., 2006; Ruepp et al., 2005; Steiner et al., 2004) indicating that gene-based classifiers can be used to predict the future onset of toxic changes, at least in the liver of rats exposed to NCEs.

Predictive gene expression signatures also have been successfully developed for more specific toxic endpoints in the liver. For example, a multigene biomarker for bile duct hyperplasia in rats has been derived in the laboratory of one author (Blomme et al., 2009) using liver transcript profiles from the DrugMatrix toxicogenomic database (https://ntp.niehs.nih.gov/drugmatrix/index.html). The objective was to define an algorithm that could predict within a few days of dosing the occurrence of bile duct hyperplasia in rats, a change that typically becomes detectable microscopically after a few weeks of continued dosing. The signature was evaluated using 10 compounds naïve to the training set and administered to rats for 1, 5, or 28 days. Liver gene expression profiles were generated from the 1- and 5-day time points, while histopathologic results from the 28-day time point represented the phenotypic anchor (i.e., demonstration of bile duct hyperplasia as the endpoint being predicted). Overall, the signature had a correct prediction 16 out of 20 times (80%). Interestingly, while this signature performed perfectly using the 5-day profiles, results were more discordant with the 1-day gene expression profiles. This discordance likely reflects the higher interindividual variability with respect to early adaptive transcriptomic changes observed after a single dose and the fact that steady-state tissue concentrations of the test articles had not been reached after a single dose.

Similar approaches have been used for the kidney, another frequent target organ of chemically induced toxicity, with comparable predictive performances. For example, a predictive gene expression signature of renal tubular toxicity in rats (Fielden et al., 2005) was derived with the DrugMatrix database using large training and testing sets (64 nephrotoxic and 21 nonnephrotoxic agents). The signature correctly predicted the future presence or absence of renal tubular injury for 76% of the test articles in the testing set. Likewise, a classifier predicted with 100% selectivity and 82% sensitivity the occurrence of proximal tubular injury in rats (Thukral et al., 2005) treated with various prototypical nephrotoxic test articles.

It is noteworthy that toxicogenomics can be used in predictive toxicology without the need for gene expression classifiers. For example,

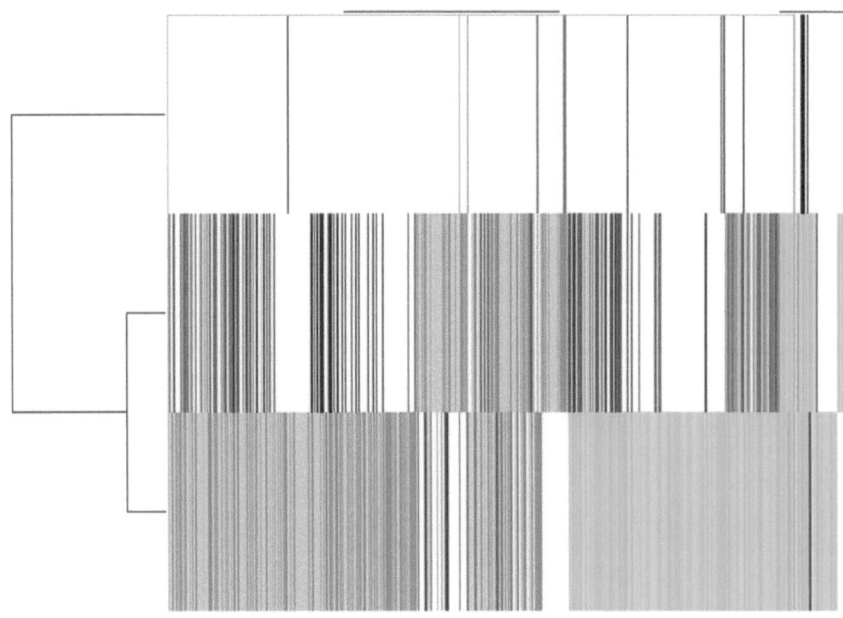

FIGURE 15.11   Heat map for mouse cecal ligation and puncture (CLP model) comparing wild-type CLP versus control (bottom row), gp130 knock-out CLP versus control (middle row), and gp130 knock-out control versus wild-type control (top row). Columns represent 978 mRNA transcripts that meet a criterion for a change substantial enough to be of interest (i.e., t-test $P<.01$ and fold change>5 in at least one comparison); light blue represents decreased abundance, light pink is increased abundance, and white means no change relative to control at $P<.01$. Visually, there are more transcripts changed by CLP in wild-type animals than in gp130 knock-out mice. These changes rarely occur in comparisons of controls from the two genotypes. Microarray data used in this analysis are publicly available in the Gene Expression Omnibus (GEO) data repository, http://www.ncbi.nlm.nih.gov/geo/ under accession GSE22009. *Figure modified from Haschek WM, Rousseaux CG, Wallig MA, editors. Haschek and Rousseaux's Handbook of Toxicologic Pathology, ed 3, 2013, Academic Press, Figure 11.7, p. 371, with permission.*

a retrospective evaluation of studies with 33 agents showed that a simple evaluation of the number of global transcriptional changes in rat livers was already a good indicator of toxic changes (Foster et al., 2007). Interestingly, in this analysis, the transcriptional changes were often observed prior to changes in traditional study endpoints (e.g., anatomic lesions and functional alterations) and could be used to confirm the intended pharmacology or infer mechanisms of toxicity (Foster et al., 2007). Similarly, another approach to analyze toxicogenomic data in a predictive mode is to use unsupervised procedures, such as clustering or PCA to seek similarities with profiles from a database. This "guilt by association" approach assumes that closely similar transcriptomic profiles are likely to reflect similar toxic or pharmacologic outcomes in the liver. Obviously, this is only possible if a sufficiently large database of reference profiles in the appropriate tissue is

available. As an illustration, gene expression profiles from male Sprague–Dawley rats treated with 15 different prototypical hepatotoxic compounds (Waring et al., 2001) causing a range of liver toxicities were clustered, showing a strong correlation of the molecular data with histopathologic and serum chemistry evidence of liver damage. This clustering approach is a simple, nonquantitative method for hazard identification that can be applied to prioritize agents for further development since test articles that are more similar to reference toxicants also are assumed to be relatively more toxic.

How can these predictive gene expression–based biomarkers be used to improve the toxicologic characterization of test articles? As will be discussed later, potential applications have been proposed to better predict and characterize the carcinogenic potential of xenobiotics. In addition, in the pharmaceutical industry, toxicogenomics assessment can be quite useful during

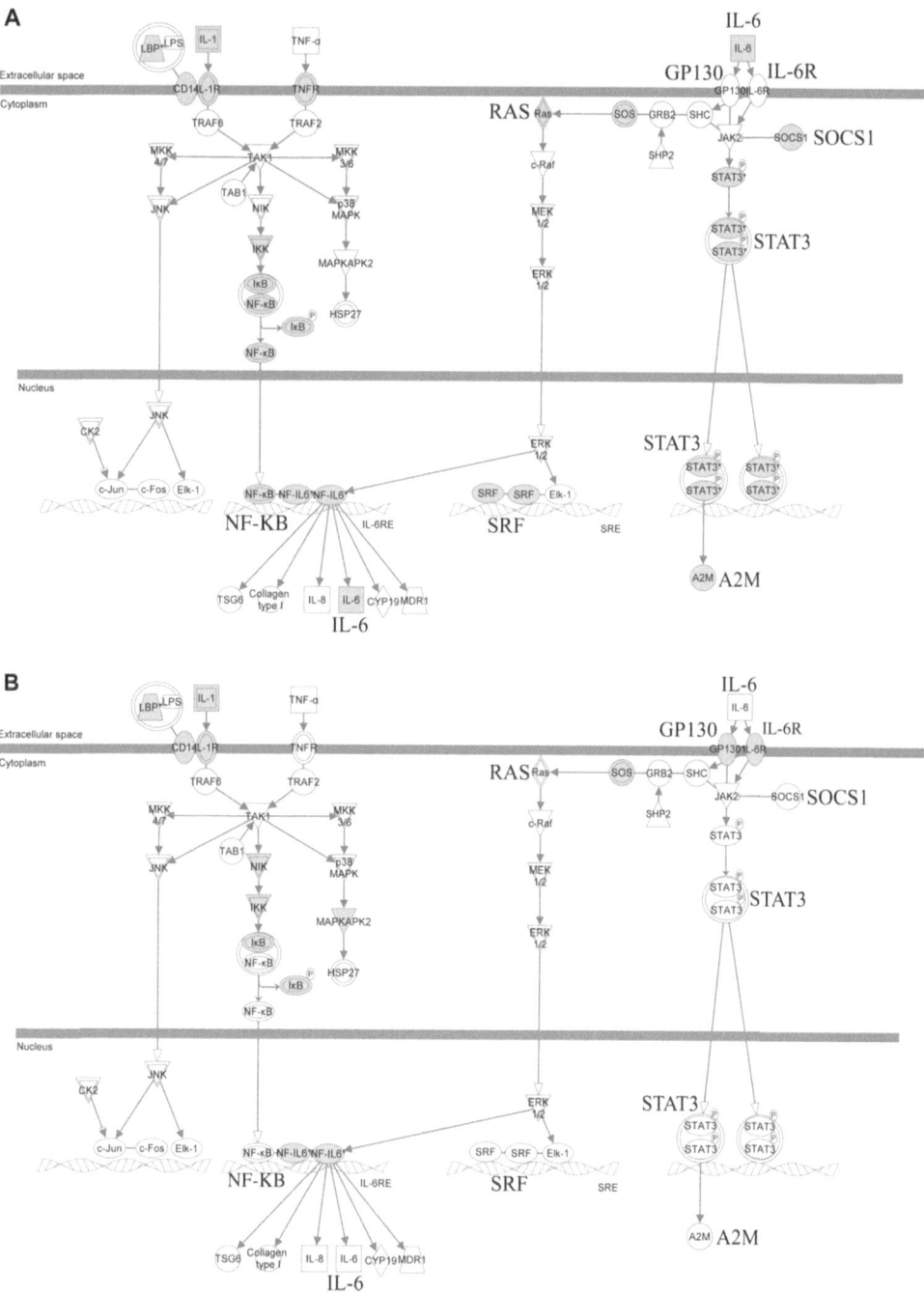

FIGURE 15.12 Diagrams comparing interleukin (IL)-6 pathways in control mice and animals with cecal ligation and puncture (CLP). Panel A is the response in wild-type mice, while panel B is the response in gp130 knock-out mice. Products of genes shown in gray have an mRNA abundance change that is twofold or greater different relative to control (t-test $P<.01$). Gene symbols are included within the icons for pathway members and also in larger font adjacent to icons for some transcripts that change relative to control. The pathway map for the CLP response in gp130 knockouts shows fewer changes in transcript abundance downstream of gp130 than in wild-type animals, including signal transducer and activator of transcription 3 (STAT3) and alpha-2-macroglobulin (A2M). The gp130 transcript is represented as being upregulated in the knock-out animals, indicating that the microarray probes do not target the deleted region of the gene (exon 16, the transmembrane domain) and suggesting that an adaptive upregulation of gp130 transcript generation occurs in the knockout. Diagrams were generated through the use of Ingenuity Pathway Analysis (IPA; Ingenuity Systems, www.ingenuity.com). Microarray data used in this analysis are publicly available in the Gene Expression Omnibus (GEO) data repository, http://www.ncbi.nlm.nih. gov/geo/under accession GSE22009. *Figure modified from Haschek WM, Rousseaux CG, Wallig MA, editors. Haschek and Rousseaux's Handbook of Toxicologic Pathology, ed 3, 2013, Academic Press, Figure 11.8, p. 372, with permission.*

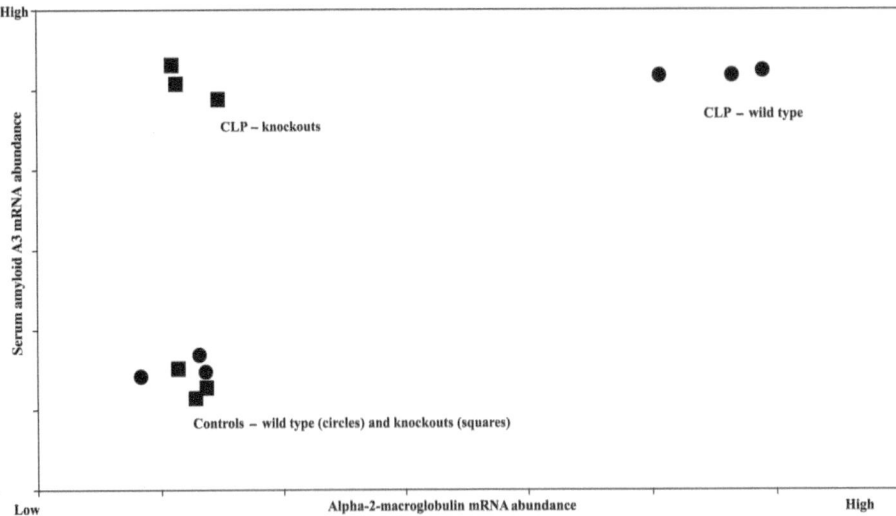

FIGURE 15.13   Hepatic abundance of two established acute phase markers (serum amyloid A3 mRNA, *y*-axis, alpha-2-macroglobulin mRNA, *x*-axis) across all mice in the cecal ligation and puncture (CLP) study (as opposed to clustering of mice across all genes as shown in Figures 15.9 and 15.10). Both analytes are elevated in the wild-type CLP mice, but only serum amyloid A3 is elevated in the gp130 knock-out mice. A "multidimensional" classifier based on these two markers (e.g., a line based on weights for the abundance of the two transcripts, a plane if three transcripts, or a "hyper plane" if many analytes) could be constructed to separate the wild-type response from the knockout (or from the responses invoked by a gp130 inhibitor or by inhibitors of other inflammatory processes). For these two analytes, there are many potential lines that can complete the separation. With tens of thousands of analytes measured, there are many possible combinations of assays (e.g., two at a time, three at a time, etc.) for which classifiers could be created and evaluated for the ability to separate or classify responses. Thus, there is no certainty from a limited set of studies that a classifier that performs well in initial testing will generalize to other situations, such as different strains of mice or other toxicant classes or the presence of potentially confounding effects like immune suppression associated with generalized toxicity. Microarray data used in this analysis are publicly available in the Gene Expression Omnibus (GEO) data repository, http://www.ncbi.nlm.nih.gov/geo/ under accession GSE22009. *Figure modified from Haschek WM, Rousseaux CG, Wallig MA, editors.* Haschek and Rousseaux's Handbook of Toxicologic Pathology, *ed 3, 2013, Academic Press, Figure 11.9, p. 374, with permission.*

the lead optimization and early development stages in the context of providing mechanistic and safety information during non-GLP studies. Specifically, gene expression–based predictive markers can bring value when used in short-term exploratory rodent toxicity studies for multiple reasons. First, they increase the probability of detecting future toxic changes, especially when used as a complement to other endpoints (**predictive value**). Second, they are helpful to confirm weak signals indicating the potential for toxicity detected through other endpoints (e.g., small elevations in serum hepatic transaminase activities) and to make better data-driven decisions in studies where animal numbers per group typically are low and the duration of dosing is short. As a matter of fact, hepatic gene expression profiles often display lower interindividual variability than traditional endpoints, which enables the use of fewer animals for -omics endpoints (**interindividual variability**). Beyond the obvious and beneficial impact of decreased animal usage on animal welfare and the replacement, reduction, and refinement, lower amounts of test article are needed, which in turn facilitates the characterization of novel entities earlier in the discovery process. Third, gene expression profiles can be used to understand mechanisms of test article toxicity (**mechanistic clarity**). For example, simple clustering analyses can be employed to understand the similarity in gene expression changes induced by an NCE compared to those in a database or to identify deregulated pathways. Likewise, gene expression analysis is a straightforward approach to identify induction of drug metabolizing enzymes, a frequent effect of xenobiotics.

7.2. Mechanistic Toxicology

Transcriptomics data can be especially useful to formulate hypotheses about mechanisms of toxicity. Because -omics data are rich in content and can be generated rapidly if tissues are available, they represent an excellent start in any mechanistic toxicity investigation. However, as a note of caution, gene expression data generally are not sufficient to confirm a mechanism of toxicity, and follow-up functional experiments using other endpoints (e.g., histopathology) typically will be needed to confirm or refute the hypothesis.

The literature contains several good illustrations of the utility of gene expression profiling to explore mechanisms of toxicity. For reasons already mentioned, most published examples have focused on hepatotoxicity mechanisms. Hepatic hypertrophy, a frequent observation in rodent toxicity studies, is a straightforward example to illustrate how toxicogenomics can be leveraged to rapidly link a phenotypic change (i.e., liver enlargement) to a specific molecular pathway of physiologic function (Hamadeh et al., 2002). There are several well-characterized mechanisms of hepatic hypertrophy in rodents: induction of cytochromes P450 (CYP) monooxygenase enzymes, peroxisome proliferation, hypertrophy of mitochondria, Nrf2 (nuclear factor erythroid 2–related factor 2)-mediated oxidative stress signaling, and glycogen or lipid accumulation (Boitier et al., 2011). In particular, CYP enzyme induction and peroxisome proliferation commonly result from the interaction of xenobiotics with nuclear receptors (e.g., aryl hydrocarbon receptor [AhR], pregnane X receptor [PXR], constitutive androstane receptor [CAR], peroxisome proliferator–activated receptor alpha [PPAR-α]), which act as transcription factors regulating gene expression and hence generate clear and specific transcriptional changes that are easily characterized using gene expression profiling (Dickinson et al., 2004). As a matter of fact, the gene expression profiles induced by nuclear receptor agonists are so specific that they can be reproduced with high confidence in *in vitro* hepatocyte-based systems (Yang et al., 2006). As an illustration of the utility of gene expression profiling, a rat study to characterize the off-target interactions of an experimental inhibitor of acetyl CoA carboxylase (ACC2) was conducted to compare the liver gene expression profiles to the Drug-Matrix gene expression reference database (Waring et al., 2008). This comparison demonstrated a high degree of similarity for the new entity's profile to those of a variety of known PPAR-α agonists, indicating that the test article was likely a PPAR-α agonist, which was further confirmed by demonstrating an increase of peroxisomes in hepatocytes using transmission electron microscopy and IHC for the peroxisome membrane protein PMP70. Toxicogenomics can also be used to investigate more complex mechanisms of liver toxicity, such as glutathione depletion, mitochondrial effects, hypoxia, oxidative stress, or disruption of fatty acid β-oxidation and lipid metabolism (Blomme et al., 2009).

There are not as many literature reports of toxicogenomics to support mechanistic toxicity investigations with tissues other than liver. However, the tool can be useful with any tissue in the context of properly designed studies, with the caveat that a smaller amount of reference data may make interpretation more challenging. The investigations of the intestinal changes in rats induced by experimental gamma-secretase inhibitors (GSIs), which were being developed as potential therapeutic agents for Alzheimer's disease, are a good illustration of the utility of gene expression profiling in mechanistic toxicology (Citron, 2004). These test articles were shown to not only to inhibit the cleavage by gamma-secretase of amyloid precursor protein but also to inhibit the processing of other gamma-secretase substrates such as Notch and a subset of cell-surface receptors and proteins involved in embryonic development, hematopoiesis, cell adhesion, and cell–cell contacts (Evin et al., 2006). In particular, they blocked the cleavage of the cell fate regulator Notch-1, which plays an important role in the differentiation of the immune system and gastrointestinal tract (Milano et al., 2004). In rats, experimental GSIs from various chemical series were associated with increased gastrointestinal weight, distended stomach and small and large intestines, and a mucoid enteropathy characterized by goblet cell hyperplasia (Milano et al., 2004; Searfoss et al., 2003). Gene expression analysis of the small intestine suggested a perturbation in Notch signaling as the primary pathway driving this toxic event and also identified fecal adipsin, a serine protease, as a potential biomarker of this metaplastic intestinal change. These findings were confirmed by an independent study that demonstrated a correlation between inhibition of Notch processing and intestinal goblet cell metaplasia as well as a comparable increase in fecal adipsin (Milano et al., 2004). Altogether, these studies indicated that the metaplastic intestinal changes observed in rats were not related to the intended mechanism of action but were instead the result of an off-target undesirable inhibitory effect on Notch signaling.

Multiple examples can be found on the use of toxicogenomics to address toxic mechanisms in a variety of tissues. For example, the structure cardiac toxicity relationship of a series of experimental ACC2 inhibitors and their inactive enantiomers was evaluated in rats using gene expression profiles generated after a short-term dosing period (3 days) to confirm that the cardiac toxicity was associated with the presence of a specific alkyne linker in the molecules (Gu et al., 2007). The gene expression profiles also showed strong correlations with a number of reference expression profiles from DrugMatrix for other cardiotoxicants or cardiotonic agents (i.e., agents that increase the efficiency and strength of myocardial contraction), such as cyclosporine A, haloperidol, or norepinephrine. Altogether, these data confirmed that the cardiotoxicity of this series of drugs was structurally based and not due to the intended inhibition of the target. Several -omics studies have also been conducted to understand the mechanism of testicular toxicity. For example, dibromoacetic acid (DBAA) is known to alter spermatogenesis in rats through defective spermiation based on microscopic evaluation, but the exact mechanism of the defective spermiation is unknown. A microarray analysis of testes from DBAA-treated rats showed that a small number of genes were altered following DBAA exposure, including a mild downregulation of cytochrome P450c17α (CYP17) mRNA, an enzyme expressed by Leydig cells that is essential for the production of testicular androgens (Carr et al., 2011). Further evaluations confirmed that testicular CYP17 protein was decreased and that testicular testosterone levels were reduced in DBAA-dosed rats, confirming that DBAA downregulates CYP17 expression in Leydig cells, resulting

in decreased testicular testosterone production and failed spermiation (Carr et al., 2011). Likewise, toxicogenomics has been used to understand the mechanisms of testicular toxicity of phthalate compounds, which are ubiquitous environmental contaminants and have been associated with a gradual but substantial decline of human male fertility, especially in developed countries (Latini et al., 2006). For example, dipentyl phthalate, a widely used plasticizer, has antiandrogenic effects (Mylchreest, Cattley, & Foster, 1998) including downregulation of several steroidogenic enzymes in fetal rat testes exposed in utero (Shultz et al., 2001) and modulation of steroidogenesis- and spermatogenesis-related genes in the testes of immature rats (Lehmann et al., 2004; Ryu et al., 2007).

Finally, toxicogenomics represents a useful addition to the toolbox available for characterization of animals as models of test article efficacy and toxicity. For example, idiosyncratic toxicity, especially in the liver, is a major concern for drug developers. Because of the overall lack of understanding of the mechanisms of idiosyncratic DILI, there has been a strong desire by many groups and companies to develop animal models that can be employed to derisk this unique toxicity. A classic model is the lipopolysaccharide (LPS)-potentiated rat model. The quinolone antibiotic trovafloxacin, which inhibits bacterial DNA gyrase and DNA topoisomerase IV, was evaluated in this model. Although quinolone antibiotics usually are well tolerated in humans, trovafloxacin has been associated with DILI characterized by hepatic parenchymal necrosis in rare patients, restricting its use to life-threatening situations (Bertino and Fish, 2000). The normal laboratory rat is not susceptible to trovafloxacin-induced hepatic injury. In contrast, trovafloxacin does induce hepatotoxicity in the LPS-potentiated rat model with elevations of serum ALT activity and histopathological evidence of multifocal coagulative hepatocellular necrosis (Waring et al., 2006), a response that is consistent with the idiosyncratic toxicity noted in humans. This toxicity was not reproduced in rats with levofloxacin, a fluoroquinolone drug with no known DILI liability in humans. Microarray analysis of the rat livers revealed interesting changes, including upregulation of leukotropic chemokines; this liver -omics profile was consistent with the hepatic accumulation and activation of neutrophils demonstrated by IHC and the increased serum levels of cytokine-induced neutrophil chemoattractant-1 and macrophage inflammatory protein-2. Altogether, these data formed the basis of the hypothesis that neutrophils play a crucial role in the development of the toxicity. This mechanism was confirmed by depleting neutrophils with serum containing antineutrophil antibodies prior to trovafloxacin treatment, which considerably attenuated the liver microscopic changes (Waring et al., 2006). A similar investigation with the nonsteroidal antiinflammatory drug diclofenac in the same LPS–rat model led to a different mechanistic hypothesis, suggesting that idiosyncratic DILI results from multiple mechanisms. Gene expression analysis of livers of the diclofenac/LPS-dosed rats revealed upregulation of multiple genes and pathways related to inflammation, cell death, and stress. Similar to trovafloxacin, prior neutrophil depletion protected rats against liver toxicity (Deng et al., 2006). However, data from rats treated with high doses of diclofenac without LPS also showed a similar pattern of gene regulation, leading to the hypothesis that at these higher doses diclofenac may cause DILI through gastrointestinal injury and endotoxin translocation from the intestine to the liver (Banks et al., 1995; Seitz and Boelsterli, 1998). Consistent with this hypothesis, prior sterilization of the intestinal microflora with oral treatment using a mixture of polymyxin B (150 mg/kg/day) and neomycin (450 mg/kg/day) for 4 days alleviated the hepatotoxicity induced by high doses of diclofenac (Deng et al., 2006).

7.3. Carcinogenicity Assessment

When required by regulatory guidelines, the carcinogenic potential of xenobiotics (e.g., small-molecule therapeutic agents, industrial chemicals, pesticides, or food additives) is assessed using a combination of in vitro genotoxicity assays and/or in vivo rodent models (e.g., two-year carcinogenicity bioassays in rodents; abbreviated [six-month] studies with genetically engineered mouse models). Readers are referred to the International Council for Harmonisation of Technical Requirements for Pharmaceuticals for Human Use carcinogenicity guidelines (S1A-S1C) (ICH, 2020) and Organisation for Economic Co-operation and Development (OECD, 2018) for the requirements and study design recommendations for carcinogenicity studies (see also *Carcinogenesis: Mechanisms and Evaluation*, Vol 1, Chap 8).

In vitro genotoxicity assays will not be discussed in detail here, as they are beyond the scope of this chapter. However, it is worth mentioning that the use of transcriptional profiling with in vitro systems can be useful to better define the genotoxic potential of molecules. For example, transcriptomic profiling has been proposed to distinguish direct from indirect genotoxic mechanisms (e.g., effects on the mitotic spindle, protein synthesis, nucleotide misincorporation) of genotoxicity (Dickinson et al., 2004; Newton et al., 2004). Likewise, transcriptomic profiles can be used to distinguish genotoxic from nongenotoxic carcinogens using cell lines (Doktorova et al., 2014; van Delft et al., 2004).

The utility of genomic technologies in the context of in vivo carcinogenicity studies is most relevant to the toxicologic pathologist. These technologies can be useful for three main reasons: (1) to predict with better accuracy the outcomes of the chronic bioassays, or even more useful, the carcinogenic potential of chemicals; (2) to evaluate whether the tumors observed are related to test article administration or are spontaneous in origin; and (3) to understand the molecular mechanism(s) of carcinogenesis (or MOA [which is the functional or structural change in cells resulting from the altered molecular pathways]). These aspects are discussed in more detail below.

Prediction of the Carcinogenic Potential of Compounds

Conventional lifetime carcinogenicity studies in mice and rats are extremely resource intensive (estimated cost $2–4 million), time consuming (2 years of dosing and at least 3 and as many as 4 years for a final report overall), pathology heavy (over 40 tissues per animal evaluated by histopathology), and utilize a large number of animals (>800 rodents/study). Hence, it is clearly not possible to assess all chemicals using lifetime (two-year) rodent bioassays. For example, it is estimated that only around 2%–3% of commercial chemicals have been evaluated in long-term bioassays (CPDB, 2020; Fitzpatrick, 2008). Furthermore, while these studies are required for most small-molecule pharmaceutical agents, their results are available only during the later phases of clinical development after exposure of significant numbers of patients or healthy volunteers. Finally, as will be discussed later, the results from these studies are not highly reproducible, and their utility for human risk assessment has and continues to be debated (Doe et al., 2019). Therefore, access to predictive models that might be used reliably for larger numbers of chemicals and earlier for pharmaceutical agents would be very valuable. Even if it is unlikely that a good predictive model for carcinogenicity would replace, at least in the near future, traditional carcinogenicity studies for pharmaceutical agents, potential carcinogenic hazards could be recognized earlier or more streamlined carcinogenicity assessment packages could be justified in some situations (e.g., negative results could provide a scientific rationale for conducting only one rodent bioassay instead of two for a pharmaceutical agent). Likewise, a predictive model could be used for better prioritization of commercial chemicals that should be tested in rodent bioassays. For example, chemicals that are identified as carcinogens based on gene expression analysis would be prioritized in the rodent bioassay.

Toxicogenomics applied in smaller and short-term studies has the potential to identify carcinogens at earlier stages in drug development. There is an abundant and well-annotated historical dataset of carcinogenicity study results (e.g., hundreds of chemicals tested in chronic rodent bioassays by the U.S. NTP), the availability of which is a prerequisite to developing robust predictive models. Furthermore, large numbers of transcriptomic data induced by well-annotated chemicals and complemented by thorough phenotypic annotation of nonproliferative and proliferative (preneoplastic and neoplastic) findings are now available, especially for liver, which is a tissue of high interest because it is the most common target organ for neoplasia in rodents. Therefore, over the years, several groups have attempted to identify hepatic carcinogens by using transcriptomics in general toxicity studies of relatively short duration (several days or weeks).

The first published -omics studies in this context were focused on finding molecular markers of hepatic carcinogenicity in short-term (e.g., 5 days

of daily dosing) rat studies (Kramer et al., 2004). Single molecular markers (e.g., transforming growth factor-beta stimulated clone 22 [TSC-22] and NAD(P)H cytochrome P450 oxidoreductase) were proposed as possible biomarkers because of their plausible mechanistic role in hepatic carcinogenesis (i.e., cell growth and differentiation and oxidative stress) and the correlation of their mRNA expression changes with the estimated carcinogenic potential of the tested agents (Kramer et al., 2004). However, these early studies mostly revealed the challenges of developing robust predictive models. First, relatively few test articles with a narrow range of carcinogenic mechanisms were used, such that several MOAs were not investigated. Second, the biostatistical algorithms used at that time did not possess sufficient performance. Third, the initial hypothesis that very few candidate genes could be used as biomarkers of chemically induced carcinogenicity risk was too simplistic. For example, on the one hand, TSC-22 was confirmed to be consistently downregulated in other studies using rats and mice exposed to nongenotoxic carcinogens, as well as in spontaneous rodent liver tumors, consistent with its role in tumor suppression generally (Iida et al., 2005, 2007; Michel et al., 2005). On the other hand, not all carcinogens were shown to downregulate TSC-22 mRNA in the liver of rodents, indicating an inability to cover all MOAs with a single or few markers.

Subsequent studies have investigated hepatic transcriptomic responses to generate predictive signatures for hepatic genotoxic carcinogens (Ellinger-Ziegelbauer et al., 2004) or to differentiate nongenotoxic from genotoxic carcinogens (Ellinger-Ziegelbauer et al., 2005). These studies showed that combinations of pathway-associated gene expression profiles could be used to identify genotoxic and nongenotoxic hepatic carcinogens in short-term rat or mouse studies (Eichner et al., 2013; Furihata and Suzuki, 2019; Kossler et al., 2015). However, because of the relatively limited set of reference transcriptomic profiles, it was not possible to estimate the predictive accuracy of these markers. When large toxicogenomics databases became freely available (essentially DrugMatrix and TG-GATEs), later efforts were able to generate predictive gene classifiers for genotoxic and nongenotoxic hepatic carcinogens using more sophisticated statistical algorithms

(Ellinger-Ziegelbauer et al., 2008) and larger repositories of gene expression profiles induced by a wider variety of structurally and mechanistically diverse compounds (Thomas et al., 2009). Not surprisingly, these studies showed more convincing predictive accuracy for their gene expression signatures during robust validation exercises consisting of independent transcript profiles (Fielden et al., 2007).

Taken together, these efforts have demonstrated many important considerations with respect to toxicogenomics data and their utility in predicting carcinogenicity.

1. Prediction is tissue-dependent, and, not surprisingly, tissue-agnostic ("universal") classifiers are not feasible (Gusenleitner et al., 2014).

2. Carcinogens, regardless of their MOA, are associated with larger numbers of differentially expressed genes (mostly exhibiting upregulation) than are noncarcinogens, with nongenotoxic carcinogens inducing the largest numbers of transcriptomic changes.

3. Classifiers offer some level of mechanistic understanding of carcinogenicity based on their MOAs (e.g., regulation of DNA damage, apoptosis and DNA repair pathways by genotoxic carcinogens; and regulation of specific pathways and processes, such as lipid metabolism, tubulin polymerization, oxidative stress, gap junction–mediated cell–cell communication, apoptosis suppression, or cell proliferation for nongenotoxic carcinogens).

4. While changes in individual genes bring some degree of mechanistic clarity, pathway-associated gene expression profiles evaluating constellations of genes are more advantageous for accurate predictions and classification.

5. The performance of classifiers is more dependent on the dose level being evaluated than the duration of exposure. In other words, short-term studies are appropriate, but it is critical to consider the cumulative level of exposure for prediction: using dose levels in short-term studies that are much higher than the highest dose levels used in the rodent bioassay can lead to false-positive predictions. Conversely, using doses similar to those used in the rodent bioassay may also lead to false-negative predictions.

Alternative approaches have combined gene expression changes with various biomarkers or parameters to improve carcinogenic predictivity. For example, structural features (i.e., 3D chemical structure) of test articles have been shown to be complementary, albeit only marginally, to transcriptomic data (Gusenleitner et al., 2014). Similarly, DNA adducts in isolation are not good predictors of carcinogenesis, but the combined analysis of DNA adducts and time-matched gene expression changes exposed to the DNA-alkylating carcinogen methylazoxymethanol acetate was promising to predict genotoxicant-induced carcinogenesis in the kidney of Eker rats (Klaus et al., 2017). While this last example represents a single chemical, similar approaches can be used to complement gene expression profiles. For example, several retrospective evaluations have shown that histopathologic endpoints (or lack of them), such as with hepatocellular hyperplasia or hypertrophy as well as atypical cell features (e.g., altered hepatic foci) in subchronic or chronic rodent toxicity studies, are good predictors of the lack of tumor induction in lifetime rodent carcinogenicity bioassays (Jacobs, 2009; Reddy et al., 2010). However, not all chemicals inducing hepatocellular hyperplasia or hypertrophy ultimately cause liver tumors, and transcriptomic profiles may provide additional experimental and mechanistic evidence to support a decision that there is no need for concern. For example, a recent study demonstrated the utility of gene expression profiles to distinguish between hepatocellular hypertrophy associated with carcinogenesis and adaptive hypertrophy (Liu et al., 2017). Aside from xenobiotic metabolism–related pathways, amino acid biosynthesis and oxidative stress responses have been shown to be relevant to hypertrophic hepatocarcinogenesis (Liu et al., 2017).

Although the liver is a primary organ of carcinogenicity, other tissues are also frequent targets of carcinogenesis. In fact, the five most common target organs of chemically induced carcinogenicity include the liver, lung, mammary gland, kidney, and hematopoietic system (chiefly leukocyte lineages). Therefore, having an -omics-based predictive model that addresses only the liver would not be sufficient to evaluate all chemicals. Discovery of tissue-agnostic classifiers (i.e., predicting target organs of tumorigenicity using transcripts from a single tissue such as liver) is likely not feasible (Gusenleitner et al., 2014), so there is a need for a tissue-specific models that could be used concurrently for a battery of organs to provide an accurate evaluation of a chemical. Very few studies have evaluated tissues other than liver for that purpose, and those studies have been limited by small -omics training sets, such that it has been difficult to build robust models that can be properly validated using independent testing sets and to confirm that the encouraging results shown with liver will translate to other tissues. In addition, in contrast to liver, other tissues may be more heterogeneous in nature, leading to increased variability of the transcriptomic data. For example, a set of genes (which was not selected using advanced statistical classifiers) was evaluated as a predictor of chemically induced renal carcinogenicity in rats; the study used dissected renal cortices and a training set of only 12 carcinogens and 10 noncarcinogens (Matsumoto et al., 2017). Whether this gene set will predict chemically induced renal carcinogenesis under slightly different experimental conditions (e.g., different durations of dosing, dose level selection methods, sampling of the kidney, or different expression profiling platforms) and for compounds with different MOAs is unclear.

Development of models for other tissues, such as mammary gland, will be associated with similar or even greater challenges. For example, the number of reference compounds for these tissues (e.g., numbers of chemicals clearly associated with mammary gland tumors) may be too low to even generate any useful and validated models. In other words, it is difficult to fathom that predictive genomic models will replace current lifetime carcinogenicity bioassays any time soon. However, their most immediate utility resides as tools to prioritize the most appropriate industrial chemicals and pesticides to test, to derisk pharmaceutical agents, and to better design those studies.

Spontaneous Versus Test Article–Related Tumors

Carcinogenicity studies are conducted to evaluate whether there is any increased incidence of neoplasms; increased proportion of malignant neoplasms, particularly in vulnerable target organ(s) of carcinogenicity; and any reduction

in the latency (time of appearance) for neoplasms in test article–treated groups versus concurrent control groups. Tumors occur spontaneously in aging rodents, and their relationship to the test article is not always clear. Genomic technologies can be particularly helpful to confirm the relationship of a tumor to a treatment. For example, spontaneous mesotheliomas are observed in carcinogenicity studies using F344/N rats at a low incidence in males (3.2% of NTP historical controls, 2011) (Blackshear et al., 2015). Gene expression profiling was shown to help differentiate spontaneous mesotheliomas from those induced by vinylidene chloride, a comonomer widely used in the manufacture of synthetic polymers, despite indistinguishable morphology of tumors resulting from these two different causes (Blackshear et al., 2015). PCA and hierarchical clustering illustrated significant differences in transcriptomes between the two categories (Figure 15.14A and B). Not surprisingly, multiple pathways associated with tumorigenesis were commonly regulated in both spontaneous and chemically induced mesotheliomas. However, multiple differences in pathway regulation could also be demonstrated between the two categories, such as overrepresentation of pathways associated with DNA replication, recombination or repair, and with inflammation and immune dysfunction in the chemically induced tumors (Blackshear et al., 2015).

Mechanism of Carcinogenicity

The ultimate objective of carcinogenicity assays is to understand the possible health hazards associated with exposure of humans to the agents that were tested in rodents. However, results of the traditional rodent bioassay can be challenging to interpret in terms of extrapolating risks to humans. For example, a tumor may be demonstrated in one rodent species (mice or rats), but it is not always clear whether the response is simply a model organism-specific response rather than a real carcinogenic risk for humans (Jacobs, 2009). Furthermore, rodent bioassays are not very reproducible in spite of the relatively large number of animals being used: there is a concordance of only 57% between results from studies conducted by the U.S. National Cancer Institute/NTP and those reported in the literature for studies run by other institutions that tested the same agents

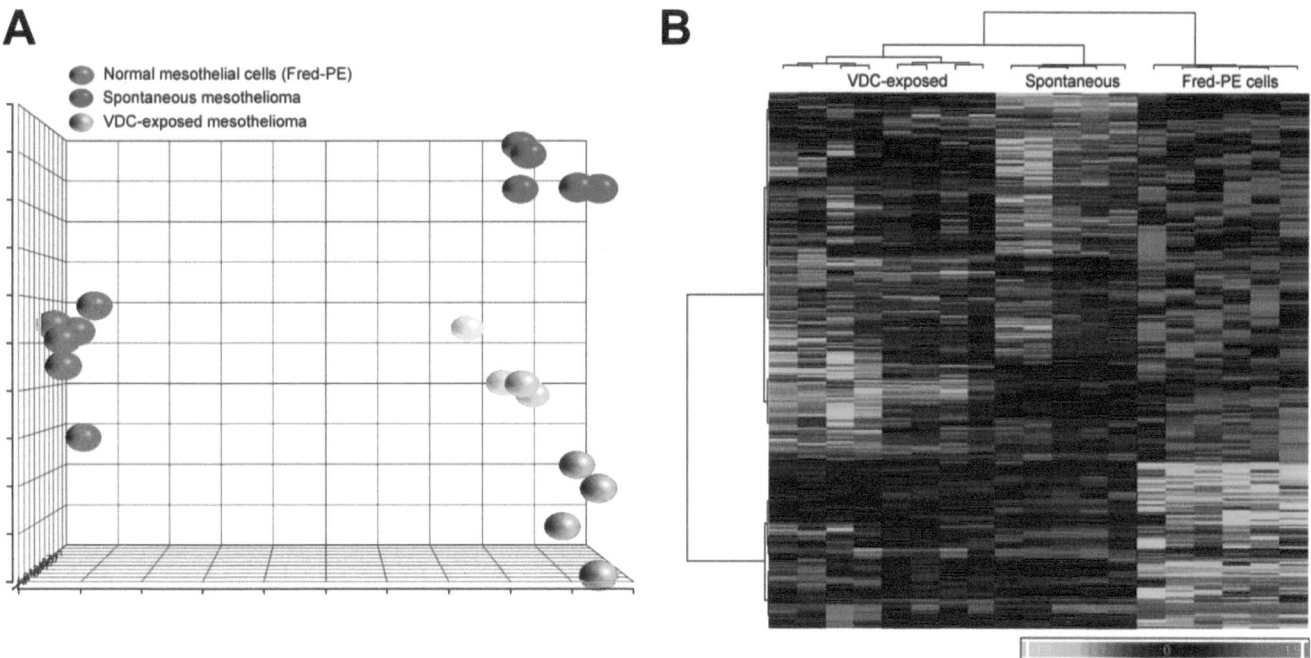

FIGURE 15.14 Principal component analysis (PCA) comparing gene expression profiles of cultured Fred-PE immortalized, nontransformed F344/N rat mesothelial cell line, spontaneous mesotheliomas from control rats, and mesotheliomas from vinylidene chloride (VDC)–exposed rats for differentially expressed probe sets. (A) PCA shows intergroup similarities in gene expression and clear separation of experimental groups in space, indicating differences among groups in terms of their gene expression profiles. (B) Hierarchical cluster analysis (HCA) comparing global gene expression profiles of Fred-PE mesothelial cells, spontaneous mesotheliomas, and vinylidene chloride–associated mesotheliomas. HCA clusters experimental samples based on global gene expression and shows relative expression levels across the genome for each of the three experimental groups. *Reproduced from Blackshear PE, Pandiri AR, Nagai H, et al: Gene expression of mesothelioma in vinylidene chloride-exposed F344/N rats reveal immune dysfunction, tissue damage, and inflammation pathways,* Toxicol Pathol 43:171–185, 2015, by permission.

(Gottmann et al., 2001). The vast majority of known human carcinogens (based on the classification of the International Agency for Research on Cancer) are genotoxic and typically induce tumors in multiple tissues and often in both mice and rats; in such instances, lifetime rodent bioassays can be justified as an appropriate means for human risk assessment (Waters et al., 1999, 2010). However, there are frequent situations where the tumor response in rodent studies is not so clear, particularly if mechanistic investigations have not been conducted and the MOAs are not understood. In these situations, chemicals inducing tumors are by default considered carcinogens.

Hemangiosarcoma in rodents is often used as an example of a rodent response to chemicals that has questionable relevance to humans. This tumor definitely is associated with specific genotoxic carcinogens (e.g., vinyl chloride and vinyl bromide) in both humans and rodents (Kielhorn et al., 2000). However, a broad range of non-DNA reactive chemicals and pharmaceuticals (e.g., calcium channel blockers, antipsychotics, phosphodiesterase-5 inhibitors, dipeptidyl peptidase-4 inhibitors, antiarrhythmic drugs, gonadotropin receptor antagonists, antisense oligonucleotides, nitric oxide releasers, hemolytic compounds, and vascular endothelial growth factor inducers) can cause hemangiosarcomas in rodents (mostly in mice and affecting the liver, spleen, heart, and subcutaneous adipose tissue) that are of questionable relevance to humans (Cohen et al., 2009; Jacobs, 2009; Nyska et al., 2002). Ultimately, an understanding of the mechanism of carcinogenesis is necessary to determine the relevance of chemically induced hemangiosarcomas in mice to humans (Cohen et al., 2009).

Transcriptional profiling of tumors can provide useful insights into the MOA of a test article and can help guide experimental activities to better understand the relevance of rodent responses to humans. For example, transcriptomic profiles generated as part of shorter-term toxicity studies can be compared to a database of transcriptomic profiles induced by various test articles for which mechanistic information is available (Fielden et al., 2007). There are well-known MOAs associated with induction of hepatic neoplasms in rodents by nongenotoxic compounds, which may have limited relevance to humans when a threshold effect can be demonstrated (Cohen, 2010). These include mostly receptor-mediated hepatocyte proliferation (e.g., activation of hepatic nuclear receptors such as AhR, CAR, PXR, or PPAR-α) and hepatocyte cytotoxicity associated with secondary regenerative proliferation. Activation of nuclear receptors is particularly easy to confirm since it is associated with increased CYP450 mRNA, protein, and activity. In particular, transcriptomic evaluation of liver is quite useful to identify test article and dose levels that are associated with nuclear receptor activation (Blomme et al., 2009). The ability of transcriptomic profiling to detect nuclear receptor activators can be useful for human risk assessment. For example, tetrahydrofuran (THF) is often used as a chemical intermediate or solvent, and there are inconsistent conclusions by regulatory agencies regarding its carcinogenic potential (Dekant, 2019). Inhalation of THF has been associated with a marginal increase in the incidence of liver tumors (e.g., hepatocellular adenomas and carcinomas) in female mice. Quantitative weight of evidence supports a CAR-mediated MOA for the induction of these liver tumors. Consequently, the relevance of these tumors for humans should be assessed using a threshold of toxicological concern (i.e., through establishment of an exposure [or dose] level for all chemicals below which there is no real risk to human health).

Results of rodent bioassays are still mostly interpreted in a binary mode: carcinogenic or not. However, there is clear experimental evidence of a threshold effect for nongenotoxic

carcinogens (see *Carcinogenesis: Mechanisms and Evaluation,* Vol 1, Chap 8), but more recent data suggest that a threshold effect is also relevant to at least some genotoxic carcinogens that are currently evaluated for risk assessment under the linear nonthreshold dogma (i.e., by assuming that all doses are carcinogenic). By providing more sensitive evaluation of cell perturbation, toxicogenomics can define with higher accuracy the threshold level for nongenotoxic agents and may provide further experimental evidence for a threshold for genotoxic agents.

8. REGULATORY CONSIDERATIONS

Results of a recent industry survey indicate that toxicogenomics is only rarely used in the pharmaceutical industry for regulatory decision-making (Vahle et al., 2018). In fact, toxicogenomics is infrequently used in regulatory-type repeat-dose GLP toxicity studies, and most companies do not even routinely bank tissue samples for potential future use with toxicogenomics in these studies (Vahle et al., 2018). The GLP toxicity studies that are the pivotal studies in regulatory filings generally use conventional endpoints that are well understood and can be interpreted with confidence by toxicologists and toxicologic pathologists. In this context, the value proposition of toxicogenomics is limited. In the cases where a toxicogenomics analysis is conducted as part of a GLP toxicity study, the objective is usually to investigate a mechanism of toxicity and the -omics endpoints are of secondary importance to the routine toxicity parameters that represent the primary purpose of the study. While these toxicogenomics data may be part of a regulatory submission, they typically are integrated with other data to confirm a proposed mechanism and as such are one component of an overall weight-of-evidence approach.

While toxicogenomics technology was positioned by some around 2 decades ago as revolutionary, it is fair to acknowledge that it has had relatively limited impact on the practice of toxicology in drug development in contrast to its impact on drug discovery. There are several reasons to explain the slow adoption of toxicogenomics in the context of drug development. First, the gene expression–based signatures that were described earlier in this chapter have been mostly developed within specific organizations to predict changes that might occur in GLP studies. Consequently, their use in GLP studies is irrelevant since they have not been developed nor have the resulting molecular databases been constructed for use in that context. In addition, generation of such signatures by a single organization cannot build broad scientific consensus regarding their validity. Protocols for toxicogenomics assays as applied to GLP toxicity studies need to be standardized for any biomarker and sufficient cross-institutional data need to be collected such that the reliability of these molecular signatures as predictive tools achieves widespread acceptance (Jacobs, 2009). Attempts at cross-validation within consortia have been disappointing for the most part and indicate that signatures obtained using current -omics platforms are not really suitable for regulatory decision-making (Fielden et al., 2008). Second, to be useful in a regulatory setting, gene expression data need to be generated and interpreted in a reproducible way. Again, efforts by various consortia have been made to ensure reproducibility of data generation and interpretation across institutions (Chen et al., 2011), but technologies have been evolving very rapidly and are not implemented consistently within industry or academia. Third, interpretation of these large molecular datasets is challenging and somewhat biased by the analyst (Vahle et al., 2018). There is not a unique approach to analyze these data, and no accepted rules have been devised regarding what is relevant or not in terms of scientific importance and regulatory decision-making (Liu et al., 2019). The toxicological significance of most gene expression changes is acknowledged by the scientific community to be incompletely understood. As a result, there are concerns from drug developers that such supportive molecular data may be interpreted differently by regulatory reviewers (Qin et al., 2016). This is compounded by the facts that (1) although large databases are available, they do not cover all tissues extensively, and (2) novel gene expression profiling platforms are being used that may or may not deliver the data that can be integrated with other elements of study data sets (Liu et al., 2019). Studies to date have shown that the interpretation of data sets generated by different profiling platforms support similar interpretations (Rao et al., 2018) and that -omics data are reciprocally transferable between transcriptomic platforms (Xu et al., 2016), but the different data formats still present some challenges for several aspects of data analysis. Finally, the traditional methods for general toxicity assessment of therapeutic agents have been very robust in enabling clinical trials to proceed safely, so there is little incentive to modify these known methods by adding potentially powerful but unproven innovations like toxicogenomics (Monticello et al., 2017).

In 2004, a "safe harbor" concept was established to promote the submission of genomics data by companies with the understanding that regulatory decisions would not be impacted by these exploratory datasets (i.e., voluntary exploratory data submission) (Goodsaid et al., 2010). The objective was to encourage the use of this novel technology and expose regulatory agencies to these data sets that, with more experience, might bolster the confidence in data-drive regulatory decisions. However, this voluntary submission process is not widely used at present due to twin impediments of added cost and uncertain interpretation. Toxicogenomics data can be useful in addressing queries from regulatory agencies, such as confirming the mechanism of liver weight increases in rodents or providing supportive evidence in early submissions that a specific toxic effect does not represent a safety concern for humans (Vahle et al., 2018). For example, thyroid gland hyperplasia in rodents due to test article–induced induction of drug metabolizing enzymes in hepatocytes is well understood as a rodent-specific response of no relevance to humans. This mechanism can be easily confirmed using transcriptomic data (Yang et al., 2012). In our experience, another acceptable use for -omics data is to provide context for tumor findings in carcinogenicity studies (e.g., thyroid gland tumors in rodents are a nongenotoxic finding of no concern to humans).

Finally, opportunities exist for incorporating toxicogenomics technology in some GLP settings, especially for carcinogenicity testing. As discussed earlier, transcriptomic data offer a unique opportunity to improve the current approach to carcinogenicity risk assessment. Molecular signatures provide insights into the

MOA of a compound and the relevance of rodent responses to humans, as already mentioned for liver and thyroid gland neoplasms (Cohen, 2010; Yang et al., 2012). These additional insights will ultimately lead to a better assessment of the carcinogenic risk to humans posed by novel test articles. There are on-going efforts focused on leveraging all available information regarding the test article's target, its specific toxicologic profile, and any class effects in a weight-of-evidence evaluation of carcinogenic risk prior to determining the need to conduct money- and time-consuming lifetime rodent bioassays (Avila et al., 2020). The use of alternative data, such as transcriptomic data, may in the future play an important role in developing a robust argument for not conducting lifetime rodent bioassays.

Beyond their use in drug regulatory submissions, evidence suggests that toxicogenomics data are rarely used in the chemical Industry. For example, a recent survey of Canadian human risk assessors indicated that the application of toxicogenomics data for human health risk assessment was marginal with 85% of respondents reporting that they never or rarely used these data (Vachon et al., 2017). Importantly, 68% of the respondents were not at all or only slightly familiar with the concept of using these data for human health risk assessment (Vachon et al., 2017). This clearly highlights not only the need for broader familiarization with -omics data among regulatory authorities but also the critical need for regulatory guidelines that describe how such data might be applied both to aid in study interpretation and quality assessment. Likewise, another survey by the European Centre for Ecotoxicology and Toxicology of Chemicals revealed that -omics technologies were not yet broadly applied during regulatory hazard identification and risk assessment and that their use was largely limited to serving as an ancillary part of a weight-of-evidence approach to investigate an MOA, somewhat similar to what is done for pharmaceutical agents (Sauer et al., 2017). Again, lack of standardization, methods for validation, and established best practices have been recognized as major hurdles to the use of -omics technology for regulatory decision-making (Sauer et al., 2017). However, there is enthusiasm for promoting the use of gene expression data to accelerate the development of adverse outcome pathways (AOPs, i.e., a conceptual framework intended to enhance the utility of pathway-based data for assessing hazards to human health and the environment) with guidance detailing internationally accepted approaches for describing and documenting AOPs for regulatory application (Bal-Price and Meek, 2017; Liu et al., 2019). These high-content molecular data (i.e., having many more data points than may be examined simultaneously by low throughput routine molecular methods like RT-PCR and Western blots) are particularly useful as screens to determine the initiating events and the subsequent cascade of downstream events that lead to phenotypic manifestations of toxicity (Alexander-Dann et al., 2018). Likewise, transcriptomic data have been proposed to enhance the specificity, reliability, and reproducibility of read-across assessments (i.e., using available data from a molecule [the source] as a basis for a safety assessment of another molecule [the target] that is considered similar enough to the source substance). The REACH (Registration, Evaluation, Authorization and Restriction of Chemicals) regulation clearly states that toxicogenomics approaches are appropriate in risk assessment (Liu et al., 2019; Reach, 2006; Sauer et al., 2017). However, no formal guidance exists, so at present toxicogenomics data only represent a complement to more conventional approaches (Kinaret et al., 2020).

9. CONCLUSIONS

Over 2 decades ago, the field of toxicogenomics began with a promise to revolutionize the field of toxicology. Significant developments have been made in developing novel technologies, bioinformatics approaches, and technical reproducibility across platforms leading to the generation of widely available reference databases to aid in the biological interpretation of -omics data. It is now apparent that the field of toxicogenomics has not revolutionized but rather evolved as a means for contributing to the mechanistic investigation of toxicity and chemical carcinogenesis, development of testable hypotheses, understanding of the translational relevance of findings in model organisms, and development of predictive biomarkers associated with test article exposure and disease. Today, -omics tools are being used increasingly for initial screening of chemical libraries for prioritization of chemicals for further testing in more biologically complex models.

Development of novel technologies and applications such as NGS; the explosion of information on transcriptomes including alternative splicing, lncRNA, and small RNA; and advances in high-throughput methods of WGS/WES are helping to better understand mechanisms of chemical-induced toxicity and carcinogenicity. In addition, generation of validated functional genomic databases provides greater confidence in the biological interpretation of toxicogenomic data, thereby providing a path to the use of toxicogenomic data for risk assessment. Toxicogenomics has not replaced traditional toxicity or carcinogenicity studies, and it is still implemented only on a case-by-case basis in risk assessment to investigate a possible mechanism of action. However, with generation of multiple validated reference databases and validated gene or molecular signatures that can robustly predict an apical endpoint, opportunities for the risk assessment community to integrate toxicogenomics into routine practice should continue to expand over time.

GLOSSARY

Adverse outcome pathways (AOPs) are a conceptual framework for assessing hazards to human health in which a sequence of "key events" essential for a biological outcome are identified starting with a molecular initiating event and eventually leading to an adverse effect or an apical endpoint.

Apical endpoints are measurable outcomes in whole organisms that have been exposed to toxicants which generally reflect the final outcomes of toxicity (e.g., cancer, death, reproductive failure, or any other defined clinical or morphologic alteration).

Array-based technology consists of densely organized probes (nucleotides or proteins) arranged in spots on a glass or plastic surface to increase the throughput of the assay. Examples include DNA microarrays to identify differential gene expression or single-nucleotide polymorphism (SNP) arrays used in genome wide association studies (GWAS).

Batch effect is an avoidable, artifactual end result produced by non-randomized (biased) sample collection or processing (e.g., all control animals assessed in the morning and all high-dose animals in the afternoon or on another day, different reagent lots used to process specimens from control and treated animals).

Benchmark dose (BMD) is the exposure level corresponding to a specific adverse change.

Bioinformatics is the utilization of analysis tools, statistics, computation, and biological resources to store, analyze, interpret, and disseminate large-scale biological data sets that are most often obtained from high-output assays of DNA, RNA, amino acid sequences, and proteins.

Comparative genomic hybridization (CGH) is a cytogenetic technique to compare copy number variations in the DNA of test and reference samples.

Electropherogram is a graphical representation of the pattern produced by charged nucleotides or nucleic acid (DNA/RNA) fragments migrating within an electric field and is used to refer to the data obtained from a DNA sequencer or from a bioanalyzer, respectively.

Epigenetics is the study of heritable phenotypes (e.g., histone modifications, nucleotide methylation) that alter gene expression but not the underlying DNA sequence (genotype).

Epigenomics is the study of epigenetics at the cellular or whole organism level using a variety of -omics approaches such as whole-genome bisulfite sequencing and RNA-Sequencing.

Error propagation is the accumulation of uncertainty when estimations of measurements from experiments are used to calculate additional valuations.

Exome is the part of the genome that codes for proteins. During RNA splicing, all the introns in mRNA transcripts are removed, leaving mRNA consisting of the exons that encode for the protein from that gene. Sequencing of the exome is much faster and cheaper than whole-genome sequencing since the exome consists of about 1% of the genome.

Exposome is the sum of all exposures an individual experiences over their lifetime (starting from conception) and the effect of these exposures on the individual's health. Sources of these exposures include the environment, occupation, and/or lifestyle choices.

Genome includes all the genetic material (DNA) in an organism. The human genome is comprised of about 3 billion nucleotides, while the mouse genome is slightly smaller, about 2.5 billion nucleotides. However, the numbers of protein-coding genes are about 20,000 in both species.

Genomics is the study of an individual's genome and its interplay between the constituent genes and its interactions with the individual's environment, in health, and/or disease conditions.

Genotoxic carcinogens are chemicals (or their metabolites) that are DNA reactive (i.e., that produce nuclear DNA damage and potentially irreversible changes in the genome). Genotoxic carcinogens are usually detected in genotoxicity assays (in vitro and/or in vivo) and typically induce tumors in more than one organ and more than one species.

Glycomics evaluates glycan modifications (i.e., sequences of carbohydrates conjugated to proteins [at serine, threonine, or asparagine residues] and lipids [ceramides]). The glycome (entire complement of glycans in the body) is more complex and dynamic than the genome, transcriptome, or proteome.

Histone modification consists of posttranslational modification of DNA-associated histone proteins by acetylation, methylation, phosphorylation, ubiquitination, SUMOylation (addition of small ubiquitin-like modifiers [SUMOs]), and ADP-ribosylation. These modifications alter chromatin structure and influence gene expression.

Lipidomics evaluates the structure and function of the complete set of lipids (the lipidome) produced in a given cell or organism as well as their interactions with other lipids, proteins, and metabolites. It is often considered as a subdiscipline of metabolomics.

Luminex technology is a bead-based multiplexed immunoassay system in a microplate format. These beads have different color codes and can simultaneously detect as many as 500 targets in a single sample. This system is used in the L1000 gene expression platform based on 978 landmark genes designed to capture alterations in molecular pathways. L1000 uses ligation-mediated amplification of RNA sequence-specific probes combined with Luminex-based detection.

Next-generation sequencing is a high-throughput technique employed to define part or all of the nucleotide sequence for an individual's genome.

Nongenotoxic carcinogens are chemicals that do not directly react with DNA but that are tumorigenic through other cellular effects, such as cytotoxicity- or receptor-induced cell proliferation, epigenetics mechanism, inhibition of cell–cell communication, or oxidative stress. Nongenotoxic carcinogens typically induce tumors only in a single tissue and often in one rodent species unless they are associated with systemic effects (e.g., hormonal modulation through interaction with hormonal receptors).

Phenotype (in the context of biology) is an organism's observable attributes (e.g., anatomy, biochemistry, behavior).

Phenotype anchoring is the process whereby morphologic endpoints are linked to molecular alterations.

Point of departure (POD) is a point on the toxicological dose–response curve that corresponds to an estimated low or no effect level. PODs are used for extrapolation to toxic reference doses or reference concentrations in the field of chemical risk assessment.

Read (plural: Reads) is an output from a genome sequencer that represents the inferred nucleotide sequence corresponding to a portion of DNA or RNA.

Read-across is a technique for predicting endpoint information for novel test articles based on characteristics of another chemically similar reference substance (e.g., sharing the same structure or active functional groups). Endpoints assessed by read-across may include mutagenicity, toxicity, or carcinogenicity. Read-across data are frequently used to fill gaps without running studies.

Read depth is the number of aligned sequence reads at a coordinate/reference base position of a genomic sequence. The higher the read depth, the more confidence there is in identifying a base.

Single-nucleotide polymorphism (SNP, pronounced as "snip") is a substitution of a single nucleotide at a specific position in the genome that is present in at least 1% of the population. SNPs may be associated with a disease phenotype in certain populations.

Single-nucleotide variant (SNV) is a single-nucleotide substitution in the genome of an individual that does not occur in a population. These are also called private mutations and may or may not be silent. An SNV could be an SNP if it occurs in at least 1% of the population.

Supervised and unsupervised analyses are means to either utilize external information or labels about the data in a classification analysis (i.e., supervised) or the classification analysis is performed on the data alone (unsupervised).

Systems biology is a multidisciplinary approach to understand biological processes by examining the interactions and behavior of the components of increasing biological complexity such as molecules, cells, tissues, organs, and organisms. In general, it involves integration of large high-throughput data sets such as -omics data and bioinformatics analysis to understand complex biological processes.

Systems toxicology is the integration of classical in vitro and in vivo toxicology with quantitative analysis of large networks of molecular and functional changes (such as -omics data) occurring across multiple levels of biological organization. One of the main goals of the systems toxicology approaches is to predict chemical or drug toxicity or efficacy based on -omics data.

TempO-Seq (Templated oligo detection assay) is a sequencing technology that enables quantification of targeted transcripts. Detector oligonucleotides ("oligos") are designed to hybridize to predefined RNA targets. Correctly hybridized detector oligos are ligated, and then amplified through primer landing sites that are shared among all probes. This approach allows multiplexing of up to 6144 samples in one sequencing library. S1500+, the high-throughput targeted transcriptomic platform from the U. S. National toxicology program, is based on the Temp-O-Seq technology.

Toxicogenomics investigates the adverse effects of chemicals and other potential toxic entities on animal or human health using high-throughput approaches such as genomics, transcriptomics, proteomics, and metabolomics.

Whole-genome sequencing (WGS) is a technique whereby the entire genome is sequenced.

Acknowledgments

We would like to acknowledge the work of the authors in the previous edition of this chapter "The Application of Toxicogenomics to the interpretation of Toxicologic Pathology" by William R. Foster, Donald G. Robertson, and Bruce D. Car in 3rd ed. W. M. Haschek, C. G. Rousseaux and M. A. Wallig, eds. (2013) Academic Press. We would also like to express our appreciation for the critical review by Stacey Fossey and Brad Bolon as well as for the assistance provided by the image editor Beth Mahler.

REFERENCES

Alexander-Dann B, Pruteanu LL, Oerton E, et al.: Developments in toxicogenomics: understanding and predicting compound-induced toxicity from gene expression data, *Mol Omics* 14:218–236, 2018.

Alexandrov LB, Kim J, Haradhvala NJ, et al.: The repertoire of mutational signatures in human cancer, *Nature* 578:94–101, 2020.

Altelaar AF, Munoz J, Heck AJ: Next-generation proteomics: towards an integrative view of proteome dynamics, *Nat Rev Genet* 14:35–48, 2013.

Anastasiadou E, Jacob LS, Slack FJ: Non-coding RNA networks in cancer, *Nat Rev Cancer* 18:5–18, 2018.

Angel TE, Aryal UK, Hengel SM, et al.: Mass spectrometry-based proteomics: existing capabilities and future directions, *Chem Soc Rev* 41:3912–3928, 2012.

Avila AM, Bebenek I, Bonzo JA, et al.: An FDA/CDER perspective on nonclinical testing strategies: classical toxicology approaches and new approach methodologies (NAMs), *Regul Toxicol Pharmacol* 114:104662, 2020.

Bal-Price A, Meek MEB: Adverse outcome pathways: application to enhance mechanistic understanding of neurotoxicity, *Pharmacol Ther* 179:84–95, 2017.

Balasubramanian S, Gunasekaran K, Sasidharan S, et al.: MicroRNAs and xenobiotic toxicity: an overview, *Toxicol Rep* 7:583–595, 2020.

Bamford S, Dawson E, Forbes S, et al.: The COSMIC (Catalogue of Somatic Mutations in Cancer) database and website, *Br J Cancer* 91:355–358, 2004.

Banks AT, Zimmerman HJ, Ishak KG, et al.: Diclofenac-associated hepatotoxicity: analysis of 180 cases reported to the food and drug administration as adverse reactions, *Hepatology* 22:820–827, 1995.

Bereman MS: Proteomics. In Smart RC, Hodgson E, editors: *Molecular and biochemical toxicology*, 2018, John Wiley & Sons, pp 91–114.

Berrino E, Annaratone L, Miglio U, et al.: Cold formalin fixation guarantees DNA integrity in formalin fixed paraffin embedded tissues: premises for a better quality of diagnostic and experimental pathology with a specific impact on breast cancer, *Front Oncol* 10:173, 2020.

Bertino Jr J, Fish D: The safety profile of the fluoroquinolones, *Clin Therapeut* 22:798–817, 2000. discussion 797.

Blackshear PE, Pandiri AR, Nagai H, et al.: Gene expression of mesothelioma in vinylidene chloride-exposed F344/N rats reveal immune dysfunction, tissue damage, and inflammation pathways, *Toxicol Pathol* 43:171–185, 2015.

Blomme EAG, Yang Y, Waring JF: Use of toxicogenomics to understand mechanisms of drug-induced hepatotoxicity during drug discovery and development, *Toxicol Lett* 186:22–31, 2009.

Boitier E, Amberg A, Barbie V, et al.: A comparative integrated transcript analysis and functional characterization of differential mechanisms for induction of liver hypertrophy in the rat, *Toxicol Appl Pharmacol* 252:85–96, 2011.

Bujak R, Struck-Lewicka W, Markuszewski MJ, et al.: Metabolomics for laboratory diagnostics, *J Pharmaceut Biomed Anal* 113:108–120, 2015.

Bushel PR, Caiment F, Wu H, et al.: RATEmiRs: the rat atlas of tissue-specific and enriched miRNAs for discerning baseline expression exclusivity of candidate biomarkers, *RNA Biol* 17:630–636, 2020.

Calvier FE, Bousquet C: Integrating the comparative toxicogenomic database in a human pharmacogenomic resource, *Stud Health Technol Inf* 270:267–271, 2020.

Carr TL, Ciurlionis R, Milicic I, et al.: Role of cytochrome P450c17alpha in dibromoacetic acid-induced testicular toxicity in rats, *Arch Toxicol* 85:513–523, 2011.

Chen M, Shi L, Kelly R, et al.: Selecting a single model or combining multiple models for microarray-based classifier development?–a comparative analysis based on large and diverse datasets generated from the MAQC-II project, *BMC Bioinf* 12(Suppl 10):S3, 2011.

Chou JW, Zhou T, Kaufmann WK, et al.: Extracting gene expression patterns and identifying co-expressed genes from microarray data reveals biologically responsive processes, *BMC Bioinf* 8:427, 2007.

Chung FF, Herceg Z: The promises and challenges of toxicoepigenomics: environmental chemicals and their impacts on the epigenome, *Environ Health Perspect* 128:15001, 2020.

Citron M: Strategies for disease modification in Alzheimer's disease, *Nat Rev Neurosci* 5:677–685, 2004.

Cohen SM: Evaluation of possible carcinogenic risk to humans based on liver tumors in rodent assays: the two-year bioassay is no longer necessary, *Toxicol Pathol* 38:487–501, 2010.

Cohen SM, Storer RD, Criswell KA, et al.: Hemangiosarcoma in rodents: mode-of-action evaluation and human relevance, *Toxicol Sci* 111:4–18, 2009.

CPDB (Carcinogenic Potency Database): *Download carcinogenic potency database (CPDB) data*, 2020.

Cui L, Lu H, Lee YH: Challenges and emergent solutions for LC-MS/MS based untargeted metabolomics in diseases, *Mass Spectrom Rev* 37:772–792, 2018.

Dai X, He YD, Dai H, et al.: Development of an approach for ab initio estimation of compound-induced liver injury based on global gene transcriptional profiles, *Genome Inform* 17:77–88, 2006.

Darwiche N: Epigenetic mechanisms and the hallmarks of cancer: an intimate affair, *Am J Cancer Res* 10:1954–1978, 2020.

Davis AP, Grondin CJ, Johnson RJ, et al.: The comparative toxicogenomics database: update 2019, *Nucleic Acids Res* 47: D948–D954, 2019.

Dekant W: Tetrahydrofuran-induced tumors in rodents are not relevant to humans: quantitative weight of evidence analysis of mode of action information does not support classification of tetrahydrofuran as a possible human carcinogen, *Regul Toxicol Pharmacol* 109:104499, 2019.

Delfour C, Roger P, Bret C, et al.: RCL2, a new fixative, preserves morphology and nucleic acid integrity in paraffin-embedded breast carcinoma and microdissected breast tumor cells, *J Mol Diagn* 8:157–169, 2006.

Dempsey JL, Cui JY: Long non-coding RNAs: a novel paradigm for toxicology, *Toxicol Sci* 155:3–21, 2017.

Deng X, Stachlewitz RF, Liguori MJ, et al.: Modest inflammation enhances diclofenac hepatotoxicity in rats: role of neutrophils and bacterial translocation, *J Pharmacol Exp Therapeut* 319:1191–1199, 2006.

Dickinson DA, Warnes GR, Quievryn G, et al.: Differentiation of DNA reactive and non-reactive genotoxic mechanisms using gene expression profile analysis, *Mutat Res* 549:29–41, 2004.

Doe JE, Boobis AR, Dellarco V, et al.: Chemical carcinogenicity revisited 2: current knowledge of carcinogenesis shows that categorization as a carcinogen or non-carcinogen is not scientifically credible, *Regul Toxicol Pharmacol* 103:124–129, 2019.

Doktorova TY, Yildirimman R, Ceelen L, et al.: Testing chemical carcinogenicity by using a transcriptomics HepaRG-based model? *EXCLI J* 13:623–637, 2014.

Eichner J, Kossler N, Wrzodek C, et al.: A toxicogenomic approach for the prediction of murine hepatocarcinogenesis using ensemble feature selection, *PLoS One* 8: e73938, 2013.

Ellinger-Ziegelbauer H, Gmuender H, Bandenburg A, et al.: Prediction of a carcinogenic potential of rat hepatocarcinogens using toxicogenomics analysis of short-term in vivo studies, *Mutat Res* 637:23–39, 2004.

Ellinger-Ziegelbauer H, Stuart B, Wahle B, et al.: Characteristic expression profiles induced by genotoxic carcinogens in rat liver, *Toxicol Sci* 77:19–34, 2005.

Ellinger-Ziegelbauer H, Stuart B, Wahle B, et al.: Comparison of the expression profiles induced by genotoxic and nongenotoxic carcinogens in rat liver, *Mutat Res* 575:61–84, 2008.

Evin G, Sernee MF, Masters CL: Inhibition of gamma-secretase as a therapeutic intervention for Alzheimer's disease: prospects, limitations and strategies, *CNS Drugs* 20:351–372, 2006.

Fielden MR, Brennan R, Gollub J: A gene expression biomarker provides early prediction and mechanistic assessment of hepatic tumor induction by nongenotoxic chemicals, *Toxicol Sci* 99:90–100, 2005.

Fielden MR, Eynon BP, Natsoulis G, et al.: A gene expression signature that predicts the future onset of drug-induced renal tubular toxicity, *Toxicol Pathol* 33:675–683, 2007.

Fielden MR, Nie A, McMillian M, et al.: Interlaboratory evaluation of genomic signatures for predicting carcinogenicity in the rat, *Toxicol Sci* 103:28–34, 2008.

Fitzpatrick RB: CPDB: carcinogenic potency database, *Med Ref Serv Q* 27:303–311, 2008.

Forbes SA, Bhamra G, Bamford S, et al.: The catalogue of somatic mutations in cancer (COSMIC), *Curr Protoc Hum Genet*, 2008:11, 2008. Chapter 10, Unit 10.

Foster WR, Chen SJ, He A, et al.: A retrospective analysis of toxicogenomics in the safety assessment of drug candidates, *Toxicol Pathol* 35:621–635, 2007.

Foster WR, Robertson DG, Car BD, editors: *The application of toxicogenomics to the interpretation of toxicologic pathology*, 2013, Academic Press.

Furihata C, Suzuki T: Evaluation of 12 mouse marker genes in rat toxicogenomics public data, open TG-GATEs: discrimination of genotoxic from non-genotoxic hepatocarcinogens, *Mutat Res Genet Toxicol Environ Mutagen* 838:9–15, 2019.

Ganter B, Snyder RD, Halbert DN, et al.: Toxicogenomics in drug discovery and development: mechanistic analysis of compound/class-dependent effects using the DrugMatrix database, *Pharmacogenomics* 7:1025–1044, 2006.

Gao XH, Li J, Gong HF, et al.: Comparison of fresh frozen tissue with formalin-fixed paraffin-embedded tissue for mutation analysis using a multi-gene panel in patients with colorectal cancer, *Front Oncol* 10:310, 2020.

Garcia EP, Minkovsky A, Jia Y, et al.: Validation of OncoPanel: a targeted next-generation sequencing assay for the detection of somatic variants in cancer, *Arch Pathol Lab Med* 141:751–758, 2017.

Goodsaid FM, Amur S, Aubrecht J, et al.: Voluntary exploratory data submissions to the US FDA and the EMA: experience and impact, *Nat Rev Drug Discov* 9:435–445, 2010.

Goodwin S, McPherson JD, McCombie WR: Coming of age: ten years of next-generation sequencing technologies, *Nat Rev Genet* 17:333–351, 2016.

Gottmann E, Kramer S, Pfahringer B, et al.: Data quality in predictive toxicology: reproducibility of rodent carcinogenicity experiments, *Environ Health Perspect* 109:509–514, 2001.

Grixti JM, Ayers D: Long noncoding RNAs and their link to cancer, *Noncoding RNA Res* 5:77–82, 2020.

Gu YG, Weitzberg M, Clark RF, et al.: N-{3-[2-(4-alkoxyphenoxy)thiazol-5-yl]-1-methylprop-2-ynyl}carboxy derivatives as acetyl-coA carboxylase inhibitors-

improvement of cardiovascular and neurological liabilities via structural modifications, *J Med Chem* 50:1078–1082, 2007.

Guo X, Zhang W, Ren J, et al.: LncRNA-OBFC2A targeted to Smad3 regulated Cyclin D1 influences cell cycle arrest induced by 1,4-benzoquinone, *Toxicol Lett* 332:74–81, 2020.

Gusenleitner D, Auerbach SS, Melia T, et al.: Genomic models of short-term exposure accurately predict long-term chemical carcinogenicity and identify putative mechanisms of action, *PLoS One* 9:e102579, 2014.

Gwinn WM, Auerbach SS, Parham F, et al.: Evaluation of 5-day in vivo rat liver and kidney with high-throughput transcriptomics for estimating benchmark doses of apical outcomes, *Toxicol Sci* 176:343–354, 2020.

Haider S, Black MB, Parks BB, et al.: A qualitative modeling approach for whole genome prediction using high-throughput toxicogenomics data and pathway-based validation, *Front Pharmacol* 9:1072, 2018.

Hamadeh HK, Bushel PR, Jayadev S, et al.: Gene expression analysis reveals chemical-specific profiles, *Toxicol Sci* 67:219–231, 2002.

Head SR, Komori HK, LaMere SA, et al.: Library construction for next-generation sequencing: overviews and challenges, *Biotechniques* 56:61–64, 2014, 66, 68, passim.

Hombach S, Kretz M: Non-coding RNAs: classification, biology and functioning, *Adv Exp Med Biol* 937:3–17, 2016.

Huang Q, Liu Y, Dong S: Emerging roles of long non-coding RNAs in the toxicology of environmental chemicals, *J Appl Toxicol* 38:934–943, 2018.

ICH: *S1A-S1C carcinogenicity studies*, 2020, International Council for Harmonisation of Technical Requirements for Pharmaceuticals for Human Use.

Igarashi Y, Nakatsu N, Yamashita T, et al.: Open TG-GATEs: a large-scale toxicogenomics database, *Nucleic Acids Res* 43:D921–D927, 2015.

Iida M, Anna CH, Gaskin ND, et al.: The putative tumor suppressor Tsc-22 is downregulated early in chemically induced hepatocarcinogenesis and may be a suppressor of Gadd45b, *Toxicol Sci* 99:43–50, 2007.

Iida M, Anna CH, Holliday WM, et al.: Unique patterns of gene expression changes in liver after treatment of mice for 2 weeks with different known carcinogens and non-carcinogens, *Carcinogenesis* 26:689–699, 2005.

Irwin RD, Boorman GA, Cunningham ML, et al.: Application of toxicogenomics to toxicology: basic concepts in the analysis of microarray data, *Toxicol Pathol* 32:72–83, 2004.

Irwin RD, Parker JS, Lobenhofer EK, et al.: Transcriptional profiling of the left and median liver lobes of male f344/n rats following exposure to acetaminophen, *Toxicol Pathol* 33:111–117, 2005.

Jacobs A: An FDA perspective on the nonclinical use of the X-omics technologies and the safety of new drugs, *Toxicol Lett* 186:32–35, 2009.

Jaksik R, Iwanaszko M, Rzeszowska-Wolny J, et al.: Microarray experiments and factors which affect their reliability, *Biol Direct* 10:46, 2015.

Jeffries MA: The development of epigenetics in the study of disease pathogenesis, *Adv Exp Med Biol* 1253:57–94, 2020.

Jones W, Greytak S, Odeh H, et al.: Deleterious effects of formalin-fixation and delays to fixation on RNA and miRNA-Seq profiles, *Sci Rep* 9:6980, 2019.

Kaplowitz N: Drug-induced liver injury, *Clin Infect Dis* 38:S44–S48, 2004.

Karu N, Deng L, Slae M, et al.: A review on human fecal metabolomics: methods, applications and the human fecal metabolome database, *Anal Chim Acta* 1030:1–24, 2018.

Kenyon GL, DeMarini DM, Fuchs E, et al.: Defining the mandate of proteomics in the post-genomics era: workshop report, *Mol Cell Proteomics* 1:763–780, 2002.

Kielhorn J, Melber C, Wahnschaffe U, et al.: Vinyl chloride: still a cause for concern, *Environ Health Perspect* 108:579–588, 2000.

Kinaret PAS, Serra A, Federico A, et al.: Transcriptomics in toxicogenomics, part I: experimental design, technologies, publicly available data, and regulatory aspects, *Nanomaterials* 10, 2020.

Klaus V, Bastek H, Damme K, et al.: Time-matched analysis of DNA adduct formation and early gene expression as predictive tool for renal carcinogenesis in methylazoxymethanol acetate treated Eker rats, *Arch Toxicol* 91:3427–3438, 2017.

Kossler N, Matheis KA, Ostenfeldt N, et al.: Identification of specific mRNA signatures as fingerprints for carcinogenesis in mice induced by genotoxic and nongenotoxic hepatocarcinogens, *Toxicol Sci* 143:277–295, 2015.

Kramer JA, Curtiss SW, Kolaja KL, et al.: Acute molecular markers of rodent hepatic carcinogenesis identified by transcription profiling, *Chem Res Toxicol* 17:463–470, 2004.

Kuo B, Webster AF, Thomas RS, et al.: BMDExpress data viewer - a visualization tool to analyze BMDExpress datasets, *J Appl Toxicol* 36:1048–1059, 2016.

Kurien BT, Everds NE, Scofield RH: Experimental animal urine collection: a review, *Lab Anim* 38:333–361, 2004.

Latini G, Del Vecchio A, Massaro M, et al.: Phthalate exposure and male infertility, *Toxicology* 226:90–98, 2006.

Lea IA, Gong H, Paleja A, et al.: CEBS: a comprehensive annotated database of toxicological data, *Nucleic Acids Res* 45:D964–D971, 2017.

Lehmann KP, Phillips S, Sar M, et al.: Dose-dependent alterations in gene expression and testosterone synthesis in the fetal testes of male rats exposed to di (n-butyl) phthalate, *Toxicol Sci* 81:60–68, 2004.

Levy SE, Myers RM: Advancements in next-generation sequencing, *Annu Rev Genom Hum Genet* 17:95–115, 2016.

Li J, Bushel PR: EPIG-Seq: extracting patterns and identifying co-expressed genes from RNA-Seq data, *BMC Genom* 17:255, 2016.

Li S: *Computational methods and data analysis for metabolomics*, New York, NY, 2020, Humana.

Lippa KA, Duewer DL, Salit ML, et al.: Exploring the use of internal and externalcontrols for assessing microarray technical performance, *BMC Res Notes* 3:349, 2010.

Liu S, Kawamoto T, Morita O, et al.: Discriminating between adaptive and carcinogenic liver hypertrophy in rat studies using logistic ridge regression analysis of toxicogenomic data: the mode of action and predictive models, *Toxicol Appl Pharmacol* 318:79–87, 2017.

Liu Z, Huang R, Roberts R, et al.: Toxicogenomics: a 2020 vision, *Trends Pharmacol Sci* 40:92–103, 2019.

Machtinger R, Bollati V, Baccarelli AA: miRNAs and lncRNAs as biomarkers of toxicant exposure. In McCullough SD, Dolinoy DC, editors: *Toxicoepigenetics: Core Principles and Applications*, 2018, Academic Press, pp 237–247.

Mardis ER: The impact of next-generation sequencing on cancer genomics: from discovery to clinic, *Cold Spring Harb Perspect Med* 9, 2019.

Marrone AK, Beland FA, Pogribny IP: Noncoding RNA response to xenobiotic exposure: an indicator of toxicity and carcinogenicity, *Expet Opin Drug Metab Toxicol* 10:1409–1422, 2014.

Matsumoto H, Saito F, Takeyoshi M: Investigation of the early-response genes in chemical-induced renal carcinogenicity for the prediction of chemical carcinogenicity in rats, *J Toxicol Sci* 42:175–181, 2017.

Mav D, Shah RR, Howard BE, et al.: A hybrid gene selection approach to create the S1500+ targeted gene sets for use in high-throughput transcriptomics, *PLoS One* 13:e0191105, 2018.

McCombie WR, McPherson JD, Mardis ER: Next-generation sequencing technologies, *Cold Spring Harb Perspect Med* 9, 2019.

Merrick BA, Auerbach SS, Stockton PS, et al.: Testing an aflatoxin B1 gene signature in rat archival tissues, *Chem Res Toxicol* 25:1132–1144, 2012.

Michel C, Roberts RA, Desdouets C, et al.: Characterization of an acute molecular marker of nongenotoxic rodent hepatocarcinogenesis by gene expression profiling in a long term clofibric acid study, *Chem Res Toxicol* 18:611–618, 2005.

Milano J, McKay J, Dagenais C, et al.: Modulation of notch processing by gamma-secretase inhibitors causes intestinal goblet cell metaplasia and induction of genes known to specify gut secretory lineage differentiation, *Toxicol Sci* 82:341–358, 2004.

Monticello TM, Jones TW, Dambach DM, et al.: Current nonclinical testing paradigm enables safe entry to first-in-human clinical trials: the IQ consortium nonclinical to clinical translational database, *Toxicol Appl Pharmacol* 334:100–109, 2017.

Morgan KT, Jayyosi Z, Hower MA, et al.: The hepatic transcriptome as a window on whole-body physiology and pathophysiology, *Toxicol Pathol* 33:136–145, 2005.

Mylchreest E, Cattley RC, Foster PM: Male reproductive tract malformations in rats following gestational and lactational exposure to di (n-butyl) phthalate: an antiandrogenic mechanism? *Toxicol Sci* 43:47–60, 1998.

National Research Council: *Applications of toxicogenomic technologies to predictive toxicology and risk assessment*, Washington, DC, 2007, The National Academies Press.

Newton RK, Aardema M, Aubrecht J: The utility of DNA microarrays for characterizing genotoxicity, *Environ Health Perspect* 112:420–422, 2004.

NRC: Toxicogenomic technologies, In National Research Council (US) Committee on Applications of Toxicogenomic Technologies to Predictive Toxicology, editor: *Applications of Toxicogenomic Technologies to Predictive Toxicology and Risk Assessment*, Washington (DC), 2007.

Nuwaysir EF, Bittner M, Trent J, et al.: Microarrays and toxicology: the advent of toxicogenomics, *Mol Carcinog* 24:153–159, 1999.

Nyska A, Moomaw CR, Foley JF, et al.: The hepatic endothelial carcinogen riddelliine induces endothelial apoptosis, mitosis, S phase, and p53 and hepatocytic vascular endothelial growth factor expression after short-term exposure, *Toxicol Appl Pharmacol* 184:153–164, 2002.

OECD: Test no. 451: carcinogenicity studies, vol section 4, Paris, 2018, OECD Publishing.

Peschansky VJ, Wahlestedt C: Non-coding RNAs as direct and indirect modulators of epigenetic regulation, *Epigenetics* 9:3–12, 2014.

Phillips JR, Svoboda DL, Tandon A, et al.: BMDExpress 2: enhanced transcriptomic dose-response analysis workflow, *Bioinformatics* 35:1780–1782, 2019.

Qin C, Tanis KQ, Podtelezhnikov AA, et al.: Toxicogenomics in drug development: a match made in heaven? *Expert Opin Drug Metabol Toxicol* 12:847–849, 2016.

Raghavachari N, Garcia-Reyero N: *Gene expression analysis: methods and protocols,* New York, NY, 2018, Humana Press.

Ramaiahgari SC, Auerbach SS, Saddler TO, et al.: The power of resolution: contextualized understanding of biological responses to liver injury chemicals using high-throughput transcriptomics and benchmark concentration modeling, *Toxicol Sci* 169:553–566, 2019.

Rao MS, Van Vleet TR, Ciurlionis R, et al.: Comparison of RNA-seq and microarray gene expression platforms for the toxicogenomic evaluation of liver from short-term rat toxicity studies, *Front Genet* 9:636, 2018.

Reach: Regulation (EC) no 1907/2006 of the European Parliament and of the Council of 18 December 2006 concerning the Registration, Evaluation, Authorisation and Restriction of Chemicals (REACH), establishing a European Chemicals Agency, amending Directive 1999/45/EC and repealing Council Regulation (EEC) no 793/93 and Commission Regulation (EC) no 1488/94 as well as Council Dective 76/769/EEC and Commission Directives 91/155/EEC, 93/67/EEC, 93/105/EC and 2000/21/EC, *Off J Eur Union*, 2006.

Reddy MV, Sistare FD, Christensen JS, et al.: An evaluation of chronic 6- and 12-month rat toxicology studies as predictors of 2-year tumor outcome, *Vet Pathol* 47:614–629, 2010.

Ruepp S, Boess F, Suter L, et al.: Assessment of hepatotoxic liabilities by transcript profiling, *Toxicol Appl Pharmacol* 207:S161–S170, 2005.

Ryu JY, Lee BM, Kacew S, et al.: Identification of differentially expressed genes in the testis of Sprague-Dawley rats treated with di(n-butyl) phthalate, *Toxicology* 234:103–112, 2007.

Sauer UG, Deferme L, Gribaldo L, et al.: The challenge of the application of 'omics technologies in chemicals risk assessment: background and outlook, *Regul Toxicol Pharmacol* 91(Suppl 1):S14–S26, 2017.

Searfoss GH, Jordan WH, Calligaro DO, et al.: Adipsin, a biomarker of gastrointestinal toxicity mediated by a functional gamma-secretase inhibitor, *J Biol Chem* 278:46107–46116, 2003.

Seitz S, Boelsterli UA: Diclofenac acyl glucuronide, a major biliary metabolite, is directly involved in small intestinal injury in rats, *Gastroenterology* 115:1476–1482, 1998.

Semizarov D, Blomme E, editors: *Genomics in drug discovery and development*, Hoboken, NJ, 2008, Wiley & Sons.

Shultz VD, Phillips S, Sar M, et al.: Altered gene profiles in fetal rat testes after in utero exposure to di(n-butyl) phthalate, *Toxicol Sci* 64:233–242, 2001.

Slack FJ, Chinnaiyan AM: The role of non-coding RNAs in oncology, *Cell* 179:1033–1055, 2019.

Slatko BE, Gardner AF, Ausubel FM: Overview of next-generation sequencing technologies. In Ausubel FM, et al., editors: *Current protocols in molecular biology*, 2018. p. e59, vol. 122.

Steiner G, Suter L, Boess F, et al.: Discriminating different classes of toxicants by transcript profiling, *Environ Health Perspect* 112:1236–1248, 2004.

Subramanian A, Narayan R, Corsello SM, et al.: A next generation connectivity map: L1000 platform and the first 1,000,000 profiles, *Cell* 171:1437–1452 e1417, 2017.

Suhovskih AV, Kazanskaya GM, Volkov AM, et al.: Suitability of RNALater solution as a tissue-preserving reagent for immunohistochemical analysis, *Histochem Cell Biol* 152:239–247, 2019.

Tate JG, Bamford S, Jubb HC, et al.: COSMIC: the catalogue of somatic mutations in cancer, *Nucleic Acids Res* 47:D941–D947, 2019.

Thomas RS, Bao WJ, Chu TM, et al.: Use of short-term transcriptional profiles to assess the long-term cancer-related safety of environmental and industrial chemicals, *Toxicol Sci* 112:311–321, 2009.

Thukral SK, Nordone PJ, Hu R, et al.: Prediction of nephrotoxicant action and identification of candidate toxicity-related biomarkers, *Toxicol Pathol* 33:343–355, 2005.

Timp W, Timp G: Beyond mass spectrometry, the next step in proteomics, *Sci Adv* 6:eaax8978, 2020.

Vachon J, Campagna C, Rodriguez MJ, et al.: Barriers to the use of toxicogenomics data in human health risk assessment: a survey of Canadian risk assessors, *Regul Toxicol Pharmacol* 85:119–123, 2017.

Vahle JL, Anderson U, Blomme EAG, et al.: Use of toxicogenomics in drug safety evaluation: current status and an industry perspective, *Regul Toxicol Pharmacol* 96:18–29, 2018.

van Delft JHM, van Agen E, van Breda SGJ, et al.: Discrimination of genotoxic from non-genotoxic carcinogens by gene expression profiling, *Carcinogenesis* 25:1265–1276, 2004.

van den Tweel JG, Taylor CR: A brief history of pathology: preface to a forthcoming series that highlights milestones in the evolution of pathology as a discipline, *Virchows Arch* 457:3–10, 2010.

van Dijk EL, Auger H, Jaszczyszyn Y, et al.: Ten years of next-generation sequencing technology, *Trends Genet* 30:418–426, 2014.

Walker DI, Valvi D, Rothman N, et al.: The metabolome: a key measure for exposome research in epidemiology, *Curr Epidemiol Rep* 6:93–103, 2019.

Wang J, Zhu S, Meng N, et al.: ncRNA-encoded peptides or proteins and cancer, *Mol Ther* 27:1718–1725, 2019.

Wang X: *Next-generation sequencing data analysis*, 2016, CRC Press.

Waring JF, Jolly RA, Ciurlionis R, et al.: Clustering of hepatotoxins based on mechanism of toxicity using gene expression profiles, *Toxicol Appl Pharmacol* 175:28–42, 2001.

Waring JF, Liguori MJ, Luyendyk JP, et al.: Microarray analysis of lipopolysaccharide potentiation of trovafloxacin-induced liver injury in rats suggests a role for proinflammatory chemokines and neutrophils, *J Pharmacol Exp Therapeut* 316:1080–1087, 2008.

Waring JF, Yang Y, Healan-Greenberg CH, et al.: Gene expression analysis in rats treated with experimental acetyl-coenzyme A carboxylase inhibitors suggests interactions with the peroxisome proliferator-activated receptor alpha pathway, *J Pharmacol Exp Therapeut* 324:507–516, 2006.

Waters MD, Jackson M, Lea I: Characterizing and predicting carcinogenicity and mode of action using conventional and toxicogenomics methods, *Mutat Res* 705:184–200, 2010.

Waters MD, Stack HF, Jackson MA: Genetic toxicology data in the evaluation of potential human environmental carcinogens, *Mutat Res* 437:21–49, 1999.

Weaver RJ, Blomme EA, Chadwick AE, et al.: Managing the challenge of drug-induced liver injury: a roadmap for the development and deployment of preclinical predictive models, *Nat Rev Drug Discov* 19:131–148, 2020.

Wei LK: *Computational epigenetics and diseases*. In *Translational Epigenetics*, vol. 9. 2019, Academic Press.

Wishart DS: Emerging applications of metabolomics in drug discovery and precision medicine, *Nat Rev Drug Discov* 15:473–484, 2016.

Wishart DS: Metabolomics for investigating physiological and pathophysiological processes, *Physiol Rev* 99:1819–1875, 2019.

Xu J, Thakkar S, Gong B, et al.: The FDA's experience with emerging genomics technologies-past, present, and future, *AAPS J* 18:814–818, 2016.

Yang L, Allen BC, Thomas RS: BMDExpress: a software tool for the benchmark dose analyses of genomic data, *BMC Genom* 8, 2007.

Yang Y, Abel SJ, Ciurlionis R, et al.: Development of a toxicogenomics in vitro assay for the efficient characterization of compounds, *Pharmacogenomics* 7:177–186, 2006.

Yang Y, Ciurlionis R, Kowalkowski K, et al.: N-vinylpyrrolidone dimer, a novel formulation excipient, causes hepatic and thyroid hypertrophy through the induction of hepatic microsomal enzymes in rats, *Toxicol Lett* 208:82–91, 2012.

Zhang L, Lu Q, Chang C: Epigenetics in health and disease, *Adv Exp Med Biol* 1253:3–55, 2020.

Zubarev RA: The challenge of the proteome dynamic range and its implications for in-depth proteomics, *Proteomics* 13:723–726, 2013.

CHAPTER

16

Experimental Design and Statistical Analysis for Toxicologic Pathologists

Colin G. Rousseaux[1], Keith R. Shockley[2], Shayne C. Gad[3]

[1]Department of Pathology and Laboratory Medicine, Faculty of Medicine, University of Ottawa, Ottawa, ON, Canada, [2]Biostatistics and Computational Biology Branch, U.S. National Institute of Environmental Health Sciences, Research Triangle Park, NC, United States, [3]Gad Consulting Services, Raleigh, NC, United States

OUTLINE

1. Introduction	**546**
1.1. Observations and Measurements	547
1.2. Data Type and Statistical Methods	548
1.3. Understanding Biological Variation	549
1.4. Biological and Statistical Significance	550
2. Considerations Made Before Designing the Experiment	**553**
2.1. Differing Group Variability	553
2.2. Involuntary Censoring	553
2.3. Metaanalysis	553
2.4. Unbalanced Designs	554
2.5. Undesirable Variables	554
2.6. Experimental Unit	554
3. Experimental Design	**555**
3.1. Basic Principles of Experimental Design	555
3.2. Detecting Treatment Effects	556
3.3. Censoring	561
3.4. Impacts of Sample Size	562
4. Designs Commonly Used in Toxicologic Pathology	**562**
4.1. Completely Randomized Design	563
4.2. Completely Randomized Block Design	563
4.3. Matched Pairs Design	563
4.4. Latin Square Design	564
4.5. Factorial Design	564
4.6. Nested Design	564
5. Functions of Statistical Analyses	**565**
5.1. Hypothesis Testing and Probability (P) Values	566
5.2. Modeling	566
5.3. Dimension Reduction	567
6. Prerequisites to Statistical Analysis	**568**
6.1. Describing the Data	568
6.2. Statistical Graphics	570
6.3. Evaluating Distributional Assumptions	576
6.4. Data Processing	578
7. Statistical Methods	**582**
7.1. Statistical Analysis: General Considerations	582
7.2. Hypothesis Testing of Categorical Data	588
7.3. Hypothesis Testing in Single Factor Experiments	590
7.4. Hypothesis Testing in Multifactor Experiments	596
7.5. Analysis of Covariance	597
7.6. Modeling Trends	599
7.7. Correlation and Agreement	608
7.8. Nonparametric Hypothesis Testing	610
7.9. Quantifying Uncertainty	619
7.10. Methods for the Reduction of Dimensionality	620
7.11. Metaanalysis	624
7.12. Bayesian Inference	626
8. Interpretation of Results	**629**
8.1. Causality versus Association	629
8.2. Possible Sources of Bias	631
8.3. Use of Historical Control Data	631
8.4. Using Scientific Judgment	632
9. Data Analysis Applications in Toxicologic Pathology	**632**
9.1. Body and Organ Weights	632
9.2. Clinical Chemistry	634
9.3. Hematology	634

Haschek and Rousseaux's Handbook of Toxicologic Pathology, Fourth Edition.
https://doi.org/10.1016/B978-0-12-821044-4.00002-9

9.4. *Incidence of Histopathological Findings*	635
9.5. *Carcinogenesis*	636

10. Assumptions of Statistical Tests	638

11. Summary and Conclusions	638

Glossary	645

References	648

1. INTRODUCTION

General texts concerning statistics (Gad, 2014; Gad, 2016; Gad, 2019; Garrett, 1982; Koehler, 2012; Kotz et al., 2006; Marriott, 1990; Sokal and Rohlf, 2011; Zar, 2015) are available; however, this chapter has been written as a practical guide to common statistical problems encountered when using differing research strategies in toxicologic pathology, and to provide the methodologies available to solve them. First, core issues in mathematical decision-making are discussed, followed by details concerning some of the principles used in making mathematical inferences, and finally discussions of why a particular procedure or interpretation is recommended. Enumeration of assumptions that are necessary for procedures to be valid is described, and problems often seen in the practice of toxicology and toxicologic pathology are discussed. A glossary of terms can be found at the end of the chapter.

Since 1960, as it has evolved, the field of toxicologic pathology has become increasingly complex and controversial in both its theory and its practice. As in all other sciences, toxicologic pathology started as a descriptive science, where pathologists described morphological changes seen following accidental exposure to xenobiotics. The need to understand the dose response for adverse effects of specific xenobiotics on tissues and organisms is a core function of predictive toxicologic pathology and safety assessment.

Prediction of adverse effects in humans is most often made when animals are dosed with (or exposed to) chemical or physical agents and the resultant adverse effects are observed at a specific dose. With the accumulation of these results, it is possible to infer, and study, underlying mechanisms of action. Toxicologic pathology has now developed to the mechanistic stage, where active contributions to the field encompass both descriptive and mechanistic studies.

Statistical analysis applied in the field of toxicology has also evolved during the last 50+ years. However, it is imperative that statistical approaches be performed in a competent and ethical manner in order to ensure transparent practices, reproducibility in results, and valid interpretations (American Statistical Association, 2018). Statistical approaches are used to describe the data, conduct hypothesis testing, model observed responses, and perform dimension reduction. Attention to statistical detail should be employed at every aspect of a study, including experimental design, data collection and processing, statistical analysis, interpretation, and reporting of results (Shockley and Kissling, 2018). These considerations will be described in detail for practitioners of toxicologic pathology throughout the course of this chapter.

Studies continue to be designed and executed to generate results in the form of measurements or observations (data), which can be statistically analyzed giving a mathematical probability of significance. The toxicologic pathologist is well trained to assist in interpretation of the biological importance of analyzed data from inferential experiments. Mathematical significance is irrelevant if there is no biological significance. In addition, the peculiarities of toxicologic pathology data need to be understood before procedures are selected and employed for analysis. There are characteristics of toxicology experiments in animals that impact their extrapolation to human populations. First, relatively small sample sets of data are collected from the members of an experimental animal population, which is not actually the human or target animal population of interest. Second, sample data are often censored on a basis other than by the investigator's design. Censoring occurs when the data points are not obtained as planned. This censoring usually results from biological factors, such as death or morbidity of an animal, or from a logistical factor (e.g., equipment failure or a tissue not collected during necropsy). Third, the conditions under which experiments are conducted are extremely varied. In pharmacology, the possible conditions by which a chemical or physical agent may interact with a person are limited to a small range of doses given via a single route of exposure over a short course of treatment to a defined patient population. In toxicologic pathology, however, the investigator seeks to control all test variables, such as dose, route, time span, and subject population. Finally, time frames available to identify, assess, and give opinions regarding issues are limited by practical and economic factors. This frequently means that there is no time to repeat a critical study. Therefore, a true iterative trial-and-error approach to toxicologic pathology is not possible.

1.1. Observations and Measurements

Observationsand *measurements* are essential to all aspects of toxicologic pathology. Even when detailing a new case, descriptive observations can be collected in regard to lesion numbers and distribution as well as sample color, size, and texture. These observations are then summarized as to severity and the distribution and the disease process affecting a specific tissue can be defined as a morphological diagnosis.

All measurements and observations produce *scalar measurement*, ordered severity, or various categories. Each of these data types has implications regarding the type of statistical analysis that should be undertaken and how inference can be made using that analysis. We shall describe three types of outputs, for which an understanding of each is necessary to select the correct method to derive inference regarding the relationship between a treatment and an observed effect. Data are collected on the basis of their association with a treatment, intended or otherwise, as an effect (a property) that is measured in the experimental subjects of a study. These identifiers, i.e., treatment and effect are termed *variables*. Treatment variables previously selected and controlled by the researcher are termed *independent variables*. Effect variables, measurements, and observations such as weight, life span, and number of neoplasms that are believed to dependent on the treatment being studied are termed *dependent variables*.

All possible measures of a given set of variables in all the possible subjects that exist are termed the *population* for those variables. Such a population of variables cannot be truly measured. For example, one would have to obtain, treat, and measure the weights of all the Fischer 344 rats that were, are, or ever will be. Instead, we deal with a representative group (sample). If the *sample* of data is appropriately collected and of sufficient size, it serves to provide good estimates of the characteristics of the parent population from which it is drawn.

Regardless of the type of data, optimal design and appropriate interpretation of experiments require that the researcher understands both the biological and technological underpinnings of the system being studied and of the data being generated. From the point of view of the statistician, it is vitally important that the experimenter both knows and is able to communicate the nature of the data and understand its limitations. The types of data generated include *quantal* (e.g., dead or alive), *categorical* (e.g., morphological diagnosis), *ordinal* (e.g., lesion severity), and *interval continuous* (e.g., clinical pathology data).

Categories

Categories, also referred to as *classes*, are quintessential to toxicologic pathology. The most common category with which the toxicologic pathologist is familiar is the definitive diagnosis. Here, there may be a number of categories (diagnoses) into which the toxicologic pathologist places his or her observations (e.g., hepatocellular carcinoma, chronic interstitial nephritis). The categories only allow accumulation of "whole" events. It is not possible to have a partial diagnosis or make an "average" diagnosis. Either the diagnosis is made, or it is not. These data are grouped on the basis of name or category; hence they are usually termed "nominal" or "categorical" data.

A special type of category results in only one of two outcomes: yes or no. Typical examples include live or dead, pregnant or not, etc. These data are referred to as *dichotomous*, *quantal*, or *binary*, and are often seen in safety studies. Again, there is only one choice, as partial choices cannot be made (i.e., an animal cannot be both dead and alive).

Nonmeasured Scales

Toxicologic pathologists are also familiar with the use of scales to express degrees of severity. These qualitative scales are not measured, but the scale shows an internal relationship. For example, severity may be scored as mild (+), which is less than moderate (++), which is less than severe (+++). Because the severity is ordered, the resulting data are often called "ordinal" in nature. Nonparametric statistical analysis of such data is required to make inferences with respect to cause and effect.

Measurements

Measurements of a scalar quantity use a recognized scale (e.g., grams) to define the places of various data points. Measurements can be either *continuous*, such as length and weight, or *discontinuous*, like white blood cell (WBC) numbers and other hematological parameters. Continuous measurements are those where any value within the scale may be assigned (e.g., for weight, the scale can be registered in grams, or ever-smaller fractions of grams), while discontinuous measurements produce whole number values. For practical purposes, some discontinuous measurements can be treated as if they were continuous numbers. A partial white cell cannot be recorded, but because there are so many cells, the data approximate a continuum. Situations where discontinuous data can be considered as a continuum for the purpose of analysis will be discussed later.

Proportions and Rates

Data can be recorded as *proportions ratios* and *rates*. Examples include the percentage of subjects affected with a specific tumor, the male: female ratio, and the incidence of occurrence. These data are continuous, as fractional values are possible. However, these quantities are seldom directly measured and are not usually normally distributed. These data require distribution-free (i.e., nonparametric) statistical analysis, unless a specified mathematical distribution can be approximated for the data set. Analyses of these data will be discussed later in this chapter.

Proportions can be misleading without reference to the absolute values from which they were calculated. For example, a "50% affected" rate represents one of two animals affected, or one million affected in a population of two million. Unscrupulous allusions regarding effectiveness can be attempted using proportions without reference to the numbers contained in the study population.

A summary of data types is presented in Table 16.1.

1.2. Data Type and Statistical Methods

Continuous variables are those which can at least theoretically assume any of an infinite number of values between any two fixed points (such as measurements of body weight between 2.0 and 3.0 kg). *Discontinuous variables*, meanwhile, are those that can have only certain fixed

TABLE 16.1   Types of Variables (Data) and Examples of Each Type

Classification	Type	Example
Continuous scale	Scalar	Body weight
	Ranked (ordinal)	Severity of a lesion
Discontinuous scale	Scalar	Weeks until the first observation of a tumor in a carcinogenicity study
	Ranked (ordinal)	Clinical observations
	Attributes (nominal)	Eye colors in fruit flies
	Quantal (nominal)	Dead or alive; present or absent
Frequency distribution	Normal	Body weights
	Bimodal	Some clinical chemistry parameters
	Others	Time to capacitation

values, with no possible intermediate values (such as counts of five or six dead animals, respectively).

Statistical methods are based on specific assumptions. *Parametric statistics*, those that are most familiar to the majority of scientists, have more stringent underlying assumptions than do nonparametric statistics. Among the underlying assumptions for many parametric statistical methods (such as the analysis of variance [-ANOVA]) is that the data are continuous. Parametric statistical analyses assume that the data come from populations with distributions that can be modeled with a predetermined set of parameters. As a rule, the normal distribution is assumed for parametric statistical analyses. Independence of cases and equality of variances across groups are also required for parametric approaches. *Nonparametric* techniques should be used whenever the requirements for parametric tests cannot be verified or are not reasonably expected to be true. For example, continuous data such as cadmium concentrations in kidney tissue from an exposed versus an unexposed population could be studied using nonparametric statistics when the assumptions for parametric analysis cannot be met (Hollander et al., 2013; Siegel and Castellan, 1988). Parametric tests are more powerful than nonparametric tests, requiring smaller sample sizes.

1.3. Understanding Biological Variation

Biological variation is central to all our lives. Diversity in our own species is recognized not only as visible characteristics, such as height, but also as functional characteristics, such as biotransformation abilities. Unfortunately, biological diversity interferes with efforts to test treatment effects, even when the experiment is designed and controlled a priori. No matter how inbred study animals are, and consequently how alike their physiological responses are likely to be, there is always a range of response displayed in measurements made on these animals. This fact has been confirmed in monozygotic human twins and in genetically identical organisms (Wong et al., 2005).

The normal or *Gaussian distribution* is an essential underpinning of many commonly used statistical analyses. This distribution is described as a bell-shaped curve (Figure 16.1). This

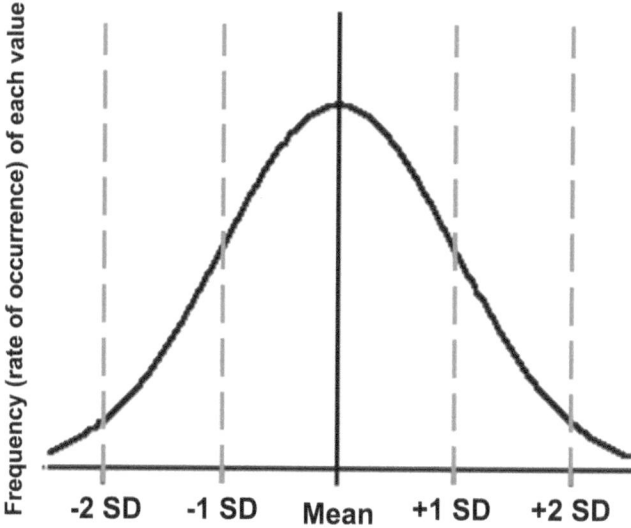

X-axis reports the frequency of the observation
Y-axis reports the measurement
SD - Standard deviation

FIGURE 16.1 **Normal biological variability—bell shaped curve.** *X*-axis reports the frequency of the observation. *Y*-axis reports the measurement. SD—Standard deviation.

distribution is the background of "noise" against which backdrop observations are made. Mathematics can help clarify whether the results seen in an experiment are a result of biological noise or a treatment-related signal. Just as the experimenter cannot be sure that the treatment did have an effect, statistical analyses do not give a definite yes or no answer, but rather renders a *probability statement* regarding the likelihood that the treatment is responsible for inducing the effect.

The mathematics used in the analysis results in a probability that the variability in results is caused by a biological variation (i.e., by chance) and not by the treatment (Figure 16.2). The experimenter can then use statistical testing to evaluate the evidence against a predetermined null effect. This decision point is referred to as rejecting the null hypothesis (H_0), where the H_0 is that the variability of effects is due to normal biological variation and not the treatment, and hence that the groups are the same. By convention, we reject this H_0 when the probability of making a false rejection is 5% or less ($P < .05$). Hypothesis testing will be discussed in more detail later.

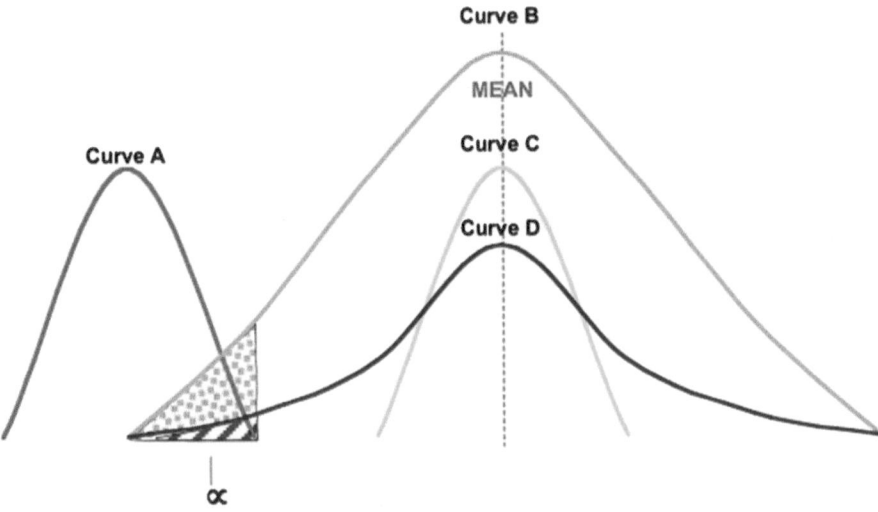

FIGURE 16.2   **Experimental outcome mixed with biological variability.** The Figure highlights the importance of biological variation. If comparison is made between curves A (e.g., the control group response) with curve C (e.g., treatment response), then the separation of the two groups is obvious. However, if curve A (e.g., response of controls) is compared with curves B or D, it is not obvious at a glance whether or the groups are truly different or merely represent subsets of biological variation within the experiment. The null hypothesis would state that all curves are part of the variability shown within the experiment and that no curve is caused by the treatment. The probability below which the experimenter is willing to reject this hypothesis is given by α (which is usually set at 5%, i.e., a P-value of <0.05).

1.4. Biological and Statistical Significance

It is essential that a professional who firmly understands statistical concepts interpret any analysis of study results. These concepts include the *nature* and *value of different types of data,* and the difference between *biological significance* and *statistical significance.*

False Negatives and Positives

To illustrate the importance of biological versus statistical significance, we shall consider the four possible combinations of these two different types of significance, which produces the relationship shown in Table 16.2.

Cases IV and I give us no problems, for the answers are the same statistically and biologically. However, cases II and III present problems. In Case II (the false positive), we have a circumstance where there is statistical significance in the measured difference between treated and control groups, but there is no true biological significance to the finding. This is not an uncommon happening, as shown by the case of clinical chemistry parameters with values falling just outside the statistically defined range. This existence of statistical significance in the absence of

TABLE 16.2   Four Possible Combinations of Biological and Statistical Significance

		Statistical significance	
		No	Yes
Biological significance	No	Case I	Case II
	Yes	Case III	Case IV

biological relevance is called a *Type I error* by statisticians, and the probability of this happening is called the *alpha* level. When this type of error occurs, the H_0 (i.e., no difference) is rejected when it is true.

In Case III (the false negative), we have no statistical significance, but the differences between groups are nonetheless biologically/toxicologically significant. Statisticians call this situation a *Type II error*, and the probability of such an error happening by random chance is called the *beta* level. In this situation, the H_0 is accepted when it is false. An example of this second situation is when a very rare tumor type is observed in a few treated animals.

In both Case II and Case III, numerical analysis, no matter how well done, is no substitute for professional judgment. Along with this, however, one must have a feeling for the different types of data and for the value or relative merit of each. Note that the two error types interact, and in determining sample size, we need to specify both α and β levels (Kraemer and Thiemann, 1987).

Statistical Power

The *power* of a statistical test, which is also known as the *sensitivity*, is the probability that a test results in rejection of a null hypothesis, H_0, when some other hypothesis, H_1, is valid. In other words, power is the probability that the test will reject H_0 when H_0 is actually false (i.e., the likelihood of not committing a Type II error [making a false-negative decision]). The probability of a Type II error (i.e., the false-negative rate) is β, while power is equal to $1 - β$. In general, power is a function of the possible distributions, often determined by a parameter, under the alternative hypothesis. Increasing the power decreases the chance of making a Type II error.

Power analysis can be used to calculate the minimum sample size required so that one can be reasonably likely to detect an effect of a given size. Power analysis can also be used to calculate the minimum sample size required so that one can be reasonably likely to detect an effect of a given size (see, for example, Table 16.3). In addition, the concept of power is useful for comparing different statistical testing procedures, such as a parametric and a nonparametric test of the same hypothesis. The larger the power required, the larger the necessary sample size. Stated another way, small sample sizes give a lower power, and heighten the chance of not detecting a true difference. Conventionally, power should be at least 80%.

True Biological Positive Effects

By now, the reader may be puzzled as to how we agree that a result is the truth. Even when it is established that an effect is of biological importance, the illustration above shows that there are always some false positive and negative outcomes based on the set false-positive level, the sample size, and the resulting false negative probability. In addition to uncertainties of biological importance based on clinical judgment and statistical probability, there are other sources of uncertainty that should be recognized.

TABLE 16.3 Sample Size Required to Obtain a Specified Sensitivity at $P < .05$

Background tumor incidence	P^a	Treatment Tumor Incidence[b]									
		0.95	0.90	0.80	0.70	0.60	0.50	0.40	0.30	0.20	0.10
0.30	0.90	10	12	18	31	46	102	389			
	0.50	6	6	9	12	22	32	123			
0.20	0.90	8	10	12	18	30	42	88	320		
	0.50	5	5	6	9	12	19	28	101		
0.10	0.90	6	8	10	12	17	25	33	65	214	
	0.50	3	3	5	6	9	11	17	31	68	
0.05	0.90	5	6	8	10	13	18	25	35	76	464
	0.50	3	3	5	6	7	9	12	19	24	147
0.01	0.90	5	5	7	8	10	13	19	27	46	114
	0.50	3	3	5	5	6	8	10	13	25	56

[a] *P = Power for each comparison of treatment group with background tumor incidence.*
[b] *Numbers indicate the minimum treatment group size necessary to detect statisitical differences among groups for a given power and alpha level.*

The generation of data through laboratory tests (particularly immunologic, hematologic and enzymatic) all inherently shows false-negative and false-positive results. These outcomes may occur because of the test itself, or because of disease classification criteria used for defining the normal and abnormal ranges for the parameter of interest. For example, an immunocytochemical stain may not label all tissues adequately or may produce too much background noise. In this example, we can detect false negative and false positives occurring not as a result of statistical error, but as a result of error inherent to the test. The concept of false negatives and false positives can be followed through reagents used in the test, etc.

The toxicologic pathologist requires knowledge of *true positives* and *true negatives* to interpret the relevance of statistical significance to biological outcomes. True positives are the probability of the test demonstrating positive findings in diseased subjects, which is termed *sensitivity*. True negatives are the probability of a negative test result in the absence of disease, which is termed *specificity*. In addition, it is important to know the ability of the test to give the same answer over a number of runs *(precision)* and also the ability to give data that correspond to the true value of a measured parameter *(accuracy)*.

If one reexamines the table given for the combinations of biological and statistical significance, the relationship between test results and disease state may be illustrated effectively.

Using the information in Table 16.4, one can now define sensitivity, specificity, and other test predictions using a series of simple equations:

Determination of the test sensitivity (probability of a positive test when the disease is present) (Eq. 16.1)

$$d/(b+d) \qquad (16.1)$$

-where b has a disease with a negative test result, and d has a disease with a positive test result.

Determination of the test specificity (probability of a negative test when the disease is absent) (Eq. 16.2)

$$a/(a+c) \qquad (16.2)$$

-where a has no disease with a negative test result, and c has no disease with a positive test result.

Determination of the test false-positive rate (probability of a positive test when the disease is absent) (Eq. 16.3)

$$c/(a+c) \qquad (16.3)$$

-where a has no disease with a negative test result, and c has no disease with a positive test result.

Determination of the test false-negative rate (probability of a negative test when the disease is present) (Eq. 16.4)

$$b/(b+d) \qquad (16.4)$$

-where b has a disease with a negative test result, and d has a disease and with a positive test result.

TABLE 16.4   Four Possible Combinations of Biological and Statistical Significance

			Disease present	
			No	Yes
Test result?	No	(a + b)	Case I (a)	Case II (b)
	Yes	(c + d)	Case III (c)	Case IV (d)
Total		(a + b + c + d)	(a + c)	(b + d)

a. Represents the number of individuals that do not have the disease and test negative (true negative).
b. Represents the number of individuals that have the disease and test negative (false negative).
c. Represents the number of individuals that do not have the disease and test positive (false positive).
d. Represents the number of individuals that have the disease and test positive (true positive).

Determination of the test positive predictive value (probability that the disease is present if the test is positive) (Eq. 16.5)

$$d/(c+d) \qquad (16.5)$$

-where c has no disease with a positive test result, and d has a disease and with a positive test result.

Determination of the test negative predictive value (probability that the disease is absent given a negative test) (Eq. 16.6)

$$a/(a+b) \qquad (16.6)$$

-where a has no disease with a negative test result, and b has a disease with a negative test result.

As precision and accuracy require data other than those given above in Table 16.2, they will not be addressed further in this chapter (See *Clinical Pathology Testing*, Vol 1, Chap 10).

Although all these values have utility, it is the *positive predictive value* (Eq. 16.5) that gives the experimenter the most information concerning the reliability of the data.

Confirmation that treatment causes an effect requires an understanding of the underlying mechanism and proof of its validity. At the same time, it is important that we realize that not finding a good mathematical correlation or suitable significance associated with a treatment and an effect does not prove that the two are not associated. In other words, failure to show a statistical correlation does not mean that a treatment does not cause an effect. At best, it gives us a certain level of confidence that under the conditions of the current test, the treatment and the effects were not associated. These points will be discussed in greater detail in the Assumptions Table (Table 16.30) at the end of this chapter, along with other common pitfalls and shortcomings associated with the method.

2. CONSIDERATIONS MADE BEFORE DESIGNING THE EXPERIMENT

Many aspects of experimental design are specific to the practice of toxicologic pathology. Before we look at general concepts for the development of experimental designs, the following aspects should first be considered.

2.1. Differing Group Variability

Frequently, the data gathered from specific measurements of animal characteristics are such that there is wide variability in the data. Often such wide variability is not present in a control or low-dose group, while variance may be inflated in an intermediate dose group. That is, the standard deviation (SD) associated with the measurements from this intermediate group may be larger than that noted for the low-dose cohort. Unequal variance across dose groups is referred to as *heteroscedasticity*. In the face of such a data set, the conclusion that there is no biological effect based on a failure to show a statistically significance effect without accounting for heteroscedasticity might well be erroneous. When working with novel endpoints, scientists should perform pilot studies in order to characterize data variability. These preliminary studies can be used to inform the primary study design. However, caution should be used when interpreting outcomes from a new endpoint when the underlying variability in the data is not well understood.

2.2. Involuntary Censoring

In designing experiments, one should keep in mind the potential effect of *involuntary censoring* on sample size. In other words, though a study might start with five subjects per group, this small size provides no margin for error should any die before the study is ended, thus precluding sample collection and data analysis. Beginning a study with "just enough" experimental units per group frequently leaves too few at the end to allow meaningful statistical analysis. Therefore, study designs should have allowances to ensure that there will be an adequate number of subjects in each group when establishing group sizes.

2.3. Metaanalysis

It is certainly possible to pool the data from several identical toxicological studies to permit a global statistical evaluation. One approach to this is *metaanalysis*, considered in detail later in this chapter. For example, after first having performed an acute inhalation study where only three treatment group animals survived to the point at which a critical measure (e.g., analysis of blood samples) is performed, there would be insufficient data to perform a meaningful statistical analysis. The protocol would then have to be repeated with new control and treatment group animals from the same source using the same experimental design and test article. At the end, after assuring (by statistical calculations) that the two sets of data are comparable, the data from survivors of the second study could be combined, or pooled, with those from survivors of the first experiment. However, this approach would require a greater degree of effort than a single up-front study with larger groups. In addition, combining samples across data sets leads to increased variability in the experimental groups and decreased statistical power compared to a single study with larger group sizes.

2.4. Unbalanced Designs

Another frequently overlooked design option in toxicology is the use of an *unbalanced design*, where various group sizes are employed for different levels of treatment. There is no requirement that each group in a study, be it control, low dose, intermediate dose or high dose, has an equal number of experimental units assigned to it. Indeed, there are frequently good reasons to assign more experimental units to some group than to others.

All the major statistical methodologies have provisions to adjust for such inequalities, within certain limits. This change in number of subjects within one or more experimental groups is done to either compensate for losses due to possible deaths during the study, to give more sensitivity in detecting subtle effects at levels close to an effect threshold, or to provide more confidence to the assertion that no effect exists. It is always good practice to make sure that there is adequate statistical power to detect an effect size of interest before conducting the experiment. Scientists should play close attention to statistical power when using unbalanced designs for groups with small sample sizes to ensure that enough samples will be available for a proper statistical analysis at the end of the experiment.

2.5. Undesirable Variables

We are frequently confronted with the situation where an undesired variable influences our experimental results in a nonrandom fashion. Such a variable is called a *confounding variable*. Its presence, as discussed earlier, makes the clear attribution and analysis of effects at best difficult, and at worst impossible. Sometimes, such confounding variables are the result of conscious design or management decisions, such as the use of different instruments, personnel, facilities, or procedures for different test groups within the same study (Morton et al., 2019). Occasionally, however, such a confounding variable is the result of unintentional factors or actions, in which case it is sometimes called a *lurking variable*. Such variables are almost always the result of standard operating procedures (SOPs) being violated. Common examples include waterers that are not connected to a rack of animals over a weekend, a set of racks not cleaned as frequently as others, or provision of rations from a contaminated batch of feed. A discussion of confounding variables can be found in Study Design and Conduct Considerations that optimize Pathology Data Generation, Reporting, and Overall Study Outcome (Vol 1, Chap 28).

2.6. Experimental Unit

The *experimental unit* in toxicology encompasses a wide variety of possibilities. It may be cells, plates of microorganisms, individual animals, litters of animals, etc. The importance of clearly defining the experimental unit is that the number of such units per group is the n, which is used in statistical calculations or analyses, because the value of n critically affects such calculations. The experimental unit is the unit that receives the treatment and yields a response that is measured and becomes a datum. A distinction should be made between biological replicates and technical replicates. Biological replicates refer to the smallest experimental unit that independently receives the treatment and are therefore sometimes referred to as "true replicates." Technical replicates represent repeated measurements of the same unit that describe the variability of the experimental protocol. In many cases, the technical replicates can be averaged over the same biological sample in order to produce the values for the biological replicates for statistical analysis.

3. EXPERIMENTAL DESIGN

Toxicological experiments generally are designed to answer two questions. The first question is whether or not an agent results in an *effect* on a biological system. The second question, never far behind, is *how much* of an effect is present. It has become increasingly desirable that the results and conclusions of studies aimed at assessing the effects of environmental agents and biopharmaceuticals be as clear and unequivocal as possible. It is essential that every experiment and study yield as much information as possible, and that the results of each study have the greatest possible chance of answering the questions for which the experiment was conducted. The statistical aspects of such efforts, so far as they are aimed at structuring experiments to maximize the possibilities of success of answering the questions above, are called experimental design.

3.1. Basic Principles of Experimental Design

The five basic statistical principles of experimental design are control, replication, randomization, concurrent (local) control, and balance (Cochran and Cox, 1992). The goal of the five principles of experimental design is *statistical efficiency* and the *economizing of resources*. The single most important initial step in achieving such an outcome is to define clearly the objective of the study, so that a clear statement can be made regarding what questions are being asked. The five principles may be summarized as follows.

Control

Control in experimentation is central to determining treatment effect. Control is the term used to describe efforts made by the researcher to remove any known systematic influence on the experiment. That is, all variables except for the independent variables under study are

removed. Failure to control for other systematic influences on the dependent variables means that the researcher cannot determine whether the effect was due to the experimental independent variable(s) or some other *source of systematic variation*. It should be noted that there are numerous sources of systematic variation ranging from the obvious, such as gender of the test species, to those that are easy to overlook, such as differences in handling by two different animal care attendants.

All inferential experiments have one or more control groups. These groups are assumed to be free of all systematic sources of variation including the independent variable(s). It may be necessary to have both negative and positive controls, where in addition to the absence of the independent variables another group is treated with a known positive outcome for the purposes of comparison. Multiple negative controls may be used where a systematic source of variation is expected. For example, a negative and pair-fed control may be used when treatment-related anorexia is known from previous studies. It is of interest that the French term for control is *temoin*, which when translates as "witness." Obviously, a witness should not be biased to the outcome of an investigation.

Replication

Any treatment must be applied to more than one experimental unit (animal, plate of cells, litter of offspring, etc.). This provides more accuracy in the measurement of a response than can be obtained from a single observation, since underlying experimental errors and biological variability tend to be averaged over the replicates. It also supplies an estimate of the experimental error derived from the variability between each of the measurements taken (or replicates). In practice, this means that an experiment should have enough experimental units in each treatment group (that is, a large enough number, or *n*) so that reasonably sensitive statistical analysis of data can be performed. The estimation of sample size is addressed in detail later in this chapter.

A distinction needs to be made between replication and duplication. *Replication* is the method of using different experimental units to increase the experimental number. An example of replication is giving the same severity rank (diagnosis, or score) to similar lesions from two mice. On the other hand, *duplication* is characterized by repeated measurements on the same experimental unit (e.g., coded ["blind"] reanalysis of lesions followed by giving a second severity rank to the same lesion). The purpose of duplication is to gain an understanding of precision of the measurements, in this case the severity rank. The distinction between replication and duplication is important to make when the toxicologic pathologist discusses the need—or not—to reassess sections of a study in a blinded manner.

Randomization

Randomization is practiced to ensure that every treatment shall have its fair share of results from among the spectrum of possible outcomes. It also serves to allow the toxicologic pathologist to proceed as if the assumption of independence is valid, meaning that there is no avoidable (i.e., known) systematic bias in how one obtains data. Animals are often randomized by body weight in most general toxicology studies. However, mechanistic studies with focused hypotheses for particular endpoints may require more and more sophisticated randomization scheme based on multiple endpoints such as resting glucose levels and bone density. More specific aspects of randomization are discussed in detail in Section B below.

Concurrent Control

Comparisons between treatments should be made to the maximum extent possible between experimental units from the same closely defined population. Therefore, animals used for the control group should come from the *same* source, lot, age, gender, etc., as test group animals. Except for the treatment being evaluated, test and control animals should be maintained and handled in exactly the same manner.

A true *concurrent control* is one that is identical in every manner with the treatment groups except for the presence of the treatment being evaluated. This means that all manipulations, including gavage with equivalent volumes of vehicle or exposure to equivalent rates of air exchanges in an inhalation chamber, should be duplicated in control groups just as they occur in treatment groups.

Balance

When several different factors are being evaluated simultaneously, the experiment should be laid out in such a way that the contributions of the different factors might be separately distinguished and estimated. Different types of experimental design help clarify the importance and interaction of the various factors. Statistical testing is less sensitive to unequal group variance, and power is greatest, when group sizes are similar. It may be tempting to place more animals in the treated group to better see the effect; after all, we know that the untreated animals will be normal. However, such an uneven weighting among control and treatment groups weakens statistical analysis of the experiment. *Counterbalancing* refers to the procedure of avoiding confounding among variables by including every possible sequence of a factor in a study. For designs in which the same subject is presented with multiple conditions over time (within subjects or repeated measures designs), it is important to control for the effects of nuisance variables through counterbalancing. In a study of the effects of two treatments on a particular outcome, by applying a treatment to half of the subjects exposed to one treatment before they are exposed to the second treatment, while the other half of the subjects are exposed to the treatments in the reverse order, the order of treatment is not a confounding factor in the study.

3.2. Detecting Treatment Effects

There are multiple facets of any study that may affect its ability to detect an effect of a treatment. The most important with respect to interpretation of toxicologic pathology data are considered here.

Choice of Species and Strain

It is important to have enough animals in the study so that a rigorous biological and statistical evaluation can be conducted. Ideally, the responses of interest should be rare in untreated and vehicle-treated control animals but should be evoked with reasonable ease by appropriate treatments. However, in practice, it is not uncommon to find a range of baseline responses in any given study. Common examples discerned by pathology evaluation include tissue degeneration and neoplasia. Some species or specific strains, perhaps because of inappropriate diets or gender-specific factors, have high background incidences of certain nonneoplastic and neoplastic conditions (e.g., chronic progressive nephropathy of F344 rats, hepatic tumors in mice) which make increases both difficult to detect and problematic to interpret. Guidelines from the Organization for Economic Cooperation and Development (OECD) recommend at least 20 animals per sex for each dose group along with a concurrent control for chronic toxicity studies. For carcinogenicity studies, there should be at least 50 animals per sex for each group (OECD, 2010).

Sampling

Sampling is an essential step upon which any meaningful experimental result depends. Sampling may involve the selection of which individual data points will be collected, which animals to collect tissue samples from, or taking a sample of a diet mix for chemical analysis.

There are three assumptions about sampling that are common to most of the statistical analysis techniques that are used in toxicology. The assumptions are that the sample is collected without bias, each member of a sample is collected independently of the others, and members of a sample are collected with replacements. Precluding bias, both intentional and unintentional, means that at the time a sample is selected from a population; each portion of that population has an equal chance of being selected. Independence means that the selection of any portion of the sample is not affected by, and does not affect, the selection of any other portion. Finally, sampling with replacement means that, in theory, after each portion is selected and measured, it is returned to the total sample pool and thus has the opportunity to be selected again. This last assumption is a corollary of the assumption of independence. Violation of this assumption, which is almost always the case in toxicologic pathology and all the life sciences (where tissue samples cannot be reattached), does not have serious consequences if the total pool from which samples are selected is sufficiently large (30 or greater) that the chance of reselecting that portion again is relatively small.

Sampling Methods

There are four major types of sampling methods: *random, stratified, systematic*, and *cluster*.

RANDOM

Random sampling is by far the most commonly employed sampling method. It stresses fulfillment of the assumption of avoiding bias. When the entire pool of possibilities is mixed (or randomized), then the members of the group are selected in the order that they are drawn from the pool.

STRATIFIED

Stratified sampling is performed first by dividing the entire pool of data into subsets (or strata) and then conducting randomized sampling from within each stratum. This method is employed when the total pool contains subsets that are distinctly different, but within each subset, the members are similar. An example is a large batch of a powdered pesticide in which it is desired to determine the nature of the particle size distribution. Larger pieces or particles are on the top, progressively smaller particles have settled lower in the container and are at the bottom, and the material has been packed and compressed into aggregates. To determine a representative answer to whether there is a particle size distribution as hypothesized, appropriate subsets from each subset (in this case, each layer) should be selected, mixed, and randomly sampled. This method is used quite commonly in diet studies.

SYSTEMATIC

In *systematic sampling*, a sample is taken at set intervals. For example, every fifth container of reagent is sampled, or a sample is collected from a fixed sample point in a flowing stream at regular time intervals. This approach is most commonly employed in quality assurance and quality control procedures.

CLUSTER

In *cluster sampling*, the pool is already divided into numerous separate groups, such as bottles of tablets. Small sets from these groups (such as several bottles of tablets) are selected, and a few individual units (i.e., tablets) from each group (i.e., bottle) are selected for analysis. The result is a cluster of measures from several groups. Like systematic sampling, this method is commonly used in quality control or in environmental studies when the effort and expense of physically collecting a small group of units is significant.

Sampling in Toxicologic Pathology Studies

In classical studies where toxicologic pathology is used, sampling arises in a practical sense in a limited number of situations. First, sampling often occurs by selecting a subset of animals or test systems to make some measurement at intervals during a study, which either destroys or stresses the measured system or is expensive. Examples include interim necropsies in a chronic study or collecting multiple blood samples from some animals during a study. Second, samples may be taken to analyze inhalation chamber atmospheres to characterize aerosol distributions with a new generation system. Third, samples of diet to which test material has been added may be collected. Fourth, quality control samples may be performed on an analytical chemistry operation by having duplicate analyses performed on some materials. In addition, duplicates, replicates, and blanks are used to ensure that the results can be relied upon; by using such samples, the specificity, sensitivity, accuracy, precision, limit of quantitation, and ruggedness can be determined. Finally, samples of selected data may be required to audit for quality assurance purposes.

Dose Levels

The *selection of dose levels* and dosing methodology is a very important and often controversial aspect of study design. In screening studies aimed at *hazard identification*, it is normal to test at dose levels higher than those to which humans likely will be exposed, but not at levels so high that overt toxicity occurs, in order to avoid requiring unreasonably large numbers of animals. One of the tested doses must elicit toxicity. A range of doses is usually tested to guard against the possibility of a misjudgment in selecting an appropriate high dose. A dose range is required because the metabolic pathways at high doses may differ markedly from those at lower doses. In studies aimed more at risk estimation, increased frequency of lower doses may be tested to obtain better information on the shape of the dose–response curve.

Unfortunately, in practice, the shape of the curve in the very low dose range often is not known. This lack is particularly important in assessing risk to cancer where the incidence of neoplasia that may be detected in a typical rodent bioassay is on the order of 2%. For the purposes of risk assessment, risk estimates applied when setting human exposure limits are at least 1000-fold lower (i.e., 10^{-5}). For this reason, carcinogenicity studies do not have much ability to characterize the shape of the curve for an assessment at lower dose (or exposure) levels.

Number of Animals

This sample size is obviously an important determinant of the precision of the findings. The calculation of the appropriate number depends on the size of the effect it is desired to detect. Very small effects may require a larger n (number of animals) per group, while obvious effects may permit smaller group sizes. The animal number is also impacted by the false-positive rate (α level or Type I error, which is the probability of an effect being detected when none exists). Similarly, the false-negative rate (β level or Type II error, or the probability of no effect being detected when one of exactly the critical sizes exists) influences the number of experimental units required. Finally, the measure of the variability of the animals' response influences the number required.

Tables relating numbers of animals required to obtaining α and β values of a given size are given in many references in the Suggested Reading. Software is also available for this purpose. As a rule of thumb, to reduce the critical difference by a factor n for a given α and β, the number of animals required will have to increase by a factor n^2.

Duration of the Study

The duration of the toxicity study is generally driven by the nature of the clinical trial that is being supported; however, some studies or dose groups have to be terminated prior to schedule sacrifice due to animal care and use considerations. It is important not to terminate a study too early, especially where the incidence of the effects of interest is strongly age related. The death datum is a powerful quantal point giving a definite answer (yes or no). However, it also important not to allow a study to continue for too long (i.e., beyond the point where further time on study likely will not provide any useful incremental information). For nonfatal conditions, the ideal stop point on average is to necropsy the animals when the prevalence of death is around 50%, as greater mortality than this often invalidates the assumptions used in the statistical analysis.

Stratification

To detect a treatment difference with accuracy, it is important that the groups being compared are as homogeneous as possible with respect to all other (nontreatment) variables, whether or not such variables are known or suspected causes of the response. Unfortunately, there are a number of reasons why groups may not be homogeneous. For example, suppose that there is another known important cause of the response for which the animals vary; in other words, there are two, not one, systematic sources of variation (factors) in the experiment, even though the experiment was designed for one source (the treatment). Such a situation may arise when the group includes a mixture of hyper- and hyporesponders to the treatment. Because the randomization scheme did not account for the hyper- and hyporesponses seen in this experiment, it is possible that the treated group may have a higher proportion of hyperresponders. This *bias* will lead to a higher response in the treatment group regardless of whether the treatment has an effect of not. Even if the proportion of hyperresponders is the same as in the controls, it will be more difficult to detect an effect of treatment because of the increased between-animal variability.

If the second factor (degree of responsiveness) is known before the experiment begins, it should be taken into account in both the design and analysis of the study. In the design, it can be used as a *blocking factor* to correct for potential *allocation bias*. This blocking factor will ensure that animals with hyper- or hyposensitivity are allocated equally, or in the correct proportion, to control and treated groups. In the analysis, the second factor should be treated as a stratifying variable, with separate treatment-control comparisons made at each level, and the comparisons combined for an overall test of difference. This is discussed later, where the *factorial design* is provided as an example of a more complex experimental design to investigate the separate effects of multiple treatments.

Randomization

Randomization is the arrangement of experimental units to simulate a chance distribution, reduce the interference by irrelevant variables, and yield unbiased statistical data. Randomization is a control against bias in assignment of subjects to test groups. If randomization is not carried out, one can never be sure whether or not treatment-control differences are due to the treatment or rather to confounding by other systematic sources of variation. In other words, unless randomization is used, we cannot determine whether the experimental treatment had an effect, or whether an observed effect was due to uneven allocation of the animals among experimental groups by chance.

The need for randomization applies not only to the allocation of the animals to the treatment but also to any method, person, or practice that can materially affect the recorded response. The same random number that is used to apply animals to treatment group can be used to determine cage position, order of weighing, order of bleeding for clinical chemistry, order of necropsy at termination, to choose the technician attending and the pathologist evaluating the gross necropsy, and so on. The location of the animal in the room in which it is kept may affect the animal's response. An example is the strong relationship between incidence of retinal atrophy in albino rats and closeness to the lighting source. Systematic differences in cage position should be avoided, preferably via randomization.

Randomization is the act of assigning a number of items (e.g., plates of bacteria or test animals) to groups in such a manner that there is an equal chance for any one item to end up in any one group. A variation on randomization is *censored randomization*, which ensures that the groups are equivalent in some aspect after the assignment process is complete. The most common example of a censored randomization is one in which it is ensured that the body weights of test animals in each group are not significantly different from those in the other groups. This is done by analyzing group weights both for homogeneity of variance and by ANOVA after animal assignment, then again randomizing if there is a significant difference at some nominal level, such as $P \leq 0.10$. The process is repeated until there is no significant difference among groups. There are several methods for actually performing the randomization process. The three most commonly used are card assignment, use of a random number table, and use of a computerized algorithm.

CARD ASSIGNMENT

For the card-based method, individual identification numbers for items (plates or animals, for example) are placed on separate index cards. These cards are then shuffled, placed one at a time in succession into piles corresponding to the required test groups. The results are a random group assignment.

RANDOM NUMBER TABLE METHOD

The random number table method requires only that one have unique numbers assigned to test subjects and access to a random number table. One sets up a table with a column for each group to which subjects are to be assigned, while randomization starts from the head of any one column of numbers in the random table. Each time the table is used, a new starting point should be utilized. As digits are found which correspond to a subject number, the subject is assigned to a group (enter its identifying number in a column) proceeding to assign subjects to groups from left to right filling one row at a time. After a number is assigned to an animal, any duplication of its unique number must be ignored, as many successive columns of random numbers are used as is required to complete the process.

COMPUTERIZED RANDOM NUMBER GENERATION

The third (and now most common) method is to use a random number generator that is built into a calculator or computer program. Procedures for generating these are generally documented in user manuals.

Adequacy of Control Group

While *historical control data* can be useful on occasion, a properly designed study demands that a relevant concurrent control group be included with which results for the test group can be compared (Elmore et al., 2009). The principle that like should be compared with like,

apart from treatment, demands that control animals should be randomized from the same source as treatment animals. An experiment involving treatment of a compound in a solvent, which included only an untreated control group, would indicate that any differences observed could only be attributed to the compound-solvent combination. To determine the specific effects of the compound, a comparison group given the solvent only, by the same route of administration, would be required.

Selecting Statistical Procedures Upfront

A priori selection of statistical methodology, as opposed to the *post hoc* approach, is as significant a portion of the process of protocol development and experimental design as any other and can measurably enhance the value of the experiment or study. Prior selection of null hypotheses and statistical methodologies is essential for proper design of other portions of a protocol such as the number of animals per group or the sampling intervals for body weight. The analysis of any set of data is dictated to a large extent by the manner in which the data are obtained.

Statistical testing relies on the probability that a particular result would be found according to chance, where the risk is referred to as the significance level. A 0.05 significance level indicates that 5% of the statistically significant results would be expected to be false positives due to chance. Therefore, it is not appropriate to repeatedly switch statistical procedures while analyzing a data set until a statistically significant or desirable result is found. This approach would have a very high probability of generating a misleading result, since it fails to acknowledge that a result obtained in this way would almost certainly be found after a large enough number of attempts. This unsound approach to data analysis is often referred to as "data dredging," "data snooping," or "*p* hacking."

Bias and the Toxicologic Pathologist

Data must be generated and recorded in an unbiased manner. It is recognized that many options exist for analysis, which will be discussed below. However, biased data generation, compiled with the knowledge of the operator, represents scientific fraud.

GOOD LABORATORY PRACTICES

Good Laboratory Practices (GLPs) have been implemented to ensure that the data analyzed represent the data generated from the experiment. GLPs have three main components: requirements for personnel, requirements for facilities, and requirements to create SOPs and records of events undertaken in the study (Volume 1: Pathology and GLPs, Quality Control and Quality Assurance in a global environment). GLP practices guard against "data snooping" by requiring that investigators conform to a pre-planned statistical analysis.

OBSERVER BIAS

Observer bias can occur when the observer is aware of the treatment. This knowledge may consciously influence the observer through true bias of observation, or unconsciously as *reading bias*, also referred to as *work-up bias*. In slide reading, or examination bias, the observer increases his or her attention to a lesion, once noted in the sections, resulting in an effect known as diagnostic drift. In some situations, it may be necessary to reread all the slides in a *blinded* fashion and in random order to be sure that diagnostic drift is avoided.

Elimination bias occurs when data are eliminated for various reasons. Usually, such protocol violations will be recorded; however, it should be noted that valid analysis could not be conducted unless one can distinguish among animals that were examined and did not have the relevant response vs. animals that were not examined. Therefore, it is important clearly to identify which data are missing and for what reason.

INFORMED ANALYSIS

In many instances, toxicologic pathologists practice an informed (nonblinded) approach to histopathological evaluation. When using an informed approach, the pathologist has full information about the dose, exposure groups, and other information pertaining to the animals in the experiment. Informed analyses may be needed in order to establish how lesions produced in response to treatment differ from the normal biology found in concurrent controls, conduct a study without exorbitant cost, or to complete evaluations in a timely manner. The danger in informed analysis would be potential subjectivity in diagnoses through observer bias and tends to contradict commonly held principles of the scientific method and statistical theory. Nevertheless, informed analysis is widely used and has become the general recommended practice in toxicologic pathology (Society of Toxicologic Pathology, 1986; Crissman et al., 2004; Burkhardt et al., 2010; Neef et al., 2012).

When informed evaluations are used, it is important to utilize procedures to diminish potential observer bias and promote reproducibility in diagnoses. For instance, an organization might utilize an independent peer review process, clear nomenclature published that has been published and broadly accepted, and incorporation of supporting data such as criteria used for experimental design, body and organ weight data, and clinical pathology results. It is important that informed approaches be performed by well-trained pathologists without any conflicts of interest.

Informed analyses have great utility when they are implemented with careful planning and conduct. Nevertheless, blinded studies should be used to the extent possible. Informed analyses should be supported by blinded evaluations on subsets of the samples and reevaluations. Blinded evaluations may be required in circumstances for which some of the conditions above cannot be met, and for evaluations of subtle lesions or when lesion severity is similar between control and treatment conditions.

3.3. Censoring

Understanding the concept of *censoring* is essential to the design of experiments in toxicologic pathology. Censoring involves the exclusion of measurements from certain experimental units, or the experimental units themselves, from consideration in data analysis or inclusion in the experiment. Censoring may occur either prior to initiation of an experiment as a planned procedure, during the course of an experiment as an unplanned procedure (e.g., through the death of animals), or after the conclusion of an experiment, when data usually are excluded because they represent some form of outlier response.

In practice, a priori censoring in toxicology studies occurs in the assignment of experimental units, usually animals, to test groups. The most familiar example is the practice of assigning test animals among groups in acute, subacute, subchronic, and chronic studies, where the results of otherwise random assignments are evaluated for body weights of the assigned members. If the mean weights are found to differ by some preestablished criterion, such as a marginally significant $(P < .10)$ difference found by ANOVA, then members are reassigned, or censored, to achieve comparability across groups in terms of starting body weights. Such a procedure of animal assignment to groups is known as a *censored randomization*.

3.4. Impacts of Sample Size

The first precise or calculable aspect encountered when designing an experiment is determining sufficient test and control group sizes to allow one to have an adequate level of confidence in the results of a study. In other words, calculations are in order to ensure the ability of the study design with the statistical tests used to detect a true difference, or effect, when it is present, where the statistical test contributes a level of power to such detection.

The power of a statistical test is the probability that a test rejects the null hypothesis, H_0, when some other hypothesis, H_1, is valid. This is termed the power of the test with respect to the alternative hypothesis H_1. If there is a set of possible alternative hypotheses, the power, regarded as a function of H_1, is termed the *power function* of the statistical test. When the alternatives are indexed by a single parameter, simple graphical presentation of the power function (a two-dimensional line graph) is possible. If the parameter is a vector, one needs to visualize a power surface (a chart describing a shape function in three dimensions). This is the significance level. A test's power is greatest when the probability of a type II error, which is the probability of missing an effect (i.e., false negative), is lowest. Specified powers can be calculated for tests in any specific or general situation.

A general rule to keep in mind is that the more stringent (lower) the significance level desired, the greater the necessary sample size. Greater protection from an incorrect conclusion requires greater effort. More subjects are needed for a 1% level test than for a 5% level test. Two-tailed tests require larger sample sizes than one-tailed tests to maintain the same power; assessing two directions at the same time requires a greater investment. The smaller the critical effect size, the larger the necessary sample size; any difference can be significant if the sample size is large enough. The larger the power required, the larger the necessary sample size. The smaller the sample size, the lower the power. The requirements and means of calculating necessary sample size depend on the desired (or practical) comparative sizes of treatment and control groups.

The sample size n can be calculated, for example, for equal-sized test and control groups, using the following equation (Eq. 16.7).

Calculation of the number of animals required for an experiment

$$n = \frac{2(z_1 + z_2)^2}{\delta^2}\sigma^2 \qquad (16.7)$$

-where z_1 is the z critical value corresponding to the desired level of confidence $1 - \alpha$ given by $z_{1-\alpha/2}$; z_2 is the z critical value corresponding to the probability of correctly rejecting the H_0 (or power) given by $z_{1-\beta}$; σ is the common variance, derived typically from historical data; and δ is the desired treatment difference ($\delta = \mu_2 - \mu_1$).

4. DESIGNS COMMONLY USED IN TOXICOLOGIC PATHOLOGY

There are six basic experimental design types used in toxicology. These are *the completely randomized, the completely randomized block, matched pairs, Latin square, factorial*, and *nested design*. Other designs that are used are really combinations of these basic designs and are very rarely employed in toxicologic pathology. However, before examining these six basic types, we must first examine the basic concept of blocking.

Blocking is the arrangement or sorting of the members of a population, such as all test animals within an available pool for the study, into treatment groups based on certain characteristics, which may, but are not sure to, alter an experimental outcome. Characteristics that are frequently selected for blocking may cause a treatment to give a differential effect. Examples include genetic background, age, sex, overall activity levels, and so on. The process of blocking attempts to evenly distribute members of each blocked group among the experimental groups.

4.1. Completely Randomized Design

A *completely randomized design* arranges experimental units to simulate a chance distribution. Here, animals are randomly assigned to any treatment group. There are no attempts made to evaluate the effects of any other source of variability except the treatment. This is the most common type of design and is particularly common in acute and subacute toxicologic pathology studies (Table 16.5).

4.2. Completely Randomized Block Design

Randomization is aimed at spreading out the effect of undetectable or unsuspected characteristics in a population of animals, or some portion of this population. The *completely randomized block design* merges the two concepts of randomization and blocking to produce the first experimental design that addresses sources of systematic variation other than the intended treatment.

This type of design requires that each treatment group have at least one member of each recognized group (e.g., animals of certain ages), the exact members of each block being assigned in an unbiased random fashion. In toxicologic pathology studies where the application of the treatment may take some time, the experiment may be blocked so that the first group of animals is randomly assigned in equal numbers to each and every treatment group. For example, the duration of surgery required to implant an experimental medical device may be such that blocking is necessary to account for systematic variation caused by the exact time of implantation (Table 16.6).

TABLE 16.5 Diagrammatic Representation of Treatment Allocation in a Completely Randomized Design

Treatment	
Placebo	Test substance
50	50

TABLE 16.6 Diagrammatic Representation of Treatment Allocation in a Randomized Block Design

	Treatment	
Gender	Placebo	Test substance
Male	250	250
Female	250	250

4.3. Matched Pairs Design

A *matched pairs design* is a special case of the randomized block design. It is used when the experiment has only two treatment conditions, allowing participants to be grouped into pairs based on some blocking variable. Within each pair, participants then are randomly assigned to different treatments.

Table 16.7 shows a matched pairs design for an experiment. The 1000 participants are grouped into 500 matched pairs. Each pair is matched based on two factors, age and gender. For example, Pair 1 could be two women aged 21, Pair 2 might be two women aged 22, and so on.

Like the completely randomized design and the randomized block design, the matched pairs design uses randomization to control for confounding factors. However, the matched pairs design is an improvement over the completely randomized design and the randomized block design. Of the three options, only the matched pairs design explicitly controls for the potential effects from two lurking (extraneous) variables: age and gender.

TABLE 16.7 An Example of Treatment Allocation in a Matched Pairs Design

	Treatment	
Pair	Placebo	Test substance
1	1	1
2	1	1
—	—	—
499	1	1
500	1	1

4.4. Latin Square Design

The *Latin Square Design* is the second experimental design that addresses sources of systematic variation other than the intended treatment. It assumes that one can characterize treatments, whether intended or otherwise, as belonging clearly to separate sets. These categories are arranged into two sets of rows. An example would be a developmental toxicity study in which the rows give the source litter of the test animal (with the first litter as row 1, the next as row 2, etc.), while the columns define a secondary category like the ages of the test animals (with 6–8 weeks as column 1, 8–10 weeks as column 2, and so on). Experimental units are then assigned so that each major treatment, such as control, low dose, intermediate dose, etc., appears once and only once in each row and each column. If one denotes test groups as *A* (control), *B* (low), *C* (intermediate), and *D* (high), such an assignment would resemble that shown in Table 16.8. Here, it can be seen that randomized experimental units are assigned to a treatment group, and then randomly assigned to a place in the Latin square.

4.5. Factorial Design

The fifth type of experimental design that addresses sources of systematic variation other than the intended treatment is the *factorial design*. Two or more clearly understood factors, such as exposure level to test chemical, animal age, or temperature, are considered in the design. The classical approach to this situation is to hold all but one of the treatments constant, and at any one time to vary just that one factor. If it is suspected that the two factors are independent so that each will have an effect on the outcome, a factorial design may be used to obtain greater information regarding the effect of each factor, and to determine the extent of the *interaction* (if any) between the factors with respect to altering the outcome.

In the factorial design, all levels of a given factor are combined with all levels of every other factor in the experiment. Consider two factors, 1 and 2. When a change in factor 1 produces a different outcome in the response variable (e.g., incidence or severity of a disease) at one level of factor 2 than occurs at other levels of the factor, then there is an interaction between the two factors being tested, which can then be analyzed as an interaction effect. The terminology used to describe a factorial design is (number of levels of factor 1) × (number of levels of factor 2) (Table 16.9). For example, one can make, design, and evaluate the dose response on two different strains off mouse. If four dose levels are used in three strains of mouse, then a 4 × 3 factorial design could be used to show the dose effect, the strain effect, and—if an effect is seen—whether there is an interaction between dose and strain (Table 16.9).

4.6. Nested Design

The last of the major varieties of experimental design are the *nested designs* (Tables 16.10 and 16.11), where the levels of one factor are nested within, or are subsamples of, another factor (i.e., a subfactor). A factor *A* is nested within another factor *B* if the levels or values of *A* are different for every level or value of *B*. Each subfactor is evaluated only within the limits of its

TABLE 16.8　Diagrammatic Representation of Treatment Allocation in a Latin Square Design

Source litter	Age at necropsy			
	6–8 weeks	8–10 weeks	10–12 weeks	12–14 weeks
1	A	B	C	D
2	B	C	D	A
3	C	D	A	B
4	D	A	B	C

TABLE 16.9   An Example of a 2 × 2 Factorial Design

		Severity of lesions (median ± IQR)	
		Dose 1	Dose 2
Mouse Strain	CD-1	1+ (±0.5)	3+ (±1.0)
	TGAC	4+ (±0)	4+ (±0)

-where IQR is the interquartile range.

single larger factor at each level except the first, or highest. For example, the influence of cumulative dose level when duration of exposure is the largest factor would be examined only within that context of that factor, and not within the context of frequency of dosing, a lesser factor.

Nested designs can be balanced or unbalanced. In an unbalanced nested design, the numbers of subfactors and observations may not be the same for each factor. In addition, there may be a number of stages, depending on the

number of subsamples selected. For example, in the tiered screening approach for selecting drug candidates for development, early stages will look at larger numbers of possibilities, and therefore examine fewer factors (an aspect of a drug's property) than is the case in later stages, where only a successively smaller number of the early candidate drugs are evaluated more extensively (that is, more factors are considered).

An example of the output of a nested design can be seen in the Table below.

5. FUNCTIONS OF STATISTICAL ANALYSES

In addition to describing the data, statistical methods may serve to do any combination of three other possible tasks: hypothesis testing, modeling, and reduction of dimensionality. The

TABLE 16.10   An Illustration of a Two-Stage Nested Design

Factor	1				2				3			
Subfactor	1	2	3	4	1	2	3	4	1	2	3	4
Observation												
	Y111	Y121	Y131	Y141	Y211	Y221	Y231	Y241	Y311	Y321	Y331	Y341
	Y112	Y122	Y132	Y142	Y212	Y222	Y232	Y242	Y312	Y322	Y332	Y342
	Y113	Y123	Y133	Y143	Y213	Y223	Y233	Y243	Y313	Y323	Y333	Y343

TABLE 16.11   Tabular Representation of Nested PCR Results From a Nested Design

Nested PCR	PCR		
	Positive ($n = 37$)	Negative ($n = 91$)	Total ($n = 128$)
GROUP I			
Positive	24	12	36
Negative	0	8	8
Total	24	20	44
GROUP II			
Positive	13	13	26
Negative	0	58	58
Total	13	71	84

one function most readers will be most familiar with is *hypothesis testing* (i.e., determining if two or more groups of data differ from each other at a predetermined level of significance). The construction and use of *models* is important for helping to predict future outcomes of chemical–biological interactions. The most common use of models is linear regression or the derivation of some form of correlation coefficient. Model fitting allows us to relate one variable (typically a treatment or "independent" variable) to another. The third function, *reduction of dimensionality*, is less commonly utilized than the first two. This final category includes methods for decreasing the number of variables in a system while only minimally reducing the amount of information, therefore making a problem easier to visualize and to understand. Examples of such techniques are *factor analysis* and *cluster analysis*. A subset of this last function, discussed later under descriptive statistics, is the reduction of raw data to single expressions of central tendency and variability.

5.1. Hypothesis Testing and Probability (P) Values

A relationship of a given treatment to some toxicological endpoint is often stated to be *statistically significant* ($P < .05$). What does this really mean? First, statistical significance need not necessarily imply biological importance, if the endpoint under study is not relevant to the animal's well-being. Second, the statement will usually be based only on the data from the study in question and will not take into account prior knowledge. In some situations (e.g., when one or two of a very rare tumor type are seen in treated animals), statistical significance may not be achieved but the finding may be biologically quite important, especially if a similar treatment was previously found to elicit a similar response. Third, the P-value does not describe the probability that a true treatment effect exists. Rather, a P-value describes the probability that the observed response, or one or more extremes, will occur by chance alone. A P-value that is not significant is consistent with a treatment having a small effect, or that was not detected with sufficient certainty in the study. Finally, there are two types of P-values. A *one-tailed* (or one

sided) P-value is the probability of getting by chance a treatment effect in a specified direction, like as great as or greater than that observed. A *two-tailed* P-value is the probability of getting, by chance alone, a treatment difference in either direction that is as great as or greater than that observed. By convention, P-values are always two tailed unless a one-tailed P-value is specified.

It is not preferable, when presenting results of statistical analyses, to mark results (as do some laboratories) simply as significant or not significant at one defined probability level (usually $P < .05$) by an asterisk or some other symbol. This practice does not allow the reader any real chance to judge whether or not the effect is a true one.

The criterion $P < .05$ implies a false-positive incidence of 1 in 20, and though now embedded in regulation, practice, and convention, was somewhat an arbitrary choice to begin with. In interpreting P-values, it is important to realize they are only an aid to judgment to be used in conjunction with other available information. One might validly consider a $P < .01$ increase as chance when it was unexpected, occurred only at a low-dose level with no such effect seen at higher doses, and was evident in only one subset of the data. In contrast, a $P < .05$ increase might be convincing if it occurred in the top dose and was for an endpoint one might have expected to be increased from known properties of the chemical or closely related chemicals.

5.2. Modeling

In toxicologic pathology, modeling is of prime interest in seeking to relate a treatment variable (e.g., the test article) with an effect variable (e.g., hepatic centrilobular necrosis). The resulting model can then be used to predict ("model") values of the effect variable for different values of the treatment variable and vice versa, where only a few such values have been determined experimentally in advance in producing the model. Note that interpolative models can only accurately predict effects within the range of experimentally derived data points.

There are models for extrapolation that can be used to predict effects where data cannot be obtained, such as the probability of carcinogenesis responses following low-dose exposures. In such cases, the model may readily predict an outcome that cannot be verified by experiment. Models are also used to estimate how good our predictions are, and occasionally, simply to determine if a pattern of effects is related to a pattern of treatment.

Interpolation is the term used to describe efforts made to establish a pattern between several data points. This pattern may be in the form of a line or a curve. It is possible for any given set of points to produce an infinite set of lines or curves which pass near (for lines) or through (for curves) the data points. In most cases, the actual pattern is not known. Therefore, a basic principle of science—Occam's razor—is applied. This principle recognizes that the simplest explanation, or in this case model, that fits the facts or data is most likely to be the correct explanation. A straight line is, of course, the simplest pattern to describe, so fitting the best line using linear regression is the most common model used in toxicologic pathology.

It should be clearly understood that a *P*-value does not give direct information about the size of any effect that has occurred. A compound may elicit an increase in response by a given amount, but whether a study finds this increase to be statistically significant will depend on the size of the study and the dispersion of the data. In a small study, a large and important effect may be missed, especially if the endpoint is imprecisely measured. In a large study, on the other hand, a small and unimportant effect may emerge as statistically significant.

Hypothesis testing tells us whether an observed effect can or cannot be reasonably attributed to chance, but not how large the effect is. Although much statistical theory relates to hypothesis testing, currently, medical statistics are trending toward confidence interval (CI) estimation with differences between test and control groups expressed in the form of a best estimate, coupled with the 95% confidence interval (95% CI). A CI is used to estimate the uncertainty of a population parameter, such as a population mean, from observed data and represents the range of values in which the true population parameter is likely to be found. In screening studies of standard design, the tendency has been to concentrate mainly on hypothesis testing.

However, presentation of the results in the form of estimates with CIs can be a useful adjunct for some analyses and is very important in studies aimed specifically at quantifying the size of an effect.

Contrasted with these continuous data, however, there are discontinuous (or discrete) data, which can only assume certain fixed numerical values. In these cases, the choice of statistical tools or tests is, as described later, more limited.

5.3. Dimension Reduction

Each measured variable in a statistical analysis or a graphic presentation can also be considered as a vector for the variable—a line with an ordered array of values for the variable. In general, we can better visualize the relationship in a two-dimensional system (a flat surface) than in more complex multidimensional systems.

Dimension reduction is a way of devising one or two variables to summarize the information contained in a number of other variables. Decreasing the dimensionality of the data set reduces the data (exploratory multivariate statistics). This reduction step pertains to analytic methods that involve decreasing the dimensionality of a data set by extracting a number of underlying factors, dimensions, clusters, etc., which can account for the variability in the (multidimensional) data set.

Techniques for reducing dimensionality are those that simplify the visual or numerical aspects of data to improve an understanding of patterns while causing only minimal reductions in the amount of information present. These techniques typically operate primarily by pooling or combining groups of related variables into single variables. However, these methods may also entail the identification and elimination of variables that are irrelevant or provide little informative content.

Descriptive statistics (calculations of means, SDs, etc.) are the simplest and most familiar form of reducing dimensionality. Other forms of reduction require the general conceptual tools of *classification*. Classes provide means of exploring identities, quantities, similarities, and differences among groups of things that have more than a single linear scale of measurement in common. Accordingly, classification tools are required for stratification of data. All classes essentially have to be *mutually exclusive* and *mutually exhaustive*, so that data can be placed in only one class.

Multidimensional scaling (MDS) is a set of techniques for quantitatively analyzing similarities, dissimilarities, and distances between data in a display-like manner. *Nonmetric scaling* is an analogous set of methods for displaying and relating data when measurements are nonquantitative (i.e., either categorical [nominal] or ordinal). In such a case, attributes or ranks describe the data.

Principal components analysis (PCA) refers to procedures that can reduce a large set of variables, many of which may be correlated, to a much smaller set of variables that can still explain a large portion of the total variance in the data. The new variables, called principal components, are arranged according to order of importance according to the amount of variance explained, where the principal components are uncorrelated with each other. Accordingly, PCA permits a way to interpret the main patterns in the data by examination of a small number of principal components.

Cluster analysis is a collection of graphic and numerical methodologies for classifying things based on the relationships between the values of the variables that they share.

The final pair of methods for reducing dimensionality, which will be addressed later in this chapter, are *Fourier analysis* and *Life Table analysis*. Fourier analysis seeks to identify cyclic patterns in data and then analyzes either the patterns in the data or the nature of the residuals after the patterns are subtracted. *Life table analysis* is directed to identifying and quantifying the time course of certain risks (e.g., death, occurrence of tumors, etc.).

6. PREREQUISITES TO STATISTICAL ANALYSIS

Statistical analyses are tools that aid us in inferring whether experimental manipulations caused an effect, or that potential associations between putative risk factors and outcomes are likely. As statistical analysis is a supportive tool to assist in

decision-making, it is not always necessary to analyze data. If all events occur in one group, but not in any other, it is obvious where treatment effect lies (subject, of course, to reasonable sample sizes and appropriate conduct of experiments). Unfortunately, biology is rarely this simple. Usually, events of interest are seen in most, if not all, experimental groups. The question that statistical analysis attempts to answer is whether the difference in the frequency or severity (or a combination of frequency and severity) observed in different groups is due to chance or is instead a result of the experimental manipulation.

6.1. Describing the Data

Many of the variables studied in toxicology are in fact continuous. Examples of these are lengths, weights, concentrations, temperatures, periods of time, and percentages. These data usually have a distribution, which may or may not be normal in nature. Regardless of the type of distribution, efforts should be made to describe the data using visible inspection and comparison to a hypothetical normal distribution or a skewed distribution. The number that summarizes a data set is termed a descriptive statistic.

Descriptive statistics are used to summarize the location or *central tendency* of the data, and to provide a measure of the *dispersion* of the data in and about this central location. The *mean* (i.e., the average), the *median* (the number at the 50th percentile [i.e., the "middle"]), and the *mode* (the most common result) give a description of the location. In contrast, the *standard deviation* (SD), the *standard error of the mean* (SEM), the *interquartile range* (IQR or dQ), the *coefficient of variation* (CV), and the *range* give descriptions of dispersion. It should be noted that the choice of descriptive statistic can imply a particular type of distribution for the data.

Mean and Standard Deviation

Most commonly, *location* or *central tendency* is described by giving the (arithmetic) mean and dispersion by giving the SD or the SEM. The statistics that we are most familiar with are the mean, denoted by the symbol $\overline{X}$ (also called the arithmetic average); the SD, which is denoted by the symbol σ; and the SEM. The SD can be calculated as in the following equation (Eq. 16.8).

Formula for calculating the standard deviation (SD)

$$SD = \sqrt{\frac{1}{n-1}\sum\left(X-\overline{X}\right)^2} \qquad (16.8)$$

-where X is the individual datum, $\overline{X}$ is the mean of the X values, and n is the total number of data in the group.

Similarly, the SEM can be calculated using the following equation (Eq. 16.9):

Formula for calculating the standard error of the mean (SEM)

$$SEM = \frac{SD}{\sqrt{n}} \qquad (16.9)$$

-where SD is the standard deviation and n is the total number of data in the group.

The SD and the SEM are related to each other, but yet are quite different. The SEM is quite a bit smaller than the SD, making it very attractive to use in presenting data. This size difference is because the SEM actually is an estimate of the error (or variability) involved in measuring the means of samples, and not an estimate of the error (or variability) involved in measuring the data from which the means are calculated. The Central Limit Theorem implies this difference for a sufficiently large sample size. First, the Central Limit Theorem states that the distribution of sample means will be approximately normal regardless of the distribution of values in the original population from which the samples were drawn. Second, it defines the mean value of the collection. Finally, the theorem states that the SD of the collection of all possible means of samples of a given size, called the SEM, depends on both the SD of the original population and the size of the sample. The SEM should be used only when the uncertainty of the estimate of the mean is of concern, while the SD is reserved for describing the variability in the data.

The use of the mean with either the SD or SEM implies, however, that there is reason to believe that the samples of data being summarized are from a population that at least approximates normal distribution. If this is not the case, then it is preferable to use a set of statistical descriptions that do not require a normal distribution of data to be adequately described (or characterized) by mean and SD. These are the median,

for location, and the semiquartile distance (or IQR or dQ), for a measure of dispersion. Another situation can arise sometimes when data are distributed in a log-normal manner, which can be relatively easily transformed to give a normal distribution and therefore make the use of mean and SD or SEM appropriate. For log-normal data, the geometric mean and geometric SD are appropriate descriptors of central tendency and dispersion. Calculations performed on the geometric scale can be back transformed to the natural scale for presentation of the data.

Median and Interquartile Range

When the data in a group are arranged in a ranked order (that is, from smallest to largest), the median is the middle value, i.e., the 50th percentile. If there are an odd number of values in a group, then the middle value is obvious; for example, for a list of 13 values, the 7th largest is the median. When the number of values in the sample is even, the median is calculated as the midpoint between the $(n/2)^{th}$ and the $([n/2]+1)^{th}$ number. For instance, in the series of numbers 7, 12, 13, and 19, the median value would be the midpoint between 12 and 13, which is 12.5.

When data are ranked, a quartile of the data contains one ordered quarter of the values. Typically, the borders of the middle two quartiles $Q1$ and $Q3$, which together represent the semiquartile distance, and which contain the median as their center, describe dispersion. Given that there are N values in an ordered group of data, the upper limit of the jth quartile (Q_j) may be computed as being equal to the $[j(N+1)/4]^{th}$ value. Then the value can be computed for the IQR with the formula $IQR = Q_3 - Q_1$. For example, for the fifteen-value data set 1, 2, 3, 4, 4, 5, 5, 5, 6, 6, 6, 7, 7, 8, and 9, the upper limits of Q_1 and Q_3 can be calculated as follows (Eq. 16.10):

Calculation of the semiquartile distance (QD)

$$Q_1 = \frac{1(15+1)}{4} = \frac{16}{4} = 4$$
$$Q_3 = \frac{3(15+1)}{4} = \frac{48}{4} = 12 \qquad (16.10)$$

-where Q_1 is the first quartile and Q_3 the last quartile.

The 4th and 12th values in this data set are 4 and 7, respectively.

Mode and Range

The mode and range can be considered as descriptive statistics in assessing data sets from toxicologic pathology studies when the data are very skewed or may have a different distribution from normal. The mode describes the most common event, whereas the range describes the distance between the lowest and highest measurement.

Coefficient of Variation

There are times when description of the relative variability of one or more sets of data is desired. The most common way of doing this is to compute the CV, which is calculated as the ratio of the SD to the mean (Eq. 16.11).

Formula for calculating the coefficient of variation (CV)

$$CV = \frac{SD}{\overline{X}} \qquad (16.11)$$

-where SD is the standard deviation and X *bar* is the mean of the data.

A CV of 0.2 or 20% would mean that the SD is 20% of the mean. Due to the inherent variability of biological responses in toxicologic pathology studies, the CV is frequently between 20% and 50%, and may exceed 100%.

6.2. Statistical Graphics

The use of graphics in one form or another in statistics is the single most effective and robust tool in the analytical arsenal (Chambers et al., 2018; Cleveland, 1994; Gad and Taulbee, 1996; Schmid, 1983; Tufte, 2005). At the same time, graphics as a statistical tool is one of the most poorly understood and improperly used techniques. Graphs are used for one of four major purposes. Each of the four is a variation on the central theme of making complex data easier to understand and use. These four major functions are exploration, analysis, data communication and display, and graphical aids.

Exploration, simply summarizing data or trying to expose relationships between variables, shows the characteristics ("behavior") of data sets, allowing visual representation of the data and hypothesis generation. Data visualization may be performed by constructing a plot for a single variable, a scatterplot comparing two variables, or a multiple-study display such as a heat map (Troth et al., 2018). In studies with small sample sizes, it is very important to visualize the raw data points rather than rely on summary statistics since different data distributions can lead to the same summary statistics (Weissgerber et al., 2015). Also, visualization of a response variable over a time course can be an effective way to begin to understand important patterns of response. An example of an exploratory statistical graph is the scatter plot or scatter gram, an example of which is shown in Figure 16.3.

Analysis is the use of graphs to formally evaluate some aspect of the data, such as whether or not outliers are present or if an underlying assumption of a population distribution is fulfilled. Table 16.12 presents a summary of major graphical techniques that are available for this purpose. An example of graphic analysis can be seen in Figure 16.3.

Communication and *display* of data is the most commonly used function of statistical graphics in toxicologic pathology. These graphics are used for internal reports, presentations at meetings, and/or formal publications in the literature. In communicating data, graphs should not be used to duplicate information that is presented in tables, but rather to show important trends and/or relationships in the data. Though such communication most commonly represents a quantitative compilation of actual data, graphs can also be used to summarize and present the results of statistical analysis as well.

Graphical aids to calculation are graphs that are becoming outdated as microcomputers become more widely available. This fourth and final function of graphics includes *nomograms* and extrapolating and interpolating data graphically based on plotted data. The classic example of a nomogram in toxicology is that presented by Litchfield and Wilcoxon for determining median effective doses.

There are many forms of statistical graphics (a partial list, classified by function, is presented in Table 16.12), and a number of these, such as *scatter plots* and *histograms* (Figure 16.4), can be used for each of a number of possible functions. Most of these plots are based on a Cartesian

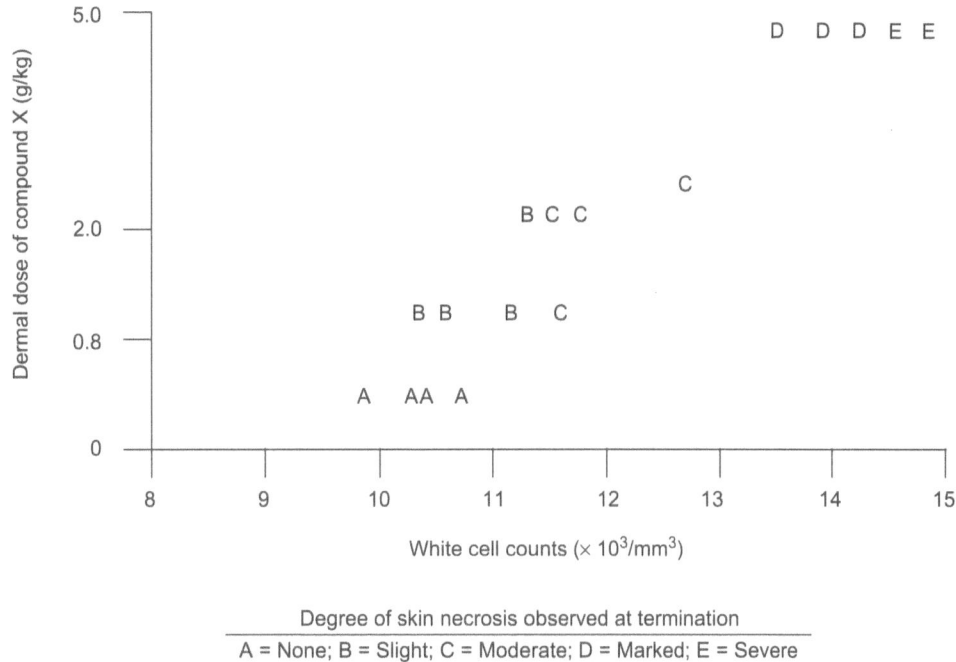

Degree of skin necrosis observed at termination
A = None; B = Slight; C = Moderate; D = Marked; E = Severe

FIGURE 16.3   **Descriptive scatterplot for dermal irritation study.**

system, i.e., they use a set of rectangular coordinates for plotting data. Our review of construction and use will focus on these forms of graphs.

Construction of a rectangular graph of any form starts with the selection of the appropriate form of graph followed by the laying out of the coordinates, or axes. Even graphs that are going to encompass *multivariate data* (i.e., more than two variables) generally have as their starting point two major coordinates. The horizontal axis (or *abscissa*, also called the *X*-axis) is generally used to present an independent variable, e.g., dose. The vertical axis (or *ordinate*, also called the *Y*-axis) is used to present a dependent variable, e.g., response. Each of these axes is scaled in the units of measure that will most clearly present the trends of interest in the data. The range covered by the scale of each axis is selected to cover the entire region for which data are presented. The actual demarcating of the measurement scale along an axis should allow for easy and accurate assessment of the coordinates of any data point, yet should not be cluttered (Table 16.13).

There are some rules that apply to diagrammatic representation of data. Data points should be presented by symbols that present the appropriate indicators of location. If symbols represent a summary of data from a normal data population, some indication of the variability, or uncertainty, associated with that population should be used. An example would be inclusion of error bars to represent the SD, or standard error, of the mean. It should be noted that error and variability are not synonymous. Both represent uncertainty, but variability is inherently irreducible, while error can be reduced through design and analysis. If the data are not normal or continuous, location should be represented by the median with the range or semiquartile distance showing the variability estimates. Symbols used to present data points can also be used to present a significant amount of additional information.

The three other forms of graphs that are commonly used are histograms, pie charts, and contour plots. *Histograms* are graphs of simple frequency distribution. The abscissa (*X*-axis) contains the independent variable of interest, such as life span or litter size, and is generally shown as classes or intervals of measurements (e.g., age ranges of 0–10, 10–20, etc., in weeks). The ordinate (*Y*-axis) displays the incidence or frequency of observations. The result is a set of vertical bars, each of which represents the incidence of a particular set of observations. Measures of error or variability about each incidence are reflected by some form of error bar on

TABLE 16.12   Forms of Statistical Graphs by Function Used for Preliminary Assessment of Data

Exploration

Data summary	Two variables	Three or more variables
Box and whisker plot	Autocorrelation plot	Biplot
Histogram	Cross-correlation plot	Cluster trees
Dot plot	Scatter plot	Labeled scatter plot
Frequency polygon	Sequence plot	Glyphs and metroglyphs
Ogive		Face plots
Stem and leaf diagram		Fourier plots
		Similarity and preference maps
		Multidimensional scaling displays
		Weathervane plot

Analysis

Distribution assessment	Model evaluation and assumption verification	Decision making
Probability plot	Average versus standard deviation	Control charts
Q–Q plot	Component plus residual plot	Cusum chart
P–P plot	Partial residual plots	Half normal plot
Hanging histogram	Residual plots	Ridge trace
Rootagram		Youden plot
Poissonness plot		

top of, or within, the frequency bars. The size of class intervals may be unequal (in effect, one can combine, or pool, several small class intervals), but it is proper in such cases to vary the width of the bars to indicate differences in interval size. Bias can be introduced by not addressing interval size as the appearance of a distorted volume of the bars gives the view an incorrect impression of the data distribution.

Pie charts are the only common form of quantitative graphic representation that is not rectangular. The figure is presented as a circle, out of which several slices are delimited (Figure 16.5). The pie chart presents a breakdown of the components of a group. Typically, the entire set of data under consideration, such as total body weight, constitutes the pie, while each slice represents a percentage of the whole, such as the organ weight as a percent of total body weight. The total number of slices in a pie should be small for the presentation to be effective. Variability or error can be readily

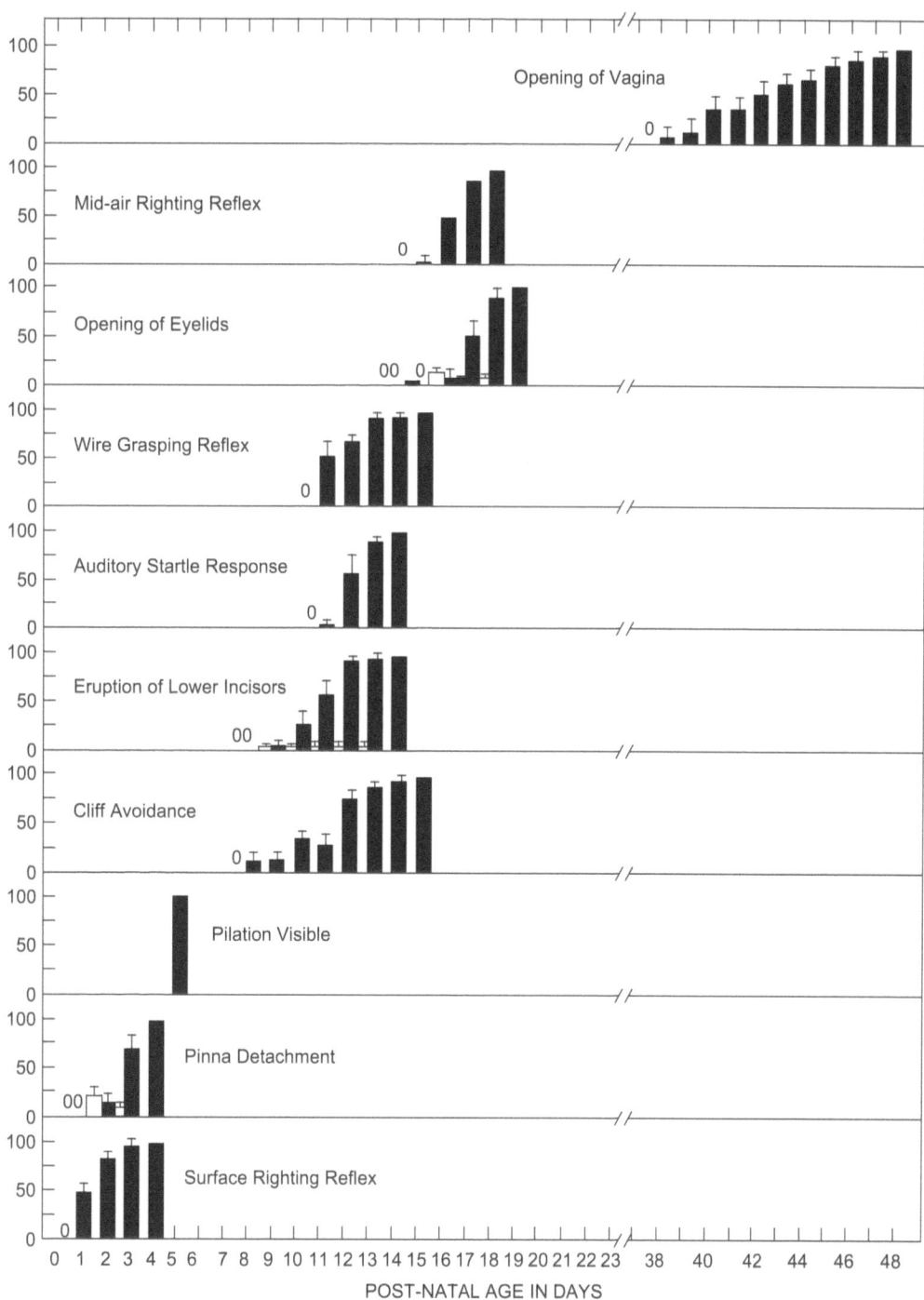

FIGURE 16.4 Acquisition of postnatal development landmarks in rats (histogram).

presented by creating a subslice of each sector shaded and labeled accordingly.

Finally, the *contour plot* (Figure 16.6) is used to depict the relationships in a three-variable, continuous data system. A contour plot visually portrays each contour as a locus of the values of two variables associated with a constant value of the third variable. An example would be a relief map that gives both latitude and longitude of constant altitude using contour lines.

The most common misuse of graphs is to either conceal or exaggerate the extent of differences by using an inappropriately scaled or ranged axis. There is a statistic for evaluating

TABLE 16.13   Forms of Statistical Communication and Display of Data

Quantitative graphics	Summary of statistical analyses	Graphic aids
Line chart	Means plot	Confidence limits
Pictogram	Sliding reference distribution	Graph paper
Pie chart	Notched box plot	Power curves
Contour plot	Facto space/response	Nomograms
Stereogram	Interaction plot	Sample size curves
Color map	Contour plot	Trilinear coordinates
Histogram	Predicted response plot	
	Confidence region plot	

the appropriateness of scale size, called the lie factor. This statistic is calculated as the ratio of the shown effect size to the range of potential change or effect. An acceptable range for the lie factor is within 0.95–1.05. If the lie factor is less than 0.95, the size of an effect is being understated, whereas a lie factor greater than 1.05 suggests that the effect is being exaggerated.

Data from toxicology studies should always be previewed before any formal statistical analysis commences. The preliminary review should determine whether the data are suitable for analysis, and if so what form the analysis should take. If the data as collected are not suitable for analysis, or if they are only suitable only for low-powered analytical techniques, one may wish to use one of many forms of *data transformation* to change the data characteristics so that they are more amenable to a robust analysis. There are a number of tools available to aid in data examination and preparation.

**Medicare Benefit Payments
By Type of Service, 2010**

Outpatient Prescription Drugs

Hospital Inpatient

Part A
Part B
Part A and B
Part D

Hospital Outpatient/ Other Part B   9%

11%

27%

Physicians and Other Suppliers   18%

5%   Skilled Nursing Facilities
3%   Hospice

Home Health   4%   24%

Durable Medical Equipment <

Medicare Advantage (Part C)

Total Benefit Payments = $504 billion

FIGURE 16.5   **Pie chart of medicare benefit payments for 2010.**

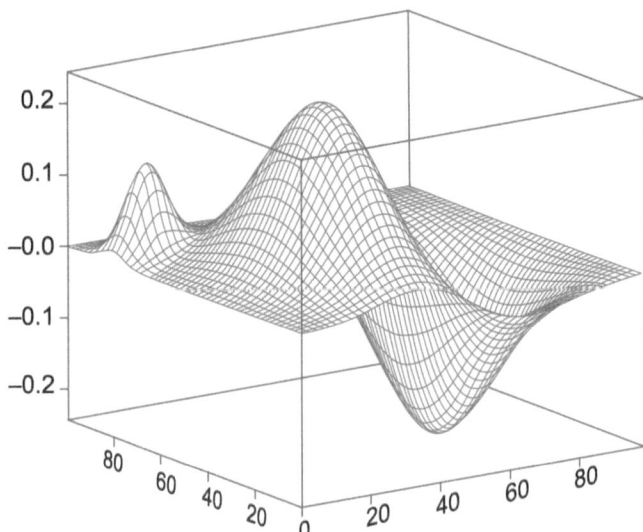

FIGURE 16.6   **An example of a contour plot.** where the bottom axes are x (left side) and y (right side) variables, while the vertical axis shows the third variable, z.

Following the preview, *exploratory data analysis* (EDA) can be done (Hoaglin et al., 2000; Tukey, 2019). EDA is a broad collection of techniques and approaches to "probe" data to both examine and to perform some initial, flexible analysis of the data. Two major points made throughout this section are the use of the appropriate statistical tests, and the effects of small sample sizes (as is often the case in experimental groups slated for toxicologic pathology assessment), on the selection of statistical techniques. The reader should plan statistical comparisons *before* conducting the experiments. The desired conclusion must not direct the choice of test to evaluate the data.

Displays visually reveal the distribution, variance, and trends of a data set. These approaches are sometimes referred to as the behavior of the data. They suggest a framework for analysis. The scatterplot is an example of this approach. *Reexpression* involves "redrawing" data to different scales to visualize which scale would serve best to simplify and improve the analysis of the data. Simple transformations are used to simplify data behavior and clarify analysis (e.g., linearizing or normalizing data).

Parameters of the population can be computed, in particular kurtosis (discussed below) and skewness (discussed below), using large groups of data. From these parameters, it is possible to determine if the population is normally distributed with respect to the parameter of interest with a certain level of confidence. If concern is especially marked with respect to the normality of the data, a Chi-square (χ^2) *goodness-of-fit* test will determine normality. When each group of data consists of 25 or fewer values, then kurtosis, skewness, and χ^2 goodness of fit are not accurate indicators of normality. For smaller groups of data, preparation and evaluation of a *scattergram* will help give a visual estimate of the normality.

The scattergram procedure is a simple histogram of the data followed by a visual appreciation of its location and distribution (Figure 16.7). The abscissa (horizontal scale) should be in the same scale as the values and should be divided so that the scale of the abscissa covers the entire range of observed values. Across such a scale we then simply enter symbols for each of our values.

Current technology allows us to add significantly more graphical information to scatterplots by means of graphic symbols for the plotted data points. An example of this approach is shown in Figure 16.3. Here dermal dose, dermal irritation, and WBC count are presented. This graph quite clearly suggests that as dose (variable x) is increased, dermal irritation (variable y) also increases; furthermore, as irritation becomes more severe, the WBC count (variable z, an

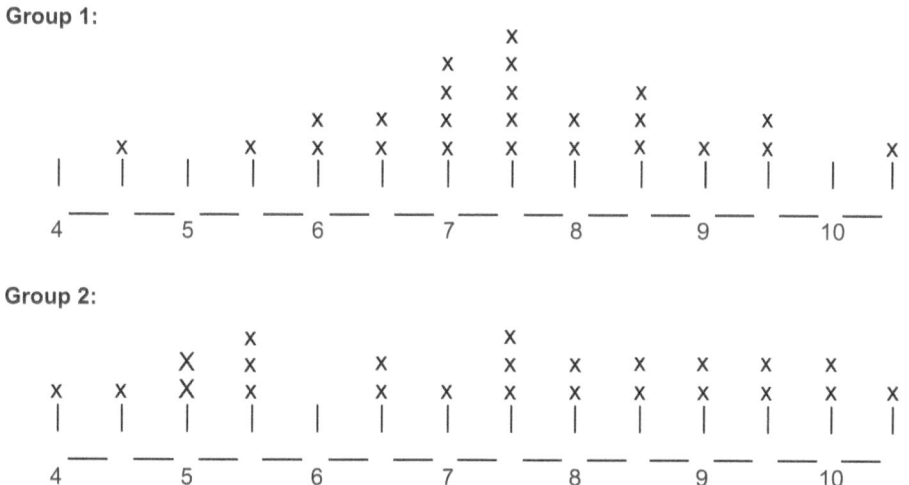

FIGURE 16.7 **Scattergram derived from the data in Table 16.19.** Group 1 approximates a normal distribution; therefore, the appropriate parametric tests can be performed on such data. In contrast, group 2 clearly does not appear to be normally distributed. In this case, the appropriate nonparametric techniques must be used.

indicator of immune system involvement, suggesting infection or persistent inflammation) also increases. However, there is no direct association of variables x (dose) and z (WBC count).

6.3. Evaluating Distributional Assumptions

It is important that the distributional assumptions of statistical tests are appropriate for the data. Violating distributional assumptions might lead to false significance, failure to detect a true difference, or biased estimation. Parametric assumptions include normality, equality of variances between experimental groups, and independent errors. When parametric assumptions of normality or equality of variances are violated, nonparametric approaches should be used instead of parametric approaches. Nonparametric tests do not rely on a specific probability distribution function.

Normality

Residuals are data remnants, or data filtered out, following construction of a fitted model for the larger portion of the data set. The residuals are the error terms and refer to the differences between the observed values and the predicted values. Residuals provide an expression of the extent to which a model does not fit to the actual data in a specific region. The analysis has removed these residuals, as residuals are the remnants of error or variability that remain following the fitting of a model. These residuals are seen as deviation from a linear plot in a linear regression; if the regression model is an adequate representation of the data set, the remnants should be without structure (i.e., they should present no pattern). The evidence of a pattern indicates an area on regression in which the model's function is not optimal.

Homogeneity of Variance

The *F-test* can be used as a test for the equality of variance in two samples (i.e., control and one test group). Bartlett's test and Levene's test are used to compare the variances among three or more groups of data, where the data in the groups are continuous sets. Examples of such data sets are body weights, organ weights, red blood cell (RBC) counts, or diet consumption measurements. Tests for the equality of variance between groups of data do not test for normality, but rather homogeneity of variance (also called equality of variances or homoscedasticity). *Homoscedasticity* is an important assumption for several statistical tests including *Student's t-test*, ANOVA, and *analysis of covariance* (ANCOVA). It is often expected that data with homogeneous variance between data groups will be suitable for parametric methods when normality of the data can be assumed.

Bartlett's test is more sensitive to departures from normality than Levene's test. Bartlett's test is based on the calculation of the corrected χ^2 value by the following formula (Eq. 16.12):

Formula for Bartlett's test

$$\chi^2_{corr}$$

$$= 2.3026 \frac{\sum df \left(\log_{10} \left[\frac{\sum [df(S^2)]}{\sum df} \right] \right) - \sum [df(\log_{10} S^2)]}{1 + \frac{1}{3(K-1)} \left[\sum \frac{1}{df} - \frac{1}{\sum df} \right]}$$

(16.12)

-where:

$$S^2 = \text{variance} = \frac{n \sum X^2 - (\sum X)^2}{\frac{n}{n-1}}$$

X = individual datum within each group.
n = number of data within each group.
K = number of groups being compared.
df = degrees of freedom for each group = $(n-1)$.

The corrected χ^2 value yielded by the above calculations is compared to the values listed in the χ^2 table according to the numbers of degrees of freedom (df), where the df refers to the number of independent units of information in a sample used in the calculation of a statistic. Bartlett's test has better performance if there is strong evidence that the data come from a normal distribution. However, because it is less sensitive to departures from normality, Levene's test is frequently preferred as a test for the assumption of equivalent variances. Levene's test statistic W is compared to the upper critical value of the F statistic at significance level a with

$k-1$ and N-k df, where W is calculated as follows (Eq. 16.13):

Formula for Levene's test

$$W = \frac{(N-k)}{(k-1)} \frac{\sum N_i (Z_i. - Z..)^2}{\sum\sum \left(Z_{ij} - Z_i.\right)^2} \qquad (16.13)$$

-where

k = number of different groups being compared.

N = total sample size.

N_i = number of data within the ith group.

Y_{ij} = the data value for the ith group and jth sample.

Y-bar_i. = the mean value for the ith group.

Z_{ij} = $\mid Y_{ij} - Y$-bar_i. $\mid$.

$Z_i.$ = mean value of the Z_{ij} for the ith group.

Z. = mean value of the Z_{ij}.

A statistical table can be consulted in order to determine if the calculated value of a test statistic exceeds a critical value. If the calculated value of the calculated χ^2 or W is smaller than the table value at the selected P-level, traditionally 0.05, the groups are considered homogeneous and the use of ANOVA is assumed to be proper (subject, or course, to the verification of normality of the distributions to be compared). If the calculated χ^2 or W is greater than the table value, the groups are considered to be heterogeneous. In the case of heterogeneity, statistical tests that are not based on assumption of homoscedasticity should be used. ANOVA is considered robust for moderately small differences in variance between data groups. In practice, a four-fold difference in variance between the group with the largest variance and the group with the smallest variance can usually be accommodated in ANOVA-based approaches.

Statistical Goodness-of-Fit Tests

A *goodness-of-fit test* is a statistical procedure for comparing individual measurements to a specified type of statistical distribution. For example, a normal distribution is completely specified by its arithmetic mean and variance (the square of the SD). The H_0, that the data represent a sample from a single normal distribution, can be tested by a statistical goodness-of-fit test. Various goodness-of-fit tests have been devised to determine if the data deviate significantly from a specified distribution.

Another goodness-of-fit method is the *maximum likelihood test*. If a significant departure occurs, it indicates only that the specified distribution can be rejected with some assurance. This does not necessarily mean that the true distribution contains two or more subpopulations. The true distribution may be a single distribution, based upon a different mathematical relationship, e.g., log normal. In the latter case, logarithms of the measurement would not be expected to exhibit by a goodness-of-fit test a statistically significant departure from a log-normal distribution. A sample size of 200 or more is required to conduct a valid analysis of mixtures of populations, which would be prohibitively large in many toxicology settings. When the calculated means of subpopulations are less than three SDs apart and sample sizes are less than 300, the maximum likelihood method should be used with extreme caution, or not at all.

None of the available goodness-of-fit methods conclusively establish bimodality. Bimodality may occur when separation between the two means (modes) exceeds two SDs. Conversely, separations in histograms of *less than* two SDs may arise from genetic differences in test subjects.

Fisher's Skewness Statistic and Engelman and Hartigan Test

Skewness is a measure of the degree of asymmetry of a distribution. If the data are plotted along a horizontal axis and the left tail (tail at small end of the distribution) is more pronounced than the right tail (tail at the large end of the distribution), the function is said to have negative skewness. If the reverse is true, the distribution has positive skewness. If the two tails are equal, it has zero skewness.

Fisher's skewness statistic is preferable when one component comprises less than 15% of the total distribution. An example would be those individuals in a Caucasian population who lack a specific isoenzyme of the cytochromes P450 complement. However, when the two components comprised more nearly equal proportions (35%–65%) of the total distribution, then the *Engelman and Hartigan test* is preferable. For other proportions, the maximum likelihood ratio test is best. Thus, the maximum likelihood ratio test appears to perform very well, with only a small loss from optimality, even when it is not the best procedure.

Maximum Likelihood Ratio Test

The likelihood ratio test answers this question: are the data significantly less likely to have arisen if the H_0 is true than if the alternate hypothesis is true? The *maximum likelihood ratio test* provides estimators of a parameter that are usually quite satisfactory. These estimators have the desirable properties of being consistent, asymptotically normal, and asymptotically efficient for large samples under quite general conditions. Maximum likelihood estimators also have another desirable property: *invariance*. The estimators are often biased, but the bias is frequently removable by a simple adjustment. Other methods of obtaining estimators are also available, but the maximum likelihood ratio test is the most frequently used.

These maximum likelihood methods can be used to obtain *point estimates* of a parameter, but one must remember that a point estimate is a random variable distributed in some way around the true value of the parameter, where the true parameter value actually may be higher or lower than the estimate. It is often useful to obtain an interval within which one is reasonably confident the true value will lie. The generally accepted method to generate such an interval is to construct *confidence limits*.

The mathematical description of the maximum likelihood estimator is as follows: Let us denote the maximum likelihood estimator of the parameter θ, where x is a random variable, by the function $f(x;\theta)$. Then, if $f(x,\theta)$ is a single-valued function of θ, the maximum likelihood estimator of $f(\theta)$ is $f(x_1;\theta) * f(x_2;\theta) * f(x_3;\theta)$ … $f(x_n;\theta)$, i.e., the product of each of the component probabilities. The principle of maximum likelihood tells us that we should use as our estimate that value which maximizes the likelihood of the observed event. For example, in a carcinogenesis study of two test compounds where one is known to have a genotoxic effect, the maximum likelihood ratio test addresses whether there is a difference in carcinogenic response between the two test compounds.

6.4. Data Processing

Preparing the data for statistical evaluation requires cleaning it. First, data should be checked for completeness, and numbers should be rounded to the correct number of significant figures for the procedure that generated the data. In addition, data points that appear to be *outliers* (see below) should be evaluated for inclusion or exclusion, using the methods described above. Once the data have been evaluated for outliers, it may be necessary to transform the data before analysis commences.

Outlier Detection

The sensitivity of techniques such as ANOVA is reduced markedly by the occurrence of outliers (i.e., either extreme high or low values, including hyper- and hyporesponders) that serve to markedly inflate the dispersion of data points, and hence the variance, of the sample. Such variance inflation is particularly common in small groups of experimental units (i.e., low n) that are exposed or dosed around a threshold level. This exposure, or dosing, results in detection of a small number of hypersensitive individuals in the sample who respond markedly.

Such a situation is displayed in Figure 16.8 below showing a plot of the mean and SDs of methemoglobin levels in a series of groups of animals exposed to successively higher levels of a hemolytic agent.

Though the mean level of methemoglobin in group C is more than double that of the control group (A), no hypothesis test will show a significant difference because of the large variance of the data. This inflated variance exists because a single individual has such a pronounced response. The occurrence of *variance inflation* is certainly an indicator that the data need to be examined closely for potential outlying events. Indeed, all tabular raw data in toxicologic pathology should be visually inspected for both trend and variance inflation, as summary statistics may hide important information concerning the existence of these distortions in the data.

Missing Data

Missing data are a common problem in toxicologic pathology. Missing tissues and inadequate blood samples for analysis are not uncommon, even under GLP conditions. How missing data are handled in statistical evaluation is critical to obtaining a valid interpretation of results.

Animals with missing data can simply be removed from the analysis. There are, however, some situations where removal of the experimental unit can be inappropriate. Particularly

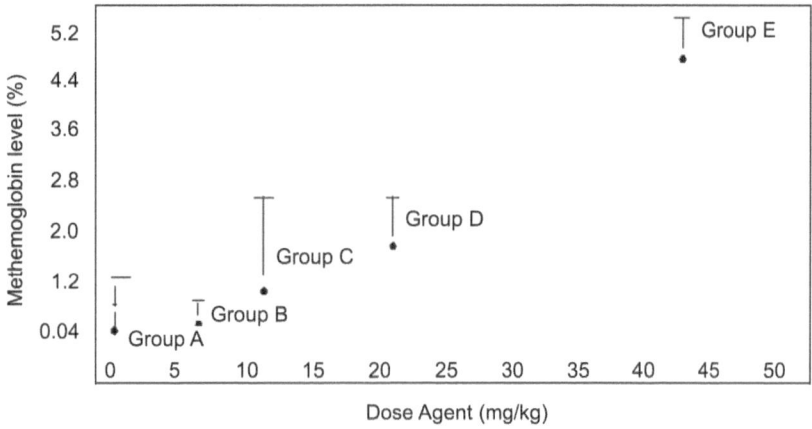

FIGURE 16.8 **Variance inflation (Mean + SD).**

of note is the situation when a lesion assumed to have caused the death of the animal is analyzed. For example, an animal dies at week 83 of a carcinogenicity bioassay for which the appropriate section to detect the lesion in question was unavailable for microscopic examination. This animal cannot contribute to the group comparison at week 83. However, as it was alive in previous weeks, it should contribute to the denominator of the calculations in all previous weeks.

Missing observations also occur when histopathological evaluation is only done when an abnormality is seen at postmortem (Table 16.14). In such an experiment, the hypothetical data may appear as in Table 16.15.

TABLE 16.14 Data Generated From a Hypothetical Experiment Where Histopathological Evaluation Is Only Done in Animals Where Gross Lesions Were Seen

Animals	Control group	Treated group
Number in group	50	50
Number with gross lesions	2	15
Histopathological evaluation	2	15
Classified neoplasm	2	14

TABLE 16.15 Hypothetical Data

Data	Time points											
Time	1	2	3	4	5	6	7	8	9	10	11	12
Control	4.5	5.4	5.9	6.0	6.4	6.5	6.9	7.0	7.1	7.0	7.4	7.5
Tx	4.0	4.5	5.0	5.1	5.4	5.5	5.6	6.5	6.5	7.0	7.4	7.5
Time	13	14	15	16	17	18	19	20	21	22	23	24
Control	7.5	7.5	7.6	8.0	8.1	8.4	8.5	8.6	9.0	9.4	9.5	10.4
Tx	7.5	8.0	8.1	8.5	8.5	9.0	9.1	9.5	9.5	10.1	10.0	10.4

Tx = treatment.
Time is given in weeks. The data represent abnormalities at necropsy.

The following statistics could be derived for these data. Ignoring animals with no microscopic sections, one would compare $2/2 = 100\%$ with $14/15 = 93\%$ and conclude treatment nonsignificantly decreased incidence. This is likely to be a false conclusion, and it would be better here to compare the percentages of animals that had a postmortem abnormality that turned out to be a tumor: $2/50 = 4\%$ of controls versus $14/50 = 28\%$ of treated animals. Unless some aspect of treatment made tumors much easier to detect at postmortem, one would then conclude that treatment did have an effect on tumor incidence.

Particular care has to be taken in studies where the procedures for histopathological examination vary by group. Otherwise, observer bias will affect the data. The protocol often requires a full microscopic examination of a given tissue list in decedents in all groups, and in terminally killed controls and high-dose animals. In other animals (e.g., terminally killed low- and mid-dose animals), microscopic examination of a tissue is only conducted if the tissue is found to be grossly abnormal at postmortem. In pharmaceutical practice, for rodent studies, the intermediate doses are evaluated if a test article elicits a histological effect at the high dose.

Such a protocol is designed to save money but can lead to invalid comparisons among treatment groups. Suppose, for example, responses in terminally killed animals are $8/20$ in the controls, $3/3$ (with 17 unexamined) in the low-dose animals, and $5/6$ (with 14 unexamined) in the mid-dose animals. Is one supposed to conclude that treatment at the low- and mid-doses increased the response, based on a comparison of the proportions examined microscopically (40%, 100%, and 83%)? Or should one conclude that it decreased the response, based on the proportion of animals in the group that were affected (40%, 15%, and 25%)? It could well be that treatment had no effect, but that some small tumors were missed at postmortem. In this situation, a valid comparison can only be achieved by ignoring the low- and mid-dose groups when carrying out the comparison for the age stratum at the terminal kill. This may seem wasteful of data, but actually represents the appropriate use of relevant data.

Transformations

If initial inspection of a data set reveals an unusual or undesired set of characteristics, or a lack a desired set of characteristics such as normality, there is a choice of three courses of action. First, a method or test may be selected that is appropriate to the present conditions that are based on *assumptions not violated* by these conditions. Second, analysis may not be attempted on the grounds that the data cannot be analyzed using the planned techniques. Finally, attempts can be made to transform the variable(s) under consideration in such a manner that the resulting transformed variates (X' and Y', for example, as opposed to the original variates X and Y) meet the assumptions of the test to be employed or have the characteristics that are desired.

The key to transformation is recognizing that the scale of measurement for most (if not all) variables is arbitrary. In other words, the relationship of each variable or variate to one another is important, whereas the actual unit of measurement is arbitrary. For example, a linear scale of measurement may have been used to record the data; however, this scale could have been changed to a logarithmic scale to represent the data. Often such scales are used because they are easier to read (e.g., pH values and the Richter earthquake intensity, in which linear data with very large values have been converted to simple logarithmic scales). Transforming a set of data (converting X to X') is really as simple as *changing a scale of measurement*. Transformation does not alter the relationship of variables, just their representation. Common transformations are presented in Table 16.16.

Data transformation is commonly done to normalize the data. As the assumptions for the common statistical analyses require normality, transformation is necessary to permit analysis by our most common parametric statistical techniques that will be discussed later in the chapter (e.g., ANOVA). However, transformation does not guarantee normally distributed data. Quantile-normal quantile plots provide a test of normality. Visualizing the spread of the data in boxplots allows assessment of equal variance. The transformed data then can be analyzed.

TABLE 16.16 Common Data Transformations

Transformation	How calculated[a]	Example of use
Arithmetic	$x' = \frac{x}{y}$ or: $x' = x + c$	Organ weight/Body weight
Reciprocals	$x' = \frac{1}{x}$[b]	Linearizing data, particularly rate phenomena
Arcsine (also called angular)	$x' = \text{arcsine } \sqrt{x}$	Normalizing dominant lethal and mutation rate data
Logarithmic	$x' = \log x$	pH values
Probability (probit)	$x' = \text{probability } X$	Percentage responding
Square roots	$x' = \sqrt{x}$	Surface area of animal from body weights
Box Cox	$x' = (x^v - 1)v$: for $v \neq 0$ $x' = 1nx$: for $v = 0$	A family of transforms For use when one has no prior knowledge of the appropriate transformation to use
Rank transformations	Depends on nature of samples	As a bridge between parametric and nonparametric statistics

[a] *x and y are the original variables; x' and y' are transformed values for x and y, respectively. C stands for a constant.*
[b] *Plotting a double reciprocal (that is, $\frac{1}{x}$ vs. $\frac{1}{y}$) will linearize almost any data set, so will plotting the log transforms of a set of variables.*

The second reason to transform data is to create a *linear relationship between a paired set of data*, such as dose and response. This transformation is commonly used in toxicologic pathology and is discussed in more detail in the section below for probit/logit plots.

Third, transformation of the data may be done to adjust for the influence of another variable. This procedure is an alternative in some situations to the more complicated process of ANCOVA which will be discussed later in this chapter. An example of where this transformation is used is the calculation of organ weight to body weight ratios for in vivo toxicity studies. Here, the resulting ratios serve as the raw data for an ANOVA performed to identify possible target organs, provided that the assumption of the ANOVA is met. If these ratios need to be normalized, the data can be transformed again to achieve normality.

Finally, transformation of the data may be undertaken to *make the relationships between variables clearer*. Removing, or adjusting for, interactions among other uncontrolled variables that may influence the pair of variables to be analyzed achieves this clarification. This case is discussed in detail in the section below for time series analysis.

Combination of Lesions

Four main situations warrant *combining pathology terms* for morphological alterations when organizing data for statistical analysis (see Nomenclature and Diagnostic Resources in Anatomic Toxicologic Pathology Vol 1, Chap 25). The first is when essentially the same lesion has been recorded under two or more different names, or even under the same name in different places. Here, failure to combine these conditions in the analysis may severely limit the chances of detecting a true treatment effect. It is best practice to record the same lesion using consistent terminology within the same experiment. The implementation of harmonized nomenclature and peer review should minimize the need to combine terms. It should be noted, however, that grouping together conditions that are actually different might also result in the masking of a true treatment effect, particularly if the treatment has a very specific effect.

The second situation is when separately recorded lesions form successive steps on the pathway of the same process. The most important example of this phenomenon is for the incidence of related types of malignant tumor, benign tumor, and focal hyperplasia. It will normally be appropriate to carry out analyses for the (1) incidence of malignant tumor, (2) incidence of benign or malignant tumor, and, where appropriate, (3) incidence of focal hyperplasia, benign, or malignant tumor.

The third situation for combining data is when the same pathological condition appears in different organs as a result of the same common underlying process. Examples of this are the multicentric tumors, such as myeloid leukemia, reticulum cell sarcoma, and lymphosarcoma, or certain nonneoplastic conditions, such as arteritis/periarteritis and amyloid degeneration. Here, analysis will normally be carried out only for the lesion's incidence combined among all sites.

The final situation where an analysis of combined pathology findings is appropriate occurs when analyzing the overall incidence of malignant tumors at any site, of benign or malignant tumors at any site, or of multiple tumor incidences. While analyses of tumor incidence at specific sites are normally more meaningful, as treatments often affect only a few specific sites, these additional analyses are usually performed to guard against the possibility that the treatment had some weak but general tumor-enhancing effect, which would not be otherwise evident. In some situations, one might also envisage analyses of other combinations of specific tumors, such as tumors at related sites (e.g., endocrine organs if the compound demonstrates a hormonal effect) or of similar histopathological type.

7. STATISTICAL METHODS

One approach for the selection of appropriate techniques to employ in a particular situation is to use a *decision tree* method. Figure 16.9 is a decision tree that leads to the choice of one of other trees to assist in technique selection, with each of the subsequent trees addressing one of the three functions of statistics that were defined earlier in this chapter. Figure 16.10 is a decision tree for the selection of hypothesis testing procedures, Figure 16.11 represents a decision tree for modeling procedures, and Figure 16.12 shows a decision tree for reduction of dimensionality procedures. For the vast majority of situations,

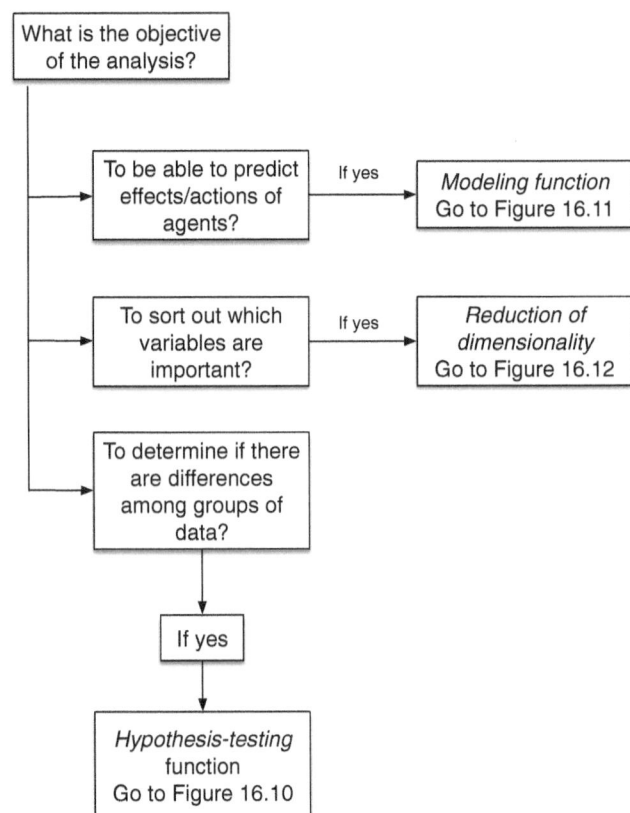

FIGURE 16.9 **Overall decision tree for selecting statistical procedures.**

these decision trees will guide the user's choice of the appropriate technique. The tests and terms in these trees will be explained subsequently.

7.1. Statistical Analysis: General Considerations

Variables to be Analyzed

Although some toxicologic pathologists still regard their discipline as providing qualitative rather than quantitative data, it is abundantly clear that pathology has to be quantitative to at least some degree. When applied to routine screening of animal toxicity and carcinogenicity studies, quantitative data generation is necessary so that statistical inferences and statements can be made about possible treatment effects. Inevitably, there will be some descriptive text that will not be appropriate for statistical analysis. However, an important objective of the toxicologic pathologist should be to provide

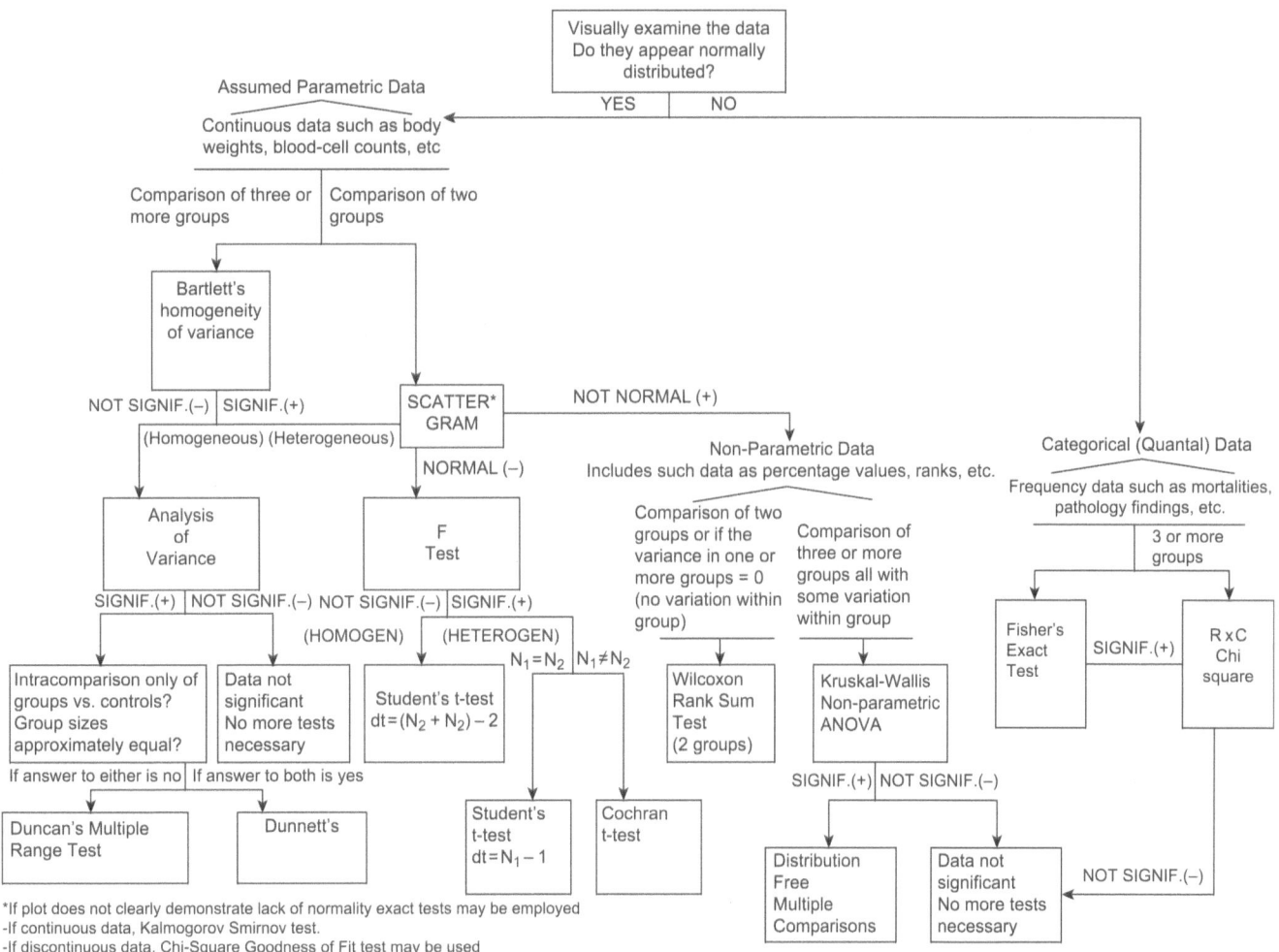

FIGURE 16.10 **Decision tree for the selection of hypothesis-testing procedures.**

information on the presence or absence, with severity grade or size where appropriate, of a list of conditions. These lesions should be consistently recorded from animal to animal and classified by well-defined criteria, which can be validly used in a statistical assessment (Vol 1, Chap 25: Nomenclature and diagnostic resources in anatomic toxicologic pathology). Toxicologic pathology data based on a tiered grading system (e.g., within normal limits, or minimal, mild, moderate, or marked lesions) is semiquantitative in nature, and not merely qualitative.

Statistical analysis is primarily applied to tumor incidence in carcinogenicity studies and hypothesis-driven studies such as pharmacology studies of microscopic data. Histopathology data are still not routinely subjected to statistical analysis for regulatory repeat-dose toxicity studies.

Study endpoints, including morphologic endpoints, need to be tailored to scientific objectives of the study. The endpoints to be studied should be specified in the study plan so that if that endpoint is to be statistically analyzed the method should be defined in the study plan.

The toxicologic pathologist can generate a plethora of data. Should one then analyze all endpoints, including those not included in the plan but are recorded, in a particular study? Some arguments have been put forward against analyzing all the endpoints; in the opinion of the authors, however, none of these arguments justify exclusion of endpoints from the statistical analysis. Nevertheless, these arguments and corresponding counterarguments are presented here to make the reader familiar with them.

One argument is that some endpoints are not of interest. Perhaps the study is essentially

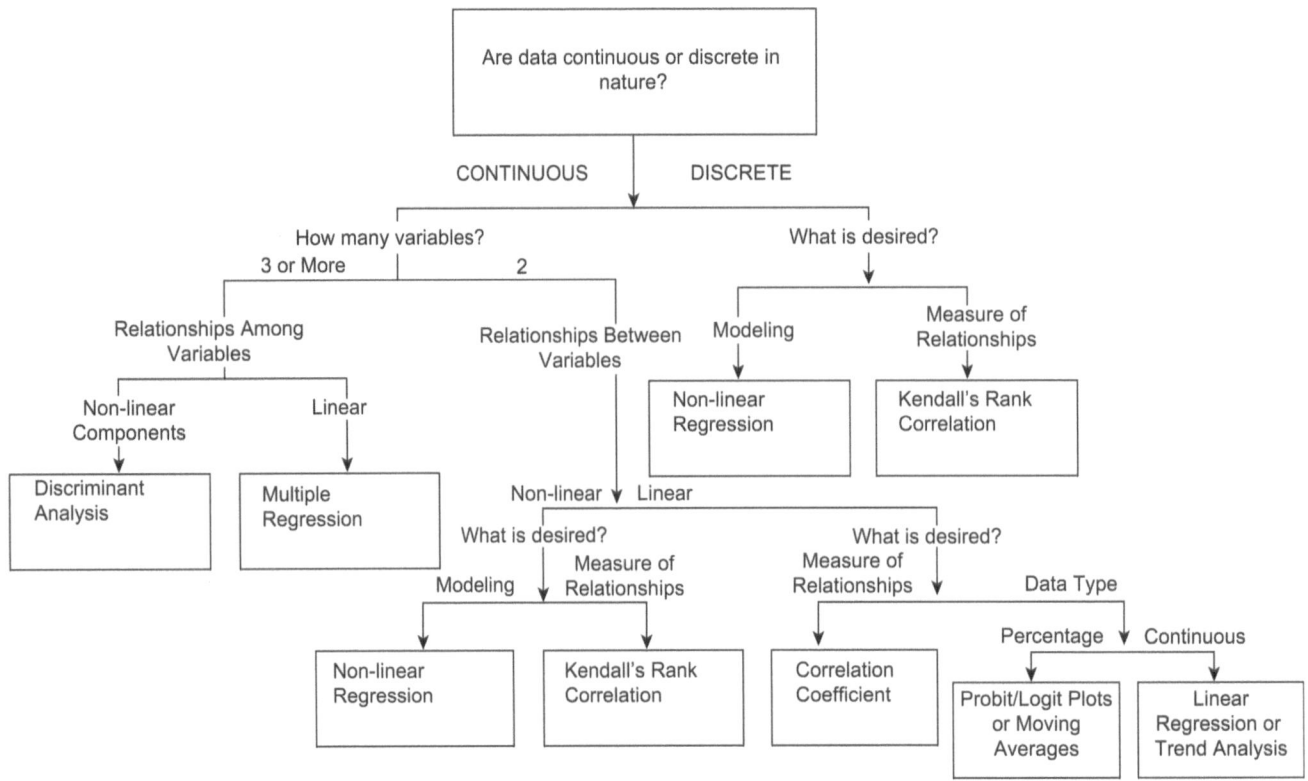

FIGURE 16.11   **Decision tree for modeling procedures.**

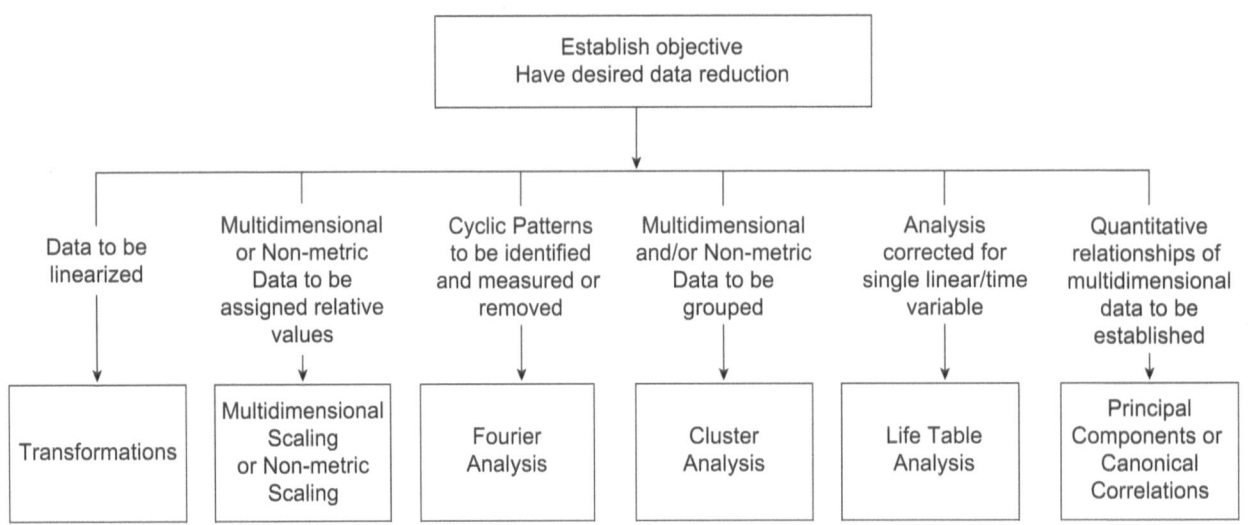

FIGURE 16.12   **Overall decision tree for reduction of dimensionality procedures.**

a carcinogenicity study, so that nonneoplastic endpoints are not considered as important. In fact, nonneoplastic findings often are considered to be "background pathology" and almost per se unrelated to treatment.

Another argument put forward against doing multiple analyses on data generated by the toxicologic pathologist is that it may by chance yield many significant *P*-values that have to be considered and evaluated for biological significance in the context of the entire set of available data. The global context of dose response, as summarized in Table 16.17, must be kept in mind when deciding whether to exclude any

TABLE 16.17   The Three Dimensions of Dose Response

Dose	Response
Increasing dose (↓)	Incidence of responders in an exposed population increases
	Severity of response in affected individuals increases
	Time to occurrence or progression of the response decreases

data from analysis. A detailed look (including appropriate statistics) at the data can only aid interpretation, provided that one is not hidebound by the false argument that statistical significance necessarily equates with biological importance and definitely indicates a true effect of treatment.

Finally, some endpoints rarely occur. One must then be clear what can be considered for classification as a rarely occurring event. For a typical study with a control and three dose groups of equal size, one would compute a significant trend if all three cases of a rarely observed morphological alteration occurred in the top dose level or in the control group. In this case, a total of three cases will normally be enough for statistical analysis. Endpoints occurring once or twice only are not worth analyzing formally, although they may be worth noting in the report if only seen in the top dose group. This is especially true if such lesions are rarely reported.

Taking Lesion Severity into Account

If the pathologist chooses to grade a condition for severity, the *grade* should be taken into account as part of the statistical considerations. There are two ways to analyze grade data. In one, data are analyzed when the animal has a condition and the condition is defined as at least grade 2, or at least grade 3, etc. In the other approach, nonparametric methods utilizing ranked data are used. The latter approach is more powerful as it uses all the information in one analysis. Note that *consistent grading* is necessary for meaningful analyses based on grade.

Using Simple Methods that Avoid Complex Assumptions

Different statistical methods can vary considerably in their complexity and in the number of assumptions they make. Regardless, such analyses should be used for data clarification (i.e., the relationship between a treatment and some effect) rather than being performed only to obtain a *P-value*. Wherever possible, statistical methods utilized should be simple, robust, and make few assumptions. The use of more complicated statistical models has its place, however, in studies of complex design.

There are three reasons for preferring simple, robust statistical tests. First, the toxicologic pathologist usually understands simpler methods, and hence she/he can justify the outputs. Second, consumers of pathology data (e.g., toxicologists, corporate managers, health and regulatory officials) also appreciate simple analyses. Third, adequate data are seldom available in practice to validate fully the assumptions of any formal statistical model. Even if particular models are shown to be suitable for use, the loss of power in using an appropriate, simpler method is often very small.

When evaluating the relationship of treatment to incidence of a well-defined pathological finding and adjusting for other factors (in particular age at death, which might bias the comparison), methods involving stratification are recommended (see discussion above). These should be used in preference to a multiple regression approach, or time-to-tumor models.

ANOVA methods can be useful for estimating treatment effects when continuously distributed data are obtained. However, the appropriateness of ANOVA as a tool depends on the validity of the fundamental assumptions of normally distributed model residuals and equal variability in each group. If these assumptions are violated, or cannot be reasonably demonstrated or assumed, nonparametric methods are more appropriate for hypothesis testing. These nonparametric tests may be based on the rank of observations, rather than their actual value, and do not depend on the assumptions common to the parametric methods.

Using all the Data

There are situations where, in addition to evaluating treatment and effect relationships, determination of the effect of other sources of systematic differences among individuals is warranted. For example, gender differences, differing times of sacrifice, and differing secondary treatments may be considered. A source of systematic difference is considered a *factor* (see discussion of factors above). It is often important to evaluate the effect of these factors so that a more powerful analysis of the specific treatment effects can be made. These factors can be evaluated for relationships within each level of the factor (e.g., factor = sex; level = male, female) and in combination to see whether data can be pooled. Some scientists consider that conclusions for males and females should always be drawn separately, but in many instances there are strong statistical arguments for a joint analysis.

Combining, Pooling, and Stratification

The following is a hypothetical study of a toxic agent that induces tumors without shortening the lives of tumor-bearing animals. The hypothetical data for the number of animals with tumor out of the total number of animals examined are shown in Table 16.18.

This example shows that if the time of death is ignored, and the *pooled* data are evaluated, the incidence of tumors is the same in each group. This leads to the *false* conclusion that treatment had no effect. However, by evaluating the *time to death* of animals on treatment, an increased incidence of death in the exposed groups can be seen. An appropriate statistical method would *combine* a measure of difference between the groups based on the early deaths and a measure of difference based on the late deaths, and conclude correctly that incidence, after adjustment for time of death, is greater in the exposed groups.

In this example, time of death is the stratifying variable (or factor) with two strata (or levels): early deaths and late deaths. The essence of the methodology is to first make comparisons only within strata so that one is always comparing like with like except in respect of treatment. Then, the differences are combined over strata. Stratification can be used to adjust for any variable, or combinations of variables.

Some studies are of factorial design, in which combinations of treatments are evaluated. The simplest such design is one in which four equal-sized groups of animals receive either no treatment, treatment *A* only, treatment *B* only, or both treatments *A* and *B*. The basic assumption for analysis of this type of experiment is that the effects of the two treatments *A* and *B* are *independent*. In this factorial experiment, one can use stratification to enable more powerful tests to be conducted to reveal any possible individual treatment effects. For example, to test for effects of treatment A, one conducts comparisons in two strata, the first consisting of groups 1 and 2 (animals not given treatment *B*) and the second consisting of groups 3 and 4 (those given treatment *B*). Combination of results from the two strata is based on twice as many animals and is therefore markedly more likely to detect possible effects of treatment *A* than is a simple comparison of groups 1 and 2. There is also the possibility of identifying *interactions*, such as synergism and antagonism, between the two treatments.

In some routine long-term screening studies, the study design involves 5 groups usually comprised of 50 animals of each sex, 3 groups of which are treated with increasing doses of a compound and 2 of which are untreated controls. Assuming that there is no systematic difference between the control groups (e.g., the second control group is housed in a different room or was populated from a different batch of animals), the main analyses will pool both control groups to produce a single group of 100 animals. Pooling the control groups should only occur following a preliminary analysis to show that there is no difference in the incidence of effects in these control groups. If there is a difference between control groups, the cause of the difference needs to be evaluated to determine how this cause may have affected, or not,

TABLE 16.18 Sample Data From a Hypothetical Carcinogenicity Study

Death	Control	Exposed	Combined
Early deaths	1/20 (5%)	18/90 (20%)	19/110 (17%)
Late deaths	24/80 (30%)	7/10 (70%)	31/90 (34%)
Total	25/100 (25%)	25/100 (25%)	50/200 (25%)

the experimental groups. Once this has been determined, the most appropriate method of analysis for the situation is used.

Experimental and Observational Units

Animals in a study are often both the *experimental unit* and the *observational unit*, but this is not always so. A common example in the toxicology field is the assessment of developmental toxicity. Prenatal exposures occur by treating the mother. In monoparous species (i.e., gestation of only one fetus at a time), the fetus is the experimental unit and the observational unit, but in multiparous species, the entire litter is the experimental unit even though toxicity endpoints are observed individually in all fetuses (Table 16.19).

In many feeding studies, where the cage is assigned to a treatment, it is the cage (and its several inhabitants) rather than any single animal that is the experimental unit. In contrast, histopathological observations for a tissue may

TABLE 16.19 An Example of a Table Addressing the Experimental Unit, Offspring, and Hepatic Pathology

Hepatic necrosis (two sections) in dog pups exposed during gestation to compound abc01

Animal number	Treatment	Pup number	Hepatic necrosis score
E-9991	B	1	0
		2	0
		3	0
		4	0
E-9992	A	1	3
E-9993	D	—	—
E-9994	A	1	3
		2	1
		2	1
E-9995	C	1	1
		2	0
		3	1
E-9996	D	—	—
E-9997	B	1	0
		2	0
		3	0
		4	0
		5	0
E-9998	C	1	1
		2	0
		3	1
		4	2

be based on multiple sections per animal. In this case, the section is the observational unit, whereas the animal is the experimental unit. Similarly, in reproduction and teratology studies, the dam is the experimental unit, while all the fetuses in a litter are the observational units. Multiple observations per experimental unit should be combined in some suitable way into an overall average for that unit before analysis. Often these multiple observations are not normally distributed, hence the median and semi-quartile range are commonly used for describing the multiple observation data for an experimental unit.

Statistical Bias

BIAS OF ESTIMATION

Statistical inference is of two types: estimation and hypothesis testing. Both methods of inference involve assumptions and systematic procedures, which may introduce bias. Bayesian methods may be used that incorporate prior information or convictions into the analysis (Box and Tiao, 1992; Gelman et al., 2004). This approach may detect a "wished" effect rather than a real effect if not carefully scrutinized. *Bias of estimator* occurs when a systematic procedure is used to make the best estimate of a true value (which is not known). This usually occurs when the mean of the sample is assumed to approximate the mean of the population. We make this assumption with all our statistical methods and have no way of testing whether or not the estimate is a true representation unless we measure the whole population. Variance is the sum of squares (SS) of the deviations of observed values from the sample mean divided by the number of observations. It does not represent the true variance of the population, but instead is a representative sample. In addition, the sample estimate of the mean is subject to sampling error, so $n-1$ is used for df (instead of n) in calculations in an attempt to remove knowledge bias of the last event to be probabilistically tested. In other words, there is a probability associated with all units taken from a sample except the last: the last sample is known.

Additional forms of bias may impact the estimate. *Bias in the assumptions* underlying the statistical analysis, such as different estimates obtained from different models, may occur. One has to assume either that these biases do not exist in the analysis, or that they have little ability to bias the endpoint. *Description bias* can occur when the wrong descriptor is used to describe a population or sample (e.g., mean vs. median and SD vs. range for normal vs. skewed data). *Prior conviction bias* may exist with respect to how to handle outliers, or data that may bias the results because the value is so large or small in comparison to the other data points.

BIAS IN HYPOTHESIS TESTING

Violation of assumptions of a test introduces bias into probabilistic testing. *Postfactor hypothesis bias* occurs in testing a hypothesis: when one is committed to accept/reject a conjecture on experimental evidence using an appropriately applied statistical procedure, failure to do so is an obvious bias, if not fraud. *Goodness-of-fit tests* are weak and can only show a good fit. They cannot demonstrate a *lack of fit*.

7.2. Hypothesis Testing of Categorical Data

Categorical data presented in a contingency table contain any single type of data. The contents of the contingency table are classified treatment and control groups, with the members of each group classified with respect to one of two or more response categories (e.g., tumor/no tumor, or normal/hyperplastic/neoplastic). In these cases, two forms of analysis can be used: *Fisher's Exact Test* for the 2×2 *contingency table* and the $R \times C$ χ^2 *test* for large tables. It should be noted, however, that there are versions of both tests that permit the analysis of any size of contingency table.

Nonparametric statistical analysis of ranked data is an exact parallel of the more traditional parametric methods. There are methods for a single comparison, similar to Student's *t*-test, and for the multiple comparisons, similar to ANOVA, followed by appropriate *post hoc* tests for exact identification of the significance within a set of groups. The following describes four tests for these situations: the *Wilcoxon rank-sum test*, *distribution-free multiple comparisons*, *Mann–Whitney U test*, and the *Kruskal–Wallis nonparametric ANOVA*. For each of these tests, tables of distribution values for the evaluations of results can be found in any of a number of reference volumes. It should be noted that for data that do not fulfill the necessary assumptions for parametric analysis, these nonparametric methods may be as powerful as the equivalent parametric test.

Fisher's Exact Test

Fisher's exact test should be used to compare two sets of discontinuous, quantal data (i.e., all or none measurements such as live or dead). Contingency data tables can check small sets of quantal data. Larger data sets, however, require computation (e.g., incidences of mortality or certain histopathological findings, etc.). These data also can be expressed as ratios. These data do not fit a continuous scale of measurement but usually involve numbers of responses classified as either negative or positive. The analysis is started by setting up a 2 × 2 contingency table to summarize the numbers of positive and negative responses as well as the totals of these responses, as shown in Table 16.20.

Using the above set of symbols, the formula for the Fisher's probability P appears as follows (Eq. 16.14):

Calculation of Fisher's P

$$P = \frac{(A+B)!(C+D)!(A+C)!(B+D)!}{N!A!B!C!D!} \quad (16.14)$$

-where P is the probability of the exact test, which is the sum of the above calculation repeated for each possible arrangement of the numbers in the above cells (that is, A, B, C, and D)

$A!$ is A factorial. For example, 4! would be (4)(3) (2) (1) = 24.

The exact test produces a probability (P) which is the sum of the above calculation repeated for each possible arrangement of the numbers in the above cells (that is, A, B, C, and D) showing an association equal to or stronger than that

TABLE 16.20   An Example of a 2 × 2 Contingency Table

Group	Positive	Negative	Total
Group I	A	B	A + B
Group II	C	D	C + D
Totals	A + C	B + D	A + B + C + D = N_{total}

between the two variables. The P resulting from these computations will be the exact one- or two-tailed probability, depending on which of these two approaches is being employed. This value shows whether the groups differ significantly (e.g., probability less than 0.05) and provides a value for the degree of significance.

Fisher's exact test must be used in preference to the χ^2 test when there are small cell numbers (i.e., less than six per cell). Tables are available that provide individual exact probabilities for small sample size contingency tables (Finney et al., 1963). Fisher's probabilities are not necessarily symmetric. Although some analysts will double the one-tailed P-value to obtain the two-tailed result, this method is usually overly conservative. However, the probability resulting from a two-tailed χ^2 test is exactly double that of a one-tailed from the same data.

2 × 2 Chi-Square

Though Fisher's exact test is preferable for analysis of most 2 × 2 contingency tables in toxicologic pathology, the χ^2 *test* is still widely used and is preferable in a few unusual situations. χ^2 is used when cell sizes are large, yet only limited computational support is available (Eq. 16.15).

Formula for Chi-square (χ^2) for an R × C contingency table

$$\chi^2 = \frac{(O_1 - E_1)^2}{E_1} + \frac{(O_2 - E_2)^2}{E_2}$$
$$= \sum \frac{(O_i - E_1)^2}{E_i} \quad (16.15)$$

-where O is the observed numbers (or counts) and E is the expected numbers (or counts).

The common practice in toxicologic pathology is for the observed figures to be tested or treatment group counts. The expected statistic is calculated for each box or cell in the contingency table as follows (Eq. 16.16):

Summary equation for an R × C (Row × Column) contingency table: summary

$$\sum = \frac{(column\ total)(row\ total)}{grand\ total} \quad (16.16)$$

The df for this statistic are $(R-1)(C-1) = (2-1)(2-1) = 1$. Looking at a χ^2 *table* for one df, we can see where our test statistic lies at the 0.05 and 0.01 probability levels. There are a number of assumptions for this contingency table. Data should be univariate and categorical, from a multinomial population, and have been collected by random, independent sampling, and from groups of approximately the same size, particularly for small group sizes.

χ^2 and $R \times C$ contingency tables can be used, when the data are of a categorical or frequency nature and fit the assumptions above, to test the goodness to fit to a known form of distribution when cell sizes are large. These methods should not be used when the data are continuous rather than categorical, samples are small and very unequal, and for any 2×2 comparison. In these instances, Fisher's exact test should be used instead.

$R \times C$ Chi-Square

The $R \times C$ χ^2 test can be used to analyze discontinuous frequency type data as in the Fisher's exact or 2×2 χ^2 tests. However, in the $R \times C$ test (R = row, C = column), we wish to compare three or more sets of data. An example would be comparison of the incidence of tumors among mice on three or more dose levels of a test article. We can consider the data as positive (tumors) or negative (no tumors). The expected frequency for any box is (row total) (column total)/(n_{total}). As in the Fisher's exact test, the initial step is setting up an $R \times C$ contingency table as shown in Table 16.21.

Using these symbols, the formula for χ^2 is as follows (Eq. 16.17):

The (χ^2) equation for calculating an $R \times C$ contingency table

$$\chi^2 = \frac{N_{tot}^2}{N_A N_B N_K}\left(\frac{A_1^2}{N_1}+\frac{A_2^2}{N_2}+\cdots\frac{A_K^2}{N_K}-\frac{N_A^2}{N_{tot}}\right) \quad (16.17)$$

-where N_A is the total of the positives, N_B the total of the negatives, N_K the last observation, A_1 the total of the positives for group I, A_2 the total of the positives for group II, A_K ... N_1 the sum of the positive and negative data for group I, N_2 the sum of the positive and negative data for group II, and N_{tot} is the total of all groups.

The resulting χ^2 value is compared to table values according to the number of df, which is equal to $(R-1)(C-1)$. If χ^2 is smaller than the table value at the 0.05 probability level, the groups are not significantly different. If the calculated χ^2 is larger, there is a difference among the groups. A $2 \times R$ χ^2 or Fisher's exact tests will have to be undertaken to determine which group(s) differ.

Some attributes of the $R \times C$ χ^2 test are that none of the expected frequency values should be less than 0, as it is always one tailed; the results must be a positive number; and the order of the cells is independent. It can be used to test the probability of validity of any distribution. Without some form of correction, the test becomes less accurate as the differences in group size increase, and it is weak with either small sample sizes or when the frequency in any cell is less than 5.0.

7.3. Hypothesis Testing in Single Factor Experiments

Univariate case data (i.e., each datum is defined by one treatment and one effect variable) from normally distributed populations generally have a higher information value associated with them than do nonnormal and nonparametric data sets. However, the traditional hypothesis testing techniques are generally affected by the presence of outliers. All data analyzed by these methods must be continuous, so that any number may represent data given datum and

TABLE 16.21   A Typical $R \times C$ Contingency Table

	Positive	Negative	Total
Group I	A_1	B_1	$A_1+B_1=N_1$
Group II	A_2	B_2	$A_2+B_2=N_2$
	↓	↓	
Group R	A_R	B_R	$A_R + B_R=N_R$
Totals	N_A	N_B	N_{total}

each such number has a measurable relationship to other numbers in the data.

Student's "t"-Test (Unpaired t-Test)

Pairs of groups having continuous, randomly distributed data are compared via *Student's t-test*. This test can be used to compare three or more groups of data, but they must be compared by examination of two groups taken at a time, and thus are preferentially compared by ANOVA. Usually, the *t*-test is used to compare a test group versus a control group, although two test groups may be compared as well.

To determine which of the three types of *t*-tests described in this chapter should be employed, the F-test is usually performed first. This test will reveal whether the variances of the data are approximately equal, which is a requirement for the use of the parametric *t*-tests. If the *F*-test indicates homogeneous variances and the numbers of data within the groups (*N*) are equal, then the Student's *t*-test is the appropriate procedure. On the other hand, if the *F* is significant (i.e., the data are heterogeneous) and the two groups have equal numbers of data, the modified Student's *t*-test is applicable. The value of *t* for Student's *t*-test is calculated using the following formula (Eq. 16.18).

Formula for calculating Student's *t*

$$t = \frac{\overline{X}_1 - \overline{X}_2}{\sum D_1^2 + \sum D_2^2} \sqrt{\frac{n_1 n_2}{n_1 + n_2}(n_1 + n_2 - 2)}$$

$$(16.18)$$

-where the value of $\sum D^2 = \dfrac{n \sum X^2 - (\sum X)^2}{n}$ -where *n* represents the number of data within groups, *X bar* is the mean of each group, and *D* is the pooled SD of the sets.

The value of *t* obtained is compared to the values in a *t*-distribution table according to the appropriate number of df, from standard statistical texts (If the *F* value is not significant, i.e., variances are homogeneous, the df = $n_1 + n_2 - 2$. If the *F* is significant and $n_1 = n_2$, then the df = $n - 1$.

Even though a nonrandom distribution may exist, the modified *t*-test is still valid. If the calculated value is larger than the *t*-distribution table value at *P* = .05, it may then be compared to the appropriate values for lower *P*-values in order of decreasing probability to determine the degree

of significance between the two groups. The test assumes that the data are univariate, continuous and normally distributed, and are collected by random sampling.

This *t*-test should not be used when the data are ranked, when the data do not approximate a normal distribution, or when there are more than two groups to be compared. This method also should not be used for paired observations. This test is the most commonly misused test method.

The main difference between the Z-test and the *t*-test is that the Z-statistic is based on a known SD, σ, while the *t*-statistic uses the sample SD, *s*, as an estimate of σ. With the assumption of normally distributed data, the variance σ^2 is more closely estimated by the sample variance s^2 as *n* gets large. It can be shown that the *t*-test is equivalent to the Z-test for infinite df. In practice, a large sample is usually considered to represent $n \geq 30$.

Cochran t-Test

The *Cochran t-test* should be used to compare two groups of continuous data when the variances, as indicated by the *F*-test, are heterogeneous and the numbers of data within the groups are not equal ($n_1 \neq n_2$). This is the situation when randomly distributed data are expected to not exhibit such a distribution. Two *t* values are calculated for this test, the observed *t* (t_{obs}) and the expected *t* (*t*). The t_{obs} is obtained by using the formula in Eq. (16.19).

Formula for the Cochran test

$$t_{obs} = \frac{\overline{X}_1 - \overline{X}_2}{\sqrt{W_1 + W_2}} \qquad (16.19)$$

-where *W* is the SEM^2 (standard error of the mean squared) = S^2/n.

S (variance) can be calculated as follows:

$$S = \frac{\dfrac{n \sum X^2 - (\sum X)^2}{n}}{n - 1}$$

The value for *t'* is obtained from the following:

$$t' = \frac{t_1' W_1 + t_2' W_2}{W_1 + W_2}$$

-where t_1' and t_2' are values for the two groups taken from the *t*-distribution table corresponding to $n-1$ df (for each group) at the 0.05 probability level (or such other significance level one may select), n is the number of observations, and $\bar{X}$ bar is the mean of the observations.

The calculated t_{obs} is compared to the calculated t' value (or values, if t' values are prepared for more than one probability level). If t_{obs} is smaller than a t', the groups are not considered to be significantly different at that probability level.

The Cochran t-test assumes that the data are univariate, continuous, and normally distributed, and that group sizes are unequal. It is robust for moderate departures from normality, and very robust for departures from equality of variances.

Multiple Comparison Tests

A wide variety of *post hoc* tests are available to analyze data after finding a significant result from an ANOVA. Each of these tests has advantages and disadvantages and proponents and critics. Four of the tests commonly used in toxicologic pathology include *Duncan's multiple range test*, *Scheffe's multiple comparisons*, *Dunnett's t-test*, and *Williams' t-test*. If ANOVA reveals no significance, it is inappropriate to perform a *post hoc* test to find differences. To do so would result in multiple comparisons for the same data set, which increases the possibility of a type I error rate (i.e., false positive) beyond the desired level.

DUNCAN'S MULTIPLE RANGE TEST

Duncan's multiple range test is used to compare groups of continuous and randomly distributed data (body weights, organ weights, etc.). The test is used to determine where significant differences exist among three or more groups and is performed by evaluating one pair at a time. This test, as with other *post hoc* tests, should only follow observation of a significant F value in the ANOVA. It serves to determine which group (or groups) differs significantly from some other group (or groups).

There are two alternative methods of calculation. The selection of the proper one is based on whether the number of data (n) in each group is equal or unequal.

GROUPS WITH EQUAL NUMBERS OF DATA Two sets of calculations must be carried out. First, the determination of the difference between the means of pairs of groups must be determined. Second, a probability rate must be prepared against which each difference in means is compared.

The means are determined (or taken from the ANOVA calculation) and ranked in either decreasing or increasing order. If two means are the same, they take up two equal positions in the rank. Thus, for four means, we could have ranks of 1, 2, 2, and 4 rather than 1, 2, 3, and 4. The situation for this parametric ANOVA differs from that of nonparametric tests, where the average rank assigned to ties in this case would be 1, 2.5, 2.5, and 4.

The groups are then taken in pairs, and the differences between the means ($\bar{X}$ bar) when they have been expressed as positive numbers are calculated: $(\bar{X}_1 - \bar{X}_2)$. Usually, each pair consists of a test group and the control group, through multiple tests groups may be compared if so desired. The relative rank of the two groups being compared must be considered. If a test group is ranked "2" and the control group is ranked "1," then we say that there are two places between them; if the test group were ranked "3," then there would be three places between it and the control. To establish the probability table, the SEM must be calculated as shown in Eq. (16.20).

Calculating the standard error of the mean

$$\text{SEM} = \sqrt{\dfrac{\sqrt{\dfrac{error\ mean\ square}{n}}}{\sqrt{\dfrac{mean\ square\ within\ group}{n}}}} \qquad (16.20)$$

-where n is the number of animals or replications per dose level.

The mean square within groups (MS_{wg}) can be calculated from the information given in the ANOVA procedure (refer to the earlier section on ANOVA). The SEM is then multiplied by a series of table values to set up a probability table. The table values used for the calculations are chosen according to the probability levels (note that standard tables for this purpose have sections for 0.05, 0.01, and 0.001 significance levels) as well as the number of places separating the means for the groups being compared and the number of error df. The error df is the number of df within the groups, and can be taken from ANOVA output. For some values of df, the table values are not given and should thus be interpolated.

GROUPS WITH UNEQUAL NUMBERS OF DATA- This procedure is very similar to that discussed above. As before, the means are ranked and the differences between the means are determined $(\overline{X}_1 - \overline{X}_2)$. Next, weighting values (a_u) are calculated for the pairs of groups being compared.

Formula for determining weighting values

$$a_u = \sqrt{\frac{2n_i n_j}{(n_i + n_j)}} = \sqrt{\frac{2n_1 n_2}{(n_1 + n_2)}} \quad (16.21)$$

-where a_u is the weighting value, $n_i \ldots n_j \ldots, n_1 \ldots, n_2 \ldots$ are observations.

This weighting value for each pair of groups is multiplied by $(\overline{X}_1 - \overline{X}_2)$ for each value to arrive at a "t" value. It is the t that will later be compared to a probability table (Beyer, 1982). The probability table is set up as described before except that instead of multiplying the appropriate table values by SEM, the multiplier SEM^2 is used. This result is equal to $\sqrt{MS_{wg}}$ as calculated previously during the ANOVA.

For the desired comparison of two groups at a time, the $(\overline{X}_1 - \overline{X}_2)$ value (if $n_1 = n_2$) is compared to the appropriate probability table. Each comparison must be made according to the number of places between the means. If the table value is larger at the 0.05 level, the two groups are not considered to be statistically different. If the table value is smaller, the groups are different, and the comparison is repeated at lower levels of significance. Thus, the degree of significance may be determined. We might have significant differences at 0.05 but not at 0.01, in which case the probability would be represented as $.05 > P > .01$.

Duncan's multiple range test assures a set α level (or Type I error rate) for all tests when means are separated by approximately regular intervals. Preserving this α level means that the test is less sensitive than other *post hoc* tests, such as the Student–Newman–Keuls test. Duncan's test is inherently conservative and not resistant or robust.

SCHEFFE'S MULTIPLE COMPARISONS TEST

Scheffe's multiple comparison test is another post hoc comparison method for groups of continuous and randomly distributed data. It compares three or more groups and is widely considered a more powerful significance test than Duncan's. Each *post hoc* comparison is tested by comparing an obtained test value (F_{contr}) with the appropriate critical F value at the selected level of significance (i.e., table F value multiplied by $K-1$ for an F with $K-1$ and $n - K$ df^2, where K = the number of groups and n = number of observations). F_{contr} is calculated as follows: compute the mean for each sample (group), calculate the residual mean squares by MS_{wg} (performed during the ANOVA), and then compute the F_{contr} as shown in Eq. (16.22).

Method for Scheffe's multiple comparisons

$$F_{contr} = \frac{\left(C_1 \overline{X}_1 + C_2 \overline{X}_2 + \cdots + C_k \overline{X}_k^{12} \right)}{(K-1)MS_{wg}\left(C_1^2/n_1 + \cdots + C_K^2/n_k \right)} \quad (16.22)$$

-where C_k is the comparison number such that the sum of C_1, $C_2 \ldots C_k = 0$, n is the number of observations, MS_{wg} is the mean square within groups, X *bar* is the means of observed values for groups, K the number of groups, and k the last observation.

The *Scheffe's procedure* is robust to moderate violations of the normality and homogeneity of variance assumptions. It is not formulated for groups with equal numbers (as one of Duncan's procedures is), and if $n_1 \neq n_2$, no separate weighting procedure is necessary.

The Scheffe's procedure is powerful because of it robustness, yet it is very conservative. Type I error (the false-positive rate) is held constant at the selected test level for each comparison. It assesses all linear contrasts among the population means, while the other three *post hoc* methods confine themselves to pair-wise comparison, except that they use a mathematical correction for multiple comparisons, such as the Bonferroni procedure. The Bonferroni method is a simple approach to control the Type I error when multiple comparisons are made. In order to perform the Bonferroni correction, the original alpha level is divided by the total number of analyzes that are conducted.

DUNNETT'S *T*-TEST

Dunnett's t-test assumes that what is desired analytically is a comparison of each of several means with one other mean and only that one other mean. In other words, it assumes that one wishes to compare every treatment group with a control group, but not compare treatment groups with each other. This approach will cause a problem if comparison of a treatment group with another treatment group is required. However, if one does want only to compare treatment groups versus a control group, Dunnett's *t*-test is a useful approach.

To illustrate the method, let us evaluate a study with K groups (one of them being the control) where one wishes to make $K-1$ comparisons (since the control does not have to be compared to itself). In such a situation, one wants to have a P-level for the entire set of $K-1$ decisions (not for each individual decision), as the Dunnett's distribution is predicated on this assumption. The parameters for utilizing a Dunnett's table, such as found in his original article (Dunnett, 1955), are K (the number of groups) and the number of df for MS_{wg}. The test value can be calculated as shown in Eq. (16.23).

Formula for calculating Dunnett's *t*-test

$$t = \frac{|T_j - T_i|}{\sqrt{2MS_{wg}/n}} \qquad (16.23)$$

-where n is the number of observations in each of the groups. The MS_{wg} is derived from the ANOVA as we have defined previously, T_j is the control group mean, and T_i is the mean of each successive test group observation.

Note that one uses the absolute value resulting from subtraction of T_i from T_j to ensure a positive number for t. Dunnett's *t*-test seeks to ensure that the Type I error rate will be fixed at the desired level by incorporating correction factors (CFs) into the design of the test value table. It is assumed that the treated group sizes must be approximately equal.

WILLIAMS' *T*-TEST

Williams' t-test is designed to detect the highest level in a set of dose/exposure levels at which there is no significant effect; in essence, it helps define the no observed effect level (NOEL). The test assumes that the response of interest, such as change in body weights, occurs only at higher dose levels and that the responses are monotonically ordered so that $X_0 \leq X_l$ ... $\leq X_k$. However, this arrangement is frequently not the case, such as occurs in the case of U-shaped dose–response relationships for essential nutrients. The Williams' technique handles the occurrence of such discontinuities in a response series by replacing the offending value at level K and the value immediately preceding it with weighted average values. The test also is adversely affected by any mortality at high dose levels. Such mortalities impose a severe penalty, reducing the power of detecting an effect not only at level K but also at all lower doses. Accordingly, it is not generally applicable in toxicologic pathology studies.

F-Test

The *F-test* for the *homogeneity of variances* between *two groups* of data is used in two separate instances. The first is when Bartlett's test indicates heterogeneity of variances among three or more groups (i.e., it is used to determine which pairs of groups are heterogeneous). Second, the *F*-test is the initial step in comparing two groups of continuous data that one would expect to be parametric (i.e., two groups not usually being compared using ANOVA), with the results indicating whether the data are from the same population and whether subsequent parametric comparisons would be valid. The F statistic is calculated by dividing the larger variance (S_1^2) by the smaller one (S_2^2). S^2 is calculated as follows (Eq. 16.24):

Formula for calculating S^2

$$S^2 = \frac{\dfrac{n\sum X^2 - (\sum X)^2}{n}}{n-1} \qquad (16.24)$$

-where n is the number of data in the group and X represents the individual values within the group.

Frequently, S_2 values may be obtained from ANOVA calculations. The calculated F value is compared to the appropriate number in an F value table for the appropriate df $(n-1)$ in the numerator (along the top of the table) and in the denominator (along the side of the table). If the calculated value is smaller, it is not significant, and the variances are considered homogeneous; the Student's t-test would be appropriate for further comparison. If the calculated F value is greater, F is significant, and the variances are heterogeneous. In this setting, the modified Student's t-test would be appropriate if $n_1 = n_2$, while the Cochran t-test should be used if $n_1 \neq n_2$.

The F-test could be considered as a two-group equivalent of the Bartlett's test and assumes normality and independence of data. If the test statistic is close to 1.0, the results are not significant.

One-Way Analysis of Variance

The *parametric ANOVA* is used for comparison of three or more groups of continuous data when the variances are homogeneous, and the data are independent and normally distributed (Scheffe, 1999). A series of calculations are required for ANOVA, starting with the values (X) within each group being added $(\sum X)$ and then these sums being added $(\sum\sum X)$. Each datum within the groups is squared (X^2), then these squares are then summed $(\sum X^2)$, and these sums added $(\sum\sum X^2)$. Next a CF can be calculated as shown in Eq. (16.25).

Formula for calculating the correction factor

$$CF = \frac{\left(\sum_1^K \sum_1^n X\right)^2}{n_1 + n_2 + ...n_k} \qquad (16.25)$$

-where n is the number of values in each group, X represents the individual values within the group, and K is the number of groups.

The *total SS* is then determined as defined in Eq. (16.26):

Formula for calculating the sum of squares (SS)

$$SS_{total} = \sum_1^K \sum_1^n X^2 - CF \qquad (16.26)$$

-where n is the number of values in each group, K is the number of groups, and CF is the correction factor from Eq. (16.28).

In turn, the SS between groups (SS_{bg}) is derived as shown in Eq. (16.27):

Formula for calculating the within group sum of squares

$$SS_{wg} = SS_{total} - SS_{bg} \qquad (16.27)$$

-where SS_{wg} is the sum of squares within groups, SS_{bg} is the sum of squares between groups, and SS_{total} is the total sum of squares for the experiment.

The SS within group (SS_{wg}) is then the difference between the last results obtained in Eqs. (16.26) and (16.27), as calculated in Eq. (16.28).

Formula for calculating the between groups sum of squares (SS_{bg})

$$SS_{bg} = \frac{\left(\sum X_1\right)^2}{n_1} + \frac{\left(\sum X_2\right)^2}{n_2} + ...\frac{\left(\sum X_k\right)^2}{n_k} - CF$$

$$(16.28)$$

-where SS_{bg} is the sum of squares between groups, CF is the correction factor, n the number of observations, k is the last observation, and X represents the individual values within the group.

There are three types of df to determine when ANOVA is calculated. The appropriate df for the first equation (no. 29), *total* df, is the total number of data within all groups under analysis, minus one (i.e., $n_1 + n_2 + ... n_k - 1$, where k is the last measurement). For the second equation (no. 30), the df *between groups* is the number of groups (K) minus one ($K-1$). In the last equation (no. 31), the df *within groups* (or error df) is the difference between the first two figures (df_{total} - df_{bg}).

The next set of calculations requires determination of the two *mean squares* (MS_{bg} and MS_{wg}). As $MS = SS/df$, these are the respective sum of square values (SS_{bg} and SS_{wg}, respectively) divided by the corresponding df figures (df_{bg} and df_{wg}). The final calculation is that of the F ratio. For this calculation, the MS between groups is divided by the MS within groups: $F = MS_{bg}/MS_{wg}$.

For interpretation, the F value obtained in the ANOVA is compared to a table of F values. If $F \leq 1.0$, the results are not significant and comparison with the table values is not necessary. The df for the greater mean square (MS_{bg}) are indicated along the top of the table. Then, read down the side of the table to the line corresponding to the df for the lesser mean square

(MS_{wg}). The figure shown at the desired significance level (traditionally 0.05) is compared to the calculated F value. If the calculated number is smaller, there are no significant differences among the groups being compared. If the calculated value is larger, there is some difference among two or more groups. However, further (*post hoc*) testing will be required to determine which groups differ significantly.

The one-way ANOVA is the workhorse of statistical testing for conventional toxicity studies (with one control and two or more treatment groups). The test is robust for moderate departures from normality if the sample sizes are large enough. If the sample sizes are approximately equal, ANOVA is often robust for moderate inequality of variances (as determined by in advance by Bartlett's test or Levene's test).

It is inappropriate to use a *t*-test as a two-groups-at-a-time substitute for a formal ANOVA when attempting to identify where significant differences exist among the groups. Instead, a multiple comparison *post hoc* method must be used, as discussed in the next section.

7.4. Hypothesis Testing in Multifactor Experiments

While one-way ANOVA is appropriate when testing for differences between three or more levels of a single factor (e.g., three or more treatment groups), more complicated experimental designs can be constructed using multiple levels of more than one factor. For these cases, multifactor ANOVA models can be used.

Multifactor ANOVA

Multifactor ANOVA models can be used to decompose responses into a sum of terms representing the contributions of two or more experimental factors. Suppose an experiment was designed to measure body weight in rats across three levels of treatment and two different ages. The main effects ANOVA model below could be employed: (Eq. M1)

$$\text{Body weight} = \mu + \text{DOSE} + \text{AGE} + \varepsilon \quad \text{(M1)}$$

where μ is the overall mean body weight, DOSE is a three-level factor representing three treatment doses (say, 0.1 mg/kg, 2 mg/kg, and 10 mg/kg), AGE is a two-level factor

representing the two different ages (say, 14 weeks and 2 years), and ε represents residual error. The significance of each model term (DOSE or AGE) can be tested by comparing the F value for the model term with standard F-distribution tables just as with one-way ANOVA.

ANOVA model terms can be fixed or random. A *fixed effects* term has units that can be placed into a well-defined category, so that the units of analysis vary between categories (e.g., male or female, defined levels of a treatment, young or old). On the other hand, a *random effects* term contains units of analysis that vary within a category (e.g., subjects within a population). Random effects capture the dependency among units of a variable.

A *mixed model* ANOVA has more than one random source of variability and is appropriate for experimental designs with at least one fixed effect independent variable and at least one random effects independent variable. For instance, designs in developmental and reproductive toxicology may include measured responses from multiple pups per litter across multiple litters. Biological responses from pups in the same litter may tend to be more correlated with each other than responses from pups in different litters due to shared genetics or a shared maternal environment. When looking for differences in a response due to dose level, litter clustering can be taken into account using a random effect for litter in a mixed model. By including a random variable in the model in addition to the random error, a mixed modeling approach permits the conclusions of statistical analysis to generalize to contexts beyond the current study. Failure to model random effects appropriately could lead to misleading inferences.

Model Selection

When an experimental design involves more than one factor, multiple ANOVA models can be constructed from the same data set. Adding more terms to a model will result in a more complicated model which fit the data better. However, increasingly complex models could result in overfitting, where the model begins to describe the random error instead of the relationship between factors. It is possible that one of the factors is not important in a given analysis. An appropriate model should fit the data well, be interpretable, and also be as simple as possible for its purpose. For instance, the same data set used to construct M1 above could also be used to construct the alternative models below (Eq. M2, M3 and M4):

$$\text{Body weight} = \mu + \text{DOSE} + \varepsilon \qquad \text{(M2)}$$

$$\text{Body weight} = \mu + \text{AGE} + \varepsilon \qquad \text{(M3)}$$

$$\text{Body weight} = \mu + \text{DOSE} + \text{AGE} + \text{DOSE}$$
$$* \text{AGE} + \varepsilon$$
$$\text{(M4)}$$

-where only the DOSE factor was not considered in model M2, only the AGE factor was not considered in model M3, and an interaction between DOSE and AGE was considered in model M4. Which of these models (M1–M4) is most appropriate? Model selection can help to answer this question.

Model selection can be used to compare two ANOVA models in order to determine whether a more complicated ANOVA model is justified given the data. Many different procedures have been developed for model selection, but the most common approaches are based on the *F*-test, the Akaike information criterion (*AIC*) and the Bayesian information criterion (*BIC*). The *AIC* information criterion (Akaike, 1974) and *BIC* information criterion (Schwarz, 1978) reward good fitting models but include a penalty for the number of parameters in each model when comparing two models. The *BIC* information criterion tends to penalize the selection of complex models more heavily than the *AIC* information criterion, and *BIC* is considered more appropriate when the true model is found among one of the models to be selected. When more than two models are compared, the order of comparisons between models must be considered. *Forward selection* starts with a model with no factors and adds the best unselected factor to the model in successive steps. This process continues until the best model is selected according to the predetermined criterion (*F*-test, *AIC*, or *BIC*). In contrast, *backward selection* starts with the most complicated model (containing all terms) and works backward in successive steps by comparing the most complicated model with the model constructed without the least important term until the process ends with the best model selected using the *F*-test, *AIC*, or

BIC criterion. Modified versions of selection include *stepwise selection* which start with a full model and successively move "backward" and then "forward and then backward" (etc.) until the best model is reached.

While model selection can aid in the process of choosing the most appropriate model, it is important to keep in mind that there are limitations to this procedure. First, the model selection approach is automated and therefore is based on mathematical criteria and not scientific knowledge. Model selection may result in a final model that is unrealistic or not scientifically meaningful. Furthermore, the results of stepwise selection may not result in the optimal model with very complicated data sets since the final model may depend on which model is used as the starting model. The toxicologic pathology should always employ scientific judgment as part of the model selection process.

7.5. Analysis of Covariance

This method compares sets of data that consist of two variables (treatment and effect, with the effect variable being called the *variate*), when a third variable (called the *covariate*) also exists. This covariate can be measured but not controlled and has a definite effect on responses to the variable of interest. In other words, ANCOVA provides an indirect type of statistical control, allowing us to increase the precision of a study and to remove a potential source of bias.

One common example of this approach is in the analysis of organ weights in toxicity studies. One usually wishes to evaluate the effect of dose or exposure level on the specific organ weights, but most organ weights also increase in proportion to increases in animal body weight. As the primary interest is not in the effect of the body weight covariate, body weight is measured to allow for adjustment. However, care must be taken before using ANCOVA to ensure that the underlying nature of the correspondence between the variate and covariate is such that it can be relied on as a tool for adjustments.

The ANCOVA calculation is performed in two steps. The first is a type of linear regression between the variate Y and the covariate X. This regression, performed as described under the linear regression section below, gives the model defined in Eq. (16.29).

Linear regression model

$$Y = a_1 + BX + e \qquad (16.29)$$

-where
a_1 = the intercept value for the Y-axis.
B = the slope factor
e = the statistical error term.
Y = the variate.
X = the covariate.

This model in turn allows us to define adjusted means ($\overline{Y}$ and $\overline{X}$) such that $\overline{Y}_{1a} = \overline{Y} - (\overline{X}_1 - \overline{X}*)$. If we consider the case where K treatment groups are being compared such that $K = 1, 2, ...k$, and we let X_{ik} and Y_{ik} represent the predictor and predicted values for each individual in group k, we can let X_k and Y_k be the means. Then, we define the between-group (for treatment) SS and cross-products as shown in Eq. (16.30).

Calculation of the between and within treatment group sum of squares and cross products for the analysis of covariance

$$T_{xx} = \sum_{k-1}^{K} n_k \left(\overline{X}_K - \overline{X} \right)^2$$

$$T_{yy} = \sum_{k-1}^{K} n_k \left(\overline{Y}_K - \overline{Y} \right)^2 \qquad (16.30)$$

$$T_{xy} = \sum_{k-1}^{K} n_k \left(\overline{X}_k - \overline{X} \right) \left(\overline{Y}_k - \overline{Y}_k - \overline{Y} \right)$$

-where T_{xx}, T_{yy} and T_{xy} denote the source of variation for the variables X and Y; X bar and Y bar are adjusted means for the variate and covariate; n is the number of observations; K is the number of groups; and k is the last observation.

In a like manner, within-group sums of squares and cross-products are calculated as follows:

$$\sum xx = \sum_{k=1}^{k} \sum_i (X_{ik} - X_k)^2$$

$$\sum yy = \sum_{k=1}^{k} \sum_i (Y_{ik} - Y_k)^2$$

$$\sum xy = \sum_{k=1}^{k} \sum_i (X_{ik} - X_k)(Y_{ik} - Y_k)$$

-where i indicates the sum from all the individuals within each group; K is the number of groups, k is the last observation, n is the number of observations, and X and Y are adjusted means for the variate and covariate, respectively.

$$S_{xx} = T_{xx} + \sum_{xx}$$

$$S_{yy} = T_{yy} + \sum_{xx}$$

$$S_{xy} = T_{xy} + \sum_{xy}$$

With these in hand, calculate the residual mean squares of treatments (St^2) and error (Se^2) as defined in Eq. (16.31).

Formula for the residual mean of squares of treatments and error for the analysis of covariance

$$St^2 = \frac{Tyy - \dfrac{S^2xy}{Sxx} + \dfrac{\sum^2 xy}{\sum xx}}{lc - 1}$$

$$Se^2 = \frac{\left(\sum yy - \dfrac{\sum^2 y}{\sum xx} \right)}{f - 1}$$

(16.31)

-where St^2 is the residual mean squares of treatment, and Se^2 is the error.

These can be used to calculate an F statistic to test the H_0 that all treatment effects are equal.

Formula for calculating the F statistic for analysis of covariance (Eq. 16.32)

$$F = \frac{St^2}{Se^2} \qquad (16.32)$$

-where St^2 is the residual mean squares of treatment, Se^2 is the error, and F is the F statistic.

The B statistic for ANCOVA can then be calculated as follows (Eq. 16.33):

Formula for calculating the B statistic for analysis of covariance

$$B = \frac{\sum xy}{\sum xx} \qquad (16.33)$$

-where B represents the estimated regression coefficient of Y or X.

The estimated standard error for the adjusted difference between two groups can also be calculated as follows (Eq. 16.34):

Formula for calculating the standard error for analysis of covariance

$$SD = SE \frac{1}{n_j} + \frac{1}{n_j} + \frac{\left(X_i - X_j\right)^2}{\sum xx} \qquad (16.34)$$

-where n_0 and n_1 are the sample sizes of the two groups, SD is the standard deviation, SE the standard error, and X_I and X_j are variate values.

A test of the H_0 that the adjusted difference between the groups is zero can now be determined (Eq. 16.35):

Formula for calculating the t statistic for analysis of covariance

$$t = \frac{Y_1 - Y_0 - B(X_1 - X_0)}{SD} \qquad (16.35)$$

-where Y_0 and Y_1 are covariate values, SD is the standard deviation, X_1 and X_2 are variate values, and B is the B statistic for ANCOVA.

The test value for the t is then looked up in the t-distribution table with $n-1$ df. Although this is a complex procedure, computation is markedly simplified if all the groups are of equal size.

The underlying assumptions for ANCOVA are fairly rigid and restrictive. First, the slopes of the regression lines of a Y and X must be equal from group to group. This can be examined visually (i.e., by graphing) or formally (i.e., by a statistical test). If this condition is not met, ANCOVA cannot be used. Next, this test assumes that the relationship between X and Y is linear and that there are no unmeasured confounding variables. Third, the errors inherent in each variable must be independent of each other. Lack of independence effectively (but to an immeasurable

degree) reduces sample size. Therefore, the method assumes that the variances of the errors within groups are equivalent among groups and that the measured data that form the groups are normally distributed. ANCOVA is generally robust to departures from normality.

7.6. Modeling Trends

The mathematical modeling of biological systems is an extremely large and vigorously growing area. Broadly speaking, modeling is the principal conceptual tool by which toxicologic pathology seeks to develop as a mechanistic science. In such an iterative process, models are developed or proposed, tested by experiment, and refined in a continuous cycle.

Trend analysis is a collection of techniques dating back to the mid-1950s that have been employed in toxicology applications since the mid-1970s. These methods are a variation on the theme of regression testing. While comparisons of individual treated groups with the control group are important, a more powerful test of a possible effect of treatment is a test for a dose-related trend. *Trend tests* use all the data in a single analysis to evaluate the effects of treatment that result in a positive or negative dose–response relationship.

Trend tests seek to evaluate whether there is a monotonic tendency in response to a change in treatment. The best example of a monotonic tendency is the direction of the dose response for induction of tumors, which is absolute; as the dose goes up, the incidence of tumors should always increase. Thus, the test loses power rapidly in response to the occurrence of reversals—for example, when a low-dose group has a decreased tumor incidence. There are methods that smooth the bumps of reversals in long data series.

Low-Dose Extrapolation and NOEL Estimation

In interpreting the results of trend tests, it should be noted that a significant trend does not necessarily imply a significant biological effect at lower doses (Clewell et al., 2019).

Conversely, a lack of a significant increase at lower doses does not necessarily indicate evidence of a threshold, i.e., a dose below which no increase occurs.

Testing for a trend is a *more sensitive method* than simple pair-wise comparisons of treated and control groups for showing a possible treatment effect. Attempting to estimate the magnitude of effects at low doses, typically below the lowest positive dose tested in the study, is a much more complex procedure, and is heavily dependent on the assumed functional form of the dose–response relationship.

Low-dose extrapolation is typically conducted for tumors caused by a genotoxic agent. Given severe limits in our current biological understanding of low-dose genotoxicity, and the inability to generate data in the very low-response range of the dose–response curve, no threshold is ordinarily assumed in making such extrapolations. This assumption is based on a current understanding of initiation and a lack of evidence for a less conservative (i.e., protective) approach. However, some, but by no means all, scientists believe these tumors have no threshold. For other types of tumors, and for many nonneoplastic endpoints, a threshold cannot be estimated directly from data at a limited number of dose levels.

A *NOEL* can be estimated by finding the highest dose level at which there is no significant increase in treatment-related effects. It should be noted that the NOEL addresses any treatment-related effect, whereas the no observable adverse effect level defines whether or not the effect was detrimental. The other statistic of great importance to understanding where on the dose curve the treatment-related response occurs is the *lowest observed effect level* (LOEL), or lowest observed adverse effect level. These levels are the lowest dose at which an effect or adverse effect occurred. The true threshold for the effect of *interest under the conditions of the study* is bracketed by the NOEL and LOEL (i.e., the threshold t is given by NOEL < t < LOEL).

Trend Test for Tumor Rates

In 1985, the United States (U.S.) *Federal Register* recommended that the analysis of tumor incidence data be carried out with a *Cochran–Armitage trend test*. Since then, controversy exists as to the test(s) to be used for analysis of tumor

incidence and there are competing approaches. The current version of the discussion here is consistent with the draft Food and Drug Administration (FDA) guidelines in that the Peto method should not be used when it is not possible to accurately determine whether a tumor is incidental, fatal, or mortality independent (Lin and Rahman, 2018). In this case, the FDA references survival-adjusted methods that do not require that information. Below we mention one such approach that has been probably the most widely used, the Poly-k approach.

COCHRAN–ARMITAGE TEST

The test statistic of the Cochran–Armitage test is defined in Eq. (16.36).

Calculation of the test statistic T_{CA} of the Cochran–Armitage trend test

$$T_{CA} = \sqrt{\frac{N}{(N-r))r'} , \frac{\sum\limits_{i=0}^{k}\left(R_1 - \frac{n_1}{N}r\right)d_1}{\sqrt{\sum\limits_{i=0}^{k}\frac{n_i}{N}d_i^2 - \left(\sum\limits_{i=0}^{k}\frac{n_i}{N}d_1\right)^2}}}$$

(16.36)

-where dose scores are represented by d_i. T represents the test statistic (for the condition carcinogenicity, CA), and the maximum likelihood estimator represented by n/N, where N is the number of tests, n are group sizes, R is the number of groups, and r is the Dawson correlation coefficient.

Armitage's test statistic is the square of this term (T^2_{CA}). As one-sided tests are carried out for an increase of tumor rates, the square is not considered. Instead, the above-mentioned one-sided T_{CA} test statistic is used. The Cochran–Armitage test is asymptotically efficient for all monotonic alternatives, but this result only holds asymptotically. Tumors are rare events; therefore, the binomial proportions are small. In this situation, approximations may become unreliable.

To address this potential unreliability, exact tests can be performed using conditional and unconditional approaches. In the conditional approach, the total number of tumors r is regarded as fixed. As a result, the null distribution of the test statistic is independent of the common probability *P*. The exact conditional null distribution is a multivariate hypergeometric distribution. In contrast, the unconditional model treats the sum of all tumors as a random variable. Then, the exact unconditional null distribution is a multivariate binomial distribution. The distribution depends on the unknown probability.

NEED FOR AGE ADJUSTMENT

Where there are marked differences in survival among treated groups, there generally is a need for an age adjustment (i.e., an adjustment for age at death or onset) when organizing the data for analysis. This is illustrated in the example above where, because of the greater number of deaths occurring early in the treated group, the true effect of treatment disappears if no adjustment is made. Thus, a major purpose of age adjustment is to avoid *temporal bias*.

It is not always recognized that, even where there are no survival differences, an age adjustment can increase the power to detect group differences. This is illustrated by the example in Table 16.22 below.

In this example, treatment results in an earlier onset of a condition causing mortality, which eventually occurs in all animals. Failure to age adjust will result in a comparison of 29/50 deaths in the exposed animals with an incidence of 21/50 in the controls, which is not statistically significant. Age adjustment will essentially ignore the early and late deaths, which contribute no comparative statistical information, and instead base the comparison on the midterm deaths—9/10 for the exposed versus 1/10 for controls—which is statistically significant. By avoiding diluting the data that are capable of detecting treatment effects with data that are of little or no value for this purpose, age adjustment sharpens the contrast while still avoiding bias.

PETO METHOD FOR CONTEXT OF OBSERVATION

Age adjustment cannot be used unless the context of the endpoint is clear. There are three relevant contexts, the first two relating to the situation where the condition is only observed at death (e.g., an internal tumor) and the third where it can be observed during life (e.g., a skin tumor). In the first context, the condition is assumed to have caused the death of the animal, i.e., to have been *fatal*. Here, the incidence rate for a time interval and a group is calculated as the number of animals dying because of the lesion during the interval divided by the number of animals alive at the start of the interval. In the second context, the animal is assumed to have died of another cause, i.e., the internal tumor is *incidental*. In the case of incidental lesions, the rate is calculated as the number of animals with the lesion dying during the interval divided by the total number of deaths during the interval. In the third context, where the lesion is *visible*, the rate is calculated as the number of animals with the condition during the interval divided by the number of animals without the condition at the start of the interval.

The *Peto method* (Peto, 1980)—a quantal categorization as to whether a tumor is incidental or fatal—takes context of observation into account (Vol 1, Chap 8: Carcinogenesis: Mechanisms and Evaluation). Sometimes the nature of the lesion does not always allow the toxicologic pathologist to decide whether a condition is fatal or incidental. However, in experiments where marked survival differences are seen, the toxicologic pathologist should attempt to decide upon the context of the lesion. Failure to do so may result in the inability to conclude reliably whether a treatment is beneficial or harmful.

For those individuals who evaluate carcinogenicity studies, the definition of what constitutes a fatal tumor sometimes conflicts with the needs of the statistician regarding hard measurable endpoints. Here, we have a paradox: the statistician requires mutually exclusive groups of fatal versus nonfatal tumors for the analysis, whereas the pathologist rarely is able to judge without

TABLE 16.22   The Effect of Age Adjustment on Mortality Data

	Control	Exposed
Early deaths	0/20	0/20
Midterm deaths	1/10	9/10
Late deaths	20/20	20/20
Total	21/50	29/50

question whether or not a given lesion was fatal. To demonstrate the problem, and pose a solution, examples can be used to showcase the concrete data needed by the statistician with the weak mortality data typically generated by the toxicologic pathologist.

The effect of poorly defined context, and the need to have context for statistical purposes, is well illustrated by evaluation of the alkylating (genotoxic) chemical N-nitrosodimethylamine (NDMA, also called dimethyl nitrosamine) for carcinogenicity. Early rodent studies with this agent suggested that exposed animals developed a higher incidence of pituitary gland neoplasia than would be expected. If an assumption was made that all pituitary tumors are fatal, the false conclusion was reached that NDMA was carcinogenic. In contrast, if it were assumed that these lesions were incidental, the equally false conclusion that NDMA was protective would have resulted. By using the toxicologic pathologist's contextual opinion as to which tumors were, and which were not, likely to be fatal, the resulting analysis correctly concluded that NDMA had no carcinogenic effect in the pituitary (Peto et al., 1991).

It is imperative that the toxicologic pathologist attempts to judge the context in which lesions have occurred, as she/he is the most competent to make such a judgment based on training and actual compilation of the pathology data set; in particularly complex cases, peer review of lesions by one or a group of additional pathologists may be warranted to assign context (Volume 1: Pathology peer review). Failure to put the lesions in context may result in either an erroneous conclusion or no conclusion at all.

Many toxicologic pathologists have entered the Peto variable (a quantal categorization regarding whether or not the tumor in question was incidental or fatal) whenever she/he felt that a particular neoplasm was why the animal came to necropsy that day. For example, an animal that has been slowly deteriorating in a bioassay was found to have a 10mm diameter pituitary mass at necropsy. The histological evaluation of the mass revealed that is was a *pars distalis* adenoma. The clinical history of no neurological signs with this space-occupying lesion indicates that the tumor was slow growing. It may seem that the Peto variable in

this case should be marked as fatal. However, such an action would be a mistake.

The Peto variable is collected for the purpose of determining the *duration* of the tumor's presence. A fatal classification generally is assigned to a tumor that has been interpreted as *rapidly fatal*. The pathologist classifies tumors as incidental, fatal, or mortality independent (observable). Incidental tumors are those tumors deemed not directly or indirectly responsible for the animal's death but observed at necropsy. Fatal tumors are neoplasms deemed to have killed the animal either directly or indirectly. Mortality-independent tumors are masses that are detected at times other than at necropsy.

The distinction between fatal and incidental tumors is important. This context is essential to distinguish between a chemical that reduces survival by shortening either the time to tumor onset or the time to death following tumor onset (a real carcinogenic effect) from a compound that reduces survival, but for which tumors are observed earlier simply because they are dying of competing causes (noncarcinogenic effect). In our example above, collection of a fatal rather than an incidental classification misrepresents the real findings for the Peto variable, as the tumor was present for a long time.

In fact, the problem usually resides with misinterpretations of what the Peto variable is supposed to represent, which is to answer a single question: was the tumor fatal or incidental? Obviously, dichotomous data must result from a simple yes/no question. However, in many cases, researchers attempt to use the Peto analysis to answer two questions instead: 1) was the tumor the cause for necropsy of the animal and 2) was the tumor rapidly fatal? The Peto variable represents the second question and not the first. For this reason, it has been suggested that only tumors recognized as rapidly fatal receive the "fatal" Peto variable designation. For example, to make sure that only rapidly fatal tumors are included in this category, some laboratories only mark malignant lymphomas and leukemias as fatal, whereas all other tumors typically should be marked as incidental.

It is recommended that the conservative use of the fatal Peto variable is preferable to misclassification of an incidental datum to the fatal category, to make sure that overly conservative assessments are not made in carcinogenesis studies that are already quite conservative in their output. Regardless of violating the assumptions of the test, it is preferable to record tumor-related deaths for Peto's trend test evaluation, even if occasional errors are made in the assignment, than not to have any data regarding premature mortality in a bioassay.

Although it is normally good practice for the toxicologic pathologist to ascribe factors contributing to unscheduled death for each animal, it is not strictly necessary to determine the context of observation for all conditions at the outset. An alternative strategy is to instead analyze the pathology data under differing assumptions. Multiple analyses of the data may be done using a different context for unscheduled deaths. Typically, the analyses of decedents would assume all cases are incidental and use the context categories of no case fatal, all cases fatal, or all cases of the same defined severity fatal.

If the conclusion for all scenarios is the same, or if the toxicologic pathologist states that one scenario is the most likely, it may not be necessary to have formally assigned the context of an observation for the condition in question for each individual animal. Using this alternative strategy might result in analysis cost reduction and time saving by allowing evaluations to focus on a limited number of lesions where the conclusion seems to hang on correct knowledge of the context. Finally, it should be noted that, although many nonneoplastic conditions observed at death are not the causes of death, it is in principle just as necessary to know the context of observation for nonneoplastic conditions as it is for tumors.

POLY-K APPROACH

The *Poly-k test* is a survival-adjusted quantal response approach and represents an alternative to the Peto method to test for dose-related trends in tumor rates when survival differs across dose groups. An important advantage of the Poly-k test compared to the Peto approach is that this test does not require the determination of cause of death, which is a necessary component of the Peto method. It is important to be aware of the Poly-k test because some pathologists do not feel that it is possible to accurately determine whether a lesion was the cause of death or incidental in some circumstances. The Society of Toxicologic Pathology (STP) has published a position paper regarding statistical analysis of rodent carcinogenicity studies that discusses appropriate use of the Peto method and the Poly-k test (Society of Toxicologic Pathology, 2007).

Linear Regression

Foremost among the methods for interpolating within a known data relationship is *regression* (Montgomery et al., 2012). This method is the mathematical fitting of a line or curve to a set of known data points on a graph, and the interpolation or estimation of values along this line or curve in areas where there are no experimental data points (Figure 16.13). The simplest regression model is that of *linear regression*, which is valid when increasing the value of one variable changes the value of the related variable in a linear fashion (either positively or negatively) or when data can be transformed in such a way that the transformed data show a linear relationship. Linear regression using the method of least squares will be addressed here.

Given two sets of variables, x (e.g., mg/kg of test material administered) and y (e.g., percentage of animals so dosed that die), a solution is required for a and b in the linear equation $Y_i = a + bx_i$ [where the uppercase Y_i is the fitted value of y_i at x_i, and we wish to minimize $(y_i - Y_i)^2$]. The solution is shown in Eq. (16.37).

Formulae for calculating linear regression. The linear equation is as follows:

$$Y_i = a + bx_i \qquad (16.37)$$

-where the uppercase Y_i is the fitted value of y_i at x_i, and we wish to minimize $(y_i - Y_i)^2$; a is the y intercept; and bx_i is the slope factor b multiplied by x_i

$$b = \frac{\sum x_i y_i - n\bar{x}\bar{y}}{\sum x_1^2 - n\bar{x}^2}$$

$$\text{and } a = \bar{y} - b\bar{x}$$

-where a is the y intercept, *y bar* is the mean of y variable, *x bar* is the mean of the x variable, b is the slope of the line, and n is the number of data points.

Note that in actuality, dose–response relationships are often not linear, so a transformation to linearize the data (i.e., a nonlinear regression method) must be used. Note also that the correlation test statistic (see correlation coefficient section below) can be used to determine if the

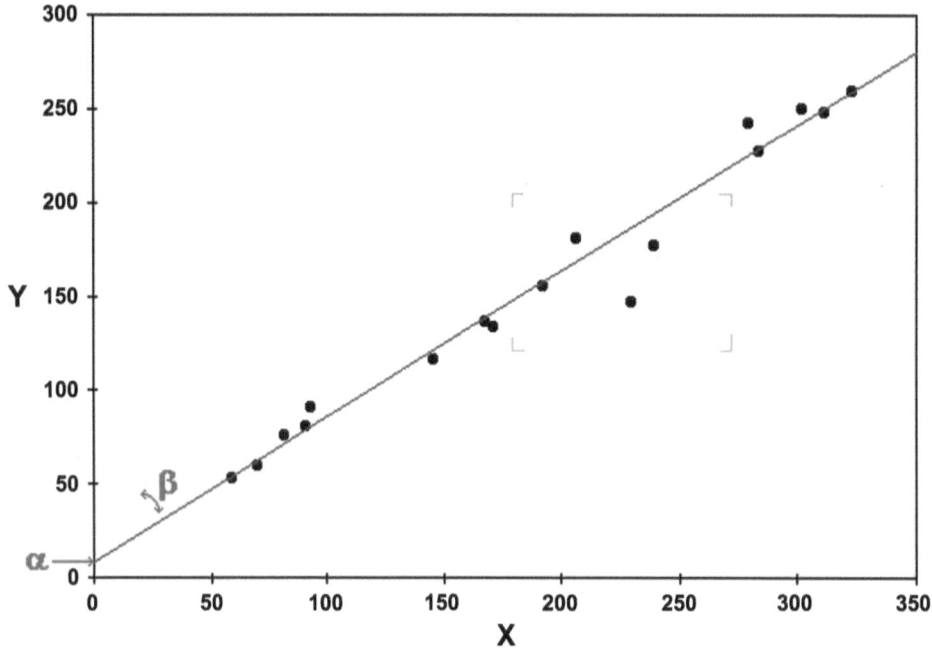

FIGURE 16.13   **A sample regression curve.**

regression is significant and, therefore, whether or not the linear model is valid at a defined level of certainty.

A more specific test for significance is the linear regression ANOVA. To do so, start by developing the appropriate ANOVA table, as previously described. Finally, determine the CIs for the regression line. In other words, given a regression line with calculated values for Y_i given x_i, within what limits at a 95% probability of certainty does the real value of Y_i lie? If the residual mean square in the ANOVA is given by s^2, the 95% confidence limits for a (denoted by A, the notation for the true—as opposed to the estimated—value for this parameter) can be calculated (Eq. 16.38):

Calculation of the 95% confidence limits for a regression line

$$t_{n-2} = \frac{a - A}{\sqrt{\dfrac{s^2\left(\sum x^2\right)}{n\sum x_1^2 - n^2\overline{x}^2}}}$$ (16.38)

-where a is the y intercept, A is true rather than estimated CI for a, s^2 is the residual mean square from ANOVA, x is the x variable, and n is the number of observations.

All the regression methods are for interpolation, not extrapolation. That is, they are valid only in the range that we have experimentally derived data, but not beyond. If such an extrapolation is made, the fact that this is a best guess must be given in the text and discussion as to the limitations of the prediction given.

The method assumes that the data are independent and normally distributed, and it is sensitive to outliers. The X-axis (or horizontal) component plays an extremely important part in developing the least squares fit. All points have equal weight in determining the height of a regression line, but extreme X-axis values unduly influence the slope of the line.

It is assumed that the treatment variable can be measured without error, that each data point is independent, that variances are equivalent, and that a linear relationship does not exist between the variables. It should be noted that a good fit between a line and a set of data (i.e., a strong correlation between treatment and response variables) does not imply any causal relationship.

Probit/Log Transforms and Regression

Dose–response relationships are among the most common interpolation problems encountered in toxicologic pathology. As noted in the preceding section, these relationships are rarely simple, so a valid linear regression often cannot be made directly from the raw data. The most common valid interpolation methods are based upon probability (*probit*) and logarithmic (*log*) value scales, with percentage responses like death and tumor incidence (Y_i) being expressed on the probit scale (generally placed on the Y-axis), while doses (X_i) are expressed on the log scale (located on the X-axis). Probit analysis is a type of regression used to analyze binomial response variables (Finney, 1971). It transforms the sigmoid dose–response curve to a straight line that can then be analyzed by regression either through least squares or maximum likelihood. A graphical representation of a probit/log transformation and regression is shown in Figure 16.14.

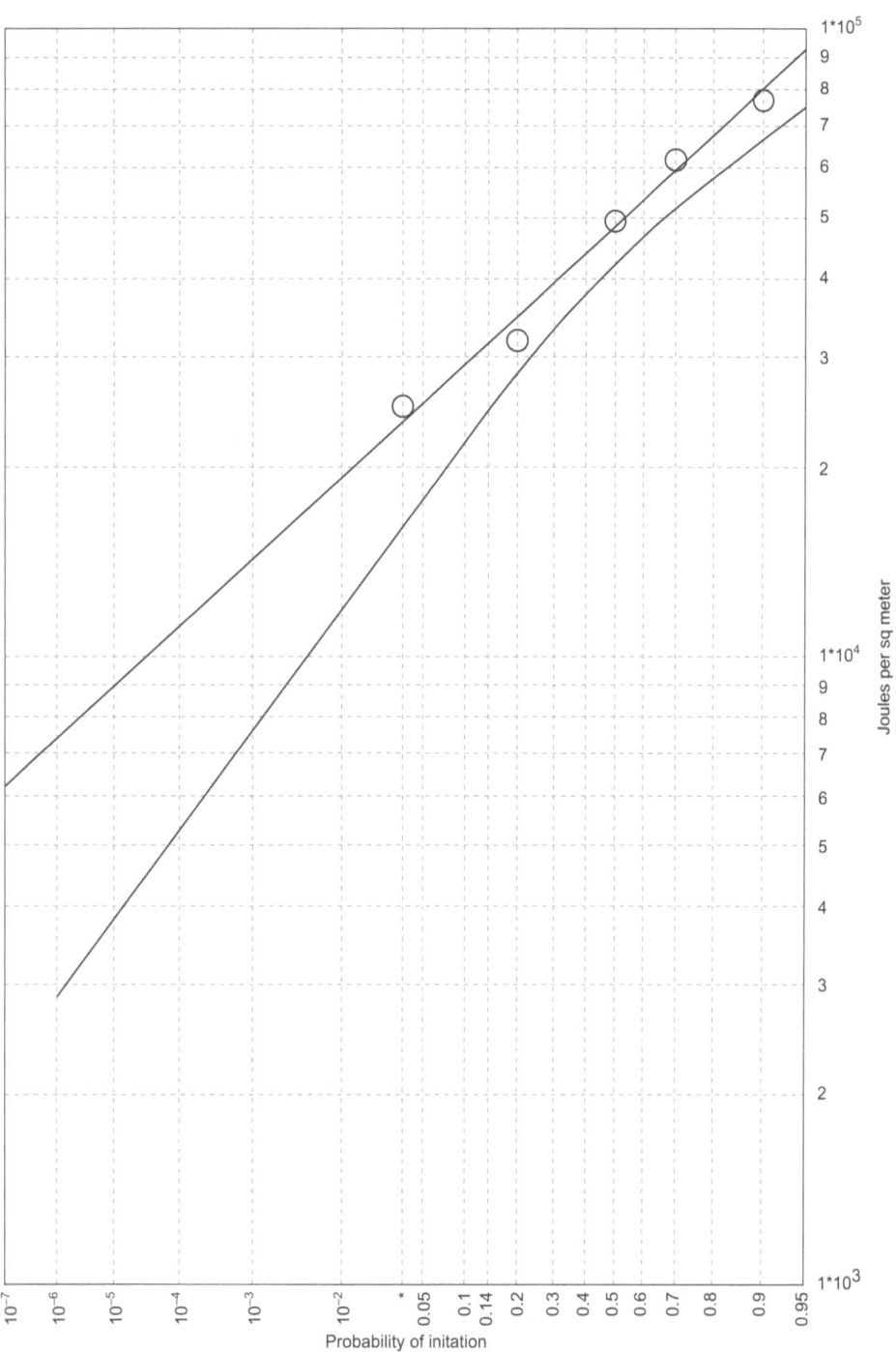

FIGURE 16.14 **A sample of a probit plot.**

There are two strategies for such a modeling approach. The first is based on transforming the data to these scales, then calculating a *weighted linear regression* on the transformed data. However, if one does not have access to a computer or a high-powered programmable calculator, it is not practical to assign weights to the data. In the absence of calculating machines, a second strategy requires the use of algorithms for the probit value and regression process. This latter technique is performed manually, and thus is extremely burdensome.

An approach to the first strategy requires construction of a table. The pairs of values of x_i and y_i are listed in order of increasing values of y_i (percentage response), and beside each of these columns, a set of blank columns remain so that the transformed values may be listed. The probits of a set value of P should be approximately linearly related to x, the measure of the treatment, and a line fitted by eye may be used to give a corresponding set of *expected probits*, Y. Then, the columns are added as described above in the linear regression procedure. Log and probit values may be taken from any of a number of sets of tables in standard texts. The remainder of the table is then developed from the transformed x_i and y_i values (denoted as x'_i and y'_i). A standard linear regression is then performed using the transformed values.

The second strategy uses methods that are computationally cumbersome. It is possible to approximate the necessary iterative computational process using the algorithms, but this process merely reduces the complexity to a point where the procedure may be readily programmed on a small computer or programmable calculator. The probit distribution then is derived from a common error function, with the midpoint (50% point) moved to a score of 5.00. A normally distributed population is assumed, and the results are sensitive to outliers.

The underlying frequency distribution used by this method becomes asymptotic as it approaches the extremes of the range. In other words, the corresponding probit values change gradually—the curve is relatively linear—in the range of 16%–84%. However, beyond this core range, the values change ever more rapidly as they approach either 0% or 100%. In fact, there are no values for either of these two limiting numbers.

Nonlinear Regression

More often than not in toxicologic pathology, relationships between two variables are *nonlinear*. Common examples include age and total body weight. In such data sets, a change in one variable (e.g., age) does not produce a directly proportional change in the other (e.g., total body weight), but some relationship between the variables is apparent. If understanding such a relationship and being able to predict unknown points is of value, two modeling options are available.

The first, which was discussed and reviewed earlier, is to use one or more transformations to render the data linear. Once converted to linear values, a linear regression can be used, but this approach has a number of drawbacks. First, not all data can be suitably transformed. Second, the transformations necessary to achieve linearity sometimes require a cumbersome series of calculations. Finally, the resulting linear regression is not always sufficient to account for the differences among sample values. For example, there may be significant deviations around the linear regression line, wherein a line may still not provide a good fit to the data or do an adequate job of representing the relationship between the variables that affect the data.

In such cases, a second option can be used: *fitting of a nonlinear function to data*, such as some form of curve. This is the general principle of nonlinear regression and may involve fitting an infinite number of possible functions to data. However, fitting curves using a polynomial function is the most commonly used technique. As the number of powers of x (the independent variable) increases, the curve becomes increasingly complex and more likely to fit a given set of data (Eq. 16.39):

The polynomial function

$$Y = a + bx + cx^2 + dx^2 + \ldots \qquad (16.39)$$

-where x is the independent variable; Y is the dependent variable; and a, b, c, d, and so on are constants.

Plotting the log of a response Y, such as body weight, versus a linear scale of doses or stimuli X results in one of four types of nonlinear curves: *exponential growth* (e.g., growth curve for the log phase of a bacterial culture), *exponential decay* (e.g., a radioactive decay curve), *asymptotic regression* (e.g., a first order reaction curve), and *logistic growth curve* (e.g., a population growth curve) (Figures 16.15–16.18). The following formulae describe these curves (Eq. 16.40, 16.41, 16.42 and 16.43). In the equations for all these cases, *A* and *B* are constants while *P* is a log transformation.

Formula for an exponential growth curve

$$\log Y = a(b^x) \qquad (16.40)$$

-where *a* is the *y* intercept and b^x is the exponential transform of the shape of the curve.

Log Y = A(Bˣ)

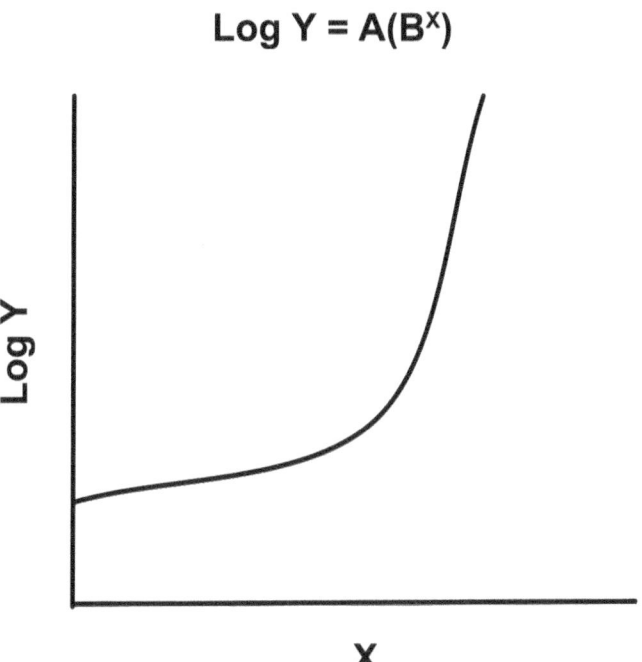

FIGURE 16.15   **Exponential growth curve.**

Log Y = A - B(pˣ)

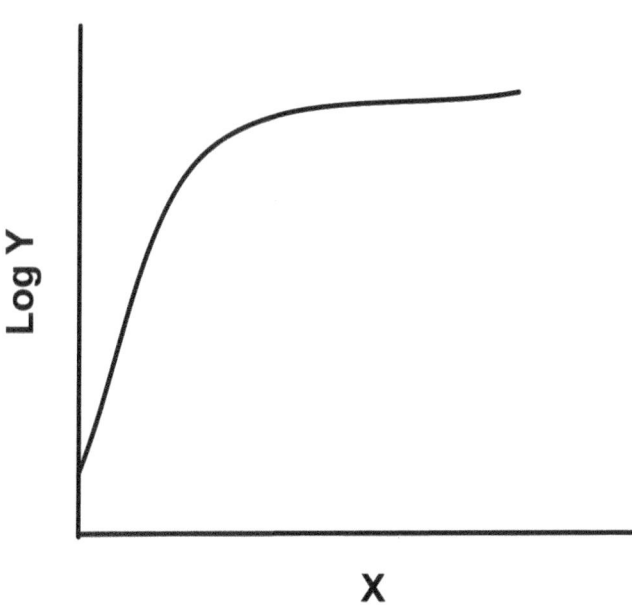

FIGURE 16.17   **Asymptotic regression curve.**

Log Y = A(B⁻ˣ)

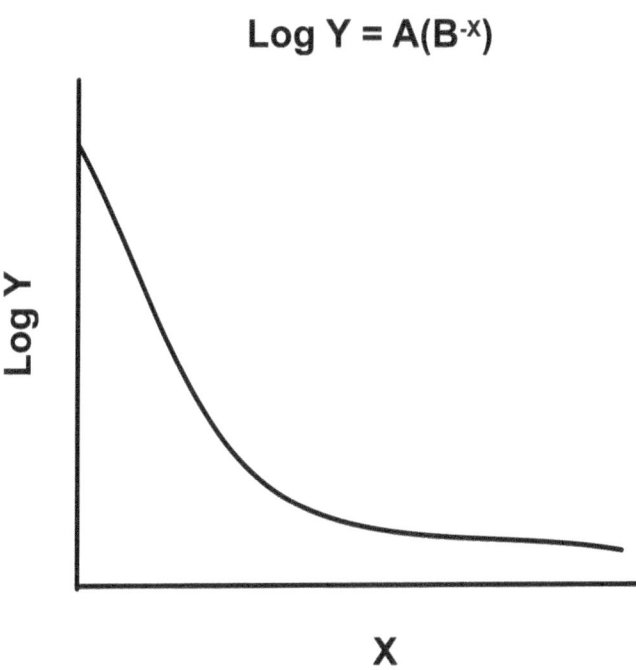

FIGURE 16.16   **Exponential decay curve.**

Log Y = A/(1 + Bpˣ)

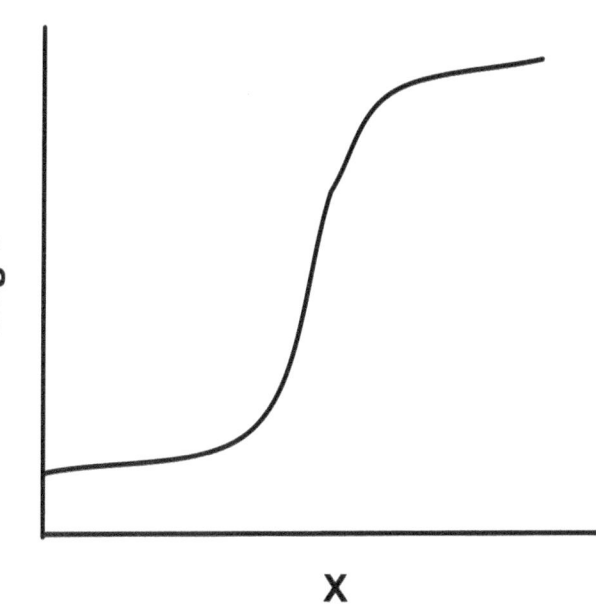

FIGURE 16.18   Logistic growth curve.

Formula for an exponential decay curve

$$\log Y = a(b^{-x}), \qquad (16.41)$$

-where a is the y intercept and b^x is the exponential transform of the shape of the curve.

Formula for an asymptotic regression curve

$$\log Y = a - b(p^x) \qquad (16.42)$$

-where p is the factor by which the rate of change in y reduces as y approaches the asymptote (log transformation), x is the primary variable on which y is defined, a is the y intercept, and b is a polynomial expression of the regression curve.

Formula for a logistic growth curve

$$\log Y = a/(1 + b * p^x) \qquad (16.43)$$

-where p is the factor by which the rate of change in y reduces as y approaches the asymptote (log transformation), x is the primary variable on which y is defined, a is the y intercept, and b is the slope factor.

Iterative processes fit all four types of curves. Thus, "best guess" numbers are initially chosen for each of the constants. After a fit is attempted, the constants are modified to improve the fit. This process is repeated until an acceptable fit has been generated. Either ANOVA or ANCOVA can be used to objectively evaluate the acceptability of the choice.

The principle of using least squares may still be applicable in fitting the best curve. Assumptions necessary to support the least squares approach include normality, independence, error-free measurement of the dose, and reasonably error-free measurement of responses. Growth curves are best modeled using a nonlinear method.

7.7. Correlation and Agreement

Both correlation and agreement are procedures used to measure the strength of association between variables. However, these two measures refer to separate concepts. Correlation describes the direction and strength of relationship between two quantitative variables, without distinguishing between explanatory and response variables. A measure of correlation may be used to describe the relationship between body weight and exposure to a pollutant. The correlation between two variables will not change when the units of the variables change. On the other hand, agreement describes the degree of concordance between two sets of measurements of one variable. A measure of agreement can be used to assess the degree to which two pathologists make the same diagnoses for the same set of lesions. Concordance can be considered a special case of correlation since two measurements that are in agreement must be correlated. Conversely, it is possible for two measurements have a strong strength of relationship (i.e., high correlation) but poor agreement.

Correlation Coefficient

The correlation procedure is used to determine the degree of linear correlation, or direct relationship, between two groups of continuous and normally distributed variables. Correlation indicates whether there is any statistical relationship between the variables in the two groups. For example, liver weights of dogs on a feeding study may be correlated with their body weights. Thus, the correlation coefficient can be calculated between liver weight and total body weight measured at necropsy to determine if there is some relationship. A formula for calculating the linear correlation coefficient (r_{xy}) is given in Eq. (16.44).

Formula for calculating the linear correlation coefficient (r_{xy})

$$r_{xy} = \frac{n \sum xy - (\sum x)(\sum y)}{\sqrt{n \sum x^2 - (\sum x)^2}\sqrt{n \sum y^2 - (\sum y)^2}}$$

$$(16.44)$$

-where x is each value for one variable, y is the matching value for the second variable, and n is the number of pairs of x and y.

Once r_{xy} has been determined, it is possible to calculate t_r, which can be used for more precise examination of the degree of significant linear relationship between the two groups. This value is calculated as shown in Eq. (16.45).

Formula for calculating the linear correlation t_r value

$$t_r = \frac{r_{xy}\sqrt{n-2}}{\sqrt{1 - r_{xy}^2}} \qquad (16.45)$$

-where r_{xy} is the linear correlation coefficient, and n is the number of observations.

It should be noted that this calculation is equivalent to $r =$ sample covariance$/(S_x S_y)$, as was seen earlier under ANCOVA.

The value obtained for r_{xy} can be compared to table values for the number of pairs of data involved, minus two (due to the two variables being tested). If the r_{xy} is smaller at the selected test probability level, the correlation is not significantly different from zero: there is no correlation. If r_{xy} is larger than the table value, there is a positive statistical relationship between the variables.

Comparisons are then made at lower levels of probability to determine the degree of relationship. Note that if r_{xy} equals either 1.0 or -1.0, there is complete correlation between the variables. If r_{xy} is a negative number and the absolute value is greater than the table value, there is an inverse relationship between the variables. In other words, a change in one variable is associated with a change in the opposite direction in the second variable.

Since the comparison of r_{xy} with the table values may be considered a somewhat weak test, it is perhaps more meaningful to compare the t_r value with values in a t-distribution table for $n-2$ df, as is done for the Student's t-test. This will give a more exact determination of the degree of statistical correlation between the two variables. Note that this method examines only possible linear relationships between sets of continuous, normally distributed data; X and Y are assumed to be independent as a H_0. The test determines whether the dependent variable (Y) depends on the independent variable (X).

The value r^2, the square correlation coefficient, is also called the coefficient of determination. It is a measure of the proportion of the variation of one variable determined by the variation of the other variable. It should be emphasized that a strong correlation does not imply a causal relationship. The distances of data points from the regression line, termed residuals, are the portions of the data not explained by the model. Poor correlation coefficients imply high residuals, which may be due to many small contributions (variations of data from the regression line) or a few large ones. Extreme values (outliers) greatly reduce correlation.

Kendall's Coefficient of Rank Correlation

Kendall's rank correlation, represented by τ (tau), should be used to evaluate the degree of association between two sets of data when the nature of the data is such that the relationship may not be linear. This situation occurs most commonly when the data are not continuous and/or normally distributed. An example of this scenario is when an attempt is made to determine if there is a relationship between the number of hydra and their survival time in a test medium measured as a range of durations in hours (e.g., 1–2 h, 2–3 h, etc.). Both variables are discontinuous, yet a relationship probably exists, as survival appears to decrease with time. Another common use of Kendall's rank correlation is to compare subjective scoring of lesions by two different toxicologic pathologists.

τ is calculated as $\tau = N/n(n-1)$, where n is the sample size and N is the count of ranks. If a second variable Y_2 is exactly correlated with the first variable Y_1, then the variates Y_2 should be in the same rank order as the Y_1 variates. However, if the correlation is less than exact, the rank order of Y_2 will not correspond entirely to that of Y. The quantity N measures how well the rank order of the second variable corresponds to the rank order of the first. It has a maximum value of $n(n-1)$ and a minimum value of $-n(n-1)$.

Each of the two variables is separately ranked, and tied ranks are assigned as shown earlier under the Kruskal–Wallis test. From this point, the original variates are disregarded, and only ranks are used to complete the test. The ranks of one of the two variables are placed in rank order, from lowest to highest, paired with the rank values assigned for the other variable. If one, but not the other, variable has tied ranks, pairs are made with the variables without ties. The resulting value of τ will range from -1 to $+1$, as does the familiar parametric correlation coefficient, r. This test is a very robust estimator that does not assume normality, linearity, or minimal error of measurement.

Cohen's Kappa

Cohen's kappa (κ) is widely used to measure the degree of agreement between two raters for categorical variables. The formula for Cohen's k is shown in Eq. (16.46).

Formula for Cohen's kappa

$$\kappa = \frac{p_0 - p_e}{1 - p_e} \qquad (16.46)$$

-where p_0 is the observed probability of success and p_e is the probability of success expected by chance.

A P-value for the estimated κ compared to $\kappa_0 = 0$ is usually regarded with little interest or not reported since it is common for κ to be found to be significantly different from zero but not be meaningfully high. Cohen's κ can range from -1 to 1, where negative values indicate that agreement is worse than expected by chance. Typical interpretations for κ include values less than 0.20 (poor agreement), $0.20 < \kappa < 0.40$ (fair agreement), $0.40 < \kappa < 0.60$ (moderate agreement), $0.60 < \kappa < 0.80$ (good agreement), and $0.20 < \kappa \le 1.00$ (very good agreement).

Intraclass Correlation Coefficient

The intraclass correlation coefficient (ICC) is used to measure the degree of agreement between two quantitative variables. An ICC value can be calculated based on a one-way random effects model using an ANOVA framework (Eq. 16.47).

Formula for ICC based on a one-way random effects model using ANOVA framework

$$Y_{ij} = \mu + s_j + \varepsilon_{ij} \qquad (16.47)$$

-where Y_{ij} represents the ith observed value (e.g., body weight) of subject j, μ is the overall mean, s_j represents the difference between μ and the true value of s_j, and Σ_{ij} is residual error for the ith observed value for subject j.

The terms s_j and ε_{ij} should each have an expected value of zero and be uncorrelated with each other, or $s_j \sim N(0, s_j^2)$ and $\varepsilon_{ij} \sim N(0, \varepsilon^2)$. For a sufficiently large number of subjects, the ICC can be calculated from the formula below: (Eq. 16.48)

Interclass correlation coefficient

$$ICC = \frac{\sigma_b^2}{\sigma_b^2 + \sigma_w^2} \qquad (16.48)$$

-where, σ_b^2 refers to the variance between subjects and σ_w^2 is the pooled variance within subjects.

The total variance between all ratings is $\sigma_b^2 + \sigma_w^2$, so that the ICC can be interpreted as the proportion of variance accounted for by the between subject differences. The ICC should range between 0 and 1, where 0 indicates no agreement and 1 indicates perfect agreement. A common approach to the interpretation of ICC value can be based on bins such that values less than or equal to 0.50 (poor reliability), $0.50 < ICC \le 0.75$ (moderate reliability), $0.75 < ICC < 0.90$ (good reliability), and $0.90 < ICC \le 1.00$ (excellent reliability). Although a P-value comparing the resulting ICC value to zero can be calculated, even very small ICC values could have a significant P-value but poor reliability. Therefore, similar to the case with Cohen's κ, P-values for ICC may be regarded with little interest.

7.8. Nonparametric Hypothesis Testing

Wilcoxon Rank-Sum Test

The *Wilcoxon rank-sum test* is commonly used for the comparison of two groups of nonparametric interval or not normally distributed data. Typically, these data are measured within certain limits on a continuum. For example, how many animals died during each hour of an acute study? How many animals had minimal versus moderate versus marked lesions? The test is also used when there is no variability (variance = 0) within one or more of the groups to be compared.

The data in both groups are initially arranged and listed in order of increasing value. Then, each number in the two groups receives a *rank value* beginning with the smallest number in either group, which is given a rank of 1.0. If there are multiples of the same numbers, called "ties," then each value of equal size will receive the median rank for the entire identically sized group. For example, if the lowest number appears twice, both figures receive a rank of 1.5. This, in turn, means that the ranks of 1.0 and 2.0 have been used, so the next highest number will be given a rank of 3.0. If the lowest number appears three times, then each tied value is given the same median rank of 2.0 (i.e., $[1.0 + 2.0 + 3.0]/3$), and the next number receives a rank of 4.0. This process continues until all of the numbers are ranked. Each of the two columns of ranks (one for each group) is totaled, giving the sum of ranks for each group being compared, as follows (Eq. 16.49):

The result should be equal to the sum of the summed ranks for both groups. The sum of rank values is compared to table values to determine the degree of significant differences, if any (Table 16.23).

Formula for the Wilcoxon rank-sum test

$$\frac{(n)(n+1)}{2} \qquad (16.49)$$

-where n is the total number of data in both groups.

The differences and affixing sign to each rank describe the data as shown in Table 16.24.

$P = .012$ indicates a significant effect.

These tables include an upper and a lower limit value that are dependent upon the probability level. If the number of data is not the same in both groups (i.e., $n_1 \neq n_2$), then the lesser sum of ranks (smaller n) is compared to the table limits to find the degree of significance. Normally, the comparison of the two groups ends here, and the degree of significant difference can be reported (Figure 16.19).

The assumptions and limitations of the test include that it can be highly biased in the

TABLE 16.23   Sample Data for the Wilcoxon Rank-Sum Test (Median Effect)

Animal	Control	Compound B	Differences
1	2.0	3.5	+1.5
2	3.6	5.7	+2.1
3	2.6	2.9	+0.3
4	7.3	9.9	−0.2
5	2.6	2.4	+2.6
6	3.4	3.3	−0.1
7	14.9	16.7	+1.8
8	6.6	6.0	−0.6
9	2.3	3.8	+1.5
10	2.0	4.0	+2.0
11	6.8	9.1	+2.3
12	8.5	20.9	+12.4
		Median	+1.65

TABLE 16.24   Difference Between Groups and Their Rank

Difference among ranks, ranks, and sign

Difference	0.1	0.2	0.3	0.6	1.5	1.5	1.8	2.0	2.1	2.3	2.6	12.4
Rank	1	2	3	4	5.5	5.5	7	8	9	10	11	12
Sign	−	−	+	−	+	+	+	+	+	+	+	+

Sum of the negative ranks, W− = 1 + 2 + 4 = 7.
Sum of the positive ranks,
W+ = 3 + 5.5 + 5.5 + 7 + 8 + 9 + 10 + 11 + 12 = 71.

presence of censored data, and that too many tied ranks increase the false-positive results (i.e., rejection of the H_0 may occur at less than 5%, even though the alpha level is set at 0.05).

Distribution-Free Multiple Comparison Tests

The *distribution-free multiple comparison test* or Dunn's test should be used to compare three or more groups of nonparametric data when a subset of all possible comparisons is desired. We often employ this test for mutagenicity studies where we wish to compare genotoxic effects in the control group to genotoxic effects in treated groups.

Two values must be calculated for each pair of groups, namely the difference in mean ranks and the probability level value against which the difference will be compared. To determine the difference in mean ranks, one must first arrange the data within each of the groups in order of

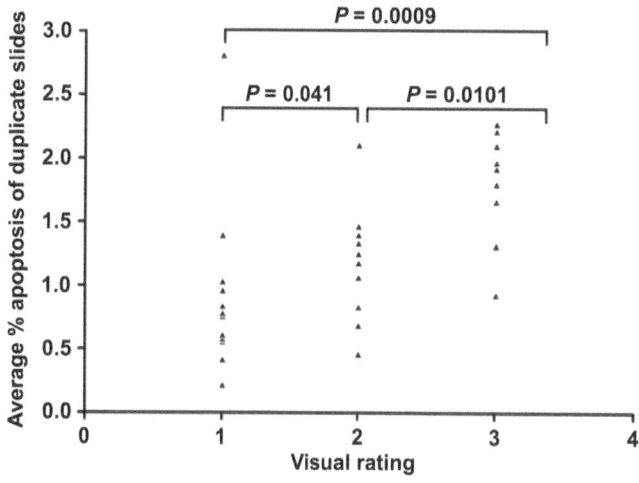

FIGURE 16.19   **An example of probabilities for the Wilcoxon rank-sum test.**

increasing values, after which rank values are assigned, beginning with the smallest overall figure. Note that this ranking is similar to that in the Wilcoxon test except that it applies to more than two groups. The ranks are then added for each of the groups. (Eq. 16.50)

Adding the ranks for distribution-free multiple comparisons

$$\frac{n_{tot}(n_{tot}+1)}{2} \qquad (16.50)$$

-where n_{tot} is the total number of data points for all groups, and n is the number of data points in a group.

Next, we can find the mean rank (R) for each group by dividing the sum of ranks by the number of data points (n) in the group. These mean ranks are then used in those pairs to be compared (usually each test group vs. the control), and the differences are found by subtraction. This value is expressed as an absolute figure $|R_1 - R_2|$, so that it is always a positive number. The second value for each pair of groups, the probability value Z, is then calculated as shown below: (Eq. 16.51)

Equation for calculating the Z statistic for distribution-free multiple comparisons

$$Z_{\alpha/[k(k-1)]}\sqrt{\frac{n_{tot}(n_{tot}+1)}{12}\left(\frac{1}{n_1}+\frac{1}{n_2}\right)} \qquad (16.51)$$

-where α is the level of significance for the comparison (usually 0.05, 0.01, 0.001, etc.), K is the total number of groups, n is the number of data points within each group, n_{tot} is the total number of data points for all groups, and Z is a figure obtained from a normal probability table used for determining the corresponding Z-score.

The result of the probability value calculation for each pair of groups is compared to the corresponding mean difference $|R_1 - R_2|$. If $|R_1 - R_2|$ is smaller than Z, then there is no significant difference between the groups. If the difference is larger than Z, the groups are different and $|R_1 - R_2|$ must be successively compared to the calculated probability values to find the degree of significance.

As with the Wilcoxon rank-sum test, too many tied ranks inflate the likelihood that a false-positive result will be obtained. Modifications of Dunn's test can be used when tied ranks are present.

It is possible to conduct a distribution-free trend test that uses the information in the rank order of groups in order to test for differences between the control and treated groups. Shirley's test is a nonparametric version of the Williams' test that was discussed earlier, where the observations are replaced by the ranks across all the groups. A modification of Shirley's test was proposed by Williams, in which observations are reranked at each stage of a sequential procedure after removing all observations at higher dose levels with significant effects. This modified Shirley–Williams' test improves the power of the original Shirley's test and is currently the most widely used version of Shirley's test for comparing control and dose groups when selecting a trend-sensitive test.

Mann–Whitney U Test

The *Mann–Whitney U test* is a nonparametric test in which the data in each group are first ordered from lowest to highest. Values in the entire data set, from both the control and treated groups, then are ranked, with the average rank being assigned to tied values as it is for the Wilcoxon rank-sum test. The ranks are then summed for each group, and U is determined. (Eq. 16.52)

Formula for Mann–Whitney U statistic

$$U_t = n_c n_t + \frac{n_t(n_t+1)}{2} - R_t$$

$$(16.52)$$

$$U_c = n_c n_t + \frac{n_c(n_c+1)}{2} - R_c$$

-where n_c, n_t are the sample size for control and treated groups, respectively; R_c, R_t are the sum of ranks for the control and treated groups; and U_c is the Mann–Whitney statistic for controls and U_t is the Mann–Whitney statistic for treated animals.

For the level of significance for a comparison of the two groups, the larger value of U_c or U_t is used. This is compared to critical values as found in appropriate tables. The Mann–Whitney U test is employed for discontinuous count data, but the choice of test to be employed for percentage variables should be decided on the same grounds as described later under reproduction studies.

The test statistic from a Mann–Whitney U test is linearly related to that of the Wilcoxon rank-sum test, and the two tests will always yield the same result. The Mann–Whitney U test is presented here for historical completeness, as it has been much favored in reproductive and developmental toxicology studies. Although it does not matter whether the observations are ranked from smallest to largest or vice versa, this test should not be used for paired observations.

Kruskal–Wallis One-Way ANOVA

The *Kruskal–Wallis nonparametric one-way ANOVA* should be the initial analysis performed when three or more groups of nonparametric data are evaluated. Typically, data are either not normally distributed, or are discontinuous, or all the groups to be analyzed are not from the same population, but they are not of a categorical, or quantal, nature. Commonly, these data are either rank-type evaluation data, such as behavioral toxicity observation scores, or reproduction study data.

The analysis is initiated by ranking all the observations from the combined groups. Ties are given the average rank of the tied values. For example, if two values tie for 12th rank—and therefore would be ranked 12th and 13th—both would be assigned the average rank of 12.5. The sum of ranks of each group (r_1, r_2, ...r_k) is computed by adding all the rank values for each group, and then the test value H is computed. (Eq. 16.53)

Formula for Kruskal–Wallis H-statistic

$$H = \frac{12}{n(n+1)} \sum \left(r_1^2/n_1 + r_2^2/n_2 + ... + r_k^2/n_k\right)$$
$$-3(n+1) \tag{16.53}$$

-where n, n_1, n_2, ... n_k are the number of observations in each group, and their values are ranked in an ordered list; r is the sum of ranks of each group (r_1, r_2, ...r_k); and k is the last observation.

The test statistic is then compared with a table of H values, available in a number of statistical texts or computer software. If the calculated value of H is greater than the table value for the appropriate number of observations in each group (df), there is significant difference between the groups. However, further testing using the distribution-free multiple comparisons

method (see above) is necessary to determine which groups are different from one another.

The test statistic H is used for both small and large samples, and data must be independent for the test to be valid. When one finds a significant difference, one does not know which groups are different. It is incorrect to then perform a Mann–Whitney U test on all possible combinations. Instead, a multiple comparison method must be used, such as the distribution-free multiple comparisons (see above). In addition, too many tied ranks will decrease the power of this test and also lead to false-positive results.

The Kruskal–Wallis test is identical to the normal approximation used for the Wilcoxon rank-sum test. When $k = 2$, the Kruskal–Wallis χ^2 value has 1 df. A χ^2 with 1 df can be represented by the square of a standardized normal random variable, which in the case of $k = 2$, the H-statistic, represents the square of the Wilcoxon rank-sum (without the continuity correction). The effect of adjusting for tied ranks is to slightly increase the value of the test statistic, H. Therefore, omission of this adjustment results in a more conservative test.

Jonckheere–Terpstra Test for Trend

The Jonckheere–Terpstra test for trend (Jonckheere's test) compares the H_0 of no difference in between k groups to the alternative hypothesis of an ordered alternative hypothesis of across k groups, where k > 2. This test is more powerful than the Kruskal–Wallis test, which does not assume a priori ordering of groups. The test statistic for Jonckheere's test follows a standard normal Z distribution (mean = 0 and variance = 1) for a sufficiently large total sample size across groups provided that the number of observations in each group is not too small. That is, the Jonckheere's test statistic is (Eq. 16.54).

Formula for Jonchheere–Terpstra test for Trend

$$Z = \frac{\sum J_{XY} - E(J)}{\sqrt{\text{Var}(J)}} \tag{16.54}$$

-where JXY is the number of observations in group Y that are greater than all observations in group X, and $E(J)$ is the expected value of J and Var(J) is the variance of J as shown below

$$E(J) = \frac{N^2 - \sum n_i}{4}$$

$$\text{Var}(J) = \frac{N^2(2N+3) - \sum n_i^2(2n_i+3)}{72}$$

-where N is the total sample size and n_i is the number of samples in each group.

Time to Event Analysis

Trend may correspond to sustained and systematic variations over a long period of time. It is associated with the structural causes of the phenomenon in question; for example, population growth, technological progress, new ways of organization, or capital accumulation. The identification of trend has always posed a challenging statistical problem. The difficulty is not one of mathematical or analytical complexity but rather of conceptual complexity, as one uses nonobservable variables. In this case, the extrapolation is made without the support of measured data.

Assumptions must be made on these latent, or unmeasured, variables as to their behavioral pattern. The trend is generally thought of as a smooth and slow movement over a long term. The concept of long in this connection is relative; what is identified as trend for a given series over a given span might well be part of an even longer cycle once the series is considerably augmented. Often, a long cycle is treated as a trend because the length of the observed time series is shorter than one complete face of the longer type of cycle.

The ways in which data are collected in toxicologic pathology studies frequently serve to complicate trend analysis. This complication occurs because the features of the experimental design frequently act to artificially censor the length of time available for the phenomenon underlying a trend to be manifested. To avoid the complexity of the problem posed by a statistically vague definition, statisticians have resorted to two simple solutions. First, trend and cyclical fluctuations can be estimated together, resulting in a combined movement *trend cycle*. Second, the trend can be defined in terms of the series length, denoting it as the longest nonperiodic movement.

Within the large class of models identified for trend, we can distinguish two main categories:

deterministic trends and stochastic trends. Deterministic trend models are based on the assumption that the trend of a time series can be approximated closely by simple mathematical functions of time over the entire span of the series. Stochastic trend models are models of nonstationary time series, which are series whose first and second moments (means and covariances) are functions of time. Classical estimation methods, however, are valid for stationary series. Therefore, such time trends must be removed from nonstationary series (thus making them stationary) before applying the methods of Box and Jenkins. Removal, however, depends on identifying the type of trend first. Generally, stationarity is achieved through differencing the series or through removal of a deterministic trend by first estimating that trend in a separate regression. We will look at both methods. First, however, let us consider what nonstationarity means.

These tests can be thought of as special cases of regression or correlation tests, in which association is sought between the observations and their ordered sample index such as a change in close magnitude or change in duration of observation. They are also related to ANOVA, except that the tests are tailored to be powerful against the subset of alternatives H_1 instead of the more general set $\{F_i \neq F_j, \text{ some } i \neq j\}$. Different tests arise from requiring power against specific elements or subsets of this rather extensive set of alternatives.

LIFE TABLES

Chronic in vivo studies (e.g., a lifetime [2 year] rodent carcinogenicity studies) are among the most complex and expensive toxicity studies. Answers to a multitude of questions are sought in such a study, particularly if a material results in a significant increase in either mortality or the incidence of tumors in those animals exposed to it. The time course of these adverse effects is an essential part of the evaluation. The classic approach to assessing these age-specific hazard rates is the use of *life tables*, also called *survivorship tables*.

It may readily be seen that during any selected period of time (t_i) there are a number of risks, or adverse events, which may affect an animal. These main adverse events that usually must be considered are *natural death*, death induced by a *direct or indirect action of the test compound,* and *death due to occurrences of interest* (e.g., tumors). Of particular interest is whether or not, and when, the last two of these risks (which may be affected by one or more doses of the treatment) become significantly different from the natural risks (which are defined by events seen in the control group). Life table methods enable such determinations as the duration of survival or the time until the onset of tumors as well as the probability of survival or developing a tumor during a selected period of time.

To use *life table analysis,* the interval length (t_i) for examination within the study must first be determined. As the interval is shortened, the information gained becomes more exact. However, as interval length is decreased, the number of intervals increases, and calculations become more cumbersome; furthermore time-related trends become less indicative of major differences because random fluctuations become more apparent. For a lifetime rodent study, an interval length of 1 month is commonly employed. Some life table methods, such as the *Kaplan–Meier* table, display each new event, such as a death, as the start of a new interval (see Figure 16.20).

Once the time interval length has been established, the data are tabulated. A separate table is created for each group of animals (e.g., each sex and each dose level). The following columns generally are recorded in each life table:

1. Interval of time selected (t_i);
2. Number of animals in the group that entered that interval of the study alive (l_i);

3. Number of animals withdrawn from study during the interval (such as those taken for an interim necropsy) (ω_i);
4. Number of animals that died during the interval (d_i);
5. Number of animals at risk during the interval, $l_i = l_i - ½\,\omega_I$, or the number on study at the start of the interval minus one half of the number withdrawn during the interval;
6. Proportion of animals that died $D_i = d_i/l_i$;
7. Cumulative probability of an animal surviving until the end of that study interval, $P_i = 1 - D_i$, or one minus the number of animals that died during that interval divided by the number of animals at risk;
8. Number of animals dying prior to the start of that interval (M_i);
9. Animals found to have died during the interval (m_i);
10. Probability of dying during the study interval, which is $c_i = 1 - (M_i + m_i/l_i)$, or the total number of animals dead prior to the start of that interval plus the animals discovered to have died during that interval, with that sum divided by the number of animals at risk through the end of that interval;
11. Cumulative proportion surviving, p_i, is equivalent to the cumulative product of the interval probabilities of survival (i.e., $p_i = p_1 \cdot p_2 \cdot p_3 \cdot \cdots \cdot p_x$); and
12. Cumulative probability of dying, C_i, equal to the cumulative product of the interval probabilities to that point (i.e., $C_i = c_1 \cdot c_2 \cdot c_3 \cdot \cdots \cdot c_x$).

Once the tables have been produced for each group in a study, the hypotheses can be tested. Examples of such hypotheses are that each of the treated groups has a significantly shorter duration of survival, or that individuals in the treated groups died more quickly. Note that plots for the total numbers of dead and alive animals will give one an appreciation of the data but can lead to no statistical conclusions. There are many methods for testing significance in life tables. The main consideration in selecting a test is to ensure acceptable statistical power, keeping in mind that where the power of the analysis is increased so does the difficulty of computation.

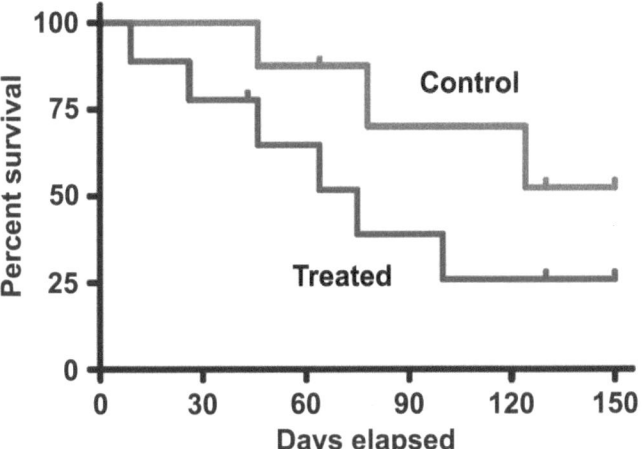

FIGURE 16.20 **An example of a Kaplan–Meier survival curve.**

The significant effects of different variables are evaluated during life table analysis using a series of calculations. These are shown sequentially in Eq. (16.55). In these calculations, the following definitions apply to these symbols: D is the proportion of animals that died, d is the proportion of animals that died during the interval in question, K is the entire period of the study, k is the last interval in study, and P is the proportion of animals surviving to that interval.

Calculations for seeking significant effects in life tables.

First, the standard error of the K interval survival rate is derived as follows:

$$S_K = P_k \sqrt{\sum_1^k \left(\frac{D_i}{l'_x - d_x} \right)} \qquad (16.55)$$

-where D is the number of deaths at a specific time, d_x is number of deaths between time x and time $x-1$, K is survival rate, k is number of groups, P_D is the probability of survival, P_1 is the survival rate for group 1, P_2 is the survival rate for group 2, S_D is the standard error of the difference between the groups, P_D is the difference in survival probabilities, t' is the test statistic, and l_1 is the sample size.

The effective sample size (l_1) can be calculated in accordance with the following:

$$l_1 = \frac{P(1-P)}{S^2}$$

-where S denotes the standard error.

Compute the standard error of difference (S_D) for any two groups (1 and 2) as follows:

$$S_D = \sqrt{S_1^2 + S_2^2}$$

The difference in survival probabilities (P_D) for the two groups is then calculated as follows:

$$P_D = P_1 - P_2$$

The test statistic (t') is then computed as follows:

$$t' = \frac{P_D}{S_D}$$

-where D is the number of deaths at a specific time, d_x is number of deaths between time x

and time $x-1$, K is survival rate, k is number of groups, and P_D is the probability of survival, P_1 the survival rate for group 1, P_2 the survival rate for group 2, S_D is the standard error of difference, P_D is the difference in survival probabilities, t' is the test statistic, and l_1 is the sample size.

This is then compared to the z distribution table. If $t' > z$ at the desired probability level, it is significant at that level.

Life table analysis has become a mainstay in chronic studies (Tarone, 1975). An example is the reassessment of the ED_{01} study, in which long-term exposure of rats to low doses of potential carcinogens was undertaken to assess the curve shape at the lower end of the dose response curve. This reassessment radically changed interpretation of the results and subsequent understanding of the underlying statistical methods that are suitable for making adjustments with respect to time on study. The increased importance and interest in the analysis of survival data has not been restricted to toxicologic pathology, but rather has encompassed all disciplines among the life sciences (Society of Toxicology, 1981; Lee, 2003).

LOG-RANK TEST

The *Log-rank test* is a statistical method for comparing the distribution of time until the occurrence of an event of interest in independent groups. In toxicologic pathology, the most common events of interest are death or onset of a tumor, but it could be any other event that occurs only once in an individual. The elapsed time from initial treatment or observation until the *event* is the *event time*, often referred to as survival time, even when the *event* is not death.

The Log-rank test provides a method for comparing *risk-adjusted* event rates, which is useful when test subjects in a study are subject to varying degrees of opportunity to experience the event. Such situations arise frequently in studies due to the finite duration of the study, early termination of the animal, or interruption/cessation of the treatment before the event occurs.

The Log-rank test might be used to compare survival times in carcinogenicity bioassay animals given a new treatment with those in the control group. Another example is comparison of time to liver failure for several dose levels of a new drug where the animals are treated for 10 weeks, or until cured, whichever comes first. If every animal were followed until the event occurred, the event times could be compared between two groups using the Wilcoxon rank-sum test. However, some animals may die or otherwise complete the study before the event occurs. In such cases, the actual time to the event is unknown since the event does not occur while under study observation. The event times for these animals are based on the last known time of study observation and are called *censored observations* since they represent the lower bound of the true, unknown event times. The Log-rank test is preferable in this case as the Wilcoxon rank-sum test can be highly biased in the presence of censored data.

The H_0 tested by the Log-rank test is that of equal event time distributions among groups. Equality of the distributions of event times implies similar event rates among groups not only for the clinical trial as a whole but also for any arbitrary time point during the trial (Eq. 16.56). Rejection of the H_0 indicates that the event rates differ among groups at one or more time points during the study.

Formula for determining the Log-rank statistic Chi-square

$$\chi^2 = \frac{\left(|O_1 - E_1| - \frac{1}{2}\right)^2}{E_1} + \frac{\left(|O_2 - E_2| - \frac{1}{2}\right)^2}{E_2}$$

(16.56)

-where O is the observed data (or counts), and E is the expected data.

The principle behind the Log-rank test for comparison of two life tables is that if there are no differences between the groups, the total deaths occurring at any time should split between the two groups at that time. For example, if the numbers at risk in the first and second groups in the sixth month of a study were 70 and 30, respectively, and 10 deaths occurred in that month, we would expect

$$10 \times \frac{70}{70 + 30} = 7$$

of these deaths to have occurred in the first group, and

$$10 \times \frac{30}{70 + 30} = 3$$

of the deaths to have occurred in the second group.

A similar calculation can be made at each time of death (in either group). By adding together for the first group the results of all such calculations, we obtain a single number, called the extent of exposure (E_1), which represents the expected number of events (in this case, deaths) in that group, if the two groups shared the same distribution of survival time. An extent of exposure (E_2) can be obtained for the second group in the same way. Let O_1 and O_2 denote the actual total numbers of deaths in the two groups. A useful arithmetic check is that the total number of deaths $O_1 + O_2$ must equal the sum $E_1 + E_2$ of the extents of exposure. The discrepancy between the O's and E's can then be measured.

χ^2 is the actual Log-rank statistic underlying distribution and hypothesis test. An approximate significance test of the H_0 (i.e., that survival times in the two groups will have identical distributions) is obtained by comparing the calculated χ^2 to a χ^2 distribution on 1 df. It has been suggested that as χ^2 is conservative, the approximation in treating the null distribution of χ^2 will tend to understate the degree of statistical significance.

In the formula for χ^2, the continuity correction of subtracting ½ from $|O_1 - E_1|$ and $|O_2 - E_2|$ is used before squaring. The endpoint of concern is (or is defined so that it is) "right censored"—once it happens, it does not reoccur. Examples are death or a minimum or maximum value for an enzyme or physiologic function (such as respiration rate). Life tables can be constructed to provide estimates of the event time distributions. Commonly used estimates of this type typically are known as *Kaplan–Meier curves* (Figure 16.20).

The Log-rank test makes no assumptions regarding distribution of the data set. Many variations of the Log-rank test exist for comparing survival distributions. The most common variant has the following form (Eq. 16.57):

Alternative formula for determining the Log-rank statistic Chi-square

$$X^2 = \frac{(O_1 - E_1)^2}{E_1} + \frac{(O_2 - E_2)^2}{E_2} \qquad (16.57)$$

-where O_i and E_i are computed for each group, as has been shown previously.

This statistic also approximates a χ^2 distribution with 1 df under H_0.

A continuity correction can also be used to reduce the numerators by 1/2 before squaring. Use of such a correction leads to a more conservative test statistic and may be omitted when sample sizes are moderate or large (i.e., n is equal to or greater than 15 per cell). The Wilcoxon rank-sum test could be used to analyze such event times in the absence of censoring. A *Generalized Wilcoxon test* (sometimes called the *Gehan test*) based on an approximate χ^2 distribution has been developed for use in the presence of censored observations.

Both the Log-rank and the Wilcoxon rank-sum tests are nonparametric tests and require no assumptions regarding the distribution of event times. When the event rate is greater early in the trial than toward the end, the Generalized Wilcoxon test is the more appropriate method since it gives greater weight to the earlier differences.

Survival and failure times often follow an exponential distribution. If such a model can be assumed, a more powerful alternative to the Log-rank test is the *likelihood ratio rest*. This parametric test assumes that event probabilities are constant over time. In other words, the chance that a patient becomes event positive is independent of t. A plot of the negative log of the event time distribution showing a linear trend through the origin is consistent with exponential event times.

The *Cox proportional hazards model* can be used to assess differences in survival with multiple covariates such as dose and weaning weight. The Log-rank test is restricted to comparing survival distributions of two groups without consideration of other covariates and is essentially a special case of the Cox proportional hazards model. Categorial or continuous predictor variables can be accommodated in the Cox proportional hazards model, while only categorical predictor variables are appropriate for the Log-rank test. The hazard, or probability of death given that a subject has survived to a given point in time, represents the response variable in proportional hazards modeling. No assumption needs to be made about the probability distribution of the hazard, but Cox proportional hazards modeling does assume that the hazard ratio between different treatment groups stays constant over time.

TARONE'S TEST

The National Cancer Institute (NCI) uses *Tarone's trend test* in the analysis of carcinogenicity data. Tarone's trend test is most powerful at detecting dose-related trends when tumor onset hazard functions are proportional to each other. A hazard function is the probability that an experimental animal dies at time t (provided that it has survived to that time). The hazard function represents the instantaneous death rate for an animal surviving to time t.

A simple, but efficient alternative to this test is the *Cox and Stuart test*, which is a modification of the sign test. For each time point at which a measurement is made (such as the incidence of animals observed with tumors), a pair of observations is prepared: one from each of the groups to be compared. In a traditional NCI bioassay, this would mean pairing control with low-dose data and low dose with high-dose data to explore a dose-related trend. In each time period, observations in a dose group (except the first) are commonly compared with the prior observation to which it is paired to evaluate the presence of any time-related trend. When the second observation in a pair exceeds the earlier observation, a plus sign for that pair is recorded. When the first observation is greater than the later one, a minus sign for that pair is used. A preponderance of plus signs suggests a downward trend, while an excess of minus signs suggests an upward trend. A formal test at an a priori selected confidence level can then be performed.

After defining the trend to test, first match the pairs as $(X_1 - X_{1+c})$, (X_2, X_{2+c}), ... $(X_{n'-c}, X_{n'})$ where $c = n'/2$ when n' is even and $c = (n'+1)/2$ when n' is odd (where n' is the number of observations in a set). Comparing the resulting number of excess positive or negative signs against a sign test table then tests the hypothesis that a trend exists over time. Combination of a number of observations allows active testing for a set of trends, such as the existence of a trend of increasing differences between two groups of animals over a period of time.

7.9. Quantifying Uncertainty

Confidence Intervals

Calculation of the upper and lower 95% *CI* defines a range that will include the true value of the parameter of interest 95% of the time, with only a 5% probability that the interval will not include the true value of the parameter. Calculating the upper and lower 95% confidence limits involves the following steps: Choose a (test) statistic involving the unknown parameter of interest and no other unknown parameter, and then place the appropriate sample values in the statistic. Next, obtain an equation for the unknown parameter by equating the test statistic to the upper 2½ percent point of the relevant distribution, where the solution of the equation gives one limit. Finally, repeat the process with the lower 2½ percent point to obtain the other limit.

The 95% CI for normally distributed data with *n* data values has the following form (Eq. 16.58):

Calculation of the 95% confidence interval for normally distributed data

$$95\% \text{ CI} = \text{mean} \pm t_{0.025} x\ s\ x\ \text{sqrt}(1\ /\ n) \quad (16.58)$$

-where mean is the population mean, $t0.025$ is the critical value for the t distribution with $n-1$ df, and $s/\text{sqrt}(n)$ is the sample standard error, where s is the sample standard deviation.

It is usually best to have a confidence interval as narrow as possible. With a symmetric distribution such as the normal or t, this is achieved using equal tails of 2½ percent. One can also construct 95% confidence intervals using unequal tails (e.g., using the upper 2% point and the lower 3% point). The same procedure very nearly minimizes the confidence interval with other nonsymmetric distributions, e.g., χ^2, and has the advantage of avoiding rather tedious computation.

When the appropriate statistic involves the square of the unknown parameter, both limits are obtained by equating the statistic to the upper 5% point of the relevant distribution. The use of two tails in this situation would result in a pair of nonintersecting intervals. When two or more parameters are involved, it is possible to construct a region within which the true parameter values will most likely lie. Such regions are referred to as *confidence regions*.

Prediction Intervals

The upper and lower 95% *prediction interval* (95% PI) for a new response has a similar interpretation to a 95% CI. That is, the 95% PI will contain the new observation with a probability of 95%. The 95% PI for normally distributed data with *n* data values must account for the uncertainty in estimating the population mean as well as the variation related to the individual observations, and has the following form: (Eq. 16.59)

Calculation of the 95% prediction interval for normally distributed data

$$95\% \text{ CI} = \text{mean} \pm t_{0.025} x\ s\ x\ \text{sqrt}(1 + 1/n)$$

$$(16.59)$$

-where mean is the population mean, $t0.025$ is the critical value for the t distribution with $n-1$ df, and $s/\text{sqrt}(1 + n)$ is the sample standard error, where s is the sample standard deviation.

It is important to note the distinction between a confidence interval and a prediction interval. The formula for the 95% PI differs from the formula of the 95% CI according to the addition of the 1 inside of the square root which accounts for the variability of an individual data point around the mean. As $n \to \infty$, the 95% CI $\to 0$. However, this would not happen for the 95% PI because of the extra term inside the square root.

The difference between formulas demonstrates that the 95% PI will always be larger than the 95% CI. While the mean would fall into the 95% CI 95% of the time, this would not be true for the individual observations in the population. The 95% PI is often confused with the 95% CI, but it would be inappropriate to construct a 95% CI for a mean and use it to predict a future observation. To illustrate this concept, it is possible that a 95% CI would only contain 20% of the individual observations. It is common to use prediction intervals to define reference intervals for clinical chemistry endpoints such as serum chemistry parameters (e.g., cholesterol, triglycerides) and hematological parameters (e.g., neutrophils, monocytes).

7.10. Methods for the Reduction of Dimensionality

Reduction of Dimensionality Through Classification

Classification is both a basic concept and a collection of techniques, which are necessary prerequisites for further analysis of data when the members of a data set are, or can be, described by several variables. At least some degree of classification is necessary prior to any data collection so that members of a given treatment group may be subcategorized appropriately in accordance with a set of decision rules. Such rules should be established when designing the experiment (i.e., prior to collection).

Whether formally or informally, an investigator has to decide which characteristics are similar enough to be counted as the same and develop rules for governing collection procedures. Such rules can be as simple as "measure and record body weights only of live animals on study," or as complex as the scheme demonstrated below (Table 16.25) by the expanded weighting classification procedure. Such a classification also shows that the selection of specific variables to measure will determine the final classification of data. Classification needs to be balanced against the numbers of individuals within each class. As classes must be mutually exclusive and mutually exhaustive, excessive classification (particularly when the group size is small) can reduce numbers of individuals within the subgroups. The comical extreme of such activity may result in each individual residing in a different class, thereby resulting in zero df for statistical analysis.

Classification of data has two purposes: *data simplification*, which is also a descriptive function, and *prediction*. Simplification is necessary because there is a conceptual limit to both the volume and complexity of data that the human mind can comprehend. Classification allows us to provide a name for each category (i.e., group of data); hence, these data are sometime referred to as *nominal* data. Classification also permits creation of a summary of the data (i.e., in assigning individual elements of data to groups, and in characterizing the population of the group). Finally, it helps the scientist define the relationships among groups (i.e., develop taxonomy).

In contrast to simplification, prediction is the use of data summaries and one's knowledge of the relationships among groups to develop hypotheses regarding what will happen when further data are collected. Classification is necessary to predict risks a priori, as required in risk characterization. For example, as more individuals (animals or people) are exposed to an agent

TABLE 16.25   Example of Data Classification From a Toxicologic Pathology Experiment

Decision criteria	Quantal output	Nominal (class output)
Is animal of desired species?	Yes/No	
Is animal member of study group?	Yes/No	
Is animal alive?	Yes/No	
Which group does animal belong to?		A. Control
		B. Low dose
		C. Intermediate dose
		D. High dose
What sex is animal?	Male/Female	
Is the measured weight in acceptable range?		Yes/No

under a given set of defined conditions, a predicted outcome can be derived (e.g., number of tumors). By creating mutually exclusive classes, mechanisms can be investigated with respect to how such relationships develop.

Indeed, classification is the prime device for discovering mechanisms in all of science. A classic example of classification's utility is Darwin's realization that there are reasons (the theory of evolution) behind the differences and similarities among species. Similarly, this diversity led Linnaeus to develop his initial modern classification scheme (taxonomy) for animals and plants based on variations in morphological features.

Expanded Weighting Procedure

To develop a classification, one first sets bounds wide enough to encompass the entire range of data to be considered. This is typically done by selecting some global variables and limiting the range of data from each group so that it just encompasses all the cases on hand. Such global variables are those that every datum has in common. Next, a set of local variables that can differentiate among groups is selected. These local variables have characteristics that are shared by only some of the cases (e.g., the occurrence of certain tumor types, enzyme activity levels, or dietary preferences).

Data are then collected, and a system for measuring differences and similarities is developed. Such measurements are based on some form of measuring the distance between two cases (x and y) in terms of each single variable's scale. If the variable is a continuous one, then the simplest measure of distance between two pieces of data is the Euclidean distance as defined in Eq. (16.60).

Description of the Euclidean distance

$$d(x, y) = \sqrt{(x_i - y_i)^2} \qquad (16.60)$$

-where d is the distance, x and y are the two data points in a line, x_i and y_i are the location of two points, and $X_1 - Y_1$ is the distance between them.

For categorical or discontinuous data, the simplest measure of the distance between the two data is the matching distance, defined as follows (Eq. 16.61):

Equation for the matching distance

$$d(x, y) = \text{number of times where } x_i \neq y_i. \quad (16.61)$$

-where d is the matching distance for a data set with points X (treatment one or the control group) and Y (treatment two).

After developing a table of such distance measurements for each of the local variables, some weighting factor is assigned to each variable. A weighting factor gives greater importance to those variables that are believed to have more relevance or predictive value (e.g., relative organ weights rather than absolute organ weights). These weighted variables are then used to assign each datum to a group. The actual act of developing numerically based classifications and assigning data members to them is the realm of cluster analysis, which is discussed later in this chapter.

Relevant examples in which classification techniques are employed range from the simple to the complex. For example, toxicological pathologists grading the severity of various morphological findings commonly use a simple classification scheme (e.g., within normal limits, or minimal, mild, moderate, or marked lesions) to categorize the response. At the other end of the spectrum, mathematically based systems are used to classify complicated data sets (e.g., genomic array data).

Multidimensional and Nonmetric Scaling

MDS is a collection of analysis methods for data sets that have three or more variables, which define each data point. MDS displays the relationships of three or more dimensions in a manner analogous to that of statistical graphics as previously described.

MDS presents the structure of a set of objects (in a visual format to facilitate comprehension) from data that approximate the distances between pairs of the objects, where the data contain some mixture of similarities, dissimilarities, distances, or proximities. These data must be presented in such a form that a value portrayed as distance between two points (which may be easily measured and handled) can be used to define the degree of similarities and differences among the pairs of objects, each of which represents a real-life data point. The reader is referred back to the discussion of measures of distances under the classification section above. Similarity is a matter of degree. Objects with small differences show a high degree of similarity, while objects with large differences are considered to be dissimilar.

In addition to the traditional human subjective judgments of similarity, data can be grouped based on an objective similarity measure (e.g., the difference in body weights between a pair of animals). An index can be used to calculate similarity from multivariate data, such as the proportion of agreement in the results obtained from of a number of carcinogenicity studies. However, the data must always represent the degree of similarity of pairs of objects.

A point in a multidimensional space represents each object or data point. Plots of these projected points are arranged in the selected space so that the distances between pairs of points have the strongest possible relation to the degree of similarity among the pairs of objects. In other words, two points that are close together represent two similar objects, and a pair of points that are far apart represents two dissimilar objects. The spaces used for this purpose are usually two- or three-dimensional Euclidean spaces, but non-Euclidean spaces (including those with more dimensions) may be used.

MDS is a general term that includes a number of different techniques. However, all methods seek to allow geometric analysis of multivariate data (Harris, 2001). The forms of MDS can be classified (according to the nature of the similarities in the data) as qualitative, nonmetric (or quantitative), and metric procedures. The MDS types can also be classified by the number of variables involved and by the nature of the model used. For example, in classical MDS, there is only one data matrix, and no weighting factors are used. In replicated MDS, more than one matrix is used, but no weighting is applied. In weighted MDS, more than one matrix is used, and at least some of the data are weighted.

MDS can be used in toxicologic pathology to analyze the similarities and differences between effects produced by different agents. The objective of such an analysis is to understand the mechanism underlying the actions of one agent as it impacts the mechanisms of other agents.

Nonmetric scaling is useful for reducing dimensionality. The primary objective of nonmetric scaling is to arrange a set of objects (usually a number of related observations) graphically in a few dimensions; the graphical methods are closely related to those of MDS. This is done while retaining the maximum possible fidelity to the original relationships between members (i.e., values that are most different from each other are portrayed as furthest apart). This scaling is not a linear technique, as it does not preserve linear relationships. In other words, data point A is not depicted as being twice as far from point C as from point B, even though its value difference may be twice as great. The spacing, or interpoint distance, is kept such that if the distance of the original scale between members A and B is greater than that between C and D, the distances on the nonmetric model scale is greater between A and B than between C and D.

This technique functions by taking observed measures of similarity or dissimilarity between every pair of M objects (where the objects are shown as points in a multidimensional display), then finding a representation of the objects as points in Euclidean space such that the interpoint distances match the observed similarities or dissimilarities.

Principal Component Analysis

PCA is another dimension reduction approach that is commonly used to interpret the variability in large datasets with a minimal amount of information loss. PCA operates by finding new variables (or principal components) that are linear combinations of the variables in the original dataset, where these new variables are uncorrelated with each other. The new variables are arranged in increasing order of importance, where importance is defined as the amount of variance explained in the dataset. For instance, the first principal component is orthogonal (uncorrelated) with all the other principal components and explains the most variance in the data. The second principal component is orthogonal to the first principal component and all other principal components and explains the second most amount of variance in the data. There are as many principal components as there are variables in the original data set.

The PCA approach is advantageous in circumstances in which the original variables in the dataset are highly correlated with each other.

Since the principal components, by definition, are uncorrelated with each other and collectively explain all the variance in the data, the principal components can be examined to potentially uncover the predominant patterns in the data. It may be particularly useful to examine the first two or three principal components, or a subset of the principal components that explain a predefined amount of variance.

Consider an experiment in which there are four groups of five male mice each, and two groups of mice are from strain A and two groups of mice are from strain B. Each strain had a control and treated group. A gene expression DNA microarray dataset consists of 45,000 rows corresponding to different gene transcripts and 20 columns corresponding to strain A control (columns 1–5), strain A treated (columns 6–10), strain B control (columns 11–15), and strain B treated (columns 16–20). A PCA analysis could be used to generate 20 principal components from the original 20 variables. In an experiment with large treatment effects, it is not uncommon from the first two principal components to explain over 50% of the variance.

Examining the first two principal components may reveal that most of the variance in global gene expression is related to treatment effects, with much less difference between strains. On the other hand, it is possible that the genetic differences between strains lead to global gene expression patterns that indicate that the difference between strains and treatment is equally prominent in the data, or that there is an interaction between strain and treatment such that one strain responds strongly to the treatment, while the other strain does not respond at all. Perhaps the differences between strains dominate any treatment effects. Of course, it is also possible that there is no large-scale treatment or strain signal detectable in the data, or that an unexpected signal which is uncorrelated with treatment or strain would be found. All of this information would be readily apparent from the evaluation of the results of the PCA approach.

The toxicologic pathologist should note that unexpected patterns manifesting as prominent features that explain a large amount of variance in such a high dimensional dataset should serve as a mechanism for quality control to ensure that the patterns did not arise due to sample mislabeling or systematic error in sample processing or data generation. However, finding unexpected patterns through the PCA procedure may lead to new lines of hypothesis generation and eventually even a new discovery.

Cluster Analysis

Cluster analysis is a quantitative form of classification (Everitt et al., 2011). It serves to help develop decision rules and then to apply these rules to assign a heterogeneous collection of objects to a series of related data subsets (clusters). This is almost entirely an applied rather than a theoretical methodology. The final result of cluster analysis is a graphical display of classifications and a set of decision rules for the assignment of new members into the classifications.

The classification procedures used in cluster analysis are based on either density of population or distance between members. These methods can serve to generate a basis for the classification of large numbers of dissimilar variables. Examples of such dissimilar variables include behavioral observations, compounds with distinct but related structures (i.e., homologs or analogs) and mechanisms of toxicity, and tumor patterns caused by different etiologies (i.e., a treatment vs. old age).

There are four types of clustering techniques with relevance to toxicologic pathology. In *hierarchical techniques*, classes are subclassified into groups, with the process being repeated at several levels to produce a tree, with the defined groups as branches. Related groups arise from a common branch. In *optimizing techniques*, clusters are formed by optimization of a clustering criterion (e.g., analysis of multicenter research, where each site is considered a separate cluster). The resulting classes are mutually exclusive where the objects are partitioned clearly into sets, so the clusters will not overlap in graphic projections. In *density- or mode-seeking techniques*, clusters are identified and formed by locating regions in a graphical representation that contain concentrations of data points. Finally, in *clumping techniques*, a variation of density-seeking techniques is used in which assignment to a cluster depends on the weighting assigned to some variables, so the clusters may overlap in graphic projections. An example is given in Figure 16.21.

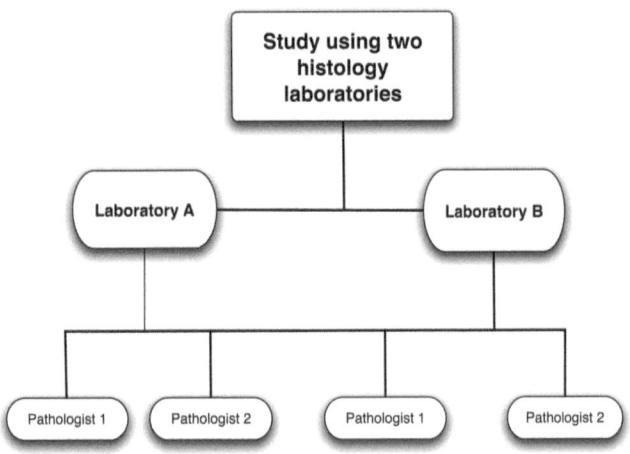

FIGURE 16.21 **Clustering nested within histopathology laboratories A and B.**

Fourier or Time Analysis

Fourier analysis is used most frequently as a univariate method for either simplifying data or for modeling, though it can also be used as a multivariate technique for data analysis (Bloomfield, 2000). In a sense, Fourier analysis is similar to trend analysis, but the Fourier method evaluates the relationship among members of data sets from a different perspective. Fourier analysis resolves the time dimension variable in the data set. The method allows one to identify, quantify, and remove the time-based cycles in data.

At the simplest level, Fourier analysis assumes that many events are periodic in nature, and that the variation in other variables due to this periodicity can be removed by using Fourier transforms. Fourier analysis allows one to evaluate the amplitudes, phases, and frequencies of data using the Fourier transform. More powerful analysis can be done on the Fourier transformed data using the remaining (i.e., time independent) variation from other variables. Unfortunately, Fourier analysis may not be appropriate when there may be several overlapping cyclic, time-based periodicities, or if time cycle event analysis is required. Details regarding the calculations employed in this technique are beyond the scope of this chapter but are available in reference texts on the subject.

7.11. Metaanalysis

Metaanalysis, meaning "analysis among," is being used increasingly in biomedical research to try to obtain a qualitative or quantitative synthesis of the research literature on a particular issue. The technique is usually applied to the synthesis of data reported for several separate but comparable studies. The process of metaanalysis has three main components: systematic review and selection of studies, quantitative analyses, and qualitative analyses.

Selection of the Studies to be Analyzed—Systematic Reviews

The issue of study selection is perhaps the most problematic for those investigators doing metaanalysis. The criteria for selection may vary from project to project. However, there are several factors concerning selection that must be addressed before an analysis commences. Each choice made by the investigator must be carefully weighed with respect to the likely effect of selection bias versus the perceived bias that the selection is designed to remove. Reports of metaanalyses should define the selection criteria in detail to ensure that this critical question was suitably designed.

USE OF THE NONPEER REVIEWED LITERATURE

The current dogma among many scientists is that only peer-reviewed literature is valuable for inclusion in reviews, and therefore, by inference, in systematic reviews. Many producers and consumers of toxicologic pathology data also hold this belief. This tenet deserves closer examination. Should studies be limited to those that are peer reviewed or published? It is well known that negative studies, or those that report little or no benefit from following a particular course of action, are less likely to be published than are positive studies. Therefore, the published literature may be biased toward studies with positive results, and a synthesis of these studies would give a biased estimate of the impact of pursuing some course of action.

When a systematic review is planned, a plethora of industrial, academic, and government research papers have often been prepared which deal with the issue under consideration. Unfortunately, access to this unpublished or hard to find "gray" literature is limited, although there are search engines now available for attempting to discover this information. These studies may give a less biased report on the topic in question, or at least provide one or more additional points of data or interpretation for consideration. That said, a number of these unpublished studies may be of lower quality than the peer-reviewed materials. Quality is of the essence as poor research methods sometimes can produce reported results that underestimate the impact, hence providing an opposite bias to that described above for the peer-reviewed literature.

PEER REVIEW

As mentioned above, peer review is considered the primary method for quality control in scientific publishing (Vol 1, Chap 26: Pathology peer review). Should publications in a systematic review and metaanalysis be limited to peer-reviewed articles? If so, what journals should be included, or excluded? The choice of journal may be used as another filter, based on the rigor of review and editorial latitude given to fill the journal. Some investigators recommend that only those studies that are published in peer-reviewed publications be considered in metaanalysis. Although this may seem an attractive option, it might produce an even more highly biased selection of studies for systematic review.

QUALITY CONTROL

Peer review is not the only method of confirming quality control and quality assurance has been applied to data chosen for metaanalysis. Additional quality control and assurance criteria may be used to select the best and most reliable data during systematic review. The rhetorical question we really have to ask is, "Should studies included in metaanalyses be limited only to those that meet additional quality control criteria?" If investigators, undertaking a systematic review, impose an additional set of criteria before including a study in the metaanalysis, the average quality of the studies that are used should be improved. Contrary to the quality issue is the concern about selection bias. In fact, by placing specific quality "filters" on the

data, the investigators may introduce more bias than would have been created by including data of lesser quality. Moreover, different investigators might use dissimilar criteria to identify a "valid" study, and therefore would select divergent groups of studies for metaanalysis. The result is likely to be a conflicting outcome of these competing metaanalyses.

STUDY DESIGN

Some investigators insist that systematic reviews should be limited to randomized controlled studies. Such a limitation produces a variant of the above potential bias. At one time, rigid quality standards were more likely to be met by randomized controlled studies than by observational studies, but this is no longer necessarily the case. Observational methods are often used in current practice to evaluate naturally occurring effects, particularly those that are uncommon. It is quite possible that more important issues, such as combining data from studies performed in different laboratories and using different strains of a single animal species, may result in more systematic error than the nature of the study design.

METHODOLOGY

Different methodologies can cause differing degrees of systematic bias on output data. This begs the following question: should studies selected for use in any given metaanalysis be limited to those using identical methods? This limitation would mean using only separately published studies from the same lab in a limited time frame, for which the methods were comprehensively monitored and determined to be identical. In practice, application of this filter would massively reduce the number of studies that could be used in metaanalyses, whose power would therefore be greatly decreased. Accordingly, the user must understand the inherent differences among studies and exercise caution and judgment in selecting and rejecting them for use.

Pooled (Quantitative) Analysis

The main purpose of metaanalysis is to provide a quantitative assessment of the similarity of responses among a number of studies. The goal is to develop better overall estimates of the degree of benefit achieved by a particular act (e.g., specific exposure and dosing techniques), based on the combining, or pooling, of estimates found in the existing studies of the interventions. This type of metaanalysis is sometimes called a *pooled analysis* because the analyst pools the observations of many studies and then calculates parameters such as risk ratios or odds ratios from the pooled data.

Because of the many decisions regarding inclusion or exclusion of studies, different meta-analyses might reach very different conclusions on the same topic. Even after the studies are chosen, there are many other methodological issues in choosing how to combine means and variances (e.g., what weighting methods should be used). For this reason, pooled analysis should report relative risks and risk reductions as well as absolute risks and risk reductions.

Methodological (Qualitative) Analysis

Sometimes the question to be answered is not how much toxicity is induced by a particular exposure but whether there is any biologically significant toxicity at all. In this case, a qualitative metaanalysis may be done, in which the quality of the research is scored according to a list of objective criteria. The analyst then examines the methodologically superior studies to determine whether or not they answer the question of toxicity consistently. This qualitative approach has been called *methodological analysis* or *quality scores analysis*. In some cases, the methodologically strongest studies agree with one another and disagree with the weaker studies. These weaker studies may or may not be consistent with one another. In such instances, the outcome supported by the superior studies is generally the one that is adopted.

7.12. Bayesian Inference

Sensitivity and specificity of a test is important to characterize and understand the accuracy and precision of data. Once a researcher decides to use a certain test to diagnose an illness, two important questions require answers. First, if the test results are positive, what is the probability that the researcher has actually uncovered the condition of interest? Second, if the test results are negative, what is the probability that the patient really does not have the disease?

Bayes' theorem provides a method to answer these two questions.

The English clergyman after whom it is named first described *Bayes' theorem* centuries ago. It is one of the most imposing statistical formulas in the biomedical sciences. Put in symbols more meaningful for researchers such as pathologists, the formula is defined in Eq. (16.62).

The definition of Bayes' theorem

$$P(D|T+) = \frac{p(T+|D+)p(D+)}{[p(T+|D+)p(D+)] + [p(T+|D-)p(D-)]}$$

(16.62)

-where p denotes a probability, $D+$ means that the animal has the effect in question, $D-$ means that the animal does not have the effect, $T+$ means that a certain diagnostic test for the effect is positive, and the vertical line ($|$) means that the value is conditional upon what immediately follows.

Most researchers who address sensitivity, specificity, and predictive values do not wish to use Bayes' theorem. However, it is a useful formula. Closer examination of the above equation reveals that Bayes' theorem is merely the formula for the positive predictive value.

The numerator of Bayes' theorem describes **cell a**, the true-positive results, in a 2 × 2 table. The probability of being in cell *a* is equal to the prevalence multiplied by the sensitivity, where $p(D+)$ is the prevalence (i.e., the probability of being in the affected column), and where $p(T+|D+)$ is the sensitivity (i.e., the probability of being in the top row) *given the fact that one is already in the affected column*. The denominator of Bayes' theorem consists of two terms, the first of which again describes **cell a**, the true-positive results, and the second of which describes **cell b**, the false-positive error rate. This rate can be represented by $p(T+|D-)$, which is multiplied by the prevalence of unaffected animals, or $p(D-)$. The true-positive results (*a*) divided by the true-positive plus false-positive results (*a + b*) give $a/(a+b)$, which yields the positive predictive value.

In genetics, an even simpler formula than Bayes' theorem is sometimes used. The numerator is the same as that employed in Bayes theorem, but the denominator is reduced to

$p(T+)$. This adaptation makes sense because the denominator in $a/(a + b)$ is equal to all of those who have positive test results, whether they are true-positive or false-positive results.

Bayes' Theorem in the Evaluation of Safety Assessment Studies

In a population with a low prevalence of a particular toxic response, most of the positive results in a screening program for that lesion or effect would be falsely positive. Although this does not automatically invalidate a study or assessment program, it raises some concerns about cost-effectiveness. Such questions can be explored using *Bayes' theorem*. An example of this premise is a study employing an immunochemistry-based test to screen tissues for a specific effect. This test uses small amounts of antibody, and the presence of an immunologically bound stain is considered to be a positive result. If the sensitivity and specificity of the test and the prevalence of the biochemical effect are known, Bayes' theorem can be used to predict what proportion of the tissues with positive test results will have true-positive results (i.e., truly show the effect).

The table below shows how the calculations are made. If the test has a sensitivity of 96%, and if the true prevalence is 1%, only 13.9% of tissues are predicted to have a positive test result that actually will be a true-positives outcome.

Pathologists and toxicologists can quickly develop a table that lists different levels of test sensitivity, test specificity, and effect prevalence and shows how these levels affect the proportion of positive results that are likely to be true-positive results. Although this calculation is fairly straightforward and is extremely useful, it seldom has been used in the early stages of planning for large studies or safety assessment programs (presumably due lack of familiarity coupled with the cumbersome appearance of the Bayes' theorem equation).

Bayes' Theorem and Individual Animal Evaluation

Uncertainty concerning the exact cause of death of an animal during a study is a problem that faces most toxicologic pathologists. Suppose a toxicologic pathologist is uncertain about an animal's cause of death (i.e., the death could be either due to treatment or some other cause) but the animal tests positive in an assay. Even if the toxicologic pathologist knows the sensitivity and specificity of the assay in question, interpretation is still problematic (Table 16.26). Even if the toxicologic pathologist knows the sensitivity and specificity of the test in question, interpretation is still problematic. In order to calculate the positive predictive value, it is necessary to know the prevalence of the specific true outcome to be used in the analysis. The prevalence typically is considered to be the expected prevalence in the population from which the animal comes. The actual prevalence generally is not known, but usually an estimate can be attempted.

When might such a situation arise? Consider the following scenario in which a pathologist evaluates a male primate observed to have fatigue and signs of renal calculi (kidney stones), which are often indicators of parathyroid disease in this species. No other clinical signs of parathyroid disease are detected on physical examination. In the typical case, the toxicologic pathologist considers the possibility of hyperparathyroidism, arbitrarily deciding that its prevalence is perhaps 2% (reflecting that in his or her experience about 2 of 100 primates with similar signs and symptoms would have the disease). This estimated disease prevalence is called the *prior probability*, reflecting the fact that it is estimated prior to the performance of laboratory tests.

Although the toxicologic pathologist believes that the probability of hyperparathyroidism is low, she/he considers the serum calcium (Ca^{++}) concentrations to "rule out" the diagnosis. Somewhat to his or her surprise, the results of the test were positive, with an elevated serum Ca^{++} level of 12.2 mg/dL. She/he could order other tests to further evaluate the possibility that the animal has parathyroid disease. However, even if disease exists, some test results may be positive and some negative, due to a number of reasons.

Under these circumstances, Bayes' theorem could be used to make a second estimate of probability, which is called the *posterior probability*, reflecting the fact that this determination is made after the test results are known. Calculation of the posterior probability is based on the sensitivity and specificity of the test that is performed (in this case the serum Ca^{++} level), and on the prior probability, which in this case was

TABLE 16.26   Use of Bayes' Theorem or a 2 × 2 Table to Determine the Positive Predictive Value of a Hypothetical Tuberculin Screening Program

Part 1. Initial data:

Sensitivity of immunohistochemical stain = 96% = 0.96

False-negative error rate of the test = 04% = 0.04

Specificity of the test = 94% = 0.94

False-positive error rate of the test = 06% = 0.06

Prevalence of effect in the tissues = 01% = 0.01

Part 2. Use of Bayes' theorem:

$$p(D + \mid T +) = \frac{p(T + \mid D+)p(D+)}{[p(T + \mid D+)p(D+)] + [p(T + \mid D-)p(D-)]}$$

$$= \frac{(Sensitivity)(Prevalence)}{[(Sensitivity)(Prevalence)] + (False - positive\ error\ rate)(1 - Prevalence)}$$

$$= \frac{(0.96)(0.01)}{[(0.96)(0.01)] + [(0.06)(0.99)]} = \frac{0.0096}{0.0096 + 0.0594} = \frac{0.0096}{0.0690}$$

$$= 0.139$$

$$= 13.9\%$$

Part 3. Use of a 2 × 2 table

Test result	True disease status Affected (%)	Not affected (%)	Total (%)
Positive	96 (96)	594 (6)	690 (7)
Negative	4 (4)	9306 (94)	9310 (93)
Total	100 (100)	9900 (100)	10,000 (100)

Positive predictive value = 96/690 = 0.139 = **13.9%**.

set at 2%. If the serum Ca^{++} test had 90% sensitivity and 95% specificity, a false-positive error rate of 5% would be expected. Note that specificity plus the false-positive error rate always equals 100%.

When this information is used in the Bayes' equation, as shown in Table 16.27, the result is a posterior probability of 27%. This means that the animal in question is now within a group of primates with a significant possibility of

parathyroid disease. In Table 16.27 (Part 3), note that the result is the same when a 2 × 2 table is used, i.e., 27%. This is true because the probability based on the Bayes' theorem is identical to the positive predictive value.

In light of the 27% posterior probability, the pathologist decides to order a parathyroid hormone radioimmunoassay, even though this test is expensive. If the radioimmunoassay had a sensitivity of 95% and a specificity of 98%

TABLE 16.27   Use of Bayes' Theorem or a 2 × 2 Table to Determine the Posterior Probability and the Positive Predictive Value

Part 1. Beginning data:

Sensitivity of the first test = 90% = 0.90

Specificity of the first test = 95% = 0.95

Prior probability of disease = 02% = 0.02

Part 2. Use of Bayes' theorem:

$$p(D+\mid T+) = \frac{p(T+\mid D+)p(D+)}{[p(T+\mid D+)p(D+)] + [p(T+\mid D-)p(D-)]}$$

$$= \frac{(0.90)(0.02)}{[(0.90)(0.02) + (0.05)(0.98)]}$$

$$= \frac{0.018}{0.018 + 0.049} = \frac{0.018}{0.067} = 0.269 = 27\%$$

Part 3. Use of a 2 × 2 table:

Test result	True disease status		
	Affected (%)	Not affected (%)	Total (%)
Positive	18 (90)	49 (5)	67 (6.7)
Negative	2 (10)	931 (95)	933 (93.3)
Total	20 (100)	980 (100)	1000 (100.0)

Positive predictive value = 18/67 = 0.269 = **27%**.

and the results turned out to be positive, the Bayes' theorem could again be used to calculate the probability of parathyroid disease. This time, however, the posterior probability for the first test (27%) would be used as the prior probability for the second test. The result of the calculation, as shown in the table of Table 16.28 below, gives a new probability of 94%. Thus, the primate in all probability did have hyperparathyroidism.

The reader may be wondering why the posterior probability increased so much the second time. One reason is that the prior probability is considerably higher in the second calculation compared to the first (27% vs. 2%), based on the fact that the first test yielded positive results. Another reason is that the specificity of the second test is high (98%), which markedly reduced the false-positive error rate and therefore increased the positive predictive value.

8. INTERPRETATION OF RESULTS

8.1. Causality versus Association

Causality is complicated to address in toxicologic pathology because of the difficulty associated with the inability to control the experimental environment. In this case, numerous factors may be associated with an observed outcome. To address the issue of causality, questions can be asked of the association(s) that may help clarify these situations. Did the *exposure precede the lesion*? What is the *strength of the association*? Do increasing doses

TABLE 16.28   Use of Bayes' Theorem or a 2 × 2 Table to Determine the Second Posterior Probability and the Second Positive Predictive Value

---

Part 1. Beginning data:

Sensitivity of the first test = 95% = 0.95

Specificity of the first test = 98% = 0.98

Prior probability of disease = 27% = 0.27

Part 2. Use of Bayes' theorem:

$$p(D+ \mid T+) = \frac{p(T+ \mid D+)p(D+)}{[p(T+ \mid D+)p(D+)] + [p(T+ \mid D-)p(D-)]}$$

$$= \frac{(0.95)(0.27)}{[(0.95)(0.27) + (0.02)(0.73)]}$$

$$= \frac{0.257}{0.257 + 0.0146} = \frac{0.257}{0.272} = 0.9449* = 94\%$$

Part 3. Use of a 2 × 2 table:

Test result	True disease status Affected (%)	Not affected (%)	Total (%)
Positive	256 (95)	15 (2)	271 (27.1)
Negative	13 (5)	716 (98)	729 (72.9)
Total	269 (100)	731 (100)	1000 (100)

[a] *The slight difference in the results for the two approaches is due to rounding errors. It is not important biologically.*
Positive predictive value = 256/271 = 0.9446[a] = **94%**.

increase the frequency and/or severity of the lesion, i.e., *dose response*? Is there a *biological explanation* for the results? Are *causal mechanisms* (i.e., mechanisms of action) for the biological outcome known?

In observational analytic studies, strength of association is measured by *relative risk* or *odds ratios*. The greater the departure of these statistics from unity (1.00), the more likely the association is causal.

Calculation of relative risk and odds ratios.
For the calculation of relative risks and odds ratios, a 2 × 2 table can be used.

	Lesion	Yes	No
Drug	Yes ($a + b$)	(a)	(b)
	No ($c + d$)	(c)	(d)
Total	($a + b + c + d$)	($a + c$)	($b + d$)

The **relative risk** can be calculated as follows (Eq. 16.63):

$$\frac{a/(a+b)}{c/(c+d)} \qquad (16.63)$$

The **population relative risk** can be calculated as follows:

$$\frac{(a+b)/n}{c/(c+d)}$$

-where n is the number of observations.

The **odds ratio** can be calculated as follows:

$$\frac{ad}{bc}$$

The **population odds ratio** can be calculated as follows:

$$\frac{d(a/c)}{c(b/d)}$$

Although no explicit statistic is used when the dependent variable is measured, the relative difference in the levels of this variable with and without a particular factor may be used to assess the likelihood of producing the observed differences. For example, the relative difference in the incidence of massive hepatic necrosis could be related to treatment (or lack of treatment) with a specific drug suspected of causing an adverse drug reaction.

Strength of association is used as an indication of a causal association. For a *confounding variable* to produce or nullify an association between the lesion and the treatment, that confounding variable must have just as strong an association with the treatment. Although the fraction and the population are not used as direct measures of strength of association, they must be borne in mind when interpreting the size of the relative risk or odds ratio. In fact, a given odds ratio could be given more credence if the population affected was large rather than small. The reasons for this credibility are the same as those given before under the discussion of proportions.

8.2. Possible Sources of Bias

Forms of bias can exist in *interpretation*, *presentation*, and *reporting* of results. One variant is the *factori argument*: "It is certainly true that the treatment group was older than the control group, but this would clearly work against the efficacy of treatment, and, had animals been comparable, the treatment would have been more effective ...." The statement may have a plausible ring to some readers, but complex biological problems are involved. For example, it is assumed that age is a monotonic trend (i.e., as time passes, the animal becomes older), and it is not assumed that drugs may act in a biphasic or polyphasic manner. It behooves the toxicologic pathologist to recognize the impacts of nonevidence–based comments made in their reports. This topic is discussed in detail (Vol 2, Chap 13: Preparation of the pathology report for a toxicology study). Acceptance of these conclusions cannot be compelled by evidence. There are many other types of biases that are more problematic in associative than inferential research. These are beyond the scope of this chapter.

8.3. Use of Historical Control Data

In some situations, particularly where lesion incidences are low, the results from a single study may suggest an effect of treatment on tumor incidence. Statistical analysis may fail to definitively demonstrate a treatment effect. The possibility of comparing treated groups' results with those of historical control groups from other recent studies in the institution is then often raised. By taking this approach, a nonsignificant incidence of 2 cases out of 50 in a treated group may seem much more significant if no cases have been seen in, say, 1000 animals representing controls from 20 similar studies. Conversely, a significant incidence of 5 cases out of 50 in a treated group as compared with 2 out of 50 in the concurrent study controls may seem far less convincing if many other historical control groups had incidences around 5 out of 50.

While not understating the importance of looking at historical control data, it must be emphasized that there are reasons why variation among studies may be greater than variation within a given study. Hence, the utility of data from historical control databases may be of lesser value than would appear on the surface. Differences in diet, duration of the studies, intercurrent mortality, and the identity of the study pathologist may all contribute to variation among studies. Statistical techniques that ignore this variation and test treatment incidence against a pooled control incidence may give results that are seriously in error and are likely to overstate statistical significance. STP guidelines discuss the use of historical control data in more detail (Keenan et al., 2009; Elmore and Peddada, 2009).

8.4. Using Scientific Judgment

P-values provide valuable information for assessing the outcomes of designed studies. However, statistical output should not substitute for scientific reasoning. The toxicologic pathologist should always keep in mind that statistical significance is distinct from biological importance. A large effect may not produce a significant *P*-value with small samples sizes. Conversely, a very large sample size may produce a significant *P*-value even when the statistical result is not biologically meaningful. A study with 80% power will still not be able to detect a real effect 20% of the time at the predetermined level of significance. For that reason, it is useful to consider the magnitude of the *P*-value and biological relevance of an observed effect size instead of relying on a "yes/no" categorization of whether a statistical test met statistical significance criterion.

Similarly, parameter estimates should be interpreted while carefully considering the context of their associated levels of uncertainty. Values inside of a 95% CI are most compatible with the data given the statistical assumptions. Nonoverlapping 95% CIs indicate a statistically significant difference between group means at the 0.05 significance level, but the converse is not necessarily true. Overlapping 95% CIs could still produce statistically significant differences between group means at the 0.05 significance level. Nevertheless, values outside of the interval may still be compatible with the data at a higher level of uncertainty. Interpretation of results should therefore involve careful consideration of the statistical outcomes, reproducibility, magnitude of changes, and biological relevance.

9. DATA ANALYSIS APPLICATIONS IN TOXICOLOGIC PATHOLOGY

Having reviewed basic principles and provided a set of methods for statistical handling

of data, the remainder of this chapter will address the practical aspects and difficulties encountered in preclinical safety assessment in the field of toxicologic pathology.

Analyses of pathology data are well defined in the literature and common practice, though they may not necessarily use the best methods available. The aim of this section is to review statistical methods on a use-by-use basis and to provide a foundation for the selection of more appropriate alternatives in specific situations. Metaanalyses and Bayesian approaches will not be addressed in detail but should be kept in mind.

9.1. Body and Organ Weights

Total body weight and the weights of selected organs are usually collected in studies where animals are dosed with, or exposed to, a xenobiotic (e.g., chemical, drug, or biomolecule). In fact, body weight is frequently the earliest and most sensitive indication of an adverse treatment effect. Considerable discussion has taken place regarding how best to analyze these data and in what form to analyze the organ weight data, e.g., absolute weights and percentages of body weight or relative weight (Sellers et al., 2007).

Both absolute body weights and rates of body weight change are best analyzed by ANOVA followed by, if called for, a *post hoc* test such as Duncan's multiple range test. Body weight change is usually calculated as the difference from a baseline measurement value, which is traditionally the animal's weight immediately prior to the first contact (dose or exposure) with the test material. To standardize body weight and facilitate statistical analysis, no group should be significantly different in mean body weight from any other group at the beginning of the study, and all animals in all groups should lie within two SDs of the overall mean body weight. Even if the groups were randomized properly at the beginning of a study, there is an advantage to formally performing the slightly more cumbersome computation required for evaluating changes in body weight. The advantage is an increase in sensitivity, because the adjustment of starting points (i.e., the setting of initial weights as a "zero" value) reduces the amount of initial variability among groups. In this case, Bartlett's test or Levene's test is performed first to ensure homogeneity of variance, after which the data are analyzed using ANOVA with a *post hoc* test such as Dunnett's test. If sample sizes are small or the normality of the data is uncertain, then nonparametric methods such as the Kruskal–Wallis ANOVA may be more appropriate. If the sample sizes are adequate (5 or more per group) and the data are near normal in distribution, however, then a classic ANOVA is the right tool.

The analysis of relative organ weights is a valuable tool for identifying possible target organs. How to perform this analysis is still a matter of some disagreement. Organ weight data, expressed as percentages of body weight, should be analyzed separately for each sex. Conclusions drawn from analyzing organ weight data of males often differ from the impressions gained by assessing females; hence such data should always be separated by gender for analysis. Other factors, such as the impact of the stage of the reproductive cycle on uterine weight, may also influence organ weights. These factors must be taken into account both in stratification of animals and in the interpretation of results. The STP has published recommendations regarding evaluation of organ weights in toxicology studies (see Suggested Reading).

Two alternative approaches are currently used most often to analyze relative organ weights. The first calls for calculating organ weights as a percentage of total body weight at the time of necropsy and then analyzing the results by ANOVA. The second undertakes a comparable evaluation but instead employs ANCOVA, with body weights as the covariates. A number of considerations should be kept in mind when the choice is made between these two approaches. First, one must recognize the difference between *biological significance* and *statistical significance*. By evaluating relative body weight, the significance of a weight change that is not proportional to changes in whole body weights should become evident. Second, the toxicologic pathologist now must interpret small changes while still retaining a similar sensitivity, i.e., the $P < .05$ level.

There are several tools that can be used to increase the power available for the analysis of all organ weight data. One is to increase the sample size by increasing the number of animals, and the other is to utilize the most powerful test

available that is appropriate to the data. The number of animals used in the groups is presently under debate with respect to the proper cohort size needed to provide sufficient power for detecting a significant change.

In the majority of cases, except for the brain, the organs of interest in conventional toxicity studies change weight in proportion to total body weight, except in extreme cases of obesity or starvation. This change is the biological rationale behind analyzing both absolute body weight and the organ weight to body weight ratio. Analytical techniques are designed to detect cases where this relative change does not occur.

Analysis of data from several hundred repeated-dose toxicity studies has shown no significant difference in the rates at which weight change occurs in common target organs (e.g., adrenal gland, gonad, heart, kidney, liver, spleen, thymus), other than the brain, compared to total body weight for healthy rats, mice, rabbits, and dogs. The ANCOVA test has limitations in analyzing body weight and related organ weight changes since a primary assumption for this method is the independence of variables. ANCOVA allows the data to determine the extent of the linear relationship between the treatment and covariable and mathematically applies the appropriate adjustment. If the chemical and body weight both affect the organ weight, then the effects of the chemical and body weight on organ weight would be confounded and difficult to separate. However, by not forcing the best-fitting regression line through the origin, the relationship between organ weight and body weight does not have to be directly proportional. Strategic investigation of the effects of body weight and dose on organ weight could potentially indicate that body weight alone and not the treatment (or vice versa) affected organ weight. While recognizing these limitations, a judicious use of covariables has been noted in the literature. Nevertheless, in toxicologic pathology, the assumption that the relationship of the two variables (e.g., relative organ weight and total body weight) is the same for all treatments is generally not true.

In cases where the differences between the error mean squares are much greater during the analysis, the ratio of *F* ratios (from ANCOVA) will diverge in precision from the result of the efficiency of the covariance adjustment. These cases occur where either sample sizes are large or where the differences between the group means themselves are great. This latter case is one that requires special attention in the toxicity study designs under discussion when attempting to use ANCOVA, because group means are very similar at the beginning of the experiment and cannot diverge markedly unless there is a treatment-induced effect. As we have discussed earlier, a treatment effect challenges a prime underpinning assumption of ANCOVA.

9.2. Clinical Chemistry

Various clinical chemistry parameters are commonly determined on blood (specifically, plasma or serum) and urine samples collected from animals in chronic, subchronic, and occasionally acute toxicity studies. In the past, and currently in some places, the accepted practice has been to evaluate these data using univariate-parametric methods, primarily t-tests and ANOVA. However, these techniques do not constitute the best approach, for several reasons. First, biochemical parameters are rarely independent of each other, nor is the focus of inquiry often limited to only one of the parameters measured in such samples. Rather, a number of parameters typically change when toxicity is seen in specific organs. For example, simultaneous elevations of creatinine phosphokinase, γ-hydroxybutyrate dehydrogenase, lactate dehydrogenase, and troponins are strongly indicative of myocardial damage. In such cases, the clinical importance of these findings is not dictated by a significant elevation in any one of these analytes. Instead, all four changes must be considered together. Second, interaction occurs among clinical chemistry parameters, indicating that they are not independent. For example, serum electrolytes (sodium, potassium, and calcium) are interconnected such that a decrease in one is frequently tied to an increase in one of the others. Finally, either because of the biological nature of the parameters or the way in which they are measured, clinical chemistry data are frequently skewed or not continuous, as is seen particularly for reference ranges of many analytes in experimental animals (e.g., creatinine, sodium, potassium,

chloride, calcium, and blood). Thus, when analyzing clinical chemistry data, the appropriate rank-based nonparametric test, such as Kruskal–Wallis nonparametric ANOVA, Dunn's test, or Shirley's test, should be used.

The Student's t-test compares the actual difference between *two means* in relation to the variation in the data. It may be used for the analysis of clinical chemistry data when one nominal variable is to be compared with the mean values of the measurement variable. The nominal variable must have only two values, such as "male" and "female" or "treated" and "untreated." If the data come from a skewed distribution, the Wilcoxon rank-sum test is more appropriate than Student's t-test.

9.3. Hematology

Much of what was said about the statistical analysis of clinical chemistry parameters holds true for the hematological measurements made in chronic, subchronic, and sometimes acute toxicity studies. Again, the usual practice in the past, and even today in some institutions, has been to examine these data using t-tests, ANOVA, and other univariate parametric techniques. Again, these approaches are not the most appropriate choice for this analysis. Choosing the correct statistical test to perform should be evaluated by use of a decision tree until one gains confidence in choosing the most appropriate method(s). It must be kept in mind that sets of values and, in some cases, population distribution vary not only among species but also among the commonly used strains of a given species. This phenomenon means that control or standard values will always tend to drift—sometimes substantially—over the course of only a few years.

Again, the majority of hematologic parameters are interrelated and highly dependent on the method used to determine them. RBC counts, mean corpuscular volume (MCV) of RBCs, and platelet counts may be determined using an automated device such as a Coulter counter to take direct measurements. A minor consideration in toxicity testing is to ensure that the analytical instrument is equipped to measure the cells of the test species. The resulting data are usually stable for analysis using parametric methods. However, the hematocrit (HCT) may actually be a value calculated from the RBC and MCV values; hence, it is dependent on them. Direct HCT measurements may be compared using parametric methods, while HCT values calculated from the RBC and MCV should be compared using nonparametric approaches like the Wilcoxon rank-sum test or Kruskal–Wallis ANOVA.

Hemoglobin is directly measured and is an independent and continuous variable. However, the distribution of values is rarely normal, but rather may be multimodal. This distribution probably occurs because several forms and conformations of hemoglobin (e.g., oxyhemoglobin, deoxyhemoglobin, methemoglobin) are typically present at any one time in blood. Here, a nonparametric technique such as the Wilcoxon rank-sum test should be employed.

Consideration of WBC counts and WBC differential counts leads to another problem. The total WBC number is typically distributed in a normal fashion, and thus is amenable to parametric analysis. However, differential cell counts are usually determined by manually counting one or more sets of 100 WBCs each. The resulting relative percentages of neutrophils are then reported as either percentages or absolute counts (which have been computed by multiplying the total WBC count by its percentage). Such data do not approximate a normal distribution, particularly in the case of eosinophils and basophils (which have low count values insufficient to provide a normally distributed sample), and therefore should generally be analyzed by nonparametric methods. It is widely believed that relative (%) differential data should not be reported if they are based on manual differential counts because they are likely to be misleading.

Finally, it must be kept in mind that a change in any single hematological parameter rarely has a clinically useful meaning. Because these parameters are so interrelated, patterns of changes affecting multiple values together (e.g., RBC and MCV and HCT) should be expected if a real effect is present. Therefore, analysis and interpretation of hematologic results instead should focus on identifying such patterns of changes. Classification analysis techniques (e.g., $N \times R \, \chi^2$) often provide the basis for a useful approach to such problems.

9.4. Incidence of Histopathological Findings

The last 4 decades have seen increasing emphasis placed on histopathological examination of tissues collected from animals in subchronic and chronic toxicity studies. Indeed, this evolution has driven the development of toxicologic pathology as a discipline. The biological significance of a statistically significant structural lesion is particularly important for the toxicologic pathologist to address.

In most cases, a statistical evaluation is the only way to determine if the morphological changes seen in treated animals really are different in number, extent, and/or severity from those seen in control animals. Particular expertise is required in cases where a change may be of such a rare type that the occurrence of only one or a few such lesions in treated animals raises a red flag or in situations in which control group sizes are very limited. Although tumors are a major concern as toxicologic pathology endpoints, nonneoplastic (background or sentinel) lesions are often of the greatest use in determining possible mechanisms of action by the test article. In addition, it is often important to determine whether or not such background changes have been impacted by some treatment. Statistical analysis can be an important tool for evaluating the potential relevance of such findings in borderline cases.

For statistical analysis, comparisons of the incidence of any one type of lesion between controls and treated animals typically are made using the multiple $2 \times 2 \, \chi^2$ test or Fisher's exact test with a modification of the numbers of animals as the denominators. In general, these tests are most appropriate for balanced study designs (i.e., the groups have equal numbers of test subjects and a group size *of n > 6*). In cases where treatment-related effects (e.g., premature deaths) result in one or more groups of a substantially reduced size, nonparametric tests often are used instead to compensate for the uneven animal numbers. Grading of lesions with respect to lesion severity results in ordinal data can produce an additional dimension in the information content of the data that would not be available by performing an analysis based only on the perceived quantal nature of a lesion being present of absent in an animal.

The traditional method of analyzing multiple, cross-classified data (e.g., an immunotoxicity study where we have within each animal both an incidence of immune responses in a range of tissues and also grades of lesions for each response) has been to combine columns and rows in the N × R contingency table over all but two of the variables. Following this data condensation, a computation of some measure of association between these variables is undertaken. For an N-dimensional table (N × R), this procedure results in $N(N-1)/2$ separate analyses (where N denotes the number of types of measures). This method results in a crude filtered analysis, where inappropriate pooling of the data yields a faulty understanding of their meaning. Though computationally more laborious, a multiway (N × R table) analysis should be utilized for such cases.

9.5. Carcinogenesis

Inferences about the potential human carcinogenicity of substances are based on experimental results obtained from two nonhuman species given the substance at a high dose or exposure level. The aim of animal carcinogenicity bioassays is to predict the possibility and probability of tumors occurring in humans at much lower levels of exposure. An entire textbook could be devoted to examining the assumptions involved in this undertaking, as well as reviewing aspects of study design and interpretation. Such detail is beyond the scope of this chapter.

In the past, the single most important statistical consideration in designing a carcinogenicity bioassay was the simple quantal response obtained for a single question: did cancer occur following exposure or did it not? Experiments were designed so that a sufficient number of animals were used so that the final data set would have a reasonable expectation of detecting an effect if one occurred. Although the primary objective of carcinogenicity bioassays today is still to determine whether the incidence of tumors is increased following exposure to the test article of interest, a much more complex model should now be considered to answer other questions pertinent to extrapolation of experimental results in animals to make inferences about risks to human health.

Many supplemental types of data may be collected in this regard. The time-to-tumor onset, patterns of tumor incidence, effects on survival rate, and age at first tumor are among the most important ancillary endpoints. The rationale for including these factors lies in concerns associated with likely planned or unplanned exposure of humans to xenobiotic and naturally occurring substances, and the potential than even minimal exposures repeated over time could generate relatively small increases in the incidence of tumors. In other words, human exposure to the substance under study will likely occur at very low levels. To statistically detect a small increase in the incidence of treatment-induced tumors over background would require the use of an impracticably large number of test animals per group.

For example (Table 16.29), only 46 animals per group are required to provide sufficient statistical power to show a 10% increase over a zero (0%) background, where the spectrum of background lesions included a rarely occurring tumor type. In contrast, to detect a 10th of a percent increase (0.1%) above a five percent (5%) background, 770,000 animals per group would be needed! As dose increases, the incidence of tumors (i.e., the response) will also increase. This increase occurs until it reaches the point where a modest increase (e.g., 10%) over a reasonably small background level (e.g., 1%) may be detected using an acceptably small group of test animals; in Table 16.29, it can be seen that 51 animals would be needed for such a situation. It also can be seen that the number of animals required to reveal a vanishingly small increase in tumor incidence (e.g., 1/100,000) above a high background level (e.g., 25%) would be very large.

There are, however, at least two potential difficulties that often occur in the group given the highest dose of a potential carcinogen. First, mortality can be higher than in other groups. This situation is problematic as there must be sufficient rodents surviving to the end of the study to allow for meaningful statistical analysis. Second, toxicologic pathologists must select the high dose level based only on the information provided by a subchronic or range-finding study, usually 90 days in length. The uncertainty in extrapolating the high dose for a long-term study

TABLE 16.29 Average Number of Animals Needed to Detect a Significant Increase in the Incidence of an Event (Tumors, Anomalies, Etc.) Over the Background Incidence at Several Expected Incidence Levels Using the Fisher Exact Probability Test ($P = .05$)

Background incidence	% Increase in tumor incidence					
	0.01	0.1	1	3	5	10
0	46,000,000[a]	460,000	4600	511	164	46
0.01	46,000,000	460,000	4600	511	164	46
0.1	47,000,000	470,000	4700	520	168	47
1	51,000,000	510,000	5100	570	204	51
5	77,000,000	770,000	7700	856	304	77
10	100,000,000	1,000,000	10,000	1100	400	100
20	148,000,000	1,480,000	14,800	1644	592	148
25	160,000,000	1,600,000	16,000	1840	664	166

[a] Number of animals needed in each group—controls as well as treated.

from such short-term data presents a difficulty to toxicologic pathologists because the correct maximum tolerated dose (MTD) may not have been defined in the previous studies.

To predict carcinogenic effects across species, it typically is necessary that the metabolism and mechanism of action of the compound at the highest level to be tested are the same as those that occur at the low levels that will be encountered during human exposures. Unfortunately, selection of an inappropriate dose can invalidate an entire lifetime carcinogenicity bioassay. Selecting a dose that is too low may render the study incapable of detecting a carcinogenic response. In contrast, if the dose is too high dose, toxicokinetic differences may alter the agent's metabolism and/or mechanism of action.

There are several solutions to this problem of in appropriate dose selection. One of these is the approach of the U.S. National Toxicology Program—Bioassay Program, which is to conduct a 3-month range-finding study with sufficient dose levels to establish a level that significantly decreases (by 10%) the rate of body weight gain. This dose is defined as the MTD and is selected as the highest dose for the lifetime carcinogenicity bioassay. Two other levels, generally one-half MTD and one-quarter MTD, are selected for testing as the intermediate and low-dose levels. In many earlier U.S. NCI

carcinogenicity studies, only one other lower dose level was used. The international conference on harmonization of technical requirements for registration of pharmaceutical for human use recommends that middle and low doses be selected after integrating human and rodent pharmacokinetic, pharmacodynamic, and toxicity data (ICH, 2008).

The dose range-finding study is necessary in most cases to establish a suitable high dose, but the suppression of body weight gain is a scientifically questionable benchmark when establishing safety factors. Physiological, pharmacological, or metabolic markers generally serve as better indicators of a systemic toxic response than body weight. Indeed, the toxicokinetic question raised above, where metabolic mechanisms for handling a compound at real-life exposure levels can be saturated or overwhelmed brings into play entirely artifactual metabolic and physiologic mechanisms.

To make sure that the metabolic profile of the test article when given at a high dose is the same as would be observed at lower doses, a series of well-defined acute and subchronic studies should be undertaken. These studies are designed to determine the chronicity factor and to study the onset of pathology. Such a series of studies typically will be more predictive for dose setting than is body weight suppression.

The regulatory response to questioning the appropriateness of the MTD as a high dose level has been to acknowledge that occasionally an excessively high dose is selected. The regulatory response also indicates that using lower doses would be expected to seriously decrease the sensitivity of detection.

10. ASSUMPTIONS OF STATISTICAL TESTS

The following table highlights the assumptions that are required for specific statistical analysis (Table 16.30).

11. SUMMARY AND CONCLUSIONS

We have attempted to highlight some of the issues that the toxicologic pathologist must address during study design and data analysis. There are many more statistical models and experimental designs that have not been addressed in this chapter, but which can be found in standard reference texts on statistics.

Regardless of the methodology used, nothing surpasses common sense and remembering that statistical analysis is a tool to aid in understanding the data rather than a prerequisite to data evaluation and interpretation. The field of biostatistics is complex and may appear

TABLE 16.30   A Summary of Assumptions Made for Some Statistical Tests

Test	Assumptions	Limitations and comments
Bartlett's test for homogeneity of variance	Homoscedasticity is an important assumption for Student's t-test, analysis of variance, and analysis of covariance Bartlett's test is designed for three or more groups Data must be normally distributed The test can be used to test normality	Bartlett's test does not test for normality, but rather homogeneity of variance (also called equality of variances or homoscedasticity) Bartlett's test is very sensitive to departures from normality. As a result, a finding of a significant Chi-square value in Bartlett's test may indicate nonnormality rather than heteroscedasticity Outliers can bring about such a finding, and the sensitivity to such erroneous findings is extreme with small sample sizes
Levene's test for homogeneity of variance	Levene's test can be used to test for equality of variance across two or more groups	Levene's test is less sensitive to departures from normality than Bartlett's test
Shapiro—Wilk test for normality	The Shapiro—Wilk test for normality is designed to test for normality of a sample	The Shapiro—Wilk test is sensitive to sample size. It tends to falsely reject normality with large sample sizes and fails to reject for normality for small sample sizes
Fisher's exact test	Fisher's exact test must be used in preference to the Chi-square test when there are small cell numbers (i.e., less than six) Fisher's probabilities are not necessarily symmetric. Although some analysts will double the one-tailed P-value to obtain the two-tailed result, this method is usually overly conservative Samples are random and independent The response is dichotomous	Tables are available which provide individual exact probabilities for small sample size contingency tables Ghent has developed and proposed a good method extending the calculation of exact probabilities to 2×3, 3×3, and R $\times$ C contingency tables. The probability resulting from a two-tailed Chi-square test is exactly double that of a one-tailed probability from the same data

(Continued)

TABLE 16.30   A Summary of Assumptions Made for Some Statistical Tests—cont'd

Test	Assumptions	Limitations and comments
2 × 2 contingency table	Fisher's exact test must be used in preference to the Chi-square test when there are small cell numbers (i.e., less than six) There are no interactions between row and column classifications The test assumes no outliers.	Fisher's probabilities are not necessarily symmetric Tables are available which provide individual exact probabilities for small sample size contingency tables The probability resulting from a two-tailed Chi-square test is exactly double that of a one-tailed probability from the same data
2 × 2 Chi-square	All expected frequencies should be 10 or greater Data are univariate and categorical Data are from a multinomial population Data are collected by random and independent sampling Groups are of approximately the same size, particularly for small group sizes If any expected frequencies are less than 10, but greater than or equal to 5, Yates' correction for continuity can be used. This is done by subtracting 0.5 from the absolute value of observed−expected values (O-E) before squaring	*Use when* the data are of a categorical (or frequency) nature The data fit the assumptions above to test goodness to fit to a known form of distribution Cell sizes are large *Do not use when* the data are continuous rather than categorical Sample sizes are small and very unequal Sample sizes are too small (for example, when total n is less than 50 of if any expected value is less than 5) For any 2 × 2 comparison, use Fisher's exact test instead
R × C Chi-square	None of the expected frequency values should be less than 5.0 Chi-square test is always one-tailed. The results from each additional column (group) are approximately additive. Due to this characteristic, Chi-square can be readily used for evaluating any R × C combination The results of the Chi-square calculation must be a positive number, which is an inevitable outcome given the other conditions Data must be independent	Without the use of some form of correction, the test becomes less accurate as the differences between group size increase The test is weak with either small sample sizes or when the expected frequency in any cell is less than 5. These limitations can be overcome by pooling—combining cells Can be used to test the probability of validity of any distribution Test results are independent of order of cells
Wilcoxon rank-sum test	Differences are assumed to be independent All data are from the same continuous population The test assumes that the distribution of signs is symmetric	Too many tied ranks increase the likelihood of a false-positive result (i.e., rejection of the null hypothesis may occur at less than 5%, even though the alpha level is set at 0.05) The Wilcoxon rank-sum test can be highly biased in the presence of censored data
Distribution-free multiple comparisons	Generally, this test should be used as a *post hoc* comparison after the Kruskal–Wallis nonparametric ANOVA	As with the Wilcoxon rank-sum, too many tied ranks inflate the likelihood of a false-positive result

(Continued)

TABLE 16.30   A Summary of Assumptions Made for Some Statistical Tests—cont'd

Test	Assumptions	Limitations and comments
Mann—Whitney U test	The test statistics from a Mann—Whitney are linearly related to those of the Wilcoxon rank-sum test. The two tests will always yield the same result. The Mann—Whitney U test has been much favored in developmental and reproductive toxicology (DART) studies It does not matter whether the observations are ranked from smallest to largest or vice versa The samples are randomly taken from a population The samples are independent within and mutually independent between samples The measurement scale is at least ordinal	This test should not be used for paired observations
Kruskal—Wallis nonparametric analysis of variance (ANOVA)	The test statistic H is used for both small and large samples Data must be independent for the test to be valid. The effect of adjusting for tied ranks is to slightly increase the value of the test statistic, H. Therefore, omission of this adjustment results in a more conservative test Within each sample, the observations are independent and identically distributed The samples are independent of each other	When we find a significant difference, we do not know which groups are different. It is incorrect to then perform a Mann—Whitney U test on all possible combinations. Rather, a multiple comparison method must be used, such as the distribution-free multiple comparisons Too many tied ranks will decrease the power of this test and also lead to false-positive results When $k = 2$, the Kruskal—Wallis Chi-square value has 1 df. This test is identical to the normal approximation used for the Wilcoxon Rank-Sum test. A Chi-square with 1 df can be represented by the square of a standardized normal random variable. In the case of $k = 2$, the H-statistic is the square of the Wilcoxon Rank-Sum (without the continuity correction)
Log-rank test	The endpoint of concern is or is defined so that it is right censored (i.e., once it happens, it does not reoccur). Examples are death or a minimum or maximum value of an enzyme activity or physiologic function (such as respiration rate) The method requires no assumption regarding the distribution of event times A continuity correction can also be used, in which the numerators are reduced by $1/2$ before squaring. Use of such a correction	The Wilcoxon Rank-Sum test could be used to analyze the event times in the absence of censoring. A "generalized Wilcoxon" test, sometimes called the Gehan test, based on an approximate Chi-square distribution has been developed for use in the presence of censored observations Both the Log-rank and the Wilcoxon Rank-Sum tests are nonparametric tests, and require no assumptions regarding

(Continued)

TABLE 16.30 A Summary of Assumptions Made for Some Statistical Tests—cont'd

Test	Assumptions	Limitations and comments
	leads to further conservatism and may be omitted when sample sizes are moderate or large (i.e., greater than or equal to 15 per cell) The subjects are randomly sampled from, or at least are representative of, larger populations The subjects were chosen independently Consistent criteria are used Baseline survival rate is not changing over time. The survival of the censored subjects would be the same, on average, as the survival of the remaining subjects	the distribution of event times. When the event rate is greater early in the trial than toward the end, the generalized Wilcoxon test is the more appropriate test since it gives greater weight to the earlier differences Life tables can be constructed to provide estimates of the event time distributions. Estimates commonly used are known as the survival rate Survival and failure times often follow the exponential distribution. If such a model can be assumed, a more powerful alternative to the log-rank test is the likelihood ratio test This nonparametric test assumes that event probabilities are constant over time. That is, the chance that a patient becomes event positive at time t given that he is event negative up to time t does not depend on t. A plot of the negative log of the event time distribution showing a linear trend through the origin is consistent with exponential event times the Kaplan—Meier estimates
Student t-test	The test assumes that the data are univariate, continuous, and normally distributed Data are collected by random sampling The test should be used when the assumptions above are met and there are only two groups to be compared The variances of the populations to be compared are equal	Do not use when the data are ranked, when the data are not approximately normally distributed, or when there are more than two groups to be compared. Do not use for paired observations This is the most commonly misused test method, except in those few cases where one is truly only comparing two groups of data and the group sizes are roughly equivalent. Not valid for multiple comparisons (because of resulting additive errors) or where group sizes are very unequal The test is robust for moderate departures from normality and, when N1 and N2 are approximately equal, robust for moderate departures from homogeneity of variances The main difference between the Z-test and the t-test is that the Z-statistic is based on a known standard deviation, σ, while the t-statistic uses the sample

(Continued)

TABLE 16.30   A Summary of Assumptions Made for Some Statistical Tests—cont'd

Test	Assumptions	Limitations and comments
		standard deviation, s, as an estimate of σ. With the assumption of normally distributed data, the variance σ^2 is more closely estimated by the sample variance s^2 as n gets large. It can be shown that the t-test is equivalent to the Z-test for infinite degrees of freedom. In practice, a "large" sample is usually considered to exist when $n \geq 30$
Cochran t-test	The test assumes normality and independence of data The blocks were randomly selected from the population of all possible blocks The outcomes of the treatments can be coded as binary responses (i.e., a 0 or 1) in a way that is common to all treatments within each block	This test could be considered as a two-group equivalent of the Bartlett's test If the test statistic is close to 1.0, the results are not significant
Analysis of variance (ANOVA)	This test is parametric If the sample sizes are approximately equal, ANOVA is robust for moderate inequality of variances (as determined by Bartlett's test) A multiple-comparison *post hoc* method must be used Samples are normally distributed There is homogeneity of variances Data are independent	The test is robust for moderate departures from normality if the sample sizes are large It is not appropriate to use a t-test (or a "2 groups at a time" version of ANOVA) to identify where significant differences are within the design group
F-test	The test assumes normality and independence of data There is homogeneity of variances	If the test statistic is close to 1.0, the results are not significant This test could be considered as a two-group equivalent of the Bartlett's test
Duncan's multiple range test	For dependent variables, the data are a random sample of vectors from a multivariate normal population In the population, the variance–covariance matrices for all cells are the same To check assumptions, homogeneity of variances tests (including Box's M) and spread-versus-level plots can be used One can also examine residuals and residual plots	Duncan's assures a set alpha level (the false positive or type I error rate) for all tests when means are separated by approximately regular intervals Preserving this alpha level means that the test is less sensitive than other similar procedures, such as the Student–Newman–Keuls test The test is inherently conservative and not resistant or robust
Scheffe's multiple comparisons	It tests all linear contrasts among the population means It is not formulated on the basis of groups with equal numbers (as one of Duncan's	The Scheffe's procedure is robust to moderate violations of the normality and homogeneity of variance assumptions The Scheffe's procedure is powerful

(Continued)

TABLE 16.30 A Summary of Assumptions Made for Some Statistical Tests—cont'd

Test	Assumptions	Limitations and comments
	procedures is), and if N1 ≠ N2 there is no separate weighing procedure In the population, the variance–covariance matrices for all cells are the same To check assumptions, homogeneity of variances tests (including Box's M) and spread-versus-level plots can be used One can also examine residuals and residual plots	because of its robustness, yet it is very conservative. Type I error (the false-positive rate) is held constant at the selected test level for each comparison
Dunnett's *t*-test	Treated group sizes must be approximately equal In the population, the variance–covariance matrices for all cells are the same To check assumptions, homogeneity of variances tests (including Box's M) and spread-versus-level plots can be used One can also examine residuals and residual plots	Dunnett's seeks to ensure that the false-positive (Type I error) rate will be fixed at the desired level by incorporating correction factors into the design of the test value table
Analysis of covariance (ANCOVA)	The slopes of the regression lines defined by a set of points (designated by X and Y coordinates) are equal from group to group. This can be examined visually or formally (i.e., by a test). If this condition is not met, ANCOVA cannot be used The relationship between X and Y is linear The covariate X is measured without error There are no unmeasured confounding variables The errors inherent in each variable are independent of each other The variances of the errors within groups are equivalent between groups The measured data that form the groups are normally and independently distributed The covariate is measured without error	ANCOVA is generally robust to departures from normality The power of the test declines as error increases Lack of independence effectively (but to an immeasurable degree) reduces sample size
Linear regression	The method assumes that the data are independent and normally distributed There is a linear relationship between dependent and independent variables There is homoscedasticity of errors All the regression methods are for interpolation, not extrapolation	The method is sensitive to outliers The X-axis (or horizontal) component plays an extremely important part in developing the least square fit. All points have equal weight in determining the height of a regression line, but extreme X-axis values unduly influence the slope of the line A good fit between a line and a set of data (i.e., a strong correlation between treatment and response variables) does not imply any causal relationship

(Continued)

TABLE 16.30   A Summary of Assumptions Made for Some Statistical Tests—cont'd

Test	Assumptions	Limitations and comments
Probit/Log transforms and regression	The probit distribution is derived form a common error function, with the midpoint (50% point) moved to a score of 5.00. A normally distributed population is assumed. Variables are discrete. The procedure is usually applied to data having a nominal scale (e.g., LD_{50})	The underlying frequency distribution becomes asymptotic as it approaches the extremes of the range. That is, in the midrange of 16%–84%, the corresponding probit values change gradually—the curve is relatively linear. But beyond this range, the probit values change ever more rapidly as they approach either 0% or 100%. In fact, there are no values for either of these numbers. The results are sensitive to outliers
Nonlinear regression	X and Y are assumed to be independent as a null hypothesis. The test determines whether the dependent variable (Y) depends on the independent variable (X). The correlation coefficient (r) is termed to calculate the coefficient of determination (r^2). r^2 is a measure of the proportion of the variation of one variable determined by the variation of the other variable. Assumes a normal distribution. Variables are measured without error (reliability). There is an assumption of homoscedasticity	A strong correlation does not imply a causal relationship. The distances of data points from the regression line are the portions of the data not explained by the model. These are called residuals. Poor correlation coefficients imply high residuals, which may be due to many small contributions (variations of data from the regression line) or a few large ones. Extreme values (outliers) greatly reduce correlation
Kendall's coefficient of rank correlation	A very robust estimator that does not assume normality, linearity, or minimal error of measurement	It is a distribution-free test of independence and a measure of independence between two variables
Trend tests	Trend tests seek to evaluate whether there is a monotonic tendency in response to a change in treatment. That is, the dose–response direction is absolute (i.e., as dose goes up, the incidence of tumors increases)	The test loses power rapidly in response to the occurrences of reversals—for example, a low-dose group with a decreased tumor incidence. The trend test will have higher power than the chi-square test when the suspected trend is correct, but the ability to detect unsuspected trends is sacrificed when a trend test is used. The trend test exploits the suspected direction of an effect to increase power, but this does not affect the sampling distribution of the test statistic under the null hypothesis
Cochran–Armitage test	The data are normally distributed	The Cochran–Armitage test is asymptotically efficient for all monotone alternatives, but this result only holds asymptotically. Tumors are rare events; therefore, the binomial proportions are small. In this situation, approximations may become unreliable

complicated to the untrained user, just as toxico-logic pathology seems incomprehensible to a number of other scientists. For this reason, we urge the reader to always discuss the design and analysis of an experiment with a biostatistician *before* execution of the experiment. Similarly, we recommend that the toxicologic pathologist understand the fundamental assumptions and limitations of the statistical models that are being used as well as the ramifications of violating these assumptions. Finally, we recommend using the most powerful test appropriate to the form, quantity, and quality of the data as this practice will provide the most robust analytical platform as well as the optimal support for risk assessment and management.

GLOSSARY

Abscissa X-axis

Absolute risk Probability of an event over a period of time, expressed as a cumulative incidence. It shows the actual likelihood of contracting the disease.

Accuracy: The match between the target population and the sample.

Adjusted odds ratio In a multiple logistic regression model where the response variable is the presence or absence of a disease, an odds ratio for a binomial exposure variable is an adjusted odds ratio for the levels of all other risk factors. It is also possible to calculate the adjusted odds ratio for a continuous exposure variable.

Alpha α α (alpha) indicates the probability of rejecting the null hypothesis tested when, in fact, that hypothesis is true. It is customary to set α at 0.05.

Alternative hypothesis The hypothesis that competes with the null hypothesis as an explanation for observed data is called the alternative hypothesis.

A priori A priori probability is the probability estimate prior to receiving new information.

Association A statistically significant correlation between exposure and a disease or condition. An association may be an artifact (random error chance, bias, confounding) or a real one.

Asymptotic Refers to a curve that continually approaches either the X- or Y-axis but does not actually reach it until x or y equals infinity. The axis so approached is the asymptote.

Asymptotic efficiency Asymptotic efficiency is the limit of its efficiency as the sample size tends to infinity.

Asymptotically unbiased In point estimation, the property that the bias approaches zero as the sample size (n) increases. Therefore, estimators with this property improve as n increases.

Balanced design An experimental design in which the same number of observations is taken for each combination of the experimental factors.

Bayesian inference An inference method that takes into account the prior probability for an event.

Beta β It is the probability of failing to reject the hypothesis tested when that hypothesis is false and a specific alternative hypothesis is true.

Bias An estimator for a parameter is unbiased if its expected value is the true value of the parameter. Otherwise, the estimator is biased.

Bimodal distribution A distribution with two modes.

Binary (dichotomous) variable A discrete random variable that can only take two possible values (success or failure).

Binomial distribution The binomial distribution gives the probability of obtaining successes in independent trials, where there are two possible outcomes one of which is conventionally called success for observed versus expected value.

Biological replicate The smallest experimental unit that independently received the treatment.

Blocks Homogeneous grouping of experimental units (subjects) in experimental design.

Causal relationship To establish a causal relationship, the following nonstatistical evidence is required: Consistency (reproducibility), biological plausibility, dose response, temporality (when applicable), and strength of the relationship (as measured by odds ratio/relative risk/hazard ratio).

Categorical (nominal) variable A variable that can be assigned to categories. A nonnumerical (qualitative) variable measured on a (discrete) nominal scale such as gender, drug treatments, disease subtypes; or on an ordinal scale such as low, median, or high dosage. A variable may alternatively be quantitative (continuous or discrete).

Censored observation Observations that survived to a certain point in time before dropping out from the study for a reason other than having the outcome of interest (lost to follow up or not enough time to have the event). Censoring is simply an incomplete observation that has ended before time to event. These observations are still useful in survival analysis.

Central limit theorem The means of a relatively large (>30) number of random samples from any population (not necessarily a normal distribution) will be approximately normally distributed. This approximation will improve as the sample increases.

Chi-squared distribution A distribution derived from the normal distribution.

Chi-squared test The most commonly used test for frequency data and goodness of fit.

Cluster sampling A sampling technique where the entire population is divided into groups, or clusters, and a random sample of these clusters are selected. All observations in the selected clusters are included in the sample.

Coefficient of variation The coefficient of variation measures the spread of a set of data as a proportion of its mean. It is often expressed as a percentage.

Confidence interval A confidence interval gives an estimated range of values, which is likely to include an unknown population parameter, the estimated range being calculated from a given set of sample data.

Confounding variable A variable that is associated with both the outcome and the exposure variable. The data should be stratified before analyzing it if there is a confounding effect.

Contingency table A contingency table is a tabular representation of categorical data.

Control group A group in an experiment that receives not treatment in order to compare the treated group against a norm.

Covariate Generally used to mean explanatory variable, less generally an additional explanatory variable is of no interest but included in the model to adjust the statistical model. More specifically, it denotes an explanatory variable which is unaffected by treatments and has a linear relationship to the response.

Covariance (covariation) It is a measure of the association between a pair of variables: The expected value of the product of the deviation of two random variables from their respective means. It is also called a measure of "linear dependence" between the two random variables.

Critical value The critical value(s) for a hypothesis test is a threshold to which the value of the test statistic in a sample is compared to determine whether or not the null hypothesis is rejected.

Cumulative frequency distribution A cumulative frequency distribution is a summary of a set of data showing the frequency (or number) of items less than or equal to the upper class limit of each class.

Data Singular—datum. Data are recorded observations made on people, objects, or other things that can be counted, measured, or quantified in some way.

Degrees of freedom (df) The number of independent units of information in a sample used in the estimation of a parameter or calculation of a statistic.

Dependability Being able to account for changes in the design of the study and the changing conditions surrounding what was studied.

Descriptive statistics Summary of available data.

Discrete variable A variable of countable number of integer outcomes.

Dispersion The variation between values is called dispersion.

Efficiency For an unbiased estimator, efficiency indicates how much its precision is lower than the theoretical limit of precision.

Empirical research The process of developing systematized knowledge gained from observations that are formulated to support insights and generalizations about the phenomena under study.

Error terms Residuals in regression models. They are assumed to be normally distributed, have equal variance for all fitted values, and independent.

Estimate An estimate is an indication of the value of an unknown quantity based on observed data.

Estimator Any quantity calculated from the sample data, which is used to give information about an unknown quantity in the population. For example, the sample mean is an estimator of the population mean.

Event A set of possible outcomes resulting from a particular experiment.

Expected value The expected value of a random variable is nothing but the arithmetic mean. For a discrete random variable, the expected value is the weighted average of the possible values of the random variable, the weights being the probabilities that those values will occur. For a continuous random variable, the values of the probability density are used instead of probabilities, and the summation operator is replaced by the integral.

Experiment Any process of observation or measurement is called an experiment in statistics.

Factor A categorical explanatory variable with small number of levels such that each item classified belongs to exactly one level for that category.

Factorial analysis of variance An analysis in which the treatments differ in terms of two or more factors (with several levels) as opposed to treatments being different levels of a single factor as in one-way ANOVA.

F distribution A continuous probability distribution of the ratio of two independent random variables, each having a Chi-squared distribution, divided by their respective degrees of freedom.

Frequency distribution A frequency distribution is a tabular summary of a set of data showing the frequency (or number) of items in each of several nonoverlapping classes (or bins).

Geometric distribution A random variable x obeys the geometric distribution with parameter p $(0 < P < 1)$.

Geometric mean $G = (x_1.x_2 \ldots xn)^{1/n}$ where n is the sample size.

Harmonic mean Harmonic mean is a measure of central location.

Hazard function The instantaneous failure rate, conditional failure, intensity, or force of mortality function, where the function that describes the probability of failure during a very small time increment (assuming that no failures have occurred prior to that time). Hazard is the slope of the survival curve.

Hazard rate It is a time-to-failure function used in survival analysis.

Heteroscedastic data Data that have nonconstant (heterogeneous) variance across the predicted values of y.

Hierarchical model In linear modeling, models which always include all the lower-order interactions and main effects corresponding to any interaction they include.

Histogram A histogram is a way of graphically showing the characteristics of the distribution of items in a given population or sample.

Homoscedasticity (homogeneity of variance) Normal theory based tests for the equality of population means such as the t-test and analysis of variance assume that the data come from populations that have the same variance, even if the test rejects the null hypothesis of equality of population means.

Hypothesis (statistical) A statistical hypothesis is an assertion or conjecture about the distribution of one or more random variables.

Independent and dependent variables Statistical models normally specify how one set of variables, called dependent variables, functionally depend on another set of variables, called independent variables. The functional relationship does not necessarily reflect a causal relationship,i.e., the independent variables do not necessarily describe the cause.

Incidence The number of newly diagnosed cases during a specific time.

Inferential statistics Making inferences about the population from which a sample has been drawn and analyzed.

Interaction If the effect of one factor depends on the level of another factor, the two factors involved are said to interact, and a contrast involving all these levels is called their interaction.

Intercept In linear regression, the intercept is the mean value of the response variable when the explanatory variable takes the value of zero (the value of y when $x = 0$).

Interpolation Making deductions from a model for values that lie between data points.

Interquartile range (IQR or dQ) IQR is a measure of spread and is the counterpart of the standard deviation for skewed distributions. IQR is the distance between the upper and lower quartiles (Q_U-Q_L).

Kurtosis Kurtosis characterizes the shape of a distribution.

Level of significance Whether observed results are consistent with chance variation under the null hypothesis, or, alternatively, whether they are so different that chance variability can be ruled out as an explanation for the observed sample.

Life tables They summarize lifetime data or, generally speaking, time-to-event data.

Life table analysis Identifies and quantifies the time course of certain risks.

Likelihood The probability of a set of observations given the value of some parameter or set of parameters.

Linear expression A polynomial expression with the degree of polynomial being 1.

Log transformation This transformation pulls smaller data values apart and brings the larger data values together and closer to the smaller data values (shrinkage effect). It is mostly used to shrink highly positively skewed data.

Main effect The effect of a factor on a dependent variable.

Mean (or average) A measure of location for a batch of data values; the sum of all data values divided by the number of elements in the distribution.

Measures of central tendency These are parameters that characterize an entire distribution. These include mode, median, and mean

Median The value that divides the frequency distribution in half when all data values are listed in order.

Metaanalysis A systematic approach yielding an overall answer by analyzing a set of studies that address a related question. Metaanalysis provides a weighted average of the measure of effect (such as odds ratio).

Mode It is a value that occurs with the greatest frequency in a population or a sample.

Model selection The selection of a statistical model from a group of possible models.

Monotonic A function or quantity varying in such a way that it never decreases or never increases.

Multidimensional scaling A set of techniques used for quantitatively analyzing similarities, dissimilarities, and distances between data in a display-like manner.

Multivariate Multivariate analysis involves more than one variable of interest.

Mutually inclusive Any two events in which one cannot happen without the other.

Mutually exhaustive Two events that cannot occur at the same time.

Negative predictive value Probability of a true negative as in a person identified healthy by a test is really free from the disease.

Nested model Models that are related where one model is an extension of the other.

Nominal variable A qualitative variable defined by mutually exclusive unordered categories.

Nonlinear curves These include exponential growth, exponential, asymptotic regression, and logistic growth curve.

Nonmetric scaling Is a set of methods for displaying and relating data when measurements are nonquantitative (i.e., either categorical [nominal] or ordinal)?

Nonparametric methods Statistical methods to analyze data from populations, which do not assume a particular population distribution.

Normal distribution (Gaussian distribution) is a model for values on a continuous scale.

Normality It is the property of a random variable that is distributed according to the normal distribution.

Null hypothesis The null hypothesis is a term that statisticians often use to indicate the statistical hypothesis tested—no effect. The purpose of most statistical tests is to determine if the obtained results provide a reason to reject the hypothesis that they are merely a product of chance factors.

Odds ratio (OR) Also known as relative odds and approximate relative risk. It is the ratio of the odds of the risk factor in a diseased group and in a nondiseased (control) group. The interpretation of the OR is that the risk factor increases the odds of the disease "OR" times.

Ordinal variable An ordered (ranked) qualitative/categorical variable.

Ordinate Y—axis

Outlier An extreme observation that is well separated from the remainder of the data.

P-value The P-value is the probability that the null model could, by random chance variation, produce a sample as extreme as the observed sample.

Parameter A numerical characteristic of a population specifying a distribution model.

Permutation A selection of objects in which the order of the objects matter.

Population It is the entire collection of items that is the focus of concern.

Positive predictive value Probability of a true positive as in a person identified as diseased by a test is really diseased.

Post hoc tests Post hoc tests (or post hoc comparison tests) are used at the second stage of the analysis of variance (ANOVA) or multiple analyses of variance (MANOVA) if the null hypothesis is rejected.

Power The power of a test is the probability that the test will reject the hypothesis tested when a specific alternative hypothesis is true.

Precision Precision is the degree of accuracy that an estimator estimates a parameter.

Prevalence The number of cases seen on a specific date.

Principal components analysis A dimension reduction technique that produces an ordered set of orthogonal variables with the first principal component explaining the most variance in the data.

Probability The ratio of the number of likely outcomes to the number of possible outcomes.

Qualitative Qualitative (categorical) variables define different categories or classes of an attribute. A qualitative (categorical) variable may be nominal or ordinal.

Quantitative Quantitative variables are variables for which a numeric value representing an amount is measured.

Quantal Dichotomous data—yes or no.

Quartile The 1st, 2nd, and 3d quartiles are the 25th, 50th, and 75th percentiles, respectively.

Random sampling A method of selecting a sample from a target population or study base using simple or systematic random methods.

Random error The random error is the fluctuating part of the overall error that varies from measurement to measurement.

Randomized (complete) block design An experimental design in which the treatments in each block are assigned to the experimental units in random order.

Range The difference between the highest and lowest values.

Ratio scale A ratio scale is a measurement scale in which a certain distance along the scale means the same thing no matter where on the scale you are, and where 0 on the scale represents the absence of the thing being measured. Thus, a 4 on such a scale implies twice as much of the thing being measured as a 2.

Reliability Reliability characterizes the capability of a device, unit, and procedure to perform without fault. Reliability is quantified in terms of probability. This probability is related either to an elementary act or to an interval of time or another continuous variable. Because the probability of failure is normally a small fraction, the reverse ratio rounded to integers is usually used.

Repeatability Repeatability is the variation of outcomes of an experiment carried out in the same conditions, e.g., by the same operator, in the same laboratory.

Reproducibility Reproducibility is the variation of outcomes of an experiment carried out in conditions varying within a typical range, e.g., when measurement is carried out by the same device by different operators, in different laboratories, etc.

Residuals Residuals reflect the overall badness of fit of the model. They are the differences between the observed values of the outcome variable and the corresponding fitted values predicted by the regression line (the vertical distance between the observed values and the fitted line).

Robustness VA statistical test or procedure is robust when violation of assumptions has little effect on the results.

Sample A subset of data from a population.

Sampling error The degree to which the results from the sample deviate from those that would be obtained from the entire population, because of random error in the selection of respondent and the corresponding reduction in reliability.

Scales of measurement The type of data is always one of the following four scales of measurement: Nominal, ordinal, interval, or ratio. Each of these can be discrete or continuous.

Sensitivity Sensitivity is the proportion of true positives that are correctly identified by a diagnostic test.

Significance level The significance level of a statistical hypothesis test is a fixed probability of wrongly rejecting the null hypothesis H_0, if it is in fact true.

Skewness The degree of (lack of) asymmetry about a central value of a distribution.

Specificity Specificity is the proportion of true negatives that are correctly identified by the test.

Standard deviation It is a measure of spread (scatter) of a set of data.

Standard error The standard error (SE) or as commonly called the standard error of the mean (SEM) is a measure of the extent to which the sample mean deviates from the true but unknown population mean.

Statistic Is a quantity that is calculated from a sample of data.

Statistical significance A finding is described as statistically significant when it can be demonstrated that the probability of obtaining such a difference by chance only is relatively low (5%).

Stochastic model A probability model that includes chance events in the form of random measurement error or uncertainty.

Symmetric distribution Distributions that have the same shape on both sides of the center are called symmetric.

Systematic error Systematic error is the error that is constant in a series of repetitions of the same experiment or observation. Usually, systematic error is defined as the expected value of the overall error.

Technical replicate A repeated measurement on the same unit.

Transformation Transformation is the conversion of a data set into a transformed data set by the application of a function. The statistical purpose of transformation is to produce a transformed data set that better conforms to the requirements of a statistical procedure. A typical use of transformation is to take the log of each value; this reduces the long right tail in a skewed distribution and produces a more normally shaped distribution.

Transformations (ladder of powers) Transformation deals with non-normality of the data points and nonhomogeneous variance. All power transformations are monotonic when applied to positive data (they are either increasing or decreasing, but not first increasing and then decreasing, or vice versa).

Treatment A treatment is what is administered to experimental units (explanatory variables).

Trends of time The change in rate over time expressed as an annual percent change.

Trend test for counts and proportions A special application of the Chi-squared test (with a different formula).

Type I error If the null hypothesis is true but we reject it this is an error of first kind or type I error (also called α error). This results in a false-positive finding.

Type II error If the null hypothesis is accepted when it is in fact wrong, this is an error of the second kind or Type II error (also called β error). This results in a false-negative result.

Uncertainty Quantification or measure uncertainty via inferential statistics. Classical statistics measures uncertainty using fundamental concepts and theories of probability and randomness.

Univariate Univariate analysis involves a single variable of interest.

Validity Validity characterizes the extent to which a measurement procedure is capable of measuring what it is supposed to measure.

Variable Some characteristic that varies among experimental units (subjects) or from time to time.

Variance The major measure of variability for a data set.

Variance inflation Outliers usually cause this.

REFERENCES

Akaike H: A new look at the statistical model identification, *IEEE Trans Automat Contr* 19:716–723, 1974.

American Statistical Association: *Ethical guidelines for statistical practice*, 2018. http://www.amstat.org/ASA/About/Ethical-Guidelines-for-Statistical-Practice.aspx. (Accessed 30 May 2020).

Beyer WH: *Handbook of tables for probability and statistics*, Florida, Boca Raton, 1982, CRC Press.

Bloomfield P: *Fourier analysis of time series: an introduction*, New Jersey, Hoboken, 2000, John Wiley & Sons Inc.

Box GEP, Tiao GC: *Bayesian inference in statistical analysis*, ed 3, New York, 1992, Wiley Classic Library Edition.

Burkhardt JE, Ennulat D, Pandher K, et al.: Topic of histopathology blinding in nonclinical safety biomarker qualification studies, *Toxicol Pathol* 38:666–667, 2010.

Chambers JM, Cleveland WS, Kleiner B, et al.: *Graphical methods for data analysis*, ed 3, Florida, Boca Raton, 2018, CRC Press.

Cleveland WS: *The elements of graphing data*, New Jersey, Summit, 1994, Hobart Press.

Clewell RA, Thompson CM, Clewell III HJ: Dose-dependence of chemical carcinogenicity: biological mechanisms for thresholds and implications for risk assessment, *Chem Biol Interact* 301:112–127, 2019.

Cochran WG, Cox GM: *Experimental designs*, ed 2, New York, 1992, Wiley Classics Library Edition.

Crissman JW, Goodman DG, Hildebrandt PK, et al.: Best practices guideline: toxicologic histopathology, *Toxicol Pathol* 32:126–131, 2004.

Dunnett CW: A multiple comparison procedure for comparing several treatments with a control, *J Am Stat Assoc* 50:1096–1121, 1955.

Elmore SA, Peddada SD: Points to consider on the statistical analysis of rodent cancer bioassay data when incorporating historical control data, *Toxicol Pathol* 37:672–676, 2009.

Everitt B, Landau E, Lease M, et al.: *Cluster analysis*, ed 5, New York, 2011, John Wiley and Sons.

Finney DJ, Latscha R, Bennet BM, et al.: *Tables for testing significance in a 2 x 2 contingency table*, New York, 1963, Cambridge University Press.

Finney DK: *Probit analysis*, ed 3, United Kingdom, Cambridge, 1971, Cambridge University Press.

Gad SC, Taulbee SM: *Handbook of data recording, maintenance and management for the biomedical sciences*, Florida, Boca Raton, 1996, CRC Press.

Gad SC: *Animal models in toxicology*, ed 3, Florida, Boca Raton, 2016, Taylor & Francis/CRC Press.

Gad SC: *Statistics and experimental design for toxicologists*, ed 4, Florida, Boca Raton, 2019, CRC Press.

Gad SC: Statistics and experimental design for toxicologists. In Hayes W, editor: *Principles and methods of toxicology*, ed 6, Florida, Boca Raton, 2014, CRC Press.

Garrett HE: *Statistics in psychology and education*, ed 6, California, Santa Barbara, 1982, Greenwood Press.

Gelman A, Carlin BJ, Stern SH, et al.: *Texts in statistical science Bayesian data analysis*, ed 2, Florida, Boca Raton, 2004, Chapman and Hall/CRC Press.

Harris J: *A primer of multivariate statistics*, ed 3, New Jersey, Mahwah, 2001, Laurence Erlbaum Associates, Inc.

Hoaglin DC, Mosteller F, Tukey JW: *Understanding robust and exploratory data analysis*, New York, 2000, Wiley Classics Library Edition.

Hollander M, Wolfe DA, Chicken E: *Nonparametric statistical methods*, ed 3, New York, 2013, John Wiley.

International Conference on harmonisation of technical requirements for registration of pharmaceuticals for human use: ICH harmonised tripartite guideline dose selection for carcinogenicity studies of pharmaceuticals S1C(R2), 2008https:// database.ich.org/sites/default/files/S1C%28R2%29% 20Guideline.pdf. (Accessed 4 September 2020).

Keenan C, Elmore S, Francke-Carroll S, et al.: Best practices for use of historical control data of proliferative rodent lesions, *Toxicol Pathol* 37:679–693, 2009.

Koehler K: *Snedecor and Cochran's statistical methods*, ed 9, New York, 2012, John Wiley & Sons Inc.

Kotz S, Read CB, Balakrishnan N, et al.: *Encyclopedia of statistical sciences*, ed 2, New Jersey, 2006, Wiley-Interscience.

Kraemer HC, Thiemann G: *How many subjects? Statistical power analysis in research*, California, Newbury Park, 1987, Sage Publications.

Lee ET: *Statistical methods for survival data analysis*, ed 3, New York, 2003, John Wiley & Sons Inc.

Lin KK, Rahman MA: Expanded statistical decision rules for interpretations of results of rodent carcinogenicity studies of pharmaceuticals. In Peace K, Chen DG, Menon S, editors: *Biopharmaceutical applied statistics symposium. ICSA book series in statistics*, Singapore, 2018, Springer.

Marriott FHC: *A dictionary of statistical terms*, United Kingdom, Essex, 1990, Longman Scientific & Technical.

Montgomery DC, Peck EA, Vining GG: *Introduction to linear regression analysis*, ed 5, New York, 2012, John Wiley & Sons Inc.

Morton LD, Sanders M, Reagan, et al.: Confounding factors in the interpretation of preclinical studies, *Int J Toxicol* 38:228–234, 2019.

Neef N, Nikula KJ, Francke-Carroll S, et al.: Regulatory forum opinion piece: blind reading of histopathology slides in general toxicology studies, *Toxicol Pathol* 40:697–699, 2012.

OECD draft guidance document no 116 on the design and conduct of chronic toxicity and carcinogenicity studies, supporting TG 451, 452, 453, 2010. Accessed online August 1, 2020: http:// www.oecd.org/chemicalsafety/testing/46766792.pdf.

Peto R, Gray R, Brantom P, et al.: Effects on 4080 rats of chronic ingestion of N-nitrosodiethylamine or N-nitroso-dimethylamine: a detailed dose–response study, *Cancer Res* 51:6415–6451, 1991.

Peto R, Pike M, Day N, et al.: *Guidelines for simple, sensitive significance tests for carcinogenic effects in long-term animal experiments, IARC monographs on the evaluation of the carcinogenic risk of chemicals to humans, supplement 2, long-term and short-term screening assays for carcinogens: a critical appraisal*, France, Lyon, 1980, International Agency for Research in Cancer.

Scheffe H: *The analysis of variance*, New York, 1999, John Wiley & Sons Inc.

Schmid CF: *Statistical graphics: design principle and practices*, New York, 1983, John Wiley & Sons Inc.

Schwarz GE: Estimating the dimension of a model, *Ann Stat* 6(2):461–464, 1978.

Sellers RS, Morton D, Michael B, et al.: Society of Toxicologic Pathology position paper: organ weight recommendations for toxicology studies, *Toxicol Pathol* 35:751–755, 2007.

Shockley KR, Kissling GE: Statistical guidance for reviewers of toxicologic pathology, *Toxicol Pathol* 44:647–652, 2018.

Siegel S, Castellan NJ: *Nonparametric statistics for the behavioral sciences*, ed 2, New York, 1988, McGraw-Hill.

Society of Toxicologic Pathologists: Society of Toxicologic Pathologists' position paper on blinded slide reading, *Toxicol Pathol* 14:493–494, 1986.

Society of Toxicologic Pathologists: The Society of Toxicologic Pathology's recommendations on statistical analysis of rodent carcinogenicity studies, *Toxicol Pathol* 30:415–418, 2007.

Society of Toxicology ED01 Task Force: Reexamination of the ED01 study-adjusting for time on study, *Fund Appl Toxicol* 1:8–123, 1981.

Sokal RR, Rohlf FJ: *Biometry: the principles and practice of statistics in biological research*, ed 4, California, San Francisco, 2011, W.H. Freeman.

Tarone RE: Tests for trend in life table analysis, *Biometrika* 62: 679–682, 1975.

Troth SP, Everds NE, Siska W, Knight B, Lamb M, Hutt J: Scientific and Regulatory Policy Committee points to consider: data visualization for clinical and anatomic pathologists, *Toxicol Pathol* 46:476–487, 2018.

Tufte ER: *Visual explanations: images and quantiles, evidence and narrative*, ed 7, Connecticut, Cheshire, 2005, Graphics Press.

Tukey JW: *Exploratory data analysis*, Massachusetts, Boston, 2019, Pearson Modern Classics.

Weissgerber TL, Milic NM, Winham SJ, et al.: Beyond bar and line graphs: time for a new data presentation paradigm, *PLoS Biol* 13:e1002128, 2015.

Wong AHC, Gottesman II, Petronis A: Phenotypic differences in genetically identical organisms: the epigenetic perspective, *Hum Mol Genet* Volume 14(suppl_1):R11–R18, 2005. https://doi.org/10.1093/hmg/ddi116.

Zar JH: *Biostatistical analysis*, ed 5, New Jersey, Englewood Cliffs, 2015, Pearson Education, Limited.

PART 3

ANIMAL AND ALTERNATIVE MODELS IN TOXICOLOGIC RESEARCH

CHAPTER

17

Animal Models in Toxicologic Research: Rodents

Peter J.M. Clements[1], Brad Bolon[2], Elizabeth McInnes[3], Sydney Mukaratirwa[4], Cheryl Scudamore[5]

[1]GlaxoSmithKline Research and Development, Ware, Hertfordshire, United Kingdom, [2]GEMpath, Inc., Longmont, CO, United States, [3]Syngenta, Bracknell, United Kingdom, [4]Boehringer Ingelheim Pharma GmbH, Biberach, Germany, [5]ExePathology, Exmouth, United Kingdom

OUTLINE

1. Introduction 653

2. Rodent Model Selection 655
   2.1. Overview of Species Selection for Toxicity Studies 655
   2.2. Rodent Species Used for Special Studies 659
   2.3. Rodent Models of Disease and Genetically Modified Animals 660

3. Issues in Extrapolation of Rodent Data for Human Risk Assessment 661
   3.1. Pharmacologic Translational Relevance and Interspecies Pathophysiologic Concordance 662
   3.2. Biological and Cell Therapies 665
   3.3. Controlling Variability and Impact of the Microbiome in Rodent Studies 665

4. Basic Biological Characteristics of Common Rodent Stocks and Strains 667

   4.1. Outbred Stocks and Inbred Strains of Mice and Rats 667
   4.2. Anatomy and Physiology of Rodents Used in Toxicologic Research 670

5. Common Pathologic Findings in Rodents 675
   5.1. Background Findings in Common Species—Mice and Rats 675
   5.2. Background Findings in Uncommon Rodent Species 680
   5.3. Considerations in Evaluating Incidental Background Findings 682

6. Conclusion 688

References 689

1. INTRODUCTION

Laboratory rodents—especially the mouse (primarily *Mus musculus*), rat (*Rattus norvegicus*), hamster (particularly the Syrian [or golden] variant, *Mesocricetus auratus*), Hartley guinea pig (*Cavia porcellus*), and Mongolian gerbil (*Meriones unguiculatus*)—are the most frequently used animal models in biomedical research. In toxicology, rodents (mainly rats and mice) are the first species to be considered for in vivo toxicity and combined efficacy/toxicity studies. Other rodent species, including chinchillas (*Chinchilla lanigera*) and many additional mouse and rat species, are also used for special kinds of biomedical studies, but at much lower frequency—and typically not in toxicological research. This chapter will consider rodents as models for toxicologic research, and thus will emphasize those species (mice, rats, hamsters, guinea pigs, and gerbils) that are utilized most commonly for this purpose.

Rodents are preferred species for biomedical and toxicological research, for economic (minor husbandry/space requirements, cost of animal and housing) but also scientific reasons.

(i) Their basic biological characteristics (e.g., small size, lifespan, short gestation period, large litter size) support study designs with larger group sizes than are possible with nonrodent species. Details on these attributes are beyond the scope of this chapter but may be obtained from many resources dedicated to biomedical applications of mice (Fox et al., 2007a, b, c, d; Hedrich, 2012); rats (Maynard and Downes, 2019; Suckow et al., 2020); hamsters (Suckow et al., 2012); guinea pigs (Suckow et al., 2012); and other laboratory rodents (e.g., chinchillas, gerbils) (Suckow et al., 2012).

(ii) A multitude of rodent outbred stocks and inbred strains have been generated, especially for mice and rats. Stocks are maintained by crossbreeding of males and females with different genetic backgrounds, thus maximizing genetic heterozygosity (making them more similar to the typical human population) and individual longevity. These features make stocks (e.g., CD-1 mice, Sprague–Dawley (SD) and Wistar Han rats) a common choice for toxicity studies. In contrast, strains are genetically identical (homozygous) at essentially all (>99%) alleles and typically less hardy; nonetheless, strains (especially mice) may be used for toxicity testing since they may be more sensitive to toxicants than stocks. Profiles of xenobiotic absorption, distribution, metabolism, and excretion (ADME), even in the outbred stocks commonly used in toxicology, make them suitable for a wide range of investigations, from acute to chronic toxicity studies as well

as abbreviated (6 month) and life-time (up to 2 year) carcinogenicity bioassays. Species- and modality-specific differences in ADME can significantly alter systemic and target tissue exposure, thereby impacting manifestations of toxicity that influence hazard identification and characterization as well as risk assessment. The expression and substrate specificity of small molecule-metabolizing enzymes differs among species (Kisui et al., 2020; Nelson et al., 2004), and for rodents may vary between males and females (Kisui et al., 2020) (see *Biochemical and Molecular Basis of Toxicity*, Vol 1, Chap 2). For example, rodents clear small-molecule test articles subject to oxidation significantly faster than do nonrodents (including humans) because cytochrome P450-dependent mixed function oxidase activity is inversely proportional to body weight; small molecules metabolized by other metabolic pathways typically do not show the same size-dependent rate variation. Similarly, species differences in the responsiveness of cytochrome P450s to xenobiotics that act as inducers or inhibitors of these enzymes may give rise to quantitative differences in exposure and potential drug interaction effects (McKillop et al., 1998). Species variability in small-molecule ADME is often explored in vitro by comparing hepatic microsomal preparations from mice and/or rats to one or more nonrodent species, including humans (see *ADME Principles in Small Molecule Drug Discovery and Development—An Industrial Perspective*, Vol 1, Chap 3). In contrast, ADME of humanized (i.e., part human and part animal) and fully human biomolecules usually exhibits significant differences in immunocompetent rodents relative to humans, especially after repeated exposure, due to the robust immune response against foreign protein or nucleic acid (see *Biotherapeutic ADME and PK/PD Principles*, Vol 1, Chap 4).

(iii) Rodent models often exhibit well-characterized phenotypes and pathophysiological alterations that can provide insights regarding disease progression and molecular mechanisms of relevance to human patients with similar diseases (Conn, 2013). Often, the model phenotypes in short-lived rodents occur quite quickly, which can increase the rate at which novel test articles may be screened for efficacy. Finally, genetic manipulation to introduce (transgenic), remove ("knock out"), or replace ("knock in") key molecules performing critical functions also allows insight into pathobiology associated with altered expression of proteins in an in vivo context, with applications ranging from target validation, humanizing targets or pathways (by substituting human genes for their mouse homologs), generating monogenic and polygenic disease models, and investigating on-target (desired or exaggerated pharmacology) and off-target ("toxic") effects (*Genetically Engineered Animal Models in Toxicologic Research*, Vol 1, Chap 23). Rodent models of disease (RMD) are essential tools for increasing our basic pathobiological knowledge, in generating efficacy-related data for new medicines, and in providing focused safety-relevant information early in product discovery and development, prior to standard toxicity studies.

Pathologic evaluation in toxicologic research is supported by extensive background data for many rodent stocks and strains. Knowledge of historical control data often informs the study pathologist's decision regarding where to set the diagnostic threshold for rodent toxicity studies. Fortunately, normal biological variation as well as spontaneous, husbandry-related, infectious, and toxicant-induced changes have been extensively characterized in mice and rats for many anatomic pathology (Barthold et al., 2016; Gopinath and Mowat, 2014; Harkness et al., 2010; Maronpot, 1999; McInnes, 2012; Mohr et al., 1992; Mohr et al., 1996; Sahota et al., 2019; Suttie, Leininger, & Bradley, 2018) and clinical pathology (Kurtz and Travlos, 2018; Weiss and Wardrop, 2010) endpoints. Knowledge of such variation is essential in distinguishing the spectra of incidental (background) versus confounding (husbandry,

experimental procedure, or infectious) versus test article–related (toxic) pathology that may be expected in a given rodent model. Knowledge regarding the "normal" (or "within normal limits") range of tissue- and fluid-based alterations may guide selection of the most suitable stock or strain for routine rodent toxicity studies and support the interpretation of pathologic findings as adverse and/or significant.

2. RODENT MODEL SELECTION

2.1. Overview of Species Selection for Toxicity Studies

Rodent species are an integral part of safety evaluation in toxicology programs to support product development and licensing. Rodent use for this purpose is detailed by various regulatory guidelines for biomolecule and small molecule therapeutics (FDA; ICH), medical devices (ISO), and agricultural and industrial chemicals (EFSA, multiple; U.S. Environmental Protection Agency, multiple). For safety assessment of small molecule and other xenobiotic therapies, additional data from nonclinical toxicity studies in nonrodent mammalian species are usually recommended for both oncology (ICH) and non-oncology (ICH) indications, but there are circumstances in which nonclinical data from a single pharmacologically relevant rodent species alone may be acceptable (e.g., for genotoxic drugs targeting rapidly dividing cells (ICH)). Pharmacologic relevance of the test species is required for regulatory toxicity studies conducted with biotechnology-derived pharmaceuticals like nucleic acids and proteins (ICH) since toxicity is generally driven by exaggerated pharmacology and/or immunogenicity to the foreign (humanized or fully human) biomolecule (Baldrick, 2017; Brennan et al., 2018). Rodents should be evaluated and a rationale for their use considered if they are selected as a species for nonclinical testing of human-origin biotherapeutic products. Regulatory guidance on rodent/nonrodent species selection is summarized in Table 17.1.

Different types of rodent toxicity studies are summarized in Table 17.2. General toxicity studies in rodents for both therapeutic xenobiotics as well as agricultural and industrial chemicals are conducted in healthy, wild-type adult animals that are housed in autoclaved containers equipped with autoclaved bedding, free access to food and water, and often with environmental enrichment materials (e.g., exercise devices, nesting materials) designed to minimize stress. The test article is given according to the route by which humans might be exposed (commonly the oral, inhalational, or intravenous routes for therapeutic agents or the oral route for agrochemicals). Study designs of increasing duration are intended to identify the maximum tolerated dose, with intermediate ("mid") and low doses to examine

TABLE 17.1   Selected Recommendations for Species Selection for Toxicity Studies

Guidance	Context for toxicity assessment	Species recommended
EMA CPMP/SWP/ 1042/99[a]	Repeat dose toxicity	Rodent; nonrodent
ICH M3 (R2)	Repeat dose toxicity (14d to 9m). Two mammalian species recommended	Rodent; nonrodent
ICH S1	Carcinogenicity	Rodent
ICH S4B	Chronic toxicity testing	Rodent (6m); nonrodent (9m)
ICH S5 (R3)	Reproduction and developmental toxicity	Rodent (rat); nonrodent (rabbit)
ICH S6 (R1)	Requirement for pharmacological relevance	Rodent; nonrodent
	Exceptions: where a single species suffices - only one relevant species - short-term toxicity findings the same in rodent and nonrodent species - Antibody to foreign, exogenous targets	Rodent considered first
	Antibody–drug conjugate (ADC): study with unconjugated toxin	Rodent preferred
ICH S9	Small molecule anticancer pharmaceuticals	Rodent; nonrodent
	Genotoxic drugs targeting rapidly dividing cells	Rodent if pharmacologically relevant
	ADCs. Payload (toxin) ± linker	
	Target not present in nonclinical species	Single species: rodent preferred
ICH S11	Small molecule pediatric pharmaceuticals	Single species, rodent preferred
FDA[b]	Short term	Rodent; nonrodent
	Subchronic	Rodent; nonrodent
	Chronic	Rodent; nonrodent
	Carcinogenicity	Rodent
	Combined chronic toxicity/carcinogenicity	Rodent
	Reproduction and developmental toxicity	Rodent (rat); nonrodent (rabbit)
	Neurotoxicity	Rodent

(Continued)

TABLE 17.1   Selected Recommendations for Species Selection for Toxicity Studies—cont'd

Guidance	Context for toxicity assessment	Species recommended
EPA Test Guidelines Pesticides and Toxic Substances: Series 870 Health Effects Test Guidelines[c]	Acute toxicity: Oral Dermal Inhalation Ocular and dermal irritation[d] Skin sensitization	Rodent (rat preferred) Rodent; nonrodent (rabbit preferred) Rodent (rat preferred) Nonrodent (if justified). Nonrodent (rabbit preferred) Rodent (mouse; guinea pig)
	Subchronic toxicity (28d; 90d)	Rodent; nonrodent (oral) Rodent (inhalation; nonrodent if justified) Rodent; nonrodent (dermal; rabbit preferred)
	Chronic toxicity	Rodent; nonrodent
	Carcinogenicity	Rodent
	Neurotoxicity	Rodent (rat preferred); nonrodent (if justified)
OECD Guidelines for the Testing of Chemicals, Section 4; Health Effects[e]	Acute toxicity: Oral; Inhalation Ocular and dermal irritation[d] Skin sensitization	Rodent (rat preferred) Nonrodent (rabbit preferred) Rodent (mouse)
	Subacute toxicity (28d)	Rodent (inhalation; rat preferred) Rodent; nonrodent (rabbit; dermal)
	Subchronic toxicity (90d)	Rodent (rat preferred); nonrodent (inhalation, oral)
	Chronic toxicity	Rodent; nonrodent
	Carcinogenicity	Rodent (nonrodent if justified)
	Neurotoxicity	Rodent (rat preferred); nonrodent (if justified)

Abbreviations: *EMA*, european medicines agency; *EPA*, U.S. environmental protection agency; *FDA*, U.S. food and drug administration; *ICH*, international council for harmonisation of technical requirements for pharmaceuticals for human use; *OECD*, organisation for economic co-operation and development.

[a] *EMA guidance refers to ICH guidelines. https://www.ema.europa.eu/en/human-regulatory/research-development/scientific-guidelines/non-clinical/non-clinical-toxicology#carcinogenicity-section. Accessed 25 April 2021.*

[b] *FDA guidance: https://www.fda.gov/regulatory-information/search-fda-guidance-documents/guidance-industry-and-other-stakeholders-redbook-2000#TOC. Accessed 25 April 2021.*

[c] *EPA guidance: https://www.epa.gov/test-guidelines-pesticides-and-toxic-substances/series-870-health-effects-test-guidelines. Accessed 25 April 2021.*

[d] *In these studies, pathological evaluation is not routinely conducted.*

[e] *OECD guidance: https://www.oecd-ilibrary.org/environment/oecd-guidelines-for-the-testing-of-chemicals-section-4-health-effects_20745788. Accessed 25 April 2021.*

dose/exposure responsiveness and establish threshold (e.g., effect and no effect) levels that can be related to estimated efficacious and/or toxic doses.

For rodent carcinogenicity testing, there are now several options. Historically, test articles were evaluated in life-time bioassays in both mice (80 weeks) and rats (104 weeks), and less

TABLE 17.2   Study Design Considerations for Rodent General Toxicity Studies

Study type; duration	Rodent species	Maximum clinical study duration supported	Typical study design[a]: n/sex/group	Pathology evaluation[b]
Dose range finding/maximum tolerated dose; 3–14 days	Rat, mouse	N/A	n = 4 Males ± Females	Evaluation restricted to key organs/tissues[c]
FTIH enabling; 14–28 days	Rat, mouse	2–4 weeks	n = 10 Males; Females	Comprehensive tissue list
Subchronic toxicity; 3 months	Rat, mouse	3 months	n = 12 Males; Females	Comprehensive tissue list
Chronic toxicity; 6 months (12 months)	Rat	6 months	n = 12 (20)[d] Males; Females	Comprehensive tissue list
Carcinogenicity; 6 months (abbreviated)[e]	Genetically altered mouse (Tg-rasH2, p53$^{+/-}$, others[f])	6 months	n = 25 Males; Females	Comprehensive tissue list
Carcinogenicity; 2-year study (life span)	Rat, mouse	N/A	n = 60 (>50) Males; Females	Comprehensive tissue list

Abbreviations: N/A, not applicable; FTIH, first time in human.

[a] Usually four groups/sex: Control (vehicle control); High dose = Maximum Tolerated Dose (MTD) from the previous study/maximum feasible dose/≥50-fold margin to estimated clinical dose; Low Dose = No Observed Effect Level (NOEL) from previous study or low multiple of estimated clinical dose; Mid Dose = generally geometric mean of the low and high doses. Numbers of animals/sex/group refer to main study groups to be terminated at the end of the specified study duration. Additional interim necropsy groups are optional. Additional animals (e.g., six per sex/group) may be added to groups (usually control and high dose) to evaluate findings following an off-dose recovery period. This is usually done for 3- or 6-month toxicity studies.

[b] Includes consideration of in-life findings, organ weights, macroscopic observations, and microscopic findings, with reference to clinical pathology endpoints (hematology and clinical chemistry). Note that clinical pathology data are not routinely generated on carcinogenicity studies. Statistical analyses on anatomic pathology data typically are restricted to carcinogenicity studies.

[c] Tissue list to include major organs (e.g., liver, heart, lungs, adrenals, thymus, stomach, intestines, eyes, gonads) plus any specific tissues indicated by prior information.

[d] Number in parenthesis refers to 12-month toxicity study (e.g., for evaluation of chemicals).

[e] Note that dose range finding studies (e.g., 7d, 28d duration) would be conducted in genetically altered strains prior to embarking on a 6-month study.

[f] Other alternative mouse carcinogenicity studies may be used (see Jacobs and Brown, 2015).

frequently in hamsters (104 weeks). These tests are characterized by large group sizes (usually 50 per sex per dose) to ensure sufficient survival for valid statistical analysis. High rates of spontaneous tumors occur in such studies for some rodent strains (Maronpot, 1999; Suttie, Leininger, & Bradley, 2018); the kinds of tumors, their frequencies, and the target organs vary by the species and among strains, but significant amounts of historical control data are available to aid data interpretation. In contrast to the traditional use of life-time mouse and rat carcinogenicity studies, assessment of carcinogenicity now often involves abbreviated (26-week) bioassays using genetically engineered mice (GEM) with intrinsic sensitivity to potential carcinogens. The two mouse strains most commonly used for this purpose are the $p53^{+/-}$ (formal strain designation: B6;129S7-$Trp53^{tm1Brd}$ N5) and Tg-rasH2 (formal strain designation: CByB6F1-Tg(HRAS)2Jic) models (*Genetically Engineered Animal Models in Toxicologic Research*, Vol 1, Chap 23 and *Carcinogenesis: Mechanisms and Evaluation*, Vol 1, Chap 8). The $p53^{+/-}$ mouse model (in which cells lack one copy of the $p53$ tumor suppressor gene [involved in DNA repair]) is carried on a mainly C57BL/6 background and is generally used to detect genotoxic agents (Storer et al., 2001). The Tg-rasH2 mouse model (which carries the c-Ha-ras oncogene plus its promotor/enhancer on a mixed BALB/c and C57BL/6 F_1 background) is widely used to identify both nongenotoxic or genotoxic agents (Bogdanffy et al., 2020; Cohen et al., 2001; Jacobs and Brown, 2015). The key advantages of GEM models for carcinogenicity testing are that they require substantially less time for the in-life phase and the rate of spontaneous background tumors therefore is very low. While these features make interpretation of the final pathology data set easier, less historical control data are available for GEM models of carcinogenicity.

Other genetically engineered rodent models are employed on occasion for toxicity testing. These systems are used for materials with particular properties (e.g., the Tg.Ac mouse is sensitive to nongenotoxic materials applied to the skin (Sistare et al., 2002)) or to investigate potential mechanisms of cell damage (e.g., *Xpa* and *Xpa/p53$^{+/-}$* mice, which have deficient DNA repair

capabilities and so are more sensitive to genotoxic chemicals (van Kreijl et al., 2001)). Engineered rodents also are growing in popularity as translational models for in vivo biomedical and toxicological research since substitution of mouse elements by insertion of human genes ("knock in") or engraftment of human tissues permits evaluation of human cells and pathways when challenged by xenobiotic exposures (Cheung and Gonzalez, 2008; Katoh et al., 2008; Shen et al., 2011; Strom et al., 2010).

2.2. Rodent Species Used for Special Studies

In addition to general toxicity studies, a number of specialized studies are performed using rodents to address particular research questions. Key studies in this regard include various developmental bioassays—mainly developmental and reproductive toxicity, developmental neurotoxicity (EPA; OECD), juvenile toxicity (ICH), and extended one-generation reproductive toxicity (OECD) studies (also see *The Role of Pathology in Evaluation of Reproductive, Developmental, and Juvenile Toxicity*, Vol 1, Chap 7)—and target organ/systemic toxicity studies (especially immunotoxicity and neurotoxicity) that require integrated functional and structural assessments. Large treatment groups are necessary in such bioassays because functional and structural testing for a given dose may need to be performed in different cohorts to avoid any impact of functional testing (i.e., environmental enrichment) on the anatomic differentiation of the organ mediating that function. For this reason, rodents (and rabbits, which are not rodents but lagomorphs, see *Animal Models in Toxicologic Research: Rabbit*, Vol 1, Chap 18) are a default test system for these specialized studies (Ema et al., 2014; FDA: Redbook; FDA: Guidance for industry: nonclinical safety evaluation of pediatric drug products; FDA: Guidance for industry: S8 immunotoxicity studies for human pharmaceuticals; OECD). Historical control data are useful when selecting and assessing the suitability of an animal model (Deschl et al., 2002; Haseman et al., 1997; Weber et al., 2011b).

Such specialized studies typically are done using outbred mice (e.g., CD-1) or rats (e.g., SD and Wistar Han). These species and stocks are utilized to mimic the heterogeneous genetic backgrounds in most human populations. Hamsters may be selected as the rodent species in some cases if the ADME profile for the test article in mice or rats differs substantially from that of humans. In general, guinea pigs are not employed for such specialized studies because the precocial offspring (i.e., born with well-developed locomotor and sensory capabilities as well as the ability to consume solid food at birth) are not good models for the developmental status of altricial (i.e., underdeveloped at birth) human infants and toddlers and because the pattern of neurotoxicity in guinea pigs for classic neurotoxicants can differ from that of other rodent species (Raboisson et al., 1997). However, guinea pigs may be used as a system for specialized studies if the test article is not pharmacologically active in other rodent species (Rocca and Wehner, 2009).

Human populations are often subject to comorbidities (e.g., cardiac and/or metabolic diseases such as hypertension, diabetes mellitus, obesity), conditions which may increase the manifestation of toxic effects. Various RMD (e.g., leptin-deficient [ob/ob] and nonobese diabetic mice for diabetes and obesity), whether spontaneous or genetically engineered, may be used to recapitulate such comorbidities in the face of toxic challenges (see Section 2.3 below). A more specific, controlled option is inclusion of a challenge (i.e., stress testing) to increase the functional activity and raise the likelihood of detecting a deficit or toxicity that is subthreshold in healthy, unstressed animals. For example, the heart may be stressed by exercise, mechanical, or pharmacologic approaches as a means to more sensitively detect cardiotoxicity. Dobutamine infusion causes beta-adrenergic stimulation, increasing heart rate, blood pressure, stroke volume, and cardiac output, with measurable echocardiographic changes (Tontodonati et al., 2011). This approach has shown to have utility in the early detection of functional cardiac effects of diesel exhaust and the functional and structural cardiotoxicity of anthracycline (Burdick et al., 2015; Hazari et al., 2012). In general, however, toxicity testing in rodents is performed in normal animals that lack comorbidities (except for spontaneous/

age-related changes) as the primary study objective is to define potential toxicity of a test article to the mainstream population rather than particularly susceptible subpopulations.

An important consideration for rodent-based testing in terms of best modeling the human population as a whole is the feeding regimen. A substantial proportion of adults in developed countries—often 40% or more—are overweight or obese. The ranges of background findings as well as the lifespans of mice and rats differ substantially depending on whether they are fed ad libitum or are given a caloric-restricted diet (Duffy et al., 2001). The responses of ad libitum versus caloric-restricted rats to toxicants also diverge (Keenan et al., 1996). Thus, the choice of feeding schedule is one factor that must be considered with care when seeking to separate the potential toxicity of test articles from confounding husbandry effects.

2.3. Rodent Models of Disease and Genetically Modified Animals

In some cases, a toxicity assessment may represent only one element of the study design. A common multipurpose study design is the combined efficacy/toxicity study, where the experiment is conducted in a RMD and the data set for the test article will address simultaneously such questions as a test article's efficacy ("Did it work?"), toxicity ("Was it safe?"), and the cellular and molecular effects underlying these responses. Such experimental designs are common for investigating monogenetic congenital diseases, many of which have reproducible and somewhat consistent disease phenotypes that may be examined using conventional anatomic pathology and/or clinical pathology methods.

The choice of RMD for use in toxicity testing depends on the experimental question(s) to be addressed. In most cases, RMD are used to test a hypothesis related to the disease pathogenesis (e.g., infection, induced surgical, metabolic, or immune-mediated pathology) and/or efficacy of a potential new therapy, while wild-type rodents are employed for standard toxicity testing to identify hazards and assess safety. This dichotomy reflects several practical factors. Many RMD exist on inbred (i.e., genetically homogeneous) backgrounds, which do not provide a good representation of more genetically diverse human populations. Second, RMD with their underlying disease manifestations may have truncated lifespans or exhibit substantial inherent anatomic, functional, and/or molecular abnormalities which have nothing to do with test article exposure and yet might be difficult to differentiate from any effects actually induced by the test article, particularly if data on spontaneous background lesions are lacking. Third, a fair percentage of RMD have limited fecundity, which will require an extended breeding program or enrollment period to produce enough healthy animals to populate multiple test groups. Fourth, for some RMD, each individual animal—especially for new spontaneous or genetically engineered lines—may be expensive to acquire and maintain. Finally, in many cases, the RMD will need to be characterized in detail prior to its use for toxicologic research due to the absence of historical control data.

Genetically engineered RMD are especially popular systems for product discovery and development, whether such mutations arise spontaneously or by deliberate engineering (*Genetically Engineered Animal Models in Toxicologic Research*, Vol 1, Chap 23). Genetically abnormal RMD are used most often to investigate a particular hypothesis, such as exploring molecular mechanisms that contribute to disease initiation and progression; to validate therapeutic targets; or to confirm the efficacy of novel drug candidates. Historically, most genetically engineered RMD have been produced in mice, for two reasons. First, transgenesis (i.e., insertion of novel DNA carrying a gene of interest) is relatively easy in mice due to the very large pronuclei in zygotes (one-celled embryos) of some strains (e.g., FVB). Similarly, mice traditionally have been preferred for gene targeting because reliable embryonic stem (ES) cell lines have been harvested from several strains (e.g., 129, C57BL/6) that permit fairly reliable albeit low-yield homologous recombination to remove ("knock out") an existing mouse gene or to replace it ("knock in") with a homologous gene from a different species (including humans). Rats have been used for transgenesis, but the absence of a reliable rat ES cell line has limited production of knockout rat models. The recent advent of nuclease-based genome engineering technology (e.g., the clustered regularly interspaced short palindromic repeats [CRISPR]/CRISPR-associated protein 9 [Cas9] platform)

will revolutionize the production of RMD since this procedure can be performed to edit genes in any species (*Genetically Engineered Animal Models in Toxicologic Research*, Vol 1, Chap 23)—and already has been so employed in many rodent (and nonrodent) species.

Various RMD are utilized for more development-oriented tasks in which the main point of the study is to describe a test article's properties (i.e., investigational toxicology) rather than to investigate a specific hypothesis. As noted above, RMD may be employed to simultaneously evaluate a test article for both predicted efficacy and undesirable toxicity, generating a therapeutic index in that model. Such models have been used to support safety assessment in a variety of disease contexts, from inborn errors of metabolism (e.g., Niemann–Pick Disease) to osteoporosis and mouse tumor models for oncolytic virus therapies, and to investigate human toxicities (e.g., Zucker diabetic fatty rats for exocrine pancreatic injury with glucagon-like peptide-1 agonists) (Blanset et al., 2020). Immunodeficient RMD, whether spontaneous or purposefully engineered, are also critical systems for evaluating human tissue responses in vivo. Such RMD typically are produced in immunodeficient mice either by introduction of viable human cells (e.g., Pdx [patient-derived xenograft] or "avatar" mice) or by chemically induced ablation of normal mouse cells bearing a toxicant-responsive gene followed by their replacement with human cells from the same tissue (e.g., "chimeric" mice with humanized bone marrow, liver, and thymus) (see *Genetically Engineered Animal Models in Toxicologic Research*, Vol 1, Chap 23). The utility of such RMD is to evaluate questions including the degree to which chemotherapeutic regimens selectively target human-origin tumor cells (Pdx model) and the ability of human metabolic enzymes to affect the pharmacokinetics and tissue manifestations of toxicity of test articles in vivo (chimeric model).

3. ISSUES IN EXTRAPOLATION OF RODENT DATA FOR HUMAN RISK ASSESSMENT

The ready availability of genetically well-defined mouse and rat strains as well as the broad translatability of rodent anatomic and physiological attributes and pathologic responses has been used for decades to identify and characterize hazards related to xenobiotic exposure. Rodents as models for human risk assessment may be more problematic since rodent pharmacology, anatomy, and pathophysiology often differ substantially from their human counterparts.

3.1. Pharmacologic Translational Relevance and Interspecies Pathophysiologic Concordance

Pharmacologic relevance of a species (i.e., whether or not the potential therapeutic being tested is active at the rodent [or nonrodent] receptor) is a major determinant (i) when selecting rodents (vs. other species; see Section 2.1) for pharmacodynamics, efficacy, and toxicity studies and (ii) in the evaluation of on-target but exaggerated pharmacologic effects in safety studies. This concept is applicable to all xenobiotics when interpreting the potential human relevance of findings in animals and is particularly important when testing the safety of biomolecule therapeutics (i.e., xenobiotics containing human-derived protein or nucleic acid sequences that are highly target-specific, metabolized differently to chemical entities, and likely immunogenic in animals Baldrick, 2017). Once pathophysiological changes have been identified and characterized in rodent models, their relevance, or translatability, to humans must be verified.

In the efficacy context, RMD (mainly in mouse and rat) are a key part of the data package to support the hypothesis that administration of a novel test article will benefit the patient population with a particular disease. It is vital to understand the comparative pathophysiology and the extent to which any pharmacologic effect in rodents may be predictive of human-relevant mechanisms and ultimately a clinically beneficial outcome. This process ideally starts by engaging the pathologist from the earliest stages of target validation and is applied through animal model selection, model characterization, and interpretation of experimental data. Relevant RMD may be engineered (e.g., via genetic manipulation), induced (e.g., by surgery), or spontaneous. In general, any given RMD only incompletely recapitulates the disease as seen in humans; this tendency is especially clear for many degenerative RMD such as engineered mouse models of Alzheimer's disease (e.g., bearing human transgenes encoding mutant forms of amyloid-β precursor protein, apolipoprotein E4, and/or presenilin 1) or osteoarthritis (e.g., null mutations in collagen 2a1 [Col2a1] or osteoprotegerin [Tnfrsf11b] genes). Key questions can help the pathologist in assessing the translational value of an RMD, and its limitations, in the context of testing mechanistic hypotheses regarding efficacy. How much is known about the cause, pathophysiological mechanisms, and progression of the human disease? How closely does the RMD recapitulate most of the major aspects of the human condition? What are the similarities and differences in the pharmacologic target and pathway biology in rodents versus people? How reproducible are the pathobiological endpoints in rodents and humans? Has a given RMD been used historically, and how well has it predicted human pharmacologic responses? The pathologist plays an essential role in both understanding comparative pathophysiological mechanisms and compiling evidence of efficacy.

In the toxicology context, evaluation of translational relevance occurs stepwise through hazard identification and characterization to subsequent risk assessment for human (and sometimes animal) populations. Hazard identification and characterization is the phase of development where effects resulting from tissue, organ, or systemic injury caused by a test article are detected (identification) and then explored with respect to their progression, impact (harmful ["adverse"] or not harmful), relationship to dose (or more accurately exposure, based on toxicokinetic data), and ability to be reversed or repaired (which collectively represent characterization). In terms of toxicologic pathology endpoints, macroscopic and histopathologic evaluation, organ weights, and clinical pathology findings (hematology, serum chemistry, and sometimes urinalysis and coagulation assays) are the main contributors to the study data set. These pathology data typically are correlated to clinical signs, physical examinations, or other allied evaluations of functional perturbation.

Biological responses in RMD to novel xenobiotics have been demonstrated over decades to be generally reasonable predictors of human responses, though translational deficiencies are recognized in their ability to predict clinical trial outcomes (van der Worp et al., 2010). Standard rodent toxicity studies typically evaluate test articles administered to achieve continuous exposure during the dosing phase, ranging up to relatively high doses (up to lifetime exposure) in normal animals. In contrast, human treatment/exposure events typically occur intermittently at lower doses over a much longer absolute period, and in the case of novel therapeutic candidates are administered to patients with a disease and sometimes one or more comorbidities. Anatomic or physiologic differences may limit the translational relevance of findings in rodents to predicting human responses. For example, the presence of lesions in the nonglandular region of the stomach of the rodent is considered to be of minimal relevance for human risk assessment. This structure in rodents may be directly affected by application of test article via gavage dosing, but the nonglandular region does not have a counterpart in humans. Similarly, thyroid follicular hypertrophy/hyperplasia associated with induction of hepatocellular enzymes (specifically uridine diphosphate–glucuronyl transferase [UGT]), leading in rodents to increased metabolism and inactivation of thyroid hormones T_3 and T_4 and upregulation of the feedback loop to increase thyroid stimulating hormone secretion, is considered to translate very poorly to humans. This divergence is due to the presence of thyroxine-binding globulin in humans, which increases the circulating half-life of T_3 and T_4. That said, substantive interspecies differences do not always minimize the utility of rodent-derived data for human risk assessment. In the brain, the numbers and organization of cerebrocortical neuron populations in the lissencephalic rodent brain differ significantly from those of gyrencephalic species like dogs and primates; similarly, the usual range of rodent behaviors is substantially less complex than the behavioral and psychological make-up of humans. Despite this, rodent neurotoxicity data acquired by toxicologic pathology analysis tend to be a suitable screen for human risk assessment. Toxicologic pathologists have a central role in determining the significance of these structural and functional differences with respect to the predictivity of toxicologic findings in rodents to responses that might occur in nonrodents and humans.

Evaluating concordance between findings in animal and human studies (and also between rodent and nonrodent species) to establish translation is therefore vital to the risk assessment enterprise. Primary goals of rodent studies are (1) to establish evidence of efficacy with greater confidence and to minimize human (or animal) risk, particularly in the context of specific modalities for treating disease, and (2) to improve the mechanistic understanding of targets/pathways responsible for toxic outcomes following exposure to potential therapeutic agents or environmental chemicals. In toxicology, undesirable findings (i.e., "toxicity") may be target-mediated ("on target") exaggerated pharmacology, side ("off target") effects due to test article activation of other biological pathways, or nonspecific ("chemical") effects associated with certain biological or physicochemical properties of a test article. Additional caveats apply when assessing the translatability of rodent data to humans, notably that true-positive results are identified infrequently in both animals and humans since

(i) most xenobiotic test articles do not progress to human exposure because development of those with significant hazards/with small safety margins is terminated as they have an unfavorable risk assessment, and
(ii) effects seen at high doses/exposures in rodent toxicity studies may not manifest at or fully recapitulate the toxicity profile observed in humans faced with much lower exposures.

The differences in exposures in rodent studies versus humans also mitigate against the establishment of true-negative outcomes for a given finding, since the presence of another/different toxicity may ethically limit human dose escalation in clinical studies. Practically, this inherently imbalanced program design limits informative data in humans to toxicities which have been shown during nonclinical safety testing in rodents to be both readily monitored using sensitive, predictive biomarkers and that are reversible, with suitably large safety margins.

Despite these limitations, various evaluations have shown the utility of rodent-derived data as a means of predicting human responses. For example, physiological responses in genetically engineered rodents where null mutations (knockouts) ablate a particular molecular pathway are good predictors of therapeutic efficacy for test articles designed to reduce the activity of that pathway in human patients (Zambrowicz and Sands, 2003). In contrast, rodent (primarily rat) toxicity data show a positive human toxicity concordance rate of only 43% compared to 71% for rodent and nonrodent species together and 63% for nonrodent species alone (Olson et al., 2000). The concordance and/or predictivity of rodent data for human responses varies with the organ system being assessed and the data set undergoing analysis, though there is general agreement among different published analyses (Clark and Steger-Hartmann, 2018; Monticello et al., 2017; Olson et al., 2000). For rodent studies, the types of human toxicity with the highest concordance—biochemical (e.g., clinical chemistry findings), cutaneous, gastrointestinal, hematological, and hepatic effects—are those best identified across all species used in regulatory toxicity studies. There are some exceptions noted among species: rodents have the highest predictivity of any test species for biochemical endpoints of toxicity, whereas cardiovascular toxicity shows better concordance in nonrodent species (Monticello et al., 2017; Olson et al., 2000).

Looking at other comparative indices, rodent toxicity findings provide a suitable screen for human risk assessment. Across all organ systems, toxicity findings in rodents have (i) a similar low sensitivity to that of nonhuman primates (NHPs), approximately 26% in rodent, versus 42% in dogs; (ii) a similar high specificity to those of both dogs and NHPs (approximately 88%); but (iii) the lowest positive predictive value for toxicity (29%) compared to approximately 39% and 47% in dogs and NHPs, respectively (Monticello et al., 2017). Conversely, the absence of target organ toxicities in rodent or nonrodent test species strongly predicts a similar outcome in humans (a negative predictive value of 86%), an important factor in risk assessment (Monticello et al., 2017). A "big data" approach to a much larger dataset (3290 approved drugs) showed that the highest proportion of "true positive" concordance between toxic responses in humans and rats for given organ systems was in endocrine, hematological and lymphatic, hepatobiliary, metabolic, renal and urinary, respiratory, and thoracic and mediastinal systems (Clark and Steger-Hartmann, 2018). For mice, the highest proportion of "true positives" with respect to predicting human toxic responses also included endocrine, hematological and lymphatic, hepatobiliary, respiratory, and thoracic and mediastinal organ systems; however, nervous system as well as skin and subcutaneous organ responses also could be extrapolated in this species (Clark and Steger-Hartmann, 2018).

Another recent review explored whether both rodent and nonrodent species are necessary for general toxicity testing as currently described by regulatory guidance seeking toxicity data from two species. Reduction to a single species for longer-term toxicity studies was only applied for 8/133 drug candidates but might have been possible for more, regardless of drug modality, as the same or similar target organ toxicity profiles (rodent vs. nonrodent, across all organ systems) were identified in the short-term studies for an average of approximately 39% of candidates (Prior et al., 2020). These data suggest that where there is concordance between rodent and nonrodent findings in shorter term toxicity studies, a single species might be sufficient to investigate chronic toxicity; at this point, it is unclear whether this single-species approach could be based on rodent testing (which would be preferable given the larger possible group sizes, lower cost, and reduced regulatory burden associated with rodent toxicity studies). Extensive further analysis of larger datasets is required to more fully understand the context-dependent benefits/risks of such an approach.

In conclusion, the translational relevance of safety assessment via rodent toxicity studies alone is variable across different organ systems and is generally less predictive than nonrodent data when each species is interpreted in isolation. However, when combined, an integrated analysis of rodent and nonrodent toxicity data improves the strength of the risk assessment in predicting human responses. Importantly, an absence of findings in rodents has a high negative predictive value for the risk of toxicity developing in subjects exposed during human clinical studies. Taken together, these data indicate that the utility of rodents as test systems depends on the nature of the scientific question, but that rodent data are vital factors in safety assessment.

3.2. Biological and Cell Therapies

Biopharmaceutical test articles such as monoclonal antibodies and peptides (*Protein Pharmaceutical Agents*, Vol 2, Chap 6) as well as antisense oligonucleotides (*Nucleic Acid Pharmaceutical Agents*, Vol 2, Chap 7) are developed for efficacy in human-specific biologic systems. Toxicity of human-derived biomolecules in animals manifests essentially as either (1) exaggerated pharmacologic activity, which is likely to be a translationally relevant effect in a pharmacologically relevant test species (Baldrick, 2017), or (2) immunologic reactions (e.g., anti-drug antibodies [ADA] and immune complex disease) as the animal immune system recognizes the human molecules as antigenic, which are less translationally relevant. Even if ADAs do not cause pathologic changes, neutralizing antibodies can limit exposure to, and pharmacologic activity of, the test article, thereby restricting assessment of toxicity. Ideally, any rodent species used in toxicity studies for biomolecules will be pharmacologically relevant; if so, then testing in a rodent species (as well as a nonrodent species) would be expected to meet current regulatory guidance (Prior et al., 2020). If the toxicity profile in short-term studies supporting Phase I clinical trials is similar in both animal species, then longer-term toxicity studies in a single species, preferably rodent, may be sufficient to support Phase II/III clinical trials for biotherapeutic candidates (ICH).

However, due to the high selectivity of biopharmaceuticals, even if there is activity of a human-derived molecule at the rodent receptor, differences in activity and knowledge of downstream [patho]biology in the rodent and human orthologs are important to account for when undertaking risk assessment. Often, only one pharmacologically relevant species, generally an NHP (due to higher DNA/amino acid sequence homology with the human protein), can be identified. In such cases, a surrogate, rodent-specific version of the human therapeutic (e.g., an antibody against the murine target) may be generated since it should have a similar impact (pharmacologic and toxic) in the rodent test system as the human-specific therapeutic candidate would in patients. However, since the intended human therapeutic is not actually being tested in rodents, it may be preferable to only use the nonrodent species to produce animal data suitable for human risk assessment.

Evaluation of toxicity for cell therapies (e.g., engineered stem cells to replace a depleted cell population or modified T-cells for tumor immunotherapy) is very challenging in rodent species (*Stem Cells and Regenerative Medicine*, Vol 2, Chap 10). Immunodeficient mouse models, where genetically altered strains with multilineage defects in leukocyte function are "humanized" by transplanting functional human immune cells (e.g., by infusing human peripheral blood mononuclear cells or seeding the bone marrow with human hematopoietic progenitor cells), can be used to explore human-specific responses to cell therapies, with the understanding that the human cells are acting in the context of a murine host system (*Genetically Engineered Animal Models in Toxicologic Research*, Vol 1, Chap 23). In efficacy models involving xenografted cells, species differences are less of an issue since the human tumor cell lines or Pdx grafts are hosted by the rodent but the pharmacologic target against which efficacy being tested is of human origin.

Testing of antibody–drug conjugate commonly involves a two-species approach for safety assessment irrespective of pharmacological relevance in the rodent (Hinrichs and Dixit, 2015). The reason for this testing paradigm is that evaluation for off-target toxicity is feasible in rodents via pathologic evaluation of tissues for toxic effects associated with the conjugated drug. Use of a pharmacologically relevant nonrodent species (usually NHPs) in which the antibody backbone is active permits assessment of both on-target and off-target toxicities (Prior et al., 2020).

3.3. Controlling Variability and Impact of the Microbiome in Rodent Studies

Comprehensive efforts are required to minimize biological variation which can confound experimental outcomes and contribute to poor experimental reproducibility (Scudamore et al., 2016). Factors that need to be considered in toxicologic research for all species include controlling genetic variation among test subjects (including purchasing replacements from a single supplier with a well-controlled breeding and testing strategy for maintaining genetic integrity); regulating the microbiological status (e.g., many rodent toxicity tests are performed with specific pathogen-free [SPF] animals); and standardizing environmental and husbandry parameters (e.g., diet, housing, bedding, temperature, water). This high degree of standardization is instrumental in planning and implementing consistent study designs. Moreover, the similar sizes and equivalent (though not identical) anatomic features of major rodent species permit the preparation of many species-agnostic standard operating procedures for in-life experimental and postmortem sampling tasks that are common to mice, rats, hamsters, guinea pigs, and gerbils.

The impact of specific pathogens on animals used in research is well documented (Nicklas et al., 1999). Maintaining SPF status of animals supplied for studies and monitoring microbiological status are well-established practices (Fox et al., 2007c; Suckow et al., 2020). Other measures to reduce microbial variability among animals include controlling genetic variation in strains (which can impact immune system effectiveness), source (supplier), and husbandry (e.g., standardizing bedding and diet lot numbers for animals on a given study). In addition to health status defined by monitoring for specific pathogens, changes in the microbial population associated with animals (mostly species considered to be commensals, principally in the gut) can impact multiple aspects of their hosts' biology (*Issues in Laboratory Animal Science that Impact Toxicologic Pathology*, Vol 1, Chap 29). These microbiome effects on systemic physiology include maturation of the immune system, immune system/inflammatory cell responsiveness, and disease phenotype in a variety of different rodent models (Cryan et al., 2019; Tomas et al., 2012; Zarate-Blades et al., 2016).

Drug–microbiome interactions have recently been shown to impact pharmacologic activity and toxicity in humans (Aziz et al., 2018). Similar effects have been demonstrated in rodents (Rosshart et al., 2019; Zitvogel et al., 2018) and could affect the translational relevance of safety findings. Despite this, the microbiota (the types of flora) and the microbiome (the large number of functional genes derived from those microorganisms) generally are not characterized or monitored in conventional

rodent toxicity studies. Since animals derive their microbiome essentially from their mother and/or the local environment (e.g., breeding house, vendor), this lack of characterization in theory could confound the reproducibility and translatability of such studies, which is a risk where business practices outsource studies for a given xenobiotic to potentially different test sites. For example, responses to the CD28 superagonist, TGN1412, which caused life-threatening T-cell activation and cytokine storms in healthy human volunteers during a Phase I clinical trial (Suntharalingam et al., 2006), had not been predicted in standard SPF laboratory rodents. However, C57BL/6 mice with a complex microbiome similar to wild mice (achieved by embryo transfer of C57BL/6 into wild mice; termed "wildling" mice) showed an inflammatory cytokine response and a lack of regulatory T-cell expansion similar to the clinical effects when given TGN1412 (Rosshart et al., 2019). For an anti-tumor necrosis factor-alpha treatment, which was efficacious in laboratory animal models but failed in the clinic due to lack of efficacy, the "wildling" mice with their complex microbiota recapitulated the human clinical response and did not prevent lethality in experimentally induced endotoxemia, whereas concurrent control laboratory mice with more restricted gut microbiomes were rescued (Rosshart et al., 2019). There are also many examples of changes in the microbiota which influence pathobiological findings via multiple mechanisms, in a wide variety of rodent (and nonrodent) models of human disease (*Issues in Laboratory Animal Science that Impact Toxicologic Pathology*, Vol 1, Chap 29).

Rodents for a given study ideally should have comparable microbial profiles. This consistency arises because animals are enrolled from a single colony (in-house or external vendor) and are exposed to similar experimental conditions. Some vendors now offer to standardize the microbiome by oral inoculation with custom microbiota to further improve consistency when the animals leave the supplier, although the flora will shift upon arrival to acquire the signature of the colony into which they are introduced. Given the complexity and cost associated with any "snapshot" characterization of the microbiome, it is challenging to decide how to monitor its status, and whether the data are of sufficient value to warrant performing the analysis on a routine basis (Hansen and Franklin, 2019). In the future, research groups may need to consider the presence or absence of a short list of defined bacterial species relevant for their models and research questions.

4. BASIC BIOLOGICAL CHARACTERISTICS OF COMMON RODENT STOCKS AND STRAINS

Rodents are widely used in toxicological and experimental pathology due to their small size, ease of breeding, regulatory acceptance, and the availability of extensive background historical control data (Gad, 2015). It is difficult to appraise the global usage of rodents due to the variations in recording data and the omission of data from rodent species in some countries (Taylor et al., 2008), but it is estimated that approximately 95% of all laboratory animal subjects in research are mice and rats. Census data from the European Union (EU) suggest that just over seven million rodents are used in the EU each year (European Commission). Home Office statistics in Great Britain reliably record that the predominant rodent species used in research are the mouse, rat, guinea pig, Syrian hamster, and Mongolian gerbil (Home Office of the United Kingdom). In the United States, mice (genus *Mus*) and rats (genus *Rattus*) bred for research are not covered by the Animal Welfare Act (USDA-APHIS), so numbers of these species used for biomedical and toxicologic studies are not reported; estimates for these species range from approximately 20 million (Sparks, 2021) to over 100 million (Carbone, 2021). In 2018, U.S. laboratories reported using about 170,000 guinea pigs and 80,000 hamsters for various research purposes (USDA-APHIS).

This section briefly introduces major species-specific attributes that toxicologic pathologists should be aware of when making their macroscopic and microscopic observations, and when interpreting anatomic pathology and clinical pathology data, for rodent species of relevance to toxicologic research. Principal anatomic and physiological attributes are given, and noninfectious spontaneous background findings that might be seen during toxicity studies are reviewed briefly. Infectious diseases that are less likely to be encountered in conventional toxicologic research facilities are not addressed here, but details on these important research confounders may be obtained elsewhere (Barthold et al., 2016; Fox et al., 2007b; Harkness et al., 2010; Suckow et al., 2020; Suckow et al., 2012).

4.1. Outbred Stocks and Inbred Strains of Mice and Rats

Rats and mice are the most commonly used rodent species and may be outbred or inbred. Outbred animals are referred to as stocks, whereas inbred animals are referred to as strains. Outbred stocks are officially defined as populations which have been closed for at least four generations and bred to maintain maximal genetic variation (heterozygosity). In contrast, inbred strains are created by brother/sister matings over a minimum of 20 generations with founder pairs used to produce experimental animals being taken from the 20th generation. Inbreeding is never absolute, but inbred strains are considered to be homozygous at approximately 99% of loci. Strategies for maintaining a consistent genetic background are outside the scope of this chapter but have been detailed exhaustively elsewhere (Flurkey et al., 2009).

Outbred stocks are traditionally preferred for safety testing as they are thought to more closely mimic the genetic diversity of human populations and therefore model the variation in phenotypic responses likely to be seen in humans. However, a recent systematic review comparing data gathered across many laboratories and protocols suggests that the genetic background of inbred or outbred mice strains is not the major contributing factor to the variation observed in many phenotypic measurements, so this distinction may not be as important as previously thought (Tuttle et al., 2018). The most common outbred rodent stocks used for safety testing in the United States and Europe are Swiss-derived CD1 mice and SD and Wistar Han rats.

Inbred rodent strains are used extensively in discovery and academic research where their defined genetic uniformity and phenotypic stability are considered to increase the statistical power (i.e., the probability in a hypothesis-driven test of finding an effect if there is an effect to be found) of experimental designs and reduce the number of animals needed for experiments. It has been suggested, but is not universally accepted, that inbred strains could also be used for toxicity studies where safety endpoints might be better determined either by using the most susceptible genetic background or for specific studies where efficacy and safety endpoints are combined in the same protocol (e.g., evaluating gene therapy test articles) (Festing, 2010). Reduced interanimal variability in inbred strains may limit divergence in responses among test animals, thereby reducing the number of animals required. The better genetic definition that is characteristic of strains also might help in more rapidly identifying and understanding any genes involved in the response to treatment or the susceptibility to toxicity (Festing, 2014).

Outbred Mice

Current outbred "Swiss" mouse stocks are originally derived from European and North American house mice (*M. musculus domesticus*) (Whary et al., 2015). Additional stocks derived from Asian (*Mus musculus castaneus*) and Mediterranean (*Mus spretus*) mice have been developed as research models but are much less commonly used in academic research and rarely if at all in toxicology. The commonly used CD-1 Swiss mouse stocks from various vendors, while described as outbred, are homozygous at many loci and do not display the genetic diversity apparent in wild-type mouse populations. Outbred mice tend to be larger than inbred strains at maturity and may have longer life spans than many inbred strains (Table 17.3).

Inbred Mice

Inbred mice are commonly used in biomedical research and are essential when knowledge of the precise genotypic background is important for modeling disease and understanding the effects of genetic alterations on biological responses. Understanding the nomenclature applied to mouse strains is critically important when evaluating the literature or choosing mice for experiments (Sundberg and Schofield, 2010). C57BL/6 mice are the most commonly used inbred strain for creating genetically engineered mouse models (Seong et al., 2004). There are multiple substrains of C57BL/6 mice, and there are significant genotypic and phenotypic differences between them which have been reported to affect a variety of experimental outcomes across many areas of biology (Selman and Swindell, 2018).

Examples of C57BL/6 strain nomenclature (Jackson; Sundberg and Schofield, 2010) will illustrate the need for due care when designing studies and interpreting published reports:

- C57BL/6J—a C57BL/6 inbred substrain distributed by The Jackson Laboratory
- C57BL/6N—a C57BL/6 inbred substrain distributed by the U.S. National Institutes of Health
- C57BL/6NTac—a C57BL/6N inbred substrain distributed by the vendor Taconic Farms Ltd.
- C57BL/6J-Apc[Min]/J—a C57BL/6 substrain distributed by The Jackson Laboratory that carries a mutant (Min) allele in the adenomatous polyposis coli (*Apc*) tumor suppressor gene, where the strain also is held at The Jackson Laboratory

Other commonly used inbred mouse strains (and associated substrains) are 129, BALB/c, C3H/He, and FVB/N. The 129 strain has historically been an important source of ES cells for the production of targeted genetic mutations in mouse models (Simpson et al., 1997). However, newer gene editing techniques can now be used on virtually any species or strain to produce genetic modifications (Burgio, 2018). BALB/c mice have been traditionally used for monoclonal antibody production and are widely used in oncology and immunology basic research. C3H/He mice are a general-purpose strain used in a variety of research areas including oncology, infectious disease, sensorineural disorders, and cardiovascular biology. FVB/N inbred mice have prominent pronuclei and have been used for generating transgenic mouse models. Descriptions of common background findings in these strains allow the rational selection among inbred genetic backgrounds when designing mouse studies (Brayton et al., 2012; Haines et al., 2001; Mahler et al., 1996; Sellers et al., 2012; Ward et al., 2000).

TABLE 17.3 Basic Biological Characteristics of Common Rodent Stocks and Strains

Species/strain or stock	Gestation length (days)	Average litter size	Age at puberty (breeding age in weeks)		Average adult body weight (g)	
			Male	Female	Male	Female
RAT – OUTBRED STOCKS						
Sprague Dawley (SD)	21–24[a]	10–11[a]	10[a]	11[a]	1400–1600[a]	900–1100[a]
Wistar Han	21–23[a]	9–10[a]	10–12[a]	8	600–1100[b]	600–700[b]
RAT – INBRED STRAINS						
F344 (Fischer)	19–21[a]	6–8[a]	10[a]	8[a]	600–900[b]	600–700[b]
MOUSE – OUTBRED STOCK						
CD1	19–21[a]	10–11[a]	10–12[a]	7–10[a]	35[c]	27[c]
MOUSE – INBRED STRAINS						
C57BL/6	19–21[a]	7.0[a]	8–10[a]	8–10[a]	22[c]	18[c]
BALB/c	19–21[a]	5.2[a]	8–10[a]	8–10[a]	21[c]	19[c]
129-elite	21[a]	5.9[a]	5–6[a]	5–6[a]	NF	NF
MOUSE – ENGINEERED MODELS						
p53[+/−] (B6; 129S7-Trp53[tm1Brd] N5)	19–21[d]	NF	8–10[d]	8–10[d]	NF	NF
Tg-rasH2 (CByB6F1-Tg(HRAS)2Jic)	19–21[d]	NF	8–10[d]	8–10[d]	32[e]	26[e]
Guinea pig (Hartley)[f]	59–72	2–5	12–16	8–12	900–1000	700–900
Hamster (Syrian)[g]	15–18	4–12	6–8	8–12	85–140	95–120
Gerbil (Mongolian)[h]	24–26	7.0	9–12	9–12	65–100	55–85

NF, information not found in publicly available databases and scientific literature.

[a] Charles River Laboratories Technical Bulletin 092619.
[b] Data obtained from Weber K, Razinger T, Hardisty JF, et al.: Differences in rat models used in routine toxicity studies, Int J Toxicol 30:162–173, 2011b.
[c] Data obtained from Gad SC, Clifford C, Goodman D: The mouse. In Gad SC, editor: Animal models in toxicology, Boca Raton, FL, 2015, CRC Press, pp. 21–152.
[d] Data obtained from Pritchett KR, Taft RA: Reproductive biology of the laboratory mouse. In Fox JG, Barthold SW, Davisson MT, et al., editors: The mouse in biomedical research, ed 2, San Diego, 2007, Academic Press (Elsevier), pp. 91–121.
[e] Data obtained from Yamamoto S, Urano K, Koizumi H, et al.: Validation of transgenic mice carrying the human prototype c-Ha-ras gene as a bioassay model for rapid carcinogenicity testing, Environ Health Perspect 106(Suppl 1):57–69, 1998.
[f] Data obtained from Shomer NH, Holcombe H, Harkness JE: Biology and diseases of Guinea pigs. In Fox JG, Anderson LC, Otto GM, et al., editors: Laboratory animal medicine, ed 3, Boston, 2015, Academic Press (Elsevier), pp. 247–285.
[g] Data obtained from Miedel EL, Hankenson FC: Biology and diseases of hamsters. In Fox JG, Anderson LC, Otto GM, et al., editors: Laboratory animal medicine, ed 3. Boston, 2015, Academic Press (Elsevier), pp. 209–246.
[h] Data obtained from Batchelder M, Keller LS, Sauer MB, et al.: Gerbils. In Suckow MA, Stevens KA, Wilson RP, editors: The laboratory rabbit, Guinea pig, hamster, and other rodents, San Diego, 2012, Academic Press (Elsevier), pp. 1131–1155.

Outbred Rats

Wistar rats include a number of substrains derived from a common lineage and include both outbred (Hannover [Wistar Han] and Unilever [Wistar WU]) and inbred strains (Kyoto [Wistar WKY] and Furth [Wistar WF]). The outbred stocks are used most commonly in safety testing. Sprague Dawley (SD) rats are an outbred stock originally developed from Wistar rats crossed with a variety of other laboratory and wild rats. Long–Evans rats are utilized occasionally for reproductive, behavioral, and dietary studies.

SD and Wistar Han rats are preferred in safety assessment studies because of the significant amount of historical data (physiological and toxicological) available for these stocks. Background data are normally compiled within laboratories, but some comparisons in the literature give an idea of the major differences between stocks (e.g., a greater maximal bodyweight is achieved by SD rats compared to Wistar rats) (Weber et al., 2011b). Other characteristics such as reduced tumor burden and increased longevity in Wistar compared to SD rats also may influence the choice of models for rat toxicity studies (Weber, 2017; Weber et al., 2011b). Significant differences in physiological and pathological data may be seen among rat stocks, especially substocks maintained by particular animal suppliers (Brower et al., 2015; Weber, 2017). These baseline variations may complicate the interpretation of results when product development programs extend across different laboratories, countries, and continents.

Inbred Rats

Inbred rat strains are employed less commonly than inbred mouse strains for toxicity testing. Historically, Fischer 344 (F344) rats have been used for safety testing in some laboratories, most notably in the United States in numerous carcinogenicity studies performed by the U.S. National Cancer Institute (NCI) and U.S. National Toxicology Program (NTP). This model has been replaced in recent years by SD rats due to the high background frequency of certain neoplasms (chiefly interstitial cell [Leydig cell] tumors, mesotheliomas of the tunica vaginalis, and large granular lymphocytic [LGL] leukemia) in the F344 strain (Maronpot et al., 2016). Other inbred rat strains include the Brown Norway (BN), Copenhagen (COP), and Lewis (LEW) strains, which have been mainly used in immunological and oncology research applications.

Genetically Engineered Rodent Strains

Genetically engineered rodent strains are extensively used in discovery and academic research based on the expectation that the genetic alteration of conserved genes, leading to over- or underexpression of function, will mimic responses in humans with similar genetic mutations or variances. They are also used in nonclinical drug development to identify and validate targets, to evaluate the likelihood that a given pharmacological intervention will predict the human response to a test article (Zambrowicz and Sands, 2003), and to detect potential toxicity and evaluate safety (Bolon, 2004; Lee, 2014). As noted above (see Sections 2.1, 2.3, and 3.1), RMD typically are used in toxicity testing for two purposes (see *Genetically Engineered Animal Models in Toxicologic Research*, Vol 1, Chap 23). The first is in combined efficacy/toxicity testing where an RMD of a particular genetic condition is treated with a test article to both evaluate its ability to ameliorate clinical and/or structural (usually histopathological) alterations characteristic of the condition and examine its toxicity in vivo. The second and more common use is as the second species for carcinogenicity testing (see Section 2.1). The two most popular models at present are the $p53^{+/-}$ mouse (Storer et al., 2001), which is sensitive to genotoxic agents, and the Tg-rasH2 mouse (Bogdanffy et al., 2020), which detects both genotoxic and nongenotoxic materials.

4.2. Anatomy and Physiology of Rodents Used in Toxicologic Research

Mouse

Mice (*M. musculus*) are the most widely used species across experimental and toxicological research making up 61% of all animals used in the EU for research purposes (including breeding and experimental protocols) (European Commission). The widespread use of genetically altered mice in nonclinical and academic studies accounts for the majority of the animals. Mice are employed less commonly in regulatory safety studies with most of the numbers being used in 2- year bioassay/carcinogenicity studies.

Mice are used extensively because of their small size, which results in reduced costs for housing; the need for low amounts of novel test articles for conducting a study relative to other test species, including rats; ease of breeding; and the availability of numerous well-characterized stocks and genetically defined strains. An abundance of tools to manipulate the mouse genome as well as molecular and immunological reagents to aid investigative approaches in vivo and in vitro permit questions to be answered easily and speedily relative to other model species.

Mice have well-characterized anatomic features that can impact the toxicologic pathology evaluation (Barthold et al., 2016; Hoyt et al., 2007). The mouse heart beats 500–800 per minute (with the higher rate at the onset of the dark cycle, when mice begin their active period). Rodents including mice have anatomically complex nasal cavities and are obligate nose breathers. The mouse lung has one major airway per lung lobe that gives off branches (where human airways tend to divide symmetrically at each junction) and lacks respiratory bronchioles. The mouse digestive tract features hypsodontic (continuously renewing) incisors but no deciduous teeth, three major salivary glands, a stomach with distinct forestomach (lined by nonglandular mucosa) and true stomach (lined by glandular mucosa), short duodenum and rectum, and a gall bladder. Hepatocytes commonly exhibit nuclear divergence including increased DNA content (polyploidy), two nuclei (polykarya), unequal size (anisokaryosis), and cytoplasmic invagination into the nucleus. Mice are coprophagic in order to optimize protein and vitamin metabolism, and about one-third of their dietary intake is nutrient-rich feces. The adrenal glands are smaller and contain less lipid in males compared to females; both sexes contain the adrenal X zone at the corticomedullary junction, which involutes at sexual maturity in males and at the time of first pregnancy in females. The spleen is a major hematopoietic organ throughout life, and extramedullary hematopoiesis (EMH) in this organ often is sufficiently prominent to yield at least some degree of splenomegaly (though EMH can also occur in other tissues, e.g., liver). The thymus does not involute, or does so incompletely, in adulthood.

Well-developed Harderian glands in mice (also in rats and hamsters) contribute lipid-rich secretion to the preocular tear film, the porphyrin component of which can increase with stress (chromodacryorrhea), resulting in staining of the muzzle and periocular regions (Olcese and Wesche, 1989). The female reproductive cycle lasts 4 days, and the uterus develops cyclic infiltrates of eosinophils as a hormonally regulated physiological response. Corpora lutea persist beyond the cycle in which they are generated. Mammary tissue is limited to females, where it is extensively distributed over the trunk and neck; its prominence in most strains waxes and wanes between bouts of lactation. Mice (and rats) also possess preputial glands (in males) and clitoral glands (in females), which may be misdiagnosed as neoplasms by those unfamiliar with their location and appearance (Rudmann et al., 2012). Compact bones lack osteons (Haversian systems) and retain active bone marrow throughout life. Sexual dimorphism is also seen in the kidney and salivary glands. In the kidney, the parietal epithelium of Bowman's capsule is cuboidal in males and flattened in females. In the submandibular salivary glands, the acinar cells and convoluted ducts of male mice contain prominent eosinophilic cytoplasmic granules that are absent in females.

Several key hematologic characteristics are important aspects of mouse biology. The circulating half-life of mouse erythrocytes is approximately 40–50 days, and reticulocyte counts are low. Lymphocytes are the principal leukocyte class in circulation (70%–80%), and the number of platelets is high compared to other rodent species. In healthy animals, EMH consists mainly of erythrocytic precursors with a few megakaryocytes, but in diseased mice the number of granulocytic precursors and sometimes plasma cells can supersede the normal erythrocytic elements. Immunodeficient mice may or may not have altered hemograms (Eugster et al., 1998; Fernandes et al., 2018) but usually do exhibit extensive attenuation of leukocyte-rich tissues (especially lymphocyte-dense regions of lymphoid organs) (Fig. 17.1).

Rat

Rats (*R. norvegicus*) make up 12% of the total animals used in the EU (European Commission) and are more often utilized in toxicity studies

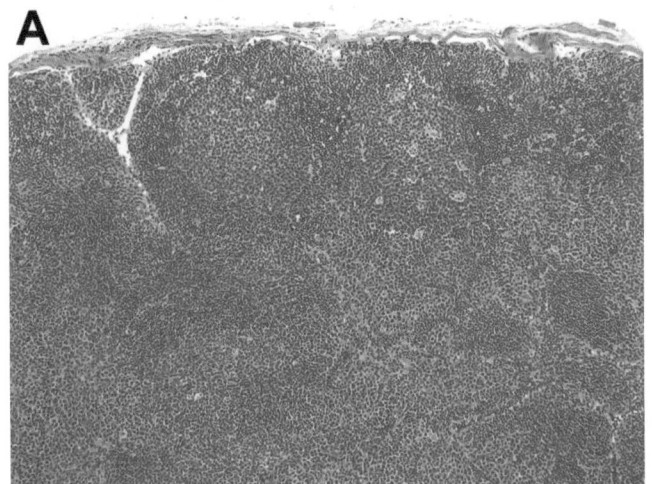

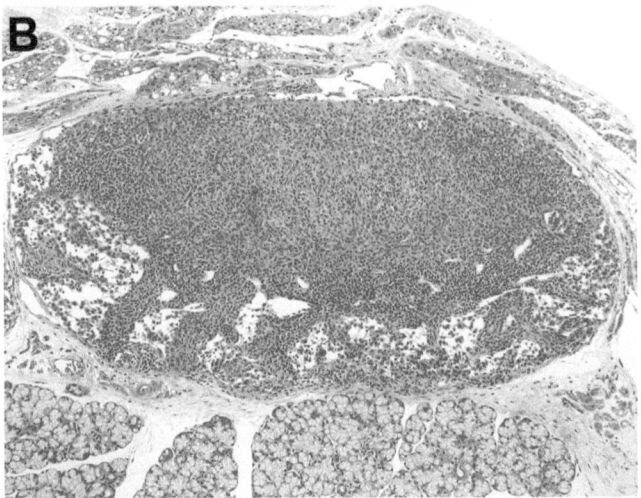

FIGURE 17.1 Comparison of lymph node architecture from adult wild-type (A) and severe combined immunodeficiency (scid) mice (B). The wild-type node exhibits prominent B-cell and T-cell domains with germinal centers, while the node from the scid mouse is depleted of lymphocytes and is greatly reduced in total size. Both nodes are shown at the same magnification. H&E.

than other rodent species, being the most common choice for acute and chronic studies. They are also the most common second species in 2-year bioassay/carcinogenicity studies. Although larger than mice, rats are still easier and cheaper to breed and maintain than larger nonrodent species. A number of well-characterized rat stocks and strains are available, including some immunodeficient models; outbred stocks typically are preferred for toxicologic research due to their genetic heterogeneity, physical hardiness, and better reproductive

success compared to inbred strains. In general, fewer immunological and molecular reagents are available for use with rat tissues, but tools for genetic manipulation are becoming more widely applied to rats (Guan et al., 2014; Ma et al., 2014). The larger body size of rats does allow sampling larger volumes of blood and tissue, permits more sampling opportunities per animal during the in-life phase of a study, and facilitates partitioning of organs for multiple analyses (e.g., molecular analysis of frozen tissue and histopathological evaluation of fixed tissue acquired from the same organ).

Rats are anatomically similar but not identical to mice (Barthold et al., 2016; Hofstetter et al., 2006). Features of the digestive, respiratory, reproductive tracts (including female cyclicity), and mammary gland as well as the skeletal system closely resemble those described above for mice apart from the absence of a gall bladder and more homogeneous hepatocyte size and nuclear morphology relative to mice. The female reproductive cycle lasts 4 days, and corpora lutea are maintained beyond the cycle in which they are generated. The mammary gland of rats shows marked sexual dimorphism with female glands having basophilic tubular ducts and males having a more abundant eosinophilic lobular alveolar pattern. The degree of EMH in rats is reduced relative to that seen in mice and is low in healthy and specific-pathogen-free animals. The thymus does involute to a considerable degree with age. The circulating half-life of rat erythrocytes is approximately 55–70 days, and reticulocyte counts are low. The majority of leukocytes in circulation are lymphocytes (60%–75%).

Syrian Hamsters

Syrian hamsters (*M. auratus*) are sometimes used in nonclinical development as an alternative rodent species for carcinogenicity studies, but the numbers used are low—approximately 0.2% of all animals used for research each year in the EU (European Commission). Historically, this choice was due to the belief that this species had a low background incidence of liver neoplasia relative to other rodents. However, increased experience with the species has challenged this assumption (McInnes et al., 2013). Other reasons for their use include the relative resistance of the hamster lung to inhaled materials which are carcinogenic in the rat (Mohr and Dungworth, 1988) and their apparent resistance to liver tumors induced by peroxisome proliferator–activated receptor alpha (PPARα) compounds (Choudhury et al., 2000).

Hamsters have some distinctive anatomic features that should not be mistaken for lesions during pathologic evaluation (Barthold et al., 2016; Murray, 2012). Hamsters have four digits on the front feet and five on the hind feet. They have hypsodontic incisors, and the shorter maxillary incisors grow approximately twice as fast (fully replaced in a week) as their longer mandibular counterparts. Hamsters are equipped with four major salivary glands and also have well-developed Harderian glands.

Syrian hamsters have prominent skin folds arising from the free edges of the lips that can distend at need to form buccal ("cheek") pouches. These compartments, which run caudally over the shoulder, have thin, highly vascularized walls that are rich in mast cells but lack lymphoid tissue and lymphatic vessels; this "immunologically privileged" site is a common system for experimental tumor implantation and vascular physiology studies. The stomach possesses distinct regions with nonglandular (forestomach) and glandular mucosae. The cecum is divided into apical and basal portions by semilunar tissue folds ("valves"). Hamsters have gall bladders and orbital venous sinuses. Compact bones lack osteons (Haversian systems).

A number of sex-related organs exhibit exceptional features in hamsters. Dorsal flank glands are modified sebaceous organs used to mark territorial boundaries. These androgen-responsive elements in the skin of the lumbar torso are large in males. The male hamster has a multipronged os penis. Unlike male mice and rats, the weights of testes and accessory sex organs in hamsters do not decline with age. The vagina of the female hamster opens much earlier (approximately 10 days of age) relative to other rodent species (where this orifice becomes patent at sexual maturity). Hamsters have a 4-day estrus cycle, but unlike mice and rats, the corpora lutea from a given cycle all regress before the next cycle begins.

Hamsters have several unusual physiological attributes. The kidney is quite responsive to estrogenic compounds, and male hamsters are a known model for evaluating renal cancer for this reason (Li et al., 1993). The liver of female hamsters undergoes substantial changes during pregnancy. The liver weight increases greatly, and bile flow is reduced by one-third at midgestation and two-thirds near term. Erythrocytes have a circulating half-life of 50–78 days (longer during hibernation) and often exhibit polychromasia and some degree of anisocytosis. Lymphocytes are the predominant circulating leukocytes (about 65%–75% of cells). The main granulocyte in circulation is termed a heterophil (functionally a neutrophil) due to its eosinophilic cytoplasmic granules.

Guinea Pigs

The use of guinea pigs (C. porcellus) in regulatory safety testing has declined significantly in the last 30 years due to the introduction of new models for testing skin sensitization. Guinea pig use in biomedical research accounts for 1.5% of animals in the EU each year (European Commission), though they typically are restricted to specific questions for which their unique physiological traits make them a sensitive species. Key areas of research in this species include investigation of respiratory allergens and anaphylaxis (including evaluation of test article efficacy in preventing these conditions), deafness, and infectious and nutritional (e.g., vitamin C deficiency) diseases (Gad and Peckham, 2015). The Hartley (Dunkin–Hartley) outbred guinea pig is most commonly used in toxicity testing.

Guinea pigs have some anatomic traits that should be recalled by pathologists during any gross and microscopic evaluation (Barthold et al., 2016; Hargaden and Singer, 2012). Some features are common to both sexes, including a fourth major salivary gland, a stomach lined almost entirely by glandular mucosa, a gall bladder, and a broad spleen (where the widest dimension is approximately 50% of the organ length in normal animals). In the lungs, numerous goblet cells are present in airway mucosa and nodular lymphocytic aggregates in the adventitia of lung vessels are common incidental findings in animals of all ages (Williams, 2012). Guinea pigs have hypsodontic incisors.

Sexual dimorphism is apparent in a few structures in guinea pigs. Only females have mammary glands. Similarly, only females have perineal sacs, a set of bilaterally symmetrical

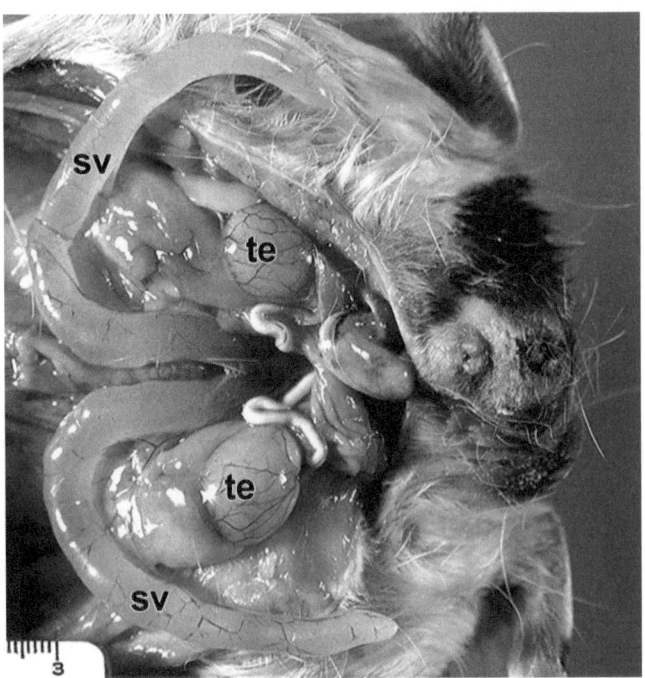

FIGURE 17.2 Caudal abdominal organs of a healthy adult male guinea pig showing the prominent seminal vesicles (sv) and testes (te). *Reproduced from Noah's Arkive (Image No. F27667) courtesy of the Davis Thompson DVM Foundation.*

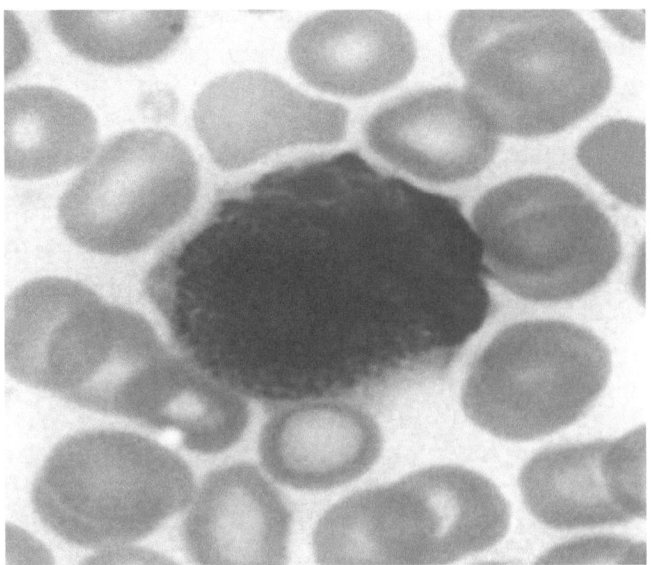

FIGURE 17.3 A Foa-Kurloff cell in a guinea pig blood smear demonstrating the very large cluster of mucopolysaccharide-laden cytoplasmic granules in this natural killer (NK) lymphocyte. Wright-Giemsa. *Reproduced courtesy of Dr. Phil Bryant from "Pathological and nonpathological bodies" (https://www.pathologicalbodies.com/).*

diverticula that extend from the anal mucocutaneous junction between the anus and vagina; fluid as well as hair fragments and skin debris may be present in the lumen as an incidental finding. In males, the glans of the penis contains a ~1-cm-long os penis bone, and the seminal vesicles fill much of the caudal abdomen (Fig. 17.2).

Guinea pigs of both sexes have a few key physiological differences compared to other rodent species used in toxicity studies (Hargaden and Singer, 2012). Compared to mice and rats, guinea pig airways are more sensitive to acetylcholine and especially histamine, making them a good model for allergic hypersensitivity (asthma) studies. Guinea pigs practice coprophagy, and interference in this practice will lead to weight loss and reduced fiber digestion. This species lacks L-gulonolactone oxidase and thus (like primates, including humans) cannot synthesize vitamin C.

Several unusual hematologic qualities are characteristics of guinea pig. Erythrocytes in this species are larger than those of other rodents and sometimes exhibit polychromasia. Guinea pigs have heterophils (which function as

neutrophils) with eosinophilic cytoplasmic granules. Lymphocytes are the most prominent class of leukocytes (about 65%–70%) in circulation and tissues, and both small and large forms are found. One lymphocyte type (Foa-Kurloff cells) unique to guinea pigs is characterized by a very large, periodic acid-Schiff (PAS)-positive granular cytoplasmic body (Fig. 17.3). These cells are especially common in pregnancy, including within the placenta, and have natural killer (NK) cell capabilities.

Mongolian Gerbils

Mongolian gerbils (*M. unguiculatus*) are used infrequently in biomedical research, representing approximately 0.05% of research animals in the EU each year (European Commission). They have been proposed as a potential alternative rodent model for toxicity testing (Homburger et al., 1985). However, gerbils are fairly long lived compared to other rodent species and develop a wide spectrum of spontaneous tumors at fairly high frequency. These factors coupled with the scarcity of historical background data relegate gerbils to a secondary status as models for toxicologic research.

Gerbils exhibit several anatomic distinctions relative to other rodent species (Barthold et al., 2016; Batchelder et al., 2012). Both sexes have adrenal glands and thymuses that are substantially larger in comparison to other rodents. The thymus persists without involuting into adulthood. Both sexes have a large pair of sebaceous glands on the midventral abdomen; these "scent" glands are larger in males. The scent glands in males will exhibit an orange hue in maturity. Both sexes lack gall bladders, and males are missing preputial glands. The incomplete arterial circle (of Willis) at the base of the brain makes gerbils a popular model for investigating cerebral ischemia ("stroke"); this anatomic variation has no impact on the health in terms of spontaneous background findings or premature death. The circulating half-life of mature erythrocytes is very short (about 10 days) compared to other rodents, so polychromasia and reticulocytes are common (especially in animals up to 20 weeks of age). Lymphocytes are the most common leukocytes (75%–80%) in circulation.

Other Rodent Species

A number of additional rodent species including chinchillas, degus, gophers, prairie dogs, voles, and other species of mice (e.g., deer mouse) and rats (e.g., kangaroo rat, naked mole rat) are used in small numbers largely for specific areas of academic and discovery research (Donnelly et al., 2015). These species are not discussed further here since they are seldom used in toxicologic research. More details on their anatomic and physiological attributes may be gained from laboratory animal science references (Harkness et al., 2010; Suckow et al., 2012).

5. COMMON PATHOLOGIC FINDINGS IN RODENTS

Due to the exhaustive nature of the literature on background findings in rats and mice, and because these are the most popular rodent species used in toxicity testing, this section will examine some of the more frequent findings in these two species and highlight major findings in the other uncommon rodent species. Photomicrographs illustrating some of these changes are provided. Common causes of death (COD) or euthanasia for older rodents on life-time carcinogenicity studies also will be discussed. Further details regarding the changes described here as well as other background findings are given elsewhere (Johnson et al., 2019; McInnes, 2012).

5.1. Background Findings in Common Species—Mice and Rats

Incidental and Spontaneous Background Findings

Background (incidental or spontaneous) lesions are defined as pathology findings that represent a change in tissue morphology outside of the range of normal variation for a particular species or stock/strain (Long & Hardisty, 2012). The presence and severity of background lesions in laboratory animals are influenced by several intrinsic factors including genetic background (stock/strain), sex, and age as well as many extrinsic factors such as environmental conditions, husbandry procedures, and the presence or absence of particular microbes (both normal flora and pathogenic agents). Examples of the most common background nonneoplastic lesions encountered when evaluating rodent toxicity studies are shown in Table 17.4. Detailed descriptions, diagnostic criteria, and interpretive information for major findings in rodents are categorized in recent INHAND (International Harmonization of Nomenclature and Diagnostic Criteria) publications and are available (along with trimming guides, terminology updates, and additional images) online in parallel through the Global Open Registry Nomenclature Information System (goRENI, hosted at https://www.goreni.org/gr3_nomenclature.php) and the Society of Toxicologic Pathology (https://www.toxpath.org/inhand.asp#pubg). Expected incidences and the range of common nonproliferative changes and spontaneous tumors in various rodent species, stocks, and strain may be gleaned from many publications (Johnson et al., 2019; Maronpot, 1999; McInnes, 2012; Mohr et al., 1992; Mohr et al., 1996; Suttie, Leininger, & Bradley, 2018); from online databases (e.g., the Mouse Tumor Biology Database, http://tumor.informatics.jax.org); and also from historical control data generated in age- and sex-matched animals of the same stock or strain for different

TABLE 17.4　Common Background Nonneoplastic Lesions of the CD-1 Mouse and Wistar Han Rat

Organ	CD-1 mouse	Wistar Han rat
Heart	Myocardial mononuclear inflammatory cell infiltration	Myocardial mononuclear inflammatory cell infiltration
	Progressive cardiomyopathy	Progressive cardiomyopathy
	Focal mineralization of pulmonary arterial walls	Atrial thrombus
Adrenal glands	Focal subcapsular cell hyperplasia	Cystic degeneration of the cortex
	Persistent X zone	Focal medullary hyperplasia
	Focal cortical hypertrophy	
Bone	Degenerative joint disease	Degenerative joint disease
	Fibro-osseous lesion	
	Chondromucinous degeneration	
Nervous system	Cerebral mineralization	Axonal degeneration of the sciatic nerve
	Axonal degeneration of sciatic nerve	Demyelination of the spinal nerve roots
	Vacuolation of white matter	Squamous cysts in the brain
Eye	Retinal atrophy	Retinal atrophy
	Lens degeneration (cataract)	Lens degeneration (cataract)
	Mineralization (iris)	Retinal folds/rosettes
	Keratitis/corneal ulceration	Keratitis/corneal ulceration
Lung	Alveolar macrophage aggregation	Alveolar macrophage aggregation
	Focal bronchioloalveolar hyperplasia	Focal bronchioloalveolar hyperplasia
	Perivascular inflammatory cell infiltration	Perivascular inflammatory cell infiltration
Testis	Seminiferous tubule degeneration/atrophy	Seminiferous tubule degeneration/atrophy
	Rete testis hyperplasia	Focal interstitial (Leydig) cell hyperplasia
		Sperm granuloma
Ovary	Follicular cysts	Follicular cysts
	Bursal cysts	Bursal cysts
	Hemorrhagic cysts	Hyperplasia, sex cord stromal
	Angiectasis	
	Hyperplasia of sex cord stroma	
Uterus	Cystic endometrial hyperplasia	Cystic endometrial hyperplasia
	Age-related atrophy	Age-related atrophy

(*Continued*)

TABLE 17.4 Common Background Nonneoplastic Lesions of the CD-1 Mouse and Wistar Han Rat—cont'd

Organ	CD-1 mouse	Wistar Han rat
Kidney	Basophilic tubules	Basophilic tubules
	Hyaline nephropathy	Corticomedullary mineralization
	Chronic progressive nephropathy	Chronic progressive nephropathy
		Cortical scars
Liver	Nonregenerative hepatocyte hyperplasia	Foci of alteration
	Hepatocyte karyomegaly and cytomegaly	Cystic degeneration
	Bile duct hyperplasia	Bile duct hyperplasia
		Hepatocyte vacuolation
		Tension lipidosis
		Necrosis, hepatocyte

vendors and research facilities. Historical control data help to support the interpretation of common and uncommon findings (Deschl et al., 2002; Keenan et al., 2009).

Background lesions in rodents can be congenital, age-related, or can be caused by trauma or infectious agents. Congenital lesions are present at birth and represent abnormalities in normal embryogenesis and organ formation of the unborn animal. Major congenital lesions (e.g., cardiac malformations, neural tube closure defects) are lethal shortly after birth, but minor anomalies have no notable functional impact and can persist into adulthood. Common asymptomatic congenital lesions observed in adult rodents include ectopic tissue (e.g., thymus present among the thyroid follicles, parathyroid islands encircled by thymus); accessory cortical tissue present outside or immediately inside the adrenal gland capsule; and squamous cysts in the stomach and central nervous system.

Chronic progressive nephropathy (CPN, Fig. 17.4) and cardiomyopathy are the most common age-related background lesions in rats and mice. They are more common in rats than mice and are more common in male rats than females. The etiology and pathogenesis for both conditions remain areas of active research (Chanut et al., 2013; Hard et al., 2009; Obert and Frazier, 2019), but their occurrence and progression is influenced by several factors including genetic background (strain), sex, age, diet, and hormones. Importantly, these two changes may be exacerbated by test article administration during toxicity studies. Other background lesions influenced by aging include spontaneous tumors, which increase in frequency and variety in older animals (Carcinogenicity Assessment, Vol 2, Chap 5). Knowledge about the incidence, correct diagnosis, and classification of these naturally occurring tumors in control animals is critical to understanding whether an external treatment has caused an increased incidence of a particular tumor type (Hardisty, 1985).

Environmental conditions can induce, exacerbate, or cause an earlier onset of some background lesions. For example, spontaneous retinal degeneration develops in many strains of albino rats and mice as an aging change. Increased incidence, severity, or early occurrence of this lesion in rats and mice have been linked to overly intense ambient light levels in animal rooms (Fig. 17.5) and may be dependent on cage location. Retinal degeneration can also be induced or exacerbated by test article administration (De Vera Mudry et al., 2013). The microscopic morphology of toxicant-induced retinal degeneration is comparable to that of spontaneous age-related and light-induced degeneration, and this similarity may complicate interpretation in toxicity studies. In ad libitum-fed

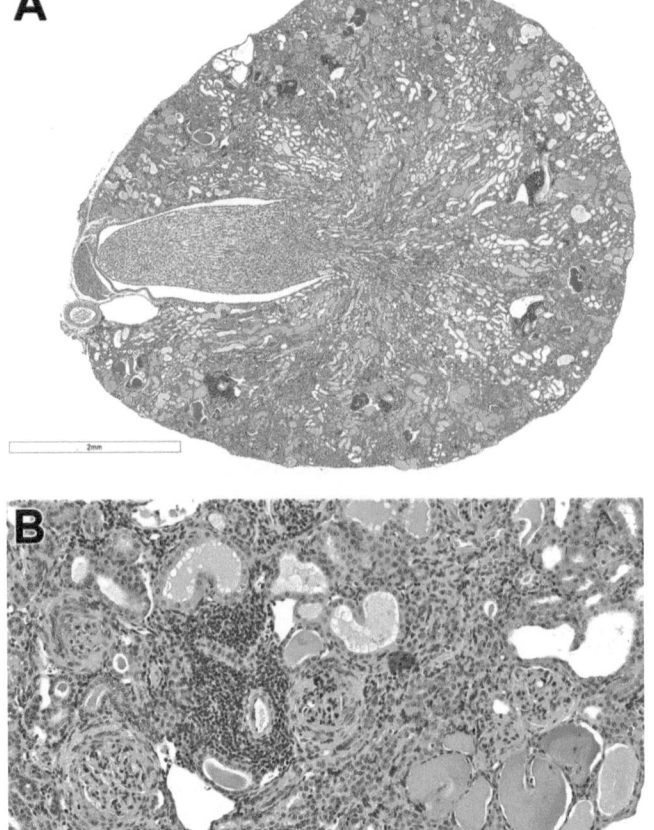

FIGURE 17.4 Age-related chronic progressive nephropathy (CPN) of the kidney in a Wistar Han rat. Low-power (A) and high-power (B) images show the characteristic thickening of the glomerular basement membranes, capillary tuft thickening, adhesions between glomerular epithelium and Bowman's capsule, glomerulosclerosis, tubular dilatation with numerous and prominent tubular casts, and inflammatory cell infiltration. H&E.

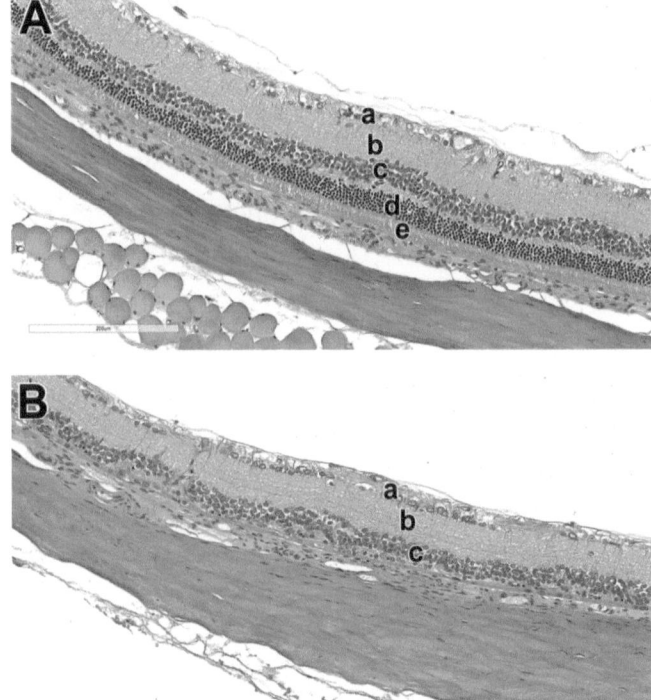

FIGURE 17.5 Relative to normal retina (A), marked retinal degeneration (B) in Wistar Han rats is characterized by complete loss of the outer nuclear layer (labeled d) and multifocal loss of the inner nuclear layer (labeled c). This incidental finding is induced by prolonged exposure to intense ambient light. Additional retinal layers: *a*, ganglion cell layer; *b*, inner plexiform layer; *e*, photoreceptor layer. H&E.

mice and rats, high caloric intake for extended periods can result in increased incidences of some spontaneous tumors including mammary gland and pituitary gland neoplasms (Keenan et al., 1996). This propensity may confound interpretation of tumor incidences in 2-year carcinogenicity studies where the test article has an influence on food intake and weight gain.

Some common background lesions in rats and mice are caused by infectious agents. For example, some immunocompetent mice such as the A/JCr strain are prone to developing chronic active hepatitis due to *Helicobacter hepaticus* infection (Ward, Fox, & Anver, 1994) (Fig. 17.6). This lesion is characterized by

perivascular, periportal, and hepatic parenchymal foci of lymphohistiocytic and plasmacytic cell infiltrates, which may induce hepatocyte necrosis and hyperplasia that can progress over time to hepatocellular adenoma and carcinoma (Ward, Fox, & Anver, 1994). Hepatocellular tumors in mice are one of the most common endpoints in bioassays for carcinogens and also are frequent age- and sex-dependent incidental findings in some mouse strains (Maronpot, 1999; Mohr et al., 1996), so the presence of pathogen-associated neoplasms superimposed on test article–related and spontaneous tumors further complicates data interpretation. Accumulation of alveolar macrophages and alveolar wall thickening in the lungs of immunocompetent, young Wistar Han rats have been shown to be associated with the presence of fungal (*Pneumocystis carinii*) DNA (Henderson et al., 2012). These lesions may

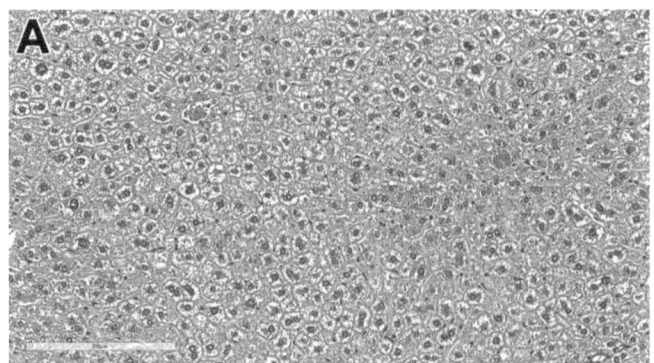

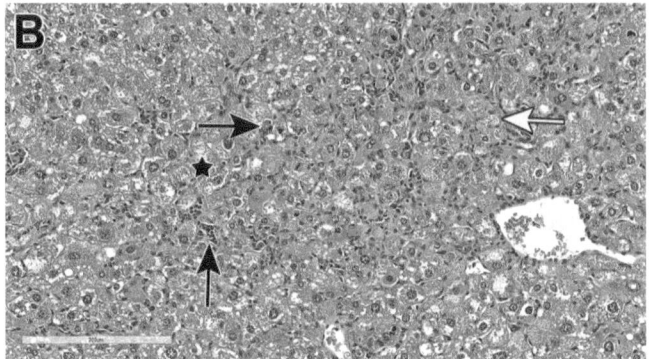

FIGURE 17.6 Relative to normal liver (A), chronic active inflammation ("hepatitis" [INHAND term: inflammatory cell infiltration, mixed], in (B) C57BL/6 mice associated with *Helicobacter hepaticus* infection features diffuse proliferation of sinusoidal lining cells, oval cell proliferation (INHAND term: oval cell hyperplasia, evident as clusters of small fusiform hepatic stem cells [white arrow]), hepatocytomegaly (hepatocyte enlargement [star]), single-cell necrosis (horizontal black arrow), and multifocal accumulation of mixed inflammatory cells (vertical black arrow). H&E.

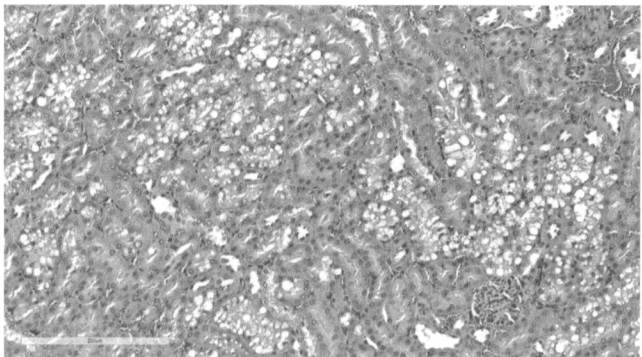

FIGURE 17.7 Incidental vacuolation in the kidney of C57BL/6 mice is characterized by clear vacuoles in the peripheral cortical tubule epithelium in the absence of any morphologic changes indicative of cell degeneration. This background finding occurs in some strains of male mice. H&E.

mask test article–related lung findings, particularly in inhalation toxicity studies.

Some background lesions may be specific to a particular rodent stock or strain and/or sex. For example, cytoplasmic vacuoles are normally present in the epithelium of peripheral renal cortical tubules of male mice in certain strains but are not typically present in female mice or rats (Fig. 17.7). This change may confound the interpretation of renal tubular vacuolation induced by some test articles such as osmotic agents, phospholipidosis-inducing cationic amphiphilic drug candidates, and cyclodextrins. Hair loss due to overgrooming (barbering, whisker trimming) occurs in some strains of mice as a social-dominant or stress-associated behavior, particularly from C57BL/6 and related

strains (Kalueff et al., 2006). These strains also are prone to developing ulcerative skin lesions (Sundberg et al., 2011).

Experimental procedures can result in some background findings that must be distinguished from test article–related lesions. For example, in inhalation studies, a higher incidence of testicular degeneration/atrophy develops in mice and rats because the animals are subjected to higher temperatures in the restraining tubes, resulting in thermal injury of the testis (Lee et al., 1993) (Fig. 17.8). Intravenous studies often produce increased numbers of foreign body granulomas in the lung as keratin and hair fragments are introduced from the skin into the blood by the injection procedure. Continuous infusion studies result in background lesions such as chronic inflammation, fibrosis, and foreign body granulomas in response to sutures and abscesses, thrombosis, and/or hemorrhage at the site of the catheter insertion into the blood vessel (Weber et al., 2011a). Blood collection from rodents using the retro-orbital venous sinus (behind the eye) or the sublingual vein (beneath the tongue) also produces areas of inflammation in the optic nerve and ventral tongue as well as occasional nerve fiber degeneration in the nearby optic nerve. Reflux of gastric contents after gavage dosing may result in nasal turbinate changes in rats including necrosis, purulent inflammation of nasal passages, and mortality (Damsch et al., 2011).

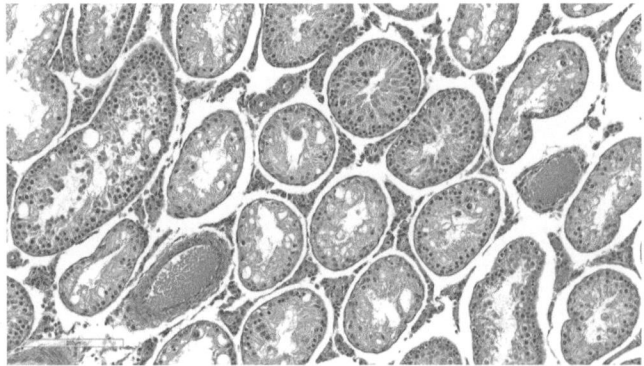

FIGURE 17.8 Testicular degeneration in Wistar Han rats is characterized by degeneration, vacuolation, exfoliation, and atrophy of the germinal epithelium present to varying degrees in multiple tubular profiles in the image. This change may be observed during inhalation studies when males are exposed to high temperatures for extended periods (e.g., 6 h a day, 5 days per week for 3 months) when they are kept in restraining tubes for chemical exposure. H&E.

Background findings in rodents may be traumatic in origin. Common effects include fractures (especially of digits and tails) and bite wounds. Gavage injury is not a background change as such but is a commonly encountered incidental finding resulting from mechanical damage to the esophagus and surrounding mediastinal and sometimes pleural tissues. This procedure-related effect results from penetration of the gavage tube through the wall of the esophagus; it is not a manifestation of test article toxicity.

Background findings may be associated with variations in physiological status, especially with sexual maturity and reproductive senescence. Substantial differences in the appearance of the reproductive organs in both sexes of mice and rats occur due to normal reproductive cyclicity or aging. Examples include estrus-associated changes in females and divergent sperm stages in seminiferous tubules of males. Normal physiological processes in rodents also result in prominent EMH in the spleen and liver, persistently open growth plates (physes) in the long bones, continuous eruption of incisor teeth, and substantial thymic involution. These changes are not lesions but rather represent expected steady-state presentations (bones, liver, spleen, teeth) or intermittent fluctuations (gonads) in organ morphology. Test articles

may alter the appearance of these findings (e.g., by inducing growth plate closure or reducing EMH or estrus cycling).

Stress is a normal physiological adaptive response, but in excess the stress-associated hormones may impact homeostatic processes in many organs. Stress during animal studies may be caused by noise, changes in environmental conditions (temperature and relative humidity), handling (frequency and roughness), dosing (frequency and route), restraint, sample collections, transport, and group housing of animals ((Everds et al., 2013) and *Issues in Laboratory Animal Science that Impact Toxicologic Pathology*, Vol 1, Chap 29). Stress alone may cause reduced total body weights or body weight gain, reduced food consumption, changed organ weights (e.g., decreased spleen and thymus weights, increased adrenal weight), lymphocyte depletion (spleen and thymus), increased or decreased leucocyte levels in the blood, gastric ulceration, and possibly reproductive organ atrophy (Everds et al., 2013). Test articles may be additive or even synergistic with stress in eliciting such changes.

5.2. Background Findings in Uncommon Rodent Species

Syrian Hamsters

Hamsters commonly develop a number of incidental nonneoplastic findings (Barthold et al., 2016; Karolweski et al., 2012). Many findings increase in frequency and severity with age, and the incidences often vary among colonies. AA amyloidosis is common in hamsters (Shtrasburg et al., 2005), occurs as early as 5 months of age, tends to affect the kidney (Fig. 17.9) and liver and to a lesser extent the adrenal gland, and is more common in females. This disease does cause mortality in animals >15 months of age, typically due to renal glomerular lesions. The rise in serum globulins associated with progressive amyloidosis suggests that chronic inflammation is a likely inciting cause for amyloid deposition in this species. Glomerulonephropathy (Fig. 17.9) is a common cause of both morbidity and mortality in aged hamsters. Typical findings of this renal disease include tubular dilation and increased interstitial connective tissue;

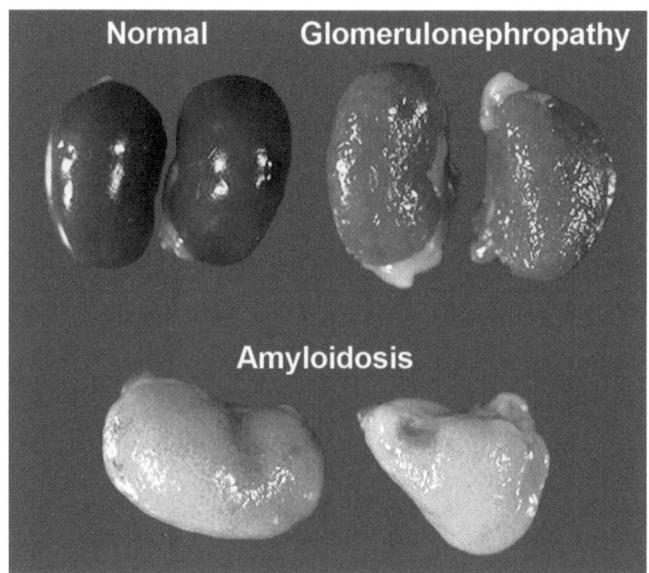

FIGURE 17.9 Montage of kidneys from adult Syrian hamsters comparing normal macroscopic features (dark red brown with smooth surface) in the kidneys in the upper left with the gross appearance of two spontaneous renal diseases: amyloidosis (pale tan with smooth surface [bottom row]) and glomerulonephropathy (pale brown with pitted surface [upper right]). *Reproduced from Noah's Arkive (Image No. F27666) by courtesy of the Davis Thompson DVM Foundation.*

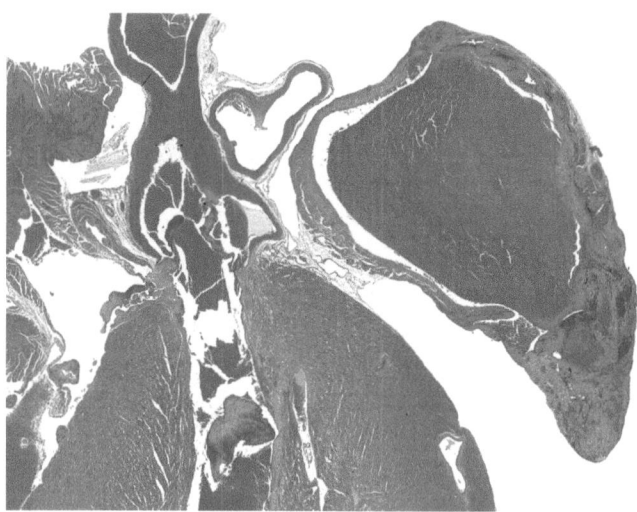

FIGURE 17.10 Thrombosis of the left atrium in the heart of a hamster. H&E. *Reproduced from Figure 4 of McInnes EF, Ernst H, Germann PG: Spontaneous nonneoplastic lesions in control Syrian hamsters in three 24-month long-term carcinogenicity studies, Toxicol Pathol 43:272–281, 2015, by permission of Sage Publications.*

glomerular changes, protein casts, and inflammation occur inconsistently. Atrial thrombosis—more often of the left atrium (Fig. 17.10)—is common in hamsters >1 year of age, ranging in frequency from 16% to 73% in reports from various colonies. Males and females are equally affected, but females tend to be affected earlier. Polycystic liver disease is often seen in hamsters >6 months of age. The origin of the cysts (hepatic sinusoids vs. bile ducts) is not clear. Interestingly, cysts are often seen in other organs including the pancreas and reproductive organs of both sexes.

Spontaneous tumors are uncommon in hamsters relative to mice and rats (Karolweski et al., 2012). Neoplasms tend to occur more often in females. The most common type is lymphoma, but adrenal tumors, intestinal adenocarcinomas, and melanomas also are well represented.

Guinea Pigs

Several classic nonneoplastic and neoplastic entities have been described in guinea pigs (Barthold et al., 2016; Williams, 2012).

Rhabdomyomatosis (sometimes called cardiac glycogenosis) occurs as well-defined pale myocardial foci in which swollen myocytes contain excessive cytoplasmic glycogen (Fig. 17.11). This change may occur anywhere in the heart but is especially prominent in the subendocardial region of the left ventricle; it may be seen in animals of all ages. In the lung, thickening of vascular musculature in arteries and arterioles as well as osseous metaplasia (including bone marrow) in the alveolar parenchyma, but with no or very little inflammation, is a common incidental finding. In the digestive tract, malocclusion of the incisors, gastric dilation and volvulus, and gastric ulcers develop with some frequency, with the latter usually arising secondary to an infection rather than from stress. Antibiotic-associated typhlocolitis is a well-documented outcome of administering broad-spectrum antibiotics; the resulting changes to the microbiota yield severe dysbiosis with overgrowth of Gram-negative bacteria, massive distension of the cecum with gas and fluid, and widespread mucosal hemorrhage and necrosis. Chronic interstitial nephritis is present in most animals 3 years of age or older, and urolithiasis is common in females. Hemorrhage is indicative of blood vessel wall fragility due to vitamin C deficiency ("scurvy") and

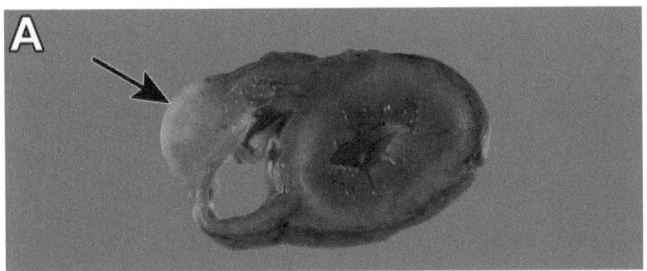

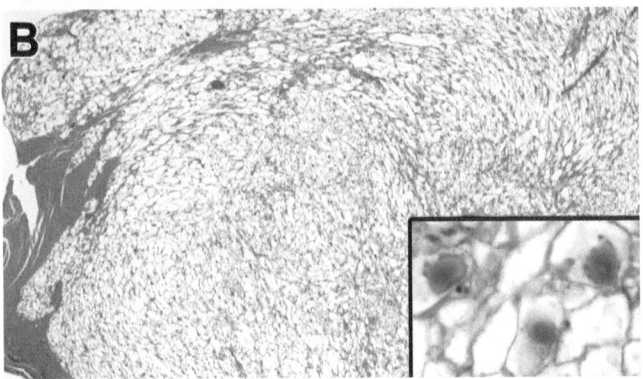

FIGURE 17.11 Macroscopic (A) and microscopic (B) appearance of rhabdomyomatosis, presenting here as a single nodule (arrow) in the right ventricular wall comprised of closely packed, vacuolated cells (H&E), some of which (inset) contain glycogen granules (stained pink by periodic acid-Schiff [PAS]). *Reproduced from Figures 1 and 2 of Kobayashi T, Kobayashi Y, Fukuda U, et al.: A cardiac rhabdomyoma in a Guinea pig,* J Toxicol Pathol 23:107–110, 2010, *by permission of the Japanese Society of Toxicologic Pathology (JSTP) under the terms of a Creative Commons BY-NC-ND license.*

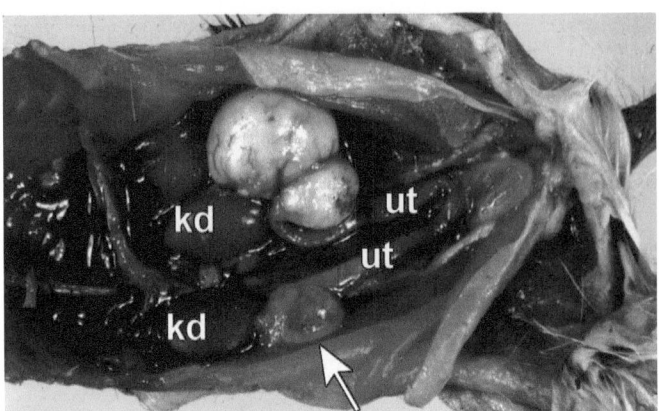

FIGURE 17.12 Caudal abdomen of an aged, adult female Mongolian gerbil showing bilateral ovarian lesions: a prominent white, multilobular granulosa cell tumor above (just caudal to the kidney [kd]) and a large cyst below (arrow). Abbreviation: ut = uterine horn. *Reproduced from Noah's Arkive (Image No. F00997) by courtesy of the Davis Thompson DVM Foundation.*

tends to develop near mobile interfaces such as the costochondral junctions and major joints. Degenerative joint disease ("osteoarthritis") appears at about 3 months of age in femorotibial (stifle or "knee") joints and progresses with age, especially in obese animals. Pododermatitis is common in heavy animals kept in unsanitary conditions, usually reflects a secondary bacterial infection, and like other chronic inflammatory conditions can lead to systemic AA amyloidosis in the kidney, liver, and spleen.

Neoplasms are rare as incidental findings in most organs of guinea pigs. Bronchogenic tumors (mainly papillary adenomas) are reported to occur in up to 35% of older animals. Skin and mammary gland tumors are also common (about 30% of older animals), with the most common variants being the trichofolliculoma (i.e., a benign epithelial neoplasm arising from the

pilosebaceous unit) and mammary gland fibroadenoma and less frequently mammary gland adenocarcinoma. Reproductive tract masses in females account for about 25% of neoplasms in this species and mainly consist of ovarian granulosa cell tumors and teratomas as well as uterine leiomyomas.

Mongolian Gerbils

Background findings in gerbils typically occur in older animals (Barthold et al., 2016; Batchelder et al., 2012) and are uncommon compared to mice and rats. Aural cholesteatomas can form in the ear canal and may be associated clinically with circling, head tilting, and scratching. Chronic interstitial nephritis often develops in older animals. Females over 1 year of age exhibit a high incidence of ovarian cysts (Fig. 17.12). The most common spontaneous tumors are granulosa cell tumors of the ovary (Fig. 17.12) and squamous cell carcinomas of the scent glands.

5.3. Considerations in Evaluating Incidental Background Findings

Terminology for Common Nonproliferative and Proliferative Findings in Rodents

The use of lexicons of standardized terms is helpful in generating incidence data for lesions encountered in toxicologic pathology

(*Nomenclature and Diagnostic Resources in Anatomic Toxicologic Pathology*, Vol 1, Chap 25). These lexicons can be established for macroscopic and microscopic data. Nomenclature conventions may be specific to an individual laboratory or contract research organization, or may adopt a more widely recognized terminology (e.g., INHAND) allowing for easier comparison between pathology studies and reports performed in different laboratories of the same company or across distant institutions or diagnostic service providers (McInnes and Scudamore, 2014). Regulatory agencies now recommend using harmonized nomenclature when feasible, and in some cases are mandating this practice (e.g., the Food and Drug Administration requirement that data sets for toxicity studies be submitted using the Standard for Exchange of Nonclinical Data [SEND] format). INHAND diagnostic terminology is available for mice and rats for all major organs and systems, and these terms are incorporated into the SEND lexicon.

Although accurate pathology reporting implies that pathologists preferentially use terms that have been harmonized among other pathologists, diagnostic terminology for incidental and test article–related findings continues to evolve (Elmore et al., 2018; Shackelford et al., 2002). Furthermore, historically several terms may exist for the same lesion, and sometimes pathologists will use different terms for a single finding within a given study ("diagnostic drift"). Such terminological shifts can confound study interpretation and make database population and the subsequent accurate retrieval of historical control data challenging. Therefore, effort should be made, at least within laboratories, to define and use a single term for each finding. For instance, cystic degeneration of various lymph nodes (observed as a background finding in rats) is also known as sinus dilatation, lymphangiectasia, cystic ectasia, lymphatic sinus ectasia, lymphangiectasis, or lymphatic cysts; the preferred INHAND term is now "dilatation, sinus" (Willard-Mack et al., 2019). A related issue is that some rodent pathologists separately diagnose the individual components of some global conditions (e.g., basophilia of tubular epithelium, thickening of peritubular basement membranes, interstitial mononuclear inflammatory cell infiltration, and hyaline casts instead

of the comprehensive term "CPN"). In most cases, diagnostic consolidation ("lumping") rather than generating separate entries for mechanistically related changes ("splitting") is preferred for rodent toxicity studies as a means of simplifying the histopathologic data set and resulting interpretation.

However, the merging of too many findings under a single term may mask a treatment-related finding, particularly in long-term studies (Shackelford et al., 2002). For instance, a pathologist may use the term "cardiomyopathy" to indicate a lesion comprised of various degrees of myocardial necrosis, myocardial fibrosis, and myocardial inflammatory cell infiltration (Fig. 17.13). If there is an increase in only one component of cardiomyopathy (e.g., myocardial necrosis), this isolated change may not be recorded separately. Therefore, there may or may not be a concomitant increase in cardiomyopathy in the treated animals, and the treatment-related finding may be missed. Such unintended combining of two lesions with mechanistically distinct pathogeneses may be minimized by employing the correct nomenclature for each finding (as stated in the most up-to-date online "List of published terms with modifications"

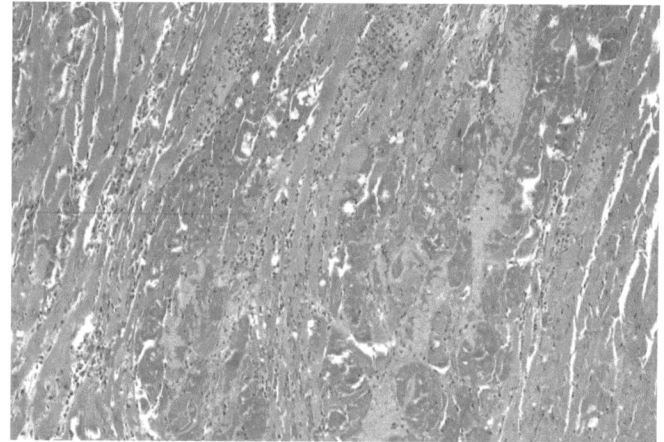

FIGURE 17.13 Chronic progressive cardiomyopathy in the heart of an adult mouse features reduced numbers of cardiomyocytes that often are necrotic (evident as hypereosinophilic [dark pink] and fragmented cells) and are associated with fibrosis (pale eosinophilic material) and mixed inflammatory cell infiltrates in the adjacent interstitium. H&E. *Reproduced from Noah's Arkive (Image No. F24955) by courtesy of the Davis Thompson DVM Foundation.*

found at https://www.goreni.org/gr3_nomenclature.php). In this regard, the diagnosis "rodent progressive cardiomyopathy" is assigned to the composite condition (Fig. 17.13) while "necrosis, cardiomyocyte" is used for the stand-alone change.

Thresholds, Diagnostic Drift, and Objectivity in Histopathological Evaluation

Although the primary goal of the toxicologic pathologist is to identify treatment-related findings, they will encounter many changes in tissues that are variations in normal tissue morphology as well as tissue artifacts and spontaneous background findings that might obscure subtle test article–induced changes (Long & Hardisty, 2012). A common means of improving the accuracy of a pathology data set by facilitating analysis and interpretation is to develop a threshold (i.e., deciding which morphologic variations are considered to be "within normal limits" and which will be recorded as diagnoses of potential consequence) prior to evaluating a set of tissue sections. Thresholds, diagnostic terminology, and severity grading of background findings should not be significantly changed from study to study in order to produce meaningful reports. Inconsistent application of thresholds will preclude accurate comparison of study results or historical control data. If the diagnostic threshold is set too high, treatment-related findings may be missed. If the threshold is set too low, complex and confusing data will be generated creating the appearance of differences where none exist (Long & Hardisty, 2012).

Consistency in reporting background variations as well as treatment- or disease-related findings is essential for accurate pathology reporting (see *Practices to Optimize Generation, Interpretation, and Reporting of Pathology Data from Toxicity Studies*, Vol 1, Chap 28). Diagnostic drift occurs when lesion nomenclature and/or severity grades gradually shift over time (Crissman et al., 2004). Diagnostic drift and inconsistent threshold application are most likely to occur during the microscopic evaluation of very long-term studies like 2-year rodent carcinogenicity bioassays where thousands of tissues from many hundreds of mice or rats require several months for the assessment. In these cases, the pathologist may start a study by ignoring a particular lesion but over

time may gradually either (i) start recording it as he/she encounters the finding more often during a study or becomes interested in the lesion (i.e., change in threshold) or (ii) give the lesion a different diagnostic term or severity grade later in the study than was assigned to similar findings seen earlier during the evaluation. If the toxicologic pathologist tends to examine the controls first (to set the threshold) and the high-dose treated animals last—a not uncommon practice when evaluating rodent toxicity studies—then a set of data may arise in which it appears that only the treated animals appear to have the particular lesion. Diagnostic drift can be avoided if the pathologist ensures that animals from various dose groups and controls are examined each day (Shackelford et al., 2002).

Sources of Variability in Rodent Lesions

Background findings are influenced by an extensive list of variables. Factors related to the in-life portion of the study include the choice of vehicle (for example, when corn oil is used as a vehicle in gavage studies, oil droplets may be seen in the lung after gastric reflux or gastric lavage); route of administration (gastric gavage administration may cause background procedure-related lesions including esophagitis and mucosal trauma); animal room environment (prolonged high-intensity lighting may cause retinal atrophy in all animals, but especially those spending more time on the top shelves near the light arrays); diet and body weight (ad libitum feeding is associated with increases in tumor numbers in mice and rats, and the incidence and severity of rodent progressive cardiomyopathy in rats); age (older animals often will have an increased number and severity of background lesions, such as CPN in male rats); and sex (group-housed male animals often have fighting wounds) (Haseman et al., 1989). Parameters during the postmortem phase also may impact the consistency of the pathology data set, including such factors as gross necropsy techniques (artifacts such as crush ["pinch"] defects in soft tissues may be caused by excessive or rough handling of tissues with forceps); pathology sampling procedures (missing tissues, or missing structures affected by trimming procedures [e.g., adrenal medulla, accessory sex organs] may affect the number of lesions recorded for one or more groups); preparation of the histology slides (creation of artifacts such as folds, tears, or inclusion of cotton lint or stain precipitate in or over tissue sections) (Haseman et al., 1989); and diagnostic drift (use of different terms for the same histopathologic lesion) (Haseman, 1995). While such issues in the pathologic analysis are not limited to rodent toxicity studies, the large number of animals per study coupled with the diminutive size of rodent organs means that even seemingly small lapses in the pathology and histology portions of the study may create fairly large gaps in rodent tissue sections. Such defects may reduce the collective quality of the tissue sections that are available for analysis, thereby damaging the accuracy of the final data set and interpretation. For more information, see *Practices that Optimize Generation, Interpretation, and Reporting of Pathology Data from Toxicity Studies*, Vol 1, Chap 28.

Many factors in the study design may influence the variability in the occurrence of spontaneous (background) tumors in control laboratory rodents. Major parameters include the animal stock or strain used (for example, F344 rats are predisposed to LGL leukemia and testicular tumors, while some 129-derived mouse substrains exhibit a high [>30%] background incidence of teratomas [Fig. 17.14]); diagnostic criteria and thresholds (e.g., inconsistency in recording certain background findings like altered hepatic foci [also termed "foci of cellular alteration"] or small areas of adrenal cortical hyperplasia because they are so common); and the extent of pathology peer review for putative proliferative findings in control animals in verifying the accuracy of the pathology data set (Hardisty, 1985). Unexpected factors such as lighting, stress of handling, and housing may alter endocrine patterns and thus affect the development of spontaneous tumors (Hardisty, 1985). Historical control tumor data may be useful for detecting rare tumors and for borderline effects (Haseman, 1995; Haseman et al., 1997).

Guides have been published for standardized organ sampling and trimming in rats and mice (Kittel et al., 2004; Morawietz et al., 2004; Ruehl-Fehlert et al., 2003) with additional information at the goRENI site (https://www.goreni.org/gr3_nomenclature.php). Efforts to

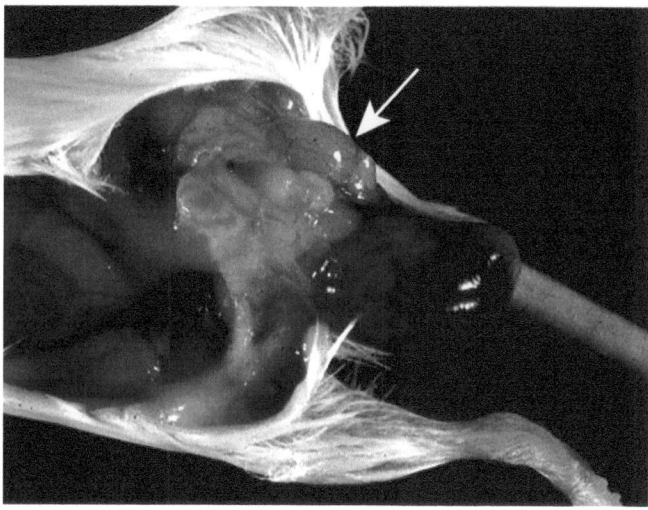

FIGURE 17.14 Testicular teratoma in an adult mouse, superimposed over the tail as a mottled, large brown mass. The opposite testis (arrow) is of normal size and pale tan color. *Reproduced from Noah's Arkive (Image No. F08447) by courtesy of the Davis Thompson DVM Foundation.*

maximize consistency in such tasks are essential since variation in background findings for rodent studies may occur due to differences in transverse or longitudinal sectioning of a given tissue (especially large, anatomically asymmetrical organs such as brain and lung). For example, a greater incidence of thyroid tumors may be detected in rodents if the organ is sectioned in a longitudinal orientation, and the number and severity of prostate lesions may increase if the gland is sectioned so that all lobes are available for evaluation rather than in a haphazard fashion (Suwa et al., 2002; Suwa et al., 2001).

Pathologist experience is a significant factor in producing variability in reporting background findings among control animals in different studies. In general, experienced pathologists recognize the range of morphological evaluation that is "within normal limits" for various rodent tissues, especially for those where the incidence and/or severity may vary among strains (such as dystrophic epicardial mineralization, which is more common in the BALB/c, C3H, and DBA/2 strains) (Keenan et al., 2009), and may record fewer background findings than less experienced pathologists. However, the context of any given study may vary, particularly if the pathologist is working with multiple laboratories with different threshold criteria for recording background findings. Pathologists may disagree regarding the diagnosis of proliferative lesions in rodents (especially those of epithelial origin where there is a continuum of progression for lesions) as hyperplasia versus benign tumor or as a benign tumor versus well-differentiated but malignant tumor (Hardisty, 1985). Ultimately, such disputed diagnoses need to be settled in order to interpret the study outcome, and close calls may need to be adjudicated by an expert pathology working group (PWG) that assigns diagnoses by coded ("blinded") histopathologic evaluation and majority vote (*Pathology Peer Review,* Vol 1, Chap 26).

Historical Control Data

Concurrent control animals are always the best comparison to assess treatment-related effects in a single study (Haseman et al., 1984). However, concurrent controls are sometimes not used as the sole reference standard for a study (Long & Hardisty, 2012). This is because considerable differences may exist among control animals in one particular study, and the pathologists and regulatory authorities may then wish to consult historical control animal data for comparison. The utilization of historical control data, while not specific to rodent disease models and toxicity studies, is particularly useful in the interpretation of studies with large numbers of animals (e.g., rodent 6-month or life-time carcinogenicity studies) and in studies with low numbers of animals (Long & Hardisty, 2012). Historical control tumor data may also be useful for detecting rare tumors and for distinguishing borderline effects (Haseman, 1995; Haseman et al., 1997).

Causes of Death or Morbidity in Rats and Mice

Animals that are found dead during the experiment or are removed from the study on welfare grounds and euthanized should have a major factor contributing to death or premature demise attributed to them by the pathologist after light microscopic examination of the tissues. It is important to establish whether the COD in any experimental study is treatment-related, a concept that is well understood in toxicity studies but may be ignored in other settings (thus contributing to poor reproducibility of data). In some instances, advanced autolysis or the absence of any obvious lesions may preclude assignment of a COD. Factors contributory to death are identified based on the most prominent major disease process that might lead to morbidity and eventually death of the animal. In most cases, these lethal lesions are either age-related, nonneoplastic conditions like CPN in male rats or neoplastic conditions such as pituitary gland adenomas in female rats and LGL leukemia in F344 rats. Common COD in outbred mice (CD-1) and rats (Wistar Han) from life-time carcinogenicity bioassays and in engineered Tg-rasH2 (specifically CByB6F1-Tg(HRAS)2Jic) mice from 26-week carcinogenicity studies are shown in Table 17.5. The incidence of these findings, including spontaneous tumors, and their age of occurrence is influenced by several factors such as strain, sex, age, diet, and hormones.

Common causes of premature death in mice result from damage in key viscera like heart and kidney. Renal pathology is one of the most common nonneoplastic COD or morbidities (McInnes and Scudamore, 2015). Murine urologic syndrome (i.e., obstructive uropathy [Fig. 17.15]) in male mice is often associated with fighting in multiple-housed male mice, while chronic nephropathy occurs in some male mice though to a lesser degree than in male rats. Other reported nonneoplastic COD in mice include degenerative lesions such as hemorrhagic cardiomyopathy or extensive inflammation (e.g., dermatitis or arteritis/periarteritis), or acute or chronic hemorrhage from ovarian and uterine lesions. Common neoplastic conditions resulting in death of mice include such malignant tumors as bronchioloalveolar carcinoma, fibrosarcoma, hemangiosarcoma, and lymphoma. Some tumors (e.g., hepatocellular carcinoma) may cause no significant clinical signs even though they may reach a very large size, while certain benign tumors may cause significant clinical signs leading to euthanasia of the moribund animal (such as Harderian gland adenomas located behind the eye, which cause protrusion of the globe and subsequent corneal and conjunctival desiccation, trauma, and infection).

Similar causes of premature death in rats impact the function of major organs like brain,

TABLE 17.5 Common Major Factors Contributing to the Cause of Death in Laboratory Rodents

CD-1 mice[a]		Wistar Han rat[a]		Tg-rasH2 (CByB6F1-Tg(HRAS)2Jic) mice[b]	
Male	Female	Male	Female	Male	Female
NEOPLASTIC					
Bronchioloalveolar tumors	Lymphoma	Pituitary adenoma/carcinoma	Pituitary adenoma/carcinoma	Squamous cell carcinoma	Bronchioloalveolar tumors
Fibrosarcoma (skin)	Fibrosarcoma (skin)	Sarcomas of the skin	Mammary adenoma/carcinomas	Hemangiosarcoma	Hemangiosarcoma
Histiocytic sarcoma	Hemangiosarcoma	Lymphoma	Astrocytoma	Bronchioloalveolar tumors	
Hemangiosarcoma	Pituitary adenoma/carcinoma	Amelanotic melanoma	Mammary fibroadenoma	Liposarcoma	
Lymphoma	Hepatocellular carcinoma	Mesothelioma	Granular cell tumor (brain)	Lymphoma	
Hepatocellular carcinoma	Harderian gland adenoma	Oligodendroglioma	Schwannoma		
Harderian adenoma	Histiocytic sarcoma	Osteosarcoma	Osteosarcoma		
	Bronchioloalveolar tumors	Thymoma			
NONNEOPLASTIC					
Urologic syndrome	Dermatitis	Chronic progressive nephropathy	Chronic progressive nephropathy	Dermatitis	Liver necrosis
Dermatitis	Nephropathy	Abscess	Pododermatitis	Urologic syndrome	
Nephropathy	Hemorrhagic cyst (ovary)	Ocular lesions	Dermatitis		
Atrial thrombosis	Uterine thrombosis	Dermatitis			
Arteritis/periarteritis	Atrial thrombosis	Preputial gland inflammation			
Atrial thrombosis	Arteritis/periarteritis				

[a] Data taken from animals found dead or euthanized prematurely due to morbidity during 104-week carcinogenicity studies.
[b] Data taken from animals found dead or euthanized prematurely due to morbidity during 26-week carcinogenicity studies.

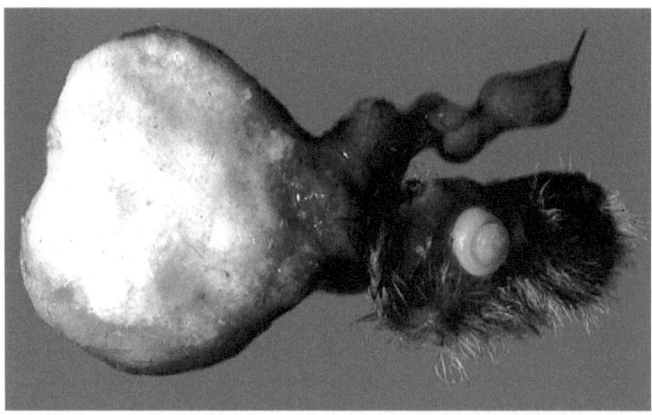

FIGURE 17.15   Mouse urologic syndrome in the lower urinary tract of an adult male mouse showing myriad white, sand-like calculi within the opened urinary bladder with markedly thickened walls (left aspect of image). The tip of the penis is extruded from the prepuce (right side of image), indicating that the animal was straining to urinate due to one or more calculi lodged within the urethra. *Reproduced from Noah's Arkive (Image No. F04224) by courtesy of the Davis Thompson DVM Foundation.*

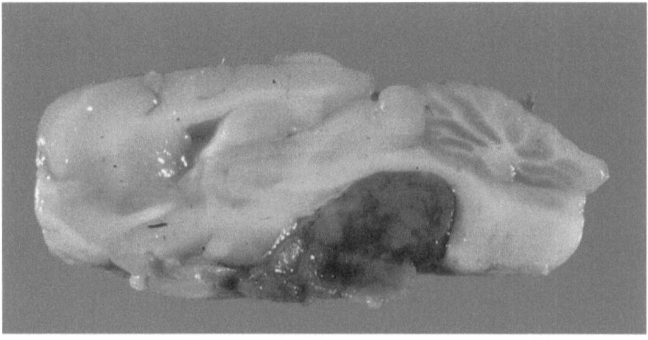

FIGURE 17.16   Pituitary gland adenoma in an adult rat, resulting in substantial compression of the ventral brain and flattening of the dorsal cerebellar surface. H&E. *Reproduced from Noah's Arkive (Image No. F25476) by courtesy of the Davis Thompson DVM Foundation.*

heart, and kidney. CPN is one of the most common causes of nonneoplastic death or morbidity in older male rats. Pituitary gland and mammary gland tumors are the most common COD in male and especially female rats in 2-year carcinogenicity studies; large adenomas of these tissues often lead to brain compression (Fig. 17.16) or ulceration and infection of the overlying skin, respectively. In many

instances, the technical COD is euthanasia due to a decision driven by impact on animal welfare (e.g., an animal with large mammary fibroadenoma) rather than because the lesion directly causes the unscheduled death of an animal in its cage.

6. CONCLUSION

Laboratory rodents, predominantly mice and rats, are the keystone animal models in biomedical research, including toxicology, where they are the first species to be considered for in vivo toxicity and combined efficacy/toxicity studies. Other rodent species, including hamsters, guinea pigs, and Mongolian gerbils, are also used on occasion to address special questions in biomedical and toxicologic research.

Rodents are preferred species for biomedical and toxicological research for many reasons. Major advantages include their basic biological characteristics (e.g., small size, accelerated lifespan, short gestation period, large litter size), which together support study designs with larger group sizes extending over more life phases than are possible with nonrodent species. A multitude of rodent outbred stocks and inbred strains have been generated, especially for mice and rats. Stocks (e.g., CD-1 mice, SD and Wistar Han rats) have increased genetic heterozygosity, making them more similar to the typical human population; this attribute makes outbred mouse and rat stocks common choices for toxicity studies. Strains are genetically identical (homozygous) and may be used (especially mice) for toxicity testing, but also are critical in efficacy/safety study paradigms that employ highly reproducible disease models. Profiles of xenobiotic ADME in rodent models commonly used in toxicology make them suitable for a wide range of investigations, from acute to chronic toxicity studies as well as abbreviated (6 month, using certain genetically engineered mouse strains) and life-time (up to 2 year) carcinogenicity bioassays. Rodent models often exhibit consistent well-characterized phenotypes and pathophysiological alterations that can provide insights in a practicable time frame regarding disease progression and molecular mechanisms of relevance to human patients with similar diseases. Finally, genetic manipulation to introduce (transgenic), remove ("knock out"), or replace ("knock in") key molecules performing critical functions also allows insight into pathobiology associated with altered expression of proteins in an in vivo context, with applications ranging from target validation, humanizing targets or pathways, generating monogenic and polygenic disease models, and investigating on-target (desired or exaggerated pharmacology) and off-target ("toxic") effects. Numerous RMD are essential tools for increasing our basic pathobiological knowledge, in generating efficacy-related data for new medicines, and in providing focused safety-relevant information early in product discovery and development, prior to standard toxicity studies.

Pathologic evaluation in toxicologic research is supported by extensive background data for many rodent stocks and strains. Knowledge of historical control data often informs the study pathologist's decisions regarding where to set diagnostic thresholds and how to interpret their relevance for changes observed in rodent toxicity studies. It is important to appreciate the multiple intrinsic (e.g., genetic) and extrinsic (e.g., environmental, procedural, commensal, and pathogenic organisms) parameters that can be confounding factors which increase the range and variability in pathological findings, influence mortality, and may affect translational relevance of model data to humans. Fortunately, normal biological variation as well as spontaneous, husbandry-related, infectious, and toxicant-induced changes has been extensively characterized in mice and rats for many anatomic pathology (Barthold et al., 2016; Gopinath and Mowat, 2014; Harkness et al., 2010; Maronpot, 1999; McInnes, 2012; Mohr et al., 1992; Mohr et al., 1996; Sahota et al., 2019; Suttie, Leininger, & Bradley, 2018) and clinical pathology (Kurtz and Travlos, 2018; Provencher Bolliger et al., 2010) endpoints. Such historical data are valuable in establishing the spectra of incidental (background) versus confounding (husbandry, experimental procedure or infectious) versus test article–related (toxicologic) pathology that may be expected in a given rodent model. Knowledge regarding the "normal" (or "within normal limits") range of tissue- and fluid-based alterations may guide selection of the most suitable stock or strain for routine rodent toxicity

studies and support the interpretation of pathologic findings as adverse and/or significant.

Acknowledgments

Noah's Arkive images are provided by courtesy of the Charles Louis Davis and Samuel Wesley Thompson DVM Foundation for the Advancement of Veterinary and Comparative Pathology (hosted at http://noahsarkive.cldavis.org/cgi-bin/show_image_info_page.cgi) and are reproduced under a Creative Commons BY-NC-SA license.

REFERENCES

Aziz RK, Hegazy SM, Yasser R, et al.: Drug pharmacomicrobiomics and toxicomicrobiomics: from scattered reports to systematic studies of drug-microbiome interactions, *Expert Opin Drug Metab Toxicol* 14:1043–1055, 2018.

Baldrick P: Getting a molecule into the clinic: nonclinical testing and starting dose considerations, *Regul Toxicol Pharmacol* 89:95–100, 2017.

Barthold SW, Griffey SM, Percy DH: *Pathology of laboratory rodents and rabbits*, 4th ed., Ames, IA, 2016, Wiley Blackwell.

Batchelder M, Keller LS, Sauer MB, et al.: Gerbils. In Suckow MA, Stevens KA, Wilson RP, editors: *The laboratory rabbit, Guinea pig, hamster, and other rodents*, San Diego, 2012, Academic Press (Elsevier), pp 1131–1155.

Blanset D, Hutt J, Morgan SE: Current use of animal models of disease for nonclinical safety testing, *Curr Opin Toxicol* 23–24:11–16, 2020.

Bogdanffy MS, Lesniak J, Mangipudy R, et al.: Tg.rasH2 mouse model for assessing carcinogenic potential of pharmaceuticals: industry survey of current practices, *Int J Toxicol* 39:198–206, 2020.

Bolon B: Genetically engineered animals in drug discovery and development: a maturing resource for toxicologic research, *Basic Clin Pharmacol Toxicol* 95:154–161, 2004.

Brayton CF, Treuting PM, Ward JM: Pathobiology of aging mice and GEM: background strains and experimental design, *Vet Pathol* 49:85–105, 2012.

Brennan FR, Cavagnaro J, McKeever K, et al.: Safety testing of monoclonal antibodies in non-human primates: case studies highlighting their impact on human risk assessment, *MAbs* 10:1–17, 2018.

Brower M, Grace M, Kotz CM, et al.: Comparative analysis of growth characteristics of Sprague Dawley rats obtained from different sources, *Lab Anim Res* 31:166–173, 2015.

Burdick J, Berridge B, Coatney R: Strain echocardiography combined with pharmacological stress test for early detection of anthracycline induced cardiomyopathy, *J Pharmacol Toxicol Methods* 73:15–20, 2015.

Burgio G: Redefining mouse transgenesis with CRISPR/Cas9 genome editing technology, *Genome Biol* 19:27, 2018.

Carbone L: Estimating mouse and rat use in American laboratories by extrapolation from Animal Welfare Act-regulated species, *Sci Rep* 11:493, 2021. https://doi.org/10.1038/s41598-020-79961-0.

Chanut F, Kimbrough C, Hailey R, et al.: Spontaneous cardiomyopathy in young Sprague-Dawley rats: evaluation of biological and environmental variability, *Toxicol Pathol* 41:1126–1136, 2013.

Cheung C, Gonzalez FJ: Humanized mouse lines and their application for prediction of human drug metabolism and toxicological risk assessment, *J Pharmacol Exp Ther* 327:288–299, 2008.

Choudhury AI, Chahal S, Bell AR, et al.: Species differences in peroxisome proliferation; mechanisms and relevance, *Mutat Res* 448:201–212, 2000.

Clark M, Steger-Hartmann T: A big data approach to the concordance of the toxicity of pharmaceuticals in animals and humans, *Regul Toxicol Pharmacol* 96:94–105, 2018.

Cohen SM, Robinson D, MacDonald J: Alternative models for carcinogenicity testing, *Toxicol Sci* 64:14–19, 2001.

Conn PM: *Animal models for the study of human disease*, San Diego, 2013, Academic Press.

Crissman JW, Goodman DG, Hildebrandt PK, et al.: Best practices guideline: toxicologic histopathology, *Toxicol Pathol* 32:126–131, 2004.

Cryan JF, O'Riordan KJ, Cowan CSM, et al.: The microbiota-gut-brain axis, *Physiol Rev* 99:1877–2013, 2019.

Damsch S, Eichenbaum G, Looszova A, et al.: Unexpected nasal changes in rats related to reflux after gavage dosing, *Toxicol Pathol* 39:337–347, 2011.

De Vera Mudry MC, Kronenberg S, Komatsu S, et al.: Blinded by the light: retinal phototoxicity in the context of safety studies, *Toxicol Pathol* 41:813–825, 2013.

Deschl U, Kittel B, Rittinghausen S, et al.: The value of historical control data-scientific advantages for pathologists, industry and agencies, *Toxicol Pathol* 30:80–87, 2002.

Donnelly TM, Bergin I, Ihrig M: Biology and diseases of other rodents. In Fox JG, Anderson LC, Otto G, et al., editors: *Laboratory animal medicine*, 3rd ed., Amsterdam, 2015, Academic Press, pp 286–330.

Duffy PH, Seng JE, Lewis SM, et al.: The effects of different levels of dietary restriction on aging and survival in the Sprague-Dawley rat: implications for chronic studies, *Aging (Milano)* 13:263–272, 2001.

EC (European Commission): *Report from the Commission to the European Parliament and the Council: 2019 report on the statistics on the use of animals for scientific purposes in the Member States of the European Union in 2015-2017*, Brussels, 2020, European Commission. https://eur-lex.europa.eu/legal-content/EN/TXT/PDF/?uri=CELEX:52020DC0016&from=EN. (Accessed 25 April 2021).

Elmore SA, Cardiff R, Cesta MF, et al.: A review of current standards and the evolution of histopathology nomenclature for laboratory animals, *ILAR J* 59:29–39, 2018.

Ema M, Endoh K, Fukushima R, et al.: Historical control data on developmental toxicity studies in rodents, *Congenit Anom (Kyoto)* 54:150–161, 2014.

EPA (U.S. Environmental Protection Agency): *Health effects test guidelines: OPPTS 870.6300: developmental neurotoxicity study*, 1998, [Listed under "Group E - Neurotoxicity Test Guidelines"]. https://www.epa.gov/test-guidelines-pesticides-and-toxic-substances/series-870-health-effects-test-guidelines. (Accessed 25 April 2021).

Eugster H-P, Müller M, Le Hir M, et al.: Immunodeficiency of tumor necrosis factor and lymphotoxin-α double-deficient mice. In Durum SK, Muegge K, editors: *Cytokine knockouts*, New York, 1998, Springer Science + Business Media, pp 103–108.

Everds NE, Snyder PW, Bailey KL, et al.: Interpreting stress responses during routine toxicity studies: a review of the biology, impact, and assessment, *Toxicol Pathol* 41:560–614, 2013.

FDA (U.S. Food and Drug Administration): *Redbook*. https://www.fda.gov/regulatory-information/search-fda-guidance-documents/guidance-industry-and-other-stakeholders-redbook-2000#TOC. (Accessed 25 April 2021).

FDA (U.S. Food and Drug Administration): *Guidance for industry: nonclinical safety evaluation of pediatric drug products*. https://www.fda.gov/regulatory-information/search-fda-guidance-documents/nonclinical-safety-evaluation-pediatric-drug-products. (Accessed 27 April 2021).

FDA (U.S. Food and Drug Administration): *Guidance for industry: S8 immunotoxicity studies for human pharmaceuticals*. https://www.fda.gov/regulatory-information/search-fda-guidance-documents/s8-immunotoxicity-studies-human-pharmaceuticals. (Accessed 27 September 2020).

Fernandes DP, Pimentel MML, Santos FAD, et al.: Hematological and biochemical profile of BALB/c nude and C57BL/6 SCID female mice after ovarian xenograft, *An Acad Bras Cienc* 90:3941–3948, 2018.

Festing MFW: Inbred strains should replace outbred stocks in toxicology, safety testing, and drug development, *Toxicol Pathol* 38:681–690, 2010.

Festing MFW: Evidence should trump intuition by preferring inbred strains to outbred stocks in preclinical research, *ILAR J* 55:399–404, 2014.

Flurkey K, Currer JM, Leiter EH, et al.: *The Jackson laboratory handbook on genetically standardized mice*, 6th, Bar Harbor, Maine, 2009, The Jackson Laboratory.

Fox JG, Barthold SW, Davisson MT, et al.: *The mouse in biomedical research, History, wild mice, and genetics*. 2nd ed., vol. 1. San Diego, 2007a, Academic Press (Elsevier).

Fox JG, Barthold SW, Davisson MT, et al.: *The mouse in biomedical research, Diseases*. 2nd ed., vol. 2. San Diego, 2007b, Academic Press (Elsevier).

Fox JG, Barthold SW, Davisson MT, et al.: *The mouse in biomedical research, Normative biology, husbandry, and models*. 2nd ed., vol. 3. San Diego, 2007c, Academic Press (Elsevier).

Fox JG, Barthold SW, Davisson MT, et al.: *The mouse in biomedical research, Immunology*. 2nd ed., vol. 4. San Diego, 2007d, Academic Press (Elsevier).

Gad SC: *Animal models in toxicology*, 3rd ed., Boca Raton, FL, 2015, CRC Press.

Gad SC, Clifford C, Goodman D: The mouse. In Gad SC, editor: *Animal models in toxicology*, Boca Raton, FL, 2015, CRC Press, pp 21–152.

Gad SC, Peckham J: The Guinea pig. In Gad SC, editor: *Animal models in toxicology*, Boca Raton, FL, 2015, CRC Press, pp 351–430.

Gopinath C, Mowat V: *Atlas of toxicological pathology*, New York, 2014, Springer.

Guan Y, Shao Y, Li D, et al.: Generation of site-specific mutations in the rat genome via CRISPR/Cas9, *Methods Enzymol* 546:297–317, 2014.

Haines DC, Chattopadhyay S, Ward JM: Pathology of aging B6;129 mice, *Toxicol Pathol* 29:653–661, 2001.

Hansen AK, Franklin C: Microbiota, laboratory animals, and research, *Lab Anim* 53:229–231, 2019.

Hard GC, Johnson KJ, Cohen SM: A comparison of rat chronic progressive nephropathy with human renal disease—implications for human risk assessment, *Crit Rev Toxicol* 39: 332–346, 2009.

Hardisty JF: Factors influencing laboratory animal spontaneous tumor profiles, *Toxicol Pathol* 13:95–104, 1985.

Hargaden M, Singer L: Anatomy, physiology, and behavior [of Guinea pigs]. In Suckow MA, Stevens KA, Wilson RP, editors: *The laboratory rabbit, Guinea pig, hamster, and other rodents*, San Diego, 2012, Academic Press (Elsevier), pp 575–602.

Harkness JE, Turner PV, Vande Woude S, et al.: *Harkness and Wagner's biology and medicine of rabbits and rodents*, 5th ed., Ames, Iowa, 2010, Blackwell.

Haseman JK: Data analysis: statistical analysis and use of historical control data, *Regul Toxicol Pharmacol* 21:52–59, 1995. discussion 81-56.

Haseman JK, Boorman GA, Huff J: Value of historical control data and other issues related to the evaluation of long-term rodent carcinogenicity studies, *Toxicol Pathol* 25:524–527, 1997.

Haseman JK, Huff J, Boorman GA: Use of historical control data in carcinogenicity studies in rodents, *Toxicol Pathol* 12: 126–135, 1984.

Haseman JK, Huff JE, Rao GN, et al.: Sources of variability in rodent carcinogenicity studies, *Fundam Appl Toxicol* 12:793–804, 1989.

Hazari MS, Callaway J, Winsett DW, et al.: Dobutamine "stress" test and latent cardiac susceptibility to inhaled diesel exhaust in normal and hypertensive rats, *Environ Health Perspect* 120:1088–1093, 2012.

Hedrich H: *The laboratory mouse*, 2nd ed., San Diego, 2012, Academic Press (Elsevier).

Henderson KS, Dole V, Parker NJ, et al.: *Pneumocystis carinii* causes a distinctive interstitial pneumonia in immunocompetent laboratory rats that had been attributed to "rat respiratory virus", *Vet Pathol* 49:440–452, 2012.

Hinrichs MJ, Dixit R: Antibody drug conjugates: nonclinical safety considerations, *AAPS J* 17:1055–1064, 2015.

Hofstetter J, Suckow MA, Hickman DL: Morphophysiology [of the laboratory rat]. In Suckow MA, Weisbroth SH, Franklin CA, editors: *The laboratory rat*, San Diego, 2006, Academic Press (Elsevier), pp 93–125.

Homburger F, Van Dongen CG, Adams RA, et al.: Hamsters and gerbils: advantages and disadvantages as models in toxicity testing, *J Am Coll Toxicol* 4:1–15, 1985.

Hoyt RFJ, Hawkins JV, St Clair MB, et al.: Mouse physiology. In Fox JG, Barthold SW, Davisson MT, et al., editors: *The mouse in biomedical research*, San Diego, 2007, Academic Press (Elsevier), pp 23–90. Normative Biology, Husbandry, and Models. 2nd ed., vol. 3.

ICH (International Council for Harmonisation of Technical Requirements for Pharmaceuticals for Human Use): *M3(R2): guidance on nonclinical safety studies for the conduct of human clinical trials and marketing authorization for pharmaceuticals.* https://database.ich.org/sites/default/files/M3_R2__Guideline.pdf. (Accessed 25 April 2021).

ICH (International Council for Harmonisation of Technical Requirements for Pharmaceuticals for Human Use): *S9: nonclinical evaluation for anticancer pharmaceuticals.* https://database.ich.org/sites/default/files/S9_Guideline.pdf. (Accessed 25 April 2021).

ICH (International Council for Harmonisation of Technical Requirements for Pharmaceuticals for Human Use): *S6(R1): preclinical safety evaluation of biotechnology-derived pharmaceuticals.* https://database.ich.org/sites/default/files/S6_R1_Guideline_0.pdf. (Accessed 25 April 2021).

ICH (International Council for Harmonisation of Technical Requirements for Pharmaceuticals for Human Use): *Safety guidelines.* https://ich.org.ich01.nine.ch/page/safety-guidelines. (Accessed 25 April 2021).

ICH (International Council for Harmonisation of Technical Requirements for Pharmaceuticals for Human Use): *S11: nonclinical safety testing in support of development of paediatric medicines.* https://database.ich.org/sites/default/files/S11_Step4_FinalGuideline_2020_0310.pdf. (Accessed 25 April 2021).

ISO (International Organization for Standardization): *Biological evaluation of medical devices.* https://www.iso.org/ics/11.100.20/x/. (Accessed 25 April 2021).

Jackson (The Jackson Laboratory): *Guidelines for nomenclature of mouse and rat strains.* http://www.informatics.jax.org/mgihome/nomen/strains.shtml. (Accessed 25 April 2021).

Jacobs AC, Brown PC: Regulatory Forum opinion piece: transgenic/alternative carcinogenicity assays: a retrospective review of studies submitted to CDER/FDA 1997-2014, *Toxicol Pathol* 43:605–610, 2015.

Johnson RC, Spaet RH, Jeppesen G, et al.: Spontaneous lesions in control animals used in toxicity studies. In Sahota PS, Popp JA, Bouchard PR, et al., editors: *Toxicologic pathology: nonclinical safety assessment*, 2nd ed., Boca Raton, FL, 2019, CRC Press (Taylor & Francis), pp 331–386.

Kalueff AV, Minasyan A, Keisala T, et al.: Hair barbering in mice: implications for neurobehavioural research, *Behav Processes* 71:8–15, 2006.

Karolweski B, Mayer TW, Ruble G: Non-infectious diseases [of hamsters]. In Suckow MA, Stevens KA, Wilson RP, editors:

The laboratory rabbit, Guinea pig, hamster, and other rodents, San Diego, 2012, Academic Press (Elsevier), pp 867–873.

Katoh M, Tateno C, Yoshizato K, et al.: Chimeric mice with humanized liver, *Toxicology* 246:9–17, 2008.

Keenan C, Elmore S, Francke-Carroll S, et al.: Potential for a global historical control database for proliferative rodent lesions, *Toxicol Pathol* 37:677–678, 2009.

Keenan KP, Laroque P, Ballam GC, et al.: The effects of diet, ad libitum overfeeding, and moderate dietary restriction on the rodent bioassay: the uncontrolled variable in safety assessment, *Toxicol Pathol* 24:757–768, 1996.

Kisui F, Fukami T, Nakano M, et al.: Strain and sex differences in drug hydrolase activities in rodent livers, *Eur J Pharm Sci* 142:105143, 2020.

Kittel B, Ruehl-Fehlert C, Morawietz G, et al.: Revised guides for organ sampling and trimming in rats and mice—Part 2. A joint publication of the RITA and NACAD groups, *Exp Toxicol Pathol* 55:413–431, 2004.

Kurtz DM, Travlos GS: *The clinical chemistry of laboratory animals*, 3rd ed., Boca Raton, FL, 2018, CRC Press (Taylor & Francis Group).

Lee H: Genetically engineered mouse models for drug development and preclinical trials, *Biomol Ther (Seoul)* 22: 267–274, 2014.

Lee KP, Frame SR, Sykes GP, et al.: Testicular degeneration and spermatid retention in young male rats, *Toxicol Pathol* 21: 292–302, 1993.

Li JJ, Gonzalez A, Banerjee S, et al.: Estrogen carcinogenesis in the hamster kidney: role of cytotoxicity and cell proliferation, *Environ Health Perspect* 101(Suppl 5):259–264, 1993.

Long GG, Hardisty JF: Regulatory Forum opinion piece: thresholds in toxicologic pathology, *Toxicol Pathol* 40:1079–1081, 2012.

Ma Y, Shen B, Zhang X, et al.: Heritable multiplex genetic engineering in rats using CRISPR/Cas9, *PLoS One* 9: e89413, 2014.

Mahler JF, Stokes W, Mann PC, et al.: Spontaneous lesions in aging FVB/N mice, *Toxicol Pathol* 24:710–716, 1996.

Maronpot RR: *Pathology of the mouse: reference and atlas*, 1st, Vienna, IL, 1999, Cache River Press.

Maronpot RR, Nyska A, Foreman JE, et al.: The legacy of the F344 rat as a cancer bioassay model (a retrospective summary of three common F344 rat neoplasms), *Crit Rev Toxicol* 46:641–675, 2016.

Maynard RL, Downes N: *Anatomy and histology of the laboratory rat in toxicology and biomedical research*, San Diego, 2019, Academic Press (Elsevier).

McInnes E: *Background lesions in laboratory animals: a color atlas*, New York, 2012, Elsevier.

McInnes EF, Ernst H, Germann PG: Spontaneous neoplastic lesions in control Syrian hamsters in 6-, 12-, and 24-month short-term and carcinogenicity studies, *Toxicol Pathol* 41:86–97, 2013.

McInnes EF, Scudamore CL: Review of approaches to the recording of background lesions in toxicologic pathology studies in rats, *Toxicol Lett* 229:134–143, 2014.

McInnes EF, Scudamore CL: Aging lesions: background versus phenotype, *Curr Pathobiol Rep* 3:107–113, 2015.

McKillop D, Butters CJ, Hill SJ, et al.: Enzyme-inducing effects of bicalutamide in mouse, rat and dog, *Xenobiotica* 28:465–478, 1998.

Miedel EL, Hankenson FC: Biology and diseases of hamsters. In Fox JG, Anderson LC, Otto GM, et al., editors: *Laboratory animal medicine*, 3rd ed., Boston, 2015, Academic Press (Elsevier), pp 209–246.

Mohr U, Dungworth DL: Relevance to humans of experimentally induced pulmonary tumors in rats and hamsters. In Mohr U, Dungworth DL, Kimmerle G, et al., editors: *Inhalation toxicology*, Berlin, 1988, Springer-Verlag, pp 209–232.

Mohr U, Dungworth DL, Capen CC: *Pathobiology of the aging rat*, Washington, D.C., 1992, ILSI Press.

Mohr U, Dungworth DL, Capen CC, et al: *Pathobiology of the aging mouse* (vol. 2). Washington, D.C., 1996, ILSI Press.

Monticello TM, Jones TW, Dambach DM, et al.: Current nonclinical testing paradigm enables safe entry to First-In-Human clinical trials: the IQ consortium nonclinical to clinical translational database, *Toxicol Appl Pharmacol* 334: 100–109, 2017.

Morawietz G, Ruehlfehlert C, Kittel B, et al.: Revised guides for organ sampling and trimming in rats and mice—Part 3. A joint publication of the RITA and NACAD groups, *Exp Toxicol Pathol* 55:433–449, 2004.

Murray KA: Anatomy, physiology, and behavior [of hamsters]. In Suckow MA, Stevens KA, Wilson RP, editors: *The laboratory rabbit, Guinea pig, hamster, and other rodents*, San Diego, 2012, Academic Press (Elsevier), pp 753–763.

Nelson DR, Zeldin DC, Hoffman SM, et al.: Comparison of cytochrome P450 (CYP) genes from the mouse and human genomes, including nomenclature recommendations for genes, pseudogenes and alternative-splice variants, *Pharmacogenetics* 14:1–18, 2004.

Nicklas W, Homberger FR, Illgen-Wilcke B, et al.: Implications of infectious agents on results of animal experiments. Report of the working group on hygiene of the Gesellschaft Fur Versuchstierkunde ("Society for Laboratory Animal Science" [GV-SOLAS]), *Lab Anim* 33:S39–S87, 1999.

Obert LA, Frazier KS: Intrarenal renin-angiotensin system involvement in the pathogenesis of chronic progressive nephropathy—bridging the informational gap between disciplines, *Toxicol Pathol* 47:799–816, 2019.

OECD (Organisation for Economic Co-operation and Development): *Test no. 426: developmental neurotoxicity study.* https://www.oecd-ilibrary.org/environment/test-no-426-developmental-neurotoxicity-study_9789264067394-en. (Accessed 25 April 2021).

OECD (Organisation for Economic Co-operation and Development): *Test no. 443: extended one-generation reproductive toxicity study.* https://www.oecd-ilibrary.org/environment/test-no-443-extended-one-generation-reproductive-toxicity-study_9789264185371-en. (Accessed 25 April 2021).

Office (Home Office of the United Kingdom): *Annual statistics of scientific procedures on living animals.* Great Britain, 2018, https://assets.publishing.service.gov.uk/government/uploads/system/uploads/attachment_data/file/835935/annual-statistics-scientific-procedures-living-animals-2018.pdf. (Accessed 25 April 2021).

Olcese J, Wesche A: The Harderian gland, *Comp Biochem Physiol A Comp Physiol* 93:655–665, 1989.

Olson H, Betton G, Robinson D, et al.: Concordance of the toxicity of pharmaceuticals in humans and in animals, *Regul Toxicol Pharmacol* 32:56–67, 2000.

Prior H, Baldrick P, Beken S, et al.: Opportunities for use of one species for longer-term toxicology testing during drug development: a cross-industry evaluation, *Regul Toxicol Pharmacol* 113:104624, 2020.

Pritchett KR, Taft RA: Reproductive biology of the laboratory mouse. In Fox JG, Barthold SW, Davisson MT, et al., editors: *The mouse in biomedical research*, 2nd ed., San Diego, 2007, Academic Press (Elsevier), pp 91–121.

Provencher Bolliger A, Everds NE, Zimmerman KL, et al.: Hematology of laboratory animals. In Weiss DJ, Wardrop KJ, editors: *Schalm's veterinary hematology*, 6th ed., Ames, IA, 2010, Wiley-Blackwell, pp 852–887.

Raboisson P, Flood K, Lehmann A, et al.: MK-801 neurotoxicity in the Guinea pig cerebral cortex: susceptibility and regional differences compared with the rat, *J Neurosci Res* 49:364–371, 1997.

Rocca MS, Wehner NG: The Guinea pig as an animal model for developmental and reproductive toxicology studies, *Birth Defects Res B Dev Reprod Toxicol* 86:92–97, 2009.

Rosshart SP, Herz J, Vassallo BG, et al.: Laboratory mice born to wild mice have natural microbiota and model human immune responses, *Science* 365, 2019.

Rudmann D, Cardiff R, Chouinard L, et al.: Proliferative and nonproliferative lesions of the rat and mouse mammary, Zymbal's, preputial, and clitoral glands, *Toxicol Pathol* 40: 7S–39S, 2012.

Ruehl-Fehlert C, Kittel B, Morawietz G, et al.: Revised guides for organ sampling and trimming in rats and mice—part 1, *Exp Toxicol Pathol* 55:91–106, 2003.

Sahota PS, Popp JA, Bouchard PR, et al.: *Toxicologic pathology: nonclinical safety assessment*, 2nd ed., Boca Raton, FL, 2019, CRC Press (Taylor & Francis).

Scudamore CL, Soilleux EJ, Karp NA, et al.: Recommendations for minimum information for publication of experimental pathology data: MINPEPA guidelines, *J Pathol* 238: 359–367, 2016.

Sellers RS, Clifford CB, Treuting PM, et al.: Immunological variation between inbred laboratory mouse strains: points to consider in phenotyping genetically immunomodified mice, *Vet Pathol* 49:32–43, 2012.

Selman C, Swindell WR: Putting a strain on diversity, *EMBO J* 37, 2018.

Seong E, Saunders TL, Stewart CL, et al.: To knockout in 129 or in C57BL/6: that is the question, *Trends Genet* 20:59–62, 2004.

Shackelford C, Long G, Wolf J, et al.: Qualitative and quantitative analysis of nonneoplastic lesions in toxicology studies, *Toxicol Pathol* 30:93–96, 2002.

Shen H-W, Jiang X-L, Gonzalez FJ, et al.: Humanized transgenic mouse models for drug metabolism and pharmacokinetic research, *Curr Drug Metab* 12:997–1006, 2011.

Shomer NH, Holcombe H, Harkness JE: Biology and diseases of Guinea pigs. In Fox JG, Anderson LC, Otto GM, et al., editors: *Laboratory animal medicine*, 3rd ed., Boston, 2015, Academic Press (Elsevier), pp 247–285.

Shtrasburg S, Gal R, Gruys E, et al.: An ancillary tool for the diagnosis of amyloid A amyloidosis in a variety of domestic and wild animals, *Vet Pathol* 42:132–139, 2005.

Simpson EM, Linder CC, Sargent EE, et al.: Genetic variation among 129 substrains and its importance for targeted mutagenesis in mice, *Nat Genet* 16:19–27, 1997.

Sistare FD, Thompson KL, Honchel R, et al.: Evaluation of the Tg.Ac mouse assay for testing the human carcinogenic potential of pharmaceuticals – practical pointers, mechanistic clues, and new questions, 21:65–79, 2002.

Sparks H: *More than 100 million rats, mice used in US labs: report (nypost.com)*, 2021, New York Post. https://nypost.com/2021/01/18/more-than-100-million-rats-mice-used-in-us-labs-report/. (Accessed 26 April 2021).

Storer RD, French JE, Haseman J, et al.: p53$^{+/-}$ hemizygous knockout mouse: overview of available data, *Toxicol Pathol* 29(Suppl):30–50, 2001.

Strom SC, Davila J, Grompe M: Chimeric mice with humanized liver: tools for the study of drug metabolism, excretion, and toxicity. In Maurel P, editor: *Hepatocytes: methods and protocols*, Totowa, NJ, 2010, Humana Press, pp 491–509.

Suckow MA, Hankenson FC, Wilson RP, et al.: *The laboratory rat*, 3rd ed., San Diego, 2020, Academic Press (Elsevier).

Suckow MA, Stevens KA, Wilson RP: *The laboratory rabbit, Guinea pig, hamster, and other rodents*, San Diego, 2012, Academic Press (Elsevier).

Sundberg JP, Schofield PN: Commentary: mouse genetic nomenclature: standardization of strain, gene, and protein symbols, *Vet Pathol* 47:1100–1104, 2010.

Sundberg JP, Taylor D, Lorch G, et al.: Primary follicular dystrophy with scarring dermatitis in C57BL/6 mouse substrains resembles central centrifugal cicatricial alopecia in humans, *Vet Pathol* 48:513–524, 2011.

Suntharalingam G, Perry MR, Ward S, et al.: Cytokine storm in a phase 1 trial of the anti-CD28 monoclonal antibody TGN1412, *N Engl J Med* 355:1018–1028, 2006.

Suttie AW, Leininger JR, Bradley AE. *Pathology of the Rat: Reference and Atlas*, 2, San Diego, 2018, Academic Press (Elsevier).

Suwa T, Nyska A, Haseman JK, et al.: Spontaneous lesions in control B6C3F$_1$ mice and recommended sectioning of male accessory sex organs, *Toxicol Pathol* 30:228–234, 2002.

Suwa T, Nyska A, Peckham JC, et al.: A retrospective analysis of background lesions and tissue accountability for male accessory sex organs in Fischer-344 rats, *Toxicol Pathol* 29: 467–478, 2001.

Taylor K, Gordon N, Langley G, et al.: Estimates for worldwide laboratory animal use in 2005, *Altern Lab Anim* 36: 327–342, 2008.

Tomas J, Langella P, Cherbuy C: The intestinal microbiota in the rat model: major breakthroughs from new technologies, *Anim Health Res Rev* 13:54–63, 2012.

Tontodonati M, Fasdelli N, Repeto P, et al.: Characterisation of rodent dobutamine echocardiography for preclinical safety pharmacology assessment, *J Pharmacol Toxicol Methods* 64:129–133, 2011.

Tuttle AH, Philip VM, Chesler EJ, et al.: Comparing phenotypic variation between inbred and outbred mice, *Nat Methods* 15:994–996, 2018 [*Corrigendum: Nat Methods* 16, 206, 2019].

USDA-APHIS (U.S. Department of Agriculture Animal and Plant Health Inspection Service): *Animal welfare act and animal welfare regulations ("Blue Book")*. https://www.aphis.usda.gov/animal_welfare/downloads/AC_BlueBook_AWA_508_comp_version.pdf. (Accessed 25 April 2021).

USDA-APHIS (U.S. Department of Agriculture Animal and Plant Health Inspection Service): *Annual report animal usage by fiscal year.* https://www.aphis.usda.gov/animal_welfare/annual-reports/Annual-Report-Summaries-State-Pain-FY18.pdf. (Accessed 25 April 2021).

van der Worp HB, Howells DW, Sena ES, et al.: Can animal models of disease reliably inform human studies? *PLoS Med* 7:e1000245, 2010.

van Kreijl CF, McAnulty PA, Beems RB, et al.: *Xpa* and *Xpa/p53*$^{+/-}$ knockout mice: overview of available data, *Toxicol Pathol* 29(Suppl.):117–127, 2001.

Ward JM, Anver MR, Mahler JF, et al.: Pathology of mice commonly used in genetic engineering (C57BL/6; 129; B6,129; and FVB/N). In Ward JM, Mahler JF, Maronpot RR, et al., editors: *Pathology of genetically engineered mice*, 1st ed., Ames, IA, 2000, Iowa State University Press, pp 161–179.

Ward JM, Fox JG, Anver MR, et al.: Chronic active hepatitis and associated liver tumors in mice caused by a persistent bacterial infection with a novel *Helicobacter* species, *J Natl Cancer Inst* 86:1222–1227, 1994.

Weber K: Differences in types and incidence of neoplasms in Wistar Han and Sprague-Dawley rats, *Toxicol Pathol* 45:64–75, 2017.

Weber K, Mowat V, Hartmann E, et al.: Pathology in continuous infusion studies in rodents and non-rodents and ITO (Infusion Technology Organisation)-recommended protocol for tissue sampling and terminology for procedure-related lesions, *J Toxicol Pathol* 24:113–124, 2011a.

Weber K, Razinger T, Hardisty JF, et al.: Differences in rat models used in routine toxicity studies, *Int J Toxicol* 30:162–173, 2011b.

Weiss DJ, Wardrop KJ, editors: *Schalm's veterinary hematology*, 6th ed., Ames, IA, 2010, Wiley-Blackwell.

Whary MT, Baumgarth N, Fox JG, et al.: Biology and diseases of mice. In Fox JG, Anderson LC, Otto GM, et al., editors: *Laboratory animal medicine*, 3rd ed., Boston, 2015, Academic Press (Elsevier), pp 43–150.

Willard-Mack CL, Elmore SA, Hall WC, et al.: Non-proliferative and proliferative lesions of the rat and mouse hematolymphoid system, *Toxicol Pathol* 47:665–783, 2019.

Williams BH: Non-infectious diseases [of Guinea pigs]. In Suckow MA, Stevens KA, Wilson RP, editors: *The laboratory rabbit, Guinea pig, hamster, and other rodents*, San Diego, 2012, Academic Press (Elsevier), pp 685–704.

Yamamoto S, Urano K, Koizumi H, et al.: Validation of transgenic mice carrying the human prototype c-Ha-ras gene as a bioassay model for rapid carcinogenicity testing, *Environ Health Perspect* 106(Suppl 1):57–69, 1998.

Zambrowicz BP, Sands AT: Knockouts model the 100 best-selling drugs — will they model the next 100? *Nature Rev Drug Discov* 2:38–51, 2003.

Zarate-Blades CR, Horai R, Caspi RR: Regulation of autoimmunity by the microbiome, *DNA Cell Biol* 35:455–458, 2016.

Zitvogel L, Ma Y, Raoult D, et al.: The microbiome in cancer immunotherapy: diagnostic tools and therapeutic strategies, *Science* 359:1366–1370, 2018.

Animal Models in Toxicologic Research: Rabbit

Lyn Miller Wancket[1], Alys Bradley[2], Lauren E. Himmel[3]

[1]Charles River, Durham, NC, United States, [2]Charles River Laboratories Edinburgh Ltd., Tranent, Scotland, United Kingdom, [3]AbbVie Inc., Preclinical Safety, North Chicago, IL, United States

OUTLINE

1. Introduction	695		5.7. Safety Studies Supporting Vaccine Development	705
2. Model Selection	696		6. Major Disease and Functional Models (Other than Safety)	705
2.1. Overview of Toxicology Model Species Selection	696		6.1. Antibody Production/Immunological Research	705
2.2. Issues in Data Extrapolation to Human	696		6.2. Oncology Disease Models	706
3. Basic Biological Characteristics and Common Breeds	696		6.3. Novel Surgical Models	706
3.1. Ethics and Animal Welfare Considerations	699		6.4. Medical Device and Regenerative Medicine—Functional Studies	706
4. Regulatory Aspects and Examples of Use of Rabbits in Biomedical Research	699		6.5. Watanabe Rabbit Model of Hypercholesterolemia	707
5. Pharmacokinetic and Toxicity Studies	701		7. Spontaneous Findings in the Experimental NZW Rabbit	709
5.1. Developmental and Reproductive Toxicity Studies	701		7.1. Normal Structures Unique to the Rabbit	709
5.2. Dermal Irritation/Toxicity Studies	701		7.2. Spontaneous Pathology Findings	712
5.3. Intracutaneous and Implantation Safety Studies	701		References	715
5.4. Cardiac Safety Studies	702			
5.5. Mucosal Irritation Studies	703			
5.6. Ocular Studies	703			

1. INTRODUCTION

Throughout modern biomedical research, the rabbit has remained a core laboratory animal species. Studies using rabbits have provided important insights into toxicology, immunology, reproduction, and other fields. Interestingly, despite their common use, many key factors about rabbit biology, physiology, and disease are either poorly documented or difficult to identify in the literature. This chapter will cover some of those lesser-documented topics, as well as recommend selected resources in the literature.

2. MODEL SELECTION

2.1. Overview of Toxicology Model Species Selection

Rabbits have an extensive history in biomedical research, extending over several centuries (Esteves et al., 2018), and continue to be utilized in emerging scientific areas, such as gene editing, including CRISPR/Cas9 (Honda and Ogura, 2017; see *Genetically Engineered Animal Models in Toxicologic Research,* Vol 1, Chap 23). Rabbits occupy an intermediate position among laboratory animals, in that they are uniquely endowed with features of both rodents and larger animal models. They are more genetically diverse than rodents and their size allows for enhanced sampling of blood and tissues, as well as being able to receive human-equivalent dose volumes and implanted articles. For rabbits, the human equivalent dose for a 60 kg human (based on surface area) is 3.1, which is the same dose adjustment as for monkeys (Aleksunes and Eaton, 2019). While larger than rodents, rabbits remain relatively small and easier to handle and house compared to larger models such as dogs, minipigs, or nonhuman primates (NHPs). A relatively long average lifespan allows rabbits to be used for interventional and recovery studies over several years, which can be highly desirable for research of chronic disease and medical devices.

There are also some key challenges when using rabbits in biomedical research. In general, many research staff are less familiar with rabbit anatomy, physiology, husbandry, and diseases compared to other common laboratory species (e.g., rodents, dogs, NHPs). For those seeking reference material on rabbits, there are fewer resources for spontaneous rabbit pathology, historical control data, and standard tissue sampling and trimming guides than for other common laboratory species. While all of these challenges can be overcome, they remain limitations on effective use of rabbits. Therefore, it is easy for individual scientists to inadvertently misattribute normal structures or background changes to a test article effect (see Spontaneous Findings, section 7).

Another important challenge encountered when working with rabbits is their propensity to respond poorly to stress. This commonly manifests as diarrhea in response to seemingly minimal stress (e.g., new personnel in a vivarium room, ambient noise) (Bradley, 2012). In addition to diarrhea, rabbits may develop cardiac lesions after routine handling (Sellers et al., 2017; see Spontaneous pathology findings section).

2.2. Issues in Data Extrapolation to Human

While rabbits are useful models for many human conditions, it is important to note where there are limitations in mimicking human physiology and disease. For example, while rabbits are generally useful for bone fusion and orthopedic device studies, the common use of autologous bone marrow at fusion sites is more challenging in rabbits than in other species, due to the relatively high bone marrow fat content in mature rabbits. Also, while rabbits have been a key resource in the field of immunology, their anatomic distribution of lymphoid tissue is very different from humans and other species. For example, in the intestine, the sacculus rotundus and vermiform appendix contain abundant lymphoid tissue, and overall the intestines comprise more than 50% of the total lymphoid tissue of the rabbit, while the spleen is relatively small compared to other species.

3. BASIC BIOLOGICAL CHARACTERISTICS AND COMMON BREEDS

Rabbits (*Oryctolagus cuniculus*, order Lagomorpha, family Leporidae) are often selected as an in vivo model system when size limitations of smaller mammals such as rodents cannot accommodate the techniques employed in a study while still representing a refinement over larger, phylogenetically higher-ranked mammalian model species (e.g., dog, pig, NHP). Refinements in rodent models have led to declining numbers of rabbits used in biomedical research (Burkholder et al., 2012). Still, the Organisation for Economic Co-operation and Development and United States Environmental Protection Agency (EPA)–preferred nonrodent species in prenatal developmental toxicity studies is the rabbit (per EPA 712–C–98–207, OPPTS 870.3700), for which the New Zealand White (NZW) is the usual strain (Burkholder et al., 2012). Other major applications include dermatological, cardiovascular, infectious disease, ophthalmological, orthopedic (including medical devices), cancer, reproductive biology, and regenerative/interventional biomedical research. Three outbred breeds predominate: the NZW (an albino large breed), the Dutch belted (a pigmented small breed), and the NZW x New Zealand Red (NZR) F1 cross (a pigmented large breed). Coat color genotypes are *cc* for the NZW, *ee* for the NZR, and *du^d du^w aa* for the black American Dutch (Weisbroth et al., 2013).

Requisite housing and husbandry conditions are stipulated by regulatory bodies. In the United States, rabbits are a United States Department of Agriculture–regulated species, elevating them above mice and rats and making them subject to standards set forth in the Guide for the Care and Use of Laboratory Animals, the Public Health Service Policy on Humane Care and Use of Laboratory Animals, and the Animal Welfare Act. One week of acclimation at a study site is generally provided prior to study recruitment. As the rabbit model is often selected for its size, adult animals are recruited within a defined body weight range. For the NZW, the minimum weight is around 2.4–2.7 kg. In the context of toxicology studies, environmental enrichment may include social noncontact enrichment and various forms of physical enrichment to enable gnawing and burrowing behavior; pen and pair housing is usually not possible for instrumented animals or those in dermatology studies (Baumans, 2005; Wyatt et al., 2017). Vendor differences have been noted to affect the incidence of background findings (Holve et al., 2011) and the strain of a rabbit breed impacts genetic composition (Alves et al., 2015). Commercially available, purpose-bred laboratory rabbit strains are regularly screened to be free from a defined set of pathogens, indicated by their vendor health reports. The importance of complete reporting on animal source, as part of the ARRIVE guidelines, cannot be overemphasized (Kilkenny et al., 2010). Rabbits are a prey species and as such have evolved with a wide visual field exceeding 330 degrees, auditory and olfactory acuity, and strong fear responses. This nervousness, combined with the high muscle mass and relatively low skeletal mass, necessitates firm and supportive handling to prevent hindleg excursions and subsequent spinal luxation or fracture.

Discussion of salient anatomic features will be limited to those relevant to test article investigation or explanation/implantation; detailed descriptions of lagomorph anatomy and physiology are well-documented in other texts (Burkholder et al., 2012; Lossi et al., 2016; Quesenberry and Carpenter 2011; Yanni 2004; Barthold et al., 2016). Notable features of general biology (Table 18.1) and reproduction (Table 18.2) are provided in tabular format below.

The gastrointestinal tract of rabbits has many unique features. The rabbit is a hindgut fermenting herbivore with commensurate large intestinal microbiota and distinctive anatomical features. Compared to other species, adult rabbits have a lower gastric pH (1.9) and higher bile flow rate (130 mL/d/kg) (Kararli, 1995). The ileum adjoins the cecum at the sacculus rotundus, a small, bulbous structure heavily laden with lymphoid tissue. An elongated appendix forms the blind end of the cecum and the cecum adjoins the colon at the ampulla cecalis coli, another small outpouching opposite the sacculus rotundus. The cecum is large, holding approximately 40% of total ingesta (Quesenberry and Carpenter, 2011). Located between the transverse and descending colon, the nonhaustrated fusus coli serves to segregate fibrous ingesta and has intestinal pacemaker function (Weisbroth et al., 2013). Gut-associated lymphoid tissue is extensive (Haines et al., 2016) comprising about 50% of the total body lymphoid mass (Quesenberry and Carpenter, 2011). Expression of rabbit intestinal CYP3A, canalicular multispecific organic anion transporter, and p-glycoprotein is reportedly similar to that in humans (Kunta et al., 2001). Cecotrophy, the ingestion of "night feces," facilitates reprocessing of protein and vitamin-rich fecal matter.

Rabbits are lissencephalic, lacking gyri and sulci on the brain surface. Rabbits are obligate nasal breathers. The olfactory ecosystem is important in rabbit behavior and physiology and includes secretion of 2-phenoxyethanol, produced from the submandibular skin gland ("chin gland") secretion from dominant rabbits (Quesenberry and Carpenter, 2011). The skin is thin and delicate. Ample subcutaneous space in the cervical and interscapular regions makes this a convenient injection site. The pinnae are highly vascular and provide thermoregulation since they represent approximately 12% total body surface area in the NZW (Quesenberry and Carpenter, 2011). In the laboratory setting,

TABLE 18.1   Basic Biometrics for the Rabbit (Burkholder et al., 2012; Lossi et al., 2016; Quesenberry and Carpenter 2011; Yanni 2004; Barthold et al., 2016)

Parameter	Value
Lifespan	5—8 years
Avg adult bodyweight	3.5—4.5 kg (NZW)
Avg adult body length	48 cm (NZW)
Vertebral formula	C7/T12-13/L6-7/S4/Ca14-16
Dental formula	I2/1 C0/0 PM3/2 M3/3; second set of maxillary incisors (peg teeth) at the lingual surface of the primary pair
Digits	5 anterior, 4 posterior
Age at skeletal maturity	8—11 months
Relative skeleton weight[a]	6%—8%
Relative heart weight[a]	0.30%
Relative total muscle mass[a]	30%—50%
Neutrophil % (min—max)	28%—44%
Lymphocyte % (min-max)	39%—68%
Mammae	8—10 (4—5 pairs)
Sexual dimorphisms	Nipples absent in males
	Large dewlap present in mature females
Lung lobation	2 left, 4 right
Midtracheal diameter	4.7×5.9 mm (NZW)
Erythrocyte lifespan	50—70 d
Urine fractional calcium excretion	45%—60%
Daily food intake	5% body weight
Daily water intake	50—150 mL/kg (10% body weight)
Water loss tolerance	48% body weight
Coprophagy	3—8 h after meal

[a] *Relative weight refers to the weight of the organ as a percentage of total body weight.*

this facilitates measurement of pulse oximetry and blood pressure, as well as blood collection/injection via the marginal ear vein. Rabbits are prone to fatal cardiac arrhythmias following prolonged exposure to halothane anesthesia (Kunta et al., 2001).

Rabbits exhibit similar clinical pathology features as other nonclinical species with some exceptions. Lymphocytes are the predominant circulating leukocyte in the baseline state with heterophils (equivalent to neutrophils in other species) superseding in periods of inflammation or infection. Basophils are more prevalent than

in most veterinary species, with upward of 30% being within normal limits (Harkness et al., 2013; Barthold et al., 2016). Heterophils should not be mistaken for eosinophils (Song et al., 1993). The cervicofacial lymph node topography of the NZW is reportedly similar to humans, numbering 12–18 in total (Dunne et al., 2003). The fractional urinary excretion of calcium for rabbits is 45%–60% as compared to less than 2% in most mammals (Quesenberry and Carpenter, 2011). Crystalluria is normal, consisting of calcium carbonate and ammonium magnesium phosphate (Barthold et al., 2016).

TABLE 18.2 Reproductive Biometrics for the Rabbit

Parameter	Value
Age at sexual maturity	5 mo (F NZW), 6–7 mo (M NZW)
Reproductive life	3 y (F), 5–6 y (M)
Testicular descent	Approximately 12 weeks of age; inguinal ring remains open (Petritz, 2012)
Mature spermatogenesis	40–70 d after puberty, 48 d spermatogenesis cycle (Morton, 1988)
Ovulation	Induced (10–13 h postcoitus)
Female receptivity	4–6 d cycle, includes postpartum estrus
Uterus structure	Bicornuate with each horn having a cervical ostia (lacks a true body)
Placenta type	Chorioallantoic placenta
Gestation	30–32 d
Litter size	4–5 (Dutch belted), 8–12 (NZW)
Birthweight	50 g
Weaning	50–60 d

3.1. Ethics and Animal Welfare Considerations

Rabbits are prey species that are easily stressed by many different changes. Methods to reduce stress and enhance environmental enrichment serve to improve the likelihood of clearer data being collected that better enables identification of potential test article–related effects. Two areas where this is manifested as clinical signs and/or pathologic changes are in the cardiac and gastrointestinal tract. Cardiomyopathy has been recognized in crowded housing (Weber and Van Der Walt, 1975) and even simple clinical procedures associated with vaccine studies (Sellers et al., 2017). Diarrhea is a common and significant clinical ailment in laboratory rabbits. Efforts to control diarrhea can backfire, such as use of antibiotics and higher levels of dietary copper given for antibacterial effects leading to hepatic copper toxicosis (Ramirez et al., 2013).

Housing environments enriched with plastic and metal toys can both reduce stress and encourage obligatory chewing to keep teeth in check, as rabbit teeth grow continuously. Stress can also be reduced through group housing (where appropriate) and limiting the scent of predators and other species. If animals will be restrained for a long period of time during treatment (e.g., ocular examinations for medical device testing, endotoxin, and sensitization testing), habituation to restraint is essential.

4. REGULATORY ASPECTS AND EXAMPLES OF USE OF RABBITS IN BIOMEDICAL RESEARCH

Many guidelines and regulations that apply broadly to use of animals in biomedical research are also relevant to studies with rabbits. There are also specific documents for more specialized studies (e.g., medical devices, regenerative medicine) for which rabbits are a disproportionally popular animal model (reviewed recently by Schuh and Funk, 2019). Key resources are summarized in Table 18.3.

While rabbits have been used extensively in studies of biopharmaceutical, industrial/environmental chemicals, and medical device products, their use in cosmetics research may be the most widely recognized use outside of research groups. Cosmetic testing involving rabbits has influenced how some regulations/guidances have developed. For example, the seventh Amendment to the European Union (EU) Cosmetics Directive states that cosmetic products and/or their ingredients are not permitted to be marketed in the EU if they underwent testing in animals including sensitization and irritation evaluations commonly still performed in rabbits in the United States. While rabbit use is being replaced with in vitro assays for specific study types (e.g., dermal irritation), these replacement assays may not be accepted by individual regulatory groups.

TABLE 18.3   Key Regulatory Documents, Databases, and Welfare Statements Pertaining to Use of Rabbits in Safety Assessment

Regulation source	References
Unites States	Animal Welfare Act https://www.nal.usda.gov/awic/animal-welfare-act-quick-reference-guides
	Registry of Toxic Effects of Chemical Substances (RTECS)
	172-C-98−207 EPA Health effects test guidelines OPPTS 870.3700. Prenatal developmental toxicity study (1998)
Europe	Animal Research Law Directive https://eur-lex.europa.eu/eli/dir/2010/63/2019-06-26
	7th Amendment to the EU Cosmetics Directive http://ec.europa.eu/DocsRoom/documents/13101/attachments/2/translations/en/renditions/pdf#:~:text=On%2027%20February%202003%2C%20Directive%202003%2F15%2FEC%20on,cosmetic%20finished%20products%20and%20ingredients.
Nongovernmental groups	
ISO (International Organization for Standardization)	10993: Biological evaluation of medical devices—Part 6 Tests for local effects after implantation (2016)
	10993: Biological evaluation of medical devices—Part 10 Tests for irritation and skin sensitization (2010)
	10993: Biological evaluation of medical devices—Part 11 Tests for systemic toxicity (2017)
ASTM (formerly known as American Society for Testing and Materials)	F2721-09 (2014) Standard Guide for Preclinical in vivo Evaluation in Critical Size Segmental Bone Defects
The Association for Research in Vision and Ophthalmology	Statement for the Use of Animals in Ophthalmic and Vision Research
ICH (International Council for Harmonisation of Technical Requirements for Pharmaceuticals for Human Use)	ICH 2017 S5R3 (Detection of toxicity to reproduction for human pharmaceuticals)
OECD	OECD guideline for the testing of chemicals. Prenatal developmental toxicity study. Test guideline 414 (2001)

5. PHARMACOKINETIC AND TOXICITY STUDIES

Many standard nonclinical studies (e.g., pharmacokinetic and general toxicity studies) are not commonly performed in rabbits in part due to limitations with rabbits compared to rodents including relatively limited historical control data, larger amounts of compound needed, and increased costs. Rabbits are more commonly used as a secondary species for toxicity studies or the primary species for specialized studies such as those for the development of vaccines, medical devices, and regenerative medicine modalities (see *Vaccines, Stem Cells and Regenerative Medicine*, and *Biomedical Materials and Devices*, Vol 2, Chap 9, 10, and 11). Specific areas of focus are discussed in more detail below. For other general references on rabbits in basic research and safety studies, the reader is directed to recent references (Kirchner and Henwood 2012; Burkholder et al., 2012).

5.1. Developmental and Reproductive Toxicity Studies

Rabbits are one of the most common nonrodent species used for developmental and reproductive toxicity (DART) studies (see *The Role of Pathology in Evaluation of Reproductive, Developmental, and Juvenile Toxicity*, Vol 1, Chap 7). Advantages of rabbits in DART studies include accuracy in the timing of conception, a longer fetal period than rodents, and easier semen collection. Additionally, some aspects of the extraembryonic membranes of the rabbit are more similar to those in humans than rodents. Disadvantages include a predisposition to spontaneous abortion, resorption when few implantations are present, and being induced ovulators.

While rabbits can be used in studies to assess effects on fertility (Segment I), embryo–fetal development (Segment II), and pre/postnatal development (Segment III), they are primarily used in embryo–fetal development studies (notably, they are a relatively sensitive species for thalidomide; Lee et al., 2011). Their larger size aids in the detection of soft tissue and skeletal alterations, as well as changes in cardiac structure.

Important guidances for using rabbits on DART studies are included in Table 18.3. For a comparison across species, please see *Embryo, Fetus, and Placenta*, Vol 4, Chap 11.

5.2. Dermal Irritation/Toxicity Studies

The overarching goal of dermal irritation testing is the early identification of materials that are potential human cutaneous and/or mucosal irritants. Primary irritants are those test articles that incite injury (e.g., inflammation and/or necrosis) through direct tissue damage. To date, rabbits remain a preferred animal model and are historically well represented in dermal irritation studies within databases and in the published literature (see Table 18.3). Rabbits are often more sensitive than other species in these tests (e.g., petrolatum; Chandra et al., 2014), although it should be noted that rabbits may overestimate absorption/penetration compared to humans (Jung and Maibach, 2015).

As part of the effort toward decreasing animal use in research, work has focused on increasing the availability of in vitro replacements for whole animal studies. There has been initial progress in decreasing whole animal testing for certain classes of test articles (e.g., neat chemicals). However, it is important to note that in vitro studies have not been validated for all potential test articles. For example, in vitro tests for skin irritation have been validated for neat chemicals, but not for extracts of medical devices (ISO 10993-10 Annex D, Table 18.3). During a period of continued validation, the reader is advised to regularly check for updates on the currently accepted models for each test article type. Some changes may involve adapting existing protocols used to produce extracts (e.g., alterations in extraction techniques or incubation times; ISO 10993-10 Annex D, Table 18.3). For a comparison across species, please see chapters in Vol 1, Part 3—Animal and Alternative Models in Toxicologic Research.

5.3. Intracutaneous and Implantation Safety Studies

Rabbits are used extensively in both biocompatibility and functional testing for medical devices. Biocompatibility refers to whether the materials in the device cause direct injury to the tissue surrounding an implanted device. Methods for testing biocompatibility are outlined in several standards (ISO 10993 series, Table 18.3). Functional testing involves evaluating whether a device is performing as designed and intended (discussed in a later section). To test general biocompatibility of a device, implantation is often performed in soft tissue (e.g., subcutaneous tissue, skeletal muscle) and compared to the tissue reaction to a control material (often high-density polypropylene is used as a negative control). The rabbit can also be used for detecting systemic effects caused by a local implant (ISO 10993-11, Table 18.3), although rats are more commonly used. For more information, refer to *Biomedical Materials and Devices, Vol 2, Chap 11.*

It is important to note that the ISO 10993 standards were originally developed with a material science focus and the scoring systems for biological responses (e.g., histopathology) may not fully incorporate or describe all of the relevant biological changes that can take place at an implantation site. It is incumbent upon the pathologist/scientist involved with the evaluation to modify standard scoring schemes or provide additional description in a narrative if the tissue response is not fully captured in a standard ISO 10993 scoring system.

Additionally, assessment of the regional draining lymph nodes for degradable implants is important (Wancket, 2019), and the larger size of rabbits and their lymph nodes is helpful for these purposes. Since polymorphonuclear cell responses are common in initial implant site reactions, it is important to remember that rabbits have heterophils rather than neutrophils.

5.4. Cardiac Safety Studies

Rabbit models of heart disease have been well described (Pogwizd and Bers, 2008). In the field of cardiac electrophysiology, rabbits have been utilized both to predict the potential arrhythmogenicity of test items and to evaluate the efficacy of antiarrhythmic agents. Safety pharmacology studies are conducted to predict arrhythmogenic liability of therapeutics, particularly torsades de pointes (TdP) that may precipitate sudden cardiac death. The effective size of the rabbit heart, calculated based on heart weight and

period of spiral wave rotation, is reportedly more similar to that of humans than the larger effective heart size of pigs and dogs; thus, it is surmised that the number of arrhythmogenic sources in ventricular fibrillation is closer to humans than pigs and dogs (Panfilov, 2006). Potassium ion channels are also similar between rabbit and human hearts, with currents I_{Kr} and I_{Ks} being predominant (Fan et al., 2015). It is reported that rabbits have similar ventricular action potential waveforms, potassium channel expression patterns, function and gating of many potassium channels, and phase 3 I_{Kr} repolarizing current to humans (Baczkó et al., 2016) and thus represent a refined, intermediate animal that is an improvement over rodents, while lower phylogenetically than dogs. Rabbits have a longer QT interval than dogs and NHPs due to a decrease in conduction velocity at the midpoint of the bundle branches (Brewer and Cruise, 1994). An alloxan-diabetic rabbit model has been used to study the effect of diabetes mellitus on ventricular repolarization, in which some have documented reduced density of various potassium channels (Baczkó et al., 2016). It has been suggested that the rabbit has a lower repolarization reserve, similar to humans, while that in dogs is higher due to stronger I_{K1} and I_{Ks}, and thus may be more predictive of test article–associated arrhythmias (Baczkó et al., 2016).

Rabbit model development since the 1990s led to the generation of the anesthetized methoxamine-sensitized rabbit model of TdP, in which the typical arrhythmia takes place in a period of bradycardia (caused by AV block) and prolonged QT interval or prolonged ventricular action potential, driven in part by alpha 1 adrenergic receptor–mediated increase in intracellular ionic calcium (Carlsson, 2008). The model has primarily been used in studies of class III antiarrhythmic drugs (Carlsson, 2008). Further investigation into the rabbit TdP model by injection of 37% formalin into the AV junction to induce AV block in anesthetized rabbits has revealed that remodeling following chronic AV block leads to intracellular calcium ion handling abnormalities that contribute to arrhythmogenic afterdepolarizations (Qi et al., 2009). Rabbit hearts are also used ex vivo in Langendorff systems to study electrophysiologic mechanisms that may be important to the development of artificial cardiostimulators (Sidorov et al., 2007) and the effects of antiarrhythmic therapies for several indications, including atrial fibrillation and cardiac ischemia (Frommeyer et al., 2013). This model may include premedication of the animals prior to cardiac harvest to attain tissue drug levels (e.g., amiodarone, dronedarone) comparable with those seen in human patients (Frommeyer et al., 2013).

5.5. Mucosal Irritation Studies

The rationale for mucosal irritation studies is that a chemical that is highly irritating/injurious to mucosa of one species will likely have a similar effect in humans (ISO 10993-10). Rabbits are used for many reproductive and urinary mucosal irritation studies (other than oral mucosa, which is typically performed in the hamster cheek pouch model). The size of the rabbit reproductive tract and lower urinary tract makes them more useful than rodents such as the rat, mouse, and hamster. Rabbit mucosa may also be more sensitive to irritants than rat mucosa, at least for the vaginal tract (Kaminsky et al., 1985). For these studies, female rabbits are generally used due to the anatomic complexity of infusing male animals.

There are limitations to using rabbits when examining the female reproductive tract. While an individual rabbit may appear to be a mature adult when determined by body weight, the vaginal tract in unbred rabbits may still be relatively small, leading to trauma during intravaginal administration. Additionally, epithelial type (stratified squamous closer to the vulva and columnar closer to the cervix) and wall thickness vary along the length of the vaginal tract (Oh et al., 2003), necessitating consistent sampling to ensure adequate microscopic evaluation.

5.6. Ocular Studies

Rabbits have been utilized in studies of ocular physiology, disease (proliferative vitreoretinopathy, PVR), and evaluation of therapeutics such as ophthalmic implants, ocular microsurgery, and ocular drug delivery modalities. Globe fixation and histologic preparation methodologies are disparate in the literature, though likely standardized within a single laboratory. We refer readers to the Society of Toxicologic Pathology position paper (Bolon et al., 2013) for optimal techniques. Conduct of ocular studies in rabbits and other animals is guided by the Association for Research in Vision and Ophthalmology statement for the use of animals in ophthalmic and vision research (Table 18.3). In addition to being used to test ocular irritancy potential (ISO 10993-10), the size and shape of the rabbit eye is uniquely suited for evaluating ocular devices as compared to other small animal models (reviewed in Alves et al., 2019 and Drevon-Gailot 2019). Rabbits can be habituated to restraint and wearing contact lenses to simulate human use. While NZW rabbits are commonly used for ocular studies, Dutch belted rabbits are also used in studies for which a pigmented eye is necessary.

Consideration of comparative anatomical features of the rabbit eye is paramount. The rabbit eye is smaller than the adult human eye but has larger anterior segment and lens (Werner et al., 2006). The rabbit globe is slightly shorter in the anterior–posterior dimension, while the human eye is roughly spherical (Lossi et al., 2016). The rabbit iris is somewhat convex, creating a curved, shallower anterior chamber than that of humans (Werner et al., 2006). The rabbit cornea is thinner than the human cornea, with the epithelium measuring 30–40 μm (Lossi et al., 2016) and lacks a Bowman's layer (Werner et al., 2006). The corneal endothelium has a notable proliferative capacity, while in humans the number of corneal endothelial cells diminishes throughout life (Werner et al., 2006). Elasticity of the anterior lens capsule in rabbits is comparable to children (Werner et al., 2006). Considerations for ocular surgery include the use of heparin to prevent disruption of the blood–aqueous barrier and protein release into the anterior chamber as well as perioperative antiinflammatory drugs, as rabbits experience more pronounced ophthalmitis than humans following ocular surgery (Werner et al., 2006). Lens nuclear hardening has been reported in older rabbits weighing >3.4 kg (Werner et al., 2006). Conscious rabbits experience an oculocardiac reflex, particularly following compression of both globes, the magnitude of which is variably dampened by different systemic and topical anesthetics (Turner Giannico et al., 2014). Fluoroscopic studies have revealed that the blood supply to the eye in most rabbits is through the external ophthalmic artery arising from the external carotid artery, but in a minority of animals, the primary arterial supply is from the internal ophthalmic artery arising from the internal carotid artery (Daniels et al., 2018). Venous drainage occurs primarily through the external jugular vein (Quesenberry and Carpenter, 2011). A retrobulbar venous plexus (orbital sinus) is present; engorgement of the plexus, due to cardiac disease, intrathoracic masses, or extreme fear, can cause exophthalmos (Quesenberry and Carpenter, 2011). Retinal vasculature in the rabbit is merangiotic, characterized by vessels traveling in a horizontal band from the optic disc, extending nasally and temporally, leaving the remainder of the retina avascular. The rabbit retina also possesses a horizontal streak (visual streak)—a region of more densely cellular retina—that runs parallel and ventral to the retinal vasculature (Lossi et al., 2016). The rabbit vitreal volume is 2–3 mL compared to 4–5 mL in human eyes (Inan et al., 2007).

The rabbit has served as a model for the testing of topical and intracameral substances. The cornea may be studied via the ex vivo corneal endothelial toxicity assay or epithelial toxicity and reepithelialization assay (Werner et al., 2006). The corneal epithelial wound healing model is established (York et al., 1988). In a study of corneal lesions generated in NZW by exposure to 4N NaOH on an 8 mm paper disc, neovascularization of the defect was monitored for 14 days to study the effect of subconjunctival injections of bevacizumab, a monoclonal antibody (mAb) against vascular endothelial growth factor on angiogenesis, as neovascularization has been associated with corneal graft rejection in humans (Ahmed et al., 2009). Rabbits may also serve as a model for glaucoma filtration surgery. In the posterior segment, PVR is modeled in Dutch belted rabbits by vitrectomy followed by injection of corneal fibroblasts, retinal pigment epithelium cells, and/or glial cells (Lei et al., 2012). Anti-PVR therapies have been tested in the rabbit (Chetoni et al., 2016). A safety study involving intravitreal injection of bevacizumab in pigmented rabbits followed for 28 days by slit lamp and fundic examination, tonometry, central corneal thickness measurements, electroretinography, visual evoked response, histopathology, and electron microscopy (EM) reported normal retinal function and structure; however, mitochondrial damage in the inner segments of photoreceptors was observed on EM, and apoptotic biomarkers (Bax, Caspase 3, Caspase 9) were increased in all treated eyes (Inan et al., 2007). NZW have been used to test the safety of docosahexaenoic acid formulated as a nanoemulsion and administered intravitreally as a putative therapeutic for retinal diseases (Dolz-Marco et al., 2014).

Historically, ocular irritancy has been studied in rabbits utilizing the low-volume eye test or Draize procedure (Maurer et al., 2001; Maurer and Parker, 1996). The former assay involves application of 10 μL test substance onto the corneal surface and is considered a refinement over the latter method, in which 100 μL test substance is deposited in the inferior conjunctival cul-de-sac. Corneal irritancy has been tested in NZW by surface application of sodium perborate monohydrate, sodium hypochlorite, 10% hydrogen peroxide, and 15% hydrogen peroxide. At 35 days postexposure, sodium perborate monohydrate and sodium hypochlorite were considered mild irritants, characterized by superficial epithelial and stromal injury; 10% and 15% hydrogen peroxide were considered severe irritants, characterized by deep stromal injury with disproportionately less severe epithelial injury. At both concentrations of hydrogen peroxide, slight to moderate keratocyte loss was still evident histologically at 35 days postinjury, though the cornea was deemed macroscopically within normal limits (Maurer et al., 2001). Surfactant-induced corneal damage has also been studied in the NZW, in which treated animals at 35 days postapplication showed corneal and conjunctival erosion, ulceration, and necrosis for all surfactants tested (cationic, anionic, nonionic), as well as keratocyte necrosis and endothelial changes with a severely irritating cationic surfactant (Maurer and Parker, 1996). Many authorities mandate that in vitro tests should be performed initially, and so the use of the Draize test in the United States and Europe has now declined and is sometimes modified so that anesthetics are administered and lower doses of the test substances are used. Chemicals already shown to have adverse effects in vitro are not currently subjected to a Draize test.

A rabbit model of intraarterial chemotherapy of the ophthalmic artery for retinoblastoma represents a refinement over nontumor–bearing pig and NHP models of the same technique and provides a novel, pediatric-scale chemosurgical model for drug delivery to the eye as well as efficacy studies. Rabbits immunosuppressed with cyclosporine A can host WERI-RB1 human xenografts injected subretinally and intravitreally (Daniels et al., 2018). Melphalan, carboplatin, and topotecan have been tested alone and in combination by the intraarterial route to achieve high local exposure while reducing the ocular and systemic side effects of periocular injection, intravitreal injection, or intravenous chemotherapy (Daniels et al., 2018). These models afford the opportunity to test the efficacy and safety of novel chemotherapeutic agents and chemosurgical approaches.

Ophthalmic devices, such as intraocular lens implantation and keratoprosthesis surgeries and substances, have been tested in the NZW and pigmented rabbits. Rabbit eyes possess comparable regenerative and scarring properties to humans in studies of intraocular lens implantation, making them a suitable model for studying pseudophakic lens designs and material biocompatibility. Owing to the regenerative capacity of rabbit lens epithelial cells, posterior capsular opacification can readily be studied in the rabbit eye at 4–8 weeks postimplantation; however, to fully encompass the spectrum of healing, the follow-up on these studies can extend into the late postoperative period of 6–8 months, particularly when new prosthetic materials are being investigated (Werner et al., 2006).

5.7. Safety Studies Supporting Vaccine Development

Rabbits have been used in vaccine research since the beginning of the field, including use by Pasteur in 1885. They have key features that have led to their continued use as one of the most common species for vaccine studies. The relatively small size (while still being large enough to receive the full human dose/dose volume via intramuscular injection) and reasonably high blood volume are advantageous compared to the rat. Rabbits also have a general tendency to mount an immune response to administered antigens, though they may have a more limited response to adjuvants that require a toll-like receptor-9 response (Liu et al., 2012). The use of rabbits in this domain and points to consider for toxicologic pathologists have been reviewed recently (Sellers et al., 2020) (see *Vaccines*, Vol 2, Chap 9).

6. MAJOR DISEASE AND FUNCTIONAL MODELS (OTHER THAN SAFETY)

6.1. Antibody Production/Immunological Research

Studies of the rabbit immune system and their immunoglobulins have established much of what is known about the structure, function, and regulated expression of antibodies (reviewed in Pinheiro et al., 2011; Weber et al., 2017).

Rabbits have a single primary immunoglobulin G (IgG) isotype (Stills, 2012) and IgGs are the most common isotypes of rabbit-derived mAbs. Rabbit-derived polyclonal antibodies have formed the backbone of numerous research tests. Additionally, rabbit mAbs are a key reagent in Food and Drug Administration–approved in vitro diagnostic tools for tumor-associated antigens, including those that detect human epidermal growth factor receptor 2, estrogen receptors, progesterone receptors, and programmed death-ligand 1. Finally, rabbit-derived mAbs are currently being tested as potential therapies in clinical trials, including as therapies for macular degeneration (Weber et al., 2017).

Rabbits uniquely develop a primary antibody repertoire through somatic diversification of Ig genes. Rabbits initially generate a limited antibody repertoire in the fetal liver and bone via B lymphopoiesis. After birth, gut-associated lymphoid tissue is the site of expansion into a more complex primary antibody collection between 4 and 8 weeks of age. As with other species, refinement of the antibody response occurs after the antigen-dependent immune response (Lanning et al., 2000).

6.2. Oncology Disease Models

An NZW rabbit model of metastatic cancer has been used to study oncologic interventional surgery and imaging. The VX2 carcinoma model provides a convenient means to study interventional oncologic surgical approaches in an intermediate size animal of metastatic cancer. The model originated from papillomaviral-associated skin cancer in cottontail rabbits and is transplantable in all domestic rabbits for the purpose of modeling human solid tumors (Aravalli and Cressman 2015). Little investigation has been done into the molecular biomarkers and drug targets in the model, though the microRNA transcriptome of VX2 tumors in the liver has recently been characterized (Aravalli and Cressman 2015). Cells are expanded subcutaneously in vivo then explanted into recipient study animals. Tumor cells or fragments can be surgically implanted (e.g., via laparotomy) or directly inoculated into a pseudometastatic site by imaging-guided injection (Vossen et al., 2008; Lee et al., 2003). Therapeutic modalities undergoing preclinical investigation include computed tomography–guided percutaneous transthoracic radiofrequency thermal ablation of lung tumors using an internally cooled electrode (Lee et al., 2003), intraarterial chemoembolization of liver tumors with the glycolysis inhibitor 3-bromopyruvate (Vossen et al., 2008), and molecular magnetic resonance imaging with targeted nanoparticles (Winter et al., 2003). Heterotopic VX2 tumors established in the liver and kidney have also been used in a limited number of studies evaluating biomarker identification and antitumor therapeutic efficacy (Zhao et al., 2015).

6.3. Novel Surgical Models

The intermediate size and phylogenetic rank of rabbits among mammalian models makes them ideal systems in which novel surgical approaches can be studied. Laboratory rodents are often too small for the required instrumentation. Rabbits represent a refinement over larger animal species (e.g., dog, pig, NHP) while still accommodating procedures using instruments and materials of a similar size to those used in humans. They may also be useful when a test article cannot yet be manufactured to the scale of a larger species.

An NZW rabbit peripheral nerve axotomy model of traumatic injury has been used to study biomaterial and cellular scaffolds, as well as test articles that promote nerve repair and regeneration. The sciatic nerve is frequently used; however, due to the potential for autotomy (self-amputation) in this model, others have chosen the common peroneal nerve (Mohammed et al., 2007) or facial nerve (Zhang et al., 2008). The traumatic injury may include crush or tension (Shen et al., 2010), neurectomy with or without repair, neurectomy with transposition (reverse autograft), or neurectomy with defect in the pelvic limb. The rabbit allows modeling gap defects greater than 2 cm, more akin to clinically affected humans, which is not possible in laboratory rodent species; nerve gaps up to 4 cm long have been studied in rabbits (Hsu et al., 2011). Rabbits in reinnervation studies are followed up to 18 months (Hsu et al., 2011) postoperatively with various functional and imaging parameters evaluated (Shen et al., 2010) as well as microscopic evaluation of scar tissue, inflammation, axon counts, myelination and regeneration, and specialized examination using EM and immunohistochemical biomarker staining (Mekaj et al., 2017; Shen et al., 2010; Zhang et al., 2008). Various therapeutic approaches have been examined in rabbits including mesenchymal stem cells with or without polylactic glycolic acid (Shen et al., 2010), hyaluronic acid with tacrolimus (Mekaj et al., 2017), keratin hydrogel (Hill et al., 2011), poly-3-hydroxybutyrate, low-level laser therapy (Mohammed et al., 2007), microporous polylactic acid conduit (Hsu et al., 2011), and neural stem cells in hyaluronic acid (Zhang et al., 2008). Nerve fiber regeneration in the rabbit is 2 mm/day, which is more comparable to the human rate of 1 mm/day than the rat at 3.5–4 mm/day (Hill et al., 2011), and has been documented to sometimes be protracted, occurring up to 2 months following tibial neurectomy in an NZW rabbit model (Shin et al., 2015).

6.4. Medical Device and Regenerative Medicine—Functional Studies

In addition to basic biocompatibility implant studies, rabbits are used for functional testing of a variety of medical devices. One key advantage of rabbits compared to rodents is their larger size, which makes them able to accommodate larger implants, including some whole devices that are sized for human use.

While rabbits are used in a wide variety of medical device and regenerative medicine testing systems, this section will focus on topics for which rabbits have a disproportionately large use.

Rabbits have several osseous properties that make them a superior small animal model compared to rodents (reviewed in Wancket, 2015), including production of substantial osteonal bone. Common models include epiphyseal implants (to model cancellous bone), diaphyseal implants (to model cortical bone), and spinal fusion. Additionally, rabbits are useful in studies evaluating cartilage regeneration, and there are rabbit-specific scoring schemes available for cartilage injury models (Laverty et al., 2010).

An NZW rabbit model of vocal apparatus damage has been used to study the anatomy, physiology, and regenerative properties of the larynx. Stimulated (evoked) and nonstimulated phonation models of phonotrauma have been developed in the rabbit to study biomechanical changes, epithelial healing, extracellular matrix remodeling in the lamina propria, and vocal fold scar (Thibeault et al., 2003). In vivo or ex vivo studies involve pulsed electrical stimulation of the cricothyroid muscles and membrane while passing a stream of compressed, humidified air to the glottis through a cuffed endotracheal tube to create phonation in the range of human hearing (Swanson et al., 2009). Modal phonation is reported in the range of 54 dB, while raised phonation occurs near 60 dB (Swanson et al., 2009). The model has allowed testing of therapeutics and tissue engineering approaches that may modulate inflammation, fibrosis, and regeneration following phonotrauma (Hirano et al., 2004). Rabbits have been utilized in vascular research applications for the study of regional ischemia and vascular engraftment. Though pigs and sheep are typically selected for long-term preclinical studies, rabbits are a reasonable model earlier in discovery, as they are smaller, less costly, and phylogenetically subordinate to the aforementioned species (Zheng et al., 2012). An NZW rabbit model of autologous vascular engraftment has been used to study intimal remodeling. In this procedure, a segment of the external jugular vein is interposed within the common carotid artery. This system models human coronary and peripheral arterial bypass surgeries, which often fail due to intimal hyperplasia of the engrafted vessel, and has provided a platform for testing therapeutics to attenuate this effect, such as selective nanoparticulate delivery of a cell-penetrating peptide-based mitogen-activated protein kinase–activated protein kinase 2 inhibitor to vascular cells (Evans et al., 2015). A rabbit model has been the basis for testing of carotid artery biomaterial engraftment (polycaprolactone plus arginine–glycine–aspartic acid coating or bilayer porcine small intestinal submucosa with heparin and dipyridamole) and femoral artery biomaterial engraftment (polyvinyl alcohol hydrogel) to study integration and the potential for revascularization (Zheng et al., 2012; Fang et al., 2020). Ischemia of the pelvic limb is modeled by segmental excision of the superficial femoral artery or femoral artery and ligation of the circumflex and deep femoral arteries, enabling the study of proangiogenic therapeutics (Rissanen et al., 2003). The caliber of vasculature in rabbits has also been leveraged in an intestinal vascular access port model for use in absorptive pharmacokinetic studies (Kunta et al., 2001).

For more information on medical devices, see *Biomedical Materials and Devices*, Vol 2, Chap 11. For more information on ocular toxicologic pathology, see *Eye*, Vol 3, Chap 10.

6.5. Watanabe Rabbit Model of Hypercholesterolemia

There are essentially 3 rabbit hypercholesterolemia models: the Watanabe heritable hyperlipidemic rabbit (WHHL), cholesterol-fed NZW or Japanese White, and transgenic rabbits (Fan et al., 2015; Yanni, 2004). The WHHL (Watanabe, 1980) laid the foundation for mechanistic investigations into low-density lipoprotein (LDL) receptor (LDLR) deficiency as the basis of human familial hypercholesterolemia (Goldstein et al., 1983) in the early 1980s and eventually the development of HMG-CoA reductase inhibitors (statins) and other hypolipidemic and cardioprotective drugs like fibrates, beta blockers, and the antioxidant probucol

(Shiomi and Ito, 2009; Fan et al., 2015; Jayo et al., 1994). The rabbit strain arose from a spontaneous deletion in exon 4 of the LDL receptor gene that was selectively bred into the colony. Compared to other available animal models, it affords the opportunity to study both lipoprotein metabolism and atherosclerosis that is most similar to that of humans (Fan et al., 2015). Atherosclerosis begins in the WHHL in utero (Yanni, 2004). The initiation and distribution of atherosclerosis in the WHHL rabbit has been documented, with mild aortic lipid deposits (fatty streaks) reliably detected by 3 months of age, particularly evident near ostia of arteries branching off the aortic arch, and coronary atherosclerosis appearing later at the 15-month-old timepoint (Buja et al., 1983). Atherosclerosis develops in the aortic arch and thoracic aorta in rabbit models, while in humans, the abdominal aorta is affected (Fan et al., 2015). Ocular lesions are also well characterized, with foamy macrophage accumulation in the choroid, sclera, iris, ciliary body, and cornea (Kouchi et al., 2006). With advanced age, WHHL rabbits also develop subcutaneous and digital xanthomas (Buja et al., 1983; Kouchi et al., 2006). Atherosclerotic lesions in the WHHL rabbit are similar to those in humans and are characterized by intimal and medial foam cells, lipid accumulation in smooth muscle and endothelial cells, extracellular matrix, and in rabbits greater than 9 months of age, development of mineral deposits, cholesterol clefts, necrotic cores, and a fibrous luminal cap (Buja et al., 1983; Yanni, 2004; Fan et al., 2015).

Since the development of apolipoprotein E and LDLR knock-out mouse models of atherosclerosis, the WHHL rabbit is less frequently used. However, critical considerations of lipid metabolism must inform appropriate animal model species selection. With regard to plasma lipoprotein composition, rabbits are very low-density lipoprotein (VLDL) and LDL predominant, with these lipids comprising approximately 40% of plasma cholesterol in chow-fed rabbits and 90% or more in WHHL rabbits, while high-density lipoprotein (HDL) predominates in mice and rats (Fan et al., 2015; Mitsuguchi et al., 2008). Rabbits also possess plasma cholesteryl ester transfer protein, while mice and rats do not (Fan et al., 2015). Substrains of WHHL rabbits, prone to atherosclerosis and coronary atherosclerosis with myocardial infarction, have also been developed (Shiomi and Ito, 2009). WHHL rabbits have very high cholesterol and LDL levels and low HDL levels, similar to humans with familial hypercholesterolemia (Shiomi and Ito, 2009). By 12 months of age, WHHL rabbits have plasma cholesterol levels of 700–1200 mg/dL (Shiomi and Ito, 2009). Other similarities between the WHHL rabbit and humans that are lacking in murine counterparts are lack of expression of apoB editing enzyme in the liver, plasma cholesteryl ester transferase activity, and apoB-containing VLDL (Shiomi and Ito, 2009). Characterization of the WHHL rabbit led to key understandings of the mechanisms of atherosclerosis, including early inflammatory events such as increased vascular cell adhesion molecule-1 expression in aortic endothelium, monocyte recruitment and transformation into foam cells, and T-cell infiltration (Fan et al., 2015). WHHL rabbits have also proven useful for imaging studies in atherosclerosis (Shiomi and Ito, 2009; Yanni, 2004). Radiolabeled flurodeoxyglucose correlates with and highlights macrophage accumulation in atherosclerotic plaques on positron emission tomography imaging in the cholesterol-fed NZW and WHHL models (Zhang et al., 2006).

NZW rabbits fed an atherogenic diet (0.1%–2% cholesterol, with or without other enhancers like corn oil or animal proteins) will develop atherosclerosis due to their inability to increase sterol excretion (Yanni, 2004) (Fig. 18.1). Plasma cholesterol rises rapidly in these animals, reaching two- to eightfold the normal value (30–90 mg/dL) (Fan et al., 2015) within 20 days (Zhang et al., 2006; Yanni 2004; Fan et al., 2015). Rabbits fed high-cholesterol diets without fat supplementation experience more severe atherosclerosis (Jayo et al., 1994). Animals may be screened for plasma cholesterol concentrations after 1 week of feeding a high-cholesterol diet prior to study recruitment in order to screen out hyporesponders (Fan et al., 2015). Atherosclerotic lesions in cholesterol-fed rabbits are foam cell predominant (Fan et al., 2015). To more closely recapitulate plaque rupture of human atherosclerosis in these animals, balloon injury of the atherosclerotic aorta may be performed (Zhang et al., 2006; Yanni, 2004). A notable difference between the cholesterol-fed NZW and WHHL rabbits is the presence of hepatocellular lipidosis and lipid-laden

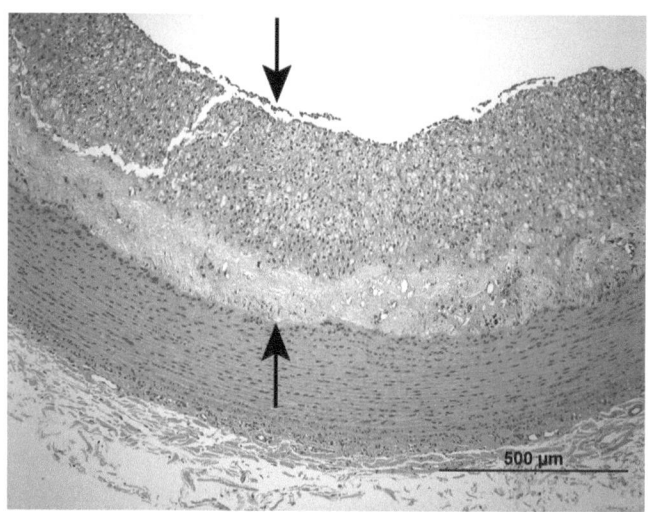

FIGURE 18.1 Atherosclerosis in a section of aorta from NZW rabbit fed a high-fat diet. Expansion of intima (between *arrows*) by macrophages containing extensive cytoplasmic lipid. Hematoxylin and eosin. *Image courtesy of Dr. Wanda Haschek.*

macrophages in the liver and spleen of the former (Buja et al., 1983). Atherosclerosis in hyperlipidemic rabbits is reportedly partially reversible when rabbits are supplemented with HDL plasma fraction (Yanni, 2004; Fan et al., 2015) but may become less so as the lesions contain increasing amounts of fibrous tissue (Jayo et al., 1994). Hepatic insufficiency secondary to lipidosis is a time-limiting factor in this model (Yanni, 2004). Alloxan-diabetic rabbits develop profound hypercholesterolemia but not atherosclerosis (Jayo et al., 1994). Cholesterol-induced atherosclerosis is inhibited in alloxan-induced diabetes mellitus because large, triglyceride-rich lipoproteins in the plasma do not penetrate the arterial wall (Fan et al., 2015).

Transgenic models of atherosclerosis with expression of human apoAI, apoAII, lecithin–cholesterol acyl transferase, hepatic lipase, or apoB-100 exist in NZW rabbits, and WHHL rabbits that express human apolipoprotein A demonstrate rapid and increased disease severity (Yanni, 2004). Additional rabbit models of hypercholesterolemia (KHC (Kurosawa et al., 1995)) and hypertriglyceridemia (e.g., SMHL, PHT, TGH) (Houdebine and Fan, 2009) exist. To date, transgenic rabbit model development has been limited by the availability of

viable methodologies and is mainly performed by pronuclear microinjection (Fan et al., 2015). CRISPR/Cas9 technology developed in recent years could provide a means for further nuanced rabbit models of atherosclerotic and dyslipidotic diseases, among others (Fan et al., 2015).

7. SPONTANEOUS FINDINGS IN THE EXPERIMENTAL NZW RABBIT

Before addressing specific spontaneous pathological findings, it is important to recognize the relative paucity of literature and references for rabbits in this area compared to other common laboratory animal species (especially rodents). One negative impact of this is that evaluation of rabbit tissue without appropriate knowledge may result in misinterpretation of normal structures unique to this species. Specialized glands, reproductive tissues, and the large intestinal tract in particular present this challenge.

7.1. Normal Structures Unique to the Rabbit

7.1.1. Specific Skin Glands and Hair Follicles

Normal rabbit fur is composed of three hair types: large central primary follicles, somewhat smaller lateral primary follicles, and much smaller and abundant secondary follicles (down hairs) (Fig. 18.2). These can be confusing if one does not routinely evaluate rabbit skin.

Rabbits also possess several specialized glands in or around the skin, most often used for social and sexual behavior activities. These include the submandibular (chin or mental) skin gland; the inguinal gland complex (brown and white glands); and the anal (rectal, perirectal) glands.

The submandibular gland is a sexually dimorphic gland positioned ventral to the mandible (Mykytowycz, 1965). In intact males, the gland contains large acini lined by columnar epithelial cells (Mykytowycz, 1965) and the oily secretions can coat the skin surface after release (Fig. 18.3). The gland may be difficult to locate in the subcutaneous tissue of female rabbits.

The paired inguinal gland complexes, also called the "preputial" and "clitoral" glands, are composed of two adjacent but morphologically

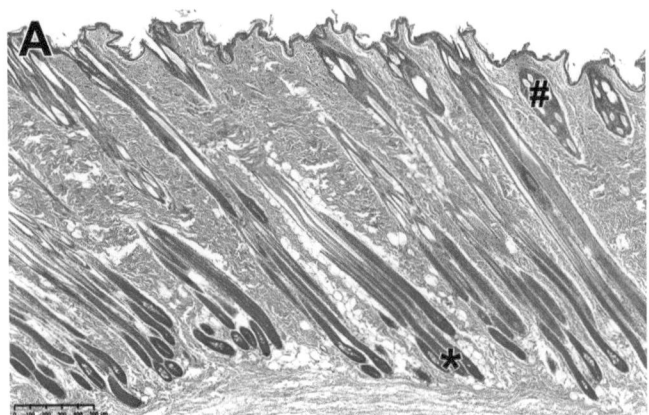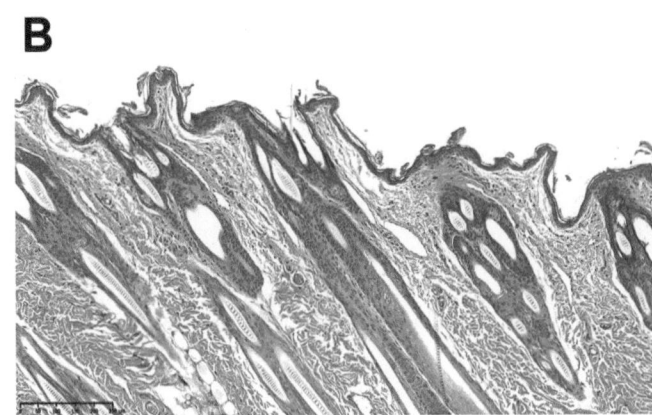

FIGURE 18.2   Section of normal skin from NZW rabbit. (A) Large central primary follicles and smaller lateral follicles (*) with smaller secondary follicles (down hairs, #). (B) higher magnification of secondary follicles. Hematoxylin and eosin.

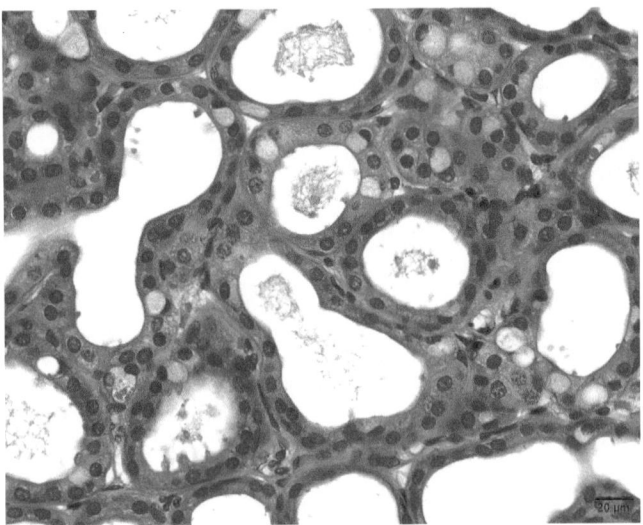

FIGURE 18.3 Section of normal submandibular (mental) gland from a male rabbit. Acini with cuboidal epithelium. Hematoxylin and eosin. *Image courtesy of Dr. Osamu Katsuta.*

different lobulated glands: the dorsolateral "white" gland and the medioventral "brown" gland. Male rabbits also have a preputial gland within the preputial dermis, which can sometimes be mistaken for portions of the inguinal gland located near the orifice of the prepuce.

Harderian Gland

The periocular Harderian gland includes two lobes that have distinct gross and microscopic appearances. The naming of the lobes can be confusing because while they are named for their gross appearance (pink and white), their microscopic appearance is the opposite of the name (Fig. 18.4). The pink lobe is the larger of the two and located ventrally (inferior) to the white lobe. The white lobe is comprised of epithelial cells with small, uniform, densely packed lipid vacuoles that stain eosinophilic with hematoxylin and eosin. In contrast, the epithelial cells in the pink lobe contain large, clear vacuoles that are poorly staining with hematoxylin and eosin.

Gastrointestinal Tract Segments

STOMACH AND SMALL INTESTINES

Unlike rodents, rabbits do not have a nonglandular region within their stomach, although its presence has sometimes, erroneously, been reported. A wide layer of Brunner's glands, containing both serous cells and mucous cells, is present in the proximal duodenum. Unlike other species where Paneth cells are most prominent in the distal small intestine, Paneth cells (with their large eosinophilic cytoplasmic granules) are easily identified in the duodenal crypts. The terminal portion of the ileum transitions to the muscular sacculus rotundus (Fig. 18.5A and B). The cecum is haustrated, tightly coiled, and terminates in the vermiform appendix. The wall of the vermiform appendix consists predominately of lymphoid follicles that protrude into the lumen.

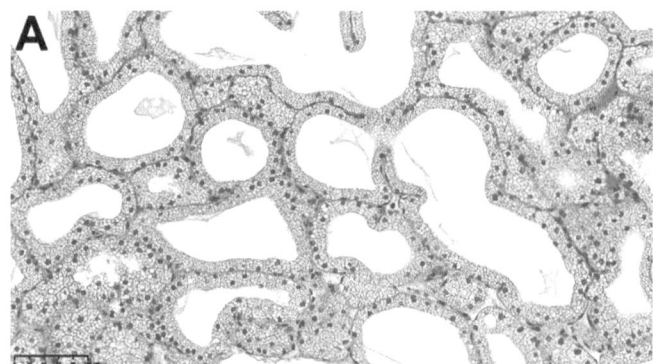
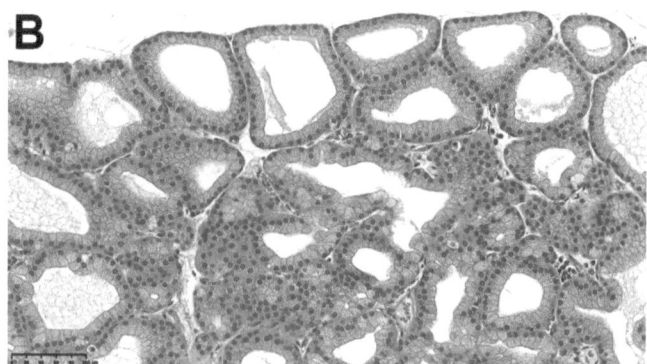

FIGURE 18.4 Section of normal Harderian gland from NZW rabbit. (A) Section of pink portion of gland where epithelial cells have fine lacy cytoplasm. (B) Section of white portion of gland where epithelial cells have eosinophilic cytoplasm with basilar nuclei. Hematoxylin and eosin.

LARGE INTESTINE

The different portions of the colon have distinct macroscopic appearances (Fig. 18.6). Adjacent to the sacculus rotundus is the muscular ampulla cecalis coli, which has wide open crypts lined by epithelium and adjacent lamina propria. The proximal part of the ascending colon has tight haustrations and prominent teniae. The proximal and distal portions of the transverse colon are demarcated by the fusus coli, a muscular spindle-shaped organ with very thick mucosa. Unlike more proximal portions of the colon, the distal ascending colon and transverse colon are not haustrated and have a relatively small diameter.

Ovary

The rabbit ovary contains two unique features that may be inadvertently misdiagnosed as a lesion: the interstitial tissue ("gland") and surface epithelial structures (Fig. 18.7). Interstitial tissue is highly developed in rabbits and is produced by theca interna cells differentiating into primary and then secondary interstitial tissue, beginning at 3 months of age (Mori and Matsumoto, 1973). The secondary tissue comprises the vast majority of the ovary by 6 months of age. The interstitial cells produce progestogens.

The ovarian mesothelium (surface epithelium) often forms short papillae lined by stratified or pseudostratified epithelium, which can be mistaken for a neoplastic process such as ovarian papillomas (Nicosia and Johnson, 1984). The papillary extensions often contain minimal stroma with rare fibroblasts, capillaries, and minimal loose connective tissue. These changes can be distinguished from a generalized mesothelial neoplastic process by their presence only on the ovary.

Male Reproductive Tract

Male rabbit sex glands include ampullae, seminal vesicles (vesicular glands), prostate (with proprostate and paraprostate), and bulbourethral glands (Fig. 18.8).

The male rabbit has three prostate-related structures: the prostate, the paraprostate, and the proprostate. The prostate and proprostate are located on the dorsal surface where the urinary bladder and urethra join. The paraprostate is microscopically identical to the prostate and is positioned ventral to the prostate gland (Fig. 18.9).

Clinical Pathology—Urine

Rabbit urine is highly variable in appearance, and multiple colors and opacities may be within normal limits. Turbidity is caused by relatively high levels of albumin, as well as fine calcium carbonate and ammonium magnesium phosphate crystals. Depending on the concentration of porphyrin pigments derived from the diet or xenobiotics (e.g., antibiotics), the urine can vary widely in color from yellow to red and it may be challenging to differentiated hematuria from a high concentration of porphyrin. For more information on urine collection and analysis, please see *Clinical Pathology in Nonclinical Toxicity Testing*, Vol 1, Chap 10.

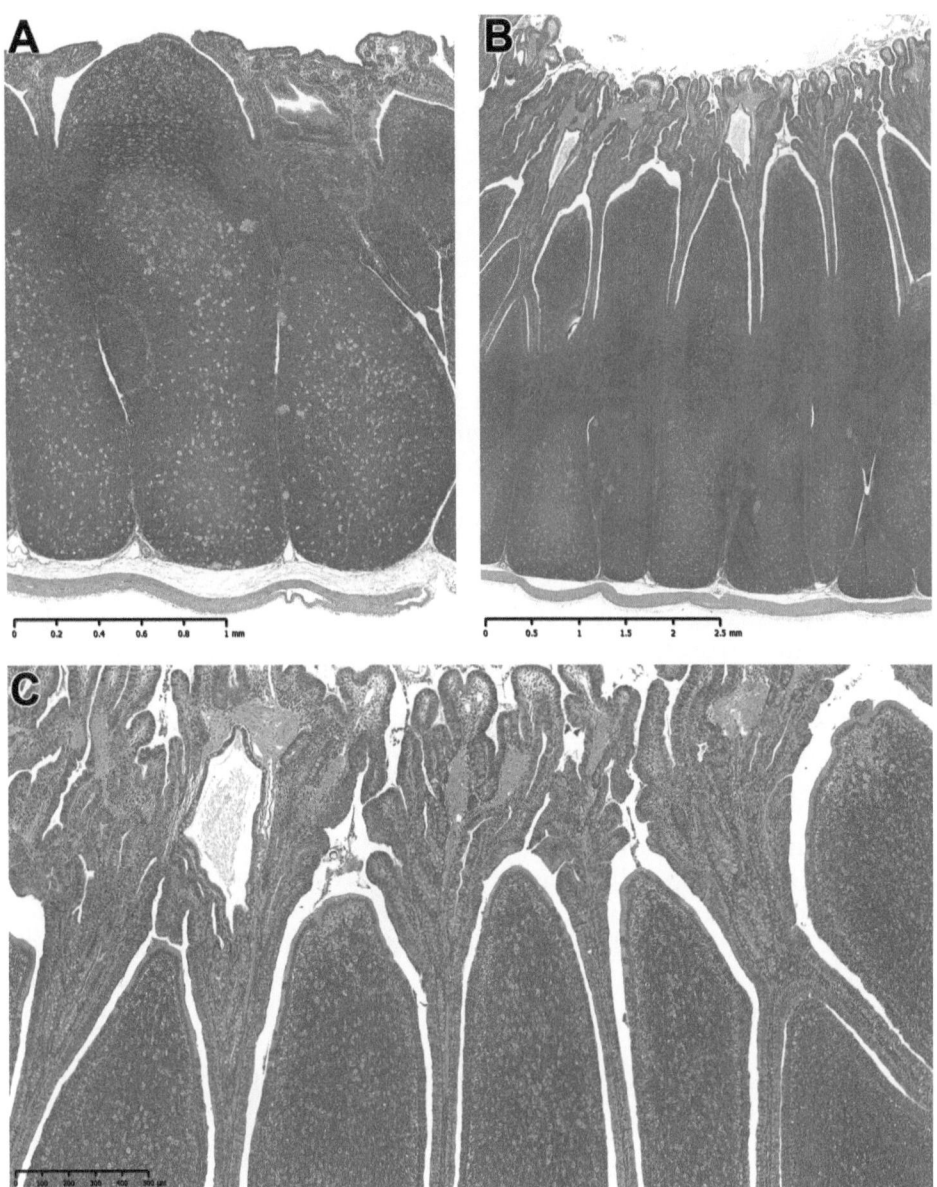

FIGURE 18.5 Section of normal appendix and sacculus rotundus from NZW rabbit. (A) The majority of the appendix consists of dense lymphoid tissue with germinal centers and minimal surface epithelium. (B) The sacculus rotundus has epithelial extensions overlying dense lymphoid tissue with germinal centers. (C) Higher magnification of (B). Hematoxylin and eosin.

7.2. Spontaneous Pathology Findings

The upcoming International Harmonization of Nomenclature and Diagnostic Criteria rabbit publication (Bradley et al., 2021) will provide specific details on a wide variety of findings, some of which have been reviewed previously in Bradley (2012), together with representative images. This section provides a highlight of the most important findings in rabbits by organ system.

Ocular

Developmental glaucoma has been reported frequently in NZW albino rabbits (Barthold et al., 2016) and can cause grossly identifiable buphthalmos.

Cardiac

A spectrum of cardiac changes has been reported in rabbits and attributed to stress

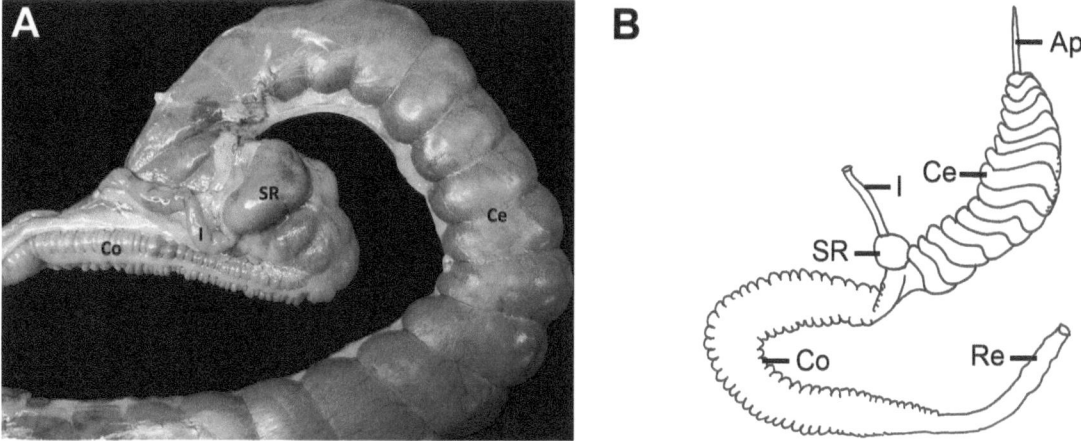

FIGURE 18.6 Distal small intestine and large intestine from a rabbit at necropsy (A) and in an illustration (B). Ileum (I), Sacculus rotundus (SR), Appendix (Ap), Cecum (Ce), Colon (Co), Rectum (Re).

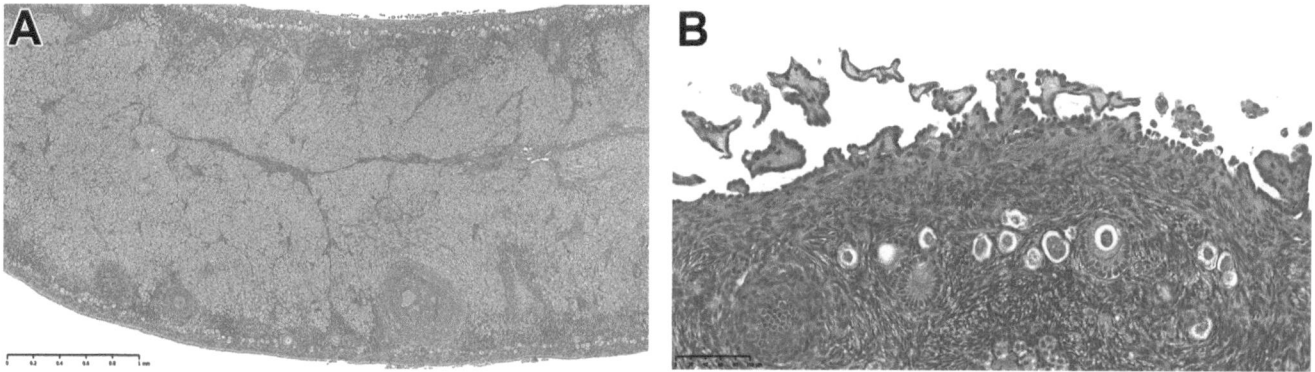

FIGURE 18.7 Section of ovary from NZW rabbit showing normal structures. (A) Interstitial tissue consisting of abundant vacuolated cells centrally (interstitial gland). (B) Surface epithelial structures consisting of fronds with fibrous core and surface epithelium. Hematoxylin and eosin.

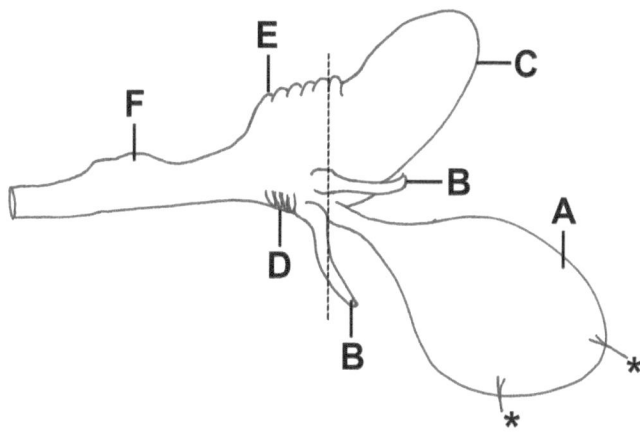

FIGURE 18.8 Illustration of male rabbit bladder and accessory sex glands. (A) Bladder with ureters (*) (B) Ampulla ductus deferens (C) Vesicular gland (D) Pro-prostate (surface extensions adjacent to the ampulae) (E) Prostate (F) Bulbourethral gland. Paraprostate not visible in image. *Dotted line* shows approximate location of histologic section in Fig. 18.9.

(catecholamine) responses (Downing and Chen, 1985; Sellers et al., 2017). Findings can include infiltration/inflammation (often macrophages and heterophils), cardiomyocyte degeneration/necrosis, interstitial edema, and/or early fibrosis (Fig. 18.10). The incidence of these findings may be highly variable, with only a few animals affected in an individual study.

Reproductive System

Mammary gland hyperplasia/dysplasia can be induced in rabbits through increased levels of prolactin. Prolactin increases are reported with both administration of cyclosporine A (Krimer et al., 2009) and prolactin-secreting pituitary acidophil adenomas in older NZW rabbits (Lipman et al., 1994).

Male rabbits can infrequently develop spontaneous focal keratinized squamous metaplasia of

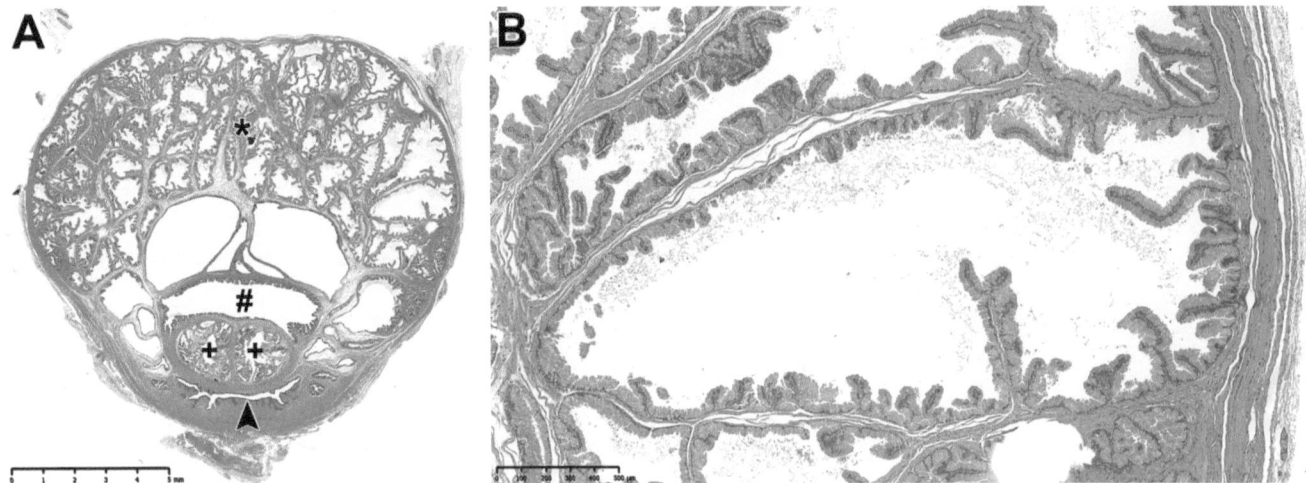

FIGURE 18.9   Section of male accessory sex glands (see Fig. 18.8 for location) from NZW rabbit. (A) Cross-section includes extensive prostate (*), vesicular gland (#), and ampulla ductus deferens (+) along with the urethra (*arrowhead*). (B) Higher magnification of prostate epithelium. Hematoxylin and eosin.

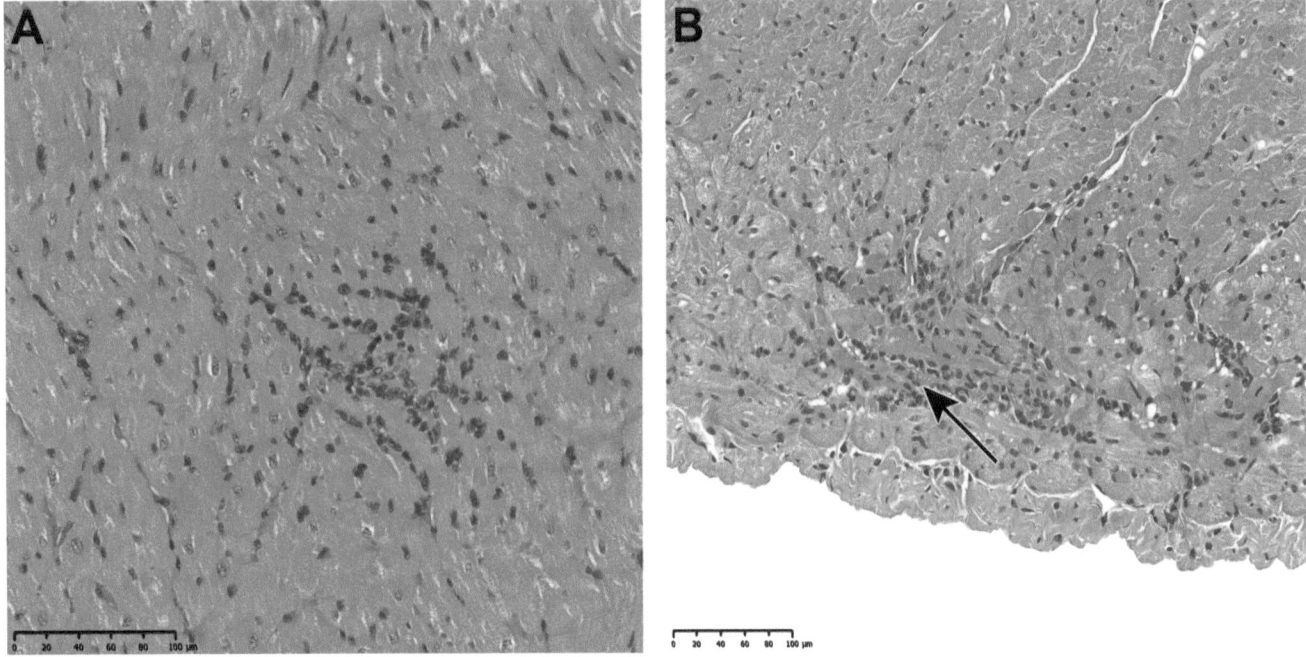

FIGURE 18.10   Cardiac inflammation and necrosis. Sections of heart from NZW rabbit showing common cardiac findings. (A) Mixed immune cell infiltrate within the ventricle. (B) Mixed inflammation and multifocal cardiomyocyte necrosis (*arrow*). Hematoxylin and eosin.

the prostate epithelium (Zwicker et al., 1985). This is notable as a rule out when a test article is being examined that has androgenic or estrogenic actions. Additionally, endometrial venous aneurysms have been reported in NZW and release of blood from the aneurysms may be mistaken as hematuria clinically.

Gastrointestinal System

Rabbits are sensitive to stress and will commonly develop diarrhea. One rabbit-specific form of gastrointestinal pathology is mucoid enteropathy, which is characterized by goblet cell hyperplasia, generally in young animals around 2–3 months old. There is an increased size and number of goblet cells more prominently in the ileum, with changes often also in the duodenum, jejunum, and portions of the large intestine. The etiology is currently unknown, but enterotoxin-induced secretory diarrhea is suspected and the finding may be induced in studies where the test article is an antibiotic.

Neoplasia

Two types of cancer are most common in rabbits and have a characteristic age distribution in incidence. Lymphoma is diagnosed in juvenile and young adult rabbits (2 years old and younger), while uterine adenocarcinoma is most common in rabbits older than 2 years.

Rabbits as young as 4 months have been diagnosed with lymphoma (Shibuya et al., 1999) and both B-cell (Gomez et al., 2002) and T-cell (Toth et al., 1990; White et al., 2000) origin tumors have been reported.

Uterine adenocarcinoma may metastasize to the lungs and mammary involvement is commonly seen. Uterine adenocarcinomas may be seen concurrently with other uterine tumors, including leiomyoma/leiomyosarcoma (Greene and Strauss, 1949) and squamous cell carcinoma (Walter et al., 2010).

Rabbits may develop deciduosarcomas, which are unique, malignant tumors that may metastasize to the lungs. It is unclear if deciduosarcomas are true neoplasms, since they are hormone dependent and can be induced in as few as 30 days after administration of estrogens and progestin and cessation of estrogen/progesterone treatment can cause disappearance of the tumor (Zook et al., 2001). Mechanistically, initial endometrial decidualization requires exogenous estrogens, while exogenous progesterones promote the development of deciduosarcoma (Janne et al., 2001).

In female rabbits, deciduosarcomas can be induced or spontaneous and arise from uterine stromal and metrial gland cells. Stromal cells can contain abundant, PAS-positive cytoplasm, and there are often numerous hypertrophied blood vessels within the tumor along with globular lymphocytes. It is important to note that deciduosarcomas can be induced in the abdominal viscera, most commonly in the spleen of castrated males treated with estrogen and progesterone.

Rabbits older than 2 years have an elevated incidence of mammary gland neoplasia (Barthold et al., 2016). The majority of neoplasms are of an epithelial origin and malignant forms (adenocarcinomas, carcinomas) are more common than adenomas (Kanfer and Reavill, 2013). Nonepithelial forms are rarely reported in rabbits (e.g., anaplastic, spindle cell, or mixed neoplasms).

A progression of changes may be seen, beginning with cystic mammary gland changes and low-grade tumors (adenoma), eventually progressing to invasive adenocarcinomas. There may be a correlation between development of uterine tumors and mammary carcinomas. The lung and regional draining lymph nodes are the most commonly reported sites for metastasis.

REFERENCES

Ahmed A, Berati H, Nalan A, et al.: Effect of bevacizumab on corneal neovascularization in experimental rabbit model, *Clin Exp Ophthalmol* 37(7):730–736, 2009.

Aleksunes LM, Eaton DL: Principles of toxicology. In Klaassen CD, editor: *Casarett and Doull's toxicology: the basic science of Poisons*, New York, 2019, McGraw Hill, pp 25–64.

Alve JM, Carneiro M, Afonso S, et al.: Levels and patterns of genetic diversity and population structure in domestic rabbits, *PLoS One* 10(12):e0144687, 2015.

Alves A, Wancket L, Metz A: Current considerations in medical device pathology. In Boutrand J, editor: *Biocompatibility and performance of medical devices*, United Kingdom, 2019, Elsevier, pp 489–543.

Aravalli RN, Cressman ENK: Relevance of rabbit VX2 tumor model for studies on human hepatocellular carcinoma: a MicroRNA-based study, *J Clin Med Res* 4(12):1989–1997, 2015.

Baczkó I, Jost N, Virág L, et al.: Rabbit models as tools for preclinical cardiac electrophysiological safety testing: importance of repolarization reserve, *Prog Biophys Mol Biol* 121(2):157–168, 2016.

Barthold SW, Griffey SM, Percy DH: *Pathology of laboratory rodents and rabbits*, Ames, IA, 2016, Wiley-Blackwell.

Baumans V: Environmental enrichment for laboratory rodents and rabbits: requirements of rodents, rabbits, and research, *ILAR J* 46(2):162–170, 2005.

Bolon B, Garman RH, Pardo ID, et al.: STP position paper: recommended practices for sampling and processing the nervous system (brain, spinal cord, nerve, and eye) during nonclinical general toxicity studies, *Toxicol Pathol* 41(7): 1028–1048, 2013.

Bradley AE: New Zealand white rabbits. In McInnes E, editor: *Background lesions in laboratory animals- A color atlas*, Edinburgh, 2012, Elsevier.

Bradley AE, Wancket LM, Rinke M, et al.: International harmonization of nomenclature and diagnostic criteria (INHAND): nonproliferative and proliferative lesions of the rabbit, *J Toxicol Pathol*, 2021 (in press).

Brewer NR, Cruise LJ: Physiology. In Manning P, Ringler D, Newcomer C, editors: *The biology of the laboratory rabbit*, San Diego, 1994, Academic Press.

Buja LM, Kita T, Goldstein JL, et al.: Cellular pathology of progressive atherosclerosis in the WHHL rabbit. An animal model of familial hypercholesterolemia, *Arteriosclerosis* 3(1): 87–101, 1983.

Burkholder TH, Linton G, Hoyt RF, et al.: Chapter 18 - the rabbit as an experimental model. In Suckow MA, Stevens KA, Wilson RP, editors: *The laboratory rabbit, Guinea pig, hamster, and other rodents*, Boston, 2012, Academic Press, pp 529–560.

Carlsson L: The anaesthetised methoxamine-sensitized rabbit model of torsades de pointes, *Pharmacol Ther* 119(2):160–167, 2008.

Chandra SA, Peterson RA, Melich D, et al.: Dermal irritation of petrolatum in rabbits but not in mice, rats or minipigs, *J Appl Toxicol* 34(8):857–861, 2014.

Chetoni P, Burgalassi S, Monti D, et al.: Solid lipid nanoparticles as promising tool for intraocular tobramycin delivery: pharmacokinetic studies on rabbits, *Eur J Pharm Biopharm* 109:214–223, December 2016.

Daniels AB, Froehler MT, Pierce JM, et al.: Pharmacokinetics, tissue localization, toxicity, and treatment efficacy in the first small animal (rabbit) model of intra-arterial chemotherapy for retinoblastoma, *Invest Ophthalmol Vis Sci* 59(1): 446–454, 2018.

Dolz-Marco R, Gallego-Pinazo R, Pinazo-Duran MD, et al.: Intravitreal docosahexaenoic acid in a rabbit model: preclinical safety assessment, *PLoS One* 9(5):e96872, 2014.

Downing SE, Chen V: Myocardial injury following endogenous catecholamine release in rabbits, *J Mol Cell Cardiol* 17: 377–387, 1985.

Drevon-Gaillot E: Ocular medical devices: histologic technique and histopathologic evaluation of the biocompatibility and performance, *Toxicol Pathol* 47(3):418–425, 2019.

Dunne AA, Plehn S, Schulz S, et al.: Lymph node topography of the head and neck in New Zealand white rabbits, *Lab Anim* 37(1):37–43, 2003.

Esteves PJ, Abrantes J, Baldauf HM, et al.: The wide utility of rabbits as models of human diseases, *Exp Mol Med* 50(66), 2018, 018-0094-1.

Evans BC, Hocking KM, Osgood MJ, et al.: MK2 inhibitory peptide delivered in nanopolyplexes prevents vascular graft intimal hyperplasia, *Sci Trans Med* 7(291):291ra95, 2015.

Fan J, Kitajima S, Watanabe T, et al.: Rabbit models for the study of human atherosclerosis: from pathophysiological mechanisms to translational medicine, *Pharmacol Ther* 146: 104–119, February 2015.

Fang Q, Gu T, Fan J, Zhang Y, Wang Y, Zhao Y, Zhao P: Evaluation of a hybrid small caliber vascular graft in a rabbit

model, *J Thorac Cardiovasc Surg March* 159(2):461–473, 2020. https://doi.org/10.1016/j.jtcvs.2019.02.083.

Frommeyer G, Milberg P, Uphaus T, et al.: Antiarrhythmic effect of ranolazine in combination with class III drugs in an experimental whole-heart model of atrial fibrillation, *Cardiovasc Ther* 31(6):e63–71, 2013.

Goldstein JL, Kita T, Brown MS: Defective lipoprotein receptors and atherosclerosis. Lessons from an animal counterpart of familial hypercholesterolemia, *NEJM* 309(5): 288–296, 1983.

Gomez L, Gazquez A, Roncero V, et al.: Lymphoma in a rabbit: histopathological and immunohistochemical findings, *J Small Anim Pract* 43:224–226, 2002.

Greene HS, Strauss JS: Multiple primary tumors in the rabbit, *Cancer* 2:673–691, 1949.

Haines RA, Urbiztondo RA, Haynes RA, et al.: Characterization of New Zealand white rabbit gut-associated lymphoid tissues and use as viral oncology animal model, *ILAR J* 57: 34–43, 2016.

Harkness JE, Turner PV, VandeWoude S, et al.: *Harkness and Wagner's biology and medicine of rabbits and rodents*, Ames, IA, 2013, Wiley-Blackwell.

Hill PS, Apel PJ, Barnwell J, et al.: Repair of peripheral nerve defects in rabbits using keratin hydrogel scaffolds, *Tissue Eng. Part A* 17(11–12):1499–1505, 2011.

Hirano S, Bless DM, Rousseau B, et al.: Prevention of vocal fold scarring by topical injection of hepatocyte growth factor in a rabbit model, *Laryngoscope* 114(3):548–556, 2004.

Holve DL, Mundwiler KE, Pritt SL: Incidence of spontaneous ocular lesions in laboratory rabbits, *Com Med* 61(5):436–440, 2011.

Honda A, Ogura A: Rabbit models for biomedical research revisited via genome editing approaches, *J Reprod Dev* 63: 435–438, 2017.

Houdebine L-M, Fan J: *Rabbit biotechnology: rabbit genomics, transgenesis, cloning and models*, Netherlands, 2009, Springer Science & Business Media.

Hsu S-H, Chan S-H, Chiang C-M, et al.: Peripheral nerve regeneration using a microporous polylactic acid asymmetric conduit in a rabbit long-gap sciatic nerve transection model, *Biomaterials* 32(15):3764–3775, 2011.

Inan UU, Avci B, Kusbeci T, et al.: Preclinical safety evaluation of intravitreal injection of full-length humanized vascular endothelial growth factor antibody in rabbit eyes, *Invest Ophthalmol Vis Sci* 48(4):1773–1781, 2007.

Janne OA, Zook BC, Didolkar AK, et al.: The roles of estrogen and progestin in producing deciduosarcoma and other lesions in the rabbit, *Toxicol Pathol* 29:417–421, 2001.

Jayo JM, Schwenke DC, Clarkson TB: *Atherosclerosis research in the biology of the laboratory rabbit*, San Diego, 1994, Elsevier, pp 367–380.

Jung EC, Maibach HI: Animal models for percutaneous absorption, *J Appl Toxicol* 35:1–10, 2015.

Kaminsky M, Szivos MM, Brown KR, et al.: Comparison of the sensitivity of the vaginal mucous membranes of the albino rabbit and laboratory rat to nonoxynol-9, *Food Chem Toxicol* 23:705–708, 1985.

Kanfer S, Reavill DR: Cutaneous neoplasia in ferrets, rabbits, and Guinea pigs, *Vet Clin North Am Exot Anim Pract* 16:579–598, 2013.

Kararli TT: Comparison of the gastrointestinal anatomy, physiology, and biochemistry of humans and commonly used laboratory animals, *Biopharm Drug Dispos* 16(5):351–380, 1995.

Kilkenny C, Browne WJ, Cuthill IC, et al.: Improving bioscience research reporting: the ARRIVE guidelines for reporting animal research, *PLoS Biol* 8(6):e1000412, 2010.

Kirchner D, Henwood S: Chapter 12: toxicity and safety testing. In Suckow MA, Stevens KA, Wilson RP, editors: *The laboratory rabbit, Guinea pig, hamster, and other rodents*, Boston, 2012, Academic Press, pp 275–300.

Kouchi M, Ueda Y, Horie H, et al.: Ocular lesions in Watanabe heritable hyperlipidemic rabbits, *Vet Ophthalmol* 9(3):145–148, 2006.

Krimer PM, Harvey SB, Blas-Machado U, et al.: Reversible fibroadenomatous mammary hyperplasia in male and female New Zealand white rabbits associated with cyclosporine administration, *Vet Pathol* 46:1144–1148, 2009.

Kunta JR, Perry BA, Sutyak JP, et al.: Development of a novel intestinal and vascular access port (IVAP) rabbit model to study regiospecific oral absorption pharmacokinetics, *Comp Med* 51(4):349–356, 2001.

Kurosawa T, Kusanagi M, Yamasaki Y, et al.: New mutant rabbit strain with hypercholesterolemia and atherosclerotic lesions produced by serial inbreeding, *Lab Anim Sci* 45(4):385–392, 1995.

Lanning D, Zhu X, Zhai S, et al.: Development of the antibody repertoire in rabbit: gut-associated lymphoid tissue, microbes, and selection, *Immunol Rev* 175:214–228, 2000.

Laverty S, Girard CA, Williams JM, et al.: The OARSI histopathology initiative - recommendations for histological assessments of osteoarthritis in the rabbit, *Osteoarthritis Cartilage* 18(Suppl 3):S53–S65, 2010.

Lee JM, Jin GY, Li CA, et al.: Percutaneous radiofrequency thermal ablation of lung VX2 tumors in a rabbit model using a cooled tip-electrode: feasibility, safety, and effectiveness, *Invest Rad* 38(2):129–139, 2003.

Lee CJ, Gonçalves LL, Wells PG: Embryopathic effects of thalidomide and its hydrolysis products in rabbit embryo culture: evidence for a prostaglandin H synthase (PHS)-dependent, reactive oxygen species (ROS)-mediated mechanism, *FASEB J* 25:2468–2483, 2011.

Lei H, Rheaume M-A, Cui J, et al.: A novel function of p53: a gatekeeper of retinal detachment, *Am J Pathol* 181(3):866–874, 2012.

Lipman NS, Zhao ZB, Andrutis KA, et al.: Prolactin-secreting pituitary adenomas with mammary dysplasia in New Zealand white rabbits, *Lab Anim Sci* 44:114–120, 1994.

Liu J, Xu C, Liu YL, et al.: Activation of rabbit TLR9 by different CpG-ODN optimized for mouse and human TLR9, *Comp Immunol Microbiol Infect Dis* 35:443–451, 2012.

Lossi L, D'Angelo L, De Girolamo P, et al.: Anatomical features for an adequate choice of experimental animal model in biomedicine: II. Small laboratory rodents, rabbit, and pig, *Ann Anat* 204:11–28, March 2016.

Maurer JK, Parker RD: Light microscopic comparison of surfactant-induced eye irritation in rabbits and rats at three hours and recovery/day 35, *Toxicol Pathol* 24(4):403–411, 1996.

Maurer JK, Molai A, Parker RD, et al.: Pathology of ocular irritation with bleaching agents in the rabbit low-volume eye test, *Toxicol Pathol* 29(3):308–319, 2001.

Mekaj AY, Manxhuka-Kerliu S, Morina AA, et al.: Effects of hyaluronic acid and tacrolimus on the prevention of perineural scar formation and on nerve regeneration after sciatic nerve repair in a rabbit model, *Eur J Trauma Emerg Surg* 43(4):497–504, 2017.

Mitsuguchi Y, Ito T, Ohwada K: Pathologic findings in rabbit models of hereditary hypertriglyceridemia and hereditary postprandial hypertriglyceridemia, *Comp Med* 58(5):465–480, 2008.

Mohammed IFR, Al-Mustawfi N, Kaka LN: Promotion of regenerative processes in injured peripheral nerve induced by low-level laser therapy, *Photomed Laser Surg* 25(2):107–111, 2007.

Mori H, Matsumoto K: Development of the secondary interstitial gland in the rabbit ovary, *J Anat* 116:417–430, 1973.

Morton D, The use of rabbits in male reproductive toxicology, *Environ Health Perspect* 77:5–9, 1988. https://doi.org/10.1289/ehp.88775.

Mykytowycz R: Further observations on the territorial function and histology of the submandibular cutaneous (chin) glands in the rabbit, *Oryctolagus cuniculus* (L.), *Anim Behav* 13:400–412, 1965.

Nicosia SV, Johnson JH: Surface morphology of ovarian mesothelium (surface epithelium) and of other pelvic and extrapelvic mesothelial sites in the rabbit, *Int J Gynecol Pathol* 3:249–260, 1984.

Oh S, Hong S, Kim S, et al.: Histological and functional aspects of different regions of the rabbit vagina, *Int J Impotence Res* 15:142–150, 2003.

Panfilov AV: Is heart size a factor in ventricular fibrillation? Or how close are rabbit and human hearts? *Heart Rhythm* 3(7):862–864, 2006.

Petritz OA, Sanchez-Migallon GD, Gandolfi RC, et al.: Inguinal-scrotal urinary bladder hernia in an intact male domestic rabbit (*Oryctolagus cuniculus*), *J Exotic Pet Med* 21(3):248–254, 2012.

Pinheiro A, et al.: Molecular bases of genetic diversity and evolution of the immunoglobulin heavy chain variable region (IGHV) gene locus in leporids, *Immunogenetics* 63:397–408, 2011.

Pogwizd SM, Bers DM: Rabbit models of heart disease, *Drug Discov Today Dis Models* 5(3):185–193, 2008.

Qi X, Yeh Y-H, Chartier D, et al.: The calcium/calmodulin/kinase system and arrhythmogenic afterdepolarizations in bradycardia-related acquired long-QT syndrome, *Circ Arrhythm Electrophysiol* 2(3):295–304, 2009.

Quesenberry K, Carpenter JW: *Ferrets, rabbits and rodents - E-book: clinical medicine and surgery,* Elsevier Health Sciences.

Ramirez CJ, Kim DY, Hanks BC, et al.: Copper toxicosis in New Zealand White rabbits (*Oryctolagus cuniculus*), *Vet Pathol* 50:1135–1138, 2013.

Rissanen TT, Markkanen JE, Arve K, et al.: Fibroblast growth factor 4 induces vascular permeability, angiogenesis and arteriogenesis in a rabbit hindlimb ischemia model, *FASEB J* 17(1):100–102, 2003.

Schuh JCL, Funk KA: Compilation of international standards and regulatory guidance documents for evaluation of biomaterials, medical devices, and 3-D printed and regenerative medicine products, *Toxicol Pathol* 47:344–357, 2019.

Sellers RS, Pardo I, Hu G, et al.: Inflammatory cell findings in the female rabbit heart and stress-associated exacerbation with handling and procedures used in nonclinical studies, *Toxicol Pathol* 45:416–426, 2017.

Sellers RS, Nelson K, Bennet B, et al.: Scientific and regulatory policy committee points to consider*: approaches to the conduct and interpretation of vaccine safety studies for clinical and anatomic pathologists, *Toxicol Pathol* 48:257–276, 2020.

Shen J, Zhou C-P, Zhong X-M, et al.: MR neurography: T1 and T2 measurements in acute peripheral nerve traction injury in rabbits, *Radiology* 254(3):729–738, 2010.

Shibuya K, Tajima M, Kanai K, et al.: Spontaneous lymphoma in a Japanese white rabbit, *J Vet Med Sci* 61:1327–1329, 1999.

Shin K-J, Yoo J-Y, Lee J-Y, et al.: Anatomical study of the nerve regeneration after selective neurectomy in the rabbit: clinical application for esthetic calf reduction, *Anat Cell Biol* 48(4):268–274, 2015.

Shiomi M, Ito T: The Watanabe heritable hyperlipidemic (WHHL) rabbit, its characteristics and history of development: a tribute to the late Dr. Yoshio Watanabe, *Atherosclerosis* 207(1):1–7, 2009.

Sidorov VY, Woods MC, Baudenbacher F: Cathodal stimulation in the recovery phase of a propagating planar wave in the rabbit heart reveals four stimulation mechanisms, *J Physiol* 583(Pt 1):237–250, 2007.

Song BZ, Donoff RB, Tsuji T, et al.: Identification of rabbit eosinophils and heterophils in cutaneous healing wounds, *Histochem J* 25:762–771, 1993.

Stills HF: Chapter 11: polyclonal antibody production. In Suckow MA, Stevens KA, Wilson RP, editors: *The laboratory rabbit, Guinea pig, hamster, and other rodents,* Boston, 2012, Academic Press, pp 259–274.

Swanson ER, Abdollahian D, Ohno T, et al.: Characterization of raised phonation in an evoked rabbit phonation model, *Laryngoscope* 119(7):1439–1443, 2009.

Thibeault SL, Bless DM, Gray SD: Interstitial protein alterations in rabbit vocal fold with scar, *J Voice* 17(3):377–383, 2003.

Toth LA, Olson GA, Wilson E, et al.: Lymphocytic leukemia and lymphosarcoma in a rabbit, *J Am Vet Med Assoc* 197:627–629, 1990.

Turner Giannico A, de Sampaio MOB, Lima L, et al.: Characterization of the oculocardiac reflex during compression of the globe in beagle dogs and rabbits, *Vet Ophthalmol* 17(5):321–327, 2014.

Vossen JA, Buijs M, Syed L, et al.: Development of a new orthotopic animal model of metastatic liver cancer in the rabbit VX2 model: effect on metastases after partial hepatectomy, intra-arterial treatment with 3-bromopyruvate and chemoembolization, *Clin Exp Metastasis* 25(7):811–817, 2008.

Walter B, Poth T, Bohmer E, et al.: Uterine disorders in 59 rabbits, *Vet Rec* 166:230–233, 2010.

Wancket LM: Animal models for evaluation of bone implants and devices: comparative bone structure and common model uses, *Vet Pathol* 52(5):842–850, 2015.

Wancket LM: Regional draining lymph nodes: considerations for medical device studies, *Toxicol Pathol* 47:339–343, 2019.

Watanabe Y: Serial inbreeding of rabbits with hereditary hyperlipidemia (WHHL-Rabbit): incidence and development of atherosclerosis and xanthoma, *Atherosclerosis* 36(2):261–268, 1980.

Weber HW, Van Der Walt JJ: Cardiomyopathy in crowded rabbits, *Recent Adv Stud Cardiac Struct Metab* 6:471–477, 1975.

Weber J, Peng H, Rader C: From rabbit antibody repertoires to rabbit monoclonal antibodies, *Exp Mol Med* 49(3):e305, 2017.

Weisbroth SH, Flatt RE, Kraus AL: *The biology of the laboratory rabbit,* San Diego, 2013, Academic Press.

Werner L, Chew J, Mamalis N: Experimental evaluation of ophthalmic devices and solutions using rabbit models, *Vet Ophthalmol* 9(5):281–291, 2006.

White SD, Campbell T, Logan A, et al.: Lymphoma with cutaneous involvement in three domestic rabbits (*Oryctolagus cuniculus*), *Vet Dermatol* 11:61–67, 2000.

Winter PM, Caruthers SD, Kassner A, et al.: Molecular imaging of angiogenesis in nascent vx-2 rabbit tumors using a novel αvβ3-targeted nanoparticle and 1.5 tesla magnetic resonance imaging, *Cancer Res* 63(18):5838–5843, 2003.

Wyatt JD, Moorman-White DM, Ventura D, et al.: Sequelae of occult aggression disqualifying young, socially housed, female New Zealand white rabbits (*Oryctolagus cuniculus*) from participation in dermal toxicology studies, *Comp Med* 67(5):430–435, 2017.

Yanni AE: The laboratory rabbit: an animal model of atherosclerosis research, *Lab Anim* 38(3):246–256, 2004.

York KK, Miller S, Gaster RN, et al.: Polyvinylpyrrolidone iodine: corneal toxicology and epithelial healing in a rabbit model, *J Ocular Pharmacol* 4(4):351–358, 1988.

Zhang H, Wei YT, Tsang KS, et al.: Implantation of neural stem cells embedded in hyaluronic acid and collagen composite conduit promotes regeneration in a rabbit facial nerve injury model, *J Trans Med* 6:67, November 2008.

Zhang Z, Machac J, Helft G, et al.: Non-invasive imaging of atherosclerotic plaque macrophage in a rabbit model with F-18 FDG PET: a histopathological correlation, *BMC Nucl Med* 6(1):3, 2006.

Zhao S, Yu H, Du N: Experimental study of doxorubicin interventional chemotherapy in the treatment of rabbit VX2 renal transplantation carcinoma, *Int J Clin Exp Med* 8(7): 10739–10745, 2015.

Zheng W, Wang Z, Song L, et al.: Endothelialization and patency of RGD-functionalized vascular grafts in a rabbit carotid artery model, *Biomaterials* 33(10):2880–2891, 2012.

Zook BC, Jänne OA, Abraham AA, et al.: The development and regression of deciduosarcomas and other lesions caused by estrogens and progestins in rabbits, *Toxicol Pathol* 29:411–416, 2001.

Zwicker GM, Killinger JM, McConnel RF: Spontaneous vesicular and prostatic gland epithelial squamous metaplasia, hyperplasia, and keratinized nodule formation in rabbits, *Toxicol Pathol* 13:222–228, 1985.

Animal Models in Toxicologic Research: Dog

John R. Foster[1], Vasanthi Mowat[2], Bhanu P. Singh[3],
Jennifer L. Ingram–Ross[4], Dino Bradley[4]

[1]ToxPath Sciences Ltd, Congleton, Cheshire, United Kingdom, [2]Labcorp Clinical & Preclinical Services Ltd, Huntingdon, United Kingdom, [3]Gilead Sciences, Foster City, CA, United States, [4]Janssen Research & Development, McKean Road, Spring House, PA, United States

OUTLINE

1. Introduction 722

2. History and Derivation of Beagles 722
   2.1. Genetics of Canines and Background for Their Use in Toxicity Testing 722
   2.2. The Evolution of the Laboratory Beagle 723
   2.3. Basic Biological Characteristics 723
   2.4. Housing and Care of the Beagle Dog 726

3. Use of Dogs in Biomedical Research 727
   3.1. Drug Metabolism, Disposition, and Excretion of Drugs/Chemicals in the Dog—Comparison with Other Species 727
   3.2. Genetic Variability within Beagles and Impact on Testing 727
   3.3. Use of the Dog in Drug Discovery and Development 728
   3.4. Duration of Studies/Age at Start of Studies in Dogs 728
   3.5. Use of the Dog for Assessing Clinical Pathology and Pharmacokinetic Changes 729
   3.6. Safety Pharmacology Studies in Dogs 730
   3.7. Use of Dogs in Developmental Toxicity Studies 731

4. Predictivity of Dog Toxicity Data to Humans 731

5. Comparative Toxicology of the Dog 732
   5.1. Toxic Responses of the Dog Compared to Other Species 732
   5.2. Small-Molecule Kinase Inhibitors 733
   5.3. Caffeine 733

5.4. Theobromine 734
5.5. Acetaminophen (Paracetamol) 734
5.6. Aspirin and Ibuprofen 735
5.7. Vasoactive Drugs 735

6. Spontaneous Background Pathology in the Beagle 735
   6.1. Spontaneous Nonneoplastic Diseases in Laboratory Beagles 735
   6.2. Spontaneous Neoplastic Diseases in Laboratory Beagles 737

7. Use of the Dog as a Model of Human Diseases 737
   7.1. The Dog as an Animal Model of Human Cardiovascular Disease 737
   7.2. The Dog as an Animal Model of Human Cancer 737
   7.3. The Dog as an Animal Model of Human Neurological Diseases 739

8. Regulatory Considerations for Toxicity Studies 742
   8.1. Pesticide and Drug Development—Need for One-Year Dog Study? 742

9. Ethics of Use of the Dog as a Laboratory Animal Species 743

10. Summary 744

References 744

1. INTRODUCTION

In order to develop new agrochemicals, industrial chemicals, and pharmaceutical products, regulatory agencies worldwide require preclinical safety evaluation trials in order to determine toxicity and pharmacokinetics. International guidelines typically recommend studies in at least two species, one rodent and one nonrodent. These studies establish target organ toxicity and are used to set acceptable exposure limits of chemicals for subsequent risk assessment and management of human exposure. In terms of regulatory requirements, the Organisation for Economic Co-operation and Development (OECD) guidance document 409 (OECD, 1998) states that "The commonly used nonrodent species is the dog, which should be of a defined breed," while the US Environmental Protection Agency's (EPA) Office of Prevention, Pesticides and Toxic Substances (OPPTS) Harmonized test guidelines 870–3150 (US EPA, 1998) states that "The commonly used nonrodent species is the dog, preferably of a defined breed; the beagle is frequently used. If other mammalian species are used, the tester should provide justification/reasoning for his or her selection." Beagle dogs are therefore the most commonly used nonrodent laboratory animal species with an estimated 18,000 used annually in the United Kingdom (UK Home Office, 2018), 29,000 across the European Union (European Union, 2013), and 65,000 in the United States of America (USDA, 2017), representing 0.5%, 0.25%, and 8%, respectively, of the total numbers of experimental animals used. In 2013, approximately 80% of this use was as the nonrodent species in the evaluation of pharmaceutical safety and efficacy (Bailey et al., 2013). Beagles are ideal laboratory animals due to their size, temperament, reproductive features, and trainability. The size of the dog allows procedures designed to facilitate and reduce the invasiveness of dosing and data collection, which simply are not amenable, or are technically difficult, in rodents.

2. HISTORY AND DERIVATION OF BEAGLES

The beagle, as the breed is known today, is thought to have originated in Ancient Greece and Britain from small hunting dogs that could fit into the hunter's pocket. Interbreeding led to the development of larger dogs that were more desirable for hunting larger game. During the eighth century, the St. Hubert Hound, a large scent hound bred by French monks, was bred to create the Talbot Hound, a tall yet slow running dog that was a poor hunter. During the 11th century, the Talbot Hound was brought to England where it was bred with the Greyhound in order to increase the breed's speed. This new breed, the Southern Hound, is thought to be one of the ancestors of the modern beagle.

During the 1700s, the Southern Hound and North Country or Northern Beagle were bred with the Foxhound to develop a hunting dog with improved speed and scenting abilities (Fleischer et al., 2008). Breed qualities were improved through established breeding programs in the 1800. In the 1870s, General Richard Rowett of Carlinville, Illinois, was one of the first individuals to import the Beagle to the United States from England. General Rowett's beagles are thought to be the models for the first American standard Beagle. In 1884, the breed was accepted into the American Kennel Club.

2.1. Genetics of Canines and Background for Their Use in Toxicity Testing

The domestic dog, *Canis familiaris*, is a direct descendant of the gray wolf, *Canis lupus*. DNA analysis suggests that the modern-day dog is derived from multiple regional wolf populations (Cagan and Bass, 2016). The genome sequence of a 35,000 years old ancient Siberian Taimyr wolf fossil represents the most recent common ancestor of modern wolves and dogs.

There are small changes in the genome that distinguishes the various breeds. Based on genome data, the majority of dog breed diversity has taken place within the last 200 years. Results of the Dog Genome Project indicate that dog breeds are generally closed populations, and a given dog is more closely related to others within that breed than to dogs of other breeds. Variations among breeds accounts for more than 27% of the total genetic diversity observed in dogs. The dog breed variation is much higher than that reported within human populations (5%–10%). Across domesticated animal species, the dog has the greatest physical diversity, based upon differences in the ranges of appearance, size, and weight. Some differences in size have been traced to a single gene encoding insulin-like growth factor 1 which is common to all small breeds yet is practically absent from giant breeds (Sutter et al., 2007).

94% of the dog genome is in the same order within individual chromosomes as is present in the human, mouse, and rat. There are many similarities when comparing the genome of domesticated dogs and humans, as suggested by over 360 genetic diseases that are observed in both humans and the domesticated dog (Fleischer et al., 2008). Although first identified in humans, many of these genetic defects involve a mutation of the same, or in an analogous gene, in the dog (Ostrander, 2005).

2.2. The Evolution of the Laboratory Beagle

Dogs are used as a model in animal research primarily due to their size, friendly disposition, and ease of handling. Randomly sourced canines have an unknown genetic background which could potentially increase the variability of data collected from the study subjects. The purpose-bred beagle has become the dog breed of choice for in vivo research, although other breeds or breed mixes are also purpose bred for investigative work (Anderson, 1970).

The first US laboratory beagle colony was established in Utah in 1952. Most likely, these dogs were derived from champion stock based on their hunting performance. In the Utah colony, 18 dogs accounted for 98% of the colony's genetic pool. The prevalence of congenital defects would be amplified with such a restricted gene pool as evidenced by spontaneous seizures being reported in several laboratory beagle colonies in the late 1960s (Bielfelt et al., 1971). As a result, breeding practices across the industry were refined to reduce these occurrences. Commercial breeders of purpose-bred dogs manage their facilities based on governmental regulations and industry guidelines. This includes maintaining a breeding program to track the health and behavior of colony progeny, providing housing units allowing normal species-specific behavior and socialization, access to environmental enrichment,

regularly scheduled husbandry, access to a clean home environment, appropriate nutrition, and adequate veterinary care.

2.3. Basic Biological Characteristics

Beagle dogs are medium-sized members of the domestic dog family, *C. familiaris*, with a lifespan of between 11 and 15 years with an average age of 12 years when kept under "controlled" conditions (Anderson and Rosenblatt, 1974). Their chromosome number is 39 pairs, 38 diploid pairs and 2 sex chromosomes. Male adult beagles have a body weight range of 10–12 kg at 1 year, while females are smaller, ranging between 9 and 10 kg at the same age. There appears to be two basic sizes of beagles in the literature (https://www.akc.org/dog-breeds/beagle/), the smaller size reaching 13 inches at the shoulder with the larger breed being between 13 and 15 inches. These sources state that pups of both sizes can be born within the same litter.

The rectal temperature varies between 38 and 39°C (100–102.5° F) in adults, with pups having a lower temperature at birth and during the first week (37°C; 94–97°F), increasing to 36–38°C (97–100°F) during the second and third weeks. The respiration rate for puppies varies between 15 and 40 breaths/min, while adults have a lower rate, with a normal range of 10–30 breaths/min (Haggerty, 2008).

Beagles mature between 6 and 12 months, with the majority reaching maturity by 10 months of age (James and Heywood, 1979; Kawakami et al., 1991; Creasy, 2012). Females show a wide range of maturation times, with puberty beginning around 6 months of age and the first "cycle" occurring between 8 and 14 months (Wildt et al., 1981). Body weight, strain, geographical location, and housing, as well as many other factors, can affect the age of maturity in both sexes. The Covance laboratories (Covance Laboratories, Huntingdon, UK) have noted that Harlan sourced beagles of both sexes mature sooner than Marshall beagles, at least partially related to their higher body weights at equivalent ages. At a laboratory in France (Charles River Laboratories—formerly MDS Pharma Services, Saint-Germain-sur-L'Arbresle, France), Dorso et al. (2008) noted that males sourced from Harlan breeders in France grew faster, and reached a higher body weight sooner, than males from Marshall Farms, USA. They also noted that 90% of Harlan males aged between 31 and 40 weeks were sexually mature, whereas only 10% of Marshall males had reached sexual maturity at this age. Rehm (2000), however, noted that 11 dogs from Marshall Farms, USA, aged between 8 and 11 months, were all sexually mature, reflecting the variability of this parameter and the need for caution especially where reproductive parameters may be important in the study.

Beagles are cyclical reproducers, with one cycle occurring roughly every 7–8 months. Despite this, they cannot be classified as either seasonal or continuous breeders given the highly variable timings found across geographical locations and interindividual variability seen in the species, at least in a laboratory setting. Each individual cycle comprises proestrus and estrous phases, followed by a long diestrus period. Whereas proestrus and estrus each lasts between 1 and 2 weeks, diestrus lasts between 2 and 3 months although this duration can be highly variable. This cycle is then followed by a variable period of anestrus, which can last between 3 and 5 months.

The reproductive system of the male and female dog is routinely examined as part of the screen incorporated into routine toxicity studies for the evaluation of the safety of pharmaceutical products. For practical purposes, most safety assessment studies are conducted with prepubescent dogs and because of this there can be wide variability in maturity status at the termination of a 1 or 3 month study. Evaluation is also complicated by the variable breeding cycle, with females often being at different stages of the estrus cycle in longer-term studies. Combined with the small group sizes used in dog toxicity studies, this can make a thorough evaluation of effects on the estrus cycle problematic but not impossible. The gestation period is between 60 and 65 days, with an average litter size of five to six puppies. Puppies weigh between 140 and 280 g at birth and are toothless. Eyes which are closed at birth open at approximately 2 weeks, although vision is not completely developed until week 8 postpartum. They are also deaf at birth due to closed ear canals, with hearing beginning between week 2 and 3 postpartum as the ear canal opens. Deciduous teeth begin to erupt at approximately 3 weeks and eruption is complete by the end of the fifth week following birth (Shabestari et al., 1967). The dental formula for deciduous teeth is 3/3 incisors, 1/1 canines, and 3/3 premolars. The dental formula of the adult dog is 3/3 incisors, 1/1 canines, 4/4 premolars, and 2/3 molars, and permanent teeth are generally complete and functional by 7 months of age. Incisors and canines have single roots, premolars have one to three roots (only the carnassial teeth have three roots), and molars have three roots (Table 19.1).

TABLE 19.1   Physiological Parameters in the Beagle Dog

Physiological parameter	Value
Lifespan	11–15 years
Chromosome number	38 diploid pairs + 2 sex chromosomes
Body weight	Males: 10–12 kg; females: 9–10 kg
Height at shoulder	13–15 inches (large); <13 inches (small)
Rectal temperature - adult	38–39°C (100–102.5°F)
Rectal temperature - pup	At birth - 37°C (94–97°F); by 3rd week - 36–38°C (97–100°F)
Age at maturity	6–12 months
Frequency of cycling in females	Every 7–8 months
Duration of estrus	1–2 weeks

(*Continued*)

TABLE 19.1 Physiological Parameters in the Beagle Dog—cont'd

Physiological parameter	Value
Duration of proestrus	1–2 weeks
Duration of diestrus	2–3 months
Duration of anestrus	3–5 months
Gestation period	60–65 days
Average litter size	5–6 pups
Weight of pups at birth	140–280 gm
Time following birth of eye opening	2 weeks
Time following birth of opening of ear canal	2–3 weeks
Time following birth of eruption of teeth	3–5 weeks
Dental formulae – deciduous teeth	3/3 incisors; 1/1 canines; 3/3 premolars
Dental formulae – permanent teeth	3/3 incisors; 1/1 canines; 4/4 premolars; 2/3 molars
Time of completion of permanent teeth	~7 months
Food consumption	25–40 gm/kg/day
Capacity of stomach	~1 L
Average pH of stomach	1.5–2.1
Length of small intestine	3–4 m
Average pH of small intestine	~7
GI tract total transit time	24 h
Transit time for stomach	3–5 h
Transit time for small intestine	1 h
Transit time for large intestine	>10 h
Heart weight	0.84% of body weight
Heart rate	70–90 beats/min
Liver weight – puppies	~7% of body weight
Liver weight - adults	~4% of body weight
Liver lobes	6; left and right lateral, left and right median, quadrate, caudate
Lung weight (6 month old)	1% of body weight
Lung lobes	7; left cranial, left caudal, right cranial, right middle, right caudal, right accessory
Kidney weight (6 month old)	0.5% of body weight

Adult beagles consume between 25 and 40 gms of food per kg body weight each day. Unlike most other animal species, the dog's saliva lacks α-amylase (Smeets- Peeters et al., 1998) even though, as in most other species, beagles possess mandibular, parotid, and sublingual salivary glands, lying in close proximity to each other. In addition, they possess a pair of smaller salivary glands known as the zygomatic glands. These are present more anteriorly than the other salivary glands and are located below the orbit representing a combination of the dorsal buccal glands present in other animals (Hermanson and de Lahunta, 2019). These zygomatic glands are composed of long, branching, mucous cell-lined tubules with occasional small, poorly developed serous demilunes (Hermanson and de Lahunta, 2019). As in other animal species, the primary function of saliva in dogs is lubrication of food and protection of the oral mucosa, but as opposed to the case in other species, digestion within the oral cavity plays a very minor role overall because dog saliva does not contain amylase.

The esophagus is lined by squamous epithelium which, like that of humans, is nonkeratinized. The capacity of the adult beagle's stomach is approximately 1 L, with lipase and pepsin being the main digestive enzymes in the gastric juices. The resting pH can vary between one and eight depending upon the dog breed (Smeets-Peeters et al., 1998; Tibbitts, 2003), although the average gastric pH of laboratory beagle dogs is reported to range from pH 1.5 to 2.1 within a couple of hours of consuming a meal (Lui et al., 1986). A further complication is that the dog stomach has a very high capacity for acid secretion, with the fed stomach pH reported to be equal to or even lower than that of the resting stomach depending upon the nature of the meal. The small intestines measure between 3 and 4 m in length and have a pH close to neutral. The total gastrointestinal transit time is usually reported as 24 h, while the individual transition times in the stomach, small intestines, and large intestines are reported as being 3–5 h, 1 h, and greater than 10 h, respectively.

The beagle's heart weight is approximately 0.84%–0.85% of the body weight in young adults (Keenan and Vidal, 2006), the age used in most safety assessment studies. The heart rate for a young adult beagle is between 70 and 90 beats per minute. In females, the heart rate increases during early pregnancy, reaching a peak shortly before parturition, and remaining above normal throughout lactation (Olsson et al., 2003). Spontaneous cardiac arrhythmias in laboratory beagles are reported to be rare, with <2% showing irregularities of the electrocardiogram (ECG) (Gauvin et al., 2009).

The beagle's liver weight is approximately 7% of the body weight in young puppies reducing to 4% in adults. The liver consists of six lobes, left lateral and left medial, right lateral and right medial, and quadrate and caudate, of which the left lateral is the largest (Singh, 2017). The lung and kidney weight of 6-month-old male and female beagle dogs is reported as being approximately 1% and 0.5% of body weight, respectively, with females generally having slightly lower organ weights than male dogs (Choi et al., 2011). There are seven lobes in the lung of the dog which are divided into left and right sides. The left lung is further divided into a cranial lobe and a caudal lobe, while the right lung is divided into cranial, middle, caudal, and accessory lobes. Other organs are essentially the same as those present in other laboratory animals.

The reader is referred to the excellent publication by McDonough and Southard (2017) for a complete listing of organ weights and a description of the gross anatomy of the dog.

2.4. Housing and Care of the Beagle Dog

In terms of housing of dogs used for laboratory animal toxicity studies, minimal requirements have changed significantly over the last 10 or so years and are fairly precisely defined in various guidelines (for example, UK Home Office, 2014; US National Academy of Sciences, 2011). Institutions are mandated to house all research animals in clean, well-maintained enclosures that allow enough space for the animals to exhibit normal behavior and activities. Access to species-appropriate food and clean water is a primary component of daily animal husbandry. Dogs require room to exercise and to have the opportunities to interact socially with both other dogs and humans. Exercise and enrichment programs are expected components of each institution's husbandry program along with timely access to veterinary care. Proper housing conditions include the appropriate environmental temperature, humidity, ventilation and air quality, and room illumination. The ultimate objective is to provide an environment that supports animal welfare, which can have a direct effect on study conduct. Findings in laboratory animal studies from dogs with compromised welfare have been shown to be misleading as a result of reduced sensitivity, reduced reliability, and inability to repeat data due to the complex physiological effects induced by the stress responses (Prescott et al., 2004). The imperative to enforce the scientific method has led to improved conditions of care for laboratory animals as a whole, and dogs in particular, and has led to substantial improvements in the value of the data obtained (UK Home Office, 2014, see *Issues in Laboratory Animal Science that Impact Toxicologic Pathology*, Vol 1, Chap 29).

3. USE OF DOGS IN BIOMEDICAL RESEARCH

In 1965, the US Food and Drug Administration (FDA) introduced the two-species paradigm, with rodent and nonrodent species required in drug discovery and development. Data collected from the nonrodent species can provide information on drug effects that may not be evident in the rodent species. While the dog is probably the most commonly used nonrodent species, other large laboratory animals may also be used for translational research including the cynomolgus macaque and minipig. For more information on these species, refer to *Animal Models in Toxicologic Research: Nonhuman Primate*, Vol 1, Chap 21, and *Animal Models in Toxicologic Research: Pig*, Vol 1, Chap 20.

As the most commonly used nonrodent species for toxicity studies, the size of the dog does provide an advantage for collecting certain types of data from studies. An example of this is in the collection of blood for hematology and clinical biochemistry or in pharmacokinetic studies where larger volumes, or multiple samples, can be taken in the beagle without negatively affecting the health of the animal. Noninvasive diagnostic tests and behavioral observations can also be more easily performed with dogs as compared to rodents. Ophthalmologic and auditory examinations can be more reliably performed on dogs than rodents to assess compounds that could potentially affect vision and hearing functions.

3.1. Drug Metabolism, Disposition, and Excretion of Drugs/Chemicals in the Dog—Comparison with Other Species

Potential species-specific differences in drug metabolism need to be taken into consideration when selecting any animal model for toxicology testing since significant differences from the human situation can seriously affect the extrapolation of any data derived from experimental studies. The rate of metabolism by cytochrome P450 (CYP)–dependent mixed-function oxidase has been shown to be inversely proportional to the subject's body weight with rodents clearing compounds at a considerably faster rate than larger animals including human beings. In contrast, for compounds that are not metabolized by oxidation, the results would be expected to be very different. The function of other organs affecting exposure to administered drugs also differs between different animal species, sometimes in a protective way and occasionally increasing the subsequent toxicity of a given drug/chemical. For example, renal function in the dog is considerably less affected by high concentrations of sulfonamide drugs in comparison to humans (Fleischer et al., 2008). In contrast, dogs are extremely susceptible to nabilone and tolbutamide metabolites, suggesting that other animal models would make more appropriate test subjects to predict safe application of these agents for humans.

3.2. Genetic Variability within Beagles and Impact on Testing

Numerous dog breeds, including the beagle, are reported to have a genetic predisposition for idiopathic epilepsy (Kandratavicious et al., 2014). Spontaneous seizure activity was first reported in laboratory beagle colonies in 1969 with subsequent research identifying the ADAM23 gene as a risk factor in the development of epilepsy in dogs (Koskinen et al., 2015). While the risk remains within the gene pool of the beagle and other dog breeds, recognition of the underlying cause has highlighted the need to monitor breeding to identify and remove susceptible individuals from the gene pool, thus keeping the problem under control for laboratory-bred animals. However, the complex interaction of the gene and the relatively low penetrance of the seizure predisposing variant in ADAM23 have made it difficult to eliminate entirely (Koskinen et al., 2015).

Immunogenicity distinctions have been identified between pet beagles and purpose-bred laboratory beagles with the latter showing a different haplotype frequency of the dog leukocyte antigen when compared to the more diverse population of pet beagles. For those laboratory-bred beagles involved in establishing safety and efficacy during vaccine trials, the results obtained from a relatively closed breeding colony involved in providing dogs for laboratory animal studies may not accurately reflect the responses that might occur with clinical use in the genetically diverse dog breeds in the general population.

Beagles are generally considered a good animal model for testing drug toxicity although certain strains may present a higher risk than others when evaluating contraceptive steroids (Johnson, 1989). Gastric motility in beagles appears to be more affected by anticholinergic and prokinetic drugs than other breeds such as Labradors. Within strains of purebred beagles, there are subpopulations of fast and slow metabolizers of celecoxib, a nonsteroidal antiinflammatory drug (Paulson et al., 1999). This genetic polymorphism is associated with isoenzymes CYP2D15 and CYP3A12, resulting in strain-related differences in drug responses.

3.3. Use of the Dog in Drug Discovery and Development

In 2015, the US FDA finalized their guidance entitled "Product Development Under the Animal Rule." The premise of this document was to provide a path forward for drug development when human efficacy studies were not ethical or feasible. This guidance provided information on the use of animal models of disease from an efficacy perspective, but there were no guidelines describing the use of animal models in general toxicology studies. As described by Boelsterli (2003), the use of animal models of disease in routine toxicology studies may be a beneficial approach but is not without its drawbacks. The use of disease models would permit evaluation of efficacy and toxicity in the same animals. A drawback to this approach is

that efficacy is usually assessed at dose levels that are relevant multiples of the anticipated human dose, whereas safety is normally evaluated at significantly higher doses. The combination of efficacy and safety in single studies could also allow for the detection of rare or unexpected adverse safety events in human disease/patient populations, thus increasing the value of such models. In addition, the effects of compounds in development could be compared directly in normal and diseased animals, thus facilitating the investigation of mechanisms of toxicity. However, the use of animal models of disease in safety studies could also result in unexpected findings that could be difficult to interpret, particularly as robust historic control databases for such models generally do not exist. Several considerations should be taken into account when considering the utility of disease models in safety assessment: (1) a clearly defined scientific rationale should be established, (2) a determination should be made as to whether the model will replace or accompany traditional toxicity studies, (3) the impact of safety findings on compound development should be understood, (4) the endpoints should be clearly defined, and associated tests should be qualified and/or validated for that species/model, and (5) it should be determined whether the safety endpoint(s) of interest can be evaluated appropriately in an efficacy study (Morgan et al., 2013).

3.4. Duration of Studies/Age at Start of Studies in Dogs

The duration of any toxicity study is determined by the scientific objective. Dogs are commonly used for both single and multiple administration for periods up to 12 months (Jacobs and Hatfield, 2013) by any of the major exposure routes: oral (both gavage and feeding), injection (intravenous, intramuscular, or subcutaneous), inhalation, or dermal although the latter route is rarely used. Where studies require intravenous administration of test items, indwelling catheters can readily be placed and maintained in superficial veins for administration of test compounds and for subsequent blood collection (Fillman-Holliday and Landi, 2002). The guidelines describe the use of

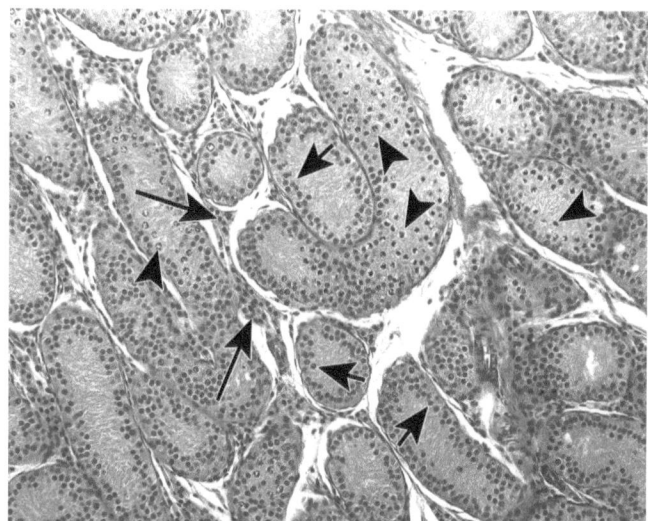

FIGURE 19.1 Immature testes from six-month old beagle dog. The seminiferous tubules are hypospermatogenic with large numbers of round spermatids (*short arrows*) and mitotic cells (*arrowheads*) with very few large spermatocytes or elongate spermatids. Normal Leydig cells are present in the interstitial tissue (*long arrows*). H&E stain. ×2.5 microscope magnification.

In terms of the numbers of dogs per sex per group, there are different recommendations dependent upon which guidelines are referenced. While most regulatory guidance, including that of the OECD guideline, for the repeat dose 90-day oral toxicity study in nonrodents (OECD, 1998) recommends that a minimum of four dogs/sex/group should be used with four dose groups (including the control group), a more typical protocol utilizes a minimum of three dogs/sex/dose group (Fillman-Holliday and Landi, 2002). Clearly, the use of even four dogs/sex/group places severe limitations on the value of statistical analysis on data such as body weight, organ weight, clinical chemistry, and hematology. While analysis of mean changes among these parameters is still recommended on a per group and per sex basis, analysis of individual animal data, utilizing scatter plots, is invaluable in identifying changing trends in parameters with increasing doses which a simple analysis of the mean changes by statistical analysis might conceal (OECD, 1998).

sexually mature animals for standard toxicity studies, but the precise definition of "sexually mature" has been a contentious one with regards to dogs in particular but is also pertinent to the use of nonhuman primates. Until recently, dosing was initiated in dogs aged 4–6 months, when the vast majority of the male, laboratory-bred, beagle dogs were still immature (Fig. 19.1). This led to questions regarding the ability of such studies to evaluate potential chemical-induced effects on fertility and prompted a Society of Toxicologic Pathology survey that resulted in a recommendation that the degree of sexual maturity be routinely documented when examining the dependent organ systems such as the reproductive and associated organs (Halpern et al., 2016). As a consequence of this concern, current recommendations and most common practices are to use both male and female dogs of approximately 12 months of age (Faqi, 2016). Since dogs can mature at different relative rates, there still exists the possibility, albeit less than in younger dogs, that some of the individuals may be immature at the end of a 1-month toxicity study, but concern is less for longer duration toxicity studies.

3.5. Use of the Dog for Assessing Clinical Pathology and Pharmacokinetic Changes

The dog has considerable advantages for taking serial samples of blood for serum chemistry, hematology, and drug kinetics assessments. Large peripheral veins and a large blood volume permit multiple sampling timepoints for the conduct of longitudinal studies on the toxicity and fate of drugs and industrial chemicals following administration to laboratory animals (Kesisoglu, 2014; Lees et al., 2015; Giorgi et al., 2012). Inclusion of a predosing blood sample in the dog also provides an intraanimal reference value against which to compare subsequent drug/chemical-induced changes in the respective parameters, a protocol that is not available to studies in rodents. For pharmacokinetic studies in particular, the dog is probably the most widely used animal species in drug development (Zhang et al., 2012). There has been criticism of the use of the dog for ADME-type studies (absorption, disposition, metabolism, and excretion), because of significant qualitative and quantitative differences in the presence of hepatic CYP450 between those present in dog liver and those present in human liver (Court, 2013; Bogaards et al., 2000). Since this enzyme group constitutes the main metabolic system for drugs and chemicals, these differences have the potential to mislead attempted extrapolations from dog studies to subsequent human trials (Tibbitts, 2003; Martignoni et al., 2006). A clear understanding of these differences does exist and it is therefore incumbent upon the scientist to determine which CYPs are responsible for metabolizing the particular chemical, and then to use appropriate judgment in determining whether or not the dog can satisfy these requirements. Clearly, for some chemicals, the dog will not be the appropriate species to use.

One major concern in utilizing any laboratory animal species is the existence of good background data that can be used to understand the normal variations in hematological and serum chemistry data with age, gender, and strain. There is extensive published information on a vast range of reference data for the dog (Ishii et al., 2013; Matsuzawa et al., 1993; Choi et al., 2011), whereas this is not always the case for the alternative nonrodent species. As with all experimental data obtained from animal studies, the experiments need an expert interpretation, with a knowledge of the vagaries and species differences present in the model. Despite these reservations, the results of a recent survey from Monticello et al. (2017) confirmed the value of the dog in predicting specific human safety concerns in subsequent clinical trials for drugs. Exceptions to the simple direct extrapolation of dog data to humans clearly exist, but the knowledge of which toxicities are predictive, and which are not, has been gained over many decades of dog use for safety evaluation. It has been clearly demonstrated that canines are a reliable model provided the necessary caveats for interpretation are understood and rigorously applied (Greaves et al., 2004).

3.6. Safety Pharmacology Studies in Dogs

Preclinical studies for potential new drugs prior to first in human clinical trials have been conventionally divided into those of primary pharmacology, safety (secondary) pharmacology,

toxico-/pharmacokinetics, and toxicology (Greaves et al., 2004). There are few prescribed guidelines for assessing primary pharmacology, but standardized regulatory guides, both Good Laboratory Practice (GLP) and non-GLP, generally inform the conduct of the remaining study types (For GLP information, see *Pathology and GLPs, Quality Control and Quality Assurance*, Vol 1, Chap 27). Safety pharmacology studies are concerned with the physiological monitoring of vital organs or organ systems and while mainly carried out in vivo, with the dog playing a major role as the animal model for cardiovascular and respiratory function studies. Increasingly, the introduction of in vitro cell systems has allowed more moderate throughput screening to eliminate the more risky chemicals before the conduct of whole animal studies (Wakefield et al., 2002; Whitebread et al., 2005). Despite the undoubted success of cell alternatives to whole animal studies, the dog for many reasons is the preferred animal species for carrying out many of the in vivo safety pharmacology studies although the minipig and nonhuman primate are also used (Prescott et al., 2004; Prior et al., 2016). In order to minimize stress and normalize the assessed physiological parameters, refinement of safety pharmacology studies has involved group housing, extensive training of the dogs prior to dosing, and "noninvasive" methods of monitoring physiological function (e.g., jacketed telemetry). For more details on the training methods applied to condition dogs and lessen any stress involved in subsequent experimental procedures, the reader is referred to the publication by Guth (2007). Before the initiation of a study, dogs can be surgically implanted with vascular access ports and telemetry devices that will facilitate test compound administration, blood collection, and collection of physiological data such as blood pressure, heart rate, specific vessel and cavity pressures, body temperature, and other measurements without hampering the dog's activity or causing it stress or pain.

An analysis of the available data for safety pharmacology endpoints obtained from dog studies showed that there was a 90% chance of predicting subsequent QT findings in human clinical trials (Vargas et al., 2015), albeit in a relatively small set of examples.

3.7. Use of Dogs in Developmental Toxicity Studies

For ease of use, short gestation period, large litter size, ease of breeding, and low cost, developmental toxicity studies have traditionally been carried out in rodents and rabbits. Under certain specific circumstances when metabolism, pharmacology, and/or pharmacokinetics in the dog may be more similar to that expected in man (Robertson et al., 1979), or alternatively when these characteristics are so different in the rodent and rabbit to warrant using an alternative species, the dog may be considered for use in these studies. The dog has a relatively short gestation period (~64 days) in comparison to alternative nonrodent species (~112 days in minipig), with a pregnancy rate of approximately 70%–90% (as opposed to the rate in cynomolgus monkey being around 45%) with a mean litter size of four to six pups and a low spontaneous malformation rate. These characteristics all favor the dog as a viable nonrodent, nonlagomorph species for developmental toxicity studies. Clearly, scientific rationale would have to be apparent not to use rodents or rabbits for these types of studies but the dog is a viable second species given the attributes above.

4. PREDICTIVITY OF DOG TOXICITY DATA TO HUMANS

In general, concordance between nonclinical and clinical safety findings is better for nonrodent than for rodent data. Olson et al. (2000) reviewed 150 compounds (from 12 pharmaceutical companies) which resulted in 221 significant human toxicities (i.e., those findings responsible for dose limitation, drug level monitoring, dose adjustment, restricted target patient population, and/or termination of development). The compounds included in the survey were distributed across several therapeutic areas and the authors indicated that concordance between human and animal findings was seen in 63% of nonrodent studies, which were conducted primarily in the dog, as opposed to 43% of rodent studies. Of 29 studies in which there was an animal correlate for cardiovascular toxicity, and 35 studies in which there was an

animal correlate for gastrointestinal toxicity, 16 studies contained findings in nonrodents only, whereas only one study contained findings that were only apparent in the rodent. 25 of 36 cardiovascular toxicities, mainly arrhythmias, electrocardiographic abnormalities, hypotension, and vasodilatation, were observed in dog studies.

Monticello et al. (2017) reviewed 182 compounds that were evaluated in animal toxicology and safety pharmacology studies as well as completed Phase I human studies in order to characterize true-positive, false-positive, true-negative, and false-negative findings. These compounds included both biologicals and small molecules and were distributed across a number of therapeutic areas. The results of this evaluation demonstrated that sensitivity (the proportion of positive findings in humans that also were positive in animals) was highest in dogs compared to rodents or nonhuman primates for several organ systems, most notably cardiovascular (87%) and gastrointestinal (54%), although dogs had markedly lower sensitivity for other organ systems such as respiratory system (0% compared to 17% in rodents and 33% in nonhuman primates). This did not correlate with positive predictive value (the proportion of positive findings in animals that also were positive in humans), which was highest in nonhuman primates for most organ systems with the exception of cardiovascular, which, again, was highest in dogs. Specificity (the proportion of negative findings in humans that also were negative in animals) was highest in nonhuman primates and generally equivalent between dogs and rodents, while negative predictive value (the proportion of negative findings in animals that also were negative in humans) was similar across species.

Two papers, designed to evaluate the use of animals, and dogs in particular, in predicting the safety of drugs in humans (Bailey et al., 2013, 2014), demonstrated a 70% rate of true positives, suggesting that dog studies were a good predictor of human toxicity. Furthermore, the majority of both positive and negative predictive values for dogs was greater than 50%, suggesting that findings in dog studies often match those seen in humans.

Greaves et al. (2004) reviewed several published studies (Litchfield, 1961; Owens, 1962;

Schein et al., 1970; Grieshaber and Marsoni, 1986) to evaluate concordance between animal and human toxicity findings and again concluded that the dog was a good predictor of subsequent human toxicity liabilities. Several reviews of data from anticancer agents demonstrated a good correlation in the responses of dogs with subsequent results in humans, especially with regard to the gastrointestinal toxicity that frequently accompanies anticancer therapies. The authors suggested that the physiology of the dog gastrointestinal tract, as well as their propensity for vomiting, may contribute to the favorable correlation with subsequent adverse events in human subjects. Reviews of data from anticancer, and antimitotic, agents also showed good concordance between both rodents and humans and dogs and humans, especially for myelotoxicity. Given the totality of the data, the author (Greaves et al., 2004) concluded that toxicity in dogs was a better predictor of human toxicity than that in other species, including nonhuman primates even though the number of studies with the latter was relatively few.

Clark and Steger-Hartmann (2018) performed a review of data in the Elsevier PharmaPendium database, which contains both animal toxicity and human safety observations as reported in FDA and EMEA drug approval packages. At the time of analysis, the database contained over 1.3 million observations for humans, 150,000 observations for rats, and approximately 50,000 observations for dogs and mice, with lesser numbers noted for other animal species. The authors analyzed the rate of true positives for toxicity findings and classified them according to species and organ system. Their analysis indicated that concordant events were not distributed evenly among either animal species or organ class with the greatest number of true positive correlations in dogs being noted for cardiac (~39%) and gastrointestinal (40%) disorders, whereas the highest number of true positives in rats, for example, was noted for renal (~52%) and hepatobiliary (~46%) disorders.

Likewise, Vargas et al. (2015) reviewed data for 40 compounds from a range of therapeutic areas, 23 of which prolonged the QT interval in humans, and again noted a high rate of concordance in animal studies (91% sensitivity and 88% specificity). Although the authors did not differentiate between nonrodent species when performing their analyses, they did note that dogs were the most frequently used animal model in nonclinical studies of QT evaluation and hence would constitute the greatest influence on the good concordance shown in respect to safety concerns for this organ. Ewart et al. (2014) reviewed conscious dog telemetry data for 113 small-molecule compounds (from seven pharmaceutical companies) which had completed human Phase I single ascending dose studies and their analysis showed that there was good concordance between the dog model and human data for compound-induced effects on the QTc interval such that at exposure multiples of $10\times$, sensitivity was 88% with specificity being 76%. Following their review of the literature, Greaves et al. (2004) suggested that ECG assessment in dogs, particularly at the times of peak plasma concentrations of administered drugs, provided the most useful data to allow physicians to effectively monitor patients in clinical studies.

5. COMPARATIVE TOXICOLOGY OF THE DOG

Metabolic studies in the beagle have shown dramatic changes in the hepatic Phase I and Phase II metabolism as the animals mature (Martignoni et al., 2006). This is exemplified by studies with caffeine and trimethadione where CYP metabolism and total body clearance of both drugs was low at 1 week postpartum, increased rapidly from the third week of life, peaked and then decreased gradually until reaching a stable level in the adult dog (Tanaka et al., 1998). Other substrates including those using the proton pump inhibitor, pantoprazole, showed an increase in metabolism with age, reaching a peak by 15 weeks with little or no decrease occurring by the age of 3 years (Foster, 2005; Kil et al., 2010; Graham et al., 2003).

5.1. Toxic Responses of the Dog Compared to Other Species

The concept of both qualitative and quantitative differences in the response of different animal species to chemical-induced toxicity is one that has driven the development of investigative toxicology and underpins the inclusion of multiple animal species when evaluating chemicals for human safety evaluation (Martignoni et al., 2006). The factors that determine sensitivity or resistance to toxicity are complex and multifactorial, and the study of the variability in these factors has provided the basis for the observed species differences in response to chemicals and drugs. Hence, most regulatory guidelines recommend the use of a rodent and a nonrodent species, commonly the dog, in evaluating hazard assessments for novel drugs and consumer products. When the lowest observed adverse effect level (LOAEL) was evaluated in animal species, the dog was found to be the most sensitive in approximately 15% of the studies. While commonly the dog is a more sensitive species to the acute toxic effects of herbicides than are the rat and mouse, with lower no observed adverse effect levels (NOAELs) on shorter duration studies, this was not the case for chronic studies where the no observed effect level (NOEL) in the rat was lower than that in the dog (Box and Speilman, 2005; Dellarco et al., 2010). There are well-understood physiological processes to explain the altered responses of the dog and a major reason revolves around differences in the basal gastric acid secretion, which is lower than that of humans, pigs, or nonhuman primates. The canine gastric pH also shows large interanimal variability and, in some cases, the gastric pH may be high enough to mirror that normally present in the duodenum. Clearly, interanimal differences in gastric acid secretion can lead to considerable variability in drug dissolution and absorption, and hence toxicity, particularly for drugs whose solubility is strongly pH dependent. Thiamine is one such drug, and studies in dogs with low gastric pH showed significantly greater absorption of thiamine than predicted, with gastric pH ranging from 3–6 and absorption varying from 5 to 50 h-ng/mL (Aoyagi et al., 1986).

The following sections illustrate the effects of a variety of drugs and industrial chemicals on the dog and their relationship to changes occurring in other animal species including rodents and humans.

5.2. Small-Molecule Kinase Inhibitors

Dose optimization for kinase inhibitors in the clinical setting has proven challenging, and patients treated with the recommended therapeutic dose of some approved targeted drugs frequently have to undergo subsequent dose reductions due to toxicity, with further dose optimization being needed in the postmarketing setting. Since the dog has been the most common nonrodent species employed in defining the safe starting doses for clinical trials, this species has been implicated as directing doses inappropriate for subsequent safety in humans. This has been especially true for cardiovascular adverse events (Dambach et al., 2016). In contrast, some publications have described the dog as being a specific and sensitive model for the cardiotoxicity associated with some small-molecule tyrosine kinase inhibitors (Mellor et al., 2011).

Acute cardiovascular and lymphoid toxicity was observed in the dog with a small-molecule p38 MAP kinase inhibitor which was not subsequently seen in either rodents or cynomolgus macaques treated with the same compound at equivalent and higher dose levels (Morris et al., 2010). These data led the authors to conclude that the dog was exquisitely sensitive among the species evaluated, demonstrating an unusual sensitivity to the inhibition of this particular target in this particular species. They ended the manuscript with the recommendation that the dog was not a suitable preclinical species in which to evaluate safety for subsequent human trials with this class of target.

5.3. Caffeine

Caffeine is present in a large number of consumer products including coffee, chocolate and chocolate products, over-the-counter stimulants, drinks, and herbal weight loss supplements containing guarana (*Paullinia cupana*). It is the most widely consumed psychostimulant taken by human beings in the world with a rough estimate of consumption of up to 89% of the United States population. A lethal dose of caffeine to humans is estimated to be between 10 and 50 gm which equates to a dose of between 140 and 715 mg/kg body weight

(Bioh et al., 2013). The toxicity of caffeine to dogs was demonstrated early on, and the lethal dose of caffeine in this species varies from 110 to 200 mg/kg of body weight with a median lethal dose of around 140 mg/kg body weight (Carson, 2006).

The mechanism of action for the toxicity of caffeine includes its competitive antagonism of the adenosine and benzodiazepine receptors, an inhibition of cyclic nucleotide phosphodiesterase, and the release of calcium from intracellular stores (Myers et al., 1999). The inhibition of adenosine receptors by caffeine explains its stimulatory effect on cognitive function while its inhibition of phosphodiesterase activity is considered to be responsible for its cardiostimulatory effects. Toxic doses of caffeine lead to positive inotropic, chronotropic, and dromotropic effects on the heart, cerebral vasoconstriction, renal vasodilation, smooth muscle relaxation in the gastrointestinal tract, and stimulation of gastric secretion (Ooms et al., 2001).

While caffeine is extremely bitter, dogs readily consume products containing it. Considering its widespread distribution, the chances of accidental poisoning of companion dogs are high considering the propensity for dogs to eat almost anything. However, the most common cause of poisoning in the United States of America is reported to be intentional, with pure caffeine being incorporated into meat (Tawde et al., 2012). The acute cause of death is considered to be cardiac failure or tetanic seizures, and this is common to both human and canine poisoning cases with little qualitative differences although humans appear to be more resistant to toxicity.

5.4. Theobromine

Chocolate is derived from the roasted seeds of the plant *Theobroma cacao*, and the main toxic components are the methylxanthine alkaloids, theobromine, and caffeine. Whereas humans can easily digest and excrete methylxanthines, theobromine has been shown to be acutely and chronically toxic to dogs. The half-life of theobromine in humans is 2–3 h, whereas absorption in dogs is relatively slow, with metabolism in the liver and extrahepatic recirculation, before excretion in the urine, which results in a half-life in dogs of approximately 18 h. Theobromine poisoning results in acute effects on the central nervous, cardiovascular, and respiratory systems, as well as diuresis. The first signs of poisoning include vomiting, hematemesis, and polydipsia. These effects may progress to cardiac arrhythmias, seizures, and death. Most symptoms will begin to appear within 2 h of ingestion but, as theobromine is metabolized slowly, symptoms could take as long as 24 h to appear, and up to 3 days for complete recovery. With chronic dosing and at relatively low doses, theobromine produces atrophy and degeneration of the seminiferous tubules of the testes. Dogs have been shown to be considerably more sensitive than rodents to these effects, probably as a consequence of the increased exposure to the compound (EFSA, 2008).

5.5. Acetaminophen (Paracetamol)

Acetaminophen is one of the most commonly used analgesics in human medicine, and as a consequence, dog poisoning cases are also relatively common. Dogs are appreciably more sensitive to acetaminophen overdose than are humans; toxicity will generally occur at doses that are therapeutic in humans, with a toxic dose to dogs being between 150 and 200 mg/kg (Judge, 2018; MacNaughton, 2003; Villar et al., 1998; Schlessinger, 1995). As in other animals, the liver is the primary target of toxicity in dogs with clinical evidence of elevations in alanine aminotransferase, alkaline phosphatase, and total bilirubin; although high, single dose mortality is generally not a consequence of hepatic damage but of systemic effects such as methemoglobinemia. Dogs will normally exhibit the early effects of acetaminophen toxicosis within 4–12 h with progressive cyanosis, tachypnea, and dyspnea, depending on the degree of methemoglobinemia which occurs. Signs attributable to hepatic necrosis usually occur approximately 36 h after the ingestion of acetaminophen and the necrosis is predominantly centrilobular in distribution (Francavilla et al., 1989) with the degree and pattern of necrosis being similar to that seen in other laboratory animal species.

5.6. Aspirin and Ibuprofen

Chronic exposure to therapeutic doses of aspirin and ibuprofen in dogs has been shown to lead to the development of gastric ulcers and analgesic nephropathy which is qualitatively similar, in terms of pathogenesis and location to that seen in humans although at increased sensitivity in the dog with the changes occurring at considerably lower dose levels (Villar et al., 1998). Gastric mucosal adaptation can occur with repeated therapeutic doses of aspirin, but some animals will nevertheless develop gastric ulcers. Acute overdose following ingestion of either analgesic can cause death through metabolic acidosis (Hunter et al., 2011).

5.7. Vasoactive Drugs

Several vasoactive drugs like minoxidil, hydralazine, and nicorandil are known to cause cardiovascular toxicity in dogs (Dogterom et al., 1992). These drugs have comparable pharmacological effects (hypotension, vasodilation, and reflex tachycardia) and cause a spectrum of changes in the heart which includes hemorrhages in the right atrium, subendocardial and papillary muscle necrosis, and necrosis/hemorrhages of the coronary vessels. These cardiovascular effects in dogs are considered secondary to exaggerated pharmacologic, or profound hemodynamic, effects rather than a direct toxicity of these chemicals on the heart (Mesfin et al., 1995). The pathogenesis of cardiovascular toxicity in dogs, and its unique susceptibility, induced through these modes of action, is not fully understood (Greaves, 1998). Several mechanisms have been postulated such as impaired myocardial perfusion (ischemia) due to a drop in systemic blood pressure leading to papillary and myocardial necrosis, or direct or compensational stimulation of contractile force to satisfy the myocardial oxygen demand.

These changes tend to occur at high doses in dogs and these cardiovascular findings have been shown not to be relevant at therapeutic doses in humans. These drugs have been widely used in the clinic without any evidence of cardiovascular events in humans (Ettlin et al., 2010). Since many of these drugs in humans have low, or even negative, preclinical to clinical safety margins, the absence of cardiac effects in humans is unlikely to be due solely to difference in systemic exposure and is more likely down to, as yet unknown intrinsic species differences that lead to dogs being especially sensitive to the cardiac events occurring (Sobota, 1989).

6. SPONTANEOUS BACKGROUND PATHOLOGY IN THE BEAGLE (REFER TO WOICKE ET AL., 2021)

6.1. Spontaneous Nonneoplastic Diseases in Laboratory Beagles

There are several excellent reviews documenting the background nonneoplastic pathology in a range of tissues/organs of the laboratory beagle (Sato et al., 2012; McInnes, 2012; Johnson et al., 2019; Barnes et al., 2016; Kobayashi et al., 1994; Maita et al., 1977; Hattendorf and Hirth, 1974). Generally, the incidences of nonneoplastic lesions are low and, unlike the situation in rodents, they rarely pose a diagnostic problem in distinguishing these changes from those induced by chemicals or drugs (Woicke et al., 2021). In addition to those reviews describing tissue changes in general, there are also several reviews of organ specific pathologies that describe both spontaneous and drug/chemically induced changes such as those occurring in the liver (Foster, 2005), the heart (Fig. 19.2) (Herman and Eldridge, 2019), and the lung (Mukaratirwa et al., 2016). In a retrospective study of spontaneous nonneoplastic pathology in the laboratory beagle, the highest incidences of findings were present in the kidneys, lung, lymph nodes, parathyroid, pituitary gland, and prostate (Johnson et al., 2019). Some common findings are listed here. The findings in the prostate consisted of lymphocytic cell infiltrations (Fig. 19.3). In the pituitary gland, cysts arising from the remnants of the craniopharyngeal pouch were primarily in the pars distalis. Inflammatory cell infiltrates were also commonly recorded in the lungs,

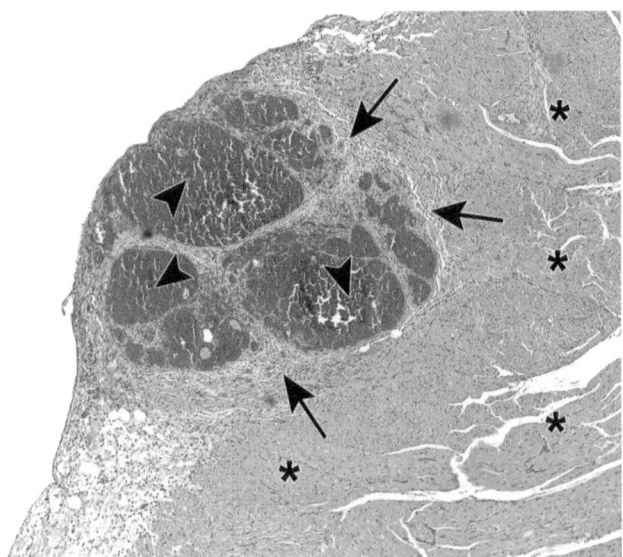

FIGURE 19.2   Hematocyst from the heart of a beagle dog. The hematocyst consists of multiple pools of red staining, amorphous, material (*arrowheads*) surrounded by, and infiltrating between, a thin layer of inflammatory cells and fibrous tissue (*arrows*). Normal cardiac tissue is present on the right hand side of the section (*). H&E stain. ×2.5 microscope magnification.

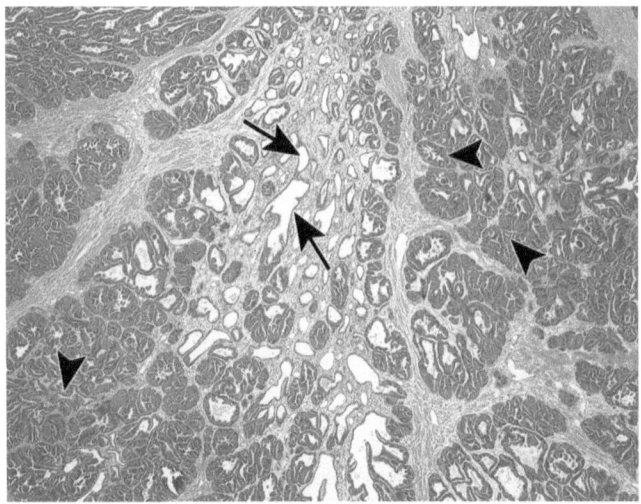

FIGURE 19.3   Prostate from a 9-month old beagle dog. In one area, dilated acini are lined by atrophic epithelium and surrounded by fibrous tissue (*arrows*) as compared to normal, compact, prostatic acini (*arrowheads*). H&E stain. ×2.5 microscope magnification.

salivary glands, and liver, while multifocal mineralization was the most common observation recorded in the kidney. The reported incidences of spontaneous inflammation of the coronary artery within the heart are variable in

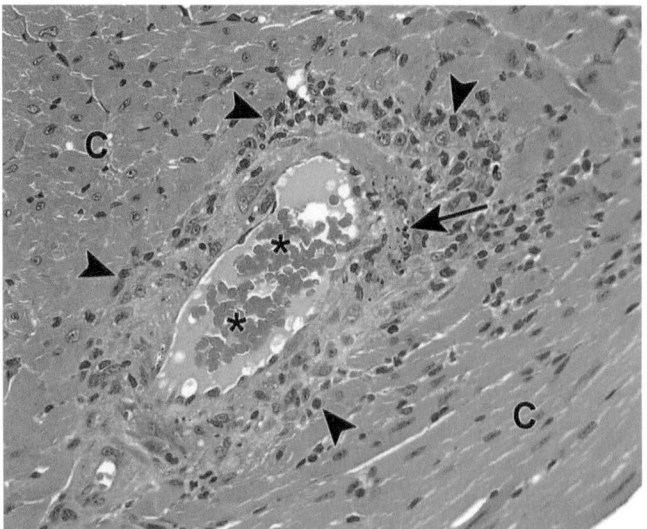

FIGURE 19.4   Intramural branch of the coronary artery of the heart from a 12-month old beagle dog. Necrosis and inflammation of the media, artery. There is fibrinoid necrosis characterized by smudgy eosinophilic staining and necrotic cell debris within the media of the arteriole (*arrow*). The lumen of the arteriole contains red blood cells (*). Mononuclear cells surround and infiltrate the vessel wall (*arrowheads*). Normal cardiomyocytes (C) are present at the periphery. H&E stain. ×20 microscope magnification.

the beagle dog (Fig. 19.4) and have caused difficulties in distinguishing spontaneous from drug-induced arteritis at this site (Clemo et al., 2003).

The spontaneous arteritis that occurs in beagles is more commonly referred to as "beagle pain syndrome" (Hayes et al., 1989). Etiologically, it is considered that the syndrome is a latent condition, the expression of which can be precipitated in predisposed dogs by stress such as that resulting from treatment with experimental compounds. Occasionally, in such cases, its incidence can be dose related and as such could complicate the interpretation of toxicity studies. In severe cases, dogs demonstrate pain on opening their mouth or, when lifted, may stand with an arched back, extended neck, and lowered head. The body temperatures are also elevated to between 104 and106°F and affected dogs may display a hunched stance and a stiff gait. Affected dogs show a number of hematological changes including neutrophilia, elevated platelet count, decreased hemoglobin and hematocrit, decreased albumin, and increased acute phase proteins such as alpha 2 globulins (Hayes et al., 1989). Histologically, arteritis is observed either in several organs (polyarteritis) or in a single organ, the most commonly reported being the coronary arteries of the heart. There is considerable variation in the extent and severity of the arteritis between dogs with similar clinical pictures ranging from minimal medial fibrinoid necrosis and inflammatory cell infiltrates affecting a single artery to extensive necrosis and a severe inflammatory cell reaction affecting multiple organs (Snyder et al., 1995). While the coronary arteries of the heart are the most commonly affected vasculature, the arteritis can occur in almost all organs of the body in severe cases.

There are a number of organs and tissues that are affected by the age and maturity status of the dog. Changes can be seen in the reproductive organs (James and Heywood, 1979; Goedken et al., 2008; Lowseth et al., 1990), the eyes (Heywood et al., 1976), and the lymphoid system (Oghiso et al., 1982; Barnes et al., 2016) with age-related involution of the thymus being the most common finding even in relatively young dogs (Fig. 19.5).

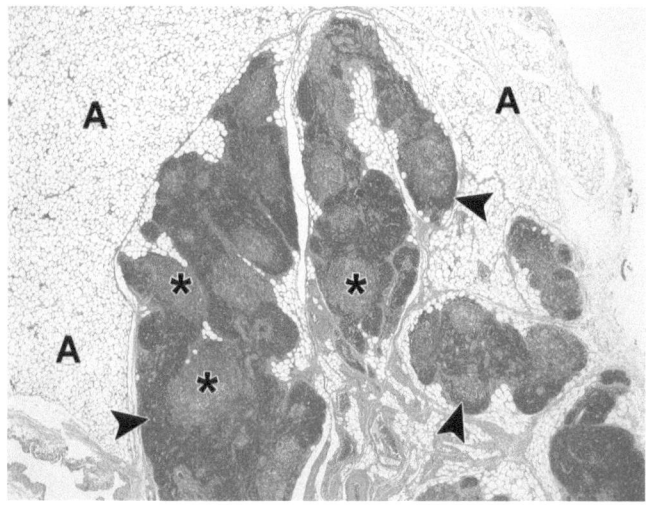

FIGURE 19.5 Thymic involution from a beagle dog on a three-month feeding study. There is a decrease in the corticomedullary ratio. The thymic medulla is seen as the pale blue staining regions (*). The thymic cortex, appearing as dark blue staining regions, is considerably thinner than normal (*arrowheads*). The involuted thymus is frequently surrounded by greater amounts of adipose tissue (A) than would normally be expected in this age of dog. H&E stain. ×2.5 microscope magnification.

6.2. Spontaneous Neoplastic Diseases in Laboratory Beagles

While sporadic incidences of neoplastic disease have been reported in laboratory beagles (Foster, 2005; Madewell, 1981; Matsushima et al., 1998; Taylor et al., 1976), the incidences are so low and their occurrences so rare, likely due to the age of animals typically on nonclinical toxicity studies, that no further detail will be covered in this chapter.

7. USE OF THE DOG AS A MODEL OF HUMAN DISEASES

7.1. The Dog as an Animal Model of Human Cardiovascular Disease

No ideal animal model of human cardiovascular disease exists. Due to commonalities of body weight, heart weight, and heart rate, dogs are used as a model for human cardiac contractility. A similar response to exercise in humans makes the dog a good model for these studies in cardiovascular research. The size of the dog heart makes it conducive for studies involving chronic instrumentation, and the introduction of noninvasive or minimally invasive monitoring technology makes the dog an ideal animal model for these studies (Fish et al., 2017). In addition, the beta-myosin heavy chain isoform is predominant in both dog and human hearts.

Although certain breeds are prone to spontaneously develop cardiovascular disease (Milani-Nejad and Janssen, 2014; Dixon and Spinale, 2009), beagle dogs can be utilized as a surgical model for myocardial infarction and the possible effects of therapy on the progression/regression of cardiac injury. However, because of significant collateral circulation in the dog myocardium, the response to infarction may not be as severe as in the human condition (Table 19.2).

7.2. The Dog as an Animal Model of Human Cancer

The average rate of successful translation of potential chemotherapies from rodent models of cancer to human clinical trials is less than 8% (Mak et al., 2014). These rodent models include human cancer xenografts and orthotopic human

TABLE 19.2 Dog Models of Human Cardiac Disease

Cardiac disease	Procedure	Dog breed	Reference
Chronic ischemic heart failure	Ligation of left anterior descending (LAD) coronary artery	Mongrel	Wei et al. (2007)
Chronic ischemic heart failure	Injection of latex beads into left circumflex artery	Mongrel	Evans and Vanoli (2001)
Sudden cardiac death	Atrioventricular block achieved by ligation of the LAD	Mongrel	Lai et al. (2000)
Arrhythmogenic right ventricular cardiomyopathy (ARVC)	Spontaneous - chromosome 17 mutation induces disease phenotype	Boxer	Meurs et al. (2010).
Nonischemic heart failure (HF)	Induction of right ventricular tachycardia with a pacemaker	Boxer	Belevych et al. (2011)
Duchenne Muscular Dystrophy	Spontaneous - point mutation on the X-linked dystrophin gene mimics the human disease	Golden retriever	Cassano et al. (2012)
Chronic valvular disease	Spontaneous	Cavalier King Charles Spaniel, Dachshunds, Miniature/toy Poodles, Chihuahuas, Terriers	Freeman et al. (2006)
Dilated cardiomyopathy	Spontaneous	Doberman Pinscher - deletion in the PDK4 gene. Doberman and Boxers - ventricular arrhythmias, Irish Wolfhounds, Newfoundlands, and other giant breeds, Cocker Spaniels - atrial premature arrhythmias	Freeman and Rush (2007)

cancers in immunodeficient mice as well as syngeneic, chemically induced, and spontaneous cancers in rodents (Tong et al., 2011). Utilizing animal models other than mice and rats has the potential to provide information that is more comparable to the human condition. With approximately 6 million dogs being diagnosed with cancer annually in the United States, companion dogs can be studied as a model of spontaneous cancer development and may be amenable to assessing the efficacy of potential therapeutic agents (Rowell et al., 2011).

The frequency of cancer in dogs in general is twice that of humans, with spontaneous cancer developing at an average age of ~8.4 years in the dog in comparison to ~50 years in humans. As a spontaneous model, these tumors are, in general, histologically similar to those that develop in humans with a reported similar progression and response to established therapies. The development of drug resistance, cancer recurrence, and/or tumor metastasis is also observed in canine cancers. Recent studies have shown that there are also greater similarities between dog and human genome as compared with the mouse genome. In addition, the same tumor oncogenes and suppressor genes that contribute to cancer development in humans (e.g., p53, Rb, MDM2, BRCA1, and BRCA2) also affect dogs (Lutful Kabir et al., 2015; Alvarez, 2014; Grosse et al., 2014). A summary table of the available canine cancers and their use as models of human cancer is given in Table 19.3.

7.3. The Dog as an Animal Model of Human Neurological Diseases

The domestic dog displays a range of neurological diseases that closely mimic those found in the human population and as such has considerable potential to help us better understand the pathogenesis and develop potential therapies (Partridge and Rossmeisl, 2020).

Epilepsy

Naturally occurring epilepsy is the most common neurologic disease in dogs (Charalambous et al., 2014; Patterson, 2014). The prevalence of epilepsy in domestic dogs is between 0.6% and 1%, while the estimated prevalence in humans is 1%–3% (Ekenstedt and Oberbauer, 2013). The similarities of electroencephalograph patterns between dog and human seizure activity suggest similar etiological factors are involved and these hold promise for testing therapeutic interventions in the management, if not the treatment, of the human condition (Potschka et al., 2013).

Stroke

There were an estimated 800,000 cases of stroke diagnosed in the human population in the United States of America in 2017 (Benjamin et al., 2017). The potential for prevention and therapeutic intervention for individuals suffering from stroke is a goal that would pay dividends in improving the quality of life, preventing subsequent episodes, and ultimately saving lives. Various experimental models of canine stroke have been developed and include occlusion of the vasculature by the injection of substances such as microfibrillar collagen (Purdy et al., 1989) and by ligation of various cerebral arteries (Yatsu et al., 1972), as models of inducing focal or global cerebral ischemia, respectively (Bacigaluppi et al., 2010). While rodent models of stroke have been more widely used than those of larger laboratory animals, the dog remains an important model system with many more features in common with those in human stroke.

Lysosomal Storage Disease

Lysosomal storage diseases are heritable errors of metabolism. The most severe manifestation of storage diseases, neurodegeneration, is the least tractable to therapy. There are over 70 separate diseases that make up the spectrum of lysosomal storage disorders in humans and many have a progressive neurodegenerative clinical course that varies depending upon the particular mutation involved. The mutations affect the function of lysosomes and cause the intracellular accumulation of sphingolipids, such as cerebrosides, gangliosides, and sphingomyelin, and mucopolysaccharides such as glycogen (Platt et al., 2018). The affected genes encode different lysosomal proteins, including lysosomal enzymes and lysosomal membrane proteins (Sun, 2018).

Gaucher disease is an example of a sphingolipidosis-type lysosomal storage disease that

TABLE 19.3   Canine Cancers as Models for Human Diseases

Canine tumor	Characteristics and comparison to human disease	Reference
Head and Neck (HNC)	• 20% of all oral malignancies in dogs • Associated with exposure to tobacco smoke and papillomavirus in dogs and humans • Used to evaluate radiation therapies for humans	Cekanova and Rathore (2014) Liu et al. (2015) Dow (2020)
Lung	• <1% spontaneous incidence of one-degree lung cancer; metastasis is more common than in humans • 80% of one-degree tumors are malignant with the same environmental risk factors as humans • Used to study disease development; immuno-compromised dog model is used to assess new chemotherapeutic agents	Ahrar et al. (2002) Cekanova and Rathore (2014) Miller (2005) Moulton et al. (1981)
Lymphoma	• Most common type of cancer in dogs • Similar to non-Hodgkin's lymphoma in humans in development, histology, behavior, and response to treatment • Used to develop new chemotherapeutic regimens	Cekanova and Rathore (2014) Sanchez et al. (2019)
Mammary and prostate	• Gender-specific, hormone-dependent cancers in both species • Chemotherapeutic treatments rarely used in dogs; early ovariohysterectomy or castration are preventative • Deregulation BRCA1 and BRCA2 genes play a role in mammary tumor development in both • Dogs and humans are the only large animals that spontaneously develop prostate cancer • Dogs used to evaluate disease progression and new treatments	Canadas-Sousa et al. (2019) Cekanova and Rathore (2014) Keller et al. (2013) Pinho et al., (2012) Abdelmageed and Mohammed (2018).
Melanomas	• ~7% of all cancers in dogs • Behavior, morphology of dog oral/cutaneous tumors similar to human • Etiology in dogs is unknown; sun exposure is the one-degree risk factor in humans • Same genetic mutations (NRAS and PTEN) in both species • Used to study disease pathogenesis, treatment	Cekanova and Rathore (2014) Prouteau and Andre (2019)
Osteosarcomas	• Most common bone cancer in children, adolescents, and dogs • Incidence of occurrence is greater in dogs than in humans; 80% reported in large and giant breeds • Similar disease progression in dogs and humans • Dog is the model of choice for establishing limb salvage procedures	Anfinson et al. (2011) Cekanova and Rathore (2014) Simpson et al. (2017) Tuohy et al. (2019)

(Continued)

TABLE 19.3 Canine Cancers as Models for Human Diseases—cont'd

Canine tumor	Characteristics and comparison to human disease	Reference
Urinary bladder (transitional cell carcinoma)	• Similar development in both species • Etiology unknown in dogs; genetic predisposition, environmental risk factors contribute as in humans • Used to develop and evaluate new diagnostic techniques, treatments	Cekanova and Rathore (2014) Knapp et al. (2014), (2020)
Glioma	• Naturally occurring, translationally relevant animal model of human glioma. • Some genetic similarities to equivalent human neoplasms • Natural history of canine gliomas is not well understood • Used to develop and evaluate new diagnostic techniques and treatment	Hubbard et al. (2018); Koehler et al. (2018) Miller et al. (2019).

results in an accumulation of glucosylceramide in the lysosomes of macrophages and is caused by a mutation in the β-glycosidase gene. On the other hand, Von Gierke disease is a mucopolysaccharidosis-type lysosomal storage disease that results in the accumulation of glycogen in the liver as a consequence of a mutation in the glucose-6-phosphatase gene that inhibits the conversion of glycogen to glucose within the liver.

A wide variety of lysosomal storage disease occur naturally/spontaneously in the dog including Krabbe's disease (beagle, poodle), Niemann–Pick disease (boxer), fucosidosis (English springer spaniel), Gaucher disease Type 1, Pompe disease (Lapland dog) and galactosidase mutation 1 (beagle, English springer spaniel), galactosidase mutation 2 (pointer), and gangliosidosis (Gurda and Vite, 2019; Jolly and Walkley, 1997). These canine diseases have provided invaluable insights into the progression of the various lysosomal storage diseases and the development of therapies for managing the diseases, as these animal models can be studied in detail throughout the development of clinical disease including any responses following intervention therapy and evaluation of potential efficacy (Bradbury et al., 2015). The characteristics of the disease, the mutations involved, and the clinical progression of the diseases closely mimic the human conditions and have provided invaluable insights into potential treatments (Skelly and Franklin, 2002).

Alzheimer's Disease

There are a limited number of animal models with which to study and predict the clinical outcomes related to Alzheimer's Disease (AD). Aged dogs develop cognitive learning changes and memory loss that are consistent with early Alzheimer's changes observed in aged humans (Youssef et al., 2016). Common pathological changes associated with AD and aged dogs include the deposition of amyloid plaques surrounded by dystrophic neurites and the presence of intraneuronal neurofibrillary tangles (NFTs) in the hippocampus, cerebral cortex, and other areas of the brain involved in cognitive function (Araujo et al., 2017). Both species share an identical amino acid sequence of the β-amyloid peptide (Aβ) that forms the amyloid plaques, and the location of these plaque deposits is similar in both species (Head, 2013). While humans develop both diffuse and dense core plaques, the aged dog primarily shows the diffuse form of the protein. Dogs generally develop the same pathology, associated with Aβ, as is present in human AD and some, but not all, of the effects of tau abnormalities without the presence of full-blown NFTs.

Studies have shown that the protein levels of Aβ42 in the cerebrospinal fluid decline with age in dogs and this change parallels that seen in humans, where decreasing levels of this protein are associated with increasing levels of amyloid deposition. There is great potential for using the levels of Aβ42 and tau in the cerebrospinal fluid as biomarkers in monitoring the progression of AD. Positron emission tomography imaging studies, examining fluorodeoxyglucose uptake into the brain, show a reduction in older dogs that is consistent with the reduced uptake seen in human AD patients.

Geriatric beagles have been used as a model of AD as their cognitive function declines with age as it does in the human disease. A set of tasks can be used to assess therapeutic interventions for both AD progression and canine cognitive dysfunction which usually occurs in later stages of the disease.

8. REGULATORY CONSIDERATIONS FOR TOXICITY STUDIES

Repeat-dose toxicity studies with rodents and nonrodents are required for the registration of new products, whether they be pesticides or pharmaceuticals. The goal of these studies is to identify toxicities associated with exposure to the chemical in accordance with international guidelines for informing human risk. For the reasons outlined in the previous sections of this chapter, the dog fits the requirements of an ideal laboratory animal species in many if not all of these aspects.

Dogs are used at all stages of the development of novel drugs and agrochemicals for defining organ/tissue toxicity in a nonrodent animal species, in studying the dose–response relationship for the organ or tissue toxicity, and in helping to establish NOEL and NOAELs for use in subsequent human risk assessment. Dogs have been used in a regulated fashion in this role for over 50 years and are embedded into OECD guidelines as the most commonly used, nonrodent, animal species for both pharmaceutical and plant protection products with rigorous guidelines as to how, and under what

conditions, they are to be used (OECD, 1998; EMEA, 2008). This guidance states that in selecting a laboratory animal species in which to assess the toxicity of a compound, the species chosen should ideally be based upon a similar pharmacokinetic profile to humans with similar metabolic conversion and generation of the same major human metabolites. Should this requirement be unachievable due to the generation of an unusual metabolite in humans, studies in which animals are dosed with the appropriate human metabolite(s) would be carried out in addition to studies with the parent compound.

8.1. Pesticide and Drug Development—Need for One-Year Dog Study?

The need for both 3-month (subchronic) and 1-year (chronic) toxicity studies using dogs has long been debated for pesticide registration (Kobel et al., 2010). Several retrospective analyses have been published on whether the requirement for both subchronic and chronic studies is scientifically justified for risk assessment. Findings of retrospective analyses of dog toxicity studies submitted for pesticide registration in Germany, United States, and Japan arrived at similar conclusions (Box and Spielmann, 2005; Dellarco et al., 2010; Ono et al., 2018) and supported the continued use of the dog as the most sensitive species for a significant number (>15%) of compounds analyzed.

In consideration of the 3Rs initiative (replacement, reduction, and refinement - Tornquist et al., 2014), the potential contribution of the one year dog study in informing subsequent risk assessment decisions for pesticides was investigated in a number of publications (Spielmann and Gerbracht, 2001; Doe et al., 2006; Baetcke et al., 2005). These publications concluded that, with a small number of exceptions, a chronic dog study did not influence the derivation of the reference doses [e.g., acceptable daily intake, acceptable operator exposure level] derived from NOAELs for the pesticides in the respective surveys. Baetcke et al. (2005) showed that of 77 pesticides analyzed from the US EPA database, in only 4% of all cases (3 studies) would the NOAEL/LOAEL be lower when derived from the 1-year dog rather than the 13-week study. In essence, the 1-year dog study did not provide different conclusions compared to that obtained from a 13-week study when both studies were conducted at similar dose levels. The US EPA carried out a similar but considerably larger review that confirmed this conclusion (US EPA, 2007).

As a direct consequence of these retrospective analyses, the one-year dog study is no longer required in Europe (EU Commission, 2013), the United States (US Federal Register Notice, 2007), and Canada (Health Canada PMRA, 2016) although a small number of exceptions exist when a chemical shows slow elimination or higher potential for accumulation. However, certain countries still require the 1-year dog study (e.g., Japan, South Korea), which means that sponsors must still submit data from the 1-year dog study in order to register pesticides in these countries. Clearly, there is an imperative for harmonization in order to avoid the unnecessary use of dogs for pesticide registration globally.

The duration of chronic toxicity studies in dogs and their contribution in supporting longer-term human clinical trials of pharmaceuticals has also been reviewed and evaluated in the past (Lumley et al., 1992; Parkinson et al., 1995; DeGeorge et al., 1999). Current International Committee of Harmonization guidance ensures that study designs are acceptable across Europe, North America, and Japan. With few exceptions, as listed in the guidance (ICH, 2009), data from the nine-month repeat-dose dog toxicity study are required to support human clinical trials longer than 6 months in duration or a marketing authorization request for a drug in which the duration of treatment is longer than 3 months. Similar to the previously discussed review of chronic dog toxicity studies for pesticides, initiatives have been undertaken to review the value of the one-year dog study for estimating "first-in-human" dose levels for pharmaceuticals (Contrea et al., 1993; DeGeorge et al., 1999) with the aim of eliminating the scientific need for the 1-year dog study and reducing its requirements by relying on data from the 3- and 6-month dog studies. However, the conclusions from the subsequent analyses of the toxicity data were contrary to

those arrived at from the pesticide work and actually supported the need for the longer duration studies in identifying additional organ system toxicity that was not observed in the shorter duration studies and that developed only with longer dosing.

9. ETHICS OF USE OF THE DOG AS A LABORATORY ANIMAL SPECIES

As a human companion animal, the use of the dog in laboratory research of all types has the potential to evoke considerable emotional and ethical considerations, mostly centered upon concerns for how the animals are treated. While these considerations are present for all animal species used in laboratory animal studies, they are particularly so with regard to the use of the dog and nonhuman primate (Hasiwa et al., 2011). Concerns are also raised by the fact that in most cases the animal is humanely euthanized at the end of a procedure. There are clear guidelines for housing, treatment, and care of laboratory animals that are set forth by organizations such as the Association for Assessment and Accreditation of Laboratory Animal Care International, which has accredited thousands of laboratories in approximately 50 countries throughout the world, while individual countries such as the United Kingdom also have their own national bodies (MAFF, 2006) that accredit the use of animals in laboratory studies (NRA, 2004). The US Department of Agriculture provides regulatory oversight for research involving all warm-blooded animals except mice, rats, and birds based on the Animal Welfare Act. For federally funded research involving laboratory animals, The Office of Laboratory Animal Welfare provides additional oversight. Enforcement of these standards has resulted in significant improvements in terms of housing and socialization of dogs over the last 30 or so years with the recognition that dogs housed in pairs or group housed generally exhibit less stereotypic behaviors. It is recommended that dogs be pair- or group housed even while on toxicology studies although in these circumstances special attention needs to be given to food consumption, an important toxicological parameter. Typically, pair- or group-housed dogs will be separated at the time of feeding due to individual differences in feed consumption rate and the possibility for fighting. Additionally, environmental enrichment has been addressed in recent years and it is common to include toys in the enclosures although the propensity for dogs to chew and swallow the constituent parts of toys necessitates their being made of innocuous materials. Enrichment in the form of interaction between humans (e.g., animal technicians) and dogs is also especially important as it enables training, reduces stress during experimental procedures, and permits acclimatization for study-related needs such as blood sampling and safety pharmacology procedures such as electrocardiography (Hubrecht, 1995; Loveridge, 1998).

For more information on this topic, see *Issues in Laboratory Animal Science that Impact Toxicologic Pathology*, Vol 1, Chap 29.

10. SUMMARY

Dogs play an integral part in establishing safety for subsequent human exposures in the development of pharmaceuticals and agrochemicals, and in protecting workers in occupational settings. They have been addressed in international guidelines, as the nonrodent species of choice, for over 50 years and have proven to be a sensitive and specific model in helping to define subsequent human risk and in many cases have been shown to be more so than the corresponding alternative laboratory animal species especially in the case of certain organ toxicities such as the heart and GI tract. They have an essential role in drug discovery and the increasing use of dog diseases as models of the human equivalent promises to pay dividends in terms of providing a better understanding of the progression of many human diseases as well as more precise monitoring of potential new therapies in clinical trials. Clearly, their role as a companion species for humans has provoked some objection to their use as a model laboratory animal species. However, until greater refinement and higher specificity in terms of available alternative methods for predicting potential human risk are introduced, the dog will continue to play an important role in informing risks associated with the introduction of new pharmaceuticals and agrochemicals (Vamathevan et al., 2013).

REFERENCES

Abdelmageed SM, Mohammed S: Canine mammary tumors as a model for human disease (Review), *Oncol Lett* 15(6): 8195–8205, 2018.

Ahrar K, Madoff DC, Gupta S, et al.: Development of a large animal model for lung tumors, *J Vasc Intervent Radiol* 13(9 Pt 1):923–928, 2002.

Alvarez CE: Naturally occurring cancers in dogs: insights for translational genetics and medicine, *ILAR J* 55(1):16–45, 2014.

Anderson AC: *The beagle as an experimental dog*, Ames, IA, 1970, Iowa State University Press.

Anderson AC, Rosenblatt LS: Survival of the beagle under natural and laboratory condition. In , New York, 1974, MSS Information Corp, pp 19–25. Anderson AC, Boyden EA, Dougherty JH, editors: *Dogs and other large mammals in aging research*, vol. 1. New York, 1974, MSS Information Corp, pp 19–25.

Anfinsen KP, Grotmol T, Bruland OS, et al.: Breed-specific incidence rates of canine primary bone tumors — a population based survey of dogs in Norway, *Can J Vet Res* 75: 209–215, 2011.

Aoyagi N, Ogata H, Kaniwa N, et al.: Bioavailability of sugar-coated tablets of thiamine disulfide in humans. II. Correlation with bioavailability in beagle dogs, *Chem Pharm Bull (Tokyo)* 34:292–300, 1986.

Araujo JA, Baulk J, de Rivera C: The aged dog as a natural model of Alzheimer's disease progression. In Landsberg G, Maďari A, Žilka N, editors: *Canine and Feline dementia: molecular basis, diagnostics and therapy*, New York, London, 2017, Springer Publications, pp 69–92.

Bacigaluppi M, Comi G, Hermann DM: Animal models of ischemic stroke. Part Two: modelling cerebral ischemia, *Open Neurol J* 4:34–38, 2010.

Baetcke KP, Phang W, Dellarco V: *A comparison of the results of studies on pesticides from 12- or 24-month dog studies with shorter duration.* https://archive.epa.gov/scipoly/sap/meetings/web/pdf/dogstudymay05.pdf.

Bailey J, Thew M, Balls M: The use of dogs in predicting human safety, *ATLA* 41:335–350, 2013.

Bailey J, Thew M, Balls M: An analysis of the use of animals in predicting human toxicology and drug safety, *Altern Lab Anim* 42:181–199, 2014.

Barnes JR, Cotton PT, Robinson S, et al.: Spontaneous pathology and routine clinical pathology parameters in aging beagle dogs, *Vet Pathol* 53(2):447–455, 2016.

Belevych AE, Terentyev D, Terentyeva R, et al.: The relationship between arrhythmogenesis and impaired contractility in heart failure: role of altered ryanodine receptor function, *Cardiovasc Res* 90:493–502, 2011.

Benjamin EJ, Blaha MJ, Chiuve SE, et al.: Heart disease and stroke statistics-2017 update: a report from the American Heart Association, *Circulation* 135:e146–603, 2017.

Bielfelt SW, Redman HC, McClellan RO: Sire- and sex-related differences in rates of epileptiform seizures in a purebred beagle colony, *Am J Vet Res* 32(12):2039–2048, 1971.

Bioh G, Gallagher MM, Prasad U: Survival of a highly toxic dose of caffeine, *Case Rep* 2013, 2013. bcr2012007454–bcr2012007454.

Boelsterli U: Animal models of human disease in drug safety assessment, *Toxicol Sci* 28:109–121, 2003.

Bogaards JJP, Betrand M, Jackson P, et al.: Determining the best animal model for human cytochrome P450 activities: a comparison of mouse, rat, rabbit, dog, micropig, monkey and man, *Xenobiotica* 30(12):1131–1152, 2000.

Box RJ, Spielmann H: Use of dog the dog as non-rodent species in the safety testing schedule associated with the registration of crop and plant protection products (pesticides): present status, *Arch Toxicol* 79:615–626, 2005.

Bradbury AM, Gurda BL, Casal ML, et al.: A review of gene therapy in canine and feline models of lysosomal storage disorders, *Hum Gene Ther Clin Dev* 26:27–37, 2015.

Cagan A, Bass T: Identification of genomic variants putatively targeted by selection during dog domestication, *BMC Evol Biol* 16(10), 2016.

Canadas-Sousa A, Santos M, Leal B, et al.: Estrogen receptors genotypes and canine mammary neoplasia, *BMC Vet Res* 15:325, 2019.

Carson TL: Methyxanthines. In Peterson ME, Talcott PA, editors: *Small animal toxicology*, St. Louis, 2006, Saunders/Elsevier, pp 845–851.

Cassano M, Berardi E, Crippa S, et al.: Alteration of cardiac progenitor cell potency in GRMD dogs, *Cell Transplant* 21:1945–1967, 2012.

Cekanova M, Rathore K: Animal models and therapeutic molecular targets of cancer: utility and limitations, *Drug Des Dev Ther* 8:1911–1922, 2014.

Charalambous M, Brodbelt D, Volk HA: Treatment in canine epilepsy – a systematic review, *BMC Vet Res* 10:257, 2014.

Choi S-Y, Hwang J-S, Kim IH, et al.: Basic data on the hematology, serum biochemistry, urology, and organ weights of beagle dogs, *Lab Anim Res* 27(4):283–291, 2011.

Clark M, Steger-Hartmann T: A big data approach to the concordance of the toxicity of pharmaceuticals in animals and humans, *Regul Toxicol Pharmacol* 96:94–105, 2018.

Clemo FAS, Evering WE, Snyder PW, et al.: Differentiating spontaneous from drug-induced vascular injury in the dog, *Toxicol Pathol* 31(Suppl.):25–31, 2003.

Contrera JF, Aub D, Barbehenn E, et al.: A retrospective comparison of the results of 6 and 12 month non-rodent toxicity studies, *Adverse Drug React Toxicol Rev* 12:63–76, 1993.

Court MH: Canine cytochrome P450 (CYP) pharmacogenetics, *Vet Clin North Am Small Anim Pract* 43(5):1027–1038, 2013.

Creasy DM: Reproduction of the rat, mouse, dog, non-human primate and minipig. In McInnes EF, editor: *Background lesions in laboratory animals*, Elsevier.

Dambach DM, Simpson NE, Jones TW, et al.: Nonclinical evaluations of small-molecule oncology drugs: integration into clinical dose optimization and toxicity management, *Clin Cancer Res* 22(11):2618–2622, 2016.

DeGeorge JJ, Meyers LL, Takahashi M, et al.: The duration of non-rodent toxicity studies for pharmaceuticals, *Toxicol Sci* 49:143–155, 1999.

Dellarco VL, Rowland J, May B: A retrospective analysis of toxicity studies in dogs and impact on the chronic reference dose for conventional pesticide chemicals, *Crit Rev Toxicol* 40:16–23, 2010.

Dixon JA, Spinale FG: Large animal models of heart failure: a critical link in the translation of basic science to clinical practice, *Circ Heart Fail* 2(3):262–271, 2009.

Doe JE, Boobis AR, Blaker A, et al.: A tiered approach to systemic toxicity testing for agricultural chemical safety assessment, *Crit Rev Toxicol* 36:37–68, 2006.

Dogterom P, Zbinden G, Reznik GK: Cardiotoxicity of vasodilators and positive inotropic/vasodialting drugs in dogs. An overview, *Crit Rev Toxicol* 22:203–241, 1992.

Dorso L, Chanut F, Howroyd P, Burnett R: Variability in weight and histological appearance of the prostate of beagle dogs used in toxicology studies, *Toxicol Pathol* 36:917–925, 2008.

Dow S: A role for dogs in advancing cancer immunotherapy research, *Front Immunol* 10:2935, 2020. https://doi.org/10.3389/fimmu.2019.02935.

EFSA: Theobromine as undesirable substances in animal feed, *The EFSA J* 725:1–66, 2008.

Ekenstedt KJ, Oberbauer: Inherited epilepsy in dogs, *Top Compan An Med* 28:51–58, 2013.

EMEA/CHMP/SWP/488313/2007, *EMEA guideline on repeated dose toxicity*, 2008.

Ettlin RA, Kuroda J, Plassman S, et al.: Successful drug development despite adverse preclinical findings part 1: processes to address issues and most important findings, *J Toxicol Pathol* 23:189–211, 2010.

European Union: *Seventh report on the statistics on the number of animals used for experimental and other scientific purposes in the member states of the European Union*. https://eur-lex.europa.eu/legal-content/EN/TXT/PDF/?uri=CELEX:52013DC0859&from=EN.

Evans PB, Vanoli E: Early autonomic and repolarization abnormalities contribute to lethal arrhythmias in chronic ischemic heart failure: characteristics of a novel heart failure model in dogs with postmyocardial infarction left ventricular dysfunction, *J Am Coll Cardiol* 37:1741–1748, 2001.

Ewart L, Aylott M, Deurinck M, et al.: The concordance between nonclinical and phase I clinical cardiovascular assessment from a cross-company data sharing initiative, *Toxicol Sci* 142:427–435, 2014.

Faqi AS: *A comprehensive guide to toxicology in nonclinical drug development*, New York, 2016, Academic Press, p 523.

Fillman-Holliday D, Landi MS: Animal care best practices for regulatory testing, *ILAR J* 43(Suppl.1):S49–S58, 2002.

Fish RE, Foster ML, Gruen ME, et al.: Effect of wearing a telemetry jacket on behavioral and physiologic parameters of dogs in the open-field test, *J Am Ass Lab An Sci* 56(4): 382–389, 2017.

Fleischer S, Sharkey M, Mealey K: Pharmacogenetic and metabolic differences between dog breeds: their impact on canine medicine and the use of the dog as a preclinical animal model, *AAPS J* 10(1):110–119, 2008.

Foster JR: Spontaneous and drug-induced hepatic pathology of the laboratory beagle dog, the cynomolgus macaque and the marmoset, *Toxicol Pathol* 33:63–74, 2005.

Francavilla A, Makowka L, Polimeno L, et al.: A dog model for acetaminophen-induced fulminant hepatic failure, *Gastroenterology* 96(2 Pt 1):470–478, 1989.

Freeman LM, Rush JE, Markwell PJ: Effects of dietary modification in dogs with early chronic valvular disease, *J Vet Intern Med* 20:1116–1126, 2006.

Freeman LM, Rush JE: Nutrition and cardiomyopathy: lessons from spontaneous animal models, *Curr Heart Fail Rep* 4:84–90, 2007.

Gauvin D, Tilley LP, Smith FWK, et al.: Spontaneous cardiac arrythmias recorded in three experimental laboratory species (canine, primate, swine) during standard pre-study screening, *J Pharmacol Toxicol Methods* 59:57–618, 2009.

Giorgi M, Portela DA, Breghi G, et al.: Pharmacokinetics and pharmacodynamics of zolpidem after oral administration of a single dose in dogs, *Am J Vet Res* 73(10):1650–1656, 2012.

Goedken MJ, Kerlin RL, Morton D: Spontaneous and age-related testicular findings in beagle dogs, *Toxicol Pathol* 36:465–471, 2008.

Graham MJ, Bell AR, Crewe HK, et al.: mRNA and protein expression of dog liver cytochromes P450 in relation to the metabolism of human CYP2C substrates, *Xenobiotica* 33(3): 225–237, 2003.

Greaves P, Williams A, Eve M: First dose of potential new medicines to humans: how animals help, *Nat Rev Drug Discov* 3:226–236, 2004.

Greaves P: Patterns of drug-induced cardiovascular pathology in the beagle dog: relevance for humans, *Exp Toxicol Pathol* 50:283–293, 1998.

Grieshaber CK, Marsoni S: Relation of preclinical toxicology to findings in early clinical trials, *Cancer Treat Rep* 70:65–72, 1986.

Grosse N, van Loon B, Rohrer Bley C: DNA damage response and DNA repair – dog as a model? *BMC Cancer* 14:203, 2014. https://doi.org/10.1186/1471-2407-14-203.

Gurda BL, Vite CH: Large animal models contribute to the development of therapies for central and peripheral nervous system dysfunction in patients with lysosomal storage diseases, *Hum Mol Genet* 28(R1):R119–R131, 2019.

Guth BD: Preclinical cardiovascular risk assessment in modern drug development, *Toxicol Sci* 97:4–20, 2007.

Haggerty GC: The dog. In Gad SC, editor: *Animal models in toxicology*, New York, 2008, Informa Healthcare.

Halpern WG, Ameri M, Bowman CJ, et al.: Inclusion of reproductive and pathology endpoints for assessment of reproductive and developmental toxicity in pharmaceutical drug development, *Toxicol Pathol* 44(6):789–809, 2016.

Hasiwa N, Bailey J, Clausing P, et al.: Critical evaluation of the use of dogs in biomedical research and testing in Europe, *Altern Anim Exp* 28(4):326–340, 2011.

Hattendorf GH, Hirth RS: Lesions of spontaneous subclinical disease in beagle dogs, *Vet Pathol* 2:240–258, 1974.

Hayes TJ, Roberts GKS, Halliwell WH: An idiopathic febrile necrotizing arteritis syndrome in the dog: beagle pain syndrome, *Toxicol Pathol* 17:129–137, 1989.

Head E: A canine model of human aging and Alzheimer's disease, *Biochim Biophys Acta* 1832(9):1384–1389, 2013.

Herman E, Eldridge S: Spontaneously occurring cardiovascular lesions in commonly used laboratory animals, *Cardio-Oncology* 5:6, 2019. https://doi.org/10.1186/s40959-019-0040-y.

Hermanson J, de Lahunta A: *Miller and Evans anatomy of the dog*, 5th Ed., St Louis, Missouri, 2019, Elsevier.

Heywood R, Hepworth PL, Van Abbe NJ: Age changes in the eyes of the beagle dog, *J Small Anim Pract* 17:171–177, 1976.

Hubbard ME, Arnold S, Bin Zahid A, et al.: Naturally occurring canine glioma as a model for novel therapeutics, *Cancer Invest* 36(8):415–423, 2018.

Hubrecht RC: Enrichment in puppyhood and its effects on later behaviour in dogs, *Lab Anim Sci* 45:70–75, 1995.

Hunter LJ, Wood DM, Dargan PI: The patterns of toxicity and management of acute nonsteroidal anti-inflammatory drug (NSAID) overdose, *Open Access Emerg Med OAEM* 3:39–48, 2011.

ICH Topic M 3 (R2) Non-Clinical Safety Studies for the Conduct of Human Clinical Trials and Marketing Authorization for Pharmaceuticals. Note for Guidance on Non-Clinical Safety Studies for The Conduct of Human Clinical Trials and Marketing Authorization for Pharmaceuticals (CPMP/ICH/286/95). https://www.ema.europa.eu/en/documents/scientific-guideline/ich-m-3-r2-non-clinical-safety-studies-conduct-human-clinical-trials-marketing-authorization_en.pdf. (Accessed April 3 2020).

Ishii T, Hori H, Ishigami M, et al.: Background data for hematological and blood chemical examinations in juvenile beagles, *Exp Anim* 62(1):1–7, 2013.

Jacobs AC, Hatfield KP: History of chronic toxicity and animal carcinogenicity studies for pharmaceuticals, *Vet Pathol* 50: 324–333, 2013.

James RW, Heywood R: Age-related variations in the testes and prostate of Beagle dogs, *Toxicology* 12:273–279, 1979.

Johnson AN: Comparative aspects of contraceptive steroids—effects observed in beagle dogs, *Toxicol Pathol* 17(2): 389–395, 1989.

Johnson RC, Spaet RH, Jeppersen G, et al.: Spontaneous lesions in control animals used in toxicity studies. In Sahota PS, Popp JA, Hardisty JF, Gopinath C, Bouchard PR, editors: *Toxicologic pathology: non-clinical safety assessment*, 2nd Ed, Boca Raton, London, New York, 2019, CRC Press.

Judge PR: *Protocol for management of paracetamol/acetaminophen toxicity in dogs and cats.* https://veteducation.com.au/wp-content/uploads/2018/05/Paracetamol-Toxicity-Protocol.pdf.

Lutful Kabir FM, Alvarez CE, Bird RC: Canine Mammary Carcinomas: a Comparative analysis of altered gene expression, *Vet Sci* 3(1):1, December 25, 2015. https://doi.org/10.3390/vetsci3010001.2015.

Kandratavicius L, Balista PA, Lopes-Aguiar C, et al.: Animal models of epilepsy: use and limitations, *Neuropsych Dis Treat* 10:1693–1705, 2014.

Kawakami E, Tsutsui T, Ogasa A: Histological observations of the reproductive organs of the male dog from birth to sexual maturity, *J Vet Med Sci* 53:241–248, 1991.

Keenan C, Vidal JD: Standard morphologic evaluation of the heart in the laboratory dog and monkey, *Toxicol Pathol* 34: 67–74, 2006.

Keller JM, Schade GR, Ives K, et al.: A novel canine model for prostate cancer, *Prostate* 73(9):952–959, 2013.

Kesisoglou F: Use of preclinical dog studies and absorption modelling to facilitate late stage formulation bridging for a BCS II drug candidate, *AAPS PharmSciTech* 15(1):20–28, 2014.

Knapp DW, Ramos-Vara JA, Moore GE, et al.: Urinary bladder cancer in dogs, a naturally occurring model for cancer biology and drug development, *ILAR* 55(1):100–118, 2014.

Knapp DW, Dhawan D, Ramos-Vara JA: Naturally occurring invasive urothelial carcinoma in dogs: a unique model to drive advances in managing muscle invasive bladder cancer in humans, *Front Oncol* 9:1493, 2020. https://www.frontiersin.org/article/10.3389/fonc.2019.01493.

Kobayashi K, Hirouchi Y, Iwata H, et al.: Historical control data of spontaneous lesions in beagle dogs, *J Toxicol Pathol* 7:329–343, 1994.

Kobel W, Fegert I, Billington R, et al.: A 1-year toxicity study in dogs is no longer a scientifically justifiable core data requirement for the safety assessment of pesticides, *Crit Rev Toxicol* 40(1):1–15, 2010.

Koehler JW, Miller AD, Miller CR, et al.: A revised diagnostic classification of canine glioma: towards validation of the canine glioma patient as a naturally occurring preclinical model for human glioma, *J Neuropathol Exp Neurol* 77(11): 1039–1054, 2018.

Koskinen LLE, Seppälä EH, Belanger JM, et al.: Identification of a common risk haplotype for canine idiopathic epilepsy in the ADAM23 gene, *BMC Genom* 16(1):465, 2015.

Jolly RD, Walkley SU: Lysosomal storage diseases of animals: an essay in comparative pathology, *Vet Pathol* 34:527–548, 1997.

Kil DY, Vester Boler BM, Apanavicius CJ, et al.: Age and diet affect gene expression profiles in canine liver tissue, *PLoS One* 5(10):e13319, 2010.

Lai AC, Wallner K, Cao JM, et al.: Colocalization of tenascin and sympathetic nerves in a canine model of nerve sprouting and sudden cardiac death, *J Cardiovasc Electrophysiol* 11:1345–1351, 2000.

Lees P, Pelligand L, Elliott J, et al.: pharmacodynamics, toxicology and of mavacoxib in the dog: a review, *J Vet Pharmacol Therapeut* 38(1):1–14, 2015.

Lichfield JT: Forecasting drug effects in man from studies in laboratory animals, *J Am Med Assoc* 177:104–108, 1961.

Liu D, Xiong H, Ellis AE, et al.: Canine spontaneous head and neck squamous cell carcinomas represent their human counterparts at the molecular level, *PLoS Genet* 11(6): e1005277, 2015. https://doi.org/10.1371/journal.pgen.1005277.

Loveridge GG: Environmentally enriched dog housing, *Appl Anim Behav Sci* 59:101–113, 1998.

Lowseth LA, Gerlach RF, Gillett NA, et al.: Age-related changes in the prostate and testes of the beagle dog, *Vet Pathol* 27:347–353, 1990.

Lui CY, Amidonx GL, Amidon GL, et al.: Comparison of gastrointestinal pH in dogs and humans: implications on the use of the beagle dog as a model for oral absorption in humans, *J Pharmacol Sci* 75(3):271–274, 1986.

Lumley CE, Parkinson C, Walker SR: An international appraisal of the minimum duration of chronic toxicity studies, *Hum Exp Toxicol* 11:155–162, 1992.

MAAF: *Assessment and accreditation Project for laboratory animal care and use,* 2006. http://www.jhsf.or.jp/English/animal_TOP.html. (Accessed 10 January 2020).

MacNaughton SM: Acetaminophen toxicosis in a dalmatian, *Can Vet J* 44:142–144, 2003.

Madewell BR: Neoplasms in domestic animals: a review of experimental and spontaneous carcinogenesis, *Yale J Biol Med* 54(2):111–125, 1981.

Maita K, Masuda H, Suzuki Y: Spontaneous lesions detected in the beagles used in toxicity studies, *Jikken Dobutsu* 26(2): 161–167, 1977.

Mak IWY, Evaniew N, Ghert M: Lost in translation: animal models and clinical trials in cancer treatment, *Am J Transl Res* 6(2):114–118, 2014.

Martignoni M, Groothuis GMM, de Kanter R: Species differences between mouse, rat, dog, monkey and human CYP-mediated drug metabolism, inhibition and induction, *Expert Opin Drug Metab Toxicol* 2(6):875–894, 2006.

Matsuzawa T, Nomura M, Unno T: Clinical pathology reference ranges of laboratory animals, *J Vet Med Sci* 55(3):351–362, 1993.

Matsushima S, Maruyama T, Torii M: Peripheral neuroblastoma in a young Beagle dog, *Toxicol Pathol* 26(6):806–809, 1998.

McDonough SP, Southard T: *Necropsy guide for dogs, cats and small mammals,* John Wiley & Sons Inc.

McInnes EF: *Background lesions in laboratory animals,* Edinburgh, London & New York, 2012, Saunders Elsevier.

Mellor HR, Bell AR, Valentin J-P, et al.: Cardiotoxicity associated with targeting kinase pathways in cancer, *Toxicol Sci* 120(1):14–32, 2011.

Mesfin GM, Robinson FG, Higgins MJ, et al.: The pharmacological basis of the cardiovascular toxicity of minoxidil in the dog, *Toxicol Pathol* 23:498–506, 1995.

Meurs KM, Mauceli E, Lahmers S, et al.: Genome-wide association identifies a deletion in the 30 untranslated region of striatin in a canine model of arrhythmogenic right ventricular cardiomyopathy, *Hum Genet* 128:315–324, 2010.

Milani-Nejad, Janssen PML: Small and large animal models in cardiac contraction research: advantages and disadvantages, *Pharmacol Ther* 141(3):235–249, 2014.

Miller YE: Pathogenesis of lung cancer - 100 year report, *Am J Respir Cell Mol Biol* 33(3):216–223, 2005.

Miller AD, Miller CR, Rossmeisl JH: Canine primary intracranial cancer: a clinicopathologic and comparative review of glioma, meningioma, and choroid plexus tumors, *Front Oncol* 9:1151, 2019. https://www.frontiersin.org/article/10.3389/fonc.2019.01151.

Monticello TM, Jones TW, Dambach DM, et al.: Current nonclinical testing paradigm enables safe entry to First-In-Human clinical trials: the IQ consortium nonclinical to clinical translational database, *Toxicol Appl Pharmacol* 334:100–109, 2017.

Morgan SJ, Elangbam CS, Berens S, et al.: Use of animal models of human disease for nonclinical safety assessment of novel pharmaceuticals, *Toxicol Pathol* 41:508–518, 2013.

Morris DL, O'Neil SP, Devraj RV, et al.: Acute lymphoid and gastrointestinal toxicity induced by selective p38a map kinase and map kinase–activated protein kinase-2 (MK2) inhibitors in the dog, *Toxicol Pathol* 38:606–618, 2010.

Moulton JE, Von Tscharner C, Schneider R: Classification of lung carcinomas in the dog and cat, *Vet Pathol* 18:513–528, 1981.

Mukaratirwa S, Garcia B, Isobe K, et al.: Spontaneous and dosing route–related lung lesions in beagle dogs from oral gavage and inhalation toxicity studies, *Toxicol Pathol* 44(7):962–973, 2016.

Myers JP, Johnson DA, McVey DE: Caffeine and the modulation of brain function. In Gupta BS, Gupta U, editors: *Caffeine and behavior: current views and research trends*, Boca Raton, FL, 1999, CRC Press, pp 17–30.

NRA: The development of science-based guidelines for laboratory animal care: proceedings of the november 2003 international workshop. In *International workshop on the development of science-based guidelines for laboratory animal care program committee, national research council*, Washington, D.C, 2004, The National Academies Press. ISBN: 0-309-54532-3, 264 pages, 6 x 9, https://www.ncbi.nlm.nih.gov/books/NBK25397/pdf/Bookshelf_NBK25397.pdf.

OECD: Guideline for the Testing of Chemicals: *Repeated dose 90-day oral toxicity study in non-rodents*. 409. https://www.oecd-ilibrary.org/docserver/9789264070721-en.pdf?expires=1578137894&id=id&accname=guest&checksum=35FCCEBBE542F651AFE164EB8187827F.

Oghiso Y, Fukuda S, Iida H: Histopathological studies on distribution of spontaneous lesions and age changes in the Beagle, *J Vet Med Sci* 44:941–950, 1982.

Olson H, Betton G, Robinson D, et al.: Concordance of the toxicity of pharmaceuticals in humans and in animals, *Regul Toxicol Pharmacol* 32:56–67, 2000.

Olsson K, Agerstedt A-S, Bergstrom A, et al.: Change of diurnal heart rate patterns during pregnancy and lactation in dogs (*Canis familiaris*), *Acta Vet Scandin* 44, 2003. Article 105.

Ono A, Yoshizawa T, Matsumoto K: Evaluation of necessity of 1-year toxicity study in dogs - development of the new tiered approach for toxicity studies of pesticide considering species difference in "toxicity profile" and "toxicity dose-response", *Food Saf (Tokyo)* 6:109–117, 2018.

Ooms TG, Khan SA, Means C: Suspected caffeine and ephedrine toxicosis resulting from ingestion of an herbal supplement containing guarana and ma huang in dogs: 47 cases (1997–1999), *J Am Vet Med Assoc* 218(2):225–229, 2001.

Ostrander EA: Wayne: the canine genome, *Genome Res* 15:1706–1716, 2005.

Owens AH: Predicting anticancer drug effects in man from laboratory animal studies, *J Chron Dis* 15:223–228, 1962.

Parkinson C, Lumley CE, Walker SR: The value of information generated by long-term toxicity studies in the dog for the nonclinical safety assessment of pharmaceutical compounds, *Fundam Appl Toxicol* 25:115–123, 1995.

Partridge B, Rossmeisl Jr JH: Companion animal models of neurological disease, *J Neurosci Methods* 331:108484, 2020.

Patterson EE: Canine epilepsy: an underutilized model, *ILAR J* 55(1):182–186, 2014.

Paulson SK, Engel L, Reitz B: Evidence for polymorphism in the canine metabolism of the cyclooxygenase 2 inhibitor, celecoxib, *Drug Metab Dispos* 27(10):1133–1142, 1999.

Pinho SS, Carvalho S, Cabral J, et al.: Cancer tumors: a spontaneous animal model of human carcinogenesis, *Transl Res* 159(3):165–172, 2012.

Platt FM, d'Azzo A, Davidson BL: Lysosomal storage diseases, *Nat Rev Dis Primers* 4:27, 2018.

Potschka H, Fischer A, von Ruden E-L: Canine epilepsy as a translational model? *Epilepsia* 54(4):571–579, 2013.

Prescott MJ, Morton DB, Anderson D, et al.: Refining dog husbandry and care, *Lab Anim* 38(1):1–94, 2004.

Prior H, Bottomley A, Champéroux P, et al.: Social housing of non-rodents during cardiovascular recordings in safety pharmacology and toxicology studies, *J Pharmacol Toxicol Methods* 81:75–87, 2016.

Prouteau A, André C: Canine melanomas as models for human melanomas: clinical, histological, and genetic comparison, *Genes* 10(7):501, 2019.

Purdy PD, Devous MDS, Batjer HH, et al.: Microfibrillar collagen model of canine cerebral infarction, *Stroke* 20(10):1361–1367, 1989.

Rehm S: Spontaneous testicular lesions in purpose-bred beagle dogs, *Toxicol Pathol* 28:782–787, 2000.

Robertson RT, Allen HL, Bokelman DL: Aspirin: teratogenic evaluation in the dog, *Exp Teratol* 20(2):313–320, 1979.

Rowell JL, McCarthy DO, Alvarez CE: Dog models of naturally occurring cancer, *Trends Mol Med* 17(7):380–388, 2011.

Sánchez D, Sánchez-Verin R, Corona H, et al.: Canine lymphoma: pathological and clinical characteristics of patients treated at a referral hospital, *Vet México OA* (2), https://doi.org/10.22201/fmvz.24486760e.2019.2.495.

Sato J, Doi T, Wako Y, et al.: Histopathology of incidental findings in beagles used in toxicity studies, *J Toxicol Pathol* 25:103–134, 2012.

Schein PS, Davis RD, Carter S, et al.: The evaluation of anticancer drugs in dogs and monkeys for the prediction of qualitative toxicities in man, *Clin Pharmacol Ther* 11:3–40, 1970.

Schlesinger DP: Methemoglobinemia and anemia in a dog with acetaminophen toxicity, *Can Vet J* 36:515–517, 1995.

Shabestari L, Taylor GN, Angus W: Dental eruption pattern of the Beagle, *J Dent Res* 46:276–278, 1967.

Simpson S, Dunning MD, de Brot S, et al.: Comparative review of human and canine osteosarcoma: morphology, epidemiology, prognosis, treatment and genetics, *Acta Vet Scand* 59:71, 2017. https://doi.org/10.1186/s13028-017-0341-9.

Singh B: *Dyce, sack, and Wensing's textbook of veterinary anatomy*, 5th Ed, Missouri, USA, 2017, Elsevier Inc. ISBN: 978-0-323442640.

Skelly BJ, Franklin RJM: Recognition and diagnosis of lysosomal storage diseases in the cat and dog, *J Vet Intern Med* 16:133–141, 2002.

Smeets- Peeters M, Watson T, et al.: A review of the physiology of the canine digestive tract related to the development of in vitro systems, *Nutr Res Rev* 11:45–69, 1998.

Snyder PW, Kazacojs EA, Scott-Moncrief C: Pathologic features of naturally occurring juvenile polyarteritis in beagle dogs, *Vet Pathol* 32:337–345, 1995.

Sobota JT: Review of cardiovascular findings in humans treated with minoxidil, *Toxicol Pathol* 17:193–202, 1989.

Spielmann H, Gerbracht U: The use of dogs as second species in regulatory testing of pesticides, *Arch Toxicol* 75:1–21, 2001.

Sun A: Lysosomal storage disease overview, *Ann Transl Med* 6(24):476, 2018. https://doi.org/10.21037/atm.2018.11.39.

Sutter NB, Bustamante CD, Chase K, et al.: A single IGF1 allele is a major determinant of small size in dogs, *Science* 316(5821):112–115, 2007.

Tanaka E, Narisawa C, Nakamura H, et al.: Changes in the enzymatic activities of beagle liver during maturation as assessed both in vitro and in vivo, *Xenobiotica* 28(8):795–802, 1998.

Tawde SN, Puschner B, Albin T, et al.: Death by caffeine: presumptive malicious poisoning of a dog by incorporation in ground meat, *J Med Toxicol* 8:436–440, 2012.

Taylor GN, Shabestari L, Williams J: Mammary neoplasia in a closed beagle colony, *Cancer Res* 36:2740–2743, 1976.

Tibbitts J: Issues related to the use of canines in toxicologic pathology—issues with pharmacokinetics and metabolism, *Toxicol Pathol* 31(Suppl.):17–24, 2003.

Tong Y, Yang W, Koeffler HP: Mouse models of colorectal cancer, *Chin J Can* 30(7):451–462, 2011.

Törnqvist E, Annas A, Granath B, Jalkesten E, Cotgreave I, et al.: Strategic focus on 3R principles reveals major reductions in the use of animals in pharmaceutical toxicity testing, *PLoS One* 9(7):e101638, 2014.

Tuohy JL, Shaevitz MH, Garrett LD, et al.: Demographic characteristics, site and phylogenetic distribution of dogs with appendicular osteosarcoma: 744 dogs (2000–2015), *PLoS One* 14(12):e0223243, 2019. https://doi.org/10.1371/journal.pone.0223243.

UK Home Office: *Guidance on the operation of the animals (scientific procedures) Act 1986. Presented to parliament pursuant to section 21 (5) of the animals (scientific procedures) Act 1986.* ISBN 9781474100281, https://assets.publishing.service.gov.uk/government/uploads/system/uploads/attachment_data/file/662364/Guidance_on_the_Operation_of_ASPA.pdf.

UK Home Office: *Statistics of scientific procedures on living animals great Britain.* In *https://assets.publishing.service.gov.uk/government/uploads/system/uploads/attachment_data/file/835935/annual-statistics-scientific-procedures-living-animals-2018.pdf.*

USDA animal and plant health inspection service: annual report animal usage by fiscal year 2017. https://www.aphis.usda.gov/animal_welfare/downloads/reports/Annual-Report-Animal-Usage-by-FY2017.pdf. (Accessed January 4 2020).

*US EPA OPPTS harmonised test guidelines series 870 – health effects*https://nepis.epa.gov/Exe/ZyPDF.cgi/901B0A00.PDF?Dockey=901B0A00.PDF.

USEPA, 40 CFR parts 9, 152, 156, 159, et al.: *Pesticides; data requirements for conventional chemicals, technical amendments, and data requirements for biochemical and microbial pesticides; final rules, federal register/Vol. 72, No. 207/Friday, October 26, 2007/Rules and Regulations*, p 60976. https://www.federalregister.gov/documents/2005/03/11/05-4466/pesticides-data-requirement-for-conventional-chemicals.

US Federal Register Notice—Pesticides: Data requirements for conventional chemicals, technical amendments, and data requirements for biochemical and microbial pesticides, *Final Rules*, October 26, 2007.

US National Academy of Sciences: Guide for the care and use of laboratory animals. In *Committee for the update of the guide for the care and use of laboratory animals. Institute for laboratory animal research. Division on Earth and life studies*, 8th Ed, Washington, D.C, 2011, The National Academies Press. https://grants.nih.gov/grants/olaw/guide-for-the-care-and-use-of-laboratory-animals.pdf.

Vamathevan JJ, Hall MD, Hasan S, et al.: Minipig and beagle animal model genomes aid species selection in pharmaceutical discovery and development, *Toxicol Appl Pharmacol* 270:149–157, 2013.

Vargas HM, Bass AS, Koerner J, et al.: Evaluation of drug-induced QT interval prolongation in animal and human studies: a literature review of concordance, *Br J Pharmacol* 172:4002–4011, 2015.

Villar D, Buck WB, Gonzalez JM: Ibuprofen, aspirin and acetaminophen toxicosis and treatment in dogs and cats, *Vet Hum Toxicol* 40(3):156–162, 1998.

Wakefield ID, Pollard C, Redfern WS, et al.: The application of in vitro methods to safety pharmacology, *Fund Clin Pharmacol* 16(3):209–218, 2002.

Wei YJ, Tang Y, Li J, et al.: Cloning and expression pattern of dog SDF-1 and the implications of altered expression of SDF-1 in ischemic myocardium, *Cytokine* 40:52–59, 2007.

Whitebread S, Hamon J, Bojanic D, et al.: In vitro safety phar-macology profiling: an essential tool for successful drug development, *Drug Discov Today* 21(10):1421–1433, 2005.

Wildt DE, Seager SW, Chakraborty PK: Behavioral, ovarian and endocrine relationships in the pubertal bitch, *J Anim Sci* 53:182–191, 1981.

Woicke J, Al-Haddawi MM, Bienvenu J-G, et al.: International Harmonization of Nomenclature and Diagnostic Criteria (INHAND): Non-proliferative and proliferative lesions of the dog, *Toxicol Pathol* 49(1):5–109, 2021. https://doi.org/10.1177/0192623320968181.

Yatsu FM, Diamond I, Graziano C, et al.: Experimental brain ischemia: protection from irreversible damage with a rapid-acting barbiturate (methohexital), *Stroke* 3:726–732, 1972.

Youssef SA, et al.: Pathology of the aging brain in domestic and laboratory animals, and animal models of human neurodegenerative diseases, *Vet Path* 53(2):327–348, 2016.

Zhang D, Luo G, Ding X, et al.: Preclinical experimental models of drug metabolism and disposition in drug discovery and development, *Acta Pharmaceut Sin B* 2(6):549–561, 2012.

Animal Models in Toxicologic Research: Pig

Kristi Helke[1], Keith Nelson[2], Aaron Sargeant[3]

[1]Medical University of South Carolina, Charleston, SC, United States, [2]Charles River Laboratories, Mattawan, MI, United States, [3]Charles River Laboratories, Spencerville, OH, United States

O U T L I N E

1. Introduction   751

2. Genetics of Pigs and Background for Their Use in Research   752
   2.1. Breeds   752
   2.2. Basic Biological Characteristics   753
   2.3. Husbandry Considerations   753

3. Use of Pigs in Toxicological Studies   755
   3.1. Study Design Considerations   755
   3.2. Oral Toxicity Studies   756
   3.3. Intravenous Toxicity Studies   756
   3.4. Subcutaneous Dosing Toxicity Studies   757
   3.5. Dermal Toxicity Studies   757
   3.6. Other Routes of Dose Administration   759
   3.7. Embryo—Fetal Toxicity Studies   759
   3.8. Juvenile Toxicity Studies   760

4. Pigs as Organ Source for Xenotransplantation   761

5. Spontaneous Background Pathology in Swine   761
   5.1. Macroscopic Observations   762
   5.2. Microscopic Findings   764

5.3. Neoplasia in Research Swine   769

6. Use of the Pig as a Model System for Medical Devices and of Human Diseases   770
   6.1. Cardiovascular   770
   6.2. Skin   770
   6.3. Renal   771
   6.4. Metabolic Syndrome/Diabetes   771
   6.5. Eye   771
   6.6. Brain   771
   6.7. Immune System   772
   6.8. Cancer   772
   6.9. Genetically Modified Pigs   772

7. Regulatory Aspects   772

8. Ethics and Animal Welfare   773

9. Summary   773

References   774

1. INTRODUCTION

The choice of animal species in nonclinical research should always be carefully considered and justified. Pigs and minipigs are considered good models for humans because they share many important characteristics. Swine exhibit particularly close resemblance to humans with respect to the anatomy of the skin, cardiovascular system, the majority of the gastrointestinal tract, and urogenital system (Swindle and Smith, 2016). In addition, similarities are often found in the metabolism of drugs and in physiological parameters, with many genes having better homology in the pig than the rat relative to humans, even though the rat is one of the most commonly used nonclinical animal models in toxicologic research.

Haschek and Rousseaux's Handbook of Toxicologic Pathology, Fourth Edition.
https://doi.org/10.1016/B978-0-12-821044-4.00001-7

In drug development, the intended clinical route of dosing should be applied in nonclinical studies, wherever possible. All general routes of product administration [i.e., dermal (topical and intradermal), intramuscular and intravenous, oral, and subcutaneous] are feasible in pigs and minipigs (Heining and Ruysschaert, 2016). Furthermore, all generally required durations of dosing can be completed, with up to 12 months of daily dosing, depending on the route of administration. For regulatory toxicity studies, the minipig in particular should always be considered as a relevant test species and is fully accepted by regulatory authorities worldwide.

For long-term studies (or any study with animals over 6 months of age), minipigs offer an advantage over conventional pigs as their smaller size requires a markedly reduced amount of test article to perform a study. Other advantages of minipigs are that they are easier to handle and reach sexual maturity at a younger age. Some of the larger minipigs, such as the Hanford, or the domestic pig breeds are better suited for device studies as their size more closely approximates the human. Today, several breeds of minipigs exist globally. In addition, pigs have a sparser hair coat than other animals and the skin of several minipig breeds is nonpigmented, which facilitates gross observations for adverse reactions in dermal toxicity and wound healing studies. The information given in this chapter will provide uses of minipigs and pigs in toxicologic research, background information on pigs including spontaneous pathology, and how they have been utilized as models of human disease.

2. GENETICS OF PIGS AND BACKGROUND FOR THEIR USE IN RESEARCH

2.1. Breeds

All pigs used in research and agriculture are *Sus scrofa*. Similar to the dog, certain traits have been selected for creating different breeds. Cross-breeding with wild pigs has led to the development of pigs with smaller stature which are more manageable in a research setting.

Interbreeding of domestic or agricultural pigs has allowed selection for a nonpigmented or white skin phenotype in some breeds. Selection for outward visible phenotypes has led to variability in other genetic traits such as background changes being more common in some breeds or differences among breeds in xenobiotic metabolizing enzymes. Because of these differences among breeds, it is important to examine the gene atlas from the specific breed being used if conducting a xenobiotic study (Heining and Ruysschaert, 2016).

Minipigs

Several minipig breeds exist worldwide. Some are naturally occurring (e.g., Yucatan and Wuzhishan) and others such as the Göttingen minipig have been bred and selected for attributes such as size and coat color that facilitate their use in biomedical research. The predominant breeds of minipigs used in biomedical research are the Göttingen, Hanford, Sinclair, and Yucatan in North America and Europe (McAnulty et al., 2012; Swindle and Smith, 2016). In Asia, several different breeds are used including Bama, Clawn, Microminipig, Ohmini, and Wuzhishan (Gutierrez et al., 2015). Body weight ranges (fully grown animals) vary among the different breeds (Figure 20.1). For the Yucatan micropig and the Göttingen minipig, the adult body weight range is 35–55 kg, for Sinclair and Hanford minipigs, it is 50–60 kg, and for the Yucatan minipig and the Hormel minipig, the weight range is 70–90 kg. Presently, the Göttingen is

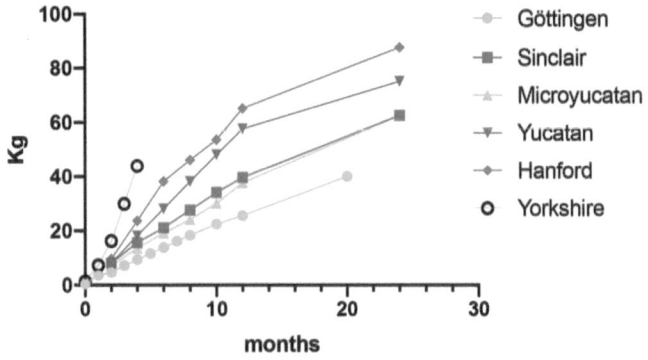

FIGURE 20.1 Comparison growth chart of several breeds. *Adapted from resource data (Bouchard et al., 2019; Ellegaard Göttingen Minipigs; Midwest Research Swine).*

the only minipig breed that is bred and available worldwide for research purposes. The other minipig breeds may be available from local breeders or via shipping. All minipigs obtained from vendors have a defined health status. Vendors regularly test for pathogens to identify if any are present in their colonies and to confirm negative status for selected pathogens. Animals with defined flora are preferred for product registration studies, especially those that must be conducted according to GLP (Good Laboratory Practice) principles, to decrease confounding findings.

Conventional/Domestic Pigs

Several breeds of larger size typically used in agriculture are used in biomedical research studies, especially those of short duration (less than 3 months). All of these breeds are bred to grow quickly; hence, their use for chronic or long-term biomedical research studies (i.e., greater than several months duration) is often limited by space and personnel. Conventionally, sized pigs are good models for conducting surgical procedures including the development of medical devices since they are closer in size to an adult human versus a minipig (Schomberg et al., 2016). Common breeds include Large White, Duroc, Landrace, and Yorkshire. The breed chosen by the investigator for these types of studies is commonly based on availability in the geographical location. There are no commercial vendors of conventional swine exclusively for research use with closed breeding and defined health status as compared to the availability of this resourcing for minipigs. These vendors typically offer research animals in addition to animals for agricultural use.

2.2. Basic Biological Characteristics

The lifespan of swine ranges from 15 to 25 years depending on the breed. Litter sizes also vary from 4 to 20 piglets, with minipigs having smaller litters (e.g., four to nine offspring) (Table 20.1). Many biomedical studies use pigs of different ages to correlate with different human life stages (Table 20.2).

Part of the pig's natural behavior is rooting. This may lead to foreign material or small particles being inhaled resulting in inflammation of the airways. Pigs have been reported to have nutritional deficiencies in the research setting, especially conventional breeds (Helke et al., 2016a). Conventional breed vendors may mix their own feed on the farm, and it is not tested as rigorously as the minipig vendors pelleted feed. This has resulted in Vitamin E and selenium deficiencies in at least one study (Helke et al., 2016a). Minipigs have suffered from water deprivation (salt toxicity) shortly after shipping (Bouchard et al., 2019). Pigs used for research are prone to all of the diseases that occur in conventional pigs, and these diseases are occasionally seen in research settings.

Sexual maturity occurs at 3–7 months depending on the breed, with minipig breeds maturing at approximately 4–6 months. Maturity in pigs is defined by some as the age at which the first estrus or mature sperm is noted, whereas others refer to the age of physeal closure (Kim et al., 2017). As such, it is difficult to designate an age of the onset of maturity without an agreed upon definition; however, most regulatory agencies require sexual maturity for safety studies, not physeal closure or skeletal maturity. Physeal closure happens sooner in smaller breeds (Swindle and Smith, 2016).

There are a few anatomical differences in the pig compared to other species. Pigs have a laryngeal diverticulum which may make intubation or gavage more difficult. They have a fibromuscular protrusion at the pyloric outflow of the stomach, known as the torus pyloricus. The colon is organized into centripetal coils in the pig, an anatomical but not functional difference (Swindle and Smith, 2016).

2.3. Husbandry Considerations

Not only do pigs grow very quickly, there are a wide range of breeds, all with different adult weights. This necessitates that the guide for animal care and use is consulted to ensure correct area needs are met when housing the animals (National Research Council, 2011). Housing guidelines may vary depending on the country in which studies are conducted. There are different guidelines that can vary greatly for housing of pigs depending on whether they are being used for biomedical or agricultural research (USDA, 2020).

Pigs have a tendency to root, and this rooting behavior often results in spillage of water and

TABLE 20.1 Normal Biological Data for Conventional (Yorkshire or Landrace) Pigs Compared to Minipig (Göttingen)

Physiological parameter	Yorkshire/Landrace	Göttingen
Lifespan	6–10 years	8–15 years
Chromosome number	18 pair plus 2 sex chromosomes	
Body weight (2 year)	296 kg	30–35 kg
Body temperature (adult)	101.6–104 F (38.7–40 C)	
Age at sexual maturity	5–6 months (F)	4–5 months (F)/ 3–4 months (M)
Frequency of cycling in females	21 days	
Gestation period	114 days	
Average litter size	13	6–8
Weight at birth	1.3 kg	0.42 kg
Dental formulae—deciduous teeth	3 + 3 (incisors); 1 + 1 (canines) 3 + 3 (premolars) (28)	
Dental formulae—permanent teeth	3 + 3 (incisors); 1 + 1 (canines); 4 + 4 (premolars) 3 + 3 (molars) (44)	
Heart weight (% of body weight)	0.5% in young, 2.5%–2.9% in older	0.412%–0.524%
Heart rate	116 ± 8 beats per minute	92 ± 7 beats per minute
Liver lobes	6	
Lung lobes	7	

food. For this reason, food and water dishes are often firmly attached to the sides or floor of caging and water can be provided via an automatic system. There is currently no consensus on the best type of caging for pigs, as most facilities require flexibility for different species. Pigs require flooring that allows secure footing and it is helpful if the flooring also helps in keeping hooves from becoming overgrown.

Pigs are intelligent and can be trained using clickers and often are amenable to extended periods in a sling. Placing a pig in a sling allows prolonged humane restraint without the need for anesthesia.

TABLE 20.2 Equivalent Ages in Pigs Compared to Human Life Stages

Age in pigs	Approximate equivalent age in human
1 week	Newborn
4 weeks	2-year-old
2 months	6-year-old
4 months	14-year-old
2 years	Sexually mature adult

Adapted from (Hood, 2012).

Pigs are social animals and, if not group housed due to study requirements, should be allowed to see or touch snouts with neighbor animals through cage walls. Pigs can be destructive, and enrichment should be sturdy enough to not be broken or chewed into smaller pieces.

3. USE OF PIGS IN TOXICOLOGICAL STUDIES

Pigs are increasingly being used for safety studies due to their similarity to humans (Henze et al., 2019; Swindle et al., 2012). This includes oral availability, dermal toxicity, immunotoxicity, juvenile studies, and others (Descotes et al., 2018; Feyen et al., 2016; Henze et al., 2019; Stricker-Krongrad et al., 2017).

3.1. Study Design Considerations

Prior to study initiation, the animals should be acclimated at the facility for a minimum of 7–10 days, during which time they are observed clinically in order to evaluate their general health status prior to start of dosing. Baseline evaluations such as collection of blood for clinical pathological analyses may also be taken, as well as electrocardiograms to examine heart function. Training for study-related procedures, such as dermal dosing, should be started during the acclimation period to both facilitate a successful start of treatment and help familiarize the animals with their handlers by daily close contact.

Minipigs are typically 4–5 months of age at start of dosing on toxicity studies, which is considered the age of sexual maturity in minipigs. Use of sexually mature animals is essential for any nonclinical toxicity studies evaluating male reproduction (see *Male Reproductive Tract*, Vol 4, Chap 9). Certain study types require older (and especially larger) animals at the start of treatment. This is the case for continuous infusion studies, where the ambulatory infusion equipment is of such a size and weight that the animal must be large enough to handle the apparatus. Larger animals are also needed for embryo–fetal studies, where sows with more

fully mature reproductive systems are needed, for wound healing studies where larger body surfaces will enable establishment of sufficient wounds without having to use more animals, and for certain studies investigating local tolerance. Younger pigs are required for juvenile toxicity studies.

There are some differences in the metabolizing enzymes between humans and pigs, between sexes, and even among different pig breeds. Many studies looking at sex differences in xenobiotic metabolizing enzymes (e.g., cytochrome (CYP) P540s, UGT, and SULT) have shown that once castrated, the differences between the sexes decrease, suggesting that the levels are dependent on testosterone. Different breeds have been shown to have different testosterone levels and subsequent differences in CYP levels (Gillberg et al., 2006; Kojima and Degawa, 2016; Puccinelli et al., 2011; Puccinelli et al., 2013; Rasmussen et al., 2019; Skaanild, 2006; Skaanild and Friis, 1999). Age-related changes in these enzymes are commonly reported as well, specifically that CYP activity increases with age in juveniles, but then decreases into adulthood. It appears that these changes coincide with puberty (increased CYP enzyme activity) and adulthood (decreased activity relative to puberty but increased from prepuberty). Due to these variables, it is recommended that there be standardization of breed, sex, and age of animals tested.

If the drug being tested is metabolized by aldehyde oxidase, *N*-acetyltransferase, or CYP2C9, the minipig should be the preferred large animal model as activity of these enzymes in the pig most closely mimics those in humans compared to other nonclinical large animal model options (e.g., dog, nonhuman primate [NHP]) (Dalgaard, 2015). The enzyme 3-phospho-adenosyl-5-phosphosulphate sulphotransferase is not effective in pigs (Dalgaard, 2015). As with selecting any relevant animal species for toxicity studies, it is best to determine if the test article being administered is metabolized in the pig if it is being considered.

According to guideline requirements for nonclinical toxicity studies across all species, systemic exposure [i.e., the pharmacokinetic profile] should be evaluated as well as other parameters (e.g., clinical observations, food consumption, body and organ weights, clinical chemistry and hematology, urinalysis, and macroscopic and microscopic pathology evaluation) (Andrade et al., 2016). In addition, ophthalmologic and electrocardiographic evaluation may be included, as well as more specialized evaluations such as dermatologic scoring or cytokine responses. Specific protocols for evaluating these parameters should be included in the study design. All of these procedures can easily be performed in minipigs under each of the dosing conditions described in this chapter.

For detailed evaluation of specific clinical parameters, the minipig may serve as an excellent test species. For example, in evaluation of cardiovascular function in specific safety pharmacology studies, use of implanted devices to measure heart rate, body temp, movements, and other parameters can greatly facilitate collection of key electrocardiographic data (Markert et al., 2018). In such studies, electrodes may be implanted subcutaneously in the chest and detailed electrocardiographic recordings generated on a continuous basis or at designated intervals, without handling the animals. In addition, blood pressure may be measured using a transducer implanted into a branch of the femoral artery.

For each parameter measured, it is important to build a historical control database for comparison with information from current and future studies. This database is essential as group sizes in nonrodent studies are typically small (e.g., 4–5/sex/group). Historic data provide support for evaluation and interpretation of data and additional assurance of data quality by showing consistency among groups and across time. While there are several retrospective review papers that discuss findings in control minipigs (Helke et al., 2016b; Jeppesen and Skydsgaard, 2015; Stricker-Krongrad et al., 2016), it is still important that each facility has an ongoing internal database developed for reference purposes.

3.2. Oral Toxicity Studies

Anatomically, the upper part of the gastrointestinal tract (e.g., esophagus, stomach, and small intestine) of pigs is very similar to the same

regions in humans (Kararli, 1995; Ziegler et al., 2016). Pigs have similar gastric cell types, intestinal villous structure, and intestinal secretions as do humans (Ziegler et al., 2016). Furthermore, the changes in pH along the small intestine, as well as the transit time in the small intestine, are very similar in pigs when compared to humans. In contrast, the porcine large intestine is arranged in a series of coils, while in humans the large intestine is organized as a linear organ with several sharp angles. Despite these physical differences, the functions of the human and pig large intestine are comparable. These facts, combined with a high degree of similarity in metabolism and in the microbiome, make the minipig an ideal species for testing orally dosed drugs (Schomberg et al., 2016).

Oral dosing of liquids (e.g., solutions or suspensions) by gavage in the minipig is a straightforward procedure that can easily be handled by two trained technicians using a swine dosing chair or sling. Volumes up to 20 mL/kg (single dose) or 10 mL/kg (multiple doses) can be administered using this procedure.

Like oral gavage dosing, administration of capsules or tablets can be accomplished with the animal in an upright position in a swine dosing chair or restrained in a sling. Alternatively, tablets can be administered hidden in a small portion of moist diet. This is also possible for capsules; however, there is a high risk that the animals will chew the capsules, resulting in an undesirable premature release of the entire dose. To minimize this risk, capsules can be placed at the caudal part of the tongue using water to help the animal to swallow the capsule.

3.3. Intravenous Toxicity Studies

Minipigs are also suitable as a nonrodent species for test articles intended for intravenous use. Intravenous dosing via both bolus and infusion is feasible in minipigs. However, access to peripheral veins is limited; the auricular (external ear) veins can be used for single intravenous bolus injections but are not recommended for repeated injections or continuous infusion. This lack of available reusable superficial vessels necessitates surgical implantation of catheters to be used when repeated intravenous dosing is required.

For repeated intravenous bolus injections or for infusion of short durations (maximum 30 min), a vascular access port (VAP) can be used. For intravenous infusions greater than 30 min, a cannula/catheter is recommended to limit irritation. The VAP is implanted subcutaneously and connected to the bloodstream via a catheter implanted in a major blood vessel. In principle, the VAP can be implanted at almost any site. However, for practical reasons it is best implanted in the region of the neck or cranial aspect of the back, with the catheter inserted into the external jugular vein allowing easy dosing in the conscious animal (Barka et al., 2010). Dosing is performed by locating the VAP externally (accomplished by palpation of the VAP through the skin), followed by skin puncture and puncture of the silicone membrane of the VAP, through which there is direct intravenous access via the catheter. For this purpose, a hypodermic needle is used. A VAP can be implanted in a minipig beginning at 7 days after birth. Growth of the animals should be taken into account when implanting the catheters and the VAPs into younger animals, or for any study during which the animal may grow.

Due to the weight and size of the equipment used (the combined weight of the ambulatory infusion pump plus counterbalance is approximately 2 kg), animals used for continuous infusion studies should be at least 10 kg. In order to allow for free movement of the animals within their pen, the preference is to use ambulatory infusion pumps, which can be carried by the animals in specially designed jackets. However, a tethered system in which a wall or pen-top mounted pump not carried by the animal delivers the dosing solution via a long overhead tube can also be considered; in this conformation, the animals are often confined to a relatively small area for the time of dosing to prevent detachment or kinks in the catheter that might disrupt the infusion. Various infusion pumps are commercially available, and it is important to consider size and weight (including the filled infusion reservoir) when choosing equipment. The infusion pump is connected to a central vein via an implanted catheter.

Using the correct techniques, patency of catheters can be maintained for several weeks without any problems, thereby enabling continuous infusion studies of approximately 4 weeks duration.

3.4. Subcutaneous Dosing Toxicity Studies

The pig is a relevant nonrodent species to be considered for test articles intended for subcutaneous administration. The sparse hair coat and lack of pigmentation of many breeds facilitate clinical evaluation needed to detect potential reactions after dosing. Although there is firm dermal attachment to the underlying tissues, the dose volume that can be applied is generally not different than that which is applied to dogs in single or repeated dose toxicity studies. Typical dose volume that can be delivered is 0.5 mL/kg and may go as high as 2.0 mL/kg (maximum of 20 mL per site not to exceed 2 sites per animal).

Subcutaneous dosing is best performed in the lateral aspect of the neck. Due to potential local reactions caused by the injection procedure, and in some cases also by the test article, daily subcutaneous injections are usually performed at different sites, alternating between both sides of the neck. The injection sites to be used during a study can be indicated by tattooing, making it possible to rotate the injections according to a planned scheme as well as identify all sites to be collected at necropsy for subsequent histopathological evaluation.

3.5. Dermal Toxicity Studies

The similarity between the skin of humans and pigs makes the pig an ideal model for use in nonclinical dermal studies (Willard-Mack et al., 2016). Features of swine skin that are similar to that of humans include sparse hair cover, a firm attachment to underlying structures, relatively thick epidermis, dermal to epidermal thickness ratios, similar dermal collagen and elastin content, formation of rete ridges, and variance in cutaneous pigment (Monteiro-Riviere and Stromberg, 1985). Other species used for dermal toxicity testing do not have all of these features, particularly including dermal to epidermal thickness ratios, sparse hair, and a firm dermal to subcutis to underlying muscle attachment. Additionally, pigs tolerate occlusive bandages well and have limited ability to manipulate, remove, or ingest material applied dorsally. There are some key differences between the pig and human skin, including a lack of eccrine sweat glands across much of the skin of pigs, decreased dermal and follicular vascularity, and variances in physiochemical response in vascular endothelium, but these are outweighed by the similarities (Stricker-Krongrad et al., 2017). Indeed, for pharmaceutical products intended for dermal application, it is difficult to justify using any nonrodent species other than the pig for these studies.

As a general practice for dermal toxicity studies in pigs, the test item is applied to an area corresponding to approximately 10% of the total body surface area. Normally, the skin on the back is used, as this area is protected from self-inflicted injuries and oral ingestion of test material and is easy to cover with protective bandages. Furthermore, this area is not normally subjected to external contamination with urine and feces. Doses up to 1 gram per kilogram body weight can be applied on the area described. Certainly, administration in this area bears certain limitations, as this is one of the areas of the thickest dermis and has more dense and coarse hair than the ventrum or axillae (Khiao In et al., 2019). However, it is still more readily translatable than a species with a dense haircoat such as the dog, rabbit, or even NHP, in which the dermis is much thinner and less similar to humans.

Selection of an appropriate intraspecimen control site for histological evaluation is an important aspect of study design, particularly as there is pronounced variance in histologic appearance and character of the skin from site to site within a given animal (Khiao In et al., 2019). The most appropriate control site is one that shares location and/or histologic features with the test article–dosed site. For example, the dermis on the flanks and shoulders of the minipig is significantly thicker than that of the ventral, inguinal, or axillary regions and even thicker than that of the mid or lower back. Additionally, the density of hair follicles, glands, and other adnexal structures varies significantly from one site to another. The epidermis overall is approximately the same thickness across most regions of minipig skin, but variance of other features, such as collagen and elastin composition or distribution of resident leukocytes, may also be a factor in evaluation of potential test article–related effects (Figure 20.2).

During dosing, the treated area is usually covered by a gauze dressing, held by a net-like bandage covering the thorax and abdomen. It is of great importance to allow a daily treatment/bandage-free period, as the risk of dermal irritation and infections otherwise increases due to the moist, warm, semiocclusive environment. As a standard practice, a daily dosing period of 6 h is often used, although other durations are possible. At the termination of the dosing period, any occlusive dressing and remaining test substance are removed, and the treated area of skin is washed or swabbed to remove residual material.

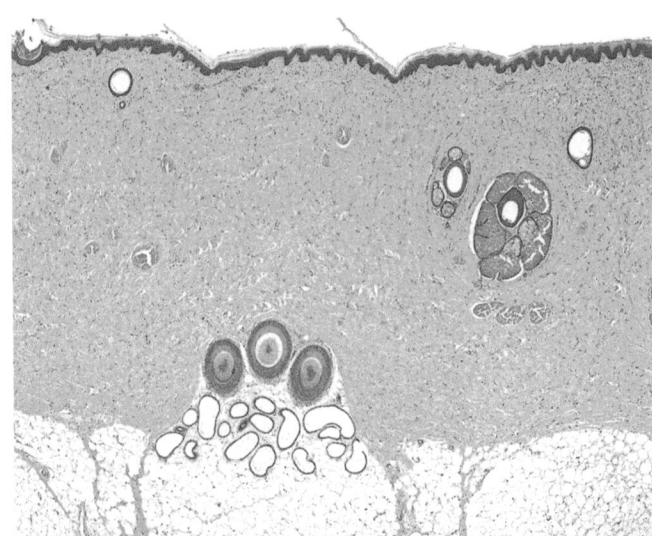

FIGURE 20.2 Histological section of Göttingen minipig skin, showing the epidermis, dermis, and upper part of the subcutis. Hematoxylin and eosin. *Figure reproduced from Haschek and Rousseaux's:* Handbook of toxicologic pathology, *ed 3. In Haschek WM, Rousseaux CG, Wallig MA, editors: Academic Press, 2013, p 464. Figure 13.2, with permission.*

Dermal Local Tolerance Studies

During a drug development program, it is a requirement to test for local dermal tolerance to determine if there is a reaction to the formulation being used when applying test articles to the skin. In some instances, this element can be integrated into single or repeat-dose studies. However, if more detailed observations need to be made (including sampling of tissue at different time points in relation to dosing), a separate study with local tolerance as the major objective may be performed.

For screening purposes of dermal compounds, it is possible to test several formulations using the same animal, if the size of the animal is fairly large. In this manner, interanimal variation can be minimized. Test sites are usually indicated by tattooing and each site is treated and bandaged as described for dermal toxicity studies. During the study, the same test site is treated with the same test item. If the various test items require different vehicles, then separate control sites must be included for each vehicle. Each treated area is covered by its own bandage to prevent migration of test materials among sites. Care in avoiding migration of materials among sites is critical in this sort of screening study. Inclusion of untreated spaces around and between test sites and control sites may facilitate this. An occlusive bandage should be applied to the control sites, even if no vehicle is applied, both to fully mimic the mechanical effects of the dosing and bandage coverage and to prevent test material contamination of control skin.

3.6. Other Routes of Dose Administration

In addition to the dosing procedures described previously, other nontraditional routes of dose administration are also possible in the minipig. The dosing procedures described below should not be seen as a complete list of possible routes in the minipig, but as examples of nonroutine options which may be utilized.

Vaginal dosing may be needed for local tolerance testing of liquid or gel formulations of test articles intended for intravaginal use in humans. Alternatively, medical devices intended for intravaginal use may also be tested. Use of sexually mature animals will ensure that any potential

effects on cyclic changes will be able to be evaluated. Care should be taken during dosing procedures not to induce iatrogenic damage of the vaginal mucosa. Aseptic principles should be applied at dosing in order to avoid procedure-related infections. When performing intravaginal dosing, physical restraints such as slings, in conjunction with preconditioning and training, may serve to limit potential iatrogenic effects, or animals may be sedated or anesthetized to provide chemical immobilization.

Repeated intravesicular dosing into the urinary bladder or even into the renal pelvis can be performed in female minipigs via a urinary catheter inserted through the urethra under surgical anesthesia. This route is not possible in males due to the anatomical course of the urethra. Intravesicular dosing can also be performed in both males and females by use of a pig-tail catheter introduced surgically into the bladder. The catheter may either be exteriorized through the abdominal wall or attached to an Access Port (AP), which is typically implanted on the back. Similarly, direct evaluation of intestinal absorption of liquid formulations or suspensions can be performed via a surgically implanted duodenal catheter. This route is used to avoid the impact of the stomach secretions on the test article. Again, the catheter can either be exteriorized through the abdominal wall or attached to a subcutaneous AP.

Topical, intravitreal, and subretinal dosing has been performed in the minipig eye in nonclinical safety assessment of pharmaceuticals. Diagnostic techniques include electroretinograms, optical coherence tomography, and histopathology.

3.7. Embryo–Fetal Toxicity Studies

Traditionally, rats and rabbits are the species of choice for developmental toxicity (embryo–fetal) studies (see *Embryo, fetus and placenta*, Vol 4, Chap 11). If these species are found unsuitable, the choice of an alternative can be difficult. In such instances, the use of the minipig as a nonrodent species of choice in developmental toxicity is increasing (Forster et al., 2010a). Studies have shown that the minipig is susceptible to teratogens known to have potential teratogenic effects in humans (e.g., tretinoin and thalidomide). Their gestation length is shorter (113 days) than the NHP and their larger number of progeny (average of 7 fetuses per litter) are well suited to the preferred design of developmental toxicity studies. In particular, minipig reproductive traits are more useful for embryo–fetal toxicity assessment than the corresponding values for common NHP species, which have longer gestation lengths [typically 165 days for macaques (cynomolgus and rhesus macaques) and 180 days for baboons] and generally carry a single conceptus.

A standard study design for minipig developmental toxicity studies is comprised of 14–18 minipigs per group, using primiparous sows that are 6–8 months of age at the start of the study. The animals are dosed during the entire length of organogenesis, which corresponds to days 11–35 of gestation. All routes of dose administration can be used (e.g., oral, subcutaneous, intravenous) without inducing any increase in the incidence of adverse developmental events that might be attributed to handling-associated maternal stress. In general, if repeat-dose intravenous injections are to be given, a VAP is suggested and the surgical procedure to implant it should be performed at least a week before mating, which will give sufficient time for healing, avoid potential adverse effects of anesthetics and analgesics during pregnancy, and which will prevent any stress to the animal during mating and the early part of pregnancy.

The fetuses are collected near term by caesarean section on gestation days 109–111. The dams are terminated, and the implantation sites are evaluated. Examination of fetuses includes the same observations and measurements that are used for rodents and rabbits, e.g., external and visceral macroscopic examination of fresh tissue at necropsy (all fetuses) and for half of the fetuses chosen at random, skeletal examination of Alizarin-stained bones. Heads from the other half of the fetuses are fixed by immersion in Bouin's fixative, sectioned, and examined for abnormalities (see also *The Role of Pathology in Evaluation of Reproductive, Developmental, and Juvenile Toxicity*, Vol 1, Chap 7).

3.8. Juvenile Toxicity Studies

Recently, increased regulatory requirements for new chemical entities have been implemented with respect to products designated for pediatric indications. By default, in the European Union, a Pediatric Investigational Plan, including nonclinical juvenile toxicity studies, should be undertaken in such circumstances (European Medicines Agency, 1995). Juvenile studies are also required in the United States for pediatric formulations (U.S. Department of Health and Human Services et al., 2006). Nonrodent juvenile animal models have been developed to meet this requirement.

The minipig constitutes an ideal juvenile animal model due to the relatively long developmental period following birth, which enables investigations during several phases of pediatric life (see Table 20.2). Approximate break points for various stages in this breed are up to 4 weeks for the neonatal period (with weaning between 21 and 28 days of age), between 4 and 8 weeks for the infant period, from 8 weeks to 3 months for the childhood, and between 3 and 5 months for adolescence. The average litter size of 6–8 offspring reduces the number of sows required to perform a study. Since administration of the test article occurs after birth, cross-fostering of the offspring among various sows should be considered in order to reduce the genetic relationship between individuals included in the same dose group. This practice will also eliminate the potential risk for chemical contamination between groups that might arise if pigs given different doses were left with their birth mother.

Attention to the developmental phase is important in determining the appropriate age for use in a given study. Additionally, the length of the study and the potential effects of the test article on maturation, both skeletal and reproductive, should be considered. For test articles intended for oral, subcutaneous, intramuscular, or intravenous administration, dosing can be commenced from day 7 of age. At this age, repeated intravenous doses are delivered through a VAP, implanted 2 days before the intended use in the same manner as described under the section discussing intravenous toxicity studies. Nutritional studies may be performed at any age, with infant formula studies beginning on postnatal Day 1, following animals receiving colostrum. For compounds administered on the skin, it is not practically feasible to begin dosing before weaning, so the start date is typically delayed until 5–6 weeks of age. By this time, the animals can be housed individually during dosing, which eliminates the risk of bandage destruction and oral ingestion of test article by littermates. In order to cover test article administration during earlier phases of life, dosing may be started using another route, with a switch to cutaneous application after weaning. Pathology evaluation of juveniles requires special considerations (see *The Role of Pathology in Evaluation of Reproductive, Developmental, and Juvenile Toxicity*, Vol 1, Chap 7).

4. PIGS AS ORGAN SOURCE FOR XENOTRANSPLANTATION

Pigs have been considered a potential animal model for xenotransplantation because of the similarities between pigs and humans (Lu et al., 2019). Heart valves from pigs have been transplanted into humans since the 1960s, but these xenotransplants invariably fail due to immune reactions and calcification (Manji et al., 2015). With the advent of technologies to more easily create transgenic pigs, this is becoming closer to reality (Sykes and Sachs, 2019). While the mechanisms involved in graft rejection may be overcome by genetically engineering pigs to express human proteins/epitopes, there is still need to reduce the porcine endogenous retroviruses (PERVs) expressed by all pigs and pig cell lines. There are breed differences in the copy number and PERVs expressed. Not all breeds express PERVc, and it is PERVa and PERVc which are of most concern for infecting human cells. Clustered regularly interspaced short palindromic repeats (CRISPRs)/CRISPR-associated protein (Cas) 9 has recently been used to generate PERV-free pigs which increases the feasibility of using pigs in xenotransplantation (Niu et al., 2017). Some examples of organs under current exploration for xenotransplantation include the kidney, heart, lung, and cartilage (Lu et al., 2019).

5. SPONTANEOUS BACKGROUND PATHOLOGY IN SWINE

The minipig breed most commonly used for biomedical research today is the Göttingen minipig, although there are numerous breeds available. Minipigs are bred in barrier facilities to maintain a defined microbial flora, and their health is monitored on a regular basis. Accordingly, untreated minipigs are generally quite healthy.

Clinical disease is uncommon in minipigs unless they are housed together with pigs obtained from a different breeder and with a dissimilar health status. Minipigs can be infected by the same pathogens as conventional production pigs, so this issue has to be considered if the laboratory uses both minipigs and conventional pigs for experimental procedures. In particular, researchers must recall that conventional pigs, even if they originate from a specific pathogen-free breeding facility, are not monitored for pathogens as extensively as minipigs.

Tissue sampling guidelines are available specifically for the pig that describe methods for different levels of testing (Albl et al., 2016). When contact with other pigs is avoided, healthy minipigs generally exhibit a narrow spectrum of relatively minor clinical diseases and subclinical conditions. This fact is evident from tissue samples of untreated animals subjected to histopathological examination, which generally have few if any incidental background lesions. Some clinical diseases and spontaneous microscopic findings, which may be encountered when using pigs in nonclinical safety testing, are discussed briefly below. There are several references that review incidence and provide descriptions of these findings in different minipig breeds (Helke et al., 2016b, 2020; Jeppesen and Skydsgaard, 2015; Kangawa et al., 2019; McInnes and McKeag, 2016; Stricker-Krongrad et al., 2016). The International Harmonization of Nomenclature and Diagnostic criteria publication also reviews all accepted nomenclature for these findings and has numerous images (Skydsgaard et al., 2021). This publication is freely available at the Society of Toxicologic website, www.toxpath.org, and additional information is available at www.goreni.org.

There are a few histological findings in pigs that are often associated with dosing and testing before study endpoint. These changes include hemorrhage and potential subsequent fibrosis in the cervical region from blood sampling of the jugular vein. Organs affected can include the thymus, thyroid, and trachea (Bouchard et al., 2019; Helke et al., 2016a). Subendocardial hemorrhages can be seen in the heart if the euthanasia period is prolonged (Helke, 2015).

5.1. Macroscopic Observations

Spontaneous Cutaneous Purpura/Erythema Multiforme/Dippity Pig Syndrome

Acute dermatitis is the most commonly used name for the condition described below, but it is also known as spontaneous cutaneous purpura, erythema multiforme, and "dippity pig" syndrome. It is worth noticing that erythema multiforme is generally used to imply a hypersensitivity reaction in the skin, while the cause of the acute dermatitis is unclear. Stress has been implicated as playing a role in the pathogenesis. The syndrome is also well known in the potbelly pig (Dijkhorst et al., 2018; Tynes, 1996).

Bleeding, oozing sores appear in a series of parallel transverse lesions located in skin folds on the caudal back, neck, or rump of affected animals (Figure 20.3) (McInnes and McKeag, 2016). The minipig kneels or sits, arches it back, and may vocalize when someone attempts to touch it as the condition is often painful. Variants of the syndrome may be encountered; thus, the pig may show signs of severe pain (e.g., arching of the back and squealing) with no visible lesions, or it may show moderate lesions on the back which do not appear to be painful to

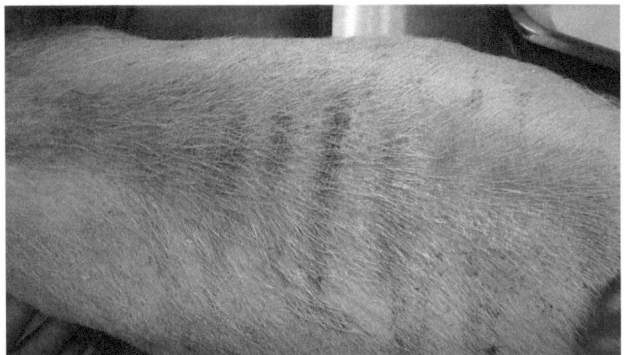

FIGURE 20.3　Gross image of transverse lesions on the back of a pig consistent with "dippity pig." *Image used with permission from McInnes and McKeag, 2016. Figure 10A.*

the touch. The onset is acute, and the typical signs are characteristic.

An infectious agent has not been identified, and based on the authors' experience, antibiotic treatment is not necessary. The syndrome is self-limiting, and the lesions will completely heal in a relatively short period (a few days to 2 weeks) with no scarring. Routine analgesic treatment should be administered in cases where evidence of pain is observed. In Göttingen minipigs, the syndrome is recognized in all age groups, whereas in potbelly pigs it has been described as more commonly affecting pigs less than one year old.

Dermatitis/Exudative Epidermitis/Eczema/ Hyperkeratosis in Göttingen Minipigs

In the Göttingen minipig, a condition resembling exudative epidermitis of production swine is well known. In the Göttingen minipig, the condition is sometimes called eczema or hyperkeratosis of the Göttingen minipig to differentiate it from the exudative epidermitis caused by *Staphylococcus hyicus*. It is recommended that the name hyperkeratosis should not be used unless a histological diagnosis of hyperkeratosis has been confirmed.

The condition is most often seen in younger minipigs (3–4 months or younger); however, it is sometimes encountered in older minipigs as well. Black scabs usually develop on the head initially and may or may not progress to become more generalized.

Exudative epidermitis in conventional pigs is caused by toxin-producing *S. hyicus*, but it has not been possible to associate the condition seen in Göttingen minipigs with any primary infectious agent to date. Furthermore, the general health of the minipigs is rarely affected, whereas piglets with exudative epidermitis caused by *S. hyicus* often show signs of clinical disease. *Candida albicans* may sometimes be isolated from the lesions, but it is a part of the normal cutaneous flora of the Göttingen minipig and is not always isolated in these cases. Therefore, *Candida* is not considered to be the cause of the condition. However, in some cases, the involvement of *Candida* may cause the clinical condition to become more severe.

In the minipig, the condition is normally self-limiting, and the lesions often heal more or less completely within a couple of months. The skin in the affected areas may be slightly red after recovery. Minipigs with a history of dermatitis and a difference in skin color due to the condition typically should be excluded from dermal toxicity and wound healing studies.

Fungal Dermatitis

As noted above, *C. albicans* is often isolated from the skin of Göttingen minipigs, at an incidence of up to 40%. Lesions associated with cutaneous *Candida* infection can be observed as white scabs around the eyes; it is much less frequently observed as a generalized skin condition. In the localized periocular form, the changes rarely present a clinical problem. However, in immunocompromised animals (e.g., due to either treatment with a test article or a concurrent systemic disease), the condition may progress, and white to gray raised, firm adherent scabs may be seen at multiple, randomly located sites on the body of the minipig as well, with underlying erythema. Cultures of the affected areas may often have multiple infectious organisms evident, including bacteria and *Candida* spp. rendering determination of the proximate infectious organism difficult (Ramot et al., 2017). Empirical treatment with antifungal agents and eventual clearance of the lesions is often the clearest evidence of cutaneous candidiasis. In the generalized form, the condition can compromise skin integrity so severely that clinical illness may ensue from secondary causes. When generalized, the condition is often difficult to treat, but antimycotic agents administered either locally (usually as a topical cream) or systemically may be effective.

Diarrhea

As with conventional pigs, barrier-bred Göttingen minipigs routinely harbor rotavirus. The pathogen typically causes clinical disease in piglets within the first 2 weeks of life, resulting in gross evidence of a profuse, watery, yellow diarrhea. Villus atrophy is a consistent lesion on histopathological examination.

If no other agents causing porcine diarrhea are expected in the facility, this virus should be suspected when uncomplicated diarrhea is observed, even if the affected animals are older than 14 days. Normally, the minipigs are otherwise unaffected and eat well. If no other agents complicate the condition, the diarrhea will subside within 2–4 days. If the minipig develops a fever, stops eating, or becomes depressed, secondary infections by other agents (usually bacteria) should be suspected. *Escherichia coli* (*E. coli*) may complicate the diarrhea in otherwise clean laboratory facilities, and *Lawsonia intracellularis* and *Clostridium* spp. have been known to act as secondary infectious agents, with attendant increased morbidity and mortality. Mortality due to secondary *E. coli* infection may be severe (Zimmerman, 2012). If a secondary bacterial infection is diagnosed, antibiotics directed at the causative agents should be administered. Otherwise, uncomplicated cases of rotaviral diarrhea are treated symptomatically.

Other common causes of diarrhea in swine include coccidiosis (*Isospora suis* and *Cryptosporidium* spp.), coronaviruses such as porcine epidemic diarrhea virus and transmissible gastroenteritis virus, *Clostridium* spp., porcine circovirus-2, *L. intracellularis*, *Salmonella* spp., *Brachyspira* spp., *Yersinia* spp., and larger parasites (Zimmerman, 2012). These are not generally seen in the laboratory minipig unless there have been significant breaks in biosecurity and cross-contamination between the minipig colony and infected standard swine breeds. This is particularly true for the viruses, coccidia, and parasites, which are readily excludable. The extensive efforts to provide microbiologically defined animals through caesarean rederivation, enactment of strict barrier conditions, and isolation of minipig stock colonies from farm swine by the various providers have resulted in research populations largely free from the diarrhea-causing organisms prevalent in conventional swine. Thus, while monitoring of laboratory colonies for some of these diseases may be routinely done, they are rarely, if ever, seen in the laboratory minipig; however, these agents are still occasionally seen in conventional pigs in research settings.

Thrombocytopenic Purpura-Like Syndrome/ Hemorrhagic Syndrome

This condition is rare (0.1% incidence) and has been associated with a type III hypersensitivity reaction, with formation of immune complexes in smaller blood vessels leading to compromised mural integrity and vascular leakage (Beal et al., 2019; Carrasco et al., 2003; Maratea et al., 2006).

Hemorrhages are observed subcutaneously and may also be pronounced in some viscera, such as the kidneys and heart. Hematologic analysis typically shows a very low platelet count in these pigs, and anemia may also be present. The condition often arises very rapidly but may in some cases develop more slowly and can be more difficult to recognize. Euthanasia is advised if the syndrome is diagnosed, as the condition is typically fatal due to widespread, intractable internal bleeding. There is suspicion that it is an inherited disorder, but the specific gene has not yet been determined.

5.2. Microscopic Findings

Cardiovascular

Spontaneous changes in the heart are few and in general are of minimal severity and focal character. Inflammatory cell infiltrates are the most common spontaneous findings, with focal myocardial infiltration by mononuclear cells, focal pericarditis/myocarditis, and arteritis/periarteritis seen occasionally. Arteritis/periarteritis may be present in one or more small- to medium-sized arteries of one or many organs (Figure 20.4) (Dincer et al., 2018). The myocardial inflammation is rarely associated with myofiber degeneration or necrosis. Myocardial interstitial hemorrhage and mineralization are seen occasionally. Mesothelial hypertrophy and hyperplasia of the epicardium can be seen in older animals (over 6 months of age).

Kidneys

In general, the incidental lesions observed in the kidneys are minimal. The most common are focal interstitial infiltration of mononuclear cells, focal cytoplasmic basophilia of tubular epithelium, focal mineralization in the papilla (typically confined within tubules), tubular dilation or cysts, and vacuolation of the urothelial cytoplasm. Occasionally, a few glomeruli with glomerulosclerosis can be seen and are often located at the corticomedullary junction; special stains indicate that the increased matrix likely represents deposition of connective tissue rather than accumulation of immune complexes (McInnes and McKeag, 2016; Vezzali et al., 2011). Glomerulonephritis is rarely observed and may overlap with nephropathy or

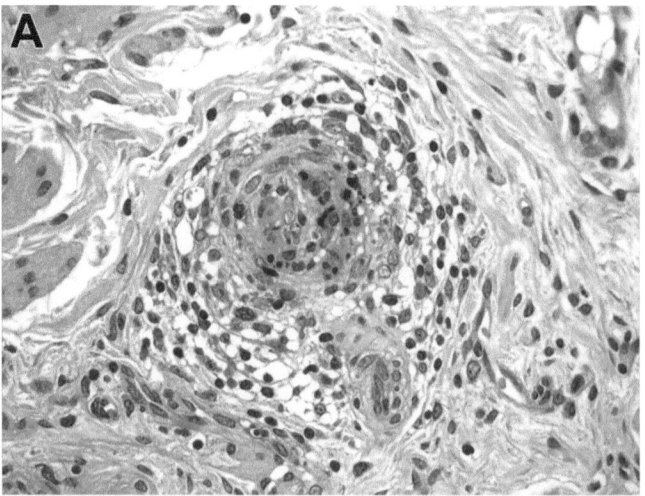

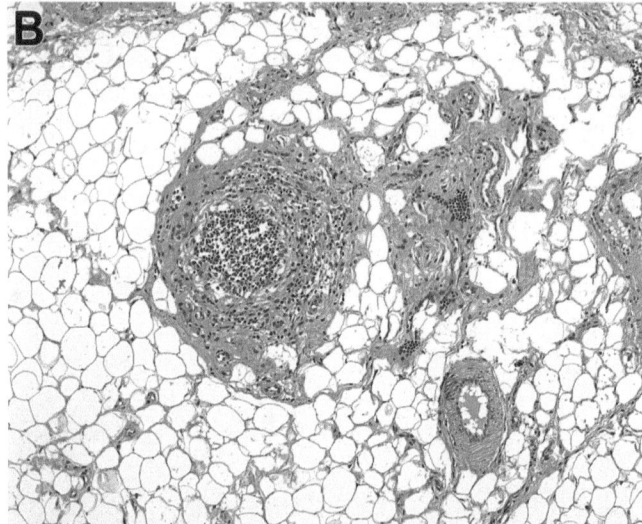

FIGURE 20.4 Vascular inflammation in Gottingen minipigs. (A) Spontaneous fibrinoid necrotic arteritis/periarteritis in the mesentery of a Göttingen minipig. There are inflammatory cell infiltrates within and surrounding the artery with necrosis and fibrin within the vessel wall. (B) Spontaneous chronic arteritis/periarteritis in the intestinal serosa of a Göttingen minipig. The arterial wall is thickened by accumulations of connective tissue and inflammatory cells. Hematoxylin and eosin. *Images used with permission from (Dincer et al., 2018). Figures 1 and 2.*

interstitial nephritis. The morphology of glomerulosclerosis covers a spectrum from acutely affected membranous to membranoproliferative glomerular changes to more chronic changes with fibrosis and adhesion of the glomerular tuft to the capsule. Glomerulonephritis may include a variable degree of nephropathy-like findings of tubular basophilia, hyaline casts, fibrosis, and interstitial/tubular accumulation of inflammatory cells (Figure 20.5). Glomerulonephritis or nephropathy may be seen in association with hemorrhagic syndrome of Göttingen minipigs.

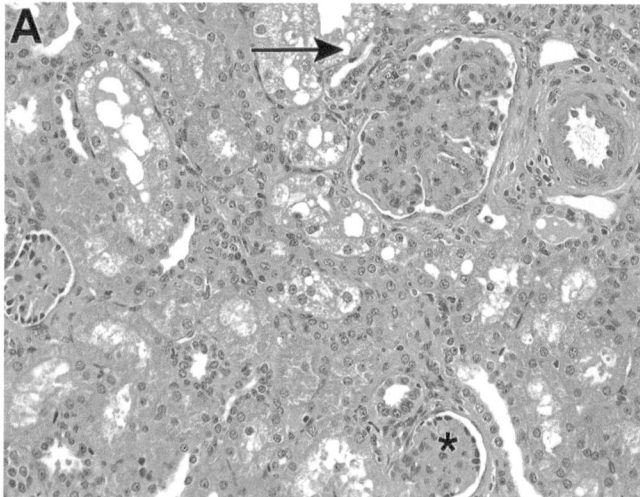

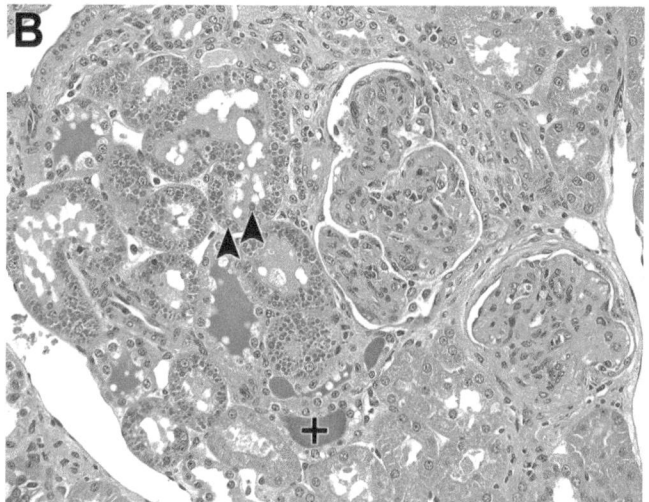

FIGURE 20.5 Kidney from a Göttingen minipig demonstrating various aspects of spontaneous glomerulonephritis. (A) Glomerulonephritis, glomerulosclerosis (*), as well as tubular vacuolation (arrow) are present. (B) Tubular intraluminal hyaline casts (+) and hyaline droplets (arrowheads) in the tubular epithelium are observed. Hematoxylin and eosin. *Figure adapted from Haschek and Rousseaux's:* Handbook of toxicologic pathology, *ed 3. In Haschek WM, Rousseaux CG, Wallig MA, editors: Academic Press, 2013, p 472. Figure 13.7, with permission.*

Liver and Gallbladder

Few spontaneous changes are found in the liver of minipigs. A characteristic normal histological feature is the marked amount of interlobular connective tissue in both conventional pigs and minipigs. The most common background changes observed include inflammatory cell infiltration and increased pigment within macrophages or Kupffer cells (Helke et al., 2016b). Minimal single-cell hepatocellular necrosis, which is often localized in the subcapsular area, and random, minimal interstitial infiltration with mononuclear cells may also be observed. Focal mild hypertrophy and marked vacuolation of hepatocytes are described rarely (Helke et al., 2016b).

Necrotizing cholecystitis of the gallbladder is a breed-specific and common lesion in the Göttingen minipig (Figure 20.6). This is a background finding observed at necropsy without clinical signs of gallbladder disease. The organ grossly appears to be decreased in size, has a thickened wall, and the contents may be inspissated. The microscopic examination most often reveals necrotic epithelium and submucosa, typically combined with regeneration, increased fibroblast numbers, and/or fibrosis in the submucosa and mineralization depending on the chronicity of the lesion. In chronic cases, the only lesion may be fibrosis with scant amounts of gallbladder mucosal epithelium remaining. Macrophages with brownish granulated cytoplasm can be observed in the submucosa/muscular layer or within the lumen. Hypoplasia/aplasia of the gall bladder, where the gallbladder is small or not apparent grossly, is occasionally observed in the Göttingen minipig. This may be a true developmental anomaly or, in some instances, may represent sequelae to chronic cholecystitis (described above).

Lung

The porcine lung is well demarcated by fibrous septae between and within lung lobes. Proper inflation of the lung allows for adequate examination of lung free from artifact. Göttingen minipigs have very few spontaneous changes. The most common changes are minimal focal accumulation of alveolar macrophages (some cell aggregates may surround small foci of mineralization), alveolar accumulation of mixed

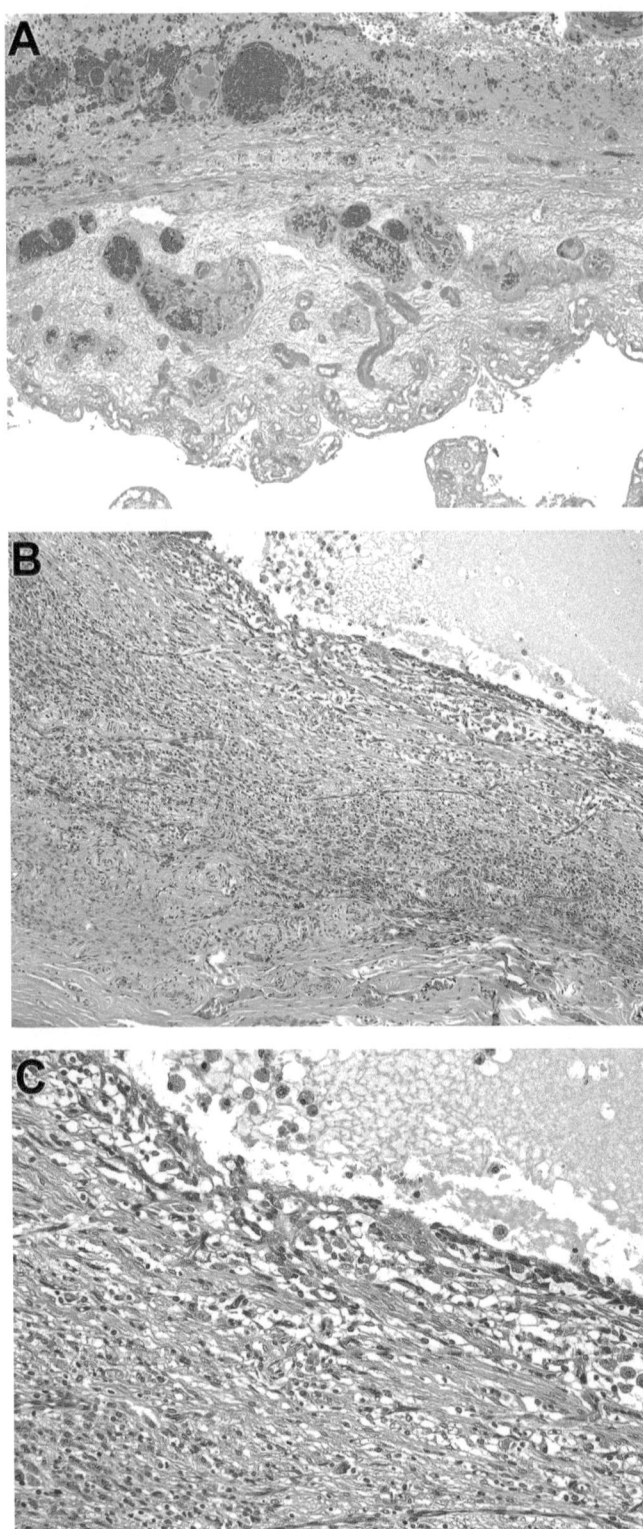

FIGURE 20.6 Gall bladder from Göttingen minipigs demonstrating acute and chronic cholecystitis, a clinically silent but pronounced finding in animals of this breed. (A) Acute hemorrhagic necrotizing cholecystitis showing marked necrosis of the mucosa/submucosa, hemorrhage, and congestion. (B) and (C) Chronic regenerating cholecystitis revealing macrophages with brownish granulated cytoplasm and clear regeneration of the epithelium and submucosa. Magnification: (A) and (B) 10× and (C) 20×. Hematoxylin and eosin. *Figure reproduced from Haschek and Rousseaux's: Handbook of toxicologic pathology, ed 3. In Haschek WM, Rousseaux CG, Wallig MA, editors: Academic Press, 2013, p 473. Figure 13.8, with permission.*

inflammatory cells, occasional granulomas, congestion and alveolar hemorrhage, and rarely focal pneumonia and adhesions (Helke et al., 2016b). Foreign material may be present in areas of inflammation and within granulomas as a result of the rooting behavior that is common in pigs. Conventional pigs used in research may have inflammatory lesions consistent with common infectious diseases such as *Mycoplasma* spp.

Eye

Posterior lenticular degeneration can occasionally be observed (Figure 20.7). Focal accumulation of inflammatory cells and focal inflammation in the cornea–scleral junction has also been described.

Ovary

Minipig reproductive maturation has been reported to occur as early as 3 months of age in the female, but full histological maturation of reproductive organs does not consistently occur until animals are 5–8 months of age (Howroyd et al., 2016). The overall reproductive maturity of the animal should be taken into consideration during evaluation of the ovary and reproductive tract.

Interstitial hemorrhage and hemorrhagic cysts have been described in the ovary of the Göttingen minipig. Polyovular follicles, with two or more oocytes per follicle, have been reported in some strains of minipig, as well as in conventional domestic swine, and are of higher incidence in younger animals (Stankiewicz et al., 2009). Mineralization of the ovaries in a multifocal pattern is a common incidental finding in the ovary. Paraovarian cysts, considered remnants of the mesonephric duct, are occasionally seen in the oviducts of minipigs, with other cystic structures associated with the ovaries or uterus also rarely observed. A putative teratoma of the ovary has been described, though no other neoplasms have been reported (Figure 20.8).

Skeletal Muscle

Commonly observed microscopic findings in skeletal muscle include degeneration or degeneration/regeneration of myofibers and inflammatory cell infiltrate. Focal to multifocal acute to chronic myositis is a well-known spontaneous change observed in a single, a few, or several

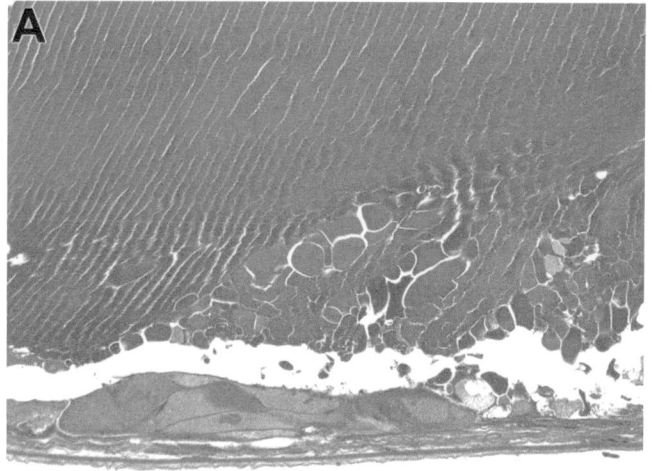

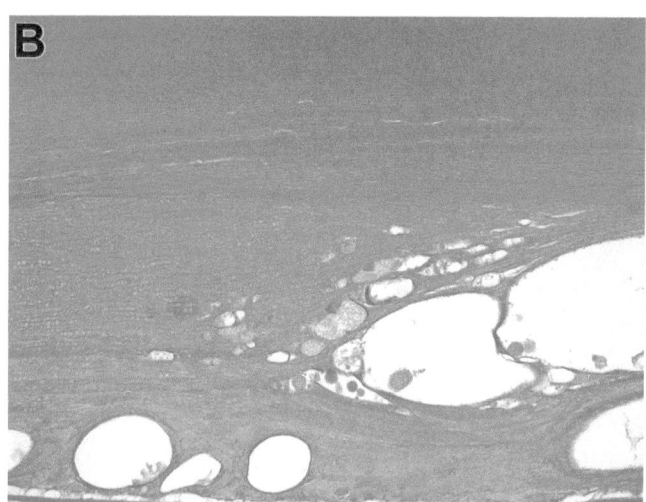

FIGURE 20.7 Eye from a Göttingen minipig demonstrating posterior lenticular degeneration with swollen and vacuolated lenticular fibers. Magnification: (A) 20×, (B) 40×. Hematoxylin and eosin. *Figure reproduced from Haschek and Rousseaux's:* Handbook of toxicologic pathology, *ed 3. In Haschek WM, Rousseaux CG, Wallig MA, editors: Academic Press, 2013, p 473. Figure 13.9, with permission.*

muscles. When observed at necropsy, the lesion is described as pale focus/foci. Microscopy often reveals both foci with acutely affected necrotic myofibers and chronic areas with mineralization and regeneration of myofibers.

Skin

The skin of healthy minipigs typically exhibits few background lesions which are typically focal and minimal. The more common findings include hyperkeratosis and epidermal hyperplasia. Crusts (i.e., collections of fibrin, keratin,

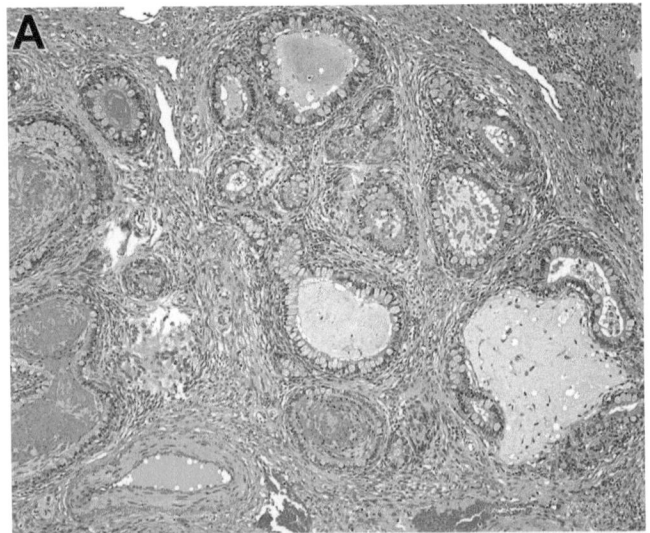

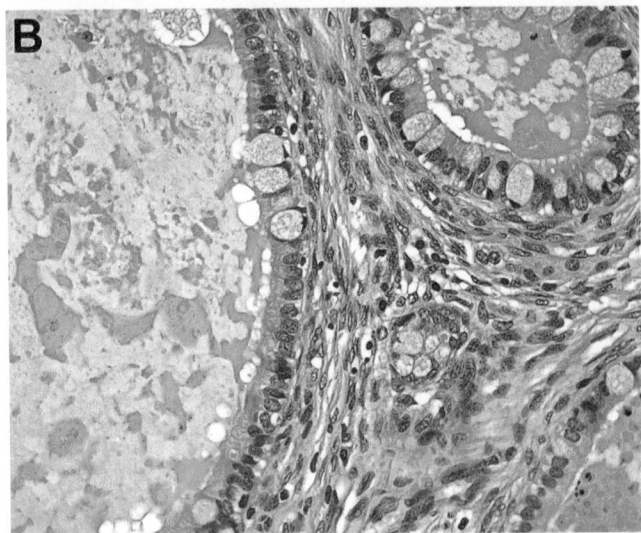

FIGURE 20.8 Ovary showing a putative teratoma from a Göttingen minipig. The ovary contained cystic spaces lined by ciliated epithelium and goblet cells with some containing hyaline material. Magnification: (A) 10×, (B) 40×. Hematoxylin and eosin. *Figure reproduced from Haschek and Rousseaux's:* Handbook of toxicologic pathology, *ed 3. In Haschek WM, Rousseaux CG, Wallig MA, editors: Academic Press, 2013, p 474. Figure 13.10, with permission.*

and degenerating neutrophils) correlating macroscopically with scabs and epidermal/subepidermal mixed inflammatory cells are occasionally seen, often in association with edema and folliculitis. Focal dermatitis is rarely observed. Folliculitis has been reported in association with highly viscous materials applied dermally.

Bone Marrow

One characteristic change seen in the bone marrow of the minipig is serous atrophy of the adipose tissue. This observation is most likely a physiological response to a normal degradation of adipose tissue under conditions where the minipig needs additional energy. Göttingen minipigs develop this change without being affected by disease or being in poor condition otherwise, as this observation is in most cases seen in apparently healthy minipigs. The morphologic appearance is varying degrees of adipocyte reduction combined with accumulation of intercellular eosinophilic material (Figure 20.9). This condition is reported widely in Europe but is extremely rare in the North American minipig stocks, perhaps suggesting variance in either the genetically isolated colonies of Gottingen minipigs on these continents or in husbandry practices (Helke et al., 2016b).

Stomach

In the gastric cardia, infiltration with neutrophils and minimal to slight erosions are occasionally observed in the nonglandular part of the stomach, with areas of separation of the

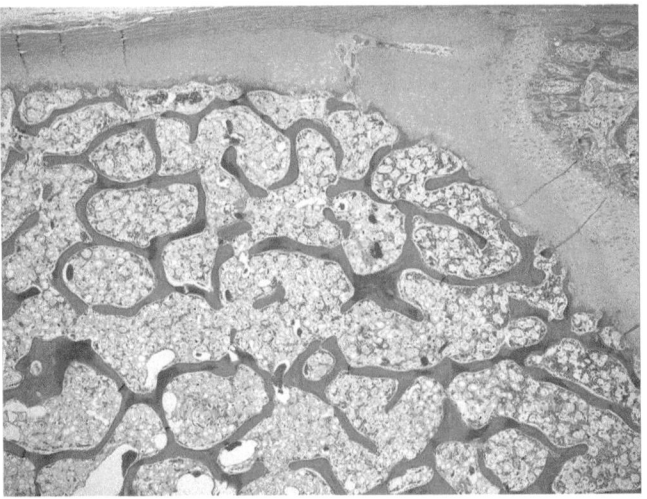

FIGURE 20.9 Bone marrow from a Göttingen minipig showing serous atrophy of adipocytes with reduction of adipocytes and accumulation of intercellular eosinophilic material. Hematoxylin and eosin. *Figure reproduced from Haschek and Rousseaux's:* Handbook of toxicologic pathology, *ed 3. In Haschek WM, Rousseaux CG, Wallig MA, editors: Academic Press, 2013, p 474. Figure 13.11, with permission.*

keratinized mucosa. In the fundic glandular region, the only common incidental finding is subepithelial hemorrhage. In the pyloric region, minimal to slight (occasionally moderate) mucosal erosions are observed from time to time, usually close to the duodenal papilla.

Testes and Epididymides

Minipig reproductive maturation has been reported to occur as early as 2 months of age in the male, but full histological maturation of the testes and other reproductive organs does not consistently occur until animals are 5–8 months of age. Evaluation of the testes and male reproductive tract should take into consideration the overall reproductive maturity of the animal, particularly in assigning pathological findings, as they may be normal for that particular stage of maturation. Additionally, if effects on reproductive organs are anticipated, use of males at the appropriate stage of development should be encouraged.

Tubular hypoplasia/atrophy (hypospermatogenesis) is a common (up to 70% incidence) spontaneous finding in the testes of Göttingen minipigs (Thuilliez et al., 2014) (Figure 20.10). This finding is characterized by variable numbers of tubules

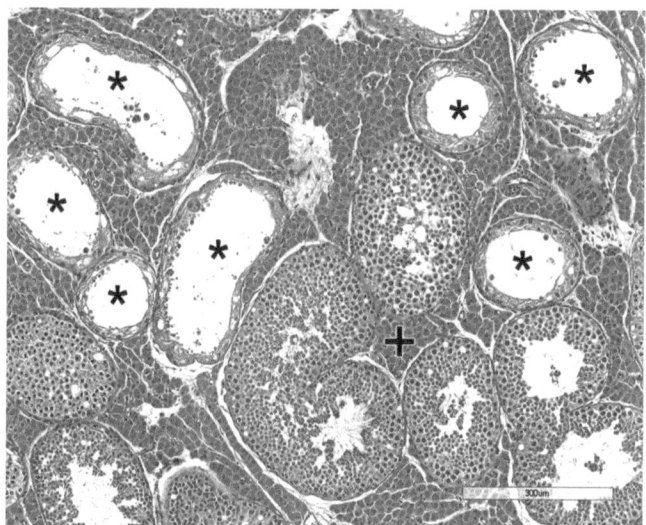

FIGURE 20.10 Testes with seminiferous tubular hypoplasia/atrophy in a minipig. Tubules contain decreased numbers of germ cells and lack maturation of spermatids (*). Most of the remaining tubules appear normal. Pigs have abundant Leydig cells which are prominent between seminiferous tubules (+). This is normal in the pig, but appears more prevalent with the decreased cells in some of the seminiferous tubules. Hematoxylin and eosin.

with vacuolated seminiferous epithelium and decreased spermatogonia, spermatocytes, and/or spermatids. Affected tubules may be scattered throughout the testis or in a focal area, with one or both testes affected. Based on the number of affected tubules, the change is normally graded as minimal to mild, but occasionally the severity is moderate to marked. Epididymal luminal sperm may be decreased in conjunction with this finding, with increased luminal round or multinucleated germ cells. Tubules immediately adjacent to the testicular rete may often be atrophied in appearance but are not considered to be part of this finding. The number and size of interstitial (Leydig) cells in the minipig testis normally exhibits great variability, which should be taken into consideration if Leydig cell hyperplasia is suspected. Age-matched control animals may have seemingly wide variance in the prominence and number of Leydig cells. Minimal arteritis/periarteritis (acute to chronic) can occasionally be observed in the tunica albuginea. In the epididymides, in addition to decreased luminal sperm and/or increased germ cell debris, epididymal cysts may be seen infrequently. Findings in other male reproductive organs are less frequent, but the prostate may have luminal mineralization or concretions as well as inflammatory cell infiltrates of the interstitium and glands, as might the seminal vesicles.

5.3. Neoplasia in Research Swine

There are several reports of tumors in pet minipigs (Ilha et al., 2010; Mozzachio et al., 2004). Many of the minipigs in use for research today have Vietnamese potbelly pigs in their lineage, and so these pet reports may be relevant. There are also reports of tumors in conventional swine which are also in the lineage of many minipigs. Lymphosarcoma, nephroblastoma, and melanoma are the most common tumors seen in young pigs (6-month-old conventional breeds). Other tumors include rhabdomyoma and nephroblastoma (Jagdale et al., 2019). An interstitial cell adenoma (Leydig cell) has been described in the testes, and interstitial cell tumors are reported in conventional and pot-bellied domestic swine, but no other reports of neoplasia in the male reproductive tract of the minipig have been made.

6. USE OF THE PIG AS A MODEL SYSTEM FOR MEDICAL DEVICES AND OF HUMAN DISEASES

6.1. Cardiovascular

The porcine heart is similar to the human heart as there are no anastomoses between vascular branches of the coronary circulation, and the hearts are of similar size. The vessel sizes of the porcine heart make the pig a good choice for modeling stents and cardiac devices such as pacemakers (Zuo et al., 2020). The heart valves of pigs are of similar size and number as humans and pigs are often used to evaluate bioprosthetics and have also been used in xenotransplantation.

Myocardial Infarction

The pig is also used for studies evaluating acute or chronic myocardial infarction due to the blood flow similarity to human. Pigs also are good models for hypertrophic cardiomyopathy (Schomberg et al., 2016).

Atherosclerosis

Pigs have a similar lipoprotein profile to that of humans and therefore represent a useful model of atherosclerosis. Pigs have low low-density lipoprotein and high high-density lipoprotein lipid profiles, but only develop mature atherosclerotic lesions on a high fat and cholesterol diet. The Rapacz pig has mutations in several apolipoprotein genes and develops spontaneous hypercholesterolemia more quickly than other models (Daugherty et al., 2017).

6.2. Skin

The similarity between the skin of humans and pigs makes the pig an ideal model for use in nonclinical dermal studies (Stricker-Krongrad et al., 2017). Features of swine skin that are similar to that of humans include sparse hair cover, a firm attachment to underlying structures, relatively thick epidermis, dermal to epidermal thickness ratios, similar dermal collagen and elastin content, formation of rete ridges, and variance in cutaneous pigment. Other species used for dermal toxicity testing do not have all of these features, particularly including dermal to epidermal thickness ratios,

sparse hair, and a firm dermal to subcutis to underlying muscle attachment. Additionally, pigs tolerate occlusive bandages well and have limited ability to manipulate, remove, or ingest material applied dorsally. There are some key differences between the pig and human skin, including a lack of eccrine sweat glands across much of the skin of pigs, decreased dermal and follicular vascularity, and variances in physiochemical response in vascular endothelium, but these are outweighed by the similarities.

Wound Healing Studies

For wound healing studies, the pig, with its human-like cutaneous anatomy and physiology, is a much better model than all other animal species. In the pig, as opposed to other species such as the rat, the wound healing process consists of the same phases that occur in humans (e.g., inflammation, contraction, proliferation, reepithelialization, and remodeling) (Seaton et al., 2015). Furthermore, wound contraction occurs quite differently in species in which the skin is firmly attached to the underlying structures, such as humans and pigs, compared with species like rats, rabbits, dogs, and NHPs whose skin has decreased attachment to underlying tissue. Finally, the overall size of the pig facilitates the use of reduced numbers of animals compared with most other species, as multiple test sites are possible on each individual.

In wound healing studies, the wounds are generally established on the back of the animal, for the same reasons as previously stated for dermal toxicity studies. Furthermore, this area is supported by the vertebrae and the ribs, with limited skin tension, thereby reducing the potential interference of skin mobility with wound contraction. Depending on the size of the animals at the start of a study, up to eight wounds can be made on each pig. Full-thickness wounds involve removal of epidermis, dermis, and some subcutaneous tissue, whereas only part of the epidermis is removed in split-thickness wounds. One method of making full-thickness wounds, which heal by granulation and reepithelialization with underlying scar tissue formation, is to make a circular defect. The circular shape provides the most uniform wound contraction, which reduces the variation in healing seen with full-thickness wounds of other shapes. The split-thickness wounds heal by reepithelialization with no contraction or scarring. Other wound types include a full-thickness incisional wound, which may be used for wound closure or hemostatic evaluations, or burn wounds, though these are both less common than the excisional wound models.

Following their creation, the wounds are treated with the test article (e.g., creams, gels, ointments, or dressings) and further covered by a secondary dressing to preclude detachment of the treatment. During the wound healing phase, the wounds and surrounding skin are subjected to detailed macroscopic evaluation, including planimetric recordings (i.e., area measurements of the various tissue types present based on software analysis of drawings or photographs of each wound). Terminal observations may include gross examination of all organs and a detailed microscopic evaluation of tissues sampled. All wounds are evaluated microscopically, with or without the use of special stains such as Masson's trichrome to assess the extent of collagen deposition or von Willebrand's Factor, vascular endothelial growth factor, or CD31 stains for evaluation of angiogenesis. Additional evaluations may also be included as needed, such as indirect measurement of the amount of newly formed collagen within the repaired tissue by analysis of 4-hydroxyproline concentration in the homogenized tissue from the wound site or mRNA analysis of relevant healing factors from frozen tissue from the wound site (Holt et al., 2013).

Pigs have been shown to be good models for skin flap studies, skin transplant studies, and are also being used for studies of reconstructive surgery (Etra et al., 2019; Kerrigan et al., 1986). Beyond the skin similarities, there are similarities in cranio-maxillary bone and attachments which make pigs a relevant model for face transplants as well (Al-Rakan et al., 2014). Pigs are commonly used in studies evaluating allergic contact dermatitis (Stricker-Krongrad et al., 2016).

6.3. Renal

The porcine kidney is more similar to the human kidney than most other species, including many NHPs. The pig has a true multireniculate and multipapillate kidney as does the human. It has a similar size, physiology, and development to humans, and is commonly used for both vascular and transplant studies.

The vascular size of swine renal arteries is advantageous as they are similar in diameter to those of many human vessels and can thus be used to model coils and other vascular devices. The vasculature of the porcine kidney branches into cranial, middle, and caudal renal arteries, and up to four of these can be occluded in a study with no ill effects on the animal, allowing multiple products or designs to be tested in one animal.

6.4. Metabolic Syndrome/Diabetes

Ossabaw, Yucatan, and Göttingen minipigs are all susceptible to diet-induced obesity and are appropriate models for studying metabolism and metabolic syndrome (Zhang and Lerman, 2016). They all develop dyslipidemia, hypertension, but do not have an overt diabetic phenotype. Diabetes can be induced via partial or total pancreatectomy, with beta cell toxins, dietary interventions, or genetic engineering (Renner et al., 2020).

6.5. Eye

Similarities in ocular anatomy between Gottingen minipigs and humans have been described (Shrader and Greentree, 2018). Reasons for the use of minipigs in ocular research include similarity in the size of globes and vitreal volume/composition (Shrader and Mowry, 2019). Pigs lack a macula but have an area centralis and visual streak and concentrated cone photoreceptor areas that confer high visual acuity.

6.6. Brain

The porcine brain is gyrencephalic and the distribution of white matter and gray matter, the ratio of white to gray matter, and the changes during development most closely mimic the human (Conrad et al., 2012). Due to the similarities in the structure of the brain, pigs are a good model for stroke, but creating the model requires direct access to the vessels as the rete mirabile (or intercarotid plexus) of the internal carotid prevents access to specific vessels commonly occluded in stroke models (Nanda, 1975). Pigs are more frequently being used for cognitive testing.

6.7. Immune System

The composition of the leukocyte fraction as determined by white blood cell types (e.g., percent lymphocytes, neutrophils, etc.) in the circulation of pigs is more similar to humans than that of NHPs or mice (Rubic-Schneider et al., 2016). There are fewer differences immunologically between the pig and human versus other species, and mucosa associated lymphoid tissue is more similar to humans than other species (Descotes et al., 2018; Schomberg et al., 2016). The pig has similar reactions to septic shock and lipopolysaccharide as do humans.

6.8. Cancer

Melanoma models have been developed in swine on three different minipig backgrounds (e.g., the Sinclair pig, Munich miniature Troll, and the Melanoma Libechov minipig) (Horak et al., 2019). Genetically engineered pigs are also being developed to study different types of cancer. So far, models for breast cancer, colorectal cancer, pancreatic cancer, and osteosarcoma have been developed using transgene methodologies (Kalla et al., 2020).

6.9. Genetically Modified Pigs

The past 2 decades have seen the advancement of gene target methodologies which are effective in the pig, as well as the porcine genome (Groenen et al., 2012). Somatic cell nuclear transfer, Adeno-associated virus targeting vectors, bacterial artificial chromosomes, zinc finger nucleases, Transcription activator-like effector nucleases, and the CRISPR/Cas systems have all been used successfully for gene modification in the pig (Klymiuk et al., 2016). These strategies have led to porcine models of Duchenne muscular dystrophy, and cystic fibrosis. These technologies are also being used to create pigs with only human vessels, making xenotransplants closer to reality (Das et al., 2020).

7. REGULATORY ASPECTS

For nonclinical safety studies, relevant guideline requirements should be consulted prior to study design and initiation. ICH M3 (R2) —

Guideline on Nonclinical Safety Studies for the Conduct of Human Clinical Trials and Marketing Authorization for Pharmaceuticals—is of major importance in relation to development of small molecules. For biotechnology-derived substances, ICH S6 (R1)—Non-clinical Safety Evaluation of Biotechnology-Derived Pharmaceuticals—should be consulted (US Food and Drug Administration, 2011; U.S. Department of Health and Human Services, 2010). Guidance for the specific study designs can be gained from relevant Organisation for Economic Co-operation and Development guidelines (Organization for Economic Cooperation and Development OECD, 2020). In general, these guidelines do not deal with specific aspects of minipig use as test subjects, but they do give broad recommendations for inclusion of nonrodent species. These remarks are readily extrapolated to studies with swine.

For safety testing of medical devices, requirements given by the International Organization for Standardization (ISO) in ISO 10993 should be carefully considered when designing these studies (International Organisation for Standardization ISO, 2018). In this respect, the use of the minipig may also be relevant, especially for subacute/subchronic toxicity testing of wound care products, using a porcine wound healing model. Another relevant guidance document is the guidance for developing products for treatment of chronic cutaneous ulcer and burn wounds, issued by the U.S. Food and Drug Administration in 2006 (U. S. Department of Health and Human Services et al., 2006). This rule is aimed for development of drugs, biological treatments and devices, and also includes nonclinical considerations. Porcine studies are specifically mentioned in this guidance as valid nonclinical models for testing products to promote skin repair.

While proof-of-concept studies do not need to be conducted in compliance with GLP, nonclinical studies required for marketing drugs and studies aimed to support product safety and efficacy for clinical trial initiation must be in compliance. This requirement applies to studies undertaken with minipigs.

The suitability of minipigs as models in regulatory toxicity testing and their use as it contributes to replacement, refinement, and reduction of animal testing have been analyzed extensively by the RETHINK project (Forster et al., 2010b).

Briefly, close similarity to humans with regards to anatomy, physiology, and biochemistry, especially with regards to the cardiovascular, integumentary, and digestive systems, provides the scientific justification for their use. From a practical standpoint, the small size of minipigs, some strains more than others, their adaptability to laboratory housing, and ease of handling and dosing makes the minipig a suitable model for nonclinical safety assessment. A growing number of reagents and biomarkers are available which broaden the utility of minipigs beyond their well-established use in dermal toxicity testing (Heining and Ruysschaert, 2016). Indeed, considering that the porcine immune system resembles humans for more than 80% of analyzed parameters, minipigs are a preferred animal model even for the nonclinical safety assessment of immune-modulating compounds (Pabst, 2020).

8. ETHICS AND ANIMAL WELFARE

Pigs and minipigs are highly intelligent animals and should be housed in an enriched environment. An adequate floor area should be provided, taking the size of the animals into consideration; national legislative housing requirements should always be consulted for this purpose. Whereas female minipigs can be group housed, this is normally not possible for noncastrated male minipigs after sexual maturity due to aggressiveness toward other males. For some study types (e.g., dermal studies and continuous infusion studies), group housing will not be possible as the animals are bandaged or wear equipment which potentially can be damaged by pen-mates. However, visual, auditory, and olfactory contact can still be maintained by keeping animals together in a single room and should be made a priority.

Materials placed in the pen can also provide additional enrichment. Absorbent bedding material (e.g., sawdust) may be offered in order to provide a clean and dry environment as well as to provide some protection to delicate body surfaces from flooring-induced abrasions. In addition, hay can be provided, not only as a dietary supplement but also as an excellent enrichment tool, as the animals enjoy chewing it, moving it, and using it for nest building. Various plastic toys may be provided, but in most cases, the animals will lose interest within a short period of time. Therefore, if implemented, it is important to switch to new toys frequently. Finally, for cognitive enrichment, the animals may be trained (by use of positive reinforcement) for different study-related procedures, such as weighing and placement in slings during ophthalmoscopy and electrocardiographic recordings. Pigs and minipigs are easy learners and will be stimulated when challenged to learn new things. The contact with humans will also be strengthened during the training sessions.

Analgesics must always be used during the postoperative period if surgery is required (as is the case when implanting catheters for continuous infusion studies). A pain management program should be individually based, which makes frequent and detailed observations of each animal very important. Clinical signs, such as reduced food consumption, aggressiveness, vocalization, and reluctance to move, may be indicators of inadequate pain treatment and corrective actions must be taken immediately. As surgery in relation to experimental procedures is a planned process, treatment with analgesics should always be started prior to surgery (preemptively), resulting in less activation of the pain sensory system. The body temperature is in most cases decreased with anesthesia, and, therefore, it is important to use heating pads or other method of warming (e.g., Bair Hugger) during surgery and to provide a warm recovery area after surgery.

9. SUMMARY

Overall, the pig recapitulates much human anatomy and is useful in developing devices and procedures to be used in humans. Porcine skin is more similar to human skin than other animals used in biomedical research. There are many similarities in xenobiotic metabolism, but there are also deficiencies in the pig. Knowledge of these similarities and differences will aid in selection of the most appropriate model for the study.

REFERENCES

Al-Rakan M, Shores JT, Bonawitz S, et al.: Ancillary procedures necessary for translational research in experimental craniomaxillofacial surgery, *J Craniofac Surg* 25:2043–2050, 2014.

Albl B, Haesner S, Braun-Reichhart C, et al.: Tissue sampling guides for porcine biomedical models, *Toxicol Pathol* 44:414–420, 2016.

Andrade EL, Bento AF, Cavalli J, et al.: Non-clinical studies required for new drug development - Part I: early in silico and in vitro studies, new target discovery and validation, proof of principles and robustness of animal studies, *Braz J Med Biol Res* 49:e5644, 2016.

Barka N, Rakow N, Lentz L, et al.: Surgical approaches to vascular access for large-caliber devices in preclinical research models, *J Am Assoc Lab Anim Sci* 49:472–474, 2010.

Beal K, Helke KL, Navratil N, et al.: Serum ADAMTS13 levels in Göttingen minipigs with thrombotic thrombocytopenia purpura are not different than their unaffected parents. In *Society of toxicologic pathology annual symposium: environmental toxicologic pathology and one health, Raleigh, NC*, 2019.

Bouchard GF, Brown LD, Liu J, et al.: *Miniature swine book of normal data 2019*, 2019, Sinclair Bio Resources, LLC and Sinclair Research, LLC. https://www2.sinclairresearch.com/bon.

Carrasco L, Madsen LW, Salguero FJ, et al.: Immune complex-associated thrombocytopenic purpura syndrome in sexually mature Gottingen minipigs, *J Comp Pathol* 128:25–32, 2003.

Conrad MS, Dilger RN, Johnson RW: Brain growth of the domestic pig (*Sus scrofa*) from 2 to 24 weeks of age: a longitudinal MRI study, *Dev Neurosci* 34:291–298, 2012.

Dalgaard L: Comparison of minipig, dog, monkey and human drug metabolism and disposition, *J Pharmacol Toxicol Methods* 74:80–92, 2015.

Das S, Koyano-Nakagawa N, Gafni O, et al.: Generation of human endothelium in pig embryos deficient in ETV2, *Nat Biotechnol* 38:297–302, 2020.

Daugherty A, Tall AR, Daemen M, et al.: Recommendation on design, execution, and reporting of animal atherosclerosis studies: a scientific statement from the American Heart Association, *Arterioscler Thromb Vasc Biol* 37:e131–e157, 2017.

Descotes J, Allais L, Ancian P, et al.: Nonclinical evaluation of immunological safety in Gottingen minipigs: the CONFIRM initiative, *Regul Toxicol Pharmacol* 94:271–275, 2018.

Dijkhorst M, Stolte S, Meijer F: What is known about the dippity pig syndrome? *Tijdschr Diergeneeskd* 143:28, 2018.

Dincer Z, Piccicuto V, Walker UJ, et al.: Spontaneous and drug-induced arteritis/polyarteritis in the Gottingen minipig-review, *Toxicol Pathol* 46:121–130, 2018.

Ellegaard Göttingen Minipigs. Available from: https://minipigs.dk/fileadmin/_migrated/content_uploads/Growth_Data.pdf. (Accessed 1 August 2020).

Etra JW, Grzelak MJ, Fidder SAJ, et al.: A skin rejection grading system for vascularized composite allotransplantation in a preclinical large animal model, *Transplantation* 103:1385–1391, 2019.

European Medicines Agency: *Scientific guidelines: paediatrics*, 1995–2020, EMA.

Feyen B, Penard L, van Heerden M, et al.: "All pigs are equal" does the background data from juvenile Gottingen minipigs support this? *Reprod Toxicol* 64:105–115, 2016.

Forster R, Bode G, Ellegaard L, et al.: The RETHINK project on minipigs in the toxicity testing of new medicines and chemicals: conclusions and recommendations, *J Pharmacol Toxicol Methods* 62:236–242, 2010a.

Forster R, Bode G, Ellegaard L, et al.: The RETHINK project-minipigs as models for the toxicity testing of new medicines and chemicals: an impact assessment, *J Pharmacol Toxicol Methods* 62:158–159, 2010b.

Gillberg M, Skaanild MT, Friis C: Regulation of gender-dependent CYP2A expression in pigs: involvement of androgens and CAR, *Basic Clin Pharmacol Toxicol* 98:480–487, 2006.

Groenen MA, Archibald AL, Uenishi H, et al.: Analyses of pig genomes provide insight into porcine demography and evolution, *Nature* 491:393–398, 2012.

Gutierrez K, Dicks N, Glanzner WG, et al.: Efficacy of the porcine species in biomedical research, *Front Genet* 6:293, 2015.

Heining P, Ruysschaert T: The use of minipig in drug discovery and development: pros and cons of minipig selection and strategies to use as a preferred nonrodent species, *Toxicol Pathol* 44:467–473, 2016.

Helke KL: Necropsy on research swine. In Swindle MM, Smith AC, editors: *Swine in the laboratory: surgery, anesthesia, imaging, and experimental techniques*, Boca Raton, 2015, CRC Press, pp 489–521.

Helke KL, Nelson KN, Sargeant AM, et al.: Background pathological changes in minipigs: a comparison of the incidence and nature among different breeds and populations of minipigs, *Toxicol Pathol* 44:325–337, 2016a.

Helke KL, Nelson KN, Sargeant AM, et al.: Pigs in toxicology: breed differences in metabolism and background findings, *Toxicol Pathol* 44:575–590, 2016b.

Helke KL, Wolfe AM, Smith AC, et al.: Mulberry heart disease and hepatosis dietetica in farm pigs (*Sus scrofa* domesticus) in a research setting, *Comp Med* 70(4):376–383, 2020.

Henze LJ, Koehl NJ, O'Shea JP, et al.: The pig as a preclinical model for predicting oral bioavailability and in vivo performance of pharmaceutical oral dosage forms: a PEARRL review, *J Pharm Pharmacol* 71:581–602, 2019.

Holt BM, Betz DH, Ford TA, et al.: Pig dorsum model for examining impaired wound healing at the skin-implant interface of percutaneous devices, *J Mater Sci Mater Med* 24:2181–2193, 2013.

Hood RD: *Developmental and reproductive toxicology: a practical approach*, 3rd, London, 2012, Informa Healthcare.

Horak V, Palanova A, Cizkova J, et al.: Melanoma-bearing Libechov minipig (MeLiM): the unique swine model of hereditary metastatic melanoma, *Genes* 10, 2019.

Howroyd PC, Peter B, de Rijk E: Review of sexual maturity in the minipig, *Toxicol Pathol* 44:607–611, 2016.

Ilha MR, Newman SJ, van Amstel S, et al.: Uterine lesions in 32 female miniature pet pigs, *Vet Pathol* 47:1071–1075, 2010.

International Organisation for Standardization (ISO): *Biological evaluation of medical devices*, 2018, ISO.

Jagdale A, Iwase H, Klein EC, et al.: Incidence of neoplasia in pigs and its relevance to clinical organ xenotransplantation, *Comp Med* 69:86–94, 2019.

Jeppesen G, Skydsgaard M: Spontaneous background pathology in Gottingen minipigs, *Toxicol Pathol* 43:257–266, 2015.

Kalla D, Kind A, Schnieke A: Genetically engineered pigs to study cancer, *Int J Mol Sci* 21, 2020.

Kangawa A, Nishimura T, Nishimura T, et al.: Spontaneous age-related histopathological changes in microminipigs, *Toxicol Pathol* 47:817–832, 2019.

Kararli TT: Comparison of the gastrointestinal anatomy, physiology, and biochemistry of humans and commonly used laboratory animals, *Biopharm Drug Dispos* 16:351–380, 1995.

Kerrigan CL, Zelt RG, Thomson JG, et al.: The pig as an experimental animal in plastic surgery research for the study of skin flaps, myocutaneous flaps and fasciocutaneous flaps, *Lab Anim Sci* 36:408–412, 1986.

Khiao In M, Richardson KC, Loewa A, et al.: Histological and functional comparisons of four anatomical regions of porcine skin with human abdominal skin, *Anat Histol Embryol* 48:207–217, 2019.

Kim NN, Parker RM, Weinbauer GF, et al.: Points to consider in designing and conducting juvenile toxicology studies, *Int J Toxicol* 36:325–339, 2017.

Klymiuk N, Seeliger F, Bohlooly YM, et al.: Tailored pig models for preclinical efficacy and safety testing of targeted therapies, *Toxicol Pathol* 44:346–357, 2016.

Kojima M, Degawa M: Sex differences in constitutive mRNA levels of CYP2B22, CYP2C33, CYP2C49, CYP3A22, CYP3A29 and CYP3A46 in the pig liver: comparison between Meishan and Landrace pigs, *Drug Metab Pharmacokinet* 31:185–192, 2016.

Lu T, Yang B, Wang R, et al.: Xenotransplantation: current status in preclinical research, *Front Immunol* 10:3060, 2019.

Manji RA, Lee W, Cooper DKC: Xenograft bioprosthetic heart valves: past, present and future, *Int J Surg* 23:280–284, 2015.

Maratea KA, Snyder PW, Stevenson GW: Vascular lesions in nine Gottingen minipigs with thrombocytopenic purpura syndrome, *Vet Pathol* 43:447–454, 2006.

Markert M, Trautmann T, Krause F, et al.: A new telemetry-based system for assessing cardiovascular function in group-housed large animals. Taking the 3Rs to a new level with the evaluation of remote measurement via cloud data transmission, *J Pharmacol Toxicol Methods* 93:90–97, 2018.

McAnulty PA, Dayan PA, Ganderup N-C, et al.: *The minipig in biomedical research*, Boca Raton, 2012, CRC Press/Taylor & Francis.

McInnes EF, McKeag S: A brief review of infrequent spontaneous findings, peculiar anatomical microscopic features, and potential artifacts in Gottingen minipigs, *Toxicol Pathol* 44:338–345, 2016.

Midwest Research Swine. Available from: https://midwestresearchswine.com/herd-health/growth-rate-chart/. (Accessed 1 August 2020).

Monteiro-Riviere NA, Stromberg MW: Ultrastructure of the integument of the domestic pig (*Sus scrofa*) from one through fourteen weeks of age, *Anat Histol Embryol* 14:97–115, 1985.

Mozzachio K, Linder K, Dixon D: Uterine smooth muscle tumors in potbellied pigs (*Sus scrofa*) resemble human fibroids: a potential animal model, *Toxicol Pathol* 32:402–407, 2004.

Nanda BS: Blood supply to the brain. In Sisson S, Grossman JD, Getty R, editors: *Sisson and Grossman's the anatomy of the domestic animals*, Philadelphia, 1975, Saunders, pp 1315–1320.

National Research Council: *Guide for the Care and Use of laboratory animals*, Washington (DC), 2011, National Academies Press (US), National Academy of Sciences.

Niu D, Wei HJ, Lin L, et al.: Inactivation of porcine endogenous retrovirus in pigs using CRISPR-Cas9, *Science* 357:1303–1307, 2017.

Organization for Economic Cooperation and Development (OECD). *OECD guidelines for the testing of chemicals, section 4*, 2020, OECD.

Pabst R: The pig as a model for immunology research, *Cell Tissue Res* 380:287–304, 2020.

Puccinelli E, Gervasi PG, Longo V: Xenobiotic metabolizing cytochrome P450 in pig, a promising animal model, *Curr Drug Metab* 12:507–525, 2011.

Puccinelli E, Gervasi PG, Pelosi G, et al.: Modulation of cytochrome P450 enzymes in response to continuous or intermittent high-fat diet in pigs, *Xenobiotica* 43:686–698, 2013.

Ramot Y, Obaya A, McNamara A, et al.: Cutaneous candidiasis in a Gottingen minipig: a potential pitfall in preclinical studies, *Toxicol Pathol* 45:1032–1034, 2017.

Rasmussen MK, Scavenius C, Gerbal-Chaloin S, et al.: Sex dictates the constitutive expression of hepatic cytochrome P450 isoforms in Gottingen minipigs, *Toxicol Lett* 314:181–186, 2019.

Renner S, Blutke A, Clauss S, et al.: Porcine models for studying complications and organ crosstalk in diabetes mellitus, *Cell Tissue Res* 380:341–378, 2020.

Rubic-Schneider T, Christen B, Brees D, et al.: Minipigs in translational immunosafety sciences: a perspective, *Toxicol Pathol* 44:315–324, 2016.

Schomberg DT, Tellez A, Meudt JJ, et al.: Miniature swine for preclinical modeling of complexities of human disease for translational scientific discovery and accelerated development of therapies and medical devices, *Toxicol Pathol* 44:299–314, 2016.

Seaton M, Hocking A, Gibran NS: Porcine models of cutaneous wound healing, *ILAR J* 56:127–138, 2015.

Shrader SM, Greentree WF: Gottingen minipigs in ocular research, *Toxicol Pathol* 46:403–407, 2018.

Shrader SM, Mowry RN: Histomorphometric evaluation of the Gottingen minipig eye, *Vet Ophthalmol* 22:872–878, 2019.

Skaanild MT: Porcine cytochrome P450 and metabolism, *Curr Pharm Des* 12:1421–1427, 2006.

Skaanild MT, Friis C: Cytochrome P450 sex differences in minipigs and conventional pigs, *Pharmacol Toxicol* 85:174–180, 1999.

Skydsgaard M, Dincer Z, Haschek-Hock WM, Helke K, Jacob B, Jacobsen B, Kato A, et al.: International Harmonization of Nomenclature and Diagnostic Criteria (INHAND): Nonproliferative and proliferative lesions of the minipig. *Toxicol Pathol.* 49(1):110–228, 2021, https://doi.org/10.1177/0192623320975373.

Stankiewicz T, Blaszczyk B, Udala J: A study on the occurrence of polyovular follicles in porcine ovaries with particular reference to intrafollicular hormone concentrations, quality of oocytes and their in vitro fertilization, *Anat Histol Embryol* 38:233–239, 2009.

Stricker-Krongrad A, Shoemake CR, Liu J, et al.: The importance of minipigs in dermal safety assessment: an overview, *Cutan Ocul Toxicol* 36:105–113, 2017.

Stricker-Krongrad A, Shoemake CR, Pereira ME, et al.: Miniature swine breeds in toxicology and drug safety assessments: what to expect during clinical and pathology evaluations, *Toxicol Pathol* 44:421–427, 2016.

Swindle MM, Makin A, Herron AJ, et al.: Swine as models in biomedical research and toxicology testing, *Vet Pathol* 49:344–356, 2012.

Swindle MM, Smith AC: *Swine in the laboratory : surgery, anesthesia, imaging, and experimental techniques*, 3rd, Boca Raton, 2016, CRC Press.

Sykes M, Sachs DH: Transplanting organs from pigs to humans, *Sci Immunol* 4, 2019.

Tynes V: Common dermatologic conditions in Vietnamese potbellied pigs - Part I: dry skin, mange, and dippity pig syndrome, *Exotic Pet Pract* 1:1–2, 1996.

Thuilliez C, Tortereau A, Perron-Lepage MF, et al.: Spontaneous testicular tubular hypoplasia/atrophy in the Gottingen minipig: a retrospective study, *Toxicol Pathol* 42:1024–1031, 2014.

U. S. Department of Health and Human Services Food and Drug Administration Center for Drug Evaluaion and Research (CDER), Center for Biologics Evaluation and Research (CBER), Center for Devices and Radiological Health (CDRH), et al.: *Guidance for industry: chronic cutaneous ulcer and burn wounds - developing products for treatment*, 2006.

U.S. Department of Health and Human Services, Food and Drug Administration Center for Drug Evaluation and Research (CDER). In US DHHS, FDA, (CDER), et al., editors: *Guidance for Industry: Nonclinical safety evaluation of pediatric drug products*, Silver Spring, MD, 2010, U.S. Department of Health and Human Services.

USDA: housing, care and welfare. 2020. Available from: https://www.nal.usda.gov/awic/housing-care-and-welfare.

US Food and Drug Administration: *ICH S6(R1) preclinical safety evaluation of biotechnology-derived pharmaceuticals*, 2011, US DHHS.

Vezzali E, Manno RA, Salerno D, et al.: Spontaneous glomerulonephritis in Gottingen minipigs, *Toxicol Pathol* 39:700–705, 2011.

Willard-Mack C, Ramani T, Auletta C: Dermatotoxicology: safety evaluation of topical products in minipigs: study designs and practical considerations, *Toxicol Pathol* 44:382–390, 2016.

Zhang X, Lerman LO: Investigating the metabolic syndrome: contributions of swine models, *Toxicol Pathol* 44:358–366, 2016.

Ziegler A, Gonzalez L, Blikslager A: Large animal models: the key to translational discovery in digestive disease research, *Cell Mol Gastroenterol Hepatol* 2:716–724, 2016.

Zimmerman JJ: *Diseases of swine*, 10th, Chichester, West Sussex, 2012, Wiley-Blackwell.

Zuo K, Koh LB, Charles CJ, et al.: Measurement of the luminal diameter of peripheral arterial vasculature in Yorkshire×Landrace swine by using ultrasonography and angiography, *J Am Assoc Lab Anim Sci* 59(4):438–444, 2020.

C H A P T E R

21

Animal Models in Toxicologic Research: Nonhuman Primate

Jennifer A. Chilton[1], Steven T. Laing[2], Alys Bradley[3]

[1]Charles River Safety Assessment, Reno, NV, United States, [2]Genentech Safety Assessment, South San Francisco, CA, United States, [3]Charles River Laboratories Edinburgh Ltd., Tranent, Scotland, United Kingdom

O U T L I N E

1. Introduction 777

2. History and Biological Characteristics of Nonhuman Primates 778
    2.1. The Cynomolgus Macaque (Macaca fascicularis) 778
    2.2. The Rhesus Macaque (Macaca mulatta) 778
    2.3. The Common Marmoset (Callithrix jacchus) 780
    2.4. The Baboon (Papio sp.) 780
    2.5. The Squirrel Monkey (Saimiri sp.) 781
    2.6. The Tamarins (Saguinus sp.) 781
    2.7. The Vervet and Green Monkeys (Chlorocebus aethiops ssp. sabaeus and pygerythrus) 781
    2.8. The Capuchin Monkey (Cebus sp.) 781

3. Selection of Nonhuman Primates for Toxicologic Research and Study Design Considerations 782
    3.1. Ethics and Welfare Considerations 782
    3.2. Regulatory Considerations 783
    3.3. Source, Origin, and Genetic Variation 784
    3.4. Relevance and Feasibility for Use in Drug Development 785

3.5. Study Design 786

4. Predictivity of Nonhuman Primate Toxicity Data to Humans 787

5. Nonhuman Primate Models in Biomedical Research 787
    5.1. Nonhuman Primate Models of Human Disease 788
    5.2. Models in Pharmacology and Toxicology Research 790

6. Background Findings in Nonhuman Primates and Use of Historical Control Data 796
    6.1. Incidental Findings in Nonhuman Primates 796
    6.2. Environmental, Endemic, and Contagious Pathogens 797
    6.3. Findings due to Antidrug Antibodies 798
    6.4. Historical Control Data 800

7. Conclusion 801

References 801

1. INTRODUCTION

At the time of writing this chapter, the Coronavirus (COVID-19/SARS CoV-2) pandemic of 2020 was in full progress without vaccines or viable treatments available to the public. Meanwhile, multiple research and toxicology studies involving nonhuman primates (NHPs) were already underway in the race to fill this unmet medical need. This situation emphasized use of the NHP as an essential element to the advancement of human medicine. NHPs are essential

Haschek and Rousseaux's Handbook of Toxicologic Pathology, Fourth Edition.
https://doi.org/10.1016/B978-0-12-821044-4.00014-5

components of the current development of human cell-based and gene-based therapies as well. No other animal models approximate the human genotype or phenotype as closely as NHPs and efforts continue to map the genomes of the various species (Rogers et al., 2019; Nonhuman Primate Genome projects at https://www.hgsc.bcm.edu/non-human-primates). In this chapter, the origins of NHPs utilized in research are described and their essential nature to the advancement of medical and toxicological science, application as animal models, and background pathology are summarized.

2. HISTORY AND BIOLOGICAL CHARACTERISTICS OF NONHUMAN PRIMATES

2.1. The Cynomolgus Macaque (*Macaca fascicularis*)

The cynomolgus macaque (syn: crab-eating macaque; long-tailed macaque) is the NHP species most commonly used in regulatory toxicology studies today (Mullan, 2019). Cynomolgus macaques belong to the family Cercopithecidae, genera *Macaca* alongside the rhesus macaque, also commonly used in biomedical research. Following the ban on exportation of rhesus macaques from India in 1978, the biomedical research community sought an NHP species that was easy to source, house, and breed in support of the growing demand for NHPs in biomedical research that continued from the previous decades (Southwick and Siddiqi, 1994). The cynomolgus macaque was selected over the rhesus macaque for its smaller size, resulting in lower compound requirements in toxicity studies, its less aggressive temperament, and nonseasonal breeding characteristics (Weinbauer et al., 2008).

Cynomolgus macaques have red-brown to gray fur with lighter underparts and tail that is considerably longer than their body length; however, there is considerable variation in both the coat color and tail length depending on the origin of particular animals (Rowe et al., 2016;

Villano et al., 2009). Males and females are sexually dimorphic, with males being larger than females and having much larger maxillary canine teeth. The skin of the face and perineum is typically pink, except in females during estrous when there is swelling and red coloration of the perineal skin, known as "sex skin." All macaques have prominent ischial callosities: thick keratinized regions of skin overlying the ischial tuberosities. Additional biological characteristics of the cynomolgus macaque are summarized on Table 21.1.

The natural habitat of cynomolgus macaques is expansive and covers much of the islands and mainland of South East Asia (Bonadio, 2000). Two major natural subgroups of cynomolgus macaque have been described: insular (originating in the Philippines and Indonesia) and Indochinese/"Asian" (originating in Vietnam, Cambodia, Thailand, Laos, and the Malaysian Peninsula) (Harihara et al., 1988). Mauritian animals represent a third subgroup that expanded from a small number of founder animals introduced to the island from mainland Asia (Sussman and Tattersall, 1981).

2.2. The Rhesus Macaque (*Macaca mulatta*)

Rhesus macaques are commonly used NHPs in biomedical research and, based on research awards, the most commonly utilized macaque for general research purposes (Feister et al., 2018). They have been critical in our understanding of many fields of human development and disease.

Rhesus macaques have a thick brown to auburn pelage and, compared to the cynomolgus macaque, are considerably larger with relatively shorter tails (Fooden, 2000). Skin is red to pink on both the face and perineal region, which are predominantly hairless. Females exhibit similar reddening and swelling of the perineal region during the menstrual cycle as cynomolgus macaques. Like other macaque species, rhesus monkeys have ischial callosities and males are larger than females with prominent maxillary canines. Additional biological characteristics of

TABLE 21.1 Biological Characteristics of the Cynomolgus Macaque, Rhesus Macaque, and Common Marmoset

Biological characteristic or parameter	Cynomolgus macaque (*Macaca fascicularis*)	Rhesus macaque (*Macaca mulatta*)	Common marmoset (*Callithrix jacchus*)
Life span	31 years	25 years	12 years
Adult body weight	Male: 4.7—8.3 kg Female: 2.5—5.7 kg	Male: 7.7 kg Female: 5.34 kg	Male: 0.25 kg Female: 0.23 kg
Adult height (head and body)	Male: 41.2—64.8 cm Female: 38.5—50.3 cm	Male: 48—63.5 cm Female: 47—53.1 cm	Male: 18.8 cm Female: 18.5 cm
Tail length	40.0—65.5 cm	18.9—30.5 cm	29—30.5 cm
Social groups	Large groups (~30) with females outnumbering males Smaller groups of bachelor males Both female and male dominance hierarchy	Very large groups (10 hundreds) with females outnumbering males Smaller groups of bachelor males Both female and male dominance hierarchy	Small groups of 3—15 individuals Dominance hierarchy not related to sex; breeding pairs are codominant Cooperative childcare involving mother, father, and other group members
Sexual maturity	Male: 1544 days (~4.5 years) Female: 1238 days (~3.5 years)	Male: 2007 days (~4 years) Female: 1231 days (~3 years)	Male: 382 days Females: 477 days
Ovarian cycle length	29.4 days	26.6 days	28.6 days
Menstruation	Overt	Overt	Absent
Placentation type	Interstitial, hemochorial villous	Interstitial, hemochorial villous	Superficial, hemochorial trabecular
Breeding season	Year round	October—December (strongly seasonal)	Year round
Fertility rate	35%—45% per cycle	35%—45% per cycle	70%—80% per cycle
Gestation length	5.5 months (165 days)	5.5 months (165 days)	5 months (145 days)
Litter size	1	1	2
Infant weight	320 g	450 g	29 g
Age at weaning	375 days	279 days	76 days
Interbirth interval	13 months	12 months	6 months

All values are approximate. There is considerable variation in values, especially age of onset of sexual maturity due to origin, environment, and social status. Presence of sperm in semen samples (males) and observation of two consecutive menstrual bleedings (females) are advised to confirm sexual maturity in macaques. Values and data adapted from "Primate Factsheets," http://pin.primate.wisc.edu/factsheets (Cawthon Lang KA. 2005–06); Chapters 8 and 19 in "Non-human primates in biomedical research" (Tardif et al., 2013); Animal Diversity Web (Bonadio, 2000) https://animaldiversity.org; "The Neuroendocrinology of Primate Maternal Behavior" (Saltzman and Maestripieri. Prog Neuropsychopharmacol Biol Psychiatry 2011 Jul 1; 35(5):1192–204).

the rhesus macaque are summarized in Table 21.1.

Rhesus macaques have the largest natural habitat of any primate, other than humans, which covers most of Asia (Fa and Lindburg, 1996).

2.3. The Common Marmoset (*Callithrix jacchus*)

Common marmosets are arboreal New World monkeys of the family Callitrichidae that are native to Brazil (Cover, 2000). Their use in biomedical research was the subject of a recently published textbook "The Common Marmoset in Captivity and Biomedical Research" to which the reader is referred for more in-depth data (Fox, 2019).

The fur of the common marmoset is a mixture of brown, gray, and yellow over the body. They have conspicuous white ear tufts, a blaze of white fur on the forehead, and long banded tails. Unlike Old World monkeys (e.g., macaques), common marmosets have wide, flat noses with laterally placed nostrils, do not have opposable thumbs or ischial callosities, and have claws rather than nails except on the first digit of the hindlimb. They do not exhibit apparent sexual dimorphism (Rowe, 1996). Additional biological characteristics of the common marmoset are summarized in Table 21.1.

2.4. The Baboon (*Papio* sp.)

Several species of baboon are commonly utilized in general research associated with reproductive biology, evolutionary biology, and ecology (Bauer, 2015; Fleagle, 2013; Jolly, 2001; Rogers et al., 2019). Up to the mid-1960s, use of baboons as laboratory subjects was relatively low in the United States, with most successful colonies existing in the Soviet Union (Johnsen et al., 2012). Largely due to National Institute of Health (NIH) support, captive breeding programs in the United States began to grow in the 1970s. Today the baboon has gained in popularity and reached a high level of utility. The genus *Papio* originates from the plains and savannas of sub-Saharan Africa and the Arabian Peninsula. Although hybridization between species under natural conditions can blur the

distinction between them, there are currently five species commonly recognized including the Guinea baboon (*Papio papio*), the Olive baboon (*Papio anubis*), the Yellow baboon (*Papio cynocephalus*), the Chacma baboon (*Papio ursinus*), and the Hamadryas baboon (*Papio hamadryas*). A sixth species, the Kinda baboon (*Papio kindae*), is recognized and noted to hybridize with Chacma baboons in Zambia (Jolly et al., 2011). Each of these species has distinguishing features, primarily hair coat color and body size, but also shares features of the genus including a long sloping hairless muzzle and medium-short tails. There are sexual dimorphisms among baboons including differences in body size (e.g., males are larger than females), dentition (e.g., males having larger canine teeth), and ischial callosities (e.g., males having fused ischial callosities below the anus and females having separate ischial callosities) (Fleagle, 2013; Groves and Wolfe-Coote, 2005; Magden et al., 2015).

Female baboons reach puberty at approximately 3–4 years of age, cycle continuously throughout the year, and are able to reproduce in any season. Changes in turgor and color of the female perineal skin (sexual swelling of the sex skin) signal changes in hormonal levels, onset of the periovulatory period, and reproductive receptivity to the male (Bauer, 2015; Higmam et al., 2009). The female baboon has an approximately 33-day estrus cycle. The rise in urinary oxytocin content during the periovulatory period may initiate or maintain intersexual relationships with the consort males during peak receptivity (Moscovice and Ziegler, 2012). Gestation is approximately 6 months for baboons and the infant is usually born at night. Female baboons generally approach menopause in their late 20s or early 30s, as defined by 6 months without vaginal bleeding or evidence of cycling (Amboseli Baboon Research Project, https://amboselibaboons.nd.edu).

Male baboons reach puberty at approximately 5–6 years of age, but successful breeders are usually over 6 years of age when they are able to maintain control of the harem (Tardif et al., 2012). In general, baboons may reach an age of over 40 years in captivity. For additional information on the baboon, access The Animal Diversity Web (https://animaldiversity.org).

2.5. The Squirrel Monkey (*Saimiri* sp.)

The squirrel monkey was a standard and popular lab animal species prior to the 1970s, as they were small and relatively easy to keep in colonies, but their reproduction in captivity remained poor, so that additional animals needed to be obtained from wild stocks (Abee, 2000). As South and Central American countries began to limit or ban the exportation of these monkeys in the 1970s, it became more urgent to develop successful captive breeding colonies in order to support the ongoing research for which they were commonly utilized. Colonies were established in the United States and Caribbean, but as the resource had become more limited, other monkeys, namely the macaques, were substituted to meet the needs of the NIH and other research establishments. Today, most of the squirrel monkeys are provided to research facilities from breeding colonies, with low numbers imported each year (Magden et al., 2015).

The breeding season for squirrel monkeys is approximately 3 months long, with females cycling approximately every 9–10 days (9–10 and 10–12 days reported in various sources) accompanied by high circulating steroid hormones and behavioral changes (increased genital investigation and sexual invitation) (Diamond et al., 1984; Ghosh et al., 1982; Magden et al., 2015; Williams et al., 2002). For additional information on the Squirrel monkey, access The Animal Diversity Web (https://animaldiversity.org).

2.6. The Tamarins (*Saguinus* sp.)

The tamarins are members of the subfamily Callitrichinae, along with marmosets, and are a diverse group of NHPs found throughout the Amazon, Guianas, Colombia, and Central America. There are multiple species within the genus *Saguinus*; perhaps the best-known tamarin in biomedical research is the cotton-top tamarin (*Saguinus oedipus*), as it is the most commonly utilized member of its genus. They are small monkeys, averaging 260–380 g and are famous for having white shaggy fur on their head. Cotton-top tamarins breed twice yearly, and generally produce nonidentical twins. They are sexually mature at 18 months for females and 24 months for males. For more information, access The Animal Diversity Web (https://animaldiversity.org).

2.7. The Vervet and Green Monkeys (*Chlorocebus aethiops* ssp. *sabaeus* and *pygerythrus*)

The Vervet and Green monkeys belong to the genus *Chlorocebus;* however, the terms green monkey, vervet monkey, or grivet are often applied interchangeably to the members of the subspecies and both have been extensively used in biomedical research. These monkeys originate from Ethiopia, including most of West Africa from Senegal to Ghana and in the Northeast to the Red Sea. Both monkeys have green-tinted golden fur by which they acquired the name green monkey. They differ in facial coloration, with *Chlorocebus aethiops sabaeus* having a dark blue hairless face and *Chlorocebus aethiops pygerythrus* having a sooty-black face. For additional information on the green monkey, access The Animal Diversity Web (https://animaldiversity.org).

2.8. The Capuchin Monkey (*Cebus* sp.)

Carl Linnaeus denoted the capuchin monkey as *Cebus* with two species, *apella* and *capucinus,* based on differences in appearance, and in years that followed, the monkeys were separated into additional species (Linnaeus, 1758). However, the phylogenetics of the capuchin monkey has come under scrutiny in recent years, with dissent over the single genus "*Cebus.*" Some primatologists prefer to split capuchin monkeys into two species, the commonly used "*Cebus*" and the recently proposed "*Sapajus*" (Lima et al., 2018). Regardless, most databases currently refer to six species under the genus of "*Cebus*" (Anderson, 2003; Long, 2009; Mijal, 2001; Schober, 2003; Song and Moses, 2009; Welch, 2019; ITIS partners). These neotropical monkeys inhabit the forests of Central and South America. They are polygynous and without a true breeding season. Females have a 150–160-day gestation period and generally give birth to one infant per year, with twins rarely reported. Females and males are considered mature at 4 and 7 years of age, respectively

(Anderson, 2003). For additional information on the Capuchin monkey, access The Animal Diversity Web (https://animaldiversity.org).

3. SELECTION OF NONHUMAN PRIMATES FOR TOXICOLOGIC RESEARCH AND STUDY DESIGN CONSIDERATIONS

3.1. Ethics and Welfare Considerations

Use of NHPs in biomedical research has always been a difficult choice and requires careful consideration. In a time when researchers strive to meet the 3Rs (replace, reduce, refine), or the additonal R (refuse) in toxicity study design, the use of NHPs has grown substantially (Mullan, 2019). Despite efforts to reduce or replace NHPs in research, the actual numbers of animals used are expanding due to specific demands of recent biomedical research (Grimm, 2018). This growth stems from the blossoming of target-specific test articles that only cross-react with highly homologous primates (human and nonhuman) that express the target epitope. For example, multiple test species express the Programmed Death-1 (PD-1) receptor that is pivotal for immune system recognition and defense against viral and bacterial infections and against multiple tumor types (Qin et al., 2019). However, the close structural homology of the NHP PD-1 results in comparable binding and potency of biologics (products made from living organisms or contain components of living organisms) in the human and NHP, while in other species (e.g., rodents, dogs, pigs) the biologic may only bind weakly, not all, and/or produce no pharmacologic effect. This makes other species less relevant to the prediction of human risk and first-in-human dose calculations. Another consideration with many biologics, such as humanized antibodies, is the potential for induction of an antidrug immune response (immunogenicity). In general, the risk of immunogenicity is expected to be lower in NHPs compared to other species (although this is not always the case). Increased use of NHPs is also due to the large number of new therapeutic products and modalities currently being developed. These new products include RNA-based, cell-based, viral-vectored, and nanoparticle-encapsulated therapeutics targeting homologous proteins

and pathways shared between NHPs and humans. With the greatest structural match of organ-specific cellular components and highest likelihood of comparable toxicity, the NHP is often the species of choice for these modalities. For example, recently reported is a cynomolgus macaque model for studying the transfer of PD1-modified T-cells. The authors modified NHP T-cells to lack PD-1 via electroporation of plasmids encoding sgRNA and Cas9, resulting in knock-out NHP-specific T-cells (PD1-KO T). These cells were adoptively transferred into cynomolgus monkeys without overt toxicity demonstrating their utility in expanding PD1-KO T-cells and evaluating the safety of this immunotherapy (Gao et al., 2020).

Today, the research community stands at the intersection of medical/preclinical research, emerging technologies, and ethical issues. In years past, housing of NHPs for toxicological research often addressed only containment and feeding of the animals, resulting in stress and poor health and thus poorly reproducible data. Higher utilization of NHPs in research today reflects the improvement in husbandry. The health and well-being of the NHP in captivity has greatly improved, allowing for better common ground between use and care; however, discussions are ongoing as to what constitutes improvements and how to implement them. The NIH workshop "Optimizing Reproducibility in Nonhuman Primate Research Studies by Enhancing Rigor and Transparency" was pending at the time of writing this chapter, but the NIH states the program will include "thinking through how welfare considerations (such as housing enrichment, long-term care needs, social engagement, etc.) might clarify—or confound—research findings, as well as discussing whether the intersection of cutting-edge science, like neuroscience or gene editing, might present unique ethical considerations for NHP research."(NIH website: https://osp.od.nih.gov/2019/09/16/update-nih-workshop-optimizing-reproducibility-nonhuman-primate-research-studies-enhancing-rigor-transparency/).

At modern facilities, multiple aspects of NHP welfare are addressed both before and during study assignment. These aspects, to include housing consideration, social and environmental enrichment, medical and nutritional needs, and individual temperament assessment, are key elements to stress reduction and resiliency for each NHP and the colony in general. For example, group or paired housing results in reduced abnormal behaviors as compared to single housing (Koyama et al., 2019) and providing elevated space for perching is preferred by most NHPs (MacLean et al., 2009). The facilities must meet the physical needs of the NHP housed within, providing adequate space of appropriate design, and this often means strict regulation and monitoring of heat and humidity for enclosed areas. For additional information, see the National Center for the Replacement, Refinement and Reduction of Animals in Research website at https://www.nc3rs.org.uk/macaques/captive-management/housing/.

3.2. Regulatory Considerations

There are multiple guidance documents that have been created by the US Food and Drug Administration (FDA) and other agencies that provide essential information for the appropriate use of NHPs in biomedical research. Additionally, there are a number of industry publications addressing the use of NHPs (Hobson, 2000; Weatherall, 2006). These publications describe the considerations necessary when constructing studies. For instance, NHPs should be selected only when they are the most relevant species that may reflect potential toxicity in humans with novel therapeutics. The number and sex of animals may have direct bearing on the ability to detect a toxicity; therefore, the sample size must be large enough to observe toxic events while utilizing the least number of animals necessary for these observations. For pharmaceuticals with metabolic profiles indicative of possible abuse liability, and for which the rodent model is inadequate for predictivity of this in humans, the NHP model may be selected (Guidance for industry, M3 (R2) Nonclinical Safety Studies for the Conduct of Human Clinical Trials and Marketing Authorization for Pharmaceuticals, 2010). For biologics, safety assessment should be conducted in NHPs when they are the most relevant species when the specificity and cross-reactivity of a biotechnology-derived pharmaceutical is demonstrated between NHP and human, and lack of cross-reactivity or pharmacologic effect in other species has been demonstrated (Guidance for Industry. S6

Preclinical Safety Evaluation of Biotechnology-Derived Pharmaceuticals, 2012). For the approval of new drugs when human efficacy studies are not ethical and field trials are not feasible, the FDA guidance approves the use of NHPs under the "Animal Rule." This states that "for drugs developed to ameliorate or prevent serious or life-threatening conditions caused by exposure to lethal or permanently disabling toxic substances, when human efficacy studies are not ethical and field trials are not feasible, FDA may grant marketing approval based on adequate and well-controlled animal efficacy studies when the results of those studies establish that the drug is reasonably likely to produce clinical benefit in humans" (Product Development under the Animal Rule Guidance for Industry, 2015). The Animal Rule has been applied to a handful of products, including levofloxacin for treatment of plague and raxibacumab for anthrax. As of the writing of this chapter, the FDA has approved the application of this rule for the development of COVID-19 therapeutics (Jackson and Engelhardt, 2020). Cases in which administration of the test article was to precede or be followed by exposure of the animals to the virus were under consideration. The goals of these studies were to investigate humoral and cellular immune responses and establish preventions and treatments for COVID-19 (Johansen et al., 2020; van Doremalen et al., 2020).

The shipment of NHPs and specimens from these animals into and out of the United States is highly regulated and involves multiple agencies. The US Fish and Wildlife Service in conjunction with the Convention on the International Trade in Endangered Species of Wild Fauna and Flora dictates and enforces the Lacey Act and the Endangered Species Act, which serve to protect NHPs from illegal transportation or sale and from threat of extinction. The US Department of Health and Human Services and the Centers for Disease Control and Prevention regulations are in place to address health risk to humans that NHPs may pose. Therefore, they dictate importation and quarantine mandates, set fines for violations and specify that NHPs may be imported into the United States only for science, education, or exhibition purposes (42 Code of Federal Regulations Part 71.53). The US Department of Agriculture regulates interstate transportation of live NHPs. These agencies ensure that these animals have appropriate documentation of acquisition and transportation.

3.3. Source, Origin, and Genetic Variation

The selection of NHPs for toxicity studies should have consideration for the source (where the animal was born and raised), origin (where the original stock for the genus and species was obtained), and any known associated genetic variation that may impact study outcomes. While these parameters are often known, particularly for animals from long-standing closed colonies with well-maintained records, in other situations this may not be the case. For example, cynomolgus monkeys have multiple countries of import with known genetic variation between these sources and origins, which may impact toxicity study design or outcome. The most northerly range of Indochinese cynomolgus macaques overlaps with that of the rhesus macaque and there is evidence of significant introgression of rhesus genes into the cynomolgus genome in animals from this region (Kanthaswamy et al., 2009; Tosi et al., 2002). As a consequence, there are genotypic and phenotypic differences in monkeys of different origins. Most cynomolgus macaques used for biomedical research in the United States up to 2019 were purpose bred and of Asian origin (Blancher et al., 2008). Despite this, there may still be significant genotypic and phenotypic diversity in animals within and between different vendors (Day et al., 2018; Kozlosky et al., 2015). Many animals are exported to the United States from China, where cynomolgus macaques are not native, and are the offspring of a diverse breeding stock, the true origin of which is generally not recorded and differs between vendors (Zhang et al., 1990). Mauritian cynomolgus macaques are considerably less genetically diverse than those of Asian origin due to the small number of founder animals (Blancher et al., 2008; Bonhamme et al., 2008; Kondo et al., 1993; Lawler et al., 1995; Smith and McDonough, 2005). These animals appear to have fewer microscopic spontaneous background lesions in tissues, suggestive of reduced inflammatory processes and significant differences in immunological parameters such as B-cell and CD4 T-cell number (Kozlosky et al., 2015). The reduced inherent variability of Mauritian macaques is preferred by many in biomedical research and has allowed detailed characterization of immune gene diversity, including major histocompatibility complex, immunoglobulin-like receptors, and Fc gamma receptors (Bimber et al., 2008; Haj et al., 2019; Wiseman et al., 2013). However, this reduced variability does not reflect the diversity of the human population modeled in toxicity studies and Mauritian macaques may provide data that are not relevant to patients. For example, Mauritius-origin macaques appear to be considerably more sensitive to the acute toxicity of vildagliptin, a dipeptidyl peptidase-4 inhibitor for the treatment of diabetes, than animals of Asian origin (Hoffmann et al., 2017). This toxicity does not appear to be relevant to humans based on the available clinical data (Mathieu et al., 2017; Williams et al., 2019).

At the time of writing this chapter, ongoing supply and airline transportation issues, particularly for sexually mature animals, were exacerbated by the international expansion in medical research and travel restrictions in response to the COVID-19 pandemic. This forced many institutions to consider the interchangeability of cynomolgus macaques of different origins and source in order to support ongoing drug development programs. Overall, the subtle differences between animals originating from different areas within Indochina (e.g., Cambodia vs. China) should not preclude a switch from one source of Asian macaques to another if necessary (Debien et al., 2019), but it is prudent to ensure that all studies supporting the development of a particular test article are carried out in macaques of the same origin when possible. Additionally, switching from Asian macaques to Mauritian macaques should be approached with caution, particularly when the test item is an immunomodulator.

Rhesus macaques are genetically diverse and there are several subspecies; however, they are generally described as being of Indian or Chinese origin. Indian-origin animals in the United States are derived from founder colonies imported prior to the ban on exportation from India. Chinese-origin animals may still be imported from vendors and are more genetically diverse (Satkoski et al., 2008; Smith and McDonough, 2005). Furthermore, some breeding colonies in the United States have purposely hybridized Indian- and Chinese-origin animals to increase genetic diversity within the population (Kanthaswamy et al., 2009). Several differences in morphology, disease susceptibility, and spontaneous lesions have been associated with origin and/or pedigree (Champoux et al., 1997; Clark and O'Neil, 1999; Lowenstine, 2003). For example, Simian Immunodeficiency Virus (SIV) progression is known to be faster in animals of Indian versus Chinese origin, and there is a strong genetic predisposition toward the development of spontaneous left ventricular hypertrophic cardiomyopathy in rhesus macaques (Kanthaswamy et al., 2014; Reader et al., 2016; Trichel et al., 2002). Therefore, potential genotypic and phenotypic differences in animals of different origin or source should be considered when designing and interpreting studies utilizing rhesus macaques. Published data describing toxicologic endpoints of interest and background findings in rhesus macaques are referenced, but appropriate controls and baseline assessments should be included in each study (Chamanza et al., 2006; Lowenstine, 2003; Sasseville et al., 2012; Simmons, 2016).

Similar to the Mauritian macaque, there was a genetic "population bottleneck" due to low numbers of founder animals in the populations of green monkeys in the Caribbean following their arrival on the islands in the 1800s. The isolation resulted in extinction of viral pathogens that are endemic in their African relatives, including SIV and simian pegivirus (Kapusinsky et al., 2015). These Caribbean animals are preferred for research purposes for this reason.

Compared to macaques, less is known about the genetic and phenotypic variation of marmosets from different sources and how this may affect study interpretation. However, the genomes of marmosets from three different colonies were easily separated by principal component analysis and functional variants of cytochrome P450 genes were identified (Uno et al., 2018).

Genomic data for NHPs provide valuable insight into genetic similarities and differences among species used as models for disease-related research. The genomes for cynomolgus macaques and Indian and Chinese rhesus macaques have been published (Ebeling et al., 2011; Yan et al., 2011). Chimerism made sequencing of the marmoset genome more challenging than other primate species, but the draft genome was published in 2014 (Marmoset Genome Project at https://www.hgsc.bcm.edu/non-human-primates). The chimerism is due to extensive anastomosis of placental blood vessels in marmosets resulting in litter mates that are hematopoietic chimeras and mutually immune tolerant (Sweeney et al., 2012). Whole-genome sequences from several baboon species have been generated and, in recent years, there has been great progress deciphering the genome of green monkeys (C. aethiops sabaeus) (Jasinska et al., 2007; Warren et al., 2015). The breeding of Specific Pathogen-Free Olive baboons has circumvented natural infections and provided great insight into functions of the immune system and immunosuppression, particularly in regard to differences in the innate and adaptive immune responses. These differences should be considered in study design, as they may have ramifications when there are immunological endpoints (Magden et al., 2020).

3.4. Relevance and Feasibility for Use in Drug Development

Prior to initiating any drug development program, it is important that the pharmacologic relevance and feasibility of the selected NHP population is assessed. Selecting a relevant species for conducting safety assessment should be in accordance with the International Conference for Harmonization S6 and Q11 (Food and Drug Administration, HHS, 2012a,b) guidance documents. Due to the genetic variation discussed above, screening of individual animals and selection based on appropriate target binding and pharmacodynamic (PD) response upon dosing of the test item (pharmacological responsiveness) may be required in some instances (Tuntland et al., 2014). While reference ranges for endpoints of interest in toxicity studies, including clinical pathology and immunotoxicology assays, have been published for macaques of specific origin, it is apparent that these are insufficient to assess test item–related effects in the small number of animals used in toxicity studies (Choi et al., 2016; Rosso et al., 2016). Appropriate controls in addition to baseline individual animal data, such as clinical pathology, are requirements in definitive toxicity studies. Due to closer phylogeny to humans compared to other animal species, NHPs often provide the greater target sequence homology and relative target binding affinity and/or ligand occupancy and kinetics, especially for biologics, that may increase their relevance for use in toxicity studies and safety assessment (see *Protein Pharmaceutical Agents,* Vol 2, Chap 6).

Rhesus macaques are considerably larger than cynomolgus macaques and are seasonal breeders with regular menstrual cycles only occurring in fall. These biological differences result in larger amounts of test article being required for studies and make development and reproductive toxicity studies challenging; thus, rhesus macaques are less frequently used in contemporary toxicity studies. Despite these drawbacks, rhesus macaques may be the most pharmacologically relevant model for a given test article and have been used in the development programs for several therapeutics, most notably vaccines (Dowd et al., 2016; Martin et al., 2019).

Adult common marmosets are approximately one tenth the body weight of cynomolgus macaques meaning they are easier and less expensive to house, maintain in biosecure facilities, handle, and require smaller quantities of test article to undertake toxicity studies (Korte and Everitt, 2019). Quantitative absorption, distribution, metabolism, and excretion studies, whole-body imaging, and inhalation studies in marmosets are more feasible due to their smaller size compared to such studies in macaques. In addition, unlike the macaques, common marmosets become sexually mature at a relatively young age, reproduce in captivity, and frequently produce dizygotic twins, making sibling-controlled experiments possible. However, the physiology and endocrinology of the marmoset reproductive system is sufficiently different from humans and macaques as to reduce the relevance of marmosets as a model of reproductive toxicology (Abbott et al., 2003; Zuhlke and Weinbauer, 2003). The small size, and thus blood volume, of the marmoset may be a disadvantage as it may be difficult to collect sufficient blood for all the endpoints of interest typically incorporated into toxicity studies. Additionally, some routes of administration are more challenging in such a small animal (e.g., intravitreal injection), but certain laboratories have developed experience with these techniques (Korbmacher et al., 2017). Another consideration for the use of common marmosets is their complex dietary requirements (Flurer and Zucker, 1989). Marmosets are specialist gummivores (omnivores that feed primarily on sap and tree gum) and require a diet that is high in energy, vitamin C, and D3. Vitamin C requirements are increased during periods of stress, which may be common in these smaller, less robust animals when included in toxicity studies (Flurere et al., 1987). Clearly, selection of a laboratory with experience in handling common marmosets is critical if they are selected as the nonrodent species for drug development.

In comparison to other cercopithecines, baboons are exceptionally large animals which present challenges in handling and housing in the laboratory; however, they are generally considered docile in captivity and, due to heartiness, are able to withstand extreme weather for outdoor troop housing and breeding. Additionally, in comparison to macaques, baboons are considered to have fewer abnormal behaviors when in a captive setting (Lutz, 2018). Viruses that occur spontaneously in baboons (Cercopithecine herpesvirus 2, Papiine herpesvirus 2, polyomavirus papionis 1 and 2, etc.) can cause confounding results in test systems; thus, careful screening prior to study assignment is essential.

Less commonly used NHPs have some traits that make them amenable for study use. For example, squirrel monkeys have been desired in research settings, due to their small size, ease of handling without chemical restraint, and the low zoonotic potential of disease transmission to the human handlers.

3.5. Study Design

In years past, NHPs were primarily utilized in GLP-compliant toxicity testing for late-stage pharmaceutical development, and often were the final test species prior to conducting clinical trials. The test articles were mostly small molecules manufactured to bind targets resulting in inhibition or enhancement of function. While these goals are generally still maintained today, the rise of large molecule (biological) test articles has changed the landscape of NHP use in toxicology. Many of these newer agents are not suitable for testing in other species, due to immunogenicity or lack of homologous protein structure of the targets; therefore, NHPs have increasingly been the species of choice for discovery and early test article candidate selection.

The number of NHPs assigned to a study is a balance between cost, animal conservation, regulatory guidance, and statistical power (Hobson, 2000). For Good Laboratory Practice (GLP)–compliant studies up to 28 days, a minimum of three NHPs per sex/dose group, including a control and a recovery cohort, is a standard study design to produce statistically significant results while using the fewest number of animals, but many companies choose to increase this number of animals, based on the pharmacological characteristics of their test article, and to increase confidence in identifying any test article–related findings. There is controversy as to whether three animals/sex truly produces values that are statistically reliable, but selection of animals that are age and weight matched has been used for many years and, for most instances, is a good indicator of comparative changes over the course of a study. For GLP-compliant studies of longer duration, there may be four or more animals per sex/dose group. Investigational studies typically have few animals per dose group, and in some cases, may have only one animal in the dose group. For additional information on study design considerations, references are available (Burbacher and Grant, 2001).

4. PREDICTIVITY OF NONHUMAN PRIMATE TOXICITY DATA TO HUMANS

While lack of efficacy accounts for much of the attrition of drug candidates in late stages of pharmaceutical development, consideration of the translation of preclinical toxicity findings from animals to human is a critical component of early drug development decisions. The accuracy of toxicity data in animal models to predict human adverse events has been subject to debate. Recently, there has been extensive research conducted examining the relevance of NHP preclinical data to clinical outcomes; however, interpretation of these studies varies when concordance of true positive events (i.e., animal

finding correlated to human finding) is discussed and efforts continue to elucidate predictivity of NHP toxicity data to clinical adverse events (Monticello et al., 2017). One study conducted with "Big Data" (PharmaPendium, Reed Elsevier Properties SA, 2014, https://www.pharmapendium.com) concluded that several species utilized in preclinical safety studies, including macaques, have a high likelihood of animal–human concordance of adverse findings (Clark and Steger-Hartmann, 2018). For the cynomolgus monkey, the authors concluded that the likelihood ratio (statistical indicator of human risk implied by an animal observation) was ≥ 10 (strong concordance) for many parameters calculated, including clinical pathology (e.g., white blood cell counts, aspartate aminotransferase, alanine aminotransferase), dehydration, diarrhea, and hepatobiliary and skin findings. However, similar to previous studies, the authors concluded that the lack of toxicity in macaques had limited predictivity for lack of adverse events in humans (Bailey et al., 2014; Clark, 2015; Clark and Steger-Hartmann, 2018; Olsen et al., 2000).

5. NONHUMAN PRIMATE MODELS IN BIOMEDICAL RESEARCH (SEE ALSO (ABEE, MANSFIELD, TARDIF, & MORRIS, 2012)

NHPs are important models in many fields of research including neurodevelopment and neuroscience; addiction; Alzheimer's and Parkinson's disease; immunology; aging; and genetic and infectious diseases (such as tuberculosis (TB), rabies, and Zika and Ebola virus) (Bennett et al., 2017; Dudley et al., 2019; Emborg, 2017; Estes et al., 2018; Friedman et al., 2017; Messaoudi et al., 2011; Pena and Ho, 2016; Van Damn and De Deyn, 2017; Van Rompay, 2017). The cynomolgus macaque, rhesus macaque, and common marmoset are generally the most commonly utilized NHPs in pharmacology and toxicology research today, while the lesser utilized species (e.g., baboon, squirrel monkey, green monkey, capuchin monkey) are more commonly utilized for other types of studies. This section discusses the traditional and more recent uses of these genera.

5.1. Nonhuman Primate Models of Human Disease

Most NHPs are valuable as models of human disease. Of the macaques, cynomolgus macaques are less frequently used as models of human disease than the rhesus macaque (Feister et al., 2018). For instance, the Indian rhesus macaque is considered the model of choice for human immunodeficiency virus/acquired immunodeficiency syndrome research, but cynomolgus monkeys have also been utilized to a lesser extent (Antony and MacDonald, 2015; O'Connor, 2006; Reimann et al., 2005). The baboon is used for studies of alcohol and drug addiction (Platt and Rowlett, 2012) and, as a natural host for Cercopithecine herpesvirus 12 (baboon herpesvirus), serves as a research model for Epstein–Barr virus in humans (Jenson et al., 2000). Their susceptibility to Flaviviruses (Zika, West Nile, Dengue, Yellow Fever, and Japanese and St. Louis encephalitis viruses) has made them popular for the study of these viruses and for development of vaccines (Gurung et al., 2018; Valdes et al., 2013; Wolf et al., 2006). Baboons are a natural model for epilepsy induced by photic stimulation, first discovered in the 1960s (Killam et al., 1967). Since then, numerous studies investigating the pathogenesis of epilepsy have used these animals as test subjects (VandeBerg et al., 2009). Owing to the availability of data from genetic characterization, the baboon is highly utilized for genetic and epigenetic studies of complex diseases, including diabetes, dyslipidemia, hypertension, and osteoporosis (Cox et al., 2013; Karere et al., 2020). It develops spontaneous atherosclerosis in a manner similar to humans and has been a popular experimental model for this condition since the late 1950s when the first colonies were established in the United States for biomedical research (VandeBerg et al., 2009). The role of diet in atherosclerosis is commonly investigated using baboons (Karere et al., 2019; Karere et al., 2020). Although the cynomolgus monkey is more prone to develop atherosclerosis than the rhesus monkey (Getz and Reardon, 20123; Peluffo et al., 2014), it is the baboon, and to lesser extent, the squirrel monkey, that has long dominated this field of research. Atherosclerosis and cerebral amyloid angiopathy are common spontaneous aging changes for squirrel monkeys, modeling that in humans and providing a laboratory model of arteriosclerosis and Alzheimer's disease (Mackic et al., 1998; Middleton et al., 1964). The squirrel monkey is still popular for the investigation of cardiovascular disease, including cardiomyopathy which occurs spontaneously in aging squirrel monkeys, and central nervous system (CNS) disorders, such as Alzheimer's disease (Abee, 2000; Bading et al., 2002; Brady et al., 2003; Huss et al., 2015).

Investigations into the pathogenesis of parasitic diseases, such as malaria, often utilize squirrel monkeys as test subjects, due to their high susceptibility to infection by multiple species of *Plasmodium* (Gysin et al., 1980; Gysin et al., 1982). Other parasitic diseases for which the squirrel monkey is utilized in research include toxoplasmosis, encephalitozoonosis, filariasis, and trypanosomiasis (Galland, 2000).

The common marmoset has also been considered an animal model that reflects human disease. With regard to their susceptibility to infectious agents, marmosets are excellent NHP models for viral, protozoan, and bacterial agents, as well as prions (Carrion and Patterson, 2012) and have been used in the investigation of conditions in the immunology, neuroscience, and aging fields (Prins et al., 2017; Tardif, 2019).

Cotton-top tamarins are popular laboratory subjects as models of Crohn's disease or ulcerative colitis due to the spontaneous colitis that this NHP often develops in captivity. This appears to be a condition uncommon in their wild counterparts, as is the high incidence of colonic adenocarcinoma in captive animals (Wood et al., 1998). More recently, a connection between coronavirus and *Helicobacter* sp. in human and tamarin colitis has been suggested, making this species the prime model for research into the disease pathogenesis and treatment (Clapp, 1993; David et al., 2009).

The vervet monkey is prized in the research of behavior, metabolism, and of the immune system, and its use in biomedical research has been increasing, as it is often considered a suitable replacement for the rhesus macaque. Similar to other NHPs, green and vervet monkeys are prone to atherosclerosis, making them useful animal models of the disease (Jasinska et al., 2013; Shelton et al., 2012).

The capuchin monkey has had a wide range of utilization in the biomedical industry. It is a naturally occurring reservoir for *Trypanosoma cruzi*, making it an ideal model for Chagas disease research (de Souza et al., 2018).

Select Models of Neurodegeneration (See Also Nervous System, Vol 3, Chap 9)

The use of NHPs as models of neurodegeneration is growing, primarily due to the close similarity between NHPs and humans with respect to cognitive function, complex motor skills, and neuroanatomy, which make them ideal subjects for studies focused on neurodegeneration and associated therapies. Currently, modeling focuses heavily on addressing deficits in therapies for Alzheimer's disease, Parkinson's disease, and Huntington's disease.

Aging NHPs often develop behavioral and neurodegenerative abnormalities that resemble Alzheimer's and Parkinson's diseases noted in humans. Alzheimer-type changes include amyloid plaques and dropout/atrophy of monoaminergic neurons, while Parkinson's type changes include dysfunction of the nigrostriatal system and resultant motor impairments (Emborg, 2007; Albert, 2002; Peters, at al. 1996; Price et al., 1991). Similar to humans, obese macaques develop type II diabetes which has been associated with Alzheimer's disease in humans (Grizzanti et al., 2016). Experiments with caloric restriction and exercise in macaques have demonstrated how these factors may be altered to offset risk by improving glucose regulation and cerebral blood flow, and by greater preservation of the frontal and parietal cortices of the brain (Rhyu et al., 2010; Kastman et al., 2012).

These models require older animals that must be housed for an extended period of time and carefully screened for any neurodegenerative features. In younger animals, intracerebral delivery of β-amyloid plaques and neurofibrillary tangles into strategic locations of the brain are used to mimic spontaneous Alzheimer's neurodegeneration and stereotactic injections of cytotoxins or neurotoxins are used to mimic Parkinson's, Alzheimer's, and Huntington's diseases (Baker et al., 1993; Beal et al., 1986; Burns et al., 1995; Ridley et al., 2006; Philippens et al., 2017). Precise delivery of materials to specific regions of the brain has been challenging but necessary to accomplish development of the disease characteristics in NHPs (Figure 21.1). Improvements in stereotactic and intracerebral methods have made both modeling of diseases and delivery of therapeutic agents more feasible.

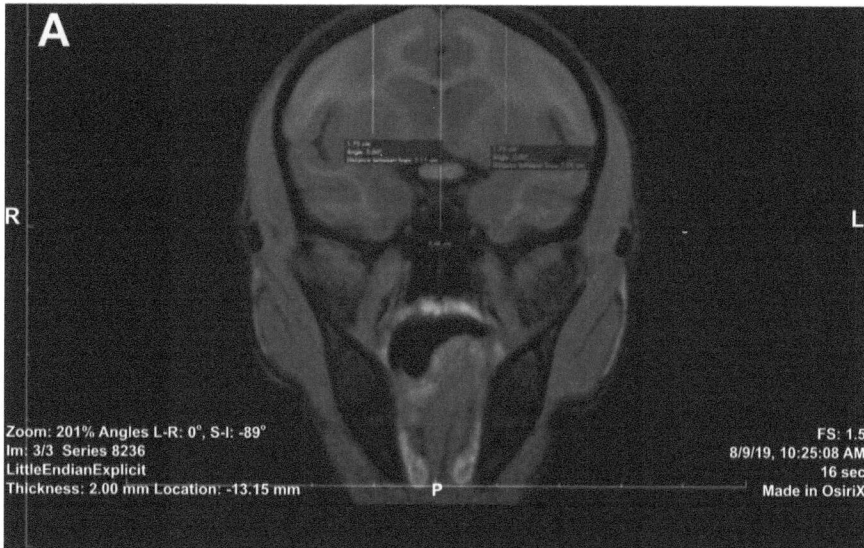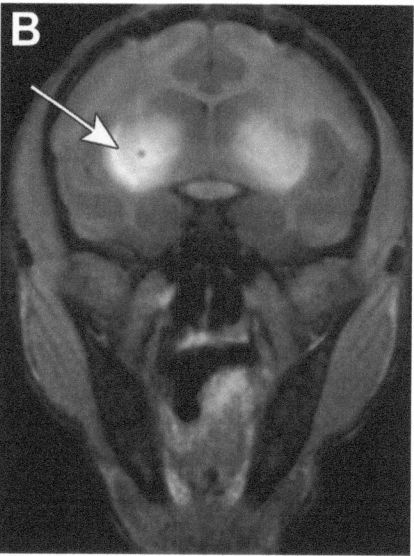

FIGURE 21.1 Stereotactic delivery of test article in a cynomolgus monkey. Images of brain from a cynomolgus macaque. MRI-assisted, stereotactic, bilateral intracerebral administration of test article to the putamen nucleus before (A) and after (B) injection. The injected media is visible as white substance (arrow) in the putamen nucleus. *Images courtesy of Barak Gunter, Charles River, Mattawan, MI.*

5.2. Models in Pharmacology and Toxicology Research

The cynomolgus macaque is the NHP that is primarily utilized in pharmacology and toxicology research today and the year-round breeding season of the cynomolgus monkey makes it a useful model for developmental and reproductive toxicology. Although rhesus monkeys are seasonal breeders, making them unsuitable for some reproductive toxicology studies, they have considerable similarity in the reproductive tracts and endocrinology to that of humans and continue to be used extensively for this purpose (Friedman et al., 2017; Stouffer and Woodruff, 2017). Following the discovery of efficient gene-editing techniques such as CRISPR–Cas 9, there is excitement in the biomedical research community as to the potential of genetic knock-out NHPs (see *Genetically Engineered Animal Models in Toxicologic Research,* Vol 1, Chap 23). Due to their shorter duration of gestation and larger litter sizes, the common marmoset is poised to become an important model in which to exploit this advancement (Kishi et al., 2014). The baboon's larger size makes it a good model for medical device implantation testing, especially spinal implants (Sheng et al., 2010). Of note, studies that confirmed that fibrate-induced hepatic neoplasia in rodents was not relevant to humans were conducted in the common marmoset (Corton et al., 2018).

Select Models for Nonclinical Toxicology and Safety Pharmacology Studies

The FDA, in conjunction with the Center for Drug Evaluation and Research and the Center for Biologics Evaluation and Research, has provided recommendations in order to "help protect clinical trial participants in patients receiving marketed products from potential adverse effects of pharmaceuticals" (Guidance for Industry, S7A Safety Pharmacology Studies for Human Pharmaceuticals, 2001). In order to better comply with FDA guidance, several models have been developed in NHPs to address the need for evaluation of critical vital organ function within the cardiac, respiratory, and neurologic systems. Additionally, models addressing immune function have become increasingly utilized for preclinical studies.

Many of these models employ technologies and methodologies with sound scientific principles to better define alterations in biologic functions. Selected models are discussed below.

TELEMETRY MODELS OF CARDIAC AND RESPIRATORY FUNCTION

At the time of writing this chapter, the FDA guidance document "E14 and S7B Clinical and Nonclinical Evaluation of QT/QTc Interval Prolongation and Proarrhythmic Potential—Questions and Answers" was under construction; however, the draft document made clear that assessment of high-quality cardiac data is essential in nonclinical studies where effects on cardiac function may occur.

Jacketed external telemetry (JET) allows for noninvasive cardiac and respiratory monitoring of NHPs by means of an external telemetry device and respiratory inductive plethysmograph (RIP), both in a reusable form. Leads from the unit to the animal's skin are usually secured to snap electrodes. The data can be continuously or intermittently collected as the study design dictates, and the JET device batteries have a long life (most over 6 months) or rapid recharge rate. The transponders usually have the capacity to add blood pressure data collection via a minimally invasive catheter placed into an appropriate vessel. Electrocardiogram (ECG) data collection may occur without physical or chemical restraint of the animals, thus cardiovascular changes due to handling and test article administration that may confound data interpretation are avoided (Derakhchan et al., 2014). ECG and RIP data can be collected at any time point in a 24-hour cycle with JET. RIP is an indirect means of evaluating pulmonary function based on movement of the chest wall, thus can be used to gather validated data on a number of parameters including respiratory rate, tidal volume, and minute ventilation. Additional nonvalidated parameters that may be evaluated include peak inspiratory and expiratory flow.

There are some disadvantages to JET. Many units are analogue, and there may be "crosstalk" between units requiring individual housing of animals to prevent interference with data collection. However, this obstacle has been overcome in more recent models which are digitalized, Bluetooth enabled, and allow for group housing and socialization of animals. The addition of blood pressure monitoring to JET requires anesthesia and minor surgery, and in some cases, the animals must be temporarily isolated to obtain accurate blood pressure readings. Animals must be acclimated to the JET jacket and leads, increasing time needed prior to study start to ensure the animals will tolerate the device and the data produced will be reliable (Figure 21.2).

Implantable telemetry units are rapidly becoming popular in NHP studies. These units provide means of collecting cardiovascular and respiratory data, but in some cases, have increased sensitivity as compared to JET. The disadvantage of implantable telemetry units is the necessity of surgery with recovery time. The units are typically implanted either within the abdominal body wall muscle, or fixed intraperitoneally on the body wall, with leads and/or catheters placed strategically for data collection, such as on the diaphragm for respiratory data collection, and within the aorta or jugular vein for cardiovascular monitoring. Based on evaluation of a small number of animals following 7 months of implantation, these units were well tolerated (Charles River internal study).

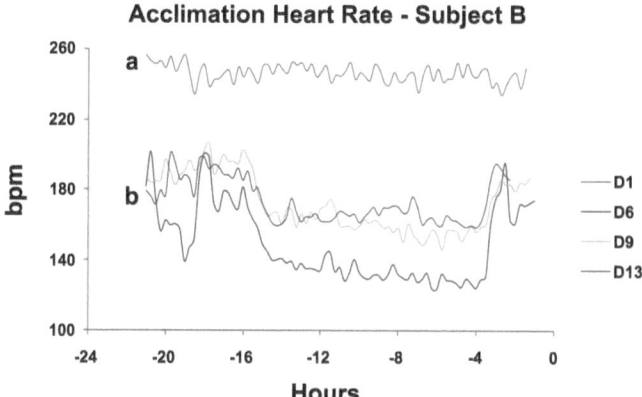

FIGURE 21.2 Graph of experimental validation data for implanted telemetry in NHPs. Heart rate alterations during JET acclimation period for an individual cynomolgus macaque (Subject B). On Day 1, the animal has increased heart rate due to the introduction of the jacket (a), Days 6 through 13, animal's heart rate returns to normal, prejacketed baseline values (b). These data demonstrate the need to ensure proper acclimation to the apparatus prior to study data acquisition.

OTHER TELEMETRY MODELS

OCULAR TELEMETRY Implantable telemetry devices have been employed to gather data from other organs in addition to the cardiovascular and respiratory systems. Researchers at the University of Alabama at Birmingham have recently developed an implantable telemetry device to monitor the transluminal pressure (TLP) in the NHP eye (Jasien et al., 2020). These researchers discovered that cynomolgus monkeys have a 56% increase in TLP while awake as opposed to sleeping, which is similar to that noted for humans, and confirms the cynomolgus monkey as an appropriate model of glaucoma.

TELEMETRY FOR NEUROLOGIC ASSESSMENT Approximately 6.1% of new-onset seizures in humans are drug related (Pesola and Avasarala, 2002); therefore, recognition of seizure activity in preclinical studies may be beneficial for risk assessment and mitigation of possible adverse events in clinical trials. Additionally, age-related epilepsy is increasing in incidence (Loiseau, 1990) necessitating development of mechanisms to study the disorder in animal models. While there have been methods available for some time to monitor the CNS in NHPs, this has been greatly limited to observations of behavior or overt clinical signs. The ability to monitor CNS activity, in real time or at scheduled time points and without sedation or restraint, has been a more recent invention using telemetered electroencephalography. Changes suggestive of altered seizure threshold or frank seizure, including increased synchrony, repetitive sharp waves, slow-wave complexes or spike trains, can be detected by electroencephalography monitoring (Authier, 2019). In one study, the authors successfully implanted the telemetry unit into the musculature of the abdominal body wall, and extended the leads subcutaneously to the skull. Following recovery, the authors collected and analyzed data from NHPs with drug-induced seizure activity and determined that NHPs represent an important model in seizure liability assessments due to their high translational potential (Bassett, 2014).

MODELS OF IMMUNE FUNCTION (SEE ALSO IMMUNE SYSTEM, VOL 4, CHAP 6)

The efforts of researchers to harness the immune system, especially through development of therapeutics directed to treat cancer and chronic diseases, continue to increase in the pharmaceutical industry. Many biologics and other test articles intended to alter specific aspects of immune function are reliant on the NHP as a test system for PD evaluation, especially those for which the NHP shares greatest cross-reactivity compared to other nonclinical species. This homology of protein sequences between humans and NHPs allows target recognition by test articles more often in NHPs, and this may limit development of immunogenicity against the test article that precludes the use of other species in toxicity studies (Swanson and Bussiere, 2012). Recent successes of biologic therapies in clinical trials have stimulated increased development of biopharmaceuticals, thus the greater utilization of NHPs. For example, immune checkpoint inhibitors have been extensively tested in NHPs and have demonstrated efficacy previously unknown against certain cancers, including malignant melanoma and non-small cell lung cancer (Ottaviano et al., 2019).

Evaluation of immune function within the NHP has become essential given the advancement of immunomodulatory therapeutic agents entering preclinical evaluation; therefore, assays to assess immune function and immunotoxicity have been added more frequently to nonclinical safety studies. T-cell–dependent antibody response (TDAR) and immunophenotyping remain the most common assays employed in nonclinical studies for evaluation of immune competence; however, delayed-type hypersensitivity (DTH) assays are gaining in popularity. Additionally, there has been increased interest in the NHP as a model of age-related changes in the immune system. These models are summarized here.

T-CELL–DEPENDENT ANTIBODY RESPONSE AND DELAYED-TYPE HYPERSENSITIVITY Both TDAR and DTH can be induced in the macaque, with intramuscular injection of Keyhole Limpet Hemocyanin (KLH). Additional antigens utilized for TDAR and/or DTH include tetanus toxoid (TT), Bacillus Calmette–Guérin (BCG),

hepatitis antigen, and sheep red blood cells. There are multiple publications addressing TDAR immunization protocols in NHPs (Caldwell et al., 2007; Haggerty, 2007; Kirk et al., 2008; Piccotti et al., 2005; Tichenor et al., 2010) but fewer addressing DTH induction in NHPs (Bleavins and de la Iglesia, 1995; Bouchez et al., 2012).

The induction of TDAR in macaques has been shown to occur at similar rates between sexes and between macaques of various origins, with a good primary IgM and IgG response by 7–10 days that generally peaks at 21 days after immunization. Both IgG and IgM responses can usually be promoted with the addition of an adjuvant to the antigen immunization (Lebrec et al., 2011).

The antigen used and dose, age of the animal, and the assay format should be considered as variables when addressing protocols for TDAR (Figure 21.3). Additionally, it is advised to survey the NHPs assigned to study for preexisting anti-KLH antibodies. Anti-KLH antibodies may form due to previous infection with *Schistosoma* sp. (flatworm infection), which shares a carbohydrate epitope with the KLH. These preexisting antibodies may result in cross-reactivity which may impact the TDAR response; therefore, KLH-naïve animals should be used (Lebrec et al., 2014).

In general, KLH produces a more robust primary immunoglobulin response in the macaque compared to TT and there is a dose-responsive change in immunoglobulin levels up to approximately 1 mg of KLH. Aged animals may have a reduced immunoglobulin response compared to younger animals.

The DTH assay is a validated platform for the assessment of in vivo T-cell trafficking and function. This assay has been gaining popularity as a means of evaluating tissue-specific immune cell alteration. Similar to TDAR, DTH in NHPs is induced with scheduled immunization of an appropriate antigen (e.g., KLH or BCG). Following induction, the DTH reaction is challenged by administration of a subcutaneous or intradermal antigen into designated locations (usually the dorsum), which are then sampled at specified time points and evaluated microscopically. Subsets of inflammatory cells within the DTH reaction of the skin section may be further elucidated with immunohistochemistry

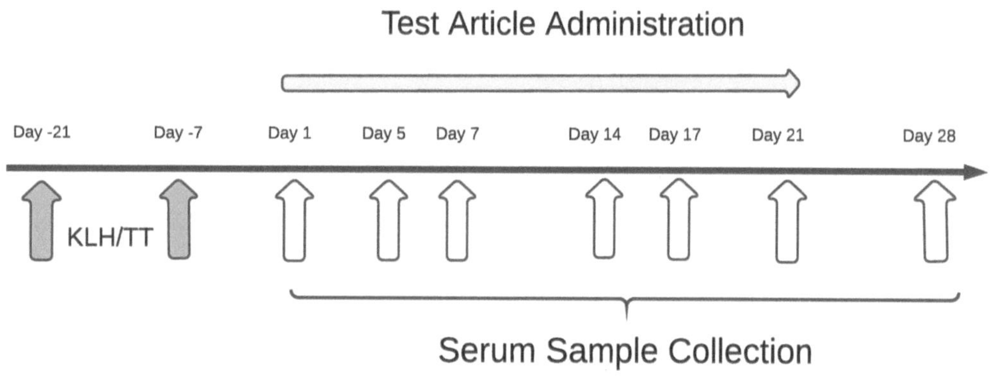

Test Article Administration

FIGURE 21.3 Hypothetical program for induction of TDAR in a 28-day NHP study: KLH/TT (Keyhole Limpet Hemocyanin/Tetanus Toxoid) is injected intramuscularly to induce TDAR in the animal. Following induction of TDAR and start of study with administration of the test article, serum samples are collected and assayed for antigen-specific IgG and IgM responses, which may be compared between control article and test article dosed animals.

(IHC) and digital image analysis applied for quantification. There are considerations that should be addressed in the protocol prior to initiation of DTH studies. Unlike TDAR, which requires only routine blood collection, the DTH assay requires surgical biopsy collection if data points are desired during the in-life phase, necessitating sedation and pain control for the animals. Ideally, the study design should incorporate skin collection at necropsy time points avoiding the need for in-life collection; however, collection time points are dictated by the study design and kinetics of the test article. The DTH response in the NHP occurs most robustly in the adipose-rich layers of the skin (e.g., subcutis/panniculus), so efforts to ensure these layers are included in the skin collection will improve assessment. There can be variation or "migration" of the challenge material through tissue within any given injection site; therefore, there should be ample space between the challenge sites to prevent overlap. Test articles, induction article, or other substances delivered via subcutaneous or dermal administration may induce inflammation and should be given in body regions other than the DTH challenge area to avoid confounding of histologic findings. For any given challenge site, serial sectioning of the skin is recommended to maximize capture of the full DTH response present; however, this approach may greatly increase the number of slides evaluated per challenge site. Diagnostic "drift" in nomenclature or severity grading of lesions is a potential issue (Crissman et al.,

2004; *Nomenclature and Diagnostic Resources in Anatomic Toxicologic Pathology*, Vol 1, Chap 25). To avoid "diagnostic drift," a suggested DTH challenge site scoring method based on a subjective five-point graded scale is presented (Figure 21.4). With serial sectioning of the skin, the severity grade for each challenge site may be an average of all the serial sections examined. Across study, the challenge sites versus dose levels and control animals may be compared to elucidate comparative test article–induced alterations in immune response (Table 21.2).

IMMUNE SENESCENCE As more of the human population survives to older ages, there is incentive to develop therapies that address immune senescence. The rhesus macaque undergoes immune senescence similar to humans (Jankovic et al., 2003). Physiologic thymic involution coincides with onset of sexual maturity in both humans and macaques (Snyder et al., 2016). Both humans and macaques experience age-related loss of naïve T-cells due to thymic involution and decreased lymphopoiesis with increased age. Increased turnover of naïve T-cells to memory T-cells in the aged primate further depletes the supply (Cicin-Sain et al., 2007). Along with the loss of naïve T-cells, there is increased frequency of T-cell–secreted interferon gamma and tumor necrosis factor alpha in aged macaques similar to that of humans (Messaoudi et al., 2011). With this knowledge, studies have been conducted to elucidate possible interventions in age-related immune senescence. For

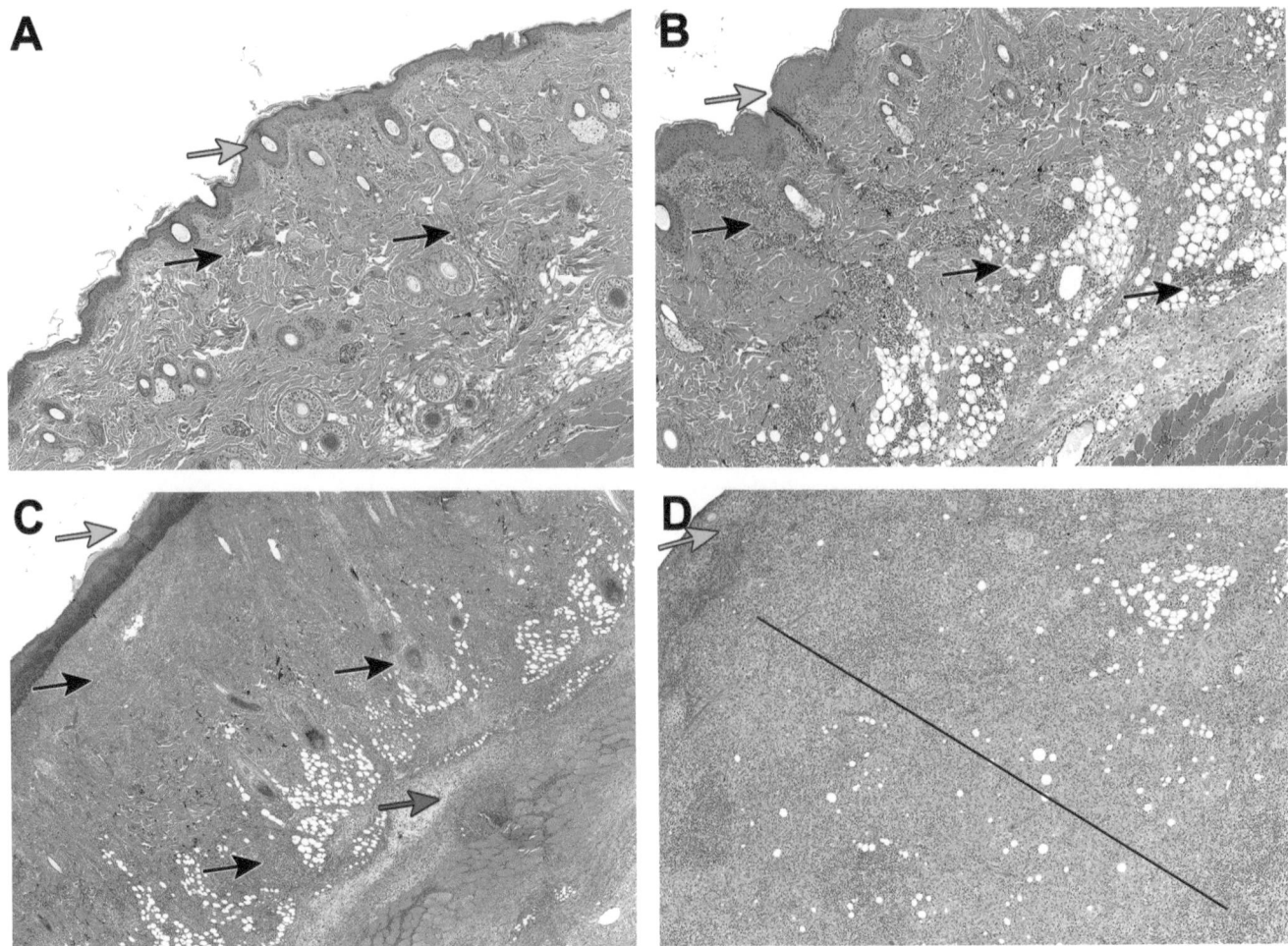

FIGURE 21.4 Delayed-type hypersensitivity (DTH) features in skin of a cynomolgus macaque. Grade 0: Normal skin without inflammation, not pictured. (A) Grade 1: Minimal perivascular inflammation of the subcutis and/or dermis is present but generally limited to scattered dermal vessels with small collections of perivascular inflammatory cells (black arrows). The inflammatory cells consist predominantly of mononuclear cells with fewer granulocytes. Minimal acanthosis and hyperkeratosis of the epidermis (green arrow) may be present, but the architecture is well preserved. (B) Grade 2: Mild perivascular inflammation of the subcutis and/or dermis is present with easily identifiable perivascular cuffs of inflammatory cells (black arrows) and limited infiltration into surrounding tissues and may also have inflammatory cell cuffing of adnexa and minimal to mild acanthosis and hyperkeratosis of the epidermis (green arrow). Ulceration is rarely present, and the architecture is well preserved. (C) Grade 3: Moderate perivascular inflammation of the subcutis and dermis is present. Consistently includes large collections of inflammatory cells that cuff and invade adnexa and multifocally replace or obscure adipose tissue (black arrows). The subcutis is consistently affected, commonly with small areas of effacement in the superficial muscle layer, may have minimal to mild edema, hemorrhage, and/or necrosis of the subcutis and/or dermis (red arrow), and may have minimal to moderate acanthosis and hyperkeratosis of the epidermis and ulceration may be present (green arrow). (D) Grade 4: Marked inflammation of the subcutis and/or dermis. The architecture is partially or completely effaced by the inflammation (black line), and may have minimal to marked edema, hemorrhage, and/or necrosis of the subcutis and/or dermis. Moderate acanthosis and hyperkeratosis of the epidermis and ulceration are common (green arrow); Hematoxylin and Eosin (H&E).

example, caloric restriction had been shown to have beneficial effects on immune senescence of several species, including rodents and yeast (Masoro, 2005), but there appears to be an age-specific timeframe for caloric restriction to have benefits in NHPs, application too early (juveniles) may lead to diminished immune response (Messaoudi et al., 2011).

TABLE 21.2 Example of Skin Section Grade Averaging for a Delayed-Type Hypersensitivity Study

Animal no.	Test article	Challenge material	Day of challenge	Day of skin collection	Challenge site	Serial section	Severity grade	Average severity grade/site
1001	PBS	Tub	Day 1	Day 3	1	1A	2	2.00
						1B	1	
						1C	3	
					2	2A	2	2.33
						2B	3	
						2C	2	
2001	Dex	Tub	Day 1	Day 3	1	1A	1	1.00
						1B	0	
						1C	2	
					2	2A	0	0.33
						2B	1	
						2C	0	

Example of grade averaging following induction of Delayed-Type Hypersensitivity (DTH) in NHPs. PBS (saline control article), Dex (dexamethasone) as an immunosuppressive test article. Tub (tuberculin) was utilized as the challenge material. In this example, the animals have two challenge sites. Animal 1 is administered PBS as a negative control article, while Animal 2 is administered an immunosuppressant agent (Dex) on Day 1 of the study. Each challenge site (site 1 and 2) is collected on Day 3, and then serial sectioned into three samples processed to three slides (A–C). Each site is evaluated for inflammation microscopically and assigned a severity grade based on a 5-point scale (normal = 0, minimal = 1, mild = 2, moderate = 3, marked = 4). Serial section grades may be averaged and compared between animals and test articles for the study.

6. BACKGROUND FINDINGS IN NONHUMAN PRIMATES AND USE OF HISTORICAL CONTROL DATA

6.1. Incidental Findings in Nonhuman Primates

Incidental (not commonly reported) or background findings (known to occur in the species) in NHPs commonly utilized in biomedical research have been the subject of multiple publications which have been compiled into "Spontaneous Pathology of the Laboratory Non-Human Primate," Bradley and Chilton, eds., (in press). Terminology associated with these findings in NHPs is currently being harmonized by the societies of toxicologic pathology's International Harmonization of Nomenclature and Diagnostic Criteria (INHAND) NHP working group, and will be accessible at https://www.toxpath.org/inhand.asp.

The most common incidental microscopic finding is the presence of small foci of mononuclear cell infiltrates within various organs (Figure 21.5). Extramedullary hematopoiesis in multiple organs is a common background finding in marmosets and may be exacerbated by blood sampling–induced anemia. Similar to the macaques, clinical pathology and background lesion data have been published for marmosets recently, but appropriate within-study controls are required (David et al., 2009; Kaspareit et al., 2006; Korte and Everitt, 2019; Kramer and Burns, 2019; Teng et al., 2018). Common incidental findings in NHPs rarely present an issue for interpretation of study data.

Findings which cause most distress when interpreting study results are those for which there is little or no published information. With low numbers of animals typically assigned to toxicity studies with NHPs, incidental findings of low frequency may not be represented in the control animal cohort. Some findings may be dismissed as incidental, "isolated" occurrences, without repetition in study animals, and considered unrelated to the test article. Other findings may be so rare that the occurrence in control animals is virtually unrecognized; therefore, it remains to be decided whether a test article–related effect was present. There are some findings in NHPs which do not currently appear in the literature. For example, rarely, cynomolgus

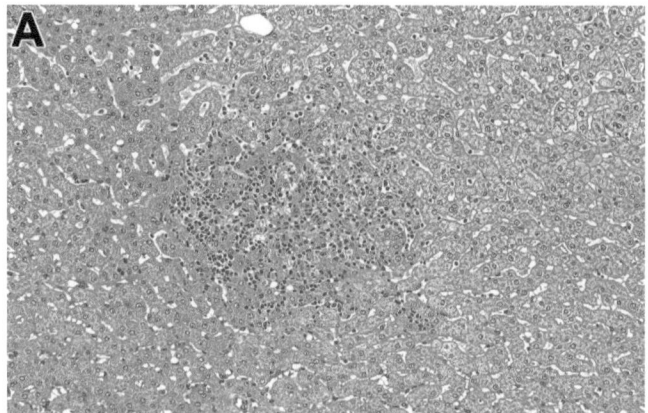

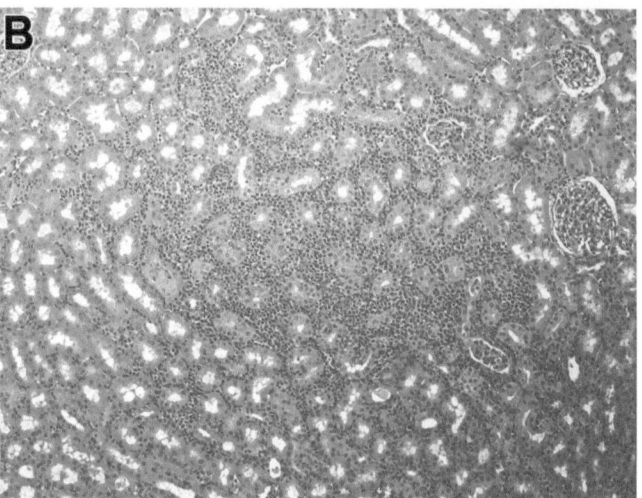

FIGURE 21.5 Mononuclear cell infiltrates, liver, and kidney. Mononuclear cell infiltrates are common background found in the liver (A) and kidney (B) of nonhuman primates. The infiltrates have little or no associated tissue disruption and are primarily interstitial in location; Hematoxylin and Eosin (H&E).

macaques may have infiltrates of large cells with abundant pale eosinophilic cytoplasm within the lamina propria of the colon or cecum, usually near the junction of the muscularis mucosa. The morphologic character of these cells is similar to that found in intestinal TB; therefore, they deserve careful evaluation in NHPs; similar cells are reported from human rectal or colon biopsies as "muciphages" (Azzopardi and Evans, 1966; DePetris and Leung, 2010). Similar to those in humans, the cells are negative with acid fast staining, variably positive for mucin with Periodic acid–Schiff staining, have abundant cytoplasmic vacuolation in electron micrographs, and are primarily confined to the large intestine (Figure 21.6), although the

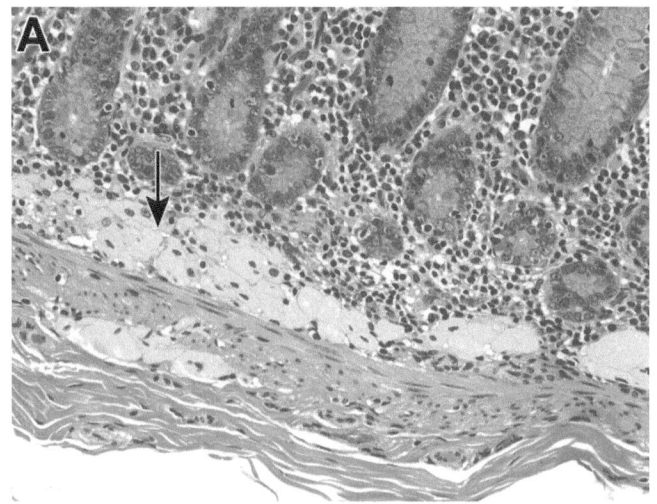

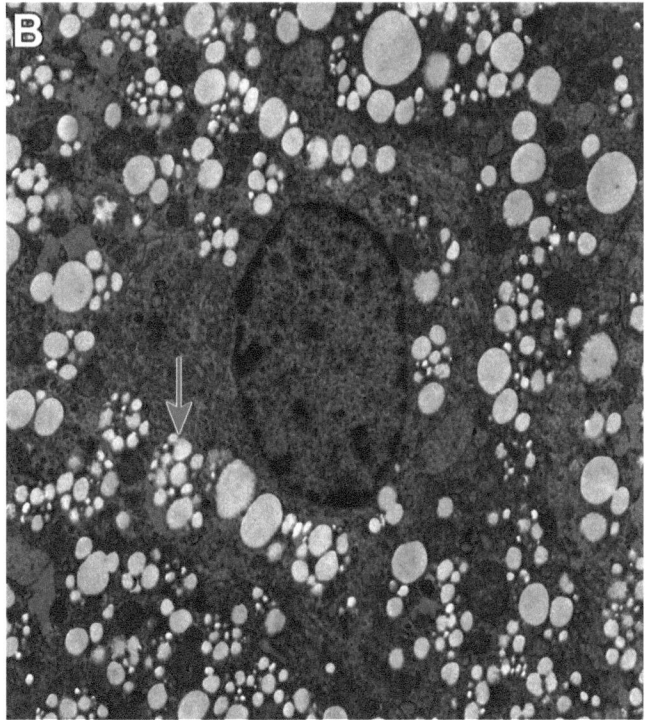

FIGURE 21.6 Muciphages in the colon of a nonhuman primate. (A) Muciphages (large, round to polygonal cells with abundant pale cytoplasm) within the cecal lamina propria and submucosa of a macaque (black arrow); Hematoxylin and Eosin (H&E). (B) Electron micrograph demonstrating cytoplasmic vacuoles (red arrow) of a muciphage. *Electron micrograph courtesy of Mersana Therapeutics.*

author has identified them rarely within the muscularis of the colon or cecum and in the mesenteric lymph node. These animals have negative TB tests.

Although there are no true background findings in clinical pathology parameters for NHPs,

there are variations between NHPs and other laboratory animals that result in changes that may be noted. For instance, macaques have increased central pallor of red cells, which results in a lower mean corpuscular hemoglobin concentration, and they have very broad and high ranges for total protein and globulin as compared to other laboratory animals. There may be changes in clinical pathology prestudy as compared to poststudy that are procedurally related. For example, increased creatine kinase activity due to minor muscle injury from injections and/or handling is exceptionally common among all NHPs (Hall and Everds, 2003).

6.2. Environmental, Endemic, and Contagious Pathogens

NHPs are generally not pathogen-free animals, and they are exposed to environmental conditions that may contain infectious agents. Zoonotic, endemic, environmental, parasitic, and contagious or food-borne diseases are all of concern for the health of NHP colonies and present challenges for the human caretaker (Sasseville and Mansfield, 2010). Old world monkeys (e.g., cynomolgus and rhesus macaques) may carry several diseases that are potentially communicable to humans. These include bacterial enteriditis such as *Shigella sp.* *and Salmonella sp.*, TB, and several viruses. Additionally, human diseases may be transmitted to immunosuppressed macaques and cause clinical observation findings that interfere with drug trials. Cases of Methicillin-resistant *Staphylococcus aureus* have been observed in young adult cynomolgus macaques with a case reported in an animal administered an anticancer therapeutic that developed immunosuppression and skin lesions. A similar presentation has been reported with Methicillin-resistant *Staphylococcus* non-*aureus* in a rhesus macaque (Kolappaswamy et al., 2008).

Macacine herpesvirus 1 (B-virus) is endemic in macaques and is a particular concern, as zoonotic human infections may be fatal if treatment is not instituted promptly after exposure (Hobson, 2000; Rohman, 2016). The common marmoset is exceptional for its freedom from zoonotic agents such as *Herpesvirus simiae* (B-virus). Old and new world primates are susceptible to diseases transmitted from humans, including TB and measles virus (Jones-Engel et al., 2006). Outbreaks of measles in NHP colonies can cause severe morbidity and mortality in addition to long-lasting effects on the immune system that would significantly affect experimental outcomes (Auwaerter et al., 1999; Christe et al., 2019).

NHPs are not immune to environmental pathogens, particularly bacterial and fungal organisms. Commonly reported environmental fungal diseases include coccidioidomycosis and aspergillosis, but new entities are reported on occasion, such as talaromycosis reported in 2018 (Iverson et al., 2018). It should be noted that some acid-fast, environmental pathogens may mimic TB in macaques with granulomatous lymphadenitis and acid-fast positive bacteria in tissue. These animals will continue to have negative TB skin tests because the environmental forms do not share the tuberculin antigen. Negative TB status should be confirmed in these animals (e.g., with PCR or other appropriate diagnostic method). Additionally, food-borne illnesses may occasionally be encountered, such as hepatitis A from contaminated produce (Figure 21.7). Careful attention to biosecurity by means of appropriate quarantine, screening, monitoring, treatment, and vaccination is essential in NHP colonies.

While parasites are generally kept under control in NHPs through the routine use of anti-parasitic drugs, they often remain present at low levels, and have potential to become a significant threat to the animal's health under certain conditions or the influence of some test articles. For example, *Balantidium coli* is an exceptionally common protozoal parasite of the NHP colon and cecum, surviving in the lumen by feeding off intestinal content. NHPs with a large burden of these parasites may have mild signs of diarrhea or may be completely asymptomatic. But with the administration of immunosuppressants or mucosal damaging agents, or under stressful conditions, the parasites may become opportunistically invasive, burrowing through the compromised intestinal mucosa, or in some cases, becoming transmural, leading to morbidity and mortality.

6.3. Findings due to Antidrug Antibodies

The development of antidrug antibodies (ADAs) is exceptionally common when biologics

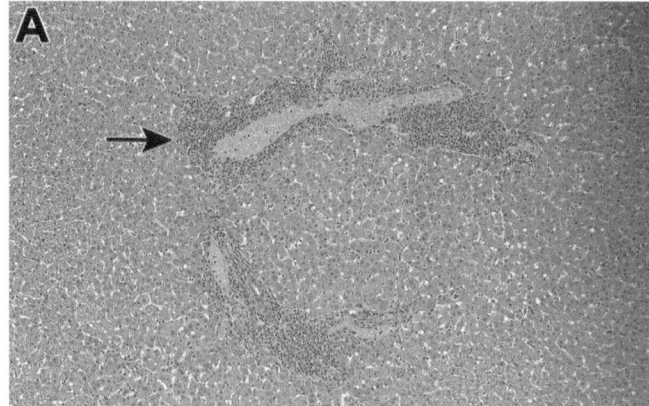

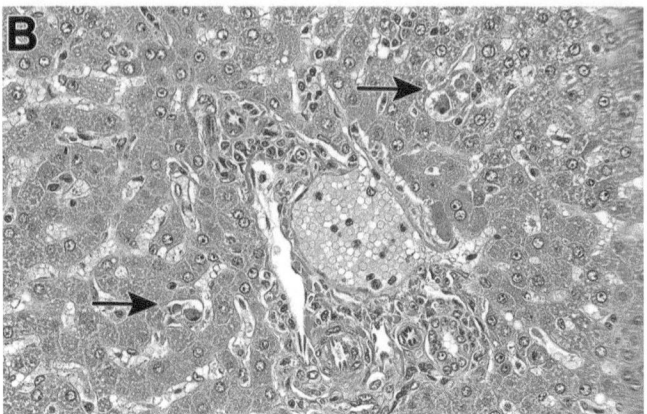

FIGURE 21.7   A case of food-borne viral hepatitis A infection in the liver of a cynomolgus macaque. (A) Viral hepatitis A infection is characterized by portal infiltrates of mononuclear and polymorphonuclear cells (black arrow) and (B) scattered apoptotic cells (Councilman bodies, black arrows); Hematoxylin and Eosin (H&E).

are administered to NHPs but may occur with the administration of nearly any foreign protein. ADAs are associated with hypersensitivity responses such as acute infusion reactions, which are not uncommonly reported in NHPs. Most mild acute hypersensitivity reactions can be managed clinically; however, more severe cases may be life threatening or require euthanasia. Immune complex (IC) formation with tissue deposition may occur due to ADA, leading to cytokine release and vascular injury. Microscopically, there may be findings in vascular tissues with ADA-associated IC deposition, but these should be differentiated from spontaneous changes that might occur in macaques, occasionally referred to as "Polyarteritis Nodosa" (Porter et al., 2003) (Figure 21.8). IC deposition may be

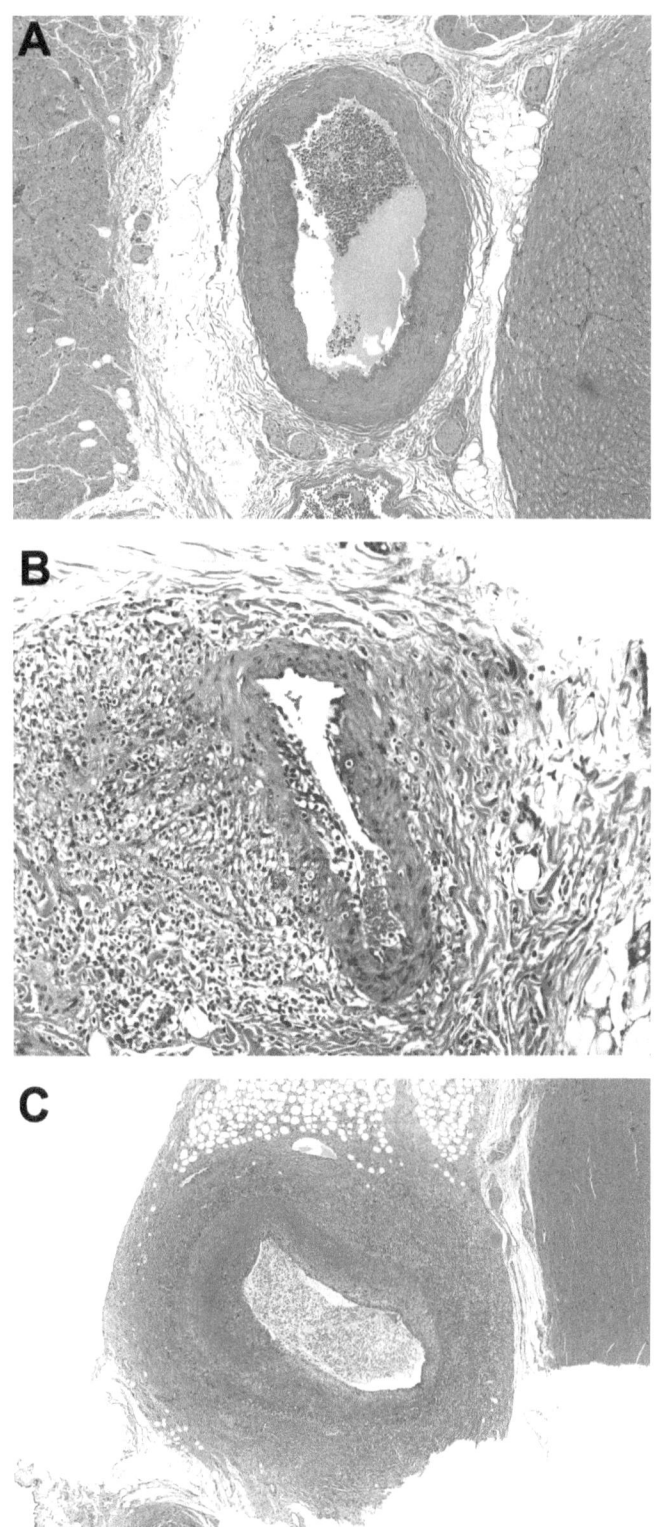

FIGURE 21.8 Examples of inflammation in arteries of cynomolgus macaques. (A) Normal coronary artery. (B) Spontaneous coronary artery inflammation, referred to as "polyarteritis nodosa" in a control animal administered PBS (saline) and (C) coronary artery inflammation with intimal proliferation due to immune complex (IC) deposition following test article–associated, antidrug antibody (ADA) development; Hematoxylin and Eosin (H&E).

demonstrated by IHC (Leach et al., 2014; Rojko, 2014). ADA responses in NHPs due to foreign protein immunogenicity are poorly predictive of similar outcomes in humans (Leach, 2013; Leach et al., 2014; *Protein Pharmaceutical Agents, Vol 2, Chap 6*).

6.4. Historical Control Data

The use of concurrent control animals for the assessment of test article–induced changes is standard practice; however, with the generally low number of animals assigned to NHP studies, concurrent controls may not completely reflect incidental or background findings for the species (Long and Hardisty, 2012). Additionally, investigative and non-GLP studies may not have any control animals. In order to supplement information gleaned from concurrent controls or supply data for studies without controls, historical control data (HCD) is often employed. HCD is not without flaws and should be used appropriately (see *Practices to Optimize Generation, Interpretation, and Reporting of Pathology Data from Toxicity Studies*, Vol 1, Chap 28). The recording of incidental findings may be variable, based on the experience and decision of the recorder, which may influence incidence rate and proportion of findings in the HCD at any given facility. The incidence rate of some common findings of NHPs may not be accurately reflected in HCD because many pathologists may not record them. Examples include parasites, such as *Trichuris* sp. (whipworm) in the large intestine, and congenital findings such as ectopic thymus within the thyroid gland. Bergmeister's papilla (remnant of the hyaloid artery) is reported as the most common congenital finding of the optic nerve head in cynomolgus monkeys from Mauritius (Denk et al., 2020) but was unaccounted for in an HCD search of 748 Mauritius animals from the author's database (Figure 21.9). Additionally, exceptionally rare incidental findings may not be reflected in HCD unless very large numbers of animals are available for survey.

A common morphology of "degeneration" in HCD is not defined but commonly applied to some NHP tissues. For example, a diagnosis of "degeneration" is not uncommon for the heart of NHPs. It is not clear from this diagnosis what specific finding was encountered and "degeneration" might apply to a variety of changes, including cardiomyocyte atrophy or hypertrophy, individual cell necrosis, fibrosis, fatty infiltration, cellular vacuolation, or a combination of these changes which may be similar to that of spontaneous cardiomyopathy of macaques (Konishi et al., 2018) (Figure 21.10,

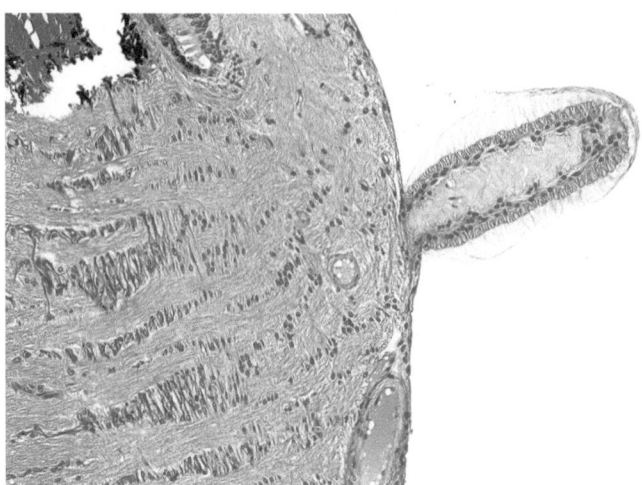

FIGURE 21.9 Bergmeister's papilla in the eye of a cynomolgus macaque (Mauritius sourced). A remnant of the hyaloid artery of the eye, "Bergmeister's papilla," on the optic nerve head; Hematoxylin and Eosin (H&E).

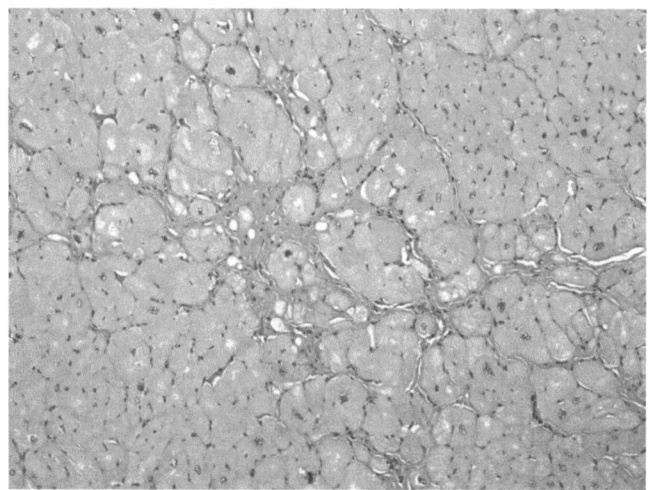

FIGURE 21.10 Cardiomyopathy in a cynomolgus macaque. Spontaneous degeneration of the myocardium, or "cardiomyopathy" characterized by cardiomyocyte disarray and karyomegaly with cytoplasmic pallor, vacuolization of the perimysial connective tissue and fibrosis that effaces and replaces cardiomyocytes; Hematoxylin and Eosin (H&E).

TABLE 21.3   Incidence of Cardiac Degeneration in Cynomolgus Macaques

	Female			Male		
	Age of animal (years)			Age of animal (years)		
	≤2.4	2.5–3.5	≥3.6	≤2.4	2.5–3.5	≥3.6
DIAGNOSIS						
Degeneration	–	4	3	–	4	3
Necrosis	–	1	–	–	–	–
Degeneration/necrosis	–	–	–	–	–	2
Karyomegaly	–	–	–	–	–	2
Number of positive recordings	0	5	3	0	4	7
Number of animals examined by sex/age	0	167	144	6	176	132

Total number of males examined = 314

Total number of females examined = 311

Total number of animals examined = 625

Incidence of cardiac degenerative findings in cynomolgus macaques of Chinese origin. Lesions are separated into three age ranges. Data collected September 15, 2020, Charles River Labs Nevada Historical Control Database.

Table 21.3). With the advent of guidance documents being developed by the INHAND nonrodent working groups, NHP nomenclature entered into the HCD should become standardized over time, replacing the myriad of terms in the database; currently, the guidance document for NHPs is available at www.GoRENI. org and will soon be published and publicly available at toxpath.org (see *Nomenclature and Diagnostic Resources in Anatomic Toxicologic Pathology*, Vol 1, Chap 25). Thresholds for lymphoid content of the spleen and lymph nodes can be highly subjective based on the pathologist's experience and are best compared to concurrent controls if possible. Additionally, HCD use should take into consideration the age of the animals because age-related changes may inappropriately skew the data as applied to the finding of concern.

Despite some drawbacks, HCD remains a powerful tool for assessing findings that occur in NHPs assigned to toxicologic studies. Ultimately, HCD should be conjoined with a "weight-of-evidence" approach and peer review scrutiny for interpretation of findings.

7. CONCLUSION

As the closest phylogenic relative to humans, NHPs are an invaluable research resource providing a means of investigating disease pathogenesis and treatment. Therefore, the number of NHPs associated with biomedical research has increased in recent years. But the contribution of NHPs to human medical advances comes with great responsibility on the part of investigators and caretakers. Caring for these intelligent and sensitive animals means providing the absolute best conditions and supplying them with an environment that is beyond their basic needs in captivity. In return, they are the key to many of the biomedical discoveries today. It is a relationship that will likely be working for many years to come.

REFERENCES

Abbott DH, Barnett DK, Colman RJ, Yamamoto ME, Schultz-Darken NJ: Aspects of common marmoset basic biology and life history important for biomedical research, *Comp Med* 53(4):339–350, 2003.

Abee CR: Squirrel monkey (Saimiri spp.) research and resources, *ILAR J* 41(1):2–9, 2000.

Abee CR, Mansfield K, Tardif S, Morris T. *Nonhuman Primates in Biomedical Research*, 2012, Elsevier.

Albert MS: Memory decline: the boundary between aging and the age-related disease, *Neurol* 51(3):282–284, 2002.

Anderson R: *Cebus apella* (On-line). 2003, Animal Diversity Web, https://animaldiversity.org/accounts/Cebus_apella/. (Accessed 5 September 2020).

Antony J, MacDonald K: A critical analysis of the cynomolgus macaque, *Macaca fascicularis*, as a model to test HIV-1/SIV vaccine efficacy, *Vaccine* 33(27):3073–3083, 2015.

Authier Simon, et al.: EEG: Characteristics of drug-induced seizures in rats, dogs and non-human primates, *Journal of Pharmacological and Toxicological Methods* 97:52–58, 2019.

Auwaerter PG, Rota PA, Elkins WR, Adams RJ, DeLozier T, Shi Y, Bellini WJ, Murphy BR, Griffin DE: Measles virus infection in rhesus macaques: altered immune responses and comparison of the virulence of six different virus strains, *J Infect Dis* 180(4):950–958, 1999.

Azzopardi JG, Evans DJ: Mucoprotein-containing histiocytes (muciphages) in the rectum, *J Clin Pathol* 19(4):368–374, 1966.

Bading JR, Yamada S, Mackic JB, Kirkman L, Miller C, Calero M, Ghiso J, Frangione B, Zlokovic BV: Brain clearance of Alzheimer's amyloid-beta40 in the squirrel monkey: a SPECT study in a primate model of cerebral amyloid angiopathy, *J Drug Target* 10(4):359–368, 2002.

Bailey J, Thew M, Balls M: An analysis of the use of animal models in predicting human toxicology and drug safety, *Altern Lab Anim* 42(3):181–199, 2014.

Baker HF, Ridley RM, Duchen LW, Crow TJ: Evidence for the experimental transmission of cerebral beta-amyloidosis to primates, *Int J Exp Pathol* 74(5):441–454, 1993.

Bassett Leanne, et al.: Telemetry video-electroencephalography (EEG) in rats, dogs and non-human primates: methods in follow-up safety pharmacology seizure liability assessments, *Journal of Pharmacological Toxicoligic Methods* 70:230–240, 2014.

Bauer C: The baboon (Papio sp.) as a model for female reproduction studies, *Contraception* 92(2):120–123, 2015.

Beal MF, Kowall NW, Ellison DW, Mazurek MF, Swartz KJ, Martin JB: Replication of the neurochemical characteristics of Huntington's disease by quinolinic acid, *Nature* 321(6066):168–171, 1986.

Bennett RS, Huzella LM, Jahrling PB, Bollinger L, Olinger GG, Hensley LE: Nonhuman primate models of Ebola virus disease, *Curr Top Microbiol Immunol* 411:171–193, 2017.

Bimber BN, Moreland AJ, Wiseman RW, Hughes AL, O'Connor DH: Complete characterization of killer Ig-like receptor (KIR) haplotypes in Mauritian cynomolgus macaques: novel insights into nonhuman primate KIR gene content and organization, *J Immunol* 181(9):6301–6308, 2008.

Blancher A, Bonhomme M, Crouau-Roy B, Terao K, Kitano T, Saitou N: Mitochondrial DNA sequence phylogeny of 4 populations of the widely distributed cynomolgus macaque (*Macaca fascicularis* fascicularis), *J Hered* 99(3):254–264, 2008.

Bleavins R, A de la Iglesia F: Cynomolgus monkeys (*Macaca fascicularis*) in preclinical immune function safety testing: development of a delayed-type hypersensitivity procedure, *Toxicology* 95:103–112, 1995.

Bonadio C: *Macaca fascicularis* (On-line). 2000, Animal Diversity Web, https://animaldiversity.org/accounts/Macaca_fascicularis/. (Accessed 17 September 2020).

Bonhomme M, Blancher A, Cuartero S, Chikhi L, Crouau-Roy B: Origin and number of founders in an introduced insular primate: estimation from nuclear genetic data, *Mol Ecol* 17(4):1009–1019, 2008.

Bouchez C, Gervais F, Fleurance R, Palate B, Legrand JJ, Descotes J: Development of a delayed-type hypersensitivity (DTH) model in the cynomolgus monkey, *J Toxicol Pathol* 25(2):183–188, 2012.

Brady AG, Watford JW, Massey CV, Rodning KJ, Gibson SV, Williams LE, Abee CR: Studies of heart disease and failure in aged female squirrel monkeys (Saimiri sp.), *Comp Med* 53(6):657–662, 2003.

Burbacher TM, Grant KS: Nonhuman primates as animal models for toxicology research, *Curr Protoc Toxicol*, 2001, https://doi.org/10.1002/0471140856.tx0101s00. Chapter 1.

Burns LH, Pakzaban P, Deacon TW, Brownell AL, Tatter SB, Jenkins BG, Isacson O: Selective putaminal excitotoxic lesions in non-human primates model the movement disorder of Huntington disease, *Neuroscience* 64(4):1007–1017, 1995.

Caldwell R, Guirguis M, Kornbrust E: Evaluation of various keyhole limpet hemocyanin dosing regimens for the cynomolgus monkey TDAR assay, *Toxicologist*, 2007. Abstract #1723.

Carrion R, Patterson JL: An animal model that reflects human disease: the common marmoset (*Callithrix jacchus*), *Curr Opin Virol* 2(3):357–362, 2012.

Cawthon Lang KA: *Primate factsheets*, 2005–2006. http://pin.primate.wisc.edu/factsheets. (Accessed 29 October 2020).

Chamanza R, Parry NM, Rogerson P, Nicol JR, Bradley AE: Spontaneous lesions of the cardiovascular system in purpose-bred laboratory nonhuman primates, *Toxicol Pathol* 34(4):357–363, 2006.

Champoux M, Higley JD, Suomi SJ: Behavioral and physiological characteristics of Indian and Chinese-Indian hybrid rhesus macaque infants, *Dev Psychobiol* 31(1):49–63, 1997.

Choi K, Chang J, Lee MJ, Wang S, In K, Galano-Tan WC, Jun S, Cho K, Hwang YH, Kim SJ, Park W: Reference values of hematology, biochemistry, and blood type in cynomolgus monkeys from Cambodia origin, *Lab Anim Res* 32(1):46–55, 2016.

Christe KL, Salyards GW, Houghton SD, Ardeshir A, Yee JL: Modified dose efficacy trial of a canine distemper-measles vaccine for use in rhesus macaques, *J Am Assoc Lab Anim Sci* 58(3):397–405, 2019.

Cicin-Sain L, Messaoudi I, Park B, Currier N, Planer S, Fischer M, Tackitt S, Nikolich-Zugich D, Legasse A, Axthelm MK, Picker LJ, Mori M, Nikolich-Zugich J: Dramatic increase in naive T cell turnover is linked to loss of naive T cells from old primates, *Proc Natl Acad Sci U S A* 104(50):19960–19965, 2007.

Clapp NK: *A Primate model for the study of colitis and colonic carcinoma : the cotton-top tamarin* (Saguinus oedipus*), Boca Raton, 1993, CRC Press.

Clark M: Prediction of clinical risks by analysis of preclinical and clinical adverse events, *J Biomed Inf* 54:167–173, 2015.

Clarke MR, O'Neil JA: Morphometric comparison of Chinese-origin and Indian-derived rhesus monkeys (*Macaca mulatta*), *Am J Primatol* 47(4):335–346, 1999.

Clarke M, Steger-Hartmann T: A big data approach to the concordance of the toxicity of pharmaceuticals in animals and humans, *Regul Toxicol Pharmacol* 96:94–105, 2018.

Corton JC, Peters JM, Klaunig JE: The PPARα-dependent rodent liver tumor response is not relevant to humans: addressing misconceptions, *Arch Toxicol* 92(1):83–119, 2018.

Cover S: *Callithrix jacchus* (On-line). 2000, Animal Diversity Web, https://animaldiversity.org/accounts/Callithrix_jacchus/. (Accessed 17 September 2020).

Cox LA, Comuzzie AG, Havill LM, Karere GM, Spradling KD, Mahaney MC, Nathanielsz PW, Nicolella DP, Shade RE, Voruganti S, VandeBerg JL: Baboons as a model to study genetics and epigenetics of human disease, *ILAR J* 54(2): 106–121, 2013.

Crissman JW, Goodman DG, Hildebrandt PK, Maronpot RR, Prater DA, Riley JH, Seaman WJ, Thake DC: Best practices guideline: toxicologic histopathology, *Toxicol Pathol* 32(1): 126–131, 2004.

David JM, Dick EJ, Hubbard GB: Spontaneous pathology of the common marmoset (*Callithrix jacchus*) and tamarins (*Saguinus oedipus, Saguinus mystax*), *J Med Primatol* 38(5): 347–359, 2009.

Day GQ, Ng J, Oldt RF, Houghton PW, Smith DG, Kanthaswamy S: DNA-based determination of ancestry in cynomolgus macaques, *J Am Assoc Lab Anim Sci* 57(5):432–442, 2018.

Denk N, Maloca PM, Steiner G, et al.: Retinal features in cynomolgus macaques (*Macaca fascicularis*) assessed by using scanning laser ophthalmoscopy and spectral domain optical coherence tomography, *Comp Med* 70(2):145–151, 2020. https://doi.org/10.30802/AALAS-CM-19-000088.

Derakhchan K, Chui RW, Stevens D, Gu W, Vargas HM: Detection of QTc interval prolongation using jacket telemetry in conscious non-human primates: comparison with implanted telemetry, *Br J Pharmacol* 171(2):509–522, 2014.

De Petris G, Leung ST: Pseudoneoplasms of the gastrointestinal tract, *Arch Pathol Lab Med* 134(3):378–392, 2010.

de Souza AB, Rodrigues RPS, Pessoa GT, da Silva AB, Moura LS, Sousa FC, da Silva EG, Diniz AN, Barbosa MA, Araújo JR, Santos IC, Guerra PC, Alves JJ, Macedo KV, Diniz BL, Marques DC, Alves FR: Standard electrocardiographic data from capuchin monkeys, *J Am Assoc Lab Anim Sci* 57(1):13–17, 2018.

Debien E, Wilcox A, Reim D, Bulera S: *Interchangeability of mainland Southeast Asian sourced non-human primates and comparitive pathology, clinical pathology, and immunology data from the main sources of non-human primates*, 2019, Charles River Laboratories International, Inc.

Diamond EJ, Aksel S, Hazelton JM, Jennings RA, Abee CR: Seasonal changes of serum concentrations of estradiol and progesterone in Bolivian squirrel monkeys (*Saimiri sciureus*), *Am J Primatol* 6(2):103–113, 1984.

Dowd KA, Ko SY, Morabito KM, Yang ES, Pelc RS, DeMaso CR, Castilho LR, Abbink P, Boyd M, Nityanandam R, Gordon DN, Gallagher JR, Chen X, Todd JP, Tsybovsky Y, Harris A, Huang YS, Higgs S, Vanlandingham DL, Andersen H, Lewis MG, De La Barrera R, Eckels KH, Jarman RG, Nason MC, Barouch DH, Roederer M, Kong WP, Mascola JR, Pierson TC, Graham BS: Rapid development of a DNA vaccine for Zika virus, *Science* 354(6309):237–240, 2016.

Dudley DM, Aliota MT, Mohr EL, Newman CM, Golos TG, Friedrich TC, O'Connor DH: Using macaques to address critical questions in Zika virus research, *Annu Rev Virol* 6(1):481–500, 2019.

Ebeling M, Küng E, See A, Broger C, Steiner G, Berrera M, Heckel T, Iniguez L, Albert T, Schmucki R, Biller H, Singer T, Certa U: Genome-based analysis of the nonhuman primate *Macaca fascicularis* as a model for drug safety assessment, *Genome Res* 21(10):1746–1756, 2011.

Emborg ME: Nonhuman primate models of Parkinson's disease, *ILAR J* 48(4):339–355, 2007.

Emborg ME: Nonhuman primate models of neurodegenerative disorders, *ILAR J* 58(2):190–201, 2017.

Estes JD, Wong SW, Brenchley JM: Nonhuman primate models of human viral infections, *Nat Rev Immunol* 18(6):390–404, 2018.

Fa JE, Lindburg DG: *Evolution and ecology of macaque societies*, Cambridge; New York, 1996, Cambridge University Press.

Feister AJ, DiPietrantonio A, Yuenger J, Ireland K, Rao A: *Nonhuman primate evaluation and analysis part 1: analysis of future demand and supply*, 2018, National Institutes of Health Office of Research Infrastructure Programs.

Fleagle JG: *Primate adaptation and evolution*, San Diego, CA, 2013, Elsevier/AP.

Flurer CI, Kern M, Rambeck WA, Zucker H: Ascorbic acid requirement and assessment of ascorbate status in the common marmoset (*Callithrix jacchus*), *Ann Nutr Metab* 31(4):245–252, 1987.

Flurer CI, Zucker H: Ascorbic acid in a new world monkey family: species difference and influence of stressors on ascorbic acid metabolism, *Z Ernahrungswiss* 28(1):49–55, 1989.

Food and Drug Administration: *HHS. International conference on harmonization; S6 (R1) preclinical safety evaluation of biotechnology-derived pharmaceuticals*, May 2012.

Food and Drug Administration: *HHS. International conference on harmonization; guidance on Q 11 development and manufacture of drug substances*, November 2012.

Fooden J: Systematic review of the rhesus macaque, *Macaca mulatta* (Zimmermann, 1780), *Fieldiana Zool* 96, 2000.

Fox JG: *The common marmoset in captivity and biomedical research*, London, United Kingdom ; San Diego, CA, 2019, Academic Press, an imprint of Elsevier.

Friedman H, Ator N, Haigwood N, Newsome W, Allan JS, Golos TG, Kordower JH, Shade RE, Goldberg ME, Bailey MR, Bianchi P: The critical role OF nonhuman primates in medical research, *Pathog Immun* 2(3):352–365, 2017.

From the cradle to the grave, Amboseli Baboon Research Project University of Notre Dame copyright © 2020 University of Notre DameNotre Dame, IN 46556. https://amboselibaboons.nd.edu/about-baboons/from-the-cradle-to-the-grave/. (Accessed 8 August 2020).

Galland GG: Role of the squirrel monkey in parasitic disease research, *ILAR J* 41(1):37–43, 2000.

Getz BS, Reardon CA: Animal models of atherosclerosis, *Arterioscler Thromb Vasc Biol* 32(5):1104–1115, 2012.

Gao CE, Song Q, Zhang M, Li J, Miao Y, Li Z, Dong J: Generation, ex vivo expansion and safety of engineered PD1-knockout primary T cells from cynomolgus macaques, *Mol Immunol* 124:100–108, 2020 Aug.

Ghosh M, Hutz RJ, Dukelow WR: Serum estradiol 17 beta, progesterone, and relative luteinizing hormone levels in *Saimiri sciureus*: cyclic variations and the effect of laparoscopy and follicular aspiration, *J Med Primatol* 11(5):312–318, 1982.

Grizzanti J, Lee HG, Camins A, Pallas M, Casadesus G: The therapeutic potential of metabolic hormones in the treatment of age-related cognitive decline and Alzheimer's disease, *Nutr Res* 36(12):1305–13015, 2016.

Grimm D: U.S. labs using a record number of monkeys, *Science* 362(6415):630, 2018.

Groves C: The taxonomy of primates in the laboratory context. In Wolfe-Coote S, editor: *The laboratory primate*, 2005, Elsevier Academic Press.

Guidance for industry, M3 (R2) nonclinical safety studies for the conduct of human clinical trials and marketing authorization for pharmaceuticals, 2010 https://www.fda.gov/regulatory-information/search-fda-guidance-documents/m3r2-non clinical-safety-studies-conduct-human-clinical-trials-and-marketing-authorization. (Accessed 4 November 2020).

Guidance for industry, S7A safety pharmacology studies for human pharmaceuticals, 2001 https://www.fda.gov/regulatory-information/search-fda-guidance-documents/s7a-safety-pharmacology-studies-human-pharmaceuticals. (Accessed 4 November 2020).

Gurung S, Preno AN, Dubaut JP, Nadeau H, Hyatt K, Reuter N, Nehete B, Wolf RF, Nehete P, Dittmer DP,

Myers DA, Papin JF: Translational model of Zika virus disease in baboons, *J Virol* 92(16), 2018.

Gysin J, Dubois P, Pereira da Silva L: Protective antibodies against erythrocytic stages of Plasmodium falciparum in experimental infection of the squirrel monkey, *Saimiri sciureus, Parasite Immunol* 4(6):421–430, 1982.

Gysin J, Hommel M, da Silva LP: Experimental infection of the squirrel monkey (*Saimiri sciureus*) with Plasmodium falciparum, *J Parasitol* 66(6):1003–1009, 1980.

Haggerty HG: Immunotoxicity testing in non-rodent species, *J Immunotoxicol* 4(2):165–169, 2007.

Haj AK, Arbanas JM, Yamniuk AP, Karl JA, Bussan HE, Drinkwater KY, Graham ME, Ericsen AJ, Prall TM, Moore K, Cheng L, Gao M, Graziano RF, Loffredo JT, Wiseman RW, O'Connor DH: Characterization of Mauritian cynomolgus macaque FcγR alleles using long-read sequencing, *J Immunol* 202(1):151–159, 2019.

Hall RL, Everds NE: Factors affecting the interpretation of canine and nonhuman primate clinical pathology, *Toxicol Pathol* 31, 2003.

Harihara S, Saitou N, Hirai M, Aoto N, Terao K, Cho F, Honjo S, Omoto K: Differentiation of mitochondrial DNA types in *Macaca fascicularis, Primates* 29:117–127, 1988.

Higham JP, Semple S, MacLarnon A, Heistermann M, Ross C: Female reproductive signaling, and male mating behavior, in the olive baboon, *Horm Behav* 55(1):60–67, 2009.

Hobson W: Safety assessment studies in nonhuman primates, *Int J Toxicol* 19(2):141–147, 2000.

Hoffmann P, Martin L, Keselica M, Gunson D, Skuba E, Lapadula D, Hayes M, Bentley P, Busch S: Acute toxicity of vildagliptin, *Toxicol Pathol* 45(1):76–83, 2017.

Huss MK, Ikeno F, Buckmaster CL, Albertelli MA: Echocardiographic and electrocardiographic characteristics of male and female squirrel monkeys (Saimiri spp.), *J Am Assoc Lab Anim Sci* 54(1):25–28, 2015.

International harmonization of nomenclature and diagnostic criteria (INHAND) on-line access. https://www.toxpath.org/inhand.asp. (Accessed 4 November 2020).

Integrated taxonomic information system on-line database, http://www.itis.gov.

Iverson WO, Karanth S, Wilcox A, Pham CD, Lockhart SR, Nicholson SM: Talaromycosis (Penicilliosis) in a cynomolgus macaque, *Vet Pathol* 55(4):591–594, 2018.

Jackson BF, Engelhardt JM: *The FDA regulatory landscape for covid-19 treatment and vaccine (updated)*, 2020. https://www.biologicsblog.com/the-fda-regulatory-landscape-for-covid-19-treatments-and-vaccine. (Accessed 15 November 2020).

Jasien JV, Samuels BC, Johnston JM, Downs JC: Diurnal cycle of translaminar pressure in nonhuman primates quantified with continuous wireless telemetry, *Invest Ophthalmol Vis Sci* 61(2):37, 2020.

Janković V, Messaoudi I, Nikolich-Zugich J: Phenotypic and functional T-cell aging in rhesus macaques (*Macaca mulatta*): differential behavior of CD4 and CD8 subsets, *Blood* 102(9):3244–3251, 2003.

Jasinska AJ, Schmitt CA, Service SK, Cantor RM, Dewar K, Jentsch JD, Kaplan JR, Turner TR, Warren WC, Weinstock GM, Woods RP, Freimer NB: Systems biology of the vervet monkey, *ILAR J* 54(2):122–143, 2013.

Jasinska AJ, Service S, Levinson M, Slaten E, Lee O, Sobel E, Fairbanks LA, Bailey JN, Jorgensen MJ, Breidenthal SE, Dewar K, Hudson TJ, Palmour R, Freimer NB, Ophoff RA: A genetic linkage map of the vervet monkey (*Chlorocebus aethiops* sabaeus), *Mamm Genome* 18(5):347–360, 2007.

Jenson HB, Ench Y, Gao SJ, Rice K, Carey D, Kennedy RC, Arrand JR, Mackett M: Epidemiology of herpesvirus papio infection in a large captive baboon colony: similarities to Epstein-Barr virus infection in humans, *J Infect Dis* 181(4): 1462–1466, 2000.

Johansen MD, Irving A, Montagutelli X, Tate MD, Rudloff I, Nold MF, Hansbro NG, Kim RY, Donovan C, Liu G, Faiz A, Short KR, Lyons JG, McCaughan GW, Gorrell MD, Cole A, Moreno C, Couteur D, Hesselson D, Triccas J, Neely GG, Gamble JR, Simpson SJ, Saunders BM, Oliver BG, Britton WJ, Wark PA, Nold-Petry CA, Hansbro PM: Animal and translational models of SARS-CoV-2 infection and COVID-19, *Mucosal Immunol* 13(6): 877–891, 2020.

Johnsen DO, Johnson DK, Whitney RA: History of the use of nonhuman primates in biomedical research. In Abee CR, Mansfield K, Tardif S, Morris T, editors: *Nonhuman Primates in Biomedical Research*, vol. 1. 2012, Elsevier.

Jolly CJ: A proper study for mankind: analogies from the Papionin monkeys and their implications for human evolution, *Am J Phys Anthropol* (Suppl 33):177–204, 2001.

Jolly CJ, Burrell AS, Phillips-Conroy JE, Bergey C, Rogers J: Kinda baboons (Papio kindae) and grayfoot chacma baboons (*P. ursinus* griseipes) hybridize in the Kafue river valley, Zambia, *Am J Primatol* 73(3):291–303, 2011.

Jones-Engel L, Engel GA, Schillaci MA, Lee B, Heidrich J, Chalise M, Kyes RC: Considering human-primate transmission of measles virus through the prism of risk analysis, *Am J Primatol* 68(9):868–879, 2006.

Kanthaswamy S, Gill L, Satkoski J, Goyal V, Malladi V, Kou A, Basuta K, Sarkisyan L, George D, Smith DG: Development of a Chinese-Indian hybrid (Chindian) rhesus macaque colony at the California national primate research center by introgression, *J Med Primatol* 38(2):86–96, 2009.

Kanthaswamy S, Reader R, Tarara R, Oslund K, Allen M, Ng J, Grinberg C, Hyde D, Glenn DG, Lerche N: Large scale pedigree analysis leads to evidence for founder effects of hypertrophic cardiomyopathy in rhesus macaques, *J Med Primatol* 43(4):288–291, 2014.

Kapusinszky B, Mulvaney U, Jasinska AJ, Deng X, Freimer N, Delwart E: Local virus extinctions following a host population bottleneck, *J Virol* 89(16):8152–8161, 2015.

Karere GM, Dick EJ, Galindo S, Martinez JC, Martinez JE, Owston M, VandeBerg JL, Cox LA: Histological variation of early stage atherosclerotic lesions in baboons after prolonged challenge with high-cholesterol, high-fat diet, *J Med Primatol* 49(1):3–9, 2020.

Karere GM, Mahaney MC, Newman DE, Riojas AM, Christensen C, Birnbaum S, VandeBerg JL, Cox L: Diet-induced leukocyte telomere shortening in a baboon model for early stage atherosclerosis, *Sci Rep* 9(1):19001, 2019.

Kaspareit J, Friderichs-Gromoll S, Buse E, Habermann G: Background pathology of the common marmoset (*Callithrix jacchus*) in toxicological studies, *Exp Toxicol Pathol* 57(5–6): 405–410, 2006.

Kastman EK, Willette AA, Coe CL, Bendlin BB, Kosmatka KJ, McLaren DG, Xu G, Canu E, Field AS, Alexander AL, Voytko ML, Beasley TM, Colman RJ, Weindruch RH, Johnson SC: A calorie-restricted diet decreases brain iron accumulation and preserves motor performance in old rhesus monkeys, *J Neurosci* 32(34):11879–11904, 2012.

Killam KF, Killam EK, Naquet R: Studies on the epilepsy induced by photic stimulation in *Papio papio*, *Electroencephalogr Clin Neurophysiol* 23(1):91, 1967.

Kirk SA, Fraser SR, Gordon D, Templeton A: Evaluation of the T-cell dependent antibody response (TDAR) to tetanus toxoid (TT), in the cynomolgus monkey, in the presence of a known immunosuppressant, *Toxicologist*, 2008. Abstract #2134.

Kishi N, Sato K, Sasaki E, Okano H: Common marmoset as a new model animal for neuroscience research and genome editing technology, *Dev Growth Differ* 56(1):53–62, 2014.

Kolappaswamy K, Shipley ST, Tatarov II, DeTolla LJ: Methicillin-resistant Staphylococcus non-aureus infection in an irradiated rhesus macaque (*Macaca mulatta*), *J Am Assoc Lab Anim Sci* 47(3):64–67, 2008.

Kondo M, Kawamoto Y, Nozawa K, Matsubayashi K, Watanabe T, Griffiths O, Stanley MA: Population genetics of crab-eating macaques (*Macaca fascicularis*) on the island of Mauritius, *Am J Primatol* 29(3):167–182, 1993.

Konishi S, Kotera T, Koga M, Ueda M: Spontaneous hypertrophic cardiomyopathy in a cynomolgus macaque (*Macaca fascicularis*), *J Toxicol Pathol* 31(1):49–54, 2018. https://doi.org/10.1293/tox.2017-0027. Epub 2017 Oct 22. PMID: 29479140; PMCID: PMC5820103.

Korbmacher B, Atorf J, Fridrichs-Gromoll S, Hill M, Korte S, Kremers J, Mansfield K, Mecklenburg L, Pilling A, Wiederhold A: Feasibility of intravitreal injections and ophthalmic safety assessment in marmoset, *Primate Biol* 4(1):93–100, 2017.

Korte S, Everitt J: The use of the marmoset in toxicity testing and nonclinical safety assessment studies. In Marini R, Wachtman L, Tardif S, Mansfield K, editors: *The common marmoset in captivity and biomedical research*, 2019, Elsevier Science.

Koyama H, Tachibana Y, Takaura K, Takemoto S, Morii K, Wada S, Kaneko H, Kimura M, Toyoda A: Effects of housing conditions on behaviors and biochemical parameters in juvenile cynomolgus monkeys (*Macaca fascicularis*), *Exp Anim* 68(2):195–211, 2019.

Kozlosky JC, Mysore J, Clark SP, Burr HN, Li J, Aranibar N, Vuppugalla R, West RC, Mangipudy RS, Graziano MJ: Comparison of physiologic and pharmacologic parameters in Asian and Mauritius cynomolgus macaques, *Regul Toxicol Pharmacol* 73(1):27–42, 2015.

Kramer R, Burns M: Normal clinical and biological parameters of the common marmoset (*Calithrix jacchus*). In Marini R, Wachtman L, Tardif S, Mansfield K, Fox J, editors: *The common marmoset in captivity and biomedical research*, 2019, Elsevier Science.

Lawler SH, Sussman RW, Taylor LL: Mitochondrial DNA of the Mauritian macaques (*Macaca fascicularis*): an example of the founder effect, *Am J Phys Anthropol* 96(2):133–141, 1995.

Leach MW: Regulatory forum opinion piece: differences between protein-based biologic products (biotherapeutics) and chemical entities (small molecules) of relevance to the toxicologic pathologist, *Toxicol Pathol* 41(1):128–136, 2013.

Leach MW, Rottman JB, Hock MB, Finco D, Rojko JL, Beyer JC: Immunogenicity/hypersensitivity of biologics, *Toxicol Pathol* 42(1):293–300, 2014.

Lebrec H, Cowan L, Lagrou M, Krejsa C, Neradilek MB, Polissar NL, Black L, Bussiere J: An inter-laboratory retrospective analysis of immunotoxicological endpoints in nonhuman primates: T-cell-dependent antibody responses, *J Immunotoxicol* 8(3):238–250, 2011.

Lebrec H, Molinier B, Boverhof D, Collinge M, Freebern W, Henson K, Mytych DT, Ochs HD, Wange R, Yang Y, Zhou L, Arrington J, Christin-Piché MS, Shenton J: The T-cell-dependent antibody response assay in nonclinical studies of pharmaceuticals and chemicals: study design, data analysis, interpretation, *Regul Toxicol Pharmacol* 69(1):7–21, 2014.

Lima MGM, Silva-Júnior JSE, Černý D, Buckner JC, Aleixo A, Chang J, Zheng J, Alfaro ME, Martins A, Di Fiore A, Boubli JP, Lynch Alfaro JW: A phylogenomic perspective on the robust capuchin monkey (Sapajus) radiation: first evidence for extensive population admixture across South America, *Mol Phylogenet Evol* 124:137–150, 2018.

Linnaeus Carl. *Systema Naturae*: Sweden, 1758, International Commission on Zoological Nomenclature, 1.

Loiseau Jean-Chrostophe, et al.: A survey of epileptic disorders in southwest France: seizures in elderly patients. *Ann Neurol* 27(3):232–237, 1990.

Long GG, Hardisty JF: Regulatory forum opinion piece: thresholds in toxicologic pathology, *Toxicol Pathol* 40(7):1079–1081, 2012.

Long J: *Cebus capucinus* (On-line). 2009, Animal Diversity Web, https://animaldiversity.org/accounts/Cebus_capucinus/. (Accessed 5 September 2020).

Lowenstine LJ: A primer of primate pathology: lesions and nonlesions, *Toxicol Pathol* 31(Suppl):92–102, 2003.

Lutz CK: A cross-species comparison of abnormal behavior in three species of singly-housed old world monkeys, *Appl Anim Behav Sci* 199:52–58, 2018.

Mackic JB, Weiss MH, Miao W, Kirkman E, Ghiso J, Calero M, Bading J, Frangione B, Zlokovic BV: Cerebrovascular accumulation and increased blood-brain barrier permeability to circulating Alzheimer's amyloid beta peptide in aged squirrel monkey with cerebral amyloid angiopathy, *J Neurochem* 70(1):210–215, 1998.

MacLean EL, Prior SR, Platt ML, Brannon EM: Primate location preference in a double-tier cage: the effects of illumination and cage height, *J Appl Anim Welfare Sci* 12(1):73–81, 2009.

Magden ER, Mansfield KG, Simmons JH, Abee CR: Nonhuman primates. In Fox JG, Anderson LC, Otto GM, Pritchett-Corning KR, Whary MT, editors: *Laboratory animal medicine*, 2015, Elsevier.

Magden ER, Nehete BP, Chitta S, Williams LE, Simmons JH, Abee CR, Nehete PN: Comparative analysis of cellular immune responses in conventional and SPF olive baboons, *Comp Med* 70(2):160–169, 2020.

Marmoset genome project. https://www.hgsc.bcm.edu/nonhuman-primates. (Accessed 5 September 2020).

Martin ML, Bitzer AA, Schrader A, Bergmann-Leitner ES, Soto K, Zou X, Beck Z, Matyas GR, Dutta S: Comparison of immunogenicity and safety outcomes of a malaria vaccine FMP013/ALFQ in rhesus macaques (*Macaca mulatta*) of Indian and Chinese origin, *Malar J* 18(1):377, 2019.

Masoro EJ: Overview of caloric restriction and ageing, *Mech Ageing Dev* 126(9):913–922, 2005.

Mathieu C, Kozlovski P, Paldánius PM, Foley JE, Modgill V, Evans M, Serban C: Clinical safety and tolerability of vildagliptin - insights from randomised trials, observational studies and post-marketing surveillance, *Eur Endocrinol* 13(2):68–72, 2017.

Messaoudi I, Estep R, Robinson B, Wong SW: Nonhuman primate models of human immunology, *Antioxidants Redox Signal* 14(2):261–273, 2011.

Middleton CC, Clarkson TB, Lofland HB, Prichard RW: Atherosclerosis IN the squirrel monkey. Naturally occurring lesions of the aorta and coronary arteries, *Arch Pathol* 78:16–23, 1964.

Mijal M: *Cebus albifrons* (On-line). 2001, Animal Diversity Web, https://animaldiversity.org/accounts/Cebus_albifrons/. (Accessed 5 September 2020).

Monticello TM, Jones TW, Dambach DM, Potter DM, Bolt MW, Liu M, Keller DA, Hart TK, Kadambi VJ: Current nonclinical testing paradigm enables safe entry to first-in-human clinical trials: the IQ consortium nonclinical to clinical translational database, *Toxicol Appl Pharmacol* 334:100–109, 2017.

Moscovice LR, Ziegler TE: Peripheral oxytocin in female baboons relates to estrous state and maintenance of sexual consortships, *Horm Behav* 62(5):592–597, 2012.

Mullan RJ: *Nonhuman primate importation and quarantine: United States fiscal year 2018*, The 42nd Meeting of the American Society of Primatologists, 2019, University of Wisconsin.

Nonhuman primate genome project. https//www.hgsc.bcm.edu/non-human-primates. (Accessed 5 September 2020).

O'Connor D: Chinese rhesus and cynomolgus macaques in HIV vaccine and pathogenesis research, *Future Virol* 1(2):165–172, 2006.

Olson H, Betton G, Robinson D, Thomas K, Monro A, Kolaja G, Lilly P, Sanders J, Sipes G, Bracken W, Dorato M, Van Deun K, Smith P, Berger B, Heller A: Concordance of the toxicity of pharmaceuticals in humans and in animals, *Regul Toxicol Pharmacol* 32(1):56–67, 2000.

Ottaviano M, De Placido S, Ascierto PA: Recent success and limitations of immune checkpoint inhibitors for cancer: a lesson from melanoma, *Virchows Arch* 474(4):421–432, 2019.

Peluffo MC, Stanley J, Braeuer N, Rotgeri A, Fritzemeier KH, Fuhrmann U, Buchmann B, Adevai T, Murphy MJ, Zelinski MB, Lindenthal B, Hennebold JD, Stouffer RL: A prostaglandin E2 receptor antagonist prevents pregnancies during a preclinical contraceptive trial with female macaques, *Hum Reprod* 29(7):1400–1412, 2014.

Peña JC, Ho WZ: Non-human primate models of tuberculosis, *Microbiol Spectr* 4(4), 2016.

Pesola GR, Avasarala J: Bupropion seizure proportion among new-onset generalized seizures and drug related seizures presenting to an emergency department, *J Emerg Med* 22(3):235–239, 2002.

Peters A, Rosene DL, Moss MB, Kemper TL, Abraham CR, Tigges J, Albert MS: Neurobiological basis of age-related cognitive decline in the rhesus monkey, *J Neuropathol Exp Neurol* 55(8):861–874, 1996.

PharmaPendium, reed elsevier properties SA, 2014. https://www.pharmapendium.com.

Philippens IH, Ormel PR, Baarends G, Johansson M, Remarque EJ, Doverskog M: Acceleration of amyloidosis by inflammation in the amyloid-beta marmoset monkey model of Alzheimer's disease, *J Alzheimers Dis* 55(1):101–113, 2017.

Piccotti JR, Alvey JD, Reindel JF, Guzman RE: T-cell-dependent antibody response: assay development in cynomolgus monkeys, *J Immunotoxicol* 2(4):191–196, 2005.

Platt DM, Rowlett JK: Nonhuman primate models of drug and alcohol addiction. In Abee CR, Mansfield K, Tardif S, Morris T, editors: *Nonhuman primates in biomedical research* vol. 2.

Porter BF, Frost P, Hubbard GB: Polyarteritis nodosa in a cynomolgus macaque (*Macaca fascicularis*), *Vet Pathol* 40(5):570–573, 2003. https://doi.org/10.1354/vp.40-5-570.

Price DL, Martin LJ, Sisodia SS, Wagster MV, Koo EH, Walker LC, Koliatsos VE, Cork LC: Aged non-human primates: an animal model of age-associated neurodegenerative disease, *Brain Pathol* 1(4):287–296, 1991.

Prins NW, Pohlmeyer EA, Debnath S, Mylavarapu R, Geng S, Sanchez JC, Rothen D, Prasad A: Common marmoset (*Callithrix jacchus*) as a primate model for behavioral neuroscience studies, *J Neurosci Methods* 284:35–46, 2017.

Product development under the animal rule guidance for industry, 2015. https://www.fda.gov/regulatory-information/search-fda-guidance-documents/product-development-under-animal-rule. (Accessed 4 November 2020).

Qin W, Hu L, Zhang X, Jiang S, Li J, Zhang Z, Wang X: The diverse function of PD-1/PD-L pathway beyond cancer, *Front Immunol* 10:2298, 2019 Oct 4.

Reader JR, Canfield DR, Lane JF, Kanthaswamy S, Ardeshir A, Allen AM, Tarara RP: Left ventricular hypertrophy in rhesus macaques (*Macaca mulatta*) at the California national primate research center (1992–2014), *Comp Med* 66(2):162–169, 2016.

Reimann KA, Parker RA, Seaman MS, Beaudry K, Beddall M, Peterson L, Williams KC, Veazey RS, Montefiori DC, Mascola JR, Nabel GJ, Letvin NL: Pathogenicity of simian-human immunodeficiency virus SHIV-89.6P and SIVmac is attenuated in cynomolgus macaques and associated with early T-lymphocyte responses, *J Virol* 79(14):8878–8885, 2005.

Rhyu IJ, Bytheway JA, Kohler SJ, Lange H, Lee KJ, Boklewski J, McCormick K, Williams NI, Stanton GB, Breenough WT, Cameron JL: Effects of aerobic exercise training on cognitive function and cortical vascularity in monkeys, *Neuroscience* 167(4):1239–1248, 2010.

Ridley RM, Baker HF, Windle CP, Cummings RM: Very long-term studies of the seeding of beta-amyloidosis in primates, *J Neural Transm* 113(9):1243–1251, 2006.

Rogers J, Raveendran M, Harris RA, Mailund T, Leppälä K, Athanasiadis G, Schierup MH, Cheng J, Munch K, Walker JA, Konkel MK, Jordan V, Steely CJ, Beckstrom TO, Bergey C, Burrell A, Schrempf D, Noll A, Kothe M, Kopp GH, Liu Y, Murali S, Billis K, Martin FJ, Muffato M, Cox L, Else J, Disotell T, Muzny DM, Phillips-Conroy J, Aken B, Eichler EE, Marques-Bonet T, Kosiol C, Batzer MA, Hahn MW, Tung J, Zinner D, Roos C, Jolly CJ, Gibbs RA, Worley KC, Consortium BGA: The comparative genomics and complex population history of papio baboons, *Sci Adv* 5(1):eaau6947, 2019.

Rohrman M: Macacine Herpes virus (B virus), *Workplace Health Saf* 64(1):9–12, 2016.

Rojko Jennifer, et al.: Formation, clearance, deposition, patholgenicity, and identification of biopharmaceutical-related immune complexes: review and case studies, *Toxicological Pathology* 42:725–764, 2014.

Rosso MC, Badino P, Ferrero G, Costa R, Cordero F, Steidler S: Biologic data of cynomolgus monkeys maintained under laboratory conditions, *PloS One* 11(6):e0157003, 2016.

Rowe N: *The pictorial guide to the living primates*, East Hampton, N.Y., 1996, Pogonias Press.

Rowe N, Myers M, Goodall J, Mittermeier RA, Rylands AB, Groves CP: *All the world's primates*, Charlestown, Rhode Island, 2016, Pogonias Press.

Sasseville VG, Mansfield KG: Overview of known non-human primate pathogens with potential to affect colonies used for toxicity testing, *J Immunotoxicol* 7(2):79–92, 2010.

Sasseville VG, Mansfield KG, Mankowski JL, Tremblay C, Terio KA, Mätz-Rensing K, Gruber-Dujardin E, Delaney MA, Schmidt LD, Liu D, Markovits JE, Owston M, Harbison C, Shanmukhappa S, Miller AD, Kaliyaperumal S, Assaf BT, Kattenhorn L, Macri SC, Simmons HA, Baldessari A, Sharma P, Courtney C, Bradley A, Cline JM, Reindel JF, Hutto DL, Montali RJ, Lowenstine LJ: Meeting report: spontaneous lesions and diseases in wild, captive-bred, and zoo-housed nonhuman primates and in nonhuman primate species used in drug safety studies, *Vet Pathol* 49(6):1057–1069, 2012.

Satkoski J, George D, Smith DG, Kanthaswamy S: Genetic characterization of wild and captive rhesus macaques in China, *J Med Primatol* 37(2):67–80, 2008.

Schober N: *Cebus olivaceus* (On-line). 2003, Animal Diversity Web. at, https://animaldiversity.org/accounts/Cebus_olivaceus/baldba. (Accessed 5 September 2020).

Sheng SR, Wang XY, Xu HZ, Zhu GQ, Zhou YF: Anatomy of large animal spines and its comparison to the human spine: a systematic review, *Eur Spine J* 19(1):46–56, 2010.

Shelton KA, Clarkson TB, Kaplan JR: Nonhuman primate models of atherosclerosis. In Abee CR, Mansfield K, Tardif S, Morris T, editors: *Nonhuman primates in biomedical research*, vol. 2. 2012, Elsevier.

Simmons HA: Age-associated pathology in rhesus macaques (*Macaca mulatta*), *Vet Pathol* 53(2):399–416, 2016.

Smith DG, McDonough J: Mitochondrial DNA variation in Chinese and Indian rhesus macaques (*Macaca mulatta*), *Am J Primatol* 65(1):1–25, 2005.

Snyder PW, Everds NE, Craven WA, Werner J, Tannehill-Gregg SH, Guzman RE: Maturity-related variability of the thymus in cynomolgus monkeys (*Macaca fascicularis*), *Toxicol Pathol* 44(6):874–891, 2016.

Song J, Moses E: *Cebus xanthosternos* (On-line). 2009, Animal Diversity Web. at, https://animaldiversity.org/accounts/Cebus_xanthosternos/. (Accessed 5 September 2020).

Southwick CH, Siddiqi MF: Population status of nonhuman primates in Asia, with emphasis on rhesus macaques in India, *Am J Primatol* 34(1):51–59, 1994.

Stouffer RL, Woodruff TK: Nonhuman primates: a vital model for basic and applied research on female reproduction, prenatal development, and women's health, *ILAR J* 58(2):281–294, 2017.

Sussman RW, Tattersall I: Behavior and ecology of *macaca fascicularis* in Mauritius: a preliminary study, *Primates* 22:192–205, 1981.

Swanson SJ, Bussiere J: Immunogenicity assessment in non-clinical studies, *Curr Opin Microbiol* 15(3):337–347, 2012.

Sweeney CG, Curran E, Westmoreland SV, Mansfield KG, Vallender EJ: Quantitative molecular assessment of chimerism across tissues in marmosets and tamarins, *BMC Genom* 13:98, 2012.

Tardif S, Carville A, Elmore D, Williams LE, Rice K: Reproduction and breeding of nonhuman primates. In Abee CR, Mansfield K, Tardif S, Morris T, editors: *Nonhuman primates in biomedical research*, 2012, Elsevier.

Tardif SD: Marmosets as a translational aging model-Introduction, *Am J Primatol* 81(2):e22912, 2019.

Tardif, et al.: *Non-human primates in biomedical research*, 2013.

Teng Y, Cong R, Liu Y: Detection and analysis of hematological and serum biochemical indices of thirty common marmosets, *Chin J Comp Med* 28(5):70–74, 2018.

The Macaque Website, National Center for the Replacement, Refinement and Reduction of Animals in Research.

https://www.nc3rs.org.uk/macaques/captive-management/housing/. (Accessed 29 October 2020).

Tichenor JN, Dumont C, Coletti KS, LeSauteur L, Calise DV, Christn-Piche MS, Satterwhite C: A 6-week study to determine the antibody response to FK-506-immunosuppressed cynomolgus monkeys following the subcutaneous administration of keyhole limpet hemocyanin and tetanus toxoid in the presence or absence of incomplete Freud's adjuvant, *Toxicologist*, 2010. Abstract # 1989.

Tosi AJ, Morales JC, Melnick DJ: Y-chromosome and mitochondrial markers in *Macaca fascicularis* indicate introgression with indochinese M. Mulatta and a biogeographic barrier in the Isthmus of Kra, *Int J Primatol* 23(1):161–178, 2002.

Trichel AM, Rajakumar PA, Murphey-Corb M: Species-specific variation in SIV disease progression between Chinese and Indian subspecies of rhesus macaque, *J Med Primatol* 31(4–5):171–178, 2002.

Tuntland T, Ethell B, Kosaka T, et al.: Implementation of pharmacokinetic and pharmacodynamic strategies in early research phases of drug discovery and development at Novartis Institute of Biomedical Research, *Front Pharmacol* 5:174, 2014.

Uno Y, Uehara S, Yamazaki H: Genetic polymorphisms of drug-metabolizing cytochrome P450 enzymes in cynomolgus and rhesus monkeys and common marmosets in preclinical studies for humans, *Biochem Pharmacol* 153:184–195, 2018.

Update on the "NIH workshop on optimizing reproducibility in nonhuman primate research studies by enhancing rigor and transparency". https://osp.od.nih.gov/2019/09/16/update-nih-workshop-optimizing-reproducibility-nonhuman-primate-research-studies-enhancing-rigor-transparency/. Accessed 29 October 2020.

Valdés I, Gil L, Castro J, Odoyo D, Hitler R, Munene E, Romero Y, Ochola L, Cosme K, Kariuki T, Guillén G, Hermida L: Olive baboons: a non-human primate model for testing dengue virus type 2 replication, *Int J Infect Dis* 17(12):e1176–1181, 2013.

Van Dam D, De Deyn PP: Non human primate models for Alzheimer's disease-related research and drug discovery, *Expet Opin Drug Discov* 12(2):187–200, 2017.

van Doremalen N, Lambe T, Spencer A, Belij-Rammerstorfer S, Purushotham JN, Port JR, Avanzato V, Bushmaker T, Flaxman A, Ulaszewska M, Feldmann F, Allen ER, Sharpe H, Schulz J, Holbrook M, Okumura A, Meade-White K, Pérez-Pérez L, Bissett C, Gilbride C, Williamson BN, Rosenke R, Long D, Ishwarbhai A, Kailath R, Rose L, Morris S, Powers C, Lovaglio J, Hanley PW, Scott D, Saturday G, de Wit E, Gilbert SC, Munster VJ: ChAdOx1 nCoV-19 vaccination prevents SARS-CoV-2 pneumonia in rhesus macaques, *bioRxiv*, 2020 [Preprint]. Nature. May 2020 Jul 30.

Van Rompay KKA: Tackling HIV and AIDS: contributions by non-human primate models, *Lab Anim* 46(6):259–270, 2017.

VandeBerg JL, Williams-Blangero S, Tardif SD: *The baboon in biomedical research*, New York, 2009, Springer.

Villano JS, Ogden BE, Yong PP, Lood NM, Sharp PE: Morphometrics and pelage characterization of longtailed macaques (*Macaca fascicularis*) from Pulau Bintan, Indonesia; Singapore; and Southern Vietnam. *J Am Assoc Lab Anim Sci* 48(6):727–733, 2009.

Warren WC, Jasinska AJ, García-Pérez R, Svardal H, Tomlinson C, Rocchi M, Archidiacono N, Capozzi O, Minx P, Montague MJ, Kyung K, Hillier LW, Kremitzki M, Graves T, Chiang C, Hughes J, Tran N, Huang Y, Ramensky V, Choi OW, Jung YJ, Schmitt CA, Juretic N, Wasserscheid J, Turner TR, Wiseman RW, Tuscher JJ, Karl JA, Schmitz JE, Zahn R, O'Connor DH, Redmond E, Nisbett A, Jacquelin B, Müller-Trutwin MC, Brenchley JM, Dione M, Antonio M, Schroth GP, Kaplan JR, Jorgensen MJ, Thomas GW, Hahn MW, Raney BJ, Aken B, Nag R, Schmitz J, Churakov G, Noll A, Stanyon R, Webb D, Thibaud-Nissen F, Nordborg M, Marques-Bonet T, Dewar K, Weinstock GM, Wilson RK, Freimer NB: The genome of the vervet (*Chlorocebus aethiops* sabaeus), *Genome Res* 25(12):1921–1933, 2015.

Weatherall D: The use of non-human primates in research. In *A working group report from the acadamy of medical sciences and the royal society*, 2006, Wellcome Treust and the Medical Research Council.

Weinbauer GF, Niehoff M, Niehaus M, Srivastav S, Fuchs A, Van Esch E, Cline JM: Physiology and endocrinology of the ovarian cycle in macaques, *Toxicol Pathol* 36(7S):7S–23S, 2008.

Welch N: *Cebus nigritus* (On-line). 2019, Animal Diversity Web, https://animaldiversity.org/accounts/Cebus_nigritus/. (Accessed 5 September 2020).

Williams LE, Brady AG, Gibson SV, Abee CR: The squirrel monkey breeding and research resource: a review of Saimiri reproductive biology and behavior and breeding performance, *Primatologie* 5:303–334, 2002.

Williams R, Kothny W, Serban C, Lopez-Leon S, de Vries F, Schlienger R: Association between vildagliptin and risk of angioedema, foot ulcers, skin lesions, hepatic toxicity, and serious infections in patients with type 2 diabetes mellitus: a European multidatabase, noninterventional, post-authorization safety study, *Endocrinol Diabetes Metab* 2(3):e00084, 2019.

Wiseman RW, Karl JA, Bohn PS, Nimityongskul FA, Starrett GJ, O'Connor DH: Haplessly hoping: macaque major histocompatibility complex made easy, *ILAR J* 54(2):196–210, 2013.

Wolf RF, Papin JF, Hines-Boykin R, Chavez-Suarez M, White GL, Sakalian M, Dittmer DP: Baboon model for West Nile virus infection and vaccine evaluation, *Virology* 355(1):44–51, 2006.

Wood JD, Peck OC, Tefend KS, Rodriguez-M MA, Rodriguez-M JV, Hernández-C JI, Stonerook MJ, Sharma HM: Colitis and colon cancer in cotton-top tamarins (*Saguinus oedipus* oedipus) living wild in their natural habitat, *Dig Dis Sci* 43(7):1443–1453, 1998.

Yan G, Zhang G, Fang X, Zhang Y, Li C, Ling F, Cooper DN, Li Q, Li Y, van Gool AJ, Du H, Chen J, Chen R, Zhang P, Huang Z, Thompson JR, Meng Y, Bai Y, Wang J, Zhuo M, Wang T, Huang Y, Wei L, Li J, Wang Z, Hu H, Yang P, Le L, Stenson PD, Li B, Liu X, Ball EV, An N, Huang Q, Fan W, Zhang X, Wang W, Katze MG, Su B, Nielsen R, Yang H, Wang X: Genome sequencing and comparison of two nonhuman primate animal models, the cynomolgus and Chinese rhesus macaques, *Nat Biotechnol* 29(11):1019–1023, 2011.

Zhang R, Guoqiang Q, Tigong Z, Southwick CH: Distribution of macaques (Macaca) in China, *Acta Theriol* 11:171–185, 1990.

Zuhlke U, Weinbauer G: The common marmoset (*Callithrix jacchus*) as a model in toxicology, *Toxicol Pathol* 31:123–127, 2003.

Animal Models in Toxicologic Research: Nonmammalian

Debra A. Tokarz[1], Jeffrey C. Wolf[2]

[1]Experimental Pathology Laboratories, Inc., Durham, NC, United States, [2]Experimental Pathology Laboratories, Inc., Sterling, VA, United States

OUTLINE

1. Introduction	811	4. Study Design Considerations	841
		4.1. Study Design and Implementation	841
2. Nonmammalian Animal Taxa	815	4.2. Subclinical Disease	844
2.1. Invertebrates	815		
2.2. Fish	818	5. Data Extrapolation	847
2.3. Amphibians	825	5.1. Results Extrapolation and Risk Assessment	847
2.4. Birds	828	5.2. Interspecies Variability	848
2.5. Reptiles	830	5.3. Knowledge Gap	850
		5.4. Reliability of Published Histopathology Data	851
3. Utilization of Nonmammalian Animals	831		
3.1. Animal Models of Human Diseases	831	6. Conclusions	851
3.2. Drug Discovery and Toxicity Screening	834		
3.3. Target Animal Safety Studies	837	References	853
3.4. Ecotoxicological Testing and Environmental Monitoring	838		

1. INTRODUCTION

In toxicological investigations, the decision to utilize a nonmammalian animal model is almost always a matter of exigency, wherein the selection of the test species and experimental system is directed at a particular scientific question to be addressed. As is the case in traditional toxicological research, investigations that employ nonmammalian models are conducted for the ultimate benefit of human health, environmental health, and/or the health and well-being of the test species itself. However, nonmammalian animal models, such as birds, amphibians, fish, and invertebrates, have unique attributes and offer specific advantages that may be difficult or impossible to replicate using conventional mammalian research subjects. Included among these qualities are specialized anatomic or physiologic features that may be particularly suited to the investigation of certain toxicologic modes/mechanisms of action, biotransformation and elimination pathways, or exposure routes. For example, amphibians have become preferred research subjects for toxicological studies involving the thyroid gland because the process of metamorphic transformation from larva to adult is tightly controlled by thyroid hormone activity. Birds are used to monitor air quality due to the inherent sensitivity of these animals to particular airborne toxicants (e.g., polytetrafluroethylene [PTFE]), and anatomic and physiological differences between the avian lung–air sac respiratory system and the bronchoalveolar lung of mammals can be exploited to study the systemic effects of inhaled toxic gases or aerosolized particulate matter. Fish species that inhabit opposing extremes of temperature, pH, and/or salinity are ideal candidates for toxicokinetic studies. And as filter feeders, bivalve mollusks are natural sentinels in aquatic ecosystems because they are adept at bioconcentrating toxic substances that may exist at large in the aquatic environment.

Nonmammalian vertebrates and invertebrates have been used as toxicological test subjects for well over a century; however, it is only in recent decades that nonlethal, morphologic endpoints have been incorporated into bioassays that involve nonmammalian subjects. The current surge in the use of nonmammalian animal models can be ascribed to the intersection of several interrelated factors that increase the feasibility and need for their use. Nonmammalian animal models are more approachable due to improved breeding and husbandry practices, the increased availability of genetic information for numerous species, recognition of the extent that genetic material is conserved across taxa, the ability to create transgenic animals, and the development of specialized histopathologic, immunohistochemical, and ultrastructural procedures. Concurrently, the need for nonmammalian models in toxicity studies has increased due to guidance for testing pharmaceutical products designed for aquaculture and poultry (VICH, 2008) and regulatory requirements to perform environmental risk assessments on human and veterinary pharmaceuticals (VICH, 2004; U.S. Food and Drug Administration, 1998).

There are a number of reasons why a toxicologist might opt to employ a nonmammalian animal model for scientific investigation (Table 22.1). Advantages of small fish, amphibians, and invertebrates as study animals include the following: the ability to house a relatively large number of test animals in a small space and at low cost; high fecundity and short generation times; and the comparative ease by which aquatic animals may be exposed to toxicants via the water bath route. From the viewpoint of the pathologist, the ability to evaluate multiple organ systems in a comparatively small number of histologic sections is of great benefit (Figure 22.1). Nonmammalian models are common subjects of ecotoxicological investigations, and a particular model may be the very species in which a certain environmentally related lesion or syndrome was initially discovered. For example, it turns out that the optimum subject for studying contaminant-induced neoplastic development and reproductive effects of endocrine disruption in the North American estuarine fish mummichog *Fundulus heteroclitus* is actually the mummichog itself. This fish possesses a number of characteristics that make it especially suitable for scientific investigation: in the field, it is an abundantly available coastal species that has limited migration, economic importance as a bait fish, and the ability to reside and persist in heavily contaminated waters; in the laboratory, it is a small, hardy, and easily cultivated experimental animal for which a wealth of information is available on topics as wide ranging as osmoregulatory and reproductive physiology, carcinogenesis, and evolutionary genetics (Burnett et al., 2007; Lister et al., 2011). Alternatively, a selected model may serve as a surrogate for a toxicologically impacted species, especially if the latter is threatened or endangered. A prime example would be the intensively cultivated and ubiquitous rainbow trout *Oncorhynchus mykiss*, which has been used extensively in toxicologic bioassays as a substitute for at-risk species such as the bull trout *Salvelinus confluentus*, Lahontan cutthroat trout *Oncorhynchus clarkii henshawi*, and other threatened salmonids (Fairchild et al., 2009). Rainbow trout are particularly useful as surrogate tumorigenesis models for a number of reasons, including a low level of spontaneous neoplasms, enzymatic systems for procarcinogen metabolism, limited capacity for DNA repair, documented induction of oncogenic Ki-*ras* gene mutations, and the ease to which various tumors can be induced by diethylnitrosamine, polycyclic aromatic hydrocarbons (PAHs), N-methyl-N'-nitrosoguanidine, 7,12-dimethylbenz[a]anthracene, aflatoxin B1 (AFB1), and other carcinogens (Williams et al.,

TABLE 22.1 Applicability of Various Taxa for Use in Toxicological Bioassays

Taxa	Applicability for toxicological assays				Representative species (listed alphabetically)
	Animal models of human diseases	Drug discovery and toxicity screening	Target animal safety studies	Ecotoxicological testing and environmental monitoring	
Invertebrates	+	++	+	+++	*Aplysia californica* (California sea hare), *Caenorhabditis elegans* (nematode), *Daphnia magna* (water flea), *Drosophila melanogaster* (common fruit fly)
Fish	++	+++	++	+++	*Carassius auratus auratus* (goldfish), *Cyprinodon variegatus* (sheepshead minnow), *Danio rerio* (zebrafish), *Fundulus heteroclitus* (mummichog), *Gasterosteus aculeatus* (three-spined stickleback), *Oncorhynchus mykiss* (rainbow trout), *Oryzias latipes* (medaka), *Pimephales promelas* (fathead minnow), *Poecilia reticulata* (guppy)
Amphibians	++	+++	−	+++	*Xenopus laevis* (African clawed frog), *Xenopus (Silurana) tropicalis* (Western clawed frog), *Rana pipiens* (leopard frog)
Reptiles	+	−	−	+	*Alligator mississippiensis* (American alligator); *Terrapene carolina carolina* (Eastern box turtle)
Birds	++	++	++	++	*Anas platyrhynchos* (mallard duck), *Colinus virginianus* (Northern bobwhite), *Coturnix japonica* (Japanese quail), *Gallus gallus domesticus* (domestic chicken), *Meleagris gallopavo* (wild turkey)
Mammals	+++	++	+++	+	*Canis lupus familiaris* (domestic dog), *Cavia porcellus* (Guinea pig), *Felis domesticus* (domestic cat), *Macaca fascicularis* (cynomolgus macaque), *Mus musculus* (laboratory mouse), *Rattus norvegicus* (laboratory rat)

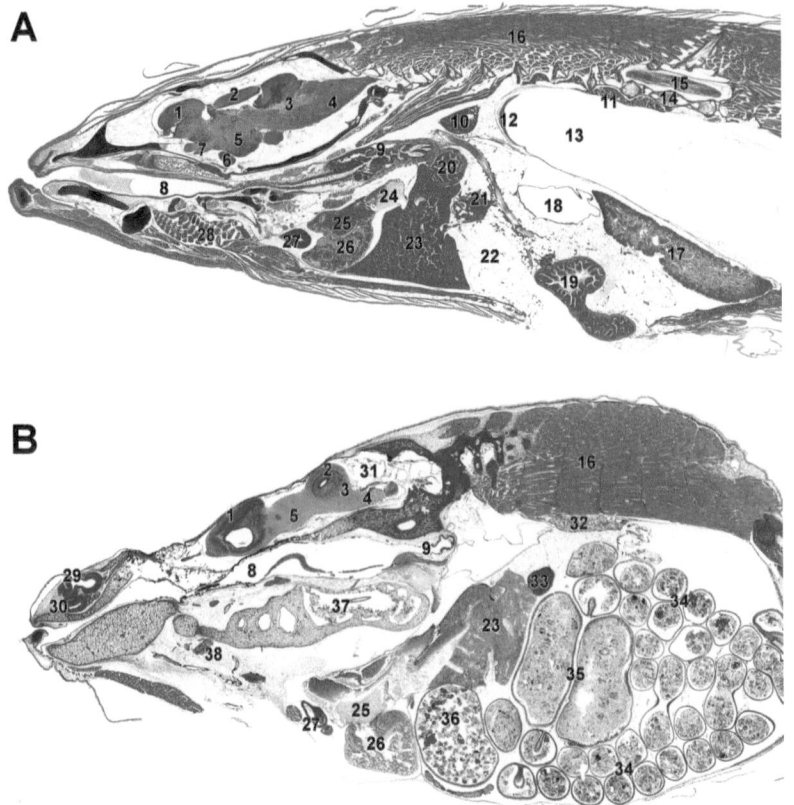

FIGURE 22.1   Sagittal histologic sections of an adult Japanese medaka *Oryzias latipes* (A) and a *Xenopus laevis* tadpole (B). A diverse array of tissue types can be appreciated in whole-body sections. Key: 1, telencephalon; 2, mesencephalon (optic tectum); 3, metencephalon; 4, medulla oblongata; 5, diencephalon; 6, pituitary gland; 7, optic nerves; 8, oropharynx; 9, esophagus; 10, anterior kidney; 11, posterior kidney; 12, gas gland of the swim bladder; 13, swim bladder; 14, notochord; 15, spinal cord; 16, epaxial musculature; 17, testis; 18, gallbladder; 19; distal intestines; 20; proximal intestines; 21; Brockman body (pancreatic islet); 22, adipose tissue; 23, liver; 24, sinus venosus; 25, cardiac atrium; 26, cardiac ventricle; 27, bulbus arteriosus; 28, gills; 29, olfactory organ; 30, vomeronasal organ; 31; inner ear; 32, kidney; 33, spleen; 34, ileum; 35, colon; 36, duodenum; 37; internal gills; 38, thyroid gland. H&E. *Figure reproduced from Haschek WM, Rousseaux CG, Wallig MA, editors:* Haschek and Rousseaux's handbook of toxicologic pathology, *ed 3, 2013, Academic Press, Figure 14.1, p 480, with permission.*

2003). Further studies are needed to determine if the sensitivity of certain surrogate species to contaminants is comparable to the sensitivity of the indigenous animals they represent.

Toxicologic pathologists who are intimidated by the prospect of evaluating nonmammalian animal studies should take some comfort in the fact that the pathologic processes of tissue damage and repair, inflammation, metabolic alterations, and tumorigenesis are evolutionarily well conserved. For example, with obvious exceptions such as mammary gland neoplasms, most broadly defined types of toxicant-induced tumors that one might find in a rodent, dog, or nonhuman primate have been observed at one

time or another in birds or poikilothermic vertebrates, and in these species, the morphologic appearance of preneoplastic and neoplastic lesions tends to be surprisingly characteristic (Figures 22.2 and 22.3). Furthermore, despite the profound degree of macroanatomical discordance that exists between vertebrates and invertebrates, it is reassuring to observe that the tissues such as skeletal muscle, sensory organs, gonads, neuropil, digestive glands, and gut are histologically similar among diverse representatives of the animal kingdom. One of the most challenging aspects of examining histologic specimens from unfamiliar species is distinguishing true pathologic changes from

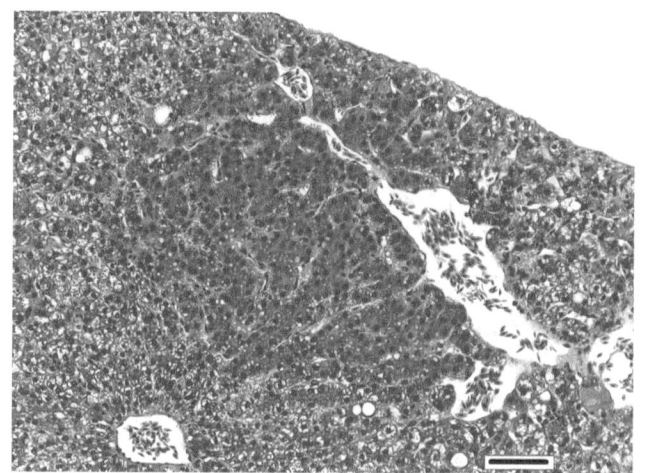

FIGURE 22.2 Liver from an adult female quail *Coturnix japonica*. Eosinophilic focus of cellular alteration in an untreated control bird. Foci in quail are comparable in appearance to those of rodents, and similar foci have also been observed in fish such as medaka. H&E, Bar = 50 μm. *Figure modified from OCSPP 890.2100: Avian two-generation toxicity test in the Japanese Quail, U. S. Environmental Protection Agency, EPA Pub no. 740-C-15-003, 2015, Figure 102, p. 96, with permission.*

background lesions, tissue processing artifacts, or differences attributable to individual animal variation. A distinct advantage for pathologists who evaluate toxicologic studies, as opposed to those who do primarily diagnostic work, is the ability to identify morphologic abnormalities by comparing treated or contaminant-exposed animals to negative controls or animals collected from relatively unspoiled reference sites. Table 22.2

provides a listing of reference materials that may be useful for pathologists who are unfamiliar with nonmammalian animal microanatomy. The forthcoming International Harmonization of Nomenclature and Diagnostic Criteria (INHAND) guide for fish will provide an additional resource. Unfortunately, a number of additional references are out of print or are otherwise difficult to obtain.

Volumes of text have been written on many of the topics broached in this chapter (risk assessment, for example); therefore, a truly comprehensive treatise on nonmammalian models is beyond the scope of this narrative. Instead, the goal here is to provide a high-level overview of the many roles that nonmammalian species play in toxicologic pathology, to describe at least a small fraction of the models that are available, and to discuss some of the special considerations that are inherent in the use of these nontraditional research subjects. For a more thorough review, readers are advised to consult the references listed at the end of the chapter.

2. NONMAMMALIAN ANIMAL TAXA

2.1. Invertebrates

Basic Biologic Characteristics and Common Species

Aquatic invertebrates such as hydra and water fleas *Daphnia magna* have been used for centuries as subjects for basic biological research. Until

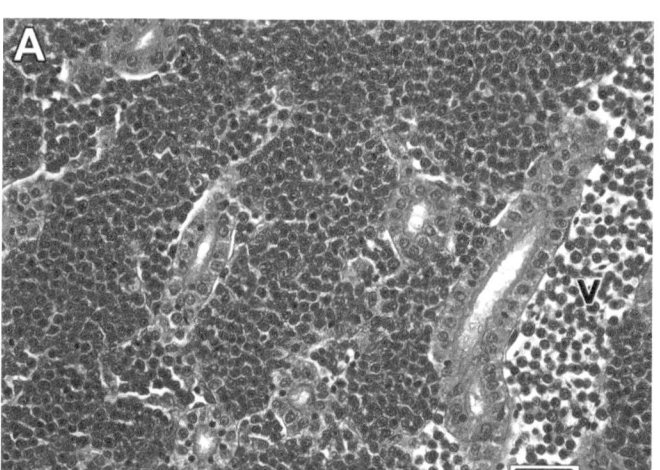
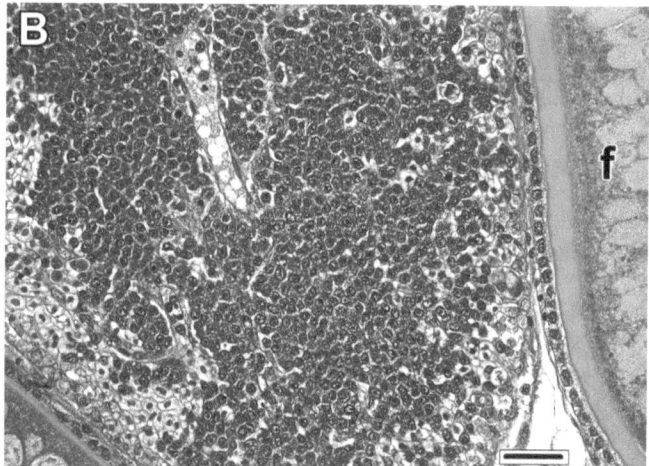

FIGURE 22.3 Multicentric lymphoma and lymphocytic leukemia in an adult fathead minnow *Pimephales promelas*. (A) Neoplastic lymphocytes expand the renal interstitium and are additionally evident within a large renal vein (v). H&E, Bar = 250 μm. (B) Lymphoma in the ovarian interstitium of the same fish. f = ovarian follicle. H&E, Bar = 100 μm. *Figure reproduced from Haschek WM, Rousseaux CG, Wallig MA, editors:* Haschek and Rousseaux's handbook of toxicologic pathology, *ed 3, 2013, Academic Press, Figure 14.3, p 481, with permission.*

TABLE 22.2   Microanatomy Resources for Nonmammalian Animal Models

INVERTEBRATES

Anderson DT: *Atlas of invertebrate anatomy,* Sydney, Australia, 1996, University of New South Wales Press.

Bayer FM, Grasshoff M, Verseveldt J, editors: *Illustrated trilingual glossary of coral morphological and anatomical terms applied to Octocorallia.* E.J. Brill, Dr. W. Backhuys, Leiden, The Netherlands, 1983.

Stachowitsch M: *The invertebrates: an illustrated glossary,* New York, NY, USA, 1992, Wiley-Liss.

FISH

Genten F: *Atlas of fish histology,* Enfield, NH, USA, 2009, Science Publishers.

Menke AL, Spitsbergen JM, Wolterbeek AP, Woutersen RA: Normal anatomy and histology of the adult zebrafish. *Toxicol Pathol* 39:759–775, 2011.

Morrison CM, Fitzsimmons K, Wright JR Jr.: *Atlas of tilapia histology,* Baton Rouge, LA, USA, 2006, World Aquaculture Society.

AMPHIBIANS AND REPTILES

Aughey E, Frye FL: A *color handbook of comparative veterinary histology and clinical correlates,* Ames, IA, USA, 2001, Iowa State University Press.

Hausen P, Riebesell M: *The early development of Xenopus laevis,* Santa Clara, CA, USA, 1991, Springer-Verlag TELOS.

Wiechmann AF, Wirsig-Wiechmann CR: *Color Atlas of Xenopus laevis Histology,* Norwell, MA, USA, 2003, Kluwer Academic Publishers.

BIRDS

Fitzgerald TC: *The Coturnix Quail: anatomy and histology,* Ames, IA, USA, 1969, Iowa State Press.

McLelland J:. *A color atlas of avian anatomy,* Philadelphia, PA, USA, 1991, W.B. Saunders Company.

Randall CJ, Reece RL, Randall C: *Color atlas of avian histopathology,* London, UK, 1996, Mosby-Wolfe.

recently, however, toxicological testing in invertebrates often involved simple exposure studies in which behavioral changes and percent mortality were the predominant endpoints. Today, this is no longer the case, as exemplified by the ever-expanding use of invertebrates such as *Drosophila melanogaster* fruit flies and *Caenorhabditis elegans* nematodes for both mechanistic and high-throughput screening studies in the areas of neurotoxicology, environmental toxicology, and genetic toxicology. In fact, representatives from many invertebrate phyla are currently used in pharmaceutical and environmental toxicological research, and examples include Porifera (e.g., marine sponges), Cnidaria (e.g., hydra, corals and anemones), Nematoda (*C. elegans*), Mollusca (e.g., snails, bivalves, and cephalopods such as *Octopus vulgaris* and squid), Platyhelminthes (e.g., planaria), Arthropoda (e.g., fruit flies, horseshoe crabs, and crustaceans such as daphnia and mysid shrimp), and Echinodermata (e.g., sea urchins) (Wilson-Sanders, 2011).

The potential for health threats to native and cultivated bee populations and other pollinators to impact commercial agriculture is becoming ever more apparent. Nontoxic threats to these insect populations include infectious agents such as Varroa destructor mites, Nosema apis microsporidian organisms, hive invaders such as *Aethina tumida* beetles, and losses to starvation, queen failure, and the poorly understood and likely multifactorial condition known as "colony collapse disorder" (Ferrier et al., 2018). Additionally, however, there is concern that exposure of bees to natural and anthropogenic substances such as insecticides (e.g., neonicotinoids, acetylcholinesterase inhibitors), herbicides (e.g., paraquat), fungicides (e.g., chlorothalonil), and other environmental contaminants (Johnson, 2015) [see *Agro/Bulk Chemicals,* Vol 2, Chap 12 and *Environmental Toxicologic Pathology,* Vol 2, Chap 18] may have negative health effects, and may be especially hazardous for native pollinators, which, unlike commercially reared honey bees (*Apis mellifera*), cannot be readily replenished. Bees may be exposed to such chemicals intentionally or inadvertently via a variety of mechanisms, including the deliberate use of insecticides to control bee pests, products used to maintain the structural integrity of hives (e.g., tin- and arsenic-based wood preservatives), pesticide overspray, and contamination of pollen and dusts transported to the hive by resident or visiting bees (Johnson, 2015). The list of potential bee toxicants that have been investigated to date is long and continues to grow (Heard et al., 2017). Although bee histopathology is still far from routine, recommended techniques for processing tissues from these and other insects have been recently published (Hidemi, 2014).

There are a number of intuitive advantages to the use of invertebrates as test subjects, which include the relatively low cost of the animals, housing, equipment, and amounts of test reagents, small space requirements, rapid generation times, exquisite sensitivity to many toxicants (e.g., metals), and comparatively less animal use concern. Additionally, many invertebrate models offer unique anatomical or physiological attributes that can be exploited in toxicological investigations, such as the giant axons of squid, the retinal neurons and well-characterized immune systems of horseshoe crabs, the regenerative capability of planarians, and ability of bivalve mollusks to filter and bioaccumulate contaminants. For example, the inability of efflux transporters belonging to the ATP Binding Cassette superfamily to recognize and export perfluorocarbons has been studied in mussels (Gómez et al., 2011), and potential links have been investigated between contaminants such as dioxins and unusually high regional prevalences of gonadal tumors in *Mya arenaria* soft-shell clams (Peters et al., 1994).

A primary limitation of invertebrate models is their relative genetic, anatomic, and physiologic distance from humans. For example, some phyla lack complex organs comparable to those of the mammalian immune, cardiovascular, and urinary systems. However, in many cases, this shortcoming is eclipsed by the lower cost and distinctive features of many invertebrate models, and the opportunity they provide for institutions to meet their goals of "reducing, refining, and replacing" mammalian assays.

Background Findings with Examples of Target Tissue Toxicities

Lists of background findings have not yet been compiled for the multitude of currently used and potential invertebrate test subjects. In contrast to traditional toxicologic bioassays, histopathology is less commonly employed in invertebrate toxicity testing, where typical endpoints have traditionally included lethality, behaviors such as stimulus avoidance, and biochemical, electrochemical, or molecular analyses. Morphologic studies that are performed in invertebrate studies may instead rely on external visualization of internal tissues, or, because of the minute nature of some invertebrate organs, ultrastructural evaluation. Histopathology is more likely to be used to investigate outbreaks of infectious disease in economically important invertebrates, such as edible shellfish, and ecologically pivotal animals such as corals, in which secondary bacterial or fungal infections are often indirect consequences of toxicologic insult. An additional challenge for many toxicological pathologists is the unfamiliarity of invertebrate gross and microscopic anatomy, and the morphologic responses of such organisms to chemical challenge. For example, the convoluted internal organization of cnidarians such as corals and anemones can be quite daunting to the uninitiated, not to mention the uncharacteristic appearance of many inflammatory and neoplastic lesions. However, it is likely that histopathology will become an increasingly utilized tool for investigating the toxicological fallout of pollution in fragile invertebrate populations, as exemplified by the apparent sensitivity of marine corals to the toxic effects of environmental contaminants such as oil dispersants.

Major Disease Models

In another example, it has become evident that sea urchin embryos (SUEs) are suitable models for developmental neurotoxicity in mammals, due to conservancy of brain neurotransmitters such as acetylcholine, serotonin, dopamine, and norepinephrine, which are utilized in the SUE as growth regulatory signals (Qiao et al., 2003). SUEs have also been used to investigate multidrug efflux transporter activity (Cole et al., 2013). A further interesting model is the California sea hare, *Aplysia californica*, which was the first mollusk to be genomically sequenced. The central nervous system of *Aplysia* contains only 20,000 neurons, as compared to the 10^{12} neurons present in mammals, and some of their largest neurons approach 1 mm in diameter, which makes them the largest somatic cells in animals. The size of *Aplysia* neurons provides several advantages for neurotoxicity research: these cells can be easily manipulated via dissection or injection, the behavioral functions of individual neurons can be mapped, and they can even be cultured for the purpose of generating in vitro neural networks (Zhao et al., 2009).

To date, one of the most convincing models of reproductive endocrine disruption is the occurrence of "imposex" in marine snails that have

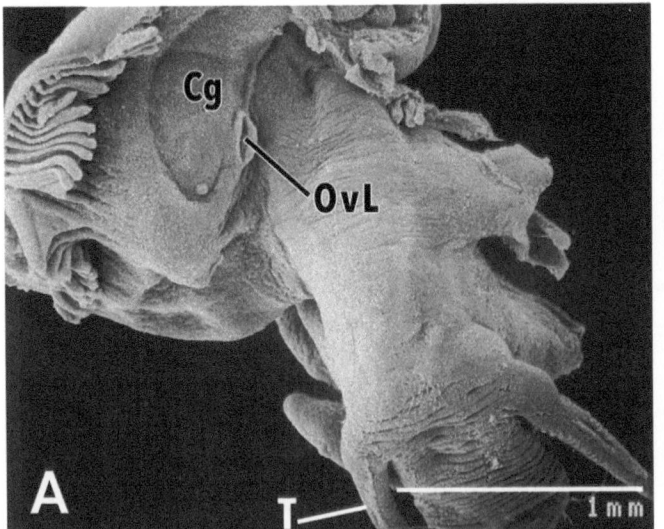
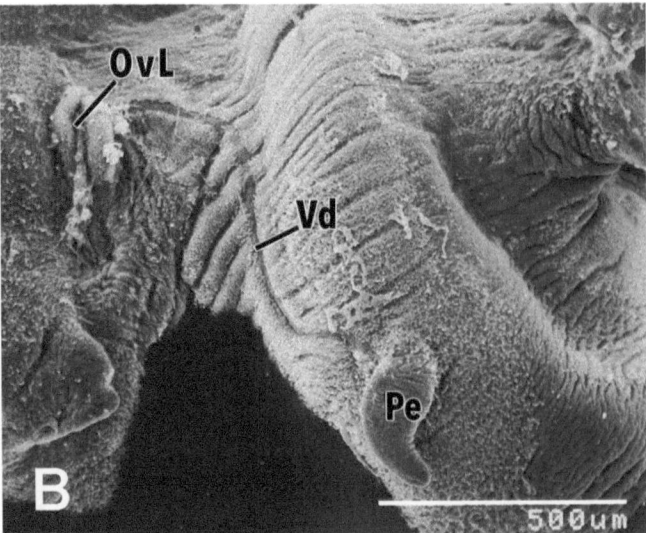

FIGURE 22.4 Scanning electron micrographs of two wild-caught, sexually mature, female marine mudsnails *Hydrobia ulvae*. (A) Normal female collected in the North Sea at a comparatively uncontaminated reference station. Evident in the image are the slit-like vagina (OvL), the capsule gland (CG), and the ocular tentacles (T). (B) Imposex female obtained near Wismar Harbor in the Baltic Sea, a shipping port known historically to have high levels of tributyltin (TBT) contamination. This female has developed a rudimentary penis (Pe) and a vas deferens (Vd), the latter of which is a tubular structure that extends from the base of the penis along the floor of the mantle cavity toward the vagina (OvL). In this example, the vaginal opening has been occluded by proliferating vas deferens tissue, thus preventing egg capsule release and rendering this female functionally sterile. *Images courtesy of Jörg Oehlmann, Goethe University Frankfurt am Main, Institute for Ecology, Evolution and Diversity, Department of Aquatic Ecotoxicology, Frankfurt, Germany.*

had environmental or experimental exposure to organotin compounds. The term "imposex" refers to a condition in which the male genitalia (penis, vas deferens) are irreversibly superimposed on the genitalia of female marine gastropods (Figure 22.4). Exposure to tributyltin (TBT), a biocide ingredient in antifouling paints applied to the undersides of ships and other marine installations, is considered to be the predominant cause of this particular reproductive tract malformation. There are numerous lines of evidence linking TBT to imposex formation, including the following: (1) the historical onset of imposex coincides with earliest utilization of TBT; (2) strong correlations exist between ambient concentrations of TBT and the prevalence and/or severity of imposex, and between the severity of imposex and tissue concentrations of TBT; (3) sex ratios are skewed to male and juvenile recruitment is reduced in TBT-impacted locations; (4) snails transplanted from clean sites to TBT-contaminated harbors absorb TBT and develop imposex; (5) the occurrence of imposex in laboratory-reared snails and those from pristine habitats is very low or nonexistent; and (6) snail populations have recovered from imposex and reemerged in at least some of the areas where TBT has been partially

banned (Oehlmann et al., 2007). Several mechanisms have been proposed for imposex induction, including inhibition of testosterone excretion, interference with testosterone esterification, neuropeptide-like effects on genital development, inhibition of aromatase, and agonistic activation of the retinoid X receptor. Imposex frequency in certain prosobranch snails has been used as a biomonitoring tool for TBT contamination, facilitated by standardized systems of imposex severity measurement such as the vas deferens sequence index and the relative penis size index (Anastasiou et al., 2016).

2.2. Fish

Basic Biologic Characteristics and Common Species

As with the other nonmammalian animal species, the use of fish in toxicology varies widely, from field research in ecotoxicology to target animal safety (TAS) studies for aquaculture to laboratory-based chemical screening and basic research. Accordingly, the fish species used are widely diverse in terms of their biological characteristics. However, those species most commonly used in a laboratory setting typically offer the advantages of small size, high fecundity, and rapid external development of embryos (Cassar et al., 2020; Katsiadaki et al., 2007; Lieschke and Currie, 2007). While the zebrafish *Danio rerio* has become the all-around workhorse among fish species in biomedical research and drug discovery, several other fish species maintain their utility in laboratory toxicology investigations, particularly for endocrine disruption studies. Some of the most commonly used species include the Japanese medaka *Oryzias latipes* (Shima and Mitani, 2004) and the fathead minnow *Pimephales promelas* (Ankley et al., 2001; Palace et al., 2002). The rainbow trout *O. mykiss* is used in endocrine disruption studies and is a frequently employed tumorigenesis model (Williams et al., 2003).

Background Findings

While a detailed discussion of background findings in fish is beyond the scope of this chapter, it is worth reviewing features of certain key tissues (liver, gill, kidney, and gonads) pertinent to toxicologic investigations in fish. It should be noted that, as is the case in mammals, toxicologic effects in fish are not restricted to these tissues. Spontaneous neoplasms in fish will be briefly discussed as these may be encountered in ecotoxicological research or aquaculture.

The liver is the most frequent site for chemically induced primary tumors in fish, and in company with the gills and kidneys, it is a preferred target for noncarcinogenic toxicity. Compared to the mammalian liver, the fish liver is generally less sensitive to hepatotoxicants, and several anatomical and physiological factors may be responsible for relative differences in susceptibility (Wolf and Wolfe, 2005). For example, because fish hepatocytes are arranged as a system of blind-ended, anastomosing, and branching tubules rather than cords, exposure to toxicants may be reduced because sinusoidal perfusion is limited to only the basal and basolateral aspects of hepatocytes. Fish livers are also smaller than mammalian livers relative to body weight and they are 25%–50% less perfused; these factors may further limit toxicant exposure. Additionally, because hepatic lobules are not sharply defined and biotransformation enzymes tend to be homogenously distributed, toxic effects tend to occur diffusely, as opposed to the more concentrated centrilobular, midzonal, or periportal patterns of hepatocellular change that are often seen in mammalian livers. Physiologically, hepatic monooxygenase cytochrome enzymes such as CYP1A appear to be less consistently induced by xenobiotics in fish livers. However, fish livers are certainly susceptible to a variety of hepatotoxicants, including classic examples such as carbon tetrachloride, acetaminophen, and microcystins (blue-green algal toxins) (Wolf and Wolfe, 2005). Compared to mammals, the regenerative ability of fish livers following toxicant-induced damage is, in some cases, nothing short of phenomenal (Choi et al., 2014).

As previously stated, the gills are another preferred site for toxic responses in fish, especially in terms of morphologic effects. Undoubtedly, the inherent vulnerability of the gill tissue to chemical trauma is due in part to the continuous exposure of the single-layered lamellar epithelium to the water environment. Additionally, the gills have a high level of metabolic activity and diverse physiological responsibilities, as they play major roles in respiratory gas exchange, ionic and acid–base balance, and the excretion of nitrogenous waste substances, and a contributing role in the extrahepatic biotransformation of xenobiotics (Evans, 1987). A consequence of this multiplicity of physiological demands is that the gills provide numerous targets for waterborne toxins that include carrier-based ionic exchange mechanisms, paracellular pathways of fluid and ion exchange, molecular transport enzymes, and vascular hormone receptors (Evans, 1987). Morphologic responses of the gills to toxic insults are varied but not infinite, and include the following: necrosis or desquamation of epithelial pavement cells (squamous cells covering the lamellar surface) or pillar cells (modified endothelial cells supporting gill lamellae); epithelial cell hyperplasia and hypertrophy; adhesion or fusion of (secondary) lamellae or filaments; lamellar edema; hemorrhage within filaments or lamellae; lamellar telangiectasis and/or thrombosis; increased leukocyte infiltration; changes in chloride cell numbers; increased rodlet cells; mucus cell hyperplasia; and excessive mucus production. Although patterns of histopathologically evident effects may suggest certain etiologies (for example, lamellar adhesions are often sequelae to metal toxicity or bacterial gill disease induced by *Flavobacterium* spp.), changes in the gills are most often nonspecific. Additionally, it may be difficult to differentiate cases of targeted gill toxicity from chemical "irritation" (e.g., caused by pH extremes) or osmotically induced stress, especially if the toxic effects become complicated by opportunistic bacterial or fungal infections, uncommon but potentially confounding factors in toxicity studies (Evans, 1987; Mallat, 1985; Wood, 2001). Nonneoplastic proliferative responses to chemically induced injury can occur with such rapidity in the gills that the term "chronic" is often not used as a temporal modifier in histopathologic diagnoses, and similar to the liver, the regenerative capacity of gill tissue can be remarkable if the fish survives the initial insult. Among the ever-expanding list of natural and man-made substances that cause gill toxicity in fish are metals (e.g., aluminum, copper, zinc, cadmium, cobalt, silver, and mercury), organochlorines, organophosphates and carbamates, herbicides, petroleum compounds, detergents, chemotherapeutic agents, and nitrogenous waste materials such as ammonia (for comprehensive lists, see Mallatt, 1985, and Wood, 2001).

Anatomically and functionally, the fish kidney differs from the mammalian kidney in a number of respects. Adult fish have a mesonephric (= opisthonephric) kidney that is primitive relative to the metanephric kidney of mammals, and as such, it contains far fewer nephrons (10–50 as compared to approximately one million in higher vertebrates), and the renal parenchyma is not organized into distinct cortical and medullary regions. Nephrons generally lack a loop of Henle; consequently, most fish cannot increase the solute concentration of their urine. Reductionism is a trend in saltwater fishes (which are evolutionarily more advanced than freshwater fishes), and nephrons in some marine species lack distal tubular segments and/or glomeruli (Larsen and Perkins, 2001). Blood flow to the fish kidney approaches that of the entire cardiac output due to the existence of a renal portal system (Pritchard and Miller, 1980). Structural elements of the hemopoietic, immunologic, and endocrine systems are located in the kidney, usually in the anterior portion; therefore, in addition to supplementing the gills in the elimination of nitrogenous wastes, the fish kidney also participates in activities as diverse as hematopoiesis, lymphopoiesis, antigen processing, calcium regulation, and the production of corticosteroid and adrenergic hormones. From a toxicologic standpoint, the excretory kidney and the interstitial hematopoietic/lymphopoietic tissue are probably the two most common targets for microscopically visible effects. Consequences of toxicologic insult to the fish nephron are qualitatively similar to the types of effects that occur in mammals, and commonly observed changes include the following: renal tubular vacuolation; degeneration and necrosis; thickening of glomerular membranes and mesangium; dilation of glomerular capillary loops; glomerular vascular thrombosis; alterations in the size of Bowman's space; periglomerular fibrosis; and secondary interstitial inflammation. As in mammals, the proximal tubule is particularly susceptible to injury as it bears primary responsibility for the renal excretion of xenobiotics and their metabolites (Larson and Perkins, 2001). There is evidence that proximal tubule damage may be at least partially mediated by endothelin-induced decreases in the multidrug resistance protein 2–associated transport of toxic substances into the urine (Masereeuw et al., 2000). The adult fish kidney has the ability to wholly regenerate nephrons following injury, as demonstrated, for example, in a study in which goldfish were exposed experimentally to the nephrotoxic compound hexachlorobutadiene (Reimschuessel et al., 1990). It is perhaps because of this regenerative ability, and the fact that the gills are the primary site for the elimination of nitrogenous wastes, that fish appear able to tolerate a proportionally greater amount of renal tissue damage as compared to mammals. Additional substances known to be nephrotoxic in fish include metals such as cadmium (for which the kidney is the primary target organ) and mercury; organophosphate, carbamate, and organochlorine pesticides; and aminoglycoside antibiotics (Larson and Perkins, 2001). Effects suggestive of immunotoxicity and/or impaired hematopoiesis have been observed in the renal hematopoietic tissue. Substances considered to be immunotoxic in fish include PAHs, halogenated aromatic hydrocarbons, metals, and organometals (Burnett, 2005). In several fish species, the administration of high doses of certain antibiotics (e.g., oxytetracycline, florfenicol) has been associated with decreases in numbers of lymphopoietic and/or hematopoietic cells located in the interstitium of the anterior kidney, with or without overt evidence of individual cell necrosis or apoptosis (Gaikowski et al., 2003). Expansion in the size and/or number of pigmented macrophage aggregates (clusters of constituent histiocytic phagocytes that function as reservoirs for cell breakdown products and as sites of antigen presentation) in the kidney, and other tissues, has also been used as a marker of prior toxicologic insult (Fournie et al., 2001).

Histopathology can be a valuable tool in reproductive endocrine disruption compound (EDC) studies involving fish because piscine gonads are quite labile during early development and even in the adults of some gonochoristic species in which the gonadal sex does not normally change during the animal's lifespan. In addition to intersex (the presence of opposite sex tissue in the gonads), characteristic microscopic changes in the gonads in response to EDCs can include the following: malformations of the gonadal efferent duct system; variations in the proportions of different gametogenic precursors (e.g., estrogenic exposure has been associated with increased spermatogonia relative to other cell stages); altered gametocyte production; gametocyte degeneration (e.g., excessive or inappropriate ovarian follicular atresia); decreased yolk formation in ovarian follicles (a consequence of aromatase inhibitors); and the increased prominence of somatic cells such as Leydig (interstitial) cells in testes or granulosa cells in ovaries. Histopathologic changes caused by the exogenous administration of reproductive hormones or their anthropogenic mimics are not restricted to the gonads. During periods prior to spawning, the livers of reproductively mature female fish typically generate a phospholipoglycoprotein called vitellogenin that is a required ingredient for egg yolk production. Vitellogenesis is associated with an upregulation of organelles (e.g., rough endoplasmic reticulum) in hepatocytes that often imparts a noticeable basophilic coloration to the cytoplasm of the liver cells in hematoxylin-stained histologic specimens. Excessive amounts of vitellogenin protein in the plasma of fish exposed to potent estrogenic substances, for example, can be visualized in histologic sections as dark pink homogenous material within the vasculature at various systemic sites. Furthermore, in male fish (which normally have minimal measurable circulating vitellogenin), chemically induced production of vitellogenin by the liver has been linked to profound renal glomerular and tubular damage (Figure 22.5), which is presumably caused by protein overload of the renal excretory system (Palace et al., 2002).

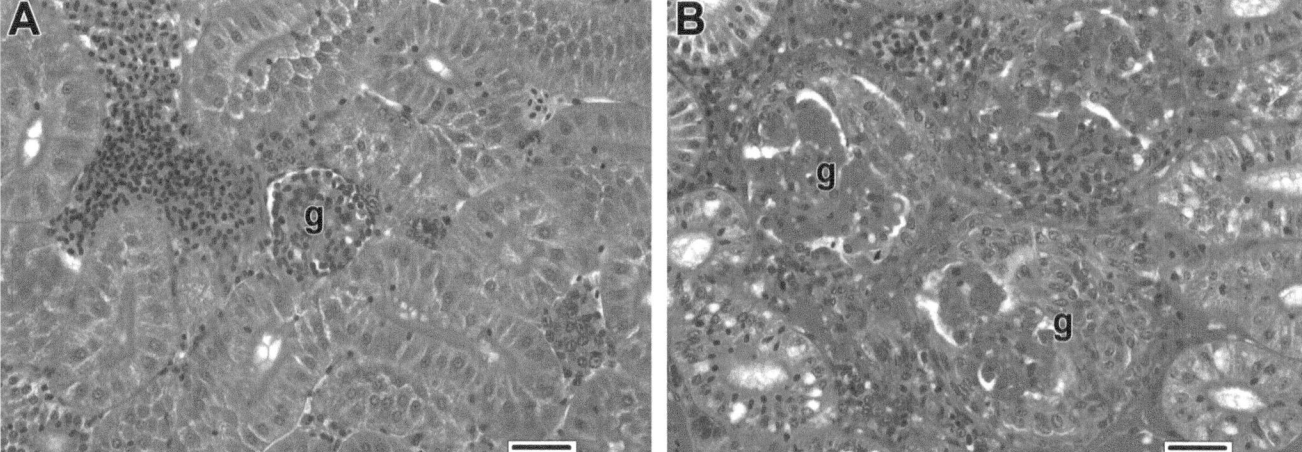

FIGURE 22.5 Estrogen toxicity. Kidneys from adult male fathead minnow *Pimephales promelas*. H&E, Bar = 250 µm. (A) Control. (B) Experimental exposure to an estrogenic chemical. Estrogen stimulates the liver to produce vitellogenin, a phospholipoglycoprotein required for egg yolk formation in females. Renal changes induced by excess vitellogenin in male fish include marked glomerulomegaly, protein droplet accumulation, and tubular epithelial vacuolation. *g*, glomerulus. *Figure reproduced from Haschek WM, Rousseaux CG, Wallig MA, editors: Haschek and Rousseaux's handbook of toxicologic pathology, ed 3, 2013, Academic Press, Figure 14.12, p 498, with permission.*

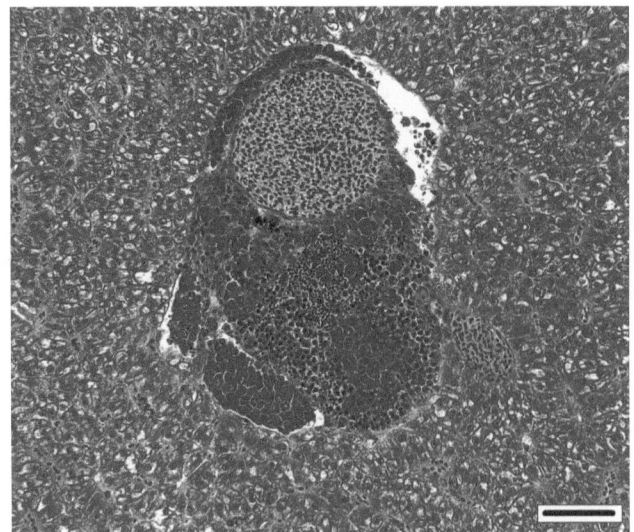

FIGURE 22.6   Liver, untreated medaka *Oryzias latipes*, metastatic spermatocytic seminoma. Multiple stages of spermatogenic development are evident in the neoplastic tissue, which partially occupies a large hepatic vein and extends into the hepatic parenchyma. Tumor metastasis is typically uncommon in fish relative to mammals. H&E, Bar = 50 μm. *Figure reproduced from Haschek WM, Rousseaux CG, Wallig MA, editors: Haschek and Rousseaux's handbook of toxicologic pathology, ed 3, 2013, Academic Press, Figure 14.11, p. 495, with permission.*

Although the background incidence of neoplasia in most fishes tends to be low, many pathologists may be surprised to learn that most of the same types of epithelial, mesenchymal, and round cell tumors found in mammals have been observed to occur spontaneously in fish, and the histomorphology of many preneoplastic and neoplastic proliferative lesions is often strikingly familiar. Distal or localized spread of malignant neoplasms occurs less commonly in fish than in mammals, but when tumor tissue does travel, it often localizes in the liver (Figure 22.6). Species predilections exist (Table 22.3) and, in some, oncogenic viruses have been shown or suspected to cause neoplasms (Coffee et al., 2013; Feitsma and Cuppen, 2008; Vergneau-Grosset et al., 2017). Spatial associations have been recognized between the presence of some other types of infectious organisms and the formation of hyperplastic lesions and tumors, and examples include the cooccurrence of pseudocapillaria nematodes and intestinal and ductal (pancreatic or biliary) carcinomas in zebrafish (Kent et al., 2002), and microsporidian organisms and ovarian granulosa cell tumors in longjaw mudsuckers

Gillichthys mirabilis (Boorman et al., 2012). However, despite the recognized ability of viruses, parasites, and various carcinogenic chemicals to cause cancer in fish, at least by experimental exposure, for most naturally occurring piscine neoplasms, the reasons for tumor formation are unknown.

Major Disease Models

The earliest known toxicological tests in fish primarily involved acute studies and lethal outcomes, in which one of several common species of freshwater carps, minnows, or salmonids was exposed to anthropogenic compounds to determine the relative toxicity of various substances found in natural waterways. During the last several decades of the 20th century, however, scientists began to fully recognize and appreciate the ability of fish to form a variety of proliferative lesions in apparent response to environmental chemical exposure. In the United States, field investigations of certain nonmigratory and benthic fishes that inhabit coastal waters known to be contaminated by industrial or sewage effluents provided seminal results (Law, 2003). In impacted Pacific coast sites such as Puget Sound, Washington, San Francisco Bay, and others, the discovery of neoplastic and preneoplastic liver lesions in bottom-dwelling fishes such as the English sole *Pleuronectes vetulus* and starry flounder *Platichthys stellatus*, and the potential association between the prevalence of these lesions and polychlorinated biphenyls (PCBs), PAHs, and other nonnatural contaminants prompted US Congressional hearings and legislative activity (Myers et al., 1994). Further impetus for toxicologic research was provided by the decades-old discovery of contaminant-associated liver and pancreatic neoplasms in mummichogs *F. heteroclitus* (an estuarine killifish) in the Elizabeth River, Virginia, USA (Burnett et al., 2007), and liver and dermal tumors in brown bullhead catfish *Ameiurus nebulosus* in the Great Lakes, its tributary rivers, and other Midwestern and Northeastern US waterways (Baumann and Harshbarger, 1995). The impact that these discoveries, and those of other fish tumor epizootics, have had on environmental research can hardly be overstated. In fact, fish from many of these locations are still being monitored for tumor burden to document the effects of contaminant site remediation, and reductions

TABLE 22.3   Common Neoplasms in Fish with Species Predilections

Species	Neoplasm	Associated etiology
Goldfish (*Carassius auratus auratus*)	Chromatophoroma	
Goldfish x Carp (*Cyprinus carpio*) hybrids	Gonadal stromal tumor	
Hawaiian butterflyfishes (*Chaetodon* spp.)	Chromatophoroma	
Zebrafish (*Danio rerio*)	Seminoma, Ultimobranchial gland tumor	
Zebrafish (*Danio rerio*)	Intestinal carcinoma	*Pseudocapillaria tomentosa*
Esox spp.	Lymphoma	Viral etiology suspected
Mangrove snapper (*Lutjanus griseus*)	Subcutaneous nerve sheath tumor	
Oncorhynchus spp.	Papilloma, Basal cell tumor	Herpesvirus
Chinook salmon (*Oncorhynchus tshawytscha*)	Ameloblastoma	Viral etiology suspected
Chinook salmon (*Oncorhynchus tshawytscha*)	Plasmacytoid leukemia	Viral etiology suspected
Bicolor damselfish (*Pomacentrus partitus*)	Nerve sheath tumors	
Freshwater angelfish (*Pterophyllum scalare*)	Lip fibroma/odontoma	Viral etiology suspected
Walleye (*Sander vitreus*)	Dermal sarcoma	Walleye dermal sarcoma virus (retrovirus)
Platyfish (*Xiphophorus maculatus*) x Swordtail (*Xiphophorus helleri*) hybrids	Melanoma	

in the concentrations of carcinogens in the water, sediment, and fish tissues have been associated with declines in tumor incidence at some impacted sites (Baumann and Harshbarger, 1995).

The emphasis of environmental research in fish over time has shifted gradually from studies that primarily involved known or suspected carcinogens and heavy metals to those focused on various agricultural, industrial, and pharmaceutical chemicals that have been associated, at least circumstantially, with nonneoplastic toxicity and endocrine disruption. As with invertebrates, toxicity testing in fish has become a critical part of environmental impact assessments required for certain new drug applications (VICH, 2004; U.S. Food and Drug Administration, 1998) and a mainstay in EDC studies (Ankley et al., 2001). Some of the most widely used fish species in EDC experiments include Japanese medaka *O. latipes*, zebrafish *D. rerio*, fathead minnow *P. promelas*, three-spined stickleback *Gasterosteus aculeatus*, guppy *Poecilia reticulata*, sheepshead minnow *Cyprinodon variegatus*, and rainbow trout *O. mykiss*. Each of these species has its own intrinsic benefits and drawbacks as a model organism for EDC studies. For example, one advantage of using fathead minnows is that reproductively active males develop macroscopically evident, external secondary sex characteristics that include specialized coloration, nuptial tubercles (a bilaterally symmetrical pattern of small, wart-like protuberances on the face), and enlargement of the dorsal nape pad (a subcutaneous deposition of loose collagenous tissue along the dorsal aspects of the head and neck). The development of these features is androgen dependent, and conversely, their phenotypic expression can be reduced or eliminated in a dose-dependent manner by exposure of the fish to exogenous estrogens or substances with estrogen-like activity (Ankley et al., 2001). Alternatively, a different set of advantages is offered by use of the three-spined stickleback model. Male sticklebacks produce a glue-like protein in their kidneys called spiggin that is essential for nest building, and spiggin production is under the control of androgens. Female sticklebacks normally do not produce this protein; consequently, the induction of measurable concentrations of renal spiggin in female sticklebacks that were exposed experimentally to contaminated effluents has been used as a biomarker for exogenous androgenic activity (Katsiadaki et al., 2007). In a similar fashion, the potential antiandrogenic activity of xenobiotic substances can be determined by the extent to which they inhibit spiggin production in males (Katsiadaki et al., 2007). A further advantage of using *G. aculeatus* is the existence of DNA markers that can be used to determine the genotypic sex of individual fish (Katsiadaki et al., 2007). Because most fish species do not have heteromorphic sex chromosomes, the existence of genetic markers for sex is a plus for experiments in which exogenous hormone administration results in an intersex condition, i.e., the genetic sex can be determined in instances where the phenotypic sex is ambiguous. Thus, the results of nonmorphologic endpoints such as these can aid the pathologist by providing context for understanding the relevance and potential mechanism(s) of action associated with certain pathologic findings.

Currently, any in-depth discussion of nonmammalian animals used in toxicological bioassays and drug screening would have to acknowledge the dominance of the zebrafish as a biomedical research model. A contemporary testament to the importance of this model, in addition to the mountain of published work that has accumulated over the past decade, is the ubiquitous presence of zebrafish colonies in the laboratories of universities, human medical centers, pharmaceutical companies, and the research arms of government agencies across the globe. Some of the medical research areas in which zebrafish have made the greatest contribution, or shown the most promise, include embryogenesis, immunology,

hemostasis, cardiology, functional anatomy of ocular and auditory organs, endocrine disruption, developmental neurology, angiogenesis, oncology, and aging. As experimental subjects, zebrafish possess all of the advantages that are typically associated with other species of small ornamental aquarium fish, such as high fecundity, short generation time, ease of culture, hardiness, small volume dosing, the ability to administer test compounds via water bath exposure, the capacity to house large numbers of animals in a small space, and the capability of viewing multiple organ systems in relatively few histologic sections. However, zebrafish have a number of bonus attributes that have caused them to vault past other fishes in terms of research utility. Consequently, they have become a universal model for many types of toxicologic studies, including those involving basic biomedical research, drug development and screening, toxicity testing (acute, developmental, or organ specific), and ecotoxicologic investigations (Cassar et al., 2020). Zebrafish spawn year round and are oviparous (the eggs are scattered and externally fertilized), and the unparalleled transparency of their early stage embryos allows visualization of several rapidly emerging organ systems, full development of which occurs by 96 h postfertilization, which is roughly equivalent to that of a 3-month-old human embryo. The period of transparency can be extended by adding the tyrosinase inhibitor 1-phenyl-2-thiourea to the growth medium, or alternatively, the *casper* mutant strain of apigmented zebrafish can be utilized (Garcia et al., 2016). Transparency also facilitates a wide variety of manipulations that involve, for example, microinjections of nucleic acid materials or the microsurgical removal or transplantation of specific embryonic cell lines. A vast array of mutant strains is available (Cornet et al., 2018; Lieschke and Currie, 2007). Some of these manipulated strains have been found to mimic genetically based human diseases, not only molecularly but also phenotypically in some cases, whereas other transgenic zebrafish are employed in studies of gene function, efficacy screening of pharmaceutical compounds, and toxicity testing (Cornet et al., 2018). The fact that zebrafish embryos can be reared in 96-well plates for up to 5 days, without requiring supplemental feeding due to their attached yolk sacs, allows them to be used in whole-animal high-throughput assays for screening drugs or toxic chemicals. Imaging platforms specifically designed for these zebrafish embryo setups facilitate rapid, automated evaluation of in vivo morphologic endpoints relevant to cardiotoxicity and neurotoxicity, among others. In one of the most efficient uses of such assays, anesthetized transgenic zebrafish embryos that expressed a green fluorescent protein (GFP) marker were combined with automated imaging and analysis to screen for compounds that modulated the FGF/RAS/MAPK intracellular signaling pathway (Saydmohammed et al., 2018).

Similar to laboratory rodents, there are several strains of zebrafish commonly in use. Mapping of the zebrafish genome has been completed for the Tuebingen strain. An annotated assembly of this reference genome is maintained and periodically updated (https://www.ncbi.nlm.nih.gov/grc/zebrafish), facilitating comparative genomics and other genetic-based research. Studies to characterize strain differences and their potential impacts on research are ongoing.

2.3. Amphibians

Basic Biologic Characteristics and Common Species

Amphibians, especially frogs, are excellent subjects for toxicological studies. Frog experiments can be conducted in the laboratory, in the field, or in intermediate enclosed systems known as "mesocosms," which offer advantages of controlled experiments with "real-world" variables. Not only are they small animals with short generational times, their aquatic phases can be exposed to test agents continuously via water bath, and exposure can occur simultaneously through multiple absorption routes (i.e., via the gills, skin, and gastrointestinal tract). Amphibians typically have complex life cycles in which the juvenile stages (egg, embryo, and larva) are particularly sensitive to a variety of toxicants, and chemically induced disturbances in these developing animals often produce dramatic morphologic changes. The potential for exposure to environmental contaminants is very high in amphibians for a number of reasons: they lay permeable eggs in water; their skin is permeable to fluids and gases; most have

both aquatic and terrestrial phases in their life cycle, plus a physiologically demanding metamorphic period; the algal diet of young amphibians and carnivorous diet of adults enhance the opportunity to ingest contaminated food; and they hibernate in sediment, which is a well-documented repository for a variety of anthropogenic pollutants (Venturino et al., 2003). The elaborate life cycles and well-characterized behavioral traits of frogs ensure that a wealth of endpoints, some universal and others uniquely amphibian (e.g., hind limb resorption), are available for toxicologic bioassays. Tumor development, whether spontaneous, virally induced (e.g., Lucke's herpesvirus [ranid herpesvirus 1]), or caused by other factors, occurs in all major organ systems of both anurans (frogs and toads) and urodeles (tailed amphibians) (Stacy and Parker, 2004); in general, responses to chemical carcinogens in amphibians tend to parallel those of mammals.

Based on recent literature reviews (Sievers et al., 2019; Slaby et al., 2019), the most utilized amphibians for contaminant-based research are members of the Ranidae (true frogs), followed by the tongueless *Xenopus* spp. African clawed frogs, bufonids (true toads), caudate (urodele) amphibians (salamanders and newts), and hylids (tree frogs). Although it is often desirable to simulate authentic ecotoxicological conditions by using amphibians that are native to a particular region of interest, native species can be challenging research subjects for a number of reasons: they may only spawn seasonally and they often have low laboratory survival; it may be difficult to capture adequate numbers of specimens for testing; standardized protocols may not be available for certain species; and collection of animals in the wild may place added pressure on at-risk populations. Presently, the premier amphibians for many types of laboratory research are *Xenopus* spp. frogs, including, in particular, *Xenopus laevis*, and the closely related *Xenopus* (*Silurana*) *tropicalis*. Unlike many other amphibians that have terrestrial phases, defined breeding seasons, and require several years of development to attain sexual maturity, laboratory-cultured *Xenopus* frogs are entirely aquatic, they can be induced to spawn year round, and they attain reproductive maturity in 1–2 years or less, depending on the species (Kashiwagi et al., 2010). Additionally,

Xenopus has long been a preferred model for early developmental and gene expression studies due to the large size and sturdiness of their embryonic cells and eggs, and the amenability of their external embryos to surgical manipulation. Although *X. laevis* is by far the most studied of the 19 members in the genus, the smaller *X. tropicalis* has advantages that include a more rapid generation time and the ability for researchers to determine the genotypic sex of individual frogs (Kashiwagi et al., 2010). While polyploid genomes are common among many amphibian species (Schmid, Evans, & Bogart, 2015), *X. tropicalis* offers the additional advantage of a diploid genome that is also fully sequenced (https://uswest.ensembl.org/Xenopus_tropicalis/Info/Index?db=core).In terms of ecotoxicological experiments, the major criticism of *Xenopus* as a surrogate test animal is that they are behaviorally, anatomically, and physiologically different from many native amphibians, and as a result, may not exhibit comparable sensitivity to toxicants. Despite that alleged shortcoming, *Xenopus* has been employed as a laboratory subject for research disciplines as diverse as tissue regeneration, drug screening, tumorigenesis, immunology, and thyroid and reproductive endocrine disruption. These frogs are now continuously available through commercial sources, and decades of research efforts have culminated in the production of various *X. tropicalis* transformants through the use of a variety of elegant transgenesis procedures (Chesneau et al., 2008). Standardized criteria developed for the visual staging of *Xenopus* embryologic development (Nieuwkoop and Faber, 1994) have allowed investigators to assess the effects of toxicants on the timing and completeness of amphibian metamorphosis, which is a process that is known to be highly thyroid hormone dependent (Figure 22.7).

Background Findings

While captive-bred *X. laevis* and *X. tropicalis* can be readily obtained from commercial suppliers, wild-caught specimens are frequently employed in environmental monitoring, ecotoxicology, and biomedical research settings. As such, infectious diseases may act as confounding factors in toxicological research utilizing amphibians. A variety of protozoan and metazoan parasites may be encountered as either asymptomatic or symptomatic infections (Densmore and Green, 2007). Septicemia caused by bacteria, including but not limited to *Aeromonas hydrophila*, is not uncommon. Outbreaks of *Mycobacterium* spp. and *Chlamydia* spp. have been reported in both wild-caught and captive-reared colonies (Densmore and Green, 2007). Ranaviruses are well-described pathogens of both amphibians and reptiles. Yet the amphibian pathogen that has received perhaps the most attention over the past 2 decades is the chytrid fungus *Batrachochytrium dendrobatidis*. Numerous amphibian species are susceptible to this chytrid fungus that infects keratinized skin, disrupting skin physiology and increasing susceptibility to secondary infections (Densmore and Green, 2007).

Many amphibian species have fastidious dietary and environmental requirements. Such requirements may not be well characterized for less commonly used species. Nutritional deficiency or excess and other husbandry-related issues are major factors affecting the health of the amphibians in captivity (Densmore and Green, 2007).

Major Disease Models

Amphibians are widely distributed and located on all continents except Antarctica. However, due to a number of factors that include habitat destruction, climate change, environmental pollution, infectious disease, and the impacts of introduced competitors or predators, worldwide numbers of amphibians appear to be declining and selected populations are threatened, endangered, or have become extinct. Wild amphibian populations as well as surrogate species in laboratory settings have been studied extensively to elucidate the causes of this global decline. Man-made pollutants are frequently identified as reasons for this decline, and yet the evidence for causal associations is not always conclusive. For example, careful experimentation has revealed that the two major types of limb malformations in frogs, extra limbs/digits and missing limbs/digits, are more likely to be a direct result of trematode metacercarial infection and nonlethal predation, respectively, rather than pollution (Johnson and Sutherland, 2003). Other well-documented threats to amphibian

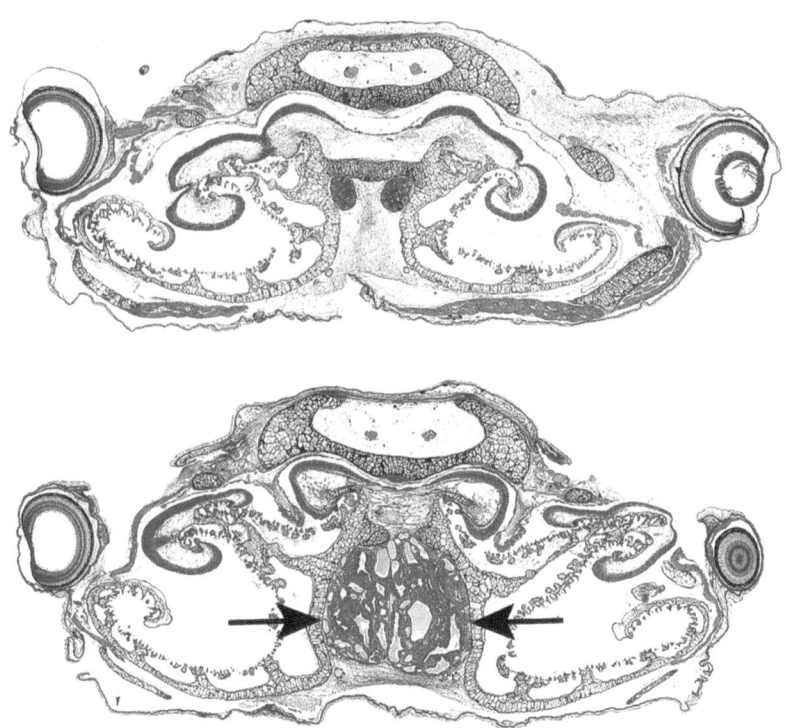

FIGURE 22.7 Cross-sections through the heads of two *Xenopus laevis* tadpoles. The upper image is from an untreated control frog, and the lower image is from a frog that was exposed to 20 mg/L 6-propylthiouracil (PTU) for 21 days. PTU-related changes included severe, diffuse enlargement of the thyroid glands (*arrows*), moderate follicular distension, marked hyperplasia of thyroid follicular cells, and pale foamy colloid. From a study conducted by the United States EPA. H&E, 12.5× magnification. *Figure reproduced from Haschek WM, Rousseaux CG, Wallig MA, editors:* Haschek and Rousseaux's handbook of toxicologic pathology, *ed 3, 2013, Academic Press, Figure 14.13, p. 501, with permission.*

populations include infections with *B. dendrobatidis* fungi or ranaviruses. However, pollution may still play a role in these scenarios. For example, eutrophication caused by agricultural runoff may provide favorable habitat for the snail intermediates of trematode infections, and other chemicals may act as immunotoxicants and thus impair resistance to bacterial and fungal infections (Johnson and Sutherland, 2003).

Because toxicological testing in amphibians tends to be environmentally motivated, investigations in amphibians often involve potential effects of anthropogenic substances found in surface waters or sediments, which serve as the ultimate sink for such contaminants (Venturino et al., 2003). Whereas early studies focused on effects of metals or organochlorine compounds, test articles of recent emphasis have included thyroid or reproductive hormones, pharmaceutical agents, and human personal care products.

They have also become frequent subjects for endocrine disruption research, both due to findings of intersex in wild frog populations (Slaby et al., 2019) and the demonstrated ease by which the thyroid and reproductive hormonal axes can be influenced by experimental chemical manipulation (Furlow and Neff, 2006). As part their two-tier Endocrine Disruptor Screening Program (EDSP), the U.S. Environmental Protection Agency (EPA) has developed a multiparameter test using *X. laevis* larvae that interrogates the hypothalamic–pituitary–gonadal (HPG) and hypothalamic–pituitary–thyroidal axes (U.S. EPA, 2015). The facility with which developmental aberrations can be assessed in frog embryos has also made them an attractive model for high-throughput screens evaluating for genotoxicity and teratogenic potential of compounds. The Frog Embryo Teratogenesis Assay—*Xenopus* (FETAX) is a 96-h bath assay developed in the 1980s and still in use today (Hoke and Ankley, 2005). More recently, assays that evaluate left–right asymmetry during gastrulation in the *Xenopus* embryo have been employed to identify drugs that modulate the Wnt/β-catenin pathway (Maia et al., 2017). Similar to zebrafish, automated platforms for analyzing behavior in *Xenopus* larvae have been developed to facilitate evaluation of small-molecule effects on cognitive development.

2.4. Birds

Basic Biologic Characteristics and Common Species

Avian toxicological studies have involved subjects ranging from the albatross *Phoebastria nigripes* to the zebra finch *Taeniopygia guttata*, but the mainstays in avian laboratory research have been the domestic chicken *Gallus gallus domesticus*, the turkey *Meleagris gallopavo*, and the mallard duck *Anas platyrhynchos*. The chicken is also a frequently employed embryogenesis model, and the turkey and mallard duck additionally serve as laboratory surrogates

and field sentinels for wild terrestrial birds and waterfowl, respectively. The surge of endocrine disruption research has spiked an interest in bird models for the testing of known or suspected hormonally active compounds (Figure 22.8) (Touart, 2004; Halldin et al., 2005). Not only are wild birds likely susceptible to toxic perturbations of the endocrine system, the unique aspects of avian physiology (they are homeothermic, oviparous, and the males are the homogametic sex) suggest that results of toxicological testing in other taxa may not necessarily be predictive of effects in birds (Scanes and McNabb, 2003). As of late, several species of quail have risen to the forefront as models for reproductive endocrine toxicity studies; these include the Japanese quail *Coturnix japonica* (Phasianidae) and unrelated new world species such as the Northern bobwhite *Colinus virginianus* (Odontophoridae). Advantages of quail relative to other galliformes or anseriformes (waterfowl) include the precocial development of the chicks (they are relatively mature and require little parental care posthatch), and the fact that they have photoresponsive breeding cycles, which means that they

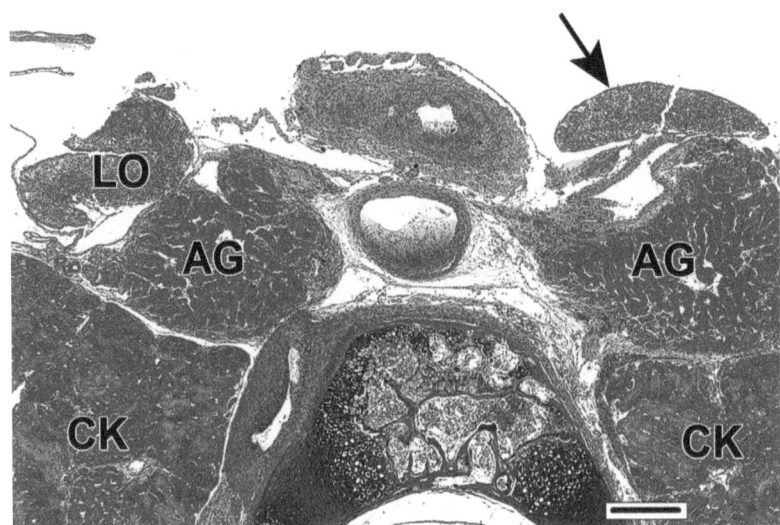

FIGURE 22.8 Transverse section through the anterior abdominal region of a hatchling female Japanese quail *Coturnix japonica*. Apparent spontaneous occurrence of a retained right ovary (*arrow*) in an untreated bird. This type of finding has been associated with exposure to exogenous estrogenic substances. *AG*, adrenal gland, *CK*, cranial kidney; *LO*, left ovary. H&E, Bar = 250 μm. *Figure modified from OCSPP 890.2100: Avian two-generation toxicity test in the Japanese Quail, U.S. Environmental Protection Agency, EPA Pub no. 740-C-15-003, 2015, Figure 118, p. 110, with permission.*

can be artificially induced to lay eggs year round through the manipulation of lighting conditions (Touart, 2004). Such advantages are especially important for studies designed to evaluate potential multigenerational effects of reproductive toxicants. As compared to new world quail, *Coturnix* spp. may be the preferred model because their egg incubation and chick maturation intervals are more rapid, they have higher egg production, and their reproductive physiology and behavioral patterns have been well characterized. Japanese quail also have a couple of sexually dimorphic features that can be exploited (Halldin et al., 2005). Located in the dorsal wall of the proctodeum, the foam-producing cloacal glands are androgen-responsive tissues, and thus the cloacal glands of reproductively active male *Coturnix* quail are measurably larger and more developed than those of females (Figure 22.9). Conversely, inhibition of cloacal gland development in males has been a demonstrated consequence of experimental exposure to estrogenic substances or nonaromatizable androgens such as trenbolone. A further gender-specific feature of *Coturnix* involves a region of the brain known as the medial preoptic nucleus. This cluster of neuronal cell bodies, which surrounds the third ventricle in the hypothalamus, is associated with vocalization in males. It has been reported that the size and number of these neurons is greater in male *Coturnix* relative to females, and that exposure of juvenile males to estrogen inhibits the development of this nucleus in the adults. However, because the magnitude of size differences between the sexes is small (only approximately 20%), morphometric techniques may be required to demonstrate treatment effects.

Background Findings

The structurally and physiologically unique avian lung–air sac respiratory system (Brown et al., 1997) is often perceived to be especially sensitive to airborne toxicants and inhaled particulate matter when compared to the bronchoalveolar lung of mammals. This impression is likely fueled by the historical use of canaries in British coal mines to detect early buildups of toxic gases and the well-known susceptibility of birds such as pet psittacines to vapors released by PTFE (Teflon, SilverStone) when

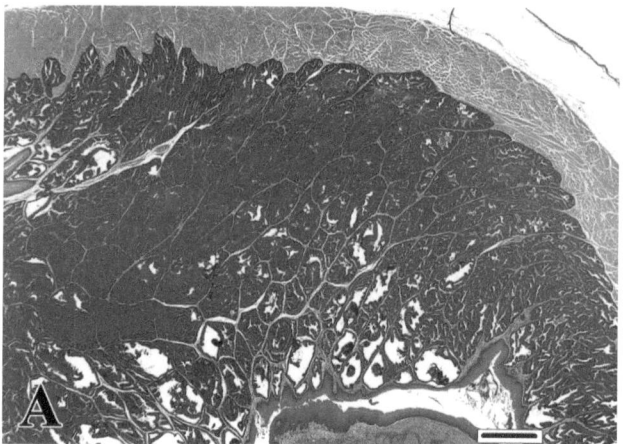
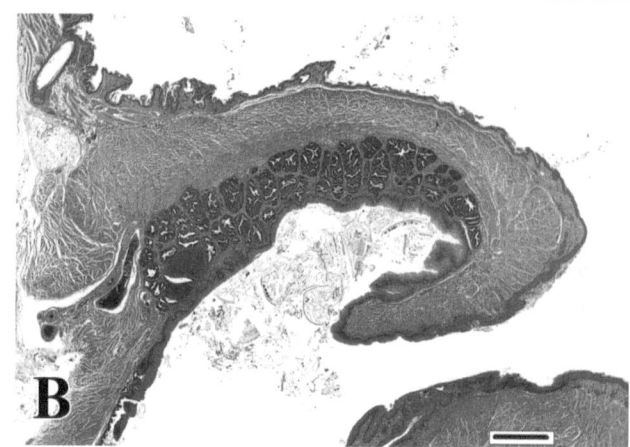

FIGURE 22.9 Sagittal section through the cloacal region of glands of adult Japanese quail *Coturnix japonica*. H&E, Bar = 800 μm. (A) Reproductively active male. The deeply basophilic, androgen responsive, cloacal glands are well developed (B) Female quail. Cloacal glands are less developed. *Figure reproduced from Haschek WM, Rousseaux CG, Wallig MA, editors: Haschek and Rousseaux's handbook of toxicologic pathology, ed 3, 2013, Academic Press, Figure 14.10, p. 503, with permission.*

nonstick cooking vessels coated with this synthetic solid fluorocarbon are overheated inadvertently. Toxic effects of inhaled PTFE degradation products in accidentally exposed broiler chicks consisted of severe pulmonary edema and congestion, but the mechanism of toxicity has not been determined. However, despite the apparent increased susceptibility of birds to the toxic effects of substances such as PTFE and carbon monoxide (the latter is attributed to the relatively high avian metabolic rate), experimental testing in domestic fowl has revealed that birds are inconsistently sensitive to toxic gases and particulates when compared to other taxa (Brown et al., 1997). As examples, study results suggest that ammonia exposure is similarly toxic to birds and mammals, and birds are actually less sensitive than mammals to hydrogen sulfide. Thus, despite the common wisdom, birds are not necessarily superior models for respiratory toxicosis research, and the results of inhaled toxicant studies conducted in mammals cannot be automatically extrapolated to birds, and vice versa.

Major Disease Models

The field of avian toxicology is heavily indebted to research performed in support of the poultry industry and to studies of environmental toxicants in wild birds. A classic example of toxicosis in domestic fowl is the liver damage caused by ingestion of feed contaminated with aflatoxins. Initially discovered as the cause of disease outbreaks in turkey poults in the early 1960s, aflatoxins are heterocyclic metabolites synthesized by *Aspergillus* spp. fungi (specifically, *Aspergillus flavus* and *Aspergillus parasiticus*). Subsequently, it was determined that the extreme sensitivity of poultry to the most potent representative, AFB1, is a result of the ability of birds to efficiently bioactivate AFB1 via cytochrome p450 mixed function oxidases, and their relative inability to detoxify AFB1 via glutathione S-transferases (Rawal et al., 2010). During the same approximate time period, additional interest in avian toxicology was triggered by associations that were drawn between pollutants such as the agricultural organochlorine pesticide dichlorodiphenyltrichloroethane (DDT) and adverse effects in raptors that included egg shell thinning and early embryonic mortality. During the past several decades, additional toxicants of special interest in birds have included: mycotoxins such as fumonisins, ochratoxins, and T-2 toxin; organochlorine compounds such as PCBs; polyhalogenated aromatic hydrocarbons; organophosphates, carbamates, and other pesticides; petroleum-based compounds; selenium derived from mining, manufacturing, and agricultural applications; and components of acid rain such as aluminum (Scanes and McNabb, 2003). Toxic effects of these substances vary, but many on this list are suspected or widely considered to be endocrine disruptors.

Although birds are frequent subjects for environmental toxicological research, there is one particular avian condition that closely models a human disease. It has been established that, unlike rodents and other laboratory mammals, the laying hen develops spontaneous ovarian tumors that are strikingly similar to ovarian cancers of women. Remarkably, this resemblance extends to four subtypes of primary epithelial carcinomas that include serous, endometrioid, mucinous, and clear cell categories (Barua et al., 2009). As in humans, putative precursor lesions have been observed in the ovaries of hens, and metastatic behavior and tumor staging results are also comparable. Additional similarities that have been demonstrated in hen ovarian carcinomas include the protective effects of progesterone and increased expression of molecules such as E-cadherin adhesion proteins and the sphingosine-1 phosphate receptor that controls human lymphocyte trafficking (Bradaric et al., 2011). Because human ovarian cancers are not often diagnosed until the late stages of the disease, the value of this preclinical model is that it allows for the study of early stage changes in a readily available animal subject: in one study, approximately 20% of laying hens had primary ovarian carcinomas that were detectable at least microscopically if not grossly (Barua et al., 2009).

2.5. Reptiles

When compared to other vertebrates and invertebrate taxa, reptiles offer few advantages as nonmammalian animal models for toxicologic bioassays. Less-than-desirable features of reptiles include opaque leathery eggs, relatively impermeable skin, periodic inactivity, extended generational cycles, demanding dietary and husbandry requirements, and a limited knowledge base and sparse genetic information for most species. Accordingly, reptile toxicology studies are typically motivated by observed or suspected effects of environmental contamination in particular species. For example, the periodic observation of aural abscesses in eastern box turtles *Terrapene carolina carolina* was the impetus for an investigation in which the potential cause was postulated to be squamous metaplasia of the inner ear caused by toxicant-induced vitamin A deficiency (Holladay et al., 2001).

One example of reproductive endocrine disruption in wildlife that has received a great deal of attention involved a dramatic decades-long decline in the American alligator *Alligator mississippiensis* population in Lake Apopka, Florida. This particular lake is located adjacent to an EPA superfund site that, in addition to experiencing a DDT and dicofol spill in 1980, was also the recipient of sewage treatment facility effluents and greater than 40 years of agricultural runoff. Investigators were able to make comparisons between findings in Lake Apopka and the nearby Lake Woodruff National Wildlife Refuge, which, although part of the same watershed, was subject to minimal if any direct agricultural or developmental impact. The suggestion that the dwindling alligator population in this lake may have been the result of contaminant-induced perturbations of the endocrine system is supported by several lines of evidence including the following: the detection in collected eggs of contaminants such as p,p'-DDE at concentrations that have been demonstrated to cause sex reversal in reptiles; decreased egg viability; altered sex ratios; single- or multifold differences in plasma concentrations of reproductive hormones when compared to male and female reference animals; abnormal ovarian, testicular, and genital morphology; elevated bone density in juvenile females; and altered gonadal steroidogenic gene expression (Guillette et al., 2007). However, the evidence on this topic remains mixed, as other lines of research have failed to demonstrate causal relationships between organochlorine exposure and embryonic mortality or clutch viability, for example (Schoeb et al., 2001).

There are many additional examples of reptile toxicological studies that could be cited here; however, most of these tend to concern population-relevant, species-specific health issues that have been linked putatively to environmental pollutant exposure. An example would be the potential immunotoxic effects of organochlorine compound exposure in loggerhead sea turtles *Caretta caretta* (Keller et al., 2006).

3. UTILIZATION OF NONMAMMALIAN ANIMALS

3.1. Animal Models of Human Diseases

Animal models are used to investigate molecular, cellular, and physiological mechanisms of human diseases, test for potential therapeutic candidates, characterize physiochemical and pathological responses to pharmaceuticals and toxic chemicals, and to confirm or elucidate the precise role of disease-causing agents. Animal models may be categorized by the extent to which they have been altered from their original phenotype and/or genotype. Such categories include the following: (1) *natural models*, (2) *manipulated models*, and (3) *genetically engineered models*. One example of a natural model involves the unique propensity of laying hens *G. domesticus* to spontaneously develop ovarian tumors that mimic different types of human ovarian cancer (Barua et al., 2009). In another example, it has been determined that the pronephric kidney of *Xenopus* spp. tadpoles may be useful for investigating human heritable disease mechanisms, because the nephrons of frogs and humans have a number of orthologous solute carrier genes (Burggren and Warburton, 2007). Similarly, certain evolutionarily advanced fishes that are aglomerular or lack other nephron components are used to model toxicologic effects that target various renal tubular segments. Thus, the marine toadfish *Opsanus tau*, whose kidneys lack glomeruli, was found to be exquisitely sensitive to proximal tubular injury caused by experimental administration of the aminoglycoside gentamicin (Reimschuessel et al., 1996). As opposed to natural models, manipulated models consist of wild-type subjects that require either chemical, surgical, or other (e.g., radiation-induced immune compromise) treatment in order to reasonably represent a particular human disease condition. Examples include animals whose tissues have been chemically or surgically ablated and xenograft recipients. The third model category comprises animals that possess biologically relevant genetic alterations as a result of chemical- or radiation-induced mutagenesis or transgenic modification. Each model category features its own set of advantages and drawbacks. For example, shortcomings of mice with human tumor xenografts include the amount of time and expense involved in creating the model, and the artificial nature of host responses because immunodeficient or humanized mice must be used as graft recipients. Understandably, a single animal model is rarely capable of portraying a human disease condition in its entirety. Thus, a certain model may mimic the human response in terms of efficacy, but not toxicity, or vice versa, or the model may only replicate a fraction of the clinical symptoms or other phenotypic disease characteristics.

Although manipulated or genetically engineered rodents currently represent the lion's share of human disease models (see *Genetically Engineered Animal Models in Toxicologic Research*, Vol 1, Chap 23), there is frequently a need for lower cost, more rapid, and more easily produced alternatives, especially in assays used to screen for potential therapeutic agents, genetically based disorders, and infectious diseases. First described scientifically in 1846, the hardy and versatile Japanese medaka (also known as ricefish) *O. latipes* was the foremost fish in which Mendelian inheritance patterns were described, and also the initial fish in which sex reversal was artificially induced (Shima and Matani, 2004). Certain advantages that medaka have over the highly popular zebrafish *D. rerio*, for example, include a smaller genome, shorter generation time, broader temperature range, and inbred strains that are permissive for tumor cell transplantation without the need for immunosuppression. During the latter part of the 20th century, medaka were tested extensively with direct-acting carcinogens such as N-methyl-N'-nitro-nitrosoguanidine and a variety of other potent tumor-inducing compounds (DEN, ethylene dibromide, dibenzo[a,l]pyrene, to name but a few) in an attempt to investigate the potential of this species to serve as a natural model for tumor induction (Brown-Peterson et al., 1999; Schartl and Walter, 2016). At one time, it was thought that teleost fish might be poised to supplant traditional experimental animals as premier subjects for carcinogenesis research; however, despite the proclivity of medaka to develop a variety of neoplasms following relatively low-dose exposure to carcinogens, their comparatively rapid onset of tumor formation, and the low background incidence of spontaneous tumors in this species, the early enthusiasm for medaka and other fish as models for human cancer waned for a time. Apparently, researchers found it difficult to reconcile various performance discrepancies between fish and rodent carcinogenesis studies, in which the target organs (e.g., gill vs. lung), routes of exposure (immersion vs. dietary), relative stage of organogenesis (juvenile vs. mature), and sensitivity to chemical challenge often differed (Brannen et al., 2016). However, medaka are mounting a comeback as a cancer model, due in large part to a novel anatomical feature in selective-bred mutant strains that gives this species a distinct advantage over the use of mice and other mammals: transparent skin (Hinton et al., 2005). The benefit of transparent skin is that it allows many internal anatomic features to be viewed in vivo in real time (Figure 22.10). Thus, treatment-related morphologic changes in internal organs may be assessed by nonlethal methods in the same animal at various time points during the study, including both the exposure and recovery phases, which allows the temporal occurrence of effects in various tissues to be chronicled. Additionally, the visualization of specific internal anatomic structures, organogenesis, and physiochemical processes may be further enhanced through the use of transgenic medaka in which the GFP gene has been fused to the regulatory regions of certain genomic sequences (Hinton et al., 2005). Alternatively, the GFP gene can be incorporated into exogenous cells that are injected into "see-through" medaka; examples include the in vivo observation of tumor cell proliferation and metastasis in medaka that have been transplanted with GFP transgenic melanoma cells (Schartl and Walter, 2016) and a tuberculosis model in which transparent medaka were infected with transgenic *Mycobacterium marinum* that express GFP or other fluorescent proteins (Broussard et al., 2009). The GFP construct has also been incorporated into a wide variety of other species including mice, *Caenorhabditis elegans* nematodes, *X. laevis* frogs, and zebrafish.

One of the earliest animal models of human cancer, first documented in the 1920s, concerns the formation of melanomas in hybrid poeciliid

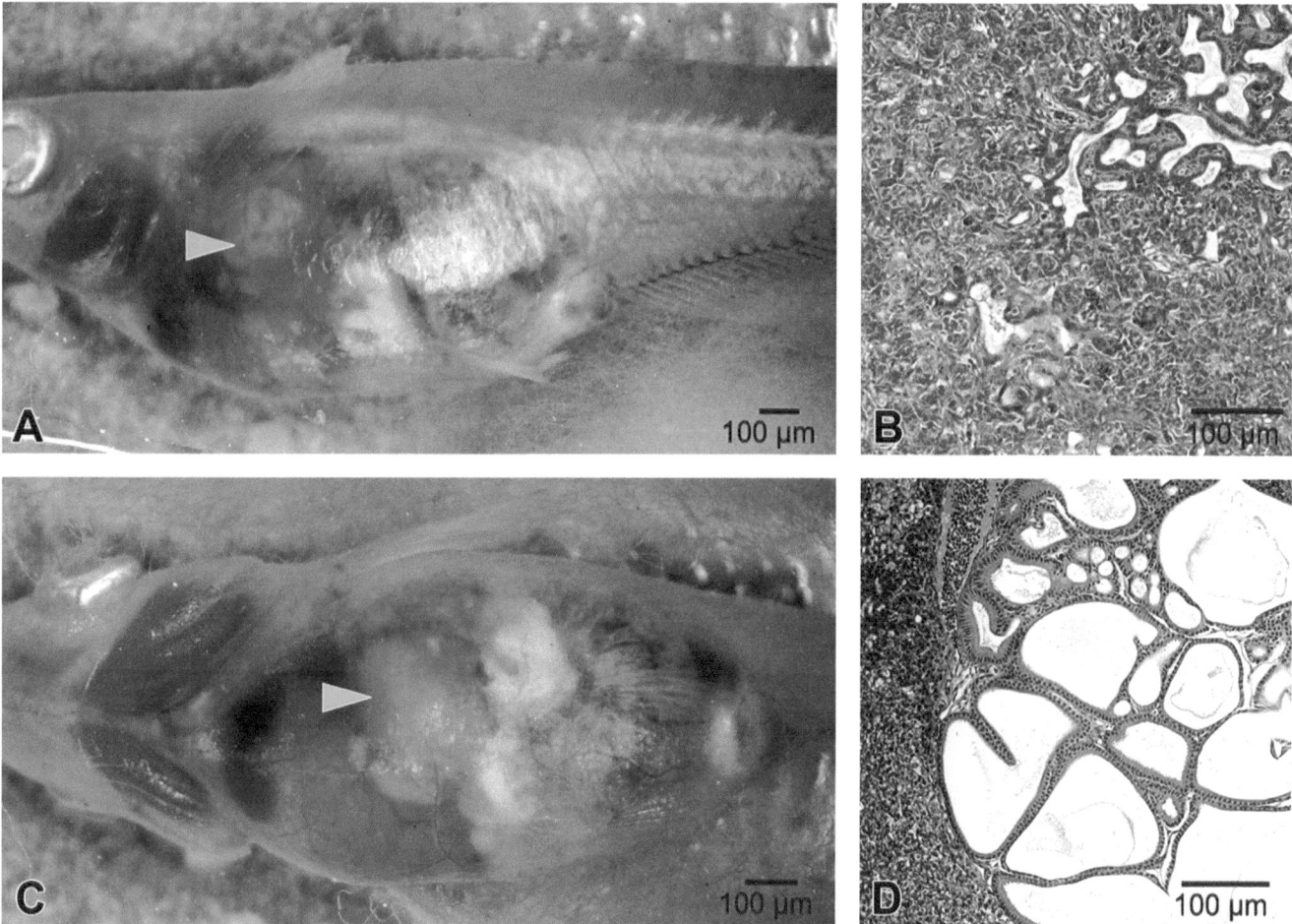

FIGURE 22.10   Proliferative hepatobiliary lesions visualized externally in transparent Japanese medaka (*Oryzias latipes*). Medaka were treated with 100 ppm diethylnitrosamine in water for 24 h, rinsed, and maintained for 10 months. (A) Intact, living female medaka in right lateral incumbency. *Arrowhead* indicates a pale, irregular liver mass. (B) Histology of liver mass is consistent with mixed hepatobiliary carcinoma. H&E. (C) Same individual in dorsal recumbency, with a second liver lesion denoted by the *arrowhead*. (D) Histology of the second liver lesion indicated biliary hyperplasia. H&E. Fish obtained originally from Yuko Wakamatsu, Nagoya University, Nagoya, Japan. Images courtesy of David Hinton, Duke University, Durham, North Carolina, USA. *Figure reproduced from Hardman RC, Kullman SW, Hinton DE: Noninvasive in vivo investigation of hepatobiliary structure and function in STII medaka* (Oryzias latipes*): methodology and applications. Comparative Hepatol 7:7, 2008; licensee, BioMed Central Ltd., Figure 1, with permission.*

aquarium fishes of the genus *Xiphophorus* (Schartl and Walter, 2016; Walter and Kazianis, 2001). At that time, it was observed that the mating of wild-type platyfish *Xiphophorus maculatus* females with wild-type swordtail *Xiphophorus helleri* males generated F1 generation hybrid females, that, when backcrossed with wild-type swordtail *X. helleri* males, produced progeny with a 25% frequency of melanomas. More recent experimentation and molecular analyses have revealed that tumor formation can be attributed to the activity of a dominant-acting sex-linked oncogene, *Xmrk* (*Xiphophorus* melanoma receptor kinase), which is considered to be a fish ortholog of the human epidermal growth factor receptor gene. Full expression of this oncogene occurs when it is no longer inhibited by the suppressor gene *Diff*, which, in accordance with Mendelian genetics, is not passed down to one quarter of the F2 generation fish. Through a number of separate signaling pathways (phosphatidylinositol 3-kinase, Ras–Raf–MAPK, and activation of the Fyn tyrosine kinase), *Xmrk* expression can impart certain capabilities that contribute to melanoma formation, including hyperproliferation of pigment cells, suppression of pigment cell apoptosis, and the differentiation, metastasis, and survival of tumor cells at metastatic sites. Numerous parallels exist between the *Xiphophorus* model and human melanomas, including shared signaling pathways activated by *Xmrk*, and a probable link between *Diff* and the human tumor suppressor gene known as *CDKN2*. In addition to these similarities, the *Xiphophorus* model is important because there are no naturally occurring translatable melanoma models in mice, due to the fact that murine pigment cells are present in hair follicles as opposed to the interfollicular dermis. Furthermore, melanoma formation in hybrid *Xiphophorus* can be induced by carcinogens or ultraviolet light exposure, and due to the fact that *Xmrk*-activated pathways are central to the development of many different tumors, the *Xiphophorus* model is also used to study other types of neural crest neoplasia (Walter and Kazianis, 2001). Finally, because poeciliids are livebearers and thus cannot be made transgenic, scientists have engineered transgenic medaka that express the *Xmrk* gene, and the resulting medaka melanoma model is currently used for screening small molecules as potential anticancer compounds (Schartl and Walter, 2016).

Serendipitous discoveries of natural models such as *Xiphophorus* are rare, and the rapid pace of modern-day research requires a variety of targeted strategies. One answer has been the development of genetically modified animals, which can be used to accelerate the detection of novel candidate compounds for the pharmaceutical and agrochemical pipelines. Among nonmammalian animal species used in toxicology, genetic engineering to create new models of human disease reaches its apex in zebrafish. Although zebrafish have fewer anatomic and molecular similarities to humans than rodents, they are closer in these aspects to humans than are invertebrates such as *D. melanogaster* and *C. elegans*, and zebrafish are less expensive and more amenable to high-throughput drug screening than are mice and rats. Genetically modified zebrafish can be produced according to a number of different methods, including forward genetic approaches such as random mutagenesis induced by ethylnitrosourea exposure or retroviral gene insertion (Lieschke and Currie, 2007). Unlike rodents, the phenotypic results of these modifications can be visualized in intact embryos using simple optical microscopy. Transient genetic changes induced by injection of mRNA or morpholino oligonucleotides can also be used to study the effects of specific gene modifications. More recently, the CRISPR/Cas9 system, a rapid and accurate method of genome editing, has accelerated the creation of transgenic zebrafish with targeted genetic mutations or reporter gene insertions (Cornet et al., 2018; see also *Genetically Engineered Animal Models in Toxicologic Research*, Vol 1, Chap 23). These manufactured mutations can confer either gain or loss of gene function. Accordingly, genetically engineered zebrafish have been developed to model a host of human conditions (Table 22.4). The list of human disease models that utilize zebrafish, and other nontraditional vertebrate and invertebrate species, has been expanding exponentially, and readers are encouraged to consult the References section for more comprehensive reviews (Cornet et al., 2018; Feitsma and Cuppen, 2008; Kain et al., 2014; Lieschke and Currie, 2007; Naert and Vleminckx, 2018; Segalat, 2007).

3.2. Drug Discovery and Toxicity Screening

Due to the degree of anatomical and evolutionary divergence that exists among animals that have fur, feathers, fins, or exoskeletons, nonmammalian animal models are not yet situated to replace conventional mammals as test subjects in traditional preclinical toxicological studies that are designed to detect and/or characterize potential human health hazards. However, it should be recognized that so-called "lower" animals can be efficient alternatives for screening studies that assess the efficacy or safety of pharmaceutical compounds, or the potential toxicity of agricultural and industrial use chemicals. Screening bioassays can be used in a "shotgun" approach, in which libraries of well-characterized compounds are administered to wild-type animals to identify novel targets or therapeutic approaches, investigate chemical mechanisms of interest, or produce biologically relevant phenotypes (Cornet et al., 2017; Segalat, 2007). Alternatively, potential candidate compounds can be applied to genetically altered animals in which a defined drug target has already been established (Cornet et al., 2018; Naert and Vleminckx, 2018). One demonstration of the latter strategy

TABLE 22.4 Genetically Engineered Zebrafish Models of Human Disease Used in Drug Discovery

Gene target	Disease/Phenotype	Reference
abcb11b	Progressive familial intrahepatic cholestasis	Naert and Vleminckx (2018)
apc	Familial adenomatosis polyposis	Feitsma and Cuppen (2008)
atp6v1h	Osteoporosis	Naert and Vleminckx (2018)
dmd	Duchenne muscular dystrophy	Santoriello and Zon (2012)
hey2 (grl)	Aortic coarctation	Lieschke and Currie (2007); Wheeler and Brandli (2009)
kcnh6a (zerg)	Long QT syndrome	Santoriello and Zon (2012)
lamb1a, pax2a	Coloboma	Santoriello and Zon (2012)
mbl2b (bmyb)	Genomic instability	Feitsma and Cuppen (2008); Lieschke and Currie (2007)
NOTCH1[a], bcl2a	Acute lymphoblastic leukemia	Santoriello and Zon (2012)
rps14	5q-deletion Syndrome	Cornet et al. (2018)
scn1a	Dravet syndrome	Baraban et al. (2013)
sod1	Amyotrophic lateral sclerosis	Da Costa et al. (2014)

[a] Human NOTCH1 transgene expressed in zebrafish.

would be the discovery of chemicals that were newly found to upregulate vascular endothelial growth factor through their ability to ameliorate an aortic malformation in zebrafish that have the *gridlock* mutation (Lieschke and Currie, 2007; Wheeler and Brandli, 2009).

Attributes of an ideal drug screening assay include low cost, rapid turnaround, high-throughput capability, the ability to produce effects in a variety of organ systems, genetic programmability for specific targets, and physiologic applicability to humans. *In vitro* assays that use cell cultures or tissue preparations are indisputably fast and comparatively inexpensive, but they may be based on transformed cells that do not necessarily replicate normal tissues, and multiple complementary tests may be required due to the limited repertoire of each individual assay. Additionally, it is usually not possible to recapitulate the temporal aspects of disease progression in an in vitro model or to test for efficacy and toxicity simultaneously. It is clear that whole organism models are required to screen for more complex cell–cell or cell–matrix interactions, for disease conditions that affect entire organs or multiple tissue types, or for the toxicologic effects of metabolites. Whole animal alternatives for drug screening include selected species of mammals, birds, amphibians, fish, and invertebrates (Table 22.1). Higher vertebrates such as rodents and chickens have a strong evolutionary connection to humans relative to less advanced species; however, the cost per animal for testing large numbers of compounds may be prohibitive, they have internal fertilization (mammals and birds) or internal embryogenesis (mammals) which limits access to their earliest developmental stages, and they are not as amenable as lower life forms to automated, high-throughput screening systems. Conversely, invertebrate and aquatic vertebrate models have advantages of large brood size, rapid organogenesis, and the capability of assaying embryonic or larval forms in 48- or 96-well plates.

Low cost and some degree of genetic and physiologic relevancy are advantages of whole animal screens that employ veteran invertebrate models such as *D. melanogaster* fruit flies and *C. elegans* nematodes. Genomic sequencing was completed more than a decade ago for both *D. melanogaster* and *C. elegans*, and subsequent research has revealed that mammalian genes and biological processes are conserved to a surprisingly high degree in many invertebrates (there is approximately 50% gene homology between humans and each of these two organisms (Leung et al., 2008; Segalat, 2007). For example, overactivation of the receptor tyrosine kinase/Ras signaling pathway is known to occur in many cancers, and experiments have confirmed the existence of that pathway in *C. elegans* (Segalat, 2007). Genetically modified versions of these animals are available that express fluorescent proteins as markers for target- and tissue-specific gene expression (Leung et al., 2008), and systems that employ video cameras and image analysis software can be used to automatically detect phenotypic changes among organisms arrayed in multiwell plates (Segalat, 2007). In this manner, invertebrate models have been used to screen for a variety of therapeutic candidates, including drugs that have the potential to treat heritable myopathies (e.g., muscular dystrophy), neurodegenerative disorders (e.g., Parkinson's disease), and certain cancers (Behl et al., 2019; Leung et al., 2008; Segalat, 2007).

Despite the benefits that invertebrates offer as drug screening models, there are negative aspects that serve to decrease the utility of invertebrates when weighed against lower vertebrates such as zebrafish *D. rerio* and *Xenopus* spp. frogs (Table 22.1). These include the relative taxonomic distance between invertebrates and humans, the physical impermeability of the invertebrate integument to small molecules, and the lack of an embryonic stage that can be micromanipulated (Wheeler and Brandli, 2009). Compared to *Xenopus*, zebrafish are by far the more proven screening model due to the availability of many chemically produced mutant strains that mimic genetically based human diseases, and the ability to maintain the transparent phenotype past the earliest embryonic stages by applying chemicals to the medium or through the use of apigmented transgenic fish (Garcia et al., 2016). Zebrafish embryos have been used to screen for agents with potential activity against diseases of virtually all major organ systems, including cardiovascular, hematopoietic, and hemostatic, developing neural, sensory, integumentary, musculoskeletal, endocrine, gastrointestinal, hepatobiliary, and urinary systems (Cassar et al., 2020) (Figure 22.11). In one specific example, a screening model that simulated puromycin aminonucleoside renal glomerular toxicity was produced by injecting zebrafish embryos with

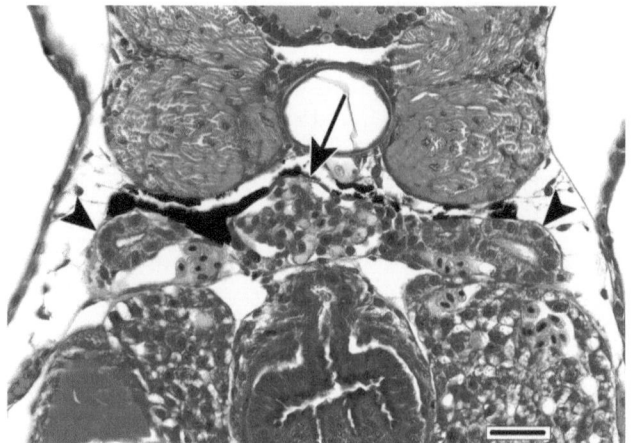

FIGURE 22.11   Transverse section through the trunk region of an embryonic zebrafish *Danio rerio*. Evident at this developmental stage is the pronephric kidney, which consists of a single central glomerulus (*arrow*) and two lateral pronephric ducts (*arrowheads*). This simplified design of two fused nephrons is an ideal model for renal drug screening. H&E, Bar = 25 μm. *Figure reproduced from Haschek WM, Rousseaux CG, Wallig MA, editors:* Haschek and Rousseaux's handbook of toxicologic pathology, *ed 3, 2013, Academic Press, Figure 14.6, p. 487, with permission.*

morpholinos (chemically altered oligonucleotides) designed to knock down the genes that code for cluster of differentiation 2–associated protein and podocin, which are known to participate in podocyte differentiation in mammals (Hentschel et al., 2007). Compromise to the integrity of the pronephric glomerular slit diaphragm was confirmed qualitatively via ultrastructural analysis and quantitatively in vivo by injecting embryos in 96-well plates with fluorescent-labeled dextran and measuring the intensity of fluorescence over time using photomicroscopy and image analysis (for more information, see *Digital Pathology and Tissue Image Analysis*, Vol 1, Chap 12 and *In Vivo Small Animal Imaging: A Comparison to Gross and Histopathologic Observations in Animal Models*, Vol 1, Chap 13). In addition, zebrafish embryos are a key component of emerging approaches for screening chemicals for developmental neurotoxicity (Behl et al., 2019; Brannen et al., 2016) and are used in the Zebrafish developmental toxicity assay for evaluating teratogenic potential of pharmaceutical compounds (Ball et al., 2014).

Although zebrafish are currently the preferred nonmammalian animal species for drug discovery and toxicity screening, it is a fact that frogs are phylogenetically, anatomically, and physiologically closer to humans, and this evolutionary proximity may be critical for studies that involve the respiratory, cardiac, renal, or immune systems, aspects of which are less effectively modeled in teleosts relative to amphibians. *Xenopus* frogs have been used to screen for compounds that have the potential to affect angiogenesis, lymphangiogenesis, pigmentation disorders, and cancer growth (Wheeler and Brandli, 2009; Maia et al., 2017). Though amphibian-based screens are not yet employed routinely for drug discovery, standardized assays that make use of *Xenopus* embryos for toxicity and teratogenicity screening have been available for almost 30 years. These include FETAX, which is a 96-hour test that incorporates endpoints of mortality, embryo growth, quantitation of abnormal embryos, and morphologic characterizations of abnormalities (Hoke and Ankley, 2005), and AMPHITOX, which offers a suite of experiments that are designed to assess the effects of acute, short-term chronic, or chronic compound exposures (Herkovits and Perez-Coll, 2003). Finally, it has been recognized that whole-animal *Xenopus* and zebrafish models have demonstrated great promise for investigating structure–activity relationships, which involves characterization of the effects that chemical moieties or geometrical structure have on the biological activity of a given molecule (Garcia et al., 2016; Wheeler and Brandli, 2009). Application of these models to quantitative research is also possible (Liu et al., 2019; Zvina-vashe et al., 2009), although the extrapolation of quantitative results from these lower animals to humans may be more challenging due to anticipated pharmacodynamic and pharmacokinetic differences.

3.3. Target Animal Safety Studies

The purpose of TAS studies is to ensure that investigational veterinary pharmaceutical products (IVPPs) are unlikely to cause undue harm to the animals that they are intended to aid. More specifically, TAS studies are conducted on healthy animals to assess the safety of drugs during routine use, the potential risk of overdose, and the need for advisory labeling. The targets of such studies include companion animals, and animals that are reared for food production, broodstock, display (e.g., animals in zoos or public aquaria), recreational activities (animals stocked for hunting and fishing), and wildlife conservation efforts (threatened and endangered species). Although it is acknowledged that most production animals will eventually be sacrificed, it is considered humane, economically beneficial, and necessary for food safety to maintain the health and well-being of livestock prior to the designated date of slaughter. Regulations in the United States require that TAS studies be performed before an IVPP can be approved for use, and regulatory agency oversight for such studies is provided by the US Food and Drug Administration Center for Veterinary Medicine (https://www.fda.gov/about-fda/fda-organization/center-veterinary-medicine). Internationally, efforts by representatives of the United States, Europe, and Japan to standardize TAS requirements resulted in publication of The International Cooperation on Harmonization of Technical Requirements for Registration of Veterinary Medicinal Products Guideline 43 (VICH, 2008). Benefits of these recommendations include avoidance of duplicate studies and minimization of the numbers of animals used in experiments.

A key element of TAS studies is the margin of safety concept (Schofield, 2011). As a result, TAS studies are typically conducted using test article concentrations that are multiples (e.g., $1\times$, $3\times$, and $5\times$) of the recommended therapeutic dose, and are administered for periods that are often two or three times the proposed duration of use. The recommended dose and duration of treatment are typically based on pharmacodynamic and pharmacokinetic data gleaned from pilot experiments or prior published reports. TAS studies may include laboratory and/or field experiments, and attempts may be made to approximate actual use conditions. In addition to gross and microscopic pathology, TAS studies generally incorporate standard toxicologic bioassay endpoints such as in-life observations, morbidity and mortality results, and body weight data. There are three primary reasons for the inclusion of anatomic pathology (gross and histopathologic examination) as an essential component of TAS experiments: (1) the cause(s) of clinically observed findings (e.g., general malaise) can often be elucidated; (2) it may be the sole mechanism for detecting certain types of subclinical effects; (3) it can provide clues to the pathogenesis of adverse responses.

Of the nonmammalian models discussed in this chapter, the most likely targets for the development of IVPP formulations are animals that are raised for production, and these include poultry, finfish, and shellfish invertebrates (e.g., lobsters and shrimp). Common types of pharmaceutical compounds tested in these animals include antibiotics, parasiticides, anesthetic and analgesic agents, feed supplements to improve performance, and synthetic hormones used for reproductive synchronization. In most cases, veterinary pharmaceuticals are approved for a narrowly defined combination of animal species, therapeutic or production need, and application conditions, and as a consequence, TAS studies are designed to meet very specific objectives. For example, in an experiment designed to test the safety of a commercial formulation of neomycin sulfate powder in turkeys, the test article was administered orally in drinking water to the 28-day-old poults, at test concentrations equivalent to 3×, 5×, and 10× the therapeutic dose, for three times the anticipated duration of treatment required to combat *Escherichia coli* infections (colibacillosis) (Marrett et al., 2000). Often, multiple experiments are initiated to ensure that a compound is consistently safe in the various animal species for which the product is intended. For example, commercial preparations of oxytetracycline have been tested independently in a number of fishes, including, in one study, walleye *Sander vitreus*, yellow perch *Perca flavescens*, and hybrid striped bass (striped bass *Morone saxatilis* X white bass *Morone chrysops*) (Gaikowski et al., 2003). Interestingly, treatment-related histopathologic findings occurred at the highest dose tested in walleye, but similar changes were not observed in either of the other two fish species. One of the most unique TAS studies to date examined the potential effects of transgenic growth hormone modification and triploid chromosome status on the health of Atlantic salmon *Salmo salar* (Tibbetts et al., 2013). These genetically modified, sterile salmon were developed for more rapid growth and feed efficiency in aquaculture for the food supply. In that set of experiments, the effects of transgenesis and triploidy were tested independently against nontransgenic and diploid controls, and because transgenic salmon grow far faster than their nontransgenic counterparts, both size-matched and age-matched controls were utilized.

For both humane and economic reasons, efforts have been made to minimize the number of animals used in TAS studies according to the doctrine of replacement, reduction, and refinement as advocated by Russel and Burch in 1959 (Flecknell, 2002). Although it is possible, if not likely, that bioassays such as TAS studies will eventually become obsolete, the fact remains that in vitro approaches are not yet able to simulate the myriad potential physiochemical interactions that may occur when a veterinary pharmaceutical compound is administered to a living production or companion animal.

3.4. Ecotoxicological Testing and Environmental Monitoring

Concern for the environment and its inhabitants exists on a number of levels that include the following: the well-being of the ecosystem as a whole; population-wide threats to economically important species that are harvested for food or pursued for sport; the vulnerability of at-risk species to various stressors; and potential effects of environmental perturbations on human health. One metric used to gauge environmental health is the extent to which certain forms of disease exist in the fauna, and changes in the occurrence of these disease forms with respect to time and location. In terms of toxicant-induced disorders, nonmammalian animal species, especially those with aquatic or semi-aquatic life stages, are particularly suited to environmental monitoring. This is because the ultimate destinations for many toxicants, especially those of anthropogenic origin, are surface waters and their subjacent sediments. Important contributors to contamination of the aquatic environment include surface runoff from municipalities and agricultural operations, industrial and wastewater treatment plant effluents, tailings from mining operations, and leakage from munitions dumps, among other man-made sources of pollution. The types of substances that tend to be of most concern are those that are found in widespread occurrence, those that make chronic intermittent appearances in the environment, and those that tend to accumulate and persist. Categories of contaminants that have received the most attention include metals, organochlorines, hormones and hormonal mimics, pharmaceuticals (antibiotics, antineoplastic agents, cardiovascular drugs, birth control hormones), industrial and consumer applications (e.g., the per- and polyfluoroalkyl "forever chemicals"), and personal care products. Another recent focus has involved potential effects of nanoparticles and microplastics on the health of fish and other aquatic animals. Aquatic invertebrates, fish, and most amphibians are uniquely positioned to bear the burden of these types of contamination. These animals not only inhabit polluted aquatic environs, many are obligated to do so on a continuous basis, through multiple, if not all, of their life-cycle stages. Contaminant exposure in aquatic animals can occur simultaneously through multiple routes, including absorption through skin, respiratory, and gastrointestinal tissues, the latter by way of drinking water and diet. In fact, the complexity of the food web chains of many aquatic organisms virtually ensures that prey items on the lower rungs of the food ladder will be likewise contaminated.

Initial discoveries of tumor-bearing fish in coastal waters in the US Pacific Northwest and other locations, and the apparent relationship that was found to exist between the occurrence of hepatic neoplasia and levels of certain environmental contaminants, alerted the scientific and lay community to the potential for contaminant-induced carcinogenesis to occur at sites that had not necessarily experienced a specific discharge episode (Myers et al., 1994). More recently, attention has been focused on reports of various wild fish and amphibians that possess reproductive tissues of both sexes (intersex). It has been theorized that these developmental anomalies might be caused by substances that mimic, antagonize, or otherwise functionally interfere with reproductive hormones; such substances have been termed EDCs. The increasingly active field of endocrine disruption has since expanded to include compounds that may affect not only the HPG axis but also the axes that maintain thyroid and adrenal gland homeostasis (HPT and HPA, respectively). The list of potential EDCs contains a vast array of primarily lipophilic compounds of both man-made and natural origin, with representatives that include organochlorine insecticides, phthalate plasticizers, nonylphenol and other alkylphenols, TBT, PCBs, PAHs, steroid pharmaceuticals, and phytoestrogens (naturally existing hormone-like substances derived from plants).

Although there appears to substantial evidence that certain endocrine disruptor substances exist in the environment at locally elevated concentrations that could cause adverse consequences in exposed wildlife, surprisingly few convincing links have been established between the presence of EDCs and pathogenic effects at the individual animal or population level. Much evidence has been compiled, for example, between the occurrence of intersex in the roach *Rutilus rutilus*, a fish that is widespread and abundant in European rivers, and wastewater treatment facility (WWTF) effluents that contain estrogens and other estrogenic compounds of lesser potency (Tyler et al., 2007). In the United Kingdom, intersex in male roach (which manifests as oocytes in the testes and testes with ovarian-like cavities) was detected in 86% of the 45 sampled river sites, with proportions of affected males reaching 100% in some locations that were downstream from WWTF (Jobling et al., 2006). Not only has a strong connection been demonstrated between the prevalence and severity of intersex and environmental estrogen concentrations, experimental exposure of male roach to effluent water from WWTF under laboratory conditions has induced both intersex and the production of hepatic vitellogenin. Additional evidence for toxicological induction of intersex is the finding of sex ratios that are skewed toward female in impacted natural populations, and the reportedly low frequency of spontaneous intersex (<0.5%) in chemically untreated, tank-reared, male roach. However, there are still insufficient data to determine whether the existence of these morphologic reproductive abnormalities has had any type of substantial negative effect on roach population dynamics. Perhaps the strongest association between environmental EDCs and population effects in wildlife is the well-documented ability of organotin compounds to cause reproductive anomalies in certain marine snail populations (see "Nonmammalian Animal Taxa—Invertebrates"). In other cases, arguments for associations between intersex and environmental contamination are less compelling. For example, in the United

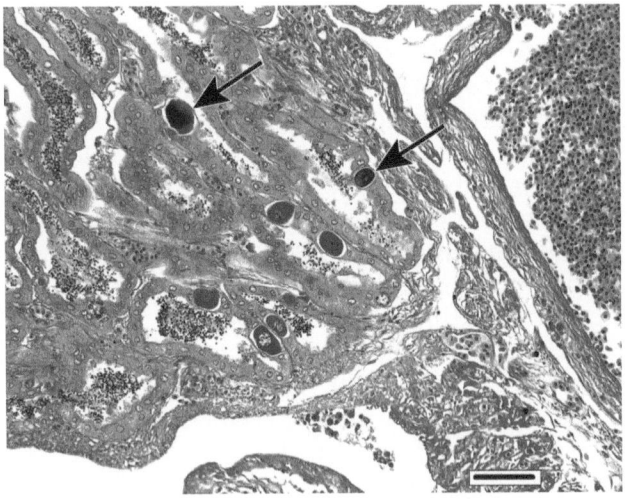

FIGURE 22.12 Oocytes (*arrows*) in the testis of a male smallmouth bass *Micropterus dolomieu* caught in 1932 in New York. There is no evidence that this particular fish was exposed to endocrine disruptive compounds. H&E, Bar = 50 μm. *Case courtesy of John Friel, Cornell University Museum of Vertebrates, Ithaca, New York, USA.*

States, studies to date have been unable to confirm that the widespread occurrence of intersex in *Micropterus* spp. black basses (Figure 22.12) is related to environmental contamination (Hinck et al., 2009; Iwanowicz et al., 2009). Additionally, attempts to establish causative relationships between certain agricultural compounds and endocrine disruptive effects in fish and amphibians have often yielded mixed results (see *Agricultural Chemicals*, Vol 2, Chap 28 and *Endocrine Disruptors*, Vol 2, Chap 29). In some situations, failures to connect intersex with environmental pollutants may be due to the unappreciated degree to which spontaneous reproductive anomalies that may exist in certain species or populations; more often, it is likely that an inability to prove causality can be attributed to the complex interaction between the convoluted chemical mixtures that are found in aquatic environments and the intricate physiological processes of biological organisms. Furthermore, although survey studies are essential for detecting potential contaminant-related health issues, for monitoring site remediation efforts, and for suggesting associations between contaminant exposure and negative consequences in wildlife, the vast array of uncontrolled variables in any natural environment makes it difficult to draw firm conclusions

regarding cause-and-effect relationships from field study data.

While it is clear that wild aquatic animals are positioned to play a pivotal role as sentinels for environmental contamination, it is for similar reasons that cultivated aquatic invertebrates, fish, and amphibians are also ideal subjects for ecotoxicological testing in the laboratory. First, in some cases, a species of animal known to encounter the contaminant of interest in a natural setting can also be adapted or reared for bioassays conducted in controlled laboratory environments (Lister et al., 2011), or if this is not possible, a taxonomically close relative may be employed as a surrogate. In either event, the results are more likely to be relevant than if a nonrelated, traditional laboratory species is used to determine the extent and manifestations of toxicity in wildlife. Second, a major benefit of the aquatic milieu is that water bath exposure allows for the continuous administration of toxicants through natural routes such as skin absorption, gill absorption, and dietary ingestion. By comparison, periodically dosing terrestrial subjects by gavage or skin application is a labor-intensive and artificial means of administering waterborne test substances, and there is an inherent risk that certain toxicants may be inactivated by enzymatic activity in the gastrointestinal tract.

It is evident that the many advantages of using nonmammalian models in laboratory experiments for ecotoxicological testing are appreciated by environmental regulatory organizations such as the USEPA, the European Organisation for Economic Co-operation and Development, and the Japanese Ministry of the Environment. For example, in addition to rats, the USEPA's two-tiered EDSP (https://www.epa.gov/endocrine-disruption/endocrine-disruptor-screening-program-edsp-overview) utilizes nonmammalian animals in laboratory experiments that range from short-term exposures to multigenerational assays, and species that have been selected include fathead minnows *P. promelas*, Japanese medaka *O. latipes*, African clawed frogs *X. laevis* (Figure 22.13), and Japanese quail *C. japonica*. Histopathological examination is either a required or proposed endpoint for the in vivo assays that involve each of these species. In addition to general laboratory animal requirements such as availability, hardiness, and ease of culture, the selection of laboratory species

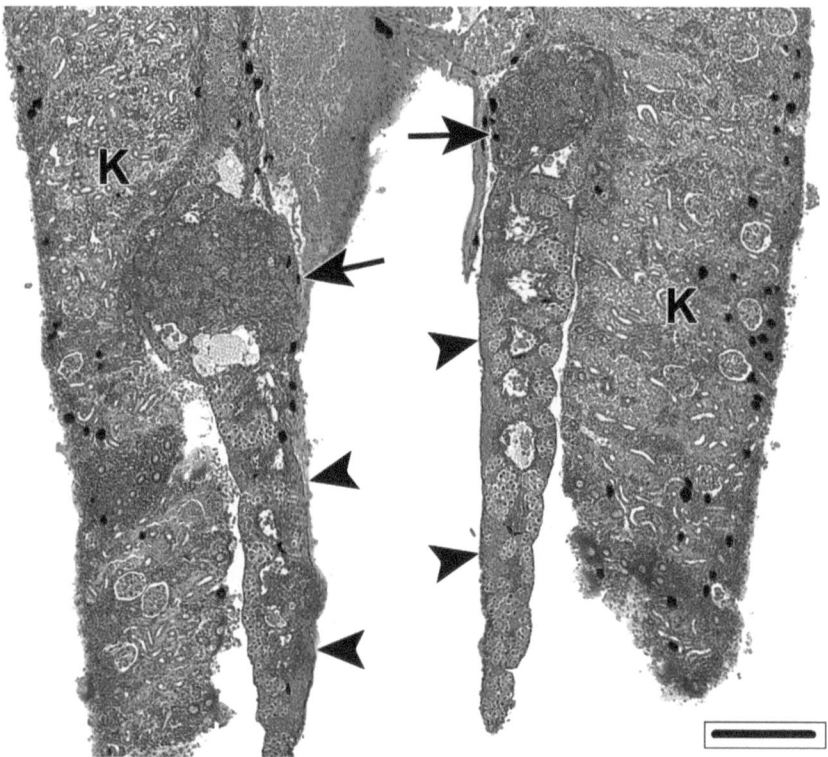

FIGURE 22.13 Longitudinal sections through the gonads and kidneys (K) of a postmetamorphic *Xenopus laevis* frog exposed to 0.2 µg/L β-estradiol continuously by water bath since approximately 8 days postfertilization. Exposure to exogenous estrogen has resulted in a mixed-sex phenotype in which the bulbous cranial portion of the gonads is testicular (*arrows*) and the caudal portion is ovarian (*arrowheads*). H&E, Bar = 250 µm. *Figure reproduced from Haschek WM, Rousseaux CG, Wallig MA, editors:* Haschek and Rousseaux's handbook of toxicologic pathology, *ed 3, 2013, Academic Press, Figure 14.9, p. 492, with permission.*

for environmental testing must take into account the degree to which the subjects represent their wildlife counterparts, and the ability of the test animals to respond in meaningful ways to known or suspected modes of toxicologic activity.

4. STUDY DESIGN CONSIDERATIONS

4.1. Study Design and Implementation

Compared to experiments that utilize conventional laboratory animals, the design and implementation of projects that involve nonmammalian animal models can be either considerably simpler or exponentially more complex. At the simple end of the spectrum are toxicological experiments in which minute invertebrates, such as *D. magna*, are exposed acutely to various concentrations of test compounds delivered in glass beakers. Conversely, some research systems designed for fish or larval amphibians may feature elaborate assemblages of diluters, dosimeters, heaters or chillers, aerators, purifying filters, ozonators or other sterilizers, lighting timers, automatic feeders, chemical reactors, and electronic devices for measuring pH, temperature, and other water quality parameters; these types of systems probably represent the epitome of complexity (Figure 22.14). Additionally, nonmammalian animal research may be conducted in the field, either via collection of wild specimens or through the placement of caged animals in contaminated environments; in laboratory cages, tanks, or other containers; or in hybrid mesocosm systems (e.g., outdoor ponds or pools) in which selected environmental conditions may

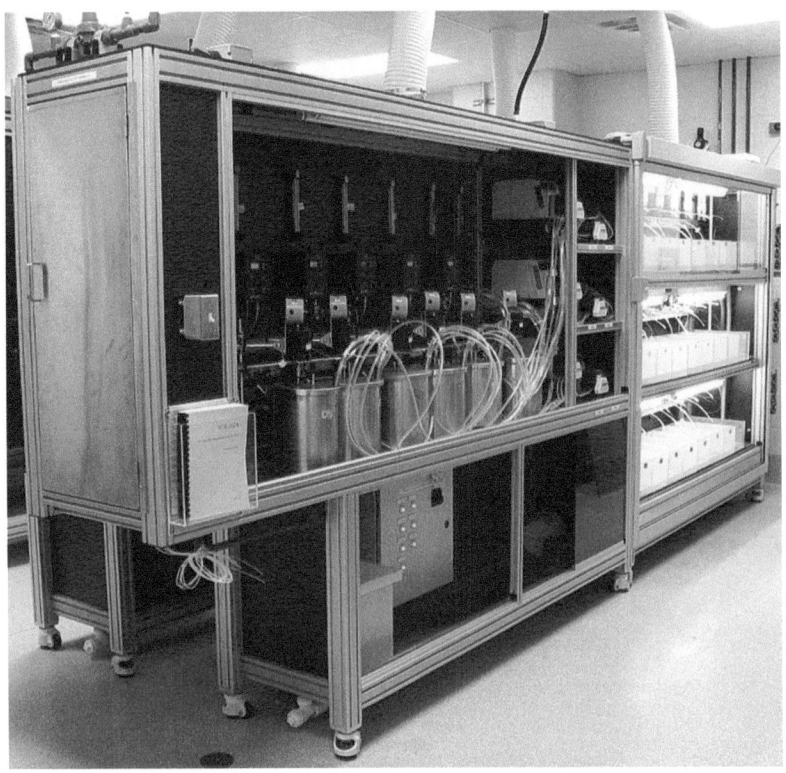

FIGURE 22.14   A complex, contemporary, state-of-the-art diluter system used to provide for the accurate, continuous delivery of various test article concentrations to the treatment aquaria (far right). *Image courtesy of Hank Krueger, Wildlife International Laboratories, Ltd., Easton, Maryland, USA.*

be reproduced while simultaneously permitting certain critical variables to be controlled. Systems created for aquatic animals can have static, recirculating, semiclosed, or flow-through designs. Common experimental exposure routes for nonmammalian animal models include oral (via diet or gavage), water bath (aquatic invertebrates, fish, and amphibians), inhalation (birds), or injection (intraova, intra-embryo, subcutaneous, intramuscular, or intra-peritoneal). Compounds delivered by water bath can be added once, replenished periodically, or dosed continuously throughout the exposure period. The aqueous solubility of a test compound must be considered when planning delivery by water bath. If the test substance is to be administered via injection, it is important to recognize that lower vertebrates have renal portal systems, in which blood from the caudal portion of the animal passes through the kidneys prior to reaching the heart and remainder of the systemic circulation. As a result, the toxicodynamic and toxicokinetic properties

of a compound can differ depending on the anatomic injection site (Holz et al., 1997); consequently, anterior body locations are typically selected for subcutaneous or intramuscular injections. Similar to mammalian species, toxicokinetic studies in nonmammalian vertebrates typically measure plasma concentrations of parent compounds and metabolites. Compound concentrations may also be measured in tissues, most often skeletal muscle, and/or tissue homogenates, particularly in ecotoxicology studies and in small organisms, such as larvae or small fish (Huerta et al., 2012; Kuhnert, Vogs, Altenburger, & Kuster, 2013).

In laboratory experiments that involve aquatic animals, subjects within a particular treatment group are generally housed and dosed as a unit, and the ambient test conditions within the local aquatic environment (e.g., a fish tank) have the potential to profoundly influence the results of most endpoints. Because of this intimate interdependence between aquatic animals and their environment, it is essential to establish that positive study results are a function of the toxicological treatment as opposed to differences in local environmental conditions (Wolf and Wolfe, 2003). For example, in a study conducted using juvenile rainbow trout *O. mykiss*, it was determined that growth indices were significantly affected by the proximity of the fish tanks to common-use walkways in the experimental facility (Speare et al., 1995). Consequently, the investigators concluded appropriately that the experimental unit (i.e., the unit used for statistical analysis) was the entire tank rather than the individual fish. This is analogous to developmental reproductive studies in mammals in which it is often the case that the litter, versus the individual offspring, is the experimental unit. However, the ramifications of treating the tank or litter as the experimental unit are not trivial. For example, if a fish study was designed so that the four treatment groups were each housed separately in single tanks at 25 fish per tank, this would mean that the study results would need to be analyzed on the basis of n = 1 instead of n = 25, and in that situation, it would be impossible to distinguish any treatment effects from "tank effects." Using the fish tank model as an example, studies are therefore often designed so that each type or level of treatment is replicated among multiple (three or more) tanks. This design method allows the investigator to determine *post hoc* if the results were influenced by tank effects. If it can be demonstrated in a particular study that tank effects truly did not occur, then the fish (rather than the tank) can be legitimately considered the experimental unit for that study. The ability to consider the fish as the experimental unit is especially desirable for histopathological investigations, because potential treatment effects may be lost (i.e., not supported statistically) if it becomes necessary to analyze lesion prevalence and severity on a per tank basis. As a final word of caution, failure to understand or acknowledge the identity of the experimental unit when analyzing data can result in an interpretive error that has been termed "pseudoreplication" (Hurlbert, 1984), which by itself has caused many manuscripts to be rejected for publication.

There are further considerations that an investigator might encounter during the design phase of a nonmammalian animal study. Although

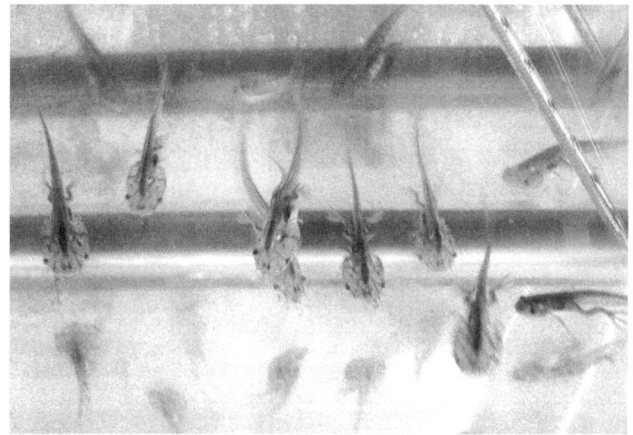

FIGURE 22.15 *Xenopus laevis* tadpoles. Larval test subjects such as these are usually not tagged individually for identification; instead, the container is labeled to indicate the treatment group and replicate. *Image courtesy of Tim Springer, Wildlife International Laboratories, Ltd., Easton, MD, USA.*

various devices such as tags, colored dyes, and electronic transponders are available for labeling larger fish, reptiles, and amphibians, individual animal identification may be impractical or impossible for bioassays that employ more diminutive subjects, e.g., small invertebrate species or larval aquatic vertebrates (Figure 22.15). Consequently, in such cases, it is typical to label the enclosures rather than individual animals, and for studies that involve lethal endpoints, to first assign each animal its own unique identification number as it is selected randomly at the time of sacrifice (Wolf and Wolfe, 2003). Similarly, for some nonmammalian animal species, the sex of individual animals may not be readily ascertained in vivo, and thus definitive determination may ultimately depend on findings gleaned from the postmortem examination of internal reproductive organs. As compared to domesticated experimental subjects, handling tends to be more stressful for many nonmammalian species, and therefore experiments should be designed to take handling stress into account. For example, the number of times animals are captured to obtain body weights and other measurements may have to be limited, and sampling may require chemical sedation to mitigate the stressful effects of physical manipulations. Aquatic containment systems are often constructed with lids to prevent cross-contamination by aerosol or splash, excessive evaporation, predation if systems are located outdoors, and escape of test subjects, or as a worst-case scenario, comingling of subjects across treatment groups.

There are several widely accepted methods for fish sedation and euthanasia (plus many other techniques that are generally considered unacceptable) (Chatigny et al., 2018; American Veterinary Medical Association, 2013), and selection of the most appropriate methods for a particular study often depends on several factors that include humane considerations, rapidity, cost, and potential confounding effects on tissue histomorphology (for a review, see Neiffer and Stamper, 2009). It is important to recognize that studies that utilize "lower" vertebrates are subject to the same types of animal care and use considerations as traditional laboratory mammals. Investigators are encouraged to consult the National Research Council's "Guide for the Care and Use of Laboratory Animals." The latest eighth edition (NRC, 2011) contains recommendations for the management, housing, and veterinary care of aquatic animals. Although invertebrates were not incorporated into these specific guidelines, evidence exists that many of these organisms, such as cephalopods, likely feel pain. As of this writing, some European countries have introduced regulatory guidelines that address the use of certain classes of invertebrates (notably cephalopods) in scientific research (Drinkwater et al., 2019).

Tissues collected from aquatic animals tend to decompose rapidly; therefore, it is especially imperative for those species that histological samples be placed promptly in fixative, and that body cavities be opened to fully preserve internal organs. Although 10% neutral buffered formalin is the standard fixative for most mammalian bioassays, empirical evidence suggests that certain aquatic vertebrate tissues (e.g., gills, kidneys, testes) may exhibit fewer artifacts if fixed initially in modified Davidson's or Bouin's solutions (Miki et al., 2018). These two solutions provide the added benefit of partial decalcification, which may be necessary for whole-body specimens, or for excised samples of bony tissues such as gill arches, scales, or ocular sclerae. Special preservation and decalcification procedures are also available for preparing histologic sections of aquatic invertebrates such as corals (Price and Peters,

2018) and bivalve mollusks (Howard et al., 2004). From a histopathological standpoint, an important study design issue may be to establish if the tissues will be harvested individually, or if the entire animal will be embedded in toto. The latter option is usually only feasible for diminutive invertebrates, larval organisms, or small aquarium fish species. If the whole-body option is elected, then the investigator needs to choose the embedding plane (e.g., sagittal, frontal, or transverse) that will provide optimal visualization of the target tissues. For example, sagittal sectioning of fish usually allows access to the most organ types (Wolf and Wolfe, 2003), but the sagittal approach is obviously not ideal for viewing bilateral tissue changes.

4.2. Subclinical Disease

Due to the advent of specific pathogen-free (SPF) laboratory mammals, subclinical disease is rarely a concern in most modern toxicologic bioassays. Exceptions still occur on occasion, however, either due to lapses in biosecurity or use of non-SPF stocks or wild-caught subjects. However, subclinical (and overt) disease, caused by infectious agents or noninfectious disorders, tends to occur far more commonly in projects that use nonmammalian animal species. In addition to an almost complete lack of SPF livestock (exceptions include some types of poultry and one current source of SPF zebrafish D. rerio), nonmammalian animal models are especially susceptible to subclinical disease for a number of reasons, and these include the following: stress-induced disease related to the demanding nature of habitat and husbandry requirements for many unconventional species; research projects that utilize wild-collected or pet trade animals; insufficient economic impetus to eliminate endemic diseases from captive livestock; absent or ineffective biosecurity practices; and study designs that incorporate limited or no histopathologic evaluation.

Because wild animals are seldom entirely free of infestations and infections, subclinical disease is an inevitable consequence of field survey studies. In most toxicological surveys (as opposed to disease outbreak investigations), collected wildlife tend to be overtly healthy, and the predominant subclinical health problems generally involve various forms of ecto- and/or endoparasitism. Low-grade parasitism is often well tolerated by the host; however, for causes that are not always immediately apparent, massive parasitic infections may be observed from time to time in individuals or populations. When this occurs, there may be a reflex tendency to ascribe heavy parasite burdens to some form of contaminant-induced immunotoxicity. While this may be true in some cases, it should be recognized that chemical contaminants are frequently more toxic to parasitic invertebrates than they are to their vertebrate hosts; consequently, animals in polluted habitats are often found to harbor fewer parasites than those collected in pristine surroundings (Burnett et al., 2007; Sures et al., 2017). It should be recognized that environmental contamination may also favor increased parasite loads through nonimmunologic mechanisms. For example, agricultural nutrient runoff into streams can promote the proliferation of snails and oligochaete worms, which are common intermediate carriers of parasitic trematodes and myxozoan organisms, respectively (Sures et al., 2017).

The situation is somewhat different for captively reared livestock, in which a combination of stress due to handling, overcrowding, and suboptimal ambient conditions, coupled with a buildup of opportunistic infectious agents over time (among animal populations and within containment systems), tends to result in periodic outbreaks of bacterial or fungal disease. Because meticulous observation of some types of nonmammalian animals can be difficult (catfish, for example, are usually reared in dark containers or muddy ponds), and because many hardy species can tolerate modest levels of infection, some disease outbreaks in their early stages may remain clinically undetected throughout the entire course of an experimental trial. Alternatively, certain infectious agents persist endemically in particular laboratory animal populations, and if so, a chronic, smoldering disease state may ensue. This is the most frequent presentation of one of the most common scourges of piscine, amphibian, and avian research: mycobacteriosis. Depending on numerous factors, such as the species of mycobacterium, the host species, the immune status of the individual, ambient conditions, and the stress of handling or treatment, mycobacteriosis may or may not present clinically (Densmore

and Green, 2007; Kent et al., 2004). These same types of factors may also govern the relative severity of subclinical mycobacterial infections and the resulting inflammatory response. For example, medaka O. latipes seem to tolerate a surprisingly advanced degree of diffuse granulomatous inflammation without exhibiting noticeable clinical signs. Not only can this extent of systemic infection interfere with the histopathologic interpretation of tissue changes, it is likely that the presence of the disease could have other untoward effects. As an example, it was demonstrated that chronic M. marinum infection acted as a tumor promotor in medaka that had been exposed experimentally to low concentrations of the mutagen benzo[a]pyrene (Broussard et al., 2009).

Although mycobacteriosis is a universal problem that affects many nonmammalian animal species, it is only one of a number of possible agents that can cause subclinical disease, and some of the most frequently employed nonmammalian models have their own distinctive pathogen issues. For example, captive-raised zebrafish D. rerio are plagued by a neurotropic microsporidian Pseudoloma neurophilia that is notoriously difficult to eradicate from affected populations (Murray et al., 2011), and an enteric nematode Pseudocapillaria tomentosa that has been associated with the formation of gastrointestinal neoplasms (Kent et al., 2002) (Figure 22.16). The ovaries of female fathead minnows may be infected by microsporidian organisms; such infections cause granulomatous oophoritis in a fish species that is often used for reproductive endocrine disruption research (Ruehl-Fehlert et al., 2005). In medaka, a trichodinid parasite of the urinary tract has been associated with renal tubular epithelial hypertrophy that appears to cause little distress to affected fish (Kinoshita et al., 2009) but may be easily misinterpreted as a treatment effect (Figure 22.17). Xenopus spp. frogs are subject to infections of A. hydrophila bacteria (the causative agent of "red leg"), mycosis caused by chytrids and other fungi, and necrotizing lesions caused by the toxin-secreting Mycobacterium liflandii (Densmore and Green, 2007). Endemic viruses may represent the ultimate stealth infections, because currently, the extent to which such viral infections may cause subclinical disease in nontraditional laboratory species is not well

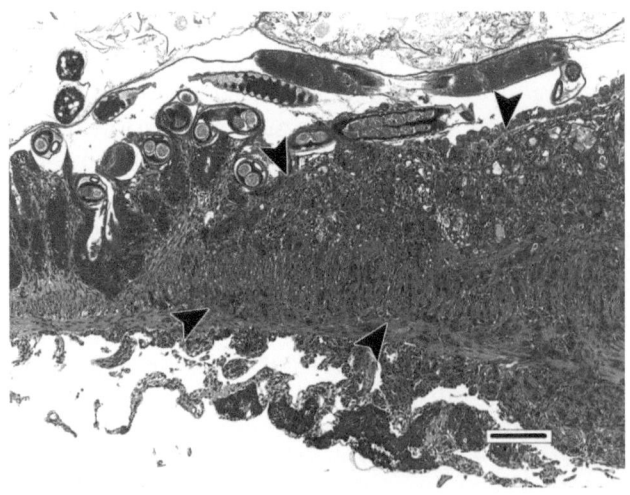

FIGURE 22.16 Longitudinal section through the proximal intestine of an adult zebrafish *Danio rerio*. Intestinal adenocarcinoma associated with the presence of pseudocapillaria parasites, which are present within the lumen and mucosa above the tumor mass. The arrowheads indicate the extent of the adenocarcinoma. H&E, Bar = 100 μm. *Figure reproduced from Haschek WM, Rousseaux CG, Wallig MA, editors:* Haschek and Rousseaux's handbook of toxicologic pathology, *ed 3, 2013, Academic Press, Figure 14.18, p. 508, with permission.*

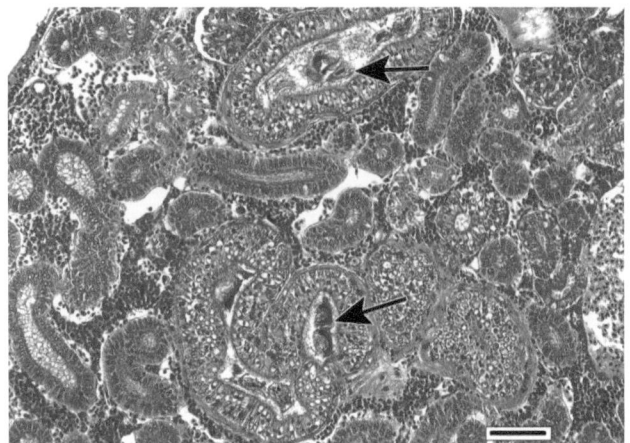

FIGURE 22.17 Kidney of a Japanese medaka used as a control in a toxicological study. There is extensive hyperplasia of the collecting duct epithelium due to the incidental presence of intraluminal trichodinid parasites (*arrows*). These lesions could potentially confound treatment-related tubular effects. H&E, Bar = 50 μm. *Figure reproduced from Haschek WM, Rousseaux CG, Wallig MA, editors:* Haschek and Rousseaux's handbook of toxicologic pathology, *ed 3, 2013, Academic Press, Figure 14.19, p. 508, with permission.*

understood. It should be recognized that subclinical disease may also be of a noninfectious variety. Examples in aquatic containment systems include gas bubble disease (formation of gas bubbles in the tissues of fish due to supersaturation caused by a rapid rise in temperature or pressure) and electrical shock resulting from power surges or faulty grounding.

The potential effects of subclinical disease on experimental outcomes are often underappreciated. Under some circumstances, subclinical diseases may mask or dampen treatment effects, or they may generate lesions that are subsequently misinterpreted as treatment-related findings. The stress of experimental manipulation may cause low-grade endemic infections to manifest clinically during the course of an experiment, resulting in sufficient morbidity or mortality to render treatment group sizes statistically inadequate. Finally, the mere existence of subclinical disease, as discovered ex post facto by histopathologic examination for example, may cause the validity of the entire study to be called into question. Curiously, many researchers seem unaware or unconcerned of the propensity for subclinical disease to exert bias on their study results. Other scientists appear to accept the existence of subclinical disease as a matter of course, especially if clinical signs of disease are generally restricted to broodstock animals as opposed to the younger experimental subjects. This last attitude is particularly prevalent when the most feasible recourse for resolving a particular disease problem is depopulation, or when a chronic disease only becomes clinically apparent in the broodstock. However, even if a specific disease agent cannot be realistically eradicated from a population, there are usually steps that can be taken to mitigate the spread and severity of subclinical infections. Furthermore, it is only through periodic monitoring for pathogens, either by histopathology or other diagnostic means, that the potential effects of subclinical disease on experimental outcomes can truly be determined. This is certainly a case of "what you do not know can hurt you." For further information on nonmammalian colony management, the reader is referred to Lawrence et al. (2018) and O'Rourke et al. (2018).

5. DATA EXTRAPOLATION

5.1. Results Extrapolation and Risk Assessment

Many toxicological studies that use nonmammalian animal species are conducted to predict the potential effects of drug administration or toxicant exposure in people. Despite the acknowledged value of preclinical research, the validity of extrapolating results from animal studies to humans is questioned periodically, and particularly in the rare instances when the results of preclinical (animal) bioassays are found to differ substantially from those of clinical (human) trials. It is acknowledged that species-specific effects have been demonstrated to occur in animals; for example, the tendency of peroxisome proliferator–activated receptor gamma agonists such as pioglitazone to induce bladder tumors in male rats is thought to involve a mode of action that is not relevant to human health (nor is it applicable to mice, for that matter). However, it has also been shown that incongruities between animal and human studies may be caused by factors that are not truly species dependent. For example, discrepancies may occur when compounds are tested in a narrowly defined animal population (e.g., a single gender, a restricted age range, or only healthy specimens) that does not adequately represent the most (or least) sensitive individuals encountered in a human trial (Olson et al., 2000).

In any event, it is understood that a degree of uncertainty always exists when the results of animal experiments are applied to human health. Added to this is the long-held perception that nonmammalian species are less toxicologically similar to humans when compared to rodents and other mammalian laboratory subjects. Nevertheless, studies designed to specifically test the strength of that assumption remain limited. Instead, the evidence can be pieced together from multiple disparate sources of information. For example, it has been estimated that the degree of genetic conservation from the zebrafish to humans is approximately 75%, and it has been determined that there is 80% conserved synteny (i.e., genes and expressed sequence tags are physically colocalized on the same chromosome) between the zebrafish and human genomes (Barbazuk et al., 2000). Other investigations have also demonstrated a relatively high level of synteny between the genomes of various fishes, *Xenopus* frogs, chickens, and humans. However, in addition to genetic compatibility, it is helpful to know whether the orthologous genes of different species govern comparable phenotypic attributes. For example, it has been shown that mutations of *PAX6* gene orthologs cause morphologically similar (although not identical) ocular malformations in fruit flies *D. melanogaster*, zebrafish *D. rerio*, mice, and humans (Nakayama et al., 2015).

Other paradigms have been created in which multispecies relationships are linked to common genetic alterations by using a system of ontological phenotypic equivalents (van der Worp et al., 2010). Alternatively, if a common mechanism of action for a family of compounds is understood, it may be possible to derive toxic equivalency factors (TEFs) that can be applied across various taxa (Van den Berg et al., 1998). Such TEFs have been established for dioxin-like compounds, for example.

Although it is useful to establish phylogenetic and mechanistic relationships, in reality empirical evidence is required to justify the extrapolation of toxicological outcomes from lower animals to humans. This can be obtained through retrospective studies that are designed to explore the concordance between the results of animal bioassays and anticipated effects in humans. For example, a 6-day duration assay that used zebrafish embryos to test for cardiotoxicity, hepatotoxicity, and neurotoxicity was found to have a positive predictive value of 88% when tested against 24 reference chemicals (Cornet et al., 2017). In another study in which zebrafish were exposed to 17 established cell cycle inhibitors, only 2 compounds were not active in vivo or in vitro, which indicates that the targets were conserved between zebrafish and mammals for the other 15 drugs. Sensitivity to a variety of thyroid active compounds such as methimazole, 6-propylthiouracil, and thyroxine has been demonstrated in screening assays that use *Xenopus* tadpoles (Degitz et al., 2005). Finally, as compared to rats, it has been determined that trout are more like humans in their resistance to hepatic peroxisome proliferation (Tilton et al., 2008). However, adequate concordance between nonmammalian animal results and those of humans can hardly be assumed. For instance, in one study, the investigators concluded that, under specific exposure conditions, fish such as medaka *O. latipes* and guppies *P. reticulata* were less sensitive than rodents for detecting the effects of the three known rodent carcinogens: nitromethane, propanediol, and 1,2,3-trichloropropane (Kissling et al., 2006). Consequently, mammalian in vivo studies remain the standard for toxicity assessment among regulatory guidelines, with few exceptions. For example, current draft guidance from the ICH for detection of reproductive toxicity [ICH S5(R3); https://www.fda.gov/regulatory-information/search-fda-guidance-documents/s5r3-detection-toxicity-reproduction] would allow for nonmammalian in vivo studies in lieu of mammalian studies, but only provided there is appropriate scientific justification. Further work will be needed to determine the degree, if any, to which nonmammalian animal studies can be used to inform human risk assessment.

5.2. Interspecies Variability

Currently, there are approximately 5500 known species of mammals. This seemingly sizable figure pales in comparison, however, when one considers that the numbers of nonmammalian animal species comprise approximately 1.2 million invertebrates, 32,000 fish, 14,000 amphibians and reptiles, and 10,000 birds. Given the wide variety of potential nonmammalian models, it is fortunate that research subject selection (i.e., species, age, sex, and source) can be narrowed by assessing a matrix of factors that include the following: availability; cost; potential for contaminant exposure; ease of cultivation and/or utilization; reproductive fecundity; hardiness to disease; sensitivity to toxicants in general or to a particular toxicant; special anatomical and physiological attributes; propensity for tumor development; type and extent of common background lesions; access to genetic information and/or genetically modified animals; research precedence; and prior experience of the investigator.

Although certain toxicologic effects may transcend taxonomical hierarchies (Figure 22.18), the remarkable degree of anatomic, physiologic, and genetic diversity that exists among nonmammalian models virtually guarantees that interspecies differences will be observed in the nature and extent of pathological responses to toxicants. Thus, for example, it is essentially meaningless to state that exposure to contaminant X causes a particular effect in "fish." Even among closely related animal species, reactions

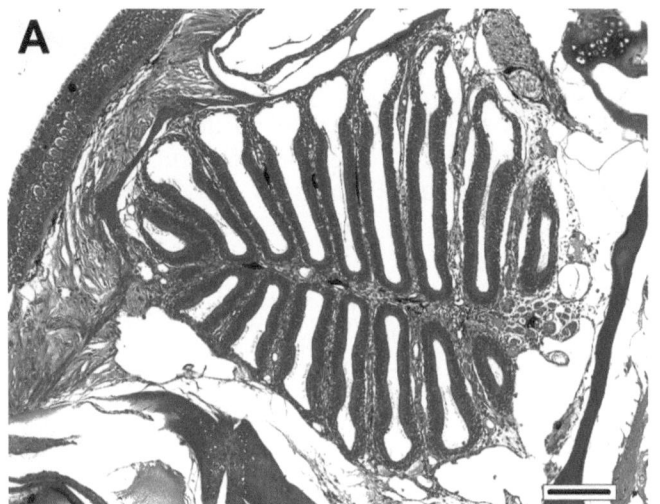
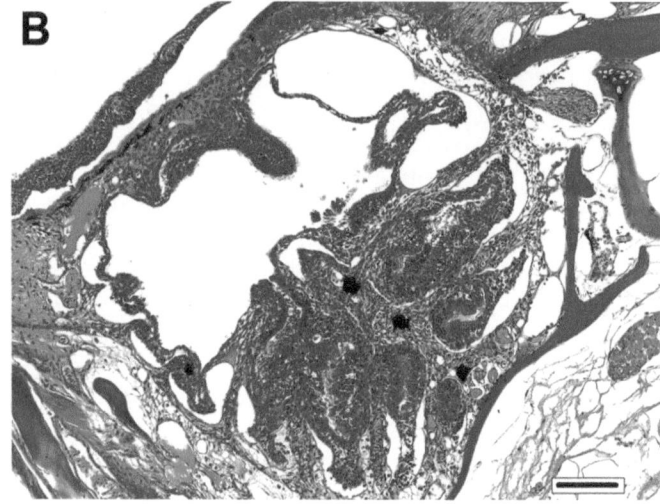

FIGURE 22.18   Cobalt toxicity in zebrafish *Danio rerio*. H&E, Bar = 100 μm. (A) Sagittal section of olfactory organ from a control fish. (B) Olfactory organ from a fish treated with 30 mg/L cobalt in tank water for 24 h. Toxicity is characterized by lamellar necrosis, interstitial collapse, lymphocytic inflammation, and reactive hyperplasia. Such changes mirror reported effects of cobalt toxicity in rodents, in which treatment-related changes are limited to the respiratory tract, and nasal lesions include degeneration of the olfactory epithelium, squamous metaplasia of the respiratory epithelium, and inflammation. *Figure modified from Hussainzada N, Lewis JA, Baer CE, Ippolito DL, Jackson DA, Stallings JD: Whole adult organism transcriptional profiling of acute metal exposures in male Zebrafish. BMC Pharmacol Toxicol 15:15, 2014, Figure 1.*

may vary as a result of differences in chemical absorption, distribution, metabolism, and elimination; receptor ligand concentration, distribution, and binding affinity; serum protein binding affinities; the presence or absence of endogenous agonists or antagonists; immunologic factors; and anatomical and microanatomical characteristics. The fact that such species differences exist should not be surprising news for pathologists, as, for example, it has been demonstrated that the approximate concordance between the results of rat and mouse carcinogenicity studies is only approximately 75% (Haseman and Seilkop, 1992). Analogously, anurans (frogs and toads) are known to develop spontaneous and chemically induced neoplasms far more readily than urodeles (salamanders and newts), and exposure to exogenous androgens can reportedly have opposite effects in anurans (masculinization or no response) versus urodeles (feminization or no response) (Eroschenko et al., 2002; Fort et al., 2004).

However, it is imperative to recognize that for many published accounts, interspecies differences in reported results may actually be interstudy differences, i.e., the results would have been similar if a number of experimental variables had been kept truly constant across studies. Such variables include experimental design elements such as test article formulation, exposure route and exposure (dose, duration, and frequency), actual versus nominal concentration, age, developmental stage, and gender. Aquatic animal studies are particularly sensitive to test condition variability, as even small discrepancies in parameters such as temperature, pH, and salinity can have profound effects on the experimental results. Additionally, interstudy differences that seem qualitative may in reality be quantitative, wherein differential responses to chemical exposure are purely a function of test article concentration (i.e., the expected effect is not observed until the compound dose is raised above a certain threshold). A concept called the "molecular equivalent dose" has been used to compare quantitatively the responses of fish and rodents to similar toxicant doses (Hobbie et al., 2009). For example, when both lambda cII transgenic Japanese medaka *O. latipes* and lambda cII transgenic (Big Blue(R)) rats were exposed to several progressive concentrations of dimethylnitrosamine, the medaka displayed mutation frequencies that were up to 20 times higher than those of the rats. Furthermore, studies that incorporate histopathologic endpoints may be affected by variation in postmortem factors that include specimen preservation, histologic preparation, diagnostic criteria and terminology, and the inherent subjectivity of observational evaluation and interpretation. Consequently, in some cases, it may be difficult or impossible to determine whether interspecies differences are real or artifactual based solely on a review of the published literature.

True interspecies differences can be exploited for the benefit of scientific inquiry. For example, new insights into the effects of growth hormone on skeletal muscle growth and regeneration may be elucidated by comparing opposing physiological characteristics of two closely related fish species, one of which, the giant danio *Devario aequipinnatus*, grows continuously throughout its lifespan by forming new muscle fibers via satellite cell recruitment, whereas the other species, the zebrafish *D. rerio*, loses this capability after reaching the postlarval stage. However, in certain areas of toxicological research, interspecies variability can also be an impediment. For example, the ability of one species to serve as a surrogate test subject for other, less readily assayed species is highly desirable for ecotoxicological investigations in which the designated species of interest may be endangered or threatened, or notoriously difficult to maintain in captivity (Sappington et al., 2001). Unfortunately, the capacity of a surrogate species (e.g., *X. laevis* frogs) to adequately represent various target species (e.g., ranid frogs) in all aspects of toxicological response may be limited by interspecies variability. Interspecies variability is also a problem for the development of pharmaceutical compounds whose purpose is to enhance the growth or well-being of farmed animals (e.g., shellfish, finfish, and poultry). Often it is not economically worthwhile for drug manufacturers to develop compounds that are only approved for use in a single species. On the other hand, the cost of performing efficacy and safety testing in multiple species is also not financially attractive. Thus, the anticipated degree of interspecies variability can influence the number and types of studies that must be performed.

5.3. Knowledge Gap

It should be evident from the preceding narrative that nonmammalian models are involved in areas of cutting-edge research that are on par with the most sophisticated experiments performed in laboratory mammals. And yet despite such advanced developments, there remain fundamental knowledge gaps relevant to toxicologic pathology. Zebrafish embryos/larvae are increasingly used in screening assays for teratogenicity and developmental neurotoxicity, yet metabolism in the developing zebrafish remains incompletely characterized (Brannen et al., 2016). Complete genomic information may not be available for less commonly used nonmammalian animal models, and biological reagents, notably immunohistochemical antibodies, are often lacking.

Studies performed in traditional subjects such as rodents, dogs, and nonhuman primates benefit from a decades-long history of targeted refinement, institutional support, and knowledge sharing by organizations such as the National Toxicology Program and the Society of Toxicologic Pathology. Meanwhile, texts such as the Pathology of the Fischer Rat: Reference and Atlas and Pathology of the Mouse: Reference and Atlas along with the INHAND initiative have provided toxicologic pathologists with a solid foundation of standardized diagnostic criteria and terminology. By comparison, there are few authoritative reference materials that

depict pathologic changes in nonmammalian species, and those that do exist tend to focus on infectious disease diagnostics or problems related to the captive rearing of animals (e.g., nutritional disorders). Due to evaporating financial and/or institutional support, other pathology resources may be less accessible than in the past, and examples include archival tissue collections such as those of the Armed Forces Institute of Pathology (now the Joint Pathology Center) and the Registry of Tumors in Lower Animals. However, there is some evidence that the knowledge gap may gradually be shrinking (Figure 22.19). As a consequence of the increased attention paid to nonmammalian animal research by government regulatory agencies, more of these studies are being performed in accordance with Good Laboratory Practice standards than in previous years, and formal peer review assessments of histopathology findings are becoming more commonplace. Continued refinement of culture and husbandry procedures for nonmammalian animals has allowed a wider variety of test species to be utilized effectively and should help to minimize intersubject variability and the occurrence of stress effects. Progress made in the development and adaptation of diagnostic procedures for lower vertebrates, including various immunohistochemical, molecular, and "omic" techniques, has furnished investigators with a wealth of tools that may facilitate the interpretation of histopathology

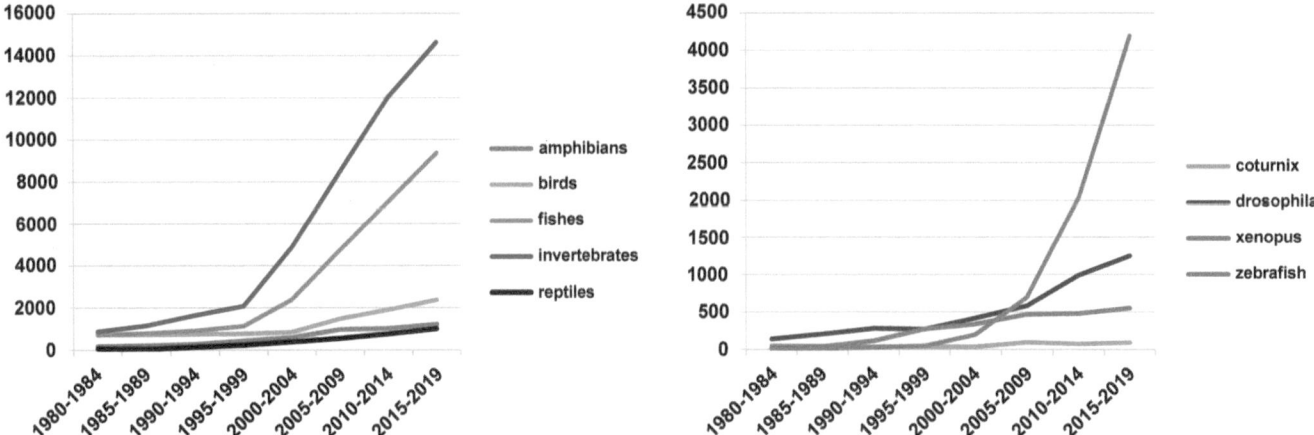

FIGURE 22.19 Chronologic trends in nonmammalian animal research. Represented are numbers of journal articles or online books involving toxicological studies, by taxonomic classification and 5-year time period, as available online through PubMed, U.S. National Library of Medicine, National Institutes of Health (http://www.ncbi.nlm.nih.gov/pubmed/, accessed 27 June 2020).

data. Scientific and technical requirements for the publication of histopathology results in journals that feature nonmammalian animal experiments have become more stringent. Projects involving fish, amphibians, birds, or invertebrates are appearing with greater frequency in posters and presentations at general pathology conferences, and ecotoxicologists are increasingly becoming aware of the value of histopathology as an endpoint. Training workshops, such as the University of Pennsylvania and Cornell University-sponsored Aquavet II program, continue to provide quality anatomic pathology instruction for professionals who have an interest in aquatic vertebrates and invertebrates (Spitsbergen et al., 2009). Finally, the past several years have witnessed the creation of numerous journal publications, guidance documents, and texts that have established standardized diagnostic criteria and terminology for nonmammalian animal studies. An INHAND guide for fish is currently being drafted.

5.4. Reliability of Published Histopathology Data

As is the case in most scientific fields, the quality and accuracy of journal articles pertaining to non-mammalian species can be quite variable. Compared to preclinical studies in mammals, nonmammalian animal research tends to be conducted by scientists from a broader range of background disciplines; consequently, morphologic interpretations are not always made by individuals who have had comprehensive training in comparative pathology, extensive experience with toxicologic bioassays, and complete familiarity with the anatomical and physiological idiosyncrasies of the target species. The same caveat may apply to volunteers who serve as manuscript reviewers prepublication.

It is unfortunate that the reliability of published histopathology data from toxicologic bioassays conducted in nonmammalian animal species is frequently less than desirable. In fact, two recent audits of peer-reviewed journal articles that involve the use of fish and other species as test subjects in environmental endocrine disruption studies uncovered substantial credibility issues in a large proportion of the reviewed papers (Wolf and Maack, 2017; Wolf and Wheeler, 2018). Common problems identified included inadequate sample sizes, poor sample preservation or preparation, absence of measures used to mitigate sampling or observer bias, insufficient detail in the methods sections and/or poorly presented data in the results, biologically implausible effect outcomes, and morphologic findings that were either questionable or patently inaccurate based on examination of the included photomicrographic images. Most often, misdiagnosed lesions were found to be artifacts of tissue collection or preparation, or the erroneous identification of normal anatomic structures as pathologic changes. Although many errors can be attributed to inexperience or inadequate opportunity for advanced training, another driver that should be acknowledged is the intense pressure that exists in many research institutions (and science in general) to generate and publish studies with positive results. Ramifications of unreliable histopathology data are extensive, and include economic costs, waste of animal resources, the miseducation of young scientists, pursuit of futile research based on misinterpreted findings, and the use of incorrect study outcomes as the basis for hazard or risk assessment and regulatory decision-making (Wolf, 2018). Early career investigators who do not possess extensive expertise in the morphologic evaluation of tissue specimens from nonmammalian animal species may need to scrutinize and consider reported journal findings with extra caution and avoid citing automatically or relying on uncertain results that cannot be confirmed through independent sources or verified by more experienced pathologists.

6. CONCLUSIONS

Indicators point to an increasing role for nonmammalian animal models in multiple research avenues. As the drive to understand the pathogenesis of both common and rare afflictions intensifies, and the availability of research funding continues to remain uncertain, investigators will endeavor to search for animal models that most closely portray specific human disease phenotypes, and assays that optimize the use of valuable biotic and monetary resources. Toward those ends, there are several reasons why nonmammalian species are poised to become progressively more attractive as subjects for toxicological research. These include ongoing efforts to reduce the numbers of laboratory and

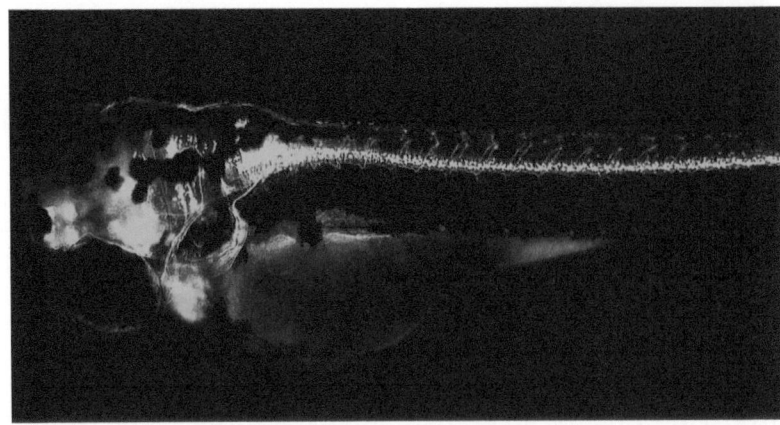

FIGURE 22.20　Live larval transgenic zebrafish engineered to express green fluorescent protein (GFP) in cranial motor neurons. GFP sequences were fused to *Islet-1* promotor/enhancer sequences, and germline transmission of the gene was established. Such fish may have application in studies involving developmental neuroanatomy, genetic mapping of neuron development, and neurotoxicity. *Image courtesy of Robyn Tanquay, Sinnhuber Aquatic Research Laboratory, Oregon State University, Corvallis, Oregon, USA. Higashijima S, Hotta Y, Okamoto H: Visualization of cranial motor neurons in live transgenic zebrafish expressing green fluorescent protein under the control of the* islet-1 *promoter/enhancer. J Neurosci 20:206–218, 2000.*

wild-caught mammals used in toxicologic bioassays, as a result of both ethical and cost considerations; the need to develop rapid and inexpensive animal systems for high-throughput drug discovery and toxicity screening; the ability of certain nonmammalian animal species to uniquely model particular human diseases; the mounting pressure exerted on wildlife populations by environmental stressors such as habitat transformation, pollution, climate change, and natural and man-made disasters; and the challenge of producing safe and effective therapeutic agents for use in poultry, finfish, and shellfish culture.

A host of clinical parameters, such as survival, growth, heart rate, swimming behavior, or spawning success, may serve as the primary endpoints of toxicologic experiments that involve nonmammalian animals, and many such projects do not include histopathology in the study design. One example of a revolutionary nonhistologic approach to internal phenotypic evaluation has been the development of unpigmented (transparent) adult zebrafish and medaka, in which morphologic changes in organ systems, cell lineages, or grafted tumors can be visualized spatially and temporally in vivo, either in unlabeled fish, or in fish that have been programmed to generate GFP or other reporter molecules (Figure 22.20). However, these and other technically advanced approaches, such as in vitro assays and genomic screens, almost inevitably require histopathological validation of empirical observations and measurements at some stage in the process. Currently, histopathology remains the most efficient, versatile, and comprehensive tool for the detection and characterization of toxicologic disease, and it continues to serve as an essential bridge between pathogenesis investigations conducted at the molecular and biochemical level, and apical effects in individuals or populations.

Acknowledgments

The authors would like to sincerely thank the following for their assistance in obtaining and preparing materials presented in this chapter: John Friel, Cornell University Museum of Vertebrates, Ithaca, New York, USA; Christiana Grim, OSCP/EPA, USA; Shelley Gruntz, EPL, Inc., Sterling, Virginia, USA; Ron Hardman, Duke University, Durham, North Carolina, USA; David Hinton, Duke University, Durham, North Carolina, USA; Michael Kent, Oregon State University, Corvallis, Oregon, USA; Hank Krueger, Wildlife International Laboratories, Ltd., Easton, Maryland, USA; Jennifer Matysczak, USFDA, USA; Jörg Oehlmann, Goethe University Frankfurt am Main, Institute for Ecology, Evolution and Diversity, Department of Aquatic Ecotoxicology, Frankfurt, Germany; Esther Peters, George Mason University, Manassas, Virginia, USA; Heather Shive, The Ohio State University, Columbus, Ohio, USA; Timothy Springer, Wildlife International Laboratories, Ltd., Easton, Maryland, USA; Robyn Tanguay, Oregon State University, Corvallis, Oregon, USA; Les Touart, OSCP/EPA, USA; and Eric Wolf.

REFERENCES

American Veterinary Medical Association: *AVMA guidelines for the euthanasia of animals: 2013 edition*, Schaumburg, 2013, AVMA.

Anastasiou T, Chatzinikolaou E, Mandalakis M, Arvanitidis C: Imposex and organotin compounds in ports of the Mediterranean and the Atlantic: is the story over? *Sci Total Environ* 569–570:1315–1329, 2016.

Ankley GT, Jensen KM, Kahl MD, Korte JJ, Makynen EA: Description and evaluation of a short-term reproduction test with the fathead minnow (*Pimephales promelas*), *Environ Toxicol Chem* 20:1276–1290, 2001.

Ball JS, Stedman DB, Hillegass JM, Zhang CX, Panzica-Kelly J, Coburn A, Enright BP, Tornesi B, Amouzadeh HR, Hetheridge M, Gustafson A, Augustine-Rauch KA: Fishing for teratogens: a consortium effort for a harmonized zebrafish developmental toxicology assay, *Toxicol Sci* 139: 210–219, 2014.

Baraban SC, Dinday MT, Hortopan GA: Drug screening in Scn1a zebrafish mutant identifies clemizole as a potential Dravet Syndrome treatment, *Nat Commun* 4:2410, 2013.

Barbazuk WB, Korf I, Kadavi C, Heyen J, Tate S, Wun E, Bedell JA, McPherson JD, Johnson SL: The syntenic relationship of the zebrafish and human genomes, *Genome Res* 10:1351–1358, 2000.

Barua A, Bitterman P, Abramowicz JS, Kirks AL, Bahr JM, Hales DB, Bradaric MJ, Edessary SL, Rotmensch J, Luborsky JL: Histopathology of ovarian tumors in laying hens, a preclinical model of human ovarian cancer, *Int J Gynecol Cancer* 19:531–539, 2009.

Baumann PC, Harshbarger JC: Decline in liver neoplasms in wild brown bullhead catfish after coking plant closes and environmental PAHs plummet, *Environ Health Perspect* 103: 168–170, 1995.

Behl M, Ryan k, Hsieh J-H, Parham F, Shapiro AJ, Collins BJ, Sipes NS, Birnbaum LS, Bucher JR, Foster PMD, Walker NJ, Paules RS, Tice RR: Screening for developmental neurotoxicity at the National toxicology program: the future is here, *Toxicol Sci* 167:6–14, 2019.

Boorman G, Crabbs TA, Kolenda-Roberts H, Latimer K, Miller AD, Muravnick KB, Nyska A, Ochoa R, Pardo ID, Ramot Y, Rao DB, Schuh J, Suttie A, Travlos GS, Ward JM, Wolf JC, Elmore SA: Proceedings of the 2011 national toxicology program satellite symposium, *Toxicol Pathol* 40: 321–344, 2012.

Bradaric MJ, Barua A, Penumatsa K, Yi Y, Edassery SL, Sharma S, Abramowicz JS, Bahr JM, Luborsky JL: Sphingosine-1 phosphate receptor (S1p1), a critical receptor controlling human lymphocyte trafficking, is expressed in hen and human ovaries and ovarian tumors, *J Ovarian Res* 28(4), 2011.

Brannen KC, Chapin RE, Jacobs AG, Green ML: Alternative models of developmental and reproductive toxicity in pharmaceutical risk assessment and the 3Rs, *ILAR J* 57:144–156, 2016.

Broussard GW, Norris MB, Schwindt AR, Fournie JW, Winn RN, Kent ML, Ennis DG: Chronic *Mycobacterium marinum* infection acts as a tumor promoter in Japanese medaka (*Oryzias latipes*), *Comp Biochem Physiol C Toxicol Pharmacol* 149:152–160, 2009.

Brown RE, Brain JD, Wang N: The avian respiratory system: a unique model for studies of respiratory toxicosis and for monitoring air quality, *Environ Health Perspect* 105:188–200, 1997.

Brown-Peterson NJ, Krol RM, Zhu Y, Hawkins WE: N-nitrosodiethylamine initiation of carcinogenesis in Japanese medaka (*Oryzias latipes*): hepatocellular proliferation, toxicity, and neoplastic lesions resulting from short term, low level exposure, *Toxicol Sci* 50:186–194, 1999.

Burggren WW, Warburton S: Amphibians as animal models for laboratory research in physiology, *ILAR J* 48:260–269, 2007.

Burnett KG: Impacts of environmental toxicants and natural variables on the immune system in fishes, *Biochem Molec Biol Fishes* 6:231–253, 2005.

Burnett KG, Bain LJ, Baldwin WS, Callard GV, Cohen S, Di Giulio RT, Evans DH, Gómez-Chiarri M, Hahn ME, Hoover CA, Karchner SI, Katoh F, MacLatchy DL, Marshall WS, Meyer JN, Nacci DE, Oleksiak MR, Rees BB, Singer TD, Stegeman JJ, Towle DW, Van Veld PA, Vogelbein WK, Whitehead A, Winn RN, Crawford DL: Fundulus as the premier teleost model in environmental biology: opportunities for new insights using genomics, *Comp Biochem Physiol D Genomics Proteomics* 2:257–286, 2007.

Cassar S, Adatto I, Freeman JL, Gamse JT, Iturria I, Lawrence C, Muriana A, Peterson RT, Van Cruchten S, Zon LI: Use of zebrafish in drug discovery toxicology, *Chem Res Toxicol* 33:95–118, 2020.

Chatigny F, Creighton CM, Stevens ED: Updated review of fish analgesia, *J Am Assoc Lab Anim Sci* 57:5–12, 2018.

Chesneau A, Sachs LM, Chai N, Chen Y, Pasquier LD, Loeber J, Pollet N, Reilly M, Weeks DL, Bronchain OJ: Transgenesis procedures in Xenopus, *Biol Cell* 100:503–521, 2008.

Choi T, Ninov N, Stainier DYR, Shin D: Extensive conversion of hepatic biliary epithelial cells to hepatocytes after near total loss of hepatocytes in zebrafish, *Gastroenterol* 146:776–788, 2014.

Coffee LL, Casey JW, Bowser PR: Pathology of tumors in fish associated with retroviruses: a review, 50:390–403, 2013.

Cole BJ, Hamdoun A, Epel D: Cost, effectiveness and environmental relevance of multidrug transporters in sea urchin embryos, *J Exp Biol* 216(Pt 20):3896–3905, 2013.

Cornet C, Calzolari S, Miñana-Prieto R, Dyballa S, van Doornmalen E, Rutjes H, Savy T, D'Amico D, Terriente J, ZeGlobalTox: An innovative approach to address organ drug toxicity using zebrafish, *Int J Mol Sci* 18:E864, 2017.

Cornet C, Di Donato V, Terriente J: Combining zebrafish and CRISPR/Cas9: toward a more efficient drug discovery pipeline, *Front Pharmacol* 9:703, 2018.

Da Costa MMJ, Allen CE, Higginbottom A, Ramesh T, Shaw PJ, Dermott CJ: A new zebrafish model produced by TILLING of SOD1-related amyotrophic lateral sclerosis replicates key features of the disease and represents a tool for in vivo therapeutic screening, *Dis Mod Mech* 7:73–81, 2014.

Degitz SJ, Holcombe GW, Flynn KM, Kosian PA, Korte JJ, TietgeJE: Progress towards development of an amphibian-based thyroid screening assay using xenopus laevis. organismal and thyroidal responses to the model compounds 6-propylthiouracil, methimazole, and thyroxine, *Toxicol Sci* 87:353–364, 2005.

Densmore CL, Green DE: Diseases of amphibians, *ILAR J* 48:235–254, 2007.

Drinkwater E, Robinson EJH, Hart AG: Keeping invertebrate research ethical in a landscape of shifting public opinion, *Methods Ecol Evol* 10:1265–1273, 2019.

Eroschenko VP, Amstislavsky SY, Schwabel H, Ingermann RL: Altered behaviors in male mice, male quail, and salamander larvae following early exposures to the estrogenic pesticide methoxychlor, *Neurotoxicol Teratol* 24:29–36, 2002.

Evans DH: The fish gill: site of action and model for toxic effects of environmental pollutants, *Environ Health Perspect* 71:47–58, 1987.

Fairchild JF, Feltz KP, Sappington LC, Allert AL, Nelson KJ, Valle J: An ecological risk assessment of the acute and chronic toxicity of the herbicide picloram to the threatened bull trout (*Salvelinus confluentus*) and the rainbow trout (*Onchorhyncus mykiss*), *Arch Environ Contam Toxicol* 56:761–769, 2009.

Feitsma H, Cuppen E: Zebrafish as a cancer model, *Mol Cancer Res* 6:685–694, 2008.

Ferrier PM, Rucker RR, Thurman WN, Burgett M: *Economic effects and responses to changes in honey bee health, ERR-246,* March 2018, U.S. Department of Agriculture, Economic Research Service.

Flecknell P: Replacement, reduction and refinement, *ALTEX* 19:73–78, 2002.

Fort DJ, Thomas JH, Rogers RL, Noll A, Spaulding CD, Guiney PD, Weeks JA: Evaluation of the developmental and reproductive toxicity of methoxychlor using an anuran (*Xenopus tropicalis*) chronic exposure model, *Toxicol Sci* 81:443–453, 2004.

Fournie JW, Summers JK, Courtney LA, Engle VD: Utility of splenic macrophage aggregates as an indicator of fish exposure to degraded environments, *J Aquat Anim Health* 13:105–116, 2001.

Furlow JD, Neff ES: A developmental switch induced by thyroid hormone: *Xenopus laevis* metamorphosis, *Trends Endocrinol Metab* 17:40–47, 2006.

Gaikowski MP, Wolf JC, Schleis SM, Gingerich WH: Safety of oxytetracycline (terramycin TM-100F) administered in feed to hybrid striped bass, walleyes, and yellow perch, *J Aquat Anim Health* 15:274–286, 2003.

Garcia GR, Noyes PD, Tanguay RL: Advancements in zebrafish applications for 21st century toxicology, *Pharmacol Ther* 161:11–21, 2016.

Gómez C, Vicente J, Echavarri-Erasun B, Porte C, Lacorte S: Occurrence of perfluorinated compounds in water, sediment and mussels from the Cantabrian Sea (North Spain), *Mar Pollut Bull* 62(5):948–955, 2011.

Guillette Jr LJ, Edwards TM, Moore BC: Alligators, contaminants and steroid hormones, *Environ Sci* 14:331–347, 2007.

Halldin K, Axelsson J, Brunström B: Effects of endocrine modulators on sexual differentiation and reproductive function in male Japanese quail, *Brain Res Bull* 65:211–218, 2005.

Haseman JK, Seilkop SK: An examination of the association between maximum-tolerated dose and carcinogenicity in 326 long-term studies in rats and mice, *Fundam Appl Toxicol* 19:207–213, 1992.

Heard MS, Baas J, Dorne JL, Lahive E, Robinson AG, Rortais A, Spurgeon DJ, Svendsen C, Hesketh H: Comparative toxicity of pesticides and environmental contaminants in bees: are honey bees a useful proxy for wild bee species? *Sci Total Environ* 578:357–365, 2017.

Hentschel DM, Mengel M, Boehme L, Liebsch F, Albertin C, Bonventre JV, Haller H, Schiffer M: Rapid screening of glomerular slit diaphragm integrity in larval zebrafish, *Am J Physiol Renal Physiol* 293:F1746–F1750, 2007.

Herkovits J, Pérez-Coll C: AMPHITOX: a customized set of toxicity tests employing amphibian embryos. In Linder G, Krest S, Sparling D, Little E, editors: *Multiple stressor effects in relation to declining amphibian populations,* West Conshohocken, PA, 2003, ASTM International, pp 46–60.

Hidemi A: Preparation of honey bee specimens for histopathological studies, including a technique for the preparation of whole sections, *J Apicultural Res* 53:385–391, 2014.

Hinck JE, Blazer VS, Schmitt CJ, Papoulias DM, Tillitt DE: Widespread occurrence of intersex in black basses (Micropterus spp.) from U.S. rivers, 1995–2004, *Aquat Toxicol* 95:60–70, 2009.

Hinton DE, Kullman SW, Hardman RC, Volz DC, Chen PJ, Carney M, Bencic DC: Resolving mechanisms of toxicity while pursuing ecotoxicological relevance? *Mar Pollut Bull* 51:635–648, 2005.

Hobbie KR, Deangelo AB, King LC, Winn RN, Law JM: Toward a molecular equivalent dose: use of the medaka model in comparative risk assessment, *Comp Biochem Physiol C Toxicol Pharmacol* 149:141–151, 2009.

Hoke RA, Ankley GT: Application of frog embryo teratogenesis assay-Xenopus to ecological risk assessment, *Environ Toxicol Chem* 24:2677–2690, 2005.

Holladay SD, Wolf JC, Smith SA, Jones DE, Robertson JL: Aural abscesses in wild-caught box turtles (*Terrapene carolina*): possible role of organochlorine-induced hypovitaminosis A, *Ecotoxicol Environ Saf* 48:99–106, 2001.

Holz P, Barker IK, Burger JP, Crawshaw GJ, Conlon PD: The effect of the renal portal system on pharmacokinetic parameters in the red-eared slider (*Trachemys scripta elegans*), *J Zoo Wildlife Med* 28:386–393, 1997.

Howard DW, Lewis EJ, Keller BJ, Smith CS: *Histological techniques for marine bivalve mollusks and crustaceans*. 2nd ed (vol. 5). 2004, NOAA Technical Memorandum NOS NCCOS.

Huerta B, Roriguez-Mozaz S, Barcelo D: Pharmaceuticals in biota in the aquatic environment: analytical methods and environmental implications, *Anal Bioanal Chem* 404:2611–2624, 2012.

Hurlbert SH: Pseudoreplication and the design of ecological field experiments, *Ecol Monogr* 54:187–211, 1984.

Iwanowicz LR, Blazer VS, Guy CP, Pinkney AE, Mullican JE, Alvarez DA: Reproductive health of bass in the Potomac, USA, drainage: Part 1. Exploring the effects of proximity to wastewater treatment plant discharge, *Environ Toxicol Chem* 28:1072–1083, 2009.

Jobling S, Williams R, Johnson A, Taylor A, Gross-Sorokin M, Nolan M, Tyler CR, van Aerle R, Santos E, Brighty G: Predicted exposures to steroid estrogens in U.K. rivers correlate with widespread sexual disruption in wild fish populations, *Environ Health Perspect* 114:32–39, 2006.

Johnson PTJ, Sutherland DR: Amphibian deformitites and Ribeiroia infections: an emerging helminthiasis, *Trends Parasitol* 19:332–335, 2003.

Johnson RM: Honey bee toxicology, *Annu Rev Entomol* 60:415–434, 2015.

Kain KH, Miller JWI, Jones-Paris CR, Thomason RT, Lewis JD, Bader DM, Barnett JV, Zijlstra A: The chick embryo as an expanding experimental model for cancer and cardiovascular research, *Dev Dyn* 243:216–228, 2014.

Kashiwagi K, Kashiwagi A, Kurabayashi A, Hanada H, Nakajima K, Okada M, Takase M, Yaoita Y: *Xenopus tropicalis*: an ideal experimental animal in amphibia, *Exp Anim* 59:395–405, 2010.

Katsiadaki I, Sanders M, Sebire M, Nagae M, Soyano K, Scott AP: Three-spined stickleback: an emerging model in environmental endocrine disruption, *Environ Sci* 14:263–283, 2007.

Keller JM, McClellan-Green PD, Kucklick JR, Keil DE, Peden-Adams MM: Effects of organochlorine contaminants on loggerhead sea turtle immunity: comparison of a correlative field study and in vitro exposure experiments, *Environ Health Perspect* 114:70–76, 2006.

Kent ML, Bishop-Stewart JK, Matthews JL, Spitsbergen JM: Pseudocapillaria tomentosa, a nematode pathogen, and associated neoplasms of zebrafish (*Danio rerio*) kept in research colonies, *Comp Med* 52, 2002, 354-348.

Kent ML, Whipps CM, Matthews JL, Florio D, Watral V, Bishop-Stewart JK, Poort M, Bermudez L: Mycobacteriosis in zebrafish (*Danio rerio*) research facilities, *Comp Biochem Physiol C* 138:383–390, 2004.

Kinoshita M, Murata K, Naruse K, Tanaka M, editors: *Medaka – biology, management, and experimental protocols*, Ames, 2009, Wiley-Blackwell.

Kissling GE, Bernheim NJ, Hawkins WE, Wolfe MJ, Jokinen MP, Smith CS, Herbert RA, Boorman GA: The utility of the guppy (*Poecilia reticulata*) and medaka (*Oryzias latipes*) in evaluation of chemicals for carcinogenicity, *Toxicol Sci* 92:143–156, 2006.

Kuhnert A, Vogs C, Altenburger R, Kuster E: The internal concentration of organic substances in fish embryos - a toxicokinetic approach, *Environ Toxicol Chem* 32:1819–1827, 2013.

Larsen BK, Perkins Jr EJ: Target organ toxicity in the kidney. In , London, 2001, Taylor & Francis, pp 90–140. Schlenk D, Benson WH, editors: *Target organ toxicity in marine and freshwater teleosts*, vol. 1. London, 2001, Taylor & Francis, pp 90–140.

Law J: Issues related to the use of fish models in toxicologic pathology: session introduction, *Toxicol Pathol* 31:49–52, 2003.

Lawrence C, Sanders GE, Wilson C: Aquatics. In Weichbrod RH, Thompson GAH, Norton JN, editors: *Management of animal care and use programs in research, education, and testing*, 2nd ed, Boca Raton, 2018, CRC Press, pp 559–578.

Leung MCK, Williams PL, Benedetto A, Au C, Helmcke KJ, Aschner M, Meyer J: *Caenorhabditis elegans*: an emerging model in biomedical and environmental toxicology, *Toxicol Sci* 106:5–28, 2008.

Lieschke GJ, Currie PD: Animal models of human disease: zebrafish swim into view, *Nat Rev Genet* 8:353–367, 2007.

Lister AL, van der Kraak GJ, Rutherford R, MacLatchy D: *Fundulus heteroclitus*: ovarian reproductive physiology and the impact of environmental contaminants, *Comp Biochem Physiol C Toxicol Pharmacol* 154:278–287, 2011.

Liu Y, Zhang X, Zhang J, Hu C: Construction of a quantitative structure activity relationship (qsar) model to predict the absorption of cephalosporins in zebrafish for toxicity study, *Front Pharmacol* 10:31, 2019.

Maia LA, Velloso I, Abreu JG: Advances in the use of Xenopus for successful drug screening, *Expert Opin Drug Discov* 12:1153–1159, 2017.

Mallatt J: Fish gill structural changes induced by toxicants and other irritants: a statistical review, *Can J Fish Aquat Sci* 42:630–648, 1985.

Marrett LE, Robb EJ, Frank RK: Efficacy of neomycin sulfate water medication on the control of mortality associated with colibacillosis in growing turkeys, *Poult Sci* 79:12–17, 2000.

Masereeuw R, Terlouw SA, van Aubel RA, Russel FG, Miller DS: Endothelin B receptor-mediated regulation of ATP-driven drug secretion in renal proximal tubule, *Mol Pharmacol* 57:59–67, 2000.

Miki M, Ohishi N, Nakamura E, Rurumi A, Mizuhashi F: Improved fixation of the whole bodies of fish by a double-fixation method with formalin solution and Bouin's fluid or Davidson's fluid, *J Toxicol Pathol* 31:201–206, 2018.

Murray KN, Dreska M, Nasiadka A, Rinne M, Matthews JL, Carmichael C, Bauer J, Varga ZM, Westerfield M: Transmission, diagnosis, and recommendations for control of pseudoloma neurophilia infections in laboratory zebrafish (*Danio rerio*) facilities, *Comp Med* 61:322–329, 2011.

Myers MS, Stehr CM, Olson OP, Johnson LL, McCain BB, Chan S-L, Varanasi U: Relationships between toxicopathic hepatic lesions and exposure to chemical contaminants in English sole (*Pleuronectes vetulus*), starry flounder (*Platichthys stellatus*), and white croaker (*Genyonemus lineatus*) from selected marine sites on the Pacific Coast, USA, *Environ Health Perspect* 102:200–215, 1994.

Naert T, Vleminckx K: CRISPR/Cas9 disease models in zebrafish and Xenopus: the genetic renaissance of fish and frogs, *Drug Disc Today Technol* 28:41–52, 2018.

Nakayama T, Fisher M, Nakajima K, Odeleye AO, Zimmerman KB, Fish MB, Yaoita Y, Chojnowski JL, Lauderdale JD, Netland PA, Graingera RM: Xenopus pax6 mutants affect eye development and other organ systems, and have phenotypic similarities to human aniridia patients, *Dev Biol* 408:328–344, 2015.

National Research Council (US): *Committee for the update of the guide for the care and use of laboratory animals: guide for the care and use of laboratory animals*, 8th ed, Washington, DC, 2011, National Academies Press.

Neiffer DL, Stamper MA: Fish sedation, analgesia, anesthesia, and euthanasia: considerations, methods, and types of drugs, *ILAR J* 50:343–360, 2009.

Nieuwkoop PD, Faber J, editors: *Normal table of Xenopus laevis (Daudin)*, New York, NY, 1994, Routledge.

Oehlmann J, Di Benedetto P, Tillmann M, Duft M, Oetken M, Schulte-Oehlmann U: Endocrine disruption in prosobranch molluscs: evidence and ecological relevance, *Ecotoxicology* 16(1):29–43, 2007.

O'Rourke DP, Cox JD, Baumann DP: Nontraditional species. In Weichbrod RH, Thompson GAH, Norton JN, editors: *Management of animal care and use programs in research, education, and testing*, 2nd ed, Boca Raton, 2018, CRC Press, pp 579–597.

Olson H, Betton G, Robinson D, Thomas K, Monro A, Kolaja G, Lilly P, Sanders J, Sipes G, Bracken W, Dorato M, Van Deun K, Smith P, Berger B, Heller A: Concordance of the toxicity of pharmaceuticals in humans and in animals, *Regul Toxicol Pharmacol* 32:56–67, 2000.

Palace VP, Evans RE, Wautier K, Baron C, Vandenbyllardt L, Vandersteen W, Kidd K: Induction of vitellogenin and histological effects in wild fathead minnows from a lake experimentally treated with the synthetic estrogen, ethynylestradiol, *Water Qual Res J Canada* 37:637–650, 2002.

Peters EC, Yevich PP, Harshbarger JC, et al.: Comparative histopathology of gonadal neoplasms in marine bivalve molluscs, *Dis Aqat Org* 20:59–76, 1994.

Price KL, Peters EC: *Histological techniques for corals, digital book*, 2018, Price and Peters.

Pritchard JB, Miller DS: Teleost kidney in evaluation of xenobiotic toxicity and elimination, *Fed Proc* 39:3207–3212, 1980.

Qiao D, Nikitina LA, Buznikov GA, Lauder JM, Seidler FJ, Slotkin TA: The sea urchin embryo as a model for mammalian developmental neurotoxicity: ontogenesis of the high-affinity choline transporter and its role in cholinergic trophic activity, *Environ Health Perspect* 111(14):1730–1735, 2003.

Rawal S, Kim JE, Coulombe Jr R: Aflatoxin B1 in poultry: toxicology, metabolism and prevention, *Res Vet Sci* 89:325–331, 2010.

Reimschuessel R, Bennett RO, May EB, Lipsky MM: Development of newly formed nephrons in the goldfish kidney following hexachlorobutadiene-induced nephrotoxicity, *Toxicol Pathol* 18:32–38, 1990.

Reimschuessel R, Chamie SJ, Kinnel M: Evaluation of gentamicin-induced nephrotoxicosis in toadfish, *J Am Vet Med Assoc* 209:137–139, 1996.

Ruehl-Fehlert C, Bomke C, Dorgerloh M, Palazzi X, Rosenbruch M: Pleistophora infestation in fathead minnows, *Pimephales promelas* (rafinesque), *J Fish Dis* 28:629–637, 2005.

Santoriello C, Zon LI: Hooked! Modeling human disease in zebrafish, *J Clin Invest* 122:2337–2343, 2012.

Sappington LC, Mayer FL, Dwyer FJ, Buckler DR, Jones JR, Ellersieck MR: Contaminant sensitivity of threatened and endangered fishes compared to standard surrogate species, *Environ Toxicol Chem* 20:2869–2876, 2001.

Saydmohammed M, Vollmer LL, Onuoha EO, Maskrey TS, Gibson G, Watkins SC, Wipf P, Vogt A, Tsang M: A high-content screen reveals new small-molecule enhancers of ras/Mapk signaling as probes for zebrafish heart development, *Molecules* 23:1691–1705, 2018.

Scanes CG, McNabb FMA: Avian models for research in toxicology and endocrine disruption, *Avian Poult Biol Rev* 14:21–52, 2003.

Schartl M, Walter RB: Xiphophorus and medaka cancer models. In , Cham, 2016, Springer, pp 531–552. Langenau D, editor: *Cancer and zebrafish: Advances in experimental medicine and biology*, vol. 916. Cham, 2016, Springer, pp 531–552.

Schmid M, Evans BJ, Bogart JP: Polyploidy in amphibia, *Cytogen Genome Res* 145:315–330, 2015.

Schoeb TR, Brown MB, Gross TS, Klein PA: *Final report: endocrine disruptors and host resistance in Lake Apopka alligators*. Available from: https://cfpub.epa.gov/ncer_abstracts/index.cfm/fuseaction/display.abstractDetail/abstract/174/report/F. (Accessed 24 January 2020).

Schofield JS: Animal-health pharmaceuticals: research responsibilities and laboratory animal welfare, *Future Med Chem* 3:851–854, 2011.

Segalat L: Invertebrate animal models of diseases as screening tools in drug discovery, *ACS Chem Biol* 2:231–236, 2007.

Shima A, Mitani H: Medaka as a research organism: past, present and future, *Mech Develop* 121:599–604, 2004.

Sievers M, Hale R, Parris KM, Melvin SD, Lanctot CM, Swearer SE: Contaminant-induced behavioural changes in amphibians: a meta-analysis, *Sci Total Environ* 693:133570, 2019.

Slaby S, Marin M, Marchand G, Lemiere S: Exposures to chemical contaminants: what can we learn from reproduction and development endpoints in the amphibian toxicology literature? *Environ Pollut* 248:478–495, 2019.

Speare DJ, MacNair N, Hammell KL: Demonstration of tank effect on growth indices of juvenile rainbow trout (*Oncorhynchus mykiss*) during an ad libitum feeding trial, *Am J Vet Res* 56:1372–1379, 1995.

Spitsbergen JM, Blazer VS, Bowser PR, Cheng KC, Cooper KR, Cooper TK, Frasca Jr S, Groman DB, Harper CM, Law JM, Marty GD, Smolowitz RM, St Leger J, Wolf DC, Wolf JC: Finfish and aquatic invertebrate pathology resources for now and the future, *Comp Biochem Physiol C Toxicol Pharmacol* 149:249–257, 2009.

Stacy BA, Parker JM: Amphibian oncology, *Vet Clin Exot Anim* 7:673–695, 2004.

Sures B, Nachev M, Selbach C, Marcogliese DJ: Parasite responses to pollution: what we know and where we go in 'Environmental Parasitology', *Parasites Vectors* 10:65–78, 2017.

Tibbetts SM, Qall CL, Barbosa-Solomieu V, Bryenton MD, Plouffe DA, Buchanan JT, Lall SP: Effects of combined 'all-fish' growth hormone transgenics and triploidy on growth and nutrient utilization of Atlantic salmon (Salmo salar L.) fed a practical grower diet of known composition, *Aquaculture* 406-407:141–152, 2013.

Tilton SC, Orner GA, Binninghoff AD, Carpenter HM, Hendricks JD, Pereira CB, Williams DE: Genomic profiling reveals an alternate mechanism for hepatic tumor promotion by perfluorooctanoic acid in rainbow trout, *Environ Health Perspec* 116:1047–1055, 2008.

Touart LW: Factors considered in using birds for evaluating endocrine-disrupting chemicals, *ILAR J* 45:462–468, 2004.

Tyler CR, Lange A, Paull GC, Katsu Y, Iguchi T: The roach (*Rutilus rutilus*) as a sentinel for assessing endocrine disruption, *Environ Sci* 14:235–253, 2007.

U. S. Environmental Protection Agency: *OCSPP 890.2300: larval Amphibian growth and development assay (LAGDA), EPA Pub No. 740-C-15-001*, 2015.

U.S. Food and Drug Administration: *Guidance for industry – environmental assessment of human drug and biologics applications, docket FDA-1998-D-0278*, 1998.

Van den Berg M, Birnbaum L, Bosveld AT, Brunström B, Cook P, Feeley M, Giesy JP, Hanberg A, Hasegawa R, Kennedy SW, Kubiak T, Larsen JC, van Leeuwen FX, Liem AK, Nolt C, Peterson RE, Poellinger L, Safe S, Schrenk D, Tillitt D, Tysklind M, Younes M, Waern F, Zacharewski T: Toxic equivalency factors (TEFs) for PCBs, PCDDs, PCDFs for humans and wildlife, *Environ Health Perspect* 106:775–792, 1998.

van der Worp HB, Howells DW, Sena ES, Porritt MJ, Rewell S, O'Collins V, Macleod MR: Can animal models of disease reliably inform human studies? *PLoS Med* 7:1–8, 2010.

Venturino A, Rosenbaum E, Caballero de Castro A, Anguiano OL, Gauna L, Fonovich de Schroeder T, Pechen de D'Angelo AM: Biomarkers of effect in toads and frogs, *Biomarkers* 8:167–186, 2003.

Vergneau-Grosset C, Nadeau M, Groff JM: Fish oncology diseases, diagnostics, and therapeutics, *Vet Clin Exot Anim* 20:21–56, 2017.

VICH: Environmental impact assessment for veterinary medicinal products – phase II guidance, *VICH GL* 38, 2004.

VICH: *Target animal safety for veterinary pharmaceutical products*, 2008. VICH GL 43 (Target Animal Safety) – Pharmaceuticals.

Walter RB, Kazianis S: Xiphophorus interspecies hybrids as genetic models of induced neoplasia, *ILAR J* 42:299–321, 2001.

Wheeler GN, Brändli AW: Simple vertebrate models for chemical genetics and drug discovery screens: lessons from zebrafish and Xenopus, *Dev Dynam* 238:1287–1308, 2009.

Williams DE, Bailey GS, Reddy A, Hendricks JD, Oganesian A, Orner GA, Pereira CB, Swenberg JA: The rainbow trout (*Oncorhynchus mykiss*) tumor model: recent applications in low-dose exposures to tumor initiators and promoters, *Toxicol Pathol* 31:58–61, 2003.

Wilson-Sanders SE: Invertebrate models for biomedical research, testing, and education, *ILAR J* 52:126–152, 2011.

Wolf JC, Maack G: Evaluating the credibility of histopathology data in environmental endocrine toxicity studies, *Environ Toxicol Chem* 36:601–611, 2017.

Wolf JC: Fish toxicologic pathology: the growing credibility gap and how to bridge it, *Bull Eur Ass Fish Pathol* 38:51–64, 2018.

Wolf JC, Wheeler JA: A critical review of histopathological findings associated with endocrine and non-endocrine hepatic toxicity in fish models, *Aquat Toxicol* 197:60–78, 2018.

Wolf JC, Wolfe MJ: Good laboratory practice considerations in the use of fish models, *Toxicol Pathol* 31:53–57, 2003.

Wolf JC, Wolfe MJ: A brief overview of nonneoplastic hepatic toxicity in fish, *Toxicol Pathol* 33:75–85, 2005.

Wood CM: Toxic response of the gill. In , London, 2001, Taylor & Francis, pp 1–65. Schlenk D, Benson WH, editors: *Target organ toxicity in marine and freshwater teleosts*, vol. 1. London, 2001, Taylor & Francis, pp 1–65.

Zhao Y, Wang DO, Martin KC: Preparation of Aplysia sensory-motor neuronal cell cultures, *J Vis Exp* 28:1355, 2009.

Zvinavashe E, Du T, Griff T, van den Berg HHJ, Soffers AEMF, Vervoort J, Murk AJ, Rietjens IMCM: Quantitative structure-activity relationship modeling of the toxicity of organothiophosphate pesticides to *Daphnia magna* and *Cyprinus carpio*, *Chemosphere* 75:1531–1538, 2009.

CHAPTER

23

Genetically Engineered Animal Models in Toxicologic Research

Lauren E. Himmel[1], Kristin Lewis Wilson[2], Sara F. Santagostino[3], Brad Bolon[4]

[1]AbbVie Inc., Preclinical Safety, North Chicago, IL, United States, [2]Amgen, Inc., South San Francisco, CA, United States, [3]Genentech, Inc., South San Francisco, CA, United States, [4]GEMpath, Inc., Longmont, CO, United States

OUTLINE

1. Fundamentals of Genetically Engineered Animal Models 859
   1.1. Methods for Genetic Modification 860
   1.2. Nomenclature Conventions 878
   1.3. Model Selection 879

2. Analysis of Genetically Engineered Animal Models 881
   2.1. Genotyping 881
   2.2. Phenotyping 883
   2.3. Large-Scale Phenotyping 883
   2.4. Directed Phenotypic Characterization for Product Discovery and Development 885
   2.5. Phenotypic Interpretation of Genetically Engineered Animal Models 886

3. Genetically Modified Models for Hazard Identification and Safety Assessment 888
   3.1. Basic Concepts for Using Engineered Animals in Hazard Identification and Safety Assessment 888
   3.2. Absorption, Distribution, Metabolism, and Excretion 889

3.3. Genotoxicity Testing 892
3.4. Carcinogenicity Assessment 895
3.5. Engineered Immunodeficient Models 898
3.6. Humanized Animal Models 904

4. Limitations in Using Genetically Modified Animals for Hazard Identification and Safety Assessment 913

5. Special Considerations in Safety Assessment of Products Derived from Genetically Engineered Animals 913
   5.1. Biopharming and Xenotransplantation 913
   5.2. Food Products 916

6. Summary 917

Glossary 917

References 918

1. FUNDAMENTALS OF GENETICALLY ENGINEERED ANIMAL MODELS

Spectacular advances in the understanding, diagnosis, and treatment of disease have been made possible in recent decades through the wonders of modern molecular biology. The rise of reliable genetic engineering methods has allowed the deliberate creation of new animal models that have enhanced our ability to better understand disease and advance human health.

Haschek and Rousseaux's Handbook of Toxicologic Pathology, Fourth Edition.
https://doi.org/10.1016/B978-0-12-821044-4.00024-8

Genetically engineered animals have been employed in discovery and development programs for new therapeutic products (Bolon, 2004; Boverhof et al., 2011). Discovery-stage experiments utilize genetically engineered mice (GEM) or sometimes genetically engineered rats (GERs) to define molecular mechanisms that contribute to disease, to validate therapeutic targets, and to demonstrate the efficacy of novel drug candidates (Diaz and Maher, 2016; Dunn et al., 2005). The growing use of these models is based on the premise that the activity of an animal or human gene in an animal model (i.e., one into which genetic material was introduced to alter or ablate genetic function) can predict the function of the human gene homolog. The validity of this premise is demonstrated by the fact that the biological effects of many top-selling drugs are well correlated with the *phenotypes* (i.e., the combination of biochemical, functional, and/or structural effects produced by a molecule's activity in vivo) seen in GEM lacking the murine homologs of the human molecular targets (Zambrowicz and Sands, 2003). Nonclinical safety studies also may incorporate GEM or GER models to explore the toxicity profile of new drug candidates (especially fully human or "humanized" [part human, part animal] biomolecules) (Webster et al., 2020). Therapeutic biomolecules (see *Protein Pharmaceutical Agents,* Vol 2, Chap 6; *Nucleic Acid Pharmaceutical Agents,* Vol 2, Chap 7), cells (see *Stem Cells and Regenerative Medicine,* Vol 2, Chap 10), or whole organs derived from engineered livestock are designed for introduction into human patients, and thus are subject to thorough nonclinical safety testing during the course of their development.

The widespread use of genetically engineered animal models in modern biomedical research necessitates that those engaged in nonclinical drug development become familiar with their applications and limitations. This chapter will briefly review fundamental principles and methods for genetic engineering in animals (Table 23.1), techniques used to verify that engineered models have the proper characteristics for inclusion in a product development program, and examples where genetically modified animals have been used successfully in drug discovery and development. This discussion will concentrate on modifications of the nuclear genome which are in common use, and introduce methods for manipulation of the mitochondrial genome, as such genetically engineered animals frequently are employed to provide a whole-animal context for decisions that influence the course of product discovery and development.

1.1. Methods for Genetic Modification

In 1981, Gordon and Ruddle coined the term "transgenic" to describe an animal in which an exogenous gene has been introduced into its genome (Gordon and Ruddle, 1981). The practices of introducing genes with known function and deliberately inducing genetic mutations into the genome of animals to illuminate novel phenotypes (a strategy termed "reverse genetics") were in part driven by the challenges of identifying spontaneous mutations in endogenous genes and interpreting the associated downstream events (an approach followed in "forward genetics"). Reverse genetics required less time and expense during the early days of this technological revolution. However, with the constant advances in DNA, RNA, and protein methods, forward genetics has become more feasible as a routine strategy for genetic investigations. This shift in approach must always be considered in the context of the animal model. In the late 1980s, the term "transgenic" was extended to gene-targeting experimentation and the production of chimeric or "knockout" mice in which a gene (or genes) was selectively removed from the host genome in some (for chimeras [i.e., animals with two or more genetically distinct cell populations]) or all cells (Koller and Smithies, 1992). Today, a transgenic animal can be defined as one having any specific genetic modification induced by transfer of genetic material from one organism to another. Transgenic animals are most commonly produced through one of three general approaches: (i) germline modifications of gametes; (ii) microinjection of DNA or gene constructs into the pronucleus of zygotes; or (iii) incorporating genetically modified cells, including embryonic stem cells (ES cells), into later-stage embryos (Behringer et al., 2014; Pinkert, 2014). Rodents (especially mice and rats) are the most commonly engineered species for biomedical research (see *Animal Models in Toxicologic Research: Rodents,* Vol 1, Chap 17).

TABLE 23.1 Advantages and Limitations of Major Technologies for Generating Genetically Engineered Animals

Method	Advantages	Disadvantages/Other considerations
TECHNIQUES TARGETING THE NUCLEAR GENOME[a]		
DNA microinjection techniques		
DNA microinjection of zygotes	• High frequency of generating transgenic animals • No constraint on size or type of DNA construct • Large constructs can be used to help avoid integration site-specific (i.e., positional) effects	• Potentially significant influence of the DNA integration site on expression of the transgene (positional effect) • Potential for undesired insertional mutagenesis • Promoter-driven expression must be well characterized • Time and expense
Gene knockdown and RNA interference (RNAi)	• RNAi (RNA interference) technology, such as antisense oligonucleotides (ASOs) and small interfering RNAs (siRNAs) can be synthesized directly instead of relying on a molecular DNA cloning step • Gene transfer in species where stem-cell homologous recombination has not been possible	• Variations in complimentary oligonucleotide length and composition affect the degree and duration of suppressing gene expression • Provokes degradation of specific mRNA (messenger RNA) transcripts • Alters the balance of mRNA degradation and production—potential for cytotoxicity by saturating endogenous RNAi pathways • Produces only a transient knockdown
Homologous recombination using blastocyst injection/morula aggregation techniques		
Embryonic stem (ES) cell/homologous recombination	• Gene targeting and selection of transgene integration sites occurs during in vitro culture • Provides defined, site-specific genetic manipulation (knockout, knockin) • Knockin models allow expression of foreign genes under the control of endogenous promoters • Verification of the correct targeted modification is possible before starting animal work • Multiple founders can be generated using the same targeted mutation	• Availability of correctly positioned restriction sites • Requires detailed DNA sequencing data • Requires homology arms longer than those that can be easily made by polymerase chain reaction (PCR) • Usually only one allele is affected, so several generations of breeding are required to achieve a homozygous animal • Alternative splicing (leading to hypomorphic alleles)

(Continued)

TABLE 23.1   Advantages and Limitations of Major Technologies for Generating Genetically Engineered Animals—cont'd

Method	Advantages	Disadvantages/Other considerations
TECHNIQUES TARGETING THE NUCLEAR GENOME[a]		
Conditional gene expression in space and/or time (e.g., Cre recombinase/loxP system, xenobiotic-inducible response elements)	• May allow for tissue- and/or time-specific expression of the engineered genetic mutation • Used to permit normal gene expression throughout development (to avoid embryonic lethality) • Employed to allow gene elimination in adulthood (to produce disease-causing mutations at maturity)	• Carries all of the disadvantages of both DNA microinjection and stem cell-based methods • Inducible promoter requires administration of chemicals or hormones that may confound the phenotypic analysis • Response to inducible promoter regulatory systems is not subject to dose-dependent control • Potential effects of expressing controllable gene on phenotype • Cre expression is not reversible and can reverse the mutagenic event through strand breakage • Mammalian genome contains cryptic (pseudo-loxP) sites for Cre activity • Multiple control groups are needed
Nuclear transfer		
Nuclear transfer	• Gene transfer in species where stem cell-based homologous recombination has not been possible • *In vitro* culture step allows for gene targeting opportunity • Ability to recover valuable genetically mediated traits from nonstem cell origins • Multiple founders can be generated that bear the same targeted mutation	• Lesser efficiency in generating engineered animals than other methods • Telomere shortening, leading to accelerated cellular senescence • Surgical embryo transfer skills are needed
Insertional mutagenesis techniques		
Gene trapping	• High throughput • Cost effective • Efficient and effective across a number of species • Disrupts gene function in enhancer, promoter, or gene sequence • Enables reporting of endogenous gene expression • Increasingly easy to interpret with advances in gene sequencing technology	• Alternative splicing (yielding hypomorphic alleles) • Insertional bias

Method	Advantages	Characteristics/Disadvantages
Retroviral vectors	• Efficient and effective across a number of species	• Single to low copy number integration • Effectively transduces dividing cells • Integration is random • High frequency of mosaicism • Limitations on the size of the DNA insert (i.e., must be < 15 kb) • Interference of retroviral sequences on transgene expression • Potential for oncogenesis, frequent gene instability, and recombination
Lentiviral vectors	• Efficient and effective across a number of species • High rates of gene transfer efficiency (up to 100%)	• Large proportion of founder animals may not express the integrated transgene • Varying proportions of intact integrations and functional expression in founders
Adenoviral, adenovirus-associated viral (AAV) vectors	• Gene transfer possible in adult animals	• Efficiency of adenoviral gene transfer varies • Adenovirus is highly immunogenic, often leading to an immune response sufficient to downregulate expression of the engineered gene
Chemical mutagenesis	• Efficient and effective across a number of species • Alkylating agents (e.g., N-ethyl-N-nitrosourea [ENU]) mainly induce random point mutations (about one event every 1–2 Mb)	• Mutagenesis using ENU is likely to generate hypomorphic mutations
Transposons	• Choice of retrotransposons, DNA transposons	• Variability in founder yields and expression profiles
Nuclease-based genome editing		
Targeted DNA strand breaks (zinc [Zn]-finger nuclease, integrase attB)	• Short 20 bp fragments are easily synthesized • Transfected as either DNA plasmids or mRNA into zygotes by microinjection • Useful for generating knockout animals where stem cells are not available for homologous recombination • Integrase attB permits high-frequency, single copy insertion into a known locus • A given Zn-finger specifies a particular target site; multiple Zn-fingers increase specificity	• Nonhomologous end joining (NHEJ) results in mutations • Homologous recombination results in replacement of the Zn-finger • Short regions of deletion may be insufficient to block gene expression • Difficult to target G nucleotide-rich sequences

(Continued)

TABLE 23.1   Advantages and Limitations of Major Technologies for Generating Genetically Engineered Animals—cont'd

Method	Advantages	Disadvantages/Other considerations
TECHNIQUES TARGETING THE NUCLEAR GENOME[a]		
Transcription activator-like effector nucleases (TALENs)	• FokI endonuclease fused to TALE domains that interact with target DNA; one TALE domain recognizes one DNA base pair • Modular assembly; fusing multiple TALE domains has no effect on binding specificity • Generates double strand breaks at a targeted site in the genome to knockin mutations or knockout genes • Many TALE repeat arrays can be quickly designed and synthesized	• 5′ base of TALEN target site must be a thymine • Off-target mutagenesis can occur at similar sequences • cDNA for TALENs is ~3× larger than for ZFN • Highly repetitive nature can impair viral packaging and delivery • NHEJ can result in mice with different mutations from the same target constructs • TALEN binding is negatively impacted by DNA methylation
Clustered, regularly interspersed, short, palindromic repeats (CRISPR)/CRISPR-associated system (Cas)	• Cas endonuclease recruited to DNA via guide RNA (gRNA) • Target specificity based on ribonucleotide complex formation; 20 bp gRNAs are readily designed • Multiple mutations can be introduced in multiple genes through injection of multiple gRNAs • Efficient system since gRNA and Cas protein injected directly into developing mouse embryos	• Variable concern for off-target effects since single mismatches are well-tolerated and multiple mismatches can be tolerated • Cas9 protein is quite large (~4.2 kb coding sequence); can impair delivery as an RNA molecule or via viral vector • NHEJ can result in mice with different mutations from the same target constructs • A protospacer-adjacent motif (PAM) sequence adjacent to target site is required • Binding efficacy impacted by chromatin accessibility
Techniques for manipulating the male germline		

Sperm-mediated and spermatogonial-mediated transfer	• Allows gene transfer in species where ES cell/homologous recombination technologies are not yet possible
	• Sperm-mediated transfer obviates the need for skill in microinjection and surgical transfer
	• Spermatogonial stem cells allow long-term maintenance and proliferation
		• Few laboratories perform the techniques
		• Sperm-mediated transfer:
		  ∘ Identification of suitable male donors is difficult
		  ∘ Large quantities of purified genetic material are needed per ejaculate/experiment
		• Spermatogonial-mediated transfer: intricate transfection/cell culture requirements

TECHNIQUES TARGETING THE MITOCHONDRIAL GENOME

Mitochondrial transfer	• Mitochondrial genome (mtDNA) is highly conserved across species, with a unique code, structure, transcriptional and translational apparatus, and tRNA (transfer RNA) • Current techniques reflect nuclear transfer modeling (e.g., ES cell transfer using ρ° ES cells and cybrid[a] fusions; mitochondrial microinjection into zygote cytoplasm)	• Few laboratories perform the technique • Mammalian embryos may carry from 50,000 to 500,000 copies of the mtDNA, thus needing more than one haplotype (heteroplasmy) in sufficient quantity to induce a phenotype • ES cell transfer is the most common technique for generating high levels of mitochondrial homoplasmy • ρ° ES cell treatment and cybrid fusion add additional cell trauma • Overall efficiencies lower compared to nuclear gene transfer
Allotopic expression	• Recoding mitochondrial genes for integration or expression within the nucleus • Takes advantage of existing techniques targeting the nuclear genome	• Mitochondrial codon usage must be replaced for proper transcription and translation in the nucleus • Mitochondrial localization signaling is required • Endogenous mitochondrial gene expression is still a factor

[a] Cybrids are cells that have had their native mitochondrial DNA (mtDNA) deleted and replaced by mtDNA from another source.
Table adapted in part from Haschek WM, Rousseaux CG, Wallig MA, editors: Haschek and Rousseaux's handbook of toxicologic pathology, ed 3, 2013, Academic Press, Table 12.1, pp 407–411, with permission.

These technologies are employed in many species beyond mice and rats, including bacteria, fungi, plants, nematodes, insects, amphibians, fish, poultry, rabbits, ruminants, swine, and nonhuman primates. For more information on these species, refer to other chapters in this volume on various animal models employed for product discovery and development (see *Animal Models in Toxicologic Research: Nonmammalian*, Vol 1, Chap 22; *Animal Models in Toxicologic Research: Rabbit*, Vol 1, Chap 18; *Animal Models in Toxicologic Research: Dog*, Vol 1, Chap 19; *Animal Models in Toxicologic Research: Pig*, Vol 1, Chap 20; *Animal Models in Toxicologic Research: Nonhuman Primate*, Vol 1, Chap 21).

Pronuclear/nuclear microinjection of DNA is a basic physical technique for transgenic technology today (Pritchett-Corning and Landel, 2015). Microinjection of DNA into zygotes (fertilized one-cell embryos) typically involves the use of micromanipulators and a microinjection apparatus to introduce a solution containing recombinant DNA into the nuclear genome on a permanent basis (Figure 23.1). Injections usually are made into the larger (derived from the male) of the two pronuclei, originally for the simple reason that it is a bigger target; thus, the FVB strain of mouse with its very large pronuclei has been a favored platform for engineering the nuclear genome by direct DNA microinjection (Brinster et al., 1985). After injection, zygotes then are implanted into the oviduct or uterus of hormone-primed pseudopregnant recipients. The resulting progeny are tested for their transgene status by genotyping a tissue biopsy (usually an ear punch or tail snip), typically at or shortly after weaning (Pinkert, 2003). "Transgene-positive" founder animals (F_0) are retained for later phenotypic analysis and/or breeding to generate F_1 and other generations of progeny that bear the desired genetic modification. Most transgene-negative littermates of the F_0 animals are culled, but some individuals of both sexes usually are kept to serve as age-matched "wild-type" controls for the underlying genetic background.

The "constructs" (i.e., DNA vectors, usually a linearized viral plasmid) that are used to carry the transgene have been engineered to contain several different components that promote efficient transgene expression. The most important components are (i) a promoter, a specific DNA sequence that binds the transcription factors needed to recruit RNA polymerase and drive transcription of the engineered gene; (ii) the DNA sequence for the transgene of interest; and (iii) a polyadenylation (polyA) sequence that signals when to terminate transgene transcription (Figure 23.1). It is essential that the spatial (tissue location) and temporal (timing) effects of the promoter be well characterized in advance, often through utilizing reporter genes in place of the transgene, prior to introducing the desired transgene in order to investigate the potential for "off-target" effects arising from unexpected expression of the transgene in time or tissues. The transgene sequence may be obtained by isolating specific sequences from an organism's endogenous gene complement (i.e., genomic DNA) or by reverse-engineering RNA transcripts to recover the gene sequence from which it was generated (i.e., complementary DNA [cDNA]). Transgenes may be designed to increase their expression in response to xenobiotics by engineering them to contain a xenobiotic response element in correct association with the promoter. Alternatively, cell ablation may be achieved using a toxicogenic approach, in which the promoter-directed expression of a toxin gene results in intracellular toxin production and cell death.

Following microinjection, DNA typically integrates randomly into the nuclear DNA (nDNA) of the zygote, generally in a single chromosomal location. The exact site of integration will differ for each F_0 animal, indicating that each line will have to be analyzed individually for the extent of transgene expression and the existence of a reliably transmitted, transgene-mediated phenotype. Transgene integration may occur as a single copy or as concatemers (many copies connected in series) containing from two or three up to several hundred copies of the transgene. When multiple copies are introduced, they are organized predominantly in a head-to-tail fashion. Several different engineered transgenes may be assembled in a single construct to link their expression in vivo. Similarly, the tendency for transgenes to integrate at a single site may be used to link the functions of two or more independent transgenes carried on different constructs. In such cases, after simultaneous coinjection, the constructs integrate randomly but in the same site, yielding coordinated expression of several transgenes.

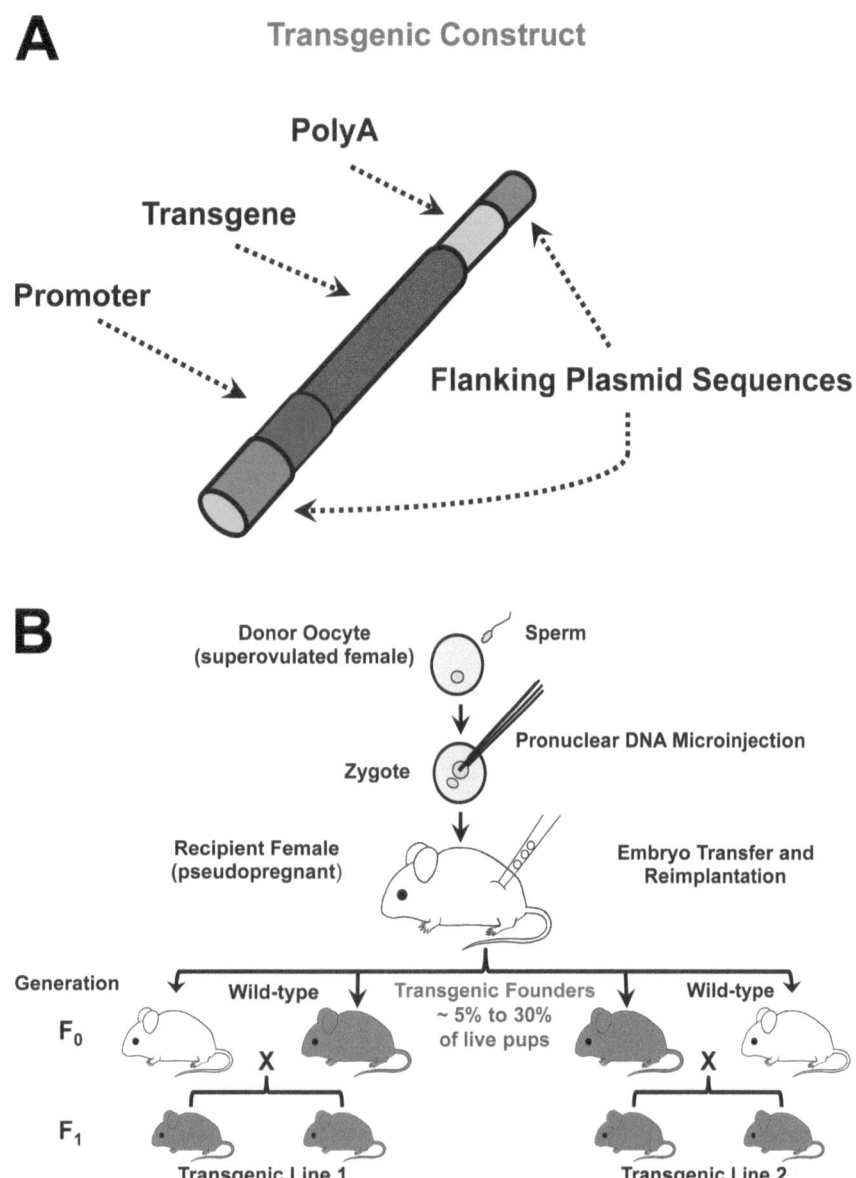

FIGURE 23.1 **Generation of transgenic animals by pronuclear microinjection.** (A) The targeting construct is assembled from three DNA sources. The foreign transgene (pink) and its associated promoter (lavender) is inserted into a plasmid (green) along with a polyadenylation sequence (polyA, yellow). The promoter drives transgene transcription, while the polyA sequence acts as the signal to stop transcription. (B) Oocyte donor females treated with gonadotropic hormones to induce superovulation are mated with males. Each zygote (i.e., single-cell fertilized embryo) receives a microinjection of engineered DNA into one pronucleus (i.e., the genetic material from one parent) with a few picoliters of fluid containing the engineered DNA construct, after which one or more copies of the transgene may insert at random into the pronuclear genome. The injected embryos are implanted in the oviduct of a pseudopregnant recipient female, which carries the litter to term. The offspring of this founder (F_0) generation will include transgenic offspring (founders) as well as wild-type progeny. Individual founders (ideally three or more per transgene) are used to establish distinct transgenic lines (the F_1 generation and beyond) as any phenotype due to incorporation of the transgene should be reproducible across all the lines. Expression of the transgene may be subject to upregulation in response to xenobiotics if the construct is engineered to contain an appropriate xenobiotic response element. *Figure modified from Haschek WM, Rousseaux CG, Wallig MA, editors:* Haschek and Rousseaux's handbook of toxicologic pathology, *ed 3, 2013, Academic Press, Figure 12.1, p 412, with permission.*

Since DNA microinjection is usually undertaken in individual zygotes (one-celled embryos), the transgene is anticipated to be present in all cells arising from the zygote. However, occasionally, the integration of the microinjected DNA into the host genome is delayed, as when incorporation of the transgene does not occur until after blastomeres (i.e., the totipotent cells that comprise early embryos) have begun dividing. With delayed integration, some, but not all, embryonic cells will contain the transgene; such embryos, in which transgene-positive and transgene-negative cells are intermingled, are termed "mosaic." These mosaic F_0 animals will have transgene expression when genotyped, and thus are technically transgenic, but they will only be able to produce transgenic progeny if the engineered gene is present in their germ cell progenitors. Therefore, the offspring (F_1 generation) of transgenic F_0 must be tested again to ensure that expression of the transgene is heritable.

Expression of a randomly inserted transgene may induce a phenotype in several fashions. First, the transgene may elicit an effect of its own that represents the inherent function of the protein that is specified by the newly introduced gene. Second, the transgene may function in a "dominant-negative" manner to inactivate or regulate the actions of endogenous genes. Third, the transgene may lead to "insertional mutagenesis" if its site of random insertion disrupts the sequence and function of an existing gene (Woychik et al., 1985); in essence, this outcome leads to an accidental gene deletion, or "knockout," the unintended phenotype of which will need to be differentiated from any true phenotype resulting from expression of the transgene. For all three of these mechanisms, host DNA near sites of random integration often undergoes sequence duplication, deletion, or rearrangement as a consequence of transgene incorporation. Furthermore, the regulatory elements in the host DNA near the site of insertion, and the general availability of that chromosomal region for transcription, appear to have major roles in affecting the location and expression level of the incorporated transgene. This "positional effect" may partially explain why expression of the same transgene can vary dramatically among individual F_0 animals and their progeny. In particular, the positional effect

may differentially affect the function of the promoter sequences used to direct transgene expression to different cell types and organs. Thus, when characterizing transgenic animals that were generated with any method where random integration of the transgene occurs, it is essential to keep in mind that cell type- or tissue-specific expression of the transgene depends not only on the specificity of the promoter sequence but also on the positional influence of the integration site. For this reason, any phenotype identified using transgenic animals must be similar in at least two lines derived from different F_0 founders before it can be concluded that the engineered gene is responsible for producing the effect (Figure 23.1).

Viral-mediated gene transfer represents an alternative means of inserting transgenes permanently into the nuclear genome (Jayant et al., 2016; Robbins et al., 1998). This technique may be utilized to explore molecular pathways or as a therapeutic modality (see *Gene Therapy/ Gene Editing*, Vol 2, Chap 8). In this approach, a retroviral or lentiviral vector is incubated with mammalian cells, commonly an ovum or zygote so that the genetic material will be present in essentially all adult cells. This technique is efficient and effective across a number of species, although species- and strain-specific differences in the efficiency of transgenesis have been reported. Infection with retroviruses commonly leads to insertion of a single transgene copy at a single integration site. Potential problems with the use of retroviral vectors include mutagenicity, oncogenicity, the limited size of the transgene payload, and the common occurrence of gene instability and recombination (Murnane et al., 2011). Lentiviral vectors provide significantly better integration efficiency and transgenic animal yields relative to both retroviruses and microinjection methods for transgenesis. Furthermore, lentiviruses permit a larger payload, promote stable integration of multiple gene copies, and do not induce mutagenic and oncogenic events. The main drawbacks to their use are the potential for transgene silencing, genetic mosaicism, and vector-related toxicity resulting in a variable percentage of the F_1 generation with transgene expression. Viral vectors must be handled using appropriate biocontainment procedures and work areas, particularly if replication competent, to avoid any

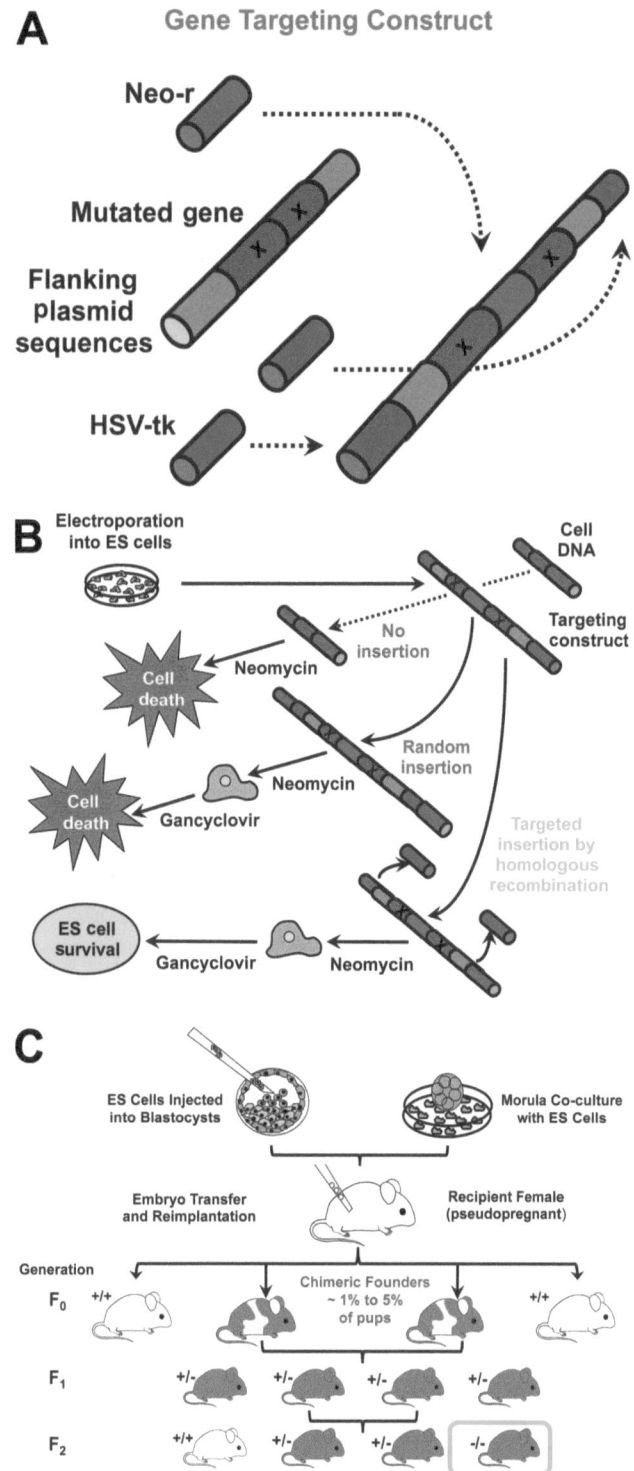

FIGURE 23.2   **Generation of gene-targeted (knockout or knockin) animals by homologous recombination.** (A) The targeting construct is assembled from four DNA sources. The mutated gene (pink cylinders denoted by X) is inserted into a plasmid (green), after which sequences are added for two xenobiotic selection markers: neomycin resistance (Neo-r [blue]) and herpes simplex type I thymidine kinase (HSV-tk [purple]). (B) Next, the engineered DNA is introduced into cultured embryonic stem (ES) cells by electroporation. The ES cells are incubated to allow homologous recombination between the similar sequence of the mutated gene and the endogenous gene (pink cylinder without an X, flanked by gray). The ES cells then are tested for the proper introduction of the engineered

potential for infecting the scientific staff. In practice, both the vector construction and in vivo experiments are conducted using conditions suitable for Biosafety Level (BSL) 2.

Systemic gene delivery ("gene therapy") into adult animals using viral vectors is a commonly used method to overexpress transgenes after an individual's development is entirely or nearly complete. The main drawback to this strategy is that persistence of the transgene is impacted by the nature of the vector. For example, adenovirus (AdV) is more immunogenic than are both adenoviral-associated viral (AAV) and retrovirus, so transgene levels are likely to be higher for a longer period if the transgene is introduced using one of the latter two options. Furthermore, the inflammatory reaction to AdV vectors may induce confounding functional and/or structural changes in the infected cells which in some circumstances may overlap with or obscure the phenotype exerted by the transgene. These viral vectors (especially AAVs and retroviruses) are common test articles in human clinical trials for gene therapy products, and now are being approved for use ex vivo and in vivo to correct diseases caused by single-gene mutations in human patients (see *Gene Therapy/Gene Editing*, Vol 2, Chap 8).

RNA interference (RNAi) is a useful means for transiently repressing the expression and function of targeted nuclear genes (Khan, 2019). The most common means for producing this effect is to introduce antisense oligonucleotides (ASOs) or small interfering RNAs (siRNAs). Delivery of these inhibitors may be done by pronuclear/nuclear microinjection (typically employed for embryos) or by parenteral injection (usually employed in adults). This approach typically elicits a partial decrease (i.e., "knockdown") rather than complete loss ("knockout") of gene function. In this regard, RNAi is gaining popularity as a means for investigating the functional consequences of innovative drug candidates, as pharmacological intervention reliably reduces but seldom completely halts activity of the targeted molecular pathway.

When using the RNAi approach, it must be remembered that variations in complimentary oligonucleotide length and composition may affect the degree and duration of suppressed gene expression. Furthermore, it has been shown that saturation of endogenous RNAi pathways can overwhelm the balance of mRNA degradation and production, thereby creating the potential for cytotoxicity. Strategies to manage this balance during therapeutic interventions are continuing to evolve (see *Nucleic Acid Pharmaceutical Agents*, Vol 2, Chap 7).

Gene targeting by homologous recombination is another routine technique used to produce genetically engineered animals (Pritchett-Corning and Landel, 2015). For this procedure, the permanent insertion of an engineered gene of interest may inactivate expression of the normal gene, thereby creating a null mutation (i.e., "knockout"). Alternatively, the insertion may replace the endogenous gene with a different functional gene (i.e., "knockin") to evaluate its role in a given disease or examine the function of a similar gene from another species (including human). In general, gene targeting by homologous recombination is undertaken in vitro by introducing the modified gene sequence into ES cells, confirming that recombination has produced the correctly engineered genotype, and then inserting the modified ES cells either by microinjection into a blastocyst

---

gene by addition of exogenous selection agents. Any ES cell in which the targeting construct was not inserted at all lacks Neo-r and will die when treated with neomycin. Those ES cells in which the construct was incorporated at random contain both the Neo-r and HSV-tk cassettes; therefore, they will survive exposure to neomycin but subsequently expire when treated with gancyclovir (an anti-HSV agent). Only ES cells that correctly performed homologous recombination will contain Neo-r but lack HSV-tk, and thus will survive exposure to both neomycin and gancyclovir. (C) Correctly generated ES cells (orange) are added to embryos by either direct blastocyst injection in the vicinity of the inner cell mass (green) or coculture with morulae (pale blue), after which the embryos are transferred into pseudopregnant recipient females. The resulting founding generation (F_0) consists of chimeric founders (i.e., where targeted ES cells were integrated into some embryonic tissues) and wild-type animals (+/+, where ES cells did not incorporate into embryonic tissues). Chimeric founders with germ-line transmission are bred to produce an F_1 generation composed entirely of heterozygous (+/−) offspring. Mating of +/− animals will yield an F_2 generation that includes targeted (−/−, denoted by the green box), +/−, and +/+ progeny (at a Mendelian ratio of approximately 1:2:1 if the mutation is not lethal). *Figure modified from Haschek WM, Rousseaux CG, Wallig MA, editors:* Haschek and Rousseaux's handbook of toxicologic pathology, *ed 3, 2013, Academic Press, Figure 12.2, pp 414–415, with permission.*

(a multicelled, cavitated embryo) or by coaggregation with a morula (a multicelled, noncavitated embryo) (Figure 23.2). For most mouse studies, the ES cells of choice are derived from one of two strains, C57BL/6 or 129 (which includes a variety of substrains with minor but nonetheless essential differences in their genetic backgrounds) (Seong et al., 2004; Simpson et al., 1997). The introduction of engineered ES cells into the multicelled embryos results in the production of chimeric F_0 animals in which the engineered gene is expressed in only a portion of the embryonic tissues. Crossing of F_0 in which the mutated gene is present within the germ cell precursors will produce one or more lines of offspring (F_1) possessing the modified gene in all cells on a permanent and heritable basis.

Typical constructs used to target genes by homologous recombination (Figure 23.2) are more complex than those designed to deliver transgenes that will be randomly inserted (Figure 23.1). The most important components in gene-targeting constructs are (i) the mutated gene of interest, (ii) DNA sequences for genes encoding selection markers, and (iii) identification and accurate construction of the 5′ and 3′ end regions of homology that will allow the correct insertion and replacement of the mutated gene in place of the endogenous gene. After introduction of the assembled construct into ES cells, homologous sequences between the specific endogenous gene of interest and its engineered counterpart carried by the construct can bind to each other as the nuclear DNA (nDNA) is being replicated. A small fraction of the time, binding of the construct to the gene of interest will result in reciprocal recombination so that the engineered mutation is exchanged into the host genome at its proper site and the endogenous gene is transferred into the plasmid. Subsequent treatment of ES cell cultures with the xenobiotic selection agents will spare only those ES cells in which homologous recombination introduced the appropriate pattern of xenobiotic response and resistance genes (Figure 23.2).

Since ES cells with gene-targeting constructs are deployed in multicelled embryos, the mutant gene always will be integrated in only a portion of embryonic cells. Confirmation of the gene integration can be performed in ES cells prior to their introduction into embryos. Ideally, most members of the founding generation (F_0) will be chimeras without needing to exploit host embryo engineering (i.e., manipulations to ablate the host blastomeres in the developing embryos). However, only some will carry the engineered gene in the germ cell precursors because the altered ES cells may or may not form germ cells in a given animal. If a founder's gametes bear the mutant gene, cross-mating with wild-type animals will produce a heterozygous (F_1) generation in which animals derived from gametes arising from the engineered ES cells will bear one copy of the mutant gene and one copy of the wild-type gene. Breeding F_1 animals will yield an F_2 generation in which approximately 25% of the progeny will be anticipated to carry two mutant genes at the targeted site (i.e., homozygous knockouts or knockins), 50% will be heterozygotes with one mutant copy and one wild-type copy, and 25% will have two wild-type genes. However, this predicted 1:2:1 Mendelian ratio may be absent when the F_2 progeny are genotyped (typically at weaning, or shortly thereafter) if the double dose of mutant gene results in death during gestation (i.e., "embryonic lethality"), at or soon after birth (i.e., "perinatal lethality"), or at any juvenile stage prior to weaning. In general, some age-matched wild-type and heterozygous littermates of both sexes should be retained as control animals for subsequent studies of knockout phenotypes (Bourdi et al., 2011).

Induced pluripotent stem (iPS) cells (or iPSCs) represent an alternative source of stem cell-like elements into which modified genetic material may be inserted (Okita et al., 2008; Paquet et al., 2016; Takahashi and Yamanaka, 2006). In this approach, differentiated cells (commonly fibroblasts in mice and rats) can be reprogrammed to enter a more embryonic-like (pluripotent) functional state when cultured by using a cocktail of embryonically expressed factors. The morphology and growth characteristics of iPS cells resemble those of totipotent ES cells. Importantly, like ES cells, following injection into blastocysts iPS cells can contribute to embryonic development for multiple cell lineages and also support the generation of genetically modified founder animals.

Nuclease-based genome editing is an enzyme-mediated method of generating nuclear gene modifications that can be adapted to many different species including plants, invertebrates, and vertebrates (both small laboratory animal species and livestock) that lack readily available, validated ES cell sources (Gupta and Musunuru, 2014; Joung and Sander, 2013). Genome editing may be undertaken to explore basic biological mechanisms or to produce therapeutic alterations to mutant genes (see *Gene Therapy/Gene Editing*, Vol 2, Chap 8). Four options have been identified and evaluated: homing endonucleases ("meganucleases"), transcription activator-like effector nucleases (TALENs), zinc finger nucleases (ZFNs), and the clustered regularly interspaced short palindromic repeats (CRISPR)/CRISPR-associated nuclease (Cas) system. Large recognition sites make meganucleases perfect for genome engineering; however, the number of naturally occurring meganucleases is finite, limiting their overall utility (Khan, 2019; Silva et al., 2011). Accordingly, they will not be discussed further here. TALENs are nonspecific DNA-cleaving nucleases composed of a FokI nuclease domain (that generates a double strand break with cohesive, staggered ends) fused to a custom-made DNA-binding domain that is composed of highly conserved repeats derived from transcription activator-like effectors (TALEs) present naturally in *Xanthomonas* proteobacteria. Most of the engineered TALE repeat arrays use four domains with hypervariable regions (designated HD, NG, NI, NN) that specifically recognize C, T, A, and G bases, respectively. A single TALEN pair is commonly used to generate nonhomologous end joining (NHEJ)–induced knockout mutations, and the use of two TALEN pairs can generate deletions and/or inversions of large chromosomal segments. The TALENs can target any DNA sequence and have been employed to alter genes in many eukaryotic cells, including yeast, plants, invertebrate, and vertebrate animals as well as human somatic and pluripotent stem cells. In contrast, ZFNs are artificial restriction enzymes formed by fusion of the FokI nuclease domain to a zinc finger DNA-binding domain. In most projects, ZFNs are transfected as either DNA plasmids or mRNA into zygotes by microinjection. Upon ZFN cleavage of their target site, endogenous cell processes are harnessed to produce targeted mutations (e.g., point mutations, deletions, insertions, inversions, duplications, and translocations) that result in gene knockouts.

The CRISPR/Cas system is a ribonucleoprotein complex developed by reverse engineering of elements involved in the prokaryotic adaptive immune response (Barrangou and Doudna, 2016; Gupta et al., 2019; Gupta and Musunuru, 2014; Khan, 2019; Meek et al., 2017; Ormond et al., 2017; Zhang et al., 2015). The CRISPR sequences are a family of DNA direct repeats that are present naturally in many prokaryotic (archaeal and bacterial) genomes. The CRISPR repeats represent residual viral sequences that serve as the "memory" sequences for prior episodes of bacteriophage invasion. Subsequent bacteriophage infections lead to transcription of the CRISPR repeats into RNA transcripts, and the small RNAs then interact with a Cas endonuclease to form a complex that binds to and degrades viral gene sequences. When employed to modify the genome in eukaryotic cells, the CRISPR/Cas system requires both an engineered guide RNA (gRNA) to target the desired gene sequence and a Cas (or equivalent) endonuclease to produce targeted DNA cleavage, thereby producing a site wherein modified genetic material may be introduced (Figure 23.3).

The CRISPR/Cas system has become the genome editing method of choice in the last half-decade because it has several key advantages over both the other nuclease-based genome editing approaches (specifically TALENs and ZFNs) and conventional gene targeting by homologous recombination. The first and foremost improvement is target design simplicity. Both TALENs and ZFNs require complex protein engineering steps to produce molecules that recognize the target DNA, which is both costly and relatively slow. In contrast, the gRNAs utilized in CRISPR/Cas editing are based on simple complementary RNA–DNA interactions, and synthesis of gRNA oligonucleotides (oligomers) is inexpensive and fast. Second, using the CRISPR/Cas system is undertaken easily by introducing (by microinjection or viral transfection) genetic material encoding the gRNA and Cas protein into embryos. This direct approach bypasses the processes of transfecting and selecting mouse ES cells that are needed for the homologous recombination gene targeting technique described above, thereby greatly expediting the speed of animal model generation (typically taking 6–12 months for homologous recombination but reduced to 2–4 weeks for CRISPR/Cas). Third, CRISPR/Cas readily supports the introduction of multiplexed (multiple gene) mutations simply by injecting several gRNAs simultaneously to target several genes at once.

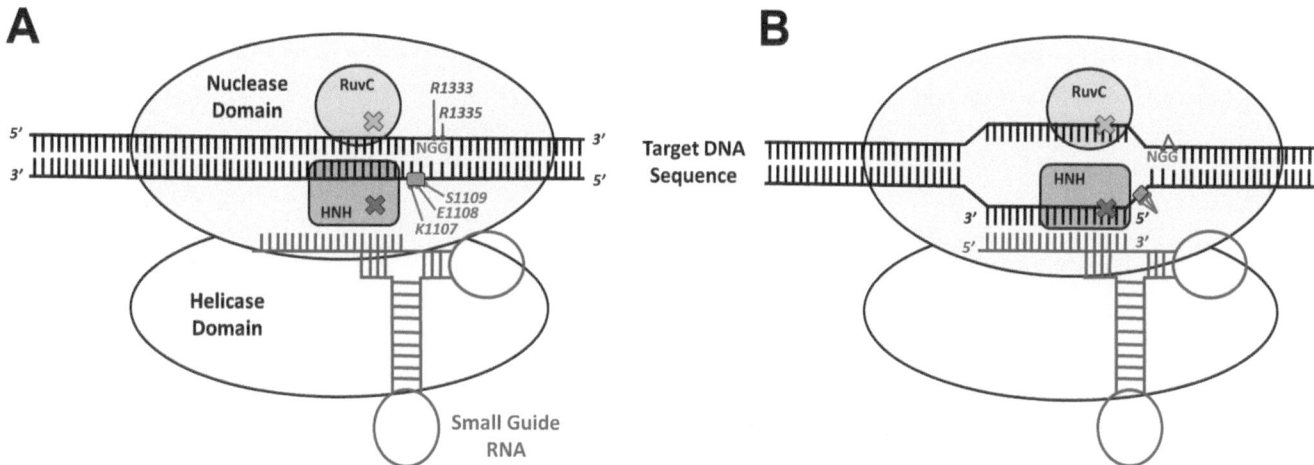

FIGURE 23.3 **Nuclease-based genomic editing with CRISPR/Cas system.** (A) The basic CRISPR/Cas9 complex consists of two elements—a Cas9 protein with distinct nuclease (yellow oval) and helicase (green oval) lobes and a small guide RNA (sgRNA, blue ladder)—associated with a length of double-stranded DNA (dsDNA, black ladder). Two arginine residues of Cas9 (R1333 and R1335) recognize the paired guanine (G) bases in the canonical "NGG" protospacer-adjacent motif (PAM, red letters) located upstream (5-prime) to the 20-bp DNA target sequence, and a "phosphate lock" (pink rectangle) forms between Cas9 lysine and serine residues and phosphate residues on the DNA lead. (B) The DNA helix melts, sgRNA binds to the complementary DNA strand, and Cas9 undergoes a conformational change that permits the HNH nuclease domain to cut the complementary DNA strand (red "X") and the RuvC nuclease domain to cut the noncomplementary strand (green "X").

Fourth, CRISPR/Cas can be used in any species with essentially no technical modifications except for defining a new gRNA sequence as microbes, plants, and animals all use DNA as their basis for transmitting genetic information. Finally, the CRISPR/Cas system provides comparable on-target gene editing efficiency and a reasonable degree of off-target gene modification compared to other currently available methods of genome modification.

"Conditional" gene modification can allow for spatial and/or temporal control of gene expression, and is most often accomplished via a combination of both gene targeting (i.e., site-specific homologous recombination) and DNA microinjection (i.e., random insertion) techniques. One example is site-specific recombinase technology, such as the use of the bacteriophage-derived Cre (cyclic recombinase) enzyme in conjunction with the small loxP sequences on DNA that serve as recognition sites for the Cre enzyme (Figure 23.4) (Belteki et al., 2005; Furuta and Behringer, 2005). When the targeted gene of interest is flanked by two separate loxP sites (i.e., "floxed") on each end of the gene, coexpression of Cre in the same cell will alter the target gene between the loxP sites. Depending on the

orientation of the loxP recognition sites with respect to one another, the action of Cre will excise, exchange, integrate, or invert the intervening targeted gene sequence; the gene alteration produced by Cre is effectively irreversible. Conditional mutagenesis in this setting requires two separate parent lines, one bearing the floxed gene of interest and the other harboring a transgene encoding Cre. The outcome of breeding these parental lines depends in large part on the promoter driving Cre expression, as the nature of the promoters defines when and where Cre will be produced.

To achieve spatially defined conditional gene modification, constitutive expression of a tissue-specific promoter is used to direct Cre expression to a particular cell population or tissue of interest. The activity of Cre will alter the targeted gene of interest only in the elements in which the promoter is active, leaving the targeted gene intact in the other tissues where Cre is not expressed. The function of a widely expressed gene in different tissues may be investigated by breeding a parental line with a floxed target gene with various established Cre lines in which Cre expression in each line is controlled by a different tissue-specific promoter.

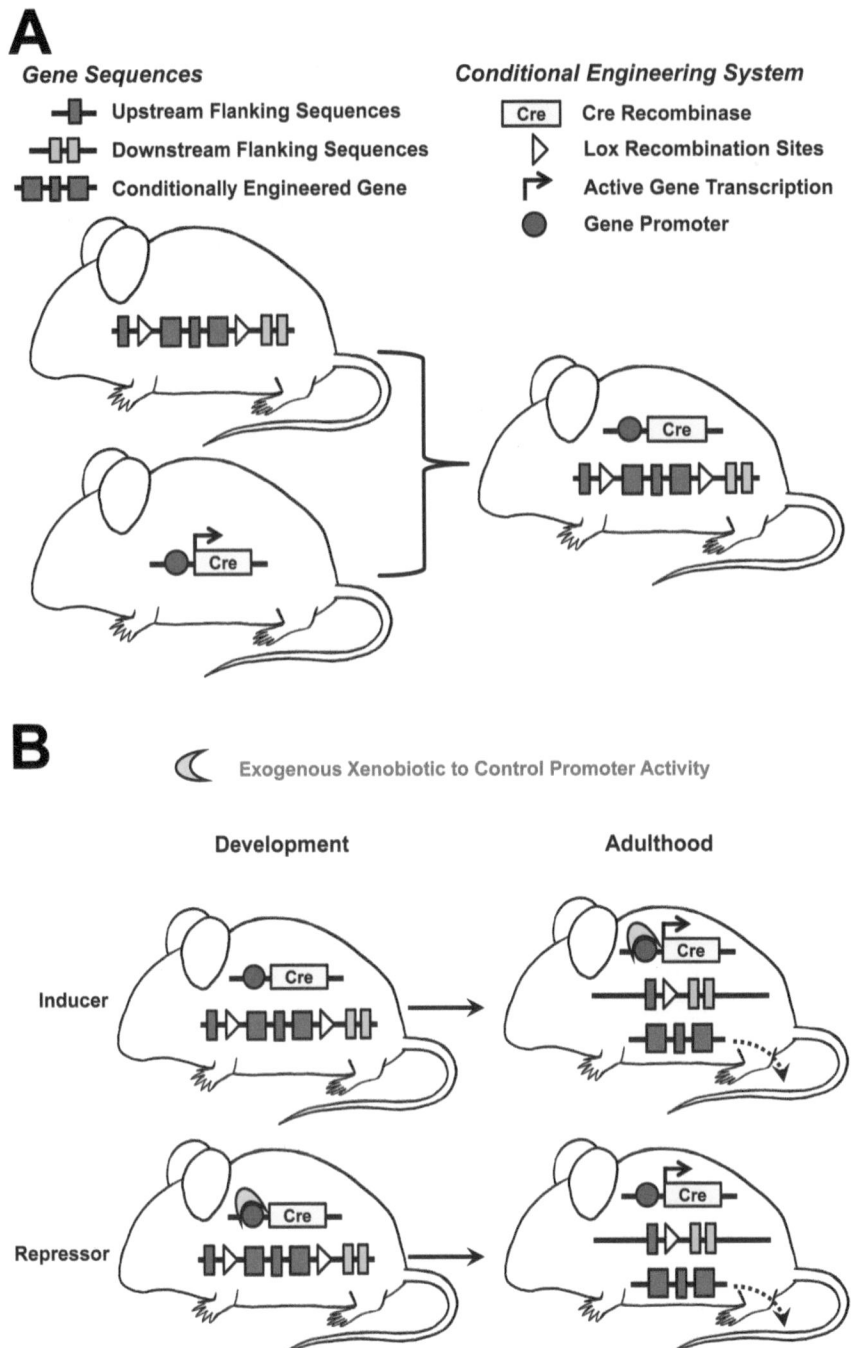

FIGURE 23.4 **Generation of conditionally gene-targeted (knockout or knockin) animals.** (A) Conditional expression requires two engineered animal lines: (i) a gene-targeted line (top left profile) bearing a functional form of the mutant gene (red boxes) sandwiched between two microbe-derived selection sites (white triangles, here as *loxP* recombination loci) and (ii) a transgenic line (bottom left profile) with a promoter (purple circles) to drive expression of the gene for a recombinase enzyme (yellow box, here representing Cre recombinase). Animals of these two parent lines are normal, but crossing them (right profile) places both the *loxP*-flanked ("floxed") mutant gene and Cre inside all cells. The action of Cre on the floxed gene will remove the DNA sequence between the selection sites. (B) Conditional mutagenesis is made possible by selecting a xenobiotic-responsive promoter (purple circle), the activity of which is subject to control by an exogenous xenobiotic (pale blue crescents), to produce expression of the recombinase (yellow box, again representing Cre). Depending on the cassettes added to the gene targeting line, the promoter is activated to either induce *Cre* transcription when the animal is exposed to the xenobiotic later in life (top profiles) or repress Cre transcription until the xenobiotic is withdrawn after development has been completed (bottom profiles). In either setting, Cre expression again will remove the engineered gene (red boxes) between the selection sites (white triangles). *Figure modified from Haschek WM, Rousseaux CG, Wallig MA, editors:* Haschek and Rousseaux's handbook of toxicologic pathology, *ed 3, 2013, Academic Press, Figure 12.3, p 417, with permission.*

Some genetic mutations can have deleterious effects when they occur in development (e.g., embryonic lethality) or over the lifetime of an animal (e.g., early-onset degenerative or neoplastic diseases). These effects can be abrogated by temporally defined conditional gene modification. For this purpose, the parental line bearing the recombinase is constructed so that an inducible xenobiotic response element capable of either enhancing or repressing recombinase expression is linked to the promoter (Figure 23.4). This design provides control over gene expression by allowing exposure to the xenobiotic to direct the onset or inhibition of expression for the targeted mutation. Tamoxifen (given in oil by parenteral injection) or tetracycline (added to the water) frequently is used for this purpose in product discovery studies (Belteki et al., 2005; Ellisor and Zervas, 2010; Schwenk et al., 1998). Literature reports suggest that the response of engineered targeted genes does not depend on the dose of xenobiotic.

Spatial and temporal control of gene expression can be conducted simultaneously for a gene of interest by combining inducible elements on promoters directing expression only in specific cell types, tissues, or organs at particular developmental time points. In the parental line carrying the recombinase, the gene for this enzyme is engineered so that its expression is controlled by both time- and tissue-specific promoters (Figure 23.5).

Although conditional targeting of gene expression using current methods is powerful for answering many questions, studies must be strategically designed for accurate interpretation (Sellers, 2012). Appropriate design of safety assessment studies with GEM must include multiple control groups; animals with and without promoters that have both received and not received the xenobiotic are necessary to differentiate whether or not the phenotype represents an effect of the engineered gene or a consequence of xenobiotic exposure. In

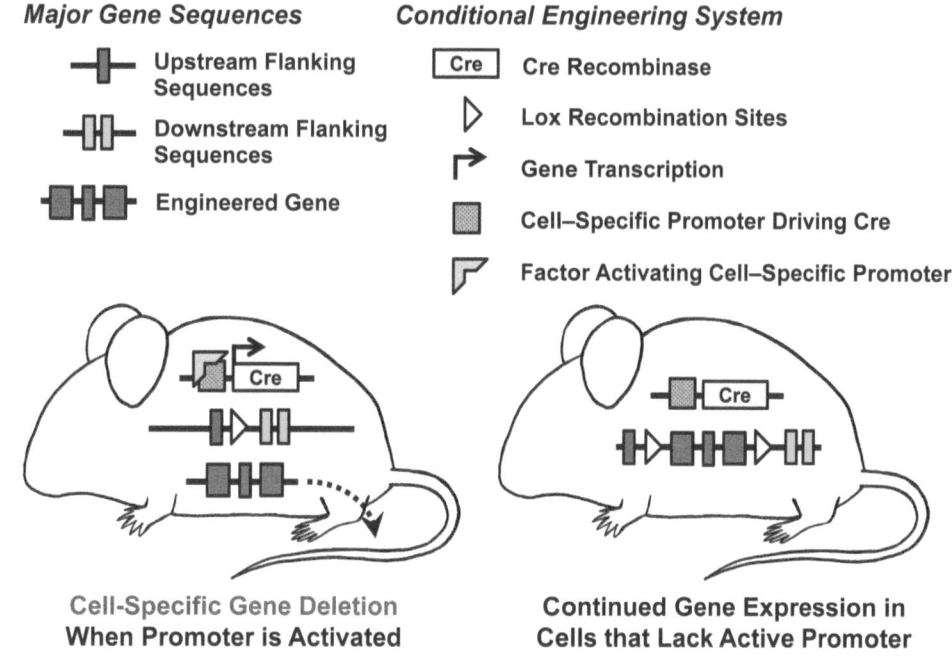

FIGURE 23.5 **Generation of tissue-specific gene-targeted (knockout or knockin) animals.** Gene expression can be deleted from a single cell type or tissue by linking the gene for the recombinase enzyme (here, Cre recombinase [yellow boxes]) to a cell-specific promoter (square brown boxes). When this Cre-bearing parent line is crossed with one carrying an engineered target gene (red boxes) that is flanked by two microbe-derived selection sites (white triangles, here as *loxP* recombination loci; see **Figure 23**.4 above for details), expression of the Cre enzyme will only delete the engineered gene in those tissues where endogenous cell-specific factors (pink angles) can bind and activate the cell-specific promoter (left profile). Cell types lacking such endogenous factors will not activate the promoter, which will prevent Cre production and gene deletion (right profile). *Figure modified from Haschek WM, Rousseaux CG, Wallig MA, editors:* Haschek and Rousseaux's handbook of toxicologic pathology, *ed 3, 2013, Academic Press, Figure 12.4, p 418 with permission.*

addition to the potential for compound-related effects of xenobiotics on the animal system, consideration should also be given to the possible presence of endogenous recombinases and the potential effects on adjacent cells of expressing exogenous gene elements (e.g., reporter genes) within the engineered gene.

Nuclear transfer (i.e., cloning) is an option employed in generating transgenic livestock. The use of this methodology in mammals captured the imagination of scientists and the general public, and received widespread press, including the successful cloning of a sheep in the mid-1990s. Importantly, nuclear transfer during that decade was particularly important for gene targeting experiments in mammalian species other than mice because pluripotent, germline-competent ES cells had not been identified and validated in nonmurine species. Thus, nuclear transfer was essential for knockout experimentation in several biologically relevant species, in particular livestock (Wilmut et al., 2015).

In this procedure (Figure 23.6), the intact nucleus of a somatic cell from a transgenic donor animal is introduced into the cytoplasm of an enucleated zygote. The most common technique involves culturing the cells from the transgenic donor animal and then either physically inserting the nucleus into the zygote by microinjection or fusing a nucleated cell from the transgenic donor with the recipient embryo. The donor cells may be either stem cells or differentiated adult cells. The reconstructed oocytes then are transferred into a pseudopregnant surrogate dam, and the resulting progeny tested for the presence of the transgene.

Insertional mutagenesis has developed into a powerful set of technologies for gene identification, even though it started out as a confounding artifact encountered in characterizing transgenic founders generated by microinjection. Techniques commonly employed today seek to alter endogenous gene activity by inserting new genetic material (DNA or DNA-targeting constructs) to directly modify endogenous

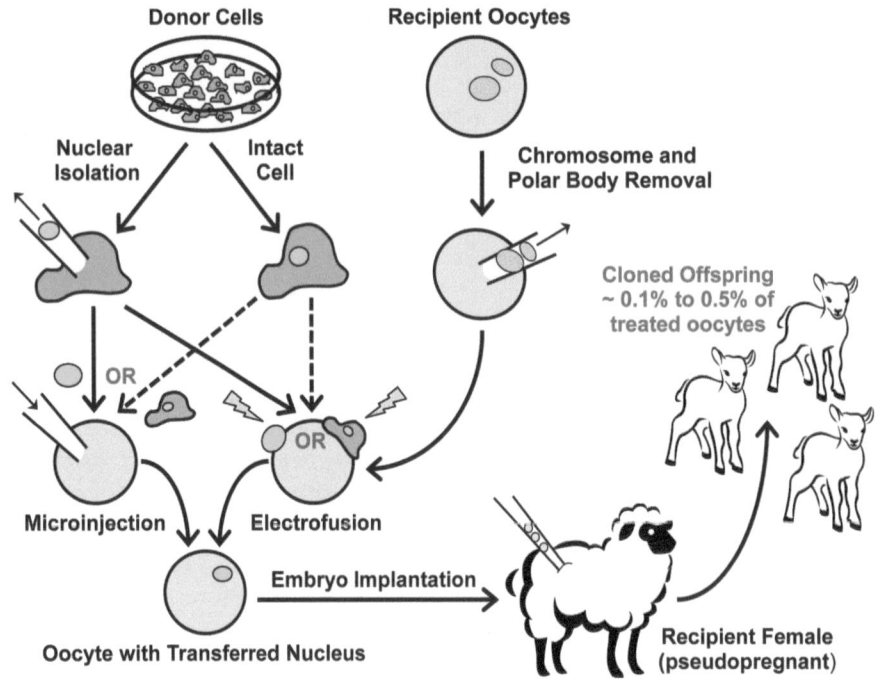

FIGURE 23.6 **Generation of cloned animals by somatic cell nuclear transfer.** For cloning, nuclei from donor cells are introduced into fertilized recipient oocytes from which the genomes (chromosomes and polar bodies) have been removed. Either isolated nuclei or intact cells can be inserted into the oocytes using either microinjection (chiefly used for nuclei) or electrofusion. The oocyte with transferred nucleus will be implanted into a pseudopregnant female, and the resulting progeny will be clones of the animal from which the donor cells were harvested. *Figure modified from Haschek WM, Rousseaux CG, Wallig MA, editors:* Haschek and Rousseaux's handbook of toxicologic pathology, *ed 3, 2013, Academic Press, Figure 12.5, p 419, with permission.*

gene sequences, thereby leading to disruption of their expression or control mechanisms. The inserted genetic material may be engineered to include regulatory sequences (e.g., promoter and enhancer traps) and reporter genes (e.g., promoter-less fluorescent protein genes) that produce phenotypic features tied to expression of the inserted construct. For example, gene trapping is a variant of insertional mutagenesis designed to disrupt gene function by randomly introducing a reporter gene construct into enhancer, promoter, or gene sequences (Evans, 1997). A "productive integration" event brings the reporter gene under the transcriptional regulation of the machinery that drives expression of an endogenous gene.

Chemical mutagenesis is a common approach to large-scale genomic investigations in mice. While other techniques for generating knockout animals often induce inactivating null mutations (i.e., total loss of an affected gene's function), mutagenesis with *N*-ethyl-*N*-nitrosourea (ENU) or similar agents is more likely to generate hypomorphic mutations (i.e., partial loss of function) (Justice et al., 1999). This difference is important as the genetic mutations found in human disease are often related to hypomorphic rather than full gene deletions. Although most mutations induced by ENU are recessive loss-of-function mutations, approximately 25% of ENU-induced events result from haploinsufficiency (i.e., presence of a single functional gene that cannot produce enough of the gene product to sustain full function) or dominant gain-of-function or dominant-negative mutations.

Transposons (transposable elements) are mobile DNA sequences that not only can integrate into the host genome but also can transfer ("jump") genetic material between the genomes of different hosts. Gene transposition can occur as a "copy and paste" event (for retrotransposons) or a "cut and paste" event (for DNA transposons); retroviruses are a variant of retrotransposon. At present, this technology seems destined to serve as a tool for phenotype-driven research ("reverse genetics") rather than a means of exploring genotype-driven processes ("forward genetics"). In comparison with ENU mutagenesis, some transposon systems have the distinct advantage that the site of mutagenesis can be rapidly identified.

Sperm-mediated DNA transfer has been demonstrated in several species as an alternative to standard transgenesis methods that modify the oocyte or zygote (Lavitrano et al., 2013). This approach uses the intrinsic ability of sperm cells to bind and internalize exogenous DNA molecules and then afterward enter the oocyte at fertilization by means of artificial insemination. Sperm-mediated DNA transfer has the advantages that neither embryo handling nor expensive equipment is required. This method has been used successfully to produce pigs bearing multiple transgenes. However, the methodology appears to work with a limited number of males and requires very large amounts of DNA vectors. Ongoing studies have attempted to identify the underlying mechanisms needed to make this technology successful on a routine basis. Interestingly, since this work was first reported, further development of spermatogonial stem cell–based technology has proven effective at generating founder transgenics and rescuing lineages through the male germline.

Any of the methods reviewed above may be used to manipulate a single nuclear gene per line or to produce a line that simultaneously expresses several modified nuclear genes. Until recently, the most common way of producing models with multiple modified genes has been to generate rodent lines having single-gene alterations and then undertake appropriate backcrossing. However, CRISPR/Cas genome editing has been demonstrated to reliably generate by a single engineering event genetically modified animals that bear multiple inserted genes; the reproducibility, rapidly, and relatively low cost of this technology for producing multi-transgenic animals now are facilitating a revolution in the speed with which new animal models of disease are being developed, especially in nonrodent species (e.g., dogs, pigs, nonhuman primates). Analysis of animal models with several engineered genes—especially "humanized" GEM and GER lines (i.e., those expressing human homologs of mouse genes or bearing human cells)—is an important translational science strategy for assessing complex metabolic interactions and mechanisms of polygenic diseases (see below).

Mitochondrial transgenesis may be employed to alter the extranuclear genome, which is harbored in the mitochondrial DNA (mtDNA). The techniques for genetic engineering of mtDNA are fairly primitive in comparison to the well-defined procedures used for traditional genetic engineering of nDNA (Dunn et al., 2012; McKenzie et al., 2004; Trounce et al., 2004; Trounce and Pinkert, 2007). Mitochondrial disorders encompass diverse disease states, affecting processes from control of cellular energy and lipid metabolism to the regulation of cell death. Although some mitochondrial disorders arise from mutations in nDNA, many instances of mitochondrial dysfunctions arise instead from abnormalities of mtDNA. The composition of mtDNA is highly conserved across vertebrate species, being 16.5 kb in length with a unique genetic code, genome structure, transcriptional and translational apparatus, and tRNAs. Relative to nDNA, mtDNA is markedly more susceptible to environmental perturbations (e.g., mutagens) and metabolic conditions (e.g., factors inducing oxidative stress), perhaps because of an absence of protective histones and/or a limited capacity for repairing mtDNA. Therefore, effects on mtDNA and mitochondrial function are of utmost importance not only for understanding the pathophysiology of heritable mitochondrial diseases but also in terms of assessing pharmaceutical activity and safety.

Early mammalian embryos may carry from tens of thousands to hundreds of thousands of copies of the mitochondrial genome. Therefore, to produce phenotypic changes, a threshold level of heteroplasmy (more than one mitochondrial haplotype) must be achieved. Both mitochondrial microinjection and ES cell transfer have been employed to modify the mitochondrial genome. Experience has shown that ES cell transfer technologies, starting with ρ° (rho zero) stem cells (i.e., cells that have been depleted of their own mtDNA by incubation in ethidium bromide, an inhibitor of mtDNA replication), are the most effective means for generating founder chimeras with high levels of mitochondrial heteroplasmy or in producing homoplasmy of the engineered mitochondrial gene (i.e., 100% of the mtDNA is derived from the ES cells) in second-generation mice. Mice engineered so that cells possess a baseline level of mitochondrial stress in the absence of other phenotypic effects have been used to model the impact of toxicant exposure on otherwise clinically silent mitochondrial disease (Boelsterli and Hsiao, 2008).

1.2. Nomenclature Conventions

A solid understanding of nomenclature conventions for gene mutations is an essential skill for scientists who work with genetically engineered animals. The nomenclature conventions have been standardized for mouse and rat strains, substrains, stocks, crosses, and genetic traits, and will be adapted in time for engineered animals of other species.

The rodent nomenclature standards are designed to succinctly and specifically identify the exact nature and origin of the model, including those that have been genetically modified. When comparing data from different publications describing mice with genetic manipulations of the same gene or genes, it is essential to understand whether or not the investigators are using the same model—including details regarding the altered gene and the genetic background—or different models. The reason for this requirement is that even seemingly subtle variations in the modified gene and/or genetic background may induce significant divergence in the ultimate phenotypes. Information on background strains, the exact genes that have been manipulated and the modifications that have been made, the method(s) of genetic manipulation, the source of the animal, and the amount of genetic uniformity based on the degree of backcrossing or inbreeding are summarized concisely when official nomenclature is used. Differences in any of these parameters may explain in part variations in experimental results among laboratories, although differences in environment, handling, and technical procedures cannot be excluded as other contributing factors.

Toxicologic pathologists and toxicologists who are not intimately involved with genetically modified rodent models often are not aware of the importance of nomenclature or how to decipher it. Glossaries and web-based resources now make this information readily available with a few computer keystrokes or clicks of a mouse. A guide to nomenclature conventions for mice is available from The Jackson Laboratory (http://www.informatics.jax.org/mgihome/nomen/). A brief glossary of essential terms in the field is presented at the end of this chapter.

1.3. Model Selection

GEM, GER, and increasingly nonrodent models are important in product discovery and development for many reasons. Key functions include to facilitate target validation, to study predicted and unexpected efficacy and toxicity, to examine biological processes leading to resistance, to evaluate pharmacokinetic/pharmacodynamic (PK/PD) characteristics, and to discover biomarkers that will predict the onset and peak of disease, monitor its progression, and/or detect subclinical disease (Boelsterli, 2003; Bolon, 2004; Bussiere, 2008; Dixit and Boelsterli, 2007; Dixit et al., 2010; Morgan et al., 2017; Morgan et al., 2013; Sharpless and Depinho, 2006; Törnell and Snaith, 2002; Wendler and Wehling, 2010). In practice, many studies conducted with GEM and GER models of disease are designed to simultaneously address multiple endpoints, especially evaluation of both product efficacy and potential toxicity.

In general, genetically engineered animal models are best used to test specific hypotheses that illuminate the relevance and/or pathogenesis of toxicities that have been observed previously in conventional ("wild type") animals or humans. The most serviceable GEMs/GERs have routine husbandry needs, which simplify colony management and handling during experimental manipulations; have been engineered to faithfully recapitulate multiple aspects (though usually not all) of a human disease; exhibit moderate or greater penetrance (i.e., a large proportion of animals bearing a mutant gene develop the expected phenotype); and show evidence of the disease following a short latent period. Model and species selection are critically important for the success of studies in terms of both efficacy and/or toxicity evaluations as well as resource management (e.g., minimizing the cost, labor, and time required to complete a study). Key biological factors in model and test species selection for biomedical product development include target specificity, potency, off-target potential, cross-species similarities in PK/PD attributes, and organ-specific anatomy and physiology. In general, if a disease model is available in multiple animal species, the best choice for routine efficacy and toxicity studies is the one lowest on the phylogenetic scale

(e.g., GEM or GER). However, for some products, the most suitable model for predicting safety liabilities may be a nonrodent, whether spontaneous or genetically engineered, due to the greater similarity in anatomy and physiology between the target organs/systems in test animals and humans (for example, nonhuman primate vs. human brains).

Therapeutic class is another key consideration during model/species selection. Small molecules generally interact with multiple cells or molecular pathways in many species, may be metabolized to toxic intermediates (although sometimes differently across species), and are not usually immunogenic. In contrast, biologics (nucleic acid- or protein-based products) generally are highly targeted to specific cellular receptors with high species specificity, are degraded to nontoxic peptides or amino acids, and can be highly immunogenic. Thus, two main issues in attempting to study biotherapeutics in GEMs/GERs are that the test article (a human-derived molecule or cell) either (1) may not bind with and/or activate rodent molecular pathways, and thus will not be pharmacologically active, or (2) may be so immunogenic in rodents that longer-term studies are not feasible due to the formation of neutralizing antibodies (see *Protein Pharmaceutical Agents*, Vol 2, Chap 6). Surrogate molecules, such as a homologous rodent protein, may be used in GEMs/GERs to estimate potential efficacy of the human test article. However, in many cases, regulators tasked with evaluating human risk will prefer evaluating the real test article using in vitro assays in human cells (see *In Silico, In Vitro, Ex Vivo, and Non-Traditional In Vivo Approaches in Toxicologic Research*, Vol 1, Chap 24) coupled with in vivo testing in nonrodents.

Animal characteristics are important during species selection (see *Issues in Laboratory Animal Science that Impact Toxicologic Pathology*, Vol 1, Chap 29). Smaller animals require less test material per subject, though significantly more animals overall may be needed on study to meet blood volume requirements for PK and clinical pathology evaluations. Compared to rodent models, large animal models of disease often are less desirable because of their relatively long gestation periods, smaller litter sizes, older age of puberty, and higher husbandry costs.

To generate GEM and GER models, several mouse and rat inbred strains are preferentially used. For mice, the most common strains are 129, C57BL/6, FVB, and BALB/c. Each strain has advantages and disadvantages. For example, 129 mice are preferentially used for gene targeting because their ES cells are relatively easy to harvest. However, 129 mice exhibit great variation among various substrains due to deliberate and accidental outcrossing (Simpson et al., 1997; Threadgill et al., 1997), have poor breeding efficiency, are susceptible to autoimmune diseases, and have a moderate overall tumor incidence (7%–21%) with a high incidence of spontaneous lung tumors (up to 46%) and testicular teratomas (up to 30%) depending on the 129 substrain. Similarly, C57BL/6 mice are desirable for gene targeting studies since their ES cells are relatively easy to manipulate, and this genetic background is considered to be a standard, disease-resistant inbred strain for basic biomedical research. Furthermore, C57BL/6 mice have good breeding efficiency, low antibody affinity, and low overall tumor incidence (1%–7%) with a low incidence of spontaneous leukemia (7%). For transgenic experiments (especially for retinal degeneration studies), FVB mice are preferred due to their large zygote pronuclei (which makes microinjection of engineered DNA simple), fully inbred background, and vigorous breeding efficiency with large litters. However, FVB mice are aggressive to cage mates, susceptible to noise-induced seizures leading to brain necrosis, have high incidences of tumors (50%–60%, especially of the mammary gland), and are highly sensitive to the B strain of Friend murine leukemia virus. The BALB/c strain is used for genetic engineering on occasion based on their routine use for other purposes such as generating monoclonal antibodies and studying infectious diseases. BALB/c mice are resistant to experimental allergic encephalomyelitis and have good breeding efficiency, but they also exhibit a high overall tumor incidence (43%) with moderate lung tumor incidence (21%). In rats, ES cells have been derived from Sprague–Dawley, Fisher 344, and other strains. In contrast to mouse ES cell development, the literature suggests that in rats the strain genetic background is not a major barrier to establishing ES cell lines; furthermore, in rats there is no evidence showing strain incompatibility between host embryo and rat ES cells for chimera generation. The advent of CRISPR/Cas technology has greatly expanded the production of GER models (Meek et al., 2017), and also genetically engineered nonrodent models (Chen et al., 2016; Wang et al., 2016; Yan et al., 2014; Zou et al., 2015).

Study designs using genetically engineered animal models differ according to the purpose. For discovery (basic biology) studies to investigate the effects of one or multiple modified genes, all genes need to be studied alone and in combination to determine their individual and collective (e.g., additive, synergistic, or competing) significance in the onset and progression of a disease phenotype. Similarly, the different genes and gene combinations may need to be studied with and without posttranslational modification. In contrast, for development (e.g., efficacy and safety) studies, only the ideal combination of genes that specifies the desired disease phenotype needs to be studied, usually both with and without the presence of the test article. Extrapolation of data from these studies must be undertaken with caution, in full consideration of the model limitations relative to the human disease. However, the basis for most studies using genetically engineered animals is that the induced genotype and phenotype provide a biological system with an enhanced degree of similarity to the proposed pathogenesis of the human condition.

In the biomedical setting, recent reports call into question the translatability of efficacy findings obtained in animal studies given the number of drug candidates that have failed in human clinical trials. For instance, xenograft studies using human tissues implanted in immunodeficient (either spontaneous or genetically engineered) rodents have several shortcomings including defects in DNA repair in severe combined immunodeficiency (*scid*) mice (which limits testing of some cytotoxicants), a profoundly narrowed capacity for mounting an immune response (which prevents testing of immunomodulatory agents), and the overall frailty of nude (*Foxn1^{nu}*) mice (which limits their capacity to tolerate novel treatments). Other disadvantages inherent in many genetically engineered rodents include differences in their telomere biology (which alters the type and frequency of secondary cytogenetic events leading to neoplastic transformation), tumor suppressor mechanisms (e.g., p53 vs. p16), cytokine biology (e.g., the lack of an interleukin-8 homolog in mice), metabolism, and chromosome expression (e.g., the tumor suppressor genes *p53* and *Brca1* are on the same chromosome in mice, so codeletion is common). Overall, many disease models in GEMs, GERs, and genetically modified nonrodents are incompletely characterized, and studies may be undertaken in strains or breeds with very little historical information on spontaneous background findings over time. Use of these models in hazard identification and characterization as well as risk and safety assessment often is plagued by a lack of concordance with the human population of interest (e.g., single inbred rodent species/strain vs. many heterogeneous populations among humans). These factors may have a negative impact on risk assessment for new products due to the presence of poorly understood findings with unknown or no (i.e., GEM/GER-specific) relevance to humans, thus leading to increased development timelines and cost.

2. ANALYSIS OF GENETICALLY ENGINEERED ANIMAL MODELS

Utilization of genetically engineered animal models for product discovery and development requires a two-stage evaluation. The first stage is validation: verifying that the model does or does not carry the gene of interest in the appropriate location (i.e., "genotype") and also expresses the predicted functional and/or structural attributes (i.e., "phenotype") that reflect the presence of the genetic modification. The second stage involves characterization: exploring how the model responds to experimental manipulation (chemical administration, etc.). Anatomic and clinical pathology methods are routine tools for phenotyping in product development to either evaluate the changes that result when test articles are administered to an engineered animal or assess the impact of materials collected from an engineered animal (e.g., cells, secreted proteins) when they have been introduced into conventional animals. This section will briefly review the experimental endpoints relevant to genotyping and phenotyping of genetically engineered animals.

2.1. Genotyping

Genotyping, the first essential datum required to validate a new engineered model, is done to confirm the presence and magnitude of expression of an engineered gene. The genotype is commonly expressed in relation to the presence or absence of the modified gene since the remainder of the genetic background is presumed to remain essentially identical across all animals in the highly inbred rodent strains favored for genetic engineering. Appropriate expression of a modified gene or absence of a native gene may be established by assaying genomic DNA, typically by real-time polymerase chain reaction and electrophoresis or Southern blot. This assessment usually is performed before or at weaning as designated by an institutionally approved animal protocol, typically through convenient tissue sampling such as a biopsy (tail snip, ear punch, digit amputation) or skin swab (Okada et al., 2017; Pinkert, 2003). In mice generated by backcrossing two or more strains, relative contributions of the strains can be elucidated via single-nucleotide polymorphism (SNP) panels, where analysis of over 94 inbred mouse strains has demonstrated the existence of 8 million SNPs (http://mouse.cs.ucla.edu/mousehapmap/full.html) (Moran et al., 2006; Petkov et al., 2004). Microsatellite (i.e., repetitive DNA sequences) and SNP profiles have become widely available for mice and rats. As few as 29 SNPs have proven to be sufficient to monitor genotypes of over 300 mouse strains (Benavides et al., 2020). Despite successes in using genome-wide association studies (GWAS) to link specific genes to various disease traits in humans, animals models such as inbred laboratory mice have a more limited genomic diversity due to their restricted genetic origin and constant selection pressure (Su et al., 2010). In fact, the majority of genetic variations observed in classical inbred mouse strains are derived from only three *Mus musculus* subspecies: *Mus musculus domesticus*, *Mus musculus musculus*, and *Mus musculus castaneus*. A large GWAS investigation of transcript abundance in 16 classical and 3 wild-derived inbred mouse strains has demonstrated the low statistical power of such studies in this species, with allelic association of various transcripts giving rise to spurious associations approaching those arising by random chance. Moreover, the genetic markers with the most significant p-values frequently fail to map to the actual expressed locations of the quantitative trait loci (QTLs) that regulate RNA expression levels. Thus, in the laboratory mouse, it appears to be necessary to combine GWAS with chromosomal linkage analysis to provide sufficient statistical power to attain higher mapping resolution, as less accuracy is achieved with either approach alone in inbred mice relative to their success as stand-alone methods in the more genetically heterogeneous human population. As an intra-species methodology, however, GWAS has demonstrated some limited utility. For instance, when investigating genetic drivers of fibro-osseous lesions in 28 strains of inbred mice, 11 candidate genes have been identified; the resulting bone changes produced by these monogenic mutations may be compared to known pheno-types in the Mouse Genome Informatics (MGI) database (Berndt et al., 2016). The synergistic power of combining GWAS with large, multi-strain compendiums of mouse data may lie in the ability to identify candidate genes that are putatively involved in complex polygenic diseases (Sundberg et al., 2016). Synthesis of GWAS data with phenotypic data from the MGI and International Mouse Phenotyping Consortium (IMPC) databases recently enabled the identification of SNPs in 23 orthologous human genes involved in metabolic disease states and 51 new metabolism-associated genes (Rozman et al., 2018). Similarly, in a study of osteoporosis and bone mass regulation, GWAS performed in a panel of inbred mouse strains elucidated a QTL (quantitative trait locus, a portion of DNA that correlates with variation in a measurable phenotypic trait) for bone mineral density that mapped to a region including the lipoma HMGIC (high-mobility-group, isoform C) fusion partner (*Lhfp*) gene. Knockout mice created to study this gene also have increased cortical bone mass, identifying *Lhfp* as a negative regulator of bone progenitor cells and osteoblast activity (Mesner et al., 2019).

Confirming a genetic alteration by genotyping (i.e., defining a DNA change) does not necessarily guarantee its magnitude of expression. An intermediary step bridging genotyping and phenotyping is transcriptomic (mRNA)

evaluation of an engineered gene. Evaluation of mRNA levels by northern blot assay, reverse transcription–polymerase chain reaction (RT-PCR), ribonuclease protection assay, and/or in situ hybridization (ISH) is required to confirm that an engineered construct is transcriptionally active. Sample selection is guided based on the anticipated distribution of gene expression (e.g., whole body vs. tissue-specific). Special care may be needed in analyzing RNA expression in certain tissues where the mRNA transcripts accrue in the cell body but the ultimate protein product is transported to a distant cell process.

Genotyping culminates with evaluation of the level of protein expression associated with the gene of interest, usually via Western blot analysis, enzyme histochemistry (EHC), and/or immunohistochemistry (IHC) (see *Special Techniques in Toxicologic Pathology*, Vol 1, Chap 11). An array-based approach to assess multiple tissue types in parallel often is useful. The apparent absence of protein detection may not reflect a lack of gene expression. Instead, protein expression levels might be sufficient to cause effects and yet not reach the sensitivity of the detection method. An example of this phenomenon is disruption of cell function or cell death that accompanies low-level expression of a biotoxin gene. Therefore, in some instances where transgene effects occur without detectable protein expression, it is necessary to use even more sensitive methods like proteomics to demonstrate very low levels of protein or RT-PCR or other transcriptomic methods to detect transgene-specific transcripts as a proxy for the extent of protein generation. As noted above, the distributions of mRNA and protein do not overlap in all tissues; for example, synaptic proteins at the neuromuscular junctions are specified by mRNA produced in neuronal cell bodies located in the central nervous system. Therefore, protein analysis is a preferred means of confirming appropriate gene expression if reliable reagents are available. Where feasible, assays that measure the levels of functionally active protein (e.g., EHC) may be preferable to tests that only establish the presence of the molecule (e.g., western blots, IHC). Expression of targeted genes may be evaluated by demonstrating the presence of an exogenous marker protein (e.g., bacterial β-galactosidase (βGal) [lacZ] or green fluorescent protein) inserted in the construct to confirm successful gene replacement (Bolon, 2008).

Maintenance of genetic fidelity in a breeding colony of genetically engineered animals is referred to as genetic quality control or genetic quality assurance. Genotyping is only part of genetic quality control, which also encompasses pedigree management and refreshing breeding stock. Genetic drift will generate one phenotypic mutation every 1.8 generations which, if breeding schemes are not properly managed, can become fixed in a colony after six to nine generations. When inbreeding mice, one impactful mutation is expected to emerge every 10 generations, and after 20 generations, a genetically distinct substrain is created. Poor genetic quality control can result in apparent loss or amplification of a desired phenotype over time that culminates in irreproducible data and degradation of the model. Further information about proper breeding practices in laboratory animals can be found in texts listed in the References section.

2.2. Phenotyping

Phenotyping is the characterization of any or all anatomic and physiological aspects of an animal model. While this often is considered in the limited sense of characterizing the effect of a specific genetic modification, a much broader approach is required to fully understand any animal model. The nature and method of genetic manipulation, the background strain (stock) and substrain, the source of the animals, husbandry practices (see *Issues in Laboratory Animal Science that Impact Toxicologic Pathology*, Vol 1, Chap 29), and microbial flora all can alter characteristics of the final animal model and should be considered when designing specific experiments. Though in the context of genotyping a transgenic animal is presumed to be genetically identical to its parental strain except at the altered gene loci, in phenotyping a genetically engineered animal—particularly in more complex models—is presumed to be different from its originating strain(s) until proven otherwise. Methods, resources, and study design considerations for phenotyping GEM and GER models are detailed elsewhere (Bolon et al., 2017; Brayton and Treuting, 2018; Crawley,

2007; Fuchs et al., 2011; Rossant and McKerlie, 2001; Zeiss, 2002; Zeiss et al., 2012).

To be useful for biomedical research, engineered animal models typically must develop a phenotype that is well correlated to the presence of the genotype. Expression of a modified gene may produce an anatomic change, functional alteration, both of these effects, or neither. However, caution must be used in deciding whether or not the engineered construct has defined the entire phenotype for a given gene. Multiple instances have been reported wherein subtle differences in the engineered gene have produced divergent phenotypes. For example, mice lacking cytochrome P450 (CYP) 1A2—a liver enzyme in humans and mice that metabolizes many exogenous chemicals and drugs—develop fatal pulmonary deficits in many but not all pups if a single exon is deleted, while the surviving single-exon knockout animals as well as mice in which four CYP1A2 exons have been removed exhibit no phenotype without the administration of a pharmacologic challenge (Liang et al., 1996; Pineau et al., 1995). In a similar manner, transgenic GEM models of Alzheimer's disease, which overexpress various mutant isoforms of amyloid precursor proteins (APPs), have been reported to develop amyloid plaques in the brain and cognitive deficits, although the extent of the anatomic and behavioral changes varies among models. For translational research purposes, the favored GEM models of Alzheimer's disease exhibit both robust functional and substantial structural abnormalities.

2.3. Large-Scale Phenotyping

Since 2002, large-scale, multicenter phenotypic screening efforts have sought to elucidate disease mechanisms by systematically generating and characterizing single-gene mouse mutant lines. An alternate name commonly applied to this analytical approach is "high-throughput" phenotyping. Foundational programs include the International Knockout Mouse Consortium, the European Union Mouse Genetics Research for Public Health and Industrial Applications, and the European Mouse Disease Clinic. Now, with advancing GWAS and PheWAS (phenome-wide association study) resources, the Mouse Genetics Project and IMPC carry on using the model of network pleiotropy (i.e., the ability of a single gene to produce two or more apparently unrelated effects) to understand the genotypic–phenotypic relationships (Brown et al., 2018). To date, the IMPC has phenotyped 5861 genes in 6255 mutant mouse lines on the C57BL/6N background; this inbred strain was chosen as the test system due to its common use in biomedical research. The large-scale phenotyping endeavor is human resource intensive, requiring tremendous parallel research efforts in numerous fields of biology, and the need to collate data for multiple different organs and endpoints from measurements undertaken in many laboratories confounded early efforts to maintain the high-throughput nature of such studies. Multidimensional datasets demand involvement of bioinformaticians in these efforts. Prediction systems that link disease genes and phenotypic attributes in GEMs have been constructed (e.g., http://combio.snu.ac.kr/targo/). Large-scale phenotyping projects often adopt strategies similar to those described in the International Mouse Phenotyping Resource of Standardised Screens (IMPReSS) guidance document, which can be accessed through the IMPC (http://www.mousephenotype.org/).

The objective of initial large-scale phenotypic screening is to rapidly identify the existence of functional and/or structural phenotypes using a defined number of tests, after which promising founders may be subjected to a more comprehensive characterization to better define the nature and mechanisms responsible for any phenotype of interest. These large-scale screening methods emphasize routine tests such as in-life functional evaluations (e.g., open field test, grip strength, electrocardiography, radiography), followed by anatomic pathology (macroscopic and microscopic analysis) and clinical pathology (e.g., hematology and serum/plasma chemistry) evaluations. Additional methods may be incorporated based on the research indication and availability of appropriate innovative technologies. Examples of such supplemental techniques include noninvasive imaging (see *In Vivo Small Animal Imaging: A Comparison to Gross and Histopathologic Observations in Animal Models*, Vol 1, Chap 13) and various "omics" platforms (see *Toxicogenomics: A Primer for Toxicologic Pathologists*, Vol 1, Chap 15).

The goal of such large-scale phenotyping studies is to find one or more easily measured biomarkers that can be used in vivo to monitor the progression of disease and candidate therapies in both animal models and human patients. This approach also advances the ideal of precision medicine by identifying ideal biomarkers that are specific for a disease, or certain subpopulations of patients with that disease (see *Biomarkers: Discovery, Qualification and Application*, Vol 1, Chap 14). In these high-throughput screening research programs, new GEM or GER models often are phenotyped as young adults (6–16 weeks of age). An obvious pitfall is that age-related phenotypes and altered survival rates are missed in this paradigm. Initial phenotyping studies may begin with two to five animals/sex/genotype, while studies designed to probe subtle phenotypes and elucidate mechanisms of disease often require higher numbers per group (often 10 or more, especially to provide adequate power for clinical pathology assessments). For transgenic animals generated through microinjection, phenotypic analysis will include the F_1 hemizygous (+) engineered animals along with age-matched controls (ideally nontransgenic littermates since they share the identical genetic background); inappropriate selection of control animals from a different substrain may confound interpretation (Bourdi et al., 2011). For gene targeting projects, individuals selected for initial screening are homozygous knockout (−/−) animals and wild-type [+/+, or "normal"] littermates. Heterozygous (+/−) littermates or other GEM lines with differing levels of expression of the modified gene also may be included as the intermediate gene dosage(s) may yield a diluted phenotype (Tohyama et al., 2000). In conditional models, additional genetic controls include animals carrying the floxed allele without recombinase and animals expressing the recombinase only. Animal numbers should be balanced in terms not only of age but also sex. In general, animals of both sexes are evaluated to be sure that sexually dimorphic phenotypes are found. Where time permits, phenotyping of gene-targeted animals may be delayed until the engineered model has been backcrossed for 10 or more generations to obtain a homogenous genetic background as phenotypes in GEM and GER lines may be magnified or masked in founders or earlier generations of progeny. Reviews that describe the common spontaneous lesions in mouse strains typically used in generating GEM models are an essential source of historical data (Brayton et al., 2012; Haines et al., 2001; Mahler et al., 1996; Mohr et al., 1996; Szymanska et al., 2014; Ward et al., 2000).

2.4. Directed Phenotypic Characterization for Product Discovery and Development

Although tiered screening approaches as outlined above have been devised for large-scale, high-throughput investigations of many gene modifications, these may not be appropriate or sufficient when subsequently attempting to use these models to support drug discovery and development. The key factor in using transgenic models for evidence-based target selection and validation decisions in drug discovery and development is the timely delivery of relevant phenotypic information for decision-making. While pharmaceutical companies may have the internal resources to generate the animal models and perform phenotypic analysis, individual pharmaceutical companies are rarely willing to commit the significant resources required to generate, breed, and characterize large numbers of genetically engineered animals in a large-scale and focused manner as a routine undertaking.

The bioinformatics revolution driven by the Human Genome Project and similar initiatives to sequence the complete genomes of common laboratory animal species has shifted the emphasis in biomedical research away from the historical disease-to-target approach to the complementary gene-to-target paradigm. Both strategies depend on researchers having a deep knowledge of both normal and disease phenotypes and their associated molecular pathways. Similar to the "omics" technologies (see *Toxicogenomics: A Primer for Toxicologic Pathologists*, Vol 1, Chap 15), genetically engineered animals provide a means to examine gene expression and to evaluate cellular pathways. When used in parallel, engineered animals and "omics" tools work together to identify modes of drug candidate action, predict aspects of potential "on-target" or "off-target" activity, and suggest paths for further mechanistic investigation. Genetically modified animal models may add an additional dimension to the full extent of nonclinical information that will be necessary

to characterize the target and test articles directed against it. In other words, the "high tech" GEM and "omics" approaches should be considered as means to enhance, not supersede, well-established toxicological parameters used to discover and develop new products.

When genetically altered animal models will be used to assess the efficacy or toxicity of an administered test article, it is critical that the model should be demonstrated to be suitable for the intended purpose. A pragmatic approach to model characterization is required in such cases. The features of the engineered model that are important for reliable data collection and interpretation should be reviewed (if already available) or generated de novo. Well-established, commercially available GEM models generally have been characterized extensively in advance of their use, while custom-made institutional models—regardless of their origin (e.g., academic, government, industrial)—may require evaluation of their basic biological status (e.g., by conventional health assessments, anatomic pathology, and clinical pathology analyses) as well as a fairly detailed assessment of the particular pathway(s) and organ(s) of interest prior to their utilization.

Ideally, initial phenotyping should be completed before studies impacting the course and/or outcome of a product development program are initiated. Frequently, however, limited numbers of valuable animals and time constraints dictate that phenotyping is performed as part of the experiment or with samples derived from animals after the experiment is over. Most discovery researchers in industry have access to sophisticated safety pharmacology, general toxicology, clinical pathology, and anatomic pathology tools and expertise only through interactions with nonclinical safety scientists. If pathologists and toxicologists conducting hazard identification and safety assessment are engaged in discussion of genetically engineered models in the planning stages of the program, they often can assist substantially in the efforts of their discovery colleagues in developing the experimental design, characterizing (phenotyping) the animals, and interpreting their responses to experimental procedures. Pathologists with advanced training in anatomic pathology or clinical pathology, particularly those with both theoretical and applied expertise in molecular pathology techniques and strategies, can contribute significantly to the optimal utilization and interpretation of efficacy and safety assessment data obtained from genetically engineered models (see *Discovery Toxicology and Pathology*, Vol 2, Chap 3).

Phenotypic assessment of GEM or GER is especially important when critical decisions for developing a new molecular entity are likely to place heavy reliance on these models for elucidating mechanisms of toxicity or for traditional hazard identification. While genetically modified alternative mouse models for carcinogenicity assessment of small molecules usually are well characterized (see *Carcinogenicity Assessment*, Vol 2, Chap 5), the GEM and GER used for mechanistic studies often are custom-made and therefore not well characterized. Accordingly, it is imperative to accurately define the appropriate pilot studies, control groups (in terms of both genetics and treatments), and overall health and pathology assessments that will be required to fully understand results that are obtained from these new models. If engineered rodent models are used to examine target organ toxicity, histopathologic assessment of the organs of interest, and in many instances other major organs as well, usually should be included in the analysis. Special pathology techniques (e.g., ISH or IHC to define the distribution of the modified gene or its product, downstream signaling pathways, cell apoptosis or proliferation; see *Special Techniques in Toxicologic Pathology*, Vol 1, Chap 11) may be appropriate both for screening purposes and to begin exploring potential mechanisms by which engineered genes may be producing their effects.

2.5. Phenotypic Interpretation of Genetically Engineered Animal Models

A stable, fairly robust, reproducible, and useful phenotype is required for a new GEM or GER line to have utility as a model in product discovery and development. The usefulness of a novel phenotype is demonstrated by showing that the change arises from a specific molecular alteration resulting from a particular gene modification. For recently discovered molecular pathways, the relevance of the biology typically is probed by making new GEM or GER lines that

modify both arms of the pathway, the target (e.g., a receptor or enzyme that is involved in a signal transduction cascade) and its ligand. Phenotypic rescue can be implemented via inducible genetic constructs (e.g., doxycycline on/off promoter function) or selective pharmacologic interventions. For instance, GEM with deletions of either the osteoclast-activating factor *RANKL* (receptor activator of NF–κB ligand, encoded by *Tnfsf11*) or its receptor *RANK* (encoded by *Tnfsf11a*) or that overexpress *OPG* (osteoprotegerin, a soluble RANKL receptor encoded by *Tnfsf11b*) develop marked osteopetrosis (Figure 23.7). In contrast, GEM with null mutations of *OPG* exhibit severe osteoporosis due to unrestrained activation of the RANKL/ RANK pathway. These GEM models are predictive of therapeutically relevant bone regulatory mechanisms, as has been shown by the ability to restore bone mass by injecting either a viral vector bearing an OPG transgene (Figure 23.7) or recombinant solubilized RANK (either human or murine) into adult wild-type mice with ovariectomy-induced osteoporosis (Bolon et al., 2002).

Considerable attention is necessary to show that a phenotype actually results from the predicted role of the engineered gene and not from one or more of the potential confounding factors that can influence or mimic a true gene-mediated phenotype. The robustness of a phenotype is strongly impacted by inherent genetic factors such as the strain (and substrain), sex, and degree of genetic homogeneity. One example of a substrain effect on a phenotype is a spontaneous null mutation of the gene for nicotinamide nucleotide translocase (*Nnt*), a mitochondrial superoxide dismutase, in C57BL/6J mice. Mutant animals on this genetic background have a decreased ability to regenerate reduced glutathione and thioredoxin under conditions of mitochondrial oxidative stress. Phenotypic differences have been found in mice in response to drug-induced liver injury (e.g., following exposure to acetaminophen or concanavalin A) or the presence of other genetic mutations (e.g., knockouts of mitochondrial antioxidant genes like manganese superoxide dismutase or glutathione peroxidase) where some animals (C57BL/6J) were of the $Nnt^{-/-}$ substrain, while other wild-type or treated animals were on the $Nnt^{+/+}$ substrain. This example highlights the

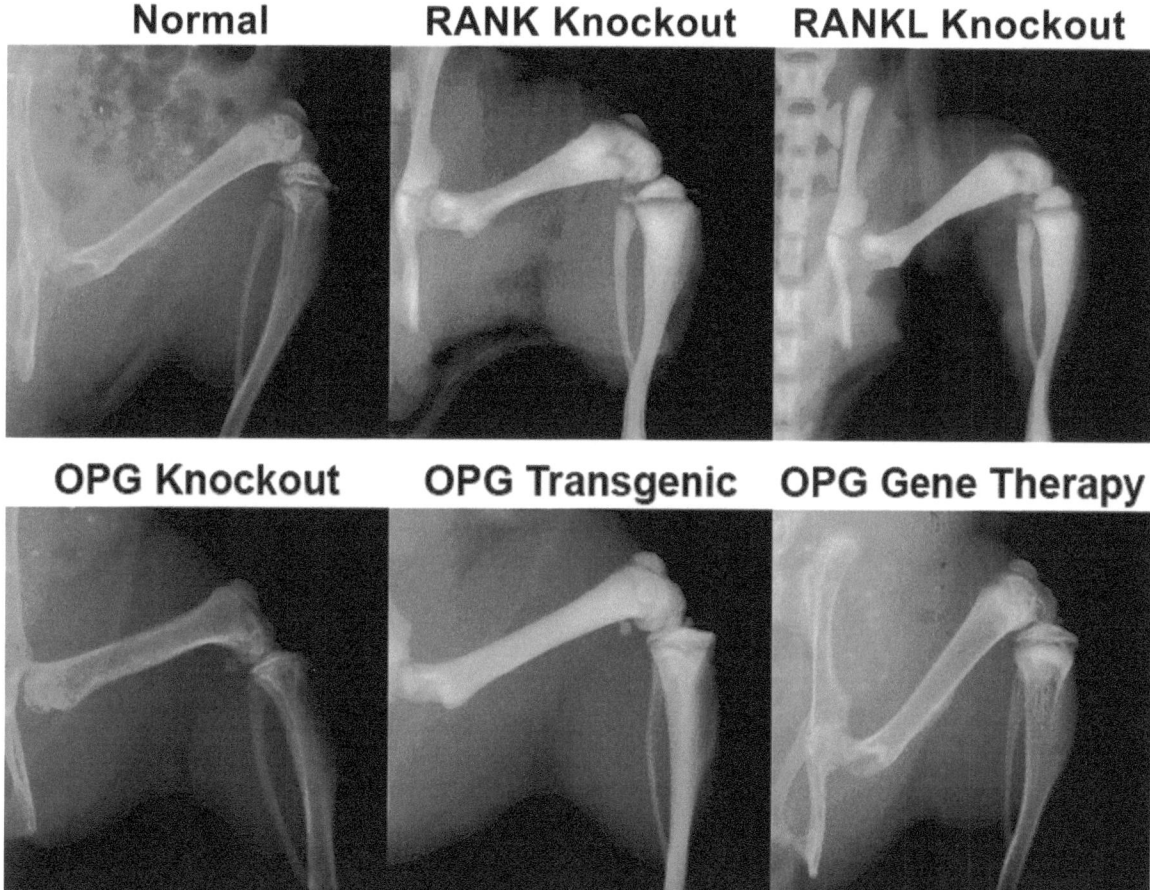

FIGURE 23.7 **Validation of novel targets uses multiple genetically engineered mouse (GEM) lines in which either a ligand or its receptor has been modified.** Similar phenotypes should result from changing multiple components of the same molecular pathway. Relative to normal mice (upper left), GEM with null mutations (knockout) of either RANK (receptor activator of nuclear factor κB [upper middle])—the main membrane-bound receptor for upregulating osteoclast activity—or its ligand RANKL (upper right) have increased bone density. In contrast, GEM harboring a deletion of OPG (osteoprotegerin [lower left]), a soluble decoy receptor for controlling RANKL levels in circulation, have reduced bone density. Lifelong transgenic overexpression of OPG (lower middle) enhances bone density by binding RANKL. Introduction of an OPG transgene into young adult, wild-type mice (lower right) increases bone density in the metaphyses. Radiographs were acquired using a bench-top system (Faxitron X-ray, Buffalo Grove, IL) set at 0.3 mA and 55 kV for 49 s. *Adapted from Bolon B, Shalhoub V, Kostenuik PJ, et al.: Osteoprotegerin (OPG): an endogenous anti-osteoclast factor for protecting bone in rheumatoid arthritis,* Arthritis Rheum 46, 3121–3135, 2002, by permission.

vital need for appropriate backcrossing and genetic analysis to ensure consistency in the substrain genetic background of both engineered animals and their genetic controls so that valid interpretations may be made for the significance of the biological response.

Other considerations also can alter the presence and extent of a phenotype. In this regard, important factors include diet, environmental conditions, microbial flora, parental care, and stress (see *Issues in Laboratory Animal Science*

that Impact Toxicologic Pathology, Vol 1, Chap 29). In instances where the engineered gene is inserted at random, the phenotype also must be shown through integration site analysis of DNA to arise from action of the introduced mutation rather than from accidental deletion or modification of an endogenous gene. Where genetic modification is undertaken in immunocompetent animals (e.g., viral gene therapy), the phenotype also must be shown to result from the action of the expressed transgene product and not from immune attack (i.e., "toxicity") against the foreign proteins (transgene and/or viral vector). For example, dose-dependent hepatic and cardiac toxicity has been documented as a consequence of injecting an AAV vector to restore function of the *survival of motor neuron 1* (*Smn1*) gene parenterally into neonatal *Smn1* null mutant mice. In another instance, long-term overexpression of OPG in mice using an adenoviral vector results in hepatitis and widespread apoptosis due to the inflammatory reaction mounted in response to hepatocyte infection with the viral vector. This effect can be attributed to antiviral immunity and not an OPG-induced phenotype because the same hepatic inflammation follows administration of an empty adenoviral vector, whereas the liver lesions do not occur when OPG is overexpressed using the less immunogenic AAV vector. Antibodies to viral capsid proteins preceding or as a result of therapy could preclude therapeutic efficacy or repeat administration.

Many novel GEM or GER exhibit no apparent phenotype even when the anticipated genotype has been achieved. In some instances, the lack of apparent phenotype may be the result of a completely unexpected or subtle phenotype that remains undetected despite rigorous but conventional investigation (Doetschman, 1999; Papaioannou & Behringer, 2005). An alternative explanation often used for a negative phenotype is that the redundancy of biologic pathways has provided one or more unknown endogenous genes that have countered the functions of the modified gene. A rare instance in which this biological phenomenon has been proven definitively involves the relationship of hippocampal long-term potentiation to the expression of nitric oxide synthase (NOS). The absence of either the neuronal variant or the endothelial version of NOS alone results in GEM with apparently normal brain function and structure, while GEM lacking both NOS forms have significant potentiation deficiencies (Son et al., 1996). In some instances, a negative phenotype is the desired outcome of a product development program. However, in most cases, the absence of an identifiable and robust phenotype in new GEM or GER lines will lead to termination of the product development effort.

3. GENETICALLY MODIFIED MODELS FOR HAZARD IDENTIFICATION AND SAFETY ASSESSMENT

Genetically modified mice are now utilized for many applications in hazard identification and characterization as well as nonclinical drug development, including research to improve mechanisms of compound exposure in the context of the whole animal. Uses include exploration of human mechanisms of small molecule absorption, distribution, metabolism, and excretion (ADME); investigation of mechanisms and potential target organs of toxicity (including genotoxicity); alternatives to conventional models for carcinogenicity assessment; immunodeficient systems for the evaluation of human cells in vivo in animals; and toxicity testing when traditional models are not appropriate. As noted above, the use of GEM models typically will represent an ancillary approach to product development rather than a replacement for conventional efficacy and safety assessments in wild-type animals.

3.1. Basic Concepts for Using Engineered Animals in Hazard Identification and Safety Assessment

Genetically engineered rodent models likely are the most common genetically altered animals used to support risk and safety assessments for novel products (Webster et al., 2020; Diaz and Maher, 2016). For example, GEM and GER models are a critical component of drug development as they can provide key insights across different stages of the product discovery and development program. Examples include identifying physiologic changes in growth, organ function (safety pharmacology), development, and reproduction; determining potential target organs and differentiating between on-target and off-target effects; and defining possible carcinogenic risks. Importantly, prospective studies to assess standard safety pharmacology endpoints can be performed using knockout animals in the absence of drug treatment. In drug development (for both biologics and small molecules), genetically engineered rodent models can be used to investigate target biology and the outcome of altered target function, with a focus on alterations that mimic pharmacological intervention. In some instances, data regarding mechanisms of action and phenotypic characterization of genetically modified animals may be gleaned from the scientific literature; in such cases, limited or no prospective studies may be required if sufficient characterization of the target is reached. However, it is important to have full knowledge of the phenotypic analysis, particularly where it was directed to focus on specific aspects of the engineered model, as selective characterization may limit the completeness—and thus the utility—of the data sets that are available in public databases. When published reports of knockout models are available and the pathophysiology of the genetic mutation in the context of the whole animal is thoroughly assessed, very early risk assessment of the target is possible even before major investments are made in chemical modeling and synthesis.

If target organ toxicity is produced or can be modeled in wild-type mice, the mechanism of toxicity involving the pathways disrupted by targeted genetic mutations can be explored using knockout mice. If a modulation of a specific target is responsible for a specific toxicity in the wild-type animals, exposure to the test article should not produce toxicity in the knockout model lacking the target. This type of study is not routine in nonclinical safety testing, and generally would only be conducted to support product development if knowledge of the mechanism is essential to advance the test article or its successors. In general, the use of these models in developing both biomedical products and chemicals should be hypothesis driven and limited to a specific context and should be supported by a thorough understanding of the strengths and limitations of the selected model. Genetically engineered rodent models are not intended to replace hazard identification and safety assessment studies in conventional (wild-type) rodents and nonrodents. Instead, GEM and GER models should be viewed as an adjunct tool to aid in the interpretation of other in vitro and in vivo data to better understand the test article, the target, and/or the disease biology.

3.2. Absorption, Distribution, Metabolism, and Excretion

For small molecules, GEM models can be used to study the ADME properties of chemicals. In particular, three genetic modification strategies, used alone or in combination, allow investigation of the potential for drug–drug interactions (DDIs) and the role of ADME on a chemical's toxicity profile (Cheung and Gonzalez, 2008; Shen et al., 2011). The first type is the targeted mutation (deletion or "knock-out") of one or more genes coding for specific mouse proteins (Zambrowicz et al., 2003). Targets include CYP450; signal transduction elements (e.g., nuclear receptors such as peroxisome proliferator–activated receptor [PPAR] complex, constitutive androstane receptor [CAR], pregnane X receptor [PXR], or other transcription factors); and membrane transporter proteins. The second strategy is random insertion of one or more human genes (often a CYP) into mice, often in a strain lacking one or more of the murine homologs to the inserted human genes. The third and more technically challenging approach involves targeted replacement ("knock-in") of specific murine genes by their human homologs, such as replacing the mouse CAR gene with the human CAR sequence. Human genes in addition to classical CYP enzymes and nuclear receptors that have been inserted into mouse models include phase II systems that conjugate chemicals to water-soluble molecules to enhance excretion (e.g., uridine 5′-phospho glucuronosyltransferase); P-glycoprotein [P-gp], also known as multidrug resistance protein 1 [Mdr1]) and related molecules as well as other specific chemical transporters.

Engineered mouse models can be useful for the qualitative study of human mechanisms of ADME and for identification of species differences in enzyme activity and metabolite formation (Cheng et al., 2011; Powley et al., 2009; Ross et al., 2010; van Waterschoot and Schinkel, 2011). Unfortunately, these models have not proven suitable for full quantitative predictions of human ADME because no mouse model currently contains all components of any given human metabolic pathway while lacking all competing mouse metabolic pathways. General features of GEM models for ADME evaluation of xenobiotics are summarized below.

- Rodents and humans differ in the expression of CYP orthologs (i.e., genes in different species that arose from a single common ancestral gene and share a conserved function) as well as in functional inhibition, substrate selectivity, and enzyme induction. As an example, none of the four human CYP3A enzymes have directly overlapping substrate activities with the six or more mouse CYP3A enzymes. Some human CYP3A substrates are also metabolized by mouse CYP2C, and mouse CYP2C enzymes in the liver (especially mouse CYP2C55) are significantly upregulated in mice that lack mouse or human CYP3A activity.

- Some mouse metabolic pathways are modified by factors that are not relevant to regulation of their human counterparts. For instance, mouse CYP3A and CYP2C enzyme activities are controlled by mouse CAR and PXR, which in turn are stimulated by natural dietary plant components (e.g., phytoestrogens) that vary in quantity within typical murine diets. Human PXR and mouse PXR have different substrate affinities, with some agents stimulating only human PXR (e.g., rifampicin), while others stimulate only mouse PXR (e.g., pregnenolone 16α-carbonitrile). Variations in the activities of mouse CYPs, CAR, and PXR will impact a broad range of metabolic pathways, and thus have the potential to impact the results of experiments based on GEM models in which specific mouse molecules have been replaced with human enzymes and receptors.

- Tissue-specific expression of human enzyme systems in mice depends on the method of insertion (random vs. targeted), the promoters used in the genetic constructs, the number of copies of the gene inserted, and other control mechanisms affecting gene expression. For example, CYP4A is important in the gastrointestinal tract and liver, and also is present in renal tubules. Models targeting organ-specific expression of human CYP3A4 in the mouse using the villin promoter for intestinal expression or the albumin promoter for liver-specific expression are useful to examine specific aspects of enzyme activity, but these models are not designed to reflect

overall human metabolism in a quantitative manner. Even when human genes are controlled by their normal human promoters or even by homologous mouse promoters, expression levels of human CYPs in mouse models may not mimic either normal mouse or normal human levels of enzyme or receptor activity.

With all of these caveats contributing to the complexity of phenotypes in GEM models used for ADME studies, investigators must clearly explore and understand the limitations of each model used and evaluate the data with these limitations in mind.

GEM models have been used to confirm in vitro data illustrating that a particular metabolic pathway contributes to a specific lesion or toxicologic mechanism. For example, in vitro studies using cultured human cells have shown that phenobarbital induces CYP3A through activation of both CAR and PXR. Wild-type mice that express normal murine CAR develop hepatocellular proliferation (hyperplasia and eventually neoplasia) when initiated with a single dose of diethylnitrosamine and then treated for 32 weeks with phenobarbital. In contrast, mice with a targeted deletion of murine CAR do not develop hepatocellular hyperplasia or neoplasms, thus demonstrating the critical role of murine CAR in the pathogenesis of phenobarbital-induced liver cancer. Mice expressing human CAR and PXR instead of mouse CAR and PXR (singly and in combination) exhibit induction of murine CYP3A11 and CYP2B10 activities only by human CAR, and not by human PXR. In contrast, mice given phenobarbital develop hepatocellular hypertrophy with induction of mouse CYP3A11 and CYP2B10 enzymes when they carry either human CAR and human PXR or mouse CAR and mouse PXR, but increased hepatocellular proliferation (hyperplasia) only occurs in mice with mouse CAR and PXR and not in mice with either human CAR and PXR or in mice lacking both human and mouse CAR and PXR. Taken together, these findings indicate that phenobarbital induces hepatocellular proliferation leading to hepatic neoplasia in mice, but does not produce this effect in humans. Therefore, GEM models were instrumental in demonstrating a species-specific mechanism of phenobarbital-induced proliferative and neoplastic responses in mice that does not translate to humans.

Similar results for other agents using GEM models further underscore the importance of understanding species-specific metabolic differences when performing risk assessments. For instance, PPAR alpha (PPARα) agonists intended for use as lipid-lowering agents in humans induce hepatocyte enlargement (associated with increased production of peroxisomes and smooth endoplasmic reticulum) and hyperplasia, eventually leading to the formation of hepatocellular adenomas and carcinomas in rodents. In contrast, epidemiologic evidence indicates that these chemicals do not cause hepatocellular proliferation or neoplasia in humans. Genetically modified mice have been used to test the hypothesis that hepatocellular neoplastic responses are rodent-specific responses to PPARα agonists. Mice with targeted deletion of the murine PPARα gene do not develop lipid reductions, hepatocytomegaly, hepatocellular proliferation, or hepatocellular neoplasms when treated with the potent PPARα agonist Wy-14643, while 100% of mice with the normal murine PPARα gene develop hepatocellular neoplasms after 11 months of treatment with Wy-14643. This outcome confirmed that the mouse PPARα pathway is responsible for hepatocellular tumor formation in mice treated with Wy-14643. Mice with targeted replacement of the murine PPARα gene with the human PPARα gene (i.e., PPARα-humanized mice) experience the expected lipid-lowering effects when treated with PPARα agonists (fenofibrate and Wy-14643) but do not develop the hepatocellular proliferation or hepatocellular neoplasms observed in wild-type mice expressing murine PPARα that have received the same agents. These experiments provided a clear explanation for the divergence in tumorigenic responses in mice and epidemiologic data obtained in humans treated with PPARα agonists. Additional work has showed that activation of PPARα by fenofibrate or Wy-14643 in mice suppresses expression of the noncoding microRNA Let-7c, resulting in stabilization of the mRNA for the oncogene *c-Myc* and increased c-Myc protein production. The c-Myc protein contributes to hepatocellular neoplasia in mice. Production of Let-7c was not altered in PPARα-humanized mice treated with PPARα agonists, again supporting the conclusion that hepatocellular neoplasia observed in wild-type mice treated with PPARα agonists results from a mouse-specific metabolic pathway and thus is not relevant to carcinogenicity risk assessment in humans.

Genetically modified mice also can be used to differentiate metabolic pathways that reduce or prevent toxicity from those that heighten toxicity. For example, docetaxel (an antimitotic drug approved for treating solid carcinomas that works by inhibiting microtubule formation) administered orally to mice lacking murine CYP3A produces higher exposures and relatively greater toxicity at lower doses than is found in wild-type mice. Furthermore, the target for toxicity is shifted from bone marrow in wild-type mice to the intestinal epithelium in animals lacking murine CYP3A. Since docetaxel is a substrate for both human CYP3A4 and human P-gp, efforts to improve the exposure of docetaxel in humans may include coadministration of agents that inhibit CYP3A4 and/or P-gp. In this light, studies in GEM lacking murine CYP3A suggest that gastrointestinal toxicity might be anticipated in humans when CYP3A4 inhibitors are coadministered with docetaxel.

Finally, GEM can be used to define the effects of membrane transport proteins that control the distribution of xenobiotics across barriers. At least 15 transporters within the blood–brain barrier can profoundly reduce the concentration of some xenobiotics within the nervous system by actively pumping chemicals from the brain parenchyma into the blood and cerebrospinal fluid. These transporters include members of the ATP-binding cassette (ABC) protein family of efflux transporters such as P-gp (also called Mdr1), breast cancer resistance protein (BCRP), the organic anion transporter, the organic anion-transporting polypeptide (OATP), the organic cation transporter, and others (see *Biochemical and Molecular Basis of Toxicity*, Vol 1, Chap 2). P-gp and BCRP use energy from the cleavage of ATP to actively transport molecules out of the brain against a concentration gradient. Mice lacking either P-gp, BCRP, or both are used to evaluate the effects of these efflux transporters on drug levels in the brain and assess transporter-mediated reductions in drug efficacy and toxicity for chemicals that are pharmacologically active in the central nervous system. Humans have a single MDR1 gene (denoted

ABCB1), while rodents have two corresponding genes (*Mdr1a* and *Mdr1b*), but the distribution of P-gp is very similar in humans and rodents. Within the brain, P-gp is located on the luminal cell membrane of capillaries as well as on the portion of the choroid plexus epithelial cell membrane facing the cerebrospinal fluid, enabling transport of chemicals into both blood and cerebrospinal fluid. P-gp is also present in intestinal and biliary epithelium, on the luminal surface of renal proximal tubular epithelial cells, and in the placenta. In mice, P-gp made from *Mdr1a* is present in the brain, while *Mdr1b* does not play a major role in the brain. Thus, for studies of drug levels in brain, mice lacking *Mdr1a* alone or both *Mdr1a* and *Mdr1b* are equally acceptable. Mice with null mutations of *P-gp* have up to 10-fold higher brain concentrations of many drugs compared to wild-type mice having the same genetic background. These drugs include opioids; human immunodeficiency virus (HIV) protease inhibitors; and many antidepressant and antipsychotic drugs, including chlorpromazine, clozapine, haloperidol, olanzapine, risperidone, and sertraline. Novel molecules may be screened in *P-gp* knockout mice and wild-type mice to assess blood-to-brain drug concentration ratios, which may be used to determine whether or not P-gp will limit drug concentrations in the nervous system. BCRP is an efflux transporter with significant substrate specificity and functional redundancy with P-gp (Chu et al., 2013; Lee et al., 2015). Similar to humans, rodent BCRP is localized in the apical plasma membrane of the intestinal tract, liver, kidney, testis, placenta, and brain capillary endothelial cells. P-gp (Mdr1) and BCRP profoundly restrict the brain penetration of palbociclib, a CDK4/6 inhibitor. In *Mdr1a/Mdr1b/Bcrp* triple knockout mice, the absence of both Mdr1 and BCRP causes a 60-fold increase in palbociclib brain-to-plasma ratio as opposed to a 19-fold increase in the absence of Mdr1 only. Therefore, knockout mice lacking Mdr1/P-gp and/or BCRP also may be useful for studying the neurotoxicity of compounds which are P-gp and/or BCRP substrates and thus do not reach high concentrations in the brain of wild-type animals. Competitive inhibition of P-gp–mediated transport is induced by certain chemicals (e.g., cyclosporine A and verapamil), but chemically mediated inhibition

of P-gp does not appear to be a significant mechanism of drug-drug interactions (DDI) or toxicity. Generally, evidence of a direct contribution of BCRP inhibition or induction to DDIs is limited due to the cross-specificity with P-gp and CYP3A substrates and inhibitors as well as the activity of other transporters (OATPs). Examples of clinical substrates for BCRP used in clinical DDI studies include oral sulfasalazine and oral rosuvastatin.

3.3. Genotoxicity Testing

Both GEM and GER models have been designed specifically to evaluate mutagenicity in vivo, and they are used occasionally as second- or third-tier tools in the safety assessment of pharmaceutical candidates and environmental chemicals (Cosentino and Heddle, 2000; Lambert et al., 2005; Mirsalis et al., 1994; Provost et al., 1993; Suzuki et al., 1994). In vivo models permit the detailed investigation of alterations to DNA in individual organs following systemic exposure to potentially mutagenic chemicals and/or their metabolites. These in vivo tests may be more predictive of human risk than standard in vitro (bacteria or cell-based) genotoxicity assays because they include all of the rodent ADME processes; even so, the limitations of using rodent ADME mechanisms to predict human risk still apply. In vivo mutagenicity models also may be used to demonstrate threshold effects that cannot be accurately determined using in vitro models. The cost and complexity of these in vivo models has generally limited their use to cases in which positive, conflicting, or equivocal results were obtained previously using the standard in vitro genetic toxicity testing battery.

The genetically modified rodent mutagenicity models (Transgenic Rodent [TGR] gene mutation assays) are established assays for genotoxicity testing that use TGRs with chromosomes in which multiple copies of plasmid or phage DNA harboring reporter genes have integrated in a stable fashion (Boverhof et al., 2011). Interaction of a genotoxic agent with one of the reporter genes produces a mutation that can be detected by introducing the altered DNA into bacteria and then observing the appearance of the resulting bacterial colonies (Figure 23.8). After treatment with a test article for periods ranging

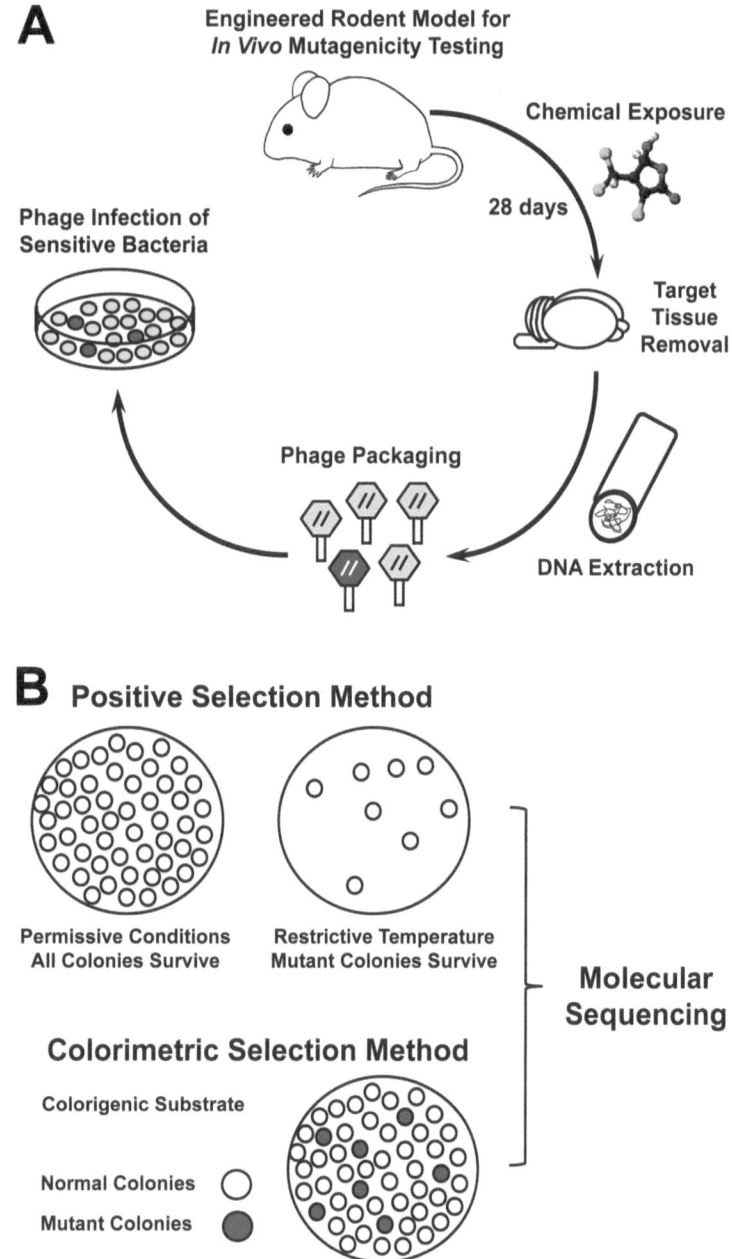

FIGURE 23.8 **Utilization of genetically engineered rodents for in vivo mutagenicity testing.** (A) Transgenic rodents bearing multiple copies of a bacterial-derived target transgene are exposed to a potential mutagen (as determined by a prior in vitro mutagenicity test, like the Ames assay). In this figure, the ball-and-stick representation depicts the environmental carcinogen 3-chloro-4(dichloromethyl)-5-hydroxy-5H-furan-2-one (also termed mutagen X), a by-product of water chlorination. (This figure is reproduced under the Creative Commons CC0 1.0 Universal Public Domain Dedication and is available at http://commons.wikimedia.org/wiki/File:Mutagen-X-3D-balls.png.) Possible target tissues are removed, and DNA is extracted. The transgene sequences are isolated and introduced into bacteriophages, which are then cultured on lawns of sensitive bacteria (commonly variants of *Escherichia coli*). (B) The presence and number of mutations can be explored using either temperature-restricted growth conditions (upper plates) or by supplementing the medium with a colorless substrate that can only be metabolized to a colored product by bacteria in which mutations permit activity of the transgene (lower plate). Once mutant colonies are identified, the bacterial DNA can be isolated so that the mutations may be sequenced to determine the nature of the genomic damage. *Figure modified from Haschek WM, Rousseaux CG, Wallig MA, editors:* Haschek and Rousseaux's handbook of toxicologic pathology, *ed 3, 2013, Academic Press, Figure 12.7, p 433, with permission.*

from 7 days to (more commonly) 28 days, the specific organs or tissues of interest are harvested from animals, the reporter DNA is isolated and packaged to form complete phage particles (for phage-based systems), and the reporter DNA within the plasmid or phage vector is incubated with bacteria. The mutation frequency is determined by the number of phage-transfected bacterial colonies that express mutations in the reporter gene compared to the total number of transfected bacterial colonies (mutated and wild-type). Genetically modified rodent models for in vivo mutagenicity testing have been utilized by the U.S. Environmental Protection Agency (EPA) to establish that a mutagenic mode of action is the explanation for the carcinogenic properties of acrylamide, cyclophosphamide, and hexavalent chromium.

The commercially available (and thus the most common) engineered models for in vivo mutagenicity testing are the Muta^{TM} Mouse, the Big Blue® mouse, and the Big Blue® rat. These models detect point mutations and small insertions, but usually fail to detect large deletions.

- The Muta^{TM} Mouse (Covance Inc., Princeton, NJ, USA) contains 40 copies of the *lacZ* reporter gene in a single locus on chromosome 3. After DNA is harvested from tissues of interest, the reporter gene is excised, inserted into phage particles, and incubated with *Escherichia coli* (*E. coli*) bacteria that lack both a functional *lacZ* gene and a functional *galE* gene (*galE−*, *lacZ−*). The bacteria are grown on selective medium that contains P-gal, a substrate that is toxic to *galE−*, *lacZ−* bacteria. Only bacteria with a back-mutated, functional *lacZ +* gene and its product (beta galactosidase [βGal]) survive on the selective medium, and these can be easily counted using automated technology. The mutation frequency can be estimated by dividing the number of bacterial colonies growing on the selective medium by the number of bacterial colonies growing on nonselective medium. The reporter DNA sequence has been shown to be stable over time even as nucleotide variants occur elsewhere in the genome (Meier et al., 2019).
- The Big Blue® mouse and Big Blue® rat (BioReliance Corporation, Rockville, MD, USA) contain the *lacI* gene with the *lacO*

operating genes and the *lacZ* gene. The *lacI* gene is the target for mutational effects. The Big Blue mouse contains about 40 copies of the construct at a single locus in each cell, and the Big Blue rat contains 30–40 copies per cell. The *lacI* gene codes for a repressor of the *lacZ* gene responsible for production of βGal. If the *lacI* gene is mutated, the repressor will not prevent production of βGal. In the presence of Xgal (a substrate for βGal that produces a blue product), bacteria with the mutated *lacI* gene and plentiful βGal will produce blue colonies, while bacteria with the intact *lacI* gene lack βGal and produce white (colorless) colonies. For this assay, the phage-infected bacteria containing the target genes isolated from chemically treated rodents are grown on medium containing Xgal. The number of blue bacterial colonies containing mutated *lacI* sequences is compared to the total number of colonies (blue mutated plus white wild-type) to determine the mutation frequency (Figure 23.8). An additional mutation assay that does not rely on plaque color has been developed using the *cII* reporter gene in the Big Blue model systems. Growth at 25°C is limited to those *E. coli* colonies that were infected by phages that had packaged chemically mutated *cII* reporter genes, while all bacteria carrying the reporter gene (mutated or not) can survive at 37°C (Figure 23.8). This *cII* system is less labor intensive than the original Big Blue® models and also can be utilized in the Muta^{TM} Mouse platform.

Safety studies for nelfinavir (an HIV protease inhibitor) offer one example of the use of the Muta^{TM} Mouse to support human risk assessment. Excess levels of ethyl methanesulfonate (EMS), an alkylating mutagen, were found in certain lots of nelfinavir produced in 2007. Treatment of the Muta Mouse model with seven different dose levels of EMS for 28 days showed that there was no mutagenic effect at doses of EMS up to and including 25 mg/kg/day, while dose-dependent mutagenic effects developed after treatment at 50 or 100 mg/kg/day. The threshold level at 25 mg/kg/day produced much higher peak exposures (C_{max}) than humans would experience at the maximum calculated human dose. The investigators also demonstrated that a single EMS dose of 350 mg/kg produced DNA damage when assessed 28 days later, while daily EMS doses of 12.5 mg/kg for 28 days (a 350 mg/kg cumulative dose) yielded no mutagenic effects. The interpretation of these data was that mechanisms for repairing alkylation damage to DNA were able to mend all mutations at doses ≤25 mg/kg/day. These findings contributed to the weight of evidence demonstrating that exposure to small quantities of EMS in standard nelfinavir doses did not pose a tangible mutagenic or carcinogenic risk to human patients.

Care must be taken when interpreting in vivo mutagenicity data for risk assessment. In most cases, xenobiotics produce comparable frequencies of mutations in both the transgene insertions and the numerous endogenous genes in the native rodent genome following acute exposure in vivo. However, chronic exposure to various low doses of ENU has been shown to selectively target the reporter transgenes while sparing endogenous loci during the early course of treatment. This effect is not specific to ENU, indicating that the rate of mutation accumulation in GEM and GER models for in vivo mutagenicity testing may not accurately reflect human risk in all cases.

3.4. Carcinogenicity Assessment

The two-year (life time) rodent carcinogenicity studies conducted in wild-type mice and rats to determine carcinogenic potential of materials to which humans may be exposed over protracted periods have significant disadvantages. Length, cost, and use of large numbers of animals do represent limitations, and it is recognized that these studies produce positive results for many chemicals that do not pose a risk for human cancer and yet fail to identify some known human carcinogens. Better animal models are needed for human carcinogenicity risk assessment. Short-term carcinogenicity testing, based on GEM models predisposed to develop chemically induced neoplasia, was introduced in 1997 as an alternative to replace one of the two standard two-year carcinogenicity studies (in wild-type mice or rats) typically required for registering chemicals and pharmaceuticals (Alden et al., 2011; Boverhof et al., 2011; Cavagnaro, 2008b;

Friedrich and Olejniczak, 2011; ICH, 1997; Mac-Donald et al., 2004; Wells and Williams, 2009; Wijnhoven and van Steeg, 2003). An added advantage of these short-term assays is that they may provide mechanistic information regarding the nature of the carcinogenic response (Gonzalez, 2001; Leder et al., 2008).

Alternative GEM models mentioned in the current International Council for Harmonisation of Technical Requirements for Pharmaceuticals for Human Use (ICH) guidance include the $p53^{+/-}$ mouse, the rasH2 mouse (also known as Tg-rasH2 or CB6F1-rasH2), the Tg.AC mouse (FVB/N-Tg.AC), and the $Xpa^{-/-}$ mouse (also denoted XPA). The genetic modifications in these models consisted of two types: deletion of DNA repair genes ($p53^{+/-}$, $Xpa^{-/-}$, and $Xpa^{-/-}$ $p53^{+/-}$ models) or insertion of multiple copies of human ras proto-oncogenes (rasH2 and Tg.AC models). These genetic modifications are considered to be appropriate because they are mechanistically relevant to the genesis of many human cancers (see Carcinogenesis: Mechanisms and Evaluation, Vol 1, Chap 8). An extensive collaboration of 48 companies plus multiple academic laboratories and government agencies initiated a multiyear effort to test these GEM models and several other alternative carcinogenicity assays with a standard set of confirmed human carcinogens, rodent-specific carcinogens (i.e., not carcinogenic for humans), and rodent noncarcinogens using uniform study protocols. These efforts were coordinated by the Alternatives to Carcinogenicity Testing Committee of the Health and Environmental Sciences Institute within the International Life Sciences Institute (ILSI HESI ACT). The tested GEM models permit carcinogenic potential to be assessed with an abbreviated (6 to 9 month) dosing duration and lower incidences of confounding spontaneous neoplasms. Due to the greater sensitivity of these GEM models to neoplastic development in response to known carcinogens, an adequate assessment of potential carcinogenicity can be performed using smaller group sizes. A positive control group often must be included to provide clear evidence of the sensitivity of the models over the period of agent administration. However, for some models (e.g., Tg.rasH2), collective experience over time has demonstrated that correctly engineered animals reliably respond to the positive control agent (Paranjpe et al., 2013), so current practice is to use genotyping quality control data (to show the presence of the predisposing genetic alteration in all study animals) as a reasonable justification for not including a positive control group (Bogdanffy, Lesniak, & Mangipudy, 2020). The spectrum and number of tumors in mouse carcinogenicity models vary with the genetic background of the GEM strain and substrains (Donehower et al., 1995; Nielsen et al., 1995).

The $p53^{+/-}$ hemizygous mouse model (B6; 129-$Trp53^{tm1Brd}$ N4; Model P53N4, Taconic Farms, Inc., Germantown, NY, USA) contains a single functional copy of the mouse $p53$ (formal gene symbol: $Trp53$) gene. The product of the $p53$ gene functions as a tumor suppressor protein. This single gene deletion increases the sensitivity of the $p53^{+/-}$ model to genotoxic agents that can inactivate the remaining functional $p53$ gene, thereby impairing gene repair and apoptosis of cells with genetic damage (French et al., 2001). The spontaneous tumor frequency for the first 36 weeks of life of these mice is low; however, after about 80 weeks, half of the animals develop spontaneous tumors including lymphomas, osteosarcomas, and hemangiosarcomas. Although this model was designed to detect mutagenic carcinogens, the $p53^{+/-}$ model also produces positive results in response to some nongenotoxic chemicals. In the ILSI HESI ACT studies, the recommended positive control chemical was p-cresidine, a potent mutagenic carcinogen that produces urinary bladder papillomas and carcinomas (Storer et al., 2001). In the ILSI studies and assays submitted to the U.S. Food and Drug Administration (FDA) to support registration of pharmaceuticals, p-cresidine inconsistently produced positive neoplastic responses in $p53^{+/-}$ mice. Therefore, a single intraperitoneal (IP) injection of N-methyl-N-nitrosourea (MNU, 75 mg/kg in citrate buffer, pH4.0) has been proposed as an alternative positive control chemical in $p53^{+/-}$ mice (Morton et al., 2008). The FDA accepts studies using the $p53^{+/-}$ model only if the chemical being tested produced positive findings in genotoxicity assays.

The rasH2 mouse model (CByB6F1-Tg(HRAS) 2Jic; Model 1178, Taconic Farms, Inc., Germantown, NY, USA) has approximately three copies of the native human Ha-ras oncogene under the control of the human Ha-ras gene promoter

inserted in tandem into the mouse genome. Overexpression of the oncogene enhances cell proliferation and predisposes the rasH2 mouse to accelerated carcinogenesis compared to wild-type littermates (Morton et al., 2002; Nambiar and Morton, 2013). In fact, while few tumors develop by 33 weeks of age, approximately 50% of mice develop tumors spontaneously by 18 months of age, including hemangiosarcomas, lymphomas, pulmonary adenocarcinomas, skin papillomas, and Harderian gland adenocarcinomas (Tamaoki, 2001). The rasH2 mouse is widely accepted for carcinogenicity assessment of genotoxic and nongenotoxic compounds administered by oral or injectable (but not topical) routes, and therefore is the current alternative carcinogenicity model of choice for most small molecules in the pharmaceutical industry. Since mice carrying the human Ha-ras transgene cannot be differentiated visually from wild-type littermates, all rasH2 mice to be used for Good Laboratory Practice (GLP)–compliant studies are genotyped by the vendor to ensure the presence of the transgene. The positive control chemical recommended by the ILSI HESI ACT Committee is MNU (75 mg/kg in citrate buffer, pH4.0), but urethane (1000 mg/kg IP on days 1, 3, and 5) also has been employed.

The Tg.AC mouse (FVB/NTac-Tg(Hba-x-v-Ha-ras)TG.ACLed/Tac hemizygote; Model TGAC, Taconic Farms, Inc., Germantown, NY, USA) contains up to 20 copies per cell of the Ha-ras oncogene linked to the ζ-globulin gene promoter. The model was developed specifically to assess the carcinogenicity of chemicals applied by the topical route of administration (i.e., skin painting) (Eastin et al., 2001; Tennant et al., 2001). The number of papillomas on the area of exposed skin of each animal can be counted easily by visual inspection, followed by microscopic confirmation of the diagnosis for each lesion. By design, the number of skin masses visible in the treated area of skin is a primary experimental endpoint. The model has demonstrated increased generation of skin papillomas and carcinomas in response to topical administration of some genotoxic (tumor inducing) and nongenotoxic (tumor promoting) carcinogens in the ILSI HESI ACT studies (Usui et al., 2001). The positive control agent for Tg.AC studies is phorbol 12-myristate 13-acetate (PMA, also known as

12-O-tetradecanoylphorbol-13-acetate [TPA]) applied topically at a dose of 2.5 µg/kg body weight on the skin of the back three times each week. However, a genotypic variant of Tg.AC mice that is nonresponsive to TPA due to spontaneous transgene rearrangements has been identified; in this substrain, 2%–5% of animals fail to respond to agents that induce tumors in other animals of the same strain. Importantly, Tg.AC mice are susceptible to skin neoplasms induced by nonspecific skin trauma and/or irritation mediated by vehicle alone. Furthermore, responses to chemicals are highly dependent on the choice of vehicle, suggesting that the Tg.AC model may produce false-positive results. Regulatory authorities have accepted studies in the Tg.AC model to replace two-year mouse carcinogenicity studies only when chemicals are applied topically. The FDA reported in 2011 that 50% (8 of 16) of Tg.AC studies submitted to support pharmaceutical registration had positive carcinogenic findings, and several of these compounds had no other evidence of carcinogenic potential. The FDA no longer recommends the Tg.AC model for carcinogenicity testing of dermal products. Caution is warranted when considering use of the Tg.AC model to support chemical hazard identification.

The $Xpa^{-/-}$ mouse models contain a mutated, nonfunctional form of the xeroderma pigmentosum (Xpa) gene that normally codes for a DNA nucleotide excision repair protein (van Kreijl et al., 2001; van Steeg et al., 2001). These mice are more susceptible than wild-type mice to mutagenic human carcinogens when treated for 9 months, while the incidence of spontaneous tumors in this strain is low. $Xpa^{-/-}$ mice exhibit an increased incidence of neoplasia following ultraviolet B irradiation and carcinogens such as 7,12-dimethylbenz(a)anthracene. In an attempt to increase the sensitivity of the $Xpa^{-/-}$ model to carcinogenic chemicals, $Xpa^{-/-}$ mice have been crossed with $p53^{+/-}$ heterozygous knockout mice to yield $Xpa^{-/-}$ $p53^{+/-}$ double knockout mice with functional deficiencies of two distinct DNA repair mechanisms. Neither model has been accepted for use in carcinogenicity risk assessment of pharmaceuticals.

The experience of the FDA with alternative mouse models for carcinogenicity testing is summarized in Table 23.2. Studies conducted in the $p53^{+/-}$ mouse, rasH2 mouse, and Tg.AC mouse are now accepted widely to support carcinogenicity hazard identification when registering new pharmaceutical products. The $p53^{+/-}$ and rasH2 models have lower positive response rates than are found in two-year bioassays in

TABLE 23.2 Alternative Carcinogenicity Studies Using Genetically Engineered Mouse (GEM) Models Submitted to Support Product Registration From 1997 to 2014[a,b]

GEM model	Number of protocols submitted	Number of final study results received	Number of inadequate studies	Number of positive studies
rasH2	134	38	2[c]	4
$p53^{+/-}$	82[d]	32	0	4[e]
Tg.AC	44	19	2[f]	9
$Xpa^{-/-}$ $p53^{+/-}$	1[g]	1	1[h]	0

[a] Studies were submitted to the Center for Drug Evaluation and Research (CDER) of the U.S. Food and Drug Administration (FDA) as of June 2014. (The data were adapted from Boverhof et al. (2011), Jacobs and Brown (2015)).

[b] Table modified from Haschek and Rousseaux's Handbook of Toxicologic Pathology, 3rd ed. W. M Haschek, C. G. Rousseaux and M. A. Wallig, eds. (2013) Academic Press, Table 12.2, p 436, with permission.

[c] One inadequate rasH2 study did not demonstrate adequate exposure for a major genotoxic metabolite.

[d] Includes older studies for compounds that were equivocally genotoxic, although now the FDA accepts the p53[+/-] model only if the drug is clearly genotoxic.

[e] Two of these four studies with positive results were also positive in wild-type animals, so p53 hemizygosity is not thought to have contributed to carcinogenesis.

[f] One negative Tg.AC study included examination only of the topical application site and is included as inadequate with a second study considered inadequate because of study execution.

[g] No studies utilizing the Xpa[-/-] p53[+/-] model had been submitted in the 10 years prior to data compilation in June 2014.

[h] This compound was not genotoxic.

wild-type rodents, produce fewer false-positive results that are irrelevant to human risk assessment, cost substantially less and require fewer animals than conventional two-year bioassays, and provide more flexibility in timing of the studies. Concerns regarding the use of these short-term GEM models include limited historical control data and fears that a positive neoplastic outcome in an alternative model could be viewed differently than a positive outcome in a standard two-year rodent study. For a more detailed discussion of study designs and interpretation for alternative GEM models for carcinogenicity testing (see *Carcinogenesis: Mechanisms and Evaluation*, Vol 1, Chap 8).

3.5. Engineered Immunodeficient Models

When stem cells or entire organs are transplanted directly from a human donor into a cross-matched human patient without in vitro propagation or activation, nonclinical safety testing is not necessary. However, if the human stem cells have been cultured, propagated, differentiated, or otherwise significantly manipulated in vitro, these products are regulated as medical products (cell therapies or medical devices, depending on the packaging) and thus require safety testing. Nonclinical safety assessment of medical therapies derived from human stem cells or other human cell–based products presents a significant challenge as the administration of such products into immunocompetent animals (e.g., mouse, rat, dog, nonhuman primate) is complicated by the immunogenic responses potentially resulting in the rejection of the administered human cells. To overcome this challenge, various models have been developed including the use of immunosuppressive agents in immunocompetent animals, genetically immunodeficient animals, or humanized animals (Cavagnaro, 2008a). Immunodeficient rodents permit in vivo assessment of biodistribution, differentiation, growth, toxicity, and carcinogenicity (teratoma formation) of products composed of human cells. While some of these immunodeficient rodent models arose spontaneously, others have been engineered deliberately through targeted deletion of genes critical to immune function and/or cross-breeding of various immunocompromised

models. Important immunodeficient rodent models are described in Table 23.3.

Investigators have reported that highly immunodeficient rodent models lacking T-lymphocyte ("T-cell"), B-lymphocyte ("B-cell"), and natural killer (NK)-cell functions are less likely to reject transplanted human cells than are models that do not lack all three cell types (Anderson and Bluestone, 2005; Ito et al., 2002, 2008; Katano et al., 2014). This principle should be considered when selecting a model to study engrafted human cells. The NOG (NOD.Cg-$Prkdc^{scid}$ $Il2rg^{tm1Sug}$/JicTac) mouse (Taconic Farms, Inc., Germantown, NY, USA) and the NSG (NOD.Cg-$Prkdc^{scid}$ $Il2rg^{tm1Wjl}$/SzJ) mouse (The Jackson Laboratory, Bar Harbor, ME) lack T-cells, B-cells, and NK cells, and also exhibit impaired cytokine production, very low lymphoma development, and a longer lifespan (approximately 1.5 years or greater) than do most other immunodeficient mouse models. Therefore, these two models may be preferable for nonclinical studies to assess chronic toxicity or carcinogenicity of human cells. However, it must be remembered that the actual lifespan of laboratory rodents depends significantly on husbandry and other environment factors as well as on specific experimental interventions. The athymic nude rat may represent a suitable option when mice are too small to be efficient models due to limitations of surgical implantation or other experimental manipulations, the volume of material that may be injected, or other factors. An important distinction is that the athymic rat model has intact B-cell and NK cell functions and may not support the growth of human cell preparations as effectively as highly immunodeficient mouse models. Commercially available immunodeficient rodent models that permit the growth of human cells are described in Table 23.4.

Immunodeficient rodents may not be as robust as conventional rodents, in part because they are exquisitely susceptible to secondary infections. The more profound the degree of immunodeficiency, the better the model serves as a host for human cells and the more vulnerable it is to infectious agents including opportunistic and uncommon pathogens. Stringent biosecurity programs and adequate husbandry procedures are required when using these animals as models. They are shipped from the vendor in

TABLE 23.3 Genetic Mutations Commonly Found in Immunodeficient Rodent Models[a]

Model, gene, and species	Immunological defect(s)
Athymic nude mouse and rat (forkhead box N1- *Foxn1^nu^*, formerly known as *Hfh11^nu^*; previously designated *nu* in mouse and *rnu* in rat)	• Lack thymus and T-cells (both CD4+ and CD8+ T-cells) in secondary lymphoid organs • May display "leakiness" (i.e., may develop low serum levels of immunoglobulins) in some strains • Normal or increased macrophage and NK activity
Severe combined immunodeficiency (*scid*) mouse—*scid* mutation/allele on *Prkdc* (protein kinase, DNA-activated, catalytic polypeptide) gene	• Lack mature T-cells and B-cells • May display leakiness as they age
Scid-beige (*bg*) mouse—autosomal recessive mutations in SCID (*Prkdc^scid^*) and beige (*Lyst^bg^*)	• Impaired function of NK cells • Decreased CD8+ T-cells, B-cells, neutrophils, and macrophages • May develop thymic lymphomas
Common γ chain of the interleukin (IL)-2 receptor (IL2R γ) mouse	• Lack NK cells and have very few T-cells and B-cells
Recombinase activating gene 1 and 2 (*Rag1* and *Rag2*) mice	• Lack mature T-cells and B-cells • Do not display leakiness
Perforin 1 (*Pfp1*) mouse	• Lack NK cell function • Decreased CD8+ T-cell activity
X-linked immunodeficiency (*xid*) mouse (*Btk^xid^*)	• Defective B-cell development, differentiation, and activation in homozygous females and hemizygous males • Profound B-cell deficiency • Impaired granulocyte maturation and function • Abnormal regulation of TLRs signaling • Defective mast cells degranulation
Beta2-microglobulin (*bm2*) mouse	• Decreased CD8+ T-cell and NK cell development/activity
Myd88 (myeloid differentiation primary response gene 88) mouse	• Decreased innate immune responses
Ticam1 Trif (Toll-like receptor adaptor molecule 1) mouse	• Decreased innate immune responses (especially when combined with Myd88-targeted mutation)

[a] *Table adapted in part from* Haschek and Rousseaux's Handbook of Toxicologic Pathology, *3rd ed. W. M. Haschek, C. G. Rousseaux and M. A. Wallig, eds. (2013) Academic Press, Table 12.3, p 438, with permission.*

carriers that prevent contamination by infectious agents. The exterior of the shipping containers should be disinfected prior to opening, and the animals should be transferred immediately to sanitized microisolators or other sterile caging systems, preferably using a class II biosafety cabinet or equivalent arrangement. Animals should be maintained in sterile caging on sterile bedding with sterile food and water for their entire lives—husbandry conditions which add greatly to the cost of long-term experiments. Careful attention must be devoted to the cleanliness of husbandry, handling, treatment, surgical procedures, and other experimental manipulations. Only terminal procedures such as euthanasia, necropsy, and large-scale blood and tissue collection may be performed using conventional (i.e., nonsterile) methods.

TABLE 23.4   Immunodeficient Rodent Models that Permit Growth of Human Cells and Tissue Xenografts[a]

Model	Immunodeficiency
Nude mouse Spontaneous mutation *nu/nu* on NCr, BALB/c, NIH Swiss, C57BL/6, and NMRI backgrounds CrTac:NCr-*Foxn1^{nu}* C.Cg/AnNTac-*Foxn1^{nu}* NE9 NTac:NIHS-*Foxn1^{nu}* B6.Cg/NTac-*Foxn1^{nu}* NE10 BomTac:NMRI-*Foxn1^{nu}* Crl:CD-1 *Foxn1^{nu}* Crl:NU(NCr)-*Foxn1^{nu}* Hsd:Athymic Nude- *Foxn1^{nu}*	Lack of T-cells
NOG mouse NOD.Cg-*Prkdc^{scid} Il2rg^{tm1Sug}*/JicTac (NOD/SCID/γc^{null}) on C57BL background	Lack of B-cells, T-cells, and NK cells Reduced complement activity, dysfunctional macrophages and dendritic cells, and deficiencies in immune signaling
SCID-Bg mouse CB17.Cg-*Prkdc^{scid}Lyst^{bg}*/Crl, or C.B-*Igh*-1b/GbmsTac-*Prkdc^{scid}-Lyst^{bg}* N7	Lack of B-cells and T-cells, neutrophils, and macrophages Impaired function of NK cells
Rag2/IL2rγ double knockout mouse B10; B6-*Rag2^{tm1Fwa} IL2rγ^{tm1Wjl}*	Lack of IL-2, IL-4, IL-7, IL-9, IL-15, and IL-21 receptor functions Lack of B-cell, T-cell, and NK cells Dysfunctional dendritic cells
NSG mouse NOD.Cg-*Prkdc^{scid} Il2rγ^{tm1Wjl}*/SzJ (NOD-*scid* IL2Rγ^{null}; albino)	Lack of IL-2, IL-4, IL-7, IL-9, IL-15, and IL-21 receptor functions Lack of B-cells, T-cells, NK cells, and complement Defective dendritic cells and macrophages
NRG, NOD Rag gamma mouse NOD.*Cg-Rag1^{tm1Mom}* *Il2rγ^{tm1Wjl}*/SzJ	Lack of B-cells, T-cells, NK cells, and complement Defective dendritic cells and macrophages
NSGS, NOD scid gamma Il3-GM-SF mouse NOD.*Cg-Prkdc^{scid}* *Il2rγ^{tm1Wjl}* Tg(CMV-IL3,CSF2,KITLG)1Eav/MloySzJ	Lacks B-cells, T-cells, NK cells, and complement Defective dendritic cells and macrophages
NOD scid mouse NOD.CB17-*Prkdc^{scid}*/J	Lacks B-cells, T-cells, and complement Defective NK cells, dendritic cells, and macrophages
Pfp/Rag2 homozygous/homozygous double knockout mouse B6.129S6-*Pfp^{tm1Clrk}Rag2^{tm1Fwa}* N12	Severe depletion of NK cell function Lack of mature T-cells and B-cells
NIH-III outbred hairless mouse (pigmented) Crl:NIH-*Lyst^{bg}Foxn1^{nu}Btk^{xid}*	Lack of mature B-cells and T-cells Defective NK cells
NIH nude rat Crl:NIH-*Foxn1^{rnu}* NTac:NIH-*Whn*	Lack of T-cells

(Continued)

TABLE 23.4 Immunodeficient Rodent Models that Permit Growth of Human Cells and Tissue Xenografts[a]—cont'd

Model	Immunodeficiency
CD34+ humanized mice hu-BLT-NSG hu-CD34-NSG NOD.Cg-*Prkdc^{scid} Il2rγ^{tm1Wjl}* Tg(CMV-IL3,CSF2, KITLG)1Eav/MloySz (hu-CD34-SGM-3 mouse) NOD.Cg-*Prkdc^{scid} Il2rγ^{tm1Sug}* Tg(SV40/HTLV-IL3,CSF2)10-7Jic/JicTac (huNOG-EXL)	Same immunodeficient phenotype as NSG and NOG mice
NSG-Tg(Hu-IL15) NOD.Cg-*Prkdc^{scid} Il2r$\gamma^{\tau m1Wjl}$* Tg(IL15)1Sz/SzJ	Same immunodeficient phenotype as the NSG mouse

[a] *Table adapted in part from* Haschek and Rousseaux's Handbook of Toxicologic Pathology, *3rd ed. W. M. Haschek, C. G. Rousseaux and M. A. Wallig, eds. (2013) Academic Press, Table 12.4, p 439, with permission.*

Biodistribution

When injected intravenously (IV), foreign cells are distributed first to the capillary beds in the lung and then to other parts of the body. The foreign cells may lodge and grow in some environments, but not in others. When cells are injected or implanted directly into a specific tissue or other site (e.g., a cavity), the potential for cell distribution and remote survival exists even if migration is not expected. Cell survival and proliferation in locations other than the intended site of action are significant safety concerns that can be partially addressed using immunodeficient rodent models. Microscopic examination of a broad list of tissues in sections stained with hematoxylin and eosin (H&E) can be used to efficiently assess abnormal colonization, proliferation, and differentiation of stem cells in a wide range of organs; however, microscopic examination of H&E-stained sections may not be sufficiently sensitive to detect single cells or small cell clusters that differentiate into normal-appearing cells at the location in which they lodge. For such small aggregates, biodistribution may be assessed using IHC, ISH, or other biochemical or molecular methods to detect antigens or mRNA found only in the engrafted (usually human) cells. For example, ISH for human-specific *Alu* DNA sequences (Batzer and Deininger, 1991) and/or human-specific pan-centromeric genomic sequences or IHC for human nuclear (HuNu) antigen (clone 235-1) can be used to identify human-derived elements, including individual cells, in rodent tissues. When biodistribution assessment is only conducted in the context of a carcinogenicity assay, additional animals should be assessed at one or more earlier time points to determine where cells migrate and survive for a period of time before gradually being lost.

Abnormal Differentiation

Products derived from differentiated stem cell precursors theoretically may not retain their intended differentiation pattern or may differentiate into unexpected phenotypes if they settle in an unanticipated location. Unexpected differentiation patterns create both efficacy and safety concerns; dedifferentiation may reduce or abrogate the cells' intended function, while an unforeseen phenotype may result in harmful functions ("toxicity"). Immunodeficient rodent models may be used to discover unexpected patterns of differentiation. If the transplanted human cells survive and propagate for long periods, their progeny and any unanticipated differentiation patterns usually can be identified in H&E-stained and IHC-labeled sections produced from routine paraffin-embedded tissues generated from studies assessing potential toxicity or carcinogenicity (i.e., teratoma formation) endpoints. For more information on stem cell–based therapies, see *Stem Cells and Regenerative Medicine*, Vol 2, Chap 10.

Toxicity

Toxicity of transplanted human cell–based products can be assessed in immunodeficient rodent models. The design of these studies may vary for each specific product and its intended use. Since each cell-based therapy has its own nonclinical and clinical safety concerns, study designs and the length of general toxicity studies should be negotiated in advance with regulatory agencies to ensure that the studies will adequately support their intended function.

In most cases, human stem cell–based products should be administered to animals in general toxicity and carcinogenicity studies by the clinical route of administration and at a frequency representing that to be used for human patients. For example, if cells are to be injected into the myocardium in humans, they should be injected into the myocardium in immunodeficient rodents. In some cases, this may mean that surgical implantation is required for each animal and that control animals should be subjected to a similar sham surgical procedure (ideally by vehicle injection, but at least by needle penetration into the myocardium). More than one "dose" level (i.e., number of cells per injection) is usually tested, and a negative control group should be included. For products designed to survive for extended periods within the patient, it may be necessary to evaluate the chronic toxicity of a product in animals prior to any human clinical testing. In these cases, the primary toxicity assessment and the carcinogenicity assessment may be combined within the same study. Shorter nonclinical studies also may be required in animals to evaluate biodistribution and toxicity when products such as mesenchymal stem cells (MSCs) are not expected to survive indefinitely in patients.

General toxicity studies supporting registration of human cell–based products should include a careful evaluation of the site of administration and any expected areas of cellular proliferation as well as a more standard general gross and microscopic assessment of all major organ systems. Routine hematology and clinical chemistry typically should be evaluated even though the leukogram and the morphology of lymphoid organs may be difficult to interpret in immunodeficient rodents due to the lack of robust historical control data for such strains. Program-specific endpoints may be added when these are appropriate.

Carcinogenicity

By definition, ES cells are totipotent and can differentiate into any tissue or organ in the body. iPSC, hematopoietic stem cells (HSCs), and MSCs have begun to differentiate along a particular precursor cell lineage and thus typically have a more limited range of differentiation. In developing medical products from human stem cells of any kind, a major concern is that the cells will proliferate without control and develop into benign teratomas (i.e., neoplasms that exhibit multi-lineage differentiation with elements resembling epithelial, mesenchymal, and neural tissues); malignant teratocarcinomas; or tumors that resemble the differentiated phenotype of the transplanted cells (Fink, 2009; Fong et al., 2010; Goldring et al., 2011; Hentze et al., 2009; Heslop et al., 2015; Lee et al., 2009; Sharpe et al., 2012). This concern is founded on the twin principles that (i) some undifferentiated stem cells capable of forming neoplasms may remain in any product derived from stem cells and that (ii) stem cells usually cannot be removed once they have been administered.

A carcinogenicity assessment strategy and study design should be tailored to each specific cell-based product and indication in collaboration with regulatory authorities. All aspects of the in vivo nonclinical safety study designs, including dose levels, the animal model, and the number of animals per group, should be discussed with regulatory authorities prior to study initiation. The goal for most cell products derived from ES cells or iPSCs is to terminally differentiate the cells in vitro prior to administration so that they do not divide and cannot form neoplasms once injected into the patient. The final form of the human cell–based product should be used for toxicity and carcinogenicity testing whenever possible. For example, the carrier, excipients, and extracellular matrix used for the final product in humans should be included in the formulation for the safety studies whenever feasible. Addition of extracellular matrix (e.g., Matrigel®), cell culture medium, and/or feeder cells should match the final composition of the clinical product as closely as possible; inclusion of Matrigel® has been shown to enhance teratoma formation (Prokhorova et al., 2009). If the cells are implanted on an organic scaffold or in a device composed of inorganic material (e.g., a semipermeable membrane), this material should be used for animal testing if possible.

Regulatory agencies have asked that negative and positive control groups be included in studies of carcinogenicity (teratoma) potential for human cell–based therapies. The negative control may be a cell-free sample of the medium used in the final product (i.e., "vehicle"). Positive control groups are intended to demonstrate that teratomas can occur in the model system selected. Since the intent of this cohort is to confirm that the animal model works (i.e., is capable of predicting the risk of tumor development for stem cell–based therapies), the positive control group need not be as large as other groups in the study if the positive control cell line readily forms teratomas. Because residual, undifferentiated pluripotent stem cells may persist in the final human cell–based product and could initiate tumor development in transplanted patients, undifferentiated stem cells from the source used to derive the differentiated cell product usually will be the most suitable positive control. These cells should be administered in the same location and manner as the differentiated final product if possible. The positive control group should be treated as similarly as possible to the groups treated with the intended human-derived product.

When feasible, several dose levels of the final cell product should be administered to explore a dose response. At least 1×10^6 stem cells often are required to enable the formation of teratomas, so at least one dose level of the product being tested should equal or exceed this number of cells. If practicable, the highest dose in the animal model should be at least 10-fold higher than the actual anticipated human dose. Orthotopic surgical injection or implantation (i.e., the location in the animal corresponding to the organ or tissue to be treated in humans) may limit the number of cells that can be engrafted into some locations in rodents, especially mice. If a maximum feasible number of cells is used as the highest dose, an explanation regarding why higher doses are not possible should be stated clearly in the product registration package.

The number of animals in each treatment group will vary depending on the product, the route of administration, and technical feasibility. Six-month $p53^{+/-}$ and rasH2 mouse studies for carcinogenicity testing of small molecules require 25 mice/sex/treatment group based on power analysis and spontaneous tumor rates of up to 5%–7% for some tumor types in most rodent strains. However, 15 or fewer animals/sex/group may be sufficient to evaluate teratoma formation by human cell–based products because spontaneous teratomas and teratocarcinomas are extremely rare in mice. When surgical transplantation to the orthotopic site is technically challenging, the numbers of animals in each dose group may be further limited. The carcinogenicity assessment may use as few as six animals/sex/group at three different time points because of such technical constraints.

The normal lifespan of the rodent model selected should be considered when determining the length of chronic studies for human cell-based products. If few pluripotential stem cells capable of teratoma formation are present, teratoma formation often takes more than 12 weeks. Thus, the duration of treatment in long-term studies exploring teratoma formation should be as long as reasonably possible, and a length of at least 12 months has been suggested as a desirable target (Carpenter et al., 2009). However, many lines of immunodeficient rodents survive for less than 1 year; six-month studies beginning at 7–8 weeks of age may encompass most of the natural lifespan of many of these immunodeficient rodent models, so two-year studies generally are not practical. Immunodeficient rodents over 6 months of age may develop spontaneous tumors that can confound interpretation of teratoma formation, biodistribution, and abnormal differentiation of the cell-based product. For these reasons, the NOG mouse strain with its average lifespan exceeding 1 year may be a suitable model for carcinogenicity testing of cell-based products, especially if studies lasting more than 6 months are deemed preferable. Consideration should be given to terminating a dose group or even the entire study when survival in one or more dose groups reaches a specific threshold (perhaps five survivors in either sex).

Formation of teratomas or differentiated neoplasms consistent with the lineage of the final cell product will be the chief parameter to be examined, but other factors should be assessed as well. In-life endpoints should include body weight, food consumption, and clinical signs as well as regular assessments to detect both teratomas and toxicity. Hematology and clinical chemistry analytes may be included if these parameters have not been adequately evaluated in prior studies. Palpation to detect masses may be worthwhile if cells in large numbers are injected at superficial locations that may produce externally detectable neoplasms. Teratomas often can be palpable within a few weeks of subcutaneous or intramuscular injection of undifferentiated (totipotent) ES cells. Typically, more differentiated (pluripotent) cell products may form teratomas much more slowly, if teratomas are formed at all. Upon study termination, a complete necropsy should be conducted on every animal in the study. The site of treatment (xenograft implantation or cell injection sites) and the full list of tissues commonly examined in routine GLP-compliant rodent toxicology studies should be collected from all animals into appropriate fixatives. For studies evaluating teratoma formation in immunodeficient rodents, all protocol tissues as well as gross lesions from vehicle control and high-dose animals should be examined microscopically to evaluate for teratoma formation at the site of treatment, the distribution and survival of transplanted cells at unexpected sites, differentiation patterns of stem cell progeny, and potential toxicity associated with the presence or function of the cell product. A reasonable addition to this standard pathology analysis would be to examine microscopically the intended site(s) of cell delivery and gross lesions in all animals in the other treated groups and in the positive control group. Microscopic examination of remaining tissues in the low and intermediate dose groups could be limited to target organs of interest based on findings in the high-dose group.

The observation of any teratomas in treated animals may raise concerns for the safety of patients. The rarity of teratomas in laboratory rodents implies that teratomas would be presumed to be derived from the human cell product. When teratomas or other neoplasms develop at any site, it may be useful to determine whether or not these neoplasms actually originate from the foreign cells (see "Biodistribution" section above). Neoplasms shown to arise from the model species should not represent a safety concern for foreign cell products.

In some cases, it may be possible to combine animal efficacy testing with in vivo nonclinical safety assessment if an appropriate disease model can be replicated in immunodeficient rodents or immune rejection of transplanted cells can be prevented in an immunocompetent model. This approach may require testing of a broad range of cell doses, several of which will exceed the therapeutic dose. Efficacy biomarkers may be incorporated into animal safety studies if the anticipated therapeutic effect can be produced and measured.

3.6. Humanized Animal Models

Nonengineered animals do not always provide a relevant platform for assessing specific mechanisms of toxicity or addressing broad general safety concerns. This shortcoming is most common for fully human protein products that have little off-target activity and cannot be studied in animals either because the candidate molecule is not pharmacologically active in nonhuman cells or because the animal model mounts an antihuman immune response that quickly limits exposure or neutralizes the activity of the foreign protein. In these cases, GEM models that have been "humanized" by introducing human molecules or cells may provide insights into mechanisms and pathways of efficacy and potential toxicity (Lin, 2008). Less commonly, specific safety issues must be studied in a genetically engineered animal model created to express molecular entities specific to a human disease because the required molecular target does not exist in normal animals or only exists in the disease state.

Engineered Models Expressing Human Molecules

When human-specific biomolecules are not pharmacologically active in rodents or exposure cannot be maintained at sufficient levels to assess toxicity, safety concerns may be addressed in nonclinical studies utilizing a "humanized" animal model. This strategy is based on genetic engineering to overexpress a human target (as a transgene or targeted knockin) for human-derived proteins that act as agonists; the opposite situation, specific ablation of the rodent target (to yield a knockout) is used if the human molecule is an antagonist, but does not introduce a humanizing DNA sequence. Such engineering usually is performed to produce expression of the human protein throughout in utero and postnatal development, so that the molecule is presented to the animal's immune system as a "self" protein. However, postnatal modification using gene therapy also may be effective for this purpose if the level of expression is sufficiently high to permit activity of the human protein even in the presence of the animal's immune response.

Genetically modified animals expressing a human target may be given the clinical candidate to assess both efficacy (i.e., pharmacology) and toxicity. Indeed, some nonclinical studies using GEMs are purposely designed to evaluate both efficacy and toxicity. Animals overexpressing the human target may provide safety information without drug administration. Most monoclonal antibodies are antagonists, so the use of knockout animals is considered more frequently for nonclinical safety assessment when designing studies for monoclonal antibody programs. Knockout models are commonly studied to define the effect of complete target inhibition without having to administer the therapeutic candidate.

In general, drug administration to "humanized" GEM models is employed as a strategy more often for efficacy evaluations than for safety assessment. The main endpoint in such efficacy studies is to ascertain whether or not the agent has a desired pharmacological effect. However, examination of key potential target organs for toxicity within the context of efficacy studies can provide very early awareness of potential nonclinical safety issues prior to the beginning of routine nonclinical safety testing. For example, perivascular edema and microhemorrhage has been observed in the brains of humans vaccinated against human amyloid beta (Aβ) peptides, a major constituent of the amyloid plaques that are thought to contribute to the neurotoxicity and cognitive deficits in patients with Alzheimer's disease. GEM models that express either human Aβ or human APP (the parent molecule from which Aβ is produced) develop numerous amyloid plaques in the cerebral cortex and hippocampus as well

as cognitive deficits similar to those in human Alzheimer's disease. These transgenic models are used as efficacy models for potential plaque-preventing or plaque-dissolving monoclonal antibody therapies; they also develop perivascular edema and microhemorrhage of the brain as an adverse response when exposed to antibodies that react with human Aβ (Kou et al., 2011). Thus, such models and others like them provide investigators with tools to simultaneously assess both therapeutic utility and undesired side effects (Esquerda-Canals et al., 2017; Jankowsky and Zheng, 2017).

A related approach to evaluating the potential toxicity of novel candidates is to use "humanized" GEM models to examine the likelihood that extended treatment will produce off-target side effects without actually administering a product candidate. For instance, transgenic mice that overexpress human APP develop large cerebrocortical plaque loads due to the action of β-secretase in cleaving the precursor protein at just the right site to produce Aβ (Figure 23.9). However, β-secretase is expressed at high levels not only in the brain but also in many peripheral tissues. Genetically engineered animals in which mouse β-secretase has been deleted do not develop anatomic, biochemical, or functional phenotypes, suggesting that extended inhibition of this enzyme would not produce adverse effects in either the brain or extraneural tissues (Luo et al., 2001). Furthermore, cross-breeding of APP transgenic mice and β-secretase knockout animals prevents the generation of Aβ plaques, indicating that β-secretase inhibition may represent an efficacious pharmacological target for treating Alzheimer's disease while producing few systemic side effects (Luo et al., 2003). To date, however, efforts to demonstrate clinical efficacy of β-secretase inhibition in humans have not fulfilled the promise suggested by the prior work in GEM models (Houlton, 2019), leading many companies to shift toward assessing test articles that are designed to impact other mechanisms proposed as drivers of Alzheimer's disease.

A further strategy for using "humanized" GEM models in efficacy and toxicity testing is to employ them to examine the likely effects of an injected biomolecule (Walsh et al., 2017). For example, artemin is a neurotrophic factor that is expressed principally in the peripheral

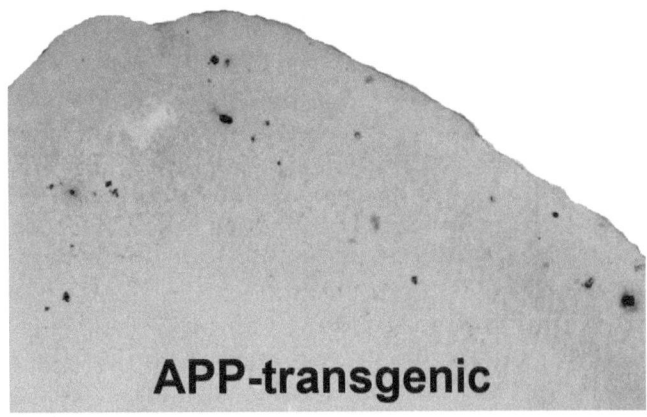

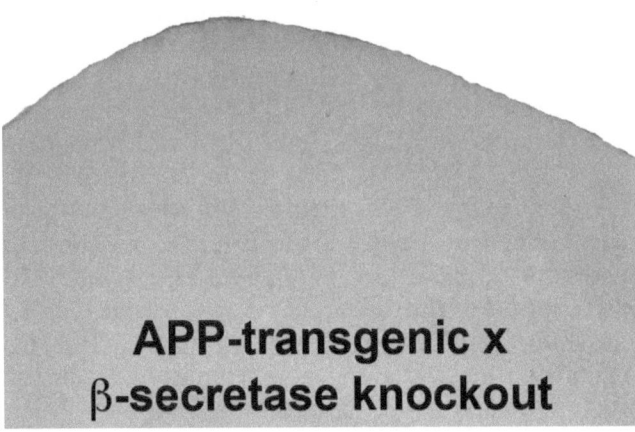

FIGURE 23.9 **Use of genetically engineered mice (GEM) for combined nonclinical assessment of efficacy and safety.** Drug discovery studies for large biomolecules often utilize GEM models to simultaneously evaluate therapeutic candidates for efficacy and toxicity. In this case, one-year-old amyloid precursor protein (APP) transgenic mice develop insoluble amyloid-β (Aβ) plaques (black deposits) in the cerebral cortex (upper panel) equivalent to those observed at this site in human patients with Alzheimer's disease. Age-matched mice both transgenic for APP and lacking the gene for β-secretase—a widely distributed enzyme that makes the critical cut in APP leading to production of Aβ in the brain—do not develop plaques (lower panel), showing that removal of β-secretase activity is a suitable means for preventing the plaques that are thought to have pathogenic significance for Alzheimer's disease. Removal of β-secretase in peripheral tissues did not induce clinical, functional, or structural phenotypes in other systems (not shown), suggesting that pharmacological inhibition of β-secretase might have a limited adverse effect profile. Stain: anti-Aβ immunohistochemistry with hematoxylin counterstain. *Adapted from Luo Y, Bolon B, Damore MA, et al.: BACE1 (β-secretase) knockout mice do not acquire compensatory gene expression changes or develop neural lesions over time, Neurobiol Dis 14, 81–88, 2003, by permission.*

nervous system, suggesting that it might be of use as a treatment for peripheral neuropathies. Parallel studies to insert a transgene for recombinant human artemin (rhArt) by embryonic microinjection or viral gene therapy in adult mice indicate that overexpression of this factor for extended periods is associated with extensive proliferation of the autonomic nervous system in many peripheral tissues, especially the adrenal gland and sympathetic ganglia. These GEM experiments predicted the outcome of studies in which repeated injection of rhArt led to neuronal metaplasia in the adrenal medulla. Unbridled proliferation of autonomic nervous system components—an undesired off-target effect ("toxicity")—coupled with the absence of clinical efficacy in rodents with tactile allodynia (i.e., heightened perception of pain peripherally after a nonpainful touch) led to termination of artemin as a therapeutic candidate without incurring the expense of a major nonclinical safety assessment effort (Bolon et al., 2004).

Similarly, GEM models with humanized immune systems have proven useful in the investigation and development of therapeutic biomolecules (Peterson, 2005; Obenaus et al., 2015). For example, human leukocyte antigen-A2 (*HLA-A2*) transgenic mice immunized with the gp100: 154–162 epitope from the gp100 melanoma–melanocyte antigen generate over time a high-avidity T-cell receptor (TCR) against the human antigen (Johnson et al., 2009). Administration of cells expressing this murine-derived TCR to patients with metastatic melanoma yielded a cancer regression in 19% of patients. Mice generated with transgenes for the entire human TCR, both T-cell receptor α (*TCRA*) and T-cell receptor β (*TCRB*), as well as for human *HLA-A*0201* but deficient for murine *TCRA* and *TCRB* possess polyclonal, fully human T-cell diversity in the circulation and thymus and have been used to generate and isolate tumor-associated antigen–specific TCRs that have superior antitumor effect in xenograft efficacy studies (Li et al., 2010). GEMs expressing the human neonatal Fc receptor in conjunction with knockout of several murine genes (i.e., the *Fcgrt* model = B6.Cg-*Fcgrt*^tm1Dcr^*Prkdc*^scid^Tg(FCGRT)32Dcr/DcrJ, The Jackson Laboratory) have been touted for use in early drug discovery to evaluate PK of therapeutic human IgG antibodies (Avery et al., 2016;

Betts et al., 2018; Proetzel and Roopenian, 2014). Numerous recombinant and fully human antibodies developed in transgenic mice carrying human immunoglobulin genes (e.g., XenoMouse® or HuMab Mouse® technology) have been successfully brought to market (Strohl, 2018).

Engineered Immunodeficient Mice with Reconstituted Chimeric or Human Organs

Although the conventional genetic engineering technologies described above provide the means to examine the effects of altering single or multiple proteins (including the addition of human molecules into animal systems), an important goal for improving the assessment of pharmaceutical efficacy and safety is to develop animal models that more fully recapitulate human organ physiology or human diseases. This feat will require engineering not of individual molecules but rather of entire cells, tissues, or organ fractions. Since human cells are not rejected after implantation into severely immunodeficient rodents, it is possible to transplant small quantities of normal, diseased, or neoplastic human tissues or cells into these animals to investigate cellular metabolism, disease mechanisms, human pathogens (which require human cells for propagation of the infectious agent), therapeutic efficacy (e.g., testing of antineoplastic agents using human tumor xenografts), and xenobiotic toxicity.

CHIMERIC ORGANS

Recent advances in engineering animals with more profound immunodeficiencies (e.g., NOG mice) have improved the ability to model human physiological conditions in vivo using animals. A major thrust of current research efforts is to manipulate the organ composition of mouse organs in such a fashion that they are capable of being reconstituted by the addition of human-derived orthotopic cells.

Chimeric human–mouse livers containing large numbers of engrafted human hepatocytes are one active area of human chimeric organ research involving engineered immunodeficient mice (Katoh et al., 2008; Strom et al., 2010). The three main chimeric liver models (briefly discussed below) may be useful for evaluating antiviral agents that target human hepatitis viruses and retroviruses, the metabolism of small molecules by human enzymatic pathways, and mechanisms of xenobiotic action in human cells. The substitution of human hepatocytes for mouse cells is accomplished by creating GEM in which the sensitivity of endogenous murine hepatocytes to toxic insults is enhanced; administration of the toxicant destroys the native mouse cells, leaving a permissive environment for colonization by engrafted human hepatocytes that have been injected into the spleen under anesthesia. The percentage of the liver reconstituted with human hepatocytes can be estimated by measuring the concentration of human albumin in the serum.

In each chimeric liver model, functional restoration with human-derived processes is variable but often substantial, while structural reestablishment is limited. Numerous human-specific molecules have been confirmed to reside in the reconstituted organs. Important examples include human CYPs; phase II metabolizing enzymes; transporter proteins; nuclear receptors, such as CAR, PPAR, and PXR; and human-specific metabolism of particular chemicals. Microscopic analysis reveals that the engrafted human hepatocytes colonize in clusters within the mouse liver, with mouse endothelial and sinusoidal cells separating and supporting human hepatocytes; normal sinusoidal and lobular architecture are incompletely restored in the human hepatocyte clusters. Cells of human and mouse origin can be distinguished based on their differing morphologies (i.e., human hepatocytes typically are smaller, contain more glycogen, and form irregular clusters rather than normal hepatic cords); IHC for human hepatocyte–specific antigens (e.g., complement C3a, cytokeratins 8 and 18, mitochondrial proteins); and/or ISH for human-specific mRNA sequences (Figure 23.10). The replacement index (i.e., the extent to which human hepatocytes replace mouse cells) varies with many factors, including the number of engrafted human cells, but currently can be adjusted to range from 5% to over 90%. An important feature of GEM chimeric liver models is that their human hepatocellular metabolic machinery more closely replicates human rather than

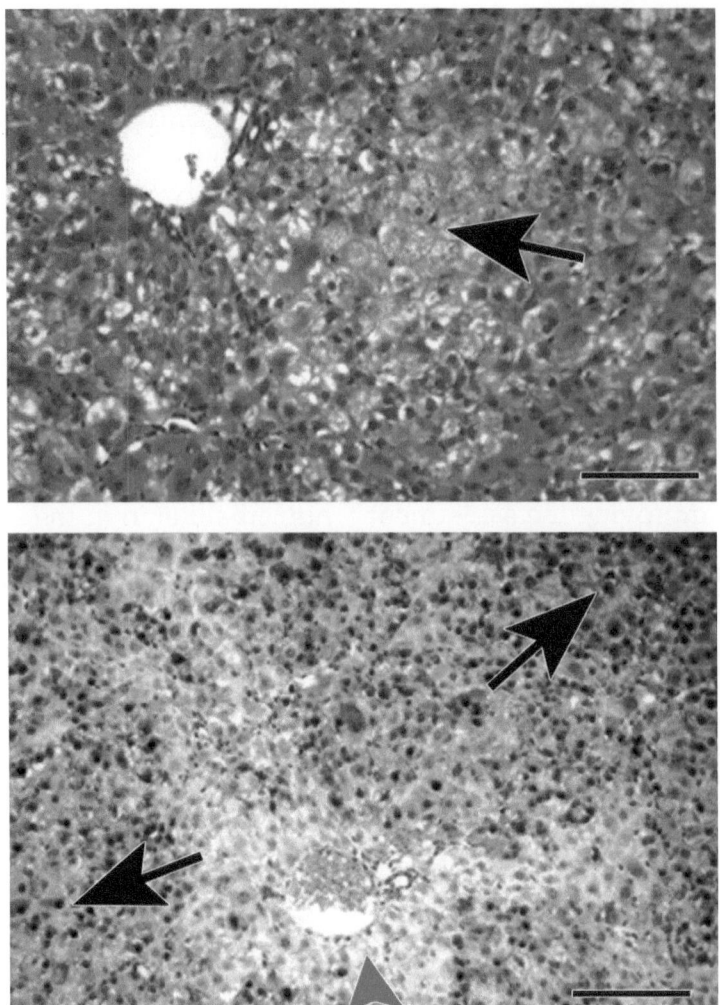

FIGURE 23.10   **Use of "humanized" genetically engineered mice (GEM) for evaluating the response of human cells in vivo.** Chimeric human–mouse organs are made by creating profoundly immunodeficient GEM in which endogenous mouse cells are deleted by a genetic manipulation leading to spontaneous or drug-induced hepatocellular toxicity and then replaced with human cells. For example, in a chimeric human–mouse liver model, the residual mouse hepatocytes (darkly eosinophilic cells in upper panel, unstained cells in lower panel; red arrowhead) can be differentiated from the colonizing human hepatocytes (pale cells in upper panel, brown-stained cells in lower panel; arrows) using routine histopathologic techniques. Anatomic restoration of hepatic cords and sinusoids is minimal by the engrafted cells, while reestablishment of organ function is substantial. Chimeric liver from a $Fah^{-/-}/Rag2^{-/-}/IL2r\gamma^{-/-}$ mouse reconstituted with human hepatocytes. Stains: H&E (upper) and anti-Fah (fumarylacetoacetate hydrolase) immunohistochemistry (lower image). *Adapted from Azuma H, Paulk N, Ranade A, et al.: Robust expansion of human hepatocytes in* Fah-/-/Rag2-/-/Il2rg-/- mice, Nat Biotechnol 25, 903–910, 2007, with permission.

mouse pathways for drug metabolism, so chimeric livers are much less susceptible to acetaminophen toxicity than are the normal livers of wild-type control mice.

The three engineered mouse–human chimeric liver models all are based on cell type–specific gene manipulation of mouse hepatocytes to selectively increase their vulnerability to hepatotoxic injury. The immunodeficient state then is superimposed by crossing animals with the modified gene with other mouse lines in which one or more leukocyte lineages is dysfunctional.

- The first chimeric mouse–human liver to be developed was the urokinase-like plasminogen activator (*uPA*) transgenic mouse model (Emoto et al., 2011). The mouse *uPA* transgene, when under control of an albumin promoter sequence, drives expression of mouse uPA in mouse hepatocytes to induce hepatocyte-specific cell death. Hepatic organization remains intact in these animals as only hepatocytes expressing the transgene are deleted; surviving mouse hepatocytes have been shown to undergo internal gene recombination that quenches expression of the transgene, thereby sparing their host cells. Subsequent crossing of *uPA* transgenic mice with immunocompromised recombination activating gene 2 (Rag2)-deficient or SCID animals results in progeny that accept transplanted human hepatocytes. The utility of this chimeric liver model is limited because human hepatocytes must be transplanted into the immunodeficient *uPA* transgenic mice prior to weaning, which is technically challenging, and because the animals are susceptible to early-onset liver failure, severe coagulopathy, and renal damage secondary to uPA expression, the combination of which commonly leads to reduced survival.

- The second GEM chimeric liver model utilizes a targeted deletion of the *Fah* (fumarylacetoacetate hydrolase) gene (Azuma et al., 2007). Crossing $Fah^{-/-}$ mice with animals lacking both Rag2 and interleukin-2 (IL-2) receptor common γ chain receptor ($Rag2^{-/-}/IL2r\gamma^{-/-}$) yields a severely immunodeficient triple knockout mouse (denoted FRG) that accepts human xenografts. The Fah protein is part of the metabolic pathway that catabolizes tyrosine, and absence of this protein leads to accumulation of a metabolite that is toxic to mouse hepatocytes. Accumulation of the toxic metabolite and resulting hepatotoxicity can be prevented by treating the mice with 2-(2-nitro-4-trifluoro-methylbenzoyl) 1,3-cyclohexedione (NTBC), allowing them to remain healthy until transplantation occurs. Withdrawal of NTBC shortly before injection of the human hepatocytes produces controlled toxicity of the mouse hepatocytes to facilitate colonization of the liver by transplanted human hepatocytes that contain the functional Fah enzyme. Transplanted mice will lose weight and eat less after 1–2 weeks without NTBC, so NTBC must be given intermittently in order to maintain transplanted mice for long periods of time and prevent the development of hepatocellular carcinoma derived from residual murine hepatocytes. The intermittent treatment with NTBC can complicate some experiments. Human hepatocytes can be identified in tissue sections using IHC for the Fah protein. The FRG model can be used to serially transplant and expand hepatocytes from a single donor.

- The third GEM chimeric liver model is the TK-NOG mouse, in which a herpesvirus simplex virus type I (HSV) thymidine kinase (TK) gene (abbreviated *HSV-tk*) controlled by a liver-specific albumin promoter has been inserted into NOD/shi mouse zygotes (Hasegawa et al., 2011). These transgenic mice then are crossed with SCID/γc^{null} mice to create severely immunodeficient TK-NOG mice. The TK-NOG animals are healthy and have normal livers. When treated with gancyclovir (a drug that treats HSV infections by utilizing the viral TK to produce a toxic metabolite), the liver-specific expression of TK protein results in selective destruction of the mouse hepatocytes; gancyclovir is not toxic to mammalian cells lacking the viral TK, so cell lineages other than hepatocytes are not affected. Gancyclovir-induced loss of mouse hepatocytes prior to transplantation primes the liver to accept the human hepatocytes. Drug treatment is not required once human hepatocytes are introduced into the mice, but further enrichment of human hepatocytes in the chimeric livers can be produced by giving an additional gancyclovir treatment after the human hepatocytes have become established. The TK-NOG model usually produces a high level of hepatocyte engraftment that persists for at least 8 months without the need for concurrent chemical treatment and does so without producing generalized toxicity in other organs and systems.

These three chimeric liver models may have value in pharmaceutical discovery and development for predicting human ADME properties and exploring mechanisms of hepatic metabolism and toxicity because they use human cells in an in vivo setting. Although these relatively new chimeric liver models have rarely been used for pharmaceutical ADME and toxicity assessments, emerging evidence suggests that these models could be very valuable in safety assessment. For example, mice with chimeric livers have been used to define the mechanism by which fialuridine, a nucleoside analogue for the treatment of hepatitis B virus infection, produced acute lethal liver failure in patients during a clinical trial after warning signs of hepatotoxicity were not observed in conventional animals during the nonclinical safety assessment program (Manning et al., 1995; McKenzie et al., 1995; Xu et al., 2014). Fialuridine-induced liver toxicity was easily reproduced in the TK-NOG mice with humanized livers, and the cause was shown to be the direct effect of the drug specifically on human hepatocytes. Despite recapitulation of several human-predominant drug-related adverse effects, outstanding questions and potential limitations remain with these chimeric liver models. Investigators should consider the variable levels of human cell engraftment, the expense and limited availability of appropriate animals (each mouse must be transplanted individually with human cells), and the uncertain behavior and tissue organization of human cells grown in a mouse when deciding whether or not to employ one of these models.

Chimeric human–mouse bone marrow models have been created to investigate normal and neoplastic human hematopoietic lineages in vivo (Ito et al., 2017; Shultz et al., 2012; Takenaka et al., 2007). These models are generated by using irradiation to ablate the existing bone marrow of highly immunocompromised mice and then giving an IV injection of human HSCs. Mice that are commonly used to generate chimeric bone marrow models, such as the $NOD.Cg\text{-}Prkdc^{scid}\ Il2rg^{tm1Wjl}/SzJ$ (NSG) mouse (The Jackson Laboratory) and the $NOD.cg\text{-}Prkdc^{scid}Il2rg^{tm1}Sug$ (NOG) mouse (Taconic Biosciences, Inc.), harbor a mutation in the IL-2 receptor γ-chain locus, which leads to severe impairment in both B-cell and T-cell development and function while completely preventing the development of NK cells. NSG mice have a NOD strain-derived polymorphism of signal regulatory protein α (*Sirpa*) that closely resembles that of human *Sirpa*, permitting appropriate recognition of human CD47 on hematopoietic cells and supporting higher levels of human HSC engraftment and survival in mice. Current commercially available models can be used in the drug development space to provide insights into drug-associated, lineage-specific toxicities. Examples of available models include hu-CD34-NSG mice (The Jackson Laboratory), triple transgenic NSG-SGM3 mice (The Jackson Laboratory), and huNOG-EXLmice (Taconic Biosciences). The hu-CD34-NSG and huNOG-EXL mice are humanized with CD34$^+$ HSCs and demonstrate a robust engraftment of human cells in the bone marrow with multi-lineage hematopoiesis of human cells. The NSG-SGM3 mice support a stable engraftment of CD33$^+$ myeloid lineages and provide cell proliferation and survival signals for engrafted cells through the production of human cytokines (e.g., stem cell factor, granulocyte–macrophage colony-stimulating factor, and interleukin-3 [IL-3]).

Multichimeric human–mouse models have been generated in recent years to aid in basic and applied research designed to evaluate the human immune response to various infective agents. For example, the BLT (bone marrow, liver, thymus) mouse is generated by surgical engraftment of human fetal and thymus tissue into immunodeficient mice—usually on the NOD/SCID, NSG, or $Rag2^{-/-}/IL2r\gamma^{-/-}$ background—followed by IV injection of human fetal CD34$^+$ HSCs to introduce human lymphoid and myeloid cells (Lavender et al., 2018). The degree of human chimerism varies among animals, but the human cells may be found in both the human xenografts and in the cell type-appropriate, homologous mouse tissues. Such models have been suggested as a potential avenue for evaluating the efficacy and safety profiles of antiretroviral cocktails and potential vaccination protocols for use in combating HIV infections (Lavender et al., 2018).

Pharmaceutical applications of chimeric organ models are limited at this time. However, while the slow rise in utility stems both from the expense of the multiengineered, immunocompromised animals and also from technical considerations—chiefly the extensive variability in replacement index among different engrafted mice—the presence of commercially available and ready-to-use chimeric models helps in mitigating some of the downsides. Despite their utility, these models are not viewed as a replacement for conventional nonclinical toxicity studies of small molecule or biologic therapeutic candidates but rather as additional investigational tools. The lack of historical control data for these models also is a deterrent for undertaking GLP-type studies using these animals. When interpreting the relevance of data acquired in these models for human risk assessment, factors such as the complexity of immunodeficient GEM systems, confounding factors of the chimeric condition, the combination of the juxtaposed human and murine cellular pathways, and the almost complete lack of immune functions always need to be considered.

HUMAN TUMOR XENOGRAFTS

Another way to assess the interaction of a drug candidate with a human target is to create an immunodeficient mouse with transplanted patient-derived tumor cells or tumor fragments, or alternatively by introduction of human-origin tumor cell lines. Collectively, these cell-based samples usually are termed "tumor xenografts," and the modified animals often are referred to as "patient-derived xenograft" (PDX) mice or "avatars." These models are based on mouse strains that have been engineered to ignore engrafted human cells (i.e., immunodeficient). Xenografts of any possible histogenesis may be evaluated, including unusual neoplasms that occur so rarely that prospective human clinical investigations are virtually impossible. An additional adjustment included in some PDX protocols is to inject both tumor cells and peripheral blood mononuclear cells (PBMCs) from the patient so that the tumor microenvironment also includes the existing immune elements that might be capable of mounting an antitumor response.

The most common pharmaceutical applications of these models are to assess the tissue penetration and/or efficacy of potential antineoplastic agents (Combest et al., 2012). Such studies generally involve multiple treatment groups which vary in terms of either the mass of implanted cells ("tumor dose") or the amount of test article that is administered ("drug dose"). Xenografts are often implanted in the subcutis of the flank or back for easier access and in-life observation, but in other cases, the human cells are placed in the orthotopic location in the mouse. Typical endpoints for evaluating efficacy in tumor xenografts are decreased growth (in terms of both the growth rate and final mass) during life as well as the extent of cell death (i.e., apoptosis or necrosis) and proliferation that can be detected by microscopic evaluation. The cell turnover parameters are valued further because they may provide mechanistic data regarding the process by which the agent is damaging tumor cells. Such studies may also be used to identify and characterize cell type–specific or prognostic markers that may be adapted for use in human patients. While carefully controlled, efficacy studies using xenografts usually are not performed in compliance with GLP guidelines. The genetic and biological correspondence of the tumor model to the human counterpart is important to increase confidence in the translation of nonclinical experimental results to clinical efficacy. Compared to tumor cell lines, PDX models maintain the heterogeneity of their parental tumors as well as a more complete human tumor microenvironment. However, the paucity of translational models that recapitulate both human tumor growth and functionality of the human immune system is an obstacle when evaluating immunotherapeutic drug candidates. While immunodeficient mice lack the intact human immune component, xenograft-bearing mouse models that have received both human tumor cells and human PBMCs allow the simulation of real patient responses and more translatable nonclinical immuno-oncology research (Choi et al., 2018; Walsh et al., 2017).

Nonetheless, nonclinical safety information also may be gathered from efficacy studies done by implanting tumor xenografts in immunodeficient GEM and GER models. The typical assessment undertaken in this regard emphasizes clinical pathology and histopathological analyses of selected fluids and tissues (e.g., blood and major viscera that are commonly targeted by antineoplastic agents, like heart, intestine, kidney, liver, and lymphoid organs) to obtain an early signal of potential target organ toxicity. Clinical pathology endpoints examining bone marrow sufficiency may be profitable as well.

Surrogate Animal Models for Human-Based Molecules

It is preferred that the actual clinical product or molecule be tested in nonclinical studies if possible. However, under certain circumstances, a suitable animal model cannot be defined. Examples of such difficulties include human-specific molecules that are not pharmacologically active in animals, or that have unexpected activities when interacting with animal signaling pathways (e.g., oncostatin M) (Juan et al., 2009); exposures that cannot be maintained at sufficiently high levels due to the animal's immunological response; or animal models that are too variable for use in GLP-type safety studies (e.g., the current generation of GEM chimeric liver models). In such instances, product safety concerns may be addressed in nonclinical studies by using species-specific (usually rodent) homologs of the human molecule as surrogate test articles for use in wild-type rodents.

Such surrogate molecules (usually a signaling molecule or antibody) specifically react with the relevant rodent homolog of the intended human target molecule (typically a cell receptor or soluble ligand) and thus are pharmacologically active in the chosen test species. Surrogate proteins are produced by conventional recombinant DNA technology, and as such typically do not involve genetic modification. However, in some cases, the surrogate may be engineered to add a "flag" (i.e., marker) that permits differentiation of the native molecule from the surrogate in analytical assays for fluid and tissue concentrations. The surrogate molecules are not the clinical candidates that will be tested in humans, but such rodent proteins (primarily monoclonal antibodies) have been used for routine reproductive toxicity conducted in wild-type animals (Bussiere et al., 2009; Clarke et al., 2004). Details for testing surrogate molecules in normal rodents are beyond the scope of this chapter, but basic procedures are detailed further in *Protein Pharmaceutical Agents* (Vol 2, Chap 6).

One of the potential innovative uses for knockout rodents is to predict the carcinogenic potential of target inhibition induced by a monoclonal antibody or other similar protein containing a complementarity-determining region. This strategy may be particularly useful when a pharmacologically relevant rodent species is not available for testing and a surrogate rodent molecule interacting with the homologous rodent target has not been produced. The assessment of potential carcinogenicity risk linked to a drug target should start early in the discovery phase. A product class for which such assessments might add value is cytokine inhibitors, especially those agents that function to downregulate immune system responsiveness. For anakinra (Kineret®), a recombinant nonglycosylated human interleukin-1 receptor antagonist (IL-1ra), IL-1ra knockout mice were utilized as supporting evidence that increased carcinogenic risk noted in animals given high IL-1ra doses were not target related. For ustekinumab (Stelara®), a targeted monoclonal antibody directed against the p40 subunit of interleukin-12 (IL-12) and interleukin-23 (IL-23), a warning of increased risk of malignancy in the product label was derived from the observation that the incidence of ultraviolet radiation–induced skin cancers was increased in mice engineered to lack p40 or treated with anti-p40 antibodies, where p40 is the common subunit essential for the activities of the proinflammatory cytokines IL-12 and IL-23 (Ergen and Yusuf, 2018; Jantschitsch et al., 2012; Maeda et al., 2006; Meeran et al., 2006). In another example, the tumor necrosis factor (TNF) blockers as a class have been given a "black box" warning due to the potential increased risk of malignancies (including lymphomas) in the adult and pediatric populations. The proposed mechanism for this class effect is that blocking master cytokines suppresses the immune system to the point that normal antitumor control mechanisms are disrupted. However, this association is confounded by the strong association between high cumulative disease activity and lymphoma development as well as by the concomitant use of other medications that also may contribute to increased malignancy risk. In *Tnf* knockout or TNF receptor knockout mice, blocking TNF at different stages of tumor growth and in different types of tumors has been associated with marked tumor inhibition. The characterization of long-term effects of TNF inhibitors on infrequent outcomes or in specific subpopulations is needed to better characterize any existing trend. This concept of using GEM models may be considered more often in the future as more biologics are developed to treat diabetes mellitus, hyperlipidemia, neurodegeneration, various inflammatory diseases, and other chronic, noncancer indications. The impetus for such studies is that treatments for noncancer indications typically are given to humans for extended periods of time, and regulatory agencies driven by mechanistic concerns require in vivo nonclinical information to better assess cancer risk.

4. LIMITATIONS IN USING GENETICALLY MODIFIED ANIMALS FOR HAZARD IDENTIFICATION AND SAFETY ASSESSMENT

Whenever animal data are extrapolated to predict human physiological responses, disease mechanisms, PK, PD, toxicity, or carcinogenic potential, there are many uncertainties and risks that the animal data may not be fully relevant to human biology. The main consideration is that any animal model will never fully replicate the human condition; a "humanized" mouse, no matter how superb the genetically engineered target or the chimeric organ restoration, fundamentally remains a mouse. As animal models become more complicated, particularly by adding human molecular pathways and/or cells, accurate interpretation and data translation to the human setting becomes ever more challenging. Genetic manipulation complicates the interpretation of animal models even if the animals appear "normal," but such manipulation also permits evaluation of questions in vivo that cannot be adequately addressed in normal wild-type animals.

Whenever genetically altered animal models are used to address nonclinical safety concerns, the effect of the genetic manipulation must be carefully considered (FDA, 1995, 2003, 2015). Proteins derived from inserted human genes may not interact with downstream rodent pathways in the same way that the proteins work in humans (Juan et al., 2009). The genetic

manipulation may adversely influence the physiology, behavior (Crawley, 2007), and morphology of the animal, so appropriate characterization (phenotyping) of the model for its intended purpose always should precede the conduct and interpretation of nonclinical safety studies. Random insertion of genetic material may produce unintentional, subtle, or striking disruption of normal gene function unrelated to the transgene's function; targeted mutations of the same gene may exhibit different phenotypes due to differences in the extent to which gene expression was altered and subtle variations in the genetic background of the resulting animals. When human cells are grafted into immunodeficient rodents, the cellular microenvironment is never equivalent in the rodent to the state that exists in the normal (or diseased) human organ. Therefore, genetically induced disease models in animals generally should be used for nonclinical safety testing only when more conventional (i.e., wild-type) animal models are not appropriate. Furthermore, such engineered disease models usually are best used to address very specific questions—such as investigating the efficacy of a therapeutic candidate that may only demonstrate activity in the disease state, comparing the nature and extent of efficacy to that of toxicity, or the possible mechanisms responsible for such effects—rather than as models for routine use in nonclinical general toxicology studies (see *Discovery Toxicology and Pathology*, Vol 2, Chap 3). Caution and skepticism should be exercised when novel genetically modified animal models are being considered for use in nonclinical safety assessment.

5. SPECIAL CONSIDERATIONS IN SAFETY ASSESSMENT OF PRODUCTS DERIVED FROM GENETICALLY ENGINEERED ANIMALS

5.1. Biopharming and Xenotransplantation

In addition to serving as models to explore basic biological pathways as well as the efficacy and toxicity of exogenous chemicals and novel drug candidates, genetically engineered animals increasingly are being used as sources for producing various "bioproducts." The most critical applications are "biopharming" (i.e., production of therapeutic proteins by their secretion into a bodily fluid) and xenotransplantation of animal-derived cells or organs into human patients. Manufacture of biopharmaceuticals in transgenic animal bioreactors relies on the availability of genetically engineered livestock (e.g., primarily cattle or goats), although other species (e.g., mice, rats, rabbits, chickens, sheep, and swine) have been utilized as well. Acquisition of donor materials for xenotransplantation typically is undertaken in transgenic swine. Examples of such products are recombinant human antithrombin III (ATryn®), which is produced in the milk of transgenic goats (Adiguzel et al., 2009), and pancreatic islet cells from pigs, which typically are implanted inside a porous membrane (resulting in fabrication of a medical device).

Genetically engineered livestock historically have been generated using standard microinjection technology (as described above), with some limitations, or more commonly via somatic cell nuclear transfer ("cloning"). The benefit of cloning relative to direct nuclear injection is that all cells in the embryo are assured of retaining the desired genotype of the donor animal—which will be a confirmed transgenic individual—including gametes needed to produce subsequent generations to expand the line. Using cattle as an example, this seemingly small advantage is of major importance in more quickly building a herd given the long generation intervals and huge costs of producing an economically viable engineered calf by traditional means (approximately USD $500,000 to $1 million and hundreds to 1000 or more embryos). Efforts to engineer other species of livestock species (e.g., goats, sheep, rabbits, chickens) typically are less expensive due to the larger number of progeny per pregnancy/cycle, the shorter interval between generations, and the potential need for fewer embryos to obtain a suitable founder. Going forward, the ease, inexpensiveness, and speed of CRISPR/Cas genome editing technology will become the chief means for generating genetically modified livestock to be used in producing biomedical products, which should greatly reduce the cost and increase the speed with which livestock may be engineered (Bertolini et al., 2016).

Biopharming to produce therapeutic biomolecules requires that the engineered livestock release the protein into a bodily fluid (Keefer, 2004). Examples of fluids that have been investigated include blood (specifically the serum or plasma component), egg white, milk, seminal plasma, and urine. Milk is a preferred substrate for several reasons. First, the rate of milk production is quite high, ensuring that a large amount of the engineered protein will be available for purification. For example, a cow can produce several thousand gallons of milk a year, yielding a harvest of dozens or hundreds of grams of raw protein; the rates at which cattle produce both milk and therapeutic protein exceed those of goats, the next species reported to have the next highest level of transgenic protein production, by at least 10-fold. Second, a number of mammary gland–specific promoters have been defined, thus ensuring that expression of the transgene is confined to the mammary gland. This limitation is important as inadvertent release of the transgene product into the circulation may impact the animal's health. Third, milk has a simpler protein complement than blood, which streamlines purification of the therapeutic molecule. Finally, proteins secreted in milk exhibit posttranslational glycosylation (carbohydrate) patterns similar to those imparted by cultured mammalian cells, but at much less cost. The presence of these carbohydrate groups often is critical to retaining any, let alone full, function of the secreted protein.

Toxicologic pathology procedures used in the safety assessment of biopharmed therapeutic proteins are comparable to those used for any other biomolecule (see *Protein Pharmaceutical Agents*, Vol 2, Chap 6). Additional considerations in evaluating biopharmed products are to ensure that the transgenic animals from which the proteins are derived retain genotypic and phenotypic stability over successive generations and to guard against inadvertent introduction of infectious agents into the milk. For example, in transgenic livestock, a possible concern is the theoretical potential for passing prions (the causative agent of transmissible spongiform encephalopathies) to human patients; prions have been detected in the milk of both cattle and goats (Franscini et al., 2006). This disquiet arises from the long incubation time for prion-induced neurodegeneration, the administration of milk-derived recombinant proteins by parenteral injections, and the lack of sensitive tools for detecting prions. This possibility cannot be explored effectively by conventional nonclinical safety studies.

Xenotransplantation is of growing interest due to the chronic, severe mismatch between the need for and the availability of suitable human organs for medical transplantation. Domestic livestock are a likely source for replacement organs, with pigs serving as a favored species because of their high fecundity and the similarity between the organ sizes and physiological processes of humans and swine (Klymiuk et al., 2010). The best porcine donors for cell and organ xenografts are animals engineered to be less susceptible to acute organ rejection by the human host. The one essential alteration is inactivation of α(1,3)-galactosyltransferase (αGT), which is found in all mammals except humans, apes, and Old World monkeys. This enzyme makes galactose-α(1,3)-galactose (αGal), an antigen that is targeted by up to 5% of circulating human IgM antibodies. Binding of IgM to αGal expressed on endothelial cells within microvessels of xenografts leads rapidly to complement activation, endothelial lysis, and rapid rejection of the engrafted organ. Inactivation of αGT has been accomplished by αGT deletion ("knockout") and by transgenic overexpression of α(1,2)-fucosyltransferase, which competes with αGT for the same substrate. In many cases, genetically engineered pigs also carry other gene modifications designed to reduce activation of complement (to further reduce endothelial damage in the xenograft) and/or the clotting cascade (which leads to thrombotic microangiopathy, a common lesion in rejected xenografts) and thus forestall acute rejection. Overexpression of cytokine inhibitors or other leukocyte-regulating molecules has been undertaken to control cell infiltration that usually is responsible for cell-mediated immunity and chronic rejection. In particular, expression of human complement regulatory proteins and antithrombotic modulators, in combination with the aforementioned modifications, has prolonged survival in pig-to-primate transplant models. CRISPR/Cas9 has improved the rapidity and complexity of generating "primatized" porcine donors (Hryhorowicz et al.,

2017). (see *Animal Models in Toxicologic Research: Pig*, Vol 1, Chap 20).

Nonclinical safety assessment for xenotransplantation products (cells and organs) typically is similar to the procedures defined above for human cell–based therapies. Guidance by the FDA regarding "Source Animal, Product, Preclinical, and Clinical Issues Concerning the Use of Xenotransplantation Products in Humans" was updated in 2016 (https://www.fda.gov/regulatory-information/search-fda-guidance-documents/source-animal-product-preclinical-and-clinical-issues-concerning-use-xenotransplantation-products). In general, studies will involve testing of donor organs in nonhuman primates that have been treated concurrently with one or several immunosuppressive drugs (e.g., corticosteroids, antithymocyte globulin, mycophenolate mofetil, abatacept, rapamycin, or the equivalent) to prevent graft rejection. The xenograft "dose" usually will be defined in terms of either mass of engrafted tissue (whether an organ piece or the entire organ) and/or the kinetics of a xenograft-derived secretory protein. Relevant endpoints will include both functional data (e.g., for pancreatic islet xenografts, a reduced need for exogenous insulin along with better responsiveness on glucose tolerance tests) and anatomic assessments (e.g., sustained viability of xenografts over time, extent of leukocytic infiltration [host-mediated rejection], or evidence of graft-versus-host disease). If the xenograft includes a device component (e.g., a semipermeable membrane to exclude cell migration in or out), connective tissue and immune reactions to the device should be investigated as well (see *Biomedical Materials and Devices*, Vol 2, Chap 11). The major parameters to note with respect to the device would be the presence of breaks or more extensive degradation of its constituents that might permit its failure, or reactions to the device itself that might cause the xenografts to malfunction or fail secondarily. Since the desired outcome of a xenotransplantation nonclinical program is an assessment of benefit and risk for patients in human clinical trials, animal models should receive the same test article, given by the same routes and dosing regimens proposed for use in the clinic. In general, the immunosuppression regimen (drugs, doses, and routes) in the nonclinical setting need not match the proposed clinical regimen for immunosuppression since the purpose of this ancillary treatment is to dampen the immune response and not to test the safety of the immunosuppression protocol.

The prime biosafety concern for xenotransplantation is the potential transfer of infectious agents from animal donors into human patients (Takeuchi et al., 2005). The concern is magnified because transplantation by necessity requires significant immunosuppression, which can permit establishment not only of natural pathogens but also of facultative pathogens and even nonpathogens. One avenue for reducing zoonotic infection is to obtain xenografts only from specific pathogen-free (SPF) donor animals. This strategy will minimize the likelihood that exogenous bacteria and viruses might be present on the surface or within extracellular spaces or retained fluids of the xenograft. However, the SPF approach cannot eliminate endogenous infectious agents stably inserted into the genome (e.g., retroviruses). Studies have shown that porcine endogenous retrovirus (PERV) can infect human cells in vitro, though transmission has not been documented in nonclinical and clinical trials (Louz et al., 2008). Routine nonclinical safety studies in nonhuman primates are unlikely to define the extent of risk for PERV transfer to a human host, so long-term follow-up of patients with xenografts appears to be the only option for evaluating this concern. Strategies to eliminate PERV have included selection of animals with low copy number and expression of PERV proviruses, selection of PERV-free animals, knockdown of PERV by RNAi, and vaccination against PERV transmembrane and surface envelope proteins. Recent advances using CRISPR/Cas9 have succeeded in inactivating PERV elements throughout the pig genome (Wolf et al., 2019).

The nonclinical testing program for xenografts also should seek to address several factors associated with the genetic engineering event other than the host's reaction to the xenografts per se. For instance, data should be gathered to confirm the stability of the genotype and phenotype (e.g., organ viability, appropriate pattern of transgene expression) in the generation of animals actually being used to produce the test article, rather than relying on information derived from the founder generation. In addition, information should be

generated to examine the potential "toxicity" that might be posed by many factors. First, possible adverse effects of the construct itself should be evaluated. Do the sequences in the engineered genes cause or exacerbate animal and/or human disease intrinsically? Could such effects arise following a genetic recombination event? Next, the risk from escape of the genetically engineered livestock needs to be evaluated. Would interbreeding with local herds result in transmission of the altered gene? If so, would its transfer be detrimental to the health of the "infected" herds, or to the local environment and its human and animal inhabitants? Finally, the impact of waste disposal (e.g., animal carcasses as well as fluid and solid excretions) needs to be assessed with respect to the likelihood that release of the engineered gene into the environment might pose a hazard to animals and humans in the vicinity. In general, nonclinical safety assessment involving toxicologic pathology analyses will be concentrated on the first of these concerns.

5.2. Food Products

Genetically engineered livestock and plants also have been modified to improve the quantity and quality of food for human use. Agricultural applications of transgenic animals (mainly fish, cattle, and pigs but also goats, sheep, rabbits, and chickens) and genome-edited plants (corn, rice, soybeans, wheat) related to food include enhanced generation of native molecules (e.g., higher milk protein levels to speed cheese manufacturing); fabrication of nutraceuticals (e.g., secretion of one or several human milk proteins for use in "humanized" infant formulas); amplified production of protein biomass (e.g., faster-growing crops, fish, and livestock); and improved disease resistance (animals and plants). Concern among various public and scientific constituencies continues to make safety testing and approval of genetically modified organisms (GMOs) as food products are a contentious issue, as indicated by application of the derogatory "Frankenfood" tag to this class of agricultural commodities. A growing body of guidance has been defined by various regulatory bodies and nongovernmental organizations to facilitate food safety testing and product qualification of GMO products

(Commission, 2008; FDA, 2015; USDA-AMS, 2020).

Fundamental attributes of toxicologic pathology as applied to the safety assessment for food products will not be covered in detail here as they have been dealt with elsewhere in this book (see *Food and Toxicologic Pathology*, Vol 2, Chap 19). A search of the literature indicates that multiple general toxicity studies in experimental animals have not discerned major differences in biology or biochemistry of meat from wild-type versus cloned cattle using standard endpoints like viability, fertility, growth rate, hormone cycling, behavior, clinical pathology (multiple chemical, hematologic, and urinary analytes), and histopathology (Heyman et al., 2007; Lee et al., 2010; Rudenko et al., 2007; Takahashi and Ito, 2004; van der Berg et al., 2019; Watanabe, 2013; Yamaguchi et al., 2007; Yang et al., 2007). Sequences of bovine endogenous retroviruses are not transcribed and thus would not represent a risk for zoonotic transmission unique to cloned livestock. Some studies suggest that subtle differences do exist between wild-type and cloned animals in terms of developmental, endocrine, metabolic, and reproductive attributes. The FDA has analyzed these data using a weight-of-evidence strategy and concluded that from a nutritional standpoint, both cloned meat and plant-based meat alternatives engineered to express animal heme (soy leghemoglobin preparation) should be safe for human consumption.

6. SUMMARY

Genetically engineered animals are important models for modern biomedical science, including product discovery and development. Basic research designed to find new targets and elucidate mechanisms of health and disease increasingly depends on the availability of GEM and GER models. GEM, and sometimes GER, may be useful for the nonclinical evaluation of the efficacy, PK (ADME) properties, and/or safety of new therapeutic candidates, especially when the materials being tested are fully human biomolecules or human cell–based products. Genetically engineered animals (mainly GEM and livestock) may be used as

factories to produce human biomolecules, to provide donor organs, or to improve food productivity. Analysis of genetically modified animals will involve the conventional armamentarium of anatomic and clinical pathology methods that are currently used for routine nonclinical testing, but will be expanded in many instances by the need for additional genotyping and phenotyping techniques to assess spatial and temporal patterns of gene and protein expression. Despite the potential advantages of such purposely created models, pathologists and toxicologists will need to keep in mind that genetically engineered animals remain animals, and that data derived from animals harboring human genes or cells should not be interpreted automatically to predict human responses.

GLOSSARY

Avatar a mouse engrafted with neoplastic cells from a specific individual (also referred to as a "patient-derived xenograft" [PDX])

Blastocyst an embryo generally with around 64–128 cells, where the inner cell mass (primordial embryo) and trophoblast layers (primordial placenta) are differentiated and a blastocoel cavity has formed

Cassette a DNA sequence carrying one or more genes that can be manipulated (and moved among DNA pieces) by using restriction enzymes to cut the fragment at specific sites

Chimera an organism carrying cell populations derived from two or more different zygotes or embryonic stem (ES) cell lineages of the same or a different species. Chimeras include animals in which only some cells contain an engineered gene, may be recipients of tissue grafts from other individuals, or may contain an organ that has been purposely damaged and then reconstituted with cells from another species.

Concatemer a continuous linear DNA sequence of considerable length comprised of multiple copies of the same DNA sequence

Conditional transgenic an animal in which the engineered gene is subject to control by an element that regulates when (at what development stage) and/or where (in what cell or organ) the gene will be expressed

Congenic a rodent strain in which continual backcrossing for 10 or more generations produces a consistent and homogenous genetic constitution at all major gene loci

Construct an assembly of DNA sequences borne on a bacterial plasmid or similar vector that is used to insert engineered genetic material into a cell

Cybrid abbreviation for "cytoplasmic hybrid" cells, which are created by introducing one or more mitochondrial DNAs (mtDNA) of interest into cells that have been depleted of their endogenous mtDNA

Dominant negative a mutation whose product overrides the function of the normal wild-type gene product within the same cell

Embryo in animals, a fertilized ovum and its descendants, which eventually become the offspring, during their period of most rapid development

Embryonic stem (ES) cell see "Stem Cell" (below)

Gamete a reproductive cell—spermatozoon for males, ovum for females—that contains the haploid set of chromosomes (i.e., only one copy of each gene)

Gene targeting the genetic engineering technique whereby a given gene is replaced specifically by homologous recombination

Gene therapy delivery of engineered genetic material in a chemical solution or by means of a viral vector (often to an adult animal)

Genome editing a site-specific method for cutting native DNA to delete a gene and/or to insert new genetic material in a defined location

Genotype the genetic makeup of an animal

Haploinsufficiency the presence of a single functional gene in a cell, which cannot alone generate enough of a gene product to sustain full function

Haplotype a group of gene sequences at adjacent positions on a DNA strand that will be transferred together during genome replication

Hemizygous an animal into which one or more copies of a non-endogenous gene have been inserted

Heterozygous an animal with differing alleles at the same gene locus on both paired chromosomes (typically denoted as HET or $+/-$)

Homozygous an animal with identical alleles at a gene locus (usually denoted as $-/-$ for knockout [KO] animals and $+/+$ for wild-type [WT] animals)

Humanized an animal into which human genetic material or human cells has been inserted, or a therapeutic molecule in which a binding site of animal derivation (commonly 10% or less of the construct) is linked to a backbone of human origin

Hypomorph a mutation in which the gene product functions at a reduced level

Induced pluripotent stem cell (iPSC) see "Stem Cell" (below)

Knockdown an animal in which a gene's function has been reduced but not deleted (sometimes designated as KD)

Knockin an animal in which a functional endogenous gene has been replaced by a foreign gene (often the human homolog) designed to restore the function of the original gene (usually designated as KI).

Knockout an animal in which an endogenous gene has been replaced by a nonfunctional engineered gene (generally denoted as KO or $-/-$)

Morula an embryo consisting of a compact ball of around 16 to 32 cells

Mosaic an individual that develops from a single zygote but which has two or more genetically different cell populations that are distinct at the level of the genotype or karyotype (i.e., at the DNA and/or chromosomal level). Mosaicism results from such events as a gene mutation or chromosomal nondisjunction during early embryogenesis. The extent of the mosaic state depends on the embryonic cleavage stage at which the genetic event occurred. See also "Chimera" (above).

Mutagenic the capacity for an agent to damage DNA

Oocyte a developing egg cell (ovum) at any stage before or after ovulation, but before fertilization

Phenotype the sum of all functional and structural changes produced by the activity of an engineered gene

Plasmid a DNA piece (or "vector"), typically of bacterial origin, that can carry engineered genes into cells and facilitate their insertion into the host genome

Pluripotent capacity of a stem cell to differentiate into many but not all possible cell lineages

Stem cell a cell that upon division replaces its own numbers and also gives rise to cells which differentiate further into one or more specialized types. Embryonic stem (ES) cells are totipotent cells obtained from an embryo in the blastocyst phase. Induced

pluripotent stem cells (iPSCs) are derived by using various growth factors to reprogram adult cells (typically hematopoietic or mesenchymal skin cells) into an embryonic-like state.

Totipotent capacity of a stem cell to differentiate into all possible cell lineages

Transgenic an engineered animal into which a specific genetic modification is induced by transfer of genetic material from one organism into another

Xenograft cells or tissue derived from a species other than the one receiving the implant

Zygote a single-cell embryo (i.e., a fertilized ovum)

Acknowledgments

Some passages in this chapter were taken directly or slightly modified from the predecessor chapter entitled "Genetically Engineered Animals in Product Discovery and Development" as printed in *Haschek and Rousseaux's Handbook of Toxicologic Pathology*, 3rd edition, by permission of the Publisher. Accordingly, the authors gratefully salute that chapter's authors—Dr. Elizabeth J. Galbreath, Dr. Carl A. Pinkert, and the incomparable Dr. Daniel Morton—for their contributions to the content of this current piece.

REFERENCES

Adiguzel C, Iqbal O, Demir M, Fareed J: European community and US-FDA approval of recombinant human antithrombin produced in genetically altered goats, *Clin Appl Thromb Hemost* 15:645–651, 2009.

Alden CL, Lynn A, Bourdeau A, et al.: A critical review of the effectiveness of rodent pharmaceutical carcinogenesis testing in predicting for human risk, *Vet Pathol* 48:772–784, 2011.

Anderson MS, Bluestone JA: The NOD mouse: a model of immune dysregulation, *Annu Rev Immunol* 23:447–485, 2005.

Avery LB, Wang M, Kavosi MS, et al.: Utility of a human FcRn transgenic mouse model in drug discovery for early assessment and prediction of human pharmacokinetics of monoclonal antibodies, *mAbs* 8:1064–1078, 2016.

Azuma H, Paulk N, Ranade A, et al.: Robust expansion of human hepatocytes in *Fah-/-/Rag2-/-/Il2rg-/-* mice, *Nat Biotechnol* 25:903–910, 2007.

Barrangou R, Doudna JA: Applications of CRISPR technologies in research and beyond, *Nat Biotechnol* 34:933–941, 2016.

Batzer MA, Deininger PL: A human-specific subfamily of Alu sequences, *Genomics* 9:481–487, 1991.

Behringer R, Gertsenstein M, Nagy KV, et al.: *Manipulating the mouse embryo: a laboratory manual*, NY, 2014, 4th Cold Spring Harbor. Cold Spring Harbor Laboratory Press.

Belteki G, Haigh J, Kabacs N, et al.: Conditional and inducible transgene expression in mice through the combinatorial use of Cre-mediated recombination and tetracycline induction, *Nucleic Acids Res* 33:e51, 2005 [Erratum in: Nucleic Acids Res. 2005; 2033: 2765.].

Benavides F, Rulicke T, Prins JB, et al.: Genetic quality assurance and genetic monitoring of laboratory mice and rats: FELASA working group report, *Lab Anim* 54:135–148, 2020.

Berndt A, Ackert-Bicknell C, Silva KA, et al.: Genetic determinants of fibro-osseous lesions in aged inbred mice, *Exp Mol Pathol* 100:92–100, 2016.

Bertolini LR, Meade H, Lazzarotto CR, et al.: The transgenic animal platform for biopharmaceutical production, *Transgenic Res* 25:329–343, 2016.

Betts A, Keunecke A, van Steeg TJ, et al.: Linear pharmacokinetic parameters for monoclonal antibodies are similar within a species and across different pharmacological targets: a comparison between human, cynomolgus monkey and hFcRn Tg32 transgenic mouse using a population-modeling approach, *mAbs* 10:751–764, 2018.

Boelsterli UA: Animal models of human disease in drug safety assessment, *J Toxicol Sci* 28:109–121, 2003.

Boelsterli UA, Hsiao CJ: The heterozygous *Sod2*$^{+/-}$ mouse: modeling the mitochondrial role in drug toxicity, *Drug Discov Today* 13:982–988, 2008.

Bogdanffy MS, Lesniak J, Mangipudy R, et al.: Tg.rasH2 mouse model for assessing carcinogenic potential of pharmaceuticals: industry survey of current practices, *Int J Toxicol* 39(3):198–206, 2020 (in press).

Bolon B: Genetically engineered animals in drug discovery and development: a maturing resource for toxicologic research, *Basic Clin Pharmacol Toxicol* 95:154–161, 2004.

Bolon B: Whole mount enzyme histochemistry as a rapid screen at necropsy for expression of β-galactosidase (LacZ)-bearing transgenes: considerations for separating specific LacZ activity from nonspecific (endogenous) galactosidase activity, *Toxicol Pathol* 36:265–276, 2008.

Bolon B, Jing S, Asuncion F, et al.: The candidate neuroprotective agent artemin induces autonomic neural dysplasia without preventing nerve dysfunction, *Toxicol Pathol* 32:275–294, 2004.

Bolon B, Newbigging S, Boyd KL: Pathology evaluation of developmental phenotypes in neonatal and juvenile mice, *Curr Protoc Mouse Biol* 7:191–219, 2017.

Bolon B, Shalhoub V, Kostenuik PJ, et al.: Osteoprotegerin (OPG): an endogenous anti-osteoclast factor for protecting bone in rheumatoid arthritis, *Arthritis Rheum* 46:3121–3135, 2002.

Bourdi M, Davies JS, Pohl LR: Mispairing C57BL/6 substrains of genetically engineered mice and wild-type controls can lead to confounding results as it did in studies of JNK2 in acetaminophen and concanavalin A liver injury, *Chem Res Toxicol* 24:794–796, 2011.

Boverhof DR, Chamberlain MP, Elcombe CR, et al.: Transgenic animal models in toxicology: historical perspectives and future outlook, *Toxicol Sci* 121:207–233, 2011.

Brayton CF, Treuting PM: Phenotyping. In Treuting PM, Dintzis SM, Montine KS, editors: *Comparative anatomy and histology: a mouse, rat, and human atlas*, San Diego, 2018, Academic Press (Elsevier, pp 9–21.

Brayton CF, Treuting PM, Ward JM: Pathobiology of aging mice and GEM: background strains and experimental design, *Vet Pathol* 49:85–105, 2012.

Brinster RL, Chen HY, Trumbauer ME, et al.: Factors affecting the efficiency of introducing foreign DNA into mice by microinjecting eggs, *Proc Natl Acad Sci USA* 82:4438–4442, 1985.

Brown SDM, Holmes CC, Mallon AM, et al.: High-throughput mouse phenomics for characterizing mammalian gene function, *Nat Rev Genet* 19:357–370, 2018.

Bussiere JL: Species selection considerations for preclinical toxicology studies for biotherapeutics, *Expet Opin Drug Metabol Toxicol* 4:871–877, 2008.

Bussiere JL, Martin P, Horner M, et al.: Alternative strategies for toxicity testing of species-specific biopharmaceuticals, *Int J Toxicol* 28:230–253, 2009.

Carpenter MK, Frey-Vasconcells J, Rao MS: Developing safe therapies from human pluripotent stem cells, *Nat Biotechnol* 27:606–613, 2009.

Cavagnaro JA: Considerations in design of preclinical safety evaluation to support human cell-based therapies. In Cavagnaro JA, editor: *Preclinical safety evaluation of biopharmaceuticals: a science-based approach to facilitating clinical trials*, Hoboken, NJ, 2008a, John Wiley & Sons, pp 749–782.

Cavagnaro JA: Preclinical evaluation of cancer hazard and risk of biopharmaceuticals. In Cavagnaro JA, editor: *Preclinical safety evaluation of biopharmaceuticals: a science-based approach to facilitating clinical trials*, Hoboken, NJ, 2008b, John Wiley & Sons, pp 399–474.

Chen Y, Niu Y, Ji W: Genome editing in nonhuman primates: approach to generating human disease models, *J Intern Med* 280:246–251, 2016.

Cheng J, Ma X, Gonzalez FJ: Pregnane X receptor- and CYP3A4-humanized mouse models and their applications, *Br J Pharmacol* 163:461–468, 2011.

Cheung C, Gonzalez FJ: Humanized mouse lines and their application for prediction of human drug metabolism and toxicological risk assessment, *J Pharmacol Exp Therapeut* 327:288–299, 2008.

Choi Y, Lee S, Kim K, et al.: Studying cancer immunotherapy using patient-derived xenografts (PDXs) in humanized mice, *Exp Mol Med* 50:99, 2018.

Chu X, Bleasby K, Evers R: Species differences in drug transporters and implications for translating preclinical findings to humans, *Expet Opin Drug Metabol Toxicol* 9:237–252, 2013.

Clarke J, Leach W, Pippig S, et al.: Evaluation of a surrogate antibody for preclinical safety testing of an anti-CD11a monoclonal antibody, *Regul Toxicol Pharmacol* 40:219–226, 2004.

Combest AJ, Roberts PJ, Dillon PM, et al.: Genetically engineered cancer models, but not xenografts, faithfully predict anticancer drug exposure in melanoma tumors, *Oncologist* 17:1303–1316, 2012.

Codex Alimentarius Commission: *Guideline for the conduct of food safety assessment for foods derived from recombinant-DNA animals.* http://www.fao.org/fileadmin/user_upload/gmfp/resources/CXG_068e.pdf. (Accessed 25 April 2021).

Cosentino L, Heddle JA: Differential mutation of transgenic and endogenous loci in vivo, *Mutat Res* 454:1–10, 2000.

Crawley JN: *What's wrong with my mouse? Behavioral phenotyping of transgenic and knockout mice,* ed 2, New York, 2007, Wiley-Liss.

Diaz D, Maher JM: The use of genetically modified animals in discovery toxicology. In Will Y, McDuffie JE, Olaharski AJ, et al., editors: *Drug discovery toxicology: from target assessment to translational biomarkers,* New York, 2016, John Wiley & Sons, pp 298–313.

Dixit R, Boelsterli UA: Healthy animals and animal models of human disease(s) in safety assessment of human pharmaceuticals, including therapeutic antibodies, *Drug Discov Today* 12:336–342, 2007.

Dixit R, Iciek LA, McKeever K, et al.: Challenges of general safety evaluations of biologics compared to small molecule pharmaceuticals in animal models, *Expet Opin Drug Discov* 5:79–94, 2010.

Doetschman T: Interpretation of phenotype in genetically engineered mice, *Lab Anim Sci* 49:137–143, 1999.

Donehower LA, Harvey M, Vogel H, et al.: Effects of genetic background on tumorigenesis in p53-deficient mice, *Mol Carcinog* 14:16–22, 1995.

Dunn DA, Cannon MV, Irwin MH, et al.: Animal models of human mitochondrial DNA mutations, *Biochim Biophys Acta* 1820:601–607, 2012.

Dunn DA, Pinkert CA, Kooyman DL: Foundation review: transgenic animals and their impact on the drug discovery industry, *Drug Discov Today* 10:757–767, 2005.

Eastin WC, Mennear JH, Tennant RW, et al.: Tg.Ac genetically altered mouse: assay working group overview of available data, *Toxicol Pathol* 29(Suppl):60–80, 2001.

Ellisor D, Zervas M: Tamoxifen dose response and conditional cell marking: is there control? *Mol Cell Neurosci* 45:132–138, 2010.

Emoto C, Iwasaki K, Murayama M, et al.: Drug metabolism and toxicity in chimeric mice with humanized liver, *J Health Sci* 57:22–27, 2011.

Ergen EN, Yusuf N: Inhibition of interleukin-12 and/or interleukin-23 for the treatment of psoriasis: what is the evidence for an effect on malignancy? *Exp Dermatol* 27:737–747, 2018.

Esquerda-Canals G, Montoliu-Gaya L, Güell-Bosch J, et al.: Mouse models of Alzheimer's disease, *J Alzheimers Dis* 57:1171–1183, 2017.

Evans MJ: Carlton MBL, and Russ AP: gene trapping and functional genomics, *Trends Genet* 13:370–374, 1997.

FDA (U.S. Food and Drug Administration): *Points to consider in the manufacture and testing of therapeutic products for human use derived from animals.* http://www.fda.gov/downloads/BiologicsBloodVaccines/GuidanceComplianceRegulatoryIn formation/OtherRecommendationsforManufacturers/UCM 153306.pdf. (Accessed 25 April 2021).

FDA (U.S. Food and Drug Administration): *Guidance for industry: source animal, product, preclinical, and clinical issues concerning the use of xenotransplantation products in humans.* https://www.fda.gov/media/102126/download. (Accessed 25 April 2021).

FDA (U.S. Food and Drug Administration): *Guidance for industry: regulation of genetically engineered animals containing heritable recombinant DNA constructs.* https://www.fda.gov/media/135115/download. (Accessed 25 April 2021).

Fink Jr DW: FDA regulation of stem cell-based products, *Science* 324:1662–1663, 2009.

Fong C-Y, Gauthaman K, Bongso A: Teratomas from pluripotent stem cells: a clinical hurdle, *J Cell Biochem* 111:769–781, 2010.

Franscini N, El Gedaily A, Matthey U, et al.: Prion protein in milk, *PloS One* 1:e71, 2006.

French J, Storer RD, Donehower LA: The nature of the heterozygous *Trp53* knockout model for identification of mutagenic carcinogens, *Toxicol Pathol* 29(Suppl):24–29, 2001.

Friedrich A, Olejniczak K: Evaluation of carcinogenicity studies of medicinal products for human use authorised via the European centralised procedure (1995–2009), *Regul Toxicol Pharmacol* 60:225–248, 2011.

Fuchs H, Gailus-Durner V, Adler T, et al.: Mouse phenotyping, *Methods* 53:120–135, 2011.

Furuta Y, Behringer RR: Recent innovations in tissue-specific gene modifications in the mouse, *Birth Defects Res* 75:43–57, 2005.

Goldring CE, Duffy PA, Benvenisty N, et al.: Assessing the safety of stem cell therapeutics, *Cell Stem Cell* 8:618–628, 2011.

Gonzalez FJ: The use of gene knockout mice to unravel the mechanisms of toxicity and chemical carcinogenesis, *Toxicol Lett* 120:199–208, 2001.

Gordon JW, Ruddle FH: Integration and stable germ line transmission of genes injected into mouse pronuclei, *Science* 214:1244–1246, 1981.

Gupta D, Bhattacharjee O, Mandal D, et al.: CRISPR-Cas9 system: a new-fangled dawn in gene editing, *Life Sci* 232:116636, 2019.

Gupta RM, Musunuru K: Expanding the genetic editing tool kit: ZFNs, TALENs, and CRISPR-Cas9, *J Clin Invest* 124:4154–4161, 2014.

Haines DC, Chattopadhyay S, Ward JM: Pathology of aging B6;129 mice, *Toxicol Pathol* 29:653–661, 2001.

Hasegawa M, Kawai K, Mitsui T, et al.: The reconstituted 'humanized liver' in TK-NOG mice is mature and functional, *Biochem Biophys Res Commun* 405:405–410, 2011.

Hentze H, Soong PL, Wang ST, et al.: Teratoma formation by human embryonic stem cells: evaluation of essential parameters for future safety studies, *Stem Cell Res* 2:198–210, 2009.

Heslop JA, Hammond TG, Santeramo I, et al.: Concise review: workshop review: understanding and assessing the risks of stem cell-based therapies, *Stem Cells Transl Med* 4:389–400, 2015.

Heyman Y, Chavatte-Palmer P, Fromentin G, et al.: Quality and safety of bovine clones and their products, *Animal* 1: 963–972, 2007.

Houlton S: *Sixth in a line of Alzheimer's drugs fails in trials.* https://www.chemistryworld.com/news/sixth-in-a-line-of-alzheimers-drugs-fails-in-trials/4010459. (Accessed 25 April 2021).

Hryhorowicz M, Zeyland J, Slomski R, et al.: Genetically modified pigs as organ donors for xenotransplantation, *Mol Biotechnol* 59:435–444, 2017.

ICH (International Council for Harmonisation of Technical Requirements for Pharmaceuticals for Human Use): *Guidance for industry: S1B testing for carcinogenicity of pharmaceuticals.* https://database.ich.org/sites/default/files/S1B_Guideline.pdf. (Accessed 25 April 2021).

Ito M, Hiramatsu H, Kobayashi K, et al.: NOD/SCID/g_c^{null} mouse: an excellent recipient mouse model for engraftment of human cells, *Blood* 100:3175–3182, 2002.

Ito M, Kobayashi K, Nakahata T: NOD/Shi-scid IL2rg^{null} (NOG) mice more appropriate for humanized mouse models, *Curr Top Microbiol Immunol* 324:53–76, 2008.

Ito R, Nagai D, Igo N, et al.: A novel in vivo model for predicting myelotoxicity of chemotherapeutic agents using IL-3/GM-CSF transgenic humanized mice, *Toxicol Lett* 281: 152–157, 2017.

Jacobs AC, Brown PC: Regulatory forum opinion piece: transgenic/alternative carcinogenicity assays: a retrospective review of studies submitted to CDER/FDA 1997-2014, *Toxicol Pathol* 43:605–610, 2015.

Jankowsky JL, Zheng H: Practical considerations for choosing a mouse model of Alzheimer's disease, *Mol Neurodegener* 12:89, 2017.

Jantschitsch C, Weichenthal M, Proksch E, et al.: IL-12 and IL-23 affect photocarcinogenesis differently, *J Invest Dermatol* 132:1479–1486, 2012.

Jayant RD, Sosa D, Kaushik A, et al.: Current status of non-viral gene therapy for CNS disorders, *Expet Opin Drug Deliv* 13:1433–1445, 2016.

Johnson LA, Morgan RA, Dudley ME, et al.: Gene therapy with human and mouse T-cell receptors mediates cancer regression and targets normal tissues expressing cognate antigen, *Blood* 114:535–546, 2009.

Joung JK, Sander JD: TALENs: a widely applicable technology for targeted genome editing, *Nat Rev Mol Cell Biol* 14:49–55, 2013.

Juan TS-C, Bolon B, Lindberg RA, et al.: Mice over-expressing murine oncostatin M (OSM) exhibit changes in hematopoietic and other organs that are distinct from those of mice over-expressing human OSM or bovine OSM, *Vet Pathol* 46: 124–137, 2009.

Justice MJ, Noveroske JK, Weber JS, et al.: Mouse ENU mutagenesis, *Hum Mol Genet* 8:1955–1963, 1999.

Katano I, Ito R, Kamisako T, et al.: NOD-*Rag2*^{null} IL-2Rγ^{null} mice: an alternative to NOG mice for generation of humanized mice, *Exp Anim* 63:321–330, 2014.

Katoh M, Tateno C, Yoshizato K, et al.: Chimeric mice with humanized liver, *Toxicology* 246:9–17, 2008.

Keefer CL: Production of bioproducts through the use of transgenic animal models, *Anim Reprod Sci* 82–83:5–12, 2004.

Khan SH: Genome-editing technologies: concept, pros, and cons of various genome-editing techniques and bioethical concerns for clinical application, *Mol Ther Nucleic Acids* 16: 326–334, 2019.

Klymiuk N, Aigner B, Brem G, et al.: Genetic modification of pigs as organ donors for xenotransplantation, *Mol Reprod Dev* 77:209–221, 2010.

Koller BH, Smithies O: Altering genes in animals by gene targeting, *Annu Rev Immunol* 10:705–730, 1992.

Kou J, Kim H, Pattanayak A, et al.: Anti-amyloid-β single-chain antibody brain delivery via AAV reduces amyloid load but may increase cerebral hemorrhages in an Alzheimer's disease mouse model, *J Alzheimers Dis* 27:23–38, 2011.

Lambert IB, Singer TM, Boucher SE, et al.: Detailed review of transgenic rodent mutation assays, *Mutat Res* 590:1–280, 2005.

Lavender KJ, Pace C, Sutter K, et al.: An advanced BLT-humanized mouse model for extended HIV-1 cure studies, *AIDS* 32:1–10, 2018.

Lavitrano M, Giovannoni R, Cerrito MG: Methods for sperm-mediated gene transfer, *Methods Mol Biol* 927:519–529, 2013.

Leder A, McMenamin J, Zhou F, et al.: Genome-wide SNP analysis of Tg.AC transgenic mice reveals an oncogenic collaboration between *v-Ha-ras* and *Ink4a*, which is absent in *p53* deficiency, *Oncogene* 27:2456–2465, 2008.

Lee AS, Tang C, Cao F, et al.: Effects of cell number on teratoma formation by human embryonic stem cells, *Cell Cycle* 8:2608–2612, 2009.

Lee CA, O'Connor MA, Ritchie TK, et al.: Breast cancer resistance protein (ABCG2) in clinical pharmacokinetics and drug interactions: practical recommendations for clinical victim and perpetrator drug-drug interaction study design, *Drug Metabol Dispos* 43:490–509, 2015.

Lee NJ, Yang BC, Hwang JS, et al.: Effects of cloned-cattle meat diet on reproductive parameters in pregnant rabbits, *Food Chem Toxicol* 48:871–876, 2010.

Li L-P, Lampert JC, Chen X, et al.: Transgenic mice with a diverse human T cell antigen receptor repertoire, *Nat Med* 16(9):1029–1034, 2010.

Liang HC, Li H, McKinnon RA, et al.: *Cyp1a2*(-/-) null mutant mice develop normally but show deficient drug metabolism, *Proc Natl Acad Sci USA* 93:1671–1676, 1996.

Lin JH: Applications and limitations of genetically modified mouse models in drug discovery and development, *Curr Drug Metab* 9:419–438, 2008.

Louz D, Bergmans HE, Loos BP, et al.: Reappraisal of biosafety risks posed by PERVs in xenotransplantation, *Rev Med Virol* 18:53–65, 2008.

Luo Y, Bolon B, Damore MA, et al.: BACE1 (β-secretase) knockout mice do not acquire compensatory gene expression changes or develop neural lesions over time, *Neurobiol Dis* 14:81–88, 2003.

Luo Y, Bolon B, Kahn S, et al.: Mice deficient in BACE1, the Alzheimer's β-secretase, have normal phenotype and abolished β-amyloid generation, *Nat Neurosci* 4:213–232, 2001.

MacDonald J, French JE, Gerson RJ, et al.: The utility of genetically modified mouse assays for identifying human carcinogens: a basic understanding and path forward, *Toxicol Sci* 77:188–194, 2004.

Maeda A, Schneider SW, Kojima M, et al.: Enhanced photocarcinogenesis in interleukin-12-deficient mice, *Cancer Res* 66:2962–2969, 2006.

Mahler JF, Stokes W, Mann PC, et al.: Spontaneous lesions in aging FVB/N mice, *Toxicol Pathol* 24:710–716, 1996.

Manning FJ, Swartz MN, U.S. Institute of Medicine Committee to Review the Fialuridine (FIAU/FIAC) Clinical Trials: *Review of the fialuridine (FIAU) clinical trials*, Washington D.C., 1995, National Academies Press. https://www.ncbi.nlm.nih.gov/books/NBK232098. (Accessed 25 April 2021).

McKenzie M, Trounce IA, Cassar CA, et al.: Production of homoplasmic xenomitochondrial mice, *Proc Natl Acad Sci USA* 101:1685–1690, 2004.

McKenzie R, Fried MW, Sallie R, et al.: Hepatic failure and lactic acidosis due to fialuridine (FIAU), an investigational nucleoside analogue for chronic hepatitis B, *N Engl J Med* 333:1099–1105, 1995.

Meek S, Mashimo T, Burdon T: From engineering to editing the rat genome, *Mamm Genome* 28:302–314, 2017.

Meeran SM, Mantena SK, Meleth S, et al.: Interleukin-12-deficient mice are at greater risk of UV radiation-induced skin tumors and malignant transformation of papillomas to carcinomas, *Mol Cancer Therapeut* 5:825–832, 2006.

Meier MJ, Beal MA, Schoenrock A, et al.: Whole genome sequencing of the mutamouse model reveals strain- and colony-level variation, and genomic features of the transgene integration site, *Sci Rep* 9:13775, 2019.

Mesner LD, Calabrese GM, Al-Barghouthi B, et al.: Mouse genome-wide association and systems genetics identifies *Lhfp* as a regulator of bone mass, *PLoS Genet* 15:e1008123, 2019.

Mirsalis JC, Monforte JA, Winegar RA: Transgenic animal models for measuring mutations in vivo, *Crit Rev Toxicol* 24:255–280, 1994.

Mohr U, Dungworth DL, Capen CC, et al.: Pathobiology of the aging mouse, vol. 2. Washington, D.C., 1996, ILSI (International Life Sciences Institute) Press. (Accessed 25 April 2021).

Moran JL, Bolton AD, Tran PV, et al.: Utilization of a whole genome SNP panel for efficient genetic mapping in the mouse, *Genome Res* 16:436–440, 2006.

Morgan SJ, Couch J, Guzzie-Peck P, et al.: Regulatory Forum opinion piece: use and utility of animal models of disease for nonclinical safety assessment: a pharmaceutical industry survey, *Toxicol Pathol* 45:372–380, 2017.

Morgan SJ, Elangbam CS, Berens S, et al.: Use of animal models of human disease for nonclinical safety assessment of novel pharmaceuticals, *Toxicol Pathol* 41:508–518, 2013.

Morton D, Alden CL, Roth AJ, et al.: The Tg rasH2 mouse in cancer hazard identification, *Toxicol Pathol* 30:139–146, 2002.

Morton D, Bailey KL, Stout CL, et al.: *N*-methyl-*N*-nitrosourea (MNU): a positive control chemical for p53+/- mouse carcinogenicity studies, *Toxicol Pathol* 36:926–931, 2008.

Murnane R, Zhang XB, Hukkanen RR, et al.: Myelodysplasia in 2 pig-tailed macaques (*Macaca nemestrina*) associated with retroviral vector-mediated insertional mutagenesis and overexpression of *HOXB4*, *Vet Pathol* 48:999–1001, 2011.

Nambiar PR, Morton D: The rasH2 mouse model for assessing carcinogenic potential of pharmaceuticals, *Toxicol Pathol* 41:1058–1067, 2013.

Nielsen LL, Gurnani M, Catino JJ, et al.: In wap-ras transgenic mice, tumor phenotype but not cyclophosphamide-sensitivity is affected by genetic background, *Anticancer Res* 15:385–392, 1995.

Obenaus M, Leitao C, Leisegang M, et al.: Identification of human T-cell receptors with optimal affinity to cancer antigens using antigen-negative humanized mice, *Nat Biotechnol* 33:402–407, 2015.

Okada M, Miller TC, Roediger J, et al.: An efficient, simple, and noninvasive procedure for genotyping aquatic and nonaquatic laboratory animals, *J Am Assoc Lab Anim Sci* 56:570–573, 2017.

Okita K, Nakagawa M, Hyenjong H, et al.: Generation of mouse induced pluripotent stem cells without viral vectors, *Science* 322:949–953, 2008.

Ormond KE, Mortlock DP, Scholes DT, et al.: Human germline genome editing, *Am J Hum Genet* 101:167–176, 2017.

Papaioannou VE, Behringer RR: *Mouse phenotypes: a Handbook of mutation analysis*, NY, 2005, Cold Spring Harbor Laboratory Press.

Paquet D, Kwart D, Chen A, et al.: Efficient introduction of specific homozygous and heterozygous mutations using CRISPR/Cas9, *Nature* 533:125–129, 2016.

Paranjpe MG, Elbekaei RH, Shah SA, et al.: Historical control data of spontaneous tumors in transgenic CByB6F1-Tg(HRAS)2Jic (Tg.rasH2) mice, *Int J Toxicol* 32:48–57, 2013.

Peterson NC: Advances in monoclonal antibody technology: genetic engineering of mice, cells, and immunoglobulins, *ILAR J* 46:314–319, 2005.

Petkov PM, Cassell MA, Sargent EE, et al.: Development of a SNP genotyping panel for genetic monitoring of the laboratory mouse, *Genomics* 83:902–911, 2004.

Pineau T, Fernandez Salgeuro P, Lee SST, et al.: Neonatal lethality associated with respiratory distress in mice lacking cytochrome P450 1A2, *Proc Natl Acad Sci USA* 92: 5134–5138, 1995.

Pinkert CA: Transgenic animal technology: alternatives in genotyping and phenotyping, *Comp Med* 53:126–139, 2003.

Pinkert CA: *Transgenic animal technology: a laboratory handbook*, ed 3, Waltham, MA, 2014, Elsevier.

Powley MW, Frederick CB, Sistare FD, et al.: Safety assessment of drug metabolites: implications of regulatory guidance and potential application of genetically engineered mouse models that express human P450s, *Chem Res Toxicol* 22:257–262, 2009.

Pritchett-Corning KR, Landel CP: Genetically modified animals. In Fox JG, Anderson LC, Otto GM, et al., editors: *Laboratory animal medicine*, ed 3, Boston, 2015, Academic Press (Elsevier, pp 1417–1440.

Proetzel G, Roopenian DC: Humanized FcRn mouse models for evaluating pharmacokinetics of human IgG antibodies, *Methods* 65:148–153, 2014.

Prokhorova TA, Harkness LM, Frandsen U, et al.: Teratoma formation by human embryonic stem cells is site dependent and enhanced by the presence of matrigel, *Stem Cell Dev* 18:47–54, 2009.

Provost GS, Kretz PL, Hamner RT, et al.: Transgenic systems for in vivo mutation analysis, *Mutat Res* 288:133–149, 1993.

Robbins PD, Tahara H, Ghivizzani SC: Viral vectors for gene therapy, *Trends Biotechnol* 16:35–40, 1998.

Ross J, Plummer SM, Rode A, et al.: Human constitutive androstane receptor (CAR) and pregnane X receptor (PXR) support the hypertrophic but not the hyperplastic response to the murine nongenotoxic hepatocarcinogens phenobarbital and chlordane in vivo, *Toxicol Sci* 116:452–466, 2010.

Rossant J, McKerlie C: Mouse-based phenogenomics for modelling human disease, *Trends Mol Med* 7:502–507, 2001.

Rozman J, Rathkolb B, Oestereicher MA, et al.: Identification of genetic elements in metabolism by high-throughput mouse phenotyping, *Nat Commun* 9:288, 2018.

Rudenko L, Matheson JC, Sundlof SF: Animal cloning and the FDA–the risk assessment paradigm under public scrutiny, *Nat Biotechnol* 25:39–43, 2007.

Schwenk F, Kühn R, Angrand PO, et al.: Temporally and spatially regulated somatic mutagenesis in mice, *Nucleic Acids Res* 26:1427–1432, 1998.

Sellers RS: The gene or not the gene—that is the question: understanding the genetically engineered mouse phenotype, *Vet Pathol* 49:5–15, 2012.

Seong E, Saunders TL, Stewart CL, et al.: To knockout in 129 or in C57BL/6: that is the question, *Trends Genet* 20:59–62, 2004.

Sharpe ME, Morton D, Rossi A: Nonclinical safety strategies for stem cell therapies, *Toxicol Appl Pharmacol* 262:223–231, 2012.

Sharpless NE, Depinho RA: The mighty mouse: genetically engineered mouse models in cancer drug development, *Nat Rev Drug Discov* 5:741–754, 2006.

Shen H-W, Jiang X-L, Gonzalez FJ, et al.: Humanized transgenic mouse models for drug metabolism and pharmacokinetic research, *Curr Drug Metabol* 12:997–1006, 2011.

Shultz LD, Brehm MA, Garcia-Martinez JV, et al.: Humanized mice for immune system investigation: progress, promise and challenges, *Nat Rev Immunol* 12:786–798, 2012.

Silva G, Poirot L, Galetto R, et al.: Meganucleases and other tools for targeted genome engineering: perspectives and challenges for gene therapy, *Curr Gene Ther* 11:11–27, 2011.

Simpson EM, Linder CC, Sargent EE, et al.: Genetic variation among 129 substrains and its importance for targeted mutagenesis in mice, *Nat Genet* 16:19–27, 1997.

Son H, Hawkins R, Martin K, et al.: Long-term potentiation is reduced in mice that are doubly mutant in endothelial and neuronal nitric oxide synthase, *Cell* 87:1015–1023, 1996.

Storer RD, French JE, Haseman J, et al.: p53$^{+/-}$ hemizygous knockout mouse: overview of available data, *Toxicol Pathol* 29(Suppl):30–50, 2001.

Strohl WR: Current progress in innovative engineered antibodies, *Protein Cell* 9:86–120, 2018.

Strom SC, Davila J, Grompe M: Chimeric mice with humanized liver: tools for the study of drug metabolism, excretion, and toxicity. In Maurel P, editor: *Hepatocytes: methods and protocols*, Totowa, NJ, 2010, Humana Press, pp 491–509.

Su W-L, Sieberts SK, Kleinhanz RR, et al.: Assessing the prospects of genome-wide association studies performed in inbred mice, *Mamm Genome* 21:143–152, 2010.

Sundberg JP, Berndt A, Sundberg BA, et al.: Approaches to investigating complex genetic traits in a large-scale inbred mouse aging study, *Vet Pathol* 53:456–467, 2016.

Suzuki T, Hayashi M, Sofuni T: Initial experiences and future directions for transgenic mouse mutation assays, *Mutat Res* 307:489–494, 1994.

Szymanska H, Lechowska-Piskorowska J, Krysiak E, et al.: Neoplastic and nonneoplastic lesions in aging mice of unique and common inbred strains contribution to modeling of human neoplastic diseases, *Vet Pathol* 51:663–679, 2014.

Takahashi K, Yamanaka S: Induction of pluripotent stem cells from mouse embryonic and adult fibroblast cultures by defined factors, *Cell* 126:663–676, 2006.

Takahashi S, Ito Y: Evaluation of meat products from cloned cattle: biological and biochemical properties, *Clon Stem Cell* 6:165–171, 2004.

Takenaka K, Prasolava TK, Wang JC, et al.: Polymorphism in *Sirpa* modulates engraftment of human hematopoietic stem cells, *Nat Immunol* 8:1313–1323, 2007.

Takeuchi Y, Magre S, Patience C: The potential hazards of xenotransplantation: an overview, *Rev Sci Tech* 24:323–334, 2005.

Tamaoki N: The rasH2 transgenic mouse: nature of the model and mechanistic studies on tumorigenesis, *Toxicol Pathol* 29(Suppl):81–89, 2001.

Tennant RW, Stasiewicz S, Eastin WC, et al.: The Tg.Ac (v-Ha-ras) transgenic mouse: nature of the model, *Toxicol Pathol* 29(Suppl):51–59, 2001.

Threadgill DW, Yee D, Matin A, et al.: Genealogy of the 129 inbred strains: 129/SvJ is a contaminated inbred strain, *Mamm Genome* 8:390–393, 1997.

Tohyama J, Vanier MT, Suzuki K, et al.: Paradoxical influence of acid β-galactosidase gene dosage on phenotype of the twitcher mouse (genetic galactosylceramidase deficiency), *Hum Mol Genet* 9:1699–1707, 2000.

Törnell J, Snaith M: Transgenic systems in drug discovery: from target identification to humanized mice, *Drug Discov Today* 7:461–470, 2002.

Trounce IA, McKenzie M, Cassar CA, et al.: Development and initial characterization of xenomitochondrial mice, *J Bioenerg Biomembr* 36:421–427, 2004.

Trounce IA, Pinkert CA: Cybrid models of mtDNA disease and transmission, from cells to mice, *Curr Top Dev Biol* 77:157–183, 2007.

USDA-AMS: *(U.S. Department of Agriculture Agricultural Marketing Service): process verified program.* In *https://www.ams.usda.gov/services/auditing/process-verified-programs.* (Accessed 25 April 2021).

Usui T, Mutai M, Hisada S, et al.: CB6F1-rasH2 mouse: overview of available data, *Toxicol Pathol* 29(Suppl):90–108, 2001.

van der Berg JP, Kleter GA, Kok EJ: Regulation and safety considerations of somatic cell nuclear transfer-cloned farm animals and their offspring used for food production, *Theriogenology* 135:85–93, 2019.

van Kreijl CF, McAnulty PA, Beems RB, et al.: *Xpa* and *Xpa/p53*$^{+/-}$ knockout mice: overview of available data, *Toxicol Pathol* 29(Suppl.):117–127, 2001.

van Steeg H, de Vries A, van Oostrom CT, et al.: DNA repair-deficient *Xpa* and *Xpa/p53*$^{+/-}$ knock-out mice: nature of the models, *Toxicol Pathol* 29(Suppl):109–116, 2001.

van Waterschoot RA, Schinkel AH: A critical analysis of the interplay between cytochrome P450 3A and P-glycoprotein: recent insights from knockout and transgenic mice, *Pharmacol Rev* 63:390–410, 2011.

Walsh NC, Kenney LL, Jangalwe S, et al.: Humanized mouse models of clinical disease, *Annu Rev Pathol* 12:187–215, 2017.

Wang X, Cao C, Huang J, et al.: One-step generation of triple gene-targeted pigs using CRISPR/Cas9 system, *Sci Rep* 6:20620, 2016.

Ward JM, Anver MR, Mahler JF, et al.: Pathology of mice commonly used in genetic engineering (C57BL/6; 129; B6,129; and FVB/N). In Ward JM, Mahler JF, Maronpot RR, et al., editors: *Pathology of genetically engineered mice*, Ames, IA, 2000, Iowa State University Press, pp 161–179.

Watanabe S: Effect of calf death loss on cloned cattle herd derived from somatic cell nuclear transfer: clones with congenital defects would be removed by the death loss, *Anim Sci J* 84:631–638, 2013.

Webster JD, Santagostino SF, Foreman O: Applications and considerations for the use of genetically engineered mouse models in drug development, *Cell Tissue Res* 380(2):325–340, 2020.

Wells MY, Williams ES: The transgenic mouse assay as an alternative test method for regulatory carcinogenicity studies—implications for REACH, *Regul Toxicol Pharmacol* 53:150–155, 2009.

Wendler A, Wehling M: The translatability of animal models for clinical development: biomarkers and disease models, *Curr Opin Pharmacol* 10:601–606, 2010.

Wijnhoven SW, van Steeg H: Transgenic and knockout mice for DNA repair functions in carcinogenesis and mutagenesis, *Toxicology* 193:171–187, 2003.

Wilmut I, Bai Y, Taylor J: Somatic cell nuclear transfer: origins, the present position and future opportunities, *Philos Trans R Soc Lond B Biol Sci* 370:20140366, 2015.

Wolf E, Kemter E, Klymiuk N, et al.: Genetically modified pigs as donors of cells, tissues, and organs for xenotransplantation, *Anim Front* 9:13–20, 2019.

Woychik RP, Stewart TA, Davis LG, et al.: An inherited limb deformity created by insertional mutagenesis in a transgenic mouse, *Nature* 318:36–40, 1985.

Xu D, Nishimura T, Nishimura S, et al.: Fialuridine induces acute liver failure in chimeric TK-NOG mice: a model for detecting hepatic drug toxicity prior to human testing, *PLoS Med* 11:e1001628, 2014.

Yamaguchi M, Ito Y, Takahashi S: Fourteen-week feeding test of meat and milk derived from cloned cattle in the rat, *Theriogenology* 67:152–165, 2007.

Yan Q, Zhang Q, Yang H, et al.: Generation of multi-gene knockout rabbits using the Cas9/gRNA system, *Cell Regen* 3(12), 2014.

Yang X, Tian XC, Kubota C, et al.: Risk assessment of meat and milk from cloned animals, *Nat Biotechnol* 25:77–83, 2007.

Zambrowicz BP, Sands AT: Knockouts model the 100 best-selling drugs - will they model the next 100? *Nat Rev Drug Discov* 2:38–51, 2003.

Zambrowicz BP, Turner CA, Sands AT: Predicting drug efficacy: Knockouts model pipeline drugs of the pharmaceutical industry, *Curr Opin Pharmacol* 3(5):563–570, 2003.

Zeiss CJ: Mutant mouse pathology: an exercise in integration, *Lab Anim* 31:34–39, 2002.

Zeiss CJ, Ward JM, Allore HG: Designing phenotyping studies for genetically engineered mice, *Vet Pathol* 49:24–31, 2012.

Zhang X-H, Tee LY, Wang X-G, et al.: Off-target effects in CRISPR/Cas9-mediated genome engineering, *Mol Ther Nucleic Acids* 4:e264, 2015.

Zou Q, Wang X, Liu Y, et al.: Generation of gene-target dogs using CRISPR/Cas9 system, *J Mol Cell Biol* 7:580–583, 2015.

Alternative Models in Biomedical Research: In Silico, In Vitro, Ex Vivo, and Nontraditional In Vivo Approaches

Jinping Gan[1,2], Brad Bolon[3], Terry Van Vleet[4], Charles Wood[5]

[1]Bristol-Myers Squibb, Princeton, NJ, United States, [2]HiFiBiO Therapeutics, Cambridge, MA, United States,
[3]GEMpath, Inc., Longmont, CO, United States, [4]AbbVie, North Chicago, IL, United States, [5]Boehringer Ingelheim,
Ridgefield, CT, United States

OUTLINE

1. Introduction	925
2. Nontraditional Models in Toxicity Research	926
2.1. Overview of In Vitro and Ex Vivo Models	926
2.2. Overview of In Vivo Models in Alternative Mammalian and Nonmammalian Species	927
2.3. Overview of In Silico Modeling	928
3. In Vitro and Ex Vivo Models	928
3.1. Cell Cultures	928
3.2. Tissue Slices	930
3.3. Bioprinted Microtissues	934
3.4. Miniorgans	935
3.5. Microphysiological Systems ("Organs On Chips")	941
3.6. Stem Cells and Genetically Modified Cells	943
3.7. Whole Embryo Culture	945
4. In Silico Models and Data Analytics	946

4.1. In Silico Predictive Structure—Activity Models	946
4.2. Pathway-Based Models of Toxicity	947
4.3. Big Data Analytics in Toxicology Pathology	948
5. In Vivo Models Using Alternative Mammalian and Nonmammalian Species	951
5.1. Genetically Engineered Animal Models	951
5.2. Non-mammalian Animal Models	952
6. Regulatory Perspective on Alternative Models	955
7. Conclusions and Perspectives	955
7.1. Integration of Pathology and Alternative Data Streams	955
7.2. Context of Use and Qualification Requirements	957
7.3. Future Directions	958
References	958

1. INTRODUCTION

In 2007, the U.S. National Research Council (NRC) formally introduced a new paradigm in safety assessment and toxicity testing on behalf of a joint consortium of U.S. federal government agencies (Krewski et al., 2010; NRC, 2007). This "Tox 21" initiative highlighted both a vision and a strategy for assessing the safety of under-evaluated agents. For example, at present, the U.S. Environmental Protection Agency (EPA) Toxic Substances Control Act (TSCA) Inventory (U.S. EPA, 2021) lists over 40,000 chemicals, most of which have little or no safety data.

Haschek and Rousseaux's Handbook of Toxicologic Pathology, Fourth Edition.
https://doi.org/10.1016/B978-0-12-821044-4.00005-4

Risk assessment of this large and diverse universe of chemicals, and their myriad complex mixtures in the environment, is simply not feasible using in vivo animal toxicity studies, which are expensive and permit a limited throughput.

The "Tox 21" vision is to increase efficiency in safety assessment by shifting away from reliance on traditional "apical" endpoints like in vivo animal studies and toward risk predictions using data derived from alternative in silico, in vitro, and ex vivo models, pathway-based biomarkers, and "big data" analytics. The strategy was to develop and validate these innovative new models, to employ computational technologies and bioinformatics to enhance the evaluation of these models, and to translate these new types of scientific information into practical readouts that can guide risk assessment decisions even if data from traditional in vivo models are limited. In a broad sense, the "Tox 21" goal was to modernize toxicity testing and, in the process, reinvent toxicology as a more prospective and mechanism-based science.

Product discovery and development requires extensive testing to define potential toxic responses in organisms that might be exposed to a given chemical, drug, food additive, gene or cell therapy, or medical device. Such testing encompasses many different systems including computer-generated predictive algorithms (in silico) for screening and prioritization, isolated tissue elements such as cultured cells and tissue slices (in vitro), and living organisms (in vivo). In general, toxicologic pathologists spend most of their time evaluating specimens acquired from in vivo studies. However, the growing interest in reducing animal use and finding more human-like test systems is accelerating the invention and validation of alternative assay systems in toxicity assessment. Going forward, the newer in silico and in vitro model systems will have important implications for the practice of toxicologic pathology.

The goals of this chapter are to summarize current alternative models for evaluating toxicity and to provide a perspective of future directions in alternative model development of particular relevance to toxicologic pathology. Alternative platforms considered here include simple and advanced in vitro models, selected less common in vivo models, and basic types of in silico

models. These models have various advantages and disadvantages, depending on the questions being asked. Models of all levels of complexity have been informative for toxicologists and toxicologic pathologists.

2. NONTRADITIONAL MODELS IN TOXICITY RESEARCH

Four main categories of nontraditional safety assessment have gained importance for hazard identification and characterization as well as risk assessment in recent years. These strategies are in vitro modeling, ex vivo modeling, in vivo modeling in alternative mammalian and nonmammalian species, and most recently in silico systems.

2.1. Overview of In Vitro and Ex Vivo Models

In vitro models consist of cells grown in isolation, while ex vivo models consist of structurally intact portions (usually small masses or thin slices) removed from a parent organ or tissue. In vitro and ex vivo models have been most successful at answering very specific questions. For example, are key proteins expressed? Are functional activities that are important for the question at hand maintained in the model? Does the model respond as predicted to known toxicants? By design, in vitro and ex vivo models address questions that relate to responses in a particular cell population and tissue without any attempt to consider other factors that contribute to toxicity in whole organisms (*ADME Principles in Small Molecule Drug Discovery and Development*, Vol 1, Chap 3, *Biotherapeutic ADME and PK/PD Principles*, Vol 1, Chap 4; *Principles of Pharmacodynamics and Toxicodynamics*, Vol 1, Chap 5).

Perhaps the simplest in vitro models use prokaryotic organisms. For example, bacterial models, such as *Salmonella typhimurium* and *Escherichia coli*, are staples in genetic toxicology as part of the Ames assay for mutagenesis (Dyrby and Ingvardsen, 1983). Bacterial strains with particular deficiencies in DNA repair have helped to elucidate mechanisms of mutagenesis, and genetic modifications (introduced via plasmids) have been useful in further sensitizing some strains (McMahon et al., 1979).

Isolated eukaryotic cells in culture are another simple in vitro model for toxicity assessment. The advantages of such models include the ability to conduct experiments using cells from multiple species, including humans, at relatively low cost and with tight control of experimental conditions. Two-dimensional (2D) cell culture models allow for complete isolation of the cell type of interest. Importantly, in vitro models can be more readily standardized than in vivo studies and therefore may be implemented with greater consistency across laboratories. Furthermore, these high-throughput models permit incredible rates of product testing due to increases in the detection sensitivity for innovative modern endpoints and the expansion of traditional 96-multiwell plates to accommodate 384 or 1536 wells per plate (Maffia et al., 1999; Titus et al., 2008). These recent advances in simple in vitro eukaryotic models are ideal for screening large libraries of chemicals or drug candidates to get an early estimation regarding efficacy or possible safety liabilities (Blomme and Will, 2016). One key criticism of 2D eukaryotic cell models is their inability to predict in vivo toxicity. This criticism often arises from poorly formulated questions (such as trying to use in vitro models to assess cellular toxicity in the absence of in vivo factors such as absorption, distribution, and metabolism in other organs) or from trying to ask questions that are too complex for a simple cell type–specific model to answer.

To improve physiological relevance and answer more complicated biological questions, more complex in vitro and ex vivo systems have been developed (Davies, 2018; Low and Tagle, 2017). These systems include cell combinations (e.g., cells of interest cocultured in 2D or three dimensions [3D] with their support cells); tissue slices; miniorgans (e.g., organoids, embryoid bodies [EBs], micromasses); and microphysiological systems (MPS) (i.e., "organs on a chip"). These more complex in vitro and ex vivo eukaryotic models have the potential to address more advanced questions because of their multiple interacting cell types and their more intact cytoarchitectural structures and microphysiological processes. Multiorgan interactions can be simulated as well (Wikswo, 2014).

Such 2D and especially 3D models can be assessed readily using conventional morphological techniques available to toxicologic pathologists, including light and electron microscopy as well as numerous molecular pathology techniques (*Special Techniques in Toxicologic Pathology*, Vol 1, Chap 11).

2.2. Overview of In Vivo Models in Alternative Mammalian and Nonmammalian Species

In vivo testing for product discovery and development traditionally relies on a limited number of mammalian species, but alternative in vivo models may offer significant advantages in certain applications. With rodents as an example, these alternatives may include less commonly used species (e.g., guinea pigs and hamsters; *Animal Models in Toxicologic Research: Rodents*, Vol 1, Chap 17) or bioengineered disease models (*Genetically Engineered Animal Models in Toxicologic Research*, Vol 1, Chap 23). In particular, genetically modified models (rodents and more recently nonrodents) have advanced the disciplines of toxicology and toxicologic pathology significantly in the last 3 decades (Kim et al., 2019a; Nagarajan et al., 2012). Alternative in vivo models of disease have been instrumental in understanding the genetic roots of disease development (Bao et al., 2018; Kim et al., 2019a; Sultan et al., 2019). Likewise, animals with genetically altered metabolic capacity have been used to identify, confirm, and characterize mechanisms of toxicity as well as to better understand clearance and distribution of novel chemical entities (Barzi et al., 2017; Heit et al., 2015; Wu et al., 2019).

The value of nonmammalian in vivo models to many scientific disciplines, including toxicology, is undisputable (*Models of Toxicity: Non-mammalian*, Vol 1, Chap 22). Key species used to gain deeper insights into genetic influences in biology and toxicology include such model organisms as nematodes (*Caenorhabditis elegans*), the fruit fly (*Drosophila melanogaster*), many fish species, and birds. For instance, zebrafish (*Danio rerio*) are a prominent non-mammalian in vivo model in toxicology (Cassar et al., 2020), valued since they share many conserved physiological processes with more traditional vertebrate models of toxicity. These alternative species have been shown to be excellent models for studying the link between genetics, toxicant-induced mechanisms of disease, and variations in sensitivity or resistance to toxicity due to their short life spans, small sizes, minimal husbandry costs, fecundity, and ease of cultivation. A primary advantage of such alternative in vivo models is that they may be maintained at very high stocking densities in petri dishes (for nematodes), multiwell plates (for fish larvae), or tanks (for adult fish), which permits much larger group sizes than can be managed for mammalian vertebrates.

2.3. Overview of In Silico Modeling

In silico methods are progressing to the point that commercially available computer software now provides substantial contributions to toxicity and safety assessments (Van Vleet et al., 2019). Quantitative structure–activity relationship (QSAR) algorithms have become a standard part of genetic toxicity screening as well as early toxicity predictions (Rao et al., 2019). Extensive and more complex toxicity databases utilizing advanced computational approaches such as artificial intelligence (AI) and machine learning are capable of identifying patterns in large datasets to build useful predictive models (Vo et al., 2020). Bioinformatics is a growing aid to toxicity testing, making major contributions to many "omics" technologies (*Toxicogenomics: A Practical Primer*, Vol 1, Chap 15). In many institutions, in silico models of toxicity are superintended by scientists with computer science or information technology backgrounds. That being said, the modern practice of toxicology requires that toxicologic pathologists and toxicologists have at least a basic comprehension of in silico strategies for evaluating toxicity.

Taken together, these trends affirm the growing importance of alternative models of toxicity as aids in hazard identification and characterization as well as safety assessment. Challenges in creating, and effectively using, more common alternative in vitro and in vivo models need to be considered in their application. Nonetheless, many standard toxicologic pathology techniques may be effectively used in their evaluation.

3. IN VITRO AND EX VIVO MODELS

In vitro and ex vivo models need to be characterized and validated carefully to confirm their appropriateness for the question being asked (Mahalingaiah et al., 2018; Van Vleet, Liguori, & Lynch, 2019). By intent, in vitro and ex vivo models focus on evaluating toxic responses in cells and tissues after they have been isolated from systemic factors (e.g., absorption, circulation, and excretion). Recent innovations have restored some of the absent systemic parameters to in vitro systems, thereby allowing them to better approximate the conditions found in cells and tissues maintained in their natural in vivo setting. The incomplete restoration of normal structural (for in vitro) and physiological (for in vitro and ex vivo) attributes means that even the best in vitro and ex vivo models are not fully equivalent to tissues in vivo. In particular, the absence of normal tissue organization may prohibit expansion of some cell populations in vitro, and may preclude analysis of processes in vitro that require a particular tissue architecture to permit effective cell interaction and function.

3.1. Cell Cultures

For decades, in vitro 2D cell cultures have been an integral part of basic biological research for the study of cellular function and metabolism, mechanisms of disease initiation and progression, and investigations of efficacy and toxicity for environmental chemicals and potential pharmaceutical candidates (Lorsch et al., 2014; Pamies et al., 2018; Zbinden, 1988). Categorically, cell cultures may be characterized as continuous cell lines or primary cell cultures. Under the right conditions, such cultures may be maintained for several weeks or a few months. Both categories are widely utilized in academic, government, and industrial research laboratories, and data from both categories have proven valuable in various regulatory settings. Each category has its advantages and shortcomings.

Continuous (immortalized) cell lines have the ability to proliferate indefinitely due to either a spontaneous and random gene mutation or by deliberate genetic alteration. Continuous cell lines have several advantages when cultured such as their indefinite proliferation, low propagation and maintenance costs, purity of cell population (vital for experimental reproducibility), and well-established culture conditions and protocols (American Type Culture Collection Standards Development Organization Workgroup, 2010; Lorsch et al., 2014). Therefore, continuous cell lines are still widely used in screening assays in drug discovery. However, such cell lines are not without problems. The inherent defects leading to immortalization mean that they do not typically resemble the native functions and metabolic pathways of the tissue from which they are derived nor are their responses to external modulations typical of their original cells. In addition, passages of continuous cell lines result, over time, in genetic drift from a growing stable of additional gene mutation that further alters their phenotype in culture. Perhaps the most problematic attribute is the wide spread contamination of continuous cell lines by other cell types (e.g., HeLa [cervical carcinoma] cells), which confounds interpretation of results from both current studies and prior scientific literature (Alge et al., 2006; American Type Culture Collection Standards Development Organization Workgroup, 2010; Lorsch et al., 2014; Pamies et al., 2018; Pastor et al., 2010).

In contrast, primary cell cultures are derived directly from freshly excised tissue or biopsy specimens harvested from humans and animals. Primary cells have a wild-type genotype (i.e., without major genetic mutations) and phenotype, so they recapitulate the attributes of their cell of origin. According to Good Cell Culture Practice, primary cell cultures are defined as *"the initial in vitro culture of harvested cells and tissue taken directly from animals and humans"* (Hartung et al., 2001). In reality, since appropriately cultured primary cells retain their genetic integrity, morphology, and native cellular functions even after limited subculture passages, certain commercially available "primary" cultures are in fact low-passage number

subcultures of the initial tissue isolation. The high structural and functional fidelity of primary cell cultures enables the study of normal physiological and biochemical processes in essentially native cells as well as the metabolic fate, chemical interaction potential, and effects (efficacy and toxicity) of environmental chemicals and drug candidates on such processes (Alge et al., 2006; Pan et al., 2009). In addition, the ability to culture primary cells from equivalent organs of animals and humans allows for direct comparison of chemical potency and toxicity across species, which aids substantially in translation of animal-derived data to guide human benefit/risk assessment. Primary cell cultures are not without their own problems. They typically have limited life spans in culture, may be relatively hard to establish and maintain in culture, and generally are more expensive than immortalized cell lines. Because of the limited yield and finite life span of freshly derived cells, primary cultures typically are obtained from multiple donors, so they have inherently divergent—and not necessarily modest—differences in function and genetic makeup based on interindividual variations among donors.

At present, primary cells used in toxicological applications are isolated from most major organs. Common sites include skin, intestine, liver, lung, kidney, eye, and brain (Aschner and Kimelberg, 1991; Berube et al., 2010; Boogaard et al., 1990; Forbes and Ehrhardt, 2005; Grant, 2020; Li, 2007; Li et al., 2018; Roguet, 1999; Ulrich et al., 1995). Tissue samples for primary cell culture may be procured from different sources, including post mortem donors, rejected transplants, surgical biopsies, and other voluntary donations such as blood, bone marrow, and skin biopsies. Mechanical and/or enzymatic processes may be necessary to dissociate the cells of interest from connective tissues. The resulting cell suspensions are typically a heterogeneous mixture of several cell types which may need to be further purified before the cell culture can be established. This additional purification can be accomplished by physical (microdissection, gradient centrifugation); immunological (antibody-specific capturing); and/or biochemical (specific media conditions to promote cell type–specific growth and proliferation) methods (Pamies et al., 2018). Purified cells can be used as a suspension (for anchorage-independent cells such as lymphocytes) or as an adherent culture (for anchorage-dependent parenchymal cells from solid organs). The composition of the culture medium is cell type-dependent and usually contains variable concentrations of many nutrients including glucose, essential amino acids, one or more growth factors, and sometimes antibiotics; the medium composition is optimized for proper growth and differentiation of the particular cell type. In some cases, extracellular matrix (ECM) protein–coated culture plates also are necessary to promote adhesion of anchorage-dependent primary cells. For example, sandwich coating of matrices is used to promote bile canaliculi formation when liver cells are being cultured (Swift et al., 2010). Such coatings may be used to impart a more 3D, quasi-organized structure to the culture that provides an environment that more closely resembles the milieu the native cells encounter within intact tissue.

Because freshly isolated cells have a finite lifespan in culture, consistency in primary cell cultures requires banking of primary cells for archiving, transportation, and future usage (Li, 2007; Pamies et al., 2018). Cryopreservation is a process to preserve living cells using ultralow temperatures. Cells are suspended in solutions containing dimethyl sulfoxide or glycerol and fetal bovine serum as cryoprotectants and then slowly frozen in a programmable controlled-rate freezer to minimize the formation of ice crystals (which can disrupt cell and organelle membranes) within the cells. The frozen cells can be stored in liquid nitrogen ($<-150°C$) for long-term preservation and transport. Cryopreserved cells can be recovered by thawing in a 37°C water bath for a few minutes.

Before their use for toxicological applications, primary cell cultures need to be characterized and qualified. Characterization usually includes the assessment of cell morphology and polarity, expression of relevant marker proteins, and demonstration of relevant functional capabilities. After satisfactory characterization, the cultures are then qualified using known toxicants (positive controls) and nontoxicants (negative controls) to ensure the recapitulation of specific cellular toxicity responses to known sets of test agents. One underappreciated aspect of qualification is to ensure that any effects seen in the toxicant-treated cells result from exposure to the test article and not to poor medium quality (due to inappropriate formulation and/or bacterial/fungal contamination). These steps are necessary to provide context to the toxicity data obtained from these cultures so that appropriate translation can be made to in vivo outcomes in the same species (e.g., in vitro rat hepatocyte cultures with in vivo liver toxicity in rats) or to similar cell populations across species (e.g., in vitro rat hepatocyte cultures to in vitro human hepatocyte cultures). An additional manipulation to assist animal-to-human translation when screening molecules for toxicity in vitro is to add the S9 (microsomal) fraction from homogenized human liver to cell cultures to add human xenobiotic-metabolizing activity (harbored predominantly in microsomes) to the system. This adaptation has been used successfully in Tox21 toxicity testing to show that metabolic activation of genotoxic agents increases their capacity to induce mutations in the DT40 (chicken cell) DNA damage response assay (Hashimoto et al., 2015).

In general, characterization and qualification consists of biochemical and functional (i.e., quantitative) endpoints. The parameters typically are preferred since they can be measured using automated, high-throughput instrumentation. Morphology of cultured cells following toxicant exposure may be undertaken by toxicologic pathologists using conventional histopathologic techniques as an additional means for characterization and qualification (Figure 24.1). Endpoints of interest subject to microscopic evaluation include culture "anatomy"—cells undergo a reproducible structural evolution as they develop—and biomarker expression (Bolon et al., 1993). These features may be assessed in live cultures throughout their life span using fluorescent or phase-contrast microscopy. In the authors' experience, toxicologic pathologists participate in evaluation of cell cultures only on an occasional basis, and chiefly during basic discovery and investigational toxicology studies.

3.2. Tissue Slices

Tissue slices have considerable attraction as ex vivo models of toxicity. Ex vivo slices consist of thin tissue slabs that have been removed from an organism for evaluation in an external

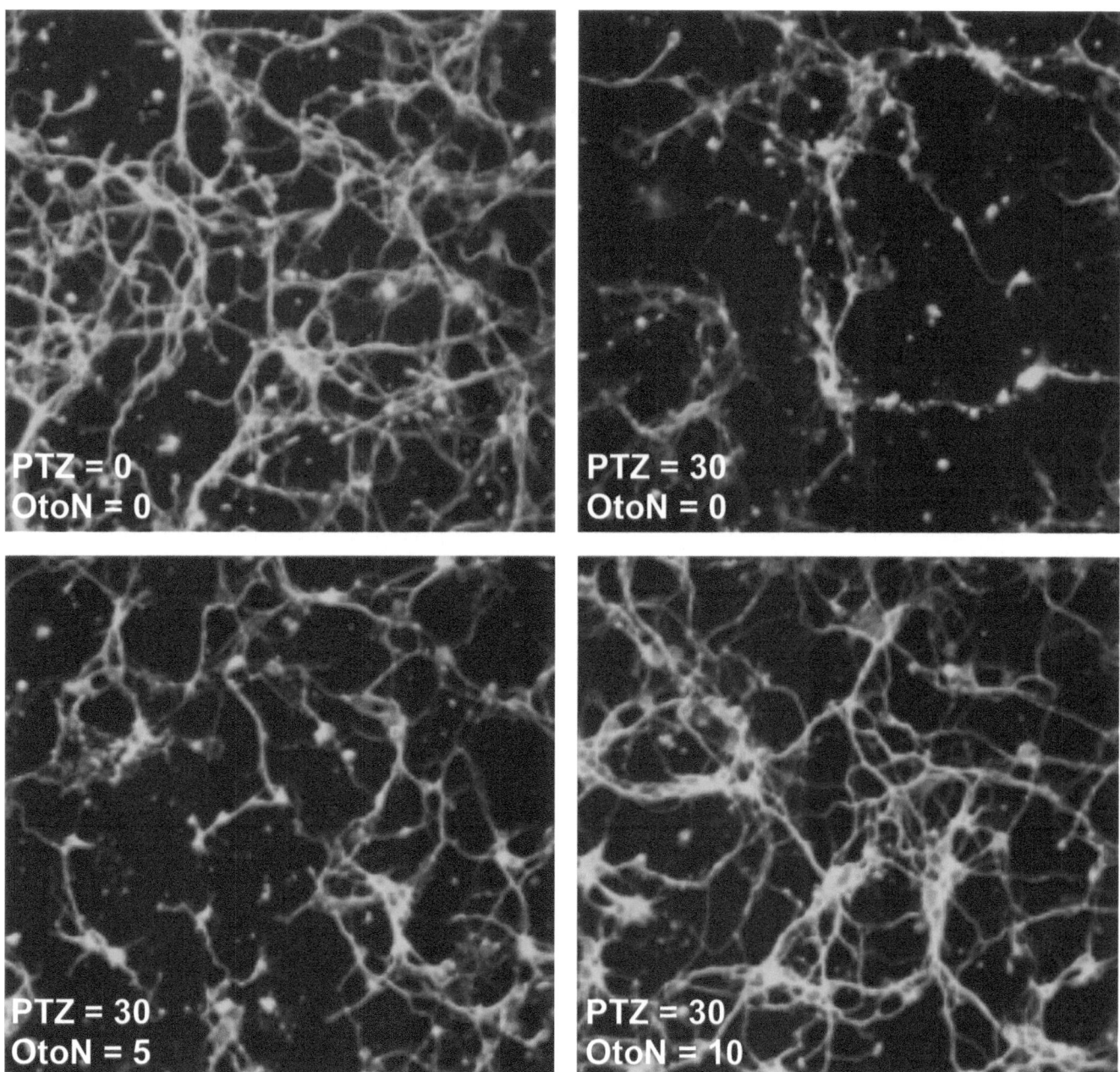

FIGURE 24.1 Neurotoxicity and its prevention in primary cerebrocortical cell cultures of near-term embryonic mice, as evaluated by fluorescent microscopy. The neurons were treated with pentylenetetrazol (PTZ, in mM), a stimulant that can induce seizures at high doses, or PTZ plus otophylloside N (OtoN, an herbal extract used to treat epilepsy, in μg/mL) for 24 h after 7 days in culture. Cells were immunostained with neuronal antiβ-tubulin marker (green) and nuclear DAPI (blue). *Reproduced from Page 4, Figure 3, Panel A (top row) in Sheng F, Chen M, Tan Y, et al.: Protective effects of otophylloside N on pentylenetetrazol-induced neuronal injury in vitro and in vivo, Front Pharmacol 7:224, 2016 under a Creative Commons Attribution License.*

environment, thereby retaining near-natural tissue architecture for cells within the piece. The key advantage of this ex vivo assay is that 3D tissue architecture is well maintained for most cells in the specimen except for those nearest the cut margins. Thus, appropriate cell–cell and cell–matrix interactions are retained, which permit such cultures to function in a more physiologically relevant setting relative to 2D monolayers or suspensions of isolated primary cells obtained from the same location. The thinness of tissue slices permits nutrients, oxygen, signaling molecules (e.g., cytokines and growth factors), and waste product levels to approximate those found in the intact organ, though over time the quantities of these constituents diverges from the norm in the deepest parts of the slices.

Tissue slices can be produced for many organs utilizing well-controlled cutting to generate thin tissue slices of reproducible thickness. The use of tissue slices (of inconsistent thickness) was first described by Otto Warburg in 1923 to measure cell metabolism in tumor tissues, and later found success in the study of amino acid metabolism by Hans Krebs in 1933 (Parrish et al., 1995). Widespread use of tissue slices was enabled in the 1980s with the development of instrumentation to allow more precise cutting of thin slices in parallel to dynamic culture methodologies to prolong the ex vivo viability of tissue slices. The use of precision-cut tissue slices (PCTS), which yields more consistent specimen characteristics, has been demonstrated in various organ types including liver, kidney, intestine, lung, heart, and brain (Baverel et al., 2013; Fischer et al., 2019; Li et al., 2016; Morin et al., 2013; Palma et al., 2019). This method is widely applied to study disease modeling, drug metabolism, pharmacologic efficacy, and toxicity (Graaf et al., 2007; Palma et al., 2019; Sewald and Braun, 2013; Westra et al., 2016).

In order to consistently obtain high-quality PCTS, tissue cores are prepared by using a sharpened metal cylinder to remove samples from isolated tissues/organs (Figure 24.2). The tissue cores are then mounted in a cylindrical tissue holder which is submerged in cold, oxygenated slicing buffer. Slices are produced by moving the tissue cylinder across a blade at the bottom of the cylinder, while a stream of cold buffer helps sweep away the slices for collection. For tissues that are difficult to cut after isolation (such as intestine and lung), prefilling the hollow spaces within the tissue core with agarose is necessary before the tissue can be cut to prevent distortion of the tissue architecture and damage to the cells that line the spaces. Freshly prepared slices are then either placed onto a titanium grid inside 25 mL glass scintillation vials containing culture media or directly introduced into tissue culture dishes; the choice of which approach to use depends on the applications. The typical thickness of slices varies with the tissue type, but normally it is from 100 (liver) to 500 (lung) μm. The viability of PCTS cultures is typically assessed by such methodologies as measuring the rate of protein synthesis, leakage of intracellular enzymes, and histopathological evaluations.

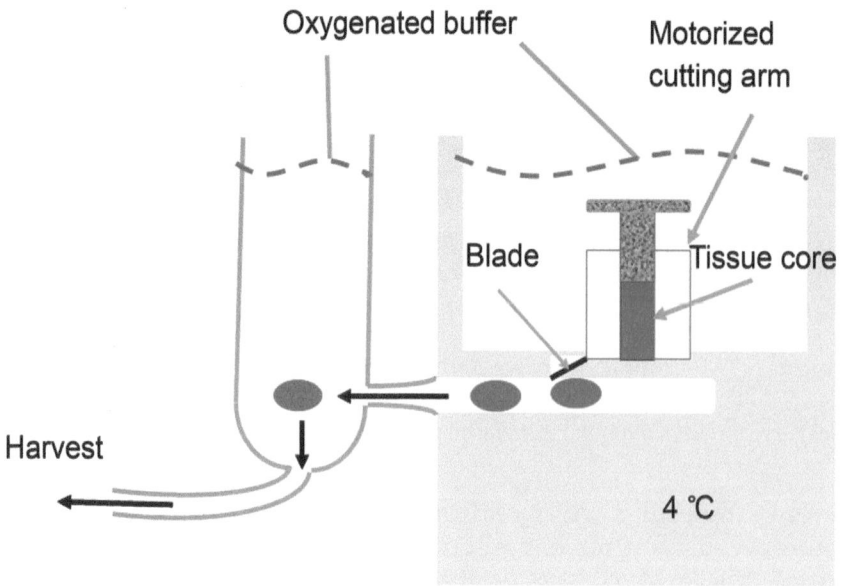

FIGURE 24.2   Representative diagram for producing precision-cut tissue slices with the Krumdieck/Alabama Research and Development Tissue Slicer.

The utility of tissue slices in toxicological research has been recently reviewed in detail. Representative reviews include liver, intestine, lung, heart, brain, and kidney (Baverel et al., 2013; Li et al., 2016; Morin et al., 2013; Palma et al., 2019). Recent trends include the incorporation of PCTS into dynamic flow devices to prolong the culture life time (Bakmand et al., 2015), the study of immunotoxicity in lymphoid organ PCTS (Sewald and Braun, 2013), the addition of physiological electromechanical stimulation for long-term functional preservation of myocardium slices (Fischer et al., 2019), and virus-assisted gene transfer studies (van Geer et al., 2009). The preservation of all cell types in their native positions and with their usual interactions makes PCTS a great model for investigating toxicities that may involve multiple cell types. Importantly, the architecture in PCTS resembles that of the intact tissue in vivo, which makes this model well suited for histopathologic evaluation; indeed, the

desire to perform a detailed microscopic assessment of a specimen that retains normal cell and tissue organization is a feature that often drives the choice to employ tissue slices rather than cell cultures as the investigational tool (Figure 24.3). The sharp margins of PCTS preserve the function of most metabolizing enzymes and transporters, which sometimes is critical in the manifestation of toxicant-induced effects.

However, the use of PCTS does have some disadvantages. First of all, the slices are typically short-lived, with viability in culture ranging from a few hours to a few days depending on the tissue type and medium. Second, because this model relies on fresh tissue isolation, both the throughput and reproducibility are limited by the availability and quality of fresh tissues—especially for human specimens—which typically come from surgical procedures. Finally, although the slices retain the native architecture of the original tissue, the ex vivo culture conditions are not representative of the tissue

Human Precision Cut Liver Slices: Heterogeneity of cell types

Hepatocytes and Kupffer cells

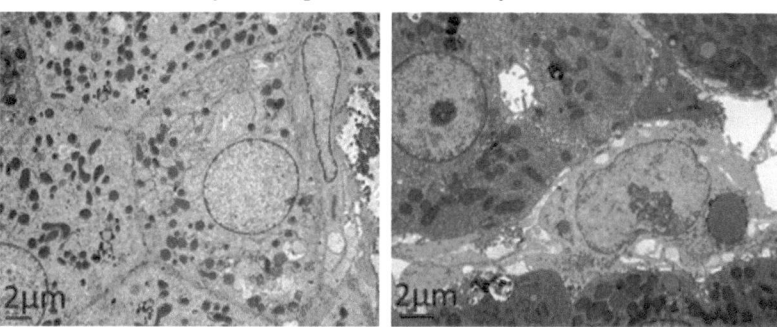

Endothelial cells

Fibroblast

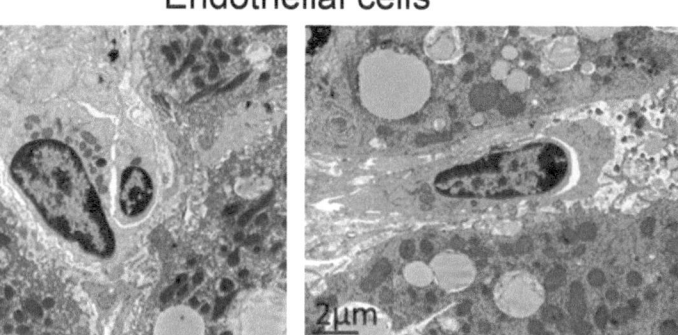
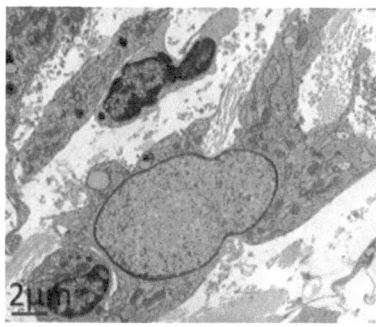

FIGURE 24.3 Cell heterogeneity in precision-cut human liver slices as assessed by transmission electron microscopy is preserved to a degree that matches that which occurs in native liver tissue. *Reproduced from Page 52, Figure 1 in Palma E, Doornebal EJ, Chokshi S: Precision-cut liver slices: a versatile tool to advance liver research,* Hepatol Int 13:51–57, 2019 *under a Creative Commons Attribution 4.0 International License.*

environment and regular molecular turnover (e.g., replenishment of blood-borne nutrients and oxygen, circulation of signaling hormones and cytokines, and removal of metabolic by-products) that occurs in vivo. By combining PCTS with microfluidic techniques (see Section 3.5), it is reasonable to anticipate that microphysiological systems ("organs on a chip") might be generated that allow for longer-term cultures under more physiological culture conditions.

3.3. Bioprinted Microtissues

Bioprinting is a technology that is driving significant innovation in several areas including tissue engineering, regenerative medicine, tissue transplantation, and the development of complex in vitro models (Bishop et al., 2017; Mekhileri et al., 2018; Murphy and Atala, 2014; Peng et al., 2016). Bioprinting tissues involves significant complexities including the selection of cell types, growth media (with differentiation factors), minimizing damage to printed cells, and the composition of extracellular scaffolds that support a defined (2D or 3D) architecture (Murphy and Atala, 2014). The proper selection and control of these factors are key to successful tissue/model construction. Bioprinting has been used to produce multiple complex in vitro models from patterned 2D-printed cultures to organoids to microphysiological systems with fluidics (Boyer et al., 2018; Knowlton and Tasoglu, 2016; Prendergast et al., 2018; Wang et al., 2018); all these have all been used for assessing toxicity. The versatility of bioprinting is further demonstrated by the wide array of microtissues that have been generated including cardiac and skeletal muscle, lung (alveolar–capillary interface), gastrointestinal villi, liver, and kidney (proximal tubules) (Benam et al., 2015; Feinberg et al., 2007; Ho et al., 2013; Huh et al., 2010; Kim et al., 2012; Park et al., 2006; Uzel et al., 2014).

Three main strategies—biomimicry, self-assembly, and microtissue approaches—have been used for creating bioprinted 3D in vitro models. Each process involves preprocessing, processing, and postprocessing stages (Bishop et al., 2017). Preprocessing encompasses the proper design and selection of appropriate materials and reagents. Processing represents the printing and assembly of microtissue models. Postprocessing generally incorporates an incubation period that allows cell attachment,

proliferation, interaction, and functioning prior to the use of bioprinted tissue in testing (Bishop et al., 2017). In addition to proper printing and assembly, other factors such as signaling molecules, structural elements, and appropriate environmental factors (e.g., temperature, pressure, sheer, and electrical forces) may need to be optimized during the processing and postprocessing stages (Bishop et al., 2017). All these factors may be addressed in the choice of bioink components (where a bioink is a complex brew of cells and/or organic materials that provide a suitable ECM environment to support the adhesion, proliferation, and differentiation of living cells).

Biomimicry

Biomimicry represents perhaps the most straightforward approach to bioprinting. This strategy assumes that proper form results in appropriate function (Bishop et al., 2017). Essentially, cells and extracellular components to support them are printed in a 3D pattern that mimics the microanatomy of a tissue or organ. However, accurate recapitulation of biologic tissue is extremely difficult. Several challenges have been noted with the biomimicry approach including incomplete and/or variable attachment, proliferation, migration, and maintenance of proper cell types and proportions (Murphy and Atala, 2014). The selection of scaffolding material is crucial in this process in order to best mimic the native structural and mechanical requirements for the target tissue being represented. The scaffold choice also significantly influences signaling through cellular interactions with the ECM component (Grayson et al., 2009). Common options for scaffolding materials include polymers of natural materials such as decellularized ECM, peptides, and DNA strands; synthetic materials such as polyethylene glycol and polyurethane; or combinations of natural and synthetic materials (Dzobo et al., 2019; Stanton et al., 2015).

Self-Assembly

The self-assembly approach to bioprinting attempts to reproduce the embryonic environmental and structural conditions so that processing will yield a tissue consistent with normal embryologic anatomy (Murphy and Atala, 2014; Steer and Nigam, 2004). With the appropriate embryonic elements in place, it is assumed that the self-assembly process will follow the natural embryogenic process in producing the appropriate cell and tissue organization characteristic of mature tissue (Steer and Nigam, 2004). Studies have demonstrated that self-assembly can result in high cellular density, improved cellular interactions, accelerated growth, and better long-term function of the bioprinted tissue (Jakab et al., 2010; Norotte et al., 2009; Takebe et al., 2013; Yu et al., 2016). This approach has been used to create the first bioengineered blood vessels from human smooth muscle and fibroblast cells (L'Heureux et al., 1998).

Microtissues

The microtissue strategy for bioprinting simplifies organ/tissue design by recognizing that tissues are constructed of many smaller functional units which contribute to the overall patterning of the whole. In this way, the smallest structural or functional units are engineered first and then combined into the desired final macrotissue model (Murphy and Atala, 2014). Tissue spheroids make ideal microtissue building blocks. Microtissue strategy for bioengineering is considered to be more efficient because the relatively small size of the building blocks lends to their easy incorporation into bioinks. Microtissue size is easily standardized, which increases the feasibility of automation and scalability in bioprinting, thereby improving the speed and efficiency of in vitro model production (Mironov et al., 2009; Zhang and Zhang, 2015).

Bioprinting Methods/Challenges

Bioprinting 3D tissues can be done with a number of different technologies, each with various strengths and weaknesses. Droplet-based bioprinting methods are common and are implemented by several inkjet printer types that use thermal and piezoelectric/acoustic printing mechanisms (Peng et al., 2016). Microextrusion-based bioprinting is likely the most common method and uses mechanical or pneumatic displacement of fluid volumes to deliver precise amounts of bioink (Murphy and Atala, 2014). Finally, laser-based bioprinting has been successfully used for tissue and model engineering, though it is less popular than droplet- or extrusion-based printing due to higher costs and lower efficiency and printing accuracy than other methods (Peng et al., 2016). Advantages and disadvantages of these

various bioprinting platforms are outlined in Table 24.1.

Bioprinters have been used to create very complex tissues/models. For example, Masaeli et al. (2019) used inkjet printing to construct a 3D multilayered model retinal tissue (Masaeli et al., 2019). The complexity of the retina reflects the resolution and precision of this bioprinting platform. Microextrusion has been used to produce several complicated tissue models such as aortic valves (Duan et al., 2013a, 2013b), vascular trees (Norotte et al., 2009), and tumor models (Xu et al., 2011).

3.4. Miniorgans

Conceptually, miniorgans are designed to approximately replicate the structure and key functions of a complete organ. Such in vitro models may exhibit either a 2D or 3D tissue architecture depending on the nature of the model fabrication process. Miniorgans may be produced from cells derived from any species, which in the future should facilitate translation of in vitro data for risk assessment via the direct comparison of comparable models from one or more animal species and humans.

Organoids

Organoid cultures are 3D multicellular masses (Figure 24.4) comprised of more than one cell type that resemble the composition of specific organs on a microscale (Little, 2017). In 2013, *The Scientist* named organoids as one of several "Advances of the Year" (Davies, 2018; Grens, 2013). More recently, *Nature Methods* designated organoids as the "Method of the Year" (Editorial, 2017).

Organoids lack the complexity of intact natural organs but represent a significant advancement in complexity relative to standard 2D monocultures. Organoids have been used to model disease, screen chemicals for efficacy and toxicity, study cell and organ development, investigate cell-to-cell interactions, and understand the process of self-organization (Dahl-Jensen and Grapin-Botton, 2017; Little, 2017). Organoids are typically derived from adult or embryonic tissue cells, embryonic stem cells (ESC), or induced pluripotent stem cells (iPSCs), which can self-organize under the right conditions (Figure 24.4) (Dahl-Jensen and Grapin-Botton, 2017). These characteristics explain their

TABLE 24.1 Bioprinting Platforms

Method	Strengths	Weaknesses	Mechanism	References
Inkjet	• Simple operating components and software • Low cost • High speed • High resolution • Compatible with most bioinks	• Nozzle clogging • Sheer stress imparted to cells (viscous bioinks) • Dilute bioinks = low cell densities	Multiple—Droplet/thermal, piezoelectric/acoustic—see below	Peng et al. (2016) Murphy and Atala (2014) Saunders et al. (2008), Xu et al. (2005) Masaeli et al. (2019)
1. Droplet/Thermal	• Widely available • Cost effective	• Thermal/mechanical stress • Less uniform droplet size, directionality, • Less reliable cell encapsulation • Nozzle clogging	Function by electrically heating the print head (exceeding 200°C) to produce pulses of pressure that force droplets of bioink from the nozzle	Goldmann and Gonzalez (2000), Okamoto et al. (2000), Xu et al. (2006) Murphy and Atala (2014)
2. Piezoelectric/ Acoustic	• Precise droplet size • Precise directionality • Lack of heat/pressure	• Cell stress from 15–25 kHz pulses • Loss of membrane integrity with viscous bioinks	Create acoustic waves in print head leading to droplet formation at regular intervals. Accomplished by applying electric current to a piezoelectric crystal, generating a rapid change in shape. Acoustic pulses eject liquid droplets from the air—liquid interface	Murphy and Atala (2014) Demirci and Montesano (2007), Fang et al. (2012) Cui et al. (2012) Kim et al. (2010)
Microextrusion	• Common • Affordable • Continuous bead droplets	• Lower cell viability (shear stress) • Slow speed • Poorer resolution	Use pneumatic or mechanical (piston- or screw like) mechanisms to control volume displacement and printing of biomaterials	Mironov et al. (2009), Smith et al. (2004) Peltola et al. (2008) Murphy and Atala (2014)

	Advantages	Disadvantages	Description	References
	• Compatible with important materials (hydrogels, cellular spheroids, copolymers, highly viscous materials) • High (biologically relevant) cell densities			Chang et al. (2011), Marga et al. (2012), Mironov et al. (2009), Duan et al. (2013a, 2013b), Norotte et al. (2009), Xu et al. (2011), Chang et al. (2008), Smith et al. (2004)
Laser	• No clogging of nozzle • No effects on cell survival	• Time consuming • Lower efficiency • Lower accuracy • Higher costs • Scale-up challenges	Laser-induced forward transfer from pulsed laser beam that is focused onto a "ribbon" with a laser-absorbing layer of gold or titanium on glass to support donor transport and a liquid layer of biological material facing the "ribbon." Focusing the laser on the absorbing layer creates a high-pressure bubble that transfers the cells and bioink matrix to the collector substrate	Barron et al. (2005, 2004), Ringeisen et al. (2004), Chrisey (2000), Colina et al. (2005), Dinca et al. (2008), Ringeisen et al. (2004), Guillemot et al. (2010), Gruene et al. (2011), Hopp et al. (2005), Koch et al. (2010), Guillotin and Guillemot (2011), Michael et al. (2013)

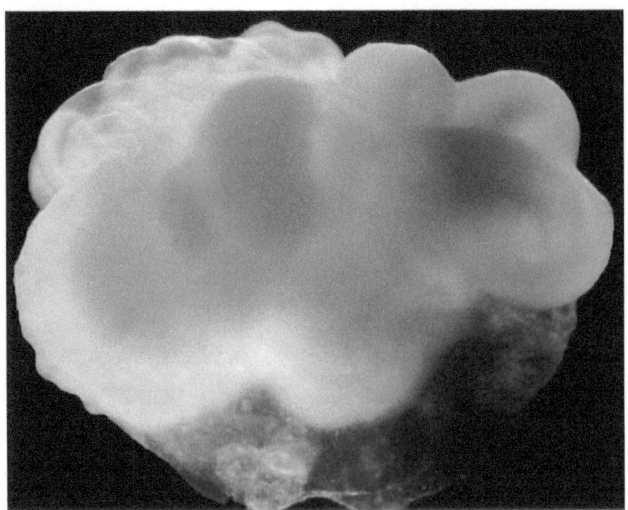

FIGURE 24.4 Representative appearance of a chimpanzee cerebral organoid. *Reproduced from Page 4, Figure 1, Panel A (left panel) in Mora-Bermudez F, Badsha F, Kanton S, et al.: Differences and similarities between human and chimpanzee neural progenitors during cerebral cortex development, Elife 5, 2016 under a Creative Commons Attribution License (CC BY 4.0).*

excellent capacities for self-renewal and ordered differentiation (Dahl-Jensen and Grapin-Botton, 2017; Fatehullah et al., 2016). Other cell sources, such as mature somatic cells, may be used in some cases to generate organoids (Davies, 2018). One example is the use of differentiated human keratinocytes mixed with fibroblasts to organize into skin organoids with a dermis-like layer (Kim et al., 1999).

Organoids contain multiple cell types that are arranged in structures resembling their organ of interest and possessing some of the biological functions of those tissues (Huch and Koo, 2015). Unlike organs in vivo, organoids are free from the influence of other organs and systems of the whole organism, allowing for highly controlled and focused experiments (Greggio et al., 2013). Other advantages to organoids are their high-throughput potential, the ability to permit histopathological evaluation by standard methods, and the opportunity to evaluate organoids over extended periods of time (Greggio et al., 2013). In many cases, due to the simultaneous presence of both progenitor and differentiated cells, organoids provide a means to evaluate the sensitivity of cells at multiple stages of development and differentiation in a single experiment (Greggio et al., 2013). Organoids can exhibit many characteristics of

differentiated cells including polarization, cell-to-cell adherence, and the formation of tubes, pits, folds, or bulges (Dahl-Jensen and Grapin-Botton, 2017). One of the biggest challenges with organoids is that small differences in the initial conditions, particularly the number of cells, create significant variability among organoid construction even under identical culture conditions (Todhunter et al., 2015; Ungrin et al., 2012). Standardization of initial seeding conditions is therefore vital to improve the consistency of organoids. One strategy to standardize organoid size and shape has been to employ 3D bioprinting technology to better control cell–cell and cell–matrix interactions as a series of organoids are being assembled (Peng et al., 2016). Cells suspended in bioink (ECM constituents) can be deposited directly onto surfaces to produce 3D cocultures with customized geometries (Yin et al., 2016).

A number of other methods have been successfully employed to generate organoids (Peng et al., 2016). The "hanging drop" method uses gravity and hydrostatic forces to culture organoids suspended in a droplet that hangs below a plate. The cells have no attachment to a substrate surface other than the membranes of adjacent cells. The "microwell plate" method serves to grow organoids in wells with nonadhesive curved floors to prevent cell attachment. A "microfluidic" method has been used to stack clustered cells ("spheroids") in layers, while a "magnetic labeling" procedure has been employed to compact spheroid structures under magnetic forces. Other methods that have been described include micromolding, Spinner flask cultures, rotary cell cultures, self-assembly on Primaria dishes, porous 3D scaffolds, poly(N-isopropylacrylamide)–based cell sheets, centrifugation of pellet cultures, and aggregation utilizing electric, magnetic, or acoustic forces (Passamai et al., 2016).

One of the greatest potential applications of organoids is to model human-specific diseases and tissue responses (Huch et al., 2017). A tremendous array of both normal and disease tissue organoids have been developed to date (Table 24.2). The expansion potential of some organoids makes autologous cell therapy via allogeneic cell transplantation a possibility (van de Wetering et al., 2015). In addition, biobanks of disease model organoids can be used as sources for testing the effects of genetic modification

TABLE 24.2 Selected Examples of Organoid Models

Tissue	Reference
Blood microvessels	Yin et al. (2016)
Brain	Lancaster et al. (2013), Schwartz et al. (2015), Wang et al. (2017)
Bone Marrow	Mahalingaiah et al. (2018)
Heart	Jang et al. (2013), Wang et al. (2018), Yin et al. (2016)
Intestine	Jung et al. (2011), Sato et al. (2011), Spence et al. (2011)
Kidney	Jang et al. (2013), Takasato et al. (2016a, 2016b), Takasato and Little (2016)
Liver	Huch et al. (2013), Huch et al. (2015), Passamai et al. (2016), Ramachandran et al. (2015), Takebe et al. (2013), Yin et al. (2016)
Pancreas/Pancreatic Cancer	Gao et al. (2014), Passamai et al. (2016)
Peritoneal Macrophages	Mohamed-Ali et al. (1995)
Prostate	Drost et al. (2016), Karthaus et al. (2014)
Skeletal muscle	Jang et al. (2013), Yin et al. (2016)
Thyroid	Ma et al. (2015)

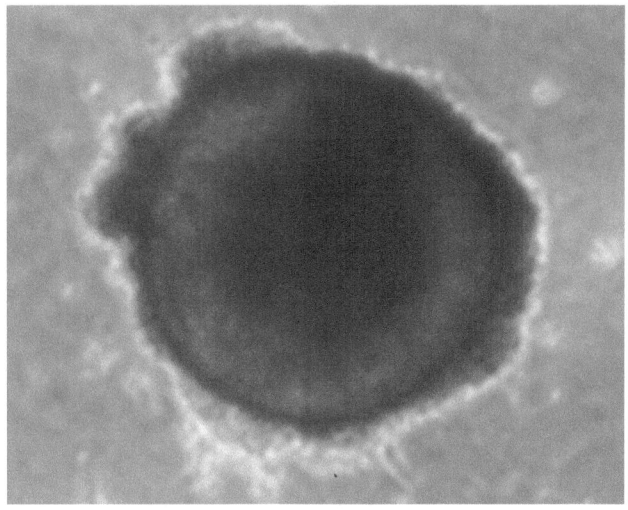

FIGURE 24.5 Morphology of a seven-day-old embryoid body derived from cardiac stem cells of a neonatal mouse. *Reproduced from Page 3, Figure 2, Day 7 (left panel) in Ou DB, Zeng D, Jin Y, et al.: The long-term differentiation of embryonic stem cells into cardiomyocytes: an indirect co-culture model,* PloS One *8:e55233, 2013 under a Creative Commons Attribution License.*

(targeting to knockout or correct a gene defect) to better understand a molecular mechanism or (in the future) optimize the function of cells destined for autologous transplantation (Schwank et al., 2013). However, the potential of transplantation is yet to be fully realized. Disease-specific organoids also have the potential to discover and validate new biomarkers of disease. Organoids are being used for toxicity testing of antineoplastic drugs and environmental toxicants as a means of assessing exposure–response relationships and mechanisms of action (Truskey, 2018; Xu et al., 2018).

Embryoid Bodies

EBs are distinct 3D organoids (Figure 24.5) to study developmental processes. EBs originate from pluripotent cell types such as ESCs or iPSCs (Dias et al., 2014; Ouyang et al., 2015; Reid et al., 2016). A distinguishing characteristic of EBs is the presence of differentiation along three specific germ cell lineages: endoderm, ectoderm, and mesoderm (Dias et al., 2014; Reid et al., 2016). These germ cell lineages comprise the origin of all somatic cell types at all life stages. EBs mimic some structures of the developing embryo and can be a source for reliable initiation of lineage-specific differentiation.

Basic research with EBs has explored key events in hematopoiesis, vasculogenesis (formation of blood vessels from differentiating endothelial cells), and angiogenesis (sprouting of capillaries from preexisting vessels). Erythroid precursors generally form from EBs by day 4 of differentiation (Karthaus et al., 2014) without the presence of any added growth factors. In suspension culture, EBs form blood islands (structures around developing embryos that contribute to many parts of the circulatory and hematopoietic systems) that differentiate into primitive blood vessels (Bautch et al., 1996; Wang et al., 1992). Similarly, EBs injected into the peritoneal cavity of mice form blood islands and subsequently undergo vasculogenesis and angiogenesis (Risau et al., 1988). Methods for in vitro differentiation of primitive blood vessels have now been described as well using EB models (Rylova et al., 2008).

Experimental conditions and methods are critical in defining the structure and organization of EBs. Seeding density in nonadhesive microwell plates can be critical for successful EB formation (Pettinato et al., 2014). Preferential differentiation of specific cell lineages is largely based on the size of the progenitor EB (Bauwens et al., 2008; Cha et al., 2015; Peerani et al., 2009; Schukur et al., 2013); if EBs are too small, they do not survive well, but if too big, they tend to develop necrotic cores. Consistency of EBs with respect to the desired size, geometry, and spatial control has been improved using laser-based bioprinting (Dias et al., 2014). Extrusion-based bioprinters have been used to create EBs that differentiated into endoderm, ectoderm, and mesodermal germ layers (Reid et al., 2016) and to biofabricate ESCs into a 3D cell-dense construct (Ouyang et al., 2015). The bioprinting process ultimately resulted in 90% viability of ESCs and proliferation in hydrogel that yielded uniform, pluripotent, size-controlled EBs at high capacity (Ouyang et al., 2015). Indeed, 3D bioprinting lends itself to better scaling for high-throughput EB production and testing (Kingsley et al., 2019).

An obvious application of EBs is the detection and characterization of teratogens (Flamier et al., 2017). EBs offer several advantages over nonclinical in vivo embryo–fetal studies in rodents and rabbits, not least of which is the ability to evaluate teratogenic potential in human-derived EBs. For example, a standardized human-derived EB model has been used successfully to assess the teratogenicity of caffeine, penicillin G, and valproic acid (Flamier et al., 2017). In addition, highly uniform EBs can be produced in large numbers to enable much higher throughput for screening than is possible with in vivo studies in animals (Flamier et al., 2017). Finally, EB research is improving our understanding of molecular and cellular events during development and permitting the elucidation of key factors that lead to differences in development among species (Weitzer, 2006). While EBs typically are produced from fresh or banked stem cells derived from normal animals, the ability to generate numerous EBs from a single sample has helped to significantly reduce the number of animal studies needed to screen pharmaceutical candidates and other chemicals for their potential impact on embryo–fetal development.

Micromass Cultures

Micromass cultures (MMCs) were initially developed using isolated hind limbs specifically to study chondrogenesis (Daniels et al., 1996) but have been adapted more recently to study other kinds of multipotent cells derived from embryonic mesoderm, including myocytes, adipocytes, and chondrocytes (Denker et al., 1995). For example, another common use for MMCs is to assess developmental events and toxic responses in embryonic heart (Hurst et al., 2007). More recently, in vitro production of MMCs has been explored as a means of producing cartilage, bone, and other mesenchymal (mesoderm-derived) cell lineages for the purpose of implantation (Handschel et al., 2009).

The main use for micromass assays in toxicology has been to study developmental toxicity (Hurst et al., 2007; Pratten et al., 2012). Indeed, rat limb bud MMCs have been validated for this purpose. For most toxicological applications, MMCs generally consist of dot (small, high density) cultures made from dissociated limb bud cells or heart fragments. Dissociation yields a 20–25-fold increase in the number of replicate cell cultures possible from an isolated limb bud (Daniels et al., 1996). These cultures form multilayered high-density mesenchyme with close cell-to-cell associations. Reaggregation (condensation) of cells is the basis for dot culture formation and requires a minimal cell number to induce differentiation along a specific mesodermal differentiation pathway (Hall and Miyake, 1992; Handschel et al., 2007). The selection of ECM scaffold material is important for MMC generation, particularly with respect to biocompatibility and biodegradability. Both natural and synthetic matrix materials have been used (Handschel et al., 2009); either origin is acceptable as long as the entrapped ECM molecules can initiate differentiation that will recapitulate the events observed in vivo during both embryogenesis and repair (Daniels et al., 1996). Alternatively, a scaffold-free approach has been reported for generating cartilage in vitro from chondrocyte spheroids cultured with human serum supplementation (Anderer and Libera, 2002). Cartilaginous tissue can be developed in only 3 days, but can be maintained for longer periods (3–5 weeks) if culture conditions are optimized (Shakibaei et al., 1993). Collagen synthesis is bolstered significantly in these cultures by the addition of transforming growth factor beta-1 (TGF-β1), a signal that regulates proliferation and differentiation of many mesoderm-derived cells (Denker et al., 1995). Extrusion-based 3D bioprinting has been used to create an automated biofabrication process for chondrogenic MMCs (Mekhileri et al., 2018).

3.5. Microphysiological Systems ("Organs On Chips")

Microfluidic microphysiological systems (MPS), or "organ-on-a-chip" platforms, are a recent innovation for advanced in vitro modeling (Figure 24.6). An MPS combines multiple cell types, and in some cases, multiple tissues, with microfluidic environmental controls to produce miniorgans that closely model the cell-to-cell and cell-to-matrix interactions as well as the 3D organization of normal structures (Wikswo, 2014). They incorporate physical cues not typical of other in vitro models, such as shear forces from media ("blood") flow or mechanical movement (to mimic breathing, peristalsis, etc.), which further replicates the conditions that pertain to intact organs in vivo (Grassart et al., 2019; Huh et al., 2010). Various fluidic approaches have replicated fluid flow by using one to several pumps or gravity (Boos et al., 2019; Uzel et al., 2014).

MPS can be generated in many different ways. Some are derived from a single organ or tissue, while others consist of interconnected sets of multiple organs/tissues. These models have been prepared from a number of cell sources including organ/tissue-specific primary cells, immortalized cell lines, and stem cells (ESC or iPSC). Although most of these models initially were made using human cells, animal cell MPS have been produced as well. Animal-derived MPS are necessary to reproduce and investigate in vitro any important species-specific findings and mechanisms that are detected in vivo, and parallel studies comparing animal to human MPS will be key for gaining confidence in the results of MPS data used in human risk assessment (Van Vleet et al., 2019). Bioprinting methods have been successfully applied to building MPS platforms (Knowlton and Tasoglu, 2016; Ma et al., 2016a; Yang et al., 2017).

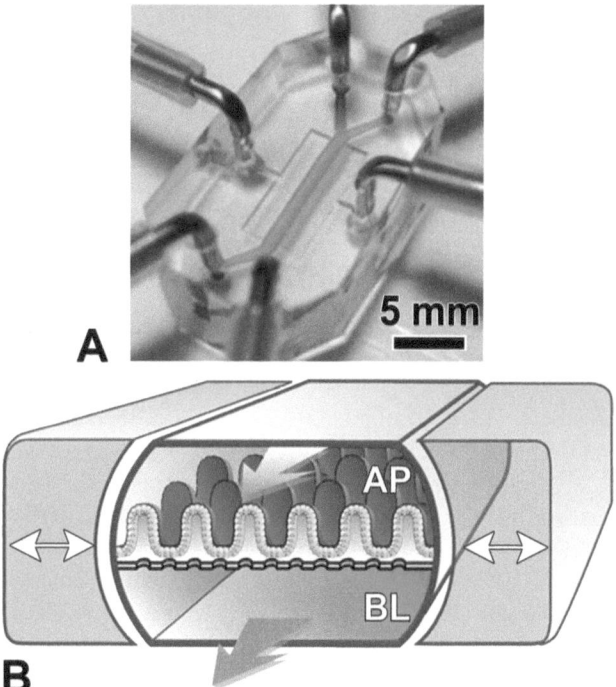

FIGURE 24.6 Microphysiological system technology, as exemplified by a microfluidic Gut Chip. Panel A: Photograph of the device showing upper (blue) and lower (red) microchannels. Panel B: The upper channel ("gut lumen" [AP = apical]) contains a layer of intestinal epithelial cells (pale green) arranged in villi-like folds atop a flexible, porous, extracellular matrix–coated synthetic membrane (black central line), while the lower channel ("vascular lumen" [BL = blood]) contains circulating media to deliver nutrients and remove metabolic waste. The broad arrows denote the direction of fluid flow in the "gut" (blue) and "vascular" (orange) lumens, while the white arrows indicate the direction of chamber deformation ("peristalsis") that can be imparted by cyclic application of suction. *Reproduced from A = Page E8, Figure 1, Panel A in Kim HJ, Li H, Collins JJ, et al.: Contributions of microbiome and mechanical deformation to intestinal bacterial overgrowth and inflammation in a human gut-on-a-chip, Proc Natl Acad Sci U S A 113:E7–E15, 2016 and (B) = cover page, upper row in Shin W, Hinojosa CD, Ingber DE, et al.: Human intestinal morphogenesis controlled by transepithelial morphogen gradient and flow-dependent physical cues in a microengineered gut-on-a-chip, iScience 15:391–406, 2019 by permission of Cell Press.*

Although their value has not been clearly defined yet, MPS have several advantages over other in vitro models. With microfluidic systems that permit the constant flow of medium (to deliver nutrients and remove waste products) as well as the potential for repeated microscopic observation, MPS systems can be monitored in real time for the development of findings representative of a disease or lesion that might result from exposure to a drug candidate or chemical (Ewart et al., 2017). The detection of sensitive biomarkers and physiological changes can also be monitored temporally in parallel to lesion formation. The presence of shear and mechanical effects has been shown to modulate the morphology, polarization, and function of cells anchored to MPS (Chang et al., 2017; da Silva et al., 2020; Jang et al., 2013). In addition, the viability of cells in MPS can be modulated by altering the composition of signaling factors (e.g., cytokines, growth factors) that are supplied in the medium (Kim et al., 2018; Park et al., 2009). Finally, the ability to link multiple tissues in sequence provides the first opportunity to assess interorgan effects of living "tissues" in vitro in response to progressive disease or intermittent encounters with drugs or chemicals.

MPS models that combine tissues have generally been designed and developed following a logical progression. For example, linked liver and gut multichip systems (Mahler et al., 2009; Tsamandouras et al., 2017a, 2017b) as well as combinations of liver and other tissues (Esch et al., 2015; Kolahchi et al., 2016; Marx et al., 2016) have been used to examine the impact of drug absorption and metabolism on tissue toxicity. For instance, toxicities in the liver related to changes in the gut have been well documented in vitro using human-derived MPS (Keshavarzian et al., 1999; Szabo and Bala, 2010). Endothelial cell MPS matched with MPS for other cell types likewise have been used to evaluate the importance of effects initiated in the endothelium in modulating the toxic effects produced in other tissue elements (Jain et al., 2016; Mathur et al., 2015; Moya et al., 2013a, 2013b). Tumor cells in liver or other common sites for metastatic seeding are also often combined to assess malignancy (Clark et al., 2014; Khazali et al., 2017; Wheeler et al., 2014).

Significant challenges remain in validating and commercializing MPS technologies for biomedical research applications, particularly with respect to the more complex, multiorgan (linked chip) models. Maintaining appropriate mechanical (i.e., stretch) and fluidic (i.e., flow rate) sheer forces for each individual tissue may present some challenges where the tolerability for such forces differs between linked tissues.

In addition, maintaining appropriate oxygenation of media that is suitable for each tissue may require significant engineering (Wikswo, 2014). One of the biggest challenges will be producing universal cell media that support optimal survival and health of the vast array of cells across each "organ" model (Wikswo, 2014). Similarly, designs that will provide viable signaling loops for paracrine factors may require either the recirculation of a portion of media back through the whole series of "organs" or alternatively a bypass of a fraction of the "conditioned" media back to various stages of the sequence so that the conditions preferred by each single-organ MPS are achieved. To date, no MPS models have been able to replicate bile production and flow. Recently, glomeruli have been replicated in MPS, and production of "urine" has been suggested as an important proof of elimination function (Allison, 2017; Musah et al., 2018; Petrosyan et al., 2019; Zhou et al., 2016). Ideally, the glomerulus chip would be able to influence vascular flow and pressure in other tissues (particularly cardiovascular tissues), which is the situation in vivo. Another challenge to creating a physiologically relevant system in vitro is the difficulty of including innervation between systems to permit normal neural control of functions. Finally, proper functional scaling that represents the normal physiological state of the various organs or functional organ units (e.g., glomeruli, hepatic lobules) that occur in an intact human or animal is extremely challenging (Wikswo, 2014).

Building MPS with cells derived from iPSCs can provide significant additional potential benefits for biomedical research. iPSCs from affected patients may form the basis of improved MPS disease models for investigating genetically based diseases (Ellis et al., 2017; Ma et al., 2016b). Such models not only may form the basis for a better mechanistic understanding but also may serve as platforms for evaluating the efficacy and safety of potential new therapies as well as discovering novel biomarkers of efficacy and disease progression. Using patient-derived iPSCs or tumor cells may be useful in optimizing treatments for individual patients (personalized medicine) or in characterizing disease-specific traits of more general relevance (Ellis et al., 2017). Another advantage in using iPSCs in MPS models is the consistency of cells across "chips" used in different experiments.

Microfluidic MPS have the potential to make dramatic changes to product discovery and development in the future (Ewart et al., 2017). With respect to drug discovery research, MPS can likely increase the speed and throughput of in vitro efficacy testing while enhancing the specificity of in vitro target identification and target validation studies. MPS also are likely to improve biomarker development and qualification as well as facilitate studies to repurpose drugs for use in other indications. Indeed, industry members are keenly interested in these categories, and some are actively pursuing a path toward adopting "organ-on-chip" models where appropriate (Ainslie et al., 2019; Baudy et al., 2020; Ewart et al., 2017; Gao et al., 2014; Hardwick et al., 2020; Jain et al., 2016; Jakab et al., 2010).

3.6. Stem Cells and Genetically Modified Cells

Stem cells are unspecialized cells that can undergo self-renewal through symmetrical cell division, and can be induced to asymmetrically divide into organ-specific cells under certain physiological and environmental conditions (Apati et al., 2019; Deshmukh et al., 2012; Kang and Trosko, 2011; Kim et al., 2019b; Liu et al., 2017b; Natale et al., 2019; Scott et al., 2013). Three classes of stem cells are used in toxicity testing: ESCs, either undifferentiated (totipotent) or partially differentiated (pluripotent), isolated from an embryo; adult stem cells isolated from adult tissues; and iPSCs that are derived from somatic adult cells by genetic "reprogramming" to attain a stem cell-like state (Kang and Trosko, 2011; Kim et al., 2019b). Similar to iPSCs, multipotent mesenchymal stem cells (MSCs) that retain a pluripotent state into adulthood have been derived from tissues including umbilical cord blood (at term), bone marrow, adipose tissue, and dental pulp, among other sources (Ibraheim et al., 2018). Figure 24.7 provides a schematic view of the generation and culturing of these three types of stem cells.

Initial work with mouse ESCs, which focused on developmental toxicities of teratogens, shows concordance and sensitivity consistent with in vivo developmental toxicity data. This agreement prompted the acceptance of the mouse embryonic stem cell test as an in vitro model for toxicity screening (Kim et al., 2019b; Liu et al., 2017b; Luz and Tokar, 2018). Human ESCs (hESCs), especially in the form of EBs (discussed in Section 3.4 above), hold tremendous potential for not only developmental toxicity testing in the broad sense but also for evaluating organ toxicities for multiple organs in EBs that have been induced to differentiate along a certain development pathway by the judicious application of various growth factor combinations (Luz and Tokar, 2018). However, ethical and regulatory restrictions related to procuring ESCs from viable embryos have limited the use of hESCs. To overcome the ethical issue, protocols have been devised for inducing iPSCs from adult somatic cells (Takahashi and Yamanaka, 2006); such cells may be obtained by nonlethal and minimally invasive biopsies. Genetic insertion of four key transcriptional factors—OCT4, SOX2, KLF4, and c-Myc—produced iPSCs that were almost identical to ESCs as indicated by their molecular signatures and morphological traits (Karagiannis et al., 2018; Takahashi and Yamanaka, 2006). The iPSC induction protocol has since been further optimized by introducing alternative transcription factors (e.g., NANOG and LIN28), insertion of other phenotype-modifying genes, or direct use of membrane-permeable proteins. Although they are restricted to producing only mesenchymal cell lineages, MSCs also are potentially useful alternative models for toxicity screening due to their availability and large number of potential adult phenotypes.

As part of characterizing pluripotent stem cell lines, the teratoma formation assay has been performed to confirm pluripotency (Nelakanti et al., 2015).This assay involves the injection of cells of interest into an organ—typically the gastrocnemius muscle of immunocompromised mice—followed by subsequent monitoring and characterization of cell growth at the injection site to verify that the introduced stem cells support the formation of cells derived from all three germ layers. Although this assay has been the "gold standard" for confirming pluripotency, alternative methods that do not require the use of animals are now gaining popularity. The alternatives include the aforementioned EB culture; monitoring genetic signatures of pluripotency such as expression of OCT4, SOX2, and other genes; and determination of

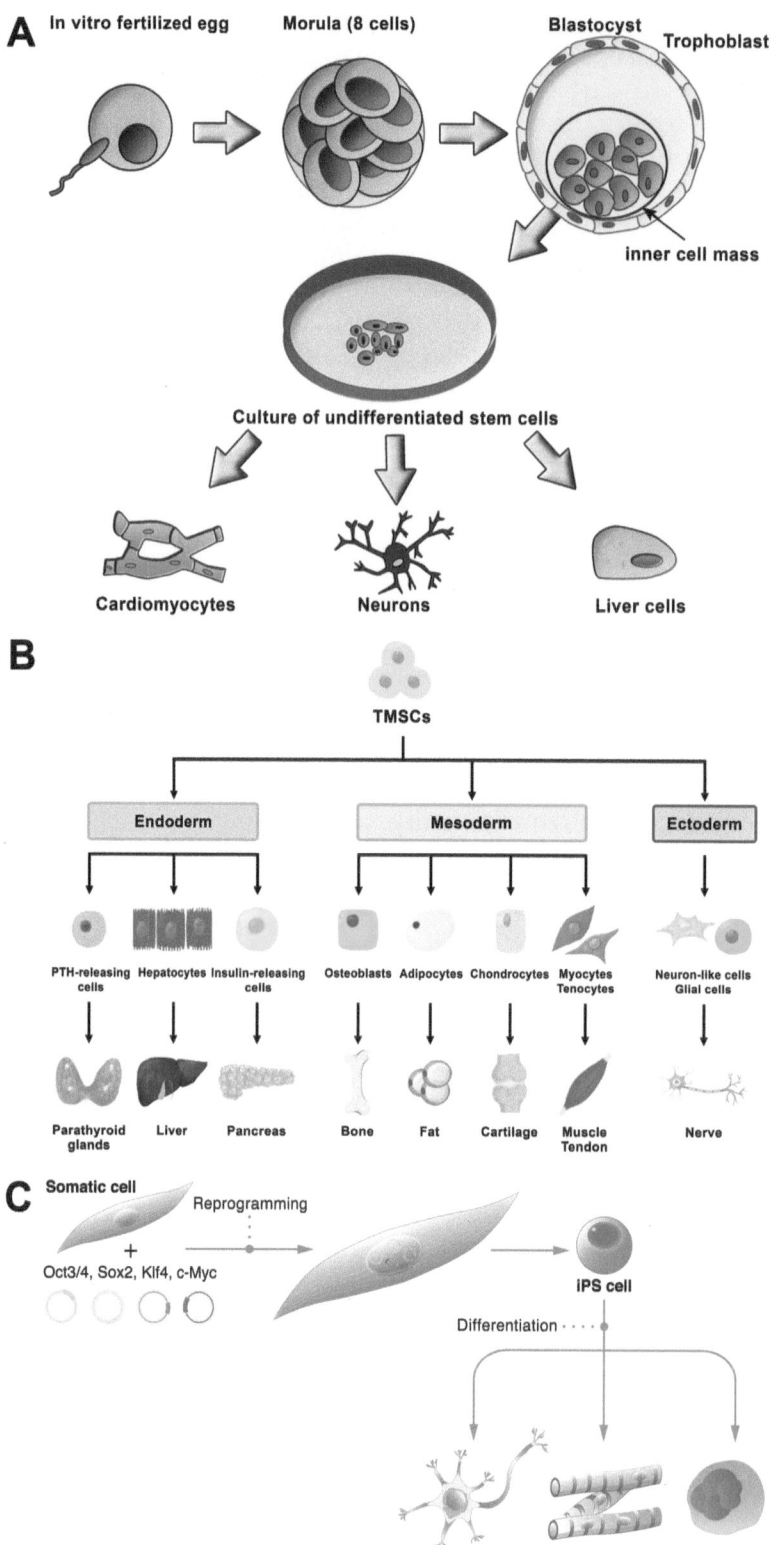

FIGURE 24.7   Sources and representative differentiation pathways for three types of stem cells used in toxicity testing. (A) embryonic stem cells (ESCs), (B) tonsil mesenchymal stem cells (MSCs), and (C) induced pluripotent stem cells (iPSCs). *Pictures are reproduced from (A) = Page 3, Figure 1 in Abou-Saleh H, Zouein FA, El-Yazbi A, et al.: The march of pluripotent stem cells in cardiovascular regenerative medicine,* Stem Cell Res Ther *9:201, 2018 (B) = Page 1254, Figure 2 in Oh SY, Choi YM, Kim HY, et al.: Application of tonsil-derived mesenchymal stem cells in tissue regeneration: concise review,* Stem Cell *37:1252–1260, 2019 and (C) = Page 7, Figure 1 in Karagiannis P; Nakauchi A; Yamanaka, S: Bringing induced pluripotent stem cell technology to the bedside,* JMA J *1:6–14, 2018 under a Creative Commons Attribution 4.0 International License.*

genome-wide fingerprints of "stemness" from microarrays and next-generation sequencing (Buta et al., 2013).

Theoretically, stem cell–derived in vitro models are ideal for efficacy and toxicity screening. Many attributes attest to their suitability for these purposes. Several advantageous properties are readily apparent:

a. Unlimited propagation because of their self-renewal and proliferation abilities, as compared to primary oligopotent (mostly differentiated) or terminally differentiated cells;

b. Generation of tissue elements from any cell lineage of any organ based on variations in environmental conditions (oxygen tension, substrate availability, medium composition, and growth factor supplementation);

c. Reasonable capability for developmental toxicity screening based on substantial cross-laboratory validation studies;

d. Opportunity (via iPSC technology) to assess population diversity and identify subpopulations that might be most vulnerable or resistant to certain toxicities;

e. Easy modification (by gene editing technology) of native cell features to facilitate the elucidation of toxic mechanisms (Schildknecht et al., 2013; Shen et al., 2015).

Toxicity has been investigated in several critical cell lineages using stem cell–derived cardiomyocytes, hepatocytes (or hepatocyte-like cells), neurons, kidney proximal tubular cells, and gastrointestinal cells (Apati et al., 2019; Deshmukh et al., 2012; Kim et al., 2019b; Liu et al., 2017b; Natale et al., 2019; Scott et al., 2013).

Stem cell–derived in vitro models are particularly suited to evaluate the relationship of potential mechanisms of action with toxicity. In exploring mechanisms of action of chemically induced toxicity, the genetic modulations of suspected pathways are very attractive in hypothesis generation and testing. By deliberate modification of certain genes, loss (or gain) of function can be produced in certain pathway proteins, which then can be assessed for their ability to confer resistance or susceptibility to toxicants. Recent advances in gene knockdown and gene editing technologies have made possible functional genomic screening across a network of pathways (Schildknecht et al., 2013; Shen et al., 2015).

Despite the potential that stem cells offer for toxicologic investigations, considerable work remains to realize the promise of this technology. First, well-characterized stem cell lines are still very limited. Second, stem cell differentiation protocols are complex, not standardized, and unvalidated. In addition, translation of in vitro toxicity data generated from stem cell–derived cultures to in vivo toxicity data acquired from whole animal testing is challenging due to multiple factors. Stem cell–derived cells typically exhibit an embryonic or fetal phenotype (i.e., abundant numbers of pluripotent cells), while organs of adult animals generally contain few stem cells and many mature (differentiated) cells; this discrepancy is particularly important for organs such as liver and heart. Moreover, the differentiation process in vitro may be subtly different from that in vivo due to differences in the tissue microenvironment (Kang and Trosko, 2011; Liu et al., 2017b; Sachinidis et al., 2019). Clearly, stem cell assays represent an increasingly important tool but not the ultimate determinant in assembling the weight of evidence (WoE) needed for risk assessment of a test article's toxicity.

3.7. Whole Embryo Culture

Whole embryo culture (WEC) of early rodent (mouse or rat) embryos is a valuable in vitro tool for investigating developmental biology toxicity (Glanville-Jones et al., 2013; Takahashi & Osumi, 2010; Tung and Winn, 2019). Briefly, rodent embryos are removed from the uterus early during organogenesis (about gestational day 8 in the mouse, which is just after the central nervous system and heart start to form). The outer placenta is removed to expose the yolk sac, and embryos are placed in individual culture vessels that contain nutrient-rich medium supplemented with adult rat serum. The embryos may be maintained in culture under conditions that mimic growth conditions in utero (approximately 37°C while culture vessels are being oscillated to encourage regular nutrient circulation) for 24–48 h, during which they continue to follow a relatively normal course of development. The culture medium may be spiked with chemicals to investigate potential mechanisms of action and dose–response relationships.

The WEC assay is a common model for developmental toxicity screening (Piersma et al., 2004,

2008; Webster et al., 1997). Key advantages are that the translucency of the yolk sac permits macroscopic examination of the embryo over time and that rodent embryos follow a well-recognized developmental sequence for which many published anatomic references are available (Behringer, 2014; Brown, 1990). Principal disadvantages are that the methodology is laborious, technically difficult (since trauma to the fragile yolk sac requires that the damaged embryo be discarded), low-throughput relative to other in vitro toxicity assays, and entails the need for regular serum collection from adult rats. An underappreciated issue is that rodent littermates vary in developmental age by up to 24 h, so scoring systems based on morphologic features must be applied and interpreted with care to avoid spurious data.

The WEC assay is one of three in vitro models—along with the aforementioned mouse ESC assay and rat limb micromass assay—that have been validated for use in developmental toxicity testing by the European Center for the Validation of Alternative Methods (ECVAM). These assays convey ~70% accuracy in the prediction of developmental toxicities (Luz and Tokar, 2018) and correctly identify non-teratogens approximately 85% of the time.

4. IN SILICO MODELS AND DATA ANALYTICS

Recent advances in bioinformatics, data science, and computational modeling have enabled major changes in the way toxicological science predicts and evaluates human health hazards. In this section, we will briefly describe some of these computer-based approaches and how they can be used to create an interface between "big data" (the "omics" disciplines) and toxicologic pathology.

4.1. In Silico Predictive Structure–Activity Models

The basic concepts underlying predictive toxicology date back at least to the mid-1800s, with the publication of early studies relating chemical structure to biological effect (Brown and Fraser,

1868). These efforts led to perhaps the earliest prospective mathematical models in toxicology, later known as QSAR analysis, which is based on the premise that structural features of a molecule determine physical, chemical, and/or biological activity, and, accordingly, that the activity of a novel entity can be inferred from structural features of related compounds with known activities. This approach is now widely used as a rapid screening tool for drugs and environmental chemicals, which may otherwise have little or no safety information (JRC, 2010; Kizhedath et al., 2017; OECD, 2014).

Structural alerts from QSAR can inform toxicologic pathology data in several ways. Historically, carcinogenicity assessment has been the most widely used application. Structural features of a drug/chemical can predict DNA reactivity and potential mutagenicity, which may in turn be used to interpret carcinogenicity study results and evaluate modes of action. Another application is drug-induced phospholipidosis (PLD), in which chemically induced enzyme inhibition leads to altered lysosomal function and lysosomal accumulation of polar phospholipids within affected tissues. The identification of PLD based on structural features may assist in the interpretation of a pathologic finding such as cytoplasmic vacuolation as adverse or not (Lenz et al., 2018). QSAR models for specific chemical classes can also provide alerts (e.g., estrogen receptor [ER] binding) related to a specific target organ or system (e.g., reproductive system toxicity) that can determine the need for and design of subsequent toxicity studies. For antibody-based therapies, the presence of specific amino acid residues and glycosylation patterns may be used to predict immunogenicity risk and the potential for antibody-dependent cytotoxicity (Kizhedath et al., 2017; Liu, 2015) and support the interpretation of immune cell infiltrates and other potential histopathologic findings as incidental or adverse.

The rapid growth of database resources and in silico prediction tools has expanded QSAR scope and application in recent years (Kizhedath et al., 2017). Large experimental data sets, including toxicologic pathology results extracted from legacy guideline studies, have now been collated within various publicly available sources and serve as an important anchor for development of computer-based predictive toxicity models. Examples include the Toxicity Reference Database (ToxRefDB) of the U.S. EPA, which contains information from more than 5000 in vivo studies conducted to support safety assessments for over 1000 agrochemicals, pharmaceuticals, and industrial agents (Watford et al., 2019) and eTOX, a shared pharmaceutical database with legacy toxicity study outcomes that intended to enable read-across and predictive modeling of safety endpoints (Sanz et al., 2017). These types of databases provide an important resource for in silico modeling, including QSAR, by assimilating diverse endpoints from multiple species and study types across large drug/chemical sets.

Current data science tools have also allowed QSAR methods to be integrated with newer types of toxicity data (Thomas et al., 2019). Broad-based initiatives are underway to link structural information with high-throughput and high-content in vitro data and toxicity pathways (Liu et al., 2017a). These large-scale integration efforts have also enabled machine learning and systematic read-across approaches, in which drug/chemical sets with a known toxicity are used to predict the likelihood of the same toxicity for a data-poor substance (Helman et al., 2018; Yang, Lou, & Li, 2020). These methods, which include bioactivity, hazard, toxicokinetic, and exposure characteristics in addition to chemical structure data, are being rapidly developed to reduce uncertainties of traditional QSAR/read-across analysis and broaden applications for drug/chemical screening and prioritization (Patlewicz et al., 2019).

4.2. Pathway-Based Models of Toxicity

A central premise of predictive toxicology is that adverse health outcomes resulting from drug or chemical exposure can be mapped to specific molecular pathways. This concept forms the basis for the **mode of action** (MOA), which organizes toxicity data for a particular pathological outcome into a sequence of key events or processes, starting with the initial interaction between a given chemical/drug and a target cell (Boobis et al., 2006; EPA, 2005; Meek et al., 2014). Each key event is a requisite and measurable precursor step (or biomarker for that step) leading to the ultimate adverse effect. The

MOA is agent-dependent and can be influenced by exposure or dose information. As designed, the MOA provides a streamlined summary of pathway information for the purposes of scientific regulatory review, in contrast to **mechanism of action**, which encompasses a more detailed understanding and description of molecular events (EPA, 2005). Review of a proposed MOA includes standardized criteria such as dose response and temporal concordance, strength, consistency, and specificity of key events, biological plausibility and coherence, and alternative MOAs. Once established, the MOA for a finding in an animal study can then be used to determine human relevance, the quantification method for risk assessment, and the susceptible populations and life stages.

Currently, the MOA has an important role in the organization and review of mechanistic data and the identification of key data gaps, particularly for cancer risk assessment. However, in practice, the application of this framework is largely retrospective (i.e., occurring after the initial observation of an adverse health effect in a guideline toxicity study). In the past decade, the **adverse outcome pathway** (AOP) has been developed as a complementary framework to the MOA to better enable predictive models (Ankley et al., 2010; Pollesch et al., 2019). Similar to the MOA, an AOP begins with a molecular-level perturbation induced by a drug/chemical stressor (called the molecular initiating event [MIE]) and proceeds through a series of obligatory and observable key events at increasing levels of biological organization (Figure 24.8). If the level of perturbation at each key event is sufficiently severe, the AOP progresses to produce the adverse outcome, which is defined as a biological change considered relevant for risk assessment or other regulatory decision-making. In contrast to the MOA, the AOP is agent-agnostic, and thus does not incorporate exposure or dose information. Rather, the AOP is intended to capture pathway information leading to predictable biological outcomes that may be applied across chemical/drug domains, potentially in a prospective manner.

An important principle of the AOP framework is that the MIE and downstream key events are necessary for toxicity but not sufficient at a qualitative level of analysis. In other words, an observed key event may not necessarily lead to the subsequent key event (or adverse outcome)

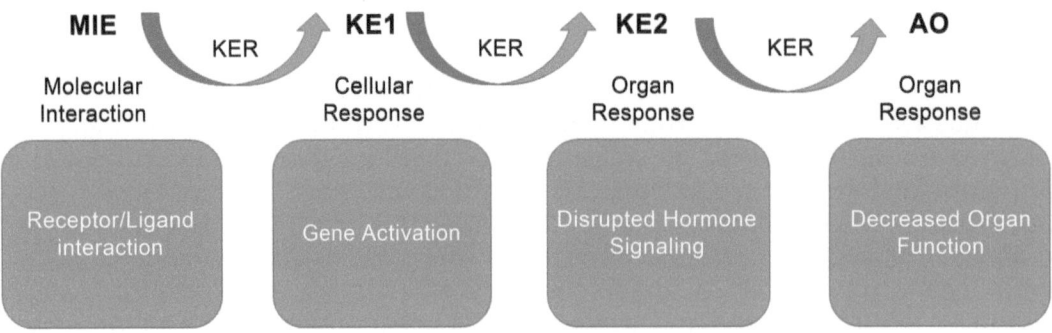

FIGURE 24.8   Schematic representation of a generic Adverse Outcome Pathway (AOP), consisting of a molecular initiating event (MIE), key events (KEs) linked by KE relationships (KERs), culminating in an adverse outcome (AO). Example events at different levels of biological organization are shown in the bottom row. *Modified from the OECD "Revised Guidance Document on Developing and Assessing Adverse Outcome Pathways," https://one.oecd.org/document/ENV/JM/MONO(2013)6/en/pdf.*

if a certain level of disruption is not reached. Key events in an AOP should thus have a probabilistic relationship. Once key event relationships (and associated modifying factors) are characterized within a given model system, a quantitative AOP (or qAOP) can be calculated (Conolly et al., 2017). These quantitative relationships would also form the basis for using precursor events in risk assessment, based on the idea that protecting against an early key event should protect against the subsequent key events and thus the putative adverse outcome. Long-term goals for qAOPs are to provide biological context around early key events or key event biomarkers, as measured during in silico, in vitro, or short-term in vivo studies, to enable greater use of alternative models and mechanistic information in risk assessment, and to build a rationale for biomarker data to be used in place of traditional measures of apical toxicity.

The development and use of qAOPs may inform interpretation of toxicologic pathology data in several ways. Pathway-based information from pharmacological, –omic, and biochemical data is routinely evaluated alongside morphologic outcomes (Palazzi et al., 2016). However, to date, there are few examples of accepted benchmark responses linking a specific precursor effect (e.g., lower serum thyroxine) with a morphologic effect (e.g., thyroid follicular cell hypertrophy and hyperplasia) or other health outcome. In the future, qAOPs may reduce arbitrary or inconsistent interpretations of pathology findings by providing greater mechanistic context. This information may also be used in determining when a marginal morphologic effect is treatment

related or not, whether a particular study is warranted or should be exempted, and what biomarkers may be useful for clinical and epidemiologic studies. The major scientific challenge here is capturing and distilling complex biological processes across large sets of drugs or chemicals. Benchmark responses between key events in the same AOP may differ widely across similar chemicals based on myriad modifying factors, even within the same model system, and it is unclear whether there will ever be enough scientific consensus around quantitative benchmark responses to use them routinely as a basis for determining points of departure in risk assessment.

4.3. Big Data Analytics in Toxicology Pathology

The rise of data science and bioinformatics has provided new analytical tools to guide prioritization of drugs/chemicals based on potential hazard, toxicity study selection and design, and interpretation of toxicologic pathology findings. Computational models, for example, are now a key part of integrated approaches to testing and assessment (IATA), an effort by the Organisation for Economic Co-operation and Development (OECD) and others to promote hypothesis-based, systematic, integrative use of hazard and exposure information (Casati, 2018). The IATA framework enables evaluation of results from different types of alternative models, which may include QSAR, read-across, in vitro, ex vivo, and omic data, and their application in risk assessment. Related aims are to improve translatability of toxicity endpoints to human health, focus testing resources on drugs/chemicals of highest concern, and support global efforts to reduce, refine, and replace animal-based models.

A major premise for this work is that adequately protecting against key precursor events in a toxicity pathway should protect against downstream apical effects. As discussed above, toxicologic pathology databases such as ToxRefDB are now commonly used to "phenotypically anchor" high-throughput and high-content bioactivity data. If successful, integrative testing approaches over time would shift regulatory focus to these short-term molecular-based biomarkers, using AOPs as the organizing scaffold, and replace at least some types of in vivo tests. Government statutes requiring toxicity studies to meet safety standards often provide flexibility in their implementation, in which health authorities can request and accept alternative assays or in some cases waive studies when they provide little additional scientific information or public health protection. Recognizing the need to reduce in vivo testing where possible, many authorities have prioritized efforts to validate alternative methods and study waiver strategies. For example, the U.S. EPA has issued several recent guidances for waiving in vivo toxicity tests for agrochemicals (EPA, 2016a) and presented a broad IATA strategy incorporating new computational and molecular tools, including read across for similar chemicals/chemical groups, predictive computer modeling including QSAR, and increased reliance on in vitro bioactivity profiles (EPA, 2016c). For regulatory scientists, this new type of assessment will require retrospective analysis of large pathology data sets to provide context and verification for new methods and assess if/when the results of a current toxicity study may impact human health risk assessment. For drug/chemical sponsors, big data resources will have an increasingly important role in establishing a rationale for alternative methods and waiver requests.

A prominent case study that is currently underway is the ER model, which was developed to support the Endocrine Disruptor Screening Program of the U.S. EPA. For this project, a battery of high-throughput in vitro screening assays were mapped to different components of the ER signaling pathway, such as receptor binding, dimerization, DNA binding, transcriptional activation, and cell proliferation (Figure 24.9) (Judson et al., 2015). Chemicals were tested in the in vitro battery, and results were assigned scores, using a computational model, into ER agonist and ER antagonist categories, which were used to assign and prioritize positive hits for further testing. When compared to the standard mouse uterotrophic assay, a classical in vivo test for estrogenic activity (EPA, 2011), this in vitro ER model showed high sensitivity and specificity, similar to that for rerunning the uterotrophic assay (Browne et al., 2015). The U.S. EPA has concluded that this ER model is a suitable replacement of uterotrophic assay requirements for environmental chemicals (EPA, 2015), illustrating how a pathway-based in vitro approach can be used as a surrogate for a required in vivo test.

The U.S. Food and Drug Administration (FDA) and other drug regulatory agencies are also investigating ways to modify testing requirements using support from big data analyses. One example is the current proposal to modify carcinogenicity testing requirements for pharmaceuticals (FDA, 2013). The proposed change is based on the premise that the absence of certain risk factors for neoplasia in shorter-term (6- or 12-month) studies can provide adequate negative predictive value for carcinogenicity outcomes to exempt certain compounds from the need for cost- and labor-intensive life-time (2-year) rat bioassays. The concept for this waiver approach originated with retrospective analyses of tumor outcomes and associated pathology findings in rat studies for two large sets of pharmaceuticals (Reddy et al., 2010; Sistare et al., 2011). Currently, the FDA is conducting a prospective study of new drug applications to evaluate this waiver concept (Bourcier et al., 2015), as part of a broader initiative by the International Council for Harmonisation of Technical Requirements for Pharmaceuticals for Human Use (ICH) to update current standard carcinogenicity study options for small-molecule pharmaceuticals (ICH, 2019).

Big data analytics also encompass emerging digital technologies, which play an increasingly important role in toxicologic pathology (*Digital Pathology and Tissue Image Analysis*, Vol 1, Chap 12). Glass slides are routinely scanned

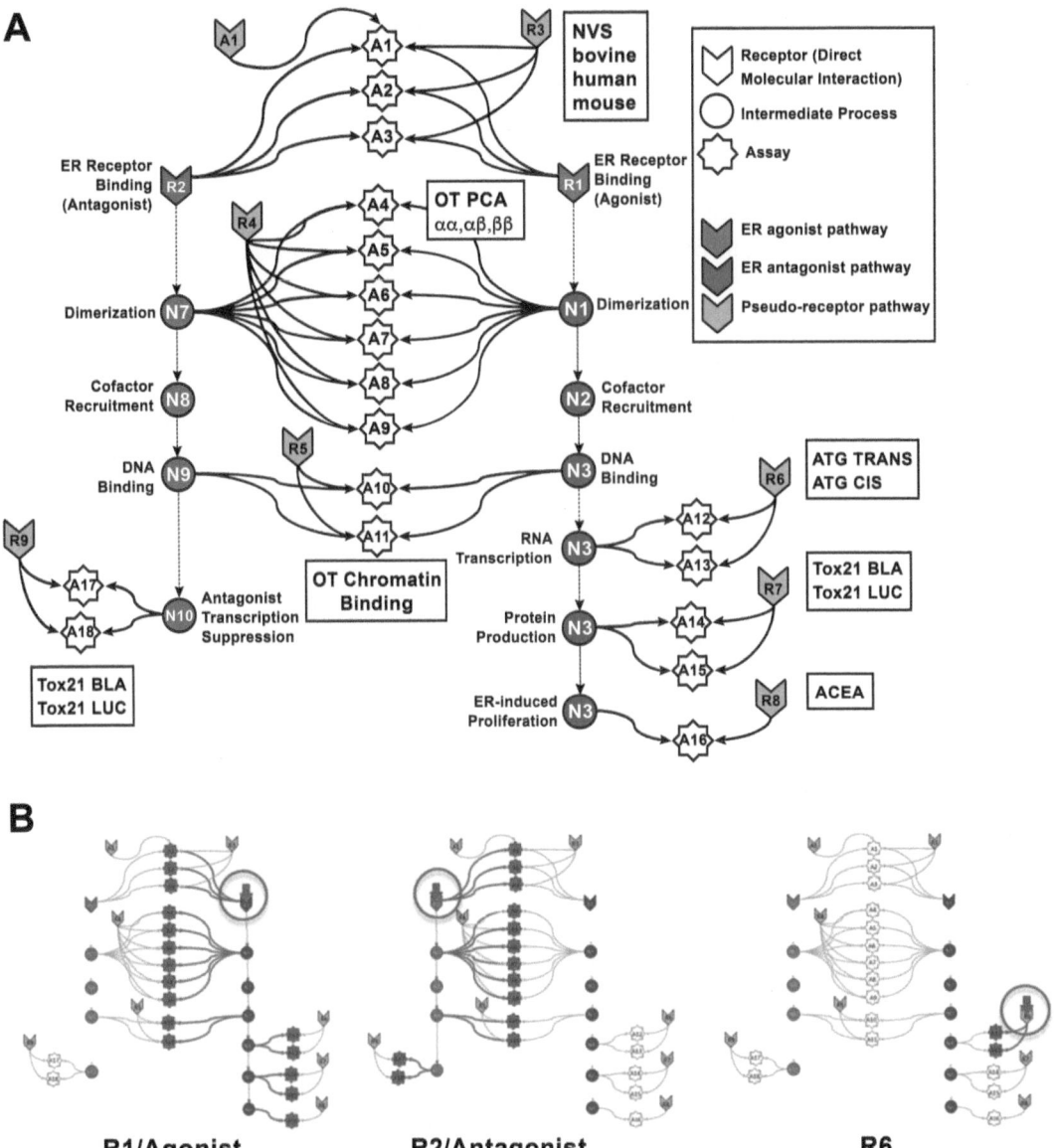

FIGURE 24.9 (A), Graphical representation of the computational network used in the *in vitro* analysis of the estrogen receptor (ER) pathway across assays and technology platforms. Colored arrow nodes represent "receptors" with which a chemical can directly interact. Colored circles represent intermediate biological processes that are not directly observable. White stars represent the in vitro assays that measure activity at the biological nodes. Arrows represent transfer of information. Gray arrow nodes are the pseudoreceptors. Each in vitro assay (with the exception of A16) has an assay-specific pseudoreceptor, but only a single example is explicitly shown, for assay A1. (B), Patterns of assays that would be activated when specific receptors are activated by the chemical, in particular R1, R2, and R6. The activating chemical in its receptor is circled in pink, and the activated assays and the pathways to them are also highlighted in pink. *Reproduced with from Page 139, Figure 1, Panel A in Judson RS, Magpantay FM, Chickarmane V, et al.: Integrated model of chemical perturbations of a biological pathway using 18 in vitro high-throughput screening assays for the estrogen receptor, Toxicol Sci 148:137–154, 2015 by permission of Oxford University Press.*

for archiving and remote review, and image analysis tools are frequently used to quantify specific morphologic features (e.g., fibrosis) and tissue-based biomarkers (e.g., apoptosis), thereby providing enhanced context to pathologic diagnoses. Artificial intelligence and machine/deep learning platforms are also being rapidly developed to add "better-than-human" value and efficiency (Turner et al., 2020). Moving forward, these types of analyses will enable various applications, from sorting normal and abnormal samples using scanned images to content-based image retrieval applications, in which regions of interest are queried across studies and databases. Ultimately, toxicologic pathologists will have an important role in translating, ground-truthing, and implementing many of these new technologies in safety assessment.

5. IN VIVO MODELS USING ALTERNATIVE MAMMALIAN AND NONMAMMALIAN SPECIES

In one sense, all animal testing is "alternative." Centuries of biological research have relied on experimentation in animals as a surrogate for understanding basic biological principles or to facilitate product discovery and development for use in humans. That said, in vivo animal models can be divided arbitrarily into "standard" and "alternative" categories. The "standard" in vivo models include such mammalian species as mice and rats (as well as their less frequently utilized rodent kindred such as guinea pigs and hamsters; *Animal Models in Toxicologic Research: Rodents*, Vol 1, Chap 17); rabbits (*Animal Models in Toxicologic Research: Rabbits*, Vol 1, Chap 18); dogs (*Animal Models in Toxicologic Research: Dogs*, Vol 1, Chap 19); pigs (*Animal Models in Toxicologic Research: Pigs*, Vol 1, Chap 20); and nonhuman primates (*Animal Models in Toxicologic Research: Nonhuman Primates*, Vol 1, Chap 21). By comparison, "alternative" in vivo models comprise such unusual animals as genetically engineered animals and nonmammalian species (e.g., invertebrates, fish, amphibians, reptiles, and birds). Methods for in vivo exploration of toxicologic pathology endpoints in these alternative species have been detailed elsewhere (*Genetically Engineered Animal Models in Toxicologic Research*, Vol 1, Chap 23; *Animal Models in Toxicologic Research: Non-Mammalian*, Vol 1, Chap 22). Therefore, the current section only briefly recapitulates some of key factors in deciding whether or not to utilize an alternative model for in vivo biological research.

5.1. Genetically Engineered Animal Models

Genetically engineered animals have been employed to address many research questions of relevance to toxicologic pathology practice. Common experimental objectives include defining molecular mechanisms that initiate and sustain disease, validating molecular and cellular targets for therapeutic intervention, and demonstrating the efficacy of novel test articles. Ample in vivo evidence shows that expression of recombinant animal and human genes in rodents effectively foretells the likely outcome of similar genetic events in humans (Zambrowicz and Sands, 2003 although the anatomic, functional, and/or molecular characteristics of such animal models in many instances recapitulate only some attributes of the human disease. Traditionally, mice, and to a lesser extent rats, have been the most common species for generating engineered disease models. This choice has reflected such practical considerations as the availability of reliable ESC lines, a broad range of desirable physiological traits (e.g., many immunodeficient strains), and extensive historical control data for many genetic backgrounds—all factors that have made the mouse a preferred species for genetic engineering. In the last decade, the discovery of the clustered regularly interspaced short palindromic repeats (CRISPR)/CRISPR-associated protein system for nuclease-based genome editing has made feasible the reliable generation of genetically engineered nonrodent models, including dogs (Zou et al., 2015), pigs (Wang et al., 2016), and primates (Chen et al., 2016). This innovation will allow investigators to choose the most appropriate genetically engineered model, balancing the need for larger group sizes (which favor the use of rodents) with the desire to maximize the physiological similarities between the test species and humans (which in many cases will dictate selection of a nonrodent species).

More recently, genetically engineered models have been adapted to permit evaluation of complex molecular and cellular events in human tissues in vivo. For example, profoundly immunodeficient mice have been engineered to accept xenografts of normal human tissues that permit investigation of human cell-to-cell interactions and metabolic systems in vivo. Examples include chimeric human–mouse livers (to assess the efficacy and toxicity of agents designed to treat hepatitis viruses and the human metabolic profiles of novel small molecule test articles) and multichimeric human–mouse models in which repopulation of hematopoietic tissues (bone marrow and thymus) is used to examine the impact of antiviral agents on human immune cell lineages. The advantage of using these alternative "humanized" models is that they provide the ability to directly investigate physiological responses of human cells and molecular pathways in the framework of an integrated ("whole organism") in vivo system.

Toxicologic pathology assessments of these vertebrate models are comparable to those done in nonmanipulated ("wildtype") animals of the same species. Standard anatomic pathology and clinical pathology techniques are applicable, and historical background data from the engineered species may be used (with caution) as a guide to the baseline physiological status of the model. Common adaptations of toxicity study design applicable to experiments with engineered animals include collection of tissue samples to confirm the presence of the engineered modification using special molecular techniques (see *Special Techniques in Toxicologic Pathology*, Vol 1, Chap 11) and collection at necropsy of additional organs that typically are not harvested during conventional general toxicity studies (e.g., dorsal root ganglia, nasal cavity) in case the results of the protocol-specified tissue battery indicate that they need to be evaluated.

5.2. Non-mammalian Animal Models

Multiple non-mammalian animals may be employed for in vivo studies. For many decades, basic biological research to discover fundamental biological principles has been conducted in several invertebrate species, most notably fruit flies (*D. melanogaster*) and nematodes (*C. elegans*) (Hunt, 2017; Peterson and Long, 2018). These organisms have relatively simple genomes and small numbers of cells (that can be identified and manipulated individually). Experiments in these invertebrates have explored such questions as defining gene functions, dissecting molecular interactions, and more recently high-throughput toxicity screening (using anatomic [pathologic] and/or functional [e.g., behavior] abnormalities). Other invertebrate species (insects,

mollusks, and snails, to name a few) also may be used, typically as sentinels for environmental contamination. Primary advantages of invertebrates as models for toxicity testing are low costs to obtain and maintain animals, short reproductive cycles, and relevance (based on their high sensitivity to environmental toxicants). Another important attribute of doing toxicity studies in non-mammalian models is that the administrative burden associated with experimentation on phylogenetically higher species is substantially reduced. The main disadvantages of invertebrates are the relatively large phylogenetic divergence from humans and other vertebrates in terms of basic anatomic, physiologic, and genetic attributes as well as the paucity of data on normal biological features (including anatomy and histology texts) and incidental background findings in most species.

Non-mammalian vertebrate models are used in toxicologic research for many purposes. Two main reasons are evaluating ecological health (where fish from the local ecosystem serve as sentinels for toxic pollutants) and chemical screening. Many species may serve as subjects for environmental testing, so investigators may be faced with a broad diversity of biological traits when designing their studies. That said, laboratory investigations typically utilize small-sized, highly fecund, freshwater species like the zebrafish (*Danio rerio*), a standard model in basic biological and applied biomedical research (Sipes et al., 2011), and medaka (*Oryzias latipes*), which serves as a common option for toxicity screening (Padilla et al., 2009). Multiple fish strains have been developed, so selection of the appropriate genetic background is an essential component of the study design. Two major benefits of these models from a pathologist's perspective are (1) their transparent embryos that undergo a defined sequence of time-dependent embryological events, which permits high-throughput developmental toxicity screening by stereomicroscopic evaluation, and (2) the ability to fit an entire adult animal into a standard tissue cassette, which allows many organs to be evaluated in a small (typically three to five) number of step sections. Additional advantages are the ability to have large group sizes, with all animals housed in a single unit; the low husbandry costs; and the relatively permissive regulatory environment.

Other nonmammalian vertebrate species may be employed in biological research (see *Animal Models in Toxicologic Research: Non-mammalian*, Vol 1, Chap 22). In terms of toxicological questions, such amphibian, reptilian, and avian species often serve as sentinels for the health of the ecosystem in which they reside. However, such models may be deployed to identify hazards of potential relevance to human risk assessment. In this regard, the Frog Embryo Teratogenesis Assay Xenopus (FETAX) assay is a recognized platform (Mouche et al., 2017). The FETAX test is a four-day developmental toxicity screen that uses the embryos and larvae ("tadpoles") of the South African clawed frog (*Xenopus laevis*). The key advantages of this assay are that it can be performed with very small quantities of test article, which is well suited to early-stage toxicity testing for drug development, and that the primary endpoints for interpreting the study are based on mortality and macroscopic analysis for malformations and behavioral abnormalities (Figure 24.10). Finally, the chick (*Gallus gallus*, subspecies *domesticus*)

embryo chorioallantoic membrane (CAM) assay is a well-characterized *ex ovo* model for toxicity testing, particularly for the impact of test articles on angiogenesis (Ribatti, 2017). The CAM test is a fairly fast, inexpensive means for high-throughput screening. Key benefits of this model include simple endpoints based on mortality and macroscopic changes in membrane structure (Figure 24.11) as well as the immuno-deficient nature of the chick embryo, which allows ready engraftment and growth of foreign tissues.

Toxicologic pathology assessments of non-mammalian models differ in some respects from conventional toxicity testing in common mammalian species: rodents, rabbits, dogs, pigs, and primates. Many studies with non-mammalian models assess toxicity relying entirely on evaluation of in-life attributes such as lethality, behavioral alterations, and macroscopic lesions (typically deformed or missing body parts) in large numbers of individuals per treatment group. This design is true for most studies (e.g., drug lead candidate screens,

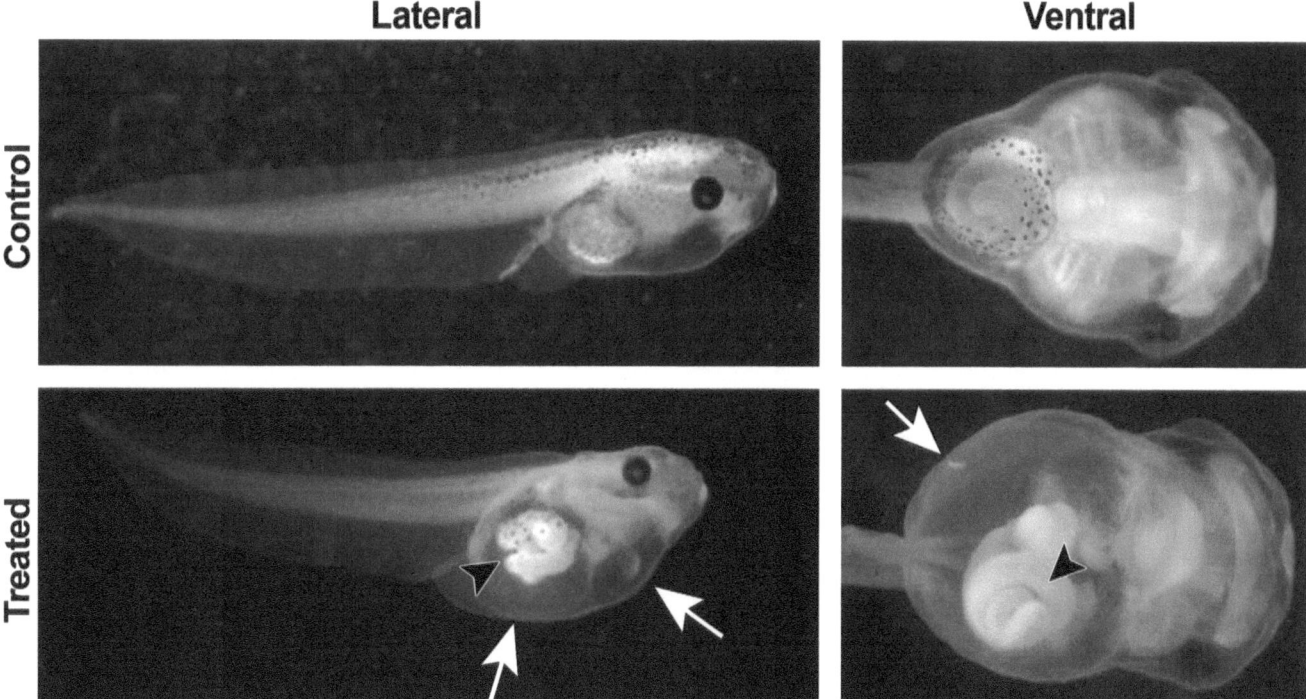

FIGURE 24.10 Developmental toxicity in the FETAX (Frog Embryo Teratogenesis Assay *Xenopus*) test as indicated by the presence of abdominal and cardiac edema (*arrows*), abnormal intestinal coiling (arrowhead), and a slight dorsal tail flexure following exposure to zinc oxide nanoparticles. *Reproduced from Page 8836, Figure 3, Panels a, b, e, and f in Bonfanti P, Moschini E, Saibene M, et al.: Do nanoparticle physico-chemical properties and developmental exposure window influence nano ZnO embryotoxicity in* Xenopus laevis*?, Int J Environ Res Publ Health 12: 8828–8848, 2015 under a Creative Commons Attribution License (CC BY 4.0).*

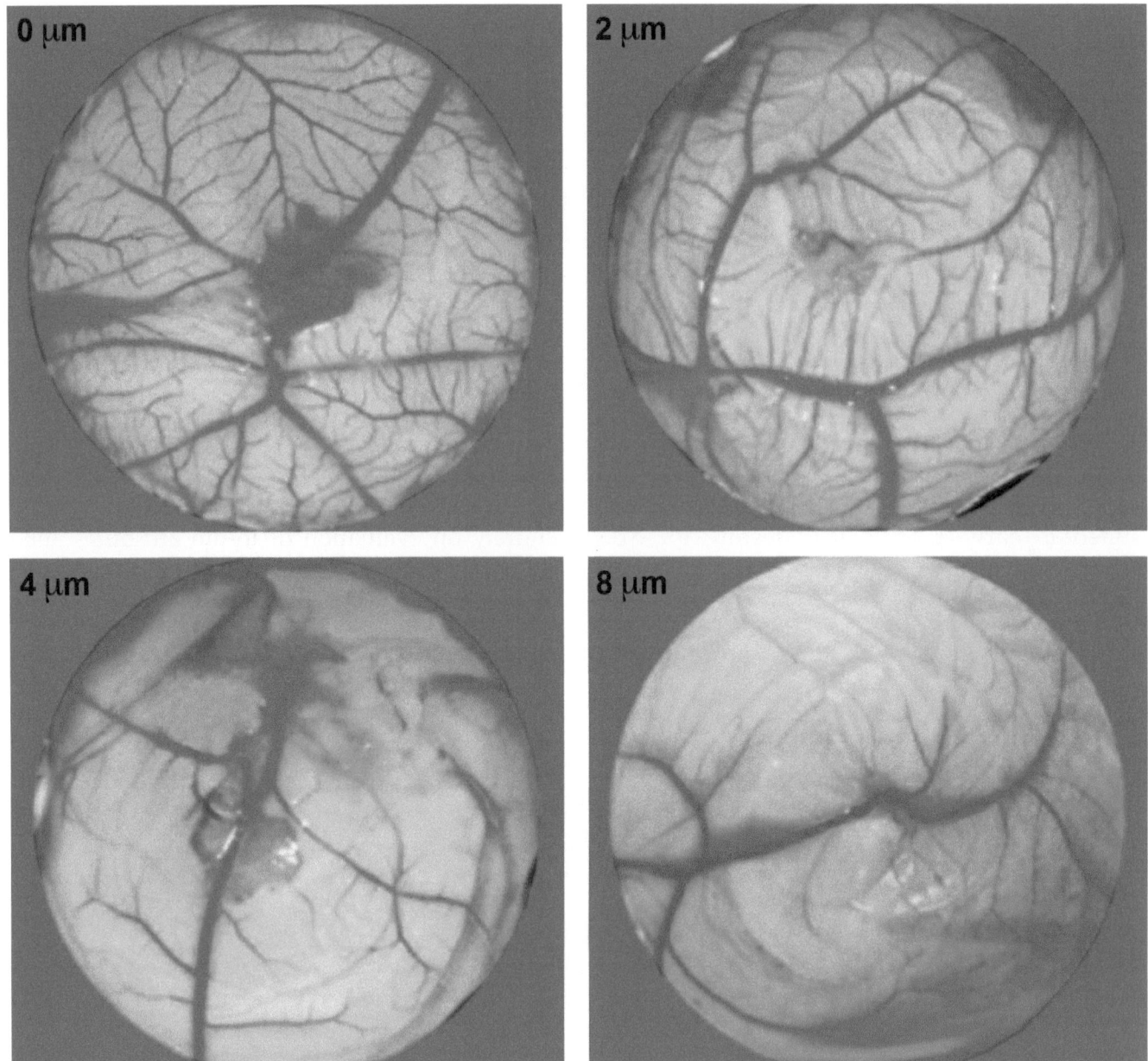

FIGURE 24.11   Reduced angiogenesis demonstrated in the chorioallantoic membrane (CAM) assay of an 11-day-old chick embryo as indicated by dose-dependent reduction in blood vessel formation and branching following application of an antidiabetic drug. *Reproduced from Page 9968, Figure 1, Panel B (top row) in Qi C, Zhou Q, Li B, et al.: Glipizide, an antidiabetic drug, suppresses tumor growth and metastasis by inhibiting angiogenesis,* Oncotarget 5:9966–9979, *2014 under a Creative Commons Attribution License (CC BY 4.0).*

environmental toxicity surveys) using invertebrates as well as toxicity screens that employ fish, frog, and chick embryos. Histopathologic evaluation is relatively uncommon for invertebrates and non-mammalian embryos and larvae since this procedure is slow compared to the high-throughput observational phase of the study—and because most pathologists have little prior exposure and limited or no access to the scarce references that describe anatomic and histologic features of invertebrate species. Histopathologic examination is a common feature of basic biological experiments where extensive characterization of new phenotypes or possible innovative models is essential for understanding. Histopathologic evaluation also is common for carcinogenicity screening, where the method is aided by the ability to embed an entire individual in one cassette for rapid assessment of multiple organs in one or a few sections. Toxicologic pathologists who provide histopathologic support for such studies in non-mammalian species will need to gain familiarity with the particular anatomic and histologic features of key organs (especially such target sites as gills, gonads, hematopoietic tissue, kidneys, and liver) as well as species-specific diagnostic nomenclature (such as the effort in progress to establish internationally recognized International Harmonization of Nomenclature and Diagnostic Criteria [INHAND] terminology for toxicant-induced lesions in fish). This learning process may be possible using online or print reference texts and atlases, but in most cases, the novice will gain significantly through apprenticeship an experienced mentor.

6. REGULATORY PERSPECTIVE ON ALTERNATIVE MODELS

Hazard identification and the assessment of risk/safety in the 21st century is a complex process (see *Risk Assessment*, Vol 2, Chap 16) Regulatory decisions regarding new products under development typically follow a WoE approach in which data acquired via many different kinds of assays are integrated in reaching the final verdict. In this regard, alternative models—whether in silico, in vitro, or in vivo—all have a place in assembling the necessary WoE. Indeed, in the current political and social environments of many regions, regulatory bodies increasingly promote the use of alternative models as a key component of product registration packages (EC, 2009; Wheeler, 2019) despite a historical preference in favor of standard in vivo mammalian models (Schiffelers et al., 2012) and remaining gaps in the knowledge base that limit the utility of in silico and in vitro data (Weaver and Valentin, 2019).

Several considerations contribute to efforts by regulatory agencies to more widely utilize data from alternative assays. One primary factor is that alternative models are a direct means for implementing 3Rs ("Replacement, Reduction, Refinement") initiatives (Schiffelers et al., 2012; Sewell et al., 2016), especially to limit the

involvement of nonhuman primates in drug discovery and development (Prior et al., 2017). In this respect, MPS such as "human-on-a-chip" cultures and organotypic in vitro models ("organoids"), especially complex 3D systems that exhibit both anatomic and functional traits similar to their native organ, represent a potent tool for mechanistic and safety studies (Hartung, 2018; Pridgeon et al., 2018). A second point is that alternative models afford an important means of understanding molecular and cellular mechanisms of toxicity, which in turn supports more science-driven data sets to use in making risk/safety assessment decisions (Dal Negro et al., 2018). A third opportunity is that human tissue—whether cultured in vitro or grown in vivo following implantation of a xenograft in a suitable animal model—may be employed in safety assessment to explore biological responses in humans without exposing any person to a substance with unknown toxic properties (Jackson et al., 2018). Indeed, an innovative "Clinical Trials in a Dish" platform proposed as a high-throughput screen for efficacy and/or toxicity is based on in vitro treatment of human iPSCs (Fermini et al., 2018). Despite these benefits, existing in silico and in vitro models, and to a lesser degree nonmammalian in vivo models, are not capable of identifying many organ toxicities that form the foundation for current regulatory decisions (McMullen et al., 2018). Furthermore, to date, many of these new technologies are not standardized or validated to a sufficient degree to accord such data a large contribution to the WoE relative to other types of in vitro and in vivo toxicity data (Adamo et al., 2018; Sauer et al., 2017).

7. CONCLUSIONS AND PERSPECTIVES

7.1. Integration of Pathology and Alternative Data Streams

Genomics, transcriptomics, proteomics, and other data-rich technologies are now routinely used in clinical medicine to predict patient outcomes and guide treatment options. For example, gene expression profiles from certain types of cancer can determine which patients are at highest risk of recurrence and will thus benefit from systemic chemotherapy, while sparing lower-risk patients who will not (McVeigh and Kerin, 2017). Increasingly, "alternative" types of data are also being used to guide safety decisions in toxicological science, by informing drug/chemical screening and prioritization, mechanisms of toxicity, model validation and read-across, and other in silico approaches, as discussed above. Despite rapid advances in big data tools, major translational challenges remain: Where is the line between hazard identification and prediction? At what point does a molecular change become biologically significant? How do we make adversity decisions based on molecular data? As translational and comparative scientists, toxicologic pathologists have an important role in navigating these issues and guiding the proper application of omic endpoints.

Several developments in recent years have helped drive the integration of pathology and molecular biology. The most obvious factors are legislative directives such as the TSCA, as amended in 2016 by the Frank R. Lautenberg Chemical Safety for the 21st Century Act (U.S. Public Law 114–182), which requires the U.S. EPA to reduce and replace animals used in chemical testing and thus promotes alternative test methods or strategies. These mandates have pushed the need to understand and apply non-morphologic endpoints. In addition, public health issues often require rapid decisions that can only be informed using integrative short-term data. An example here is the U.S. National Toxicology Program (NTP) response to the 2014 chemical spill in the Elk River of West Virginia, which included a diverse array of short-term experimental approaches, including studies in rodents, zebrafish, and worms, cell-based toxicity tests, and computer modeling (https://ntp.niehs.nih.gov/whatwestudy/topics/wvspill/index.html).

More broadly, there is a clear need for toxicology to incorporate current tools and models into the risk assessment process. Integrative testing approaches provide a way to evaluate alternative models and align them with programmatic or regulatory needs. One example is the tiered testing framework for hazard characterization outlined recently by scientists at the U.S. EPA (Figure 24.12) (Thomas et al., 2019). The first tier of this approach applies both computational read-across methods and broad coverage in vitro assays to evaluate and group chemicals based on potential health effects. In the second tier, chemicals with a predicted biological target or toxicity pathway then are evaluated using targeted follow-up assays. In the third tier, likely, toxicological effects are assessed in the context of existing AOPs or more complex culture systems, and quantitative PODs for hazard are estimated.

Pathology and molecular data streams complement each other in many ways. Target expression profiling using transcriptomic and proteomic methods may guide species selection, study design, sample collection, and biomarker options for subsequent toxicity studies. Gene expression biomarkers can be used to identify target toxicity pathways, either preemptively (e.g., in cell model screens) or retrospectively (e.g., in the interpretation of morphologic findings). Short-term –omic data, if clearly anchored to an MOA/AOP, may also serve as a surrogate basis for determining health guidance values and justifying study waivers. A recent example of this approach is the agrochemical halauxifen-methyl. The U.S. EPA determined in 2016 that increased liver expression of the $Cyp1a1$ gene in a subchronic rat study of halauxifen-methyl was a suitable biomarker for toxicity due to activation of the liver aryl hydrocarbon receptor MOA and used it for setting the point-of-departure estimates for chronic exposure, rather than requiring long-term oral studies (EPA, 2016b). Increased application of benchmark dose estimates for both morphologic and transcriptomic endpoints will continue to advance this type of integrated assessment (Lake et al., 2016; NTP, 2018).

Big data technologies such as next-generation sequencing now provide unprecedented access to biological information contained within archival tissue specimens (Hester et al., 2016). Global biorepositories, which house millions of formalin-fixed, paraffin-embedded (FFPE) blocks from nonclinical and clinical samples, have immense potential value in characterizing drug/chemical effects, without the need for de novo studies. In many cases, these FFPE samples have well-validated pathologic or phenotypic outcomes, making them a valuable resource for omic biomarker development, mechanistic studies, and dose modeling. Tissue archives thus provide an important interface between toxicologic pathology and related disciplines such as molecular toxicology and computational biology, given that morphologic context is often needed to anchor or validate omic information.

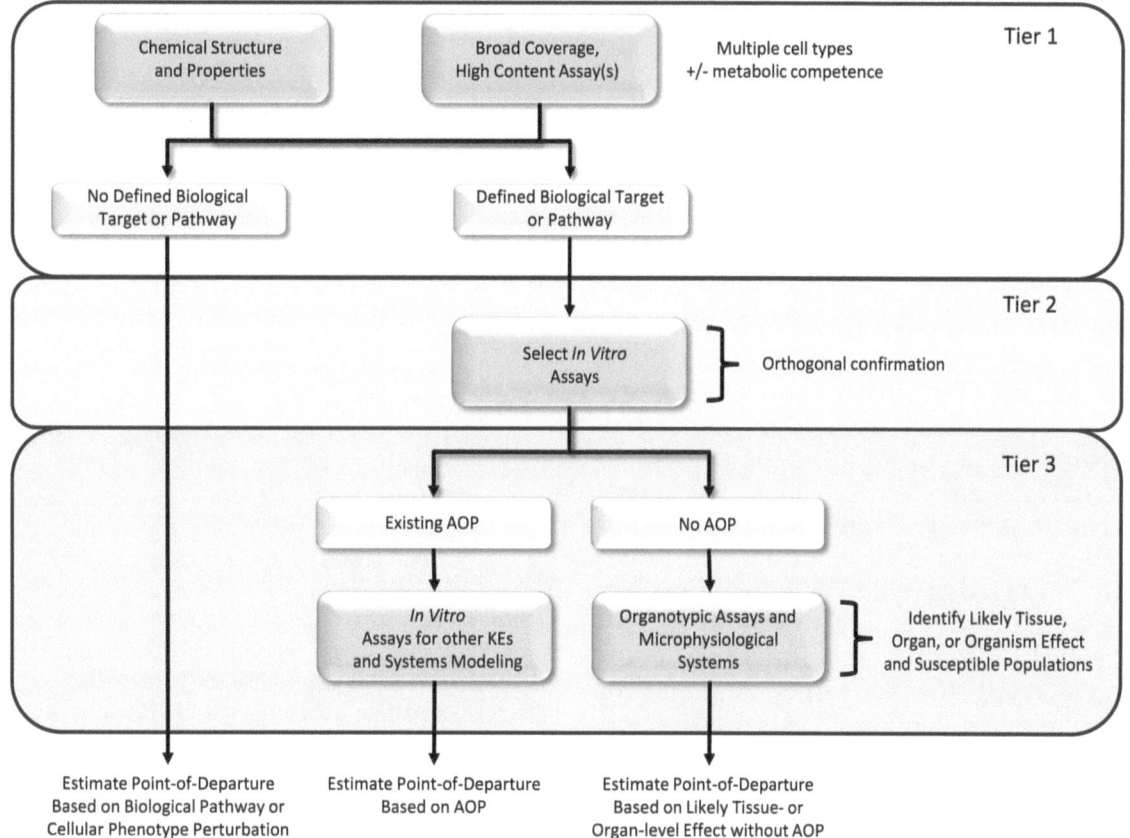

FIGURE 24.12   Tiered testing framework for hazard characterization. Tier 1 uses both chemical structure and broad coverage, high-content assays across multiple cell types for comprehensively evaluating the potential effects of chemicals and grouping them based on similarity in potential hazards. For chemicals from Tier 1 without a defined biological target/pathway, a quantitative point-of-departure for hazard is estimated based on the absence of biological pathway or cellular phenotype perturbation. Chemicals from Tier 1 with a predicted biological target or pathway are evaluated Tier 2 using targeted follow-up assays. In Tier 3, the likely tissue, organ, or organism-level effects are considered based on either existing adverse outcome pathways (AOPs) or more complex culture systems. Quantitative points-of-departure for hazard are estimated based on the AOP or responses in the complex culture system. *Reproduced from Page 323, Figure 2 in Thomas RS, Bahadori T, Buckley TJ, et al.: The next generation blueprint of computational toxicology at the U.S. Environmental Protection Agency, Toxicol Sci 169:317–332, 2019 by permission of Oxford University Press.*

7.2. Context of Use and Qualification Requirements

Each model was initially conceived for a specific purpose and brings its own unique advantages and limitations. Accordingly, it is the context in which these models are used that can take full advantage of the potential benefits, but the possible limitations need to be fully appreciated before conclusions are made with data generated from these models. If utilized appropriately, these models are expected to provide mechanistic insights into molecular pathways leading to various toxicological endpoints, can increase throughput to provide QSAR data in a time efficient manner, and will reduce, refine, and ultimately replace the use of certain in vivo animal studies.

In order to use these alternative models, prerequisite qualifications are needed to ensure the robustness of their predictive power. A test set of compounds needs to be assembled so that a database may be built that includes both positive and negative effects relative to the desired context of use. Relevant in vitro and alternative in vivo endpoints need to be established, measured, and compared with known findings from more conventional in vivo tests so that the specificity and accuracy of these alternative methods can be assessed. In addition, intra- and interlab reproducibility needs to be established.

7.3. Future Directions

Drug- and chemically-induced toxicities are often complicated. Assessing the relevance of animal-based effects to human risk assessment must consider a host of factors and the interactions of various cell types within an organ, and sometimes cells from different organs to define the drivers for such toxicities. Therefore, integrated approaches that integrate the information obtained from in silico, in vitro, and in vivo models are highly desirable for holistic assessment. These alternative models need to exhibit physiological, histological, and functional characteristics relevant to the target organ(s) of interest in more conventional test species and humans. The sources and quality of various cells and reagents will need to be established. Finally, clarity regarding this multidisciplinary approach must await further work to establish generally accepted protocols and scoring criteria so that the validity of various models for their intended uses may be confirmed. In particular, such efforts may require industry-wide consortia to provide the needed interlaboratory comparisons needed for harmonization and assay validation.

REFERENCES

Abou-Saleh H, Zouein FA, El-Yazbi A, et al.: The march of pluripotent stem cells in cardiovascular regenerative medicine, *Stem Cell Res Ther* 9:201, 2018.

Adamo JE, Bienvenu 2nd RV, Fields FO, et al.: The integration of emerging omics approaches to advance precision medicine: How can regulatory science help? *J Clin Transl Sci* 2:295–300, 2018.

Ainslie GR, Davis M, Ewart L, et al.: Microphysiological lung models to evaluate the safety of new pharmaceutical modalities: a biopharmaceutical perspective, *Lab Chip* 19: 3152–3161, 2019.

Alge CS, Hauck SM, Priglinger SG, et al.: Differential protein profiling of primary versus immortalized human RPE cells identifies expression patterns associated with cytoskeletal remodeling and cell survival, *J Proteome Res* 5:862–878, 2006.

Allison SJ: Bioengineering: kidney glomerulus-on-a-chip, *Nat Rev Nephrol* 13:382, 2017.

American Type Culture Collection Standards Development Organization Workgroup ASN-0002: Cell line misidentification: the beginning of the end, *Nat Rev Cancer* 10:441–448, 2010.

Anderer U, Libera J: In vitro engineering of human autogenous cartilage, *J Bone Miner Res* 17:1420–1429, 2002.

Ankley GT, Bennett RS, Erickson RJ, et al.: Adverse outcome pathways: a conceptual framework to support ecotoxicology research and risk assessment, *Environ Toxicol Chem* 29: 730–741, 2010.

Apati A, Varga N, Berecz T, et al.: Application of human pluripotent stem cells and pluripotent stem cell-derived cellular models for assessing drug toxicity, *Expet Opin Drug Metabol Toxicol* 15:61–75, 2019.

Aschner M, Kimelberg HK: The use of astrocytes in culture as model systems for evaluating neurotoxic-induced-injury, *Neurotoxicology* 12:505–517, 1991.

Bakmand T, Troels-Smith AR, Dimaki M, et al.: Fluidic system for long-term in vitro culturing and monitoring of organotypic brain slices, *Biomed Microdevices* 17:71, 2015.

Bao L, Yin J, Gao W, et al.: A long-acting FGF21 alleviates hepatic steatosis and inflammation in a mouse model of non-alcoholic steatohepatitis partly through an FGF21-adiponectin-IL17A pathway, *Br J Pharmacol* 175:3379–3393, 2018.

Barron JA, Krizman DB, Ringeisen BR: Laser printing of single cells: statistical analysis, cell viability, and stress, *Ann Biomed Eng* 33:121–130, 2005.

Barron JA, Wu P, Ladouceur HD, et al.: Biological laser printing: a novel technique for creating heterogeneous 3-dimensional cell patterns, *Biomed Microdevices* 6:139–147, 2004.

Barzi M, Pankowicz FP, Zorman B, et al.: A novel humanized mouse lacking murine P450 oxidoreductase for studying human drug metabolism, *Nat Commun* 8:39, 2017.

Baudy AR, Otieno MA, Hewitt P, et al.: Liver microphysiological systems development guidelines for safety risk assessment in the pharmaceutical industry, *Lab Chip* 20: 215–225, 2020.

Bautch VL, Stanford WL, Rapoport R, et al.: Blood island formation in attached cultures of murine embryonic stem cells, *Dev Dynam* 205:1–12, 1996.

Bauwens CL, Peerani R, Niebruegge S, et al.: Control of human embryonic stem cell colony and aggregate size heterogeneity influences differentiation trajectories, *Stem Cell* 26:2300–2310, 2008.

Baverel G, Knouzy B, Gauthier C, et al.: Use of precision-cut renal cortical slices in nephrotoxicity studies, *Xenobiotica* 43:54–62, 2013.

Behringer R: Summary of mouse development. In Behringer R, Gertsenstein M, Nagy KV, Nagy A, editors: *Manipulating the mouse embryo: a laboratory manual*, ed 4, NY, 2014, Cold Spring Harbor Laboratory Press, pp 23–84.

Benam KH, Dauth S, Hassell B, et al.: Engineered in vitro disease models, *Annu Rev Pathol* 10:195–262, 2015.

Berube K, Prytherch Z, Job C, et al.: Human primary bronchial lung cell constructs: the new respiratory models, *Toxicology* 278:311–318, 2010.

Bishop ES, Mostafa S, Pakvasa M, et al.: 3-D bioprinting technologies in tissue engineering and regenerative medicine: current and future trends, *Genes Dis* 4:185–195, 2017.

Blomme EA, Will Y: Toxicology strategies for drug discovery: present and future, *Chem Res Toxicol* 29:473–504, 2016.

Bolon B, Dorman DC, Bonnefoi MS, et al.: Histopathologic approaches to chemical toxicity using primary cultures of dissociated neural cells grown in chamber slides, *Toxicol Pathol* 21:465–479, 1993.

Bonfanti P, Moschini E, Saibene M, et al.: Do nanoparticle physico-chemical properties and developmental exposure window influence nano ZnO embryotoxicity in *Xenopus laevis*? *Int J Environ Res Publ Health* 12:8828–8848, 2015.

Boobis AR, Cohen SM, Dellarco V, et al.: IPCS framework for analyzing the relevance of a cancer mode of action for humans, *Crit Rev Toxicol* 36:781–792, 2006.

Boogaard PJ, Nagelkerke JF, Mulder GJ: Renal proximal tubular cells in suspension or in primary culture as in vitro models to study nephrotoxicity, *Chem Biol Interact* 76:251–291, 1990.

Boos JA, Misun PM, Michlmayr A, et al.: Microfluidic multi-tissue platform for advanced embryotoxicity testing in vitro, *Adv Sci* 6:1900294, 2019.

Bourcier T, McGovern T, Stavitskaya L, et al.: Improving prediction of carcinogenicity to reduce, refine, and replace the use of experimental animals, *J Am Assoc Lab Anim Sci* 54:163–169, 2015.

Boyer CJ, Ballard DH, Barzegar M, et al.: High-throughput scaffold-free microtissues through 3D printing, *3D Print Med* 4(9), 2018.

Brown AC, Fraser TR: On the connection between chemical constitution and physiological action; with special reference to the physiological action of the salts of the ammonium bases derived from Strychnia, Brucia, Thebaia, Codeia, Morphia, and Nicotia, *J Anat Physiol* 2:224–242, 1868.

Brown NA: Routine assessment of morphology and growth: scoring systems and measurements of size. In Copp AJ, Cockroft DL, editors: *Postimplantation mammalian embryos: a practical approach*, Oxford, 1990, IRL Press, pp 93–108.

Browne P, Judson RS, Casey WM, et al.: Screening chemicals for estrogen receptor bioactivity using a computational model, *Environ Sci Technol* 49:8804–8814, 2015.

Buta C, David R, Dressel R, et al.: Reconsidering pluripotency tests: do we still need teratoma assays? *Stem Cell Res* 11:552–562, 2013.

Casati S: Integrated approaches to testing and assessment, *Basic Clin Pharmacol Toxicol* 123(Suppl 5):51–55, 2018.

Cassar S, Adatto I, Freeman JL, et al.: Use of zebrafish in drug discovery toxicology, *Chem Res Toxicol* 33(1):95–118, 2020.

Cha JM, Bae H, Sadr N, et al.: Embryoid body sized-mediated differential endodermal and mesodermal differentiation using polyethlyene glycol (PEG) microwell array, *Macromol Res* 23:245–255, 2015.

Chang CC, Boland ED, Williams SK, et al.: Direct-write bioprinting three-dimensional biohybrid systems for future regenerative therapies, *J Biomed Mater Res B Appl Biomater* 98:160–170, 2011.

Chang R, Nam J, Sun W: Effects of dispensing pressure and nozzle diameter on cell survival from solid freeform fabrication-based direct cell writing, *Tissue Eng A* 14:41–48, 2008.

Chang SY, Voellinger JL, Van Ness KP, et al.: Characterization of rat or human hepatocytes cultured in microphysiological systems (MPS) to identify hepatotoxicity, *Toxicol In Vitro* 40:170–183, 2017.

Chen Y, Niu Y, Ji W: Genome editing in nonhuman primates: approach to generating human disease models, *J Int Med* 280:246–251, 2016.

Chrisey DB: Materials processing: the power of direct writing, *Science* 289:879–881, 2000.

Clark AM, Wheeler SE, Taylor DP, et al.: A microphysiological system model of therapy for liver micrometastases, *Exp Biol Med* 239:1170–1179, 2014.

Colina M, Serra P, Fernandez-Pradas JM, et al.: DNA deposition through laser induced forward transfer, *Biosens Bioelectron* 20:1638–1642, 2005.

Conolly RB, Ankley GT, Cheng W, et al.: Quantitative adverse outcome pathways and their application to predictive toxicology, *Environ Sci Technol* 51:4661–4672, 2017.

Cui X, Boland T, D'Lima DD, et al.: Thermal inkjet printing in tissue engineering and regenerative medicine, *Recent Pat Drug Deliv Formulation* 6:149–155, 2012.

da Silva ACG, Chialchia AR, de Castro EG, et al.: A new corneal epithelial biomimetic 3D model for in vitro eye toxicity assessment: development, characterization and applicability, *Toxicol In Vitro* 62:104666, 2020.

Dahl-Jensen S, Grapin-Botton A: The physics of organoids: a biophysical approach to understanding organogenesis, *Development* 144:946–951, 2017.

Dal Negro G, Eskes C, Belz S, et al.: One science-driven approach for the regulatory implementation of alternative methods: A multi-sector perspective, *Regul Toxicol Pharmacol* 99:33–49, 2018.

Daniels K, Reiter R, Solursh M: Chapter 12 micromass cultures of limb and other mesenchyme, *Methods Cell Biol* 51:237–247, 1996.

Davies JA: Organoids and mini-organs: introduction, history, and potential. In Davies JA, Lawrence M, editors: *Organoids and mini-organs*, Edinburgh, UK, 2018, Academic Press, Elsevier, pp 3–23.

Demirci U, Montesano G: Single cell epitaxy by acoustic picolitre droplets, *Lab Chip* 7:1139–1145, 2007.

Denker AE, Nicoll SB, Tuan RS: Formatin of cartilage-like spheroids by micromass cultures of murine C3H10T1/2 cells upon treatment with transforming growth factor-B1, *Differentiation* 59:25–34, 1995.

Deshmukh RS, Kovacs KA, Dinnyes A: Drug discovery models and toxicity testing using embryonic and induced pluripotent stem-cell-derived cardiac and neuronal cells, *Stem Cell Int* 2012:379569, 2012.

Dias AD, Unser AM, Xie Y, et al.: Generating size-controlled embryoid bodies using laser direct-write, *Biofabrication* 6:025007, 2014.

Dinca V, Kasotakis E, Catherine J, et al.: Directed three-dimensional patterning of self-assembled peptide fibrils, *Nano Lett* 8:538–543, 2008.

Drost J, Karthaus WR, Gao D, et al.: Organoid culture systems for prostate epithelial and cancer tissue, *Nat Protoc* 11:347–358, 2016.

Duan B, Hockaday LA, Kang KH, et al.: 3D bioprinting of heterogeneous aortic valve conduits with alginate/gelatin hydrogels, *J Biomed Mater Res A* 101:1255–1264, 2013a.

Duan B, Hockaday LA, Kapetanovic E, et al.: Stiffness and adhesivity control aortic valve interstitial cell behavior within hyaluronic acid based hydrogels, *Acta Biomater* 9:7640–7650, 2013b.

Dyrby T, Ingvardsen P: Sensitivity of different *E. coli* and *Salmonella* strains in mutagenicity testing calculated on the basis of selected literature, *Mutat Res* 123:47–60, 1983.

Dzobo K, Motaung K, Adesida A: Recent trends in decellularized extracellular matrix bioinks for 3D printing: an updated review, *Int J Mol Sci* 20, 2019.

EC (European Council). Regulation (EC) No 1223/2009 of the European Parliament and of the Council of 30 November 2009 on cosmetic products. https://ec.europa.eu/health/sites/health/files/endocrine_disruptors/docs/cosmetic_1223_2009_regulation_en.pdf. Published 2009. (Accessed 25 April 2021).

Editorial: Method of the year 2017: organoids, *Nat Methods* 15, 2017.

Ellis BW, Acun A, Can UI, et al.: Human iPSC-derived myocardium-on-chip with capillary-like flow for personalized medicine, *Biomicrofluidics* 11:024105, 2017.

EPA (U.S. Environmental Protection Agency): *Guidelines for carcinogen risk assessment*, EPA/630/P-03/001F, Washington, DC, 2005.

EPA (U.S. Environmental Protection Agency): *Endocrine disruptor screening Program. Uterotrophic assay, OCSPP guideline 890.1600 standard evaluation procedure (SEP)*, 2011. Washington, DC.

EPA (U.S. Environmental Protection Agency): *Use of high throughput assays and computational tools; endocrine disruptor screening program*, Notice of Availability and Opportunity for Comment, Washington, DC, 2015.

EPA (U.S. Environmental Protection Agency). In Office of Pesticide Programs, editor: *Guidance for waiving acute dermal toxicity tests for pesticide formulations & supporting retrospective analysis*, 2016a. Washington, DC.

EPA (U.S. Environmental Protection Agency). In US Environmental Protection Agency, editor: *Halauxifen-methyl; pesticide tolerances*, 2016b, Fed. Regist., 53029-53025.

EPA (U.S. Environmental Protection Agency). In Office of Pesticide Programs, editor: *Process for evaluating and implementing alternative approaches to traditional in vivo acute toxicity studies for FIFRA regulatory use*, 2016c.

EPA (U.S. Enviornmental Protection Agency). TSCA chemical substance inventory, 2021. https://www.epa.gov/tsca-inventory. Accessed 25 April 2021.

Esch EW, Bahinski A, Huh D: Organs-on-chips at the frontiers of drug discovery, *Nat Rev Drug Discov* 14:248–260, 2015.

Ewart L, Fabre K, Chakilam A, et al.: Navigating tissue chips from development to dissemination: a pharmaceutical industry perspective, *Exp Biol Med* 242:1579–1585, 2017.

Fang Y, Frampton JP, Raghavan S, et al.: Rapid generation of multiplexed cell cocultures using acoustic droplet ejection followed by aqueous two-phase exclusion patterning, *Tissue Eng C Methods* 18:647–657, 2012.

Fatehullah A, Tan SH, Barker N: Organoids as an in vitro model of human development and disease, *Nat Cell Biol* 18:246–254, 2016.

FDA (U.S. Food and Drug Administration): International conference on harmonisation; proposed change to rodent carcinogenicity testing of pharmaceuticals; request for comments. Notice; request for comments, *Fed Regist* 78:16681–16684, 2013.

Feinberg AW, Feigel A, Shevkoplyas SS, et al.: Muscular thin films for building actuators and powering devices, *Science* 317:1366–1370, 2007.

Fermini B, Coyne ST, Coyne KP: Clinical trials in a dish: a perspective on the coming revolution in drug development, *SLAS Discov* 23:765–776, 2018.

Fischer C, Milting H, Fein E, et al.: Long-term functional and structural preservation of precision-cut human myocardium under continuous electromechanical stimulation in vitro, *Nat Commun* 10:117, 2019.

Flamier A, Singh S, Rasmussen TP: A standardized human embryoid body platform for the detection and analysis of teratogens, *PloS One* 12:e0171101, 2017.

Forbes B, Ehrhardt C: Human respiratory epithelial cell culture for drug delivery applications, *Eur J Pharm Biopharm* 60:193–205, 2005.

Gao D, Vela I, Sboner A, et al.: Organoid cultures derived from patients with advanced prostate cancer, *Cell* 159:176–187, 2014.

Glanville-Jones HC, Woo N, Arkell RM: Successful whole embryo culture with commercially available reagents, *Int J Dev Biol* 57:61–67, 2013.

Goldmann T, Gonzalez JS: DNA-printing: utilization of a standard inkjet printer for the transfer of nucleic acids to solid supports, *J Biochem Biophys Methods* 42:105–110, 2000.

Graaf IA, Groothuis GM, Olinga P: Precision-cut tissue slices as a tool to predict metabolism of novel drugs, *Expet Opin Drug Metabol Toxicol* 3:879–898, 2007.

Grant RL: Primary cultures of rabbit corneal epithelial cells as an experimental model to evaluate ocular toxicity and explore modes of action of toxic injury, *Toxicol In Vitro* 64:104634, 2020.

Grassart A, Malarde V, Gobaa S, et al.: Bioengineered human organ-on-chip reveals intestinal microenvironment and mechanical forces impacting Shigella infection, *Cell Host Microbe* 26, 2019, 435–444 e434.

Grayson WL, Martens TP, Eng GM, et al.: Biomimetic approach to tissue engineering, *Semin Cell Dev Biol* 20:665–673, 2009.

Greggio C, De Franceschi F, Figueiredo-Larsen M, et al.: Artificial three-dimensional niches deconstruct pancreas development in vitro, *Development* 140:4452–4462, 2013.

Grens K: *Big advances in science*, The Scientist.

Gruene M, Deiwick A, Koch L, et al.: Laser printing of stem cells for biofabrication of scaffold-free autologous grafts, *Tissue Eng C Methods* 17:79–87, 2011.

Guillemot F, Souquet A, Catros S, et al.: Laser-assisted cell printing: principle, physical parameters versus cell fate and perspectives in tissue engineering, *Nanomedicine* 5:507–515, 2010.

Guillotin B, Guillemot F: Cell patterning technologies for organotypic tissue fabrication, *Trends Biotechnol* 29:183–190, 2011.

Hall BK, Miyake T: The membranous skeleton: the role of cell condensations in vertebrate skeletogenesis, *Anat Embryol* 186:107–124, 1992.

Handschel J, Wiesmann H, Meyer U: Prospects of micromass culture technology in tissue engineering. In Meyer U, Handschel J, Wiesmann H, et al., editors: *Fundamentals of tissue engineering and regenerative medicine*, Berlin, Heidelberg, 2009, Springer, pp 551–555.

Handschel JG, Depprich RA, Kubler NR, et al.: Prospects of micromass culture technology in tissue engineering, *Head Face Med* 3(4), 2007.

Hardwick RN, Betts CJ, Whritenour J, et al.: Drug-induced skin toxicity: gaps in preclinical testing cascade as opportunities for complex in vitro models and assays, *Lab Chip* 20:199–214, 2020.

Hartung T: Perspectives on in vitro to in vivo extrapolations, *Appl In Vitro Toxicol* 4:305–316, 2018.

Hartung T, Gstraunthaler G, Coecke S, et al.: Good cell culture practice (GCCP)–an initiative for standardization and quality control of in vitro studies. The establishment of an ECVAM Task Force on GCCP, *ALTEX* 18:75–78, 2001.

Hashimoto K, Takeda S, Swenberg JA, et al.: Incorporation of metabolic activation potentiates cyclophosphamide-induced DNA damage response in isogenic DT40 mutant cells, *Mutagenesis* 30:821–828, 2015.

Heit C, Dong H, Chen Y, et al.: Transgenic mouse models for alcohol metabolism, toxicity, and cancer, *Adv Exp Med Biol* 815:375–387, 2015.

Helman G, Shah I, Patlewicz G: Extending the Generalised Read-Across approach (GenRA): a systematic analysis of the impact of physicochemical property information on read-across performance, *Comput Toxicol* 8:34–50, 2018.

Hester SD, Bhat V, Chorley BN, et al.: Editor's highlight: dose-response analysis of RNA-seq profiles in archival formalin-fixed paraffin-embedded samples, *Toxicol Sci* 154:202–213, 2016.

Ho CT, Lin RZ, Chen RJ, et al.: Liver-cell patterning lab chip: mimicking the morphology of liver lobule tissue, *Lab Chip* 13:3578–3587, 2013.

Hopp B, Smausz T, Kresz N, et al.: Survival and proliferative ability of various living cell types after laser-induced forward transfer, *Tissue Eng* 11:1817–1823, 2005.

Huch M, Boj SF, Clevers H: Lgr5(+) liver stem cells, hepatic organoids and regenerative medicine, *Regen Med* 8:385–387, 2013.

Huch M, Gehart H, van Boxtel R, et al.: Long-term culture of genome-stable bipotent stem cells from adult human liver, *Cell* 160:299–312, 2015.

Huch M, Knoblich JA, Lutolf MP, et al.: The hope and the hype of organoid research, *Development* 144:938–941, 2017.

Huch M, Koo BK: Modeling mouse and human development using organoid cultures, *Development* 142:3113–3125, 2015.

Huh D, Matthews BD, Mammoto A, et al.: Reconstituting organ-level lung functions on a chip, *Science* 328:1662–1668, 2010.

Hunt PR: The C. elegans model in toxicity testing, *J Appl Toxicol* 37:50–59, 2017.

Hurst HS, Clothier RH, Pratten M: An evaluation of a novel chick cardiomyocyte micromass culture assay with two teratogens/embryotoxins associated with heart defects, *Altern Lab Anim* 35:505–514, 2007.

Ibraheim H, Giacomini C, Kassam Z, et al.: Advances in mesenchymal stromal cell therapy in the management of Crohn's disease, *Expet Rev Gastroenterol Hepatol* 12:141–153, 2018.

Jackson SJ, Prior H, Holmes A: The use of human tissue in safety assessment, *J Pharmacol Toxicol Methods* 93:29–34, 2018.

Jain A, van der Meer AD, Papa AL, et al.: Assessment of whole blood thrombosis in a microfluidic device lined by fixed human endothelium, *Biomed Microdevices* 18:73, 2016.

Jakab K, Norotte C, Marga F, et al.: Tissue engineering by self-assembly and bio-printing of living cells, *Biofabrication* 2:022001, 2010.

Jang KJ, Mehr AP, Hamilton GA, et al.: Human kidney proximal tubule-on-a-chip for drug transport and nephrotoxicity assessment, *Integr Biol* 5:1119–1129, 2013.

JRC. In Joint Research Center, editor: *Applicability of QSAR analysis to the evaluation of the toxicological relevance of metabolites and degradates of pesticide active substances for dietary risk assessment Prepared by Computational Toxicology Group, Institute for Health & Consumer Protection*, Italy, 2010, Ispra.

Judson RS, Magpantay FM, Chickarmane V, et al.: Integrated model of chemical perturbations of a biological pathway using 18 in vitro high-throughput screening assays for the estrogen receptor, *Toxicol Sci* 148:137–154, 2015.

Jung P, Sato T, Merlos-Suarez A, et al.: Isolation and in vitro expansion of human colonic stem cells, *Nat Med* 17:1225–1227, 2011.

Kang KS, Trosko JE: Stem cells in toxicology: fundamental biology and practical considerations, *Toxicol Sci* 120(Suppl 1):S269–S289, 2011.

Karagiannis P, Nakauchi A, Yamanaka S: Bringing induced pluripotent stem cell technology to the bedside, *JMA J* 1:6–14, 2018.

Karthaus WR, Iaquinta PJ, Drost J, et al.: Identification of multipotent luminal progenitor cells in human prostate organoid cultures, *Cell* 159:163–175, 2014.

Keshavarzian A, Holmes EW, Patel M, et al.: Leaky gut in alcoholic cirrhosis: a possible mechanism for alcohol-induced liver damage, *Am J Gastroenterol* 94:200–207, 1999.

Khazali AS, Clark AM, Wells A: A pathway to personalizing therapy for metastases using liver-on-a-chip platforms, *Stem Cell Rev* 13:364–380, 2017.

Kim BM, Suzuki S, Nishimura Y, et al.: Cellular artificial skin substitute produced by short period simultaneous culture of fibroblasts and keratinocytes, *Br J Plast Surg* 52:573–578, 1999.

Kim HJ, Huh D, Hamilton G, et al.: Human gut-on-a-chip inhabited by microbial flora that experiences intestinal peristalsis-like motions and flow, *Lab Chip* 12:2165–2174, 2012.

Kim HJ, Li H, Collins JJ, et al.: Contributions of microbiome and mechanical deformation to intestinal bacterial overgrowth and inflammation in a human gut-on-a-chip, *Proc Natl Acad Sci U S A* 113:E7–E15, 2016.

Kim JD, Choi JS, Kim BS, et al.: Piezoelectric inkjet printing of polymers: stem cell patterning on polymer substrates, *Polymer* 51:2147–2154, 2010.

Kim JH, Sim J, Kim HJ: Neural stem cell differentiation using microfluidic device-generated growth factor gradient, *Biomol Ther* 26:380–388, 2018.

Kim DH, Jang YS, Jeon WK, et al.: Assessment of cognitive phenotyping in inbred, genetically modified mice, and transgenic mouse models of Alzheimer's disease, *Exp Neurobiol* 28:146–157, 2019a.

Kim TW, Che JH, Yun JW: Use of stem cells as alternative methods to animal experimentation in predictive toxicology, *Regul Toxicol Pharmacol* 105:15–29, 2019b.

Kingsley DM, Roberge CL, Rudkouskaya A, et al.: Laser-based 3D bioprinting for spatial and size control of tumor spheroids and embryoid bodies, *Acta Biomater* 95:357–370, 2019.

Kizhedath A, Wilkinson S, Glassey J: Applicability of predictive toxicology methods for monoclonal antibody therapeutics: status Quo and scope, *Arch Toxicol* 91:1595–1612, 2017.

Knowlton S, Tasoglu S: A bioprinted liver-on-a-chip for drug screening applications, *Trends Biotechnol* 34:681–682, 2016.

Koch L, Kuhn S, Sorg H, et al.: Laser printing of skin cells and human stem cells, *Tissue Eng C Methods* 16:847–854, 2010.

Kolahchi AR, Mohtaram NK, Modearres HP, et al.: Microfluidic-based multi-organ platforms for drug discovery, *Micromachines* 7:1–33, 2016.

Krewski D, Acosta Jr D, Andersen M, et al.: Toxicity testing in the 21st century: a vision and a strategy, *J Toxicol Environ Health B Crit Rev* 13:51–138, 2010.

L'Heureux N, Paquet S, Labbe R, et al.: A completely biological tissue-engineered human blood vessel, *FASEB J* 12:47–56, 1998.

Lake AD, Wood CE, Bhat VS, et al.: Dose and effect thresholds for early key events in a PPARalpha-mediated mode of action, *Toxicol Sci* 149:312–325, 2016.

Lancaster MA, Renner M, Martin CA, et al.: Cerebral organoids model human brain development and microcephaly, *Nature* 501:373–379, 2013.

Lenz B, Braendli-Baiocco A, Engelhardt J, et al.: Characterizing adversity of lysosomal accumulation in nonclinical toxicity studies: results from the 5th ESTP international expert workshop, *Toxicol Pathol* 46:224–246, 2018.

Li AP: Human hepatocytes: isolation, cryopreservation and applications in drug development, *Chem Biol Interact* 168:16–29, 2007.

Li AP, Alam N, Amaral K, et al.: Cryopreserved human intestinal mucosal epithelium: a novel in vitro experimental system for the evaluation of enteric drug metabolism, cytochrome P450 induction, and enterotoxicity, *Drug Metab Dispos* 46:1562–1571, 2018.

Li M, de Graaf IA, Groothuis GM: Precision-cut intestinal slices: alternative model for drug transport, metabolism, and toxicology research, *Expet Opin Drug Metabol Toxicol* 12:175–190, 2016.

Little MH: Organoids: a special issue, *Development* 144:935–937, 2017.

Liu L: Antibody glycosylation and its impact on the pharmacokinetics and pharmacodynamics of monoclonal antibodies and Fc-fusion proteins, *J Pharm Sci* 104:1866–1884, 2015.

Liu J, Patlewicz G, Williams AJ, et al.: Predicting organ toxicity using in vitro bioactivity data and chemical structure, *Chem Res Toxicol* 30:2046–2059, 2017a.

Liu S, Yin N, Faiola F: Prospects and frontiers of stem cell toxicology, *Stem Cell Dev* 26:1528–1539, 2017b.

Lorsch JR, Collins FS, Lippincott-Schwartz J: Cell biology. Fixing problems with cell lines, *Science* 346:1452–1453, 2014.

Low LA, Tagle DA: Tissue chips - innovative tools for drug development and disease modeling, *Lab Chip* 17:3026–3036, 2017.

Luz AL, Tokar EJ: Pluripotent stem cells in developmental toxicity testing: a review of methodological advances, *Toxicol Sci* 165:31–39, 2018.

Ma R, Morshed SA, Latif R, et al.: Thyroid cell differentiation from murine induced pluripotent stem cells, *Front Endocrinol* 6(56), 2015.

Ma C, Zhao L, Zhou EM, et al.: On-chip construction of liver lobule-like microtissue and its application for adverse drug reaction assay, *Anal Chem* 88:1719–1727, 2016a.

Ma X, Qu X, Zhu W, et al.: Deterministically patterned biomimetic human iPSC-derived hepatic model via rapid 3D bioprinting, *Proc Natl Acad Sci U S A* 113:2206–2211, 2016b.

Maffia 3rd AM, Kariv II, Oldenburg KR: Miniaturization of a mammalian cell-based assay: luciferase reporter gene readout in a 3 microliter 1536-well plate, *J Biomol Screen* 4:137–142, 1999.

Mahalingaiah PK, Palenski T, Van Vleet TR: An in vitro model of hematotoxicity: differentiation of bone marrow-derived stem/progenitor cells into hematopoietic lineages and evaluation of lineage-specific hematotoxicity, *Curr Protoc Toxicol* 76:e45, 2018.

Mahler GJ, Esch MB, Glahn RP, et al.: Characterization of a gastrointestinal tract microscale cell culture analog used to predict drug toxicity, *Biotechnol Bioeng* 104:193–205, 2009.

Marga F, Jakab K, Khatiwala C, et al.: Toward engineering functional organ modules by additive manufacturing, *Biofabrication* 4:022001, 2012.

Marx U, Andersson TB, Bahinski A, et al.: Biology-inspired microphysiological system approaches to solve the prediction dilemma of substance testing, *ALTEX* 33:272–321, 2016.

Masaeli E, Forster V, Picaud S, et al.: Tissue engineering of retina through high resolution 3-dimensional inkjet bioprinting, *Biofabrication*, 2019.

Mathur A, Loskill P, Shao K, et al.: Human iPSC-based cardiac microphysiological system for drug screening applications, *Sci Rep* 5:8883, 2015.

McMahon RE, Cline JC, Thompson CZ: Assay of 855 test chemicals in ten tester strains using a new modification of the Ames test for bacterial mutagens, *Cancer Res* 39:682–693, 1979.

McMullen PD, Andersen ME, Cholewa B, et al.: Evaluating opportunities for advancing the use of alternative methods in risk assessment through the development of fit-for-purpose in vitro assays, *Toxicol In Vitro* 48:310–317, 2018.

McVeigh TP, Kerin MJ: Clinical use of the oncotype DX genomic test to guide treatment decisions for patients with invasive breast cancer, *Breast Cancer* 9:393–400, 2017.

Meek ME, Boobis A, Cote I, et al.: New developments in the evolution and application of the WHO/IPCS framework on mode of action/species concordance analysis, *J Appl Toxicol* 34:1–18, 2014.

Mekhileri NV, Lim KS, Brown GCJ, et al.: Automated 3D bioassembly of micro-tissues for biofabrication of hybrid tissue engineered constructs, *Biofabrication* 10:024103, 2018.

Michael S, Sorg H, Peck CT, et al.: Tissue engineered skin substitutes created by laser-assisted bioprinting form skin-like structures in the dorsal skin fold chamber in mice, *PloS One* 8:e57741, 2013.

Mironov V, Visconti RP, Kasyanov V, et al.: Organ printing: tissue spheroids as building blocks, *Biomaterials* 30:2164–2174, 2009.

Mohamed-Ali H, de Souza P, Shakibaei M, et al.: Synovial and peritoneal macrophages in organoid culture, *Histol Histopathol* 10:393–403, 1995.

Mora-Bermudez F, Badsha F, Kanton S, et al.: Differences and similarities between human and chimpanzee neural progenitors during cerebral cortex development, *Elife* 5, 2016.

Morin JP, Baste JM, Gay A, et al.: Precision cut lung slices as an efficient tool for in vitro lung physio-pharmacotoxicology studies, *Xenobiotica* 43:63–72, 2013.

Moya M, Tran D, George SC: An integrated in vitro model of perfused tumor and cardiac tissue, *Stem Cell Res Ther* 4(Suppl 1):S15, 2013a.

Mouche I, Malesic L, Gillardeaux O: FETAX assay for evaluation of developmental toxicity, *Methods Mol Biol* 1641:311–324, 2017.

Moya ML, Hsu YH, Lee AP, et al.: In vitro perfused human capillary networks, *Tissue Eng C Methods* 19:730–737, 2013b.

Murphy SV, Atala A: 3D bioprinting of tissues and organs, *Nat Biotechnol* 32:773–785, 2014.

Musah S, Dimitrakakis N, Camacho DM, et al.: Directed differentiation of human induced pluripotent stem cells into mature kidney podocytes and establishment of a glomerulus chip, *Nat Protoc* 13:1662–1685, 2018.

Nagarajan P, Mahesh Kumar MJ, Venkatesan R, et al.: Genetically modified mouse models for the study of nonalcoholic fatty liver disease, *World J Gastroenterol* 18:1141–1153, 2012.

Natale A, Vanmol K, Arslan A, et al.: Technological advancements for the development of stem cell-based models for hepatotoxicity testing, *Arch Toxicol* 93:1789–1805, 2019.

Nelakanti RV, Kooreman NG, Wu JC: Teratoma formation: a tool for monitoring pluripotency in stem cell research, *Curr Protoc Stem Cell Biol* 32, 2015, 4A 8 1–4A 8 17.

Norotte C, Marga FS, Niklason LE, et al.: Scaffold-free vascular tissue engineering using bioprinting, *Biomaterials* 30:5910–5917, 2009.

NRC (U.S. National Research Council): *Toxicity testing in the 21st century: a vision and a strategy*, Washington, DC, 2007, The National Academies Press.

NTP (U.S. National Toxicology Program): *NTP research report on national toxicology program approach to genomic dose response modeling*, National Toxicology Program.

OECD: *Guidance on grouping of chemicals*, Paris, France, 2014, OECD Publishing.

Oh SY, Choi YM, Kim HY, et al.: Application of tonsil-derived mesenchymal stem cells in tissue regeneration: concise review, *Stem Cell* 37:1252–1260, 2019.

Okamoto T, Suzuki T, Yamamoto N: Microarray fabrication with covalent attachment of DNA using bubble jet technology, *Nat Biotechnol* 18:438–441, 2000.

Ou DB, Zeng D, Jin Y, et al.: The long-term differentiation of embryonic stem cells into cardiomyocytes: an indirect co-culture model, *PloS One* 8:e55233, 2013.

Ouyang L, Yao R, Mao S, et al.: Three-dimensional bioprinting of embryonic stem cells directs highly uniform embryoid body formation, *Biofabrication* 7:044101, 2015.

Padilla S, Cowden J, Hinton DE, et al.: Use of medaka in toxicity testing, *Curr Protoc Toxicol*, 2009. Chapter 1: Unit 1.10.

Palazzi X, Burkhardt JE, Caplain H, et al.: Characterizing "adversity" of pathology findings in nonclinical toxicity studies: results from the 4th ESTP international expert workshop, *Toxicol Pathol* 44:810–824, 2016.

Palma E, Doornebal EJ, Chokshi S: Precision-cut liver slices: a versatile tool to advance liver research, *Hepatol Int* 13:51–57, 2019.

Pamies D, Bal-Price A, Chesne C, et al.: Advanced good cell culture practice for human primary, stem cell-derived and organoid models as well as microphysiological systems, *ALTEX* 35:353–378, 2018.

Pan C, Kumar C, Bohl S, et al.: Comparative proteomic phenotyping of cell lines and primary cells to assess preservation of cell type-specific functions, *Mol Cell Proteomics* 8:443–450, 2009.

Park JW, Vahidi B, Taylor AM, et al.: Microfluidic culture platform for neuroscience research, *Nat Protoc* 1:2128–2136, 2006.

Park JY, Kim SK, Woo DH, et al.: Differentiation of neural progenitor cells in a microfluidic chip-generated cytokine gradient, *Stem Cell* 27:2646–2654, 2009.

Parrish AR, Gandolfi AJ, Brendel K: Precision-cut tissue slices: applications in pharmacology and toxicology, *Life Sci* 57:1887–1901, 1995.

Passamai VE, Dernowsek JA, Nogueira J, et al.: From 3D boprinters to a fully integrated organ biofabrication line, *J Phys* 705, 2016.

Pastor DM, Poritz LS, Olson TL, et al.: Primary cell lines: false representation or model system? a comparison of four human colorectal tumors and their coordinately established cell lines, *Int J Clin Exp Med* 3:69–83, 2010.

Patlewicz G, Lizarraga LE, Rua D, et al.: Exploring current read-across applications and needs among selected U.S. Federal Agencies, *Regul Toxicol Pharmacol* 106:197–209, 2019.

Peerani R, Bauwens CL, Kumacheva E, et al.: Patterning mouse and human embryonic stem cells using microcontact printing. In Audet JSWL, editor: *Stem cells in regenerative medicine methods in molecular biology*, Humana Press.

Peltola SM, Melchels FP, Grijpma DW, et al.: A review of rapid prototyping techniques for tissue engineering purposes, *Ann Med* 40:268–280, 2008.

Peng W, Unutmaz D, Ozbolat IT: Bioprinting towards physiologically relevant tissue models for pharmaceutics, *Trends Biotechnol* 34:722–732, 2016.

Peterson EK, Long HE: Experimental protocol for using Drosophila as an invertebrate model system for toxicity testing in the baboratory, *J Vis Exp*, 2018, https://doi.org/10.3791/57450. Accessed 25 April 2021.

Petrosyan A, Cravedi P, Villani V, et al.: A glomerulus-on-a-chip to recapitulate the human glomerular filtration barrier, *Nat Commun* 10:3656, 2019.

Pettinato G, Wen X, Zhang N: formation of well-defined embryoid bodies from dissociated human induced pluripotent stem cells using microfabricated cell-repellent microwell Arrays, *Sci Rep* 4:7402–7412, 2014.

Piersma AH, Genschow E, Verhoef A, et al.: Validation of the postimplantation rat whole-embryo culture test in the international ECVAM validation study on three in vitro embryotoxicity tests, *Altern Lab Anim* 32:275–307, 2004.

Piersma AH, Janer G, Wolterink G, et al.: Quantitative extrapolation of in vitro whole embryo culture embryotoxicity data to developmental toxicity in vivo using the benchmark dose approach, *Toxicol Sci* 101:91–100, 2008.

Pollesch NL, Villeneuve DL, O'Brien JM: Extracting and benchmarking emerging adverse outcome pathway knowledge, *Toxicol Sci* 168:349–364, 2019.

Pratten M, Ahir BK, Smith-Hurst H, et al.: Primary cell and micromass culture in assessing developmental toxicity, *Methods Mol Biol* 889:115–146, 2012.

Prendergast ME, Monoya G, Pereira T, et al.: Microphysiological systems: automated fabrication via extrusion bioprinting, *Microphysiol Syst* 2:1–16, 2018.

Pridgeon CS, Schlott C, Wong MW, et al.: Innovative organotypic in vitro models for safety assessment: aligning with regulatory requirements and understanding models of the heart, skin, and liver as paradigms, *Arch Toxicol* 92:556–557, 2018.

Prior H, Sewell F, Stewart J: Overview of 3Rs opportunities in drug discovery and developmentusing non-human primates, *Drug Discov Today: Disease Models* 23:11–16, 2017.

Qi C, Zhou Q, Li B, et al.: Glipizide, an antidiabetic drug, suppresses tumor growth and metastasis by inhibiting angiogenesis, *Oncotarget* 5:9966–9979, 2014.

Ramachandran SD, Schirmer K, Munst B, et al.: In vitro generation of functional liver organoid-like structures using adult human cells, *PloS One* 10:e0139345, 2015.

Rao MS, Gupta R, Liguori MJ, et al.: Novel computational approach to predict off-target interactions for small molecules, *Front Big Data* 2, 2019.

Reddy MV, Sistare FD, Christensen JS, et al.: An evaluation of chronic 6- and 12-month rat toxicology studies as predictors of 2-year tumor outcome, *Vet Pathol* 47:614–629, 2010.

Reid JA, Mollica PA, Johnson GD, et al.: Accessible bioprinting: adaptation of a low-cost 3D-printer for precise cell placement and stem cell differentiation, *Biofabrication* 8:025017, 2016.

Ribatti D: The chick embryo chorioallantoic membrane (CAM) assay, *Reprod Toxicol* 70:97–101, 2017.

Ringeisen BR, Kim H, Barron JA, et al.: Laser printing of pluripotent embryonal carcinoma cells, *Tissue Eng* 10:483–491, 2004.

Risau W, Sariola H, Zerwes HG, et al.: Vasculogenesis and angiogenesis in embryonic-stem-cell-derived embryoid bodies, *Development* 102:471–478, 1988.

Roguet R: Use of skin cell cultures for in vitro assessment of corrosion and cutaneous irritancy, *Cell Biol Toxicol* 15:63–75, 1999.

Rylova SN, Randhawa PK, Bautch VL: In vitro differentiation of mouse embryonic stem cells into primitive blood vessels, *Methods Enzymol* 443:103–117, 2008.

Sachinidis A, Albrecht W, Nell P, et al.: Road map for development of stem cell-based alternative test methods, *Trends Mol Med* 25:470–481, 2019.

Sanz F, Pognan F, Steger-Hartmann T, et al.: Legacy data sharing to improve drug safety assessment: the eTOX project, *Nat Rev Drug Discov* 16:811–812, 2017.

Sato T, Stange DE, Ferrante M, et al.: Long-term expansion of epithelial organoids from human colon, adenoma, adenocarcinoma, and Barrett's epithelium, *Gastroenterology* 141:1762–1772, 2011.

Sauer UG, Deferme L, Gribaldo L, et al.: The challenge of the application of 'omics technologies in chemicals risk assessment: Background and outlook, *Regul Toxicol Pharmacol* 91(Suppl 1):S14–S26, 2017.

Saunders RE, Gough JE, Derby B: Delivery of human fibroblast cells by piezoelectric drop-on-demand inkjet printing, *Biomaterials* 29:193–203, 2008.

Schiffelers M-JWA, Blaauboer BJ, Hendriksen CFM, Bakker WE: Regulatory acceptance and use of 3R models: a multilevel perspective, *ALTEX* 27:287–300, 2012.

Schildknecht S, Karreman C, Poltl D, et al.: Generation of genetically-modified human differentiated cells for toxicological tests and the study of neurodegenerative diseases, *ALTEX* 30:427–444, 2013.

Schukur L, Zorlutuna P, Cha JM, et al.: Directed differnetiation of size-controlled embryoid bodies towards endothelial and cardiac lineages in RGD-modiefied poly (ethylene glycol) hydrogels, *Adv Health* 2:195–205, 2013.

Schwank G, Koo BK, Sasselli V, et al.: Functional repair of CFTR by CRISPR/Cas9 in intestinal stem cell organoids of cystic fibrosis patients, *Cell Stem Cell* 13:653–658, 2013.

Schwartz MP, Hou Z, Propson NE, et al.: Human pluripotent stem cell-derived neural constructs for predicting neural toxicity, *Proc Natl Acad Sci U S A* 112:12516–12521, 2015.

Scott CW, Peters MF, Dragan YP: Human induced pluripotent stem cells and their use in drug discovery for toxicity testing, *Toxicol Lett* 219:49–58, 2013.

Sewald K, Braun A: Assessment of immunotoxicity using precision-cut tissue slices, *Xenobiotica* 43:84–97, 2013.

Sewell F, Edwards J, Prior H, Robinson S: Opportunities to apply the 3Rs in safety assessment programs, *ILAR J* 57: 234–245, 2016.

Shakibaei M, Schroter-Kermani C, Merker HJ: Matrix changes during long-term cultivation of cartilage (organoid or high-density cultures), *Histol Histopathol* 8:463–470, 1993.

Shen H, McHale CM, Smith MT, et al.: Functional genomic screening approaches in mechanistic toxicology and potential future applications of CRISPR-Cas9, *Mutat Res Rev Mutat Res* 764:31–42, 2015.

Sheng F, Chen M, Tan Y, et al.: Protective effects of otophylloside N on pentylenetetrazol-induced neuronal injury in vitro and in vivo, *Front Pharmacol* 7:224, 2016.

Shin W, Hinojosa CD, Ingber DE, et al.: Human intestinal morphogenesis controlled by transepithelial morphogen gradient and flow-dependent physical cues in a micro-engineered gut-on-a-chip, *iScience* 15:391–406, 2019.

Sipes NS, Padilla S, Knudsen TB: Zebrafish: as an integrative model for twenty-first century toxicity testing, *Birth Defects Res C Embryo Today* 93:256–267, 2011.

Sistare FD, Morton D, Alden C, et al.: An analysis of pharmaceutical experience with decades of rat carcinogenicity testing: support for a proposal to modify current regulatory guidelines, *Toxicol Pathol* 39:716–744, 2011.

Smith CM, Stone AL, Parkhill RL, et al.: Three-dimensional bioassembly tool for generating viable tissue-engineered constructs, *Tissue Eng* 10:1566–1576, 2004.

Spence JR, Mayhew CN, Rankin SA, et al.: Directed differentiation of human pluripotent stem cells into intestinal tissue in vitro, *Nature* 470:105–109, 2011.

Stanton MM, Samitier J, Sanchez S: Bioprinting of 3D hydrogels, *Lab Chip* 15:3111–3115, 2015.

Steer DL, Nigam SK: Developmental approaches to kidney tissue engineering, *Am J Physiol Ren Physiol* 286:F1–F7, 2004.

Sultan A, Singh J, Howarth FC: Mechanisms underlying electro-mechanical dysfunction in the Zucker diabetic fatty rat heart: a model of obesity and type 2 diabetes, *Heart Fail Rev*, 2019.

Swift B, Pfeifer ND, Brouwer KL: Sandwich-cultured hepatocytes: an in vitro model to evaluate hepatobiliary transporter-based drug interactions and hepatotoxicity, *Drug Metab Rev* 42:446–471, 2010.

Szabo G, Bala S: Alcoholic liver disease and the gut-liver axis, *World J Gastroenterol* 16:1321–1329, 2010.

Takahashi K, Yamanaka S: Induction of pluripotent stem cells from mouse embryonic and adult fibroblast cultures by defined factors, *Cell* 126:663–676, 2006.

Takahashi M, Osumi N: The method of rodent whole embryo culture using the rotator-type bottle culture system, *J Vis Exp* 42:2170, 2010.

Takasato M, Er PX, Chiu HS, et al.: Generation of kidney organoids from human pluripotent stem cells, *Nat Protoc* 11:1681–1692, 2016a.

Takasato M, Er PX, Chiu HS, et al.: Kidney organoids from human iPS cells contain multiple lineages and model human nephrogenesis, *Nature* 536:238, 2016b.

Takasato M, Little MH: A strategy for generating kidney organoids: recapitulating the development in human pluripotent stem cells, *Dev Biol* 420:210–220, 2016.

Takebe T, Sekine K, Enomura M, et al.: Vascularized and functional human liver from an iPSC-derived organ bud transplant, *Nature* 499:481–484, 2013.

Thomas RS, Bahadori T, Buckley TJ, et al.: The next generation blueprint of computational toxicology at the U.S. Environmental Protection Agency, *Toxicol Sci* 169:317–332, 2019.

Titus SA, Li X, Southall N, et al.: A cell-based PDE4 assay in 1536-well plate format for high-throughput screening, *J Biomol Screen* 13:609–618, 2008.

Todhunter ME, Jee NY, Hughes AJ, et al.: Programmed synthesis of three-dimensional tissues, *Nat Methods* 12:975–981, 2015.

Truskey GA: Human microphysiological systems and organoids as in vitro models for toxicological studies, *Front Public Health* 6:185, 2018.

Tsamandouras N, Chen WLK, Edington CD, et al.: Integrated gut and liver microphysiological systems for quantitative in vitro pharmacokinetic studies, *AAPS J* 19:1499–1512, 2017a.

Tsamandouras N, Kostrzewski T, Stokes CL, et al.: Quantitative assessment of population variability in hepatic drug metabolism using a perfused three-dimensional human liver microphysiological system, *J Pharmacol Exp Therapeut* 360:95–105, 2017b.

Tung EWY, Winn LM: Mouse whole embryo culture, *Methods Mol Biol* 1965:187–194, 2019.

Turner OC, Aeffner F, Bangari DS, et al.: Society of toxicologic pathology digital pathology and image analysis special interest group article*: opinion on the application of artificial intelligence and machine learning to digital toxicologic pathology, *Toxicol Pathol* 48:277–294, 2020.

Ulrich RG, Bacon JA, Cramer CT, et al.: Cultured hepatocytes as investigational models for hepatic toxicity: practical applications in drug discovery and development, *Toxicol Lett* 82–83:107–115, 1995.

Ungrin MD, Clarke G, Yin T, et al.: Rational bioprocess design for human pluripotent stem cell expansion and endoderm differentiation based on cellular dynamics, *Biotechnol Bioeng* 109:853–866, 2012.

Uzel SG, Pavesi A, Kamm RD: Microfabrication and microfluidics for muscle tissue models, *Prog Biophys Mol Biol* 115:279–293, 2014.

van de Wetering M, Francies HE, Francis JM, et al.: Prospective derivation of a living organoid biobank of colorectal cancer patients, *Cell* 161:933–945, 2015.

van Geer MA, Kuhlmann KF, Bakker CT, et al.: Ex-vivo evaluation of gene therapy vectors in human pancreatic (cancer) tissue slices, *World J Gastroenterol* 15:1359–1366, 2009.

Van Vleet TR, Liguori MJ, Lynch 3rd JJ, et al.: Screening strategies and methods for better off-target liability prediction and identification of small-molecule pharmaceuticals, *SLAS Discov* 24(1):1–24, 2019.

Vo AH, Van Vleet TR, Gupta RR, et al.: An overview of machine learning and big data for drug toxicity evaluation, *Chem Res Toxicol* 33:20–37, 2020.

Wang R, Clark R, Bautch VL: Embryonic stem cell-derived cystic embryoid bodies form vascular channels: an in vitro model of blood vessel development, *Development* 114:303–316, 1992.

Wang X, Cao C, Huang J, et al.: One-step generation of triple gene-targeted pigs using CRISPR/Cas9 system, *Sci Rep* 6:20620, 2016.

Wang Z, Lee SJ, Cheng HJ, et al.: 3D bioprinted functional and contractile cardiac tissue constructs, *Acta Biomater* 70:48–56, 2018.

Wang Z, Wang SN, Xu TY, et al.: Organoid technology for brain and therapeutics research, *CNS Neurosci Ther* 23:771–778, 2017.

Watford S, Ly Pham L, Wignall J, et al.: ToxRefDB version 2.0: improved utility for predictive and retrospective toxicology analyses, *Reprod Toxicol* 89:145–158, 2019.

Weaver J R, Valentin JP: Today's challenges to de-risk and predict drug safety in human "Mind-the-Gap", *Toxicol Sci* 167:307–321, 2019.

Webster WS, Brown-Woodman PD, Ritchie HE: A review of the contribution of whole embryo culture to the determination of hazard and risk in teratogenicity testing, *Int J Dev Biol* 41:329–335, 1997.

Weitzer G: Embryonic stem cell-derived embryoid bodies: an in vitro model of eutherian pregastrulation development and early gastrulation, *Handb Exp Pharmacol*, 2006:21–51, 2006.

Westra IM, Mutsaers HA, Luangmonkong T, et al.: Human precision-cut liver slices as a model to test antifibrotic drugs in the early onset of liver fibrosis, *Toxicol In Vitro* 35:77–85, 2016.

Wheeler SE, Clark AM, Taylor DP, et al.: Spontaneous dormancy of metastatic breast cancer cells in an all human liver microphysiologic system, *Br J Cancer* 111:2342–2350, 2014.

Wheeler A: *Directive to prioritize efforts to reduce animal testing [at EPA].* https://www.epa.gov/sites/production/files/2019-09/documents/image2019-09-09-231249.pdf. Published 2019. (Accessed 25 April 2021).

Wikswo JP: The relevance and potential roles of microphysiological systems in biology and medicine, *Exp Biol Med* 239:1061–1072, 2014.

Wu Z, Liu Q, Wang L, et al.: The essential role of CYP2E1 in metabolism and hepatotoxicity of N,N-dimethylformamide using a novel Cyp2e1 knockout mouse model and a population study, *Arch Toxicol* 93:3169–3181, 2019.

Xu F, Celli J, Rizvi I, et al.: A three-dimensional in vitro ovarian cancer coculture model using a high-throughput cell patterning platform, *Biotechnol J* 6:204–212, 2011.

Xu H, Lyu X, Yi M, et al.: Organoid technology and applications in cancer research, *J Hematol Oncol* 11:116, 2018.

Xu T, Gregory CA, Molnar P, et al.: Viability and electrophysiology of neural cell structures generated by the inkjet printing method, *Biomaterials* 27:3580–3588, 2006.

Xu T, Jin J, Gregory C, et al.: Inkjet printing of viable mammalian cells, *Biomaterials* 26:93–99, 2005.

Yang H, Lou C, Li W, et al.: Computational approaches to identify structural alerts and their applications in environmental toxicology and drug discovery, *Chem Res Toxicol* 33(6):1312–1322, 2020.

Yang Q, Lian Q, Xu F: Perspective: fabrication of integrated organ-on-a-chip via bioprinting, *Biomicrofluidics* 11:031301, 2017.

Yin X, Mead BE, Safaee H, et al.: Engineering stem cell organoids, *Cell Stem Cell* 18:25–38, 2016.

Yu Y, Moncal KK, Li J, et al.: Three-dimensional bioprinting using self-assembling scalable scaffold-free "tissue strands" as a new bioink, *Sci Rep* 6:28714, 2016.

Zambrowicz BP, Sands AT: Knockouts model the 100 best-selling drugs - will they model the next 100? *Nature Rev Drug Disc* 2:38–51, 2003.

Zbinden G: Reduction and replacement of laboratory animals in toxicological testing and research. Interim report 1984–1987, *Biomed Environ Sci* 1:90–100, 1988.

Zhang X, Zhang Y: Tissue engineering applications of three-dimensional bioprinting, *Cell Biochem Biophys* 72:777–782, 2015.

Zhou M, Zhang X, Wen X, et al.: Development of a functional glomerulus at the organ level on a chip to mimic hypertensive nephropathy, *Sci Rep* 6:31771, 2016.

Zou Q, Wang X, Liu Y, et al.: Generation of gene-target dogs using CRISPR/Cas9 system, *J Mol Cell Biol* 7:580–583, 2015.

PART 4

PRACTICE OF TOXICOLOGIC PATHOLOGY

Nomenclature and Diagnostic Resources in Anatomic Toxicologic Pathology

Cynthia J. Willson[1], Charlotte M. Keenan[2], Mark F. Cesta[3], Deepa B. Rao[4]

[1]Integrated Laboratory Systems, LLC, Cary, Morrisville, NC, United States, [2]C.M. Keenan ToxPath Consulting, Doylestown, PA, United States, [3]U.S. National Institute of Environmental Health Sciences, Research Triangle Park, NC, United States, [4]StageBio, Frederick, MD, United States

O U T L I N E

1. Introduction	969	5.3. Diagnostic Drift	978
2. The Need for Standardized Nomenclature	970	5.4. Severity Grading	978
		5.5. Lesion Complexity	978
3. Components in Nomenclature	971	5.6. Multiple Pathologists	979
3.1. Terminology for Nonneoplastic Lesions	971	5.7. The Pathology Narrative	979
3.2. Terminology for Neoplastic Lesions	972	6. Harmonization of Nomenclature	980
4. Challenges in Standardizing Nomenclature	973	6.1. International Harmonization of Nomenclature and Diagnostic Criteria	980
4.1. Training	973	6.2. Standard for Exchange of Nonclinical Data	982
4.2. Thresholds	974	6.3. National Toxicology Program Nonneoplastic Lesion Atlas	983
4.3. Diagnostic Drift	975	6.4. Other Nomenclature Resources	983
4.4. Severity Grading	975		
4.5. Lesion Complexity	976	7. Conclusions	983
4.6. Multiple Pathologists	976	References	984
5. Recommended Practices	977		
5.1. Training	977		
5.2. Thresholds	977		

1. INTRODUCTION

In general nonclinical toxicology studies conducted for hazard evaluation and/or safety assessment, toxicologic pathologists document nonneoplastic and neoplastic morphological changes from laboratory animals to identify potential treatment-related effects of a test article (see Sahota et al. (2019); *Pathology in Nonclinical Safety*, Vol 2, Chap 4). The primary means of communicating such morphological changes is through a system of nomenclature, i.e., the terminology of diagnoses. Such terminology of diagnoses is often amenable to statistical analysis (especially for neoplasms), which is a necessary requirement in carcinogenicity assessments (see *Experimental Design and Statistical Analysis for Toxicologic Pathologists*, Vol 1, Chap 16 and *Carcinogenicity Assessment*, Vol 2, Chap 5). Since histopathological diagnoses are primarily based on subjective observations, terminology used to classify morphological changes must be standardized so that valid analysis and interpretation of data derived from nonclinical toxicology studies can be made.

Many factors can affect the application of specific diagnostic terms to morphological changes by pathologists, and such factors can contribute to the inconsistencies observed within and between toxicological studies. This chapter reviews the factors and challenges that commonly affect terminology usage in toxicologic pathology and proposes recommended practices to help minimize common challenges. Efforts undertaken to harmonize nomenclature worldwide include the Standards for Exchange of Nonclinical Data (SEND), International Harmonization of Nomenclature and Diagnostic Criteria for Lesions in Rats and Mice (INHAND), National Toxicology Program (NTP) Nonneoplastic Lesion Atlas (NNLA), and global open Registry Nomenclature Information System (goRENI).

2. THE NEED FOR STANDARDIZED NOMENCLATURE

In toxicologic pathology, the pathologist wears two hats: the diagnostic pathologist (morphological diagnosis) and the scientist (generating data). Due to inherent complexities of evaluating histopathological changes, the training and experience of the toxicologic pathologist is of primary importance, because the diagnoses provided by the pathologist are the substrate for statistical analyses. Regulatory authorities often require statistical inferences of the relationship of adverse morphological changes, toxicity, or carcinogenicity with a test article. These adverse morphological changes are often presented as a morphological diagnosis, e.g., hepatocellular carcinoma. Such morphological diagnoses (variables) must be independent to comply with the assumptions required for valid statistical analysis and inferences drawn with respect to the morphological changes and the treatment.

Standardized nomenclature is essential not only to communicate results to other colleagues but also to ensure the independence of the named variable. Standardized nomenclature should aim to provide categories that are mutually exclusive (i.e., only those morphological diagnoses placed in a specific diagnosis category, e.g., hepatocellular carcinoma) as well as mutually exhaustive, such that all cases of the category in question are included (e.g., all cases of hepatocellular carcinoma are within the named category) (see *Experimental Design and Statistical Analysis for Toxicologic Pathologists*, Vol 1, Chap 16).

When separate categories are generated from overlapping diagnostic criteria, the toxicologic pathologist should determine which categories are relevant to the study at hand before subjecting diagnoses to statistical testing. Conducting statistical tests across multiple correlated categories can lead to increased false positive rates. Subset relations between different diagnoses also challenge the independence assumption of statistical testing and further complicate the interpretation of the results. The toxicologic pathologist must be well trained and experienced in order to select the categories best suited to the scientific goals of the investigation.

Reproducibility is a growing concern in scientific research and is indispensable to regulatory practices that must compare results across studies. Nomenclature may be updated to accommodate the expansion of knowledge. However, such revisions should only be done when necessary, since even small modifications in nomenclature may complicate data management as well as the interpretation and reporting of results. Moreover, the diverse interests and focus areas of various laboratories often produce inconsistent diagnostic criteria and terminology. Basing diagnoses on published and accepted nomenclature standards will mitigate observer bias and promote consistency and objectivity in toxicology studies. The previous lack of a universally accepted and standardized system of nomenclature within toxicologic pathology has, in the past, resulted in inconsistent terminology, controversy, additional costs, and/or delays in the product review and approval by regulatory authorities. Under such circumstances, regulators are unable to evaluate the dose–response effects, and the statistical analyses from such data may violate assumptions of the test. Moreover, inaccuracies or inconsistencies in the diagnostic terminology used for morphological changes impact safety assessment and/or hazard identification, and ultimately risk assessment (see *Risk Assessment*, Vol 2, Chap 16). Diagnostic terminology should therefore be precise, reliable, consistent, and convey a clear picture of the important morphological changes to facilitate unambiguous interpretation of the pathological effects of chemicals, drugs, biologics, and/or medical devices, as well as to aid in understanding underlying mechanisms of toxicity.

3. COMPONENTS IN NOMENCLATURE

In toxicologic pathology, the morphologic diagnosis is the foundation of data collection (see *Pathology and GLPs, Quality Control and Quality Assurance*, Vol 1, Chap 27). The approach to making a morphological diagnosis is hierarchical, resulting in flexibility and variation in the range of diagnostic terminology used. Essentially, a morphologic diagnosis is made by sequentially designating the topography first (organ/tissue affected), with or without a subsite modifier, followed by a single morphological diagnosis (predominant pathological change or type of lesion), followed, where applicable, by descriptive qualifier(s) that include duration, distribution, and/or severity. Topographic designations may include as many as three hierarchical terms: (1) organ, (2) site within an organ, and, if necessary, (3) a subset of increasing specificity within sites. An example would be "brain, cerebral cortex, cingulate." Morphological diagnoses are used to describe the major pathological processes or abnormalities occurring in an organ or tissue (neoplastic or nonneoplastic). Although both nonneoplastic and neoplastic lesions may have site modifiers, most types of qualifiers (e.g., duration, distribution, and severity) are predominantly used for nonneoplastic lesions. Further, each diagnosis typically allows the inclusion of a comment to capture the intricacies of a specific lesion.

3.1. Terminology for Nonneoplastic Lesions

For nonneoplastic lesions, morphologic changes often allow the use of qualifiers that specify important characteristics of the morphological disease process (e.g., distribution, severity, and duration) to effectively convey additional information about morphologic changes. For example, "liver, infiltrate, mononuclear cells, focal, moderate" allow some degree of perspective on the distribution and severity of the morphological change noted. It should be noted that each category of qualifiers typically has a large pool of potential terms lending several possible permutations and combinations available for the capture of the final diagnosis. For example, the qualifier for distribution may include such terms as focal, multifocal, locally extensive, or diffuse.

Organ-specific site qualifiers should be used to delineate lesions based on different regional anatomical differences, tissue-specific responses, or biological significance. The choice of site qualifiers can vary with the anatomic complexity of an organ or tissue and the prevalence of treatment-related effects in an organ. For example, at different "levels" along its length, the nasal cavity is lined by squamous, transitional, respiratory, or olfactory surface epithelia. The response(s) of these epithelia to inhaled toxicants may differ by location, and the use of a site qualifier helps characterize site-specific effects. Likewise, chemically induced lesions in the larynx often have site specificity at the base of the epiglottis; thus, the designation "larynx, epiglottis" is appropriate. Other possible examples of site qualifiers include "liver, bile duct"; "nerve, sciatic"; and "kidney, renal tubule." Alternatively, in some situations, it may be best to refrain from using site qualifiers. As an example, for inflammation in hollow organs or tissues that have surface epithelia (e.g., the nose, stomach, gastrointestinal tract, or urinary bladder), the use of qualifiers that indicate specific sites (e.g., lumen, epithelium, mucosa, submucosa) may not be appropriate, because the presence of small numbers of inflammatory cells around organs associated with points of entry and/or external environment is generally considered to be within normal limits and has no biological relevance. Therefore, unless a site-specific toxicity is suspected, in such instances, characterization of a background lesion is unnecessary, and designating the overall severity of inflammation may be best used to convey differences in lesion distribution.

Distribution qualifiers are used to indicate the pattern of an effect (e.g., diffuse, locally extensive, multifocal, or focal). However, focal and multifocal qualifiers may also be addressed by the severity grade. Distribution modifiers can provide additional site specificity and indicate an inherent feature of a lesion that has a particular biological significance or reflects a specific pathogenesis. For example, centrilobular hepatic necrosis rarely has the same pathogenesis as multifocal, randomly distributed hepatic necrosis; therefore, it is important to include these types of distribution modifiers. Likewise, it may be toxicologically relevant to the interpretation of a study to know whether hyperplasia of the forestomach is focal versus diffuse. However, the use of distribution qualifiers is usually not warranted for common background, spontaneous, and/or age-related lesions specific for certain species and strains, unless an exacerbation of such lesions is suspected. Because the objective of the pathologist is to identify test article–related effects, such common background, spontaneous, and/or age-related findings may typically be cited via references in the pathology report. Severity grading of common background lesions is particularly relevant when such lesions are dose response related, where grading may be the most reliable means of effectively documenting differences between test groups and controls and among test groups, i.e., dose response. For example, certain classes of chemicals can potentiate chronic progressive nephropathy (CPN) as well as alpha$_{2u}$-globulin nephropathy in male rats. In such cases, assigning severity grades can provide important information.

Although distribution qualifiers depict the pattern of a lesion with additional specificity, the intensity or magnitude of the lesion is reflected by the use of severity grades. Severity grading is the designation of a semiquantitative score to a lesion or process (e.g., often a four- or five-point scale, depending on the software program used for data entry). It is used to reflect a combination of the amount and distribution of tissue involvement, as well as the actual degree of tissue damage. Typically, these include minimal (1), mild (2), moderate (3), and marked (4), and if a five-point scale is used, severe (5). Regardless of whether a four- or five-point scale is used, general criteria used to define each grade

should be included in the pathology report. Severity grading of nonneoplastic lesions can provide useful dose–response information in that a test article may alter incidence of a lesion or its severity, or both. Severity grades are continuous rather than discrete data representing degrees of changes relative to similar lesions in controls and other animals in a study, and thresholds for grading often vary between individual pathologists and or study types.

Severity grading (ordinal data) is reserved for nonneoplastic lesions, whereas neoplasms are considered either present or not present (nominal [diagnosis] or quantal [malignant vs. benign] data). Severity grading adds little valuable information in some nonneoplastic lesions. Examples include calculus in the urinary tract or cysts of the pituitary *pars distalis*. Severity grades are most useful when making comparisons of qualitative changes, for example, when average severity increases with increasing dose, or when comparing the relative toxicity of structurally related compounds. The generation of data allows statistical analysis and, in some instances, may be the only indication of treatment-related differences among test groups.

Duration qualifiers are more commonly used in association with particular types of inflammatory changes. The commonly used notation of "-itis" in diagnostic pathology is discouraged in toxicologic pathology and replaced with more descriptive terminology. Commonly used duration qualifiers include acute (neutrophils), subacute (lymphocytes), chronic (macrophages or mononuclear cells with or without fibrosis), and chronic active (a mixture of macrophages or mononuclear cells and neutrophils). In histopathological evaluation of toxicological studies, it is recommended to describe the cell type within the morphological description in the pathology narrative rather than duration qualifiers.

3.2. Terminology for Neoplastic Lesions

A few rules exist for the terminology applied to neoplasms. By convention, it is assumed that neoplasms not designated as metastatic are primary or arising at that site. For neoplasms in tissues distant from the primary site, the qualifier "metastatic" is added to the diagnosis, and the site of the primary lesion can be indicated parenthetically (e.g., "lung—hepatocellular carcinoma, metastatic (liver)"). For some neoplasms, the diagnosis should indicate whether the lesion is benign or malignant (e.g., "adrenal gland, medulla—pheochromocytoma, benign" and "adrenal gland, medulla—pheochromocytoma, malignant"). The occurrence of multiple and bilateral neoplasms should be indicated, especially when this occurrence appears to be a treatment-related phenomenon. Examples include "liver—hepatocellular adenoma, multiple" and "kidney, renal tubule—adenoma, bilateral."

Diagnoses for neoplasms should not contain site qualifiers unless such qualifiers serve to distinguish the histogenesis of one neoplasm from another. For example, the site qualifiers "C-cell" or "follicular cell" should be used to distinguish carcinomas of the thyroid gland.

Finally, inflammation and other types of secondary changes that may result from tissue damage associated with the presence of neoplasms (e.g., a histiocytic infiltrate in the alveoli associated with an alveolar bronchiolar carcinoma) are usually not meaningful to the study and therefore should not be recorded as separate diagnoses, but, if deemed important, they can be described in the narrative section of the pathology report (see *Preparation of the Anatomic Pathology Report for a Toxicity Study*, Vol 2, Chap 13).

4. CHALLENGES IN STANDARDIZING NOMENCLATURE

Histopathological evaluation of the tissues is one of the most resource-intensive phases of toxicity and carcinogenicity studies. Given that histopathology is a descriptive and interpretative science, the inherent complexity underlying a biological response compounded with the spectrum of subjectivity in determining selective diagnostic criteria between pathologists often underscores the lack of consistency in diagnoses within and between studies. No two pathologists independently evaluating the same study could be expected to arrive at identical findings for every tissue, organ, and animal. Factors influencing standardization of histopathological diagnoses include the training and experience level of the pathologist to select diagnostic criteria within

the spectrum of available terminology, thresholds, diagnostic drift, severity grading, lesion complexity, and involvement of multiple pathologists for a single test article. Moreover, in some pathology data collection systems, variations in the use of topographical, morphological, and/or qualifier designations may result in separate and distinct diagnosis categories when tabulated, thereby generating more than one morphologic diagnosis for the same lesion. For more information, see *Practices to Optimize Generation, Interpretation, and Reporting of Pathology Data from Toxicity Studies*, Vol 1, Chap 28.

4.1. Training

Most anatomic toxicologic pathologists are trained in a veterinary diagnostic pathology setting, usually at a college of veterinary medicine or, much less frequently, a medical college. The primary objective in diagnostic pathology is to identify the cause of disease or death for an individual animal and communicate the findings in a detailed fashion (i.e., each disease process is identified and recorded as a separate entity) to the veterinarian or clinician for that single case. In contrast to toxicologic pathology, consistency in morphologic diagnosis terminology across cases is not a major concern.

The emphasis in toxicologic pathology is on identifying changes in relation to a treatment group rather than in an individual animal—dose and response. Specifically, the goal of the toxicologic study pathologist is to determine if there are differences in the incidences and/or severities of lesions in treated groups compared to the control animals (positive and negative controls, where applicable) in order to provide dose–response data, and occasionally, where applicable, to delineate effects of test article from formulation. Study pathologists must identify the various lesions in tissues, but generally have less freedom than a veterinary or medical diagnostic pathologist in the type and number of diagnoses that they may record. For the study pathologist, it is especially important to use consistency and brevity in recording diagnoses in order to facilitate the statistical evaluation (e.g., carcinogenicity studies) and interpretation of the findings.

Diagnostic terminology is influenced by the training and experience in laboratory animal pathology that the toxicologic pathologist may have received. A histopathological diagnosis is primarily a qualitative judgment of the nature of a specific lesion and its apparent or expected biological behavior. Each diagnosis is a subjective observation, the accuracy of which depends on the pathologist's training and experience, the state of knowledge of the specific disease process, and the generally accepted diagnostic criteria and nomenclature within the profession.

The training, qualifications, and experience of the pathologist can influence how lesions are interpreted, and hence, the selection of diagnostic terminology. The majority of veterinary anatomic pathology training occurs in domestic and companion animal settings, with occasional exposure to the common background lesions of laboratory animals; trainees are less often exposed to toxicologic pathology. This may lead to selection of inappropriate terminology by pathologists with less experience evaluating rodent studies. Common issues encountered in evaluations by novice pathologists include the use of multiple morphological descriptive terms or synonyms for a lesion or disease process; inconsistencies in the designation of topography, sites, and subsites; and duplication of diagnoses, any of which may result in misinterpretation of toxicologic data.

Among experienced pathologists, nomenclature is still an issue. It is influenced by their training, as well as by individual and philosophical biases. One example includes terminology to describe inflammation composed primarily of mononuclear cells and fewer neutrophils. Some pathologists prefer the term "chronic active," while others prefer the term "chronic." Still others may use the term "cellular infiltrate" rather than "inflammation" with or without cell type modifiers.

Regardless of the chosen terminology, it is important for the study pathologist to identify such diagnostic differences and either resolve the difference, explain the reason for the use of alternate terminology in the pathology narrative, or state that the two different diagnoses reflect the same pathological process. Pathologists with experience evaluating rodents trained in a "basic" experimental research setting may be accustomed to nomenclature used for genetically engineered rodents, which may differ from that used in toxicologic pathology (Elmore et al., 2018).

Some customized Good Laboratory Practice–compliant computerized systems allow study pathologists to build a selective diagnostic vocabulary. For experienced and novice pathologists alike, the availability of a wide range of possible diagnostic terms can be a source of inconsistency due to overlapping criteria in defining subjective lesions, thus violating the assumptions for the statistical tests used. Additionally, multiple studies conducted with different pathology data capture systems for the same test article often generate nomenclature issues based on the differences in lexicon available within each data capture system. Often, this is mitigated by inclusion of a second-tier evaluation by a peer review pathologist. The peer review process allows the peer review pathologist to evaluate and compare diagnoses with the study pathologist, which results in better standardized nomenclature for the study (see *Pathology Peer Review*, Vol 1, Chap 26). Occasionally, unresolved diagnoses between the study and peer review pathologist are further examined by a Pathology Working Group (PWG) to reach a consensus. Such a process allows for consistency in diagnoses between pathologists and between studies for the same test article.

4.2. Thresholds

Training and/or experience of the pathologist can play a role in the applications of "thresholds" by individual pathologists from a diagnostic perspective. The use of "thresholds" should not be confused with use of this term by toxicologists as relevant in carcinogenicity risk assessment. Histopathology evaluation of subtle lesions poses problems when one pathologist considers a tissue to show variation within normal limits of the species/strain, while another pathologist considers the variation to be above the threshold and, therefore, a lesion. Such differences impede the dose–response assessment.

In general, there exists an inherent spontaneous biological variation in a given tissue that is expected for the species/strain, which may change with age. Pathologists use knowledge of this variation in species/strain, as well as incidence in concurrent control group animals (when appropriate), to ascertain diagnostic criteria to determine thresholds for selecting and differentiating diagnoses. Exacerbation may occur as increased incidences or severities or both. Some pathologists may choose to diagnose all changes considered to be background at the lowest severity grade, and any treatment-related changes with an increased severity grade (where applicable). Alternatively, a diagnosis may be made only when the level of variation is determined to be above a diagnostic "threshold" of the background finding when it exceeds that considered to be within normal limits. For example, peripheral nerve fiber degeneration is a common age-related finding in older rats (especially males). Because an actual treatment-related effect is not diagnostically different from background findings, an increase in severity across dose groups may be the only parameter that captures potential exacerbation at the nomenclature level. Therefore, such triggers during histopathological evaluation should spur reevaluation of the diagnostic threshold initially set for this finding to ensure that exacerbation of the background lesion due to treatment is indeed considered. Further, the pathologist must address this specific finding in the narrative within the context of what is known about background nerve fiber degeneration in rodents, potential differences between sexes, age (a one-month repeat-dose study vs. a carcinogenicity study), and other influencing factors.

4.3. Diagnostic Drift

Diagnostic drift is the phenomenon whereby variation in the application of diagnostic terminology or criteria and/or grading severity of the alteration changes during the temporal course of histopathological evaluation of a study. Essentially, diagnostic drift results when histopathological evaluation of tissues is performed over an extended time period or for a large number of animals. On finding a morphological change during the course of histopathological evaluation that is an abnormality and "new" to the study, any slide read after this recognition is evaluated with this novel knowledge; hence, those slides read in lower doses may have missed this new "knowledge" of a significant lesion. Maintaining consistency over an extended course of the histopathological evaluation within or between studies of the same test article can be a challenge since tissues for a study

are typically read in an animal-by-animal approach. Although an organ-by-organ approach allows for more consistency, the compromise is a lack of each animal's complete health status obtained by the typical animal-by-animal approach to slide reading. Regardless of the slide reading approach, terminology is subject to change given that histopathology evaluation is a dynamic and continuous process as the pathologist gains perspective across the full spectrum of treatment-related effects.

A common manifestation of diagnostic drift is the use of multiple terms or modifiers for similar lesions (for example, "heart, cardiomyopathy," and "heart, inflammation, chronic"). Diagnostic drift can result in the application of overlapping but slightly different diagnostic criteria to distinguish between closely related lesions, e.g., "hyperplasia" versus "adenoma," over the complete course of histopathological evaluation of a test article. The result of diagnostic drift is an inconsistent use of diagnostic terminology, which may falsely create or mask treatment-related effects between dose groups within a study, as well as between short-term and long-term studies.

4.4. Severity Grading

Severity grading for nonneoplastic lesions conveys important information for dose–response evaluation. Because severity grading represents ordinal data along a continuous spectrum, differences between grades are often borderline. It is not at all uncommon to note slight differences in grading between two pathologists, such as during peer review. As mentioned earlier, a four- or five-point scoring system of severity grading is commonly used to denote histopathological alterations across the continuous spectrum of changes. A description of the grading criteria for each grade should be included in the appendix or study narrative for, at least, the treatment-related lesions in the study. Criteria set for severity grades should be definable, reproducible to the extent possible, and interpretable, because undefined or overly generic criteria can lead to irreproducibility and different interpretations by regulatory reviewers.

It should be noted that not all morphological diagnoses require grading. For example, either a neoplasm is either present or absent (nominal data). Similarly, not all nonneoplastic lesions require a severity score. For example, for findings such as calculi, severity grading would add no useful information regarding the interpretation of the findings. Some findings (e.g., cysts) may be given a severity score by some institutions, but not others.

4.5. Lesion Complexity

Lesions often consist of a variety of morphological features, the complexity or composition of which may affect diagnostic terminology. In these cases, some pathologists may elect to diagnose each component of the lesion, referred to as "splitting." Others may elect to use a single general term to embrace the spectrum of changes present, referred to as "lumping." This decision is influenced by training, experience, or the objectives of a specific study. Excessive splitting of diagnoses may lead to inconsistency in diagnosis and obscuring treatment-related effects, via reducing the power of the experiment (see *Experimental Design and Statistical Analysis for Toxicologic Pathologists*, Vol 1, Chap 16).

A complex lesion that serves as an illustration is the spontaneous age-related renal disease that occurs in rats (see *Kidney*, Vol 4, Chap 3). Microscopic features include alterations of the renal tubular epithelium such as degeneration, regeneration, dilation, and the presence of protein casts, plus other components such as glomerulonephritis, glomerulosclerosis, interstitial fibrosis, basement membrane thickening, chronic inflammation, and mineralization. The histological appearance of the syndrome may vary among individual animals depending on the age of the animal and/or the degree of severity of disease. However, the vast majority of affected rats exhibit similar changes and disease progression. Thus, it has been suggested that the characteristic changes are classified under the single diagnosis of "CPN."

Diagnosing each element of nephropathy separately clutters the data, provides no additional useful information, and impedes statistical analysis and interpretation. In addition, the danger inherent in such a practice is diagnostic inconsistency. As a caveat, when using a single term such as CPN to cover a spectrum of changes, it is important to clearly define and characterize the term in the pathology narrative (see *Preparation of the Anatomic Pathology Report for a Toxicity Study*, Vol 2, Chap 13). As always, the pathology narrative should include a brief one to two sentence morphologic description for relevant treatment-related diagnoses.

4.6. Multiple Pathologists

Although every effort should be made to have one pathologist examine a single study or a series of related studies, often this is impractical. In drug development alone, animal toxicology studies span across several years differing in study type (e.g., acute studies, chronic studies, reproductive studies) or exposure route or species for the same test article.

For those studies with a long duration with interim, terminal, and recovery sacrifices, or studies with multiple target organs requiring specialized histopathology expertise (e.g., immunopathology, neuropathology, reproductive pathology) or specialized endpoints (e.g., electron microscopy, immunohistochemistry, stereology, morphometry), the primary study pathologist should be responsible for the overall histological evaluation. Subcontracted studies for specialized expertise typically designate the overseeing pathologist as the Principal Investigator for that specific endpoint evaluated.

There are a number of issues when results between different pathologists are compared or when similar lesions between species with different diagnoses are compared. These comparisons may be particularly problematic when the lesions are subtle or controversial or when there is disagreement as to the nature of the lesion(s) observed. For example, reactive or regenerative epithelial hyperplasia adjacent to treatment-induced ulceration or an area of inflammation may be recorded by one pathologist and ignored by another who considers it a component of the spectrum of lesions associated with and secondary to ulceration. With meaningful communication between pathologists, such differences for treatment-related lesions should be addressed in the overall pathology evaluation for a single study, hence the need for standardized nomenclature. Similarly, communication between pathologists and toxicologists is underscored for meaningful evaluation across all studies for the test article.

Experimental design considerations and early involvement of pathologists can alleviate this problem by simply ensuring that each pathologist looks at slides from across the treatment groups (e.g., for the study in question, each pathologist would evaluate the same number of tissues from each dose of the study).

5. RECOMMENDED PRACTICES

For more information, see *Practices to Optimize Generation, Interpretation, and Reporting of Pathology Data from Toxicity Studies*, Vol 1, Chap 28.

5.1. Training

Terminology problems originating from training may be addressed by adjusting the manner in which toxicologic pathologists are trained. Because toxicologic pathologists primarily receive training within diagnostic veterinary programs (although a few have additional graduate training in experimental pathology), training programs for toxicologic pathologists must include a solid foundation in the pathology of common laboratory animals (Bolon et al., 2010). Additionally, the knowledge of the principles of toxicology allows one to make the transition from diagnostic pathology of individual animals to toxicologic pathology that rests on treatment-related lesions within and across animal groups (Crissman et al., 2004). Ideally, from a pathology viewpoint, this includes knowledge of common tissue-specific responses to toxicants and the nature and distribution of common background and toxicant-induced lesions (Cesta et al., 2014; Maronpot et al., 1999; McInnes and Mann, 2011; Sahota et al., 2019; Suttie et al., 2017) and the terminology used in toxicological pathology (SEND, INHAND, goRENI). In addition, several journals (e.g., *Toxicologic Pathology, Journal of Toxicologic Pathology (Japan)*) have published multiple organ- and species-specific background lesions that serve as a resource for practicing toxicologic pathologists. From a toxicology viewpoint, coursework in basic principles of toxicology, pharmacokinetics, toxicokinetics (see *ADME Principles in Small Molecule Drug Discovery and Development—An Industrial Perspective*, Vol 1,

Chap 3, *Biotherapeutic ADME and PK/PD Principles*, Vol 1, Chap 4), toxicology testing (see *Basic Approaches to Anatomic Toxicologic Pathology*, Vol 1, Chap 9), experimental design in toxicity studies, and basic statistics (see *Experimental Design and Statistical Analysis for Toxicologic Pathologists*, Vol 1, Chap 16) should be included. The ability to deal effectively with many of the challenges discussed in Section 4 is in part related to the training and extent of the experience of individual pathologists evaluating toxicological studies.

For the novice pathologist entering toxicologic pathology from diagnostic or experimental pathology settings, histopathological evaluation should initially be performed in consultation with more experienced toxicologic pathologists. Familiarization with standardized terminology from harmonization efforts, described below, will be essential in training. Laboratories performing and evaluating toxicological studies should have procedures for comprehensive review and mentoring of trainee pathologists. Toxicologic pathologists should become familiar with guidance for pathology peer review from regulatory authorities (e.g., Food and Drug Administration [FDA] draft guidance, https://www.fda.gov/regulatory-information/search-fda-guidance-documents/pathology-peer-review-nonclinical-toxicology-studies-questions-and-answers) and practical, informal, and/or formal pathology peer review processes (Boorman et al., 2010; Fikes et al., 2015; Morton et al., 2010; Ward et al., 1995), including the role of PWGs to review unresolved differences in diagnoses arising from the peer review process (Mann and Hardisty, 2014). See *Pathology Peer Review*, Vol 1, Chap 26 for more information on pathology peer review and PWGs.

5.2. Thresholds

With experience, the toxicologic pathologist becomes familiar with the natural variation in tissues expected for species/strains used in toxicity studies. Examination of concurrent controls for a study is essential for determining which variations exceed the criteria for diagnostic "threshold" beyond those expected by normal variation to capture exacerbation by a test article. However, given inherent biological variation, there can be differences even in the control groups from one study to another. Therefore, determination of when a tissue exceeds normal limits must also be made based on experience or knowledge of the range of variation from other studies. This can be aided by the use of a collection of slides of tissues considered to be within historical control normal limits, as well as by knowledge of background lesions (Long and Hardisty, 2012; McInnes and Mann, 2011; Sahota et al., 2019).

5.3. Diagnostic Drift

The lapse in time between the initial histopathological examination of tissues from the control versus high-dose groups and subsequent examination of tissues from lower dose groups may be enough to allow minor differences in diagnostic and/or grading criteria for severity for a specific lesion. This diagnostic drift can be minimized. For example, the study pathologist may begin evaluation of the control group first followed by the high-dose group, then by the lower dose groups to facilitate identification of the full range of lesions. Alternatively, it is often helpful to examine a few animals from the control group and each dose group to determine the salient treatment effect(s). If possible, the various treatment groups can be evaluated in replicates of 5 or 10 starting with the controls and high-dose groups and subsequently, the mid- and low-dose groups. The overall goal is to facilitate consistent application of diagnostic terminology and criteria and to acquaint the pathologist with the range of lesion severity.

5.4. Severity Grading

In addition to establishing a diagnostic "lexicon" specific for a study, the preliminary evaluation of control and high-dose groups allows the pathologist to set thresholds and scales for severity grading. Drift in severity grading can occur when a study is evaluated over a long period of time or involves a large number of animals and/or multiple pathologists. Such drift can be mitigated by continued reference to representative examples of different severity grades, by a targeted masked review prior to finalization, or by peer review (Schafer et al., 2018). It is preferred that only one

pathologist grades the lesions to reduce interobserver variability (see *Experimental Design and Statistical Analysis for Toxicologic Pathologists*, Vol 1, Chap 16). Severity grading scales may be general for common changes (e.g., CPN). More detailed grading scales may consider lesion location, distribution, or pattern; proportion of the tissue/organ affected; or changes along a spectrum. To aid in consistency and meaningful interpretation by toxicologists and regulatory reviewers, severity grading criteria and their clear rationale should be included in the narrative of the report within the context of the study, especially for critical lesions or when severity of a lesion potentially impacts the No Observed Adverse Effect Level/Low Observed Adverse Effect Level (Schafer et al., 2018). Although other factors that are not directly part of the histologic features should not generally be considered when assigning a severity grade (e.g., organ weights, clinical pathology data, organ function, moribundity or mortality of the animal, adversity, potential human relevance, or reversibility), the interpretative narrative may relate severity grades to these factors (Schafer et al., 2018). While severity grading can provide additional useful information, severity grades are essentially subjective scores and comparing results between studies or between pathologists can sometimes be challenging. Hence, in the pathology narrative, it is imperative that pathologists define the grading criteria adequately so that another pathologist can understand the process by which they were assigned and, ideally, reproduce any result.

5.5. Lesion Complexity

Synonymous terms often exist for many lesions, and individual pathologists often have preferences based on their training and experience. In general, lesions with similar characteristics and pathogenesis at a particular site can be consolidated into as few diagnoses as possible, preferably as a single diagnosis that reflects the biological significance of the pathologic process. In situations where diagnoses are consolidated, the pathology narrative should detail the characteristics and features encompassing the grouped diagnoses. Conversely, situations exist in which diagnosing each component of a complex lesion is more appropriate. In general, multiple diagnoses should be used when important information about the pathogenesis or biology of a lesion must be conveyed. For example, squamous cell papillomas in the forestomach of rodents may occur secondary to focal ulceration that is often accompanied by chronic submucosal inflammation and squamous epithelial hyperplasia. Frequently, some component of that lesion is absent in some tissue sections; primary ulceration and inflammation along with papillomas may be the only lesions observed. In other sections, prominent squamous epithelial hyperplasia may be observed with or without ulceration or papillomas, whereas in other sections, all lesions may be observed. In this situation, it would be inappropriate to combine the nonneoplastic changes under a single diagnosis of ulceration because information critical to understanding the pathogenesis of the forestomach papillomas would be lost.

5.6. Multiple Pathologists

Ideally, one pathologist should evaluate the control and treated groups of both sexes in an individual study and for all species for a given test article so as to capture the overall treatment-related effects within and between each of the test species. Comparative assessment between species is a critical aspect in the determination of risk assessment. However, that said, implementation of a single pathologist to such a role may be impractical. In situations where this is not feasible, good communication between pathologists, and between pathologists and toxicologists, can help maintain consistency. Comparison of lesions among pathologists conducting the evaluations is important, as they must be cognizant of the exact nature of the lesions observed. By working together and with toxicologists, pathologists can lessen the potential for inconsistencies in diagnostic terminology. A complete histopathological evaluation should ideally include not only a review of the data by the initial (study) pathologist(s) but also a pathology peer review whenever practical. Due to the subjective nature inherent in histopathological evaluation, peer review and, when necessary, PWGs are often included following evaluation by the study pathologist so as to identify and resolve inconsistencies and/or inaccuracies (see *Pathology Peer Review*, Vol 1, Chap 26).

5.7. The Pathology Narrative

At the end of the initial evaluation, and at the completion of the histopathologic evaluation, the diagnostic lexicon for the study can be reviewed for duplications in terminology; the use of inappropriate terminology for topography, sites, and morphology; and for terminology that is inconsistent with previous studies performed on same or related compounds. Finally, an important means of communicating the histopathologic findings is the descriptive and interpretive pathology narrative that must accompany the tabulated data. The narrative should not include an exhaustive list of all pathology findings for every organ and tissue examined. Rather, it should include the significant pathology findings for the study and place major treatment-related lesions into context of the study objectives (see *Preparation of the Anatomic Pathology Report for a Toxicity Study*, Vol 2, Chap 13). The narrative should attempt to identify the target organs/tissues and include brief morphologic descriptions of the lesions documented. Grading criteria can be included in the narrative or as an Appendix to the Pathology Report. When tissues within a single study are subcontracted for specialized expertise, the study pathologist should integrate pathology findings across all organ systems and/or endpoints to complete evaluation. Two of the most commonly encountered problems with the pathology narrative are inadequate morphological descriptions of lesions and the lack of information regarding any pertinent baseline diagnostic thresholds for lesion diagnosis and severity grading. Communication between multiple pathologists for any given study remains paramount.

In the overall pathology narrative that includes pathology findings across multiple studies and species for a given test article, it is appropriate to describe the diagnostic terminology and criteria used for classifying lesions and treatment-related effects, as well as to note differences in terminology between studies where the lesion criteria remain consistent. Here, communication between the study pathologist and study toxicologist for any given test article remains paramount.

6. HARMONIZATION OF NOMENCLATURE

6.1. International Harmonization of Nomenclature and Diagnostic Criteria

Early initiatives to harmonize nomenclature and diagnostic criteria began in the late 1980s in the United States by the Society of Toxicologic Pathology (STP) and in Europe by the Registry of Industrial Toxicology Animal Data (RITA) database group. Both initiatives resulted in internationally recognized publications that included the Standardized System of Nomenclature and Diagnostic Criteria (SSNDC) guides for toxicologic pathology by STP and the International Classification of Rodent Tumors for the rat and the mouse by World Health Organization (WHO)/International Agency for Research on Cancer (IARC)/RITA. Additional efforts to harmonize in the mid-1990s by the Joint STPs and International Life Sciences Institute committee on INHAND in Toxicologic Pathology resulted in additional publications.

In 2005, a global collaborative project was initiated to compile a series of publications for each organ system in order to provide a standardized nomenclature and differential diagnoses for classifying microscopic lesions observed in laboratory rats and mice in toxicity and carcinogenicity studies. This initiative is referred to as INHAND (https://www.toxpath.org/inhand.asp) that has now expanded to include nonrodent species. The INHAND project is supported by the societies of toxicologic pathology from Europe (European Society of Toxicologic Pathology [ESTP]), Great Britain (British Society of Toxicological Pathologists [BSTP]), Japan (Japanese Society of Toxicologic Pathology [JSTP]), and North America (STP). A Global Editorial and Steering Committee (GESC) was formed to administer the activities of the project. The GESC is composed of toxicologic pathologists from all participating societies. Committees of expert toxicologic pathologists from each of the participating societies form Working Groups (WGs; not to be confused with PWGs associated with resolving diagnostic discrepancies) from an administrative and organizational perspective and are tasked with developing preferred nomenclature and diagnostic criteria for each rodent organ system or one of the nonrodent species used in toxicity studies (Keenan et al., 2015; Mann et al., 2012; Vahle et al., 2009).

The rodent species WGs have the responsibility to prepare the nomenclature guidelines for both proliferative and nonproliferative lesions of rats and mice for their assigned organ system—15 total organ systems. The nonrodent species WGs cover terminology specific to a species as well as noting diagnostic criteria that may be different from rodents for common lesions. The nonrodent species include nonhuman primate, dog, minipig, rabbit, and fish. Along with lesions that occur spontaneously, the WGs are tasked with determining if there are common, toxicant-induced lesions for which standardized nomenclature is needed.

WGs draw broadly from existing nomenclature documents, websites, and publications including prior work of the RITA, SSNDC Guides for Toxicologic Pathology (Streett, 1988), the WHO/IARC International Classification of Rodent Tumors, and NTP. For each diagnostic term, the WGs recommend a preferred diagnosis and suitable alternative or historical diagnoses, list diagnostic criteria and differential diagnoses, provide representative photomicrographs, and include a comment section with key references. WGs primarily develop nomenclature that is descriptive in nature.

All 15 rodent organ systems have been published (Table 25.1). To address consistent terminology for cell death, recommendations from an Apoptosis/Necrosis WG have been published (Elmore et al., 2016). The nonrodent species have been drafted and are in review at the time of writing this chapter.

An essential aspect of the INHAND project is utilization of goRENI. While systems and species terminology are being developed and shared for review, access to goRENI is restricted to members of the participating STPs (Mann et al., 2012; Vahle et al., 2009). Pathologists or regulatory scientists with accounts can navigate by organ system and select a diagnosis they would like to view along with the material described above (e.g., differential diagnoses, diagnostic criteria, images) that is generated by the INHAND WGs. Within the goRENI system, each diagnostic entity is referred to as a manuscript.

TABLE 25.1 INHAND Published Guides for Rodent Species

Organ system	Reference
Hematolymphoid System	Willard-Mack et al. (2019) Nonproliferative and Proliferative Lesions of the Rat and Mouse Hematolymphoid System
Endocrine System	Brandli-Baiocco et al. (2018) Nonproliferative and Proliferative Lesions of the Rat and Mouse Endocrine System
Special Senses (Ocular, Olfactory, Otic)	Ramos et al. (2018) Nonproliferative and Proliferative Lesions of the Rat and Mouse Special Sense Organs (Ocular [eye and glands], Olfactory, and Otic)
Cardiovascular System	Berridge et al. (2016) Non-proliferative and Proliferative Lesions of the Cardiovascular System of the Rat and Mouse
Skeletal System and Teeth	Fossey et al. (2016) Nonproliferative and Proliferative Lesions of the Rat and Mouse Skeletal Tissues (Bones, Joints, and Teeth)
Digestive System	Nolte et al. (2016) Nonproliferative and Proliferative Lesions of the Gastrointestinal Tract, Pancreas and Salivary Glands of the Rat and Mouse.
Female Reproductive System	Dixon et al. (2014) Nonproliferative and proliferative lesions of the rat and mouse female reproductive system
Soft Tissue, Skeletal Muscle, and Mesothelium	Greaves et al. (2013) Proliferative and non-proliferative lesions of the rat and mouse soft tissue, skeletal muscle and mesothelium
Integument	Mecklenburg et al. (2013) Proliferative and Non-Proliferative Lesions of the Rat and Mouse Integument
Mammary, Zymbal's, Preputial, and Clitoral Glands	Rudmann et al. (2012) Proliferative and nonproliferative lesions of the rat and mouse mammary, Zymbal's, preputial, and clitoral glands
Male Reproductive System	Creasy et al. (2012) Proliferative and nonproliferative lesions of the rat and mouse male reproductive system
Nervous System	Kaufmann et al. (2012) Proliferative and nonproliferative lesions of the rat and mouse central and peripheral nervous systems
Urinary System	Frazier et al. (2012) Proliferative and nonproliferative lesions of the rat and mouse urinary system.
Hepatobiliary System	Thoolen et al. (2010) Proliferative and nonproliferative lesions of the rat and mouse hepatobiliary system
Respiratory System	Renne et al. (2009) Proliferative and nonproliferative lesions of the rat and mouse respiratory tract

Finalized nomenclature is available to toxicologic pathologists and the broader scientific community, in both electronic (https://www.toxpath.org/inhand.asp) and print forms (Table 25.1). The print-based publications are available in the toxicologic pathology journals: *Toxicologic Pathology,* which is the official journal of STP, BSTP, and ESTP (https://journals.sagepub.com/home/tpx), and the *Journal of Toxicologic Pathology,* which is the official journal of JSTP (https://www.jstage.jst.go.jp/browse/tox). Electronic access is possible via the goRENI website (https://www.goreni.org) or other websites (https://www.toxpath.org/inhand.asp#pubg

or https://www.jstage.jst.go.jp/browse/tox). The international scope and review of the INHAND documents offer an effective framework for acceptance and application by pathologists and regulatory agencies engaged in the safety assessment of drugs, biologics, and chemicals (Elmore et al., 2018) (see *Risk Assessment*, Vol 2, Chap 16).

Although the published INHAND nomenclature for each organ system is expected to be comprehensive, it is acknowledged that additional lesions may need to be included, inaccuracies rectified as they become apparent, or changes to terminology made based on new scientific information. A formal change control process was implemented in 2013 and is available on https://www.goreni.org and through each toxicologic pathology society website. Society members are encouraged to submit proposals for changes to the nomenclature systems and provide rationale for such changes through these mechanisms. Updates will be posted on goRENI and as presentations or posters at society meetings, and this will be the source for the most current information (Keenan et al., 2015).

6.2. Standard for Exchange of Nonclinical Data

The US FDA Center for Drug Evaluation and Research is collaborating with Clinical Data Interchange Standards Consortium (CDISC) to bring harmonization to the clinical and nonclinical data submission process. CDISC standards are widely used for study planning and data collection, tabulation, analysis, and submissions to the FDA and other regulatory agencies internationally. The foundation for the standardized clinical content is the CDISC Study Data Tabulation Model (SDTM). The National Cancer Institute Enterprise Vocabulary Service (NCI EVS) codes, maintains, and publishes all CDISC-controlled terminologies including SDTM, and EVS also supports many FDA terminology standards (EVS, 2012). SDTM includes nonclinical requirements based on the SEND models that are being harmonized with the SDTM.

SEND is a standardized procedure for submitting data from nonclinical studies to FDA electronically that specifies directives to share nonclinical data in a consistent format to the FDA (Keenan and Goodman, 2014). Sponsors whose studies start after December 17, 2016, must submit data in the data formats supported by FDA and listed in the FDA Data Standards Catalog. This applies to New Drug Applications, Biologic License Applications, Abbreviated New Drug Applications, and subsequent submissions to these types of applications. For Investigational New Drugs, the requirement applies for studies that start after December 17, 2017. A SEND package consists of several components, but the main focus is on individual study endpoint data. Endpoints typically map to domains (essentially, datasets) with a number of variables (columns or fields). SEND is in production now and available for use (https://www.fda.gov/industry/fda-resources-data-standards/study-data-standards-resources). SEND is also the US FDA's required and supported format for nonclinical general toxicology and carcinogenicity study data.

The US FDA has requested the use of the INHAND nomenclature as standard terminology for SEND. INHAND GESC representatives work with the SEND Controlled Terminology (CT) committee to provide definitions for base processes and modifiers associated with the INHAND published terminology. Any issues or questions are presented to the full GESC and/or appropriate INHAND WG for resolution. The initial list for the SEND codelist of nonneoplastic (NONNEO) microscopic pathology contains terms from published INHAND organ systems. The list will continue to grow as INHAND publishes additional organ systems and nonrodent species. Some terms on the NONNEO codelist may look different from how they have been presented in the INHAND publications. Terms on the NONNEO codelist are mostly generic and can be used across tissues, where appropriate. INHAND published terms have been modified to fit the SEND standard in some cases by being broken into base process and modifiers. For example, the INHAND term "Necrosis, zonal" would be separated into NECROSIS for population in MISTRESC (Microscopic Standardized Result) and ZONAL in MIDISTR (Microscopic Distribution). Tissue-specific terms from INHAND are included on the NONNEO codelist when it is important to use the exact term representing a spectrum of tissue changes (e.g., focus of cellular alteration). As inconsistencies are noted or new terms needed, this will be addressed using the new change control process and the most current terminology will be available on the goRENI website. The most current SEND CT can be found at the NCI EVS site: https:// evs.nci.nih.gov/ftp1/CDISC/SEND/.

6.3. National Toxicology Program Nonneoplastic Lesion Atlas

Since the early 1970s, the US NTP has remained the benchmark for rodent carcinogenicity and toxicology studies. In addition to carcinogenicity evaluations, the NTP has generated and continues to maintain an expansive database of nonneoplastic endpoints. In order to facilitate cross-study comparisons, data mining, and the creation of a historical control database for some of the nonneoplastic lesions, the NTP recognized the need for more standardized terminology and a consistent approach to diagnosing nonneoplastic lesions.

To that end, the NTP created the online NNLA (Cesta et al., 2014). Although the primary users of the NNLA are the toxicologic pathologists evaluating studies for the NTP, the atlas is publicly accessible (https://ntp.niehs.nih.gov/ nnl/) and can be used by any toxicology or pathology laboratory, researchers evaluating tissues, and as a resource by trainees in toxicologic pathology.

The NNLA is an online resource that contains thousands of photomicrographs of nonneoplastic lesions across all organs and tissues routinely examined in NTP studies. Multiple magnifications of the digital, downloadable photomicrographs are included. There are recommendations on the NTP's preferred approach to diagnosing these lesions, numerous references, links to related lesions, and other useful information. As an online resource, the NNLA can be updated as needed. It is completely searchable and includes a useful guide on how to use the NNLA during review of toxicity and carcinogenicity studies. The NTP has made every effort to be consistent with the terminology presented in the INHAND in rats and mice and is a valuable supplement to the INHAND documents.

6.4. Other Nomenclature Resources

Several published texts are also excellent sources of standardized nomenclature. These include "Boorman's Pathology of the Rat" (Suttie et al., 2017) and "Pathology of the Mouse" (Maronpot et al., 1999); both are authoritative and comprehensive pathology reference texts of spontaneous and induced lesions observed in the rat and the mouse. The terminology in these texts is based on the NTP database of millions of extensively peer-reviewed histopathological slides from more than 600 short- and long-term toxicity and carcinogenicity studies. Diagnostic categories included in these texts are based on standardized diagnostic criteria for the pathology terminology utilized by the NTP. The mouse text also contains references to lesions of transgenic mouse strains and mechanistic considerations (see also *Genetically Engineered Animal Models in Toxicologic Research,* Vol 1, Chap 23). A more recent reference is the "Illustrated Dictionary of Toxicologic Pathology and Safety Sciences" that lists lesions by organ systems along with color photomicrographs for most lesions (Sahota et al., 2019). Additional reference texts include "Histopathology of Preclinical Toxicity Studies" (Greaves, 2012), "Pathobiology of the Aging Rat" (Mohr et al., 1992), "Pathobiology of the Aging Mouse" (Mohr, 1996), "Rat Histopathology" (Greaves, 1992), and "Mouse Histopathology" (Faccini et al., 1990). Finally, the World Association of Veterinary Anatomists, an international umbrella organization of the veterinary anatomy associations, has published guidelines for harmonized veterinary species terminology for gross anatomy and histology: *Nomina anatomica veterinaria* and *Nomina histologica veterinaria* that are available online (http:// www.wava-amav.org/wava-documents.html). Because histology is a vital platform upon which pathology rests, an excellent resource is "Histology for Pathologists" (Mills, 2019).

7. CONCLUSIONS

This chapter addresses the importance of and the issues involved with the application of nomenclature in toxicologic pathology. Consistent and unambiguous diagnostic terminology describing morphological changes clearly impacts interpretation and risk assessment in general nonclinical toxicology studies. The role of the toxicologic pathologist lies not only in discerning differences between control and treatment groups in order to identify potential toxicities of a test article but also to properly communicate such differences to the scientific community through nomenclature. For treatment-related histopathological findings, the toxicologic pathologist plays a critical role in the interpretation of histopathological findings and discussion of these findings with other scientists in order to inform on risk to humans. Toxicologic pathologists must consider the intended users of the data within the realms of regulatory toxicology and risk assessment who may be less familiar with pathology terminology and may approach study results with a different perspective. The goal for toxicologic pathologists is to report findings and interpretations in a clear and concise manner that facilitates comparison of data among related studies.

Since histopathological findings are embedded within nomenclature, a systematic and consistent approach to the diagnosis and documentation of lesions is highly desirable. Nomenclature comprises a hierarchical system of components for a diagnosis including topography (organ/tissue), morphology (pathological change), and modifiers (also known as qualifiers). The lexicon and components of nomenclature differ between neoplastic and nonneoplastic lesions. An overview of the challenges of assigning and managing nomenclature encountered during histopathological evaluation and recommended practices has been detailed. Due to the many variables that impact nomenclature as described in this chapter, the reporting of results with consistency and clarity remains a challenging task. Efforts toward consistent application and harmonization of a standardized system of nomenclature are essential for assessing comparative toxicologic effects of different or structurally related test articles and when applied will result in the improvement of the quality and clarity of toxicologic pathology data.

Acknowledgments

The authors acknowledge previous authors of this chapter, Drs. Amy Brix and Ron Herbert. This work was supported in part by the NIH, National Institute of Environmental Health Sciences.

REFERENCES

Berridge BR, Mowat V, Nagai H, et al.: Non-proliferative and proliferative lesions of the cardiovascular system of the rat and mouse, *J Toxicol Pathol* 29:1s–47s, 2016.

Bolon B, Barale-Thomas E, Bradley A, et al.: International recommendations for training future toxicologic pathologists participating in regulatory-type, nonclinical toxicity studies, *Toxicol Pathol* 38:984–992, 2010.

Boorman GA, Wolf DC, Francke-Carroll S, et al.: Pathology peer review, *Toxicol Pathol* 38:1009–1010, 2010.

Brandli-Baiocco A, Balme E, Bruder M, et al.: Nonproliferative and proliferative lesions of the rat and mouse endocrine system, *J Toxicol Pathol* 31:1s–95s, 2018.

Cesta MF, Malarkey DE, Herbert RA, et al.: The national toxicology program web-based nonneoplastic lesion atlas: a global toxicology and pathology resource, *Toxicol Pathol* 42:458–460, 2014.

Creasy D, Bube A, de Rijk E, et al.: Proliferative and nonproliferative lesions of the rat and mouse male reproductive system, *Toxicol Pathol* 40:40s–121s, 2012.

Crissman JW, Goodman DG, Hildebrandt PK, et al.: Best Practices guideline: toxicologic histopathology, *Toxicol Pathol* 32:126–131, 2004.

Dixon D, Alison R, Bach U, et al.: Nonproliferative and proliferative lesions of the rat and mouse female reproductive system, *J Toxicol Pathol* 27:1s–107s, 2014.

Elmore SA, Cardiff R, Cesta MF, et al.: A review of current standards and the evolution of histopathology nomenclature for laboratory animals, *ILAR J* 59:29–39, 2018.

Elmore SA, Dixon D, Hailey JR, et al.: Recommendations from the INHAND apoptosis/necrosis working group, *Toxicol Pathol* 44:173–188, 2016.

EVS N: *US national cancer institute's enterprise vocabulary services*, 2012.

Faccini JM, Abbott DP, Paulus GJJ: *Mouse histopathology: a glossary for use in toxicity and carcinogenicity studies*, Amsterdam, 1990, Elsevier.

FDA draft guidance. https://www.fda.gov/regulatory-information/search-fda-guidance-documents/pathology-peer-review-nonclinical-toxicology-studies-questions-and-answers.

Fikes JD, Patrick DJ, Francke S, et al.: Scientific and regulatory policy committee review: review of the organisation for economic co-operation and development (OECD) guidance on the GLP requirements for peer review of histopathology, *Toxicol Pathol* 43:907–914, 2015.

Fossey S, Vahle J, Long P, et al.: Nonproliferative and proliferative lesions of the rat and mouse skeletal tissues (bones, joints, and teeth), *J Toxicol Pathol* 29:49s–103s, 2016.

Frazier KS, Seely JC, Hard GC, et al.: Proliferative and nonproliferative lesions of the rat and mouse urinary system, *Toxicol Pathol* 40:14s–86s, 2012.

Global open RENI. The standard reference for nomenclature and diagnostic criteria in toxicologic pathology. https://www.goreni.org/.

Greaves P: *Rat histopathology: a glossary for use in toxicity and carcinogenicity studies*, ed 2nd rev., Amsterdam, 1992, Elsevier.

Greaves P. In Greaves P, editor: *Histopathology of preclinical toxicity studies*, ed 4, Boston, 2012, Academic Press, p 892.

Greaves P, Chouinard L, Ernst H, et al.: Proliferative and non-proliferative lesions of the rat and mouse soft tissue, skeletal muscle and mesothelium, *J Toxicol Pathol* 26:1s–26s, 2013.

https://ntp.niehs.nih.gov/nnl. (Last accessed September 2020).

https://evs.nci.nih.gov/ftp1/CDISC/SEND.

https://www.fda.gov/industry/fda-resources-data-standards/study-data-standards-resources.

https://www.fda.gov/regulatory-information/search-fda-guidance-documents/pathology-peer-review-nonclinical-toxicology-studies-questions-and-answers.

https://www.toxpath.org/inhand.asp.

https://www.toxpath.org/inhand.asp#pubg.

INHAND Manuscripts. https://www.toxpath.org/inhand.asp. (Last accessed April 2012).

Journal of toxicologic pathology which is the official journal of JSTP. https://www.jstage.jst.go.jp/browse/tox.

Kaufmann W, Bolon B, Bradley A, et al.: Proliferative and nonproliferative lesions of the rat and mouse central and peripheral nervous systems, *Toxicol Pathol* 40:87s–157s, 2012.

Keenan CM, Baker J, Bradley A, et al.: International harmonization of nomenclature and diagnostic criteria (INHAND): progress to date and future plans, *Toxicol Pathol* 43:730–732, 2015.

Keenan CM, Goodman DG: Regulatory forum commentary: through the looking glass-SENDing the pathology data we have INHAND, *Toxicol Pathol* 42:807–810, 2014.

Long GG, Hardisty JF: Regulatory forum opinion piece: thresholds in toxicologic pathology, *Toxicol Pathol* 40:1079–1081, 2012.

Mann PC, Hardisty JH: Pathology working groups, *Toxicol Pathol* 42:283–284, 2014.

Mann PC, Vahle J, Keenan CM, et al.: International harmonization of toxicologic pathology nomenclature: an overview and review of basic principles, *Toxicol Pathol* 40:7–13, 2012.

Maronpot RR, Boorman GA, Gaul BW: *Pathology of the mouse: reference and atlas*, Vienna, IL, 1999, Cache River Press.

McInnes EF, Mann P: *Background lesions in laboratory animals: a color atlas*, Saint Louis, 2011, W.B. Saunders.

Mecklenburg L, Kusewitt D, Kolly C, et al.: Proliferative and non-proliferative lesions of the rat and mouse integument, *J Toxicol Pathol* 26:27S–57S, 2013.

Mills: *SEE: histology for pathologists*, ed 5, Wolters Kluwer.

Mohr U: *Pathobiology of the aging mouse*, Washington, D.C, 1996, ILSI Press.

Mohr U, Dungworth DL, Capen CC: *Pathobiology of the aging rat*, Washington, D.C, 1992, International Life Sciences Institute.

Morton D, Sellers RS, Barale-Thomas E, et al.: Recommendations for pathology peer review, *Toxicol Pathol* 38:1118–1127, 2010.

Nolte T, Brander-Weber P, Dangler C, et al.: Nonproliferative and proliferative lesions of the gastrointestinal tract, pancreas and salivary glands of the rat and mouse, *J Toxicol Pathol* 29:1s–125s, 2016.

Nomina anatomica veterinaria and Nomina histologica veterinaria that are available online http://www.wava-amav.org/wava-documents.html. (Last accessed September 2020).

Ramos MF, Baker J, Atzpodien EA, et al.: Nonproliferative and proliferative lesions of the ratand mouse special sense organs(ocular [eye and glands], olfactory and otic), *J Toxicol Pathol* 31:97s–214s, 2018.

Renne R, Brix A, Harkema J, et al.: Proliferative and non-proliferative lesions of the rat and mouse respiratory tract, *Toxicol Pathol* 37:5s–73s, 2009.

Rudmann D, Cardiff R, Chouinard L, et al.: Proliferative and nonproliferative lesions of the rat and mouse mammary, Zymbal's, preputial, and clitoral glands, *Toxicol Pathol* 40: 7s–39s, 2012.

Sahota P, Spaet R, Bentley P, Wojcinski Z, editors: *The illustrated dictionary of toxicologic pathology and safety science*, ed 1, Boca Raton, 2019, CRC Press.

Schafer KA, Eighmy J, Fikes JD, et al.: Use of severity grades to characterize histopathologic changes, *Toxicol Pathol* 46:256–265, 2018.

Streett CS: *Standard nomenclature and diagnostic criteria in toxicologic pathology*, Los Angeles, CA, 1988, SAGE Publications Sage CA.

Suttie AW, Leininger JR, Bradley AE: *Boorman's pathology of the rat: reference and atlas*, Academic Press.

Thoolen B, Maronpot RR, Harada T, et al.: Proliferative and nonproliferative lesions of the rat and mouse hepatobiliary system, *Toxicol Pathol* 38:5s–81s, 2010.

Toxicologic pathology, the official journal of STP, BSTP and ESTP. https://journals.sagepub.com/home/tpx.

Vahle J, Bradley A, Harada T, et al.: The international nomenclature project: an update, *Toxicol Pathol* 37:694–697, 2009.

Ward JM, Hardisty JF, Hailey JR, et al.: Peer review in toxicologic pathology, *Toxicol Pathol* 23:226–234, 1995.

Willard-Mack CL, Elmore SA, Hall WC, et al.: Nonproliferative and proliferative lesions of the rat and mouse hematolymphoid system, *Toxicol Pathol* 47:665–783, 2019.

Pathology Peer Review

Frank J. Geoly[1], Bindu M. Bennet[2], James D. Fikes[3], Jerry F. Hardisty[4]

[1]Pfizer Worldwide Research, Development, and Medical, Groton, Connecticut, United States, [2]Nonclinical Safety Relay Therapeutics, Cambridge, Massachusetts, United States, [3]Biogen, Cambridge, Massachusetts, United States, [4]Experimental Pathology Laboratories, Inc., Research Triangle Park, North Carolina, United States

OUTLINE

1. Introduction	987	5. Regulatory Aspects of Pathology Peer Review	1004
2. Peer Review Timing and Pathology Raw Data	988	5.1. Regulations for Contemporaneous Pathology Peer Review in China and Japan	1006
2.1. Pathology Raw Data and Peer Review	989		
3. Peer Review Process	990	6. Use of Digital/Whole-Slide Images in Pathology Peer Review	1006
3.1. Consultation	990	6.1. Use of Whole-Slide Images for National Toxicology Program Pathology Working Groups	1007
3.2. Peer Review: Contemporaneous Peer Review	990		
3.3. Resolution of Disagreements during Contemporaneous Peer Review	997		
3.4. Documentation of Contemporaneous Peer Review	1000	7. Conclusion	1007
3.5. Peer Review: Retrospective Peer Review	1001	References	1008
4. National Toxicology Program Review Process	1003		

1. INTRODUCTION

In vivo regulatory-type animal toxicity studies that include pathology endpoints are generally *not* hypothesis-driven experiments. Instead, these studies are meant to gather information using multiple, medical diagnostic endpoints, assessed both antemortem (i.e., in life) and postmortem, to discover or characterize the toxicity profile that results from the administration of relatively high doses of a test article to animals. Characterizing the toxicity profile necessitates integration of these diagnostic endpoints that form the basis of the conclusions of the study.

Typically, the study pathologist (SP), as the principal medical diagnostician (veterinarian or physician) on the study team, is responsible not only for describing the macroscopic (gross) observations, organ weights, and microscopic pathology findings but integrating those finding with the antemortem endpoints to fully describe the toxicity profile in the pathology report; in some instances, the SP also may be asked to address clinical pathology parameters (e.g., hematologic and serum chemistry values) along with anatomic pathology endpoints. It follows that, from the perspective of the SP, a toxicity study is, in fact, a medical diagnostic exercise.

Haschek and Rousseaux's Handbook of Toxicologic Pathology, Fourth Edition.
https://doi.org/10.1016/B978-0-12-821044-4.00004-2

Diagnosis in a toxicity study goes beyond the postmortem microscopic anatomic evaluation of tissue sections from a comprehensive set of samples from bodily organs, although the SP is the contributing scientist who generates these diagnoses. Proper diagnosis requires integration of clinical endpoints; such as body weight and food consumption; clinical signs and symptoms and their time of onset (including evaluating the cause of death, if early death or unscheduled euthanasia occurs); and clinical pathology parameters (e.g., serum chemistry, hematology, urinalysis) in addition to the postmortem endpoints of organ weights and the gross and microscopic evaluation of the organs. For practical purposes, the necropsy essentially equates to a thorough, and final, physical examination.

The SP's evaluation that leads to the final diagnoses and their interpretation is perhaps the most essential component of identifying and characterizing potential hazards to human or animal health associated with exposure to the test article in most studies. Therefore, it is crucial that the SP's evaluation is thorough, and the diagnoses are accurate, for this becomes the foundation upon which the risk assessment is built. Procedures or practices should ordinarily be in place at a testing facility to ensure diagnostic accuracy and minimize misdiagnosis or inadvertent diagnostic error. The principal practice to ensure accuracy, and one that is required by the global Good Laboratory Practice (GLP) regulations and guidance documents (FDA, 1987; OECD, 1998), is assuring that SPs have sufficient pathology education, training, and experience to evaluate toxicity studies (*Pathology and GLPs, Quality Control and Quality Assurance*; Vol 1, Chap 27; Bolon et al., 2010; Morton et al., 2010). However, achieving an accurate pathology diagnosis is an iterative process of progressive diagnostic refinement that is, at its best, a collaborative activity. While the SP is ultimately responsible as the contributing scientist for the generating the pathology raw data and preparing the final pathology report, most pathologists do not reach their conclusions in isolation.

Although generally not required in the global GLP regulations, the practice of pathology peer review serves as an important quality control (QC) procedure to increase confidence in the accuracy of the pathology diagnoses and their interpretations. Pathology peer review entails having a second pathologist (known as a peer review pathologist [PRP]), or occasionally a group of three or more additional pathologists (known as a pathology working group [PWG]), evaluate a subset of the pathology postmortem findings originally identified by the SP (microscopic diagnoses as well as diagnostic terminology and severity grades) in addition to the overall interpretation of these findings in the report. This chapter will review current pathology peer review practices and their applications for the various types of animal toxicity studies conducted by industry and government research institutes as well as the current state of government regulation of peer review in industry, including appropriate documentation and reporting practices.

2. PEER REVIEW TIMING AND PATHOLOGY RAW DATA

Pathology peer review is not required by regulatory agencies, but studies in which the pathology data have undergone peer review are particularly welcome by regulatory reviewers due to the perception that the QC afforded by the additional level of review has improved the quality of the pathology raw data. Recommendations for performing an effective pathology peer review have been prepared by the Society of Toxicologic Pathology (STP); these are available both in print (Morton et al., 2010) and online (https://doi.org/10.1177/0192623310383991). These peer review best practices have been endorsed by nine other societies of toxicologic pathology from around the world as well as the American College of Veterinary Pathologists (ACVP).

There are two types of pathology peer review, and they differ in respect to timing (Figure 26.1) A **contemporaneous** (or **prospective**) peer review is conducted after the SP has generated draft or preliminary pathology diagnoses and prepared a draft narrative report but prior to signing and dating the final pathology report (i.e., prior to the creation of the pathology raw data, as discussed below). This is the most common type of pathology peer review conducted in industry and in government research institutes. During a contemporaneous peer review, the PRP works with the SP to refine the pathology diagnoses and terminology. In contrast,

Association of Peer Review & Histopathology Raw Data

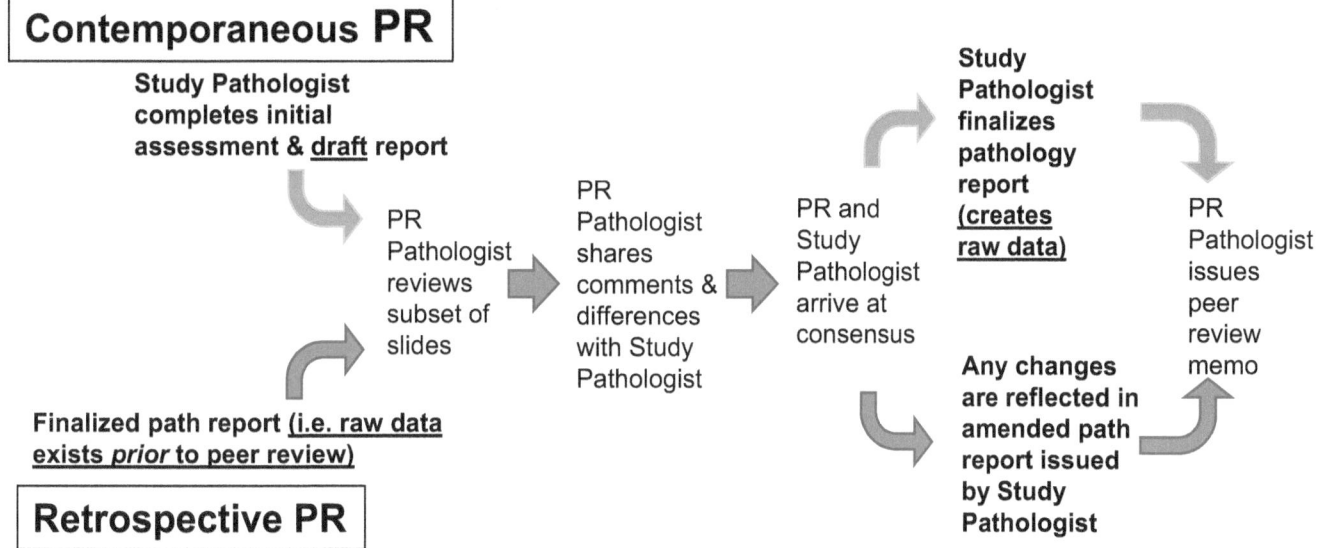

FIGURE 26.1 Summary of the differences between contemporaneous and retrospective peer review as they relate to the histopathology raw data.

a **retrospective** peer review is performed after the pathology report has been finalized, signed, and dated—often weeks, months, or years later—in order to review a specific question(s) or render a second opinion. In other words, a retrospective pathology peer review is performed on a study for which pathology raw data already exist, so the outcome of the peer review may lead to changes in existing data and the need to prepare an amended pathology report.

2.1. Pathology Raw Data and Peer Review

Understanding the difference between a contemporaneous and retrospective peer review requires an understanding of the definition of "raw data" as it pertains to histopathology diagnosis. The definition of "pathology raw data" influences why certain documentation actions are, or are not, required with contemporaneous or retrospective peer review. Pathology raw data has long been considered by the U.S. Food and Drug Administration (FDA) as *the signed and dated final report of the* SP (to include the finalized histopathology diagnoses). Importantly,

[t]he pathologist's interim notes, therefore, which are subject to frequent changes as the pathologist refines the diagnosis, are not raw data because they do not contribute to study reconstruction. Accordingly, only

the signed and dated final report of the pathologist comprises raw data respecting the histopathological evaluation of tissue specimens. **U.S. FDA, Federal Register (1987)**

In a contemporaneous peer review, the PRP is reviewing the SP's preliminary diagnoses and interpretation as recorded in the draft report, thereby serving a QC function. The PRP is not generating raw data in this peer review but merely is producing a list of suggested adjustments to hone the diagnoses, interpretation, and/or terminology—if any seem to be needed. In general, the PRP does not recommend any alteration to the preliminary diagnoses and severity grades if the impressions of the SP and PRP use diagnostic terminology from a widely recognized lexicon (e.g., International Harmonization of Nomenclature and Diagnostic Criteria [INHAND, https://www.goreni.org/gr3_download_nom.php]) and are only one severity grade apart. Discussion between the SP and PRP regarding the PRP's suggested adjustments may be used to further refine the preliminary diagnoses. The SP may accept all, some, or none of the PRP's recommendations since the SP is ultimately the sole scientist responsible for generating the final diagnoses and interpretation of the pathology portion of the study. Thus, in a contemporaneous peer review, pathology raw data are not yet established at the initiation of the peer review because the SP has only recorded preliminary pathology findings and written the draft narrative/interpretation. From the FDA General Rule, 1987 (above), it is important to note that the SP's preliminary (or "interim") notes regarding draft diagnoses are not pathology raw data; the raw data are established only when the final pathology report is signed by the SP. Logically, notes or annotations made by the PRP to the SP's preliminary histopathology diagnoses and/or draft report and then shared with the SP are also not pathology raw data. The pathology raw data are listed in the final signed pathology report, so neither the SP nor the PRP is required to retain their interim notes. The basis for this regulatory perspective is that the pathology results for the study may be recapitulated, if necessary, by the original SP or another pathologist by reviewing the tissue sections and report, without the need to review the SP's (and/or PRP's) interim notes. Thus, documentation of the peer review is limited to a statement (often called a certificate, statement, or memorandum) by the PRP of the peer review procedure. See the section below on "Documentation of Contemporaneous Peer Review" for additional detail on appropriate documentation of contemporaneous peer review.

In contrast, a retrospective peer review is conducted after the pathology report has already been finalized so that the pathology raw data already exists for the study. Therefore, any changes made as a result of the retrospective peer review will alter the original pathology raw data. Such changes will be subject to documentation in an audit trail and will require preparation of an amendment to the original pathology report. Such amended reports will not only reflect the updated pathology data and, if warranted, revised interpretation but also will incorporate an additional report subsection noting what portions of the original report were amended, how they read before and after the new data were inserted, and the reason for writing the amended report.

In certain situations, a second pathology report may be written by the retrospective PRP to address the new pathology raw data and its interpretation. This circumstance is discussed in Section 5 in the discussion of Retrospective Peer Review by an Expert. There may also be instances when the original SP is not available possibly necessitating a second report by the retrospective PRP or a report from a PWG.

3. PEER REVIEW PROCESS

3.1. Consultation

Informal consultation with colleagues is frequently utilized by the SP as part of the process of refining histopathologic diagnoses. Seeking such spontaneous opinions from colleagues is not a peer review and need not be documented in the pathology report or study file. In this regard, consultation includes seeking opinions through casual discussions with colleagues either individually or in group settings (e.g., institutional pathology rounds) and/or through mentoring by more experienced pathologists. Consultation is used routinely during the primary evaluation of the study to get opinions on complex or unusual findings. The consultation can be as simple as sharing a slide or digital image with a fellow pathologist to obtain their opinion. Slightly more elaborate input may be sought by asking a colleague to review a small set of slides to see if they can sort the slides into those with the change and those without, often using criteria suggested by the SP but sometimes using criteria developed by the person being consulted. The SP will have already gone through this same sorting exercise and made their initial commitment. Consultation serves as an excellent "reality check" for the SP since it is quick and helps reinforce or refine the SP's initial diagnosis. Regardless of how extensive the consultation may be, it can contribute to SP's confidence in their histopathologic diagnosis, attribution of changes to treatment, and assignment of adversity in the draft pathology report.

3.2. Peer Review: Contemporaneous Peer Review

General Process

Although there is generally no regulatory requirement for peer review, organizations conducting toxicity studies routinely conduct contemporaneous peer reviews to optimize the quality of the pathology data. Additional considerations for whether a peer review may be appropriate include whether a nonclinical study may be submitted to a regulatory agency or support substantial financial and/or operational decisions. This motivation may extend to include peer review of investigative toxicology studies, efficacy studies, non-GLP dose range-finding toxicity studies, and due diligence evaluations of toxicity studies of compounds that have been acquired or are being considered for acquisition.

The intent to perform a peer review (either contemporaneous or retrospective) must be documented for GLP studies (and is highly recommended for all nonclinical studies with pathology endpoints) in the protocol or in a protocol amendment. The protocol or amendment should list the reviewing pathologist's name, credentials, and affiliation. The PRP is not listed as a principal investigator since they are not creating raw data but rather as a contributing scientist. Details on how the peer review will be planned, conducted, and documented are generally included in a peer review SOP and the peer review statement rather than the protocol.

A contemporaneous peer review generally starts with a review of the relevant peer review SOP. The peer review SOP to be followed can be that of the sponsor (if the PRP is from a sponsoring organization), the testing facility, or third-party entity if the peer review is subcontracted. The SOP should provide guidelines regarding what study related material to review, the groups and number of animals for examination of full tissues, the review process for target tissues, how to proceed if there is disagreement between the PRP and SP, and how to document the peer review. Detailed considerations for the initial selection for review of animals for full tissue, target tissues, and neoplasms and proliferative changes are included in the SOP and discussed later in the section below on "Core Planning Considerations."

If a study has recovery groups or necropsies at multiple time points, conducting a single peer review at the end of a study typically is easiest administratively and logistically. This arrangement also optimizes the review across all phases of the study, thereby minimizing drift (i.e., shifts in diagnostic terminology and/or grading schemes over time) within diagnoses and severity scoring. However, development program needs may require a peer review to be

conducted with each phase of the study to keep the entire project on the fastest possible track. One of the most common times the peer review is split is for studies with a recovery cohort, when the initial peer review is conducted at the end of the dosing phase and the later peer review at the end of recovery phase. The peer review concepts are still the same for both phases regardless of whether the study is reviewed in a single defined time frame or reviewed in separate phases, and the approach to the planning, conduct, and documentation of the peer reviews is similar for all portions of a study regardless of how many phases are reviewed.

Based on the study design, peer review SOP, draft pathology report, and preliminary pathology data, the PRP designs the peer review plan. Considerations in organizing the peer review process include the initial dose groups (control and treated) to assess, the number of animals (per group) to evaluate, target tissues to review, and if relevant how extensive the review will be for systemic findings that reflect a singular mechanism of action (e.g., collection of vacuolated macrophages in numerous tissues associated with systemic antisense oligonucleotide exposure). The PRP should have access to the study protocol and protocol amendments as well as the full range of study data such as mortality information, in-life observations, clinical pathology and organ weight data, macroscopic observations and the SP's preliminary microscopic diagnoses, and other relevant information (if available) such as toxicokinetic, biodistribution, and transduction data. The PRP also may consult with the SP for input in advance of the review, but the PRP has the authority and bears the sole responsibility for designing the peer review.

The PRP then proceeds with reviewing the slides from the selected subsets of animals and target tissues and compares their diagnoses and severity scores to those generated by the SP. The PRP is tasked with checking that substantive treatment-related findings are identified. This endorsement is accomplished by confirming that microscopic diagnoses, terminology, and grading criteria are consistently and appropriately applied, recorded, and interpreted across the pathology data set that was selected for review. At this point, the PRP shares their comments with the SP. The SP considers the

PRP's suggestions and then decides through discussions with the PRP whether the suggested changes will be incorporated (fully or with modifications) in the revised report draft or ignored. Failure to reach consensus between the SP and PRP may require additional levels of peer review by other pathologists as covered in the section below on "Resolution of Disagreements."

Key Study Elements to Review

The PRP carries several responsibilities during the review. This section will highlight key elements the PRP must focus on to maximize their contribution to quality of the pathology data. The PRP will ultimately be working toward consensus on these items with the SP.

COMPLETENESS OF THE PATHOLOGY REVIEW (TARGET TISSUES IDENTIFIED)

The scope of the PRP's review will vary by the study type and may be adjusted as deemed necessary by the PRP within the guidelines of the appropriate peer review SOP.

In general, peer reviews examine all tissues from 30% of high-dose animals, tissues from control animals as deemed necessary by the PRP, all tissues from early deaths, target tissues from all animals of all dose groups, and all gross findings as well as preneoplastic and neoplastic changes (Morton et al., 2010). For this purpose, the "high-dose group" should be the highest-dose group with a sufficient number of surviving animals. The baseline review for short-term general toxicity studies may be more streamlined since few neoplasms typically will need to be reviewed. Specific options for peer review of different study types for different species are detailed below under "Core Planning Considerations."

For the reviewed tissues, the PRP must ensure that the SP's review was complete and that all treatment-related findings in target tissues were identified, diagnosed, and graded appropriately and consistently. The review includes assessment of whether key threshold levels (e.g., the no observed effect level [NOEL] or no observed adverse effect level [NOAEL]) were also properly assigned.

CONSISTENT USE OF DIAGNOSTIC TERMINOLOGY AND ASSIGNMENT OF SEVERITY GRADES

Consistent and proper use of diagnostic terminology is foundational for broad acceptance and confidence in histopathology diagnoses and their interpretation. During the primary evaluation of a large and/or complex study, the SP may drift inadvertently over time in their use of a histopathologic diagnosis and/or assignment of severity scores. The PRP should also be sensitive to potential shifts in diagnostic thresholds by the SP. In addition, the SP will routinely encounter changes that are variations in tissue morphology, tissue artifacts, and spontaneous background lesions. Therefore, an SP may choose to not record an observation (sometimes referred to as "thresholding") as a means to avoid creating an overly complex data set with the appearance of differences when none exists (Long & Hardisty, 2012). The review of control animals during a peer review helps the PRP understand the spectrum of changes that may be "thresholded out" by the SP. The PRP is perfectly situated during their focused and time-limited review to identify possible shifts in diagnostic nomenclature, severity scores, and/or thresholding.

APPROPRIATE INTERPRETATION AND CORRELATION IN THE PATHOLOGY REPORT

Once the SP generates the preliminary histopathology data set, the findings are categorized with respect to their relationship to the test article—usually as treatment related, procedure related, or incidental. These decisions should be clearly articulated in the draft pathology report. The SP typically should comment in the pathology report regarding whether or not a specific microscopic finding is adverse or nonadverse. It is essential in the peer review that the PRP ensures the appropriateness of the SP's interpretation of the findings because treatment-related histopathologic changes are the basis of the dose level assignments for setting dose/exposure levels (e.g., NOEL, NOAEL) used by regulators as a snapshot of a test article's potential for toxicity.

Once the slide review is complete, the PRPs then review the draft report to ensure it accurately describes the treatment-related microscopic observations and the dose groups affected, and that it adequately correlates the microscopic findings to other study parameters such as gross necropsy findings, organ weights, clinical signs, clinical pathology changes, morbidity, or early death. This report review is critical to ensure that ultimately, in the integrated study report, anatomic pathology changes are accurately conveyed and that the NOEL or NOAEL are assigned to the proper dose level if histopathologic changes contribute to that assignment.

Core Planning Considerations

As highlighted previously, the PRP is solely responsible for planning and executing the pathology peer review. The specific peer review process will vary based on the type of study, study design, number of animals, and study objective(s), but the PRP has wide latitude to examine whatever materials they feel are necessary to properly verify that tissue changes have been properly identified, diagnosed, and graded and to confirm threshold values (e.g., the NOAEL). In general, minimum requirements for pathology peer review reflecting current best practice differ for two different study designs: (1) general toxicity studies and (2) carcinogenicity studies. The STP recommendations for the specific pathology materials to be reviewed for various study types are listed in Table 26.1.

Peer reviews for certain specialty studies, such as tissue cross-reactivity (TCR) studies (i.e., ex vivo immunohistochemical studies for target binding of antibody or antibody-like pharmaceuticals) or investigative toxicity studies, may incorporate an alternative peer review design, and these are also discussed briefly below.

Finally, all peer reviews should include, as stated previously, review of the Pathology Report to insure agreement between the PRP and SP with regard to study findings and interpretations.

GENERAL TOXICITY STUDIES

FULL TISSUE LIST ("COMPLETE") REVIEW It is generally accepted that all diagnoses from all protocol-required tissues should be reviewed from a specified subset of animals as part of a routine pathology peer review to ensure the accuracy of the pathology diagnoses and that no subtle target organ changes were overlooked by the SP in the original evaluation. Full tissue examination is focused on a proportion of the high-dose animals (or some of the animals from the dose group that had at least a 50% survival rate, if the high-dose group had high mortality). However, the actual number of animals for which all tissues are reviewed varies, depending on the type of study and the experienced

judgment of the PRP. Though not typically undertaken, in some cases, certain tissues are sent for review to a subject matter expert for that organ or system (e.g., brain, spinal cord, ganglia, and nerves to a neuropathologist) to ensure that subtle findings are captured, while the remaining protocol-specified tissues are submitted to another PRP.

For rodent general toxicity studies with their large group sizes (usually 10 or more per sex per study), the STP recommends reviewing all tissues from at least 30% of the animals in the high-dose group (see Table 26.1). The U.S. National Toxicology Program (NTP), to achieve their specific purposes (see section below, "NTP Review Process"), currently recommends that 60% of the animals in subchronic toxicity studies (i.e., noncarcinogenicity studies) should undergo a complete review. In some instances, the PRP may decide during the review that they should review more animals than initially planned. The PRP should always extend the review as necessary to be confident that all target organs have been identified.

Nonrodent studies use many fewer animals per group (usually two to five per sex per study) when compared to rodent studies. Because of the smaller group sizes and greater individual animal variability, advice regarding the number of nonrodents for which all tissues should be reviewed has varied over time. For example, in the previous edition of this chapter, the recommended numbers for review were 75% for dogs and 100% for nonhuman primates (NHPs). STP currently recommends that peer review be undertaken for all tissues in at least 50% of the animals (minimum of two per sex) of the high-dose group.

TARGET ORGAN REVIEW Target organs are those organs identified by the SP with presumptive test article–related anatomic changes or findings. As was the case with the complete review above, the strategy for reviewing target organs varies with the preference of the PRP and sometimes the organization. For example, the STP recommends that all target tissues be examined from all control animals and all animals in the highest dose group lacking the treatment-related finding to confirm the threshold value (Morton et al., 2010). They further suggest that in some rodent studies, examination of target tissues in a subset

TABLE 26.1   STP Recommendations for Materials to Be Reviewed in a Pathology Peer Review of a Regulatory-Type Toxicity Study

Study type	Complete review of microscopic slides of all protocol organs	Review of microscopic slides of target organs	Control animals	Microscopic slides of tumors
Rodent general toxicity	30% of the high-dose animals per sex	• ≥50% of animals from affected dose groups to characterize the finding • All animals from the highest group lacking the finding[a]	All target organs	All tumors[b]
Nonrodent general toxicity	One-half of the high dose animals per sex (minimum of two animals)	• All animals from affected dose groups • All animals from the highest group lacking the finding[a]	All target organs	All tumors[b]
Rodent two-year carcinogenicity	10% of the high-dose animals per sex	• Treatment-related neoplastic findings: All target organs from all dose groups • Treatment-related nonneoplastic findings: 30% of the affected animals to characterize the finding, and all animals from the highest dose group lacking the finding[a]	All target organs for treatment-related neoplastic and nonneoplastic findings	All tumors
Mouse six-month carcinogenicity in genetically modified mice	All animals from five high-dose animals per sex	• As above for two-year rodent carcinogenicity	As above for two-year rodent carcinogenicity	All tumors

[a] Examination of all animals from the highest dose group lacking a treatment-related finding is to verify the no effect level (NOEL) for the test article.

[b] Tumors will be rare in general toxicity studies (≤1 year), but tumor diagnoses should typically be peer reviewed in all studies whether treatment related or not.

All Studies: Review of data as needed such as in-life data (body weight, food consumption, clinical signs, mortality, clinical pathology) and other postmortem data (organ weights, gross observations) in order to assess the diagnostic interpretations in the draft and final pathology report.

Adapted from Morton D., et al.: Recommendations for pathology peer review, Toxicol Pathol 38(7):1118–1127, 2010. Peer review pathologists can adapt these recommendations according to their specific institutional SOPs and their needs in order to properly verify the conclusions of the pathology report.

of high-dose animals (50% or more) may be sufficient to confirm the findings (See Table 26.1). The NTP has similar guidelines but requires that all diagnoses for all target organs be reviewed. Reviewing the target organs in all dose groups can provide a greater degree of confidence that the incidence, range of severity grades, and threshold value (e.g., NOEL or NOAEL) have been accurately determined.

If the study includes recovery groups or multiple-phase (i.e., interim and terminal or terminal and recovery) necropsies, the recommendations for target organ review in animals from all phases are the same as in the main necropsy of the study. Since many protocols have only a high-dose and control group in the recovery phase, the number of target organs to be reviewed is significantly lower at this time point. Very few organizations promote the complete review of any animals in the recovery groups since the main reason for these groups is to see if the previously diagnosed treatment-related changes have persisted or not, and if so to what degree (i.e., full or partial or no reversal). However, it should be noted that in the case of delayed onset changes that are related to treatment, it would be likely that the full spectrum of changes would not be captured in the review if only the target tissues identified by the SP at the terminal necropsy are examined by the PRP. In such cases, the design of the peer review should be guided by other indicators as warranted, including in-life clinical signs, ancillary pathology findings (e.g., gross changes, organ weights, hematologic, and/or serum chemistry values), or nature of the test article (epigenetic target, covalent inhibitors, prolonged tissue half-life, etc.).

CONTROL ANIMALS The recommendations for complete review of control animals are more varied than those for animals in the high-dose group. Reviewing a percentage of concurrent control animals allows the PRP to get a sense for the criteria used by the SP, and to appreciate the incidence and severity of background changes in the control groups. The STP in its recommendations states that the decision to review all protocol-specified tissues in a subset of control animals should be determined by the PRP (Morton et al., 2010). The determination should be based on the review of the pathology data tables, microscopic findings in treated animals, and the requirements set forth in the applicable peer review SOP. In addition, the PRP's overall familiarity with the strain/age/sex of the animal species being reviewed should be considered. In a guest editorial in the same issue of *Toxicologic Pathology* that included the STP recommendations for peer review, a group of pathologists experienced in peer review and representing both regulatory agencies (which evaluate peer-reviewed studies) and contract research organizations (CROs) (which employ many SP and PRP) recommended that a routine complete review of a subset of concurrent control animals also be performed (Boorman et al., 2010). Since it assumed that there will be no treatment-related changes in the control group, fewer control animals need to be assessed relative to the high-dose group.

If a target organ is identified as having an increase or decrease in the incidence and/or severity of a background change, it becomes important to assure that the data are accurate in this respect. In this case, the suspected target tissues may be reviewed in all control animals at the PRP's discretion.

LIFETIME (TWO-YEAR) CARCINOGENICITY STUDIES IN WILD-TYPE RODENTS

Peer review of two-year rodent carcinogenicity studies, as for general toxicity studies, also includes complete review of all organs from a subset of high-dose animals and review of non-neoplastic target organs. However, the percentage of animals and organs to be evaluated is lower because the total number of animals per group in these studies is much greater (typically 60 per sex per group) than in a general toxicity study. For complete tissue review, the STP suggests that all organs from 10% of the animals in the high-dose group per sex are sufficient (Morton et al., 2010). Nonneoplastic target organs are handled much the same as they are in general toxicity studies (see Table 26.1). The most important aspect of the peer review of a two-year rodent carcinogenicity is review of the various tumor diagnoses, both to ensure diagnostic accuracy for individual neoplasms and to verify which tumors are related to administration of the test article versus which tumors represent spontaneous age-related lesions (See Table 26.1). Once the SP and PRP have reached agreement on tumor diagnoses, the PRP in consultation with the SP and study statistician determine which tumors should be combined (i.e., benign and malignant tumors of the same histotype) for the statistical analysis phase of the study.

Both the NTP and the STP (Morton et al., 2010) recommend that all tumors diagnosed from all dose groups (including controls) should be examined. The European Medicines Agency (EMA) recommends that at least 10% of all tumors be examined (EMA, 2002). While the general consensus is clear that all the neoplastic changes diagnosed by the SP should be reviewed, the recommendation regarding possible preneoplastic proliferative lesions is less uniform. If the peer review only includes neoplastic changes, then hyperplasic changes presumed to be intermediate (i.e., preneoplastic) steps are not being verified; this omission may limit the ability to relate findings along the spectrum from hyperplastic to neoplastic diagnoses to test article exposure. Following the presumed course of tumor progression can be especially problematic for endocrine tumors, where neoplasms exhibit a continuum with few morphological differences from hyperplasia (often a nonneoplastic proliferative state) to atypical hyperplasia (usually a preneoplastic change) and to adenoma (a benign tumor). Accordingly, diagnostic verification by the PRP must be undertaken using generally accepted criteria, such as those published by the INHAND initiative (Brändli-Baiocco et al., 2018). In general, it is highly recommended that all nonneoplastic proliferative changes (i.e., diagnoses of "hyperplasia" or "atypical hyperplasia") be reviewed in an organ in which test article–related neoplasia has been detected, and this aspect of the peer review is the basis of the recommendation to review all target organs where a suspected treatment-related neoplasm is diagnosed. However, peer review of common proliferative changes (e.g., endometrial hyperplasia in mice and adrenal gland medullary hyperplasia in rats) with no evidence of association to treatment and dose generally adds little to the value of the review or the final pathology raw data, so review of these and similar common background findings should be left to the discretion of the PRP.

SIX-MONTH MOUSE CARCINOGENICITY STUDIES IN GENETICALLY ENGINEERED MICE

For six-month carcinogenicity studies using genetically modified mice, the STP recommends at least five of the high-dose animals/sex be subject to complete review (Morton et al., 2010). The STP further suggests that for six-month mouse carcinogenicity studies with a positive control group (i.e., a cohort in which a material known to induce tumors in the model is given at a proven carcinogenic dose), a minimum of all neoplasms in expected target organs (e.g., generally lung and spleen in the commonly used rasH2 model (Paranjpe et al., 2019)) should be reviewed as well.

In either two-year lifetime studies or six-month alternative carcinogenicity studies, the authors' recommendations follow those of the NTP and the STP. At minimum, all diagnoses of neoplasia by the SP should be reviewed in all dose groups, including controls.

TISSUE CROSS-REACTIVITY STUDIES (EX VIVO IMMUNOHISTOCHEMISTRY FOR TARGET EXPRESSION)

Tissue cross-reactivity (TCR) studies present a special case for pathology peer review. These studies are conducted ex vivo by performing immunohistochemistry (IHC) with a monoclonal antibody (mAb) or similar test article. The purpose of a TCR study is to screen panels of human and/or animal tissues for predicted and unexpected binding of the mAb test article to assist in characterizing potential sites in patients at which unwanted mAb binding and activity might pose a hazard (Leach et al., 2010). The purposes of the peer review for TCR studies are (1) to verify that the IHC method is valid and (2) to reach consensus with the SP (or other nonpathologist investigator) regarding the staining pattern in the panel of organs/tissues (*Protein Pharmaceutical Agents*; Vol 2, Chap 6).

No published recommendations are currently available to guide peer review of TCR studies. However, in alignment with the principles outlined above, the authors judge that peer review of a TCR study should include the following specific features:

(1) IHC Method Validation Review: Review all slides containing positive or negative control material. Control material may be tissue sections of organs or cell lines (natural or engineered) that normally express high levels of the mAb target (positive control) or that have no expression of the target (negative control). The TCR design also usually incorporates IHC staining with a positive control mAb, the negative control mAb, and one of several (usually two to three) concentrations of the test article mAb. Other controls may be included as determined by the study protocol (e.g., sections labeled with the ubiquitous endothelial cell marker anti-CD31 to confirm that tissue preservation was suitable), which the PRP may evaluate if they deem it is warranted.

(2) Staining Pattern Review: From each tissue type in each species (human and animal), at a minimum, one slide should be reviewed with the test article mAb applied at the highest concentration. As with peer review of conventional toxicity studies, the PRP should have the flexibility to also examine additional sections, as needed, to verify the conclusions of the study.

(3) Review of the draft TCR report to ensure agreement with the SP on the validity of the staining method as well as the overall tissue staining pattern and its interpretation.

Pathology peer review can also be conducted on other GLP-compliant study types that may include pathology endpoints. These include developmental and reproductive toxicity studies, juvenile toxicity studies, and studies designed to investigate a specific safety issue. Because of the variety of study, design-specific recommendations are not available, but PRPs can utilize the general principles described above to design the peer review paradigm for these specialized studies.

REVIEW OF THE DRAFT PATHOLOGY REPORT

For all in vivo toxicity studies in which pathology findings are peer reviewed, the PRP should also review the SP's draft pathology report to reach consensus on the interpretation of the key study data. In this review, the PRP will assess all aspects of the proposed interpretation including the following:

- Causes of death, if unscheduled death or euthanasia occurred in the course of the in-life phase;
- Target organs of toxicity;
- Integration, as warranted, with other data (in-life data, clinical pathology, etc.) to accurately describe the overall toxicity profile and to put the pathology findings in context;
- Threshold values (e.g., NOEL or NOAEL or both); and
- Decisions on adversity of test article–related findings.

The STP recommends that threshold values (e.g., NOAEL) generally should be included only in the fully integrated study report and not the pathology report (Kerlin, 2016), so other scientists besides the SP and PRP may be involved in setting such values. In some cases, the larger team also may decide that adversity calls made by the SP and PRP will be communicated only in the integrated study report.

3.3. Resolution of Disagreements during Contemporaneous Peer Review

Initial differences of opinion between the SP and PRP during contemporaneous pathology peer review are a part of the iterative process of refining preliminary pathology diagnoses. In the vast majority of contemporaneous peer reviews, differences between diagnoses and severity grades assigned by the SP and PRP are fairly modest and can be resolved readily during the consensus-building discussions between them. These deliberations may be verbal (e.g., by online video exchange or telephone) or written (usually an exchange of emails). They may involve real-time discussion of projected microscope fields or still images, or exchange of annotated images in emailed documents, or written descriptions of key features. As long as the SP and PRP reach agreement on the appropriate histopathologic diagnoses and their interpretations, the organization of the consensus-building process is fairly flexible.

However, sometimes there may be differences of opinion that cannot be resolved during the contemporaneous peer review. It is acceptable for the two pathologists to not achieve consensus on a diagnosis that does not have a significant impact on the overall interpretation or conclusion of the study. In such cases, the usual course is for the SP to keep the original diagnosis. However, for diagnoses that are critical to the interpretation of the study, the SP and PRP typically will consider one or more of the following options to develop consensus in a stepwise fashion: (1) informal consultation with other experienced pathologists, (2) formal (documented) consultation with other subject matter experts who are pathologists or nonpathologists, or (3) convening a PWG of experienced pathologists to review and provide a final consensus or majority diagnosis. The process to resolve differences should be defined in SOPs and/or protocol amendments. A useful wording for such additional tie-breaking review is that "Differences of opinion may be resolved through consultation with other pathologists and/or subject matter experts or by convening a PWG" (Fikes et al., 2015). For a contemporaneous peer review, these additional levels of review also must take place before the histopathology diagnoses are finalized.

Informal (Undocumented) Consultation With Other Experienced Pathologist(s)

Informal consultation during the contemporaneous peer review typically involves seeking input from one or more mutually agreed colleagues and does not typically involve any documentation. It is quick and quite commonly done in pathology groups worldwide. There are no specific rules, and this may be conducted using actual glass slides, real-time projections of slides mounted on one pathologist's microscope stage, scanned images, or printed pictures. This approach may involve seeking input on an individual finding to obtain answers to one or more questions such as whether there is a finding, what terminology should be used in the diagnosis, what severity grade should be assigned, have they seen such a finding before, and if they are aware of published references for further study of the change and its interpretation, etc. Informal consultation is also helpful to rule out bias when considering a subtle finding proposed as a potential outcome of test article exposure. Consultation may be done by informing the consulting pathologist about the potential finding they will be evaluating or by just asking for their impression of the tissue (i.e., without providing such information in advance).

Pathologists typically learn based on what they have seen in prior studies, and informal consultation is a valuable learning experience for everyone involved. Generally, the SP and PRP will reach consensus after utilizing the additional information obtained through informal consultation. The consulted pathologist(s) may have experience with the proposed target organ or a similar finding or with the class of compounds and thus are providing input based on their experience. The consulted pathologist(s) may not only provide their opinion about the finding and its interpretation but also share experience gained from other studies and/or published literature. They may ask questions regarding the study (such as species, breed/stock/strain, sex, age, compound class, pharmacology, toxicokinetics, clinical pathology data, in-life findings, etc.) to determine appropriate terminology, and these questions may help the SP and PRP to pursue relevant information that they might not have considered. The SP and PRP will consider the consulted pathologist's input to inform themselves, but the SP and PRP are not obligated to agree with the consulted pathologist or accept their opinion.

Formal (Documented) Consultation With Subject Matter Expert Pathologists and Nonpathologists

Formal consultation is not a routine part of the pathology peer review for most toxicity studies. The purpose of formal consultation is to seek expert input on a specific question(s) regarding one or more study findings and/or their interpretation and then record the expert opinions as a means of increasing confidence in the final data set. Common questions addressed by subject matter experts include the relationship of a finding to treatment, whether the change is adverse or nonadverse, the impact of the finding on the overall conclusion of the study, the predicted human relevance (if any), and possible investigative approaches for future studies. More than one subject matter expert may need to be approached if the lesion in question is very subtle or seldom (or never before) seen.

Consultants with subject matter expertise are specialists in the topic of interest. Most are veterinary medical or medical pathologists or occasionally nonmedically trained comparative pathologists from academia, government, or industry, but some are nonpathologists with knowledge of the target organ or test article class. The type of discussions during the formal consultation may be similar to those that take place during an informal consultation. Formal consultation is often conducted at the request of the sponsor or SP and can occur during either a contemporaneous peer review or a retrospective peer review. It is helpful to have the SP and PRP present during the formal consultation as they can help identify any subtle findings for the consultant's review and answer the consultant's questions about the study. Based on the consultation, the SP may modify the histopathologic diagnoses and interpretations in the draft report. It is important to note that the SP is not obligated to accept the consultant's opinion and need not modify the draft report.

Formal consultation typically involves documentation that the opinion of a subject matter expert was actively sought. Such records could take the form of the expert's signature on the peer review statement, thereby documenting consensus with the SP and PRP. Alternatively, the expert may issue an individual report of their opinion (discussed below under "Retrospective Peer Review"), the elements of which might be included in the pathology report (by SP-initiated modifications of their original findings and/or by including the expert's signed opinion as an appendix to the pathology report). If consensus regarding a question that will impact the study conclusions is still not reached between the SP and PRP following the formal consultation, then a PWG may need to be considered.

Pathology Working Group

PWGs also are not a routine part of the peer review process for toxicity studies. The purpose of a PWG is to provide an independent opinion on a specific disagreement between the SP and PRP and/or to address a particular question(s) regarding study results that may impact overall interpretation the study.

PWGs are useful to address questions that may be of potential concern by regulatory agencies, to compare results from multiple studies that may have been conducted and evaluated by different laboratories and/or pathologists, for in-depth review of complex or unique lesions, and for mediation of persistent discrepancies between the SP and PRP. PWGs can be convened to discuss an individual finding (e.g., to define if a change is neoplastic or non-neoplastic) or multiple types of findings in one or several target organs. Commonly, PWGs are called on to consider various aspects such as the diagnostic criteria and their application, the incidence and range of severity grades for findings, and their relationship (if any) to treatment and dose.

A PWG typically is composed of five voting members (sometimes ranging up to seven or nine) and a nonvoting PWG chairperson to coordinate the review and record the minutes and vote counts. PWG members are usually veterinary medical or medical pathologists or occasionally nonmedically trained comparative pathologists with expertise in the topic of interest, and may be from academia, government, or industry. Other interested parties/observers (e.g., one or more sponsor representatives) may be present during the review but have no vote in setting the final majority or consensus diagnoses. If available when the PWG convenes, the SP and PRP are generally invited to serve as voting members since they can help identify any subtle findings for the PWG review and answer the PWG's questions about the background of the study.

Pathology Working Group Procedure

The following is an example of a routinely used PWG procedure. The specific organization and procedure may vary depending on the study type and specific issue. The Chairperson organizes the PWG, identifies the expert panel members in consultation with the sponsor of the PWG, reviews all relevant data and study results before convening the PWG (thus making him or her ineligible to serve as a voting member), selects the materials (typically all sections with the diagnosis of interest and sometimes normal sections as needed to understand the background range), coordinates and prepares the data for the PWG, and ultimately chairs the session. Typically, the panel discusses the diagnostic criteria at the beginning of the PWG prior to examination of the coded slides. In most cases, all slides are then coded, and the PWG members do not know the diagnoses or treatment group during their review, discussion, and voting, though occasionally an initial unblinded review can be considered to establish the diagnostic criteria. Each PWG member reviews the coded slides on their own and records their diagnosis, severity grade, and any additional notes on worksheets provided by the chairperson. After the initial examination of the slides and initial discussion of their diagnoses, there is an option to reexamine some of the slides again. The chairperson then calls for a vote on each slide and records the consensus (if all agree) or majority vote as the final diagnosis for each slide (Ward et al., 1995). After the PWG voting is concluded, final diagnoses are established and cannot be changed. The chairperson then breaks the code and shares the outcome of the voting with the PWG; depending on the size of the slide set, this sharing may be delayed until the next day. The PWG often then discusses the implications of any findings that are subtle or contentious and how they may impact the overall study interpretation and conclusion. Most SPs find that this additional round of review and discussion is particularly helpful to them as they adjust their report narrative. The chairperson prepares a draft PWG report (typically including the SP's original diagnoses and the consensus diagnoses of the PWG along with the PWG's interpretations and conclusions). The PWG members review this draft, edit as needed to achieve a document acceptable to all signatories, and subsequently sign the piece; this document ultimately will end as an appendix to the pathology report (if submitted as part of a contemporaneous peer review) or a separate element of the study file (if undertaken as a retrospective peer review). Based on the PWG contemporaneous review, the SP may modify the draft pathology report, so including the SP as a voting member of the PWG is particularly helpful in this regard. It is important to note that the SP is not obligated to accept the PWG's opinion.

3.4. Documentation of Contemporaneous Peer Review

When peer review is conducted prior to establishing the pathology raw data in the final signed pathology report (contemporaneous peer review), the intent to perform a peer review should be stated in the study protocol or plan.

This intent may be declared in the original protocol or may be added later in a protocol amendment depending on when the decision to perform a peer review is reached. The general methods of the contemporaneous peer review should be outlined in an SOP, but the specific materials to be examined for a given study should be chosen by the PRP and then recorded in the peer review statement (sometimes called a peer review certificate or memorandum). This peer review statement typically is drafted by the PRP at the completion of the peer review but is not signed until after the pathology report has been finalized and the PRP has confirmed that the consensus diagnoses and interpretation resulting from the peer review are reflected in the final report; that said, some sponsors prefer that the statement be signed at another stage of the study (see below for options).

The peer review statement of a contemporaneous peer review functions as a record of the review process and does not include specific diagnoses or interpretations. Pathology notes and interpretations generated by the PRP do not need to be retained since only the SP generates the raw data. Accordingly, the peer review statement does not represent pathology raw data but merely verifies the quality of the raw data and their interpretation as set forth by the SP in the pathology report.

Elements of the Peer Review Statement

The peer review statement generally is a short document, typically running one or two pages, that includes the following information documenting the peer review process:

- Identification of the study (by title and study numbers);
- The microscopic specimens examined, including the following:
  - The specific animal numbers and groups (test article and dose or vehicle) for which all tissues were reviewed—this information often is segregated by the timing of the necropsy (e.g., recovery vs. terminal) and/or sex,
  - Any specific potential target organs that were reviewed and in which groups they were reviewed, and
  - Any special procedures (e.g., IHC stains, ultrastructural images) evaluated in

addition to routinely prepared (hematoxylin and eosin–stained tissue sections);

- A statement that the draft and/or final pathology report (narrative and data tables) was reviewed;
- Any ancillary data or reports that were reviewed (such as clinical signs, gross necropsy data, organ weights, body weight data, clinical pathology data, biodistribution or toxicokinetic data, the draft and/or final clinical pathology report, etc.) in order to fully understand the conclusions of the SP; and
- For some organizations, the date(s) when the peer review was conducted, which usually are different from the signature date on the final peer review statement (see below).

The peer review statement should conclude with a clear declaration that the PRP is in agreement with the diagnoses and interpretations of the SP with respect to the materials that were peer reviewed and conclude with the PRP's signature (accompanied by the date signed and a byline giving the PRP's name and professional qualifications). At the institution's discretion, an optional signature line also can be included for the SP to attest that the content of the peer review statement accurately reflects the outcome of the peer review process. Addition of the SP signature on the statement provides a further means of documenting that the two pathologists are in agreement regarding the pathology raw data.

Timing of the Signature on the Peer Review Statement

The timing of the signature(s) on the peer review statement varies among test facilities and study sponsors.

- At the earliest, the peer review statement may be signed after completion of the peer review process, when the SP and PRP have reached consensus, and any changes to the preliminary data and draft report resulting from the peer review have been made, but before quality assurance (QA) audit of the proposed final report has been undertaken.

Although convenient, signing the peer review statement immediately after the peer review process has been completed only documents consensus for the draft pathology raw data and report and not agreement on the contents of the final signed pathology report, which establishes the actual pathology raw data for the study. Any changes to the preliminary data and interpretations made as a result of the QA audit would not necessarily be reviewed and/or affirmed by the PRP. As such, many institutions have processes whereby the signature on the peer review statement occurs at a later time:

- After the draft pathology report has completed the audit, the PRP signature documents consensus on any changes that were made to the draft data as a result of the audit.
- After the final pathology report has been signed and dated by the SP, the PRP's signature on the peer review statement documents agreement with the final pathology raw data and interpretations as recorded in the signed report.

When the two pathologists have not reached consensus at the end of the peer review process, additional peer review measures (already described above) may include consultation of another expert (formal or informal) or convening a PWG. Informal consultations generally are not documented, while formal review by one or more additional pathologists and/or subject matter experts and/or a PWG is documented for inclusion in the study file or report. Documents for these additional levels of contemporaneous peer review may be signed and dated using any of the timing options described above for the PRP, but typically, documentation for these additional rounds of peer review are signed before the final pathology report has been signed and dated by the SP.

3.5. Peer Review: Retrospective Peer Review

General Process

Retrospective peer reviews, either by a single pathologist, a specialist/expert pathologist, or as part of the PWG process, are undertaken after the completion of a study (i.e., after the pathology raw data for the study have already been generated by the SP's signature). Unlike contemporaneous peer review, retrospective peer reviews require specific documentation of the changes in histopathologic diagnoses and interpretation that will be made to existing pathology raw data. These changes are implemented by amending the original pathology report and study report.

Retrospective peer reviews can be requested in one of three circumstances. The first is when a specific issue regarding a target tissue and/or one or more diagnostic criteria is identified later in the development program, perhaps after evaluation of tissues from later studies with the same test article or based on literature reports from similar agents. The second is when unexpected questions arise after a study is finalized (e.g., in response to a regulatory query) and additional work is needed to clarify the issue. Another instance is in the process of "due diligence" after the acquisition of a compound from a third party to verify the conclusions of the SP.

The process for a retrospective peer review is like that described above for a contemporaneous peer review, with one important difference: all changes in the study data must be fully documented, and an audit trail of the changes must be maintained. Since the study has already been finalized, a retrospective peer review also requires preparation and signing of both an amended pathology report once there is consensus between the SP and PRP to incorporate the changes to the pathology raw data and study conclusions. (An amended study report, prepared by the study director, will be generated once the amended pathology report has been completed; in a few institutions, the study director and SP both sign the amended study report.) If the SP is no longer available and/or if there is disagreement between the retrospective PRP and the SP concerning the final data set and conclusions, a PWG process may be used to resolve these differences.

When consensus is not reached during a retrospective peer review, a PWG is necessary to conclude the review process. The PWG is conducted as described previously, after which a stand-alone PWG report is produced to document each diagnosis that was reviewed. In such cases, the PWG report will include the SP's original diagnosis, the consensus or majority diagnosis of the PWG as determined by coded review and discussion, and a detailed description of the diagnostic criteria and interpretation

with respect to the specific issue being examined. If the SP is available and in agreement with the PWG's suggested changes, the PWG report can be used by the SP to prepare an amended pathology report.

Retrospective Review by an Expert

As discussed under contemporaneous peer review, occasionally, a sponsor or test facility may request an independent subject matter expert to formally review specific finding(s) from a study, and such requests may be made retrospectively as well. The subject matter expert is generally well recognized as possessing special knowledge in the biology and pathology of the organ that is being investigated. A retrospective expert report offers opinions following the reexamination of selected findings in a study. This may be the result of reexamination of the organ from all animals in the study, reexamination of organ from all groups for a specific sex, or reexamination of organs only from those animals in which the finding was previously diagnosed being reviewed.

The retrospective expert report should explain the reasoning for the review and logically justify the expert's conclusions. Some expert reports only contain a narrative and summary incidence tables, while others will include a detailed tabulation of the expert's diagnosis for each tissue examined. Generation of this retrospective expert opinion results, when signed and dated, in the creation of a second report that may or may not support the diagnoses and conclusions of the original finalized pathology report. Some regulatory agencies accept expert reports and use them in their deliberations. However, when there are significant differences between the expert report and the original pathology report, it is sometimes difficult for regulatory agencies to resolve these differences. In such cases, a PWG should be convened to eliminate the discordance when the data and interpretations of the expert opinion review vary significantly from those of the original pathology report. For example, in 1994, the US EPA issued Pesticide Regulation Notice 94–5: "Requests for Re-considerations of Carcinogenicity Peer Review Decisions Based on Changes in Pathology Diagnoses (EPA, 1994)." The EPA stated that the use of a PWG should be part of every reevaluation of pathology data. They believed that a procedure for obtaining consensus in pathology reevaluation improves the quality of decision-making in classifying pesticide chemicals having carcinogenic potential. The EPA further stated that unless the reevaluation has been conducted using a peer review/PWG procedure, they will base their regulatory evaluations and decisions on the pathology data in the original report.

4. NATIONAL TOXICOLOGY PROGRAM REVIEW PROCESS

The U.S. NTP is an interagency public health partnership of the U.S. National Institutes of Health, U.S. FDA, and U.S. Centers for Disease Control and Prevention (CDC) that characterizes potential hazards of chemical and nonchemical agents of human importance. The NTP conducts or sponsors toxicity studies in rodents on non-pharmaceutical chemicals and occasionally physical agents (e.g., electromagnetic radiation) that may be present in the environment and pose a potential risk to human health. Experiments range from short-term dose range-finding screens to two-year carcinogenicity bioassays to special toxicity bioassays. Most but not all studies are performed in mice or rats.

The NTP conducts contemporaneous quality assessment pathology peer review on all studies that are conducted in their bioassay testing program before the final pathology and study reports (and thus the pathology raw data) are finalized (Sills, 2019). The NTP pathology review process is more extensive than that generally performed for industry-sponsored studies that will be submitted to regulatory authorities. In addition to the contemporaneous pathology peer review steps performed by industry, the NTP peer review process for every study includes a detailed audit of the pathology specimens (necropsy records, paraffin blocks, slides [including special stains], and residual formalin-fixed ["wet"] tissues) and also a PWG review (usually by panels of seven or more voting pathologists with additional nonvoting pathologist observers) before the final pathology data and interpretation are published in a publicly available technical report. Residual wet tissue is examined to make sure all potential gross lesions have been trimmed in, that all organs have been properly incised or opened,

and that animal-specific identifiers (e.g., tail tattoos) match the identification on the wet tissue bags and on the necropsy records. Slides and blocks are examined to make sure that they are present and accounted for, to check for complete and accurate labeling, and for proper sectioning of blocks and proper preparation of slides.

After the audit of the gross pathology specimens, a contemporaneous peer review of the tissue sections for all organs is done by the primary quality assessment PRP, who is an independent contract pathologist who has had no prior interaction with the SP (another independent contractor) concerning the study. The PRP reviews all the organs and lesions. After the PRP has examined all indicated slides, he or she will prepare a peer review quality assessment report, which differs somewhat in organization from the peer review statements produced for a typical industry-sponsored study. The NTP peer review quality assessment report includes a brief narrative summary of the original study results as well as the results of the peer review by the PRP. Any differences of opinion that occur between the SP and the PRP are shown to the NTP pathologist (a third pathologist) assigned to the study. The NTP pathologist examines the slides and resolves the differences between the SP and PRP. After the NTP pathologist has addressed all the differences of opinion, the PRP and NTP pathologist decide together which slides to take to the NTP PWG.

The purpose of an NTP PWG is to confirm the diagnoses of potential treatment-related effects, to resolve any remaining differences between the SP and PRP, and to harmonize diagnostic nomenclature and criteria. Representative examples of all treatment-related lesions are examined by the PWG along with any unresolved differences and unusual or uncommon lesions. The final diagnoses in NTP studies published in the NTP Technical Report for the study thus represent a consensus among multiple, independent pathologists: the SP, the PRP, the NTP pathologist, and where needed the many voting PWG participants. The PWG Chairperson prepares a final combined peer review quality assessment/PWG report which is maintained in the study file at the NTP Archives, thereby providing detailed and fully transparent documentation of the NTP pathology peer review process.

5. REGULATORY ASPECTS OF PATHOLOGY PEER REVIEW

The concept and practice of pathology peer review was not an original consideration at the time during which the first GLP regulations were drafted in the 1970s and 1980s. The practice of pathology peer review originated later as a QC process at the behest of the global pathology profession. This tool was invented based on the practices used to refine histopathologic diagnoses and improve the quality of pathology data as performed in government research institutes (e.g., the NTP), pharmaceutical and chemical firms, and CROs. Best practices for pathology peer review have been honed over at least the last 30 years through the various global toxicologic pathology societies without a mandate by regulatory authorities, culminating in globally accepted practices that are used by pathology peer reviewers in most countries and geographic regions (Morton et al., 2010).

To date, the only government regulatory agency to comment, in the form of regulatory guidance, on contemporaneous pathology peer review is the European Agency for the Evaluation of Medicinal Products (EMEA, now supplanted by the European Medicines Agency [EMA]), specifically as it pertains to rodent two-year carcinogenicity studies. The Committee for Proprietary Medicinal Products (CPMP) included in their "Note for Guidance on Carcinogenic Potential" in 2002 (EMA, 2002) the statement that the following practices should be undertaken for such studies:

> *Peer review of slides is required for all identified target organs and for at least 10% of all tumours. A complete review of 10% of the animals in each group should also be performed. If more than one pathologist is involved more extensive peer review is needed to assure consistency. The peer review should be documented in raw data and in the study report. Board certification or equivalent should qualify pathologists.*

Aside from this EMEA guidance, and until recently, national regulatory authorities have been silent on specific peer review practices. However, in the last decade, pathology peer review in nonclinical studies in industry has received increased attention from some regulatory authorities or international consortia of regulators (e.g., the Organisation for Economic Co-operation and Development [OECD]). Specifically, two guidance documents have emerged, one from the OECD that was finalized in 2014, and the other proposed by the FDA that is still in draft form as of mid-2021 (following a public comment period in late 2019).

The OECD "Guidance on the GLP Requirements for Peer Review of Histopathology" (Guidance No. 16) first emerged in September 2014 and after feedback from outside stakeholders was finalized in December of that year (OECD, 2014). The OECD is an international, global, intergovernmental consortium of government officials from more than 30 countries that, among other functions, "meet[s] to coordinate and harmonize policies, discuss issues of mutual concern, and work together to respond to international problems." The stated purpose of the OECD guidance on histopathology peer review was "to provide guidance to pathologists, test facility management, study directors, and QA personnel on how the peer review of histopathology should be planned, managed, documented, and reported in order to meet GLP expectations and requirements." While much of the guidance is drawn from, and in line with, published professional best practices discussed previously (e.g., Morton et al., 2010), some of the sections are inconsistent with the best practices globally accepted by pathologists or are unclear. Specifically, the OECD recommendations on peer review documentation practices, when peer review is conducted prior to pathology data finalization (contemporaneous peer review), are not aligned with current best practices as devised and implemented by experienced PRPs.

As discussed above, globally endorsed best practice recommendations for pathology peer review do not suggest that specific changes to refine preliminary microscopic diagnoses that are made during the course of a contemporaneous peer review be documented or retained prior to finalization of the pathology report since the pathology raw data are established only when the pathology raw data have been signed. Therefore, best practice as devised by pathologists is that only the consensus/final diagnoses and none of the iterative adjustments need to be recorded when there is agreement between the SP and PRP. However, the OECD guidance, as stated principally in subsection 2.5, seems to disagree with this globally accepted best practice:

> 2.5 All correspondence regarding the histopathological evaluation of the slides used for peer review between the sponsor and representatives of the test facility and the PRP should be retained in the study file, including minutes of teleconferences between the sponsor and the test facility (OECD, 2014).

The definition of "all correspondence" has caused considerable confusion among the global toxicologic pathology community, so OECD issued a "frequently asked questions" document to clarify their expectations in March 2017 (OECD, 2017):

> The clarification is as follows: Correspondence refers to any communication that is needed to reconstruct how slides were selected and reviewed. This should include communications regarding the interpretation of any observations (preliminary or final) on adverse or nonadverse effects made during the review (OECD, 2017).

In 2015, an STP working group with international representation published a consensus view and interpretation regarding the 2014 OECD guidance on histopathology peer review (Fikes et al., 2015). In this publication, the authors provided line-by-line interpretation of the guidance, including for Section 2.5, regarding retention of correspondence. The pathology community maintained that "all" correspondence between the pathologists did not need be retained because "communications regarding preliminary observations (pathology diagnoses that are not "locked" or signed) and draft pathology interpretations would not be required to be maintained since these are pathology working notes" in accordance with the existing GLP regulations and definitions of pathology raw data. This publication was endorsed not only by the STP but also by 11 other global societies of toxicologic pathology as well as the ACVP.

Though this 2015 STP-generated publication by Fikes and colleagues occurred prior to the 2017 OECD clarification of what was meant by "all correspondence," the Fikes interpretation is still valid for the very common situation where the SP and PRP reach agreement by the end of the contemporaneous peer review process. When the SP and PRP are in agreement, retaining documentation of all discussions and correspondence would be cumbersome, impractical, and moreover totally unnecessary as such interim notes would not contribute to the reconstruction of the final pathology report. In contrast, if the SP and PRP cannot come to agreement on one or more findings in the study, mechanisms already in place, as detailed in each institution's peer review SOP (and reviewed above), should prove quite capable of documenting the means used to resolve the disagreements.

Following the OECD publications in 2014 and 2017, an additional regulatory document that proposes methodology to be used during pathology peer review appeared in August 2019. The FDA Office of Study Inspection and Surveillance posted a draft guidance on pathology peer review for public comment (FDA – CDER-OSIS, 2019), which represents the first time the FDA has commented on peer review practices. This question-and-answer draft guidance was intended to clarify the FDA's recommendations concerning the management, conduct, and especially the documentation of pathology peer review. Many of the documentation recommendations in the guidance mirrored the content in the OECD guidance, and thus exceeded the current expectations as stated in both the existing FDA GLP regulations and professional best practices among pathologists. The FDA received 30 formal comments on the draft guidance from individuals, corporations, and several global societies of toxicologic pathology. These comments from experienced PRPs noted (1) the potential issues arising if the draft guidance was implemented in its original form and (2) potential modifications to improve the usefulness of the FDA's proposal. As with all guidance, this FDA document is not binding on the FDA or the public (i.e., is not a legally enforceable regulation but rather a statement of current FDA thinking on the topic). It is not known when the guidance will be finalized or what form the final guidance will take.

The theme that is clearly emerging from the existing OECD guidance and the initial draft

FDA guidance is that regulatory authorities prefer increased transparency, supported by relevant documentation, of the interactions between the SP and PRP during contemporaneous peer review. This desire runs counter to current professional best practices for pathology peer review and does not acknowledge that the process of histopathologic diagnosis is an iterative process in which initial impressions need to undergo one or more additional rounds of refinement before an accurate final diagnosis can be rendered. Given these FDA and OECD perspectives, the regulatory environment on pathology peer review seems certain to evolve over the coming years. That said, hopefully these changes will be driven by constructive dialogue between the toxicologic pathology community and regulatory authorities, and adherence to science-based first principles regarding the definitions of histopathology raw data will prevail.

5.1. Regulations for Contemporaneous Pathology Peer Review in China and Japan

The regulation of contemporaneous pathology peer review in China and Japan is very similar. The China Food and Drug Administration (China) and the Pharmaceuticals and Medical Devices Agency (Japan) both require that the intent to perform a peer review be clearly stated in the original study protocol or a protocol amendment. They require that the peer review process as well as the reviewed samples and documents be recorded in detail and easily traceable. A process should be established to handle any discrepancies between the SP and PRP. If there are important changes in the SP's conclusions as a result of the peer review, they must be explained in the final pathology report. They also require that the name, affiliation, and qualifications of the PRP must be stated in the final pathology report.

As the result of these various regulatory guidance documents, sponsors and CROs in China and Japan and the laboratory QA units at the CROs have diverged in their interpretation of the degree of documentation required to provide the transparency desired by the regulatory authorities. The CRO practices range from no

retention of interim notes or worksheets (regarding agreement or differences concerning the tissues and diagnoses that were reviewed) to maintaining detailed worksheets in the study file (that provide complete documentation of the SP's initial findings, the PRP's comments, and the consensus diagnoses for each of the differences noted during the peer review).

6. USE OF DIGITAL/WHOLE-SLIDE IMAGES IN PATHOLOGY PEER REVIEW

With the maturation of high-resolution digital cameras, whole-slide imaging (WSI) technology, and high-speed data streaming to facilitate sharing and viewing digital images, it is now routine to use WSIs for informal consultation among pathologists. In addition, there is increasing use of WSIs in the formal peer review of non-GLP studies, especially for study materials that cannot be shipped between continents (e.g., slides with NHP tissue sections). The advantages of using WSIs are considered to be notable enough that some companies are only using WSIs for peer review of non-GLP studies, and there are now examples of WSI being used to facilitate PWGs; these advantages include the previously mentioned ease of moving and sharing images as well as greater field of view at the corresponding magnification, ease of image rotation, and flexibility to view two or more images simultaneously for comparison purposes (Bradley & Jacobsen, 2019). Potential disadvantages of peer review using WSI, such as slow data streaming speeds and insufficient resolution of features in the images, often can be overcome by simple technical improvements.

The approach for planning, managing, and documenting a pathology peer review using digital images largely follows those previously described when using tissue sections viewed through a microscope. The peer review would need to be documented in the protocol, and appropriate "change of custody" documentation is needed if the images are transferred using an external hard drive. When digital images are used for peer review, the STP recommends that if the SP used glass slides and the PRP uses digital images for the peer review, then any differences during the peer review should be resolved using the glass slides. The digital images used during a contemporaneous peer review by the PRP generally need not be archived after the peer review is complete since the archived original slides may be used for a later reevaluation and study recapitulation should the need arise.

Lack of regulatory guidance on the conduct of digital peer review of GLP studies has limited widespread adoption of this technology in the area of regulated nonclinical safety. European companies and regulatory agencies appear to be ahead of the United States on this issue. From unofficial discussions and meetings on the subject, it appears that regulatory authorities recognize the rapidly increasing use of digital image evaluation within the clinical and nonclinical settings and that it is already extending to pathology peer review. From these ongoing discussions, concepts on the use of WSI for pathology peer review in GLP toxicity studies are beginning to emerge (see the "Regulatory Considerations for Digital Pathology" section in *Digital Pathology and Tissue Image Analysis*; Vol 1, Chap 12). Briefly, WSIs will need to be created using a validated system, and a chain of custody process likely will need to be in place for images transferred between sites. The digital images will not meet the current definitions of specimen or raw data in GLP guidance documents. Whether a WSI must be retained as part of the study file may ultimately be linked to how it was used. If viewed as part of a contemporaneous peer review, then the WSIs are not raw data and do not need to be retained. However, if WSIs are evaluated as part of a retrospective peer review (when pathology raw data already exist), then these images may need to be saved based on the basic GLP principle that whatever was used to create (or change) the raw data must be retained.

6.1. Use of Whole-Slide Images for National Toxicology Program Pathology Working Groups

In recent years, the NTP has adopted the use of WSI for illustrative purposes to facilitate PWG discussions following the initial review of the glass slides. In this setting, the PWG Chairperson selects the glass slides to be scanned and annotated prior to the PWG meeting. The coded glass slides are then reviewed by the expert panel. The corresponding coded WSI of the glass slides that were reviewed may be projected for use by the PWG in discussing specific tissue features. This serial approach to the review allows all participants to simultaneously see the finding (which they already have viewed independently using the glass slide) for discussion to achieve a consensus diagnosis. PWG participants may also request to revisit available digital scans to review specific lesions prior to the consensus vote. In some situations, the scanned images are also shared with the SP and/or remote subject matter experts so that they can participate and/or be an observer during the PWG Meeting. Although the digital illustrations are used to facilitate the discussion and may be relied on to address terminology issues, the final consensus diagnoses are based on the findings as observed on the glass slides and not on the digital images. The images are maintained on a server, but not with the study file because no pathology raw data are generated from the images. The NTP continues to refine its use of WSI as a part of PWGs and envisions ultimately moving to fully digital PWGs using WSIs for consensus diagnosis in the next few years.

7. CONCLUSION

The diagnoses and interpretations of the SP in a regulatory-type toxicity study are often the key data on which the toxicity profile of a test article is understood, and by which the risk assessment is developed. While the SP is ultimately responsible as the Principal Investigator for generating the pathology raw data in a toxicity study, because of the importance of accuracy in their data, most pathologists do not reach their conclusions in isolation. Achieving accurate pathology diagnoses is an iterative process that is, when done well, a collaborative activity. Pathology peer review is a means to formalize this diagnostic collaboration in the context of a toxicity study and is recognized as a valuable tool for the QC of pathology raw data within the global pathology community and by government regulators.

REFERENCES

Bolon B, et al.: International recommendations for training future toxicologic pathologists participating in regulatory-type, nonclinical toxicity studies, *Toxicol Pathol* 38(6):984–992, 2010.

Boorman GA, et al.: Pathology peer review, *Toxicol Pathol* 38(7):1009–1010, 2010.

Bradley A, Jacobsen M: Toxicologic Pathology Forum: opinion on considerations for the use of whole slide images in GLP pathology peer review, *Toxicol Pathol* 47(2):100–107, 2019.

Brandli-Baiocco A, et al.: Nonproliferative and proliferative lesions of the rat and mouse endocrine system, *J Toxicol Pathol* 31(3 Suppl):1S–95S, 2018.

EMA: *Note for guidance on carcinogenic potential, 2002.* Retrieved from: https://www.ema.europa.eu/en/documents/scientific-guideline/note-guidance-carcinogenic-potential_en.pdf. (Last accessed 1 June 2021).

EPA: *PRN 94-5: requests for Re-considerations of carcinogenicity peer review decisions based on changes in pathology diagnoses.* Retrieved from: https://www.epa.gov/pesticide-registration/prn-94-5-requests-re-considerations-carcinogenicity-peer-review-decisions. (Last accessed 1 June 2021).

FDA: 1987 final rule - Good laboratory practice regulations, *Fed Regist* 52(172):33769–33770, 1987. Retrieved from: https://cdn.loc.gov/service/ll/fedreg/fr052/fr052172/fr052172.pdf. (Last accessed 1 June 2021).

FDA: *Pathology peer review in nonclinical toxicology studies: questions and answers guidance for industry – draft guidance,* CDER, OSIS. Retrieved from: https://www.regulations.gov/document?D=FDA-2019-D-2330-0002. (Last accessed 1 June 2021).

Fikes JD, et al.: Scientific and Regulatory Policy Committee review: review of the organisation for economic co-operation and development (OECD) guidance on the GLP requirements for peer review of histopathology, *Toxicol Pathol* 43(7):907–914, 2015.

https://www.ema.europa.eu/en/documents/scientific-guideline/note-guidance-carcinogenic-potential_en.pdf.

INHAND Criteria: Summarized at global open registry nomenclature information system. Retrieved from: https://www.goreni.org/gr3_download_nom.php.(Last accessed 1 June 2021).

Kerlin R, et al.: Scientific and Regulatory Policy Committee: recommended ("best") practices for determining, communicating, and using adverse effect data from nonclinical studies, *Toxicol Pathol* 44(2):147–162, 2016.

Leach MW, et al.: Use of tissue cross-reactivity studies in the development of antibody-based biopharmaceuticals: history, experience, methodology, and future directions, *Toxicol Pathol* 38(7):1138–1166, 2010.

Long GG, Hardisty JF: Regulatory Forum opinion piece: thresholds in toxicologic pathology, *Toxicol Pathol* 40(7):1079–1081, 2012.

Morton D, et al.: Recommendations for pathology peer review, *Toxicol Pathol* 38(7):1118–1127, 2010. https://doi.org/10.1177/0192623310383991. (Last accessed 1 June 2021).

OECD: *OECD series on principles of good laboratory practice and compliance monitoring number 1 OECD principles on Good laboratory practice (as revised in 1997).* Retrieved from: http://www.oecd.org/officialdocuments/publicdisplaydocumentpdf/?cote=env/mc/chem(98)17&doclanguage=en. (Last accessed 1 June 2021).

OECD: *OECD series on principles of good laboratory practice and compliance monitoring number 16 advisory document of the working group on Good laboratory practice - guidance on the GLP requirements for peer review of histopathology.* Retrieved from: http://www.oecd.org/officialdocuments/publicdisplaydocumentpdf/?cote=env/jm/mono(2014)30&doclanguage=en. (Last accessed 1 June 2021).

OECD: *OECD Good laboratory practice: frequently asked questions (FAQ).* Retrieved from: http://www.oecd.org/chemicalsafety/testing/glp-frequently-asked-questions.htm. (Last accessed 1 June 2021).

Paranjpe MG, et al.: A comparison of spontaneous tumors in Tg.rasH2 mice in 26-week carcinogenicity studies conducted at a single test facility during 2004 to 2012 and 2013 to 2018, *Toxicol Pathol* 47(1):18–25, 2019.

Sills RC, et al.: National Toxicology Program position statement on informed ("nonblinded") analysis in toxicologic pathology evaluation, *Toxicol Pathol* 47(7):887–890, 2019.

Ward JM, et al.: Peer review in toxicologic pathology, *Toxicol Pathol* 23(2):226–234, 1995.

Pathology and GLPs, Quality Control, and Quality Assurance

Kathleen Marie Heinz-Taheny

Lilly Research Laboratories – Toxicology, Drug Disposition, and PKPD, Eli Lilly and Company, Indianapolis, IN, United States

OUTLINE

1. Introduction   1009

2. Overview of Good Laboratory Practice
   Standards   1010
   2.1. History and Evolution of GLP Standards   1010
   2.2. Objective and Scope   1015
   2.3. FDA GLP General Content   1016
   2.4. Organization of 21 CFR 58 Good Laboratory
        Practice for Nonclinical Laboratory Studies   1016

3. GLP and Pathology Data   1021
   3.1. Study Pathologist Requirements   1021
   3.2. Histopathology in the GLP Environment   1021

4. Clinical Pathology Assessment in the GLP
   Environment   1024

5. Ultrastructural Assessment in the GLP
   Environment   1024

6. Noninvasive Imaging Applications in the GLP
   Environment   1024

7. In the Spirit of GLP   1025

8. GLP Criticism   1025
   8.1. Academic Research   1025
   8.2. Perspectives on GLP Limitations   1026

9. Conclusions   1026

References   1026

1. INTRODUCTION

Good Laboratory Practice (GLP) standards were authored by the United States Food and Drug Administration (FDA) to ensure sound and repeatable nonclinical safety assessment studies. They set the standard by which studies are planned, conducted, monitored, reported, and archived to assure reproducibility, accuracy, and consistency. Similar guidelines were later developed by the United States Environmental Protection Agency (EPA) and internationally by the Organisation for Economic Co-operation and Development (OECD) and regulatory organizations in other countries. The OECD, established in 1961, is an intergovernmental organization with representatives from countries in North America, Europe, and the Pacific Rim as well as the European Commission that promotes policies improving social and economic well-being by coordinating and harmonizing international policies, identification of good practices, discussion of issues of mutual concern, and working collectively to respond to international problems. Over time, the modest differences among GLP standards among various institutions have become increasingly harmonized.

Haschek and Rousseaux's Handbook of Toxicologic Pathology, Fourth Edition.
https://doi.org/10.1016/B978-0-12-821044-4.00018-2

The main goal of GLP in any venue is to assure that animal toxicity studies produce data that are reliable, repeatable, auditable, and globally acceptable. The OECD defines GLP as a "quality system concerned with the organizational process and the conditions under which nonclinical health and environmental safety studies are planned, performed, monitored, recorded, archived, and reported" (OECD, 1998). GLP attempts to assure integrity, reproducibility, verifiability, and traceability of data. Following GLP principles requires good operational management. Finally, GLP focuses on aspects of study execution including the planning, monitoring, recording, reporting, and archiving that are critical for the reconstruction of the study.

2. OVERVIEW OF GOOD LABORATORY PRACTICE STANDARDS

2.1. History and Evolution of GLP Standards

The origin of GLP standards in the United States followed the discovery of scientific misconduct in animal safety testing by pharmaceutical and industrial chemical manufacturers in the 1970s. Before the 1970s, the FDA and EPA received and accepted animal-derived safety data, trusting that the data were generated with integrity. The FDA had gained greater authority of drug safety assessment in 1962 following approval of the Kefauver–Harris Amendments to the Federal Food, Drug, and Cosmetic Act. These amendments followed the thalidomide tragedy in which a sedative widely used outside the United States to treat morning sickness in pregnant women caused birth defects in Europe, Canada, and other countries. The end result of these amendments provided for more safety and efficacy testing as well as better documentation with regular inspection of such records, and afforded the FDA additional time to review new drug applications. In subsequent years, the FDA began requiring drug efficacy data and postapproval reporting.

The United States was not the first to initiate GLP-like standards. New Zealand introduced the Testing Laboratory Registration Act in 1972, defining the "testing laboratory" to encompass staff records, procedures, equipment, and facilities and established a related registration council

"to promote the development and maintenance of GLP in testing." Denmark followed suit that same year. GLP standards in the United States were enacted later that decade following investigation of scientific misconduct.

GLP in the United States

Between 1975 and 1977 the Senate Judiciary Committee, Subcommittee on Health (chaired by Senator Edward Kennedy), and the FDA investigated multiple incidents of pharmaceutical and contract research organization (CRO) drug testing fraud. Known as the "Kennedy Hearings," the focus was "Preclinical and Clinical Testing by the Pharmaceutical Industry." During the hearings, Kennedy stated the following:

> Accurate science is the best protection the American people have from an unsafe and ineffective drug supply. Inaccurate science, sloppy science, fraudulent science—these are the greatest threats to the health and safety of the American people. Whether the science is wrong because of clerical error, or because of poor technique, or because of incompetence, or because of criminal negligence is less important than the fact that it is wrong. For if it is wrong, and if, as in this case, the FDA did not—indeed, under the current practice, could not—know it was wrong, then the protective regulatory barrier between a potentially dangerous drug and the patient is removed.

U.S. Senate (1975).

G.D. Searle and Company, one of the largest pharmaceutical companies of its time, was a central focus of the investigation. With Searle's full cooperation, the FDA investigated nonclinical safety studies conducted by Searle in house and at a CRO, Hazelton Laboratories, used by Searle. Inspection findings by the FDA investigators included the following:

- Excision of tissue masses from rodents during the study and return of those animals to the study with no report of malignant masses to the FDA,
- Long delays in reporting "alarming findings" to the FDA,
- Lack of histological examination of all collected tissues and gross lesions required by the study protocol,
- Differences between initial findings and the pathology raw data submitted in the final report,

- Lack of proper personnel training,
- Rats listed as dead were recorded later as being alive (sometimes multiple times),
- Undocumented study protocol deviations,
- Poor accuracy and timeliness of study documentation,
- Inconsistent data retention,
- No quality control of reported data,
- Statistical manipulation to reduce adversity of findings, and
- Frank omission of adverse findings from reports.

While criminal charges against employees of Searle were considered, the grand jury decided against indictment. Following the hearings, Searle authored a draft of GLP regulations, submitting it to both the FDA and the Pharmaceutical Research and Manufacturers Association of America, a large portion of which was incorporated into the FDA's draft GLP document. In 1978, the final version of FDA GLP regulations was published in the Code of Federal Regulations (CFR) under Title 21: "Food and Drugs" as Part 58: "Good Laboratory Practice for Nonclinical Laboratory Studies" (21 CFR 58, FDA, 1978), applying to all nonclinical safety studies supporting FDA-regulated products. The FDA Office of Regulatory Affairs (ORA) published "Guidance for Industry GLP Question and Answers" as assistance to research facilities in the interpretation and application of the directives (FDA, 1998). With standards set for nonclinical safety assessment conduct, the FDA made clear that violating these standards could result in criminal prosecution or disqualification of data and/or the testing facility from conducting further animal testing until violations were remedied. FDA also initiated a more formal inspection and audit program for study examination. The most recent version of FDA GLP was published in 1987 in the Federal Register as "Final Rule—Good Laboratory Practices" (FDA, 1987). Significant changes were made in the provisions with respect to quality assurance (QA), protocol preparation, test and control article characterization, and retention of specimens and samples based on FDA's experience in implementing the initial 1978 regulations.

Soon after, other agencies released GLP regulations including the EPA and OECD. In 1983, GLP regulations were published by EPA under the Federal Insecticide, Fungicide, and Rodenticide Act (FIFRA; 40 CFR 160, EPA, 2011a) and the Toxic Substances Control Act (TSCA; 40 CFR 792, EPA, 2011b). In 1981, an international body, the OECD, issued "OECD Principles of Good Laboratory Practice" (revised in 1997, OECD, 1998) and "Guidelines for the Testing of Chemicals" (Test Guidelines, which are periodically reviewed and revised, OECD, 1981). The OECD is not a regulatory agency and does not approve and register new medicines, so its GLP documents are guidelines and not regulations. While the United States is a member of the OECD, the U.S. FDA alone is the sole body for medical product registration in this country; as such, studies conducted for submission to the FDA should be conducted using the FDA GLP standards and not those outlined by the OECD. Fortunately, the increasing harmonization of GLP standards across regulatory agencies around the world over time now permits sponsors and CROs to establish procedures that comply simultaneously with GLP principles and practices of many regulatory bodies (FDA, 2004).

Following the publication of the FDA GLP standards, the agency formed the Bioresearch Monitoring Program that conducted a pilot inspection program of research facilities to understand their baseline competence level and conformity to GLP standards. The goal of this effort was to prevent fraud, reduce public risk, eliminate the unnecessary use of animals, avoid waste of time and money, avoid acceptance of false results, and ensure confidence in regulatory decisions. "Major failings" noted during the pilot evaluations included lack of QA departments, lack of testing each batch of test article, and failure to maintain standard operating procedures (SOPs) (Zhou, 2011). During the first few investigations, it was found that the industry lacked standards in animal research and testing, quality control measures and their documentation, and recording and reporting of data. Also, important nonclinical safety findings were frequently not reported to the FDA promptly and, occasionally, not reported at all.

After the Kennedy Hearings, scientific misconduct continued to occur, warranting further investigation. In particular, two examples of major scientific fraud occurring in CROs were publicized widely. Biometric Testing Inc. and

Industrial Bio-Test Laboratories (IBT) were extensively investigated by the FDA. Biometric Testing Inc. went bankrupt following the guilty pleas of two vice presidents for falsifying reports of animal tests that had not, in fact, been carried out. However, the most sensational case of scientific misconduct was that of IBT, at that time the largest CRO in the world, conducting approximately 35%–40% of all safety studies in the United States. More than 22,000 toxicity studies had been conducted during its existence, mainly supporting the assessment of pesticides and other chemicals, pharmaceuticals, and cosmetics. Violations of sound scientific conduct by IBT included the following:

- Poor animal husbandry including constant cage flooding by automatic watering systems resulting in the drowning and frequent escape of test animals,
- Faulty record keeping,
- Inadequately trained personnel,
- "Borrowing" data from control groups of loosely related studies,
- Test animals receiving incorrect doses or the wrong test article,
- Dead animals listed as alive (similar to Searle),
- Chronic studies that reported no findings in control animals despite the geriatric age of the rodents,
- Replacement of dead animals mid to late study with naïve animals, with no documentation of this replacement, and
- Fabricated data that were never collected.

After the IBT hearings, four senior administrative and technical leaders including the company president were indicted by a U.S. grand jury. Three were found guilty of mail fraud and making a false statement to the government with one sentenced to a year in prison and the other two receiving 6-month sentences. More than 70% of the over 900 studies audited at IBT were invalidated. Sales of marketed products that had been supported by invalidated studies were suspended until new studies were conducted and reviewed.

GLP Internationally

Following the institution of GLP standards by the U.S. FDA, implementation of GLP standards was broadened by the 1981 OECD decision on Mutual Acceptance of Data (MAD) among member countries (OECD, 1997) stating that "data generated in the testing of chemicals in an OECD Member country in accordance with OECD Test Guidelines (for chemical testing) and OECD Principles of GLP shall be accepted in other Member countries for purposes of assessment and other uses relating to the protection of man and the environment." By signing the decision, all OECD member countries agree to conduct all nonclinical safety studies under GLP, advance the international harmonization of GLP and monitoring compliance, and eliminate the need for study repetition to fulfill differing requirements. By instituting international guidance and requirements, international trade in chemicals would not be encumbered by removing the need for duplicative testing. The OECD GLP guidance document provided countries with a framework to implement an internationally recognized standard that still addressed the needs of their own national programs by allowing some minor nation or region-specific variation (i.e., the European Union [EU]), such as archival storage length as an example. Due to the incredible cost and labor associated with chemical testing and the burden of testing in each individual country, OECD sought a way to establish standards that, if followed, would allow acceptance across a number of countries. Barriers to economic progress and world trade were reduced. To meet the conditions of OECD's MAD,

- Data must have been produced in compliance with the OECD Principles of GLP, which is assured by the signature of the Study Director,
- A functioning regulatory authority must exist in the country where the data are produced, and
- The testing facility must be included in the GLP monitoring program of the country's regulatory authority.

Following their acceptance of the OECD GLP Principles, some countries or regions have integrated the Principles into law, as is the case for the EU which adopted the OECD GLP Principles in a European directive.

International organizations and some of their regulations involved in enforcing and modifying GLP guidelines include the following:

- Directive 2004/9/EC of the European Parliament and the Council on the inspection and verification of GLP.

- This Directive requires that the OECD Revised Guides for Compliance Monitoring Procedures for GLP and the OECD Guidance for the Conduct of Test Facility Inspections and Study Audits must be adhered to during laboratory inspections and study audits.
- Directive 2004/10/EC of the European Parliament and the Council on the harmonization of laws, regulations, and administrative provisions relating to the application of the principles of GLP and the verification of their applications for tests on chemical substances.
  - This directive specifies that Member States must designate the authorities responsible for GLP inspections in their country and outlines requirements for reporting and the internal market (i.e., MAD).
- EU: Commission Directive 1999/12/EC of March 8, 1999 adapting to technical progress for the second time the Annex to Council Directive 88/320/EEC on the inspection and verification of GLP.
- United Kingdom (UK) Statutory Instrument: "The Good Laboratory Practice Regulations 1997" replaced the existing voluntary UK GLP Compliance program.
- European Parliament and the Council of the European Union: 89/569/EEC Council Decision of July 28, 1989 on the acceptance by the European Economic Community of an OECD decision/recommendation on compliance with principles of GLP.
- Swiss (GLP/OECD) Working Group on Information Technology (AGIT).
- OECD: "OECD Principles of Good Laboratory Practice" [C(97)186(Final)] (OECD, 1998).
  - Member nations are comprised of North American, Central American, South American, Asian (including Japan and Korea), and European countries.
  - Nations currently working with OECD but not as official member countries include Russia, Brazil, China, India, Indonesia, and South Africa.
- Chinese Ministry of Science and Technology: Regulation on GLPs.
  - The initial standard was drafted in 1993, was abolished in 1999, and a new draft was issued following the current U.S. FDA policies when Chinese GLP affairs came

under the State Food and Drug Administration (SFDA).
- In 2013, the SFDA renamed itself the China Food and Drug Administration (CFDA) to reflect the advancement of the agency to ministerial level. This meant the CFDA would report directly to China's State Council with broader authority to oversee the food, drug, and medical device divisions.
- In 2018, in conjunction with China's 2018 government administration overhaul, the CFDA was renamed the National Medical Products Administration (NMPA) and merged into the newly created State Administration for Market Regulation. The NMPA issued regulatory reforms with the goal to improve the drug review process and shorten Investigational New Drug (IND) and New Drug Application (NDA) review timelines, namely by increasing the number of drug reviewers at the Chinese Center for Drug Evaluation. These reforms also aim to encourage and increase novel drug development, accelerate market authorization, and reduce drug lag.

For a complete list of national websites on GLP refer to the OECD website (OECD, 2018).

Since the February 1, 2020 withdrawal of the UK from the EU, and upon completion of a transition period lasting until the end of 2020, the UK will no longer follow the EU Directives but instead will apply the OECD "MAD" system. The UK as well as many of the EU countries are OECD members already and thus are fully adherent to the MAD system. Therefore, the UK withdrawal from the EU should not have a major impact on the acceptance of GLP data generated in UK facilities by European or other international regulatory receiving authorities.

The International Council/Conference on Harmonisation of Technical Requirements for Registration of Pharmaceuticals for Human Use

Established in 1990, the International Conference on Harmonisation (ICH), now referred to as the International Council on Harmonisation, is a collaborative effort to unify and align the drug regulatory authorities and the pharmaceutical industries of Europe, Japan, and the United

States. ICH sets forth guidelines on the types and timing of nonclinical safety assessments but does not cover aspects related to the quality or integrity of nonclinical studies as defined by GLPs (ICH, 1990). They were authored through scientific consensus of regulatory and industry experts, thereby achieving greater harmonization of international pharmaceutical product registration while reducing or obviating duplication of testing carried out during the research and development of new human drugs. The ICH guidelines offer best practices leading to a more economical use of human, animal, and material resources by preventing duplication of human clinical trials, reducing animal usage in safety testing, streamlining regulatory assessment of new drug applications, and reducing time and resources for drug development, ultimately to eliminate unnecessary delays in the availability of new medicines. ICH sets out to remove barriers to global drug development while maintaining the utmost quality, safety, and efficacy to ensure public health. ICH guidelines have been adopted as the regulatory standard in several countries, but are only used as guidance by the FDA to supplement their own existing standard; therefore, familiarity with the content of the ICH guidelines is essential. ICH has published harmonized tripartite guidelines in four areas: quality (chemical and pharmaceutical QA), safety (nonclinical safety assessment), efficacy (clinical research in human patients including Good Clinical Practice [GCP], E6), and multidisciplinary (which includes medical terminology, Medical Dictionary for Regulatory Activities or MedDRA, and Nonclinical Safety Studies, M3, among others).

In 2015, ICH underwent a reformation to extend its global influence beyond the founding regions through formation of the ICH Assembly, an overarching governing body. The Assembly is focused on international pharmaceutical regulatory harmonization that allows pharmaceutical regulatory authorities and other industry organizations to be more actively engaged in ICH's harmonization work. The reforms included the following: increasing global outreach; revamping ICH's governance structure; disseminating more information on ICH processes to a wider number of stakeholders; and establishing ICH as a legal entity to provide for a more stable operating structure.

FDA Proposed Rule on Good Laboratory Practice for Nonclinical Laboratory Studies

In December of 2010, the FDA released an Advanced Notice of Proposed Rulemaking to modernize 21 CFR Part 58, the first proposed major revision since 1987 (FDA, 2010). Incorporating the comments and suggestions of 90 responders, a proposal was opened for comments in early 2017. The proposal addressed nine specific areas of Part 58 including the GLP Quality System, Multisite Studies, Electronic/Computerized Systems, Sponsor Responsibilities, Animal Welfare, Information on QA Inspection Findings, Process-Based Systems Inspections, Test and Control Article Information, and Sample Storage Container Retention. The content of the proposal represents current thoughts and direction of the FDA, but, as a proposal, these concepts are not yet incorporated formally in the enforceable GLP standard.

Highlights of the proposed changes included enhancement of the current quality system approach called the GLP Quality System, conduct and considerations in laboratory oversight (particularly of multisite studies), and harmonization of wording with domestic and international guidelines or regulations, specifically OECD, to increase data integrity and record keeping. The regulations would expand the scope to include tobacco products and veterinary medical devices in addition to those for human use. New and modified definitions, terms, and organizational and personnel roles and responsibilities are detailed including test site, test facility with executive responsibility, attending veterinarian, contributing scientist, and principal investigator for greater clarity. These also included new directives on SOPs for developing, maintaining, and administering SOPs and clarity on management roles, responsibilities, and accountability especially regarding establishing and maintaining the quality system. Additionally, all data generated during a nonclinical study must follow the acronym "ALCOA": accurate, legible, contemporaneous, original, and attributable. Section 21 CFR 58.61 on equipment design includes computerized systems and other modern equipment used for maintenance, archiving, and retrieval of data since that is currently how most data are stored. To support and expand on the principles of humane animal research, the 3Rs (Replacement, Reduction, and

Refinement), the FDA supports the use of nonanimal models when valid alternatives are available. In acknowledgment of the prevalence of multisite studies, the new proposal would revise the Testing Facility definition to "the person responsible for, coordinating, conducting, or completing a nonclinical laboratory study, or any combination thereof" capturing all possible contractual relationships because, in a multisite study, the test facility might not be the facility that conducted the in-life portion of the study as the current definition specifies but rather a contracted or subcontracted person at another location (a satellite entity termed a Test Site). For multisite studies, new communication requirements are added to sponsor responsibilities to establish appropriate lines of communication among all persons conducting any phase of the nonclinical laboratory study as well as documentation by the sponsor. The last goal of the proposed revision is to establish consistency with current domestic and international guidelines, rules, or regulations of GLP (FDA, 2016). The proposed rule change has generated significant public comment and, as of publication, the proposed changes have not been finalized.

2.2. Objective and Scope

Studies Under GLP Jurisdiction

GLP is required only for animal studies conducted to permit safety evaluation of novel products. Categories of products where safety testing is conducted by GLP include food and color additives, human and veterinary drugs, biological products, cosmetics, medical devices, pesticides, electronic products, and cosmetics, as examples. GLPs regulate all nonclinical safety studies that support or are intended to support applications for research or marketing permits for FDA-regulated products, or by similar agencies. GLP standards do not apply to exploratory or efficacy studies, human or animal clinical studies, or chemical analysis. Additionally, repeat-dose pilot toxicity studies and dose escalation studies, while typically conducted in the "spirit" of GLP, are not formally performed under GLP guidelines.

The FDA defines nonclinical studies as any in vivo or in vitro experiment in which test articles are studied prospectively in test systems under laboratory conditions to evaluate their safety. General study types performed under GLP include single-dose toxicity, repeat-dose toxicity, developmental and reproductive toxicity, genotoxicity, carcinogenicity, toxicokinetics, and pharmacodynamics. Phototoxicity, irritation assays, sensitization studies, and abuse potential studies also fall under GLP guidelines. Recall that GLP principles are not directly concerned with study design, which is evaluated by the regulatory authorities (for example, FDA, EPA, OECD), but rather in optimizing the conditions in which the study will be conducted. GLP principles should be applied independently of the site where the study will be performed. For example, if a company outsources a nonclinical study to a CRO or university, those sites must comply with GLP standards to assure acceptance of test results. The main difference between GLP and non-GLP studies is the type and amount of documentation, not in the study design and conduct. GLP studies increase operational costs by up to 30% compared to non-GLP studies. The objective is not only to improve the quality of data but also to maximize the traceability, integrity, accuracy, and reproducibility of data. Similar to GLP studies in animals, clinical trials in humans are regulated by GCP and the production of test articles through Good Manufacturing Practice (GMP).

Differences Across GLP Standards

All GLP standards require a Sponsor-approved study plan or protocol signed by the Study Director, a Quality Assurance Unit (QAU), test article characterization, trained and qualified personnel, procedures for documenting raw data and deviations, a final report, and data archive. Minor differences exist among the standards including the party responsible for compliance (Study Director vs. Test Facility Management), a requirement of a specific statement of GLP compliance in the final report (EPA), laboratory certification and test facility inspection, and archiving process and retention length. In general, institutions that perform animal toxicity studies will design studies so that a single test will address not only the internationally recognized GLP standards but also, if feasible, the minor nation- or region-specific GLP differences that pertain to the markets in which they propose to register their product (FDA, 2004).

2.3. FDA GLP General Content

FDA GLP principles are outlined and described in 21 CFR 58. The purpose of this section is to summarize key points of the U.S. FDA regulations, but the OECD and EPA regulations have similar content (FDA, 2004). Key concepts of the FDA GLP principles include that for each study

- Responsibilities are defined for the sponsor management, study management including the study director, and the QAU,
- Experimental conduct follows written SOPs,
- Testing facilities are adequate to ensure the integrity of a study,
- Test and control articles are high quality,
- Instruments are calibrated and well maintained,
- Personnel are properly trained and educated to execute their duties, and
- Raw data are acquired, processed, documented, and archived to ensure the reliability of data.

These principles ensure the uniformity, reproducibility, quality, accuracy, and consistency of study conduct.

2.4. Organization of 21 CFR 58 Good Laboratory Practice for Nonclinical Laboratory Studies (FDA, 1987)

Subpart A—General Provisions

This section includes the scope, definitions, applicability to third-party (grant organization and CRO) studies, and test facility inspections. When a sponsor conducting a nonclinical laboratory study that is intended to be submitted to or reviewed by the FDA utilizes the services of a consulting laboratory, contractor, or grantee to perform an analysis or other services, the third party (termed a Test Facility) must be made aware that the study must be conducted in GLP compliance. The responsibility for ensuring compliance with GLP standards rests with the sponsor.

Subpart B—Organization and Personnel

Within this section, personnel, testing facility management, Study Director, and the QAU are discussed and responsibilities for the sponsor, test facility management, Study Director, and study personnel summarized. GLP requires a curriculum vitae, training records, and a detailed job description for each employee to demonstrate that staff have the education, experience, and training necessary to perform their tasks. GLP mandates sufficient staffing for a given study and explicitly requires that all personnel should understand the meaning of GLP, its importance, and how to perform their tasks in a GLP-compliant manner. Testing facility management is required to designate the Study Director and promptly replace a Study Director who can no longer fulfill their study duties. The Study Director wholly assumes responsibility for the interpretation, analysis, documentation, and reporting of results and represents the single point of study control. The Study Director must assure that the protocol is followed; that all experimental data and deviations from the protocol are documented; that incidents impacting the quality of data are reported, that corrective actions (if any) are described and documented; that GLP principles are followed; and that at study conclusion all study components are archived. The final report is approved and signed by this individual. An assistant Study Director is not permitted, but an alternate Study Director—chosen by the testing facility management—may be appointed to fulfill necessary tasks if and only if the Study Director is absent.

The QAU functions as an internal control of each study. The QAU is responsible for monitoring each study to assure the test facility management that the facilities, equipment, personnel, methods, practices, records, controls, SOPs, final reports (data integrity), and archives conform with GLP regulations. The QAU is entirely separate from, and independent of, the personnel engaged in the direction and conduct of that study. The QAU intermittently reports any potential compliance issues and suggested corrective actions to the test facility management and the study director. Internal auditing is not only limited to study-specific activities but also process-based tasks such as animal husbandry and sample handling practices as well as system inspections that holistically assess the facility's quality compliance. The FDA has access to the written procedures established for the inspection and may request testing facility management to certify that inspections are being implemented, documented, and followed-up under GLP mandates.

Subpart C—Facilities

Each testing facility must be of suitable size and construction to facilitate proper study conduct. A degree of separation is required among laboratory activities to prevent difficulties in any one function or activity from adversely impacting the entire study. This separation may be physical or by organization; for example, the establishment of defined laboratory work areas to carry out distinct activities in the same area at different times allows for cleaning and preparation between operations or maintaining separation of staff. Facility components described include animal care, animal supply, test and control article preparation, laboratory operation, and specimen and storage facilities.

Subpart D—Equipment

Study equipment must be of appropriate design, adequate capacity, and regularly calibrated to function according to the SOPs and shall be suitably located for operation and routine inspection, cleaning, and maintenance. Equipment subject to GLP includes analytical devices as well as computerized equipment used for instrument control, data capture, statistical analysis, printing, archiving, and retrieval.

Subpart E—Testing Facilities Operation

For clarity, "testing facility" refers to a site that actually conducts a nonclinical laboratory study (i.e., actually uses the test article in a test system). In contrast, "test site" has not yet been defined in 21 CFR 58 but usually is taken to mean a location where a satellite activity for the study is to be completed (e.g., the office of a contractor tasked with sample analysis). A proposed definition for "test site" is under comment and consideration in the "proposed rule" for updating FDA GLP standards (see FDA Proposed Rule on Good Laboratory Practice for Nonclinical Laboratory Studies).

This section describes the requirement for SOPs that direct daily laboratory conduct, thereby assuring quality and robustness of data produced, integrity of reagents and solutions, and animal care. SOPs encompass procedures such as animal room preparation, animal care, handling of test and control articles, test system observations, handling of moribund or dead animals, necropsy, tissue collection and processing, histopathology,

data handling and storage, data retrieval, equipment maintenance, and calibration, as examples. Each facility should have an SOP on writing an SOP to maintain consistency. SOPs are clearly written and updated on a systematic basis, and laboratory staff are required to document training as it pertains to SOPs for their area of operation. SOPs must be immediately available to study personnel. All deviations from SOPs must be documented in the study raw data. Published literature may be used as a supplement but cannot replace institution-specific SOPs. The test facility must maintain a file of current SOPs and also an archive of historical (i.e., expired) prior versions, including the dates of revisions. SOPs are frequently mentioned as deviations in FDA warning letters. The most common deviations include SOPs that are not available, not adequate, and/or were not followed.

Subpart F—Test and Control Articles

The identity, strength, purity, composition, and/or other physical attributes (for each batch or lot) that define the test or control articles as well as method of synthesis will be identified and documented. If currently marketed control articles are used, they will be characterized by their labeling. The stability of each test or control article is determined either before study initiation or concurrently with the study. Either the test facility or the sponsor will generate this information.

Control articles or reference substances are critical components of a study. These materials are necessary to calibrate instruments used to determine endpoints in a study and also to serve as a baseline against which outcomes related to test article exposure may be gauged against responses associated with various study procedures. If the control article is not of the correct material (identity), purity, or other characteristics, the test results generated from an incorrectly calibrated instrument will also be erroneous. Similarly, inappropriate composition of the control article may invalidate conclusions made regarding the impact of the test article on the animal. Provisions and documentation of proper preparation, storage, identification, receipt, and distribution of test and control articles must be established. If a test or control article is mixed with a carrier, proper consistency, stability, and concentration of the final mixture must be verified before study commencement or periodically assessed as per protocol. GMP is not required for the production of test article batches used in GLP studies since GMP is only required for the preparation of clinical trial materials and the manufacture of actual medicines. That said, late-stage GLP-compliant nonclinical studies often are conducted with GMP material to support the clinical development program and eventual licensing application.

Subpart G—Protocol for and Conduct of a Nonclinical Laboratory Study

Each nonclinical study requires a study protocol (referred to as the "study plan" in the OECD Principles of GLP) delineating the purpose, objectives, and methods. Components of the protocol include the title and purpose of the study, identification of the test and control articles, identification of the "test system" (the biological system—typically defined by such factors as species, breed or strain, sex, and age—to which the test or control article is administered), sponsor name, description of experimental design, type and frequency of tests and analyses, records to be maintained, and conduct of a study. The study protocol serves as a means of communication to staff, to provide key dates such as study start and conclusion, and to lay out general study methods. Each study must have a unique protocol, the number of which is used to identify the study data and can be cross-referenced to other studies. The Study Director is the primary author of the study protocol with collaborative input from the sponsor (if a contracted study) and study pathologist, among other contributors. Experimental design and type and frequency of endpoints are the most critical pieces of the protocol.

The study then should be conducted with rigorous adherence to the protocol. Study samples must be identified by test system, study, nature, and date of collection which will be located on the specimen container or accompany the specimen. Gross findings will be recorded and available to the pathologist when examining that specimen histopathologically. All handwritten data must be in ink, recorded promptly, and legibly. If an entry is changed, it must not be obscured but merely crossed out and

corrected. The new data point must be dated and signed and a reason provided for the change. Any deviations from the protocol as well as their impact on interpreting the resulting data must be thoroughly documented. Finally, the Study Director must indicate whether the study was GLP compliant and, if not, identify those portions that were not compliant.

Subparts H–I [Reserved]

This section is held for additions to the Code and has not been populated since the original issuance of the GLP.

Subpart J—Records and Reports

The final study report must include the name and address of the testing facility and the dates on which the study was initiated and completed. The report will state the objectives and procedures and any changes to the original protocol. The names of key personnel (e.g., Study Director and other scientists or professionals such as Principal Investigators [who, as defined by the OECD, are individuals responsible for delegated phases of the study on behalf of the Study Director]; Contributing Scientists [who are individual(s) responsible for conducting, interpreting, analyzing, or performing any service for a phase of the study]; and all supervisory personnel) are listed. Statistical methods, details about the test and control articles including stability, methods, experimental design, and dose information are defined. Data analysis and conclusions are discussed. Any deviations that may have affected the quality or integrity of the data will be stated and discussed as to their overall impact to the study. Finally, signatures and dates, archival information, and a the statement prepared and signed by the QAU, as described in Subpart B, are included.

GLP requires retention of all raw data (discussed in detail below), documentation, protocols, final reports, and specimens (except those specimens obtained from genotoxicity tests and wet specimens of blood, urine, feces, and biological fluids). Each testing facility must have an archive, maintained by an individual, that allows only authorized personnel to enter or retrieve items from the archive. All archived material must be indexed for convenient retrieval.

Important notes on the retention of records include the following:

- Minimum of 2 years retention following FDA **approval**
  - Not applicable to studies supporting IND applications or applications for investigational device exemptions (IDEs)
- Minimum of 5 years retention following FDA **submission** (for INDs and IDEs)
- When the nonclinical laboratory study does not result in the submission of the study in support of an application for a research or marketing permit, a minimum of 2 years retention following the date on which the study is completed, terminated, or discontinued
- For wet specimens, retention is shorter: they should only be retained as long as the quality does not degrade so far that evaluation would yield questionable data, but internationally, each country may have a slight variation on length

Subpart K—Disqualification of Testing Facilities

DISQUALIFICATION DEFINITION

The FDA reserves the right to exclude studies conducted at sites not compliant with GLP requirements unless the testing facility adequately proves that the noncompliance did not occur during the conduct of the study or did not affect the validity or acceptability of data. Grounds for disqualification include the following:

- The testing facility fails to comply with one or more of the GLP regulations,
- The noncompliance adversely affects the validity of the nonclinical laboratory studies, and/or
- Other lesser regulatory actions (e.g., warnings or rejection of individual studies) have not or will not be adequate to achieve compliance with GLP.

The purposes of disqualification are to permit exclusion of completed studies conducted by a testing facility which failed to comply with the GLP regulations and to exclude all studies completed after the date of disqualification until the facility can satisfy the agency that it will conduct studies in compliance with GLP regulations.

GLP ENFORCEMENT

It is the FDA's responsibility to enforce the federal Food, Drug, and Cosmetic Act to ensure the safety and effectiveness of medicines and medical devices. This is enforced through regulations, guidance documents, and FDA inspections. The FDA has the sole responsibility to inspect GLP safety studies related to all products that are marketed in the United States regardless of where the products were developed or manufactured. The Office of Regulatory Affairs (ORA) at the FDA is the lead office for all field activities, including inspections and enforcement.

The FDA executes two types of inspections. Surveillance or routine inspections occur approximately every other year and can cover all or specific units within a testing facility. Directed inspections can be instituted when an NDA is filed or on a "for cause" basis. These inspections aid in maintaining facility compliance with GLP. Directed inspections also occur as a Preapproval Inspection after submission of a marketing application—an NDA, Biologic License Application, Pre-market Approval Application, or equivalent—have been filed, and involve the review of study materials to verify reliability, integrity, and compliance. "For cause" inspections occur less frequently and constitute about 20% of all GLP inspections. Reasons for such inspections include reports or suspicion of noncompliance, a follow-up of a testing facility cited for GLP violations, or part of the reinstatement process of a disqualified site. Inspections are usually unannounced, and if the testing facility refuses inspection, the FDA will not accept study data generated by that site.

Legally, an FDA investigator providing a written notice (called a Form 482) and with appropriate credentials may enter a regulated establishment. At the conclusion of the inspection, if the investigator believes conditions deviate from FDA requirements, the investigator will issue a notice of objectionable observations relating to products, processes, or other violations of FDA requirements (called a Form 483). Concerning observations are listed in order of significance. The format of any single observation begins with a statement based on a citation of law, regulation, or Act and is followed by a statement of specific conditions observed during the inspection. During an exit meeting, the investigator reviews the Form 483 and each observation with management-level personnel and may ask management representatives for comment. About half the inspections in the United States conclude with a Form 483. Observations on a Form 483 are not a final agency judgment on a facility; therefore, a written response by the testing facility can significantly affect whether FDA takes further action after an inspection. Following the inspection, the lead FDA investigator authors a full inspection report, the Establishment Inspection Report, which is an expanded version of the Form 483.

Depending on the seriousness of the citations made on Form 483, the inspector may or may not issue a Warning Letter. The warning letter stipulates the need for corrective action, a written response, and a follow-up inspection. If a warning letter is issued, the site must respond within 15 business days delineating its proposed corrective action plan. Once the agency has completed the evaluation of corrective actions undertaken by a testing facility in response to a warning letter, the FDA may take one of two actions.

- One approach is to issue a "close-out letter" if, based on FDA's evaluation, the site has taken successful corrective action to address the violations contained in the warning letter. Corrective action is typically verified by a follow-up inspection.
- An alternative approach will be an enforcement action, which will take place if violations are observed during subsequent inspections or through other means. An enforcement action may be taken without further notice. The FDA office that issued the warning letter will also issue the closeout letter, an acknowledgment that corrective actions have satisfactorily addressed the violations identified in the warning letter, and that the office may be contacted for information on a warning letter and its resolution. Citations are maintained in a database and are reviewed, edited, and updated periodically.

Violations that impact the validity of a study can result in nonacceptance of data, either in part or in whole. Data rejection for a submission typically is not made public. Severe violations affecting multiple studies can disqualify a test facility. When a test facility is to be disqualified, the FDA Commissioner may issue a written notice proposing that the facility be disqualified, and a hearing on the disqualification is held. Upon disqualification, the Commissioner notifies the test facility of the ruling. Disqualification decisions are listed in a database that may be viewed by the public. If violations are severe enough to warrant legal action, civil or criminal charges can be directed toward the testing facility or employees.

Some of the most common GLP compliance violations listed by the FDA include the following:

- Insufficiently trained Study Directors and study personnel,
- Poorly designed protocols and failure to follow the study protocol,
- Unsatisfactory collection and documentation of raw data,
- Substandard animal husbandry,
- Inadequate characterization of test items and test systems,
- Inadequate facility resources,
- Equipment not properly calibrated or otherwise qualified,
- Reports not sufficiently verified, inaccurate account of study, or raw data, and
- Deficient archive and retrieval processes.

Following disqualification, the FDA reviews any submissions or approvals that contain nonclinical studies conducted at the disqualified testing facility to determine if any of these studies were compromised by the GLP noncompliance. If studies were impacted, then the FDA may rule those studies as unacceptable and, if critical to the application's approval, would require retesting for validity. Application approval may be terminated or withdrawn. The FDA may also choose to not accept nonclinical study data without also disqualifying the testing facility if the breach in integrity was an isolated incident and not a pervasive issue. Nonclinical studies initiated after testing facility disqualification are not considered in support of any application for a research or marketing permit unless the facility has been reinstated before the studies are started.

Disqualification of a testing facility falls under public disclosure and the FDA may choose to notify additional groups such as other government agencies that may review studies conducted at the site or the general public whenever such disclosure would further the public interest or promote compliance with the GLP regulations. In addition to site disqualification and nonacceptance of study data, the FDA may also press legal charges (civil or criminal). If a sponsor terminates a contract with a testing facility conducting a study supporting a submitted application, the sponsor must notify the FDA within 15 working days of the action and include a statement of the reasons behind the termination. However, suspension or termination of a testing facility by a Sponsor does not relieve the Sponsor of any obligation to submit the results of the study to the FDA.

To be reinstated, the testing facility must write a document to the FDA Commissioner indicating the reasons why it should be reinstated and a detailed description of corrective steps it has taken to assure that the facility is now and will remain GLP compliant in the future. The FDA will conduct a thorough inspection to verify that all corrective steps meet the FDA's expectations. Upon reinstatement, the FDA will notify the testing facility and any other organization that it had contacted at the point of disqualification and this information is available to the public under the Freedom of Information Act.

3. GLP AND PATHOLOGY DATA

3.1. Study Pathologist Requirements

GLP regulations require that the generation and interpretation of anatomic pathology and/or clinical pathology data must be by a Study Pathologist with the education, qualifications, and experience to perform these tasks. In a practical sense, the Study Pathologist also must have the expertise to integrate pathology findings with in-life findings, toxicokinetic data, and other relevant study information. The primary tasks of Study Pathologists are to characterize, describe, and tabulate alterations. In addition, the pathologist must decide which alterations are related to test article administration—and particularly which should be considered adverse or nonadverse (Kerlin, Bolon, & Burkhardt, 2016))—versus those that are spontaneous background changes and provide an interpretation of safety implications and functional consequences, all with consideration of the relevance to human safety. GLP standards do not specify precise requirements for Study

Pathologists, leaving it to sponsors and test facilities to define and confirm the proficiency of their pathology practitioners.

Toxicologic pathologists may come from different disciplines including veterinary medicine, human medicine, comparative pathology, toxicology, pharmacology, and biology, among others. Globally, significant differences exist in educational requirements, experience, and continued education of toxicologic pathologists (Bolon et al., 2010). In the United States, nonclinical safety assessments are predominantly performed by veterinary pathologists, recognizing the unique expertise in whole animal biology/ physiology/anatomy, animal diseases, animal models of disease, and comparative aspects between animal and human diseases and physiological responses. Veterinary pathology board certification is not required by GLP guidelines, but nonetheless is a benchmark of entry-level proficiency for toxicologic pathologists that is recognized by regulators who review pathology reports for animal toxicity studies.

3.2. Histopathology in the GLP Environment

Histology Processing

Histology documentation includes keeping records of the tissues procured, trimmed, embedded, sectioned, and stained as well as documentation of quality control checks such as a block to slide comparison. All materials must be uniquely identified and retrievable for future inquiries. Histology quality should assure that the same blocking pattern is used each time, no unnecessary sections exist, slide uniformity is maintained in terms of tissue thickness and orientation, and comparable hematoxylin and eosin staining intensity is achieved for control and test article–treated groups. Mixing of cassettes from multiple treatment groups or running the entire study on the same processing and staining cycle helps prevent processing artifacts that may be interpreted as a test article–related effect. Such counterbalancing is a requirement in some regulatory guidance for specific study types—and has been shown by collective experience to be a good idea in general—but is not a formal element in existing GLP standards.

Histopathological Evaluation and Pathology Peer Review

GLP regulations do not address the histopathological examination process aside from stating that all gross findings will be available to the pathologist at the time of microscopic evaluation. Pathology peer review as a quality control activity is not required by GLP regulations, but the FDA has released, at the time of writing this chapter, a *draft* guidance document (FDA, 2019). However, regulatory agencies look favorably on pathology peer review as a proven means for increasing the confidence that morphologic alterations are appropriately named and described, and that no test article–related findings have been missed or misinterpreted. Best practices for the primary and peer review pathologist are described in this book series (*Pathology Peer Review*, Vol 1, Chap 26) and various publications (Crissman et al., 2004; Morton et al., 2010).

The diagnostic lexicon for microscopic findings will vary among pathologists. Terminology standardization, such as International Harmonization of Nomenclature and Diagnostic Criteria (INHAND) (STP, 2005), attempts to establish definitions and "preferred" diagnostic terminology for common histopathologic changes. The INHAND effort (available online at https://www.goreni.org/gr3_nomenclature.php) forms the basis for nonclinical diagnostic terminology that now is required in product registration applications submitted to the FDA under its recent Standard for Exchange of Nonclinical Data initiative (*Nomenclature and Diagnostic Resources in Anatomic Toxicologic Pathology*, Vol 1, Chap 25; Mann et al., 2012,). Within the context of a study, the review of any previous study reports related to the same test article or development program assists in maintaining lexicon consistency so that reviewers are aware of the recurring findings and are not misled into thinking that a new finding has occurred. Careful consideration of terminology in earlier studies is important since this lexicon often carries forward into future studies for the same test article. If the terms used are inaccurate or constantly shifting, a disconnect may exist between earlier and chronic studies which can complicate the regulatory review process.

Pathology Report

GLP does not specify the content of the pathology report. However, recommended elements as described in an Society of Toxicologic Pathology (STP) Best Practices document (Morton et al., 2006) include a table of contents, materials, and methods, individual animal data and summary tables, interpretation and discussion of test article relatedness, text summary of morphologic findings, references, and signature of the study pathologist. More details can be found in *Preparation of the Anatomic Pathology Report for a Toxicity Study* (Vol 2, Chap 13).

The QA audit of the pathology report typically occurs after performance of a contemporaneous peer review, if one is conducted. This sequence assures that the text and tables of the final report are an accurate reflection of any refinements in diagnoses and/or severity grades implemented as a result of the peer review process. The actual conclusions and safety interpretation of the pathology report should not be called into question by the QA audit; the purpose of the audit is simply to ensure that studies meet regulatory requirements and study data are accurate. Any changes made to the study report once it has been signed and issued require the generation of an audit trail and an amended report. This revised report must indicate what changes were made, who made the alteration, the date and time of the change, and the reason for making them.

Definition of Raw Data in Pathology

The GLP definition of "raw data" is any laboratory worksheets, records, memoranda, notes, or exact copies thereof that are the results of original observations and activities of a study. This definition covers all data necessary for the reconstruction of the study report. Data must be recorded promptly, accurately, legibly, and indelibly; should be signed and dated (manually in ink, or electronically with an individual-specific code) when originally entered; and should include explicit reasons stated for any correction that might be needed later. Pathology raw data are covered by this definition.

What constitutes pathology raw data? The process of histopathologic diagnosis potentially may produce multiple changes in the preliminary diagnoses and/or their severity grades as controls are reviewed and reexamined against the treated groups. This iterative process is acknowledged in GLP by the understanding that the initial diagnoses produced by the Study Pathologist constitute "interim notes" that may change as the diagnoses are refined and the pathology report is being drafted. Introducing the element of pathology peer review presents another challenge. If changes are made to the histopathology data tables as a result of the peer review, should an audit trail be initiated? When faced with this question, the FDA has stated heretofore (FDA "Final Rule" of 1987, FDA, 1987) that to qualify as raw data, two components must be satisfied: (1) a finding is a recording of an original observation, and (2) such observations are necessary for the reconstruction of the study report. Logically, by this view, the study pathologist's interim notes do not meet the second of these criteria; instead, the current FDA perspective recognizes that the pathologist's notes are not necessary for the reconstruction and evaluation of the pathology raw data, which are defined as the list of diagnoses set forth in the final signed and dated pathology report. Since 21 CFR § 58.190(a) requires specimen retention (paraffin blocks, wet tissues, and slides), the histopathologic data in the final pathology report can be reconstructed by verification of the findings by another pathologist (pathology peer review) or a group of pathologists (pathology working group) working with the original tissue sections or newly produced sections from the archived blocks or tissues.

Pathology Imaging Compliance

PATHOLOGY IMAGES

As defined by GLP guidelines, images that are necessary for the reconstruction of a study and interpretation of the study report must be considered raw data for that study. Therefore, any image used for pathology data generation must be authenticated (annotated as raw data) and archived. In contrast, images generated for illustrative purposes to convey the characteristics of the lesion rather than as a basis for diagnosis are not considered raw data and thus need not be retained in archives.

In 2007, the STP made recommendations for the use and capture of pathology images in compliance with the 21 CFR 58 (GLP) and 21 CFR 11 (Electronic Records/Signatures, Tuomari et al., 2007). Key provisions include the following:

- Pathology images (printed, electronic, or digital) used for data generation are raw data requiring authentication and archiving.
- Physical images must be dated and signed, and electronic file images annotated in compliance with 21 CFR 11.
- Images used for raw data are subject to GLP procedures and controls ensuring data integrity including written SOPs, testing/validation of equipment, training of personnel, etc.
- Validation of imaging systems must be documented, and any exceptions must be described in the GLP Compliance Statement for the study
- Illustrative images are not raw data.
  - Accordingly, such images are not subject to GLP requirements, and
  - Images of this type should not be used to challenge or supplant the pathologist's diagnosis.

WHOLE-SLIDE IMAGING

Digital whole-slide imaging (WSI) is the generation of digital images from conventional glass microscope slides and discussed in detail in this volume (*Digital Pathology and Tissue Image Analysis*; Vol 1, Chap 12) as well as the published literature (Aeffner et al., 2019; Evans et al., 2018). While commonly used in pathology laboratories in multiple ways including for image analysis and consultation, WSI is not widely utilized for primary study evaluation in GLP nonclinical safety studies. Within the context of GLP-compliant studies, WSI is mainly used to gather second opinions from other, remotely based pathologists or to demonstrate a lesion but is not employed for primary study evaluation or formal peer review. The concern with incorporating digitized images rather than tissue sections as study materials for GLP studies is that data could be lost during the conversion process.

Several hurdles exist for the routine use of digital pathology in nonclinical safety studies. With respect to GLP compliance, validation of the whole-slide scanner (WSS) would be required in a regulated environment pertinent to study reconstruction, a time-intensive, multidisciplinary effort. Current FDA GLP regulations state that "equipment used for the generation, measurement, or assessment of data shall be adequately tested, calibrated, and/or standardized" (FDA, 1978). WSS validation would then require multiple assurances including security image file retention, inability to alter raw images, and trackable audit trails (Long et al., 2013). WSI may have archival advantages over glass slides since staining intensity of slide-mounted tissue sections fades with time and digital images remain constant. As technologies develop and the FDA is assured of image quality, scanning fidelity, and the ability of virtual imaging to conform to GLP standards, virtual pathology peer review may become a widespread practice.

4. CLINICAL PATHOLOGY ASSESSMENT IN THE GLP ENVIRONMENT

Clinical pathology laboratories are bound to GLP standards including the validation, certification, and/or qualification of all operations. These activities encompass the same attributes that must be addressed for anatomic pathology endpoints including employees, facilities, systems, equipment, methods, reagents, sampling, sample handling and testing, stability testing, and raw data management as well as the documentation, review and acceptance of test results, data generation, and reporting. All activities are SOP driven and must be well documented, traceable, and accountable. In addition to internal quality control measures, external quality control via participation in available proficiency programs, such as those administered by the College of American Pathologists (CAP) or performed according to Clinical Laboratory Improvement Amendments (CLIA) standards, can be a useful practice though they are not required under GLP. Novel biomarkers may require a GLP exemption if a GLP-compliant laboratory is not available to measure the analyte (Tomlinson et al., 2013).

5. ULTRASTRUCTURAL ASSESSMENT IN THE GLP ENVIRONMENT

Ultrastructural assessment using transmission electron microscopy (TEM) is occasionally used in nonclinical safety studies, often for confirmation of certain processes suggested by an initial light microscopic evaluation. In this regard, changes such as phospholipidosis, glomerular pathology, mitochondrial toxicity, and hepatic smooth endoplasmic reticulum proliferation due to enzyme induction are especially likely to be confirmed by TEM. The use of TEM is not addressed in regulatory guidance, and it is not specified that TEM should be conducted in compliance with GLP. The Scientific and Regulatory Policy Committee of the STP conducted a survey to understand current practices on the use of TEM in nonclinical toxicity studies, recognizing the utility of TEM on GLP-compliant nonclinical studies to support regulatory filings. The survey identified a decline in the use of TEM mainly due to a decrease in the number of external facilities or internal capabilities to perform TEM as well as the limited number of external companies executing GLP-compliant TEM. Therefore, most companies perform TEM in non-GLP fashion with emphasis on high-quality technical expertise and scientific accuracy rather than GLP compliance (Keirstead et al., 2019).

6. NONINVASIVE IMAGING APPLICATIONS IN THE GLP ENVIRONMENT

Imaging applications such as magnetic resonance imaging (MRI), computed (CT) and positron emission (PET) tomography, ultrasound, and other modalities have significantly contributed to drug discovery and development by characterization of pathophysiology of disease states and animal models of human disease. These platforms permit the longitudinal evaluation of disease progression in the same animal throughout a study while serving as a complement to histopathologic evaluation and other traditional endpoints for evaluating organ structure. Nonclinical imaging data have been used in support of regulatory submissions with GLP exemptions and can often readily translate to the clinical environment. However, the use of these modalities in a GLP-compliant regulated environment, like any unconventional endpoint, requires assurance of reliability, reproducibility, data integrity, and documentation. The electronic nature of the data lends itself to GLP compliance because the images can be fully tracked following calibration of the imaging equipment and validation of the processing software.

To achieve GLP compliance, each imaging modality would require specific SOPs for calibration, maintenance, and application of the instrument as well as software validation, retrieval, and archiving of raw and calculated data. Individuals involved in the operation of the instruments must be properly trained with appropriate management and QA oversight. Imaging biomarkers will need to be compared to a validated "gold standard" (i.e., micro-CT to assess fetal skeletons in developmental and reproductive toxicology studies validated against the standard Alizarin red stain) to assure noninferiority to current practice. Ultimately, interpretation and reporting of the images require training and experience of the evaluator and the respective peer reviewers (if applicable) in the assessments. Conclusions for such imaging data would be included in the final study report, and raw data—consistent with the situation for histopathologic raw data—would be the list of observations included in the signed image evaluation report. Given the extensive application of these modalities to address many wide-ranging research questions, broad validation under GLP would be challenging. However, GLP compliance should be attainable for repetitive, targeted, tissue-specific functional and morphological imaging procedures (Maronpot et al., 2017).

7. IN THE SPIRIT OF GLP

Many studies conducted before or concurrently with GLP-compliant studies may still be conducted "in the spirit of GLP," maintaining data integrity by following laboratory best practices though without the burdensome documentation and subsequent QA audit. Frequently, this approach means that the test article may not have all the documented purity assays in place, the QA unit does not inspect the study, and the endpoints are often more limited than with a GLP repeat-dose toxicity study. Non-GLP studies include in vitro and in vivo pharmacology studies designed to assess potential efficacy, screening ADME (absorption, distribution,

metabolism, and excretion) and toxicity studies designed to select clinical candidate molecules, and certain investigative studies. Repeat-dose pilot toxicity studies such as rodent screens, dose escalation, and investigative studies are not required to be conducted under GLP standards but typically are conducted under the same scientific integrity as GLP studies. However, submission of these studies to the FDA during the IND phase is encouraged. Other studies outside the scope of GLP include studies conducted in human subjects covered by GMP and GCP.

8. GLP CRITICISM

The GLP regulations focus on the integrity of nonclinical safety studies. Key features include assuring data reliability, integrity, and study reproducibility with thorough documentation, thereby reducing opportunities for error and fraud. GLP does not govern study design or quality of the scientific assessments.

8.1. Academic Research

Academic laboratories occasionally carry out studies for the development of pharmaceutical products. As government funding for research has become more competitive in recent years and funds for training graduate students have dwindled, academic laboratories have looked to industry as a source of income for their research efforts. Academic research, however, is not generally conducted under GLP conditions (unless they are conducting a study in partnership with a sponsor preparing a test article for submission to a regulatory agency). Best practice in academic research is covered by a series of recommended experimental and reporting procedures (Kilkenny et al., 2010; Scudamore et al., 2016), but in large part these address study design and reporting features needed for high-quality publications rather than standardizing and documenting study activities per se.

The main deterrents for academic laboratories conducting research under GLP directives are the large expense, time commitment, and infrastructure required for the extensive documentation required to carry out GLP-compliant studies. Such expenditures are prohibitive for most academic research projects or departments. Academic laboratories often exploit novel testing paradigms (for example, genetically engineered mice and identification of biomarkers) or technology to address a diverse array of biomedical research needs and only rarely produce compound-specific safety endpoints to support submissions, Additionally, academic laboratories operating in fiercely competitive grant landscape consider their methods proprietary, preventing other laboratories from competing for the same funding source. Academic research is scrutinized by granting agencies, peer reviews by leading experts in that field, and journal editors and manuscript reviewers instead of regulatory agencies. Some argue that this level of critique is as strict as that of regulatory agencies, although regulatory agencies have not been accepting of such an inconsistent system of oversight as an alternative for data to support regulatory filings.

If an academic institution chooses to initiate a GLP program, there are several options (Bolon et al., 2018). Discovery and efficacy studies typically are not performed using a GLP quality system; rather, only nonclinical safety studies intended to support initiation of human clinical trials will need to be GLP compliant. Options in an academic setting include placing the study(ies) at CROs or out-licensing the test articles to companies with experience in drug development that have existing GLP infrastructure. This approach comes with higher expenditure than in-house studies, and proprietary control of the molecule as well as much of the potential profit may need to be relinquished. Another option entails building the GLP infrastructure within the academic institution. This strategy comes at a significant cost but allows retention of intellectual control within the institution. Lastly, the institution can conduct the safety study in the "spirit" of GLP requiring establishment of SOPs, personnel training programs, and other components of GLP conduct but without the heavy commitment to documentation. The main drawback for this approach is lack of formal QA auditing.

8.2. Perspectives on GLP Limitations

GLP compliance focuses on ensuring the quality and integrity of the nonclinical data being generated. Importantly, GLP compliance does not set specific testing schemes, assays, and study designs. As such, adherence to GLP standards does not guarantee that decisions based on safety data are made correctly but merely ensures that the data used in making the decision are as trustworthy as possible. This distinction is critical.

Opponents of GLP argue that while GLP compliance assures thoroughness of documentation for reliable and valid scientific results, it cannot guarantee it. Academicians note that GLPs are guidelines and are unlike the NIH grant review process in which the quality of the research design, specific training of technicians, sensitivity of assays, and contemporary nature of the method can be reviewed, commented upon, and suggestions provided as feedback. One could argue that GLP stipulates a statement of experimental design that is agreed upon by the authors of the protocol suggesting that appropriate study design is in place to perform the safety evaluation. However, GLPs are focused on data integrity and may fall short with limitations in the model systems used.

9. CONCLUSIONS

In conclusion, GLP regulations ensure sound and repeatable nonclinical safety assessment studies. They set the standard by which studies are planned, conducted, monitored, reported, and archived to assure safety, reproducibility, and consistency in development of biomedical products. The pathologist plays an integral role in the design, conduct, and reporting of many GLP-compliant nonclinical toxicity studies. Therefore, a solid understanding of the principles of GLP assists the toxicologic pathologist in fulfilling their essential role in upholding the integrity, quality, and reproducibility of these safety defining studies.

REFERENCES

Aeffner F, Zarella MD, Buchbinder N, et al.: Introduction to digital image analysis in whole-slide imaging: a white paper from the digital pathology association, *J Pathol Inf* 10(9), 2019.

Bolon B, Barale-Thomas E, Bradley A, et al.: International recommendations for training future toxicologic pathologists participating in regulatory-type, nonclinical toxicity studies, *Exp Toxicol Pathol* 63:187–195, 2010.

Bolon B, Baze W, Shilling CJ, et al.: Good laboratory practice in the academic setting: fundamental principles for nonclinical safety assessment and GLP-compliant pathology support when developing innovative biomedical products, *ILAR J* 59:18–28, 2018.

Crissman JW, Goodman DG, Hildebrandt PK, et al.: Best practices guideline: toxicologic histopathology, *Toxicol Pathol* 32:126–131, 2004.

EPA (U.S. Environmental Protection Agency): *Title 40 - Protection of Environment Part 160—Good Laboratory Practice Standards Pesticide Programs*, 2011a. https://www.govinfo.gov/content/pkg/CFR-2011-title40-vol24/xml/CFR-2011-title40-vol24-part160.xml. (Accessed 15 May 2021).

EPA (U.S. Environmental Protection Agency): *Title 40 - Protection of Environment Part 792 Good Laboratory Practice Standards Toxic Substances Control Act*, 2011b. https://www.govinfo.gov/content/pkg/CFR-2011-title40-vol32/xml/CFR-2011-title40-vol32-part792.xml. (Accessed 15 May 2021).

Evans AJ, Bauer TW, Bui MM, et al.: US food and drug administration approval of whole slide imaging for primary diagnosis: a key milestone is reached and new questions are raised, *Arch Pathol Lab Med* 142:1383–1387, 2018.

FDA (U.S. Food and Drug Administration): *Comparison chart of FDA and EPA good laboratory practice (GLP) regulations and the OECD principles of GLP*, 2004. https://www.fda.gov/downloads/ICECI/EnforcementActions/Bioresearch Monitoring/UCM133724.pdf. (Accessed 15 May 2021).

FDA (U.S. Food and Drug Administration): *Title 21 - Food and Drugs Part 58 Good Laboratory Practice for Nonclinical Laboratory Studies*, 1978. https://www.accessdata.fda.gov/scripts/cdrh/cfdocs/cfcfr/CFRSearch.cfm?CFRPart=58. (Accessed 15 May 2021).

FDA (U.S. Food and Drug Administration): *21 CFR Part 58: Good Laboratory Practice Regulations; Final Rule*, 1987. https://www.fda.gov/media/75860/download. (Accessed 15 May 2021).

FDA (U.S. Food and Drug Administration): *Guidance Document: Good Laboratory Practice Regulations Questions and Answers*, 1998. https://www.fda.gov/regulatory-information/search-fda-guidance-documents/good-laboratory-practice-regulations-questions-and-answers. (Accessed 15 May 2021).

FDA (U.S. Food and Drug Administration): *Proposed Regulations and Draft Guidances*, 2010. https://www.federalregister.gov/documents/2010/12/21/2010-31888/good-laboratory-practice-for-nonclinical-laboratory-studies. (Accessed 15 May 2021).

FDA (US Food and Drug Administration): A Proposed Rule on Good Laboratory Practice for Nonclinical Laboratory Studies, 2016. Accessed 3 July 2020).

FDA (U.S. Food and Drug Administration): *Draft Guidance Document Pathology Peer Review in Nonclinical Toxicology Studies: Questions and Answers*, 2019. https://www.fda.gov/regulatory-information/search-fda-guidance-documents/pathology-peer-review-nonclinical-toxicology-studies-questions-and-answers. (Accessed 15 May 2021).

ICH (International Council for Harmonisation of Technical Requirements for Pharmaceuticals for Human Use): *ICH Guidelines*, 1990. https://www.ich.org/page/ich-guidelines. (Accessed 15 May 2021).

Keirstead ND, Janovitz EB, Meehan JT, et al.: Scientific and regulatory policy committee points to consider: review of scientific and regulatory policy committee points to consider: review of current practices for ultrastructural pathology evaluations in support of nonclinical toxicology studies, *Toxicol Pathol* 47:461–468, 2019.

Kerlin R, Bolon B, Burkhardt J, et al.: Scientific and Regulatory Policy Committee: recommended ("best") practices for determining, communicating, and using adverse effect data from nonclinical studies, *Toxicol Pathol* 44:147–162, 2016.

Kilkenny C, Browne WJ, Cuthill IC, et al.: Improving bioscience research reporting: the ARRIVE guidelines for reporting animal research, *PLoS Biol* 8:e1000412, 2010.

Long RE, Smith A, Machotka SV, et al.: Scientific and Regulatory Policy Committee (SRPC) paper: validation of digital pathology systems in the regulated nonclinical environment, *Toxicol Pathol* 41:115–124, 2013.

Mann PC, Vahle J, Keenan CM, et al.: International harmonization of toxicologic pathology nomenclature: an overview and review of basic principles, *Toxicol Pathol* 40:7s–13s, 2012.

Maronpot RR, Nyska A, Troth SP, et al.: Regulatory Forum Opinion Piece: Imaging Applications in Toxicologic Pathology—Recommendations for Use in Regulated Nonclinical Toxicity Studies, *Toxicol Pathol* 45:444–471, 2017.

Morton D, Kemp RK, Francke-Carroll S, et al.: Best practices for reporting pathology interpretations within GLP toxicology studies, *Toxicol Pathol* 34:806–809, 2006.

Morton D, Sellers RS, Barale-Thomas E, et al.: Recommendations for pathology peer review, *Toxicol Pathol* 38:1118–1127, 2010.

OECD (Organisation for Economic Co-operation and Development): *OECD Guidelines for the Testing of Chemicals*, 1981. https://www.oecd-ilibrary.org/environment/oecd-guidelines-for-the-testing-of-chemicals_72d77764-en. (Accessed 15 May 2021).

OECD (Organisation for Economic Co-operation and Development): *OECD Principles on Good Laboratory Practice*, 1998. http://www.oecd.org/officialdocuments/publicdisplaydocumentpdf/?cote=env/mc/chem(98)17&doclanguage=en. (Accessed 15 May 2021).

OECD (Organisation for Economic Co-operation and Development): *Links to National Web Sites on Good Laboratory Practice*, 2018. https://www.oecd.org/chemicalsafety/testing/linkstonationalwebsitesongoodlaboratorypractice.htm. (Accessed 15 May 2021).

OECD (Organisation for Economic Co-operation and Development): *Decision of the Council Concerning the Mutual Acceptance of Data in the Assessment of Chemicals,*

1997. https://legalinstruments.oecd.org/en/instruments/263. (Accessed 15 May 2021). Adopted on 5 November 1981.

Scudamore CL, Soilleux EJ, Karp NA, et al.: Recommendations for minimum information for publication of experimental pathology data: MINPEPA guidelines, *J Pathol* 238: 359–367, 2016.

STP (Society of Toxicologic Pathology): *International Harmonization of Nomenclature and Diagnostic Criteria (INHAND) Nonproliferative and Proliferative Lesions of the Rat and Mouse,* 2005. https://www.toxpath.org/inhand.asp. (Accessed 15 May 2021).

Tomlinson L, Boone LI, Ramaiah L, et al.: Best practices for veterinary toxicologic clinical pathology, with emphasis on the pharmaceutical and biotechnology industries, *Vet Clin Pathol* 42:252–269, 2013.

Tuomari DL, Kemp RK, Sellers R, et al.: Society of Toxicologic Pathology position paper on pathology image data: compliance with 21 CFR Parts 58 and 11, *Toxicol Pathol* 35:450–455, 2007.

United States Senate: *Joint hearings on preclinical and clinical testing by the pharmaceutical industry (before the subcommittee on health of the committee on labor and public welfare, and the subcommittee on administrative practice and procedure of the committee on the judiciary of the 94th congress),* Washington, D.C., 1975, U.S. Government Printing Office.

Zhou M: *Regulated bioanalytical laboratories : technical and regulatory aspects from global perspectives,* New Jersey, 2011, Wiley.

CHAPTER

28

Practices to Optimize Generation, Interpretation, and Reporting of Pathology Data from Toxicity Studies

Armando R. Irizarry Rovira[1], *David Garcia-Tapia*[1], *Daniel J. Patrick*[2]

[1]Eli Lilly & Company, Indianapolis, IN, United States, [2]Charles River Laboratories, Mattawan, MI, United States

OUTLINE

1. Introduction   1030

2. Practices that Prevent or Mitigate the Introduction of Pathology-Related Issues During Study Design and Protocol Preparation   1031
  2.1. Ensure a Deep Understanding of Regulatory Guidance and Best Practices   1032
  2.2. Clearly Define Realistic Study Goals, Design the Study to Accomplish Those Goals, and Minimize Study Complexity   1035
  2.3. Choose the Appropriate Animal Species, Genetic Background, and/or Disease Model for Toxicity Testing   1037
  2.4. Use Optimal Communication Practices   1039
  2.5. Estimate and Communicate the Number of Potential Target Tissues   1040
  2.6. Develop and Practice Novel or Nonstandard Pathology Procedures and Other Methods Prior to the Start of the Study and Use Accepted Practices for Incorporation of Nonstandard Endpoints   1040
  2.7. Ensure that Study Procedures Are Adequately Described in the Study Protocol or Standard Operating Procedures   1042
  2.8. Plan for Pathology Peer Review   1043
  2.9. Do Not Blind the Study Pathologist   1043
  2.10. Facilitate the Study and Peer Review Pathologists' Workflows   1044

3. Practices that Prevent or Mitigate the Introduction of Pathology-Related Issues Arising During the In-Life Phase   1044
  3.1. Ensure the Proper Training of Personnel, Use of Appropriate Assays, Maintenance of Required Instrumentation, and Use of Quality Assurance Programs   1045
  3.2. Ensure Awareness of Emerging Data from In-Life Time Points and Unscheduled Terminations   1046
  3.3. Mitigate the Impact of Unexpected or Significant Toxicity   1047
  3.4. Scrutinize Impromptu Requests for Samples from Ongoing Studies for Assays that Are Not Critical to the Purpose of the Study   1049
  3.5. Understand When Not to Generate Pathology Data   1049

4. Practices that Prevent or Mitigate Issues Arising from Pathology Assessment and Reporting   1050
  4.1. Ensure Proper Training, Supervision, Procedures, and Protocol Familiarity in the Necropsy, Histology, and Clinical Pathology Laboratories   1050
  4.2. Schedule Adequate Time for Processing and Evaluation   1054
  4.3. Establish Strong Lines of Communication and Freely Share Scientific and Program Information with the Study Pathologist   1057

Haschek and Rousseaux's Handbook of Toxicologic Pathology, Fourth Edition.
https://doi.org/10.1016/B978-0-12-821044-4.00016-9

4.4. *Recommended Practices for Histopathologic Assessment*   1060

4.5. *Facilitate Finalization of a Well-Constructed, High-Quality, On-Time Pathology Report*   1069

5. **Conclusions**   1072

Glossary   1072

References   1072

1. INTRODUCTION

Toxicologic pathologists fill important roles in enabling the delivery of new medicines, chemicals, and other products that improve and save lives across the world. These include serving as study pathologists, peer review pathologists, sponsor pathologists, consultants, toxicologists, and other roles. For many pathologists, postgraduate training is just the beginning of a journey of professional growth practicing toxicologic pathology at a diverse group of organizations including contract research organizations (CROs), bio/pharmaceutical companies, regulatory agencies, universities, and other institutions. In the course of our professional careers, pathologists learn a great deal via interactions with talented colleagues, on-the-job experiences, and continued study.

In this chapter, we share a series of recommended practices related to nonclinical toxicity study design and conduct. We believe that awareness and implementation of these practices by toxicologic pathologists optimizes the generation, interpretation, and reporting of pathology data and improves the overall study outcome. These practices are written from the perspective of Good Laboratory Practice (GLP)–regulated nonclinical toxicity studies supporting the development of biotherapeutics and pharmaceuticals. We will not specifically address these practices as they might apply to animal toxicity studies supporting nontherapeutic products, such as agrochemicals and occupational chemicals, and veterinary drugs. However, some, if not all, of these general principles should be applicable to these types of studies as well.

This chapter focuses on the toxicologic pathology practices that prevent or mitigate the introduction of pathology-related issues during the three main study stages: study design and protocol preparation, the live ("in life" or antemortem) phase, and the postmortem phase (necropsy through clinical pathology and histopathologic assessment and reporting). Our goal for this chapter is for the toxicologic pathologist to understand three key principles:

1. A solid understanding of study goals, regulatory expectations, and pathology best practices is foundational to successful pathology evaluations.
2. Active study oversight combined with timely and deliberate communications among the study team will facilitate prompt adjustments to unplanned events and are key factors in the success of nonclinical toxicity studies.
3. Suboptimal design and/or execution of pathology evaluations will undermine the value of nonclinical toxicity studies.

The understanding and application of these three key principles will help the toxicologic pathologist become an effective and valuable member of any organization that conducts and/or sponsors nonclinical toxicity studies. Furthermore, the toxicologic pathologist that combines these principles with a passion for learning, continuous improvement, and translational research will have a positive influence on the development of therapies or products that benefit people and animals.

2. PRACTICES THAT PREVENT OR MITIGATE THE INTRODUCTION OF PATHOLOGY-RELATED ISSUES DURING STUDY DESIGN AND PROTOCOL PREPARATION

Fundamental to all sciences is the process of investigation, commonly known as the scientific method, which is applicable to the studies performed to assess the toxicity of new chemical or biological entities. Experimentation is a key aspect of the scientific method and requires thoughtful planning and implementation of controls that allow testing of hypotheses. Therefore, successful planning of toxicity studies follows the same principles of planning for any scientific experiment. Well-planned and smoothly executed toxicity studies allow the generation of reliable data that minimize uncertainty, reduce variability in toxicologic responses, and enable effective decision-making during the development of new drugs. Careful planning and design of toxicity studies are key components of the process of risk assessment in drug development. Suboptimal study design may lead to wrong or misleading conclusions that could harm humans and hamper the progression of a new therapy or chemical by introducing poor-quality data.

The drug development process requires the conduct of nonclinical and clinical studies. Nonclinical studies include animal toxicity studies, which most of the time are regulated by GLPs (see *Pathology and GLPs, Quality Control and Quality Assurance*, Vol 1, Chap 27). During the early research and development phase, new drug candidates need to be evaluated through initial studies which help in the characterization of bioavailability; ADME (absorption, distribution, metabolism and elimination); safety pharmacology; and general toxicology. These exploratory and pilot studies are performed under stringent method controls but usually do not follow GLP regulations. However, pivotal nonclinical studies supporting the dosing of humans must be conducted under GLP standards in order to support submission of an Investigational New Drug (IND) application in the United States, or submission of marketing authorization to the European

Medicines Agency's (EMA) Committee for Advanced Therapies in the European Union, or its equivalent process in other countries or geographic regions. The study package submitted as part of the regulatory applications should provide the information needed to establish a safe starting dose level that allows the testing of drug candidates (termed "test articles" by the US Food and Drug Administration [FDA] and "test items" by the EMA) in humans. Usually, that level is based on the "no observed adverse effect level" (NOAEL), but other approaches such as the benchmark dose also can be used (see *Interpreting Adverse Effects*, Vol 2, Chap 15). Since those studies are used to set the safety parameters needed for dosing the drug candidate in humans for the first time, the nonclinical study team must assure that the planning/design, conduct, and interpretation of those studies were done under the most stringent standards. This assurance will support the safety of humans that will be administered the new drug. Once the new drug candidate is in the clinical phase of development, additional nonclinical toxicity studies of longer duration are conducted. Depending on the intended purpose of the new drug, this battery of tests may include chronic toxicity, genotoxicity, developmental and reproductive toxicity, juvenile toxicity, and/or carcinogenicity studies, all of which must be performed under GLP standards (see *The Role of Pathology in Evaluation of Reproductive, Developmental, and Juvenile Toxicity*, Vol 1, Chap 7 and *Carcinogenicity Assessment*, Vol 2, Chap 5). Careful study planning and design is an essential responsibility of the toxicologist and/or toxicologic pathologist. In particular, toxicologic pathologists are responsible for ensuring that all aspects related to pathology endpoints in a nonclinical toxicity study are thoughtfully planned.

Regardless of the stage of development, a variety of factors are of importance to designing optimal in vivo nonclinical toxicity studies. These include a thorough understanding of the overall development strategy for the test article, regulatory guidance and best practices applicable to the area of study, the intended goal(s) of the study, knowledge of the pharmacology of the test article, competitive intelligence information or data from the literature on the same or related materials, choice of animal species, availability of exploratory pharmacokinetic (PK), toxicokinetic (TK) and toxicity data, and the estimated doses to be administered in clinical trials. An understanding of the overall development strategy will influence the number and duration of nonclinical toxicity studies, permit estimation of when (or if) to include reversibility phases and define when these studies will need to be initiated within the timeline of the development program. Lynch and collaborators (Lynch et al., 2009) suggest that the development team should draft the product label before designing the toxicology package needed to achieve product registration. This working document will allow the team to agree on a common understanding of key components of the development program, such as therapeutic indication, target population, dosing regimen, duration of treatment, route of administration, formulation, potential drug combinations, etc. Once the development team has a draft of the product label, it will be easier to establish a development strategy to achieve the program goals, which will be followed by the identification of the potential animal-based pharmacology and toxicity studies that would be needed for the authorization of the first dosing in humans and eventually for the marketing authorization. Regulatory guidance sets minimum requirements and provides the general framework for development programs and nonclinical toxicity studies. Best practice recommendations, such as those published by the Society of Toxicologic Pathology (STP; https://www.toxpath.org/best-practices.asp; Table 28.1) and the American Society for Veterinary Clinical Pathology (https://www.asvcp.org/page/QALS_Guidelines), complement guidance documents provided by regulatory agencies (e.g., EMA, FDA) and international consortia (e.g., the International Council for Harmonisation of Technical Requirements for Pharmaceuticals for Human Use [ICH], the Organisation for Economic Co-operation and Development [OECD]) by providing more detailed information on the what parameters or procedures to include in toxicity studies. Clearly defining the goals of the study facilitates the design of optimal, efficient, and simple studies. Knowledge of the intended or unintended pharmacologic activity can be derived from in vitro or in vivo investigations and help the development team define potential target tissues, types of toxicity, and proposed dose levels. Published information on chemically similar test articles, research on the pharmacologic target, characterization of genetically modified animals, and other kinds of public disclosures can be very informative and allow development teams to fine-tune their study designs. Selection of the appropriate animal species is a critical deliverable for the development team prior to designing any toxicity study. As described below, the selection of animal species will be influenced by a variety of factors. Exploratory PK, TK, and toxicity data help guide formulation of the test article, define dose levels, frequency of dosing, potential tolerability, animal species selection, and possible dose–response relationships. Lastly, knowing the estimated doses to be used in clinical trials in combination with simulations of PK, TK, and pharmacodynamic (PD) profiles allows the team to estimate potential margins of exposure and safety, and set dose levels in the nonclinical toxicity studies supporting the clinical trials.

In conclusion, toxicologic pathologists play a key role in the design of nonclinical toxicity studies and their participation is of paramount importance during protocol preparation in order to prevent or mitigate the introduction of pathology-related issues during this phase.

2.1. Ensure a Deep Understanding of Regulatory Guidance and Best Practices

Governmental regulatory agencies such as the FDA in the United States and the EMA in Europe as well as international consortia like the OECD have issued GLP standards specifying that all procedures used in the toxicologic assessment of new drugs intended for human use must be clearly defined and accountability accurately documented. These guidelines should be followed when toxicity assessment is conducted in order to satisfy the regulatory requirements for the registration and marketing of new drugs.

Although each country may have unique regulatory requirements for the assessment of the safety of new chemical or biological entities, international efforts for harmonization have

TABLE 28.1   Selected Useful References Applicable to Study Design, Conduct, and Reporting

BEST PRACTICES[a]

Topic	Reference
Toxicologic clinical pathology	Tomlinson et al. (2016) Best practices for evaluating clinical pathology in pharmaceutical recovery studies
Toxicologic clinical pathology	Tomlinson et al. (2013) Best practices for veterinary toxicologic clinical pathology, with emphasis on the pharmaceutical and biotechnology industries
Toxicologic histopathology	Crissman et al. (2004) Best practices guideline: toxicologic histopathology
Reporting pathology interpretation	Morton et al. (2006) Best practices for reporting pathology interpretations within GLP toxicology studies
Adversity in nonclinical studies	Kerlin et al. (2016). Scientific and Regulatory Policy Committee: recommended ("best") practices for determining, communicating, and using adverse effect data from nonclinical studies
Best practices on recovery studies	Perry et al. (2013) Society of toxicologic pathology position paper on best practices on recovery studies: the role of the anatomic pathologist

POSITION PAPERS, RECOMMENDATIONS, AND OTHER REFERENCES[a]

Topic	Reference
Use of animal models	Morgan et al. (2013) Use of animal models of human disease for nonclinical safety assessment of novel pharmaceuticals
Interpretation of stress responses	Everds et al. (2013b) Interpreting stress responses during routine toxicity studies: a review of the biology, impact, and assessment
Organ weights	Sellers et al. (2007) Society of toxicologic pathology position paper: organ weight recommendations for toxicology studies
Blinded slide reading	STP Society of Toxicologic Pathology (1986) Society of toxicologic pathologists' position paper on blinded slide reading
Evaluation of pathology data	Burkhardt et al. (2011). Recommendations for the evaluation of pathology data in nonclinical safety biomarker qualification studies
Severity grades in histopathology	Schafer et al. (2018). Use of severity grades to characterize histopathologic changes
Pathology peer review	(Fikes, Patrick, & Francke (2015)) Scientific and Regulatory Policy Committee Review: Review of the Organisation for Economic Co-operation and Development (OECD) guidance on the GLP requirements for peer review of histopathology
Pathology peer review	Morton et al. (2010) Recommendations for pathology peer review
Carcinogenicity studies	Bregman et al. (2003) Recommended tissue list for histopathologic examination in repeat-dose toxicity and carcinogenicity studies: a proposal of the society of toxicologic pathology (STP)
Carcinogenicity studies	Nold et al. (2001) Society of toxicologic pathology position paper: diet as a variable in rodent toxicology and carcinogenicity studies
Digital pathology	Long at al. (2013). Scientific and Regulatory Policy Committee (SRPC) paper: validation of digital pathology systems in the regulated nonclinical environment.

[a] *From the Society of Toxicologic Pathology, https://www.toxpath.org/best-practices.asp.*

resulted in the publication of standardized approaches by the ICH (Table 28.2; https://www.ich.org/page/safety-guidelines). This Council is composed of representatives from regulatory authorities and bio/pharmaceutical firms.

Toxicologists and toxicologic pathologists working in the bio/pharmaceutical industry are expected to know and understand the appropriate regulatory guidelines. Understanding these guidelines is the basis for the appropriate design of studies intended to assess the safety

TABLE 28.2 Selected International Council on Harmonization of Technical Requirements for Registration of Pharmaceuticals for Human Use (ICH) Safety Guidelines[a]

S1A-S1C	Carcinogenicity Studies • S1A Need for Carcinogenicity Studies of Pharmaceuticals • S1B Testing for Carcinogenicity of Pharmaceuticals • S1C(R2) Dose Selection for Carcinogenicity Studies of Pharmaceuticals • S1(R1) EWG Rodent Carcinogenicity Studies for Human Pharmaceuticals
S2	Genotoxicity Studies • S2(R1) Guidance on genotoxicity testing and data interpretation for pharmaceuticals intended for human use
S3A-S3B	Toxicokinetics and pharmacokinetics • S3A Note for guidance on toxicokinetics: The assessment of systemic exposure in toxicity studies • S3A Q&As Questions and answers: Note for guidance on toxicokinetics: The assessment of systemic exposure-focus on microsampling • S3B Pharmacokinetics: Guidance for repeated dose tissue distribution studies
S4	Toxicity testing • S4 Duration of chronic toxicity testing in animals (rodent and nonrodent toxicity testing)
S5	Reproductive toxicology • S5(R3) Detection of reproductive and developmental toxicity for human pharmaceuticals
S6	Biotechnological products • S6(R1) Preclinical safety evaluation of biotechnology-derived pharmaceuticals
S7A-S7B	Pharmacology studies • S7A Safety pharmacology studies for human pharmaceuticals • S7B The nonclinical evaluation of the potential for delayed ventricular repolarization (QT interval prolongation) by human pharmaceuticals • E14/S7B IWG Questions and answers: Clinical and nonclinical evaluation of QT/QTc interval prolongation and proarrhythmic potential
S8	Immunotoxicology studies • S8 Immunotoxicity studies for human pharmaceuticals
S9	Nonclinical evaluation for anticancer pharmaceuticals • S9 Nonclinical evaluation for anticancer pharmaceuticals • S9 Q&As Questions and answers: Nonclinical evaluation for anticancer pharmaceuticals

(Continued)

TABLE 28.2 Selected International Council on Harmonization of Technical Requirements for Registration of Pharmaceuticals for Human Use (ICH) Safety Guidelines[a]—cont'd

S10	Photosafety evaluation • S10 Photosafety evaluation of pharmaceuticals
S11	Nonclinical paediatric safety • S11 EWG Nonclinical safety testing in support of development of paediatric medicines
S12	Nonclinical biodistribution studies for gene therapy products • S12 EWG Nonclinical biodistribution studies for gene therapy products
M3	Nonclinical safety studies • M3(R2) Guidance on nonclinical safety studies for the conduct of human clinical trials and marketing authorization for pharmaceuticals • M3(R2) Q&As (R2) Questions and answers: Guidance on nonclinical safety studies for the conduct of human clinical trials and marketing authorization for pharmaceuticals

[a] *https://www.ich.org/page/safety-guidelines or https://www.ich.org/page/multidisciplinary-guidelines.*

of new chemical and/or biological entities. For instance, for the pharmaceutical industry, the ICH guideline M3(R2) describes the nonclinical safety studies that are recommended to support human clinical trials as well as marketing authorization of bio/pharmaceuticals. It is the basis for planning safety assessment packages and the specific toxicity studies that compose those packages. Specific guidelines pertaining to various toxicity studies (e.g., genotoxicity, carcinogenicity, acute toxicity, repeated-dose toxicity, reproductive toxicity, etc.) are also available and are discussed elsewhere in this textbook (see *The Role of Pathology in Product Discovery and Safety Assessment*, Vol 2, Chap 2; *The Role of Pathology in Evaluation of Reproductive, Developmental, and Juvenile Toxicity*, Vol 1, Chap 7; and *Carcinogenicity Assessment*, Vol 2, Chap 5).

In some cases, a deep understanding of regulatory guidance and pathology best practices needs to be augmented with additional consultations to ensure that the pathology aspects of a nonclinical toxicity study will be sufficient to enable dosing in humans, predict potential risks to exposed humans, or permit registration. In these cases, proactive consultations with third-party subject matter experts and/or regulatory agencies will be helpful, if not essential. Examples of these cases include carcinogenicity studies, programs with expected complex toxicity profiles, programs with low margins of safety, or test articles with novel mechanisms of

action or unusual therapeutic modalities. The communication may include the submission of background project information and the proposed protocol or study design elements for key studies together with the key questions that the development team is submitting for advice. Such proactive consultations increase the chances that the study design is scientifically robust, will provide meaningful data to enable dosing or predict potential risk in humans, and will be acceptable to regulators. Not consulting with regulators or subject matter experts may result in nonclinical toxicity studies that are not acceptable to regulatory agencies. Communication with regulatory agencies will help the development team to incorporate the perspective and experience of regulators into study designs, especially since regulators may have knowledge of toxicity risks unique to a class of test articles. Understanding the regulatory perspective on a specific program is helpful for the most efficient allocation of time and resources as well as for the appropriate design of studies for that program.

2.2. Clearly Define Realistic Study Goals, Design the Study to Accomplish Those Goals, and Minimize Study Complexity

The study design starts with identifying the goals and objectives that the study team wants or needs to achieve with the experiment. These goals must be realistic and achievable, and the study team must understand the problem and what question(s) the study can and cannot address. It is often most efficient to start with the end in mind and then work backwards when designing the study. The identification of a hypothesis, or hypotheses, is a critical part of defining study goals and is easier to achieve if the team understands the details of the research program and the current status of the development program. For instance, knowing the pharmacologic target, the intended therapeutic indication, the proposed population to be treated, the literature reporting the biology of the target, and the potential implications of manipulating the target may guide the team as to what nonstandard endpoints must be included in the study. Understanding the current point in the development program helps determine if a short-duration or a dose-ranging study should only include survival and tolerability endpoints rather than including full batteries of in-life, clinical pathology, and anatomic pathology endpoints. Sometimes pathology endpoints, such as microscopic evaluation of tissues, are not essential to the goals of a study and avoiding inclusion of these endpoints will allow the use of nonnaïve animals to avoid the unnecessary use and termination of naïve animals. Having a clear understanding of the main goals of a toxicity study will help the toxicologist and/or toxicologic pathologist fine-tune the risk assessment of new chemical entities and avoid the conduct of unnecessary studies or the addition of unnecessary, complex, or unachievable goals or endpoints to toxicity studies.

The likelihood of ending up with an unsuccessful, confounded, invalid, or inaccurate study increases when an experiment has too many variables, requires an excessively complex design to test the hypotheses, if the goals are not sufficiently clear or specific, and/or has goals that are unlikely to be achievable. An example of the latter would be not planning for a sufficiently long reversibility period to determine whether or not complete recovery takes place for findings that require longer periods to reverse (e.g., testicular toxicity). Although being mindful of the 3Rs (Replacement, Reduction, and Refinement) in animal research is important, one should avoid the temptation to "get as much as possible" from any particular study by including too many endpoints. Currently, there is a strong push in industry for drug development teams to accelerate their research and development programs, prompting the common request for "innovative" ways to design nonclinical toxicity studies that maximize the amount of information obtained from a single study. Although innovation in such omnibus studies is welcomed and encouraged, study teams must always ensure that any novel endpoints or designs do not undermine the integrity of their studies. For example, the development team, which includes scientists outside of the toxicology or pathology disciplines, may request that the team "take advantage" of a toxicity study to answer questions regarding the pharmacology of the test article, which may greatly complicate the study design. Interest in "taking advantage" of a toxicity study is common within multidisciplinary teams that have a limited understanding of toxicology risk assessment or the limitations of nonclinical toxicity studies. If the toxicologist and toxicologic pathologist are not careful, agreeing to these requests to address side issues may introduce nonessential goals to the toxicity study, triggering the need for the collection of samples or data that are not commonly collected in standard toxicity studies. For instance, development teams may be interested in collecting tissue samples that require special surgical procedures to be performed during the in-life phase of the study in order to have special assessments of the pharmacology of the test article. Those procedures could introduce new variables into the study such as postprocedure complications, medications, and/or anesthesia that might jeopardize the interpretation of the core pathology data. Before introducing those new variables, the toxicologist and/or toxicologic pathologist must evaluate the impact on study procedures, the tissue samples, and the quality, accuracy and validity of the study. Features of an excessively complex study design may also include an unnecessarily large number of experimental groups, more than one test article, endpoints for which tests are not standardized or well understood, excessive sampling time points, and/or the collection of samples that require special procedures that have not been practiced in "production mode."

If the inclusion of any of these "extra" items is elected in a study, it is important to keep in mind that the main goal of a toxicity study is the toxicologic characterization of the test article. Therefore, study designs should emphasize acquisition of data to serve that purpose without introducing errors or external factors that may jeopardize the validity of the study. There may be times where designing separate studies rather than a single all-encompassing study will be better for the evaluation and interpretation of clinical pathology and anatomic pathology data.

2.3. Choose the Appropriate Animal Species, Genetic Background, and/or Disease Model for Toxicity Testing

The choice of which animal species to use in a nonclinical toxicity study is dictated by a number of factors including regulatory guidance, the test species' physiological and metabolic similarities to humans, the pharmacological activity (or lack thereof) of the test article in the species, availability of historical control data for the species, typical lifespan of the species (relevant mainly for chronic toxicity or carcinogenicity studies), adaptability of the species to experimental conditions, and feasibility of using the species under the intended experimental conditions. In addition to selecting the appropriate animal species for investigating the test article, the development team must select the appropriate genetic background or strain, geographic origin of animals, and/or determine if an animal model of disease will be used in the toxicity studies. The use of the appropriate animal species, genetic background, and (when necessary) disease model are key elements of a well-designed toxicity study that minimizes variability in toxicologic responses and facilitates the generation of high-quality pathology data. Irrelevant, confounding, or potentially misleading pathology data may be generated if inappropriate animal species, background, or disease models are used during the development program. For each animal species, strain, or model selected, the toxicologic pathologist must become deeply familiar with the types of spontaneous findings in the animals under investigation (McInnes, 2012). This knowledge will be increased with experience and awareness of the many scientific

publications dedicated to these topics. Armed with experience and knowledge, the toxicologic pathologist will be able to better assess if microscopic and/or clinical pathology findings are spontaneous or test article related.

The growing use of biological entities has evolved to the point of increasing the need for nonhuman primates (NHPs) as test species. This choice is dictated because such human-derived test articles may not be pharmacologically active in nonprimates, thus limiting the use of rodents as part of the safety assessment package. Alternatively, other approaches might be needed, such as surrogate molecules (e.g., a rodent-derived biomolecule with a similar pharmacologic action in rodents as the human-derived test article), nonstandard animal species such as marmosets, or genetically modified animals (e.g., which express the human molecule that is targeted by the human-derived test article) to test the potential for pharmacologically driven toxicity (Leach, 2013, and *Genetically Engineered Animal Models in Toxicologic Research*, Vol 1, Chap 23). If a biologic is not cross-reactive with rodents, the development team must also consider if assessing carcinogenicity in alternative models will be a necessary course of action (Vahle et al., 2010). The toxicologic pathologist must be aware of the limitations, complications, and influence of these alternative approaches on the generation of pathology data. For example, the use of nonstandard animal species may complicate the interpretation of test article effects because of the lack of historical experience at the test facility or lack of a robust historical control database of spontaneous findings.

The use of nonstandard animal species may also be needed for test articles that are not biotherapeutics. Rodents have many metabolic pathways, physiological processes, and pathological responses similar to those in humans. However, there are some responses in rodents that have been demonstrated to not be relevant to humans due to differences in the PK, TK, PD, metabolism, genetic differences, and other factors (see *Animal Models in Toxicologic Research: Rodents*, Vol 1, Chap 17). Furthermore, these responses may also differ among rodent species (and strains) and may result in selection of nonstandard rodent species as the appropriate rodent species for testing, such as the Syrian Golden hamster for carcinogenicity (Wang et al., 2017; FDA, 2010a, FDA Food and Drug Administration, 2015). The toxicologic pathologist must be part of the discussion when the use of nonstandard animal species is being considered and be prepared to generate pathology data without the availability of robust historical control data.

In addition to the appropriate selection of a rodent species, the selection of a proper stock or strain is an essential piece of planning for a toxicology program and ensuring that relevant pathology data are generated. Being aware of the characteristics of the rodent outbred stocks and inbred strains or genetic lines used for toxicological assessment is important, and the development team must define, based on the nature of the test article, whether chronic toxicity and/or carcinogenicity studies will be required. If the toxicology package will include chronic toxicity and carcinogenicity studies, it is highly recommended to use the same rat stock, strain, or genetic line throughout the entire toxicology program due to the differences occurring among different strains or genetic lines (Weber et al., 2011). Examples of the impact of rodent genetic background on the generation pathology data were highlighted in a recent publication (Bhaskaran et al., 2018) where pancreatic microscopic changes occurring only in rats after administration of a Bruton's Tyrosine Kinase inhibitor were strain dependent. Other strain-dependent spontaneous findings in rodents, such as aortitis in BALB/c mice (Ramot et al., 2009), can influence the assessment of test article–related effects. Similarly, genetic background can influence spontaneous tumor incidence in rodents of different stocks and strains (Weber et al., 2011). Rodent strains with high spontaneous tumor incidences in certain tissues may make the assessment of test article–related carcinogenicity in those tissues more difficult for the toxicologic pathologist.

The source of the animals is an important consideration in study design. When utilizing NHPs in toxicity studies, the geographic source (e.g., China vs. Mauritius vs. other regions of Southeast Asia) may be an important factor since it is known that there is slight genetic and phenotypic variability among populations of monkeys (Kozlosky et al., 2015; Chamanza et al., 2010; Blancher et al., 2008). The use of different geographic sources across a development program may impact the toxicologic pathologist by introducing variation in the incidence of spontaneous microscopic changes or clinical pathology parameters and thus potentially confound the interpretation of test article–related changes (Kozlosky et al., 2015; Cauvin et al., 2015). It is recommended that when possible study teams utilize animals from a consistent geographic origin across the toxicity studies supporting a drug program, and that the toxicologic pathologist be well versed in the common spontaneous findings that occur in the animals from that geographic origin (see *Animal Models in Toxicologic Research: Nonhuman Primate*, Vol 1, Chap 21). Familiarity with the common spontaneous findings will enable the pathologist to more accurately separate test article–related findings from incidental findings. For rodents, we also recommend that the study team use a consistent source and breeding facility to minimize sources of variability across studies. However, over time, continued inbreeding of rodents at a specific location likely may result in generation of a substrain (e.g., C57BL/6NCrl vs. C57BL/6NTac substrains maintained by Charles River Laboratories and Taconic, respectively) (Sellers, 2017).

Animal models of disease are not routinely used to assess the toxicity of test articles. However, the thoughtful use of these disease models can sometimes help investigate pathogeneses and inform the evaluation of test article–related findings and risk to humans (Tomohiro et al., 2019; Tirmenstein et al., 2015; Morgan et al., 2013). For example, some targets that are present only during a disease process, such as the expression of beta-amyloid (Aβ) in Alzheimer's disease patients, have prompted the use of engineered animal models of this disease, such as the PDAPP mouse model (which overexpresses mutant human amyloid precursor protein), as one of the species used to assess specific potential risks that are present only when Aβ is deposited in brain (Imbimbo et al., 2012). Similarly, spontaneous or engineered rodent and nonrodent models of many inherited genetic diseases are employed in combined efficacy/toxicity studies to examine biologic or gene therapy test articles. When a decision is made to utilize an animal model of disease, the toxicologic pathologist should be familiar with the limitations of the animal model including model-related microscopic or clinical pathology changes; inconsistency or variability in the phenotype or severity of the pathologies; different types of spontaneous findings; and limited or no historical control information (see *Genetically Engineered Animal Models in Toxicologic Research*, Vol 1, Chap 23). The toxicologic pathologist can gain experience in the typical pathologic findings in the animal model via literature reviews, microscopic evaluation of prior (e.g., efficacy or pharmacology) studies, and the use of pilot toxicity studies (Chadwick et al., 2014). Although not animal models of disease, engineered mice with enhanced vulnerability to test article–mediated carcinogenicity, such as p53 hemizygous and Tg.RasH2 mice, are used in accelerated (i.e. six month) bioassays to assess carcinogenicity of pharmaceuticals (Nambiar and Morton, 2013, *Carcinogenicity Assessment*, Vol 2, Chap 5). In determining the most appropriate carcinogenicity testing approach, study teams should assess if the test article's pharmacologic actions interfere with a molecular pathway (e.g., Ras signaling for the Tg.RasH2 mouse) in a way that could alter the sensitivity of the bioassay such that a two-year carcinogenicity study in wild-type mice would be a better test system. Understanding potential limitations of confounding factors related to the animal models used in a safety assessment program is important for ensuring that the toxicologic pathologist generates high-quality pathology data.

During the study planning phase, the age and health of the test animals are important items to consider since these can have a negative impact on the generation of pathology data. In our experience, these issues are of greater importance in studies using nonrodents. The toxicologist and toxicologic pathologist should know the most relevant age or sexual maturity state of the animals for safety assessment in any study. Sometimes this factor is not considered early enough in the planning process, and limited availability of sexually mature animals may delay the start of the study. The utilization of a sexually immature animal when a sexually mature animal should have been utilized may lead to incorrect conclusions about the reproductive safety of a test article. The prestudy health of the animals may be dependent on the source of

the animals, transportation-related stress, and other factors. Toxicologic pathologists and/or veterinary staff should assist in screening animals prior to inclusion in a study to ensure that those with suboptimal health are not included in the study. Suboptimal health of the animals may negatively impact the generation of pathology data by introducing the confounding effects of preexisting illnesses and lesions, or by altering the response of less robust animals to test articles. Some preexisting key health issues in NHPs and dogs that the authors have encountered over the years include diarrhea, inability to maintain or gain weight, and inability to maintain serum glucose concentrations within the accepted reference intervals prior to inclusion in a study.

2.4. Use Optimal Communication Practices

Proactive and collaborative communication by the entire study team is an important practice that facilitates the generation of high-quality pathology data. Suboptimal communication at the time of protocol preparation can occur due to the practices, institutional cultures, and business models of the diverse, and often complex, network of organizations involved in toxicity studies/programs (Dixon, Ripco, & Nrdo, 2011). Some bio/pharmaceutical companies conduct all or most of the toxicity studies at different test facilities operated by CROs. Thus, sponsor representatives, including sponsor pathologists, have a key role in implementing good communication practices. Good communication must start with the members of the study team, and certainly must include proactive communication between the study director, toxicologist, the study pathologist(s), peer review pathologist(s), and when applicable, sponsor representatives such as the sponsor pathologist. In outsourced studies, the sponsor and CRO must establish an effective working relationship and maintain open and proactive communications. The interactions should start before placing any studies (Irizarry Rovira et al., 2011). During the preparation of the protocol sponsors should clearly communicate their goals and expectations, including communication practices and preferred procedures/processes for when in-life findings arise such as moribundity/mortality, and the CROs should communicate to sponsors when proposed study designs and sponsor expectations are not realistic. At this stage of the study, sharing critical background information such as the nature of the test article (e.g., small vs. large molecule), intended pharmacology, pharmacologic target, potential target tissues, and data obtained from previous studies will help the study team obtain a complete understanding of the test article and the potential toxicity that might be observed. Awareness of the potential toxicity can have an impact on protocol-specified study procedures.

2.5. Estimate and Communicate the Number of Potential Target Tissues

The toxicologic pathologist plays an integral role in the identification of potential target tissues in any toxicity study, which are tissues that are expected to demonstrate test article–related changes, regardless of if these changes are direct (i.e., primary) or indirect (i.e., secondary) effects due to the test article. Indirect changes include soft tissue mineralization due to altered calcium/phosphorus ratio resulting from renal disease and atrophic changes in fat secondary to test article–induced decrements in body weight and food consumption. Providing the expected number of potential target tissues (if known) is one of the optimal communication practices that benefits the generation of pathology data and facilitates the generation of timely pathology reports. The biggest benefit of this communication during the protocol preparation phase is the ability to proactively schedule enough time for the study pathologist(s) and the peer review pathologist(s) to complete their tasks without excessive and unnecessary timeline pressure. Not communicating target tissues thoroughly and proactively could limit the ability of the timeline to absorb unexpected target tissues and may cause delays in finalization of the study report. Sometimes, delays in finalization of the study report can have a negative impact on the progression of the test article in development, such as delays to planned regulatory filings. Timely communication of the expected target tissues may also influence the scheduling of sample collections (e.g., blood),

preparation of the laboratory for nonstandard tissue collection or nonstandard procedures, or result in other modifications to protocol-specified procedures. Although not much can be done to decrease the risk of truly unexpected target tissues, it is possible to identify the likely potential target tissues at the time of the preparation of the study protocol by having a good understanding of results of previous toxicity studies with the test article or related compounds and by researching the potential toxicity risks associated with the chemical structure, excipients, chemical modifications or conjugates, and risks inherent in modulating the therapeutic target. For example, toxicologic pathologists should be aware of the potential findings related to administration of biomolecules conjugated to polyethylene glycol (Irizarry Rovira et al., 2018), some excipients such as cyclodextrins (Gad et al., 2016; Healing et al., 2016), and therapeutic platforms such as antisense oligonucleotides (Frazier, 2015); in some cases, findings associated with these materials can result in clinical pathology or microscopic findings in many tissues that are unrelated to the pharmacologic action of the test article.

2.6. Develop and Practice Novel or Nonstandard Pathology Procedures and Other Methods Prior to the Start of the Study and Use Accepted Practices for Incorporation of Nonstandard Endpoints

The use of standardized tissue lists and/or procedures across toxicity studies greatly helps maintain consistency in toxicity data sets in product development programs. Standardization also helps laboratories minimize errors, deviations, and delays. However, one of the most common dilemmas that a toxicologist or toxicologic pathologist may face during the study design phase is whether or not to include the assessment of nonstandard tissue samples, assays, or procedures in toxicity studies, particularly if these are not standard for a particular test facility or sponsor. Examples of nonstandard procedures may include perfusion fixation, immunohistochemistry (IHC) or in situ hybridization (ISH), transmission electron microscopy (TEM), in vivo assessments of immune function, and nonstandard biomarkers. As alluded to earlier, it is essential for the study team and/or for the toxicologic pathologist to ponder the true need of including those endpoints in the study and to confirm if the inclusion of those endpoints is essential for the risk assessment of the test article. If nonstandard samples, assays, or procedures are indeed needed in the study, we strongly recommend that nonstandard procedures be practiced to proficiency prior to implementation in definitive GLP toxicity studies. Such newly developed procedures may become the subjects of new standard operating procedures (SOPs), or these may be recorded as study-specific procedures.

Perfusion fixation prior to tissue collection requires planning and practice as the procedure adds significant complexity and time to necropsy workflows. Improper perfusion can easily ruin tissues due to excessive perfusion pressure or incomplete perfusion. Furthermore, perfusion fixation changes the normal postmortem appearance of tissues, which can greatly distort the appearance of highly vascular organs (e.g., lung, spleen) or interfere with the identification and collection of very small structures such as sympathetic or parasympathetic ganglia. Although assessment of ganglionic neurons or other small tissues may be important for a thorough toxicology evaluation in a particular study, it is important to define and practice how the samples will be collected, preserved, processed, and evaluated (Bolon & Butt, 2014).

In situ molecular pathology assays (e.g., IHC and ISH) and TEM are great investigative tools that toxicologic pathologists can utilize, if warranted. However, successful implementation of these procedures in toxicity studies requires planning, practice, and/or proactive method development to ensure the generation of high-quality pathology data. For example, associated with the development of new biotherapeutics, the incidence of immunogenicity-related events in nonclinical toxicity studies has increased. Characterizing these immunogenicity-related reactions may include confirmation of the occurrence of immune complex disease (ICD) with the use of ancillary tests such as IHC or TEM. Therefore, it is important to allocate additional time for sample processing and evaluation as well as to add special directions and trained personnel for

sample collection, preservation, processing, and evaluation. Starting method development as soon as possible for the special procedures will prevent undesirable delays in toxicity studies.

Inclusion of in vivo assays of the immune response in routine nonclinical toxicity studies can help demonstrate and further characterize test article–related effects and avoid the need for stand-alone studies (see *Immune System*, Vol 4, Chap 6). However, inclusion of these assays may require practice and piloting. One methodology to assess cellular immune function is by studying the influence of a test article on the immunogenic response to the administration of tuberculin in NHPs. This assessment introduces a nonstandard procedure consisting of vaccination with bacille Calmette–Guérin (BCG) vaccine before and/or during the dosing phase. The assessment of the response includes the microscopic evaluation of the cellular reaction in skin samples taken during the in-life phase. Although implementation of these ancillary methods is feasible, their application in a toxicity study may introduce additional stress to the animals and potential consequences that may affect the overall toxicity assessment in the study. Specifically, the administration of BCG in NHPs may cause the formation of microscopic granulomas in multiple organs (Al-Bhlal, 2000; Jurczyk-Procyk et al., 1976). This phenomenon, commonly known as "BCGitis," may complicate the interpretation of pathology results.

Nonstandard or novel biomarkers, such as Kidney Injury Molecule-1 (KIM-1) or Neutrophil Gelatinase–Associated Lipocalin (NGAL), can be valuable tools for the characterization of toxicity in nonclinical studies and/or can help guide the implementation of biomarkers in the clinic (see *Biomarkers: Discovery, Qualification and Application*, Vol 1, Chap 14). If the toxicologist and pathologist decide that the evaluation of those endpoints is warranted for the toxicological assessment of the test article, they must understand how and when in the study the samples must be collected, preserved, and processed in order to obtain as much accurate information as possible. Not communicating those requirements clearly in the protocol might affect the quality, accuracy, and validity of the results. A specific example on this would be the need for quantifying reproductive hormones (e.g., luteinizing hormone, follicle stimulating hormone, testosterone, and estradiol). The blood concentration of these hormones varies over different days during the estrous cycle in females or even throughout a single day in males (testosterone) and females (estradiol) (Chapin and Creasy, 2012; Anderson et al., 2013). Understanding these characteristics of the biology of the biomarkers helps in determining the number and timing of when samples need to be taken in order to have an accurate determination of the blood concentration of each hormone. Another example is the quantification of cardiac troponin I (cTnI), which is widely accepted as a biomarker for cardiac injury in several animal species, including rats, dogs, and NHPs. However, in order to have confidence in the validity of cTnI data, the study team must understand the analytical method used and craft a protocol that describes in detail appropriate sample handling procedures and the appropriate time points for sample collection. The half-life of cTnI is short, and early timepoints (e.g., 4 h or less after dosing) should be included to maximize the chances of identifying test article–related increases. The toxicologic pathologist also should be aware that simple stimuli such as restraining animals can induce stress and affect the concentrations of serum cTnI (Schultze et al., 2015).

2.7. Ensure that Study Procedures Are Adequately Described in the Study Protocol or Standard Operating Procedures

A clearly written study protocol that is easy to understand and follow greatly enables generation of pathology data and the success of nonclinical toxicity studies. The toxicologic pathologist must ensure that any procedures related to pathology endpoints are adequately, but not excessively, described in the protocol prior to initiation of the study. Protocols provide the minimum necessary amount of information to guide the collection of pathology endpoints, while detailed descriptions of standard pathology processes are generally defined in permanent institutional SOPs or a study-specific procedure document (see *Pathology and GLPs, Quality Control and Quality Assurance,*

Vol 1, Chap 27). Such documents commonly include written descriptions and, if warranted, schematic diagrams, flowcharts, photographs, or tables to facilitate understanding by the personnel responsible for performing the task. Practices that should be documented in this fashion include the processes for tissue or blood collection, sample preservation, handling, processing, and analysis. Well-written protocols and SOPs facilitate the reproducibility and accuracy of the pathology data in a study and across studies for a given development program. Study teams must be aware that procedures differ among research facilities; therefore, detailed descriptions of the methodologies to be used in the study are important for the generation of reproducible and reliable data over time.

Tissue processing is an important step in toxicity studies. It is critical to clearly define in SOPs how processing will be performed and that these processes avoid the introduction of variables that complicate the microscopic evaluation by the study pathologist. Furthermore, not following well-written tissue processing SOPs may introduce artifacts, such as tissue vacuolation, that complicate the histopathological interpretation. If the study team has decided to include special procedures such as IHC or TEM, the relevant special directions for tissue collection, preservation, and processing must be included in the study protocol and/or SOPs. Poorly detailed protocols and/or SOPs reduce the chances of obtaining high-quality samples that are suitable for interpretation.

Most toxicity studies collect data that are subjected to statistical analysis. It is recommended to define in the study protocol which endpoints will be statistically analyzed and what kind of statistical tests will be applied. In some studies, a statistician should be consulted early in the study planning process to discuss what standard statistical analysis should be performed and what modifications may be needed based on the emerging data (see *Experimental Design and Statistical Analysis for Toxicologic Pathologists,* Vol 1, Chap 16). For instance, in carcinogenicity studies, early mortality in control or experimental groups may prompt the application of different statistical methods. Discussing the application of those methods either during the planning of the study or during the conduct of the study with the study director, toxicologist, statistician, study pathologist, the peer review pathologist, and, if applicable, sponsor representatives is an essential practice.

2.8. Plan for Pathology Peer Review

Reappraisal of a portion of the study pathologist's initial histopathologic observations is a useful quality control (QC) procedure (see *Pathology Peer Review*, Vol 1, Chap 26). We recommend that study teams incorporate pathology peer review (Morton et al., 2010) in their GLP-regulated toxicity studies at the time of protocol preparation rather than waiting to see draft pathology results before deciding to add pathology peer review. Pathology peer review as set forth in a study protocol typically is performed by a single peer review pathologist. Peer review or less formal data review processes can also be utilized in non-GLP toxicity studies to increase confidence in the pathology data.

2.9. Do Not Blind the Study Pathologist

The practice of performing a histopathological assessment without knowledge of treatment and/or related demographic and clinical data, also known as an evaluation under "blinded" or "masked" conditions, can be used as a tool to reduce bias in the interpretation of findings. In product development programs, this practice is most commonly utilized in experimental studies used for standardization of biomarker identification or for assessment of efficacy of novel therapeutic entities (Burkhardt et al., 2011). However, this practice is not recommended in GLP-compliant nonclinical toxicity studies, and its use is discouraged by the STP (Neef et al., 2012; STP Society of Toxicologic Pathology, 1986). Accordingly, we recommend that study protocols for GLP nonclinical toxicity studies do not include "blinding" of the study pathologist. Since the histopathology assessment in GLP studies is performed with the goal of identifying all effects related to the administration of the test article, it is important for the pathologist to know which animals are controls since they provide context regarding the range of normal incidental findings (or "within normal limits") to be expected in the test animals under the conditions of the study that is being evaluated. The response to the administration of a test article, stress, infections, or other pathologies is variable, and may induce subtle changes that may not be possible to distinguish from test article–related effects if the pathologist does not understand what "normal" is in the animals of the study. Blinding the pathologist to treatment without the ability to define this normal range of background lesions may prevent the accurate identification of subtle test article–related changes such as atrophy, hypertrophy, increased or decreased cellularity, apoptosis, necrosis, and reproductive tissue estrous cycle abnormalities. An informed ("nonblinded" or "open") evaluation in which the treatment group and clinical observations for each animal are known allows the pathologist to have an increased sensitivity in the detection of test article–related effects, helps in developing appropriate criteria for grading the severity of microscopic findings, and permits the more efficient evaluation and documentation of changes occurring in the study. This last item is of essential importance because a diagnosis is not simply the identification of one change but a holistic understanding of its variability from animal to animal and its impact in each affected group and the interpretation of its significance under the conditions of the study. Therefore, before making a histopathologic diagnosis, the pathologist must know all information from each individual in the study, including the treatment group allocation, time of termination during the study, clinical observations, gross findings, body and organ weights, and clinical pathology findings.

Although blinded histopathologic analysis is discouraged for the primary evaluation, the STP acknowledges that it can be appropriate during the pathologist's reassessment of the slides in order to fine-tune diagnoses and severity grades, minimize diagnostic drift, and/or confirm a subtle test article–related effect and threshold value, such as a NOAEL (STP Society of Toxicologic Pathology, 1986). This masked reevaluation is performed on a case-by-case basis at the discretion of the study pathologist and usually is performed informally (i.e., by hiding the slide labels) rather than formally (i.e., by having the original slide labels covered by new coded labels).

2.10. Facilitate the Study and Peer Review Pathologists' Workflows

Study teams, including the study pathologist and peer review pathologist(s), should consider implementing other practices that facilitate efficient workflows for all personnel involved in enabling the generation of pathology data. These practices include advance agreement to allow the collection of digital images by the study pathologist, to set the format and general elements of the pathology report prior to evaluation, and to process all protocol-specified tissues from all animals in all groups to glass slides.

Illustrative/informational digital images can be utilized to consult with other colleagues, communicate to the study team or sponsor's representative regarding draft pathology findings, start an early dialogue with the peer review pathologist, and help achieve diagnostic consensus during peer review. By proactively defining in the protocol or in SOPs that digital images may be collected for informational/illustrative purposes and not used for data generation, the study pathologist does not have to wait for case-by-case approval by the sponsor or study team, and these images do not need to be included in the study report or be archived. In the fast-paced workflows of drug development, every minute counts, and the less the pathologist pauses, the more efficient data generation and reporting will be. If inclusion of images in the study report is required and/or if the images are to be used for data generation (e.g., histomorphometry), it may be helpful to include in the protocol a detailed description of how those images should be captured and presented in the results to assure the appropriate end result.

An additional consideration when writing the protocol is whether all tissues from all animals in all groups should be processed to tissue sections on glass slides. This is traditionally more of a dilemma in rodent GLP studies since processing all tissues to glass slides is common practice in nonrodent studies. The difference is that the rodent studies have many more animals (typically 10 [for toxicity studies] or ≥50 [for carcinogenicity studies] animals per sex per group) relative to nonrodent studies (usually 2–4 per sex per group per time point). Processing all tissues a priori also minimizes the possible variability in the quality or appearance of tissue sections due to differences in the batch of fixative, duration of tissue fixation or storage, processing equipment, histotechnologist (HTL) experience, batches of stain or other chemicals, and/or other additional variables. Furthermore, processing all tissues to glass slides decreases delays due to unexpected urgent requests for the histology laboratory to process newly identified potential target tissues, decreases the need for multiple rounds of tissue reviews by the study and peer review pathologists, and minimizes the potential for delays in study reporting timelines. The additional expense of processing all tissues up front is often more than offset by the invaluable savings in time experienced by the test facility, study pathologists, and peer review pathologists.

3. PRACTICES THAT PREVENT OR MITIGATE THE INTRODUCTION OF PATHOLOGY-RELATED ISSUES ARISING DURING THE IN-LIFE PHASE

The in-life phase of the study is an important study phase filled with potential issues that, if they manifest, can interfere with the generation, interpretation, and reporting of pathology data (Table 28.3). Such issues include suboptimal communication practices, unexpected toxicity, errors in study conduct procedures, potentially compromised animal models, and unexpected toxicokinetics. It is incumbent on toxicologic pathologists to be aware of these potential issues, follow best practices in all study activities, be aware of and/or engaged in the training of personnel involved in pathology activities, and have contingency plans for how to prevent, mitigate, and/or manage the impact of these issues on the generation of pathology data. Some of these issues can be prevented or mitigated by proactive, alert, and engaged toxicologic pathologists and study teams. However, many issues may not be preventable, and toxicologic pathologists must often react in the moment to the occurrence of these events. Here we offer our thoughts on practices that help minimize these issues and/or help mitigate the impact.

TABLE 28.3 Potential Issues That can Interfere With the Generation, Interpretation, and Reporting of Pathology Data in Nonclinical Toxicity Studies

Issue	Examples
Suboptimal communications within the study team	• Delays in notification of the occurrence of moribund animals • Lack of awareness of administration of medication in response to illness or injury during the study • Lack of awareness of emerging in-life observations that may impact sample (blood or tissue) collection procedures, necropsy, etc.
Unexpected toxicity of the test article or formulation	• Intended ("on target") or unintended ("off target") pharmacological activity • Hypersensitivity reactions • Unexpected vehicle toxicity—nasal injury from gavage reflux, known excipient via untested route of administration • Lack of toxicity when toxicity was expected
Errors in study procedures due to mistakes in execution, inadequately described study procedures, or unexpected events	• Failure to follow protocol, SOPs, and/or training • Gavage injury • Administration of incorrect dose level or frequency • Administration of the incorrect test article • Administration of compromised formulation (i.e., wrong pH, incorrect excipients, or buffers) • Unintentional fasting after dosing hypoglycemia-inducing drugs • Unintended intermingling of animals, including animals of different sexes • Handling injuries in animals • Errors in interpretation of protocol instructions • Suboptimal description of study procedures in protocol • Animal facility events such as excessive light intensity, flooding of cages • Block effects introduced during in-life tissue collections
Potentially compromised animal model	• Preexisting poor health of animals - diarrhea, poor glucose homeostasis • Preexisting or spontaneous systemic infections (*Plasmodium* spp., *Trypanosoma cruzi*, others) • Infected or suboptimally implanted devices • Contraindicated, excessive, and/or unbalanced administration of palliative medication (s) • Contaminated food or formulations
Unexpected toxicokinetics (TK)	• Greater than expected plasma exposures • Lower than expected plasma exposures • Inconsistent plasma exposures

3.1. Ensure the Proper Training of Personnel, Use of Appropriate Assays, Maintenance of Required Instrumentation, and Use of Quality Assurance Programs

The study pathologist, clinical and/or anatomic, generates and signs the final pathology report(s). However, the generation of pathology data begins during the in-life phases of nonclinical toxicity studies, well before reports are drafted, let alone signed. Therefore, it is important to consider training, assays, instrumentation, and quality assurance (QA) topics prior to necropsy. Data that are generated during the in-life phase may include predosing and interim clinical pathology results as well as anatomic pathology data from unscheduled deaths or terminations. The individuals involved in the study, including the toxicologic pathologists, must have the appropriate core education and task-related training to perform their responsibilities (Aulbach et al., 2019a; Schultze and Irizarry, 2017; Bolon, Barale-Thomas, & Bradley, 2010). The assays used in the study must be properly validated for the intended use, the instrumentation must be properly maintained and calibrated, and the facility must have robust SOPs and QA oversight to minimize variability or block/batch effects (Schultze, Bennet, & Rae, 2020; Arnold et al., 2019; Schultze and Irizarry, 2017; Tripathi et al., 2017; Ramos-Vara et al., 2008). A detailed discussion of these important topics is outside the scope of this chapter, and the reader is referred to other excellent resources to learn more (Aulbach et al., 2017, 2019a, 2019b; Tomlinson et al., 2013; Bolon, Barale-Thomas, & Bradley, 2010; Crissman et al., 2004; *Pathology and GLPs, Quality Control and Quality Assurance,* Vol 1, Chap 27).

3.2. Ensure Awareness of Emerging Data from In-Life Time Points and Unscheduled Terminations

Minimizing the impact of suboptimal communication practices is well within the grasp of members of study teams, including toxicologic pathologists. Emerging clinical signs in an ongoing toxicity study may drive treatment with medications, the addition or removal of protocol-specified tissues, adjustments to the frequency or number of blood collections, and/or early termination of individual animals or entire dose groups. Toxicologic pathologists must be aware of the administration of veterinary care as these procedures or medications may interfere with or confound the assessment of test article–related effects. For example, gastrointestinal side effects, including ulceration and diarrhea, may occur with the use of nonsteroidal anti-inflammatory drugs (NSAIDs) in dogs at therapeutic doses (McLean and Khan, 2018), and as such, the use of NSAIDs in toxicity studies of test articles that may cause gastrointestinal toxicity must be considered carefully. Furthermore, NSAIDs also may reduce or prevent microscopic inflammatory findings induced by some test articles and thus confound the interpretation of test article–related changes (Peter et al., 2011). Poor or delayed communication of emerging clinical signs can result in limited or no time to determine if

protocol amendments are needed to adjust in vivo collections and pathology procedures for unscheduled and/or scheduled terminations. As an integral part of the study team, the toxicologic pathologist must be aware of emerging clinical signs and be included in discussions related to veterinary medical treatment, adjustment of test article dose levels, animal moribundity, planned or unplanned terminations, and possible procedure-related deaths such as gavage errors. The study team should implement a communication plan that will promptly inform all members, including sponsor representatives such as the study monitor and sponsor pathologist in outsourced studies, of significant events in the study. However, it behooves the toxicologic pathologist to not wait to be informed but to also be proactive in seeking periodic updates on studies that they support as a study pathologist, peer review pathologist, and/or sponsor pathologist.

Optimal communication practices during the in-life phase of nonclinical toxicity studies will help study sponsors with ongoing clinical trials to abide by 21 CFR §312.32 (FDA, 2010b; IND Safety Reporting) and subsequent clarifying guidance issued after the rule was finalized (FDA, 2012). These documents focus on the responsibility of the sponsor to engage in **expedited** reporting of "potential serious risks, from clinical trials or any other source, as soon as possible, but in no case later than 15 calendar days after the sponsor determines that the information qualifies for reporting" (FDA, 2010b). Expedited safety reporting can potentially impact toxicologic pathologists since "findings from animal studies, such as carcinogenicity, mutagenicity, teratogenicity, or reports of significant organ toxicity at or near the expected human exposure are examples of the types of findings that could suggest a significant risk" (FDA, 2012). Evaluation of clinical pathology data from interim samples and/or anatomic pathology data from unscheduled terminations during the in-life phase of an ongoing toxicity or carcinogenicity study could reveal findings that portend possible serious risk. As such, the study pathologist should maintain good prompt communication with the study director, peer review pathologist, and, if the study is outsourced, with the sponsor's study monitor and the sponsor's pathologist when potentially significant pathology-related findings are identified (Irizarry Rovira et al., 2011). Prompt collaborative communication will allow the sponsor to "use judgment to decide whether the finding suggests a significant risk in humans or is too preliminary to interpret without replication or further investigation" (FDA, 2012). The sponsor will be best positioned to determine whether findings meet the criteria for expedited reporting or the determination that additional information or confirmation will be needed, such as expedited pathology peer review, additional analyses, or other actions.

3.3. Mitigate the Impact of Unexpected or Significant Toxicity

Unexpected or significant toxicity can result from a variety of factors including intended or unintended pharmacological activities of the test article, unexpected TK patterns, vehicle- or formulation-related toxicity, hypersensitivity reactions, and errors in study procedures to name a few. Some of these factors can be mitigated with careful dose selection, enhanced evaluation of clinical observations (e.g., detailed examination for effects on the central nervous system and comprehensive ophthalmologic exams), or staggered dosing initiation based on data from pilot studies, tolerability studies, PK and TK studies, thorough reviews of the literature, and a firm understanding of the test article and expected pharmacologic activity(ies). Despite excellent planning procedures, study designs, and/or utilization of ideal mitigation plans, unexpected or significant toxicity may occur during the in-life phase of a study. The toxicologic pathologist must be ready to help determine the appropriate course of action to ensure that, if warranted, pathology procedures are adjusted and implemented appropriately in ongoing studies to facilitate the interpretation and reporting of potentially complex data.

The toxicologic pathologist should promptly and routinely evaluate emerging clinical signs to determine if adjustments are needed to protocol-mandated tissue collections or other endpoints. Clinical signs may suggest a cause of moribundity or death for unscheduled deaths and early terminations, portend that microscopic changes are occurring in a nonprotocol–specified

tissue, or guide the addition of nonstandard biomarker endpoints. For example, significant respiratory clinical signs in rodents may signal gavage-related injury or the need to examine the nasal cavities and/or pharyngeal region for evidence of gavage-related reflux (Damsch et al., 2011). Discolored or broken teeth or mandibular masses may signal the need for microscopic examination of these tissues to look for evidence of test article–related injury (Irizarry et al., 2017; Fletcher et al., 2010). Incidents of bone fractures during the in-life phase may signal the possibility of a test article–related effect in bones and may help guide a more thorough examination of bones using in vivo or ex vivo imaging modalities or special histological stains. Enlarged organs (e.g., liver) or interim microscopic data may indicate that TEM evaluation of the affected organ should be added to the protocol. Interim clinical pathology data may indicate the need to expand the hematologic or clinical chemistry panels, add other nonstandard biomarkers, and/or increase the frequency of blood sampling throughout the study. For example, increases in serum total bilirubin concentrations during interim sampling may necessitate revision of the protocol to include determination of indirect and direct bilirubin in order to better characterize toxic effects on the liver. Unexpected hematologic or infusion site findings during the in-life phase may guide the addition of nonstandard biomarkers or other assays (Mease et al., 2017; Everds et al., 2013a).

When evaluating biotherapeutics, it is important to have a plan in place for adjusting protocol procedures due to hypersensitivity reactions or ICD due to antidrug antibodies (ADAs) (Mease et al., 2017; Engelhardt et al., 2015; Frazier et al., 2015), which may result in unexpected toxicity and mortality. The toxicologic pathologist involved in the testing of biotherapeutics should be familiar with the clinical signs associated with hypersensitivity and ICD (such as anaphylactic or anaphylactoid reactions), stay abreast of clinical observations and interim clinical pathology results, and have a plan in place to implement collection of extra tissues, such as kidney for TEM or blood for biomarkers, to help confirm the occurrence of hypersensitivity and ICD (Heyen et al., 2014; Rojko et al., 2014). An additional potential complication with biotherapeutics is reduced plasma drug exposure due to neutralizing ADAs. In these cases, the toxicologic pathologist should actively participate in the decision regarding if, and when, to terminate those animals or dose groups with insufficient plasma drug exposures since lack of exposure and/or the lag in time between the last dose and euthanasia will have an impact on the interpretation of pathology data.

Be aware of findings from the in-life phase or from unscheduled deaths or early terminations that suggest the occurrence of secondary infections or failure of implanted medical devices (Irizarry Rovira and Schultze, 2012), including diagnostic telemetry devices (i.e., not the test article) that assess cardiovascular safety pharmacology parameters. Disseminated infections originating from these implanted devices may be obvious and easy to see in tissue sections or the infections may be subtle. We recommend that the study protocol mandate collection and preservation of the sites where the devices were implanted and inserted. If necessary, these tissues can be evaluated microscopically to determine if infections occurred at these sites.

Prompt evaluation of emerging data as well as having a plan in place for sample collection and processing from unscheduled deaths and early terminations supports mitigation of the impact of unexpected toxicity. Moribundity and mortality in animals can be an outcome of unexpected or significant toxicity, and these animals present unique situations that may warrant special handling procedures or revisions to protocol-mandated procedures. For example, collection of organ weights from individual animals or entire dose groups terminated at unplanned intervals should be avoided unless the control group is being terminated at the same time (Sellers, Morton, & Michael, 2007). This avoids the generation of data that may be confounded by differences in fasting, time of necropsy, lack of concurrent controls, differences in age, etc. Collection of blood from animals after death is not recommended to avoid artifactual effects on results. When dealing with interim collections and unscheduled terminations, the toxicologic pathologist should also be aware of and avoid block/batch effects. Block/batch effects are effects that happen when one

or more sets of groups, animals, or specimens are handled in a different way than how all the other groups were handled in the same study (Schultze, Bennet, & Rae, 2020). A common example would be to collect blood from all control animals at the beginning of a long necropsy and from the high-dose animals at the end, resulting in artifactual effects due to prolonged fasting in the latter cohort. These effects may impact samples for clinical pathology and histology. The toxicologic pathologist should be alert to protocol-driven procedures that may introduce block effects and should be aware when these situations occur, or act to avoid or mitigate these effects in order to appropriately differentiate test article–related effects from block effects. For example, in rodent studies, the study pathologist typically evaluates all protocol-specified tissues from all animals from the control and high-dose groups and, if warranted, potential target tissues from the intermediate dose groups. However, excessive toxicity in the high-dose group may result in unscheduled/early euthanasia of individual animals or protocol-specified early termination of the entire high-dose group. In this situation, animals terminated early, or that died early, may be handled differently than others. These differences may include differences in necropsy personnel, batches of fixative, duration of tissue fixation or storage, processing equipment, HTLs, and/or batches of stain or other reagents. It is imperative that the study pathologist understand how these differences impact the identification of test–article related effects.

In studies of immunosuppressive test articles, toxicologic pathologists should anticipate and plan methods for identification of potential systemic secondary infections (Hutto, 2010; Price, 2010; Sasseville and Mansfield, 2010; Dubey et al., 2002; van Gorder et al., 1999). Immunosuppressive test articles may result in the recrudescence of preexisting infections or increased susceptibility to new secondary infections. The specific organisms or manifestations may vary due to the mechanism of immunosuppression, the animal species evaluated, and other variables. Secondary infections may manifest unexpectedly during the in-life phase of the study and ultimately confound the interpretation of test article–related effects. The toxicologic pathologist must be attentive to these manifestations and bring their biomedical and pathology training forward to help design a plan to confirm secondary infections and avoid misinterpreting the effects of a microorganism as a potential direct effect of the test article. The plan may include revising protocols to include additional samples for diagnostic testing (e.g., feces, blood, tissues) and special pathology procedures (e.g., IHC, ISH, TEM). Secondary infections may also lead to additional challenges for the toxicologic pathologist or the study team because the veterinary staff may advocate for the administration of antimicrobials, medications for pain, anti-inflammatory agents, steroids, and/or other drugs (Olivier et al., 2010; Taylor, 2010). These medications may confound the interpretation of test article effects—especially for agents with anti-inflammatory or immuno-modulatory effects—by introduction of an unknown and unbalanced treatment variable, interference with the pharmacologic or toxic effects of the test article (Peter et al., 2011), or influence the disposition, TK, or PK of the test article. The toxicologic pathologist must have a thorough understanding of the treatments administered to all the animals in the study to ensure the best possible interpretation of pathology data.

3.4. Scrutinize Impromptu Requests for Samples from Ongoing Studies for Assays that Are Not Critical to the Purpose of the Study

As alluded to above, members of a development team may request tissue samples from an ongoing study for PD or other exploratory assays. These impromptu tissue requests may include blood or tissue samples (e.g., from the brain, heart, or eyes). Some of these tissues are not subject to sharing due to the way laboratories preserve and/or process tissues, organ size, or blood volume limitations. For example, hearts in rodents and brains in all species are generally fixed whole and are less amenable for excision of fresh fragments for polymerase chain reaction

analyses or other assays; the choice to divide the unfixed brain to permit harvesting of fresh specimens for molecular assays may introduce artifacts into the other half of the brain and will present as defects in the tissue sections used for microscopic evaluation. Excessive blood sampling during a study may impact clinical pathology endpoints and/or the welfare of the animals; thus, removal of blood should not exceed recommended guidelines (IQ, 2016; see *Clinical Pathology in Nonclinical Toxicity Testing*, Vol 1, Chap 10). The toxicologic pathologist plays an important role in helping clarify the feasibility of satisfying these requests and ensuring that the generation of data by those investigators will not interfere with the pathology interpretation of the main endpoints for the ongoing toxicity study.

3.5. Understand When Not to Generate Pathology Data

Toxicologic pathologists must occasionally grapple with the question of when NOT to generate pathology data from a study, animal, and/or tissue. Knowing when not to generate pathology data is as important as focusing on how to generate high-quality pathology data. For example, there may be instances when clinical pathology or microscopic examination of animals or tissues is, at best, unlikely to yield meaningful information or, at worst, generate misleading or incorrect data (e.g., from unscheduled deaths with greatly delayed necropsies). Table 28.4 lists three key questions that toxicologic pathologists should ask when encountering unplanned situations like the listed examples. These examples are not meant to be all inclusive, and similar situations should result in case-by-case determination of suitability for generation of pathology data. These are critical determinations as the generation of severely confounded pathology data may lead to erroneous conclusions about a test article. The decision to not generate pathology data must be carefully balanced with consideration of the 3Rs, ensuring that animal resources are not unnecessarily wasted, and ensuring the scientific integrity of a toxicity study

TABLE 28.4 Pathology Considerations in Response to Unplanned Nonclinical Toxicity Study Events[a]

Key questions that the toxicologic pathologist should ask	Examples of unplanned situations
Should any, or very limited, pathology data be generated in a study?	• Sudden unexpected deaths in animals after single doses of a test article, despite clear previous evidence of lack of toxicity at the same dose levels for at least a month of dosing in previous studies • Discovery that an incorrect test article was utilized to dose animals in a study
Should pathology data be generated from an animal or group of animals?	• Deaths in rodents from satellite groups used for toxicokinetic sample collection and analysis • Errors in labeling of blood or other tissue samples prevent definitive assignment of the samples to specific study animals • Inadvertent freezing of a carcass
Should pathology data be generated from inappropriately preserved tissue or tissues?	• Inadvertent freezing of blood samples intended for clinical pathology analyses • Delayed fixation of tissue specimens slated for histopathologic evaluation • Inadvertent freezing of tissues samples intended for transmission electron microscopy evaluation

[a] These examples are not meant to be all inclusive, and similar situations should result in case-by-case determination of suitability for generation of pathology data.

(see *Issues in Laboratory Animal Science that Impact Toxicologic Pathology*, Vol 1, Chap 29).

4. PRACTICES THAT PREVENT OR MITIGATE ISSUES ARISING FROM PATHOLOGY ASSESSMENT AND REPORTING

This final section focuses on the postmortem "pathology" stages of a study, from necropsy through the histopathologic assessment and generation of the pathology report(s). These stages are critical to a high-quality pathology evaluation and successful reporting of the pathology data package for a nonclinical toxicity study. The following discussion will focus primarily on practical aspects to consider and will provide recommendations based on publications, industry standards, and lessons learned through personal experience of the authors, sometimes the hard way.

4.1. Ensure Proper Training, Supervision, Procedures, and Protocol Familiarity in the Necropsy, Histology, and Clinical Pathology Laboratories

Training and Supervision

A high-quality assessment by the pathologist is dependent on high-quality macroscopic observations and specimens (fluid and tissue). The value of well-trained necropsy, histology, and clinical pathology personnel cannot be overemphasized. Poorly trained study personnel can quickly and substantially, sometimes irretrievably, damage a study. Although robust "on-the-job" training of personnel is most important, there are also various laboratory personnel qualifications that can indicate an additional level of proficiency and certification. Some common certifications for individual contributors that serve this purpose include the Histotechnician (HT) and HTL for histology staff and the Medical Laboratory Technician (MLT) and Medical Laboratory Scientist (MLS) for clinical pathology personnel. At present, there are no directly applicable professional certifications for necropsy personnel. Ideally, necropsy procedures such as recording of macroscopic observations and collection of tissue should be conducted according to SOPs and under the supervision of the well-trained and well-informed study pathologist. However, many factors, including the timing when the study pathologist is assigned to the study and the study pathologist's histopathology assessment obligations on other studies, may present substantial challenges to this ideal scenario. Some necropsy labs employ a full-time necropsy pathologist, while others utilize a revolving "on-call" necropsy duty in order to ensure that there is always a suitable pathologist ready and available to oversee a necropsy and answer any pertinent questions regarding procedures or data entry. Complex or specialized necropsies of outsourced studies, or those requiring a detailed special assessment for the presence or absence of macroscopic changes observed on previous studies, may also benefit from the sponsor pathologist being present. It is our experience that *direct* necropsy supervision by the specific study pathologist assigned to all aspects of an individual study is usually not necessary or cost effective, especially for necropsy labs with well-trained necropsy technicians experienced in following protocols and appropriate SOPs.

Standard Operating Procedures and Study Protocol Familiarity

Every test facility or test site must determine how they confirm consistent implementation of routine procedures such as blood collection, animal euthanasia, necropsy, histology, and other procedures. Which procedures are chosen to represent the "standard" is an important decision, and organizations need to be willing to revise the chosen standards when deficiencies are identified or technical improvements can be made. Strict adherence to SOPs by study personnel markedly reduces study data variability, inaccuracies, and errors within and between studies conducted for a test article.

A deviation is an unplanned variation from a task specified in a study protocol. Such deviations are often the result of personnel performing procedures too rapidly, while distracted, or

assuming that the current study protocol is the same as other recent protocols. It is imperative that study personnel treat each study as a unique experience and invest significant time in studying the new protocol closely. Unless specifically necessary, sponsors should refrain from including nonstandard collection and/or tissue trimming methods in the protocol, as these unusual directives significantly increase the chance for errors and can also decrease tissue processing efficiency. Any necessary nonstandard study procedures require the utmost attention by study personnel, including the toxicologic pathologist, and management should be consulted before the protocol is finalized to determine if any pilot work, practice runs, or method development should be conducted before the procedures are implemented in the definitive study. These prestudy efforts can substantially prevent the chances of study deviations, errors, unforeseen complications, and delays during the actual study. Preinitiation meetings (e.g., prenecropsy, pretrimming, etc.), so that the entire team can review the study plan and procedures, are also recommended.

Necropsy

Necropsy is an important opportunity to collect meaningful macroscopic and organ weight data for assessment of test article–related effects. Protocol-specified tissues are assessed for macroscopic findings and then collected for microscopic evaluation. Special collections for fresh frozen tissues or electron microscopy are also taken if needed. Certain findings may only be ascertained during this portion of the pathology assessment including fluid accumulation in body cavities, dilatation of organ cavities, or body condition assessments. The necropsy phase of any study is a time of potential risk for inaccuracies and errors since macroscopic observations are not usually verified contemporaneously by another technician or peer reviewed by a pathologist, tissue specimens can be damaged or discarded, and/or omissions of tissue collections (formalin fixed and fresh frozen) can occur. Rodent carcass remnants can be retained in fixative for further assessments if needed, but for larger nonrodent species, necropsy is the only opportunity to collect tissues as it is not possible to retain the full carcass. If a gross abnormality is not identified at necropsy, it is unlikely that it will be examined microscopically unless it happens to be represented serendipitously in the standard tissue section or is identified in the rodent carcass during the tissue trimming phase. Sometimes gross abnormalities occur in nonstandard tissues or in areas of protocol-specified tissues that are not part of the standard collection and trimming procedures. To avoid unbalanced collections and avoid leaving the study pathologist without the appropriate control tissues, we recommend that necropsy teams consider collecting these same nonstandard tissues or areas from a few or all control animals.

Excessive or inaccurate macroscopic observations can cause confusion or unnecessary work for pathologists, sponsors, and regulatory reviewers. We strongly recommend the use of descriptive rather than interpretational or diagnostic terminology in recording such observations. For example, "decreased size" should be used instead of "atrophy," or "red discoloration" should be used instead of "hemorrhage." Macroscopic changes usually require a microscopic assessment to fully define the process creating the gross appearance, so interpretational macroscopic observations can be premature and inaccurate. Additional evaluations or discussion in the pathology report is usually required to help address inaccurate diagnostic necropsy macroscopic findings, which can create significant extra work for the study pathologist, QA staff, and regulatory reviewers.

Autolysis is the destruction of a cell or tissue through the action of its own cellular enzymes, which are released when cells or tissues decay. Autolysis begins shortly after death, so it is important to start the dissection of the animal and fixation of tissues as soon as possible (within minutes of euthanasia). This is important to consider when euthanasia stations and prosection areas are at physically separate locations. Certain tissues undergo autolysis and develop postmortem artifacts more quickly than others. Thus, tissues that are of greater toxicologic concern or that deteriorate more readily should be collected and placed in an appropriate fixative as a priority before other less labile tissues. Examples of labile tissues include, but are not limited to, the eyes, gastrointestinal tissues, liver, kidneys, pancreas, bone marrow, and brain.

Animal termination and postmortem tissue prosection, evaluation, and handling should be as consistent as possible among animals processed by different personnel to minimize introduction of technician bias. Elimination of such bias may allow for the detection of subtle test article–related effects. All animals should be equally exsanguinated to produce the most relevant organ weights and microscopic examination. All animals should also undergo uniform procedures such as lung inflation with fixative to expand the alveoli and airways, which facilitates detection of test article–related changes. Organ prosection should be consistent, and extraneous tissue or fat should also be removed in a consistent manner by the necropsy technician to avoid skewing group mean organ weights. If the organ weight technician recognizes extraneous tissues prior to weighing, such tissue should be removed, but after the weighed tissues have been fixed, additional trimming should be avoided so that the pathologist is able to correlate any abnormal organ weights with the presence of extraneous tissue. The organ weight technician should verify the accuracy of any organ weights outside the range of normal at the time of weighing and before finalization in the data set.

Missing tissues, especially small tissues from rodents, can be a significant source of protocol deviations. A tissue collection verification checklist is useful in reducing or eliminating missing tissues. An example process would be the prosecting technician placing each protocol-required tissue in a saline tray or on a saline-moistened paper towel or gauze so that a verifying technician can review the list of protocol-required tissues, after which both the prosecting technician and the verifying technician can visualize and check off each tissue before it is placed in fixative.

When blood or tissue specimens are collected from study animals at necropsy, meticulous care must be taken in following protocol directives and SOPs. Any deviations can lead to poor-quality or ruined samples which can significantly impact the study, even leading to study failures for that fluid or organ in some scenarios. Blood samples need to be collected in the correct types of collection tubes, identified with the correct animal number, and processed and analyzed expeditiously. Transport of samples to the laboratory, contamination of control animal samples with test article, and activities such as centrifugation to permit collection of supernatants for analysis all pose opportunities for error. Clinical pathology samples are especially sensitive to delayed analysis, suboptimal phlebotomy methods, and animal handling and restraint techniques.

Tissues begin to autolyze at the point of death. For this reason, animals that are found dead or euthanized early should be quickly transported to necropsy and necropsied as soon as feasible. If the necropsy cannot be started soon after death, as often occurs when death takes place after working hours and on weekends, the carcass should be refrigerated (NOT frozen!) to slow the autolysis process. Autolysis will continue even in refrigerated carcasses, so these animals should be necropsied at the earliest opportunity. Animal carcasses that have been frozen often exhibit significant tissue artifacts (e.g., destruction of normal cell features by formation of ice crystals) that may interfere with microscopic evaluation. Animals should be quickly taken to the prosection area immediately after euthanasia and exsanguinated quickly so that tissue collection may begin as rapidly as possible. The team euthanizing animals should monitor the availability of the individuals or teams prosecting animals so that the interval from euthanasia to the start of necropsy and tissue collection is minimized. The process of tissue autolysis can largely be halted when tissues are placed in fixative, so necropsy personnel should understand this and complete the collection and immersion of tissues into fixative as rapidly as possible. Larger tissues should be sectioned into smaller slabs ($\leq$0.5 cm thick) as fixative penetration is limited and thick tissues can continue to autolyze if fixative penetration is inadequate. Rodent brains in general toxicity studies typically are fixed intact by immersion to avoid "dark neuron" and other artifacts introduced by handling fresh tissue (see *Nervous System*, Vol 3, Chap 9), while nonrodent brains may be sliced in a coronal (transverse) plane to permit fixative access into the lateral ventricles, thereby facilitating preservation of deep regions. Care should be taken to make sure the correct fixatives are used for each organ. For most tissues, neutral buffered 10% formalin (NBF, approximately 3.7% formaldehyde plus about 1% methanol as a stabilizing agent in most commercial formulations) provides adequate fixation. This fixative,

however, is not optimal for eyes and testes since it is slow to penetrate the dense tissues of the capsule (testes) and sclera (eye). Alternative fixatives suitable for these special cases are Davidson's fixative for eyes and modified Davidson's fixative for testes (Latendresse et al., 2002). If tissues are collected for TEM, specialized mixtures such as Karnovsky's fixative (2% methanol-free formaldehyde—colloquially called paraformaldehyde—with 2.5% glutaraldehyde [GLUT]) are generally optimal for preservation of cellular architectural detail since GLUT penetrates slowly but cross-links molecules more effectively. Tissues slated for TEM need to be trimmed to a very small size (e.g., 1 mm^3) to allow fixative penetration with sufficient rapidity to fix subcellular structures. Using nonoptimal fixatives (such as NBF instead of modified Davidson's or Karnovsky's fixatives for testes and TEM specimens, respectively) can markedly impair tissue quality and hamper the ability of the pathologist to identify a test article–related microscopic change (Figure 28.1). Similarly, decalcification of fixed bones, a necessary step so that they can be trimmed and sectioned for histologic staining, can also allow for the creation of substantial tissue artifacts if they are left too long in decalcification reagents. Overdecalcified sections are very difficult to evaluate, particularly those of the bone marrow. An example of a catastrophic error on a study would be the accidental use of water or saline instead of a fixative, which would result in complete loss of tissue details due to severe autolysis and thus offer little or no ability to perform a useful microscopic assessment. Some organizations minimally tint their formalin solutions with a dye (e.g., phloxine) as a visual aid for prosectors to ensure that tissue collection containers contain fixative.

SOPs should be developed for all aspects of the necropsy to minimize any variables that are not of primary interest to the anatomic or clinical pathologist, such as differences in laboratory instruments, reagents, time of necropsy, or tissue staining runs. As mentioned earlier, these variables are often referred to as "nuisance factors" and may influence other groups of data and result in "block effects" or "batch effects" that complicate interpretation. Methods to lessen the occurrence of these effects include statistical blocking and utilization of study designs that incorporate randomization, employ an

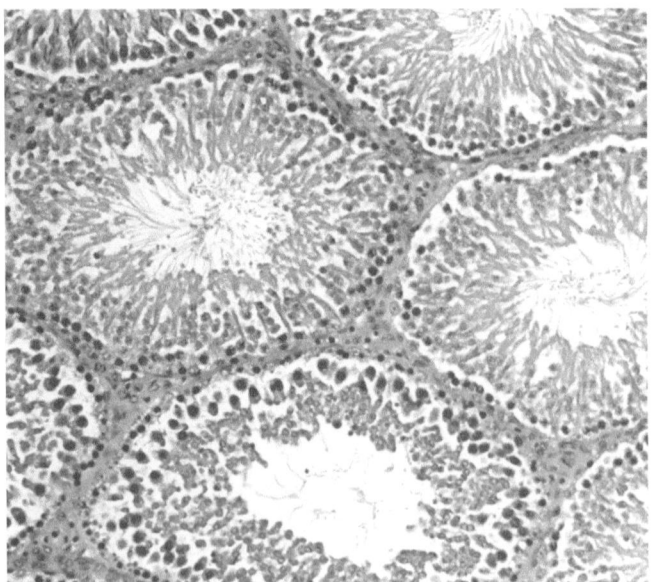
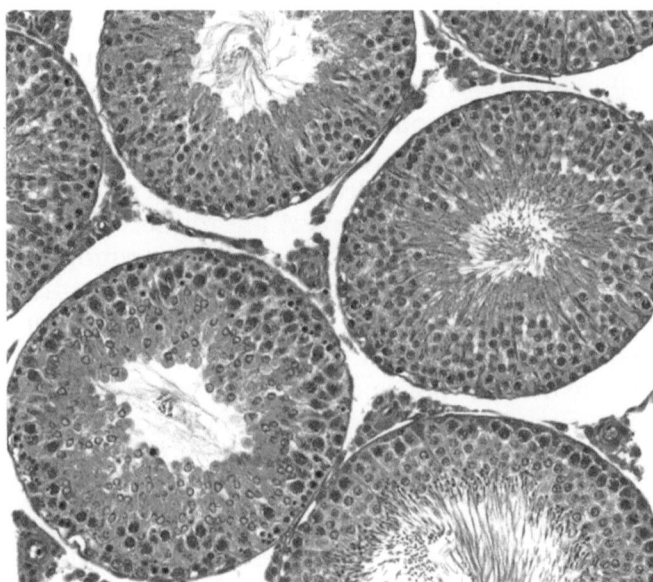

FIGURE 28.1   Rat. Testes sections demonstrating differences in the quality of fixation between neutral buffered 10% formalin (NBF) as shown on the left and modified Davidson's fixative on the right. The testes fixed in modified Davidson's fixative demonstrate superior cell and tissue preservation. Hematoxylin and Eosin (H&E). *Images courtesy of Dr. Justin Vidal.*

appropriate number of animals, or use repeated measurements of specific parameters (Schultze, Bennet, & Rae, 2020 and *Experimental Design and Statistical Analysis for Toxicologic Pathologists,* Vol 1, Chap 16).

Artifacts represent an alteration in the structure or features of a tissue due to excess handling or inappropriate processing. Artifacts can be introduced during necropsy, tissue fixation, tissue trimming, or histological processing and staining. Techniques to avoid the creation of artifacts must be utilized as these tissue alterations have the potential to substantially decrease the effectiveness and efficiency of the histopathologic assessment (Figure 28.2). The pathologist must be familiar with a range of common tissue artifacts and always be on the lookout for novel ones so that an artifactual change ("pseudo lesion") is not misinterpreted as a real antemortem change. One such alteration is vacuolation of neuronal tissues caused by prolonged immersion in an alcohol bath during tissue processing. A comprehensive review of artifacts is outside the scope of this chapter, but a description of some of the most common artifacts with illustrations is available in the outstanding atlas by McInnis (2012) and other sources (Li et al., 2003; Garman, 1990).

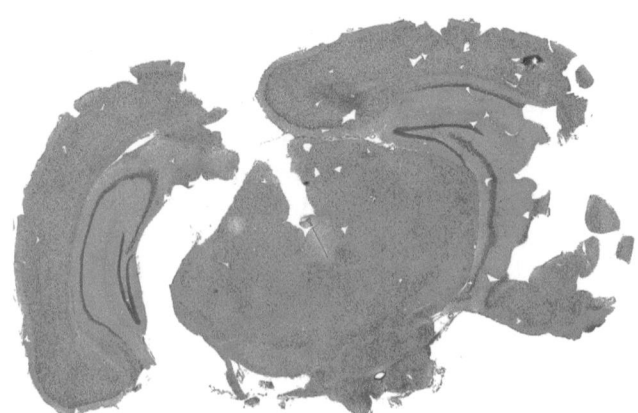

FIGURE 28.2   Mouse. Brain section with multiple artifacts due to inappropriate handling with forceps at the time of trimming, and handling-induced damage and loss of parenchyma. Artifacts include forceps-induced perforations, uneven tissue section, as well as fragmentation, separation, and loss of brain tissue. Hematoxylin and Eosin (H&E). *Image courtesy of Dr. D. Gregory Hall.*

4.2. Schedule Adequate Time for Processing and Evaluation

In the fast-paced world of drug development, getting new therapies to patients as fast as possible is paramount. All phases of a study need to be as rapid and efficient as possible without affecting quality. Not surprisingly, study pathologists are often asked by development teams or sponsors to expedite the evaluation and reporting of pathology data. However, as important as speed is to programmatic success, there are tipping points where expediting a study phase can exponentially increase the risk of errors and decrease the quality of the pathology diagnoses and interpretation. For this reason, organizations should ensure that there is always adequate time scheduled for the generation of analytical data (e.g., clinical pathology values, organ weights), preparation and microscopic evaluation of tissue sections, statistical analysis (if warranted), drafting of high-quality pathology reports, conducting pathology peer review (if specified in the protocol), undertaking QC and QA functions, and finalization of reports. Cutting time or prematurely releasing draft reports can have costly consequences. Rather than just looking at ways that time can be cut in technical steps or rushing critical steps in assessment, organizations should primarily seek creative ways to increase the *efficiency* of activities which can then be used to shorten the study timeline. There are some study activities that require specific durations and cannot be shortened, such as bone decalcification. Other activities have inherent time requirements that may not be obvious, including tissue trimming, tissue embedding, microtomy, histopathologic assessment, pathology peer review, and pathology reporting (including the QA audit). Rushing these activities can create technical errors, reduce tissue quality, and increase the likelihood of inappropriate or incomplete assessments and reporting. Like driving a car when tired, the chance for errors increases when organizations exceed the capacity limits of technical staff and pathologists (Smith and Raab, 2011; Renshaw and Gould, 2007; Raab and Grzybicki, 2006); GLP guidance by regulatory agencies (e.g., U.S. FDA) and international consortia seeking to harmonize product development practices (e.g., OECD) require preparation of a master schedule in part to prevent such overload. In outsourced studies, CROs should notify the sponsor when proposed timelines are unreasonably short to avoid having a negative impact on the quality of the pathology evaluation and study outcome (Irizarry Rovira et al., 2011).

Although there are substantial differences regarding study assignments and scheduling among organizations, we strongly recommend the following practices to increase the consistency and quality of pathology activities in toxicity studies:

1. The pathologist should be assigned by test facility/test site pathology management carefully with a goal of identifying the best fit based on a combination of factors, as described below. In contracted studies, sponsors may request the assignment of a specific pathologist with relevant subject matter expertise or selection from a short list of "preferred pathologists" of known capability. They should be aware that accommodation of such requests may, however, result in study and program delays due to the preferred pathologist's prior workload. The assignment should be made considering various factors (in order of importance) such as the pathologist's level of experience and expertise with the test article or class of the test article (e.g., monoclonal antibodies, gene therapy agents, oligonucleotides); knowledge in particular target tissues (e.g., reproductive, ocular, skeletal, nervous, etc.); or familiarity with the test species or study type (e.g., acute toxicity, carcinogenicity study). Because pathologists' schedules are ever changing due to shifting study timelines and requirements, identifying the study pathologist in the original protocol can result in the need for a protocol amendment if the study is reassigned later. There is no regulatory requirement to name the pathologist in the protocol, but the pathologist needs to be identified in the final pathology report and study report. The CRO should inform the sponsor when the assigned study pathologist is not a CRO employee but rather a contractor as this may impact the location of the pathology peer review and the communication between the study pathologist, CRO, and sponsor (Irizarry Rovira et al., 2011).

2. When possible, study pathologists should be scheduled to work on only one study at a time. If multiple studies cannot be avoided, the amount of study overlap should be

minimized. In practice, the ability of pathologists to achieve this focused time will be dependent on the scheduled delivery of data from the laboratories or slides from the histology laboratory and is complicated by reporting timelines. Adequate time should also be scheduled for drafting reports, issue resolution, internal quality reviews, peer review including discussions to reach diagnostic consensus, and finalization of the reports. At CROs, schedulers should include in their time estimates any specific experience with various sponsors or peer reviewers regarding the timeliness of their feedback, the intensity of their report reviews, and their tendency to revise draft reports. This may help mitigate the impact of frequent or major revisions of the study pathologist's schedule and the completion of an on-time final pathology report.

3. For clinical pathologists, it is important to schedule the duration of the evaluation to account for an expected number or increased complexity of findings, number of sampling times throughout the study, number of endpoints, numbers of animals, the need for bone marrow or blood smear microscopic evaluation, and the need for special tabulation or graphing of data to aid in interpretation. For example, studies of test articles that induce decrements in glucose concentrations or deficits in blood cell numbers may necessitate the inclusion of multiple sampling timepoints in the study to fully characterize the test article–related effects. Depending on the resources available, the clinical pathologist may need additional time to generate the time-course graphs of these endpoints to facilitate data interpretation.

4. As mentioned in the sections above, for anatomic pathologists, it is important to schedule the duration of the microscopic examination phase for a study by considering a variety of factors including the number of tissues and animals to evaluate and (if known) the estimated number of target tissues. This estimate should be adjusted based on findings from previous studies with the test article or related test articles with similar pharmacologic actions, from the expected or known pharmacologic and secondary effects observed during the in-life phase of the current study or in genetically modified animal models, and, if available, findings from unscheduled terminations or deaths. When faced for the first time with a completely new test article of a novel class, the authors suggest building a timeline for histopathologic evaluation using a minimum assumption of 10 target tissues.

5. Ideally, the evaluation of target tissues should be scheduled into the study pathologist's workload as stand-alone tasks. Target tissue review often involves reassessment of tissue changes in high-dose and control animals to ensure consistency and accuracy of assessments, and this review can be very time consuming. Time is necessary to define a "no observed effect level" (NOEL) for each target tissue. Time to evaluate a certain number of target tissues (e.g., 10 tissues) should be scheduled up front. This is especially important since the high dose is often set to induce toxicity and many test articles (e.g., antibody drug conjugates, oligonucleotides, and therapeutics for oncology indications) are often sufficiently potent to induce microscopic findings in multiple tissues.

6. Organizations should establish scheduling standards for the rate of slide review (e.g., evaluation of full-tissue sets—generally 60–75 tissue sections per animal—for 5 animals/day) that allows for some flexibility to address unanticipated complex patterns of toxicity, consultations with fellow pathologists, and repeat reviewing to hone data quality. Ensuring enough time for these activities also helps facilitate increased intradepartmental consistency. The exact review rate may depend on a variety of factors including the pathologist's experience/expertise, training, and evaluation style.

7. We strongly recommend a peer review of study material and data by a second pathologist as a standard practice for all studies enabling clinical trials. This recommendation applies to both GLP-compliant and non-GLP studies. After the draft diagnoses are recorded and the draft pathology narrative is written, the data tables and narrative should be reviewed by the peer review pathologist to ensure clarity, quality, and consistency; this review may also require a review of selected slides (Morton et al., 2010). This review process can be

facilitated by reserving time in advance in both the study pathologist's and peer review pathologist's calendars to permit the necessary interactions to achieve diagnostic consensus.

8. The sponsor should allow the study pathologist to finish the evaluation before preliminary results are released. Preliminary results can lead to inappropriate business decisions and are difficult to rein in or overturn once communicated. It is encouraged that sponsors limit their requests for interim updates so that the iterative process of refining the microscopic diagnoses can be focused, efficient, and thorough. Macroscopic and organ weight data can only be interpreted in the context of microscopic assessment. Draft pathology diagnoses need to be refined along the course of the microscopic evaluation and the peer review process and should not be interpreted or shared prematurely. Draft pathology data tables and draft narratives should not be submitted to regulatory agencies as they are not finalized raw data and thus are subject to change. For similar reasons, it can be costly and inappropriate to set dose levels for future studies and to make other pivotal decisions based on draft pathology data. Interim reports for various study phases can be scheduled if needed for regulatory submissions or sponsor business decisions, but findings in these reports may be altered in the final study report based on the comprehensive study assessment at the end of a study.

4.3. Establish Strong Lines of Communication and Freely Share Scientific and Program Information with the Study Pathologist

Proactive and collaborative communication with, and by, the study pathologist is an important practice that facilitates the generation of high-quality pathology data and reports. However, suboptimal communication with the study pathologist often occurs due to the practices, culture, and business models of the diverse, and sometimes complex, network of organizations (Dixon, Ripco, & Nrdo, 2011)

involved in conducting toxicity studies. Additional complications to communication arise from the transfer of ownership among companies of some test articles due to licensing, merger, and acquisition activities. Toxicologic pathologists working at bio/pharmaceutical companies are more likely to be aware of the details of the test article program and can connect many pieces of information and integrate their knowledge into the data collection, interpretation, and pathology report. In contrast, study pathologists at CROs or contract pathologists may be limited in experience with the novel therapeutic targets, modalities, or indications for the test article being tested. An understanding of this information and previous findings with the test article can shape the assessment strategy as well as the final organization and wording of the pathology report. Withholding such information from study pathologists can lead to inappropriate use of diagnostic terminology and conclusions from the assessment and can lead to considerable effort in reworking one or more pathology reports, thereby resulting in delivery delays. Sponsors that purposely or unintentionally fail to deliver important program information to the study pathologist add complexity to the process of completing thorough and meaningful assessments. Even pathology peer reviewers occasionally may be blinded to test article information, though in general pathology peer review should incorporate a nonblinded strategy. The practice of limiting how much information is shared with study pathologists may at times be driven by fears of loss of intellectual property or biasing the study pathologist's interpretation. Although these fears are frequently held by nonpathologists, it is our experience that the benefits of sharing information (i.e., nonblinded evaluation) with the study pathologist up front, including greater sensitivity and speed, far outweigh the risk of bias (Bolon et al., 2020). Sharing of test article information within the framework of an established confidentiality agreement allows the study pathologists to better identify test article–related findings and produce a more accurate and consistent pathology report that can be easily integrated into regulatory filings.

Information Needed Before the Start of the Microscopic Evaluation

Before the microscopic evaluation starts, the study pathologist should have basic information on the test article such as class, mechanism of action, any unique features of the modality/molecule, past findings with the program, and terminology used for any previous test article–related findings. Study information including the protocol with amendments, deviations in study design or conduct (e.g., dose holidays), and study mortality including any antemortem observations leading to euthanasia is also important. Additional information that is helpful when conducting evaluations includes clinical signs; clinical pathology data with interpretation (hematology, clinical chemistry, urinalysis, ± specialized biomarkers); veterinary observations; therapeutic interventions; body weights; food consumption; and other in-life assessments such as ophthalmologic examination. These pieces of information can influence the overall microscopic assessment and interpretation. It is recognized that all such information is not available at the time of slide evaluation; however, it is important to receive these data as soon as possible to minimize the potential for errors and need to repeat work. To illustrate, a pathologist benefits from knowing that an animal had seizures before they evaluate the tissues so that they may more critically evaluate that animal's neural tissues.

The most common source for study information is the Study Director, who can share what information they have and seek additional information from the sponsor as needed. TK information is usually not available during the microscopic evaluation, but it may be considered during study integration efforts or prior to finalization of the pathology report.

Sponsors occasionally have specific reporting guidelines that impact formatting and/or the order in which findings are presented. These guidelines should be agreed upon and provided to the study pathologist before the pathology report is drafted. Agreeing proactively on these guidelines helps optimize reporting by the study pathologist and minimizes back and forth disagreements with other members of the study team, including the peer review pathologist. Examples include using interpretive versus descriptive language, use of in-text summary tables, presentation of data from animals with early mortality, separating test article–related findings as primary versus secondary, extent of addressing correlates with other findings, adversity designations, and the degree of study data integration (e.g., in-life, TK, etc.) (Irizarry Rovira et al., 2011). This helps ensure that the study pathologist's report meets sponsor expectations and minimizes the need for additional rounds of revision.

Study Pathologist and Peer Review Pathologist Communication

If the study protocol includes a pathology peer review, there should be communication between the study pathologist and the peer review pathologist, ideally initiated before necropsy or at least before the microscopic evaluation commences. This can be easily accomplished through a phone call or email initiated by either pathologist. Any gaps or clarification of the information listed in the previous paragraph can also be discussed with the sponsor peer review pathologist. Other recommended discussion items include information on the logistics of the peer review (on-site or remote, scheduled start, and consensus dates) and the preferred diagnostic lexicon for both expected pathology findings and common spontaneous findings (e.g., International Harmonization of Nomenclature and Diagnostic Criteria [INHAND] terms vs. alternative nomenclature). It is important to keep the diagnostic terminology the same across studies if the findings are to be consistent. This assures consistency for the sponsor across the program, minimizes queries from regulatory reviewers, and minimizes uncertainty during regulatory reviews (see *Nomenclature and Diagnostic Resources in Anatomic Toxicologic Pathology*, Vol 1, Chap 25). The study pathologist and peer review pathologist should continue to communicate freely and directly during the primary microscopic examination in a manner analogous to an ad hoc consultation when a pathologist "walks down the hall" to talk with a colleague (Irizarry Rovira et al., 2011).

Sponsor Communication, Test Site Management Communication, and Undue Influence

Because histopathology data are only considered raw data after the pathology report is signed (FDA, 1987), preliminary or draft histopathology data have some unique considerations regarding safety reporting. In outsourced studies, CRO study pathologists should focus on providing study directors and sponsor and/or peer review pathologists with timely updates of study findings, participate in data review integration meetings with study directors and principal scientists, and deliver high-quality and timely draft reports. Study directors and study pathologists should share updates, especially any related to severe toxicities, with the sponsor as soon as possible. Communication of unexpected or new test article–related toxicities must be communicated once the relationship to test article exposure is suspected. This is particularly important if human clinical trials are ongoing. If the primary sponsor study monitor is not available, the alternate sponsor contact should be notified. Pathologists must understand the role that their communication plays and how it might ultimately result in an expedited safety reporting event between sponsor and regulators. Similar principles of communication apply to nonclinical toxicity studies that are conducted "in house" by a pharmaceutical company and not outsourced. In those situations, the study pathologist should proactively communicate to their study director, study team colleagues, and test site managers of any emerging significant toxicities that could potentially qualify for expedited safety reporting.

Undue sponsor influence in outsourced studies, especially on draft pathology data, is an oft-mentioned concern of regulators and an impetus for both CROs and sponsors to be as transparent as possible regarding sponsor comments, communication, and peer review (OECD Organisation for Economic Co-operation and Development). Undue influence may be defined as excessive, unwarranted, or unjustified manipulation or persuasion to modify data or reports to hide or minimize toxicologically significant changes. However, study pathologists at CROs should not immediately interpret any feedback from sponsor peer review pathologists as an attempt at undue influence. Pathology data and interpretation are influenced by individual experience and as such there may be different views regarding interpretation of the same pathology data set. Reasonable pathologists can be expected to disagree, and frank, clear dialogue can often prevent misinterpretation of peer review feedback. Hypothetical examples of undue influence on study pathologists might include pressuring a pathologist to improperly record, or not record, findings, intentionally raise a recording threshold to mask a potential test article effect, apply unique diagnostic or recording criteria to inappropriately alter perceptions of the data, use nonstandard terminology that obfuscates the significance of findings, and/or application of reduced severity grading criteria to inappropriately "soften" test article–related findings. Modifications of reports that disregard some or all of the weight of evidence supporting a change as being test article related or that downplay an impression of meaningful toxicity are also considered undue influence. Sponsor and/or peer review pathologist–provided feedback on data and interpretation can be considered if scientific or experiential support for such feedback is provided and relevant. To avoid the perception of undue influence, it is most helpful if peer review pathologists focus their feedback on substantive differences of opinion (e.g., emphasizing an agreement on the nature of a finding rather than minor differences in severity) and ensure that their feedback is solidly grounded in best practices, published data, digital slide historical repositories, and internal historical control data if available while avoiding unfounded or excessive speculation. Such feedback should not be coercive or compromise the integrity of the study pathologist's assessment and interpretation.

One of the best ways a study pathologist can prevent situations that may be perceived as undue influence by a sponsor is to consult with his or her colleagues and management to gather additional opinions and gain greater insight into the proposed findings and their interpretation. Sharing the outcome of these consultations can also greatly facilitate the resolution of any differences of opinion between the study pathologist and the sponsor and/or peer review pathologist.

Similar to the peer review pathologist, the study pathologist must ensure that draft pathology interpretations are solidly grounded in best practices, published data, robust experience, digital slide historical repositories, and internal historical databases (if available) while avoiding unfounded or excessive speculation. The more speculative an interpretation is, the more likely that there will be substantive disagreement that may be perceived as undue influence. A study pathologist should not compromise their integrity in any way, no matter how much pressure they may feel from other individuals within or outside their organization, and they should also have unwavering support from their manager and organizational senior leadership in order to ensure this ethical standard. When impasses occur, consultations with subject matter experts can be used to address disagreements with scientific rigor. Pathology working groups (PWGs) may also help to resolve differences (see *Pathology Peer Review*, Vol 1, Chap 26).

The principles outlined above for outsourced studies also apply to "in-house" GLP toxicity studies. For these, the pathology evaluation and report are undertaken by a sponsor pathologist and then peer reviewed by colleagues or managers at the same organization. Study pathologists in these situations may feel pressure from more senior peer reviewers or test facility management. In these cases, study pathologists will do well to follow the advice outlined above regarding consultation with colleagues to ensure that study interpretations are solidly grounded and to avoid compromising the integrity of their assessments.

4.4. Recommended Practices for Histopathologic Assessment

Prepare and Gather Materials Early

The study pathologist should know as much as possible about the test article, the purpose/objectives of the study, and findings from previous studies with the same or similar test articles. Sometimes, this information will be freely shared with the study pathologist, and sometimes the study pathologist must seek this information from the study director, sponsor representative, or scientific literature. Published

literature can be an excellent source of information if one investigates the portfolio of the sponsor on company websites or evaluates publicly available information on government archives (e.g., published patents, regulatory documents). Additionally, animal models (e.g., knock-out animals), studies with like molecules, patents, or review articles with background on the target in mind can also be useful. Much of this information is freely available online. Before evaluating tissues, the study pathologist should carefully review the macroscopic and organ weight summary tables. Many study pathologists even generate a rough outline or list of potential target tissues using these necropsy data.

Individual and summary body weights and food consumption should also be provided or made readily available to the study pathologist before the microscopic evaluation starts. Pathologists should be fully aware of the common effects that occur with decreases in food consumption, body weight, and/or with stress and use a weight-of-evidence approach in their interpretation. For example, decreased food consumption and body weights are often associated with decreased secretory material in and/or increased apoptosis of acinar cells within the pancreas and salivary glands. Stress, which can be a secondary test article–related effect, can be associated with lymphoid depletion or necrosis of the thymus and spleen, ulceration of the stomach, hypertrophy/hyperplasia of the adrenal cortex, and atrophy/degeneration/inactivity of some reproductive organs (Everds et al., 2013b). A pathologist who is not fully familiar with the physiology of stress and the associated in-life, organ weight, clinical pathology, and histopathologic changes produced by this condition could misinterpret certain stress-related changes as direct effects of test article exposure, or erroneously discount some direct test article–related findings as merely due to stress.

Ideally, clinical pathology and TK data with interpretation should be accessible before the microscopic evaluation starts. However, it is recognized there are organizational nuances in the timing of when these data and their interpretation become available. In some institutions, the anatomic pathologist also is responsible for interpretation of clinical pathology data. In other institutions, clinical pathologists conduct these assessments, while anatomic pathologists are confined to microscopic evaluation of tissues. At a minimum, the study pathologist should have the clinical pathology data or their interpretation before the scheduled pathology report is completed. Integration of clinical pathology findings with anatomic pathology findings is an important component of the pathology report, even if the initial presentation begins as separate anatomic pathology and clinical pathology sub-reports. Such correlations can let clinicians and regulators know if clinical pathology monitoring in clinical trials might signal the possibility of related histopathologic outcomes in humans. Of note, since it is sometimes overlooked and undervalued, TK data are important to the study pathologist since they often inform determination of the test article relationship based on the presence or absence of an apparent dose response in the incidence and/or severity of microscopic findings. For example, if some observations are only present in treated animals but do not increase in incidence or severity with increasing dose (i.e., a flat dose–response relationship), these observations might be considered incidental in nature if there is a dose proportional increase in exposure; however, these observations might be considered test article induced if exposure is equal across treated groups. Clinical pathology data can be equally helpful in determining the test article's involvement in questionable microscopic findings such as a small increased incidence of single-cell necrosis in the liver and the presence or absence of a test article–related increase in alanine aminotransferase activity or with bone marrow hypocellularity accompanied by or lacking a test article–related hematologic alteration.

Apply Uniform Thresholding

A key to determining test article–related effects in tissues is understanding normal background variation of tissue changes and establishing thresholds with respect to when diagnostic calls should be made. We characterize thresholding as described by Schafer et al. (2018): "a practice defined as determining which findings will be recorded as morphologic changes and which will be considered variations in normal morphology and not be recorded." Almost every tissue has a "microscopic change" that could be recorded. However, many such minor tissue changes have no relationship to treatment and no biological significance to the animal. Thresholding during study evaluation sets a practical limit on when findings in tissues will be recorded and interpreted. Pathologists often consider small but recognizable variances to be below a recordable threshold and enter an observation of "within normal limits" or "no significant lesions." Most pathologists use thresholding to reduce the overall "background noise" in the data tables and to help filter out extremely minor (i.e., unimportant, within normal limits) changes. Findings not considered to be within the limits of normal variation should be recorded utilizing globally accepted terminology (e.g., INHAND), best practice papers (especially for establishing scoring criteria and assigning severity grades; Schafer et al., 2018 and *Nomenclature and Diagnostic Resources in Anatomic Toxicologic Pathology*, Vol 1, Chap 25), and feedback from colleagues and peer review pathologists. Many early-career pathologists have extremely low recording thresholds; however, if the threshold and severity grading are consistent across the study, test article effects can still be accurately identified. Over time and with more experience and understanding of what constitutes "within normal limits," most pathologists establish slightly higher recording thresholds that reduce the number of inconsequential diagnoses and thus are more aligned with industry standards. Whenever possible, pathologists should share any thresholding criteria or practices for commonly used endpoints to ensure consistency across studies for a given test article.

Avoid Diagnostic Drift

Diagnostic drift is an unintentional shift in the nomenclature or severity grading of microscopic observations within a study over time. Diagnostic drift is typically more common in longer-duration studies, studies with multiple assessment intervals, and studies with large numbers of animals per group. A two-year carcinogenicity study is one instance where these factors can unintentionally result in impactful diagnostic drift. The drift may be due to a lack of attention, differences in accepted or published terminology, or a pathologist's increased familiarity with a lesion as the review progresses. Diagnostic drift can be minimized by not examining all of the animals from a particular group at the same time, reassessing the initial microscopic observations after the initial review (preferably in a random fashion without looking at the group number on the slide label), and/or including an informal review or formal pathology peer review at the conclusion of the histopathology evaluation phase of the study. Variability in thresholding, nomenclature, and severity grading from study to study should be expected, particularly if different pathologists evaluated these studies, due to the individual nature of experiences obtained during the course of pathology practice. For this reason, caution should be used when attempting to compare findings (severity grades or incidence of findings) or conclusions between studies evaluated by different pathologists. Diagnostic drift can also occur when more than one pathologist is assigned to evaluate a study, for example, if one pathologist evaluates a subset of tissues and another pathologist evaluates the rest. This drift can be minimized by assigning a single pathologist to evaluate a study instead of assigning multiple pathologists to complete the evaluation and reporting.

Minimize Errors in Recording

Study evaluations often include assessments of thousands of tissues from dozens to hundreds of animals. Inaccuracies can occur during the recording of data in pathology data acquisition systems. This might consist of inadvertently entering observations under the wrong animal or wrong tissue or alternatively entering the wrong diagnosis or severity grade in the proper place. The greatest chance of catching such errors is through the pathologist's own QC review of the pathology data during a rereview of the slides and checking of individual animal data and tables for inconsistencies and outliers. A review of a subset of tissues and data by a second pathologist (whether the review is formal or informal) is also an important verification check of data and conclusions. The most common process for microscopic data entry is direct computer input by the pathologist into a computer database. The advantage of a direct computer entry process is that the pathologist is directly responsible for the data entered, the diagnoses entered can be visually confirmed on the computer screen, any errors spotted can be

corrected in real time, and these data entry systems help maintain the integrity of the data. Additionally, the standard diagnostic glossary for each tissue is provided, which encourages their use, and the observations from past animals are also displayed by incidence which facilitates intrastudy and interstudy consistency. Potential disadvantages of direct computer entry are that a substantial number of computer mouse clicks and/or keystrokes are necessary, which introduce the possibility of errors. A less common process for microscopic entry is dictation or data transfer where verbally recorded or written diagnoses by the study pathologist are transcribed later into a computer database by support personnel. Advantages of this process are a faster microscopic evaluation since the pathologist does not need to pause to enter observations, less chance for keystroke errors, and the ability to perform a 100% QC of the data entry compared to the recorded observations to ensure accuracy (Mann et al., 2002). Disadvantages include the requirement for highly skilled support personnel to transcribe the data with consistency and accuracy. Some pathologists utilize notes during the initial slide review before entering findings directly into computer systems. This allows them to rapidly gather preliminary information in a survey of animals and revise inconsistent diagnostic terminology applied to the same finding before making conclusive entries into the data set. Since this process also introduces the potential for transcription errors, the pathologist should perform a QC check of the entered data against the paper notes. The pathology raw data for a study are the compilation of entries in the signed final pathology report. Therefore, any interim or draft paper notes made by the pathologists are not considered raw data and do not need to be retained or archived once the raw data are established in the final signed report.

Use Standardized Terminology and Severity Grades

In 2005, the European Society of Toxicologic Pathology (ESTP) and the Registry of Industrial Toxicology Animal-data (RITA) endorsed a proposal put forth by the STP in 2005 to create the INHAND diagnostic criteria for nonproliferative and proliferative lesions in rodents. In 2006, the British Society of Toxicological Pathology

(BSTP) and Japanese Society of Toxicologic Pathology (JSTP) joined the initiative. In recent years, the effort has been expanded to generate similar terminology for a number of nonrodent species including fish, rabbits, dogs, minipigs, and NHPs.

INHAND has improved the global harmonization of nomenclature and diagnostic criteria in toxicologic pathology. There is also an online platform for all members of the participating STPs to gain quick access to the most current INHAND nomenclature and diagnostic criteria; this searchable, regularly updated database is known as the "global open Registry Nomenclature Information System" (goRENI, www.goreni.org), and the direct nomenclature portal is https://www.goreni.org/gr3_nomenclature.php. Diagnoses can be sorted by organ system or by an alphabetical index, and many representative photomicrographs are provided. In addition to goRENI, the nomenclature is published in *Toxicologic Pathology* (the journal of the BSTP, ESTP, and STP) and/or the *Journal of Toxicologic Pathology* (the journal of the JSTP); online access to these publications is available at https://www.toxpath.org/inhand.asp. Oversight for INHAND is provided by the Global Editorial Steering Committee, which is composed of toxicologic pathologists from the four participating STPs. The nomenclature and criteria are generated and refined by dedicated Organ System Working Groups composed of individuals from all four participating STPs to ensure that they represent the consensus of international collaborators. Toxicologic pathologists are heavily encouraged to use INHAND diagnoses and criteria to help ensure consistency within studies, among studies, among different pathologists, across organizations and test sites, and across different countries (see *Nomenclature and Diagnostic Resources in Anatomic Toxicologic Pathology*, Vol 1, Chap 25). INHAND nomenclature is used as the basis for the Standardization for Exchange of Nonclinical Data (SEND) required by the FDA since 2017, and regulators likely have increased interest and confidence in this nomenclature since it is based on expert working groups providing internationally recognized terminology that is published in peer-reviewed journals. SEND controlled terminology (CT) is regularly updated and maintained by the National Cancer Institute

Enterprise Vocabulary Services and can be accessed at https://www.cancer.gov/research/resources/terminology/cdisc. However, the controlled INHAND terminology as applied in SEND does not always cover every possible microscopic change, especially for novel test article–related findings. Although study pathologists should attempt to use preferred INHAND nomenclature, if they need to use a non-INHAND term, the diagnosis can be 1) used in the submission as is and described in the Study Reviewer's Data Guide or 2) can be mapped to a related term deemed to be the most appropriate in the INHAND/SEND CT. It is important to note that the study pathologist's original diagnosis is always submitted with the SEND data, and the study pathologist should be consulted if their diagnoses need to be adjusted for mapping to SEND CT (Watanabe et al., 2017). The severity grade (i.e., minimal, mild, moderate, marked, severe) is an important part of a histopathologic diagnosis since it can be used to help distinguish treatment-related effects and determine adversity (see *Nomenclature and Diagnostic Resources in Anatomic Toxicologic Pathology*, Vol 1, Chap 25). Histopathology severity grades should not be based on organ weight differences, clinical pathology findings, test article relationship, presumed human relevance, biological impact, adversity, or reversibility (Schafer et al., 2018).

Appropriate Use of Historical Control Data and Reference Ranges

Although the concurrent control group is always the most appropriate comparator for study data, these data may not capture all changes normally observed as background variability for findings (Snyder et al., 2016). Historical control data should also be utilized to support the interpretation of nonneoplastic or neoplastic findings. Historical control data are especially helpful in interpreting rare spontaneous lesions, such as the presence of lymphoma in a young animal on a noncarcinogenicity study or increases in incidence or severity of findings that do not logically seem to represent test article–related changes based on the intended target and pharmacologic action. By proactively reviewing historical control data and appropriately referencing such data within the pathology report to support conclusions, the pathologist is often able to avert questions from regulatory reviewers that can result in significant delays to the drug development program and potentially in a "clinical hold" or halt to dosing in humans. In our experience, interest in historical control data from regulatory agencies remains very high. Because nonneoplastic data can be more readily impacted by pathologists' training, thresholding, and diagnostic criteria, neoplastic historical control data are generally considered more useful and accurate than nonneoplastic historical control data. Diagnostic criteria and terminology for tumors have historically been more standardized than criteria and terminology for nonneoplastic lesions. Therefore, the tumor data are less likely to be impacted by the variables outlined above, which increases the value of neoplastic historical data relative to nonneoplastic historical data. However, the use of harmonized nomenclature and diagnostic criteria has improved the consistency and thus comparability of nonneoplastic historical control data. The best historical control data are from the same test facility during a finite time period since there are fewer differences in variables such as animal sourcing, environmental conditions, food, water, etc. The next best historical control data are from other test sites from the same organization since they often share similar vendors and husbandry practices across sites. For a wider assessment, historical control data from the animal vendor, other organizations, or publications can be referenced. It is important to consider and match the species, strain (e.g., Sprague–Dawley vs. Wistar rats), source (e.g., Charles River vs. Harlan), sex, and animal age/study duration (e.g., 28 day vs. 3 month) as closely as possible to ensure the credibility of the data comparison. Because genetic drift over time can also influence the expression of spontaneous nonneoplastic and neoplastic lesions, the US Environmental Protection Agency recommends using historical control data within 2–3 years, and both the EMA and OECD recommend using data within 5 years. Older historical control data can be used for context but are likely to hold less weight with regulators. Pathologists should also consider establishing a digital image or a physical glass slide repository to depict the changes included in the historical control database. These visual representations can assist with the training of

new pathologists, provide organizational guidelines for recording thresholds and what comprises "within normal limits" for various tissues, and afford a readily accessible "normal control" comparison in addition to the concurrent controls or when control animals are lacking (e.g., small non-GLP and investigative studies).

For clinical pathology data, the most appropriate comparator for data from treated animals is concurrent control animal data or prestudy baseline values (where each animal will serve as its own control). Less helpful are historical or published reference intervals for clinical pathology data from the same species and strain, and their use is typically limited to studies that lack concurrent controls or studies with a small number of subjects per group. These reference intervals provide additional weight of evidence for an interpretation for or against test article relationship and provide further information on the magnitude and severity of test article–related changes. Reference intervals can also be used to identify biologic or analytical drift due to instrumentation or reagent problems within the clinical pathology laboratory (Clemo, 1997). Reference intervals are typically broad (usually representing the central 95% of the population) and should not be used exclusively to identify test article–related clinical pathologic effects (Hall, 1997, 2017). Test article–related responses can occur for data that are within these reference ranges. Statistical significance, or lack thereof, should not be utilized as the sole criterion for determination of a relationship to test article administration.

Assess Tumor Data Using a Weight-of-Evidence Approach

Tumors that arise in treated animals in noncarcinogenicity studies often quickly get the attention of sponsors, peer review pathologists, and regulatory reviewers. For this reason, they warrant special attention and discussion in the pathology report by the study pathologist. "Murphy's Law" dictates that a spontaneous tumor will most often arise in an animal in a test article–treated group. The pathologist must always provide rationale in the report for why the neoplasm is considered incidental or spontaneous, addressing such considerations as the duration of the study, limited occurrence in a study, the nature and biologic activity of the molecule (genotoxicity, hormonal activity), absence of an increase in preneoplastic lesions (e.g., hyperplasia) in the tissue, presence of the tumor in the historical control data, and ideally references to publications supporting the spontaneous nature of the tumor in a species, such as amphophilic-vacuolar renal tubular tumors in rats (Crabbs et al., 2013). A similar weight-of-evidence approach should be used and reported when assessing neoplastic incidences in carcinogenicity studies (see *Carcinogenicity Assessment*, Vol 2, Chap 5). The presence of a statistically significant p-value flag for a tumor type does not necessarily mean that the increased incidence is a test article–related event. Evidence against test article involvement includes significance in a pairwise statistical test that is not significant at a higher dose group, absence of significance in both pairwise and trend tests, lack of a dose response in the tumor's incidence, similarity to historical control animal incidences, lack of similar statistically significant findings in the other sex, and lack of a dose-related increase in similar preneoplastic proliferative findings. These are only a sample of factors to consider in appropriate risk assessments for unexpected tumors in noncarcinogenicity studies.

Seek Informal Reviews by Other Pathologists

Toxicologic pathology and pharmaceutical research are constantly evolving disciplines. New therapeutic targets, novel modalities of treatment, study designs and outputs, and evolving scientific understanding are only a few factors that add complexity to these disciplines. No single pathologist has seen all possible outcomes or study-related findings. Consultation with peers is one way to ensure that diagnostic challenges or study-related issues are handled appropriately. Many pathologists work alongside other pathologists, which provides the invaluable opportunity for informal (nonprotocol specified) reviews. This is important for pathologists at all levels of experience but is especially valuable for early-career pathologists since the skills and knowledge needed to interpret nonclinical toxicity studies require training and practice gained over a period of years working under the mentorship of experienced toxicologic pathologists (Gosselin et al., 2011). Board certification in pathology (e.g., by the American and/or European College of Veterinary Pathologists) does not automatically equate with toxicologic pathology proficiency. For this reason, early-career pathologists should actively seek and utilize the mentoring of experienced pathologists whenever possible. Informal reviews may occur by the pathologist walking next door to share slides or data, during scheduled departmental slide rounds, or during ad hoc slide review sessions. Besides the slide evaluation, other items that can benefit from review include the draft summary tables and draft pathology report narrative. With the ability to easily share computer desktops (e.g., Microsoft Teams, Cisco WebEx, Zoom) as well as captured digital images and whole-slide digital images, reviews of data and images can occur even with remote colleagues and subject matter experts. To facilitate using these reviews for refining preliminary diagnoses, the study pathologist should seek input contemporaneously during the evaluation or shortly after microscopic evaluation and allow enough time for review by another pathologist. Pathologists that participate in reviews should make sure they fully engage in the review, including a critical review of the scientific content and rationale provided for the interpretations. Specific attention should be directed to determining the cause of unscheduled deaths, establishing the diagnostic terminology and test article effect levels, and assigning adversity. Ideally, informal reviews by other pathologists should also be conducted before the formal pathology peer review. This is especially helpful for early-career pathologists employed by CROs and can ensure that a higher-quality product is available for review by the peer review pathologist. These informal consultations/reviews do not require documentation in the protocol or in the pathology report. They are an aid to the study pathologist who is ultimately responsible for data and report, and thus serve the same purpose as interim notes used to hone preliminary diagnoses.

Utilize Study Pathologist Quality Control Activities

There are many activities that the study pathologist themselves can undertake to optimize the pathology data, prevent errors, and minimize questions and concerns from regulatory reviewers. Regulatory agencies understand that draft histopathology data are often refined by the study pathologist as they progressively evaluate the tissue sections from control and treated animals and gain more perspective on both background and test article–induced lesions. This acknowledgment is reflected in the 1987 US FDA Final Rule (FDA, 1987; https://www.fda.gov/media/75860/download) stating that the raw data for histopathology for a given study are the findings listed in the final signed pathology report. This decision allows, and should even encourage, pathologists to continuously refine and improve their draft diagnoses and draft narrative up to the finalization of the pathology report.

QC endeavors that the study pathologist should consider before the report is finalized include a masked (i.e., blinded) reevaluation of subtle findings in any potential target tissues. The purposes for such a follow-on informal review are to confirm diagnoses and severity grades, a critical review of the draft microscopic observation tables to identify outlier diagnoses or potential dose responses that need to be reevaluated and/or explained, and a careful assessment of any diagnostic inconsistencies that could be corrected by additional microscopic assessment and nomenclature standardization. The decision regarding whether or not to undertake this additional review should be left to the discretion of the study pathologist. When drafting the pathology report narrative, the study pathologist should focus on writing for the primary audience who will be reading it. This audience is typically *nonpathologists* such as the Study Director, sponsor teams, and regulatory reviewers. The study pathologist should describe unique pathology diagnoses, define severity grades that determine test article relationship or adversity, provide robust interpretation for conclusions, and if warranted include citations for relevant scientific literature. The appropriate level of detail needed to describe microscopic findings should be implemented based on the study pathologist's experience and preferences balanced with the expectations of the development team or sponsor. The pathologist should not assume that the reader of the pathology report has any medical or pathology training, and highly technical terms and pathology jargon should be avoided unless explained. The pathologist should also try to

help the reader by writing succinctly and clearly. Long, verbose, or meandering descriptions may interfere with effective communication of the key points of the pathology narrative. Each section (e.g., mortality, macroscopic findings, organ weight findings, microscopic findings, clinical pathology findings) should be introduced by clearly stating tissues or systems with test article–related findings and effect levels and allow subsequent paragraphs and in-text tables to provide further detail to characterize tissue effects and severity scores (see *Preparation of the Anatomic Pathology Report for a Toxicity Study*, Vol 2, Chap 13).

Engage in Data Review and Integration Meetings

After the initial pathology evaluation is complete and the pathologist has identified test article–related effects, there should be a discussion between the key scientific contributors on the study—the study director, clinical pathologist, TK scientist, anatomic pathologist, and other contributors as needed. These discussions are an important opportunity to integrate findings so that associated data relationships can be correlated and included in the various subreports that will be included in the final study report. It also markedly improves the study director's ability to understand and effectively summarize the findings from the various contributing scientists. Discussion and input from these key study members can also assist with setting of the study's NOEL and NOAEL. This discussion should be scheduled for each study according to the availability of the scientists and data. Prior to the discussion, the scientists should review all available draft subreports. During the meeting, the study director can provide a summarized overview of the study design, test article class/indication, and any previous studies and findings. The study director then should present a summary of in-life data including clinical observations and any potential dose dependency or trends observed, mortality, and any other antemortem findings (such as from veterinary or ophthalmoscopic examinations). Body weights and food consumption should also be discussed, including potential dose dependency or trends observed. Any additional testing such as cardiovascular or neurobehavioral assessment (e.g., functional observational battery) should also be summarized. The clinical pathologist and anatomic pathologist(s) should each present their findings and make relevant correlations with other data categories. The TK scientist should provide a summary of their data including any sex differences in test article exposure, dose—exposure relationships, and any changes following repeated administration. It is also important to consider if the systemic test article exposure data correlate to any clinical observations, clinical pathology changes, or anatomic pathology findings. For example, loss of test article exposure based on TK measurements could suggest liver microsomal enzyme induction, which in turn could correlate to liver weight increases consistent with hepatocellular hypertrophy. Toward the end of the discussion, the scientists should attempt to reach consensus on the study NOEL and NOAEL. This meeting also provides an opportunity to discuss any problems that occurred during the conduct of the study that could be addressed with corrective or preventative actions as well as any study design considerations for application to future studies.

Optimize Pathology Peer Review Workflows

Although there is no GLP requirement for a second pathologist to conduct a formal pathology peer review, many regulatory authorities expect that some level of pathology peer review will be performed (OECD Organisation for Economic Co-operation and Development, 2014). Peer reviews are commonly recommended as a means of increasing confidence in the pathology data set (see *Pathology Peer Review*, Vol 1, Chap 26). Pathology peer review consists of a reevaluation of a subset of the slides (e.g., all tissues from a certain percentage of high-dose animals (commonly 30% for rodents and 50% or more for nonrodents); target tissues from all high-dose animals and intermediate-dose group animals to establish a no effect level; all neoplasms; and animals from all dose groups with early mortality) and the draft pathology narrative (Morton et al., 2010). Pathology peer review ensures that all test article—related effects are properly identified, consistently diagnosed, and correctly interpreted. It also confirms the test article—related effects and adverse findings, which helps ensure that the study NOEL and

NOAEL as well as the interpretations in the narrative are accurate. The process of pathology peer review is guided by an SOP but allows the peer review pathologist flexibility to expand their review if needed. The methods regarding the extent of the review and the conclusions of the review (i.e., whether the study pathologist and peer review pathologist have achieved consensus) are detailed in the pathology peer review statement or memorandum. This peer review memo can be included in the study report as an appendix. Pathology peer review should be considered a quality check, and suggestions provided to the study pathologist should be viewed as a means for enhancing the accuracy and clarity of the pathology raw data and report. The peer review pathologist does not generate any raw data. Typically, pathology peer reviews are prospective/contemporaneous, and the pathology report has not been finalized. Thus, there is no need for documentation of changes to unfinalized data/reports or retention of the peer review notes.

Nonstandard pathology peer reviews include targeted/focused contemporaneous peer reviews, retrospective or postfinalization peer reviews, and expert PWG reviews. Targeted or focused peer reviews are typically added to review an organ or system after a target tissue effect or concern is identified (e.g., an unexpected testicular finding) and are often conducted by a peer review pathologist with expertise in that organ system (e.g., reproductive pathology). Retrospective or postfinalization peer reviews are occasionally performed after the pathology data and reports have been finalized. These *post hoc* reviews have the potential to create new data or alter original raw data, so it is important to provide an audit trail of all changes and ensure that any changes to the original data are included in a formally amended pathology report signed by the original study pathologist.

Rarely, we have encountered situations where an additional stand-alone pathology report generated retrospectively by third-party consultants has been submitted by the sponsor in parallel to the "official" final study report to regulatory authorities without the benefit of a PWG or other reconciliation process. These circumstances place regulatory authorities in a difficult situation as they are handed two separate pathology raw data sets and interpretations of the same set of tissue slides. Unreconciled, disparate, or contradictory data sets and interpretations can create significant uncertainty and confusion for sponsors, regulators, and clinical investigators. Such uncertainty can jeopardize the progression of a drug and increase the risk to clinical trial participants.

There are various opinions and factors to consider regarding where the pathology peer review for a study should take place. In general, a review at the test facility (i.e., where the study was performed and slides were prepared) facilitates enhanced and timely communication between study and peer review pathologists, avoids slide shipping delays, and may avoid issues with shipment of regulated animal tissues (especially NHPs) across international borders (Irizarry Rovira et al., 2011). An on-site peer review also allows the peer review pathologist to "escape" from their normal daily routine (and associated distractions) and focus on the pathology peer review, which can increase the quality and efficiency of the peer review process. The SOP that will be followed for the pathology peer review should be determined ahead of time and shared with the test facility in order to support appropriate preparation and reduce delays while on site. Alternatively, a pathology peer review may be performed at other locations by shipping slides to the peer review pathologist's test site or to a different agreed upon site; for example, a different facility belonging to the Sponsor or the CRO. Digital peer review is another option to consider by providing the peer reviewer with access to high-resolution whole-slide scanned images. Advantages to this approach may include reduced cost (by avoiding charges for travel time and expenses) and stress for the peer review pathologist arising from a time-constrained review in an unfamiliar environment.

If feasible, we recommend that a peer review of the entire study, including both treatment and recovery phases, be performed at one time rather than reviewing each stage separately at different times. A single peer review is more efficient, and possibly more valuable, because it allows the peer review pathologist to better compare effects across time points and minimizes the need to repeat the evaluation of tissues from the treatment phase of the study (Irizarry Rovira et al., 2011). Peer review by interval may be disruptive and is more labor intensive for the study pathologist and support staff compared to one single peer review at the end of the microscopic evaluation.

Pathology peer review can sometimes lead to significant study delays. New findings may be uncovered during the review by a subject matter expert that require additional tissue assessments by the study pathologist to clarify no-effect levels. This may necessitate additional tissue processing and slide preparation. This generally leads to timeline delays, but these are necessary for a full and accurate assessment. Other delays in the peer review process can occur if the peer review pathologist gets "too far into the weeds" of slide, data, or report reviews that lead to multiple, often inconsequential, rounds of diagnostic and/or interpretive revision. The purpose of pathology peer review is not the confirmation of every microscopic observation or making refinements to the narrative to suit personal writing style preferences (of the peer review pathologist); rather, peer reviews should ensure that test article–related findings and effect levels are properly identified, consistently diagnosed, and correctly interpreted (Crissman et al., 2004). Therefore, peer review pathologists are encouraged to stay focused on this QC concept which also increases the chances of an on-time completion of the peer review.

One of the most important principles regarding pathology peer review, which sometimes is misunderstood, is that the peer review pathologist does not generate raw data. Instead, pathology raw data are created for a study only when the study pathologist signs the pathology subreport (or final study report). Pathology peer reviews should be considered GLP compliant when the following criteria are met, and any discrepancies with respect to these criteria may be noted in the compliance statement of the pathology and/or toxicology subreport and/or final study report.

1) The pathology peer review should utilize GLP-compliant procedures including chain of custody for transfer of study materials, and for OECD sites, be performed at a GLP facility.

2) The peer review pathologist should have received GLP training, including periodic refresher training. Documentation of this, as well as a copy of their curriculum vitae which demonstrates other training and qualifications, should be provided to the test facility/test site.

3) The peer review pathologist should follow a pathology peer review SOP, and the test facility/test site should maintain a copy of the SOP on file. Typically, the peer review pathologist follows their employer's pathology peer review SOP. Use of a different SOP should be referenced in the study protocol or peer review statement. Documentation stating that the peer review pathologist understands the SOP should be filed at the test facility/test site.

4) The peer review pathologist will issue a peer review memorandum/statement/certificate, which will be included in the study report or study file. Since the peer review pathologist is a scientist who does not have responsibility for primary generation or interpretation of data, they are not principal investigators. Further documentation of their involvement in the study, including QA inspections and compliance statements, is not required.

As of the time of writing, the FDA has been contemplating but has not released updated guidance for industry regarding the management and conduct of pathology peer review performed during GLP-compliant toxicity studies (FDA U.S. Food and Drug Administration). Final guidance may or may not impact the criteria provided above.

PWGs are uncommon but serve a critical role in safety assessment. PWGs can be added to pathology assessments of a study for several reasons. These groups are a made up of a small number of experienced or expert pathologists (typically three to seven) convened to address specific pathology issues at the bequest of the study or peer review pathologist, the sponsor, or regulators. In the authors' opinion, the study pathologist should be included in the PWG; however, the study pathologist may or may not be included in the PWG as an official member at the discretion of the sponsor. These groups can be convened before a study report is finalized, in which case their findings serve to refine the pathology raw data, or may be convened after a study is finalized, in which case the PWG findings should be incorporated in an amended final study report. These PWGs are used to establish consensus on specific meaningful safety findings when it cannot be reached during the pathology peer review process, to review and interpret disputed or questionable findings, answer questions or address concerns from regulatory agencies, generate new pathology data requested by a regulatory agency, and/or to provide additional scientific insight. PWGs can also clarify or explain if any perceived differences in findings across multiple studies for the same test article are genuine effects of the test article or are due to the use of different test facilities or pathologists' differences in training, experience, nomenclature, and/or diagnostic criteria. They are often the last recourse and are generally considered definitive since the PWG report represents the consensus interpretation of several subject matter experts and because there is a priori agreement that the PWG data will be definitive. PWGs have a robust structured review process that may include independent review of coded tissue sections (i.e., without knowledge of the treatment and dose) before voting to establish a majority or consensus diagnosis for each finding (see *Pathology Peer Review*, Vol 1, Chap 26).

4.5. Facilitate Finalization of a Well-Constructed, High-Quality, On-Time Pathology Report

Pathology Report Components

Best practices regarding the components of the pathology report and practices for assembling it have been published (Morton et al., 2006). A pathology report is comprised of both data tables and a narrative that provides an interpretation of them (see *Preparation of the Anatomic Pathology Report for a Toxicity Study*, Vol 2, Chap 13). The individual and summary data tables should always be reviewed along with the narrative since the narrative is the only location where test article–related findings are specifically defined by the study pathologist and the wording of a well-constructed narrative prevents misinterpretation of the tabular data.

The pathology report narrative should include a discussion of early deaths and their causes (if known), organ weight changes, macroscopic findings, clinical pathology correlates or findings, and microscopic findings. Many organizations also include summary, study background, and/or conclusion sections in the pathology report. The narrative should clearly describe test article–related findings and the dose levels at which they occur. Microscopic correlates for other test article–related pathology data, such as macroscopic and organ weight changes, should also be included. Rationale must be provided in the narrative for any observations that have an apparent dose response but are interpreted as incidental or spontaneous by the pathologist, including supporting references and/or historical control data that will help justify these conclusions and prevent regulatory questions later. Integration of other data such as clinical observations, clinical pathology values, and test article exposure should also be considered, but their inclusion is optional or should be agreed upon with the study team or sponsor.

Adversity determinations should be provided in the pathology report and/or the study report. Pathologists should be very careful in reporting adversity, as the improper use of "adverse" or "nonadverse" can have profound consequences. Recently, working groups from the STP and ESTP have produced well-received overviews addressing this topic (Kerlin et al., 2016; Palazzi et al., 2016). Users of the pathology data should be provided with as much weight of evidence and reasoning for the adversity determination as possible. If the study pathologist fails to clearly apply and justify their decisions, especially regarding findings of potential concern, regulatory agencies may question the interpretation and instead apply a more conservative determination of adversity. Some studies do not require adversity determinations, such as studies supporting development of anticancer therapeutics (per ICH S9) and exploratory (dose range finder) or early screening studies. In general, NOAEL and NOEL levels should not be included in the pathology subreport but should be defined only in the final study report. The rationale for this is that the most sensitive

endpoint that defines the NOAEL or NOEL for the study may not be found in the pathology data set (Kerlin et al., 2016).

Report Quality Control

Robust QC of the draft pathology report is necessary to reduce the occurrence of errors and facilitate the QA audit observations (see *Pathology and GLPs, Quality Control, and Quality Assurance*, Vol 1, Chap 27). It is important for the study pathologist to recognize that the primary responsibility for pathology data QC resides with them. They should not rely too heavily on support personnel who are focused on a secondary QC pertaining to formatting, grammar, and typographical (nonscientific) errors. The only opportunities for catching scientific errors are the study pathologist's own QC, informal reviews by pathologist colleagues and other study team members, and pathology peer review. Errors in diagnoses need to be identified and addressed as early as possible to minimize the potential impact to the interpretations of the study pathologist or study director. A robust QC effort also helps minimize the amount of reevaluation, sponsor comments, and regulatory challenges. Any necessary changes to the pathology subreport after it is finalized need to be documented in an audit trail and can only be made via an amended pathology report.

Timeliness and Signatures

There are several issues that can arise during the pathology reporting phase which, if not resolved in a timely manner, may result in delayed finalization of the study report. Other reasons to finalize pathology reports in a timely manner include reducing the amount of time for potential undue influence and reducing the chance of the study pathologist not being able to sign the report if they leave the organization. If the study pathologist is unable to sign the pathology report for any reason, the pathology evaluation needs to be reassigned to a new pathologist to rereview the study and issue a new pathology report. Rereview could include a complete reevaluation of the study or of a limited set of tissues. This reassignment can lead to lengthy reporting and program delays.

Timely pathology report finalization requires timely pathology peer reviews, sponsor reviews, and authorization from the sponsor for report finalization. Prolonged pathology peer reviews are an especially common source of schedule delays. Delays at this study phase can be minimized by conducting peer reviews at the testing facility to facilitate discussions, which avoids the need for slide shipment, and by prompt attention by the study pathologist, sponsor pathologist, and/or peer review pathologist to each other's communications, including suggestions made by the peer reviewer. Promising advancements in digital imaging technology have made the possibility of fully digital pathology peer reviews using high-resolution, whole-slide scans more feasible, which could save the time that would have been required for slide shipment (see *Digital Pathology and Tissue Image Analysis*, Vol 1, Chap 12).

During scientific review of the draft pathology report, the reviewers (in house at the test site and/or sponsor reviewers) should focus on content—data and their interpretation—rather than writing style preferences unless the writing style interferes with the clarity and readability of the report. Any suggested revisions should be focused on those that are relevant to understanding the safety assessment of the test article and should be conveyed to the study pathologist as a *proposal for consideration* rather than a demand. The reviewer should also understand that only the study pathologist can write the pathology report (since only she or he has evaluated all tissue sections), and the study pathologist maintains the sole authority to accept or reject any proposed revisions. Particularly in outsourced studies, the sponsor should avoid any editorial activity that could be perceived by a regulatory agency as undue influence. When reviewing the draft pathology report, the study director (for in-house studies) and the sponsor study monitor (for outsourced studies) should compile all comments from various reviewers into a single document before they are sent to the study pathologist (for the draft pathology report) or study director (for the draft study report) for consideration. This prevents unnecessary repetition or contradictory comments as well as multiple rounds of comments and revisions, which is an inefficient and time-consuming strategy for completing a study (Gosselin et al., 2011). The peer review pathologist

must be included in the report review process and informed of modifications made to the pathology report and/or pathology sections of the study report.

Development teams, study teams, and/or other members of the organization sponsoring the study may request draft data from organs of interest but should recognize that these draft results are subject to change within the context of the full evaluation and the iterative process of diagnostic refinement. These teams must also understand that pathologists ultimately evaluate *studies*, not individual tissues or animals (Gosselin et al., 2011). Any preliminary tables and/or summary narratives are not raw data and thus are not suitable for regulatory submission. Extreme caution must be used if considering important decisions (such as setting dose levels for future studies) based on this preliminary data.

The study pathologist, by signing the pathology report, attests that they are fully and individually accountable for all the diagnoses and interpretations within it. Study pathologists must be unwavering in their integrity and avoid circumstances or actions that suggest the potential of any undue influence from others. This is important for toxicologic pathologists in any organization, not only toxicologic pathologists working at a CRO. Use of 21 CFR part 11 (FDA Food and Drug Administration) and OECD Guidance Document 17 (OECD Organisation for Economic Co-operation and Development) compliant e-signatures (electronic signatures) can also be considered by the test facility/test site to increase the ease and speed of finalization of the reports. Numerous GLP-compliant e-signature software options exist (e.g., DocuSign), and should employ procedures and controls designed to ensure the authenticity, integrity, and confidentiality of electronic records from the point of their creation to the point of their receipt. An e-signature can usually be applied to a pathology report by the study pathologist from an internet-connected, password-protected personal computer or cell phone from anywhere in the world. Peer review memos can also employ e-signatures as a time-saving measure.

Regulatory agencies will typically reject any study reports with unsigned pathology reports because unsigned pathology reports are not considered to contain raw data. Signature-related issues can also result in observations on an FDA Form 483 (i.e., a postinspection document stating any conditions found to constitute substantive violations of the US Food, Drug, and Cosmetic Act). One example is the study report being signed on the same day that the pathology report is signed, which is not considered enough time to review and incorporate the pathology raw data into the main toxicity study report and conclusions. Another example is the pathology report being signed by the study pathologist's manager instead of the study pathologist as only the study pathologist can affirm that the report is theirs (by signing the report they authored).

The peer review pathologist is not required to sign the pathology report but should prepare and sign a peer review certificate/statement/memorandum describing the materials reviewed, the methods used in the review, and if general agreement was reached with the study pathologist regarding the interpretation of the pathology findings (Morton et al., 2006). It is unnecessary for the study pathologist to sign the pathology peer review statement although some sponsors request this step. Requiring this additional signature is a needless logistical hurdle and can present delays. The peer review pathologist should sign their statement after the pathology report is finalized and not before. This timing ensures that the peer review pathologist has had a chance to review and acknowledges the accuracy of the final pathology report.

5. CONCLUSIONS

Awareness and implementation of the practices shared here will optimize the generation and reporting of pathology data as well as the overall study outcome by preventing the introduction of pathology-related issues during the various phases of a nonclinical toxicity study. Implementation of these practices is greatly aided if the toxicologic pathologist has a solid foundation in toxicologic pathology and drug development, is actively involved in oversight and communications, particularly of the pathology portions of the study, and thoroughly understands that suboptimal design and/or execution of pathology evaluations will undermine the value of toxicity studies.

GLOSSARY

Development team A cross-disciplinary team of individuals employed by the sponsor of the study. The development team is in charge of crafting and executing the comprehensive development plan for a drug, taking it from discovery to regulatory approval. Representatives from areas such as drug chemistry, manufacturing, biology, regulatory affairs, toxicology, pathology, pharmacology, patient safety, and many others are members. The representatives from toxicology, pathology, and other nonclinical areas at the sponsor are responsible and accountable for crafting the nonclinical safety testing strategy and for the planning of and design of nonclinical toxicity studies.

Peer review pathologist A pathologist who is assigned to perform a quality control review of the draft pathology data and interpretation generated and reported by a study pathologist. This role commonly is fulfilled by reevaluation of a fraction of the tissues sections from which the histopathologic data were generated as well as the draft pathology report (consisting of text describing the main findings with interpretation, a summary, and individual animal data tables).

Sponsor pathologist A pathologist employed by the sponsor of the study. The sponsor pathologist may serve as the study pathologist, peer review pathologist, and/or as a consultant to the study and/or peer review pathologists.

Study pathologist A pathologist who is assigned to generate, interpret, and report pathology raw data in a nonclinical toxicity study. This role commonly is undertaken through histopathologic evaluation of all tissue sections followed by interpretation of the draft histopathology findings in the context of other categories of pathology data acquired at necropsy (e.g., macroscopic observations, organ weights, clinical pathology findings). Depending on the sponsor preference, a single study pathologist may integrate all pathology data in a single report or two study pathologists may prepare separate descriptions of anatomic pathology data (usually combining macroscopic observations, organ weights, and histopathology findings) or clinical pathology data.

Study team The group of individuals that is responsible for planning, designing, and executing nonclinical toxicity studies. In studies outsourced by the sponsor to a CRO, the study team includes representatives from both the sponsor (e.g., toxicologist, peer review pathologist, study monitor, and/or others) and representatives from the CRO (e.g., study director, study pathologist(s), and/or others), all of whom work together to ensure the success of nonclinical toxicity studies.

REFERENCES

Al-Bhlal LA: Pathologic findings for Bacille Calmette-Guérin infections in immunocompetent and immunocompromised patients, *Am J Clin Pathol* 113(5):703–708, 2000.

Arnold JE, Camus MS, Freeman KP, et al.: ASVCP guidelines: principles of quality assurance and standards for veterinary clinical pathology (version 3.0): developed by the american society for veterinary clinical pathology's (ASVCP) quality assurance and laboratory standards (QALS) committee, *Vet Clin Pathol* 48:542–618, 2019.

Anderson H, Rehm S, Stanislaus D, et al.: Scientific and Regulatory Policy Committee (SRPC) paper: assessment of circulating hormones in nonclinical toxicity studies III.

Female reproductive hormones, *Toxicol Pathol* 41:921–934, 2013.

Aulbach A, Provencher A, Tripathi N: Influence of study design variables on clinical pathology data, *Toxicol Pathol* 45:288–295, 2017.

Aulbach A, Vitsky A, Arndt T, et al.: Interpretative considerations for clinical pathology findings in nonclinical toxicology studies, *Vet Clin Pathol* 48:383–388, 2019a.

Aulbach A, Vitsky A, Arndt T, et al.: Overview and considerations for the reporting of clinical pathology interpretations in nonclinical toxicology studies, *Vet Clin Pathol* 48: 389–399, 2019b.

Bhaskaran M, Cornwell PD, Sorden SD, Elwell MR, et al.: Pancreatic effects of a Bruton's tyrosine kinase small-molecule inhibitor in rats are strain-dependent, *Toxicol Pathol* 46:460–472, 2018.

Blancher A, Bonhomme M, Crouau-Roy B, et al.: Mitochondrial DNA sequence phylogeny of 4 populations of the widely distributed cynomolgus macaque (*Macaca fascicularis* fascicularis), *J Hered* 99:254–264, 2008.

Bolon B, Butt MT: Fixation and processing of central nervous system tissue. In Aminoff MJ, et al., editors: *Encyclopedia of Neurological Sciences*, ed 2, San Diego, 2014, Academic Press (Elsevier), pp 312–316.

Bolon B, Caverly Rae JM, Colman K, et al.: Opinion on current use of non-blinded versus blinded histopathologic evaluation in animal toxicity studies, *Toxicol Pathol* 48:549–559, 2020.

Bolon B, Barale-Thomas E, Bradley A, et al.: International recommendations for training future toxicologic pathologists participating in regulatory-type, nonclinical toxicity studies, *Toxicol Pathol* 38:984–992, 2010.

Bregman CL, Adler RR, Morton DG, et al.: Recommended tissue list for histopathologic examination in repeat-dose toxicity and carcinogenicity studies: a proposal of the Society of Toxicologic Pathology (STP), *Toxicol Pathol* 31(2): 252–253, 2003.

Burkhardt JE, Pandher K, Solter PF, et al.: Recommendations for the evaluation of pathology data in nonclinical safety biomarker qualification studies, *Toxicol Pathol* 39(7):1129–1137, 2011.

Cauvin AJ, Peters C, Brennan F: Advantages and limitations of commonly used nonhuman primate species in research and development of biopharmaceuticals. In Bluemel J, et al., editors: *The nonhuman primate in nonclinical drug development and safety assessment*, San Diego, 2015, Academic Press (Elsevier), pp 379–395.

Chadwick KD, Fletcher AM, Parrula MC, et al.: Occurrence of spontaneous pancreatic lesions in normal and diabetic rats: a potential confounding factor in the nonclinical assessment of GLP-1-based therapies, *Diabetes* 63(4):1303–1314, 2014.

Chamanza R, Marxfeld HA, Blanco AI, et al.: Incidences and range of spontaneous findings in control cynomolgus monkeys (*Macaca fascicularis*) used in toxicity studies, *Toxicol Pathol* 38(4):642–657, 2010.

Chapin RE, Creasy DM: Assessment of circulating hormones in regulatory toxicity studies II. Male reproductive hormones, *Toxicol Pathol* 40:1063–1078, 2012.

Clemo F: Response to utility of clinical pathology reference ranges in preclinical safety studies, *Toxicol Pathol* 25(6):650, 1997.

Crabbs TA, Frame SR, Laast VA, et al.: Occurrence of spontaneous amphophilic-vacuolar renal tubule tumors in Sprague-Dawley rats from subchronic toxicity studies, *Toxicol Pathol* 41(6):866–871, 2013.

Crissman JW, Goodman DG, Hildebrandt PK, et al.: Best practices guideline: toxicologic histopathology, *Toxicol Pathol* 32:126–131, 2004.

Damsch S, Eichenbaum G, Tonelli A, et al.: Gavage-related reflux in rats: identification, pathogenesis, and toxicological implications (review), *Toxicol Pathol* 39:348–360, 2011.

Dixon J, Ripco F, Nrdo F: Vipco (website), *Nat Biotechnol*, 2011. http://blogs.nature.com/tradesecrets/2011/05/31/ripco-fipco-nrdo-fipnet-vipco. (Accessed 15 May 2021).

Dubey JP, Markovits JE, Killary KA: Cryptosporidium muris-like infection in stomach of cynomolgus monkeys (*Macaca fascicularis*), *Vet Pathol* 39:363–371, 2002.

Engelhardt JA, Fant P, Guionaud S, et al.: Scientific and Regulatory Policy Committee points-to-consider paper: drug-induced vascular injury associated with nonsmall molecule therapeutics in preclinical development: part 2. Antisense oligonucleotides, *Toxicol Pathol* 43(7):935–944, 2015.

Everds N, Li N, Bailey K, et al.: Unexpected thrombocytopenia and anemia in cynomolgus monkeys induced by a therapeutic human monoclonal antibody, *Toxicol Pathol* 41:951–969, 2013a.

Everds NE, Snyder PW, Bailey KL, et al.: Interpreting stress responses during routine toxicity studies: a review of the biology, impact, and assessment, *Toxicol Pathol* 41(4):560–614, 2013b.

FDA (U.S. Food and Drug Administration): *Pharmacology review(s). Roflumilast, application number 022522Orig1s000*, 2010a. https://www.accessdata.fda.gov/drugsatfda_docs/nda/2011/022522Orig1s000MedR.pdf. (Accessed 15 May 2021).

FDA (U.S. Food and Drug Administration): *IND safety reporting. 21CFR312.32*, 2010b. https://www.accessdata.fda.gov/scripts/cdrh/cfdocs/cfcfr/CFRSearch.cfm?fr=312.32. (Accessed 15 May 2021).

FDA (U.S. Food and Drug Administration): *Pharmacology review(s). Evolocumab, application number 125522Orig1s000*, 2015. https://www.accessdata.fda.gov/drugsatfda_docs/nda/2015/125522Orig1s000PharmR.pdf. (Accessed 15 May 2021).

FDA (U.S. Food and Drug Administration): Good laboratory practice regulations; Final rule, *Fed Regist* 52:33768–33782, 1987.

FDA (U.S. Food and Drug Administration): *Guidance for industry part 11, electronic records; electronic signatures — scope and application*, August 2003. https://www.fda.gov/media/75414/download. (Accessed 15 May 2021).

FDA (U.S. Food and Drug Administration): *Guidance for industry. Safety reporting requirements for INDs and BA/BE studies,* December 2012. https://www.fda.gov/regulatory-information/search-fda-guidance-documents/safety-reporting-requirements-inds-investigational-new-drug-applications-and-babe. (Accessed 15 May 2021).

FDA (U.S. Food and Drug Administration): *Pathology peer review in nonclinical toxicology studies: questions and answers. Guidance for industry, draft guidance,* August 2019. https://www.fda.gov/media/129533/download. (Accessed 15 May 2021).

Fikes JD, Patrick DJ, Francke S, et al.: Scientific and regulatory policy committee review: review of the organisation for economic co-operation and development (OECD) guidance on the GLP requirements for peer review of histopathology, *Toxicol Pathol* 43(7):907–914, 2015.

Fletcher AM, Bregman CL, Woicke J, et al.: Incisor degeneration in rats induced by vascular endothelial growth factor/fibroblast growth factor receptor tyrosine kinase inhibition, *Toxicol Pathol* 38(2):267–279, 2010.

Frazier KS: Antisense oligonucleotide therapies: the promise and the challenges from a toxicologic pathologist's perspective, *Toxicol Pathol* 43(1):78–89, 2015.

Frazier KS, Engelhardt JA, Fant P, et al.: Scientific and Regulatory Policy Committee points-to-consider paper: drug-induced vascular injury associated with nonsmall molecule therapeutics in preclinical development: part I. Biotherapeutics, *Toxicol Pathol* 43(7):915–934, 2015.

Gad SC, Spainhour CB, Shoemake C, et al.: Tolerable levels of nonclinical vehicles and formulations used in studies by multiple routes in multiple species with notes on methods to improve utility, *Int J Toxicol* 35(2):95–178, 2016.

Garman RH: Artifacts in routinely immersion fixed nervous tissue, *Toxicol Pathol* 18(1):149–153, 1990.

Gosselin SJ, Palate B, Parker GA, et al.: Industry-contract research organization pathology interactions: a perspective of contract research organizations in producing the best quality pathology report, *Toxicol Pathol* 39:422–428, 2011.

Hall RL: Lies, damn lies, and reference intervals (or hysterical control values for clinical pathology data), *Toxicol Pathol* 25(6):647–651, 1997.

Hall RL: Practical considerations in clinical pathology data interpretation and description, *Toxicol Pathol* 45(2):362–365, 2017.

Healing G, Sulemann T, Cotton P, et al.: Safety data on 19 vehicles for use in 1 month oral rodent pre-clinical studies: administration of hydroxypropyl-ß-cyclodextrin causes renal toxicity, *J Appl Toxicol* 36(1):140-150, 2016.

Heyen JR, Rojko J, Evans M, et al.: Characterization, biomarkers, and reversibility of a monoclonal antibody-induced immune complex disease in cynomolgus monkeys (*Macaca fascicularis*), *Toxicol Pathol* 42:765–773, 2014.

Hutto DL: Opportunistic infections in non-human primates exposed to immunomodulatory biotherapeutics: considerations and case examples, *J Immunotoxicol* 7:120–127, 2010.

Imbimbo BP, Ottonello S, Frisardi V, et al.: Solanezumab for the treatment of mild-to-moderate Alzheimer's disease, *Expet Rev Clin Immunol* 8:135–149, 2012.

IQ (*international consortium for innovation and quality in pharmaceutical development*): guidelines for blood collection for common laboratory animals, 2016. https://iqconsortium.org/images/LG-3Rs/IQ_3Rs_LG_CRO_WG_Blood_Collection_Guideline_June_2016.pdf. (Accessed 15 May 2021).

Irizarry AR, Yan G, Zeng Q, et al.: Defective enamel and bone development in sodium-dependent citrate transporter (NaCT) Slc13a5 deficient mice, *PloS One* 12(4):e0175465, 2017.

Irizarry Rovira AR, Bennet BM, Bolon B, et al.: Scientific and Regulatory Policy Committee points to consider: histopathologic evaluation in safety assessment studies for PEGylated pharmaceutical products, *Toxicol Pathol* 46:616–635, 2018.

Irizarry Rovira AR, Schultze AE: What is your diagnosis? CBC data and blood smear from a cynomolgus macaque (*Macaca fascicularis*), *Vet Clin Pathol* 41(1):162–163, 2012.

Irizarry Rovira AR, Foley GL, Clemo FA: Sponsor-CRO practices that facilitate the creation of a high-quality pathology report: a pharmaceutical sponsor's perspective, *Toxicol Pathol* 39:1013–1016, 2011.

Jurczyk-Procyk S, Martin M, Dubouch P: Toxicity studies of intravenously administered BCG in baboons, *Cancer Immunol Immunother* 1:55–61, 1976.

Kerlin R, Bolon B, Burkhardt J, et al.: Scientific and Regulatory Policy Committee: recommended ("best") practices for determining, communicating, and using adverse effect data from nonclinical studies, *Toxicol Pathol* 44(2):147–162, 2016.

Kozlosky JC, Mysore J, Clark SP, et al.: Comparison of physiologic and pharmacologic parameters in Asian and Mauritius cynomolgus macaques, *Regul Toxicol Pharmacol* 73:27–42, 2015.

Latendresse JR, Warbrittion AR, Jonassen H, et al.: Fixation of testes and eyes using a modified Davidson's fluid: comparison with Bouin's fluid and conventional Davidson's fluid, *Toxicol Pathol* 30:524–533, 2002.

Leach M: Regulatory forum opinion piece: differences between protein-based biologic products (biotherapeutics) and chemical entities (small molecules) of relevance to the toxicologic pathologist, *Toxicol Pathol* 41:128–136, 2013.

Li X, Elwell MR, Ryan AM, et al.: Morphogenesis of post-mortem hepatocyte vacuolation and liver weight increases in Sprague-Dawley rats, *Toxicol Pathol* 31:682–688, 2003.

Long RE, Smith A, Machotka SV, et al.: Scientific and Regulatory Policy Committee (SRPC) paper: validation of digital pathology systems in the regulated nonclinical environment, *Toxicol Pathol* 41(1):115–124, 2013.

Lynch CM, Hart BW, Grewal IS: Practical considerations for nonclinical safety evaluation of therapeutic monoclonal antibodies, *Monoclon Antibodies* 1(1):2–11, 2009.

Mann PC, Hardisty JF, Parker MD: Managing pitfalls in toxicologic pathology. In Haschek WM, Rousseaux CG, Wallig MA, editors: *Handbook of toxicologic pathology,* ed 2, San Diego, 2002, Academic Press, pp 187–206.

McInnes EF. *Background Lesions in Laboratory Animals: A Color Atlas,* Edinburgh, Scotland, 2012, Saunders.

McLean MK, Khan SA: Toxicology of frequently encountered nonsteroidal anti-inflammatory drugs in dogs and cats: an update, *Vet Clin N Am Small Anim Pract* 48:969–984, 2018.

Mease KM, Kimzey AL, Lansita JA: Biomarkers for nonclinical infusion reactions in marketed biotherapeutics and considerations for study design, *Curr Opin Toxicol* 4:1–15, 2017.

Morgan SJ, Elangbam CS, Berens S, et al.: Use of animal models of human disease for nonclinical safety assessment of novel pharmaceuticals, *Toxicol Pathol* 41(3):508–518, 2013.

Morton D, Sellers RS, Barale-Thomas E, et al.: Recommendations for pathology peer review, *Toxicol Pathol* 38:1118–1127, 2010.

Morton D, Kemp RK, Francke-Carroll S, et al.: Best practices for reporting pathology interpretations within GLP toxicology studies, *Toxicol Pathol* 34:806–809, 2006.

Nambiar PR, Morton D: The rasH2 mouse model for assessing carcinogenic potential of pharmaceuticals, *Toxicol Pathol* 41(8):1058–1067, 2013.

Neef N, Nikula KJ, Francke-Carroll S, et al.: Regulatory forum opinion piece: blind reading of histopathology slides in general toxicology studies, *Toxicol Pathol* 40(4):697–699, 2012.

Nold JB, Keenan KP, Nyska A, et al.: Society of toxicologic pathology position paper: diet as a variable in rodent toxicology and carcinogenicity studies, *Toxicol Pathol* 29(5):585–586, 2001.

OECD (Organisation for Economic Co-operation and Development): *OECD Series on principles of good laboratory practice and compliance monitoring: no. 16, advisory document of the working group on good laboratory practice—guidance on the GLP requirements for peer review of histopathology*, Paris, France, 2014, OECD Publishing. http://www.oecd.org/officialdocuments/publicdisplaydocumentpdf/?cote=env/jm/mono(2014)30&doclanguage=en. (Accessed 15 May 2021).

OECD (Organisation for Economic Co-operation and Development): *OECD series on principles of good laboratory practice and compliance monitoring, number 17, application of GLP principles to computerised systems*. ENV/JM/MONO(2016)13, April 22, 2016, https://www.oecd.org/officialdocuments/publicdisplaydocumentpdf/cote=env/jm/mono(2016)13&doclanguage=en. (Accessed 15 May 2021).

OECD (Organisation for Economic Co-operation and Development): *OECD series on principles of good laboratory practice and compliance monitoring, number 21, OECD position paper regarding possible influence of sponsors on conclusions of GLP studies*. ENV/JM/MONO(2020)5. May 7, 2020, https://www.oecd.org/officialdocuments/publicdisplaydocumentpdf/cote=env/jm/mono(2020)5&doclanguage=en. (Accessed 15 May 2021).

Olivier Jr KJ, Price KD, Hutto DL, et al.: Naturally occurring infections in non-human primates (NHP) and immunotoxicity implications: discussion sessions, *J Immunotoxicol* 7:138–146, 2010.

Palazzi X, Burkhardt JE, Caplain H, et al.: Characterizing "adversity" of pathology findings in nonclinical toxicity studies: results from the 4th ESTP international expert workshop, *Toxicol Pathol* 44(6):810–824, 2016.

Perry R, Farris G, Bienvenu JG, et al.: Society of toxicologic pathology position paper on best practices on recovery studies: the role of the anatomic pathologist, *Toxicol Pathol* 41(8):1159–1169, 2013.

Peter D, Göggel R, Colbatzky F, et al.: Inhibition of cyclooxygenase-2 prevents adverse effects induced by phosphodiesterase type 4 inhibitors in rats, *Br J Pharmacol* 162(2):415–427, 2011.

Price KD: Bacterial infections in cynomolgus monkeys given small molecule immunomodulatory antagonists, *J Immunotoxicol* 7:128–137, 2010.

Raab SS, Grzybicki DM: Anatomic pathology workload and error, *Am J Clin Pathol* 125:809–812, 2006.

Ramos-Vara JA, Kiupel M, Baszler T, et al.: Suggested guidelines for immunohistochemical techniques in veterinary diagnostic laboratories, *J Vet Diagn Invest* 20:393–413, 2008.

Ramot Y, Manno RA, Okazaki Y, et al.: Spontaneous aortitis in the Balb/c mouse, *Toxicol Pathol* 37:667–671, 2009.

Renshaw AA, Gould EW: Measuring errors in surgical pathology in real-life practice: defining what does and does not matter, *Am J Clin Pathol* 127:144–152, 2007.

Rojko JL, Evans MG, Price SA: Formation, clearance, deposition, pathogenicity, and identification of biopharmaceutical-related immune complexes: review and case studies, *Toxicol Pathol* 42:725–764, 2014.

Sasseville VG, Mansfield KG: Overview of known non-human primate pathogens with potential to affect colonies used for toxicity testing, *J Immunotoxicol* 7:79–92, 2010.

Schafer KA, Eighmy J, Fikes JD, et al.: Use of severity grades to characterize histopathologic changes, *Toxicol Pathol* 46(3):256–265, 2018.

Schultze AE, Bennet B, Rae JC, et al.: Scientific Regulatory Policy Committee points to consider: nuisance factors, block effects, and batch effects in nonclinical safety assessment studies, *Toxicol Pathol* 48(4):537–548, 2020.

Schultze AE, Irizarry AR: Recognizing and reducing analytical errors and sources of variation in clinical pathology data in safety assessment studies, *Toxicol Pathol* 45:281–287, 2017.

Schultze AE, Anderson JM, Kern TG, et al.: Longitudinal studies of cardiac troponin I concentrations in serum from male cynomolgus monkeys: resting values and effects of oral and intravenous dosing on biologic variability, *Vet Clin Pathol* 44(3):465–471, 2015.

Sellers RS: Translating mouse models, *Toxicol Pathol* 45(1):134-145, 2017.

Sellers RS, Morton D, Michael B, et al.: Society of Toxicologic Pathology position paper: organ weight recommendations for toxicology studies, *Toxicol Pathol* 35(5):751–755, 2007.

Smith ML, Raab SS: Assessment of latent factors contributing to error: addressing surgical pathology error wisely, *Arch Pathol Lab Med* 135:1436–1440, 2011.

Snyder PW, Everds NE, Craven WA, et al.: Maturity-related variability of the thymus in cynomolgus monkeys (*Macaca fascicularis*), *Toxicol Pathol* 44:874–891, 2016.

STP (Society of Toxicologic Pathology): Society of Toxicologic Pathologists position paper on blinded slide reading, *Toxicol Pathol* 14(4):493–494, 1986.

Taylor K: Clinical veterinarian's perspective of non-human primate (NHP) use in drug safety studies, *J Immunotoxicol* 7:114–119, 2010.

Tirmenstein M, Horvath J, Graziano M, et al.: Utilization of the Zucker Diabetic Fatty (ZDF) rat model for investigating hypoglycemia-related toxicities, *Toxicol Pathol* 43(6):825–837, 2015.

Tomlinson, et al.: Best practices for evaluating clinical pathology in pharmaceutical recovery studies, *Toxicol Pathol* 44(2):163–172, 2016.

Tomlinson L, Boone LI, Ramaiah L, et al.: Best practices for veterinary toxicologic clinical pathology, with emphasis on the pharmaceutical and biotechnology industries, *Vet Clin Pathol* 42(3):252–269, 2013.

Tomohiro M, Okabe T, Kimura Y, et al.: Toxicologic pathology forum: current status on the use of animal models of human disease in the pharmaceutical industry in Japan in nonclinical safety assessment-opinion paper, *Toxicol Pathol* 47(2):108–120, 2019.

Tripathi NK, Everds NE, Schultze AE, et al.: Deciphering sources of variability in clinical pathology, *Toxicol Pathol* 45:90–93, 2017.

Vahle JL, Finch L, Heidel SM, et al.: Carcinogenicity assessments of biotechnology-derived pharmaceuticals: a review of approved molecules and best practice recommendations, *Toxicol Pathol* 38:522–553, 2010.

van Gorder MA, Della Pelle P, Henson JW, et al.: Cynomolgus polyoma virus infection: a new member of the polyoma virus family causes interstitial nephritis, ureteritis, and enteritis in immunosuppressed cynomolgus monkeys, *Am J Pathol* 154:1273–1284, 1999.

Wang Z, Niimi M, Ding Q, et al.: Comparative studies of three cholesteryl ester transfer proteins and their interactions with known inhibitors, *PloS One* 12(8):e0180772, 2017. https://doi.org/10.1371/journal.pone.0180772.

Watanabe A, Kusuoka O, Sato N, et al.: Specific pathologist responses for standard for exchange of nonclinical data (SEND), *J Toxicol Pathol* 30(3):201–207, 2017.

Weber K, Razinger T, Hardisty JF, et al.: Differences in rat models used in routine toxicity studies, *Int J Toxicol* 30(2):162–173, 2011.

Issues in Laboratory Animal Science That Impact Toxicologic Pathology

Jeffrey Everitt[1], Angela King-Herbert[2], Peter J.M. Clements[3], Rick Adler[4]

[1]Duke University School of Medicine, Durham, NC, United States, [2]DNTP Comparative Medicine Group, National Institutes of Environmental Health Sciences, Research Triangle Park, NC, United States, [3]GlaxoSmithKline Research and Development, Ware, Hertfordshire, United Kingdom, [4]GlaxoSmithKline, Collegeville, PA, United States

O U T L I N E

1. Introduction	1078
2. Trends in Global Research Animal Care and Use	1078
3. Regulatory Issues	1081
3.1. Overview of Rules and Regulations	1081
3.2. Institutional Animal Care and Use Committee	1083
4. Euthanasia of Research Animals	1083
5. Selection of Animal Models	1084
5.1. Overview	1084
5.2. Issues of Translation in Animal Model Selection	1084
5.3. Genetic Considerations	1086
5.4. Issues to Consider When Sourcing Animals	1087
5.5. Use of Specialized Animal Models in Toxicology Research	1088
6. Animal Health Considerations	1089
6.1. Adventitious Agents	1089
6.2. Sentinel Monitoring Programs	1090
6.3. Microbial Effects on Toxicity	1090
7. Microbiome and Microbial Effects on Pathophysiology and Study Outcomes	1091
7.1. Introduction to the Microbiome	1091
7.2. Definitions, Natural History, and Characterization	1092
7.3. Association With Development, Immune Status, and Disease Phenotype—Cause or Effect?	1092
7.4. Impact on Efficacy, Biotransformation, and Toxicology	1094
7.5. Impact of Microbiome on Safety Translatability	1095
7.6. Minimizing Experimental Variability and Monitoring Microbiome Status	1095
8. Housing and Husbandry Issues	1096
8.1. Role of Environment in Lesion Production	1096
8.2. Study Design Considerations	1097
9. The Role of Diet in Toxicity Studies	1099
9.1. Introduction	1099
9.2. Types of Diets	1100
9.3. Contaminant Issues	1101
9.4. Dietary Optimization	1101
10. 3R's and In-Life Study Conduct for the Toxicologic Pathologist	1102
11. Description of Animal Studies in Scientific Publications	1103
12. Conclusion	1103
References	1103

1. INTRODUCTION

As an integral member of the preclinical study team, the toxicologic pathologist needs to have a thorough understanding of the laboratory animal model that serves as a test system for studies with pathology requirements. Genetic, microbial, experimental, and environmental factors greatly affect lesion development in laboratory animals, and an understanding of the interplay of these factors with test article–induced effects is necessary for the pathologist to correctly interpret study findings. In addition to the role of assessing compound-induced tissue findings, the toxicologic pathologist often identifies health-related issues in study animals and must be knowledgeable about the common spontaneous and infectious disease states that arise in long-term preclinical studies. The pathologist must work closely with laboratory animal science professionals who are responsible for oversight of animal colony management and care during the in-life phase of the study.

Toxicology research and testing is becoming increasingly more complex with the advent of new and exciting advances in biotechnology. This is best exemplified by the widespread use of increasingly complex genetically modified mouse and rat models in toxicology testing facilities performing safety assessment bioassays, as well as in basic research laboratories (see *Genetically Engineered Animal Models in Toxicologic Research*, Vol 1, Chap 23). There is also an increasing sophistication in animal monitoring systems such as telemetric (remote monitoring) assessment of physiological parameters and nuclear and nonnuclear preclinical imaging methods (see *In* Vivo *Small Animal Imaging: A Comparison to Gross and Histopathologic Observations in Animal Models*, Vol 1, Chap 13). These technologies utilized during in vivo studies contribute to an improved understanding of the pathogenesis of many laboratory animal diseases and lesion states, provide new and useful adjuncts to traditional pathology assessment, and may reduce the number of animals used in studies.

Laboratory animal science is a diverse and complex discipline encompassing many different types of experimental animals. The discipline is a dynamic one and is shaped in part by the regulatory landscape as well as scientific advancements. In the United States, the eighth Edition of the *Guide for the Care and Use of Laboratory Animals* (NRC, 2011) provides the basis for the care of research animals in the laboratory. There are similar guidance documents elsewhere in the world that govern the highly regulated use of research animals in laboratories (Bayne and Turner, 2019). These major guidance documents impact animal care and use programs and influence the conditions under which toxicity studies are conducted.

There are many questions in laboratory animal science that need to be considered during the planning and conduct of a toxicity study (Table 29.1), and the pathologist is an important member of the study team who should be involved in the design phase. The design of toxicity studies often requires professional judgment to balance the needs of the research animal against experimental objectives or other needs such as those of personnel safety, environmental contamination, and/or regulatory requirements (see *Practices to Optimize Generation, Interpretation, and Reporting of Pathology Data from Toxicity Studies*, Vol 1, Chap 28 and *Experimental Design and Statistical Analysis for Toxicologic Pathologists*, Vol 1, Chap 16). Selected laboratory animal science issues that pertain to the work of pathologists and that influence lesion development will be stressed in this chapter. Remarks in this chapter will be primarily focused on selected issues involving laboratory rodents, given that they are the most commonly utilized animals in toxicity studies. For more in-depth review of specific animal models, the reader is directed to other chapters in this volume (see Part 3—Animal and Alternative Models in Toxicologic Research).

2. TRENDS IN GLOBAL RESEARCH ANIMAL CARE AND USE

Laboratory animal science is a dynamic discipline and there are numerous regulatory changes that occur in response to new scientific knowledge and best practices on how animals should be cared for and used in the research laboratory. Major changes have occurred in how animals are cared for and housed in the toxicology laboratory such as types of caging and social housing arrangements. Work with laboratory animals is a highly

TABLE 29.1 Laboratory Animal Science Issues to be Addressed by the Toxicology Study Team

INSTITUTIONAL ANIMAL CARE AND USE COMMITTEE (IACUC) CONSIDERATIONS:

Plan experiment from the standpoint of optimizing animal numbers, assuring proper statistical design, and scientific justification (harm vs. benefit)

Review issues of animal pain and distress and consider methods to minimize pain or distress

Obtain IACUC review and approval of the experimental protocol

Ensure personnel are properly trained with up-to-date documentation

Define humane endpoints/criteria for euthanasia

Assure dose volumes and blood withdraw volumes comply with IACUC guidelines

STUDY ISSUES:

Assure compliance with regulatory testing guidelines

Review staffing (e.g., number of trained personnel to cover activities) and associated concerns such as blinding of personnel to allocation groups where appropriate to minimize bias

Determine methods of allocation of animals to study without bias (randomization)

Establish animal identification and cage identification methods

Define acclimation and quarantine periods (e.g., length, location, methods)

Review dosing methods and issues related to test compound (e.g., dose schedule, volume, vehicle, special monitoring needs)

Review all experimental manipulations of animals, including timing of events

Establish procedures for removing animals from study with unexpected morbidity/mortality and determine handling and disposition of animals

ANIMAL MODEL SELECTION AND USE:

Determine species and strain and review scientific rationale for model selection

Establish age, sex, weight, physiological status, and genetic requirements

Choose source or supplier

Review genetic and health history of source colony

Establish need for any prestudy health or genetic testing of supplied animals

Review strain-related causes of morbidity and mortality and institutional experience with chosen animal model

ANIMAL ENVIRONMENT:

Review animal room conditions (e.g., temperature, humidity, lighting, noise, air flow)

Establish methods and intervals for environmental monitoring

Review housing issues (e.g., group vs. single housing, type of caging, type of bedding, frequency of cage change, room allocation, and methods to prevent bias in housing and handling such as rotation of cage or rack placement)

Arrange for special housing as needed (e.g., inhalation or metabolism caging) and methods for acclimation to equipment and special procedures

Determine whether other animals (e.g., sentinel animals) or studies (e.g., microbial infections in facility) pose hazard to study animals and institute protective procedures if warranted

Establish environmental enrichment methods

(Continued)

TABLE 29.1   Laboratory Animal Science Issues to be Addressed by the Toxicology Study Team—cont'd

DIET:

Specify type (e.g., open vs. closed formula, natural vs. semipurified ingredients) and form (e.g., pelleted, powder, liquid) of diet

Review method of feeding (i.e., ad libitum vs. diet restriction)

Determine the need for certified diet or methods for contaminant analysis

Review water distribution method (e.g., bottle vs. automatic) and treatment method if any (e.g., autoclaved, filtered, acidified, chlorinated)

Determine methods and intervals for monitoring food and water consumption if needed

In the case of dosing in feed or water, review stability, mixing, and analytical issues related to the diet, and palatability

IN-LIFE:

Establish clinical parameters to be monitored as well as schedules and methods of monitoring

Determine animal health monitoring needs on study

Review sentinel monitoring program for study and test facility

Review animal manipulation, sampling, and dosing procedures with respect to circadian issues, photoperiodicity, and to minimize interventional stress

Review chemical safety issues and cage change procedures

Table modified from Haschek WM, Rousseaux CG, Wallig MA, editors: Handbook of toxicologic pathology, *ed 2, 2002, Academic Press, Table 29.1, p. 252, with permission.*

regulated endeavor in most parts of the world and those that use in vivo studies must be well versed with the rules and regulations pertaining to their work. In the United States, there are national, state, and local regulations that address many facets of the animal care and use program. In recent years, there has been a trend to examine research animal issues with a global perspective (Bayne and Turner, 2019). This is especially true for large pharmaceutical companies that work across numerous facilities located in multiple countries. In some cases, companies have global policies concerning their animal care and use so that they can assure a common best practice approach where warranted.

Over the past decade, one of the major scientific changes in the field of laboratory animal science has been the recognition of the importance of the microbiome in the pathophysiology of research animals (Silbergeld, 2017). Another important trend in laboratory animal science that has been growing and strengthening over the past several years has been the recognition of the importance of social interactions among research animals (Hannibal et al., 2017). Group housing of social

species is the normal default situation for virtually all studies now unless there are well-justified scientific reasons for exception. The ability to socially house animals in the laboratory setting may require changes in standard operating procedures so that food consumption and clinical evaluations can be obtained during the in-life conduct of toxicity studies. An additional trend in the housing of research animals that has gained favor in many laboratory settings is the recognition that cage complexity and enrichment is warranted so that animals can express species-specific behaviors. Many study directors have been reluctant in the past to incorporate these devices, citing differences in responses on study or the possibility for ingestion of contaminants leading to unwanted effects. Environmental enrichment programs are now the norm for the toxicology laboratory as they are for other research animal settings and there are many certified products available to control contaminant levels that might otherwise adversely impact results. In the past, many rodents were individually housed in barren metal wire caging suspended over bedding. Modern rodent housing methods consider the importance of social housing and the need for solid flooring with direct contact bedding that allows for normal behaviors as well as for thermoregulatory needs to be met. There is an increasing realization of the importance of thermoregulation in housing rodents and the role that this factor plays in lesion incidence and development.

A very important trend in laboratory animal science in toxicity studies has been the advancement of the so-called 3Rs (i.e., Replacement, Reduction, and Refinement) as a culture of animal use. Adherence to working in a 3Rs mode of thinking is now the norm in many countries and has been recently mandated by changes in guidance and regulations in many parts of the world. A section devoted to the 3Rs is incorporated in this chapter due to its importance regarding how animals are used in research and testing in toxicology. The toxicologic pathologist must be aware of 3Rs issues during the design and conduct of animal studies (Hukkanen et al., 2019; Sewell et al., 2016). There is strong societal pressure throughout the world for the optimization of animal care and use and many companies put high internal value on the minimization of animal use. The expertise of the toxicologic pathologist is best utilized at the design phase of studies so that animal care and use can be optimized during protocol development. There is great value in close collaboration of the toxicologic pathologist with study directors and principal investigators during the course of the in-life conduct of toxicity studies so that all unexpected findings and events can be understood at the earliest time possible to effect interventions as well as to design modifications to obtain the most data of the highest quality from study endpoints. The use of diagnostic investigation of unscheduled mortality and morbidity can be an important component of optimized animal welfare during the course of the study.

The overwhelming majority of laboratory animals used in biomedical institutions are rodents. Rodent populations are increasing in some institutions primarily due to the burgeoning use of genetically modified mouse models in basic research (see *Genetically Engineered Animal Models in Toxicologic Research*, Vol 1, Chap 23). There has been a diminution in the use of nonrodent species in many areas of toxicology research and testing, and the use of nonhuman primate

models is a particularly scrutinized area (see *Animal Models in Toxicologic Research: Nonhuman Primate*, Vol 1, Chap 21). Some pharmaceutical companies require justification for not using other nonrodent preclinical species such as dogs and minipigs prior to utilizing nonhuman primates in drug safety studies (see *Animal Models in Toxicologic Research: Dog*, Vol 1, Chap 19 and *Animal Models in Toxicologic Research: Pig*, Vol 1, Chap 20). Certain nonhuman primate models, such as chimpanzees, are no longer utilized in safety assessment studies due to regulatory restrictions.

3. REGULATORY ISSUES

3.1. Overview of Rules and Regulations

All scientists who utilize laboratory animals must be knowledgeable about government regulations and guidelines pertaining to the proper care and use of research animals. It should be noted that although regulations differ between regions and countries, there has been a trend toward globalization of animal care and use practices (Bayne and Turner, 2019). There are certain aspects of research animal use that are associated with broad societal concerns such as the use of genetically modified animals, humanized animal models, and nonhuman primate models.

Many pharmaceutical and chemical companies are multinational with laboratories in multiple countries and thus scientists must be aware of differing policies that affect animal use. Some companies have developed worldwide practices so that their studies are similar no matter where conducted. In many instances, these practices are clearly delineated in policy statements on company websites so that there is transparency to the public. In the pharmaceutical industry, there has been a trend toward increasingly complex collaborative and contract research interactions, and this has often necessitated development of common approaches to animal care and use issues. Consortia such as the IQ Consortium and the UK's National Centre for the Replacement, Reduction and Refinement of Animals in Research (NC3Rs) are entities that have attempted to address this need (Adams et al., 2019; Chapman et al., 2009). The NC3Rs is an independent scientific organization set up by the UK government to find innovative solutions to minimize animal use and improve animal welfare in research.

In the United States, oversight of animal care and use is primarily provided by two national laws, the Animal Welfare Act (7 USC 2131-2157) and the Health Research Extension Act (42 USC 289d). The latter was amended in 1985 by Public Law 99-158 to cover the care and use of animals in research. The regulations that implement the Animal Welfare Act are published in the Code of Federal Regulations (9 CFR 1-3) and are administered by the U.S. Department of Agriculture (USDA). For the purposes of this Act, animals are presently defined as "any live or dead dog, cat, nonhuman primate, guinea pig, hamster, rabbit, or any other warm-blooded animal which is being used, or is intended for use for research, teaching, testing, experimentation, or exhibition purposes, or as a pet" (9 CFR 1.1). Rats and mice bred for use in research are currently exempted from these regulations, although this exemption may be eliminated in the future.

Among the provisions of the Animal Welfare Act are (1) standards to ensure the humane care of animals being transported; (2) standards for care of animals in research facilities, including minimum requirements for housing, feeding, watering, sanitation, handling, adequate veterinary care, and the appropriate use of anesthetic, analgesic, and tranquilizing drugs to ensure the minimization of pain and distress; (3) the reporting of requirements to the USDA showing that professionally acceptable standards for the humane care and use of animals are in effect; (4) establishment of an Institutional Animal Care and Use Committee (IACUC); and (5) establishment of training for all personnel involved in the care and use of animals.

The Health Research Extension Act is implemented by the Public Health Service Policy on Humane Care and Use of Laboratory Animals (PHS Policy) and is administered by the National Institutes of Health, Office for Laboratory Animal Welfare. The policy pertains to all activities conducted and supported by the Public Health Service involving any live vertebrate animal used or intended for use in research, research training, biological testing, or related purposes. The PHS Policy requires compliance with the Animal Welfare Act and use of the *Guide for the Care and Use of Laboratory Animals (Guide)* (NRC, 2011) as a basis for developing and implementing an institutional program for activities involving animals. No activity supported by the PHS involving animals may be conducted until the institution conducting the activity has provided a written assurance of compliance with PHS Policy.

Many institutions that perform toxicology research and testing are accredited by AAALAC International. AAALAC is a nonregulatory, not-for-profit organization whose mission is to serve as a voluntary accrediting organization that enhances the quality of research, teaching, and testing by promoting humane, responsible animal care and use. Participation in the peer review accreditation program is voluntary and at the initiative of the individual institution. The AAALAC Council evaluates animal programs by conducting site visits and reviewing reports. It relies on performance standards and uses guidance such as the eighth Edition of the *Guide for the Care and Use of Laboratory Animals* (NRC, 2011) and the *European Convention for the Protection of Vertebrate Animals Used for Experimental and Other Scientific Purposes Council of Europe* for the evaluation of laboratory animal care and use programs. AAALAC accreditation demonstrates that a program has achieved a standard of excellence beyond the minimum required by law. It is presently the only accrediting body recognized by the PHS for activities involving animals.

In addition to working under the auspices of the Animal Welfare Act and in some cases PHS Policy, the work of many toxicologic pathologists is conducted under the guidance of the Good Laboratory Practice (GLP) regulations of the Food and Drug Administration or U.S. Environmental Protection Agency (Keatley, 1999). The GLP regulations contain additional provisions for the care and use of laboratory animals. Included among these are certain requirements for animal housing, separation of species, quarantine of new and sick animals, and separation of projects (Howard et al., 2004). There are also requirements for monitoring and documenting the health of research animals, as well as requirements for recording any treatments performed on research animals. There is a GLP stipulation that all animals and their enclosures be properly identified. Identification requirements and documentation methods are of particular importance to pathologists who also must track tissues and samples obtained at necropsy.

3.2. Institutional Animal Care and Use Committee

Both PHS Policy and the Animal Welfare Act require organizations using animals for research to designate an institutional official that will be responsible for the animal care and use program, and to mandate the formation of an IACUC. The IACUC is responsible for oversight of the animal care and use program. Specifically, the IACUC must assure that consideration be given to the minimization of pain and distress for all experimental animals. This is particularly important in toxicity testing, where the administration of potentially deleterious test articles can induce animal pain and distress. A specific requirement of the IACUC is to perform a semiannual review of the institution's animal care and use program as well as an inspection of the facilities where animals are housed, using the *Guide* and the standards of the Animal Welfare Act as a basis for evaluation. Reports of these reviews are sent to the designated institutional official with recommendations for programmatic improvements, if necessary, and corrective actions and timetables if deficiencies are noted. Among its various duties, the primary task of the IACUC is the review of all animal use protocols prior to study initiation to assure compliance with applicable regulations such as the Animal Welfare Act and PHS Policy.

The IACUC review of protocols requires an assurance that the animal model is appropriate and that the proposed experimental design uses a suitable number of animals in a manner likely to achieve the scientific objectives of the study. There is a requirement that investigators consider alternatives to the use of animals where possible and that every effort be made to minimize pain and distress. IACUC review also includes review of the proposed method of euthanasia. Toxicologic pathologists may be called upon to serve as members of the IACUC due to their familiarity with study design and animal care and use issues.

4. EUTHANASIA OF RESEARCH ANIMALS

The toxicologic pathologist should be involved in all facets of preclinical study design and protocol development, and special attention should be directed to laboratory science issues that affect the necropsy (see *Basic Approaches to Anatomic Toxicologic Pathology*, Vol 1, Chap 9). A very important part of the necropsy is performance of the euthanasia procedure. The pathologist needs to determine the proper method of euthanasia and to assure oversight of the procedure. In general, the euthanasia method selected should be in accordance with the recommendations of the American Veterinary Medical Association (AVMA) Panel on Euthanasia (Shomer et al., 2020). Euthanasia in the necropsy laboratory can present special challenges when it is associated with terminal surgical procedures, such as during the collection of certain samples and during the conduct of organ perfusion methods. These methods require a proper understanding of anesthetic management and monitoring procedures and involve careful description of the procedures to the IACUC for approval.

The method of euthanasia chosen should (1) have the ability to produce death without causing pain or distress to the animal; (2) be reliable; (3) be safe to personnel; (4) be nonreversible; (5) cause minimal emotional distress to necropsy personnel; and (6) be compatible with the scientific objectives of the experiment. There are many examples of untoward effects of the euthanasia method on research endpoints. Anesthetic overdose using injectable or inhalant anesthetic agents followed by exsanguination is a commonly utilized method favored by many toxicologic pathologists. This methodology is compatible with excellent tissue preservation and can be carried out efficiently. A variety of commonly used methods for rodent and nonrodent species euthanasia are associated with tissue artifacts (Grieves et al., 2008; Shomer et al., 2020). These include pulmonary hemorrhage associated with carbon dioxide (CO_2) inhalation and tissue trauma associated with decapitation and cervical dislocation methods. Histopathologic assessment of tissues is often only one of several study endpoints, and thus the pathologist must understand the needs of the entire experiment (e.g., clinical biochemistry, hematology, body fluid analysis, immunologic assessments) so that the most appropriate euthanasia method can be chosen to minimize untoward effects on the study (see *Clinical Pathology in Nonclinical Toxicity Testing*, Vol 1, Chap 10). Clinical pathology parameters may be affected by rapid acid–base shifts induced by CO_2 or terminal hypoxia. Other toxicologic endpoints such as hormone levels, neurotransmitter activity, liver metabolism, and immune function parameters can be affected by certain anesthetic regimens and euthanasia methods (Shomer et al., 2020).

Because euthanasia of research animals is so critical to the work of the pathologist, it is imperative that controversies concerning these methods be well understood. Guidance often changes over time. Even the most commonly used method of euthanasia in rodents, inhalation of CO_2, has had changes and conflicting methodology (e.g., rate of administration) during the past 2 decades and there have been changes in the AVMA guidance concerning recommendations for how to conduct the technique to minimize the occurrence of pain and distress. The latest guidance from the AVMA recommends introducing the gas into the chamber at a rate of 30%–70% of the chamber volume per minute in order to reduce distress to the rodent. There have also been controversies concerning the use of decapitation and cervical dislocation in animals. In all instances, the selection of the technique for euthanasia should be reviewed by pathologists involved with the study and discussed with the study director and institutional veterinarian to assure compatibility with research endpoints. The method must be approved by the relevant institutional animal care and use and ethical review committees. Pathologists must consider the possibility that variance in euthanasia administration, prior to necropsy and exsanguination, between animals may also contribute to biologic variation observed in research results.

5. SELECTION OF ANIMAL MODELS

5.1. Overview

The use of laboratory animal models will continue to play a critical role in toxicologic pathology. They have proven to be useful in

toxicology testing because they share many similarities with humans. Broad translation of cellular, tissue, organ, and system similarities of xenobiotic-induced toxicologic pathology findings in animals is the long-standing premise for nonclinical in vivo testing of test articles intended for administration in humans. Relative comparisons of toxicities in nonclinical species with those in humans support this continued use. There are metabolic, anatomic, and physiologic similarities that allow for comparisons in absorption, distribution, and excretion of xenobiotics, but differences in these attributes also must be appreciated that potentially impact translation (see *ADME Principles in Small Molecule Drug Discovery and Development—An Industrial Perspective*, Vol 1, Chap 3 and *Biotherapeutic ADME and PK/PD Principles*, Vol 1, Chap 4). The small size, docile nature, short life spans and gestation periods, and large litter size make rodents very economical animal models to maintain, breed, and use in the conduct of toxicology studies, including for lifelong studies used to assess carcinogenicity. Historical databases and publications on spontaneous disease characteristics of mice and rats and other laboratory animal species make them invaluable animal models for toxicology studies (Deschl et al., 2002; Keenan et al., 2009a, 2009b).

For the proper interpretation of toxicology and pathology data, the age, sex, physiologic status, microbiologic status, nutrition, and genotype of the test animals must be considered. It is also necessary to consider the environment in which they are bred, maintained, and observed. Most modern toxicology testing facilities use barrier-reared rodents with defined microbial flora, perform health surveillance on the colony, and order animals from reliable suppliers. These sources should be able to provide information concerning diet and feeding methods, breeding procedures, genetic control, caging, and husbandry as part of the source history.

5.2. Issues of Translation in Animal Model Selection

Translation of animal model toxicity to humans is a controversial topic, but nonclinical testing is codified and required by harmonized international regulatory expectations. These regulations are predicated on the known value of hazard characterization (e.g., tissue, organ, or system injury caused by the test article as evident in histopathologic evaluation, and correlative clinical signs, clinical pathology, organ weight changes, or other allied and appropriate evaluations of injury or functional perturbation). Hazard characterization is used to screen out drugs in development considered to have high risk for causing similar human toxicity. Risk assessment is used after hazard characterization to establish a risk–benefit ratio for a specific disease indication, and nonclinical safety testing is essential to establish a safe starting dose in clinical trial subjects (e.g., based on a No Observed Adverse Effect Level, or NOAEL, in animals) and to define predicted safety margins based on comparison of estimates of the test article exposure needed to provide efficacy for the disease and estimates of therapeutic index from toxicokinetic assessment of exposures in animals (see *Interpreting Adverse Effects*, Vol 2, Chap 15] and *Risk Assessment*, Vol 2, Chap 16).

Retrospective evaluation of toxicity in animal studies compared to human toxicity to determine translatability must take into account that true positives are typically not identified in both animals and humans (Monticello et al., 2017; Olson et al., 2000). Drugs showing greater toxicity in animals are typically "screened out" and not often advanced to clinical trials if the risk–benefit ratio is deemed too high for continued development. Further, toxicity in animals is often manifest at a high dose that is not pursued in clinical trials, so genuine positive concordance to human outcomes in the case of animal toxicity will generally remain undetermined unless patients are more sensitive to toxicity than nonclinical species or have contributing concomitant conditions or therapies not tested for in animals. True negatives may also not be easily determined since it would be considered unethical to escalate the human dose beyond the efficacious range to specifically test for toxicity. Instead, only drugs with low order or manageable toxicity will advance to human testing and development. Manageable toxicities are those that have suitable benefit to risk ratio for the specific indication; identifiable safety biomarkers that can measure toxicity early in the course of injury; readily reversible toxicity; a reasonable margin of safety; and/or a reaction in animals already known to be species specific. Translational knowledge for drug toxicity has grown over time and continues to be readily applied so that unnecessary toxicity testing can be avoided or minimized in animals, with cautious assessment of potential human risk, the constant overarching requirement in pharmaceutical research and development.

The increasing complexity of different drug modalities (drug tools) that are available in current pharmaceutical discovery to target human disease has brought evolution in toxicity testing approaches, along with slowly adapted regulatory expectations and guidelines for these respective modalities. Drug toxicity translation from animals to humans should no longer be collectively considered. Modality-based approaches now recognize the diversity of toxicity expression and translatability. These approaches are science driven, and in select cases, animal testing is not scientifically valid (Bailey and Balls, 2019). Small-molecule drug modalities are typically tested in animals for hazard characterization, and this can manifest as target mediated (i.e., exaggerated pharmacologic effect), off-target toxicity (i.e., receptor-like activity in a tissue, organ, or system, not expected in the desired disease pathway or expected pharmacologic target), and chemically mediated toxicity (i.e., nonpharmacologic or indirect mechanisms that are chemically induced and independent of the drug target, and often related to absorption, distribution, metabolism, and excretion). Concordance of small-molecule toxicity to human toxicity identified in subsequent clinical trials has been studied and found to have high correlation in most organ systems, particularly where comparison of rat and nonrodent testing is combined (Olson et al., 2000). This concordance is also most likely to be characterized in toxicity studies of 1-month duration or less. Biopharmaceutical compounds such as monoclonal antibodies and peptides are singularly developed for efficacy on human-specific biologic systems; their toxicity expression in animals is essentially divided into translationally relevant exaggerated pharmacologic activity in a pharmacologically relevant species (e.g., typically nonhuman primate) and less relevant antihuman drug reaction (e.g., neutralizing antibodies, immune complex disease) (see *Protein Pharmaceutical Agents*, Vol 2, Chap 6). Antisense oligonucleotides present a different challenge as these drug modalities create toxicity in rodent and nonrodents that have low translational relevance to human; however, worldwide regulatory agencies are increasingly aware of these issues through case-by-case learning, and through publications that advance collective understanding of risk translation (see *Nucleic Acid Pharmaceutical Agents*, Vol 2, Chap 7). Cellular therapies (for example, stem cell reengineering or lymphocyte effector cell reengineering) are entirely designed as human specific, and animal testing for these modalities has very limited purpose (see *Stem Cells and Regenerative Medicine*, Vol 2, Chap 10).

5.3. Genetic Considerations

There are three main classes of laboratory rodents used in research laboratories: isogenic strains (i.e., all individuals are genetically identical), outbred stocks (i.e., from parents that are not closely related), and mutants (e.g., spontaneous and genetically modified). All three groups of rodents have been extensively used in toxicology research and testing, although critical evaluation of how rodent models were historically chosen has not been well elucidated in the literature. More recently, humanized mouse models have entered the arena of therapy development to examine human tissue responses and to create surrogate human disease models (Ito et al., 2018). In some humanized mice, a mouse gene is replaced by either a human gene, genomic sequence, or regulatory element. In other models used in therapy discovery and development, immunodeficient mice are engrafted with functional human biological systems.

There has been a continuing debate concerning the choice of rodent stocks and strains most suitable for toxicity studies (Festing, 2010, 2016). This debate has intensified recently because of apparent genetic drift in certain outbred stocks of rats, leading to significant declines in life span, increased background of spontaneous disease, and changes in other parameters that impact historical data (Haseman et al., 1998; Tennekes et al., 2004). Scientific debate in favor of using multiple inbred strains within the same toxicity study to more closely mimic heterogeneity of human populations has not led to

changes in how rodents are used in safety assessment testing in the pharmaceutical industry. Outbred sources of rodents are still in broad use.

Outbred stocks of rodents are often known by generic names such as Sprague–Dawley rats or Swiss mice but should always be designated by their proper genetic nomenclature. As a result of genetic assortment, inbreeding, and selection, different colonies of outbred stocks will be genetically different from each other within a few years. It is important for scientists to understand that commercial rodent producers maintain multiple colonies of many of the important outbred stocks; therefore, the relationship between the various colonies is dependent on the breeding practices utilized. Control of these breeding practices is critical to assure uniformity, even among single suppliers. Although genetic drift can be minimized using large colony sizes and specific breeding schemes, genetic quality control of outbred stocks is difficult and expensive and requires significant supplier effort.

In general, toxicologic pathologists feel most comfortable using animal models for which they have historical data on the incidence of spontaneous and test article–induced lesions. The lesion database for any animal stock or strain is best utilized when it is based on in-house studies with animals that have a similar genetic history and are maintained under identical environmental conditions to the study being conducted. Thus, many institutions become reluctant to change the design of studies or to use new animal models if they feel that the changes will negate their ability to utilize historical data. This is particularly true when studies need to be reported to regulatory agencies. Historical data can provide an extremely valuable tool for study interpretation, but sometimes the value of these databases is overstated. Genotypic qualities of rodent models change over time due to selection procedures, alterations in breeding schemes, and genetic drift. These genetic changes have led to changes in the incidences of many neoplasms and nonneoplastic findings in both isogenic strains and outbred stocks. In addition to alterations in genetic qualities of rodents, animal husbandry practices change over time, contributing to the need to view historical databases as living documents subject to change. Animal housing, trends in stocking density, and many other aspects of animal husbandry such as diets and feeding practices contribute to significant changes in historical databases of both neoplastic and nonneoplastic lesions.

It is important to understand individual stock and strain characteristics when choosing rodent models for toxicology experiments. In some instances, anatomical, biochemical, or physiological attributes may be used to select a model for use. The longevity of the selected model is an important characteristic to consider for certain long-term studies. Regulatory requirements dictate certain survival criteria, and the decreasing longevity in certain stocks of ad libitum–fed rats in recent years has led to difficulty in some laboratories. Various approaches have been used in efforts to reverse the declining trends in survival. These efforts have included changes in breeding schemes and husbandry procedures (such as types of diets and the way in which rodents are fed) (Keenan et al., 2000). In a number of instances, institutions have changed their routine stocks and strains for chronic bioassays based on longevity issues.

A key point in properly selecting a rodent model is to understand the impact of strain-related spontaneous lesions on the proposed study endpoints. For instance, if the lung is a suspected target organ of toxicity, the Fischer 344 rat strain is probably not the animal model of choice for a long-term study. This strain has a very high incidence of leukemia, with pulmonary vascular infiltrates that would compromise the ability of the pathologist to diagnose interstitial lung disease. Similarly, if a nose-only method was the proposed route of exposure in a long-term inhalation study, one might not wish to choose a rat strain with a high incidence of spontaneous mammary tumors that would mechanically interfere with animal placement in the nose-only apparatus. In virtually all rodent stocks and strains, examples can be found of target organ compromise by a genetic predisposition to a high spontaneous background of lesions. There is no ideal rodent model for all types of toxicity studies, and one must critically evaluate model selection for each experiment. This is an area where active discussion between the study director, laboratory animal science professionals, and the toxicologic pathologist is warranted before decisions are made on specific models.

5.4. Issues to Consider When Sourcing Animals

In addition to considerations of stock and strain, it is critically important to consider the source colony of the animal model selected for toxicity studies and not just take into account the vendor from which a model is procured. Animals derived from different source colonies can have significant differences in response to xenobiotics for a variety of reasons related to differences in housing and husbandry, diet, microbiome factors, pathogens, and other nongenetic reasons (Colman, 2017; Naaijkens et al., 2014). Animals derived from differing source colonies can have varying spontaneous as well as induced lesion incidence. It is important for toxicology professionals to monitor the health and conditions of source colonies and to consider what happens to animals prior to their arrival in test facilities. The importance of procurement issues such as transport stress, quarantine procedures, and animal training and acclimation methods should not be underestimated. Animal stress is associated with both biochemical changes as well as morphological alterations in a number of organ systems, most notably the immune and endocrine systems (Everds et al., 2013).

The size of source colonies and husbandry methods used by animal vendors can have practical implications for toxicity studies. For instance, there can be issues associated with litter effects in long-term rodent bioassays used for carcinogenicity assessment. It takes many age, weight, and sex-matched animals to set up a carcinogenicity study and some vendors include entire litters in the shipment. There have been instances of hereditary cancer predispositions within source colonies leading to multiple rare tumors arising in chronic bioassays (Lanzoni et al., 2007).

Toxicologic pathologists that perform nonhuman primate pathology evaluation must pay particular attention to the source of their animals. In these species, there is far less genetic and microbial standardization within colonies and there have been many noted differences in study endpoints depending on the source of animals. For many years, the pharmaceutical industry has utilized cynomolgus monkeys from the Indian Ocean island of Mauritius due to the fact that these animals are free of a number of adventitious viral agents such as *Herpes simiae*. This relatively healthy stock of outbred animals is only 400-500 years old and is derived from original animals of Southeast Asian origin deposited on the island by Dutch traders. Because the cynomolgus monkey is not native to Mauritius and all animals from this source are derived from an original group, these animals demonstrate genetic homogeneity compared to cynomolgus monkeys of other origins (e.g., China, Indonesia, Philippines) due to a narrow genetic base. There are known immunologic variations and other differences in responses noted that can be important in certain types of studies depending on source of macaque (Colman, 2017; Vidal et al., 2010) (see also *Animal Models in Toxicologic Research: Nonhuman Primate*, Vol 1, Chap 21).

5.5. Use of Specialized Animal Models in Toxicology Research

Conventional toxicity animal models include outbred or inbred strains of rats and mice, purpose-bred beagle dogs, and nonhuman primates (e.g., cynomolgus most commonly). Minipigs have been used for dermal toxicity testing due to close alignment of porcine and human skin attributes (see *Animal Models in Toxicologic Research: Pig*, Vol 1, Chap 20). More recently, minipigs have been utilized for systemic toxicity evaluation, but extensive use can be deterred by the size these animals reach in chronic toxicity studies and the large amounts of test article needed, and by limitations of investigative reagents, such as might be applied for protein (e.g., immunohistochemistry) or genomic (e.g., transcriptomic) evaluations applied in mechanistic understanding of toxicity or in determination of species relevance to human.

It is very common for pharmaceutical discovery teams to identify a therapeutic target receptor or pathway that has broader cellular expression outside of the disease target tissue. The pursuit of novel approaches to address unmet medical needs is driving these new avenues of scientific investigation. Some receptors or mediators are nearly ubiquitous, and thus finding or suspecting high expression in other tissues or the development of off-target effects is common at early stages of drug discovery particularly where the target is unprecedented. Thus, there is an opportunity to increase understanding of potential target safety concerns by adding pathology endpoints to efficacy studies of modest duration (i.e., sufficient time to allow for steady-state evaluation), and this approach also optimizes animal use. Expanding the dose range to include higher multiples of efficacious concentration, efficacious dose, or inhibitory concentration for 50% response (EC50, ED50, or IC 50, respectively) can offer the opportunity to promote an "informed progression" where a target safety concern should be understood before classic toxicity models are used. Investigators should apply this with caution, however, since severe disease phenotype models or variant mouse strains may not have sufficient translation to humans for immunologic changes and the interpretation of toxicologic findings in the presence of overlapping disease processes can be challenging; thus, risk assessment to humans at this very preliminary stage should be conducted with prudence. Instead, informed progression with early hazard confirmation should trigger earlier investment in classic toxicity model hazard characterization where risk assessment to humans has a broader base of certainty.

There are times when specialized animal models such as disease models are used in toxicology and safety assessment laboratories. There has been an increasing reliance on the use of genetically modified rodent models, particularly mice, in toxicology as in other areas of biological science. These rodent models are getting increasingly sophisticated with exquisite genetic engineering to allow temporal and spatial control of gene expression. It is possible to insert or delete a wide variety of rodent and human genes and to customize disease models to study particular pathways and targets (see *Genetically Engineered Animal Models in Toxicologic Research*, Vol 1, Chap 23). The use of modern gene editing technology will allow the development of translational nonrodent disease models in the near future and the toxicologic pathologist will be increasingly involved with experimental discovery pathology.

Recent advances in stem cell technology have led to creation and use of humanized rodent models in toxicology research. These models are being increasingly used in the development and testing of a wide number of human therapeutics including gene therapy treatments, infectious disease drugs, and immune-oncology products. The use of these valuable models has created special challenges for the toxicologic pathologist. Lesion development in many of these immuno-deficient stem cell and immune reconstituted strains differs from those commonly used in standard toxicity bioassays. There is often a very limited published database of lesions and conditions in these animals and there are many unique immunopathologic changes that arise. Sorting biologically relevant from nonessential changes can be exceptionally challenging especially since these models often have organisms that normally do not have a clinical impact in wild-type animals but can cause pathologic changes due to the abnormal immunologic status in the genetically altered model.

6. ANIMAL HEALTH CONSIDERATIONS

6.1. Adventitious Agents

The veterinary pathologist is often the toxicology study professional who is responsible for assessing the role and impact that pathogens have on the experimental results. Thus, the pathologist must be familiar with rodent pathogens and with the microbial factors that modify toxicity. Modern toxicology research and testing facilities are relatively free of the adventitious pathogens that caused clinical disease in rodents and plagued bioassays in decades past (Baker, 1998; Everitt and Richter, 1990). This situation has come about because commercial rodent suppliers have instituted serologic screening of animals for antibodies to specific pathogens and employed subsequent elimination or cesarean rederivation of antibody positive colonies. There has been increasing awareness of the varied effects of natural pathogens in laboratory animals with ever-greater efforts to exclude these microbial agents from research subjects. Despite these efforts, microbial factors remain an important variable in toxicology research studies, and pathologists and laboratory animal science professionals must maintain a constant vigil against their untoward effects on experiments. Facilities using genetically modified mice are at particular risk for outbreaks of rodent pathogens due to the fact that many of these strains have immune dyscrasias.

Microbial infection indicates the presence of organisms that may be considered pathogenic, opportunistic, or commensal, of which the last two are most numerous. Few agents found in laboratory animal models today cause overt clinical disease; however, rodents that appear normal and healthy clinically may be unsuitable as research subjects due to the unobservable but significant effects of a microbial infection. Over the past several decades, there has been a significant shift in the spectrum of murine pathogens, and there is a constant need to refine diagnostic testing methods, microbial containment, and disease prevention strategies. In addition to shifts in the spectrum of pathogens found in the toxicology laboratory, there have been significant changes over the years in rodent husbandry and caging methods that influence the spread of rodent infections (Miller et al., 2016). Many modern facilities now have very high animal stocking densities, and facilities that produce genetically altered mice can have multiple breeding colonies present in close proximity, factors that predispose to spread of microbial diseases.

Microbial infections of laboratory rodents exert effects through a complex interplay of host and environmental factors. This is well illustrated by chronic respiratory disease of rats caused by *Mycoplasma pulmonis*. This mycoplasmal infection serves as an exemplar of how a pathogen can affect experimental results and at the same time be influenced by chemical toxicity factors and animal husbandry issues. *M. pulmonis* infection in the laboratory rat may cause overt clinical respiratory disease depending on a variety of host factors such as genotype and age. It can be exacerbated by high ammonia levels and thus influenced by husbandry conditions such as the type of bedding and caging and the schedule of cage changes. Similarly, there is a reported exacerbation of pulmonary lesions caused by the synergism of inhaled chemical compounds such as hexamethylphosphoramide with this respiratory pathogen (Overcash et al., 1976).

6.2. Sentinel Monitoring Programs

Many modern toxicology laboratories employ an ongoing microbial monitoring program during the course of subchronic and chronic studies. Animal health status can change dramatically during the course of a study. Microbial infections can enter otherwise healthy colonies via newly supplied animals, feral rodents, insect pests, contaminated food, water, or bedding, contact with technical staff carrying organisms, entry of biological materials into the colony, or stress-induced spread of low-level, undetected infections that entered with the supplied animals. Specifically, designated sentinel animals are often kept with study animals to facilitate the monitoring of the microbial status of rodent experiments. Important components of the sentinel monitoring program include a determination of the optimal number, age, strain, immune competence level, and exposure means of the sentinel animals (Mailhiot et al., 2020). These sentinel animals are most commonly exposed to experimental animals through cohousing or exposure to contaminated bedding. There is no single optimal design of a sentinel program. The design depends on study type, rodent model, microbial history, equipment, staffing, and physical layout of the laboratory.

Most rodent sentinel monitoring programs use serological assessment for common murine viral and mycoplasmal agents. Utilization of molecular diagnostic techniques such as polymerase chain reaction (PCR) for examination of feces for viral and bacterial pathogens (e.g., *Helicobacter* species) provides the laboratory animal professional with extremely sensitive and specific tools to monitor animal health.

Less frequently employed, but an important component of some animal health monitoring programs, is the use of histopathology in the screening of target tissues prior to and during the toxicity experiment. Gross and microscopic evaluation of selected colony and sentinel animals provides study personnel with the ability to detect important infectious states for which the etiology is unknown or for which there are no serologic or molecular diagnostic assays. In addition to the detection of unknown infectious agents, target organ pathology screening allows the investigator to evaluate common

environment-induced lesions. Certain target tissues in toxicity studies can be severely affected by environment-related background lesions. The rat upper airway, a common target of xenobiotic-induced toxicity, provides one such example. Poor air quality due to ammonia and cage contaminant buildup associated with insufficient cage changes can induce nasal epithelial alterations and obscure test article–induced change (Bolon et al., 1991).

6.3. Microbial Effects on Toxicity

It should be noted that a comparison of test article–treated animals with vehicle treated may not be sufficient to separate compound-induced findings from spontaneous and microbial-induced effects. It may be necessary to determine if study animals have target organs that are within normal limits and free of spontaneous conditions, so that study endpoints of interest can be evaluated. This may be performed on source animal sentinels prior to study start. The pathologist must always be cognizant of the fact that subclinical infection in dosed animals may be activated and manifested differently than in controls. Many pathogens are exacerbated by stress and these stress-associated effects can be compound induced and in a dose-dependent manner.

There are numerous ways in which pathogens can exert their effects as unwanted variables in toxicity studies. These effects can be exerted systemically on the whole animal (Table 29.2) or can be exerted through specific local changes

TABLE 29.2   Selected Systemic Effects of Microbial Agents on Toxicity Studies

Alterations in longevity

Changes in food or water consumption

Alterations in fertility and fecundity

Metabolic changes

Immunomodulation

Changes in body weight

Table reproduced from Haschek WM, Rousseaux CG, Wallig MA, editors: Handbook of toxicologic pathology, ed 2, 2002, Academic Press, Table III, p. 259, with permission.

TABLE 29.3 Microbial Alteration of the Respiratory Tract That May Influence Toxicologic Responses

Alterations in airway epithelial cells:

    Hypertrophy and hyperplasia

    Necrosis

    Syncytial cell formation

    Squamous metaplasia

    Mucous cell hyperplasia

Hyperplasia of type II cells

Altered tumor response following carcinogen

Decreased mucociliary function

Altered surfactant

Changes in airway cytokines

Alterations in pulmonary lymphocytes

Table reproduced from Haschek WM, Rousseaux CG, Wallig MA, editors: Handbook of toxicologic pathology, *ed 2, 2002, Academic Press, Table IV, p. 260, with permission.*

in the relevant target organs of toxicity (Table 29.3). Of great importance for the pathologist is the fact that subclinical infections with certain pathogens, particularly those not found on the commonly utilized serologic screening profiles, are often first detected by noting lesions in target tissues (Roediger et al., 2018). Chronic liver inflammation caused by *Helicobacter hepaticus* infection in mice has served as an excellent example of why the toxicologic pathologist is integral to evaluating colony health and providing needed input for the interpretation of study results. Depending on genotype, sex, and other host factors such as immunocompetency, this infection can influence toxic and carcinogenic responses and can modify important metabolic processes.

In some instances, experimental procedures can interact with pathogens to induce adverse outcomes. For example, Syrian golden hamsters used in chronic inhalation bioassays have developed severe enteritis and mortality secondary to growth of latent clostridial infections triggered by the stress of immobilization in nose-only restraint tubes of the inhalation exposure apparatus. Stress responses in rodents to experimental manipulations and chemical treatment must always be considered a possible trigger for the induction of pathogenicity and lesion development by opportunistic organisms. Immune modulation by chemical exposure must be considered a potential confounder in animals bearing potentially pathogenic organisms that do not induce lesions or systemic effects in the immunocompetent host. Microbial-induced lesions in the treated groups may not develop in control animals, potentially confusing the interpretation by the pathologist. In a similar manner, some test article–treated animals can have microbiome changes resultant from gut antimicrobial effects leading to secondary pathologic effects.

7. MICROBIOME AND MICROBIAL EFFECTS ON PATHOPHYSIOLOGY AND STUDY OUTCOMES

7.1. Introduction to the Microbiome

Changes in the microbial population of an animal can impact multiple aspects of their host, including maturation and responsiveness of the immune system, disease phenotype, and changes secondary to test article treatment in a variety of different animal models and in man where maintenance of a balanced, diverse microbiota has a role in many areas of human health. The diversity of the microbiome can affect immune repertoire/responses, clinical translatability of immunotoxic responses, tumor initiation, progression, and response to therapeutics. There is a growing recognition of the importance of the microbiome influencing experimental outcomes in both safety and efficacy animal studies and of the mechanisms associated with these effects, which can vary from stimulation of microorganism-associated molecular patterns, regulation of local and systemic immune responses, to alteration of therapeutics, lipids, and intermediates in energy metabolism. Despite this, the microbiome is generally not characterized or monitored in toxicity studies. This lack of characterization may confound reproducibility and translatability of animal studies, impact human risk assessment, and increase attrition in biopharmaceutical development. Given the influence on immune responses and disease states, manipulating the gut microbiome also shows therapeutic promise. Therapeutic strategies for the management or prevention of chronic inflammatory conditions and their potential side effects have been recently reviewed (Durack and Lynch, 2019; Nuzzo and Brown, 2020) and are out of scope for this chapter.

7.2. Definitions, Natural History, and Characterization

From birth, animals are colonized with diverse microorganisms. The human gastrointestinal system is inhabited by approx. 3×10^{13} microbes, representing over one million genes, which constantly interact with the body's defense system, the relationship helping to mold the immunological state.

In the environmental niches on all epithelial barriers (e.g., the gut, skin, lung, and vagina), the term microbiota denotes the community of microorganisms (e.g., bacteria, viruses, fungi, protozoa, helminths), while microbiome refers to the large number of functional genes derived from those microorganisms with this information gained via metagenomics. The metagenome is the functional genetic capacity of the microbiome, which may be a more informative characterization but is more expensive to undertake. Most of this knowledge has been obtained from studies looking at the gut microbiome, which is particularly relevant to the oral route of administration used for many therapeutics, but also potentially impacts biotransformation following biliary excretion of systemically administered drugs (Silbergeld, 2017; Zimmermann et al., 2019b).

Animals derive their microbiome essentially from their mother and/or the local environment. Microbiota from animals born by cesarean section and cross-fostered reflect that of the foster mother rather than their donor strain (Hansen et al., 2014). In addition to differences in strain of mouse (e.g., genetic factors), the environment (e.g., breeding house, vendor) can also influence variation in gut microbiota (Hufeldt et al., 2010). Specifically, interactions between caging and bedding have a strong influence on cecal microbiome composition but not on fecal microbiome, which has implications for monitoring. Data from CD-1 mice suggested that ventilated housing (i.e., compared to static, nonventilated isolators) may be more optimal for studies that require gut microbiome consistency (Ericsson et al., 2018). Variations in composition of bedding, including volatiles, lipopolysaccharide, and coliform counts, may be significant factors. Diet and transportation/stress also influence gut microbiome composition (Ericsson et al., 2018). Therefore, variation in vendor/animal facility, acclimation time, and conditions in the unit once animals have been delivered can have a significant impact on microbiome composition, metabolic function, and potentially on experimental reproducibility.

Most commonly, the bacterial microbiota composition and diversity can be measured using PCR/next-generation sequencing–based approaches (e.g., 16s ribosomal RNA) with bioinformatic-driven taxonomic identification of numbers and relative proportions of different operational taxonomic units (with a 97% similarity threshold). Unidentified taxa can be counted but not characterized and the composition represented graphically, often in a bar plot, or phylogenetic tree, with principal component analysis conducted to examine differences in these diverse populations. Accounting for actual numbers rather than proportions is considered to be more accurate (Viney, 2019). More informative characterization is experimentally complex and costly but can be achieved by measuring the following: (a) functional capacity of the microbiome by metagenomics (DNA); (b) functional gene expression by metatranscriptomics (RNA), protein expression (proteomics); and (c) metabolic productivity (metabolomics). This provides greater mechanistic insight into functional differences in microbiota populations (e.g., differences in drug metabolic capacity and biochemical consequences). These more complex methods, while more detailed, computationally intensive, or semiquantitative, still have their drawbacks including the unknown composition of host genes, origins of proteins or metabolites, and variable RNA preservation (Durack and Lynch, 2019).

7.3. Association With Development, Immune Status, and Disease Phenotype—Cause or Effect?

The impact of specific pathogens on animals used in research is well documented (Nicklas, 1999) and "intestinal dysbiosis" is well recognized as a predisposing factor for various diseases in animals and man. Transfer of the wild gut microbiome to laboratory mice induces long-lasting immune modulatory effects over several generations, which improves disease outcome against viral infection and mutagen- and inflammation-induced carcinogenesis (Rosshart et al., 2019). Alterations in the microbiome have been reported in association with multiple disease states, but whether such changes are causal, consequential, or a bystander effect are often unclear. Care must be taken when interpreting experimental data. A large "n" number of mice in a study evaluating the effects of different microbiota may actually represent a very small number of biological replicates, particularly where microbiomes from healthy and diseased individuals are pooled samples before inoculation to different experimental groups (Walter et al., 2020). This underpowers the study, may be associated with inappropriate statistical analysis, and is more likely to lead to false-positive results. Bearing in mind this cautionary note, there is abundant experimental data supporting biological interaction between microbiome, normal development, and pathological phenotypes suggesting that differences in the microbiome could influence immune and/or inflammatory responses in animals, including models used in biomedical research.

Establishment of the gut microbiota early in life appears to affect the proportions of T-cell subtypes in the lymphoid system of adult mice (Hansen et al., 2014) and different bacterial genera/species have been classified as proinflammatory (e.g., *Prevotella copri*, *Proteus mirabilis*, *Bacteroides fragilis*, *Bacteroides vulgatus*, *Alistipes* spp.) and antiinflammatory (e.g., *Akkermansia muciniphila*, *Bifidobacterium* spp, *Faecalibacterium prausnitzii*), exerting systemic effects by the secretion of antiinflammatory cytokines/chemokines, metabolites, antimicrobials, and neuropeptides (Zitvogel et al., 2018). Microbiota have also been shown to impact development of tissues outside of the immune system, for example, influencing the structural development of the brain (as assessed via magnetic resonance imaging) and behavioral responses in mice (Lu et al., 2018).

The mechanisms related to altered immune or inflammatory states are not always clear and may be multiple (Durack and Lynch, 2019). They range from competing out pathogen colonization to alterations in intestinal permeability, activation of microorganism/pathogen-associated molecular patterns (e.g., various toll-like receptors [TLRs]), lipids (e.g., short-chain fatty acids which are antiinflammatory, antiproliferative), carbohydrates, amino acids, vitamins, hormones, neuroactive molecules, and xenobiotic metabolites. These may influence local or distant organs either directly or via cytokine expression and balance of Th1, Th2, Th17 immune responses, and regulatory T-cells (Durack and Lynch, 2019).

There is evidence in animals and man to suggest that differences in the gut microbiome are associated with modulation of inflammatory phenotypes both in the gastrointestinal tract and at distant sites. Colonization of the gut with segmented filamentous bacteria (SFB; *Candidatus savagella* in mammals) induces Th17 cells to accumulate in the lamina propria of the gut, increases gene expression patterns associated with inflammation and microbial defense, and confers resistance to the pathogen *Citrobacter rodentium* (Ivanov et al., 2009). Modulation of the gut microbiota has been shown to alter susceptibility to different rodent models of colitis (Scher et al., 2013; Escalante et al., 2016). In the mouse, application of the hapten oxazolone to the surface of the pinna induces a chronic Th2 hypersensitivity reaction characterized by pinnal thickening, edema, hemorrhage, excoriation, and chronic inflammation. The gut microbiome has shown to strongly correlate with pinnal tissue levels of interferon gamma, tumor necrosis factor alpha (TNF-α), and interleukin 10. It is also possible to transfer different levels of sensitivity/inflammatory response to mice via the gut microbiome, an effect which seems to have translational parallels in patients with atopic dermatitis compared to healthy controls (Zachariassen et al., 2017).

Neuroscience models may also be influenced by the microbiota. In a mutated superoxide dismutase-1, transgenic mouse model of amyotrophic lateral sclerosis (ALS), alterations in gut microbiota (11 different commensals), and differences in metabolites (e.g., nicotinamide) were measured presymptomatically in mice and were associated with subsequent differences in the severity of the neurodegenerative phenotype associated with these models. Preliminary evidence suggests that this correlation also translated to ALS patients (Blacher et al., 2019). A similar phenomenon occurs in the PINK1 (PTEN-induced kinase 1) mutant mouse model of Parkinson's Disease, where intestinal gram-negative bacterial infection triggered autoimmune mechanisms generating CD8+ T-cells targeting mitochondria in the brain and periphery, emphasizing the importance of the gut–brain axis (Matheoud et al., 2019).

Evading host immune responses is a recognized means by which tumor survival and progression is mediated and microbial effects on immune responsiveness have also been shown to influence this area of disease biology. Similar microbial alterations are seen in the tumor microenvironment of human pancreatic ductal adenocarcinoma patients and spontaneous mouse models of this disease (e.g., KC (KrasLSL.G12D/+; PdxCretg/+) and KCP (KrasLSL.G12D/+; p53R172H/+; PdxCretg/+) mice) which promote tumor progression. Various experiments including antibiotic treatment, microbial and T-cell transfers, analysis of tumor growth, molecular histopathologic investigations of the tumor microenvironment, and flow cytometry suggest that the altered microbiome promotes the suppression of tumor-associated macrophages (toward an M2 phenotype) and infiltrating T-cell responses via signaling through selected TLR pathways, notably TLR2 and TLR5 (Pushalkar et al., 2018).

7.4. Impact on Efficacy, Biotransformation, and Toxicology

Given the evidence summarized above on how the microbiome can affect development, pathophysiology, and disease model phenotypes, microbiome variation based on animal supplier or laboratory can clearly affect experimental readouts and reproducibility in efficacy studies across multiple indications and therapeutic areas. Response to therapeutics in such studies has been shown to depend on the gut microbiota in animals and in man (e.g., in the oncology therapeutic area). Therapeutic responses can be affected via multiple mechanisms, including altered epithelial barrier function and integrity in the gut, modulation of immune responses and biotransformation of xenobiotics, and/or other metabolic substrates (Zitvogel et al., 2018). The impact of the microbiome on

biotransformation also affects toxicologic exposures and responses (Silbergeld, 2017).

Animals treated with antibiotics, germ-free animals, or those lacking microbial species known to be immune potentiators have shown reduced responsiveness in tumor models. Positive responses to antiprogrammed cell death protein 1 (PD1) therapy in cancer patients are associated with more diverse gut microbiota compared with nonresponders. Improved efficacy of anti-PD1 treatment in the clinic translated to mice when they were transplanted with fecal microbiota from responder patients and in mice supplemented with bacterial taxa including *Akkermansia, Faecalibacterium,* and *Bifidobacterium* species, which activate type-1 interferon genes in antigen-presenting cells. These bacterial taxa are known to be depleted in nonresponders (Durack and Lynch, 2019; Zitvogel et al., 2018). Efficacy of alkylating agents (e.g., cyclophosphamide) can also be decreased in germ-free mice (or those treated with antibiotics). These animals do not have mucosa-penetrating gut microbiota which are important in antitumor immunity, because they stimulate Th17 anticommensal responses, and increase Th1 cell recruitment in tumor beds (Viaud et al., 2015).

Altered efficacy may be mediated via biotransformation. Gemcitabine can be metabolized to its inactive form by intratumor gammaproteobacteria expressing an isoform of the enzyme cytidine deaminase, resulting in tumor resistance in a mouse model of colon cancer (Geller et al., 2017). Enzymes in the microbiome can also generate toxic metabolites. Specific inhibition of bacterial beta-glucuronidases in the intestinal tract protected mice treated with the anticancer drug CPT-11 (irinotecan) from colonic epithelial damage, mucosal inflammation, and bloody diarrhea (Wallace et al., 2010). Antibiotic treatment also reduced this toxicity by altering the microbiome species expressing this enzyme activity (Xu and Villalona-Calero, 2002). Understanding such mechanisms may allow the therapeutic window of certain drugs to be increased.

Alteration of the microbiome is also associated with chemical toxicity. For example, arsenic metabolism is reduced and liver toxicity increased in mice treated with antibiotics (Chi et al., 2019). Differences in microbiome can alter drug metabolism and pharmacokinetics, e.g., of brivudine and clonazepam in mice, increasing exposure to active metabolites which may be toxic (Zimmermann et al., 2019a). Alterations in the gut microbiome in aquatic species by environmental toxicants (e.g., nanomaterials and hydrocarbons) have been implicated in adverse outcome pathways culminating in decreased growth, survival, and susceptibility to bacterial infection in different fish species (Adamovsky et al., 2018). Interaction between microbiome and effects of chemical and environmental toxicants in humans are also well recognized, both from the perspective of microbial transformation of chemicals and microbial alteration as a consequence of chemical toxicity, and have been recently reviewed (Koontz et al., 2019; Tu et al., 2020).

7.5. Impact of Microbiome on Safety Translatability

Laboratory animals do not replicate the repertoire of commensal and pathogenic microbes and therefore may poorly model the diversity of gut microbiota seen in wild animals (Viney, 2019) and in man. This may also have an impact on the translational relevance of their immune repertoire and responses, specifically in preclinical safety hazard identification and risk assessment. To investigate the effects of microbiome diversity Rosshart and coworkers (Rosshart et al., 2019) created a colony of "wildling" mice while maintaining a controlled genotype by transferring C57BL/6 embryos into wild mice. The wildling microbiota and splenic/peripheral immunophenotype were much more diverse than specific pathogen-free counterparts. These wildling mice also showed greater translational relevance in their responses to superagonist (e.g., CD28 superagonist, TGN1412) and anti-TNF alpha treatment. The life-threatening T-cell activation and cytokine storm which occurred in a Phase 1 clinical trial of TGN1412 had not been predicted in standard laboratory rodents. In contrast, wildling mice showed an inflammatory cytokine response and a lack of regulatory T-cell expansion similar to the clinical effects. For anti-TNF alpha treatment, which was efficacious in laboratory animal models, but which failed for lack of efficacy in the clinic,

wilding mice recapitulated the clinical response and did not show rescue of lethal endotoxemia. (Rosshart et al., 2019). These results suggest that some animal models, for example, within immunology, would be improved if the immune system had been challenged with a more diverse microbiota, even if this included some pathogens.

7.6. Minimizing Experimental Variability and Monitoring Microbiome Status

Since microbiome variability is associated with significant alterations in normal physiology and pathologic/disease states and can impact therapeutic efficacy and evaluation of safety liabilities, such effects need to be minimized in experimental design and better understood by defining the microbiome composition and, perhaps more importantly, its function. Some vendors are offering to standardize the microbiome by oral gavage with custom microbiota to improve consistency. Given the complexity and cost associated with any "snapshot" characterization of the microbiome, it is challenging to decide how to monitor its status (Hansen et al., 2019). Modern molecular techniques have revealed that there may, depending on the research type, be equally good reasons for monitoring the colony status of some commensal bacteria that are essential for the induction of specific rodent models, such as *Alistipes* spp., *A. muciniphila*, *Bifidobacterium* spp., *B. fragilis*, *B. vulgatus*, *F. prausnitzii*, *P. copri*, and SFB (Hansen et al., 2019). In the future, research groups may need to consider the presence or absence of a short list of defined bacterial species relevant for their models. This list can be tested by cost-effective sequencing or even a simple multiple PCR approach, which is likely to be cost neutral compared to more traditional screening methods.

In summary, the microbiome is an integral component of animal biology with pleiotropic effects on health and disease susceptibility. These effects range from organ development to immune system maturation/responses, modification of disease phenotypes and therapeutic responses (efficacy and safety) influencing animal model reproducibility and translatability.

It is often not clear whether associated changes in microbiota were cause or effect, though more recent research is beginning to address this issue. Intentionally increasing the diversity of the microbiome seems to improve the translational relevance of rodent models with respect to their immunophenotype and ability to predict aberrant superantigen cytokine release responses. However, housing such animals and maintaining intact microbiological barriers in units where other animals of lower diversity, or specific pathogen-free status animals are kept, presents logistical challenges. Awareness of the effects of caging, bedding, and diet on the microbiome as well as maternal/litter effects on establishing microbial composition, plus the impact of transport and acclimation in new housing/or facilities, is important. Monitoring of the microbiota is being practiced and discussed more frequently. As more data are generated and analyzed, this will improve our understanding of the impact of microbial variation, and how to optimally monitor and control for these in our animal model efficacy and safety studies.

8. HOUSING AND HUSBANDRY ISSUES

8.1. Role of Environment in Lesion Production

Environmental factors in the animal room environment that affect studies have been well studied and extensively documented (Clough, 1982; Conour et al., 2006). They include temperature, humidity, light, photoperiod, noise, housing methods, bedding, sanitation chemicals, airflow, diet, water, cage change methods, and handling. Although control of the environment is primarily the concern of the study director, environment-associated lesions are an extremely important aspect of toxicologic pathology.

A number of laboratory rodent pathology findings that are associated in large part with environmental influence are listed in Table 29.4. Many rodent background lesions that manifest secondary to these conditions are strongly influenced by the interplay of environmental and genetic factors. For example, the development of dystrophic cardiac calcinosis, a common cardiac lesion with a known genetic basis in

TABLE 29.4   Selected Lesions in Laboratory Rodents Associated With Environmental Conditions

Lesion	Environmental condition
Phototoxic retinopathy	Light levels, photoperiodicity
Nephrocalcinosis	Diet
Cardiac calcinosis	Semipurified diet
Myocardial inflammation	Rancid dietary fat
Olfactory epithelial change	Bedding contaminants
Dental dysplasia	Powdered diet
Chronic progressive nephropathy	Dietary protein and caloric levels
Airway epithelial necrosis	High ammonia levels
Hepatic lipidosis	Semipurified diet
Obstructive genitourinary disease	Wire caging
Pododermatitis	Wire caging
Peripheral neuropathy	Wire caging
Ringtail	Temperature and humidity
Seizure-induced brain changes	Noise

Table reproduced from Haschek WM, Rousseaux CG, Wallig MA, editors: Handbook of toxicologic pathology, *ed 2, 2002, Academic Press, Table V, p. 260, with permission.*

certain mouse strains, is influenced by the type of diet. In addition to the marked interplay between environmental, microbial, and genetic factors, there can be significant interrelationships among various environmental conditions. For example, phototoxic retinal degeneration associated with high light levels and alterations in photoperiod can be exacerbated by exposure to test articles (De Vera Mudry et al., 2013; Yamashita et al., 2016).

The pathologist must carefully consider environmental conditions when comparing results from different rodent bioassays. For example, the type of housing conditions (e.g., group vs. single) and type of caging (e.g., direct contact bedding in polycarbonate shoebox style cages vs. suspended wire over indirect bedding) can dramatically influence weight gain and tumor incidence in rodents. Therefore, control of the environment and, more importantly, the documentation of environmental conditions are critical to the evaluation of rodent studies and to the establishment of rodent lesion databases. There has been much discussion about cold stress in rodents, the housing of rodents in ambient temperatures lower than their thermoneutral zone of 26–34°C for mice and 26–30°C for rats (Hankenson et al., 2018). The ambient temperature of the macroenvironment of the rodent housing room is typically held at 20–26°C as recommended by the *Guide for the Care and Use of Laboratory Animals* (Guide) (Council, 2011). Due to their small size and large body surface area, mice are particularly prone to the adverse effects of lower room temperatures. It has been shown that tumor cells grow faster in mice that have adapted to colder temperatures as compared to mice housed in temperatures of 30°C (Hylander et al., 2019).

In the design of toxicity studies, the study team must consider the use of procedures to minimize sources of environmental variation. These procedures might include cage or rack rotation at various intervals throughout the study and variation in the order of certain husbandry and manipulative procedures. To enhance animal welfare, group housing is the expectation for social animals such as rats and mice. Aggression in group-housed male mice is not uncommon and the pathologist must be made aware of situations of bite wound lesions and other injuries, and even death, that may be the result of housing socially incompatible male mice (Weber et al., 2017).

Stress responses in animals can occur as the result of many different factors on study that have already been mentioned including husbandry, handling, study procedures, room and microenvironment, social interactions with conspecifics, and/or combinations of various animal and environmental conditions. Stress is known to perturb many physiological attributes of the study animal and can result in a variety of anatomic and clinical pathology changes important to the toxicologic pathologist. These have been very nicely reviewed by Everds and colleagues (Everds et al., 2013). The most

common organ systems that manifest stress-related changes are the immune and endocrine systems.

In recent years, the laboratory animal science community has advocated a position that rodents should be housed in a manner that permits species-specific behaviors that contribute to their overall well-being. Most laboratory animal scientists believe that this is best accomplished using direct contact bedding in solid floored caging under group-housed conditions. Use of direct contact bedding can have effects in both rodent and nonrodent studies causing particulate-associated changes in the pulmonary tract. In rodents, nasal fungal lesions have been associated with contaminated bedding and certainly there have been a number of studies impacted by use of bedding contaminated by environmental chemicals or natural substances such as mycotoxins (Bolon et al., 1991). Some toxicity studies are still conducted with individually housed animals in suspended wire caging to prevent variables that can be introduced by contact with metabolites in urine or feces or from the bedding itself. Recently, the National Toxicology Program (NTP) began allowing the use of nesting material (e.g., crinkled kraft paper) and polycarbonate shelving in their short-term and long-term toxicity studies (Churchill et al., 2016). An NTP study with the enrichment devices showed that they did not impact commonly evaluated parameters in rodents (e.g., body weight gain, food and water consumption, corticosterone concentrations, organ weights) or study outcomes. The impact on the NTP historical lesion database is not yet known.

Changes in animal husbandry variables such as housing affect lesion databases used by pathologists. There is ample evidence in rodents from the experience of the NTP to realize that group versus individual housing markedly influences tumor outcome data for certain sites where body weight gain is important (Haseman et al., 2003). As has been mentioned previously, historical databases are subject to change and must be considered living documents.

8.2. Study Design Considerations

It is critical that animals be allocated to a study in a manner that minimizes bias for the endpoints of interest (see *Practices to Optimize Generation, Interpretation, and Reporting of Pathology Data from Toxicity Studies,* Vol 1, Chap 28 and *Experimental Design and Statistical Analysis for Toxicologic Pathologists,* Vol 1, Chap 16). In most instances, this is accomplished by using randomization procedures based on body weight criteria. Many rodent suppliers ship animals based on body weight and estimate age from age/body weight growth charts. For certain types of studies (e.g., cell proliferation studies in young animals), age may be an extremely important factor, and relatively rigid criteria for age as well as weight may be required. There are correlations between body weight and certain site-specific tumors. Many long-term rodent toxicity studies result in body weight differences between dosed and control groups. When such differences are large, they could have an impact on the interpretation of study results for those tumor types showing a strong correlation with body weight. For nonrodent species, the toxicologic pathologist should recognize that study randomization by body weight does not necessarily homogenize animals for other factors such as sexual maturity. If these endpoints are critical to study outcomes, randomization by body weight may introduce bias.

Acclimation of animals to environment, personnel, and equipment is an often-overlooked aspect of study design. Animals should be properly acclimated to all equipment used in a study. Rats that were not acclimated to metabolism caging prior to test article exposure were noted to have a 60-fold difference in LD_{50} to a nephrotoxic uranium compound due to differences in water intake caused by the housing change (Damon et al., 1986). In some instances, such as with nose-only inhalation exposure equipment, animal handling can have a dramatic influence on body weight gain.

At the outset of any toxicology experiment, the study director and pathologist should evaluate experimental procedures and consider whether any of the animal manipulations are likely to result in clinical or pathological effects. Numerous examples can be found in which study procedures influenced lesion development. For example, repeated prolonged immobilization of male rats in nose-only inhalation tubes is associated with testicular lesions, presumably from thermoregulatory and positional effects of blood flow on the testes. Extensive handling of mice has been associated with hepatic damage and changes in clinical chemistry parameters from thoracic compression. Similarly, bandage application in subchronic rat dermal toxicity bioassays has been associated with passive congestion of the liver leading to fibrosis. The use of continuous physiologic monitoring of rodents in their home cages using electromagnetic field (EMF) technology has expanded over the last few years. Electronic receivers are placed under the mouse or rat's home cage and parameters such as activity levels, cage environment, and the animal's physiological state can be measured. Recordati et al. recently studied the effect of low-intensity EMF in digitally ventilated cages (Recordati et al., 2019). Female mice exposed to low-intensity EMF had a decrease in neutrophils as compared to females in the control group which was found to be biologically relevant but not clinically relevant. Administration of xenobiotics by oral gavage has been associated with pulmonary deposition and other causes of mortality. Gavage-associated mortality, noted to be more prevalent in female Fischer 344 rats than in other strains, has been reported to be due to irritant exacerbation of strain-related oropharyngeal degeneration. Recently, there have been published reviews of the lesions associated with gavage-related reflux in rats and the toxicological significance (Damsch et al., 2010). The toxicologic pathologist is often called upon to contribute to the discussion to determine when respiratory lesions are related to gavage error versus reflux-induced effects from direct compound-induced toxicity. Formulations that are more viscous or irritating at higher concentration may cause more gavage issues, such as nasopharyngeal reflux, in high-dose animals compared to vehicle-treated controls.

In studies that measure cell proliferation using an exogenous label, the pathologist should be closely involved with planning in-life procedures. The method, dosing regimen, and route of label administration to animals should be carefully considered and can involve challenging decisions. For instance, the condition of the animals at the time of manipulations such as the implantation of osmotic pumps to deliver the label should be considered at the beginning of the study. Anesthetizing an 8-week-old animal at an early interim time point is often a simple procedure, but a very specialized anesthesia regimen may be required to perform the same procedure on an 18-month-old rodent with chronic renal dysfunction at time of terminal sacrifice. During protocol development, one must think through all the stages of the experiment so that the proper treatment regimens can be employed with consistency throughout the entire study. Knowledge of the target organs of toxicity is often important to consider during study design, and thus the pathologist is often critical in decision-making to eliminate sources of bias.

For the pathologist, one of the most important considerations in study design is the determination of how animals are to be removed from the study at times other than scheduled necropsy. Toxicology protocols have traditionally used the term "moribund sacrifice" to designate animals that are removed at unscheduled times. Exactly what constitutes a moribund state may differ among individuals and may not reflect the strict definition of this term (i.e., dying or at the point of death). For many years, the primary objective of the moribund sacrifice was to provide the pathologist with tissues devoid of postmortem autolytic change. More recently, with renewed emphasis on animal welfare concerns, there has been increasing pressure to replace the so-called moribund sacrifice with sacrifice for humane reasons. The primary objective of the change is a conscientious effort to reduce suffering associated with dying. Unfortunately, ascribing specific behavioral and physiological attributes that identify rodents in the process of dying is an exceedingly difficult task. Nonetheless, strict and consistent criteria and written procedures for the removal of animals from study for humane reasons should be in place. The study pathologist is well suited for interacting with the appropriate laboratory animal science personnel and the study director to develop the necessary criteria for determining removal for humane reasons. This criteria should be developed and added to the study protocol before the study begins to ensure that there is no delay in removing animals from study while safeguarding the goals of the study (OECD, 2000). Clinical and anatomic pathology findings in moribund animals in toxicity studies may reflect many secondary effects of morbidity (e.g., dehydration, electrolyte shifts, shock), and these effects may not necessarily reflect toxicity in animals that survived to scheduled termination.

9. THE ROLE OF DIET IN TOXICITY STUDIES

9.1. Introduction

The diet represents the most complex mixture of chemicals to which animals are exposed and has been said to be the most important uncontrolled variable in toxicity studies with rodents (Camacho et al., 2016; Newberne and Sotnikov, 1996). The importance of diet as a variable in rodent bioassays can be recognized by the fact that the Society of Toxicologic Pathology has generated a position paper on this issue (Nold et al., 2001). Nonetheless, rodent diets draw relatively little attention as a research variable compared with microbial agents. The ingredients, essential nutrients, contaminant concentrations, and energy density of the diet influence the physiological processes and health of rodent models and their responses to administered chemicals. Over 40 nutrients are required in the diet of rodents. The diet must be adequate for the animal's sex, physiological condition (e.g., maintenance vs. reproduction and lactation), and age (see *Animal Models in Toxicologic Research: Rodents*, Vol 1, Chap 17 and *Nutrition and Toxicologic Pathology*, Vol 2, Chap 20).

An optimal rodent diet should have adequate concentrations of all the nutrients required for growth and maintenance without excessive fats, proteins, and other high-energy and growth-enhancing nutrients. Overnutrition linked to the common practice of ad libitum feeding of rodent chow has led to increased growth and body weight of many important rodent strains used in toxicology experiments. This excessive caloric intake is associated with a number of important pathophysiologic processes that influence lesion development (Table 29.5).

Food consumption is a commonly monitored clinical parameter in short- and long-term rodent

TABLE 29.5   Health Effects Associated With Ad Libitum Feeding of Rodents

Increased growth rate

Elevated body weight

Pancreatic islet cell hyperplasia and insulin hypersecretion

Accelerated onset time for spontaneous tumors secondary to dysregulated endocrine effects

Nephropathy—increased incidence and severity

Cardiomyopathy—increased incidence and severity

Obesity

Decreased longevity

Table reproduced from Haschek WM, Rousseaux CG, Wallig MA, editors: Handbook of toxicologic pathology, *ed 2, 2002, Academic Press, Table V, p. 260, with permission.*

toxicity and carcinogenicity studies. Decreased food consumption may lead to malnutrition and this in turn may exacerbate, mimic, or mask toxic effects. Many rodent toxicity studies involve animal exposures sufficient to result in systemic toxicity, reduced food consumption, and decreased terminal body weights compared to control animals. This observation may impair the toxicologist's ability to determine whether the observed adverse health effects are due to the test article, changes in food consumption, or an interaction of these two factors. For example, these interactions may influence the interpretation of parameters for assessing neurotoxicity and growth and development. Anorexia and its accompanying weight loss are associated with a wide variety of behavioral changes in rats, including delayed pup development, increased motor activity, decreased hind limb grip strength, increased escape behaviors, and cognitive learning deficits. These results indicate that reduced food or water intake could mimic the behavioral effects of neurotoxic agents. Therefore, toxicologists reviewing study results cannot overlook the impact of reduced food consumption.

An animal's diet may also influence its response to a test article. There are numerous examples of the influence of diet on the development of both neoplastic and nonneoplastic lesions (Duffy et al., 2008). Dietary modulation of lesion development can be through direct effects of dietary constituents or through secondary mechanisms such as alteration of the microbiome as discussed above.

9.2. Types of Diets

Three major types of diets are used in rodent toxicity studies: nonpurified (natural-ingredients) diets, purified diets, and chemically defined diets. These diets can be fed in a variety of physical forms, although pelleted chow is the most commonly utilized. Nonpurified diets constitute the most widely used food in rodent toxicity studies. These diets are generally cereal based, are composed primarily of unrefined plant and animal materials, and often contain added vitamins and minerals. These diets are characterized as "open-formula" or "closed-formula diets." An open-formula diet is a diet in which the precise percentage composition of each ingredient is available to the investigator. A closed-formula diet is one that does not have the composition specified by type and amount of each ingredient by the manufacturer. Open-formula diets have been recommended for use in toxicity studies to reduce the variability in response that can arise because ingredients or their proportions are altered (Barnard et al., 2009).

Purified diets are composed primarily of refined ingredients including refined proteins, carbohydrates, and fat with added mineral and vitamin mixtures. These diets were called "semi-synthetic" or "semipurified" diets in the past. In general, purified diets are expensive, and standardized purified diets useful for long-term rodent studies have not been established. A commonly utilized purified diet has been the AIN-76A formulation by the Council of the American Institute of Nutrition (AIN). This diet has been associated with periportal hepatic lipidosis, hemorrhagic changes, and soft-tissue calcifications in rodents (Mitchell et al., 1989). The National Research Council modified their rodent nutritional recommendations and the AIN developed the AIN-93G and M diets based on those recommendations. Some of the changes to the diet included increasing the calcium to phosphorus molar ratio, adding additional ultratrace minerals, and replacing corn oil with soy oil (Lien et al., 2001). AIN-93G is used in pregnant, lactating, and growing rodents, while AIN-93M is considered a maintenance diet. Purified diets are used selectively in studies in which the role of certain dietary constituents in tissue response is being examined. Chemically defined diets are characterized by inclusion of nitrogen from pure amino acids, carbohydrate from refined monosaccharides or disaccharides, and fat from purified fatty acids or triglycerides. These diets are seldom employed in toxicity studies.

9.3. Contaminant Issues

Contaminants may be present in nonpurified diets composed of natural ingredients. For example, these diets may contain arsenic, lead, and other heavy metals, malathion and other pesticides, unintended antioxidants (e.g., BHA and BHT), phytoestrogens, mycotoxins, and other toxins (see *Heavy Metals*, Vol 2, Chap 27 and *Mycotoxins*, Vol 2, Chap 23). Whenever possible, the concentration of these contaminants should be kept as low as possible to prevent modification of the toxic response of the chemical under investigation. For example, a variety of natural ingredients such as estrogenic isoflavones in soybean meal have been shown to be chemoprotective and may prevent or decrease the development of spontaneous and experimental tumors. Estrogenic isoflavones such as genistein and daidzein may also affect the growth and development of rodents on natural-ingredient diets that use soy as a source of protein (Jensen and Ritskes-Hoitinga, 2007). Standardized rodent diets with minimal estrogenic activity are desirable for some types of bioassays and are now available commercially (Thigpen et al., 2004).

Many toxicology facilities utilize the so-called "certified diets." The toxicologic pathologist should realize that the certification process deals with the issue of contaminant levels and has nothing to do with nutrient content. There are diet-associated lesions that can arise on study using certified diets. Several years ago, for example, multiple animal facilities had simultaneous outbreaks of scurvy in nonhuman primates fed certified chow in which the ascorbic acid was inadvertently left out during processing. After lesions were noted, the diet was found to be lacking in vitamin C content (see *Nutrition and Toxicologic Pathology*, Vol 2, Chap 20).

Lesions can also be associated with diets that deteriorate. Rancid fat in rodent diets that are improperly stored and fed have been associated with myocardial degeneration and inflammation (Everitt et al., 1988).

9.4. Dietary Optimization

A decline in survival of rodents in two-year carcinogenicity bioassays has been noted in many laboratories over the past several decades. This finding closely correlates with increases in food consumption and adult body weight over this same period of time. These changes have been observed in several commonly used toxicology models, including outbred Wistar and Sprague–Dawley rats, inbred Fischer 344 rats, and B6C3F1 hybrid mice. During this period, rodent bioassays have had a steady increase in study-to-study variability, decreases in survival, and increases in the incidence, onset time, and severity of degenerative diseases such as chronic progressive nephropathy and degenerative cardiomyopathy. In addition, spontaneous tumors have increased, primarily those that are endocrine related (Keenan et al., 1996b).

Changes in body weight of these rodent stocks and strains have been influenced in large part by the breeding practices inherent in colony management. Commercial suppliers have understandably selected rodent breeding stock for more rapid growth and greater fecundity. Although genetic factors undoubtedly are at least partially responsible for strain characteristics, these changes appear to be greatly influenced by the environmental conditions under which the animals are maintained. The practice of ad libitum feeding of rodent diets and the associated extremely high caloric intake is believed to be an important factor in the alteration of these animal models (Table 29.5, and see *Nutrition and Toxicologic Pathology*, Vol 2, Chap 20). The decline in longevity and high lesion content of study animals has led some scientists and policy makers to question the utility of the rodent bioassay for studies of safety assessment (Keenan et al., 1996a). There are examples of rodent carcinogenicity studies where high-dose test articles actually decreased the high incidence of some background tumors compared to controls. The sensitivity of the rodent bioassay in distinguishing treatment effects from control requires adequate animal survival. Ironically, survival is often lower in *ad libitum*–fed control groups compared to high-dose groups administered maximum tolerated doses of compounds that induce body weight loss from both toxicologic mechanisms and secondary effects.

Diet restriction is a well-established method of extending the life span of rodents. The restriction of fat, protein, minerals, and other nutritional components without caloric restriction does not increase the overall long-term survival of animals. A number of investigators have demonstrated that moderate diet restriction (i.e., 70%-80% of ad libitum levels) can significantly improve longevity in rodents and will support the maintenance of healthier animals with a lower incidence (or later onset) of certain degenerative and neoplastic diseases (Keenan et al., 1999). Studies have shown that moderate diet restriction does not adversely affect metabolism, clinical chemistry, or toxicokinetic or toxicologic responses to pharmaceutical agents. Despite the benefits of moderate diet restriction, changing current rodent feeding practices has not received a universal endorsement as a standard of rodent husbandry. It is being employed in a number of laboratories for certain types of long-term rodent studies and studies conducted with these feeding practices have been accepted by regulatory agencies.

10. 3R'S AND IN-LIFE STUDY CONDUCT FOR THE TOXICOLOGIC PATHOLOGIST

All study scientists including toxicologic pathologists should be aware of the changes in both animal care and use regulations and societal pressures to incorporate a 3Rs culture in working practices. The 3 Rs refer to replacement, reduction, and refinement of animal use in research. The 3Rs are global principles underpinning animal research, first introduced by Russell and Burch in 1959. Toxicologists have managed to replace a number of in vivo testing approaches with nonanimal in silico and in vitro methods (see *In Silico*, In Vitro, *Ex* Vivo, *and Non-Traditional In* Vivo *Approaches in Toxicologic Research*, Vol 1, Chap 24). While most think of the concept of replacement as the

absolute substitution of animals with nonanimal methods, some think of replacement as the switching out of one model with another that is a lower phylogenetic species (see *Animal Models in Toxicologic Research: Non-mammalian*, Vol 1, Chap 22). The work of the toxicologic pathologist generally involves the use of preclinical animal models. Thus, rather than working with replacement methods, the work of the toxicologic pathologist predominantly fits closest with the goals of reducing animal use and refining how animals are used so that a minimum number of animals are used to obtain the same or more optimized data and scientific understanding. Reduction can occur through improved experimental designs and statistical analyses, sharing data and resources and implementation of techniques to obtain more or better data (Hukkanen et al., 2019). It must be noted though that the best scientific approach to animal research can mean increasing animal numbers in some situations to ultimately achieve reductions in the longer term. In all cases, the toxicologic pathologist should strive to optimize animal usage and to collaborate with statisticians and other specialists to derive the best experimental design (see *Experimental Design and Statistical Analysis for Toxicologic Pathologists*, Vol 1, Chap 16).

The toxicologic pathologist should also consistently strive to optimize experimental design to minimize animal numbers and to refine procedures to reduce pain and distress on animals to the extent possible and that are compatible with scientific objectives. There are a variety of important considerations of protocol development that should be considered by the pathologist including the use of properly sized and constituted control groups, refined methods of dose delivery, multiplexing of endpoints, and use of noninvasive in vivo imaging methods in longitudinal studies to optimize pathology data (see *In Vivo Small Animal Imaging: A Comparison to Gross and Histopathologic Observations in Animal Models*, Vol 1, Chap 13). Pathologists are ideal scientists to bridge animal issues with endpoint considerations and to provide important expertise to toxicology study teams that have a mission of refining their animal studies. A different set of 3R's has been put forward that are focused on translational science and these are the 3Rs of relevance (i.e., translatability of preclinical animal models to the clinic), robustness, and reproducibility (Everitt, 2015).

11. DESCRIPTION OF ANIMAL STUDIES IN SCIENTIFIC PUBLICATIONS

The proper description of the laboratory animal model, the animal care and use environment, and the conditions of use during in vivo studies is critically important to the work of the practicing toxicologic pathologist who may be responsible for scientific reporting and publishing. Several important guidance documents have been published to aid in this effort. Included among these are the ARRIVE guidelines (Animal Research: Reporting *In* Vivo Experiments) from the UK NC3Rs (Percie du Sert et al., 2020a, 2020b). All pathologists, as well as those serving on the editorial boards of veterinary and toxicologic pathology and toxicology journals, should strive for optimal animal reporting so that studies are reproducible and the 3Rs are promoted. Most journals and professional societies have incorporated animal use policy statements on their websites to reiterate their views on ethical animal research. In addition to the promotion of ethical animal use, proper description of animal models and care and use is critical for the comparison of studies and the formation of historical lesion databases.

12. CONCLUSION

Numerous genetic, microbial, environmental, and experimental factors work together to influence development of the lesions studied by the toxicologic pathologist. The pathologist should understand how factors associated with the laboratory animal including the microbiome, animal care and use program, research facility environment, and study conditions contribute to findings so that the results of toxicity experiments can be properly evaluated and interpreted. The toxicologic pathologist should be knowledgeable with the rules and regulations pertaining to animal research, in-life study best practices, and optimal methods for reporting animal-based data in order to contribute to high quality and reproducible nonclinical studies.

REFERENCES

Adamovsky O, Buerger AN, Wormington AM, et al.: The gut microbiome and aquatic toxicology: an emerging concept for environmental health, *Environ Toxicol Chem* 37:2758–2775, 2018.

Adams K, Clemons D, Impelluso LC, et al.: An IQ consortium perspective on the scientific committee on health, environmental and emerging risks final opinion on the need for nonhuman primates in biomedical research, production and testing of products and devices (update 2017), *Toxicol Pathol* 47:649–655, 2019.

Bailey J, Balls M: Recent efforts to elucidate the scientific validity of animal-based drug tests by the pharmaceutical industry, pro-testing lobby groups, and animal welfare organisations, *BMC Med Ethics* 20:16, 2019.

Baker DG: Natural pathogens of laboratory mice, rats, and rabbits and their effects on research, *Clin Microbiol Rev* 11:231–266, 1998.

Barnard DE, Lewis SM, Teter BB, et al.: Open- and closed-formula laboratory animal diets and their importance to research, *J Am Assoc Lab Anim* 48:709–713, 2009.

Bayne K, Turner PV: Animal welfare standards and international collaborations, *ILAR J* 60:86–94, 2019.

Blacher E, Bashiardes S, Shapiro H, et al.: Potential roles of gut microbiome and metabolites in modulating ALS in mice, *Nature* 572:474–480, 2019.

Bolon B, Bonnefoi MS, Roberts KC, et al.: Toxic interactions in the rat nose: pollutants from soiled bedding and methyl bromide, *Toxicol Pathol* 19:571–579, 1991.

Camacho L, Lewis SM, Vanlandingham MM, et al.: Comparison of endpoints relevant to toxicity assessments in 3 generations of CD-1 mice fed irradiated natural and purified ingredient diets with varying soy protein and isoflavone contents, *Food Chem Toxicol* 94:39–56, 2016.

Chapman K, Pullen N, Coney L, et al.: Preclinical development of monoclonal antibodies: considerations for the use of non-human primates, *mAbs* 1:505–516, 2009.

Chi L, Xue J, Tu P, et al.: Gut microbiome disruption altered the biotransformation and liver toxicity of arsenic in mice, *Arch Toxicol* 93:25–35, 2019.

Churchill SR, Morgan DL, Kissling GE, et al.: Impact of environmental enrichment devices on NTP in vivo studies, *Toxicol Pathol* 44:233–245, 2016.

Clough G: Environmental effects on animals used in biomedical research, *Biol Rev* 57:487–523, 1982.

Colman K: Impact of the genetics and source of preclinical safety animal models on study design, results, and interpretation, *Toxicol Pathol* 45:94–106, 2017.

Conour LA, Murray KA, Brown MJ: Preparation of animals for research–issues to consider for rodents and rabbits, *ILAR J* 47:283–293, 2006.

Council NR: *Guide for the care and use of laboratory animals*, ed 8, Washington, DC, 2011, The National Academies Press.

Damon EG, Eidson AF, Hobbs CH, et al.: Effect of acclimation to caging on nephrotoxic response of rats to uranium, *Lab Anim Sci* 36:24–27, 1986.

Damsch S, Eichenbaum G, Tonelli A, et al.: Gavage-related reflux in rats: identification, pathogenesis, and toxicological implications (review), *Toxicol Pathol* 39:348–360, 2010.

De Vera Mudry MC, Kronenberg S, Komatsu S, et al.: Blinded by the light: retinal phototoxicity in the context of safety studies, *Toxicol Pathol* 41:813–825, 2013.

Deschl U, Kittel B, Rittinghausen S, et al.: The value of historical control data-scientific advantages for pathologists, industry and agencies, *Toxicol Pathol* 30:80–87, 2002.

Duffy PH, Lewis SM, Mayhugh MA, et al.: Nonneoplastic pathology in male Sprague-Dawley rats fed the American Institute of Nutrition–93M purified diet at ad libitum and dietary-restricted intakes, *Nutr Res* 28:179–189, 2008.

Durack J, Lynch SV: The gut microbiome: relationships with disease and opportunities for therapy, *J Exp Med* 216:20–40, 2019.

Ericsson AC, Gagliardi J, Bouhan D, et al.: The influence of caging, bedding, and diet on the composition of the microbiota in different regions of the mouse gut, *Sci Rep* 8:4065, 2018.

Escalante NK, Lemire P, Cruz Tleugabulova M, et al.: The common mouse protozoa Tritrichomonas muris alters mucosal T cell homeostasis and colitis susceptibility, *J Exp Med* 213:2841–2850, 2016.

Everds NE, Snyder PW, Bailey KL, et al.: Interpreting stress responses during routine toxicity studies: a review of the biology, impact, and assessment, *Toxicol Pathol* 41:560–614, 2013.

Everitt JI: The future of preclinical animal models in pharmaceutical discovery and development: a need to bring in cerebro to the in vivo discussions, *Toxicol Pathol* 43:70–77, 2015.

Everitt JI, Olson LM, Mangum JB, et al.: High mortality with severe dystrophic cardiac calcinosis in C3H/OUJ mice fed high fat purified diets, *Vet Pathol* 25:113–118, 1988.

Everitt JI, Richter CB: Infectious diseases of the upper respiratory tract: implications for toxicology studies, *Environ Health Perspect* 85:239–247, 1990.

Festing MF: Inbred strains should replace outbred stocks in toxicology, safety testing, and drug development, *Toxicol Pathol* 38:681–690, 2010.

Festing MF: Genetically defined strains in drug development and toxicity testing, *Methods Mol Biol* 1438:1–17, 2016.

Geller LT, Barzily-Rokni M, Danino T, et al.: Potential role of intratumor bacteria in mediating tumor resistance to the chemotherapeutic drug gemcitabine, *Science* 357:1156–1160, 2017.

Grieves JL, Dick Jr EJ, Schlabritz-Loutsevich NE, et al.: Barbiturate euthanasia solution-induced tissue artifact in nonhuman primates, *J Med Primatol* 37:154–161, 2008.

Hankenson FC, Marx JO, Gordon CJ, et al.: Effects of rodent thermoregulation on animal models in the research environment, *Comp Med* 68:425–438, 2018.

Hannibal DL, Bliss-Moreau E, Vandeleest J, et al.: Laboratory rhesus macaque social housing and social changes: implications for research, *Am J Primatol* 79:1–14, 2017.

Hansen AK, Nielsen DS, Krych L, et al.: Bacterial species to be considered in quality assurance of mice and rats, *Lab Anim* 53:281–291, 2019.

Hansen CH, Andersen LS, Krych L, et al.: Mode of delivery shapes gut colonization pattern and modulates regulatory immunity in mice, *J Immunol* 193:1213–1222, 2014.

Haseman JK, Hailey JR, Morris RW: Spontaneous neoplasm incidences in Fischer 344 rats and B6C3F1 mice in two-year carcinogenicity studies: a national toxicology program update, *Toxicol Pathol* 26:428–441, 1998.

Haseman JK, Ney E, Nyska A, et al.: Effect of diet and animal care/housing protocols on body weight, survival, tumor incidences, and nephropathy severity of F344 rats in chronic studies, *Toxicol Pathol* 31:674–681, 2003.

Howard B, van Herck H, Guillen J, et al.: Report of the FELASA working group on evaluation of quality systems for animal units, *Lab Anim* 38:103–118, 2004.

Hufeldt MR, Nielsen DS, Vogensen FK, et al.: Variation in the gut microbiota of laboratory mice is related to both genetic and environmental factors, *Comp Med* 60:336–347, 2010.

Hukkanen RR, Dybdal N, Tripathi N, et al.: Scientific and regulatory policy committee points to consider*: the toxicologic pathologist's role in the 3Rs, *Toxicol Pathol* 47:789–798, 2019.

Hylander BL, Gordon CJ, Repasky EA: Manipulation of ambient housing temperature to study the impact of chronic stress on immunity and cancer in mice, *J Immunol* 202:631–636, 2019.

Ito R, Takahashi T, Ito M: Humanized mouse models: application to human diseases, *J Cell Physiol* 233:3723–3728, 2018.

Ivanov II , Atarashi K, Manel N, et al.: Induction of intestinal Th17 cells by segmented filamentous bacteria, *Cell* 139:485–498, 2009.

Jensen MN, Ritskes-Hoitinga M: How isoflavone levels in common rodent diets can interfere with the value of animal models and with experimental results, *Lab Anim* 41:1–18, 2007.

Keatley KL: A comparison of the U.S. EPA FIFRA GLP standards with the U.S. FDA GLP standards for nonclinical laboratory studies, *Qual Assur* 7:147–154, 1999.

Keenan C, Elmore S, Francke-Carroll S, et al.: Best practices for use of historical control data of proliferative rodent lesions, *Toxicol Pathol* 37:679–693, 2009a.

Keenan C, Elmore S, Francke-Carroll S, et al.: Potential for a global historical control database for proliferative rodent lesions, *Toxicol Pathol* 37:677–678, 2009b.

Keenan K, Ballam G, Soper KA, et al.: Diet, caloric restriction, and the rodent bioassay, *Toxicol Sci* 52:24–34, 2000.

Keenan KP, Ballam GC, Soper KA, et al.: Diet, caloric restriction, and the rodent bioassay, *Toxicol Sci* 52:24–34, 1996a.

Keenan KP, Laroque P, Ballam GC, et al.: The effects of diet, ad libitum overfeeding, and moderate dietary restriction on the rodent bioassay: the uncontrolled variable in safety assessment, *Toxicol Pathol* 24:757–768, 1996b.

Keenan KP, Laroque P, Soper KA, et al.: The effects of overfeeding and moderate dietary restriction on Sprague-

Dawley rat survival, pathology, carcinogenicity, and the toxicity of pharmaceutical agents, *Exp Toxicol Pathol* 48:139–144, 1999.

Koontz JM, Dancy BCR, Horton CL, et al.: The role of the human microbiome in chemical toxicity, *Int J Toxicol* 38:251–264, 2019.

Lanzoni A, Piaia A, Everitt J, et al.: Early onset of spontaneous renal preneoplastic and neoplastic lesions in young conventional rats in toxicity studies, *Toxicol Pathol* 35:589–593, 2007.

Lien EL, Boyle FG, Wrenn JM, et al.: Comparison of AIN-76A and AIN-93G diets: a 13-week study in rats, *Food Chem Toxicol* 39:385–392, 2001.

Lu J, Synowiec S, Lu L, et al.: Microbiota influence the development of the brain and behaviors in C57BL/6J mice, *PloS One* 13:e0201829, 2018.

Mailhiot D, Ostdiek AM, Luchins KR, et al.: Comparing mouse health monitoring between soiled-bedding sentinel and exhaust air dust surveillance programs, *J Am Assoc Lab Anim Sci* 59:58–66, 2020.

Matheoud D, Cannon T, Voisin A, et al.: Intestinal infection triggers Parkinson's disease-like symptoms in Pink1(-/-) mice, *Nature* 571:565–569, 2019.

Miller M, Ritter B, Zorn J, et al.: Exhaust air dust monitoring is superior to soiled bedding sentinels for the detection of pasteurella pneumotropica in individually ventilated cage systems, *J Am Assoc Lab Anim Sci* 55:775–781, 2016.

Mitchell GV, Dua PN, Jenkins M, et al.: Nutritional and pathological changes in male and female rats fed modifications of the AIN-76A diet, *Food Chem Toxicol* 27:185–191, 1989.

Monticello TM, Jones TW, Dambach DM, et al.: Current nonclinical testing paradigm enables safe entry to first-in-human clinical trials: the IQ consortium nonclinical to clinical translational database, *Toxicol Appl Pharmacol* 334:100–109, 2017.

Naaijkens BA, van Dijk A, Meinster E, et al.: Wistar rats from different suppliers have a different response in an acute myocardial infarction model, *Res Vet Sci* 96:377–379, 2014.

Newberne PM, Sotnikov AV: Diet: the neglected variable in chemical safety evaluations, *Toxicol Pathol* 24:746–756, 1996.

Nicklas W: Microbiological standardization of laboratory animals, *Berl Münchener Tierärztliche Wochenschr* 112:201–210, 1999.

Nold JB, Keenan KP, Nyska A, et al.: Society of toxicologic pathology position paper: diet as a variable in rodent toxicology and carcinogenicity studies, *Toxicol Pathol* 29:585–586, 2001.

Nuzzo A, Brown JR: The microbiome factor in drug discovery and development, *Chem Res Toxicol* 33:119–124, 2020.

OECD: *OfEC-oaD: guideline 19: guidance document on the recognition, assessment, and use of clinical signs as humane endpoints for experimental animals used in safety evaluation*, Organization for Economic Co-operation and Development [OECD].

Olson H, Betton G, Robinson D, et al.: Concordance of the toxicity of pharmaceuticals in humans and in animals, *Regul Toxicol Pharmacol* 32:56–67, 2000.

Overcash RG, Lindsey JR, Cassel GH, et al.: Enhancement of natural and experimental respiratory mycoplasmosis in rats by hexamethylphosphoramide, *Am J Pathol* 82:171–190, 1976.

Percie du Sert N, Ahluwalia A, Alam S, et al.: Reporting animal research: explanation and elaboration for the ARRIVE guidelines 2.0, *PLoS Biol* 18:e3000411, 2020a.

Percie du Sert N, Hurst V, Ahluwalia A, et al.: The ARRIVE guidelines 2.0: updated guidelines for reporting animal research, *PLoS Biol* 18:e3000410, 2020b.

Pushalkar S, Hundeyin M, Daley D, et al.: The pancreatic cancer microbiome promotes oncogenesis by induction of innate and adaptive immune suppression, *Cancer Discov* 8:403–416, 2018.

Recordati C, De Maglie M, Marsella G, et al.: Long-term study on the effects of housing C57BL/6NCrl mice in cages equipped with wireless technology generating extremely low-intensity electromagnetic fields, *Toxicol Pathol* 47:598–611, 2019.

Roediger B, Lee Q, Tikoo S, et al.: An atypical parvovirus drives chronic tubulointerstitial nephropathy and kidney fibrosis, *Cell* 175:530–543.e524, 2018.

Rosshart SP, Herz J, Vassallo BG, et al.: Laboratory mice born to wild mice have natural microbiota and model human immune responses, *Science* 365, 2019.

Scher JU, Sczesnak A, Longman RS, et al.: Expansion of intestinal *Prevotella copri* correlates with enhanced susceptibility to arthritis, *Elife* 2:e01202, 2013.

Sewell F, Edwards J, Prior H, et al.: Opportunities to apply the 3Rs in safety assessment programs, *ILAR J* 57:234–245, 2016.

Shomer NH, Allen-Worthington KH, Hickman DL, et al.: Review of rodent euthanasia methods, *J Am Assoc Lab Anim Sci* 59:242–253, 2020.

Silbergeld EK: The microbiome, *Toxicol Pathol* 45:190–194, 2017.

Tennekes H, Kaufmann W, Dammann M, et al.: The stability of historical control data for common neoplasms in laboratory rats and the implications for carcinogenic risk assessment, *Regul Toxicol Pharmacol* 40:293–304, 2004.

Thigpen JE, Setchell KD, Saunders HE, et al.: Selecting the appropriate rodent diet for endocrine disruptor research and testing studies, *ILAR J* 45:401–416, 2004.

Tu P, Chi L, Bodnar W, et al.: Gut microbiome toxicity: connecting the environment and gut microbiome-associated diseases, *Toxics* 8, 2020.

Viaud S, Daillere R, Boneca IG, et al.: Gut microbiome and anticancer immune response: really hot Sh*t!, *Cell Death Differ* 22:199–214, 2015.

Vidal JD, Drobatz LS, Holliday DF, et al.: Spontaneous findings in the heart of Mauritian-origin cynomolgus macaques (*Macaca fascicularis*), *Toxicol Pathol* 38:297–302, 2010.

Viney M: The gut microbiota of wild rodents: challenges and opportunities, *Lab Anim* 53:252–258, 2019.

Wallace BD, Wang H, Lane KT, et al.: Alleviating cancer drug toxicity by inhibiting a bacterial enzyme, *Science* 330:831–835, 2010.

Walter J, Armet AM, Finlay BB, et al.: Establishing or exaggerating causality for the gut microbiome: lessons from human microbiota-associated rodents, *Cell* 180:221–232, 2020.

Weber EM, Dallaire JA, Gaskill BN, et al.: Aggression in group-housed laboratory mice: why can't we solve the problem? *Lab Anim* 46:157–161, 2017.

Xu Y, Villalona-Calero MA: Irinotecan: mechanisms of tumor resistance and novel strategies for modulating its activity, *Ann Oncol* 13:1841–1851, 2002.

Yamashita H, Hoenerhoff MJ, Peddada SD, et al.: Chemical exacerbation of light-induced retinal degeneration in F344/N rats in national toxicology program rodent bioassays, *Toxicol Pathol* 44:892–903, 2016.

Zachariassen LF, Krych L, Engkilde K, et al.: Sensitivity to oxazolone induced dermatitis is transferable with gut microbiota in mice, *Sci Rep* 7:44385, 2017.

Zimmermann M, Zimmermann-Kogadeeva M, Wegmann R, et al.: Mapping human microbiome drug metabolism by gut bacteria and their genes, *Nature* 570:462–467, 2019a.

Zimmermann M, Zimmermann-Kogadeeva M, Wegmann R, et al.: Separating host and microbiome contributions to drug pharmacokinetics and toxicity, *Science* 363, 2019b.

Zitvogel L, Ma Y, Raoult D, et al.: The microbiome in cancer immunotherapy: diagnostic tools and therapeutic strategies, *Science* 359:1366–1370, 2018.

Index

'*Note*: Page numbers followed by "f" indicate figures, "t" indicate tables and "b" indicate boxes.'

A

Abciximab, 45—46
Abnormal differentiation, 901
Absorption, 16, 55—58
  dose volume recommendations for exposure studies, 57t
  dose-proportional, super-proportional, and dose-limited exposure relationships, 57f
  microbiome effects on, 34—35
  monoclonal antibody administration and, 84—85
  properties, 16—19
    biological membranes, 16—17
    filtration, 17
    simple diffusion, 17
    specialized transport, 17—19, 18t—19t
  reduction in exposure to auto-induction, 58f
  routes
    absorption from GI tract, 19—20
    absorption from respiratory tract, 20—21
    absorption through skin, 21
Absorption, distribution, metabolism, and excretion (ADME), 51, 177, 654, 888—892
  GEM models for, 889—890
  principles in small molecule drug discovery and development
    absorption, bioavailability, and PK/TK studies, 55—58
    derivation of PK parameters from concentration—time profiles, 53f
    development, 67—68
    discovery overview, 54f
    distribution, 59—61
    drug development paradigm, 52f
    drug disposition after oral administration, 54f
    drug metabolism studies in development, 71
    excretion, 65—67, 71—73
    mass balance studies, 68—69
    metabolism, 61—65
    PBPK modeling, 67
    specialized excretion studies, 73
    timing of development ADME studies, 73
    tissue distribution studies, 69
    wide *vs.* narrow therapeutic range, 53f
Acalabrutinib, 108—109
Accelerator mass spectrometry (AMS), 71
Accurate, legible, contemporaneous, original, and attributable (ALCOA), 1014—1015
Acetaminophen (APAP), 24, 734

Activated partial thromboplastin time (APTT), 300
Activation-induced deaminase (AID), 220—221
Active transport, 17—19
Acute idiosyncratic hepatocellular injury (AIHI), 464
Acute phase proteins (APPs), 321
Acyclovir, 31—32
Adaptation, cellular, 116—122
  atrophy, 116—120
  hypertrophy, 120—122
Adefovir, 22
Adenine nucleotide transporter (ANT), 130
Adeno-associated virus (AAV), 870
  AAV9, 342
Adenomatous polyposis coli (*APC*), 215—217
Adenosine triphosphate (ATP), 114, 442
Adenovirus (AdV), 870
Adipose tissue, 22—23
  storage, 22—23
Adipsin, 471b
ADME. *See* Absorption, distribution, metabolism, and excretion (ADME)
Adrenocorticotropic hormone (ACTH), 116
Adverse drug reaction
  action on nonreceptors, 103
  action on signal transduction receptors, 103—104
  biochemical, 102—104
  physiochemical property, 102
  types of, 104—106, 105f
Adverse outcome pathways (AOPs), 536, 947
  key event, 947—948
  molecular-initiating event, 947
  quantitative AOP (qAOP), 947—948
Adversity, 171, 955—956, 978, 1058, 1070
Aethina tumida, 816. *See also* Small hive beetle (*Aethina tumida*)
Aflatoxin, 24
Aflatoxin B1 (AFB1), 29, 206—207, 812—814, 830
Aging-related physiological factors, 6
Agonist, 106
  full, 106
  inverse, 106—107
  partial, 106—107
Alanine aminotransferase (ALT), 264, 300, 312—313, 464b
Albumin, 22, 311
  albumin/globulin (A/G) ratio, 311
  binding therapeutics, 81—82
Alcohol, 27
Alcohol dehydrogenase, 27
Aldehyde dehydrogenases, 27

Aldehyde oxidase, 27
Alexa Fluor, 337
Alkaline phosphatase (ALP), 300, 313—314, 337
Alligator mississippiensis. *See* American alligator (Alligator mississippiensis)
Allometric scaling approach, 95
Allosteric interaction, 106
α(1,3)-galactose (αGal), 915
α(1,3)-galactosyltransferase (αGT), 915
Alpha acid glycoprotein (AAG), 59, 330
α-glutathione S-transferase (α-GST), 321
Altered gene expression, 38—40
Altered organ function
  biomarkers of, 468—469
  functional markers of vascular toxicity, 469
  2.x circulating micro-RNA as biomarkers of tissue injury, 469
Alternative models in biomedical research
  context of use and qualification requirements, 957—958
  integration of pathology and alternative data streams, 955—956
  nontraditional models in toxicity research, 926—928
  regulatory perspective, 955
  in silico models and data analytics, 946—951
  in vitro and ex vivo models, 928—946
  in vivo models using alternative mammalian and nonmammalian species, 951—955
Alzheimer's disease (AD), 741—742
American alligator (*Alligator mississippiensis*), 831
American Board of Toxicology (ABT), 8
American College of Veterinary Pathologists (ACVP), 8, 988
American Institute of Nutrition (AIN), 1100—1101
American Society for Clinical Pathology (ASCP), 302
American Society for Veterinary Clinical Pathology (ASVCP), 296
American Veterinary Medical Association (AVMA), 1083
Ames test, 231—232
Amino acid conjugation, 29
[2-amino-3-(5-methyl-3-oxo-1,2-oxazol-4-yl) propanoic acid] (AMPA), 103
Aminobenzene, 29
Amphibians, 811—812, 825—828. *See also* Animal models
  basic biologic characteristics and common species, 825—826
  findings, 826
  major disease models, 826—828

AMPHITOX, 836—837

Amyloid beta peptides (Aβ peptides), 905, 1038—1039

Amyloid precursor proteins (APPs), 883

Amyotrophic lateral sclerosis (ALS), 1093—1094

Androgen receptor (AR), 225
  modulators, 228

Angiogenesis, 218—219

Angiotensin converting enzyme (ACE), 174

Animal health consideration, 1089—1091
  adventitious agents, 1089
  sentinel monitoring programs, 1090

Animal models, 238, 777—778. See also
      Genetically engineered animal
      models
  breeds, 752—753
    conventional/domestic pigs, 753
    minipigs, 752—753
  dog, 722. See also Dog
    ethics of use of dog as laboratory animal
      species, 743—744
    predictivity of dog toxicity data for
      human responses, 731—732
    spontaneous background pathology in
      beagle, 735—737
    spontaneous neoplastic diseases in, 737
    use of dog as model of human diseases,
      737—742
    use of dogs in biomedical research,
      727—731
  nonhuman primate. See also Nonhuman
     primates
    biomedical research, 787—794
    pharmacology and toxicology research,
      790—794
  nonmammalian, 811—812, 952—955. See also
     Amphibians; Birds; Fish; Invertebrates
    applicability of taxa for use in
      toxicological bioassays, 813t
    data extrapolation, 847—851
      interspecies variability, 848—849
      knowledge gap, 850—851
      reliability of published
        histopathology data, 851
      results extrapolation and risk
        assessment, 847—848
    microanatomy resources for, 816t
    study design considerations,
      841—846
      study design and implementation,
        841—844
      subclinical disease, 844—846
    utilization, 831—841
  pig. See also Pig
    ethics and animal welfare, 773
    genetics of pigs and background for use
      in research, 752—755
    as model system for medical devices and
      of human diseases, 770—772
    neoplasia, 715, 769
    as organ source for xenotransplantation,
      761
    regulatory aspects, 772—773

spontaneous background pathology in
    swine, 761—769
  in toxicological studies, 755—761
rabbit, 697. See also Rabbit
  basic biological characteristics and
    common breeds, 696—699
  gastrointestinal system, 714—715
  large intestine, 711
  major disease and functional models,
    705—709
  male reproductive tract, 711
  model selection, 696
  mucosal irritation studies, 703
  New Zealand Red (NZR), 696—697
  New Zealand White (NZW), 696—697
  ovary, 711, 767
  pharmacokinetic and toxicity studies,
    701—705
  regulatory aspects and examples of
    rabbits in biomedical research, 699
  spontaneous findings in experimental
    NZW rabbit, 709—715
  stomach and small intestines, 710
rodents. See also Mouse; Rat
  basic biological characteristics of
    common rodent stocks and strains,
    667—675
  common pathologic findings in rodents,
    675—688
  inbred mice, 668
  inbred rats, 670
  inbred strains of mice and rats, 667—670
  issues in extrapolation of rodent data for
    human risk assessment, 661—667
  nonproliferative findings, 682—684
  outbred rats, 670
  outbred stocks
    of mice and rats, 667—670
    of rodents, 1086
  proliferative findings, 682—684
  selection of species, 655—661
Antagonist, 106—107, 107f
Antibody, 78, 337
antibody-based detection systems, 486
antibody-based therapeutics, 80—82,
  80f
PK of, 90—92
availability, 352—353
production/immunological research in
  rabbits, 705
Antibody drug conjugates (ADCs), 80—81
Antibody-dependent cellular cytotoxicity
  (ADCC), 78
Antibody-dependent cellular phagocytosis
  (ADCP), 78
Antidrug antibodies (ADA), 85, 665,
  798—800, 1047—1048
Antigen binding fragment (Fab), 81
Antisense oligonucleotide (ASO)
  therapeutics, 361
Aplysia californica, 817. See also California
  sea hare (Aplysia californica)
Apoptosis, 46, 127, 133—138, 136f, 143—145,
  213, 217—218

evaluation of, 350—352
  necrosis vs., 128t
Apoptotic protease activating factor 1
  (Apaf-1), 136—137
Arachidonic acid (AA), 308
Area under curve (AUC), 52—53, 84, 466—467
Area/pixel-based measurements, 410
Artificial intelligence in tissue image
  analysis, 414—416
Aryl hydrocarbon receptor (AhR), 38,
  224—225
Aspartate aminotransferase (AST), 264, 300,
  312—313
Aspirin, 474b, 735
Atherosclerosis, 770
ATP-binding cassette (ABC), 891—892
ATP-dependent transporter, 17—18
Atrazine, 165—166
Atrial natriuretic peptides, 328
Atrophy, 116—120
  autophagic cell death, 118
  macroautophagy, 118
  microautophagy, 117—118
Autolysis, 128—129
Autophagy, 40—41, 117
Autopsy, 3—4
Avatar (patient-derived xenograft) mouse
  cancer models, 661, 911
Avidin—biotin complex (ABC), 337

B

B-cell lymphoma 2 (BCL-2), 41
Baboon (Papio sp.), 780
Bacillus Calmette—Guérin (BCG), 792,
  1041
Bacteroides species, 35
Balantidium coli, 798
BALB/c mouse strain, 880
Barrier function, 141
Base excision repair (BER), 222
Basophils, 698
BCGitis, 1041
Beagles. See Animal models; dog; Dog
Bees, 816
Benchmark dosing (BMD), 501
Benzo[a]pyrene (BaP), 220
β-adrenergic receptors (BARs), 111
Bevacizumab, 84, 704
Big Blue mouse, 894
Big Blue rat, 894
Big data
  analytics in toxicology pathology,
    948—951
  technologies, 956
Bile acids, 315
Bile acid, total, 315
Bile duct cannulated studies (BDC studies),
  64—65
Bile salt export pump (BSEP), 17—18, 315
Biliary excretion, 33, 68
Biliprotein, 314—315
Bilirubin, 314—315
Bilirubin, total, 512—513
Binding assays, 372—373

Bio-Formats toolbox, 403
Bioanalytical assays for assessing
    monoclonal antibody concentrations,
    90, 91f
Bioassay, 229
    screening, 834—835
Bioavailability, 53, 55—58
Biodistribution, 901
Bioinformatics, 928
Biologics, 77—78, 347, 665
Bioluminescence imaging, 442
Biomarkers, 264—265, 459—481
    acute phase protein (APPs), 321
    of altered organ function, 468—469
    application in nonclinical studies, 319
    assay kits, 318—319
    biologic validation, 319
    biomarkers of environmental exposure,
        472—473
    characterization, 488
    drug-induced vascular injury biomarkers,
        329—330
    drug response or pharmacodynamic,
        473—474
    female reproductive toxicity assessment,
        163
    fit-for-purpose validation, 319
    heart, 327—329
    hormones, 319—321
    liver biomarkers, 325—327
    male reproductive toxicity assessment, 157
    mechanistic, 469—472
    methods for biomarker measurement and
        quantitation, 483—487
        antibody-based detection systems, 486
        genomics, 485
        histocytomics, 486
        metabolomics, 485
        morphology-based methods, 486—487
        multiplexed assays, 486
        proteomics, 485
    novel renal biomarkers, 321—325
    organ-specific biomarkers of tissue injury,
        463—468
        cardiac injury, biomarkers of, 467—468
        drug-induced vascular injury,
            biochemical markers, 465—466
        kidney damage reversibility, biomarkers
            for, 467
        liver injury, biomarkers of, 463—465
        renal injury, biomarkers of, 466—467
        vascular toxicity, biomarkers of, 465—466
    patient/clinical trial subject selection,
        475—476
    pharmacogenomic, 478
    predictive, 474—475
    prognostic, 478—481
    qualification of, 488—489
    qualification vs. validation, 460
    strategies for discovery, 481—483
        discovery and application of panels of
            biomarkers, 483
    surrogate endpoint, 476—478
    surrogate vs., 460
    of tissue injury/damage, 460—468

urinary biomarkers in, 323t—325t
Biomedical institutions, 1081
Biomedical product development, 9—10
Biomedical research, 787—794
Biomimicry, 934
Biopharming, 913—916
Bioprinted microtissues, 934—935
Bioprinting, 934
    methods/challenges, 935
    platforms, 936t—937t
Biotherapeutics, 77—78, 372—373
    ADME and PK/PD principles
        antibody-based therapeutics, 80—82
        monoclonal antibodies, 78—80
        PD of biotherapeutics, 92—94
        PK of biotherapeutics, 83—92
        PK—PD modeling andinterspecies
            scaling, 95—96
    pharmacodynamics of, 92—94
        antibody mechanism of action, 93f
    PK of, 83—92
Biotransformation, 16, 24—25, 1094—1095
    enzymes, 348
    microbiome effects on, 34—35
Birds, 811—812
    basic biologic characteristics and common
        species, 828—829
    findings, 829—830
    major disease models, 830
Blinded evaluation, 1043
Blood urea nitrogen (BUN), 311, 460
Blood—brain barrier (BBB), 17, 23, 183
Blood—epididymis barrier (BEB), 155
Blood—testis barrier (BTB), 155
Body and organ weights, 632—634
Bone, 23
    marrow, 768
        evaluation, 317—318
Bottom-up approaches (BU-MS
        approaches), 499
Brain, 771
Brain natriuretic peptides, 328
Break-induced replication (BIR), 223
Breast cancer resistance protein (BCRP),
    17—18, 891—892
British Society of Toxicological Pathology
    (BSTP), 980, 1062—1063
Bruton's tyrosine kinase inhibitor (Btk
    inhibitor), 108—109
Bull trout (Salvelinus confluentus), 812—814

C

^{14}C-labeled drug, 68
C57BL/6 mice, 880
Cadmium (Cd), 22
Caenorhabditis elegans, 815—816
Caffeine, 733—734
Calcium, 311
California sea hare (Aplysia californica), 817
Callithrix jacchus. See Marmoset, common
        (Callithrix jacchus)
Calquence, 108—109
Cancer, 206, 772
Cancer stem cell theory (CSC theory), 207
Candida albicans, 762

Candidate identification (CI), 54
Candidate prognostic marker, 479b
Candidate selection (CS), 54
Canis familiaris. See Dog; domestic (Canis
        familiaris)
Canis lupus. See Gray wolf (Canis lupus)
Capuchin monkey (Cebus sp.), 781—782
Carbon dioxide (CO$_2$), 1083—1084
Carbon monoxide (CO), 25
Carbon tetrachloride (CCl$_4$), 39
Carbonyl sulfide (COS), 427
Carcinogenesis, 46—47, 206—207, 636—638,
        812—814, 902—904
    angiogenesis, 218—219
    apoptosis, 217—218
    assessment, 529—534, 895—898
        genotoxic carcinogens, 220
        mechanism, 532—534
        prediction of carcinogenic potential of
            compounds, 529—532
        spontaneous vs. test article—related
            tumors, 532
    carcinogenicity study data interpretation,
        242—244
    carcinogenicity testing, 234—235
        conventional rat strains for, 237
        in rodents, 235—237
    cell cycle regulation, 211f
    cell growth and proliferation, 210—213
    chromosomal aberration assay, 232
    clinical pathology, 242, 243t
    consequences of genotoxicity, 224
    DNA
        damage repair, 217—218
        DNA-based assays, 232—233
        replication and repair mechanisms,
            222—224
    evolving and new technologies, 244—245
    features of, 208—210
    hamster model, 240—241
    high-fidelity/nonmutagenic DNA repair,
        222
    histopathology, 242
    identification of carcinogens, 231—244
    in genetically modified mice, 996
    invasion, 218—219
    in vitro mutagenicity assays, 231—232
    low fidelity/mutagenic DNA repair, 222
    mechanisms of chemically induced,
        219—231
    metastasis, 218—219
    micronucleus test, 232
    mouse models of carcinogenesis, 238—240
    nongenotoxic carcinogens, 224—231
    OECD testing, 221t
    oncogenes, 213—217
    organoids, 242
    testing, 234—235
        conventional rat strains for, 237
        programs and guidelines, 233
    in rodents, 235—237
    in wild-type rodents, 995—996
        Tg.AC, 895—896
        Xpa+/-, 895—896
        Trp53+/-, 895—896

Carcinogenesis (*Continued*)
  Tg. rasH2 mouse model, 240, 895–896
  theories of, 207–208
  Tp53$^{+/-}$D/L mouse model, 240
  transgenic models for mutagenicity testing, 240
  tumor suppressor genes, 213–217
  two-year NTP bioassay, 233–234
  zebrafish, 241
Carcinogenicity Assessment Document (CAD), 236
Carcinogens
  nongenotoxic, 224–231
    AhR, 224–225
    androgen receptor modulators, 228
    CARs, 225–226
    cytotoxicity, 228–229
    epigenetic mechanisms, 229–231
    estrogen receptor agonists, 227–228
    hormonal mechanisms, 227
    immune suppression, 229
    PPARs, 226–227
    PXRs, 225–226
    receptor-mediated MOAs, 224
Cardiac injury, biomarkers of, 467–468
Cardiac safety studies in rabbits, 702–703
Cardiac troponins (cTns), 304, 327–328
  cTnI, 1041–1042
Cardiomyopathy, 683–684
Cardiovascular, 764, 770
  atherosclerosis, 770
  myocardial infarction, 770
  and pulmonary system, 180–182
Caretta caretta, 831. *See also* Loggerhead sea turtle (*Caretta caretta*)
Cas9, 871–872. *See also* CRISPR-associated nuclease (Cas)
Caspase, 137
Catalyzed reporter deposition (CARD), 337
Cationic drugs, 31–32
Cause of death (COD), 278–279, 675
Cavia porcellus. See Guinea pig (*Cavia porcellus*)
Cebus sp. *See* Capuchin monkey (*Cebus* sp.)
Cell
  apoptosis, 347
  atrophy, 117
  biodistribution of, 341–345
  cell-based measurements, 410–411
  cultures, 928–930
  cycle–related proteins evaluation, 349–350
  death mechanisms, 40–42
    apoptosis, 41
    autophagy, 40–41
    necroptosis, 41–42
    necrosis, 41
  growth and proliferation, 210–213
  immunophenotyping, 369–372
  injury, 113
  membranes, 16–17
  proliferation, 44–46, 347
    studies, 349–350
  repair and adaptation
    cell proliferation, 44–45
    fibroblasts and ECM, 45–46

swelling, 129
therapy, 82, 665
Cell injury, 127–146
  accidental cell death, 127–133
  adaptation, 116–122
  cell death terminology, 134t–135t
  consequences of, 139–146
    apoptosis, 143–145
    hyperplasia, 145
    metaplasia, 145–146
    necrosis, 139–143
  host reaction to, 116
  irreversible cell injury, 127–146
  irreversible *vs.* reversible cell injury, 122–127
  morphologic assessment in toxicologic pathology, 113–114
  programmed cell death, 133–139
  reversible cell injury *vs.*, 122–127
    cellular swelling, 124–125
    fatty change, 126–127
  structural and functional components of, 114–116
Cellular oncogene, 213
Cellular protein targets, 107
Cellular targets, interactions of toxicants with
  altered gene expression, 38–40
  covalent modification, 35–36
  mechanisms of cell death, 40–42
  stress responses in toxicity, 36–38
Central nervous system (CNS), 126–127, 163, 427, 788
Cerebrospinal fluid (CSF), 84–85
Certification, professional, 8–9
Chacma baboon (*Papio ursinus*), 780
Charged-couple device detectors (CCD detectors), 442
Chemical mutagenesis, 877
Chemokine C–C motif ligand 2 (Ccl2), 39
Chimeric antigen receptor (CAR), 82
Chimeric antigen receptor T-cells (CARTs), 339
Chimeric human–mouse, 910
  bone marrow models, 910
  liver models, 907
Chimeric organs, 907–911
China Food and Drug Administration (CFDA), 1013
Chinchillas (*Chinchilla lanigera*), 653–654
Chinese hamster ovary cells (CHO cells), 232
Chlordane, 22–23
Chloride, 312
Chlorine, 1
Chlorocebus aethiops pygerythrus. *See* Green monkeys (Chlorocebus aethiops pygerythrus)
Chlorocebus aethiops sabaeus. *See* Vervet monkeys (Chlorocebus aethiops sabaeus)
Cholecystitis, necrotizing of gall bladder, 765
Cholesterol, 310

Chorioallantoic membrane (CAM) assay, 953
Chromosomal aberration assay, 232
Chronic dosing, 110–111
  exhaustion of mediators, 111
  physiological adaptation, 111
  receptor downregulation, 111
Chronic progressive nephropathy (CPN), 677, 972
Cimetidine, 27, 31–32
Cis-platinum, 22
Citrobacter rodentium, 1093
Clara (club) cells, 25–26
Clearance (C$_L$), 85
  parameter, 85
  pathways, 52
Clinical chemistry, 634
Clinical Data Interchange Standards Consortium (CDISC), 982
Clinical pathology testing. *See also* Biomarkers
  clinical pathology laboratory, 296–302
  clinical pathology parameters, 305–318
    clinical chemistry, 310–315
    flow cytometry, 318
    hematology, 305–307
    hemostasis, 307–310
    urinalysis, 315–317
  controls, 305
  kinetics, 304–305
  nonstandard biomarkers, 318–330
  parameters in nonclinical toxicity studies, 299t
  samples to, 302–303
  test parameters, 303–304
  value of, 295–296
Cloning, 876
Clot dissolution, 309
Cloudy swelling. *See* Degeneration, ballooning
Club (Clara) cells, 25–26
Clustered regularly interspaced short palindromic repeats (CRISPR), 761, 871–872, 951
  function in bacteria, 871–872
  Cas 9, 761
  off-target effects, 872–873
Coagulation, 307–310. *See also* Hemostasis
Coagulometers, 301
Code of Federal Regulations (CFR), 258–259, 1011
Common fragile sites (CFSs), 223
Comparative genomic hybridization arrays (CGH arrays), 493–494
Comparative pathology, 3
Competitive antagonists, 106
Complement-dependent cytotoxicity (CDC), 78
Complementarity-determining region (CD), 338
Complementary DNA (cDNA), 496
Complete blood count (CBC), 296
Computational pathology, 414
Computed tomography (CT), 424, 430–434, 1024–1025

advantages, 433
basic principles, 430–432
disadvantages, 433–434
experimental procedures, 432–433
image information, 432
imaging in preclinical toxicology, 434
Conditional gene modification, 873
Confocal microscopy (CM), 336, 377–380, 419. *See also* Electron microscopy (EM)
applications in toxicologic pathology, 377–378
limitations, 380
technical considerations for, 378
Connective tissue growth factor (CTGF), 45–46
Constitutive androstane receptor (CAR), 29–30, 225–226, 889
Contract research organizations (CROs), 3, 991, 1010, 1030
Contrast-enhanced ultrasound imaging, 450–451
Control animals
concurrent control, 261, 353, 686, 800, 995
historical control, 686, 1064–1065
positive control, 996
Controlled terminology (CT), 982–983, 1063
Convolutional neural networks (CNNs), 414–415
Coronary artery disease, type 2 diabetes mellitus patients with, 474b
Cotton-top tamarin (*Saguinus oedipus*), 781
Coturnix, 828–829. *See also* Quail (*Coturnix*)
Coumarin, 45
Cre. *See* Cyclic recombinase (Cre)
Creatine kinase (CK), 304, 314
Creatinine, 311
CRISPR. *See* Clustered regularly interspaced short palindromic repeats (CRISPR)
CRISPR-associated nuclease (Cas), 871–872
Cas 9, 761
Cristolysis, 130
Cryopreservation, 930
Cutaneous purpura, 762
Cycle evaluation, female reproductive toxicity assessment, 163–164
Cyclic recombinase (Cre), 873
Cyclin, 210–212
cyclin D1, 212
cyclin E, 212
Cyclin D1, 212
Cyclin-dependent kinase (CDK), 43–44, 210–212
Cynomolgus macaque (*Macaca fascicularis*), 778
Cystatin C, discovery and qualification of, 468b
Cytochrome c, 116, 122–123, 130, 137
Cytochrome P450 (CYP), 20, 61, 755, 883
CYP1A2 exons, 883
enzymes, 25–26
Cytosolic receptors, 104
Cytotoxicity, 228–229
Cytotoxic T-lymphocyte–associated protein-4 (CTLA-4), 23

D

Damage-associated molecular pattern molecules (DAMPs), 129
Danio rerio. *See* Zebrafish (Danio rerio)
Daphnia magna, 815–816
Dark neuron artifact, 282–283
DART study. *See* Developmental and reproductive toxicity (DART)
Death-inducing signaling complex (DISC), 137
Deciduosarcomas, 715
Deep learning (DL), 414–415
Degeneration, cellular
ballooning, 124
high amplitude swelling, 130
Delayed-type hypersensitivity (DTH), 792–793, 795t
Dendritic cells, 82
Dermal absorption, 21
Dermal toxicity studies, 757–759
dermal irritation/toxicity studies in rabbits, 701
intracutaneous safety studies in rabbits, 701–702
Dermatitis, 762–763
fungal, 763
Detoxification, 24–30, 63–64
Devario aequipinnatus. *See* Giant danio (*Devario aequipinnatus*)
Developmental and reproductive toxicity (DART), 149–150, 150f
developmental immunotoxicity (DIT), 180
developmental neuropathology, 183–185
developmental neurotoxicity (DNT), 180
embryo-fetal development (EFD), 170–172
pre- and post-natal development (PPND), 172–174
regulatory guidance for, 151t
studies, 701
Diacylglycerol (DAG), 104
Diagnosis, 988
Diagnostic toxicologic pathology, 10–11
4′,6-Diamidino-2-phenylindole (DAPI), 232
Dichloro-diphenyl-trichloroethane (DDT), 22–23, 830
Diet role in toxicity studies, 1099–1102
contaminant issues, 1101
dietary optimization, 1101–1102
types of diets, 1100–1101
optimization, 1101–1102
Diethylstilbestrol, 24, 46–47
Diff gene, 832–834
Diffusion, 17
Diffusion-weighted magnetic resonance imaging (DWI), 427
4,4-Difluoro-4-bora-3a, 4a-diaza-sindacene (BODIPY), 443
Digital pathology, 336, 384, 396, 401–406
calibration, 399–400
considerations for designing pathologist's digital pathology workstation, 405–406
digital image analysis, 10–11
Digital Imaging and Communications in Medicine (DICOM), 400

other imaging modalities, 419
pathologist role in, 404–405
preanalytical variables impact on WSI, 402–403
regulatory considerations for digital pathology evaluation, 416–418
slide scan storage, retrieval, databases, and metadata, 403–404
slide viewing, 403
stereology, 418–419
3D reconstruction, 419
tissue image analysis, 406–416
whole slide imaging, 396–406
Digital technologies, 949–951
Digital tissue image analysis, 407
Dioxin-like compounds (DLCs), 225
Dippity pig syndrome, 762
Direct acting carcinogens, 220
Discovery metabolism, 64–65
comparative metabolite profiles of NME incubated in mouse, 65f
types of metabolism studies conducted during discovery, 66t
Distribution, 16, 59–61
barriers affecting distribution
blood-brain barrier (BBB), 23
gut barrier, 23
placental barrier, 23–24
estimates of blood flow in liver and kidney, 22t
microbiome effects on, 34–35
modifiers, 972
principles, 21–24
protein binding, 59
qualifiers, 972
storage of toxicants in tissues, 22–23
transporter interactions, 59–61
volume of distribution (Vd), 21–22, 59
D methotrexate, 103
DNA, 358
damage repair, 217–218
DNA-based assays, 232–233
microarray chip, 496
repair
high-fidelity/nonmutagenic, 222
low-fidelity/mutagenic, 222
replication and repair mechanisms, 222–224
DNA damage response (DDR), 212
DNA methyl transferases (DNMTs), 230
Dog, 722. *See also* Animal models; dog
comparative toxicology, 732–735
acetaminophen, 734
aspirin and ibuprofen, 735
caffeine, 733–734
small-molecule kinase inhibitors, 733
theobromine, 734
toxic responses of dog compared to other species, 732–733
vasoactive drugs, 735
domestic (*Canis familiaris*), 722
ethics of use of dog as laboratory animal species, 743–744
genetic variability within beagles, 727–728

Dog (Continued)
  Genome Project, 722–723
  history and derivation of beagles, 722–727
  juvenile toxicity assessment, 190
  as model of human diseases, 737–742
    dog as animal model of human cancer,
      737–742
    dog as animal model of human
      cardiovascular disease, 737–742
    dog as animal model of human
      neurological diseases, 739–742
  nonneoplastic diseases, 735–737
  predictivity of dog toxicity data to humans,
    731–732
  regulatory considerations for toxicity
    studies, 742–743
    pesticide and drug development,
      742–743
  spontaneous background pathology in
    beagle, 735–737
    spontaneous neoplastic diseases in
      laboratory beagles, 737
    spontaneous nonneoplastic diseases in
      laboratory beagles, 735–737
  use in biomedical research, 727–731
    dog use for assessing clinical pathology
      and pharmacokinetic changes,
      729–730
    dogs in developmental toxicity studies,
      731
    drug metabolism, disposition, and
      excretion of drugs/chemicals in dog,
      727
    duration of studies/age at start of studies
      in dogs, 728–729
    genetic variability within beagles and
      impact on testing, 727–728
    safety pharmacology studies in dogs, 730
    use of dog in drug discovery and
      development, 728
Dopaminergic neurons (DA neurons), 436
Dose levels, 558
Dose optimization, PD biomarker and, 474
Dose range-finding studies (DRF studies),
  168
Double-strand breaks (DSBs), 209
Draize test, 704
Dried blood spot (DBS), 54–55
Drosophila melanogaster (fruit fly),
  815–816. See also Fruit fly
  (Drosophila melanogaster)
Drug, 101
  action mechanism, 102–104
  development process, 51, 742–743,
    785–786, 1031
  discovery, 460–463, 834–837
    dog in drug discovery and development,
      728
  drug-induced hepatocellular injury
    biomarkers, 463–464
  drug–microbiome interactions, 666
  metabolism
    in dog, 727
    studies in development, 71
  response, 473–474

screening with in vivo or ex vivo imaging,
  453
toxicity translation, 1085–1086
Drug regulatory authorities (DRAs), 236
Drug-induced kidney injury (DIKI), 321
Drug-induced liver injury (DILI), 325,
  520–521
Drug-induced vascular injury (DIVI),
  102–104, 329
  biochemical markers of, 465–466
  biomarkers, 329–330
  seeking site-specific and selective
    biomarkers of, 466b
Drug–drug interactions (DDI), 52, 61, 889
Dubin–Johnson syndrome, 29–30
Duplex sequencing, 244–245
Duration qualifiers, 972

E

E-testing facilities operation, 1017
Eastern box turtles (Terrapene carolina
  carolina), 830–831
Ecotoxicological testing, 838–841
Ecotoxicology, 818–819
Eczema, 762–763
Efalizumab, 45–46
Eisai hyperbilirubinemic rat (EHBR), 33
Electrocardiogram (ECG), 790
Electrolytes, 312
Electromagnetic field (EMF), 1098
Electron microscopy (EM), 336, 380–382. See
  also Confocal microscopy (CM)
  applications in toxicologic pathology,
    380–381
  limitations, 382
  technical considerations for, 381–382
Electrophiles, 24
Elimination, 16
Embryo–fetal development (EFD), 167–172
  data interpretation, 170–172
  embryo–fetal toxicity studies, 759–760
  preliminary EFD (pEFD), 168–169
  testing endpoints, 169–170
Embryoid bodies (EBs), 927, 939–940
Endocrine disruption compound (EDC), 821
Endocrine Disruptor Screening Program
  (EDSP), 167, 827–828
Endocrine disruptors, 188
Endocrine effects, 348
Endocrine gland–derived vascular
  endothelial growth factor (EG-
  VEGF), 358–359
Endothelial cell (EC), 465–466
  activation and injury, 329–330
Engineered models
  expressing human molecules, 904–907
  immunodeficient mice with reconstituted
    chimeric or human organs, 907–912
  immunodeficient models, 898–904
English sole (Pleuronectes vetulus), 822–823
Enhanced pre- and postnatal
  developmental (ePPND) study, 168,
  174–176
  testing endpoints, 175–176
ENU. See N-ethyl-N-nitrosourea (ENU)

Environment role in lesion production,
  1096–1097
Environmental exposure, biomarkers of,
  472–473
Environmental monitoring, 838–841
Enzyme histochemistry (EHC), 336,
  356–358, 882–883. See also
  Immunohistochemistry (IHC)
  applications in toxicologic pathology, 357
  technical considerations for, 357
Enzyme inhibitors, 103
Enzyme-linked immunosorbent assay
  (ELISA), 90, 344–345, 467
Enzymes, 312
Epididymides, 769
Epigenetic mechanisms, 229–231
Epigenomics, 492, 494
Epilepsy, 739
Epithelial growth factor (EGF), 141
Epithelial–mesenchymal transition (EMT),
  219
Erythema multiforme, 762
Erythrogram, 306
Estrogen receptor (ER), 38, 225, 946, 949
  agonists, 227–228
Ethanol, 24
Ethyl methanesulfonate (EMS), 894–895
Ethylenediaminetetraacetic acid (EDTA),
  277, 296
European College of Veterinary Pathologists
  (ECVP), 8
European Medicines Agency (EMA), 996,
  1031
European Registered Toxicologist (ERT), 8
European Society of Toxicologic Pathology
  (ESTP), 980, 1062–1063
European Union (EU), 1012
Euthanasia techniques, 844
Exposome, 1–2
Ex vivo models, 926–946
Excision repair pathways, 223
Excretion, 16, 65–67
  microbiome effects on, 34–35
  studies, 71–73, 72f
  of toxicants, 30–34
    exhalation, 34
    fecal excretion, 32–34
    routes of elimination, 34
    urinary excretion, 30–32
Exhalation, 34
Exhaustion of mediators, 111
Exindirtrusion-based bioprinters, 940
Exposure-dependent response, 107–110
  nonmonotonic dose–effect, 109–110
  quantal dose–effect model, 109
  receptor occupancy relationship, 107–108
  turnover model, 108–109
Extended one-generation
  reproductivetoxicity study (EOGRT),
  167
Extracellular matrix (ECM), 45–46, 84, 114,
  218–219, 360, 929–930
Extracting patterns and identifying
  coexpressed genes (EPIG), 516
Extrinsic pathway, 41

Exudative epidermitis, 762–763
Eye, 767, 771

F

[^{18}F]-fluorodeoxyglucose ([^{18}F]-FDG), 435–436
Facilitated diffusion, 17–19
Fanconi anemia pathway (FA pathway), 223
Fas receptor (FasR), 115
Fatty acid binding protein (Fabp), 328–329
  Fabp3, 328
Fatty change, 126–127
Fatty degeneration. *See* Fatty change
FDA. *See* U.S. Food and Drug Administration (FDA)
Fecal excretion, 32–34
Feed restriction studies, 170
Female fertility study, 166
Female reproductive toxicity assessment, 159–166. *See also* Male reproductive toxicity assessment
  confounding factors, 160–162
  reproductive milestones across species, 161t
  sexual maturity, 160
  species selection, 159–160
  study types, 165–166
  testing endpoints, 162–165
    biomarkers, 163
    cycle evaluation, 163–164
    macroscopic and microscopic evaluation, 162–163
    mating trials, 164–165
    organ weights, 162
Ferroptosis, 138–139
Fetal exposure, 169
FFPE. *See* Formalin-fixed paraffin-embedded (FFPE)
Fibrinogen, 309
Fibrinolysis, 309
Fibrosis, 42–43
Filtration, 17
Final Rule—Good Laboratory Practices, 1011
Firefly, North American (*Photinus pyralis*), 442
Firmicutes, 35
First-in-human studies (FIH studies), 153
First-pass effect, 20, 53
Fischer 344 rats (F344 rats), 670
Fish, 811–812, 818–825. *See also* Animal models; nonmammalian
  basic biologic characteristics and common species, 818–819
  findings, 819–822
  major disease models, 822–825
  neoplasms, 823t
  sedation, 844
Fixation procedures, 272–275
Flavin monooxygenases (FMOs), 27
Flavonoid, 20
Flow cytometry, 318, 345, 365–374
  advantages and limitations of, 373–374
  in animal toxicity studies, 368–369
  applications in toxicologic pathology, 369–373

cell immunophenotyping, 369–372
  functional assays in flow cytometry, 372
  receptor occupancy and binding assays, 372–373
  basic principles of, 367–368
  common uses in nonclinical and clinical testing, 365–367
  functional assays, 372
Fluorescein isothiocyanate (FITC), 337, 443
Fluorescence imaging, 442–443
Fluorescent proteins (FPs), 443
Fluorine, 1
Fluorophores, 443
Follicle-stimulating hormone (FSH), 157
Food. *See also* Diet
  consumption, 267
  food safety, 10
  products, 916–917
Formaldehyde, 20–21, 353–354
Formalin, 273
Formalin-fixed paraffin-embedded blocks (FFPE blocks), 502, 956
Forward scatter (FSC), 367–368
Fraction unbound (fu), 59
Fragment crystallizable portion (Fc portion), 78, 81
Frog Embryo Teratogenesis Assay—*Xenopus* (FETAX), 827–828, 836–837, 953
  Xenopus, 825–826
Fruit fly (*Drosophila melanogaster*), 815–816
Fundulus heteroclitus. *See* Mummichog (*Fundulus heteroclitus*)

G

G-coupled receptor protein kinases (GRKs), 111
G-protein—coupled receptors (GPCRs), 103–104, 111
Gadolinium (Gd), 427
Galactose (Gal), 86–87
Gamma-aminobutyric acid (GABA), 103, 184
Gamma-glutamyl transferase (GGT), 300, 314, 512–513
Gastrointestinal tract (GI tract), 17, 71–73, 177–178, 182
  absorption from, 19–20
  intestinal flora, 34
  intestinal permeability, 23
Gene expression
  analysis, 244
  comparing gene expression across species, 360
  study of changes in gene expression in animal models, 359–360
Gene Expression Omnibus (GEO), 495
Gene targeting by homologous recombination, 870–871
Gene therapy, 82
  biodistribution of, 341–345
  in situ hybridization (ISH)in evaluation of, 361
Genetic modification methods, 860–878
Genetic mutations, 899t
  BRAF V600E, 476b

Genetic quality
  assurance, 883
  control, 883
Genetically engineered animal models, 831–832, 951–952
  fundamentals of, 859–881
    advantages and limitations, 861t–865t
    genetic modification methods, 860–878
    model selection, 879–881
    nomenclature conventions, 878
      genetically engineered mice (GEM), 215–217, 657–659, 860
      genetically engineered mouse models (GEMMs), 233
      genetically engineered rats (GERs), 860
      genetically engineered rodent strains, 670
      genetically modified animals, 660–661
      genetically modified pigs, 772
  ISH in study of, 360
  special considerations in safety assessment of products derived from, 913–917
  use for hazard identification and safety assessment, 888–913
    ADME, 889–892
    basic concepts, 888–889
Genetically modified cells, 943–945
Genetically modified organisms (GMOs), 916–917
Genome editing, 871–872
Genome instability, 244–245
Genome-wide association studies (GWAS), 881–882
Genomic imprinting, 230
Genomic instability, 208–210
Genomics, 485, 492–494. *See also* Toxicogenomics
Genotoxicity
  consequences of, 224
  testing, 892–895
Genotyping, 881–883
Gerbil, Mongolian (*Meriones unguiculatus*), 653–654, 674–675, 682
  granulosa cell tumor, 675
  ovarian cyst, 675
Germline DNA, 502
Giant danio (*Devario aequipinnatus*), 849
Glial fibrillary acidic protein (GFAP), 342
Global biorepositories, 956
Glomerular filtration rate (GFR), 66
Glomerular function, 468b
Glucose, 310, 316
  deprivation, 40–41
  transporters, 19
Glucuronidation, 28
Glutamate dehydrogenase (GLDH), 312–313
Glutaraldehyde (GLUT), 381
Glutathione (GSH), 61
  conjugation, 28–29
Glutathione transferases (GSTs), 28–29
Glycogen, 125

Gonadotrophin releasing hormone (GnRH), 153–155
Good Clinical Practice (GCP), 1013–1014
Good Laboratory Practice (GLP), 2, 258, 302, 337, 398, 561, 730, 787, 896, 988, 1009–1021, 1082–1083
  clinical pathology assessment, 1024
  criticism, 1025–1026
    academic research, 1025–1026
    perspectives on GLP limitations, 1026
  history and evolution of, 1010–1015
    FDA proposed rule on GLP for nonclinical laboratory studies, 1014–1015
    GLP internationally, 1012–1013
    ICH, 1013–1014
    in United States, 1010–1012
  noninvasive imaging applications, 1024–1025
  objective and scope, 1015
    differences across GLP standards, 1015
    FDA GLP general content, 1016
    studies under GLP jurisdiction, 1015
    21 CFR 58 good laboratory practice for nonclinical laboratory studies, 1016–1021
  and pathology data, 1021–1024
    histopathology in GLP environment, 1021–1024
    study pathologist requirements, 1021
  spirit of GLP, 1025
  ultrastructural assessment, 1024
Good Manufacturing Practice (GMP), 1015
Göttingen minipig (Sus scrofa domesticus), 761. See also Pig
Grading, histopathology. See Histopathology; assessment
Graphical user interface (GUI), 412
Gray wolf (Canis lupus), 722
Green fluorescent protein (GFP), 443
Green monkeys (Chlorocebus aethiops pygerythrus), 781
Guanylyl cyclase (GC), 104
Guarana (Paullinia cupana), 733–734
Guide RNA (gRNA), 872
Guinea baboon (Papio papio), 780
Guinea pigs (Cavia porcellus), 673–674, 681–682
  anaphylaxis, 673
  Foa-Kurloff cell, 674
  gastric ulcers, 673
  Hartley guinea pig, 653–654
  heterophil, 673
  rhabdomyomatosis, 673
  scurvy, 674
  typhlocolitis and antibiotics, 674
  vitamin C, 674
Gunn rat, 28
Guppy (Poecilia reticulatas), 823–824

H

Hair follicles, 709–710
Hamadryas baboon (Papio hamadryas), 780
Hamster (Mesocricetus auratus), 240–241, 653–654
  amyloidosis, 680–681
  atrial thrombosis, 680–681
  buccal pouch, 680–681
  flank gland, 680–681
  glomerulonephropathy, 680–681
  polycystic liver disease, 680–681
  Syrian hamsters, 672–673, 680–681
Haploinsufficiency, 877
Hazard identification, 3, 558
Health and Environmental Sciences Institute (HESI), 466
Health Research Extension Act, 1082
Heart rate (HR), 469
Heat shock, 38
Heat shock protein (HSP), 224–225
Heat shock protein complex (HSPC), 227
Helicobacter hepaticus infection, 678–679
Hematocrit (Hct), 304
Hematology, 296, 305–307, 634–635
Hematoxylin and eosin (H&E), 113–114, 277, 337
Hemoglobin, 635
Hemoglobin distribution width (HDW), 306
Hemorrhagic syndrome, 763–764
Hemostasis, 300, 307–310
  fibrinolysis, 309
  hypercoagulable states, 309–310
  primary, 308
  prothrombotic states, 309–310
  screening, 307
    samples for, 307–308
  secondary, 308–309
Herpesvirus simiae, 797–798
Herpesvirus simplex virus type I (HSV), 909
Heterologous desensitization, 111
High-density lipoprotein (HDL), 708
High-fidelity/nonmutagenic DNA repair, 222
"High-throughput" phenotyping, 883–884
Higher-ranked mammalian model species, 696–697
Histamine 1 (H$_1$), 107
Histocytomics, 486
Histologic techniques, 275–277
Histone acetyltransferase (HAT), 39
Histone deacetylase (HDAC), 39
Histopathology, 242
  assessment
    data review and integration meetings, 1066–1067
    diagnostic drift, 1061–1062
    errors in recording, 1062
    historical control data and reference ranges, 1063–1064
    informal reviews by other pathologists, 1065
    pathology peer review workflows, 1067–1069
    quality control activities, 1065–1066
    recommended practices for, 1060–1069
    standardized terminology and severity grades, 1062–1063
    tumor data using weight-of-evidence approach, 1064–1065
    uniform thresholding, 1061
  in GLP environment, 1021–1024
  histology processing, 1021
  histopathological evaluation, 277–282
    cause of death, 278–279
    nomenclature, 279–281
    pathology peer review, 1022
    severity grading, 281–282, 972, 975–976, 978
  histopathological interpretation, 459–460
  pathology imaging compliance, 1023–1024
  pathology report, 1022
  raw data in pathology, 1022–1023
Historical control data (HCD), 800–801
Histotechnologist (HTL), 1044
Homeostasis, 108
Homologous desensitization, 111
Homologous recombination (HR), 223
Hormonal mechanisms, 227
Hounsfield units (HU), 431–432
"Hub-and-spoke" models, 404
Human immunodeficiency virus (HIV), 891–892
Human leukocyte antigen-A2 (HLA-A2), 906–907
Human tumor xenografts, 911–912
Humanized animal models, 904–913
Husbandry-related factors, 259–260
Hyaline droplets, 124
Hydrophobic interaction chromatography (HIC), 86
Hydroxyl radical (HO•), 24, 25f
4-hydroxynonenal (HNE), 36, 37f
Hypercoagulable states, 309–310
Hyperplasia, 120, 145, 996
Hypertrophy, 120–122
Hypothalamic–pituitary–gonad axis (HPG axis), 153–155, 827–828
Hypothalamic–pituitary–thyroid axes, 827–828
Hypoxia, 126
Hysteresis loop, 101–102

I

Ibuprofen, 735
Idiosyncratic adverse drug reactions (IADRs), 61–62
Idiosyncratic mechanisms of toxicity, 42
Idiosyncratic reaction, 104–106
Imaging, non-invasive
  methods, 424
  small animal imaging
    comparison of small animal imaging modalities, 425t
    computed tomography, 430–434
    magnetic resonance imaging and magnetic resonance microscopy, 426–429
    optical imaging, 442–448
    radionuclide-based imaging, 434–441
    translational application, in or ex vivo imaging, 453
  techniques
    computed tomography (CT), 430–434
    magnetic resonance imaging (MRI), 426–429

magnetic resonance microscopy (MRM), 426–429

positron emission tomography (PET), 434–441

single-photon emission computerized tomography (SPECT), 434–441

ultrasound (US), 448–453

Image analysis workflow, pathologist's role in, 413–414

Image compression, 400–401

Image pyramids, 401

Immersion, 272

Immune complex (IC), 798–800

and complement deposition, 347–348

Immune complex disease (ICD), 1041

Immune function models, 792–794

Immune senescence, 793–794

Immune suppression, 229

Immune system, 185–186, 772

Immunodeficient rodent models, 900t–901t

Immunofluorescence microscopy for immunohistochemistry, 354

Immunoglobulin, 347

IgG, 705

Immunohistochemistry (IHC), 7, 336–356, 396–397, 466, 792–793, 882–883, 996, 1040–1041

applications in toxicologic pathology, 338–352

cell proliferation studies and evaluation of cell cycle–related proteins, 349–350

evaluation of apoptosis and necrosis, 350–352

evaluation of infectious disease agents, 352

evaluation of responses to test article administration, 345–349

lesion identification and characterization, 345

test article biodistribution, 341–345

tissue cross-reactivity studies, 338–341

chromogenic, 405

combination techniques, 354–355

method validation review, 996–997

technical considerations for

availability of antibodies, 352–353

bright-field vs. immunofluorescence microscopy, 354

controls, 354

multiplex labeling and combination techniques, 354–355

quantitative analysis, 355–356

tissue collection and fixation, 353–354

Immunophenotyping, 370, 792

example of immunophenotyping panels, 371t

Implantable telemetry units, 791

Implantation safety studies in rabbits, 701–702

Imposex, 817–818

In silico

modeling, 928

models, 946–951

predictive structure–activity models, 946–947

In situ end labeling (ISEL), 350–351

In situ hybridization (ISH), 7, 336, 358–365, 396–397, 882, 1040–1041

applications in toxicologic pathology, 358–361

comparing gene expression across species, 360

discovery research, 358–359

evaluation of gene therapy and antisense therapeutics, 361

study of changes in gene expression in animal models, 359–360

study of genetically engineered animals, 360

technical considerations, 361–364

controls for in situ hybridization, 363–364

fixation, 363

probe label selection, 362–363

probe type selection, 361–362

In situ nick translation (ISNT), 350–351

In vitro

cell culture, 7

models, 926–946

mutagenicity assays, 231–232

screening, 2

In vitro diagnostic assays (IVD), 318–319

In vitro to in vivo extrapolations (IVIVEs), 54–55

In-life

observations, 2

phase, 1044

Indole-3-carbinol (I3C), 224–225

Industrial Bio-Test Laboratories (IBT), 1011–1012

Industrial toxicologic pathology, 3, 9–10

Inflammation, 38, 42

biomarkers of, 330

Inflammatory stress, 38

Information technology (IT), 398

Inositol triphosphate (IP3), 104

Insertional mutagenesis, 876–877

Institutional Animal Care and Use Committee (IACUC), 265, 1083

Integrated approaches to testing and assessment (IATA), 948–949

Interferon-γ (IFN γ), 360

Interleukin 17E (IL-17E), 360

International Academy of Toxicologic Pathology (IATP), 8

International Agency for Research on Cancer (IARC), 206–207, 980

International Color Consortium (ICC), 399–400

International Council on Harmonisation (ICH), 149–150, 338, 1013–1014

International Harmonization of Nomenclature and Diagnostic Criteria (INHAND), 5, 675–677, 796, 814–815, 970, 980–982, 981t, 1063

International Mouse Phenotyping Consortium (IMPC), 881–882

International Organization for Standardization (ISO), 772

Intersex, 821

Interspecies

pathophysiologic concordance, 662–664

scaling, 95

variability, 848–849

Interspecies translation. See Interspecies—scaling

Interstrand cross-links (ICLs), 223

Intestinal dysbiosis, 1092–1093

Intracellular receptors, 103–104

Intramuscular administration (IM administration), 84

Intraperitoneal injection (IP injection), 896

Intrathecal administration (IT administration), 84–85

Intravenous administration (IV administration), 84

dose, 53, 53f

toxicity studies, 756–757

Intravitreal administration (IVT administration), 84

Intrinsic pathway of apoptosis, 136–137

Intrinsic reaction, 104–106

Inverse agonists, 106–107

Invertebrates, 811–812, 815–818

background findings with examples of target tissue toxicities, 817

basic biologic characteristics and common species, 815–817

major disease models, 817–818

Investigational New Drug (IND), 1013, 1031

Investigational veterinary pharmaceutical products (IVPPs), 837

Ionotropic receptors, 103

Ipomeanol, 45

Irinotecan, 34–35

Isoniazid, 29

J

Jacketed external telemetry (JET), 790

Japanese Society of Toxicologic Pathology (JSTP), 980

Joint Photographic Expert Group (JPEG), 400

Juvenile toxicity assessment, 149, 177–192

challenges in assessing neonatal period, 179

guidelines and regional legislation, 190–192

juvenile animal testing, 191t

models of disease, 188

postnatal development of specific organ systems, 180–188

practical species-specific considerations, 188–190

toxicity studies, 760–761

weaning through puberty, 179–180

K

Karyolysis, 46, 131

Karyorrhexis, 46

Kelch-like ECH-associated protein 1 (Keap1), 42–43

Keap1–Nrf2 regulatory pathway, 42–43, 43f

Keratinocytes, 21

Ketones, 316

Keyhole limpet hemocyanin (KLH), 792
Kidneys, 764–765. *See also* Renal
  biomarkers for kidney damage
    reversibility, 467
  glomerulonephritis, 764–765
Kinda baboon (*Papio kindae*), 780
Kinetics, 304–305
Klenow fragment, 351
Knock-in studies (KI studies), 60–61
Knock-out studies (KO studies), 60–61
Knockout, 868
Knudson's two-hit hypothesis, 215–217

L

Laboratory animal science, 1078,
    1079t–1080t
  animal health consideration, 1089–1091
  description of animal studies in scientific
    publications, 1103
  diet role in toxicity studies, 1099–1102
  euthanasia of research animals, 1083–1084
  housing and husbandry issues
    environment role in lesion production,
      1096–1097
    study design considerations, 1097–1099
  microbial and microbial effects on
    pathophysiology and study outcome,
    1091–1096
    association with development, immune
      status, and disease phenotype,
      1092–1094
    definitions, natural history, and
      characterization, 1092
    impact on efficacy, biotransformation,
      and toxicology, 1094–1095
    introduction to microbiome, 1091–1092
    microbiome impact on safety
      translatability, 1095
    minimizing experimental variability and
      monitoring microbiome status,
      1095–1096
  regulatory issues, 1081–1083
    IACUC, 1083
    rules and regulations, 1081–1083
  selection of animals models, 1084–1089
    consider when sourcing animals,
      1087–1088
    genetic considerations, 1086–1087
    issues of translation in animal model
      selection, 1084–1086
    overview, 1084
    specialized animal models in toxicology
      research, 1088–1089
  3R'S and in-life study conduct for
    toxicologic pathologist, 1102–1103
  trends in global research animal care and
    use, 1078–1081
Lactate dehydrogenase (LDH), 314
lacZ gene, 894
Lahontan cutthroat trout (*Oncorhynchus
    clarkii henshawi*), 812–814
Large granular lymphocytic (LGL),
    670
Large molecule therapies, biodistribution
    of, 343–345

Laser capture microdissection (LCM), 336,
    374–377, 504
  applications in toxicologic pathology, 375
  limitations, 377
  technical considerations for, 375–377
Lead, 19
Lempel–Ziv–Welch codecs (LZW codecs),
    400
Lentiviruses, 868–870
Lesions. *See also* Histopathology
  combination of, 581–582
  complexity, 976, 978–979
  identification and characterization, 345
Leucine aminopeptidase (LAP), 314
Leukocyte, 316
Leukogram, 306
Lhfp (lipoma HMGIC fusion partner),
    881–882
Ligand-activated transcription factors, 38
Light sheet fluorescence microscopy
    (LSFM), 419
Lipemia, 303
Lipid solubility, 17
Lipidosis. *See* Fatty change
Liquid chromatography–mass
    spectrometry (LC/MS), 59, 90, 499
Liquid scintillation counting methods (LSC
    methods), 68
Liver, 520–521, 765
  biomarkers of liver injury, 463–465
Locked nucleic acid (LNA), 358
Loggerhead sea turtle (*Caretta caretta*), 831
Long non-coding RNAs (lncRNAs), 494
Loss of heterozygosity (LOH), 215–217
Low-fidelity/mutagenic DNA repair, 222
Lowest observed adverse effect level
    (LOAEL), 732–733
Luciferase reporters, 442
Luteinizing hormone (LH), 157
Luteinizing hormone receptor (LHR), 360
Lymphatics
  lymphangiectasia, 683
  lymphatic cysts, 683
  lymphatic sinus ectasia, 683
Lymphocytes, 82, 698
Lymphotoxin-β, 358–359
Lysosomal storage disease, 739–741
Lysosomes, 115

M

Macaca fascicularis. *See* Cynomolgus
    macaque (*Macaca fascicularis*)
Macaca mulatta. *See* Rhesus macaque
    (*Macaca mulatta*)
Macacine herpesvirus 1, 797–798
Machine learning (ML), 412–413
  in tissue image analysis, 414–416
Macroautophagy, 118
Macrophage chemoattractant protein 1
    (MCP1), 39
Macrovesicular lipidosis, 126, 127f
Magnetic resonance imaging (MRI), 424,
    426–429
  advantages, 428
  basic principles, 426–428

correlation of MRI or MRM to gross or
    histopathological lesions, 429
  disadvantages, 428–429
Magnetic resonance microscopy (MRM),
    424, 426–429
  advantages, 428
  basic principles, 426–428
  correlation of MRI or MRM to gross or
    histopathological lesions, 429
  disadvantages, 428–429
Male reproductive toxicity assessment,
    152–159
  blood-testis barrier, 155
  confounding factors, 153–155
  fertility study, 158–159
  reproductive milestones across species,
    154t
  sexual maturity, 153
  species selection, 152–153
  study types, 158–159
  testing endpoints, 155–158
    biomarkers, 157
    macroscopic and microscopic evaluation,
      155–156
    mating trials, 157–158
    organ weights, 155
    sperm assessment, 156–157
Malondialdehyde (MDA), 36
Manganese (Mn), 19–20
Marmoset, common (*Callithrix jacchus*), 780
Mass balance studies, 68–69
  concentration–time curve of radioactivity,
    69f
Mass spectroscopy (MS), 493
Mauritian macaques, 784
Maximum concentration (C_{max}), 84
Maximum plasma concentration (C_{max}),
    52–53
Mean arterial pressure (MAP), 469
Mean corpuscular hemoglobin (MCH),
    305–306
Mean corpuscular hemoglobin
    concentration (MCHC), 305–306
Mean corpuscular volume (MCV), 305–306,
    634–635
Mean platelet volume (MPV), 307
Mechanisms of action (MOAs), 945
Mechanistic biomarkers, 469–472
  discovery and application of, 471b
Medaka (*Oryzias latipes*), 952
  Japanese medaka, 832
Median effective dosage (ED_{50}), 109
Medroxyprogesterone acetate (MPA), 165
Meriones unguiculatus. *See* Mongolian
    gerbils (*Meriones unguiculatus*)
Mesenchymal stem cells (MSCs), 82, 902,
    943
Mesocricetus auratus. *See* Hamster
    (*Mesocricetus auratus*)
Messenger RNAs (mRNAs), 39, 492
Metabolic syndrome/diabetes, 771
Metabolism, 24–30, 61–65
  discovery, 64–65
  metabolite coverage, 71
  phase I, 25–28, 61, 62f

cytochrome P450 enzymes families and general function, 26t
phase II, 28–29, 61, 62f
phase III, 29–30, 30f
reactive metabolites, 61–64
Metabolomics, 485, 492, 497, 499–500
Metadata, 403–404
Metal stress, 38
response, 44
Metallothionein (MT), 22
Metaplasia, 142–143, 145–146
Metastasis, 218–219
Metformin, 33
Methodological (qualitative) analysis, 626
Methylation, 29
3-Methylindole, 45
Methylphenidate, 109–110
Mice. See Mouse (Mus musculus)
Micro-CT, 424–425, 430–431
microscopy, 434
Micro-MRI, 424–425
Micro-PET, 424–425
Micro-SPECT, 424–425
Microarrays, 244
technologies, 495–496
Microautophagy, 117–118
Microbial infection, 1089
Microbiome, 10–11
effects on absorption, distribution, biotransformation and elimination, 34–35
impact on safety translatability, 1095
microbiome-mediated metabolism, 35
in rodent studies, 665–667
Microfluidic microphyphysiological systems, 943
Microhomology-mediated break-induced repair (MMBIR), 222, 224
Micromass cultures (MMCs), 940–941
Micronucleus test, 232
Microphysiological systems (MPS), 927, 941–943
MicroRNAs (miRNAs), 494
Microscopy with UV surface excitation (MUSE), 419
Microvesicular lipidosis, 126, 127f
Microwell plate method, 938
Minipigs, 751–753, 754t. See also Pigs
Minnow, fathead (Pimephales promelas), 822–823
Mismatch repair (MMR), 209
Mitochondrial DNA (mtDNA), 877–878
Mitochondrial permeability transition (MPT), 40, 130
Mitochondrial transgenesis, 877–878
Mitogen-activated protein kinases (MAPK), 220–221
Mitotic DNA synthesis (MiDAS), 222
Mixed lineage kinase domain-like protein (MLKL), 41–42
MNU. See N-methyl-N-nitrosourea (MNU)
Mode of action (MOA), 224, 501, 947
receptor-mediated, 224
Molecular biology techniques, 358
Molecular in vivo imaging, 424

Molecular targets, interactions of toxicants with, 35–42
Monoclonal antibody (mAb), 78–80, 165–166, 704, 996. See also Antibody
administration and absorption, 84–85
bioanalytical assays for assessing monoclonal antibody concentrations, 90
monoclonal antibody distribution, 85
monoclonal antibody elimination, 85–89
monoclonal antibody screening for acceptable PK properties, 89–90
distribution, 85
elimination, 85–89
effect of FcRn affinity modifications on mAb PK, 88f
pharmacokinetics (PK), 84–90
of antibody-based therapeutics, 90–92
of biotherapeutic modalities, 92
monoclonal antibody administration and absorption, 84–85
screening for acceptable PK properties, 89–90
structure and functions of immunoglobulin molecule, 79f
Morphology-based methods, 486–487
Mouse (Mus musculus), 653–654, 670–671. See also Animal models; rodents
background findings in common species, 675–680
incidental and spontaneous background findings, 675–680
causes of death or morbidity in, 686–688
embryonic stem cells, 943
models of carcinogenesis, 238–240
Mus musculus castaneus, 881–882
Mus musculus domesticus, 881–882
Mus musculus musculus, 881–882
outbred stocks and inbred strains of, 667–670
Mouse Genome Informatics (MGI), 881–882
Mouse Tumor Biology Database, 675–677
Muciphages, 796–797
Multichimeric human–mouse models, 910
Multidrug and toxin extrusion transporters (MATEs), 17–18
Multidrug resistance proteins (MRPs), 17–18, 59–60. See also P-glycoprotein
Mdr1a, 891–892
Mdr1b, 891–892
transporters, 33
Multiplex labeling in immunohistochemistry, 354–355
Multiplexed assays, 486
Mummichog (Fundulus heteroclitus), 812–814
Murphy's Law, 1064–1065
Muta Mouse, 894
Mutagenic DNA repair, 222
Mutagenicity, 244–245
transgenic models for mutagenicity testing, 240
Mutual Acceptance of Data (MAD), 1012
My13. See Myosin light chain 1

Mycobacteriosis, 845–846
Mycobacterium, 826
Myeloid:erythroid ratio (M:E ratio), 317
Myocardial infarction, 770
Myosin light chain 1, 328–329

N

N-acetylglucosamine residues (GlcNAc), 86–87
N-ethyl-N-nitrosourea (ENU), 220, 877
[N-Methyl-D-aspartate] (NMDA), 103
N-methyl-N-nitrosourea (MNU), 896
NAD(P)H oxidoreductase 1 (NQO1), 27–28
Naphthalene, 45
Naringin, 20
Natalizumab, 45–46
National Cancer Institute (NCI), 618
National Cancer Institute Enterprise Vocabulary Service (NCI EVS), 982
National Institute of Health (NIH), 780
National Medical Products Administration (NMPA), 1013
National Toxicology Program (NTP), 167, 233, 276–277, 970, 983, 993, 1003, 1097
Natural killer cells (NK cells), 94
functions, 898
Necropsy, 3–4, 268–272, 1051–1054
brain section, 1054f
testes sections demonstrating differences, 1054f
Necrosis, 46, 127–133, 139–143. See also Cell injury
apoptosis vs., 128t
caseous, 133
evaluation of, 350–352
pyronecrosis, 134t–135t
pyroptosis, 133
single-cell necrosis, 138–139, 765
Nelfinavir, 894–895
Neovascularization, 218–219
NETosis (neutrophil extracellular traps), 139–140
Neutral buffered 10% formalin (NBF), 273–274, 353–354
Neutrophils, 139–140
Nervous system
neurodegeneration, 789
neurons, 115
neuroscience models, 1093–1094
New chemical entity(NCEs), 234, 519–520
New Drug Application (NDA), 1013
New molecular entity (NME), 51
Next generation sequencing (NGS), 244–245, 494, 496–497, 956
NF–E2-related factor 2 (Nrf2), 42–43
Nicotinamide nucleotide translocase (Nnt), 886–887
Nitric oxide synthase (NOS), 888
Nitrites, 316
2-(2-nitro-4-trifluoromethylbenzoyl) 1,3-cyclohexedione (NTBC), 909
2,6-nitrotoluene, 27
Nivolumab, 94

No observed adverse effect level (NOAEL), 170–171, 261, 732–733, 1031
Nomenclature. *See also* International Harmonization of Nomenclature and Diagnostic Criteria (INHAND); Toxicologic pathology
challenges in standardizing nomenclature, 973–977
components in nomenclature, 971–973
conventions, 878
Global Open Registry Nomenclature Information System (goRENI), 675–677, 970
harmonization of nomenclature, 980–983
need for standardized nomenclature, 970–971
neoplastic lesions, 972–973
Standardized System of Nomenclature and Diagnostic Criteria (SSNDC), 980
Nonclinical laboratory studies
disqualification of testing facilities, 1019–1021
disqualification definition, 1019
GLP enforcement, 1019–1021
equipment, 1017
facilities, 1017
general provisions, 1016
organization and personnel, 1016
protocol for and conduct of nonclinical laboratory study, 1018
records and reports, 1018–1019
reserved, 1019–1021
test and control articles, 1017–1018
testing facilities operation, 1017
21 CFR 58 Good Laboratory Practice for, 1016–1021
Nonclinical toxicity studies, 969–970
Noncoding RNAs (ncRNAs), 229–230, 492
Noncompartmental analysis (NCA), 52–53
Noncompetitive antagonists, 106
Noncompetitive interaction, 106
Nonhomologous end joining (NHEJ), 222–223
Nonhuman primates (NHPs), 152–153, 190, 301, 339–340, 664, 777–778, 993, 1037. *See also* Animal models; nonhuman primates
antidrug antibodies, 798–800
background findings in NHPs and use of historical control data, 796–801
enhanced pre- and postnatal development study in, 174–176
environmental, endemic, and contagious pathogens, 797–798
historical control data, 800–801
history and biological characteristics of, 778–782, 779t
incidental findings in, 796–797
models in
biomedical research, 787–794
pharmacology and toxicology research, 790–794
predictivity of NHP toxicity data to humans, 787

select models for nonclinical toxicology and safety pharmacology studies, 790–794
selection of NHPs for toxicologic research and study design considerations, 782–787
ethics and welfare considerations, 782–783
regulatory considerations, 783–784
relevance and feasibility for use in drug development, 785–786
source, origin, and genetic variation, 784–785
study design, 786–787
Noninvasive imaging. *See* Imaging, non-invasive
Nonmammalian animal taxa, 815–831
invertebrates, 815–818
Nonmammalian vertebrates and invertebrates, 812. *See also* Animal models; nonmammalian
Nonmonotonic dose–effect, 109–110, 110f
Nonmutagenic DNA repair, 222
Nonneoplastic Lesion Atlas (NNLA), 970, 983
Nonneoplastic lesions, terminology for, 971–972
Nonneoplastic microscopic pathology (NONNEO microscopic pathology), 982–983
Nonquantitative image analysis, 412. *See also* Quantitative image analysis
Nonreceptors, action on, 103
Nonsteroidal antiinflammatory drugs (NSAIDs), 23, 1046
Nontraditional models in toxicity research, 926–928
in silico modeling, 928
in vitro and ex vivo models, 926–927
in vivo models in alternative mammalian and nonmammalian species, 927–928
Northern blots technique, 358
Nuclear DNA (nDNA), 871
Nuclear imaging methods, 424
Nuclear magnetic resonance spectroscopy (NMR spectroscopy), 62–63, 426, 493, 497
Nuclear receptors (NRs), 29–30, 104
Nuclear transfer, 876
Nuclease-based genome editing, 871–872
Nucleic acid-based approaches, 493
Nucleic acid-based-omics platforms, 493–500
5′ Nucleotidase (5′ NT), 314

O

Occult blood, 316
Octamethylcyclotetrasiloxane (D4), 166
Ocular studies, 703–705
Ocular telemetry, 791
Office of Prevention, Pesticides and Toxic Substances (OPPTS), 722
Office of Regulatory Affairs (ORA), 1011
Oligonucleotide probes, 362
Olive baboon (*Papio anubis*), 780
Omics disciplines, 492

Oncogenes, 213–217, 214t–215t
Oncology disease models, 706
Oncorhynchus clarkii henshawi. *See* Lahontan cutthroat trout (*Oncorhynchus clarkii henshawi*)
Oncorhynchus mykiss. *See* Rainbow trout (*Oncorhynchus mykiss*)
Optical coherence tomography (OCT), 419
Optical imaging, 424–425, 442–448
advantages, 443–444
basic principles of
bioluminescence imaging, 442
fluorescence imaging, 442–443
disadvantages, 444–445
in preclinical toxicity studies, 447–448
Oral toxicity studies, 756
Organ weight ratios, 4–5, 155, 272
Organ-on-a-chip, 941–943. *See also* Microfluidic microphysiological systems
Organic anion transporters (OATs), 17–18
Organic anion transporting polypeptides (OATPs), 17–18, 59–60, 891–892
Organic cation transporters (OCTs), 17–18, 59–60
Organisation for Economic Co-operation and Development (OECD), 7–8, 150, 258, 556–557, 722, 1009, 1031–1032
Organoids, 242, 935–939
Orphan receptors, 103
Oryctolagus cuniculus. *See* Rabbit (*Oryctolagus cuniculus*)
Oryzias latipes. *See* Medaka (*Oryzias latipes*)
Oxidative stress, 36, 38

P

P-glycoprotein (P-gp), 17–18, 59–60, 891–892. *See also* Multidrug resistance 1
p53 pathway, 43–44
p53[+/−] hemizygous mouse model, 896
Paclitaxel, 20
Palivizumab, 84
Pancreas
acinar cells, 115
islet cells, 82
Papio anubis. *See* Olive baboon (*Papio anubis*)
Papio cynocephalus. *See* Yellow baboon (*Papio cynocephalus*)
Papio hamadryas. *See* Hamadryas baboon (*Papio hamadryas*)
Papio kindae. *See* Kinda baboon (*Papio kindae*)
Papio papio. *See* Guinea baboon (*Papio papio*)
Papio sp. *See* Baboon (*Papio* sp.)
Papio ursinus. *See* Chacma baboon (*Papio ursinus*)
Paraformaldehyde (PFA), 273, 353–354
Partial agonist, 106–107
Pathanatosis, 134t–135t
Pathogen-associated molecular patterns (PAMPs), 132–133
Pathology endpoints

special pathology techniques in, 336
  confocal microscopy, 377—380
  digital pathology, 384
  electron microscopy, 380—382
  enzyme histochemistry, 356—358
  flow cytometry, 365—374
  immunohistochemistry, 337—356
  in situ hybridization, 358—365
  laser capture microdissection, 374—377
  stereology, 382—384
  traditional pathology assays, 491
Pathology imaging, 1023—1024
  whole slide imaging, 1023—1024
Pathology peer review, 987—990, 1068
  completeness of pathology review, 992
  core planning considerations, 993—997
  diagnostic drift, 975, 978, 1061—1062
    in histopathological evaluation, 684
  disagreements, during, 997—1000
    formal consultation, 998—999
    informal consultation, 998
    pathology working groups, 999—1000
    resolution of, 991—992
  documentation, 1000—1001
    peer review statement, 1000—1001
    timing of signature, 1001
  general process, 990—992
  general toxicity studies, 993—995
  interpretation and correlation in pathology
    review, 992—993
  National Toxicology Program (NTP), 1003
  peer review, 625
  peer review pathologist (PRP), 988
  peer review timing and pathology raw
    data, 988—990
    pathology raw data and peer review,
      989—990, 989f
  process, 990—1003
    consultation, 990
    contemporaneous peer review, 990—997
  regulatory aspects, 1004—1006
    regulations for contemporaneous
      pathology peer review in China and
      Japan, 1006
  retrospective, 988—990, 1001—1003
    general process, 1001—1002
    retrospective review by expert,
      1002—1003
  use of diagnostic terminology and
    assignment of severity grades, 992
  use of digital/whole-slide images in,
    1006—1007
    whole-slide images for national
      toxicology program pathology
      working groups, 1007
Pathology Working Group (PWG), 974, 988,
  999
  procedure, 999—1000
Pathway-based models of toxicity, 947—948
Patient-derived xenograft (PDX), 238—239,
  911
Patient/clinical trial subject selection,
  475—476
  discovery and application of biomarker for
    patient selection, 476b

Paullinia cupana. See Guarana
    (Paullinia cupana)
Peer review, 988—997. See also Pathology
    peer review
Pegylation, 82. See also Polyethylene glycol
    conjugation
Pembrolizumab, 94
Peptide nucleic acid (PNA), 358
Peptide transporters (PEPTs), 17—18, 32
  Pept1, 20
Perfusion, 273
  fixation prior, 1041
Peripheral blood mononuclear cells
    (PBMCs), 911
Peroxisome proliferator—activated
    receptors (PPARs), 121, 226—227
  PPARα, 38, 891
Pesticides, 742—743, 830
Pharmaceutical agents, 347
Pharmacodynamics (PD), 77—78, 101,
  260—261, 473—474, 1031—1032
  biomarkers, 473—474
    and dose optimization, 474
  of biotherapeutics, 92—94
  mechanism of drug action and adverse
    drug reaction, 102—104
    chronic dosing, 110—111
    exposure-dependent response, 107—110
    plots of concentration (PK) or effect (PD)
      over time course, 102f
    quantitative modeling for PK/PD and
      toxicodynamic data analysis, 111—112
    types of adverse drug reaction, 104—106
    types of xenobiotic—target interaction,
      106—107
  response, 785—786
Pharmacogenomic biomarkers, 478
Pharmacokinetics (PK), 16, 52, 77—78,
  260—261, 1031—1032
  analyses, 101
  of antibody-based therapeutics, 90—92
  of biotherapeutics, 83—92
    modalities, 92
    monoclonal antibody
      concentration—time profile, 83f
    monoclonal antibody PK, 84—90
  PK/PD
    characteristics, 879
    modeling and interspecies scaling, 95—96
    and toxicodynamic data analysis,
      111—112
  PK/TK studies, 55—58
Pharmacokinetics/pharmacodynamics
    (PK/PD), 77—78
Phenome-wide association study
    (PheWAS), 883—884
Phenotyping, 883
  anchoring, 492
  directed phenotypic characterization for
    product discovery and development,
    885—886
  interpretation of genetically engineered
    animal models, 886—888
  large-scale, 883—885
Phosphatase and tensin (PTEN), 215—217

Phosphatidyl serine (PS), 138
Phosphatidylcholine, 16—17
Phosphatidylethanolamine, 16—17
Phosphatidylinositol 3-kinase delta (PI3Kδ),
  220—221
3'-phosphoadenosine-5'-phosphosulfate
  (PAPS), 28
Phosphohistone H3 (PhH3), 349—350
Phospholipidosis (PLD), 946
Phosphorus, 311
Phosphorylation, 349—350
Photinus pyralis. See Firefly, North
  American (Photinus pyralis)
Photoacoustic imaging (PAI), 447
Physiochemical property reactions, 102
Physiological adaptation, 111
Physiologically based PK modeling (PBPK
  modeling), 67
PI. See Isoelectric points (PI); Prediction
  intervals (PI)
Pigs, 751. See also Animal models; pig
  ethics and animal welfare, 773
  genetically modified pigs, 772
  genetics of pigs and background for use in
    research, 752—755
    basic biological characteristics, 753
    breeds, 752—753
    husbandry considerations, 753—755
  juvenile toxicity assessment, 189
  as model system for medical devices and of
    human diseases, 770—772
  as organ source for xenotransplantation,
    761
  regulatory aspects, 772—773
  spontaneous background pathology in
    swine, 761—769
    macroscopic observations, 762—764
    microscopic findings, 764—769
    neoplasia in research swine, 769
  in toxicological studies, 755—761
    dermal toxicity studies, 757—759
    embryo—fetal toxicity studies, 759—760
    intravenous toxicity studies, 756—757
    juvenile toxicity studies, 760—761
    oral toxicity studies, 756
    routes of dose administration, 759
    study design considerations, 755—756
    subcutaneous dosing toxicity studies, 757
Placenta, 23—24
Placental barrier, 23—24
Platelet distribution width (PDW), 307
Platelet-activating factor (PAF), 308
Platichthys stellatus. See Starry flounder
  (Platichthys stellatus)
Pleuronectes vetulus. See English sole
  (Pleuronectes vetulus)
Pneumocystis carinii, 678—679
Polyadenylation sequence, 866
Polyaromatic hydrocarbons (PAHs),
  812—814
Polyarteritis nodosa, 798—800
Polychlorinated biphenyls (PCBs), 348,
  822—823
Polyethylene glycol (PEG) conjugation.
  See Pegylation

Polymerase chain reaction (PCR), 341–342, 1090
Polymerase I (Pol 1), 350–351
Polymorphisms, 42
Polytetrafluroethylene (PTFE), 811–812
Porcine endogenous retroviruses (PERVs), 761, 916
Positron emission tomography (PET), 424, 434–441, 1024–1025
    advantages, 437–438
    basic physics of, 434–436
    comparative utility of PET and SPECT, 437
    disadvantages, 438–439
Postnatal development of specific organ systems, 180–188
    assessment of growth, 186
    cardiovascular and pulmonary system, 180–182
    developmental neuropathology, 183–185
    endocrine disruptors, 188
    gastrointestinal tract, 182
    immune system, 185–186
    renal system, 182–183
    reproductive system, 186–188
Postprocessing, 934
Potassium, 312
Potential target tissues, estimate and communicate number of, 1040
Poultry, 812
Pre-and postnatal development study (PPND study), 167–168, 172–174
    data interpretation, 172–174
    enhanced PPND study, 174–176
    minimum PPND endpoints, 173t
    pregnancy, 42, 172–174
        and developmental toxicity, 167–177
            embryo-fetal development study, 168–172
            enhanced pre- and postnatal development study, 174–176
            guidelines, 176–177
        testing endpoints, 172
Preanalytical variables
    impact on image analysis, 409
    impact on whole slide imaging, 402–403
Precision-cut tissue slices (PCTS), 932–933
Preclinical toxicology
    computed tomography imaging in, 434
    fetal evaluation, 434
    magnetic resonance microscopy imaging in, 427–428
Predictive biomarkers, 474–475
Predictive toxicology, 519–526
Predictivity
    of dog toxicity data to humans, 731–732
    of nonhuman primate toxicity data to humans, 787
Pregnane X receptor (PXR), 29–30, 225–226, 889
Probe label selection, 362–363
Probe type selection, 361–362
Progesterone, 209–210
Prognostic biomarkers, 478–481
Programmed cell death (PCD), 133–139, 350
    apoptosis, 133–138, 136f

Programmed death-1 (PD-1), 782
Programmed death-ligand 1 (PDL1), 369
Prolactin, 163
Proliferating cell nuclear antigen (PCNA), 341–342
Proliferative vitreoretinopathy (PVR), 703
Promoter, 866
Pronuclear/nuclear microinjection of DNA, 866, 867f
Protein
    binding, 59
    protein-based-omics platforms, 497
Proteomics, 485, 492, 497
    technologies, 497–500
Prothrombin time (PT), 300
Prothrombotic states, 309–310
Proto-oncogene. See Cellular oncogene
Pseudoreplication, 842–843
Puberty, weaning through, 179–180
Public health, 2
Pyknosis, 46
Pyramid representation, 401

Q

Quail (Coturnix sp.), 828–829
Qualification, 460
    of biomarkers, 488–489
Quality assurance programs, 1045–1046
Quality Assurance Unit (QAU), 1015–1016
Quality control (QC), 396–397, 625, 988, 1044
Quantal dose–effect model, 109, 110f
Quantitative antibody-based assays, 486
Quantitative image analysis, 410–411
    area/pixel-based measurements, 410
    cell-based measurements, 410–411
    object-based measurements, 411
Quantitative modeling for PK/PD and TD data analysis, 111–112
Quantitative structure–activity relationship (QSAR), 928, 946
Quantitative system pharmacology (QSP), 111–112
Quantitative trait loci (QTLs), 881–882
Quantitative whole-body autoradiography (QWBA), 69
Quantum dots (QDs), 427

R

Rabbit (Oryctolagus cuniculus), 695–697
    basic biological characteristics and common breeds, 696–699
        basic biometrics, 698t
        ethics and animal welfare considerations, 699
        reproductive biometrics, 699t
    hypercholesterolemia, Watanabe rabbit model of, 707–709
    juvenile toxicity assessment, 189
    major disease and functional models, 705–709
        antibody production/immunological research, 705
        medical device and regenerative medicine—functional studies, 706–707

        novel surgical modelss, 706
        oncology disease models, 706
        Watanabe rabbit model of hypercholesterolemia, 707–709
    model selection
        issues in data extrapolation to human, 696
        overview of toxicology model species selection, 696
    pharmacokinetic and toxicity studies, 701–705
        cardiac safety studies, 702–703
        dermal irritation/toxicity studies, 701
        developmental and reproductive toxicity studies, 701
        intracutaneous and implantation safety studies, 701–702
        mucosal irritation studies, 703
        ocular studies, 703–705
        safety studies supporting vaccine development, 705
    regulatory aspects and examples in biomedical research, 699, 700t
    reproductive system, 186–188, 713–714
    small intestines, 710
    spontaneous findings in experimental NZW rabbit, 709–715
        normal structures unique to rabbit, 709–711
        spontaneous pathology findings, 712–715
    stomach, 710, 768–769
Radiofrequency (RF), 426
Radionuclide-based imaging, 434–441
    radionuclide-based imaging in preclinical toxicity studies, 439–441
Rainbow trout (Oncorhynchus mykiss), 812–814
Raman spectrography, 419
Raman spectroscopy, 448
Rat (Rattus norvegicus), 653–654, 671–672
    background findings in common species, 675–680
        incidental and spontaneous background findings, 675–680
    causes of death or morbidity in, 686–688
    chronic progressive nephropathy (CPN), 677
    outbred stocks and inbred strains of, 667–670
    rodent progressive cardiomyopathy, 660–661
Rattus norvegicus. See Rat (Rattus norvegicus)
Raw data in pathology, 1022–1023
Reactive metabolites, 61–64
Reactive oxygen species (ROS), 208
Real-time polymerase chain reaction, 244
Receiver operator characteristic curves (ROC curves), 463–464, 475b
Receptor-interacting protein kinase 1 (RIPK1), 41–42
Receptor-interacting protein kinase 3 (RIPK3), 41–42
Receptors

with associated enzymatic activity, 104
  downregulation, 111
  G protein-coupled (GPCR), 111
  kinase-linked, 104
  ionotropic, 103
  intracellular, 103
  metabotropic, 103
  occupancy, 372–373
    relationship, 107–108, 108f
  receptor-mediated modes of action, 224
Recombinant human antithrombin III
    (ATryn), 913–914
Recombinant human artemin (rhArt),
    905–906
Red blood cells (RBCs), 296, 512–513, 576
Red cell distribution width (RDW), 306
Red cell mass, 306
Red fluorescent protein (RFP), 443
Redox-sensitive transcription factors, 36
Reductive metabolism, 34
Redundant Array of Independent Disks
    (RAID), 404
Region of interest (ROI), 432
Region-specific kidney damage, 467
Registry of Industrial Toxicology Animal
    Data (RITA), 980
Regulations, 1011
Regulatory authorities, 970
Renal, 771. See also Kidney
  biomarkers of renal injury, 466–467
  glomerulus, 17
  physiology studies, 300
  system, 182–183
Renilla reniformis. See Sea pansy (Renilla
    reniformis)
Repair mechanisms
  cell repair and adaptation, 44–46
  failure to repair after toxic insult, 46–47
    carcinogenesis, 46–47
    fibrosis, 42–43
    necrosis, 46
  stress response constituents and pathways,
    42–44
Repeat-dose toxicity studies, 165–166
Replacement, reduction, and refinement
    (3Rs), 6–7, 1102
  and in-life study conduct for toxicologic
    pathologist, 1102–1103
  NC3Rs, 1081–1082
Reporter enzymes, 337
Reproducibility, 970–971
Reproductive toxicity, 149. See also
    Developmental and Reproductive
    Toxicity (DART)
  assessment, 150–167
  female, 159–166
  guidelines, 167
  male, 152–159
Reptiles, 830–831
Residual bodies, 118
Respiratory inductive plethysmograph
    (RIP), 790
Respiratory tract, absorption from, 20–21
Reticulocytes, 306
Retinoblastoma (RB), 212

Retrieval data, 403–404
Reverse genetics, 860–866
Reverse transcription–polymerase chain
    reaction (RT-PCR), 496, 882
Reversible cell injury. See also Irreversible
    cell injury
  irreversible cell injury vs., 122–127
    cellular swelling, 124–125
    fatty change, 126–127
Reversible interaction, 106
Rhesus macaque (Macaca mulatta), 778–780,
    784–785
Riboprobes, 361
Ribosomal RNA (rRNA), 497
Risk assessment
  concordance, 662–664
  predictivity, 662
  sensitivity, 662
  specificity, 662
  translational relevance, 664
Risk characterization, 3
Risk management, 3
Rituximab, 94, 369
RNA interference (RNAi), 870
RNA sequencing (RNA-Seq), 244, 494
Rodent models of disease (RMD), 660–661
Rodents, 654–655. See also Animal models;
    Mouse; Rat
  basic biological characteristics of common
    rodent stocks and strains, 667–675,
    669t
    anatomy and physiology of rodents used
      in toxicologic research, 670–675
    outbred stocks and inbred strains of mice
      and rats, 667–670
  bioassays, 5
  common pathologic findings in, 675–688
    background findings in common
      species—mice and rats, 675–680
    background findings in uncommon
      rodent species, 680–682
    considerations in evaluating incidental
      background findings, 682–688
  issues in extrapolation of rodent data for
    human risk assessment, 661–667
    biological and cell therapies, 665
    controlling variability and impact of
      microbiome in rodent studies, 665–667
    pharmacologic translational relevance
      and interspecies pathophysiologic
      concordance, 662–664
  juvenile toxicity assessment, 188–189
  populations, 1081
  selection, 655–661
    rodent models of disease and genetically
      modified animals, 660–661
    rodent species used for special studies,
      659–660
    species selection for toxicity studies,
      655–659, 656t–657t
Rough endoplasmic reticulum (RER), 114

S

Safety assessment, 3, 913
  with in vivo or ex vivo imaging, 453

Safety pharmacology studies in dogs, 730
Safety translatability, microbiome impact
    on, 1095
Saguinus oedipus. See Cotton-top tamarin
    (Saguinus oedipus)
Saguinus sp. See Tamarins (Saguinus sp.)
Saimiri sp. See Squirrel Monkey (Saimiri sp.)
Salmonella typhimurium, 926–927
Salvelinus confluentus. See Bull trout
    (Salvelinus confluentus)
scFvs. See Single-chain variable fragments
Sea pansy (Renilla reniformis), 442
Sea urchin, 815–816
Sea urchin embryos (SUEs), 817
Segmented filamentous bacteria (SFB), 1093
Selective estrogen receptor modulators
    (SERMs), 227–228
Senescence, 218
Sentinel monitoring programs, 1090
  microbial alteration, 1091t
Sequencing, 496–497
  sequencing-based technologies, 493–494
Severe combined immunodeficiency
    (SCID), 238–239
Severity grading, 281–282, 972, 975–976,
    978. See also Histopathology;
    assessment
Sex skin, 778
Sex-related physiological factors, 6
Sexual dimorphism, 287–289, 673–674
Sexual maturity
  female reproductive toxicity assessment,
    160
  male reproductive toxicity assessment, 153
Sialic acid (SA), 86–87
Side scatter (SSC), 367–368
Signal regulatory protein α (Sirpa), 910
Signal transduction receptors
  action on, 103–104
  G-protein coupled receptors, 103–104
  intracellular receptors, 104
  receptors with associated enzymatic
    activity, 104
Signal-to-noise ratio (SNR), 426
Simian immunodeficiency virus (SIV),
    784–785
Simple diffusion, 17
Single nucleotide variants (SNVs), 516
Single-chain variable fragments, 81
Single-nucleotide polymorphisms (SNPs),
    209, 493–494, 881–882
Single-photon emission computed
    tomography (SPECT), 424, 434–441
  advantages, 437–438
  basic physics of, 437
  comparative utility of PET and SPECT, 437
  disadvantages, 438–439
Single-strand breaks (SSBs), 209
Sister chromatid exchanges (SCEs), 232
Skeletal muscle, 767
  stem cells, 82
Skin, 767–768, 770–771
  absorption through, 21
  wound healing studies, 770–771
Slide preparation. See Tissues

Slide scanning. *See* Whole slide scanning
capacity and time, 398
in focus, 397—398
magnification, 398—399
modalities, 396—397
resolution, 399
Small hive beetle (*Aethina tumida*), 816
Small molecule therapies, biodistribution of, 343—345
Small-molecule drug modalities, 1085—1086
Small-molecule kinase inhibitors, 733
Smn1. *See* Survival of motor neuron 1 (Smn1)
Smooth endoplasmic reticulum (SER), 122
Snails, 815—816
Society of Toxicologic Pathology (STP), 8—9, 155, 263—264, 603, 980, 988, 1022
Sodium, 312
Solution-based assays, 336
Somatic mutation theory (SMT), 207
Sorbitol dehydrogenase (SDH), 312—313
South African clawed frog (*Xenopus laevis*), 953
Southern blots technique, 358
Specific pathogen-free animals (SPF animals), 665—666, 844, 916
Sperm assessment, 156—157. *See also* Male reproductive toxicity assessment
Sperm-mediated DNA transfer, 877
Spiggin, 823—824
Squirrel monkey (*Saimiri* sp.), 781
Standard for Exchange of Nonclinical Data format (SEND format), 682—683, 970, 982—983, 1063
Standard operating procedures (SOPs), 259—260, 301, 404—405, 554, 1011, 1051
Standardized System of Nomenclature and Diagnostic Criteria (SSNDC), 980. *See also* Nomenclature
Starry flounder (*Platichthys stellatus*), 822—823
State Food and Drug Administration (SFDA), 1013
Statistical analysis, 546, 582—588
adequacy of control group, 560
age adjustment, 601
allocation bias, 559
analysis of covariance (ANCOVA), 576, 597—599
analysis of variance (ANOVA), 509—512, 549
assumptions of statistical tests, 638, 638t—644t
Bartlett's test, 576
Bayes' theorem, 626
biological and statistical significance, 550—553
body and organ weights, 632—634
categories, 547
causality *vs.* association, 629—631
censoring, 561—562
central Limit Theorem, 569
cluster analysis, 565—566, 568, 623. *See also* Tissue image analysis

cluster sampling, 557—558
Cochran t-test, 591—592
Cochran—Armitage trend test, 600—601
coefficient of variation (CV), 568, 570
Cohen's kappa, 609—610
combining, pooling, and stratification, 559, 586—587
confidence intervals (CI), 567, 619
confounding variable, 554
contour plot, 573
correlation, 608—610
Cox and Stuart test, 618
Cox proportional hazards model, 618
data processing, 578—582
data simplification, 620
data transformation, 574, 580, 581t
data type and statistical methods, 548—549
decision tree method, 582
describing data, 568—570
description bias, 588
descriptive statistics, 567—568
detecting treatment effects, 556—561
dimension reduction, 567—568
distribution-free multiple comparison tests, 611—612
Duncan's multiple range test, 592—593
Dunnett's t-test, 592, 594
Engelman and Hartigan test, 577
expanded weighting procedure, 621
experimental unit, 554—555
exploratory data analysis (EDA), 575
F-test, 576, 594—595
factor analysis, 565—566
factorial design, 559, 564
false negatives and positives, 550—551
Fisher's exact test, 588—589
Fisher's Skewness test, 577
Fourier analysis, 568, 624
goodness-of-fit test, 575
hierarchical techniques, 623
homogeneity of variance, 576—577
hypothesis testing and probability values, 566
impacts of sample size, 562
in multifactor experiments, 596—597
in single factor experiments, 590—596
in toxicologic pathology studies, 558
independent variables, 547
interpolation, 567
interpretation of results, 629—632
interquartile range (IQR), 568—570
intraclass correlation coefficient (ICC), 610
Jonckheere—Terpstra test for trend, 613—614
Kendall's coefficient of rank correlation, 609
Kruskal—Wallis one-way ANOVA, 613
Latin square design, 564
Levene's test, 577
life table analysis, 568, 614—616
linear regression, 603—604
Log-rank test, 616—618
low-dose extrapolation, 599—600
Mann—Whitney U test, 612—613
matched pairs design, 563

maximum likelihood test, 577
metaanalysis, 553—554
missing data, 578—580
mixed model ANOVA, 596
mode-seeking techniques, 623
modeling, 566—567
multidimensional scaling (MDS), 568, 621—622
multiple comparison tests, 592—594
nested design, 564—565
nonlinear regression, 606—608
nonmeasured scales, 548
nonmetric scaling, 568, 621—622
nonparametric hypothesis testing, 610—619
observer bias, 561
outliers, 578
Peto method for context of observation, 601—603
Pie charts, 572—573
poly-k approach, 603
polynomial function, 606
pooled (quantitative) analysis, 625—626
postfactor hypothesis bias, 588
power analysis, 551
prediction intervals (PI), 619—620
principal component analysis (PCA), 513, 568, 622—623
prior conviction bias, 588
probit/Log transforms and regression, 604—606
proportions and rates, 548
quantal data, 547
R x C Chi-Square, 590
randomization, 556, 559—560, 563
reading bias, 561
reduction of dimensionality through classification, 620—621
relative risk, 631
replication, 555—556
residuals, 576
sampling, 557
Scattergram, 575
Scheffe's multiple comparisons, 593—594
selection of studies to analyzed—systematic reviews, 624—625
sensitivity, 551—552
specificity, 552
standard deviation (SD), 553, 568—569
standard error of the mean (SEM), 568—569, 592
statistical bias, 588
stratified sampling, 557
Student's t-test, 576, 591
systematic sampling, 557
Tarone's test, 618—619
time to event analysis, 614—619
transformations, 580—581
trend analysis, 599
trend test for tumor rates, 600—603
type I error, 550
type II error, 550
unbalanced designs, 554
undesirable variables, 554
unpaired t-test, 591

use of historical control data, 631—632
  Wilcoxon rank-sum test, 610—611
  Williams' t-test, 592, 594
Steatosis. *See* Fatty change
Stem cells, 943—945
  assays, 945
  embryonic stem cell (ESC), 860—866, 871,
    935—938
  hematopoietic stem cells (HSCs), 82, 902
  human embryonic stem cells (hESCs), 943
  induced pluripotent stem (iPS), 871
  induce pluripotent stem cells (iPSCs), 871,
    935—938
  mesenchymal stem cells (MSCs), 943
  stem cell—derived in vitro models, 945
  tissue-specific stem cells, 45
Stereology, 10—11, 336, 382—384, 418—419.
    See also Image analysis
Stickleback (*Gasterosteus aculeatus*), 823—824
Stress, 680
Stress response
  constituents and pathways, 42—44
    Keap1—Nrf2 regulatory pathway, 42—43
    metal stress response, 44
    p53 pathway, 43—44
  in toxicity, 36—38, 37t
Stroke, 739
Structure—activity relationship (SAR), 52
Study Data Tabulation Model (SDTM), 982
Study design, 841—846
Study pathologist (SP), 987. *See also*
    Toxicologic pathologist
  lines of communication and shared
    information with, 1057—1060
  information needed before start of
    microscopic evaluation, 1058
  sponsor communication, test site
    management communication, and
    undue influence, 1059—1060
  study pathologist and peer review
    pathologist communication, 1058
  requirements, 1021
  responsibility for generating pathology raw
    data, 988
Subcutaneous administration (SC
    administration), 84
  dosing toxicity studies, 757
Sulfamethazine, 29
Sulfation, 28
Sulfotransferases (SULTs), 28
Surface-enhanced Raman scattering (SERS),
    448
Survival of motor neuron 1 (Smn1), 887—888
Sus scrofa, 752. *See also* Pigs
Systematic uniform random sampling
    (SURS), 382—383
Systems biology, 2—3

T

T-cell receptor (TCR), 906—907
  TCRA, 906—907
  TCRB, 906—907
T-cell—dependent antigen response
    (TDAR), 175—176, 792—793
Tamarins (*Saguinus* sp.), 781

Tamoxifen, 165, 227—228
Target animal safety (TAS), 818—819
  studies, 837—838
Target organs, 993—995
  Society of Toxicologic Pathology
    recommendations, 994t
Targeted gene panels, 493—494
TdT-mediated bio-dUTP nick end-labeling
    (TUNEL), 350—351
Telemetry
  models of cardiac and respiratory function,
    790—791
  for neurologic assessment, 791
TempO-Seq technology, 495
Teratoma, 898
Terminal deoxynucleotidyl transferase
    (TdT), 350—351
Terrapene carolina carolina. *See* Eastern box
    turtles (*Terrapene carolina carolina*)
Test article biodistribution (test item, test
    substance), 2—3
  biodistribution, 879
Testes, 769
Tetanus toxoid (TT), 792
2,3,7,8-tetrachlorodibenzodioxin (TCDD),
    17, 224—225
Tetraethylammonium, 31—32
Tetramethylrhodamine (TRITC), 443
Tg.AC mouse mouse model, 896—897
Theobroma cacao, 734
Theobromine, 734
Therapeutic(s). *See also* Biotherapeutics
    class, 879
  strategies, 1091—1092
Thiostatin discovery, 484b
Three dimensions (3D), 927
  reconstruction, 419
Thresholds, 974—975, 977—978
  in histopathological evaluation, 684
Thrombin clotting time, 308—309
Thrombocytopenic purpura-like syndrome,
    763—764
Thrombogram, 306—307
Thromboxane B2, 474b
Thymidine kinase (TK), 909
Thyroid stimulating hormone (TSH), 116
Tissue cross-reactivity (TCR), 337, 993,
    996—997
  studies, 338—341
Tissue image analysis, 406—416. *See also*
    Digital pathology
  application areas, 407—409
  artificial intelligence and machine learning
    in, 414—416
  available tools, 412—413
  basics of quantitative image analysis,
    410—411
  computational pathology, 414
  manual *vs.* automated image annotations,
    409—410
  nonquantitative image analysis, 412
  pathologist's role in image analysis
    workflow, 413—414
  preanalytical variables impact on image
    analysis, 409

visual and cognitive biases of manual slide
    review, 407, 408t
Tissue list, full, 993
Tissue microarray (TMA), 399
Tissue organizational field theory (TOFT),
    207—208
Tissues preparation, 336
  collection and fixation for
    immunohistochemistry, 353—354
  distribution studies, 69, 70t
  fixation, 258
  processing, 1042
  slices, 930—934
  special stains, 277
  storage of toxicants in, 22—23
  tissue mass/slice test systems, 7
TNF-like weak inducer of apoptosis
    (TWEAK), 360
Tocilizumab (anti—IL-6R), 94
Top-down approaches, 499
"Tox 21" initiative, 925—926
Toxic Substances Control Act (TSCA),
    925—926, 956
Toxicant, 101
  elicit adverse effects, 15—16
  toxicant-induced lesions, 6
Toxicity, 901—902
  biochemical and molecular basis
    determinants of toxic outcomes, 16f
    idiosyncratic mechanisms of toxicity,
      42
    interactions of toxicants with cellular and
      molecular targets, 35—42
    principles of xenobiotic disposition,
      16—35
    protective mechanisms, repair
      mechanisms, and adaptation or failure,
      42—47
Toxicity equivalence factors (TEFs), 225
Toxicity Reference Database (ToxRefDB),
    946—947, 949
Toxicity screening, 834—837
Toxicity studies, 1030, 1081
  introduction of pathology-related issues
    arising during in-life phase, 1044—1050
    ensure proper training of personnel, use
      of appropriate assays, maintenance of
      required instrumentation, and use of
      quality assurance programs,
      1045—1046
    generate pathology data, 1049—1050
    minimize impact of suboptimal
      communication during in-life phase,
      1046—1047
    mitigate impact of unexpected or
      significant toxicity, 1047—1049
    pathology considerations in response,
      1050t
    potential issues, 1045t
  issues arising from pathology assessment
    and reporting, 1050—1072
    ensure proper training, supervision,
      procedures, and protocol familiarity in
      necropsy, histology, and clinical
      pathology laboratories, 1050—1054

Toxicity studies (Continued)
establish strong lines of communication and share scientific and program information with study pathologist, 1057—1060
facilitate finalization of well-constructed, high-quality, on-time pathology report, 1069—1072
necropsy, 1051—1054
pathology report components, 1069—1070
recommended practices for histopathologic assessment, 1060—1069
robust quality control, 1070
schedule adequate time for all processing steps and evaluations, 1054—1057
standard operating procedures and study protocol familiarity, 1051
timeliness and signatures, 1070—1072
training and supervision, 1050—1051
pathology-related issues during study design and protocol preparation, 1031—1044
appropriate animal species, genetic background, and disease model for toxicity testing, 1037—1039
develop and practice novel or nonstandard pathology procedures and methods prior to start of study and use accepted practices for incorporation of nonstandard endpoints, 1040—1042
do not blind study pathologist, 1043
ensure deep understanding of regulatory guidance and best practices, 1032—1035
ensure study procedures adequately described in study protocol or standard operating procedures, 1042—1043
communications practices, 1039—1040
estimate and communicate number of potential target tissues, 1040
facilitate study and peer review pathologists' workflow, 1044
ICH and test standardization, 1034t—1035t
plan for pathology peer review in GLP-compliant toxicity studies, 1043
realistic study goals, design study to accomplish goals, and minimize study complexity, 1035—1037
useful references, 1033t
Toxicodynamics (TD), 101, 473—474. See also Pharmacodynamics (PD)
chronic dosing, 110—111
exposure-dependent response, 107—110
mechanism of drug action and adverse drug reaction, 102—104
plots of concentration (PK) or effect (PD) over time course, 102f
quantitative modeling for PK/PD and TD data analysis, 111—112
types of
adverse drug reaction, 104—106
xenobiotic—targetinteraction, 106—107
Toxicogenomics, 492—493

applications, 519—534
carcinogenicity assessment, 529—534
mechanistic toxicology, 527—529
predictive toxicology, 519—526
conducting toxicogenomic studies, 500—501
goals and applications of toxicogenomic studies, 501—502
regulatory considerations, 534—536
sample considerations, 502—519
collection and processing of-omics samples, 503—504
controls for-omics assays, 505—507
data analysis and interpretation, 509—519
extraction of biomolecules, 504—505
software tools and databases, 509
study designs and statistical considerations, 507—509
study planning for-omics endpoints, 502—503
technologies, 493—500
metabolomics technologies, 500
microarray technologies, 495—496
next-generation sequencing technologies, 496—497
nucleic acid-based-omics platforms, 493—495
protein-and metabolome-based-omics platforms, 497
proteomics technologies, 497—500
Toxicokinetics (TK), 16, 1031—1032
analysis, 55
Toxicologic pathologists, 492, 583, 1021, 1039, 1081, 1087—1088
bias and, 560—561
GLPs, 561
informed analysis, 561
observer bias, 561
Toxicologic pathology, 1—3, 337, 395—396, 546, 981—982, 991, 1065. See also Clinical pathology testing; Digital pathology; Histopathology; Nomenclature
artifacts vs. lesions, 282—284
basis of, 3—4
diagnostic challenges in, 284—289
fixation and histologic procedures, 272—275
histological techniques, 275—277
histopathologic evaluation, 277—282
in-life evaluations, 265—268
necropsy, 268—272
practitioner of, 9—11
diagnostic toxicologic pathology, 10—11
industrial toxicologic pathology, 9—10
management roles in toxicologic pathology, 11
research in toxicologic pathology, 11
toxicologic pathology relating to environment and food safety, 10
protocol development, 258—265
recommended practices, 977—979
training and certification in, 8—9
understanding biological variation, 549
Toxin, 101
TP53 protein, 213
Trans-membrane receptors, 103

Transcription activator-like effector nucleases (TALENs), 871—872
Transcription activator-like effectors (TALEs), 871—872
Transcriptomics, 492, 494
Transducer, 450
Transepithelial/transcellular pathways, 23
Transfer RNA (tRNA), 497
Transforming growth factor (TGF), 44—45
TGF-β, 141
Transgenic animals, 860—866
Transgenic models for mutagenicity testing, 240
Transgenic rodent gene mutation assays (TGR gene mutation assays), 892—894
Translation in animal model selection, 1084—1086
Transluminal pressure (TLP), 791
Transmembrane metabotropic receptors, 103
Transmission electron microscope (TEM), 273—274, 352, 381, 1024, 1040—1041. See also Electron microscopy
Transporter interactions, 59—61
Transposons, 877
Tributyltin (TBT), 817—818
Triglycerides, 310
Trout, 847—848
Tuberculosis (TB), 787
Tubular hypoplasia/atrophy, 769
Tumor cell heterogeneity, 210
Tumor formation mechanisms, 348—349
Tumor necrosis factor (TNF), 912—913
TNF-α, 137, 1093
Tumor suppressor genes, 213—217, 216t—217t
Trp53 mouse model, 895—896
Tumor xenografts, 911
Turnover model, 108—109
Two-dimension (2D), 927
cell culture models, 927
morphometry, 382
planar images, 426—427
Two-dimensional gel electrophoresis (2D-GE), 497
Type 2 diabetes mellitus patients with coronary artery disease, 474b
Tyramide signal amplification (TSA), 337

U

U.S. Department of Agriculture (USDA), 1082
U.S Environmental Protection Agency (US EPA), 150, 258, 348, 696—697, 827—828, 925—926, 1009
U.S. Food and Drug Administration (FDA), 2, 258, 338, 407, 459—460, 600, 783, 896, 949, 989, 1009
GLP general content, 1016
UDP-glucuronic acid (UDPGA), 24—25
UDP-glucuronosyl transferases (UGTs), 28
Ultrasound, 424, 448—453
advantages, 451—452
basic physics, 448—451
disadvantages, 452
in preclinical efficacy studies, 452—453

Ultrastructural assessment, 1024. *See also* Electron Microscopy
Ultraviolet (UV), 339
Urinalysis, 300, 315—317
  quantitative, 317
  standard, 315—317
Urinary excretion, 30—32
Urobilinogen, 316
Uterine adenocarcinoma, 715

V

Vacuolar change. *See* Vacuolar degeneration
Vacuolar degeneration, 124
Vaginal dosing, 759
Validation, 460
Variability sources in rodent lesions, 684—686
Vascular access port (VAP), 757
Vascular endothelial growth factor (VEGF), 141—142
Vascular injury, drug-induced. *See* Drug-induced vascular injury (DIVI)
Vascular toxicity
  biomarkers of, 465—466
  functional markers of, 469
Vasoactive drugs, 735
Vervet monkeys (*Chlorocebus aethiops sabaeus*), 781
Very low-density lipoprotein (VLDL), 708
Veterinary pathologist, 1089
Vinclozolin, 348
Vincristine, 20
Vinyl acetate, 20—21
Viral oncogene, 213
Viral-mediated gene transfer, 868—870
Volume of distribution (Vd), 21—22, 52—53, 59
von Willebrand Factor (vWF), 465—466
vWF propeptide (vWFpp), 465—466

W

Warfarin, 22
Wastewater treatment facility (WWTF), 839—840
Watanabe heritable hyperlipidemic rabbit (WHHL), 707—709
Weight-of-evidence approach (WoE approach), 150, 945
White blood cells (WBCs), 296, 548
Whole embryo culture (WEC), 945—946
Whole genome sequencing (WGS), 245, 493—494
Whole-exome sequencing (WES), 493—494
Whole-slide imaging (WSI), 354, 395—406, 1023—1024. *See also* Digital pathology; Tissue image analysis
  color preservation, 399—400
  digital workflow, 401—406
  image compression, 400—401
  pyramid representation, 401
  scanning
    capacity and time, 398
    in focus, 397—398
    magnification, 398—399
    modalities, 396—397
    resolution, 399
Whole-slide scanner (WSS), 1023—1024
Wild-type platyfish (*Xiphophorus maculatus*), 832—834
Wild-type swordtail (*Xiphophorus helleri*), 832—834
Wildlife, 831
Women of child-bearing potential (WOCBP), 168—169
Work-up bias. *See* Reading bias
World Health Organization (WHO), 980
Wound healing studies, 770—771

X

X-ray CT, 430—431
Xenobiotics, 35, 102—103, 121, 220—221

agonist, partial agonist, antagonist, and inverse agonist, 106—107
disposition, 15
principles of, 16—35
  elimination of toxicants, 30—34
  metabolism, 24—30
  microbiome effects on absorption, distribution, biotransformation and elimination, 34—35
  principles of distribution, 21—24
  properties of absorption, 16—19
  routes of absorption, 19—21
  reversible, irreversible, noncompetitive, and allosteric interaction, 106
  transporters, 31—33, 32f
  types of xenobiotic—target interaction, 106—107
Xenopus laevis. *See* South African clawed frog (*Xenopus laevis*)
Xenotransplantation, 913—916
  pigs as organ source for, 761
Xiphophorus, 832—834
Xiphophorus helleri. *See* Wild-type swordtail (*Xiphophorus helleri*)
Xiphophorus maculatus. *See* Wild-type platyfish (*Xiphophorus maculatus*)
Xiphophorus melanoma receptor kinase (Xmrk), 832—834
Xpa$^{-/-}$ mouse models for carcinogenicity testing, 897

Y

Yellow baboon (*Papio cynocephalus*), 780
YKL-40, 479b

Z

Zebrafish (*Danio rerio*), 241, 836—837, 952
Zeiosis, 133
Zidovudine, 24
Zinc (Zn), 22
Zinc finger nucleases (ZFNs), 871—872